Clinical laboratory methods

Clinical laboratory methods

JOHN D. BAUER, M.D.

Associate Professor of Pathology, Washington University School
of Medicine; Chairman, Department of Laboratory Medicine, DePaul
Community Health Center; Director of Laboratories, Faith Hospital and
Central Medical Center, St. Louis, Missouri; St. Peters Community Hospital,
St. Peters, Missouri

NINTH EDITION

With 667 illustrations and 19 color plates

The C. V. Mosby Company

ST. LOUIS • TORONTO • PRINCETON   1982

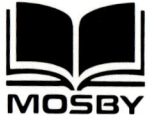

Editor: Don Ladig
Assistant editor: Rosa Kasper
Manuscript editors: Mary C. Wright, Sally Gaines
Design: Susan Trail
Production: Barbara Merritt

NINTH EDITION

The C.V. Mosby Company
11830 Westline Industrial Drive, St. Louis, Missouri 63146

Library of Congress Cataloging in Publication Data

Bauer, John D.
    Clinical laboratory methods.

    Bibliography: p.
    Includes index.
    1. Diagnosis, Laboratory. I. Title. [DNLM:
1. Diagnosis, Laboratory. QY 25 B344c]
RB37.B37   1982   616.07′5   81-16820
ISBN 0-8016-0508-3   AACR2

C/CB/MV   9   8   7   6   5   4   3   02/B/226

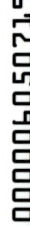

Contributors

PHILIP G. ACKERMANN, Ph.D.

Consultant in Biochemistry to Alexian Brothers Hospital; formerly Biochemist, DePaul Community Health Center, and formerly Consulting Biochemist to Faith Hospital, St. Louis, Missouri

JOHN D. BAUER, M.D.

Associate Professor of Pathology, Washington University School of Medicine; Chairman, Department of Laboratory Medicine, DePaul Community Health Center; Director of Laboratories, Faith Hospital and Central Medical Center, St. Louis, Missouri; St. Peters Community Hospital, St. Peters, Missouri

RAYMOND F. GRAY, Ph.D.

Director, Department of Microbiology, DePaul Community Health Center, St. Louis, Missouri

DAVID C. HOHNADEL, Ph.D., D.A.B.C.C.

Director of Clinical Chemistry, Department of Laboratory Medicine, The Christ Hospital, Cincinnati, Ohio

MILDRED G. HUTCHINSON, M.T., A.S.C.P.

DePaul Community Health Center, St. Louis, Missouri

LAWRENCE A. KAPLAN, Ph.D.

Associate Director, Clinical Chemistry Laboratory, Department of Pathology and Laboratory Medicine, University of Cincinnati Medical Center, Cincinnati, Ohio

KATHLEEN S. McLAUGHLIN, M.D.

Assistant Professor of Pathology, Washington University School of Medicine; Associate Pathologist, DePaul Community Health Center, Faith Hospital, and Central Medical Center, St. Louis, Missouri; St. Peters Community Hospital, St. Peters, Missouri

ALPHONSE POKLIS, Ph.D.

Director of Forensic and Environmental Toxicology Laboratory and Assistant Professor in Pathology and Pharmacology, St. Louis University School of Medicine, St. Louis, Missouri

EVAN A. STEIN, M.D., Ph.D.

Director, Clinical Chemistry; Associate Professor of Pathology and Laboratory Medicine; Associate Professor of Medicine, University of Cincinnati Medical Center, Cincinnati, Ohio

RICHARD C. TILTON, Ph.D.

Professor of Laboratory Medicine; Director of Clinical Microbiology Division, Department of Laboratory Medicine, University of Connecticut Health Center, Farmington, Connecticut

CHENG C. TSAI, M.D.

Associate Professor of Pathology; Director of Clinical Immunopathology Laboratory, St. Louis University School of Medicine; Consultant Immunopathologist, St. Louis V.A. Hospital, Cardinal Glennon Memorial Hospital, DePaul Community Health Center, St. Louis, Missouri

Preface

This, the ninth edition of *Clinical Laboratory Methods,* appears 8 years after the last edition. During the intervening years there has been a tremendous growth in all phases of laboratory medicine, spearheaded by new developments in instrumentation and technic. The present edition reflects the breadth and depth of these advances, since it is updated and almost completely rewritten by a number of expert contributors. The format and the organization of the material are new; the subject matter is grouped into units that reflect typical laboratory organization. The units are divided into chapters, each one highlighted by a short introductory outline. Outdated and infrequently used tests have been eliminated, and new chapters dealing with safety, platelets, bone marrow, immunology, and serology have been added. The chapter on toxicology and therapeutic drug monitoring is entirely new.

In Unit One quality control procedures employed in each subdivision of the clinical laboratory are summarized and are then discussed in each unit in greater detail if deemed necessary. In Chapter 2 of this unit Mildred G. Hutchinson, M.T., A.S.C.P., offers suggestions and guidelines for safety in the laboratory.

In Unit Two, Hematology, I emphasize the role of automation, including automated differential counters. The discussion of hemoglobin includes a current list of hemoglobin variants and a section on glycosylated hemoglobins and their use in the evaluation of diabetic patients. The investigation of hemoglobinopathies includes electrophoresis of globin chains and isoelectric focusing. The sections dealing with disorders of red and white cells have been expanded and include a discussion of serum ferritin and the investigation of functional disorders of polymorphonuclear leukocytes. Functional disorders of lymphocytes and complement are discussed in Unit Six. Detailed instructions in how to proceed in the investigation of hemolytic anemias are contained in Units Two and Three.

The descriptions of morphology, function, and pathology of the cellular components of blood are extended by electron-microscopic, phase-microscopic, and cytochemical investigations, which reveal not only structural details but also enzymatic and antigenic properties. The chapter on white cell disorders deals in detail with the leukemias and offers among other classifications the French, American, and British Cooperative Working Group classification of acute leukemias. Mention is made of the newly surfaced concept of preleukemia. Among the chronic leukemias, space is devoted to a discussion of hairy cell leukemia. The lymphoreticular disorders include Sézary syndrome and T and B cell malignancies. The monoclonal immunoglobulin disorders embrace heavy- and light-chain diseases as well as the rather common benign monoclonal gammopathy. Space is devoted to the role of the Epstein-Barr (EB) virus in the etiology of infectious mononucleosis and to its serologic expressions. The chapter on bone marrow has information on bone marrow culture and cytogenetic studies and their uses in the diagnosis of leukemia and preleukemia.

Three chapters of Unit Two are dedicated to hemostasis. They contain the latest information on the role of platelets in hemostasis, on the newer Fitzgerald and Fletcher factors, on the kallikrein-kinin system, and the enzyme nature of some of the coagulation factors and their complexes. Naturally occurring inhibitors, including antithrombin III, are contrasted with acquired inhibitors of coagulation factors. The assay procedures include single-factor assays and the latest methods using synthetic chromogenic or fluorescent substrates. The discussion of idiopathic thrombocytopenic purpura also mentions the Coombs' antiglobulin test to detect platelet-associated IgG and C3. A section on hypercoagulability follows the discussion of bleeding disorders.

Unit Three, by Kathleen S. McLaughlin,

M.D., reflects the new technology of blood banking and has been completely revised and reorganized into six chapters. Chapter 14 examines current biochemical data demonstrating basic differences between red cell antigens, allowing them to be categorized into families, or blood group systems. Basic serologic testing of the ABO and rhesus systems is again included with a greater discussion of discrepancies between ABO serum and cell testing; the problem of polyagglutination is discussed in detail with appropriate test procedures included. For the first time, a discussion of the complex system of tissue antigens is included with its relevance to human disease indicated. Chapter 15 discusses general basic transfusion practices and methods. It includes the newest anticoagulants that are available, with their impact on blood storage. Much greater emphasis is placed on cellular blood components and plasma fractions; the methods of preparation are included with the advantages and disadvantages of each. Newer concepts in transfusion practices are discussed for the first time, including the use of low–ionic strength solution, the elimination of some routine cross matching steps, the concept of a type and screen program, and the usefulness of autologous transfusions. Hepatitis testing has been updated with a discussion of third-generation test procedures. Chapter 16 is devoted to specialized test procedures, many of which are invaluable to current blood bank serology. The basic concepts of immunology, as they relate to blood banking, are found in Chapter 17. Chapter 18 deals primarily with clinical diseases as they pertain to erythrocyte antigen-antibody reactions. The discussion of isoimmune hemolytic disease of the newborn has been updated, and autoimmune hemolytic anemia is presented for the first time, as is the very difficult problem of drug-induced red cell sensitization, which can cause great difficulty in the interpretation of basic blood bank procedures. Chapter 19 pertains to the problem of adverse reactions to incompatible blood transfusions. A systematized approach to a workup of a transfusion reaction is included, and for the first time there is an extensive discussion of nonhemolytic transfusion reactions as well.

Unit Four, the section on clinical chemistry, is the result of my collaboration with Philip G. Ackermann, Ph.D., David C. Hohnadel, Ph.D., Lawrence A. Kaplan, Ph.D., Evan A. Stein, Ph.D., M.D., and Alphonse Poklis, Ph.D. The initial five chapters in this unit are the result of efforts by Drs. Ackermann and Hohnadel. Chapter 20, on laboratory instrumentation, has been updated to include an expanded discussion of the principles of gas-liquid and high-performance liquid chromatography. Chapter 21, on carbohydrates and nitrogen compounds, contains all tolerance tests and the current classification of glucose intolerance recommended by the National Diabetes Data Group. The manual methods presented have been updated to current, nonbiased methods that can easily be used in any but the largest laboratories requiring automated technic. In Chapter 22, on inorganic elements and blood gases, a calcium colorimetric method replaces the titration method and is joined by methods for ionized calcium. Also included are contemporary methods for copper, magnesium, zinc, serum iron, and iron binding. Newer electrolyte instrumentation is described, including those instruments using cesium internal standards, those using ion electrodes, and those using electrochemical half cells.

Chapter 23, on liver functions, now includes a direct spectrophotometric method for bilirubin for neonates and an enzymatic method for triglycerides followed by a procedure for high-density lipoprotein cholesterol and calculations for very low–density lipoprotein cholesterol and low-density lipoprotein cholesterol. Chapter 24, on enzymology, has been completely rewritten and reorganized, so that the assays for the various enzymes are grouped under the disease entities in the diagnosis of which they are primarily used. Sections have been added for lactate dehydrogenase (LDH), creatine phosphokinase (CPK), and amylase isoenzymes. Virtually all enzyme assays presented employ continuous monitoring kinetic technics.

Chapter 25, on hormone analysis, results from the collaboration of Drs. Ackermann and Kaplan and presents new concepts in the utilization of nonisotopic methods, such as enzyme-linked immunosorbent assays (ELISA) and enzyme inhibition assays (EIA), procedures that are also mentioned in Chapter 35, Immunology.

Dr. Poklis has written an entirely new chapter on toxicology and therapeutic drug monitoring. A systematic approach to toxicologic screening, which involves analysis of urine and blood and toxic metal determination, is presented. The qualitative urine screening procedures discussed include confirmatory technics for all drugs presented and require only generally available instrumentation, such as thin-layer chromatography and ultraviolet spectrophotometric and fluorometric capabilities. Using the methods presented, even a moderately sized laboratory can offer a significant toxicology service for emergency urine drug screening. Numerous new procedures for drugs not previously considered are offered, such as for acetaminophen, benzodiazepines, antidepressants, sedatives, and hypnotics. The section on thin-layer chromatography allows the technologist to choose one of several developing and extraction systems to focus on the detection of drugs of primary interest.

Chapter 27, on urinalysis, which I revised, is introduced by a section on kidney structure and formation of urine, followed by carefully revised and expanded discussions of the tests for urinary constituents.

With the welcome assistance of Dr. Kaplan, I also revised the chapter on semen analysis, pregnancy tests, and placental hormones.

The contributors are also responsible for the chapter that deals with the examination of biologic fluids. The section on spinal fluid analysis offers new insight into the use of pH, glucose, lactic acid measurements, and the IgG-albumin index. In the amniotic fluid analysis, the tests for L/S ratio are updated and the foam stability test as a screen for fetal maturity is presented.

Chapter 30, on gastric, duodenal, and pancreatic juice analysis, by Drs. Ackermann and Stein, presents the stool guaiac test as a screening procedure for colon cancer as recommended by the American Cancer Society, the serum carotene assay as a screening procedure for fat malabsorption, the serum D-xylose procedure for carbohydrate malabsorption, and the use of stool electrolyte analysis in malabsorption syndromes. An expanded discussion on gastrin increases the value of the section on gastric and duodenal juice analysis.

Unit Five, Microbiology, is the result of my collaboration with Raymond F. Gray, Ph.D., and Richard C. Tilton, Ph.D. The discussions of quality control, *Legionella, Campylobacter,* and rapid immunochemical tests for the identification of in-

fectious diseases have been expanded and updated. All taxonomy has been made current. Chapter 33, on mycology, has been carefully revised, and the taxonomy of fungi has been reviewed for correct usage. Chapter 34, on parasitology, was critically reviewed by Lynne Shore Garcia, A.B., M.T. (A.S.C.P.), and I am grateful for the improvements and additions she suggested. *Dientamoeba fragilis* is classified as an intestinal flagellate that may be responsible for attacks of gastroenteritis. The section dealing with free-living amebae is brought up to date as are the discussions of toxoplasmosis, *Pneumocystis,* babesiosis, and serologic methods in parasitology. A section on arthropods of medical importance completes the chapter.

Unit Six appears in this edition for the first time. Chapter 35, on clinical serology, spans the period between the earliest precipitation and agglutination tests and the most up-to-date enzyme immunoassays and laser nephelometry. Special thanks go to Alex C. Sonnenwirth, Ph.D., who permitted the use of material he published in Part XI of *Gradwohl's Clinical Laboratory Methods and Diagnosis,* ed. 8, edited by A.C. Sonnenwirth and L. Jarett. Chapter 36, on clinical immunology, by Cheng C. Tsai, M.D., and me, reflects the tremendous growth in this area of laboratory medicine. It includes the latest methods of lymphocyte typing, the harvesting of these cells, and a discussion of their disorders. Emphasis is placed on fractionation of antinuclear antibodies, quantitation of circulating immune complexes, and membrane receptor studies of frozen tissue sections.

I would like to acknowledge, with gratitude, the assistance of several persons, in particular, Carolyn Humphrey, Cathy Metz, Wendy Hoffman, and Nora Carlisle, whose efforts were essential. I would also like to thank Glenn Humphrey, who did the new line drawings for this edition.

To my wife, Marjorie, your patience and understanding are appreciated.

John D. Bauer

Contents

COLOR PLATES

INTRODUCTION

CHAPTER 1

Some laboratory rules and quality control

SOME LABORATORY RULES

All requests for laboratory examinations should be made in writing and should contain the patient's full name, the hospital number, the type of specimen, the clinical diagnosis, the physician's name, and the specific examination desired. Knowledge of the patient's race is helpful at times (for instance, in hematology). Three time slots on the requisition should indicate time and date when request was issued, when the specimen was obtained, and the time, date, and by whom the test was completed.

On entering a patient's room technologists should identify themselves and state the reason for their presence (e.g., blood test ordered by the patient's physician). Prior to any procedure they must identify the patient by checking his Ident-A-Band for name and hospital number. The patient must not be identified by bed number or by asking his or her name. If there is any doubt, the floor nurse should identify the patient.

Good work records are a must. They should contain not only the patient's identification, test, and results but also the procedure used to arrive at these results. For example, in biochemistry specify the dilution used; in bacteriology, include the various media used and the reactions of each.

Each laboratory should have an accession book that lists all incoming specimens, the patient's and physician's names, the date of acquisition, the final disposition, the results of the tests, and the date of completion. A number is assigned to each specimen. An adequate filing system must allow easy access to alphabetized records.

Common errors and their elimination

Quality control has as one of its objectives the elimination of errors. Errors frequently result from failure to observe basic precautions and laboratory rules. Frequent sources of error in the laboratory include the following:

1. *Improper identification of patients or specimens.* Proper identification of the patient before obtaining samples of blood or other body fluids is essential. The name on the requisition must always be checked against the name on the patient's wristband. If the patient does not have a wristband, identification must be confirmed by a member of the nursing staff. This may not seem essential if the same technician is frequently obtaining samples from the same patient, but it is good practice to always make the check. Whenever two or more patients in the hospital have identical or very similar names, a notice should be posted in the laboratory. After collection of the specimen the tube or other container must be properly labeled with the patient's full name and room number (or some other identifying number). The labels on the tubes must be such that they cannot be easily removed or fall off. The proper type of specimen must also be obtained, with the minimal amount of hemolysis. If on return to the laboratory the specimen is to be divided into two or more aliquots for different types of tests, care must be taken to ensure proper identification and labeling.

2. *Common methodologic errors.* These may include the following:
   a. Failure to adhere to established rules and procedures
   b. Use of improperly or poorly tested procedures that appear to be satisfactory in the normal range but are inadequate in the pathologic range
   c. Use of reagents that are outdated, improperly prepared, or labeled or are stored in the wrong type of container or at the wrong temperature
   d. Failure to do regular instrumentation preventive maintenance, to properly check heating bath temperatures, spectrophotometer wavelength scales, and linearity of photometric response in the spectrophotometer, and to keep all instruments free from dirt and moisture
   e. Lack of familiarity with basic arithmetic calcula-

tions (Use of an inexpensive pocket calculator may result in greater speed and accuracy.)

f. Transcription errors, which can occur at many points in the system: in writing down the actual instrument readings, results of calculations, entries into the log book or reporting system

QUALITY CONTROL

Quality control is an all-embracing concept that includes much more than the elimination of errors or standard deviation charts posted on the wall. By quality control we mean the sum of our efforts to achieve the highest degree of excellence, so that both the patient and physician obtain correct information in the shortest possible time and at a reasonable cost.[1,2]

Quality control includes the following areas, which are first discussed generally and then focused on in the individual laboratory sections.

1. All patients, laboratory personnel, laboratory equipment, and laboratory tests are involved. Specific aspects include patient preparation and identification, specimen collection, transportation and handling of the specimen, performance of the test, and the reporting of test results.

2. The laboratory's relation to other hospital departments should be expressed in writing and revised and updated at least once a year. The quality control program extends beyond the confines of the laboratory and must include many other areas, such as the nursing service, the admitting office, the outpatient department, housekeeping, public relations, purchasing, the "storeroom," the pharmacy, surgical supplies, the medical staff, and laboratory representation on appropriate committees.

3. Laboratory policies and procedures should be collected in a manual to be revised at least once a year or when procedures are changed. Copies of this manual should be available to other hospital departments.

4. A quality surveillance system should establish norms that must be met (e.g., tests must not be reported if results are outside an established limit such as ± 2 SD).

5. A correction system should be established to offer education, realization of why errors happen, and a program to remedy defects (e.g., in equipment, technic, specimen procurement, or storage of reagents).

6. Objective quality control parameters must be established to prove that corrective measures have actually brought results. Such parameters are quality control charts, standard deviation calculations, and comparison of results to internal and external standards. Internal standards are prepared by dividing known patients' sera into aliquots, which are stored at $-20°$ C and are included in the daily "run" at suitable intervals. External standards are available from many sources such as the U.S. Public Health Department, the College of American Pathologists, the American Society of Clinical Pathologists, and commercial laboratory supply houses.

For a more complete discussion of the preceding points the book by Dharan[1] is recommended.

Factors involved in quality control*

Standard: A standard is a substance of known composition, the value of which is established by an analytic procedure different from that used in the clinical laboratory. If the clinical laboratory procedure is able to duplicate the standard value, then this procedure is accurate. **Accuracy** is defined as the closeness of test results to the true value and implies freedom from error.

Control: Controls (both physical and chemical) resemble the unknown specimen, e.g., serum controls or urine controls, and contain various substances of known concentration that are assayed by the usual clinical laboratory methods. Controls are assayed daily, together with the unknown; the results of these assays form the basis for the calculation of the mean and standard deviation of a given test. The control specimens are used to measure **precision,** which is the closeness of test results to each other and implies freedom from variation. Control specimens may vary in their composition and are not constant as are standards. (See the discussion of quality control in biochemistry.)

Neither standards nor controls are stable; they must be reassayed by reference methods. In some departments of the laboratory, standards may not be available, and tests will have to be monitored by controls (e.g., control red cell and white cell suspensions used in hematology). In some laboratories negative and positive controls are the only controls available (e.g., serologic testing for syphilis, pregnancy, and infectious mononucleosis).

Continued education: Since laboratory medicine changes rapidly, the staff must be kept well informed through refresher courses, workshops, educational films, and seminars. An active program of interdepartmental postgraduate education is a valuable asset.

Motivation: The practice of laboratory medicine is a professional activity, with the primary motivation being service to the patient. Inadequate training or knowledge must not be tolerated, since very often the patient's diagnosis and treatment depend on the results of laboratory tests. The technologist should be encouraged to verify the results not only by quality control methods but by relating them to the results of tests (e.g., urine sugar, blood sugar, and urine culture tests) obtained in other sections of the laboratory.

Patients: Proper identification and preparation of patients; exact timing of tests; proper identification and dating of specimen.

Laboratory personnel: Board certification or the equivalence for laboratory director; adequate time for supervision; adequate training and number of technicians, technologists, and supervisors; record of workshops and refresher courses attended; in-service training programs; personnel policy manual; job descriptions.

Equipment: Adequate work and bench space; preventive maintenance of equipment according to written

---

*Some of the following key words and phrases are taken from Commission on Laboratory Inspection and Accreditation: Standards for accreditation of medical laboratory, Chicago, 1970, College of American Pathologists.

schedule, with defects recorded and corrective measures taken. Maintenance procedures should be followed on balances, spectrophotometers, photofluorometers, centrifuges, automated equipment, incubators, water baths, microscopes, refrigerators, thermometers, and pH meters.[3]

Laboratory tests: Speed; economy; reliability; ease with which they can be performed by personnel of various training levels.

Reagents: Identity; concentration; purpose; date of purchase or preparation; manufacturer; expiration date; initials of technician who prepared reagent; standard used to check accuracy; distilled water check.[4]

Clinical chemistry

The preceding general remarks apply to all branches of the clinical laboratory and thus to the chemistry laboratory. In addition, a number of other points apply particularly to the chemistry laboratory and are discussed here.[5,6] Among the mistakes that may cause appreciable assay errors are (1) prolonged application of the tourniquet before drawing the sample, (2) undue exposure to extremes of temperature, (3) mechanical shock or bright sunlight during transport of the specimen, (4) prolonged centrifugation (which may result in undesirable heating), (5) unduly prolonged contact between the serum and clot, and (6) keeping the samples in open tubes for many hours. (Significant evaporation can occur under some circumstances from open tubes, changing the concentration of the constituents. In addition, many enzymes and some other constituents are rather unstable, and improper storage conditions may cause rapid deterioration.)

Any discussion of quality control programs in the clinical laboratory should include certain statistical concepts.[7] For example, if a large number of assays of a single sample or of supposedly identical samples are made (as is done when daily measurements are made of aliquots of the same serum), it will be found that, because of random errors, not all measurements will yield precisely the same result. The results will tend to cluster around some particular value. Most of the re-

sults will be close to this value, some will be slightly farther from the value, and a few will be even more distant. If a large number of determinations are made, the distribution of values usually tends to follow a theoretic curve, often known as the gaussian curve (Fig. 1-1). The various values found are plotted against the frequency of occurrence. The value arbitrarily labeled "100" in this plot is the one most frequently found, and values differing appreciably from this are less frequent. This is an idealized curve; in actual practice there would not be an infinite distribution of values but a discrete distribution such as that shown in Fig. 1-2. In theory this would approach the true curve as the number of measurements is increased to a very large value. It is only an assumption that the values obtained in any actual case do follow the gaussian curve, but this assumption works out fairly well in practice, at least for the type of distributions we are considering here. If we assume that the actual data do follow the theoretic curve, we can make some interesting mathematical deductions. The true gaussian curve is determined completely by only two parameters, which are conventionally designated by the two Greek letters μ and σ.

The first parameter, μ, which is the mean value, governs the position of the maximum of the curve in reference to the range of values. In Fig. 1-1 μ is arbitrarily set at 100. The best estimate of μ from the actual data is the average value of the determinations as usually calculated. This is usually designated as

$$\mu \cong \bar{x} = \sum_{i}^{n} x_i / n$$

where x_i indicates the separate values of the series of numbers, x_1, x_2, x_3, . . . x_n, or in general x_n and $\sum^{n} x_i$ denote the sum of these n numbers. The mean or average is this sum divided by the number of observations.

The other parameter, σ, is a measure of the spread of the values. In Fig. 1-1 two curves have been plotted with different values for σ (5 and 2.5 for the solid and dashed curves, respectively). The dashed curve with the smaller value for σ has a smaller spread, with very few values under 92 or over 108; however, in the distribution indicated by the solid curve ($\sigma = 5$), an ap-

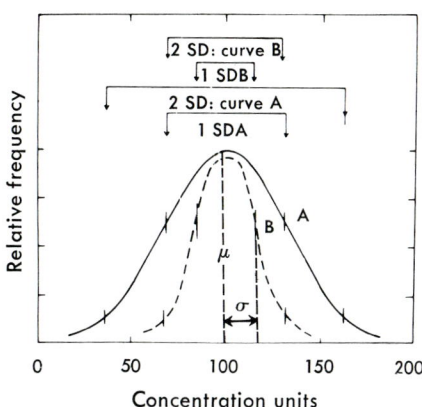

Fig. 1-1. Two typical gaussian curves. Curve A has twice the standard deviation (SD) of curve B. The ranges of 1 and 2 SD are shown for each curve.

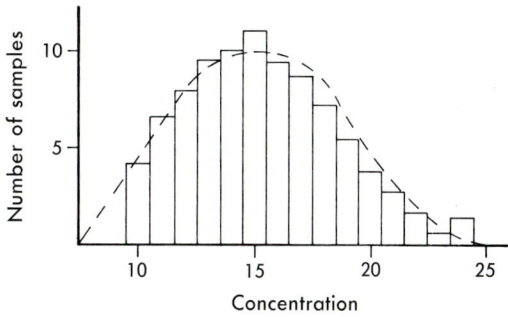

Fig. 1-2. Gaussian curve frequency histogram of hypothetical experimental results in the determination of a normal range.

preciable number of values are beyond these points. The σ value is generally termed the standard deviation (SD); an explanation of the actual method of calculating standard deviation is given later.

The Greek letters μ and σ are used for the theoretic values of the mean and standard deviation as derived from the true curve, and the English letters m and s (or M and S) refer to the calculated values from the experimental data. If the data conform closely to the theoretic curve, an average of 68.3% of the values should be within ± 1 SD of the mean and 95.5% within ± 2 SD. Furthermore, almost all of the values (99.7%) should be within ± 3 SD from the mean (Fig. 1-1). For some purposes the standard deviation is expressed as a percentage of the mean value: 100 SD/M. This is often called the *coefficient of variation* (CV), but a better term is *relative standard deviation* (RSD). The purpose of any quality control program is to check the precision of the measurements by noting whether repeated analyses of aliquots of the same material remain within certain definite limits. A limit of ± 2 SD (as calculated from a series of measurements) is often used, but other limits may be used as well.

In addition to standards for each substance being determined, a quality control program for analytic determinations requires one, or preferably two or more, control substances containing the constituent being analyzed. These are usually similar in nature to the body fluid being analyzed (serum, urine, etc.) and are analyzed with the regular samples in exactly the same way. Standards are needed whether or not a quality control program is used; therefore a discussion of standards follows.

The **standards** for use in chemical analysis may be aqueous solutions or standards in serum (or other body fluids if required). Aqueous solutions can be used for many manual testing methods (except for those testing lipids and enzymes), but the automated methods generally require standards in serum. Aqueous standards may be prepared in the laboratory or purchased, usually as stock solutions from which the actual standards can be prepared by dilution. The latter is usually preferable; however, larger laboratories may have the proper facilities for accurate weighing. Care must be taken in the dilution of aqueous stock standards. If the stock solutions are kept in the refrigerator, they must be warmed to room temperature before diluting. The stock solutions purchased are usually quite accurate, because they are prepared by weighing the proper amount of required chemical; when this is done in large batches, the error in weighing and dilution is small. Occasionally, one might suspect a stock solution to be in error. Even if the laboratory does not routinely prepare its own standards, it is helpful to be able to do so to check a purchased standard. Standard in serum are more satisfactory because they tend to compensate for the matrix elements present in the regular serum samples.

Most automated methods require a standard that is prepared in serum and contains all the constituents to be determined by the system. This is usually obtained as a lyophilized serum, which is reconstituted as needed. Most sera used for quality control are of a similar nature, and most of the following comments will apply whether the serum is used as a standard or as a quality control sample. The lyophilized material is obtained in small vials, which are stored in the refrigerator. The material usually can be obtained in several different vial sizes; the size to be used depends on the needs of the laboratory and the volume of tests requiring the serum for standard or control. The lyophilized material is reconstituted with water or, if carbon dioxide is one of the labeled constituents, with a standard ammonium bicarbonate solution. The diluting fluid should be carefully added with a volumetric pipet and the vial gently swirled; then the vial should be allowed to stand and should be occasionally swirled until the contents are completely in solution. It is not advisable to shake the vials vigorously, because this tends to inactivate some of the enzymes and the foam produced may prove troublesome. If bilirubin is one of the constituents, exposure to strong light should be avoided. The vials should be kept tightly stoppered and refrigerated when not in use. Under these conditions, many vials will be suitable for use on two consecutive days if reconstituted one morning. The stability should be checked by comparing the results from a newly reconstituted vial with one that has stood for 24-36 hr. In my experience, of the common constituents, those most likely to change under these conditions are glucose, which may decrease some 10% in value, and alkaline phosphatase, which will increase 15% or more in value. Tanishima et al.[8] have shown that reconstituting the lyophilized material with an equal-volume mixture of water and ethylene glycol will prevent changes in the level of alkaline phosphatase. This may also prevent other changes, and it might be helpful to compare the results obtained on other constituents with material reconstituted with water and with the water–ethylene glycol mixture. A serum standard prepared in a water–ethylene glycol mixture that does not require further reconstitution and is said to be quite stable under proper storage has been introduced on the market (Decision Chemistry Control Serum, Beckman Instruments, Fullerton, Calif.).

A number of different enzyme units are still in use for many of the common enzymes; when using a lyophilized serum as an enzyme standard or control, make certain that the enzyme values given on the package insert apply to the method used in the laboratory. Most of the control serums (except those made for a particular type of automated system) list the enzyme values by several different methods. Correction can be made if needed for differences in temperature, but these are not always reliable even when the appropriate factor is available.

Quality control sera can usually be purchased in different ranges: "low," "normal" "high," and "abnormal." The "high" levels are usually considerably higher than the normal values for most constituents. However, the "abnormal" values are not always higher; they may even be lower than the normal values if such lower values are of clinical significance.

When using any of the commercial control sera, a contract should be arranged with the manufacturer or supplier to set aside a sufficient amount of one lot number of each of the types of sera desired so that the same lot number can be used for at least 1 year. Frequent changes in the lot numbers of sera used in quality control add to the difficulties in implementing a good quality control program. The billing and delivery for the sera can usually be made on a monthly or bimonthly basis.

Another type of material that has been used for quality control is a pooled serum prepared in the laboratory. Excess nonhemolyzed sera without gross hyperlipemia are collected daily in the laboratory and pooled for storage in the refrigerator. When 1-2 L has been collected, the serum is centrifuged to remove gross contamination and then filtered through rapid paper. The mixed filtrate may then be divided into 5 ml aliquots, placed in tightly stoppered tubes, and stored at $-20°$ C. The aliquots are thawed as needed and mixed well before use. This material has several disadvantages. It is not as stable as the lyophilized material and requires some effort for preparation. Also it usually does not have elevated values for any constituents and may have undesirably low values for glucose and some enzymes. (A control serum with elevated levels is desirable, because the instrument may give correct values in the normal range for a constituent but may give false low or high values in the elevated range.) Attempts can be made to concentrate the serum somewhat by partially freezing the pool and pouring off the serum from the ice crystals. In addition, the serum can be "spiked" with constituents such as glucose, urea, creatinine, and the inorganic elements; however, this is not so successful with bilirubin, cholesterol, and the enzymes. Virtually the only advantage of the serum pool is that it is relatively inexpensive. It is sometimes used as a preliminary check before using the regular control serum in some types of automated equipment.

What are the proper limits for the control serum analyses? Often the limits are taken as ± 2 SD from the average determined by the analysis of a number of control serum samples by the regular method used. However, no matter how imprecise a method may be, 95% of the results will by definition fall within 2 SD of the mean, and the question of what is a "reasonable" variation remains. One of the earlier suggestions was that of Tonks,[9] who proposed that twice the coefficient of variation for repeated analyses of a constituent should not exceed one fourth of the difference between the limits of the normal range for that constituent expressed as a percentage of the midpoint of the range. For example, if the normal range for serum calcium is taken as from 8.5-10.5 mg/dl, then twice the relative standard deviation for the control serum determinations would be

$$\frac{10.5 - 8.5}{4} \times \frac{100}{9.5} = 5.3\%$$

For a control serum having a stated value of 10.3 mg/dl, the acceptable range would be

$$10.3 \ (1 + 0.0533) = 10.3 \pm 0.55$$

or from 9.75-10.85 mg/dl. If the normal range of serum sodium is from 135-145 mmole/L, then the 2 RSD for the control serum would be

$$\frac{145 - 135}{140} \times \frac{100}{140} = 1.8\%$$

and the acceptable limits for a control serum having a stated value of 138 mmole/L would be

$$138 \ (1 \pm 0.018) = 138 \pm 2.5$$

or from 135.5-140.5 mmole/L. This procedure leads to a 2 SD of 1.8% for sodium and chloride, 5% for calcium, and 7% for glucose, total protein, urea nitrogen, potassium, inorganic phosphate, and albumin. Whenever the calculated limits are greater than 10%, a value of 10% is used. (If the normal range for a constituent is narrow, this constituent must be determined more precisely to give relevant information about borderline values than when the range is large.) Although this concept has not been too widely accepted, it offers some idea as to what the standard deviation should be for control purposes. The calculations break down for substances such as creatinine and bilirubin for which the normal levels are around 1 mg/dl. A range of 2 SD calculated by the above formula would be too narrow for many procedures.

Another way to determine acceptable limits for a quality control program is to examine what limits other present-day methods obtain in the analysis of survey samples. In a survey of the 1974 ASCP program,[10] the results of the analyses of 13 common constituents in sera at various levels of concentration were subjected to computer analysis and the average relative standard deviation determined for the different analyses (Table 1-1). The methods of analysis were divided into two groups: manual methods and automated methods. Since the analyses for each constituent were made at different levels of concentration, regression equations were developed relating the relative standard deviation to the concentration level. In some instances the relative standard deviation was independent of the concentration level; in others it varied, though not necessarily in a linear manner. The equations were used to calculate the relative standard deviation for round values of the concentrations as presented in Table 1-1. Since these figures are merely intended to be guides and not absolute limits, linear interpolation can be made between the concentration limits given. Thus, for example, in an automated analysis of a serum having a total protein content of 6.5 g/dl, the relative standard deviation may be estimated to be about 2.4% and the actual standard deviation to be $6.5 \times 0.024 = 0.16$ g/dl. The values calculated from Table 1-1 should give a good approximation of a desirable standard deviation, and if in any instance the actual standard deviation found was more than about 1.2 times these calculated values, the method and procedure should be carefully examined for errors or deficiencies.

After an average or "target" value for each constituent has been established, the control serum is analyzed each day along with the regular samples. The number

Table 1-1. Average relative standard deviation values found for various analyses*

Constituent	Concentration level	Manual method (%)	Automated method (%)
Albumin	2.0 g/dl	5.6	4.9
	5.0 g/dl	5.6	2.8
Bilirubin	0.7 mg/dl	18.0	15.0
	1.0 mg/dl	14.0	13.0
	1.5 mg/dl	10.0	6.3
	2.0 mg/dl	7.5	5.0
	6.0 mg/dl	5.6	4.8
BUN	10.0 mg/dl	7.5	4.9
	50.0 mg/dl	6.5	3.6
	80.0 mg/dl	5.8	4.6
Calcium	8.0 g/dl	3.4	2.6
	12.0 g/dl	3.4	2.6
Chloride	80.0 mmole/L	2.3	1.6
	120.0 mmole/L	1.7	1.6
Cholesterol	120.0 mg/dl	4.5	4.6
	220.0 mg/dl	4.5	4.6
Creatinine	1.0 mg/dl	9.2	7.9
	1.5 mg/dl	8.3	6.2
	2.0 mg/dl	7.5	5.0
	6.0 mg/dl	5.3	3.6
Glucose	70.0 mg/dl	4.4	4.0
	160.0 mg/dl	4.4	3.1
	220.0 mg/dl	4.4	3.2
Phosphorus, inorganic	3.0 mg/dl	5.6	3.9
	8.0 mg/dl	4.0	3.9
Potassium	3.0 mmole/L	2.4	2.3
	8.0 mmole/L	2.4	1.7
Protein, total	5.0 g/dl	2.9	2.7
	8.0 g/dl	2.9	2.1
Sodium	120.0 mmole/L	1.3	1.3
	160.0 mmole/L	1.3	1.3
Uric acid	4.0 mg/dl	5.7	3.2
	11.0 mg/dl	4.5	2.3

*Data from Ross, J.W., and Fraser, M.B.: Am. J. Clin. Pathol. **68**(suppl. 1):130, 1977.

of control sera to be run depends on the number of samples. If very few samples are run by a manual method, it is necessary to run only one control serum, using a normal serum unless it is anticipated that some sample results will be high. When a number of samples are run in a batch, two control sera, one normal and one abnormal, are included. The control sera are treated the same way as the regular samples. In theory the control samples should be run "blind" (i.e., the analyst should not know which samples are the control sera). In practice this is difficult to accomplish, particularly when only a few samples are run at a time. In completely automated systems this is of less importance, because the instrument will show no bias in the analyses. In any event the control sera should not always be placed in the same position in the series, such as the first or last. When many samples are run in an automated system, the various control sera should be placed at random positions in the series. In some automated systems it may be helpful to run a few control sera at the beginning to rule out gross abnormalities. The serum pool mentioned earlier can be used for this.

When the analysis results for the different constituents of the control sera are obtained, they are checked to determine if they are within the allowable limits for each constituent. If the results are all within acceptable limits for the control sera, the results for the samples are released. If the results for the control sera are not within the acceptable limits for some or all constituents, further study is required. The analysis of the control sera serves as a basis for deciding whether the analysis of the samples is accurate enough to be released.

Plotting the daily control results helps to obtain a good picture of the whole quality control program, including the day-to-day variation. A commonly used graph is the Levey-Jennings graph (Fig. 1-3).[11] The expected average value and the $\pm$ 2 SD limits (or other limits if used) are marked off as indicated and the results for each day plotted. If more than one aliquot of a control serum is run, both values or their average may be plotted. In Fig. 1-3 the results of the analyses are in good control, with all the points within the required limits. The solid horizontal line represents the average value, and the dashed lines represent 2 SD from the mean. During days 1 to 6 at *A*, the values found all fall well within the normal control limits. On days 7 to 10 at *B*, although the values are within the normal range, they appear to be fluctuating considerably, which might indicate that somewhere in the procedure some factor (e.g., bath temperature) is fluctuating more than it should. On days 11 to 21 at *C,* we note that although the values are all within the normal range there appears to be a definite upward trend. This usually indicates a deterioration of one or more of the reagents or of the standard. At the point indicated by the arrow it is assumed that new reagents were made up. One notes a return to good control. The point on day 27 is too low. This would require immediate investigation to find the cause and a repeat analysis of the samples and control serum.

A number of other methods of plotting have also been used. One of these is the modified Youden plot[12] (Fig. 1-3). It consists of two Levey-Jennings charts placed at right angles to each other and is used when two different control sera are analyzed with each batch of samples. In order for the inner rectangular area between the two pairs of ± 2 SD lines to be approximately a square, the scales for the two axes must be different. This requires extra calculations; it may be more convenient to express the results in terms of the percentage of the average values. The results should fall along the diagonal line, clustering around the intersection of the two SD lines. Several points that are out of control are shown in Fig. 1-4. The point in the lower left-hand corner represented by the open circle indicates an analytic result in which both sera are below the lower limit. Since this point is near the diagonal, this indicates that the cause of error is effecting both sera proportionately (as would be the case if the standard gave too high a reading). The opposite would be true for the point represented by the triangle in the opposite corner. The square represents a point that shows a low value for X_1 and a high value for X_2; the point represented by * indicates a high value for X_1 and a normal value for X_2. If the results for different days are plotted, the points must be identified in some manner, such as by placing a number close to them.

When two aliquots of the same control serum are run at different times in the series, the difference between the values obtained in the two analyses can be plotted. It is preferable to use the algebraic difference, always subtracting the results obtained late in the series from those obtained earlier. Normally these points should fluctuate around the zero line. Results consistently above or below the line indicate that the results run later in the day were consistently higher or lower than those run earlier, and a search should be made for the cause.

A definite procedure should be set up to handle all instances in which the control serum analyses are outside the designated limits. The exact procedure will vary with the laboratory, but it must be sufficiently detailed so that all the analysts know what to do in every situation.

Precision and accuracy

In previously discussing errors involved in a given determination, the terms *precision* and *accuracy* were used. The terms are not synonymous. The results of repeated analyses on the same samples duplicating each other indicate **precision.** If the results of repeated analyses are all very close to each other, the method is high in precision. If the results of an analysis or of the

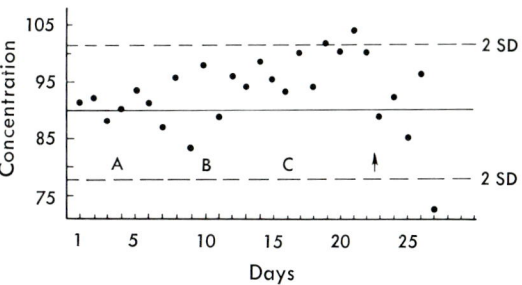

Fig. 1-3. Levey-Jennings quality control chart.

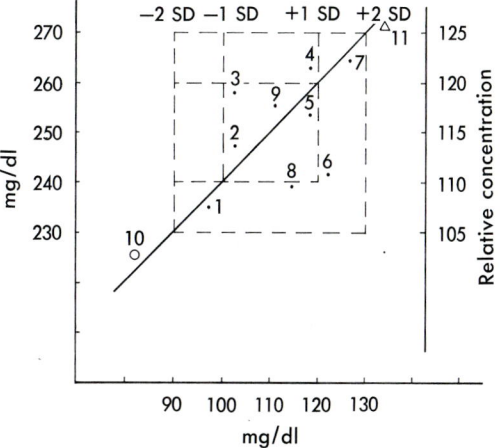

Fig. 1-4. Youden plot, modified. For explanation see text.

average of a series of analyses approach the true or correct value, then the analysis is said to be **accurate.** Precision can be readily estimated by methods that will be mentioned later. The determination of **accuracy** is not always simple, since the **true value** of the concentration of a substance in a biologic system may not be known. Usually the accuracy of a method is judged by analyzing the constituent by a number of different methods involving different types of chemical reactions; often those methods that are too long and complicated for routine use are used as reference. The problem is not always simple, as illustrated by the fact that although relatively precise blood sugar methods have been in use for nearly 40 years, there is still some discussion as to the "true" level of glucose in the blood.

In the laboratory the accuracy of a method can be checked by comparing results obtained on samples of known concentrations previously analyzed by competent workers or by using commercially available control sera. These are usually obtained in a lyophilized form and are quite stable under refrigeration, but they must be used within a short period after reconstitution. Even here, errors are possible. Care must be taken to add exactly the right amount of pure water and to make certain that the material is completely solubilized. Usually the control sera are quite reliable, but it should not always be assumed that they are absolutely correct. In cases of unexplainable discrepancies it is often advisable to try another sample from a different lot of the serum or even from a different manufacturer.

In the laboratory there is generally more interest in the **precision** of a method, or how well the results of repeated analyses are reproduced on the same sample. If, for example, the blood sugar level on one specimen is reported as 100 mg/dl and a second specimen taken at a later date is 110 mg/dl, does this represent a true change in the glucose level or is the difference within the limits of laboratory error and can significance be attached to the difference in reported levels? Obviously the more precise the method, the more meaningful are small differences.

Calculation of standard deviation: The standard deviation (SD) is a measure of the spread of values; the greater the standard deviation, the greater the differences between the individual determinations and the less the precision of the method. The mathematic formula for the standard deviation of a number of values is:

$$SD = \sqrt{\frac{\Sigma \, (\bar{x} - x_i)^2}{n - 1}} \qquad (1)$$

Expressed in words, this means to calculate the average value of the determinations $(\bar{x})$, find the difference between $\bar{x}$ and the separate values of (x_i), square these differences $(\bar{x} - x_i)^2$, and form the sum of these squares (Σ indicates the summation). This sum is then divided by one less than the number of values $(n - 1)$, and the square root of the quotient is extracted. Except

for the very simplest uses, this formula is not used in the calculations; the following equivalent formula is preferred.

$$SD = \sqrt{\frac{\Sigma(x_i)^2 - (\Sigma x_i)^2/n}{n - 1}} \qquad (2)$$

Note the difference between $\Sigma(x_i)^2$ and $(\Sigma x_i)^2$. In the former, the squares of the individual values are added; in the latter, the individual values are added, and the final sum is squared. The methods of calculation are illustrated in Table 1-2, which gives several variations. In column 1 are given the various individual values, x_i. Their sum, 1084, divided by 12 (the number of values) gives 90.33, the average value, $\bar{x}$. In column 2 the differences between the average and the separate values $(\bar{x} - x_i)$ are given. Since only the squares of these values are used, the sign of the difference need not be recorded. In column 3 the values for $(\bar{x} - x_i)^2$ are given. Their sum is 214.667. This value divided by $(n - 1)$, which is 11, gives 19,515. The square root of this last value is the standard deviation (SD = 4.42).

Column 4 gives the values for $(x_i)^2$ for use in calculating the standard deviation from equation 2. The sum of the values in this column is 98,136. From this is subtracted the square of the sum of the first column divided by the number of values, in accordance with equation 2, $(\Sigma x_i)^2/N$, to obtain 214.667, from which the standard deviation is calculated as before. With a good calculator, this method is simpler than using equation 1.

Columns 5 and 6 of the table represent a variation that is convenient when the calculations must be done

Table 1-2. Calculation of standard deviation

1 x_i	2 $(\bar{x} - x_i)$	3 $(\bar{x} - x_i)^2$	4 $(x_i)^2$	5 x'_i	6 $(x'_i)^2$
87	3.33	11.0889	7569	7	49
95	4.67	21.8089	9025	15	225
88	2.33	5.4289	7744	8	64
97	6.67	44.4889	9409	17	289
91	0.67	0.4489	8281	11	121
83	7.33	53.7289	6889	3	9
94	3.67	13.4689	8836	14	196
87	3.33	11.0889	7569	7	49
96	5.67	32.1489	9216	16	256
91	0.67	0.4489	8281	11	121
86	4.33	18.7489	7396	6	36
89	1.33	1.7689	7921	9	81
1084		214.6668	98,136	124	1496

$$\bar{x} = \frac{1084}{12} = 90.33$$

$$SD = \frac{214.667}{11} = 19.515$$

$$SD = \sqrt{19.515} = 4.418$$

$$\frac{(1084)^2}{12} = 97,921.333$$

$$\begin{array}{r} 98,136.000 \\ -\,97,921.333 \\ \hline 214.667 \end{array}$$

$$x' = \frac{124}{12} = 10.33$$

$$\bar{x} = 80 + 10.33 = 90.33$$

$$\frac{(124)^2}{12} = 1281.333$$

$$\begin{array}{r} 1,496.000 \\ -\,1,281.333 \\ \hline 214.667 \end{array}$$

manually. From the values in column 1 a convenient constant (in this illustration, 80) is subtracted to give the small positive numbers that have been designated x'_i in column 5. Column 6 contains the squares of these numbers. The average of the numbers in column 5 is 124/12, or 10.33, which, when added to the constant factor subtracted earlier (80), gives the true average of the original numbers, 90.33. Using equation 2, one again obtains from the sums of columns 5 and 6 the figure 214.667, from which the standard deviation is calculated.

Another convenient trick involves the change in decimal points. Suppose that the figures in column 1 were actually 8.7, 9.5, etc. The simplest way to proceed is to multiply all the figures by 10 to obtain the results actually shown. Then proceed as illustrated and, after all the calculations have been made, divide the final results by 10 to give an average of 9.033 and a standard deviation of 0.442. This method reduces the chances of errors resulting from misplaced decimal points.

For having a large number of determinations, many duplicate values, the simplest procedure is illustrated in Table 1-3. In column 1 of the table all the values obtained are listed in numeric order. Go through the list of actual determinations and count the number of results corresponding to each of the values in column 1 as illustrated in column 2. These figures are given in column 3 as Arabic numerals for convenience. Then subtract from each value in column 1 the lowest figure used (in the example, 85) to obtain the numbers in column 4. The figures in column 5 are then obtained by multiplying the figures in each row of columns 3 and

4. The figures in column 6 are obtained by multiplying the figures in each row of columns 4 and 5, as indicated at the top of the table. The sums of columns 3, 5, and 6 thus represent N, x_i, and $(x_i)^2$, respectively, from which the average and standard deviation can be calculated as illustrated in Table 1-2.

After the three sums, $N = 65$, $x_i = 475$, and $(x_i)^2 = 4063$ have been obtained, the final calculations can be done with sufficient accuracy for most purposes with a good 10 in. slide rule. Using a slide rule, one obtains an average of 92.32 and a standard deviation of 3.04.

Standards in clinical chemistry

In almost all determinations made in the laboratory by colorimetry, spectrophotometry, fluorometry, flame photometry, atomic absorption spectrometry, pH measurement, or titration, a comparison is made (directly or indirectly) between the results obtained on the samples and those obtained on a standard or standards of known composition. Thus the accuracy of the method can be no better than the accuracy with which the concentration of the standard is known. It is imperative, then, that the standards be as pure as possible. Very pure substances for standards can be obtained from the National Bureau of Standards (NBS). Those furnished by the NBS that are applicable to clinical chemistry include cholesterol, urea, bilirubin, creatinine, glucose, potassium chloride (for potassium and chlorine), sodium chloride, uric acid, lithium carbonate, vanillylmandelic acid, bovine serum albumin (for albumin and total protein), calcium carbonate, potassium acid phthal-

Table 1-3. Calculation of standard deviation

1 x	2	3 N_i	4 $x'_i = x_i - 85$	5 $x' \times N$	6 $x' \times x' \times N$
85	|	1	0	0	0
86		0	1	0	0
87	||	2	2	4	8
88	ﱢﱢ	5	3	15	45
89	||||	4	4	16	64
90	ﱢﱢ ||	7	5	35	175
91	ﱢﱢ |	6	6	36	216
92	ﱢﱢ |||	8	7	56	392
93	ﱢﱢ ﱢﱢ	10	8	80	640
94	ﱢﱢ |	6	9	54	486
95	ﱢﱢ ||	7	10	70	700
96	||||	4	11	44	484
97	|||	3	12	36	432
98		0	13	0	0
99	|	1	14	14	196
100	|	1	15	15	225
		$N = 65$		$\Sigma x_i = 475$	$\Sigma(x)^2 = 4063$

$$\overline{x} = 475/65 = 7.31$$
$$\overline{x} = 85 + 7.31 = 92.31$$

$$475^2/65 = 3471.2$$
$$4063.0 - 3471.2 = 591.8$$
$$SD^2 = 591.8/64 = 9.25$$
$$SD = 3.04$$

ate (acidimetric standard), tris(hydroxymethyl)amino-methane (alkalimetric standard), monopotassium phosphate and disodium phosphate (for the preparation of standard buffers), and potassium dichromate (as an absorbance standard). Others may be available in the future. These standards are too expensive for daily routine use; they are generally used to check the secondary standards, which are usually reagent-grade chemicals.

If the standards are to be made up in solution, they must usually be thoroughly dried and then weighed out on an analytic balance to at least 1 part in 5000. Stable materials such as inorganic salts and some organic chemicals can be dried for several hours in an oven at 100° C and then cooled in a desiccator over a good water absorbent such as anhydrous magnesium perchlorate. Other substances may be dried by placing them in a desiccator (preferably a vacuum type) over a desiccant for several days. No attempt should be made to dry bilirubin or urea. In making up aqueous solutions, a good grade of distilled or deionized water must be used as well as accurate volumetric flasks.

Many substances are available commercially as standards in solution that can be used directly or simply diluted to the proper concentration. Although such solutions have been generally found to vary less than 1% from the nominal value, they cannot always be assumed to be correct. If questionable results are obtained, the standards should always be checked against a solution made up in the laboratory or at least against a standard made by a different manufacturer.

One problem that sometimes arises with aqueous standards is that the biologic material being analyzed (such as serum) may contain interfering material not removed by preliminary treatment (e.g., the preparation of a protein-free filtrate) and thus may not react as it did with the pure aqueous standard. There is no simple solution to this problem. Sometimes internal standards are necessary, but usually the correct level is the one that is obtained when the determination is carefully run in comparison with the aqueous standard. The standardization of multichannel automated instruments may also present special problems. These are often standardized with commercially available lyophilized sera containing stated amounts of the desired constituents. The labeled amounts cannot always be uncritically accepted. They should be checked occasionally by running accurately prepared aqueous standards through the instrument when possible or by analyzing the standardizing serum for the constituents by a good reference method.

Serology

The field of clinical serology has rapidly expanded from the initial syphilis serology and febrile agglutination tests to present-day immunology (see Chapter 36).[13]

Quality control in serology is more difficult for the following reasons:

1. No standards are available, only controls.
2. Results obtained by one technic cannot be duplicated by another technic.
3. Some technics are more sensitive than others; e.g., the microcomplement fixation technic is more

sensitive than the agglutination technic, and the latter is more sensitive than the precipitation technic.

4. Various methods designed to detect the same antibody measure various properties of this antibody and thus vary in specificity (and sensitivity); e.g., the antinuclear antibody of lupus erythematosus can be detected by a fluorescent method, by a clot method, and by nucleoprotein precipitation. Each method further varies according to the actual technic employed.

In serology, commercial kits are frequently used. It is mandatory to always employ negative and positive controls supplied by the manufacturer and augmented by internal positive and negative controls; these consist of previously assayed clinical specimens, aliquots of which have been kept frozen and are rerun with each new kit before it is used routinely.

The list of items to be checked in a quality control program in serology follows the established outline.

Equipment: The equipment to be used includes timers, centrifuges, shakers, water baths, thermometers, fluorescence microscope (burning time of lamp), etc.

Reagents: If commercial reagents are employed, the manufacturer's instructions regarding use, storage, and outdating must be carefully followed.

Specimens: Two sterile specimens—an acute-phase specimen and a convalescent-phase specimen—are often required. Special precautions must be exercised in the collection of the specimen; e.g., cold agglutinins should not be stored in the refrigerator.

Personnel: Even though commercial kits are used, there should be a written procedure book available that adapts the manufacturer's instructions to the circumstances and equipment of the laboratory.

Commercial kits and replicate testing: Before a new serologic kit is used to test patients' specimens it is tested against the negative and positive controls employed in the old kit to determine whether the new kit's sensitivity and avidity are equal to or exceed those of the previously used kit.

Blood banking

Like all quality control programs, the program in blood banking can be divided into controls involving equipment, reagents, personnel, donor and recipient, and test procedures. Some features are unique to blood banks, because they deal with a biologic product.[12-15]

Equipment: Dated records should be kept of all maintenance and control procedures.

Centrifuges: Most laboratories use modifications of a standardized Sero-Fuge (Clay-Adams, Parsippany, N.J.) that require checking of the speed and timer. The speed should be kept at 3400 rpm and should be checked with a strobe-light tachometer. The timer should be tested against an accurate stopwatch. Vibration of the head should be checked, since it will dislodge the red cell buttons. Automated devices that wash, decant, and add Coombs serum are available. Coombs-positive control cells are used to check their efficiency.

View boxes: The use of the tube test is suggested for ABO and Rh typing, eliminating any worry about incorrect view box temperature or thermometer.

Refrigerators and freezers: Refrigerator temperature should be checked daily and should remain between 2° and 6° C. The freezer temperature should be maintained with an automated recorder and alarm system. At −20° C the storage time of most reagents is limited to 6 months. Many biologic products require storage at −80° C.

Blood storage: A refrigerator should be devoted entirely to the storage of blood, blood products, and blood bank reagents. It must be equipped with an automatic temperature recorder and an alarm system tied to a hospital station that is staffed day and night. The temperature must be kept at 4° C and must never exceed 10° C.

Water baths, heating blocks, and incubators: Certified thermometers should be used to control the temperatures and a daily log kept of the temperature readings.

Glassware: All test tubes should be made of disposable glass and should be used only once.

Reagents: The blood bank reagents (antisera, reagent test cells, enzyme preparations, etc.) are usually commercially prepared. The specificity, avidity, and potency of antisera, including Coombs sera, should be checked against specific cells. Antisera should be checked daily by the tube typing technique as follows: Anti-A_1, anti-**B,** group O, and absorbed anti-**A** sera should be tested against a panel of group A_1, A_2, B, A_2B, and O cells. Anti-**A** serum will react with A_1, A_2, and A_2B cells; anti-A_1 will react only with A_1 cells; group O will react with A_1, A_2, B, and A_2B cells; and anti-**B** will react with B and A_2B cells. Rh typing sera should be tested against Rh-positive, D^u-positive, and Rh-negative cells. Antiglobulin serum will react with sensitized cells coated with varying amounts of anti-**D.** It should not react with nonsensitized cells.

All blood banks should have at least two sets of typing sera and of Coombs sera produced by different manufacturers. Their reactions must be graded and should be 4+.

Reagent red cells: A and B cells, Rh-positive and Rh-negative cells, and Coombs-positive and Coombs-negative cells should be tested against the corresponding antisera and their reactions graded on a scale from 1+ to 4+.

The tube method is preferred for ABO and Rh typing because is prevents evaporation, allows an optimal ratio of antigen to antibody, and permits better temperature control.

Enzymes: The activity of proteolytic enzymes can be checked by their action on the gelatin layer of x-ray films.

Personnel: Well-trained technologists must have available an up-to-date outline of blood bank procedures and policies and a current copy of *Technical Methods and Procedures* by the American Association of Blood Banks.

Donor and recipient: A log book must be kept to account for every unit of blood received. The following information should be recorded: date, source and code number of donor units, result of processing (ABO and Rh typing, STS, atypical antibody screen result, hepatitis B surface antigen [HBsAg] etc.), result of compatibility testing, name of recipient, date of transfusion, and result of transfusion. Sequential numbering devices are commercially available for identification of donor blood, of pilot tubes, and of the recipient's blood samples.

If "outside" blood is used by the blood bank, the blood in the plastic segments should be used for retyping (ABO and Rh typing and antibody screening). The red cells obtained from the plastic segments must be washed in saline to remove the CPDA-1 solution before they are typed. HBsAg screen and serologic tests for syphilis do not have to be repeated.

External control systems are available from blood bank supply houses and from the American Association of Clinical Pathologists.

Urinalysis

In the urine laboratory there should be available an up-to-date procedure book that not only includes the approved procedures but also the corresponding references and source and grades of chemicals used. All chemicals and dipsticks should be appropriately stored and labeled as to date of purchase, manufacturer, and date of expiration if applicable.

Many of the erroneous results of urinalysis stem from errors in collecting and handling the urine specimen. The specimen should be an early-morning midstream sample and should be examined within 30 min of the time it was obtained. The specimen should not be subject to various delays in the patient's room, at the nurses' station, or on the laboratory bench. If delay is unavoidable, the specimen should be refrigerated. Allowing urine to stand at room temperature tends to encourage precipitation of phosphates in alkaline urine, bacterial growth with concomitant change to an alkaline pH, photodegradation, oxidation, and hydrolysis.

Before testing, mix urine specimen well and allow it to come to room temperature. The various semiquantitative tests for urinary protein, glucose, ketones, phenylpyruvic acid, occult blood, pH, etc. should be checked from time to time using solutions containing known quantities of these substances. A relatively stable urine control known as Tek-Chek (Ames Co., Elkhart, Ind.) is commercially available; this control provides a means of evaluating the daily accuracy of methods used for determining urinary pH, protein, glucose, ketones, hemoglobin, bilirubin, urobilinogen, and phenylketones.

The preparation of solutions for testing the urinalysis dipsticks and for standardization of urinometers and refractometers used in specific gravity measurements are discussed in Chapter 27.

Coagulation

All clotting procedures must be standardized to a high degree. Normal controls must be run with each test, and both test and control should be performed in duplicate.

Equipment:

Water bath and heating blocks: The thermometer temperature must be checked before each test. The thermostatic control must maintain a constant temperature of 37° C. A thermometer should be kept in the water bath and checked frequently.

Glassware: Glassware must be scrupulously clean and should not be scratched. Disposable plastic tubes are ideal for clotting procedures. Accurate, slow-emptying pipets are important, since the average amount handled varies from 0.1-0.3 ml. Test tubes should be uniform, because variation in size alone may alter the result of a coagulation test (e.g., the disintegration of a blood clot in the fibrinolysin test).

Reagents: Blood must be carefully obtained without contamination by tissue thromboplastin and without stasis. The proportion of anticoagulant to blood must be accurate (see Chapter 3). The specimen should not be exposed to temperatures of 37° C or greater for longer than 5 min. It can be kept in the refrigerator as long as 2 hr. Immediate return of a blood specimen to the laboratory is imperative. Best results are obtained if the blood is drawn in the laboratory. If this is not possible, double-walled jars with ice-water jackets are taken to the patient's room.

Method for precise visualization of clotting: An electronic clot timer is suggested for the clotting procedure.

Centrifugation: Because the number of platelets in plasma depends on the speed and size of the centrifuge, centrifugation should be carefully standardized. For many purposes a refrigerated centrifuge is advisable, or a small centrifuge can be placed in a refrigerator.

Siliconization: To preserve the number and function of platelets, contact with a rough glass surface must be prevented by a nonwettable surface such as that provided by siliconization. Smooth plastic or paraffinized surfaces closely duplicate the effectiveness of siliconization.

Technic: Details such as temperature, pH, and timing must be carefully standardized. The standard deviation of various tests should be determined after repeating the same test at least 15 times. (See discussion of quality control in clinical chemistry.)

Hematology[16,17]

The sources of error in hematology can be classified as follows[16,17]:

1. *Errors related to methods of sampling.* Capillary blood obtained from an inadequate puncture wound may yield lower counts than those obtained from venous blood because of dilution with tissue fluid when the puncture site is squeezed.

2. *Errors in preservation of the specimen.* Improper mixing, inadequate or excessive amounts of anticoagulant, and incorrect type of anticoagulant as well as a leaking stopper may lead to inaccurate counts and hematologic tests.

3. *Technical errors related to the instruments.* Inaccurate or dirty pipets, inadequately standardized automatic pipets, unmatched or dirty cuvets, and poor standards may all add up to inaccurate laboratory work.

Many of the errors related to a specific test (e.g., white count, red count, and hematocrit) are included in the discussion of the various tests.

Equipment such as centrifuges, cell counters, and diluters should be checked according to a definite preventive maintenance plan based on manufacturers' instructions.

Methods for detection of errors

Controls are available for automated and manual determinations of hemoglobin, hematocrit, white cell and red cell counts, and platelet counts.

Daily analysis results of hematology controls are plotted on a graph to show daily variations and to indicate any possible trend toward inaccurate results. All control tests are done in duplicate, and the standard deviation of duplicate tests should be calculated daily. (See discussion of quality control in clinical chemistry.)

The mean corpuscular hemoglobin (MCH) of normal blood can also be used as a control. The mean and the standard deviation can be recorded daily.

The calibration and quality control procedures for the completely automated hematology instruments are not uncomplicated. It is suggested that all determinations of the automated instruments be checked against fresh blood samples whose parameters have been determined by careful manual methods[18] or by a different automated method.

The commercial cell suspensions may be used for quality control purposes. The data obtained in this way are treated in the same way as outlined in the previous discussion of chemical determinations, using a quality control chart and calculating the standard deviation at intervals.

For quality control in chemistry it has been suggested that when a large number of determinations are made each day on patient samples, the average of all the values within the normal range be used as a control value.[19] This has been subject to some criticism[20] and is probably feasible only if the results are entered directly into a computer for the daily calculations. For hematology the daily determinations of hemoglobin, red cell count, and hematocrit vary too much for control use, but the derived quantities (mean corpuscular hemoglobin [MCH], mean corpuscular hemoglobin concentration [MCHC], and mean corpuscular volume [MCV]) appear to vary much less and to have a nearly normal distribution about the mean. Thus the daily averages of these values would serve as control values in indicating trends in the operation and results of the automated apparatus.[21] Bull et al. give examples of the use of this method in detecting changes in the output of the instrument. This method, however, involves many tedious calculations unless some computer assistance is available.

Estimation of total white cell count from stained blood smear:

No./hpf	Estimated total count
2-4	4000-7000
4-6	7000-10,000
6-10	10,000-13,000
10-20	13,000-18,000

Fragile leukemic cells may disintegrate in the Coulter counter; therefore the total white count should be estimated from the slide as a check on the Coulter counter result.

Estimation of platelets: A peripheral blood smear may be used to judge the platelet count:

Less than 1 platelet/oil-immersion field—decreased number of platelets

Several platelets with occasional clumps—adequate supply of platelets

More than 25 platelets—increased number of platelets

If the number of platelets in 10 oil-immersion fields is counted and the total figure is multiplied by 2000, the result closely approximates the platelet count as obtained by the manual method.

The standard deviation of various tests should be determined and the results of normal, high, and low controls plotted daily on graph paper. (See discussion of quality control in clinical chemistry.)

Microbiology

Safety rules. Quality control begins with a properly designed bacteriology laboratory equipped with a dedicated safety hood that pulls air from the laboratory to the outside. A number of safety rules—careful technique, the use of safety pipetting devices, and periodic washing of all equipment with 2% phenol solution—should be enforced at all times when working with bacteria. An alcohol-sand flask should be available for cleaning inoculating loops prior to flaming, which should be done in a spatter-proof Bacti-Cinerator (Scientific Products, McGaw Park, Ill.). All bacteriologic waste material must be autoclaved prior to leaving the department.

Quality control procedures must be observed in the handling of every specimen, from collection and transportation to the laboratory to handling by the technologists, plating, choice of media, recording of findings, and incorporation of the findings into the patient's record.

Collection: A representative, adequate specimen must be obtained from a suitable source or area under conditions that prevent contamination. It must be collected in sterile, labeled, covered containers that allow ready access to the material. Material may also be collected on Culturette swabs (Scientific Products, Evanston, Ill.). Anaerobic culture technics require special methods and media of collection.

The label on the specimen and the request must not only identify the patient but also state the source of the material and the time when it was obtained. The material should be sent to the laboratory immediately and not be allowed to remain at the nurses' station. After its arrival in the laboratory, it should be handled immediately.

Transportation: Transport media are not needed if the culture can be taken at the bedside or in the outpatient department and sent immediately to the laboratory for processing. When specimens are collected in areas removed from the laboratory, Culturette rayon-tipped swabs should be used. After the specimen is obtained, these are kept moist by a modified Stuart transport medium. The medium provides a moist environment for 72 hr without supplying nutrients. If *Neisseria gonorrhoeae* is suspected, the material should be streaked directly on Thayer-Martin agar; if *Shigella* is suspected, the material should be streaked directly on XLD medium.

Equipment: Written records should be kept of the carbon dioxide content (which should be from 5-10%),

of carbon dioxide incubators, and of their temperature (which should be 35-37° C, 35° C being the preferred temperature). Carbon dioxide analyzers are commercially available. Autoclaves, refrigerators, and freezers must all be kept in top working condition and monitored daily.

Handling of culture by technologist: The technologist must be adequately trained in the recognition of pathogens and normal flora and have the opportunity for further training. Detailed up-to-date laboratory manuals should be available to point out step-by-step the correct choice of media, inoculation, preparation of smears, and staining. To aid in properly identifying bacteria, mimeographed forms are suggested that list the various procedures used for identifying bacteria (including sensitivities) and allow space for recording the results of these procedures. These work sheets are filed for future reference.

Media control: Media should not be prepared (or bought) in too large quantities, as they dry out and must then be discarded.

Media control involves first the proper choice of media (i.e., the minimal number of media necessary to identify pathogenic organisms). The media must be appropriate for the type of specimen, and at least two media of different levels of selectivity and specificity should be chosen. Since errors such as incorrect weighing, incorrect measuring of water, and deteriorated stock powder occur in the preparation of media, the following characteristics must be controlled: sterility, ability to selectively support the growth of desired bacteria and/or suppression of others, and chemical reactivity.

Sterility testing: Check media for sterility after an incubation of 24 hr at 35° C in 5% carbon dioxide. There should, of course, be no growth in the uninoculated agar.

Performance of media: Test the performance of media with organisms that normally grow well on them and produce typical reactions (Table 1-4; see also Chapter 32).

Gram stain control: The Gram stain can be checked by applying a match head–sized drop of a mixture of known gram-positive and gram-negative bacteria to the slide, allowing it to dry, and then staining it and the unknown with Gram stain.

Sensitivity test controls: Using the Kirby-Bauer technic (4 mm thick, 150 × 15 mm Mueller-Hinton agar plates), monitor the reactions of a specific strain of *Escherichia coli* (ATCC 25922) and of a specific strain of *Staphylococcus aureus* (ATCC 25923) to various antibiotics. The same strains are used as controls in the tube dilution and micro-tube systems (see Chapter 32).

Stock cultures: Most of the steps just outlined employ reference cultures (Table 1-5). Such cultures are commercially available (American Type Culture Collection (ATCC), Rockville, Md., and National Collection of Type Cultures (NCTC), Central Public Health Laboratory, London). Pure cultures obtained daily in the laboratory can be carried on stock culture media for prolonged periods when stored in the refrigerator. Periodic transfer of these cultures can be arranged as

Table 1-4. Tests of performance of media and differential disks

	Test organism	Results
Media		
Blood agar	Group A *streptococcus*	β-Hemolysis 1-2 mm diameter in 18 hr at 35° C in 5% CO_2
Chocolate agar	*Neisseria gonorrhoeae*	Growth in 5% CO_2
MacConkey agar	*Escherichia coli*	Red 2 mm colonies in 24 hr at 35° C
SS agar	*Escherichia coli*	Pink colonies partially inhibited
XLD agar	*Escherichia coli*	Yellow colonies, yellow agar
TSI agar	*Escherichia coli*	Acid butt, acid slant, gas, no H_2S
Mycosel agar	*Candida albicans*	Growth
Citrate agar slant	*Escherichia coli*	No growth
	Enterobacter aerogenes	Growth, change in color of slant to blue
Urea agar slant	*Proteus*	Growth, pink color of medium
	Escherichia coli	No growth
Anaerobic system		
Blood agar	Bacteroides	Growth
Methylene blue indicator*		Reduction of dye
Differential disks		
Bacitracin disk	Group A streptococcus	Inhibition zone
	Streptococcus faecalis	No inhibition zone
Oxidase test	*Pseudomonas aeruginosa*	Positive, purple color
	Escherichia coli	Negative, no color change
Optochin test (ethylhydrocupreine hydrochloride)	*Streptococcus pneumoniae*	Growth inhibition zone 5 mm
	α-Hemolytic streptococcus	No growth inhibition zone
Differential test		
Bile solubility	*Streptococcus pneumoniae*	Loss of turbidity of fresh culture tube in 5-15 min
	Streptococcus faecalis	No loss of turbidity

*Methylene blue is superior as an indicator of anaerobiosis because, if the test culture does not grow, the fault may be in the stock culture and not in the anaerobiosis.

shown in Table 1-6. Freeze-drying equipment allows lyophilization of young cultures suspended in sterile serum. Standardized lyophilized preparations of bacteria are commercially available (Bacto-Check, Roche Diagnostics, Nutley, N.J.).

Serology: Serologic tests employed in bacteriology are only meaningful if they are accompanied by negative and positive controls. Titrated sera from the first specimen should be frozen and retitrated with the second specimen. (See discussion of quality control in serology.)

Recording and reporting of laboratory results: An accession book should show the date (and time if necessary) when the culture was received and should identify the patient (name and hospital number) and the material as well as the physician. After the bacteria are identified, the date of the test's completion and the final diagnosis are entered in the accession book. If identification requires a prolonged period of time, the reporting system must be organized so that the physician is certain to receive the results of the completed work. Many bacteriologic results only reach the record room and not the physician. If a culture requires several

weeks, an interim report should be sent to assure the physician that the laboratory is still working on the analysis.

Parasitology

Adequately trained personnel with knowledge and experience in the correct identification of parasites are essential. Supervisory personnel with extensive experience should check all positive specimens and spot-check every tenth negative specimen. Control parasitology specimens are included in several commercially available laboratory surveys.

Specimens

Specimens and material sent to the laboratory must be fresh, sufficient in amount, and properly collected (see Chapter 3). Stool specimens are unsuitable if they contain barium, oil, iron, or bismuth or are contaminated with urine, toilet paper, or water. All specimens should be brought immediately to the laboratory.

Procedures: Approved routine procedures should be arranged in the procedure book in sequence of suggested performance. No single test is satisfactory for

Table 1-5. Recommended strains of stock cultures*

Genus	NCTC	ATCC	Genus	NCTC	ATCC
Acinetobacter anitratus	7844	15308	*Proteus valgaris*	4175	13315
Aeromonas liquefaciens	7810	9071	*Pseudomonas aeruginosa*	7244	7700
Alcaligenes faecalis	655		*Salmonella typhi*	786	
Bacillus subtilis	3610	6051	*Salmonella typhimurium*	74	13311
Clostridium sporogenes	533	10000	*Shigella dysenteriae I*	4837	13313
Clostridium welchii	6719	9856	*Shigella sonnei*	8220	
Enterobacter aerogenes	10006	13048	*Staphylococcus aureus*	8532	12600
Enterobacter cloacae	10005	13047	*Staphylococcus epidermidis*	4276	
Escherichia coli	9001	1175	*Streptococcus agalactiae*	8181	13813
Klebsiella aerogenes	418	15380	*Streptococcus dysgalactiae*	4669	
Mycobacterium phlei	8151		*Streptococcus faecalis*	8213	
Mycobacterium smegmatis	8159		*Streptococcus hominis*	8618	7073
Nocardia brasiliensis	10300		*Streptococcus pneumoniae*	7465	10015
Nocardia caviae	1934		*Streptococcus sanguis*	7863	10556
Proteus morganii	10041				

*From Cowan, S.T., and Steel, K.J.: Manual for the identification of medical bacteria, London, 1965, Cambridge University Press.

Table 1-6. Conditions for maintenance of test organisms*

Genus	Medium	Incubation		Storage (°C)	Interval between subcultures (mo)
		Temp. (°C)	Time (hr)		
Acinetobacter	Nutrient agar	37	18	5-25	3
Aeromonas	Nutrient agar	37	18	5-25	3
Alcaligenes	Nutrient agar	37	18	5-25	3
Bacillus	Nutrient agar	30	48	5-25	12
Clostridium	Cooked meat	37	48	5-25	12
Enterobacter	Nutrient agar	37	18	5-25	6
Escherichia	Nutrient agar	37	18	5-25	6
Klebsiella	Nutrient agar	37	18	5-25	3
Mycobacterium	Dorset egg	37	48-72	15-25	6
Nocardia	Dorset egg	37	48-72	15-25	3
Proteus	Nutrient egg	37	18	5-25	3
Pseudomonas	Peptone water agar	30	18	5-25	3
Salmonella	Dorset egg	37	18	5-25	12
Shigella	Nutrient agar	37	18	5-25	6
Staphylococcus	Nutrient agar	37	18	5-25	3
Streptococcus	Cooked meat or	37	18	5-25	3
	blood broth	37	8	5	1

*From Cowan, S.T., and Steel, K.J.: Manual for the identification of medical bacteria, London, 1965, Cambridge University Press.

all specimens. Each specimen should be examined at least three times. Errors in diagnosis may occur if details of even the "simplest" method (e.g., the preparation of wet mounts) are not adhered to.

Continuing education: It is necessary to preserve positive specimens and to collect slides so that they are available for teaching and training. Prepared slides are commercially available (General Biological Supply House, Inc., Chicago). The U.S. Public Health Service Centers for Disease Control have many excellent teaching films available for loan.

Parasite sources: A variety of animals harbor representatives of various intestinal parasites and can be used to supply living specimens. The following are sources of parasites.

Roundworms (pinworms): Pinworms similar to human pinworms are found in the hindgut of the cockroach. Puppies may supply hookworm and whipworm eggs. Adult pig *Ascaris* is indistinguishable from that of humans. Stools from monkeys or chimpanzees contain motile *Strongyloides* larvae.

Tapeworms: Laboratory mice may harbor the dwarf tapeworm. Eggs of cat and dog *Taenia* are indistinguishable from human *Taenia*. Adult worms may also be obtained.

Trematodes: Freshwater snails harbor a variety of larval trematodes. When placed in tap water they may liberate cercariae.

Protozoa: Monkey and chimpanzee feces often contain *Balantidium coli, Entamoeba histolytica, Entamoeba coli, Iodamoeba* species, and *Trichomonas hominis*. Guinea pig feces contain *Balantidium coli, Giardia, Trichomonas,* and *Entamoeba*. Laboratory mice supply *Amoeba, Giardia, Trichomonas,* and other flagellates.

The motility of amebas can be demonstrated at room temperature using *Entamoeba terrapinae* (General Biological Supply House, Inc., Chicago), which grows readily in culture.

REFERENCES

1. Dharan, M.: Total quality control in the clinical laboratory, St. Louis, 1977, The C.V. Mosby Co.
2. Ottaviono, P.J., and DiSalvo, A.P.: Quality control in the clinical laboratory, Baltimore, 1977, University Park Press.
3. Winstead, M.: Instrument check systems, Philadelphia, 1971, Lea & Febiger.
4. Winstead, M.: Reagent grade water, Austin, Tex., 1967, American Society of Medical Technologists.
5. Whitehead, T.P.: Quality control in clinical chemistry, New York, 1977, John Wiley & Sons, Inc.
6. Anido, G., et al., editors: Quality control in clinical chemistry, Hawthorne, N.Y., 1973, Walter De Gruyter, Inc.
7. Barnett, R.N.: Clinical laboratory statistics, Boston, 1971, Little, Brown & Co.
8. Tanishima, K., et al.: Clin. Chem. **23:**1873, 1977.
9. Tonks, D.B.: Clin. Chem. **9:**217, 1963.
10. Ross, J.W., and Fraser, M.B.: Am. J. Clin. Pathol. **68**(suppl. 1.):130, 1977.
11. Levey, S., and Jennings, E.R.: Am. J. Clin. Pathol. **20:**1059, 1950.
12. Youden, W.J.: Anal. Chem. **22:**23A, 1966.
13. Neff, J.: Quality control, serology, MT-12: telephone lectures for medical technologists, Columbia, Mo., 1971, University of Missouri-Columbia Medical Center and Extension Division.
14. Quality control: a practical workshop, Chicago, 1970, American Association of Blood Banks.
15. Miller, M.: Quality control, blood bank, MT-14 and MT-15: telephone lectures for medical technologists, Columbia, Mo., 1971, University of Missouri- Columbia Medical Center and Extension Division.
16. Dorsey, D.B.: Am. J. Clin. Pathol. **40:**457, 1963.
17. Lewis, S.M., and Coster, J.F., editors: Quality control in hematology, New York, 1975, Academic Press, Inc.
18. Gilmer, P.R., Jr., et al.: Am. J. Clin. Pathol. **68:**185, 1977.
19. Hoffman, R.G.: Am. J. Clin. Pathol. **43:**134, 1969.
20. Reed, A.N.: Clin. Chem. **16:**129, 1970.
21. Bull, B.S., et al.: Am. J. Clin. Pathol. **61:**473, 1974.

CHAPTER 2

Safety in the clinical laboratory

GENERAL CONSIDERATIONS

Safety in the clinical laboratory has received increased emphasis in recent years, partly as a result of the manifold regulations of the Occupational Safety and Health Administration (OSHA).[1] Regulations concerning the physical layout of the laboratory and emergency exits will not be discussed here except to note that all personnel should know the exit routes and should be familiar with the locations of the various safety devices—fire extinguishers, emergency showers, eye washers, fire blankets, and other equipment such as respirators and goggles—and with their use and operation. This information should be carefully explained to new employees and to all employees after the acquisition of new emergency equipment. (If any information is not understood, laboratory personnel should not hesitate to ask the supervisor for clarification.) Personnel should also recognize the various auditory or visual signals for fire or other emergencies and should fully cooperate in all emergency drills.

Safety manual

Every laboratory should have a safety manual covering all safety practices and precautions, including regulations concerning the proper use of equipment and the handling of toxic or infectious materials. The references cited give further information on these points.[2-4] Material in this chapter deals in a general way with factors most common to clinical laboratories.

Warning signs

Consistent warning signs should be used to indicate the presence of hazards. The Hazards Identification System developed by the National Fire Protection As-

sociation has been adopted by some laboratories. This system consists of four small, diamond-shaped symbols grouped into a larger diamond shape (Fig. 2-1).[5] The left diamond is blue and is used to identify health hazards. The top diamond is red and indicates a flammability hazard. The diamond on the right is yellow and warns of a reactivity-stability hazard (meaning that materials capable of explosion or violent chemical change are present). The bottom diamond is white and is used to provide special hazard information. It may indicate the presence of radioactivity (Fig. 2-2), special bio-

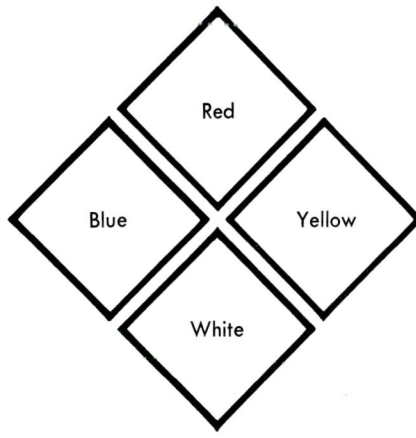

Fig. 2-1. Identification system of the National Fire Protection Association.

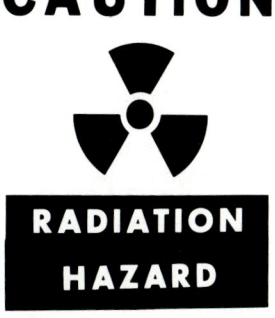

Fig. 2-2. Special hazard warning.

CAUTION

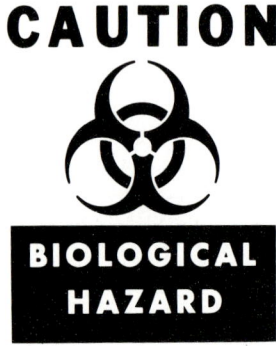

Fig. 2-3. Special hazard warning.

CAUTION

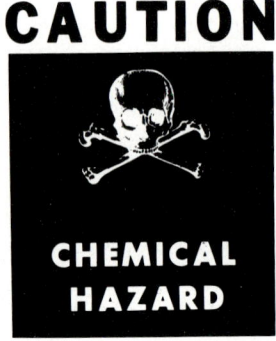

Fig. 2-4. Special hazard warning.

hazard (Fig. 2-3), corrosives, or other dangerous elements (Fig. 2-4). The severity of each hazard included in the symbol is suggested by numbers from 0 to 4, the greatest degree being 4. This simple system can provide safety information for all personnel and aid in any fire fighting as well.

Personal behavior

Smoking, eating, and drinking should be prohibited in all work areas. These activities should be carried out only in designated rest areas completely separated physically from work areas. Foot-operated drinking fountains may be allowed just outside the work areas. Although the greatest danger from eating or smoking in the laboratory is the possibility of infection from laboratory specimens, there is also the possibility that food or tobacco could contaminate test materials. For the same reasons application of cosmetics should not be done in work areas. No matter what type of work is done in the laboratory, the hands should always be washed before eating, smoking, or leaving the laboratory.[6]

Long hair must be secured so that it will not come in contact with specimens, work areas, reagents, or media or become entangled in laboratory equipment. In the microbiology laboratory it may be advisable to use the same precautions that food service workers use in regard to hair containment, since contamination may occur from shedding of long hair and beards.

VOLATILE FLAMMABLES
Storage

All refrigerators must be clearly marked on the outside as to the type of material to be placed in them, indicating whether they are explosion proof. (Under no circumstances should food or drinks be placed, even temporarily, in a refrigerator in the work area; these should be left only in designated refrigerators in the rest area.) Volatile solvents should be labeled as to their hazardous qualities and should be kept in explosion-proof refrigerators. These solvents should be kept in these refrigerators only in as small a quantity as is consistent with daily use, preferably not more than 1 week's supply. (There is some question as to the safety of storing flammable solvents such as ethyl ether under refrigeration instead of on an open shelf in a well-ventilated area. Opening a refrigerator door can release evaporation vapors, resulting in ignition and explosion.) Large amounts of such solvents must be kept in a fireproof, specially ventilated area with explosion-proof switches and lighting and a 4 in. sill or ramp at the bottom of the door to prevent the escape of heavier-than-air vapors. Flammable liquids in quantities of more than 2 L should be stored only in clearly labeled, approved red safety storage containers with pressure-relieving, spring-closing covers and flame-arrester screens. Maintaining only the minimal amount of flammables necessary is a good practice.

Handling

All flammable[7] and toxic liquids should be handled in a space with good ventilation, preferably in a fume hood. Evaporation of such liquids must be carried out in a fume hood using a water bath. Extreme caution should be taken with very volatile flammable liquids[7] such as ethyl ether, since the vapors of these liquids can be ignited by any ignition source, even a hot plate or oven. In the evaporation of larger quantities of volatile liquids, glass beads or other antibump granules should be added to prevent bumping and the sudden release of large amounts of vapors. The fume hood function may be checked easily by noting the disposal of smoke or fumes produced after cautiously bringing close together two applicator sticks whose cotton tips have been dipped in strong ammonia and hydrochloric acid, respectively (rinse the tips in running water before discarding).

COMPRESSED GAS
Handling and storage[8]

Large cylinders (200 ft^3) of compressed gases often are used in the laboratory. The most commonly used gases are oxygen with acetylene or methane (for atomic absorption or flame spectroscopy), hydrogen or helium (for gas-liquid chromatography), nitrogen, and carbon dioxide. The cylinders are color coded, but the contents must be clearly marked on the cylinder. (Otherwise it should be returned unused to the supplier marked "Contents Unknown.") All cylinders must be securely fastened to the wall or bench or placed in floor holders so that they cannot overturn. A fall can rupture the outlet valve, and the cylinder may then act like a torpedo and inflict serious injury. When transported, the cylinders must always be secured on a dolly or hand truck, and the protective caps must be on when the cylinders are not connected to equipment.

It is advisable to place a large tag on the tank indicating the date that the cylinder was put into use. Empty cylinders must be marked as such. (Note, however, that a small amount of gas must be left in the cylinder and valves closed to prevent negative pressure and drawing in of foreign contaminating materials.) Extra cylinders should be stored away from the laboratory in a secure, upright position, preferably in a locked, ventilated, fire-resistant space with the empty cylinders well separated from the full ones.

Precautions

The reduction valves for the different types of gases are not interchangeable, and no attempt should be made to interchange them. Laboratory personnel should not attempt to force or free stuck or frozen cylinder valves. When in use, all connections to the cylinders should be tested for leaks with soapy water. Very small leaks of oxygen or nitrogen are of little consequence (except for the waste of gas), but leaks of hydrogen, acetylene, or other flammable gases are not to be tolerated. When shutting down flammable gases, the gas is first turned off at the main take-in valve and the gas allowed to burn out; then the reduction valves are closed. It should be remembered that propane is heavier than air and that a little leaking gas can flow along the top of the bench to be ignited by a flame elsewhere. Many flame photometers use small cylinders of propane. These are very convenient and usually cause little difficulty. Because of potentially hazardous characteristics, only properly trained persons should handle compressed gases.

CORROSIVES
Handling

Caution must be observed when using toxic or corrosive solutions such as those of mercury salts or caustic acids or alkalis. When handling these chemicals, laboratory personnel should wear goggles or a face mask. Strong stirring should be avoided or done in a hood. If considerable stirring is needed, a magnetic stirrer can be used to avoid splashing. In preparing reagents, caution should always be taken to *slowly* add acid to water. If a small amount of any reagent gets into an eye, it should immediately be rinsed well (for at least 15 min) in the eye washer while holding the eyelids apart with the fingers and rotating the eyeball. Contact lenses should not be worn in the laboratory. They prevent proper washing of the eyes in the event a harmful solution does reach them, which could result in serious, permanent damage. Plastic lenses may be damaged by organic vapors.

Spills

All spills should be cleaned up at once. If the material is toxic or corrosive, rubber gloves and plastic apron should be donned before cleaning up. All potentially infectious materials such as serum or other body fluids should be flooded with a 5% solution of sodium hypochlorite or other disinfectant before being wiped up (wearing gloves); the waste should be disposed of with other infectious materials, not with ordinary wastes. Dilute solutions of acids or bases may be neutralized with solid sodium bicarbonate. For stronger acids, after dilution with water, solid sodium carbonate may be used with caution. For strongly basic solutions, a 1:5 dilution of acetic acid can be used. The "Space Clean-Up Kit" (Mallinkrodt Chemical Co., St. Louis) is satisfactory for laboratory use. It contains rubber gloves, towels, a scoop, and various chemicals for neutralizing and absorbing acid or alkaline spills, as well as material for absorbing organic solvents. Similar kits can be made with gloves, towel and other tools, sodium bicarbonate, an organic acid such as citric acid, and a quantity of absorbing material such as celite or diatomaceous earth. For such kits only the cheapest grade of technical chemicals need be used. These kits should be kept in strategic places in the laboratory, conspicuously labeled to indicate their use.

MERCURY

A particularly troublesome substance to recover is metallic mercury. Although it is not used so much as formerly (with Van Slyke or Natelson apparatus), it may still be used occasionally. Spilled mercury tends to break up into very fine droplets that are difficult to pick up. Even after collection disposal is a problem, since metallic mercury should not be incinerated or buried. If mercury is used in the laboratory, the "Mercury Absorption/Disposal Kit" (Aldrich Chemical Co., Milwaukee) may be helpful. It contains material that will readily absorb mercury droplets, producing a less toxic substance that may be disposed of by burial. Older benches or floors may contain fine cracks in which minute mercury globules may be lodged. These are very difficult to remove, but the cracks should be cleaned if possible, since mercury is somewhat volatile at room temperature. Rubbing powdered sulfur or sodium polysulfide into the cracks may help to change the mercury to the less volatile sulfide.

Some colorimetric methods, particularly for chloride, use mercury salts in a reagent. The disposal of large amounts of spent reagent in automated methods may be a problem, since the solution should not be disposed of in the sewer.[9] The waste material may be collected in large plastic containers and made slightly acid with acetic acid, if necessary, and with thioacetamide (about 10 g/L) added. This is stored in a ventilated area (small amounts of hydrogen sulfide may be liberated), and over a period of time the mercury will be precipitated as mercuric sulfide. The supernatant may then be decanted and disposed of in the sewer. The mercuric sulfide may be disposed of by burial.

AZIDES

Another troublesome chemical, sodium azide, was used as a preservative in the past, though its use has largely been discontinued. Azides form explosive salts with a number of metals such as copper and iron. These salts are readily detonated by mechanical shock. Although the amount used as a preservative is relatively small, continued use with disposal through the sewer can result in a buildup of the metallic salts in the sewer pipes. These salts are extremely explosive; even use of a wrench on such a drain line may result in a violent explosion. It is difficult to remove the azides from the pipes. One suggestion is to close the lower end of a section of pipe and allow a 10% solution of sodium hydroxide to stand at least 16 hr in the pipe, then rinse copiously with water (a minimum of 15 min). It is best to avoid the use of solutions containing azides, particularly since they are also said to be carcinogenic.

CARCINOGENIC HAZARDS

The use of chemicals that are possibly carcinogenic is another hazard in the laboratory.[10] Many of these are aromatic amines. One, benzidine, has been used frequently in the laboratory for testing hemoglobin (plasma hemoglobin and occult blood). Generally this can be replaced by the compound 3,3′, 5,5′-tetramethylbenzidine dihydrochloride, which is much safer. With proper precautions some potentially carcinogenic compounds can be used occasionally, if necessary. Precautions should include performing the procedure in an isolated area or in a good fume hood, wearing rubber gloves and (if dusty material is handled) a respirator, careful cleanup of the work area, rinsing the glassware with a strong acid or an organic solvent before placing it in the regular washing cycle, and using disposable equipment as much as possible. No pipetting should be performed by mouth.

PROCEDURES AND EQUIPMENT

Whenever a potentially toxic or dangerous chemical is used in a procedure, the directions in the procedure manual should include warnings of the noxious properties of that chemical. For example, it may seem superfluous to add ''Caution: Corrosive'' whenever the use of concentrated sulfuric acid is mentioned, or ''Caution: Highly Flammable'' whenever the use of diethyl ether is mentioned, but these warnings may be helpful to someone who is not familiar with the procedure or to the worker who may become careless through the routine use of a dangerous chemical.

Cracked or chipped glassware should not be used (being more likely to break during use), but should be discarded. Flasks or beakers used with corrosive or toxic substances should be rinsed well with water or alcohol (depending on the solubility) before being placed in the collection container for soiled glassware. No pipetting by mouth should be allowed. Although it may seem safe to orally pipet distilled water or saline, it is best to use a pipetting device at all times; thus an attempt to pipet a dangerous substance by mouth is less likely. For simple dilutions with water or saline, the use of a good quality buret with a Teflon stopcock (or automatic dispensing bottle) is often convenient.

HEPATITIS

The presence of hepatitis viruses in blood, tissue, urine, and feces from infected individuals constitutes a hazard to laboratory personnel.[11] Samples from known (or suspected) hepatitis patients should be noticeably marked as such. Food, beverage, and smoking restrictions, good personal hygiene, use of disposable gloves and disinfectants, and prevention of aerosols must be stringently applied. Employee education in regard to this problem is important.

SAFEGUARDS

Disposable, plastic, Pasteur-type pipets are useful for transferring serum or other samples from the collection tubes to the test tube or sample containers of many types of automated apparatus. Samples should not be poured, since this could contaminate the fingers and the outside of the tubes. The empty sample cups may first be placed in the rack, the serum samples then added to the cups with the pipets, and the rack placed in the analyzer. After analysis the cups can be dropped directly from the rack into the waste container.

Centrifuges should not be operated without the covers being completely closed. (Many of the newer models cannot be operated unless this is done.) Potentially infectious, volatile, or toxic substances should not be centrifuged in open tubes, as centrifugation may result in the formation of infectious aerosols or the volatilization of the liquid. In using older centrifuges, do not attempt to open the cover until the rotor has completely stopped. In those with hand-operated brakes, do not brake sharply. Be certain that the tubes are properly balanced and that the cushions are at the bottoms of the holders. Always use tubes of the correct size and strength for the desired application. If a tube breaks in the centrifuge, immediately turn the centrifuge off, and after donning rubber gloves and other protective clothing (if necessary), clean up. Allow any droplets in the chamber to settle for about 15 min, then wash it with an appropriate solution (dilute acid for strongly alkaline solutions, sodium bicarbonate solutions for acid solutions, and 5% sodium hypochlorite for potentially infectious material).

RADIOACTIVITY PRECAUTIONS

All precautions against eating, drinking, or smoking are particularly applicable to the radioisotope laboratory. Although the amount of radioactivity associated with the kits for radioimmunoassays is small, it can present some hazards. Radioisotopes often used for labeling are ^{125}I and ^{131}I. If either is ingested, the radioactive compound may be broken down in the body and radioactive iodine absorbed and concentrated in the thyroid gland. Thus the thyroid can receive a much larger dose of radiation than would be expected from a random distribution in the body. All personnel performing work with radioactive material should wear film badges at all times when in the isotope laboratory.

The radioactive material used in radioimmunoassays is generally so small that it can be harmlessly flushed down the sewer with copious amounts of water.[12] Plastic beads or other resins used to absorb some of the radioactivity should not be incinerated. Burial is satisfactory since the radioactivity gradually decays. All radioactive material should be stored in special refrigerators or cabinets conspicuously labeled with appropriate signs indicating the presence of radioactive elements. Generally the level of radioactivity used in a radioimmunoassay laboratory that purchases the material in the form of kits and does not prepare its own will not be sufficiently high to require lead shielding for storage.

The procedures using radioactive materials should be carried out in a separate room with a good ventilating system. The door into the room should be conspicuously marked "Radioactive Material—Authorized Personnel Only." All waste containers should be clearly marked as containing radioactive material so that the waste will not be incinerated.

MICROBIOLOGIC HAZARDS
Precautions and decontamination

The microbiology laboratory[13] should be in a separate room with a sign at the door indicating biologic hazards. Traffic should be limited to assigned personnel. It must be emphasized that there should be no smoking, drinking, or eating in the laboratory. Personal items such as eyeglasses or purses should not be placed in the work areas. If they must be carried into the room, they should be deposited in a special nonworking area. Laboratory gowns should be worn, because they give better protection than regular laboratory coats. The protective clothing should not be worn outside the laboratory.

All work with potentially highly infectious specimens should be done in clean air hoods. If contaminated material is accidently dropped, pour disinfectant over the contaminated area, cover with paper towels, let stand about 30 min, and then clean up. Use rubber gloves for the cleaning operations. All discarded material should be covered with disinfectant-soaked paper towels after it is placed in the disposal container. The container should later be autoclaved. Bacterial culture plates and tubes should be opened with care (possibly using a safety hood) and should not be "sniffed."

Fungal culture should be done in tubes as much as possible, and the cultures should be handled in a safety hood. A wetting agent should be applied to mycelial growth before direct examination to lessen chances of spore-containing aerosol.

Centrifuge tubes for microbiology use should be closed (preferably with screw caps) and opened after centrifuging only in a clean air hood. For sterilizing inoculation loops, use burners with covered heating areas that do not allow splatter or aerosolization of infectious material. Inoculation loops should be cooled in still air for 10-15 sec before using. Plunge contaminated loops into a bottle containing sand in 5% phenol before flaming to prevent scattering of microorganisms. All work areas should be cleared of cultures and wiped with disinfectant before leaving at the end of the workday. If a requisition card or slip becomes contaminated, a new one should be prepared and the old one autoclaved before discarding.

Precautions for handling material (blood, feces, or any body fluid or tissue) likely to contain highly infectious agents (viruses, bacteria, fungi, or parasites) should include covering all cuts or skin breaks with tape, wearing protective clothing and rubber gloves, and working under a safety hood if possible. Aerosol formation must be prevented. Screw-capped centrifuge tubes in an enclosed centrifuge should be used. Leaky or spilled specimens require thorough disinfecting of outer surfaces. Clearing, cleaning, and disinfecting work surfaces, as well as thorough hand washing, reduce chances of infection. Overfilled stool specimen containers should be handled with gloved hands only, and soiled requisitions must be autoclaved, discarded, and replaced.

ELECTRICAL EQUIPMENT
Safeguards

All electrical apparatus should have three-pronged grounding plugs, and sufficient grounded outlets should be available. The only exceptions may be small items such as clocks, which are totally enclosed in plastic, and microscope lamps, which are similarly enclosed. No attempt should be made to adjust any piece of electrical apparatus while it is plugged in, unless it is absolutely necessary (e.g., adjusting the lamp position in a spectrophotometer; this should be done with insulated tools). Under no circumstances should hands be placed inside an electrical instrument with the current on. Rings or jewelry along the forearms should not be worn. Preferably, rubber gloves should be worn for delicate adjustments. All electrical cords should be as short as possible and kept out of any areas where water or other solutions might contact them. Personnel should know the locations of the fuse boxes or circuit breakers for the different outlets. If electrical equipment fails to work properly (and particularly if smoke appears or sparks are seen), the apparatus should be disconnected and the maintenance department notified.

QUALITY CONTROL

Safety precautions, like all other aspects of laboratory function, must undergo a sort of "quality control." Inspection of safety equipment operation and availability must be regular. It must be determined whether warning signs are displayed where needed and whether decontamination and disposal practices are adequate, in addition to whether adherence to other safety procedures and rules is being practiced. Maintaining safe working standards may require extra effort, but risk minimization is "part of the job."

REFERENCES

1. Halper, H.R., and Foster, H.S.: Laboratory regulation manual, Germantown, Md., 1976, Aspen Systems Corp., vol. 3.
2. Flury, P.A.: Environmental health and safety in the hospital laboratory, Springfield, Ill., 1978, Charles C Thomas, Publisher.
3. Carlson, D.J.: Guidelines for laboratory safety for medical technologists: policies and procedures. In Clinical laboratory improvement seminar, Chicago, 1980, Commission on Inspection and Accreditation, American Society of Clinical Pathologists.
4. Laboratory safety at the center for disease control. HEW no. (CDC) 76-8118, Washington, D.C., 1976, U.S. Government Printing Office.
5. Moya, C., Guarda, L. and Sodeman, T.: Lab. Med. **11:**576, 1980.
6. Steere, A.C., and Mallison, G.F.: Ann. Intern. Med. **83:**683, 1975.
7. Stevens, A.: Lab. Med. **11:**598, 1980.
8. Henry, R.J., et al.: Safety in the clinical laboratory, Van Nuys, Calif., 1976, Bio-Science Enterprises.

9. Laboratory waste disposal manual, ed. 2, Washington, D.C., 1975, Manufacturing Chemists Association.

10. Christiansen, H.E., and Lugibyhl, T.T., editors: Suspected carcinogens. HEW no. (NIDSH) 75-188, Washington, D.C., 1975, U.S. Government Printing Office.

11. Snydman, D.R., Bryan, J.A., and Dixon, R.E.: Ann. Intern. Med. **83:**838, 1975.

12. Duckworth, J.K., and Von Boechman, J.: In Commission on Inspection and Accreditation: Clinical laboratory improvement seminar, Skokie, Ill., 1980, College of American Pathologists.

13. Isenberg, H.D., et al.: In Lennette, E.H., et al.: Manual of clinical microbiology, ed. 3, Washington, D.C., 1980, American Society for Microbiology.

UNIT TWO

HEMATOLOGY

CHAPTER 3

Collection and preparation of the specimen

Obtaining blood specimens
Prevention of hemolysis
Anticoagulants
Storage of specimens
Separation methods
Preparation of the specimen
Methods of microscopy

Blood collection requires skill, a professional attitude, and decorum.[1] The phlebotomist is frequently the only representative of the team of highly skilled laboratory workers that the patient ever encounters; thus the patient is apt to judge the laboratory's performance on the basis of this contact.

OBTAINING BLOOD SPECIMENS
Capillary blood

Procedure: Capillary blood is obtained from the tip of a finger in adults and from the great toe or the heel in infants. Wash area with 70% alcohol, dry with sterile gauze, and puncture skin with a sterile disposable blood lancet that is designed to penetrate no deeper than 2 mm. Use sterile gauze to wipe away the first drop of blood and collect the subsequent drops. Avoid squeezing the extremity to obtain blood, since this will alter the composition of the blood specimen. If blood is difficult to obtain, warm the extremity or allow it to remain in a hanging position for some time.

Advantages:
1. Capillary blood can be obtained with ease.
2. Capillary blood is the preferred material for making peripheral blood smears.

Disadvantages:
1. Only small amounts of blood can be obtained, and repeated examinations require a new specimen.
2. Blood in microtubes frequently hemolyzes, and hemolysis interferes with most laboratory tests.
3. Test results on capillary blood cannot be compared with test results on venous blood.
4. The finger is not only sensitive but difficult to adequately sterilize in the time usually available. In patients with a lowered resistance to infection (those with leukemia, agranulocytosis, diabetes, uremia, and immune deficiency diseases), a specimen taken from the finger is much more likely to

lead to infection than one taken from the arm. If a capillary blood specimen is necessary for these patients, the alcohol should remain in contact with the skin for at least 7-10 min.
5. Red and white cell counts and enumeration of platelets and reticulocytes should not be performed on capillary blood because of the difficulty in standardizing capillary blood flow.

Venous blood

Venous blood is necessary for most tests that require anticoagulation or larger quantities of blood, plasma, or serum than can be provided by capillary blood.

Procedure: Venous blood is usually obtained from one of the cubital fossa veins (Fig. 3-1), although other veins may be chosen. The vein is congested by placing a tourniquet on the upper arm and tightening it suffi-

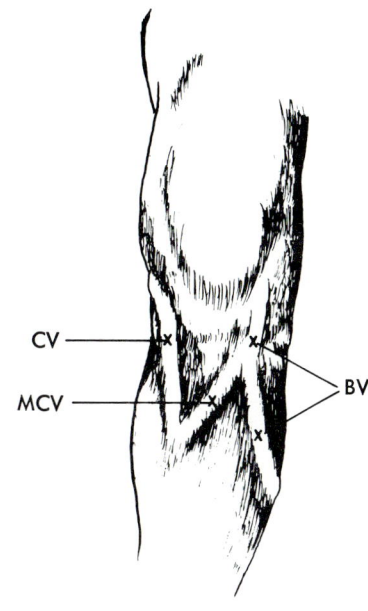

Fig. 3-1. Veins of antecubital fossa suitable for venipuncture. *CV*, Cephalic vein; *MCV*, median cubital vein; *BV*, basilic vein.

ciently to prevent venous blood return. A blood pressure cuff inflated to a level between systolic and diastolic pressure acts as an excellent tourniquet; it is also helpful for the patient to open and close the hand several times. Cleanse the puncture site with 70% ethyl alcohol, dry with sterile gauze, and cleanly puncture the vein with a sterile 1 in. needle attached to a sterile syringe. The bevel of the needle should point upward. A 20- or 21-gauge needle is adequate for 10 ml blood. For 30-50 ml an 18-gauge needle is preferable, because the 20-gauge needle may deliver blood too slowly to prevent clotting and hemolysis in the syringe. After the vein is entered, loosen the tourniquet and obtain blood by gentle suction. After the procedure is completed, use sterile gauze to apply pressure over the puncture site to stop bleeding. If oozing from the puncture site is difficult to stop, elevate the arm and apply a small pressure dressing. Remain with the patient until the bleeding has stopped. Remove the needle from the syringe, and quickly transfer blood into a test tube (which may or may not contain an anticoagulant). If an anticoagulant has been added, mix blood gently by inverting the stoppered tube several times.

If multiple blood specimens are required, the Vacutainer evacuated blood collection tube system (Becton-Dickinson & Co., Rutherford, N.J.) permits the filling of a number of test tubes with blood obtained from a single puncture. The tubes and needles are siliconized and sterile, and the gentle vacuum allows rapid filling of the test tubes without producing chemical or morphologic changes in the blood. The system eliminates the need for large tubes and needles and effectively prevents hemolysis.

Advantages:
1. Multiple and repeated examinations can be performed on the same specimen.
2. Aliquots of the specimen (plasma and serum) may be frozen for future reference.
3. There is no variation in blood values if specimens are obtained from different veins; therefore ankle veins can be used if the arm veins are being used for intravenous medication. Never draw blood for any laboratory test from the same extremity that is being used for intravenous medication (blood transfusion, glucose, etc.).

Disadvantages:
1. The venous method is a somewhat lengthy procedure that requires more preparation than the capillary method.
2. The method is technically difficult in children, obese individuals, and patients in shock.
3. Hemolysis must be prevented, because it leads to lowered red cell counts and interferes with many chemical tests. See discussion of hemolysis prevention.
4. Hematoma (or blood clot formation) inside and outside the vein must be prevented, the former by a clean needle puncture and the later by releasing the tourniquet before blood is aspirated and by applying sufficient pressure over the puncture site after completion of the procedure.
5. Prolonged stasis produced by the tourniquet must be avoided, because it produces hemoconcentra-

tion and other changes that make the blood unsuitable for gas analysis, blood counts, blood pH determination, and some clotting tests.
6. Anticoagulated blood, unless freshly obtained, should not be used for peripheral blood smears, because some anticoagulants produce changes in platelets that may cause clumping and in white cells that may make their identification difficult.
7. Since some components are not stable in anticoagulated blood, the white cell and platelet counts and sedimentation rate determinations should be performed with 2 hr after the blood has been obtained.

Two-syringe procedure: For a discussion of the two-syringe procedure and its use in blood coagulation studies, see Chapter 11.

Arterial blood

The procedure to obtain arterial blood is similar (with a few exceptions) to a venous puncture with syringe and needle. No tourniquet and no local anesthetic are required. The specimen may be obtained from the brachial artery in the cubital fossa (Fig. 3-2), The radial artery in the radial sulcus of the forearm (Fig. 3-2), or the femoral artery in the groin (Fig. 3-3). Whatever

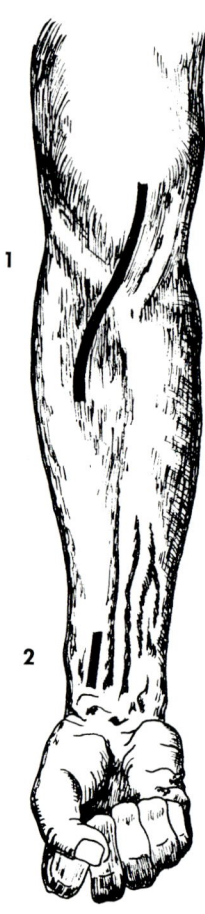

Fig. 3-2. Location of brachial *(1)* and radial *(2)* arteries.

location is used, the artery is identified by palpation of the pulse, the area is treated with povidone-iodine (Betadine),* and the needle is inserted into the pulsating vessel. Because arterial blood is under pressure, little, if any, suction is required to obtain the specimen. After the procedure a pressure dressing is applied, and the area is frequently checked for evidence of superficial or deep bleeding.

Blood specimens from infants

Capillary blood: Capillary blood is best obtained from infants by skin puncture of the heel or great toe. The baby's foot is held firmly between the thumb and second finger of the left hand, and the outer rim of the posterior aspect of the heel is punctured after suitable preparation (same as previously described for adults) (Fig. 3-4). In newborns the hemoglobin values of capillary blood are higher than values obtained from cord blood. This difference can be virtually eliminated by warming the extremity prior to the skin puncture.

The B-D Microtainer capillary blood serum separator and the capillary (anticoagulated) whole blood collector

---

*Before treating the area, ask about iodine sensitivity.

(Becton-Dickinson & Co., Rutherford, N.J.) provide a method of collecting, separating, and storing serum and plasma obtained from a capillary blood sample. The serum collecting device contains inert silicone material that, after centrifugation, forms a barrier separating serum from the blood clot, and the plasma-collecting device contains disodium EDTA. The first tube is marked at 250 and 600 µl as a filling guide and the second one at the 200 and 300 µl levels.

Venous blood:

Cord blood: Cord blood is obtained at the time of delivery. An admixture of cord jelly must be carefully avoided. The placental segment of the cord is either allowed to drain into a test tube or (preferably) the umbilical vein is aspirated with needle and syringe.

External jugular vein: Puncture of the external jugular vein is the procedure of choice for obtaining venous blood from infants and small children (Fig. 3-5). The infant is wrapped in a sheet so that the arms are immobilized alongside the body. The child is placed on the back on the examining table so that the head hangs over the edge of the table as the body is steadied by an assistant. The head is supported and turned to one side by a second assistant. When the child cries, the exter-

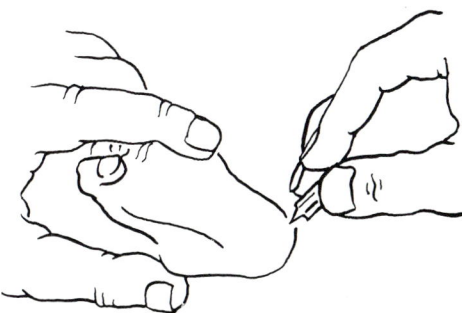

Fig. 3-4. Heel-stick method of obtaining capillary blood from infants.

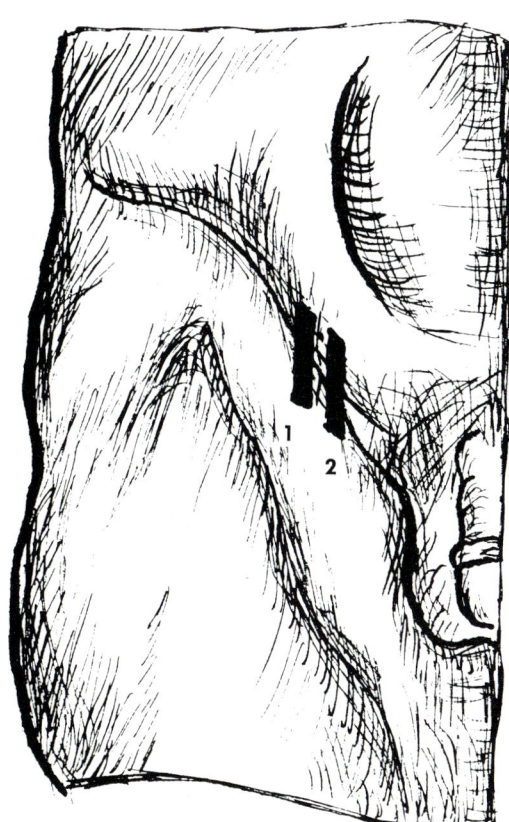

Fig. 3-3. Sketch of inguinal area to show position of femoral artery *(1; lateral)* and femoral vein *(2; medial).*

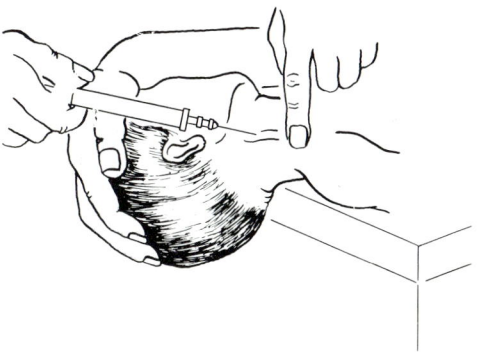

Fig. 3-5. Technic for puncture of jugular vein in infants and children.

nal jugular vein stands out distinctly, running from the angle of the mandible to the midclavicular area. The area is then disinfected, and the specimen is obtained. After completion of the procedure, the puncture site is treated as described in the discussion on obtaining venous blood in adults.

Femoral vein: This procedure should preferably be performed by a physician. The child's legs are slightly abducted, and the body and arms are immobilized by an assistant. The femoral pulse is located just below the inguinal ligament at the junction of the middle third and the outer two thirds of the ligament (Fig. 3-3). An antiseptic is applied to the skin, and the area over the pulse is stretched between two fingers and punctured with a long needle directed posteriorly and slightly medially to the maximal impulse. As soon as the needle touches bone, it is very slowly withdrawn; at the same time the plunger in the syringe is slightly raised so that blood can enter the syringe. After completion of the aspiration, pressure is applied over the puncture site using sterile gauze.

PREVENTION OF HEMOLYSIS

Hemolysis of capillary blood specimens can be prevented by using sharp 2-3 mm lancets that produce clean puncture wounds, allowing the blood to escape freely. To prevent hemolysis of venous blood, smooth, good-quality, sharp needles with a large gauge (20 or over) should be used to enter the vein without excessive trauma. The syringe must be dry, and the specimen should be obtained by gentle suction. The tourniquet must not be too tight and should be released before blood is aspirated. If serum is needed, do not ''rim'' the clot and do not centrifuge the blood until a firm clot has been formed. The needle must be removed from the syringe before the specimen is transferred to a test tube. The transfer must be slow, with minimal agitation and without formation of bubbles. If an anticoagulant is used, the blood and the anticoagulant must be mixed gently and slowly by inversion.

The use of vacuated tubes eliminates many of the factors that cause hemolysis.

ANTICOAGULANTS

Coagulation of blood can be prevented by the addition of oxalates, citrates, EDTA (ethylenediamine tetraacetate), or heparin, or by defibrination. The first three remove calcium by forming insoluble or un-ionized calcium salts; heparin inactivates thrombin and thromboplastin; defibrination removes fibrinogen converted to fibrin. The correct choice and the correct amount of anticoagulant are important. The incorrect anticoagulant may lead to distortion of cells, while an insufficient amount of anticoagulant may lead to partial clotting, and too much anticoagulant may dilute the blood sample. The ratio of anticoagulant to blood should be 1:10. If the hematocrit is high and the plasma volume low (as, for instance, in infants), the amount of anticoagulant should be decreased; if the hematocrit is low and the plasma volume high, the amount of anticoagulant should be increased. A blood sample with a hematocrit of 80 vol% (plasma volume of 20 vol%) requires 0.4 ml of anticoagulant for 10 ml of blood,

whereas a blood sample with a hematocrit of 20 vol% requires 1.4 ml anticoagulant for 10 ml blood (Fig. 3-6).

Ethylenediamine tetraacetate

One drop of any commercially available solution of ethylenediamine tetraacetate (EDTA) is enough to prevent coagulation of 5 ml blood. The material may also be dried at the bottom of the test tube. Because of the small quantity of anticoagulant, careful mixing is necessary. This anticoagulant prevents platelet aggregation and is therefore the anticoagulant of choice for platelet counts and platelet function tests. Fresh EDTA-anticoagulated blood allows the making of blood films without distortion of white cells, but platelet aggregation cannot be evaluated.

Heparin

Heparin is an antithrombic mucopolysaccharide isolated from mammalian liver or pancreas. Minute quantities of heparin that cannot be seen but adhere to the barrel of the syringe after heparin is aspirated and expelled produce excellent anticoagulation. Heparin is the anticoagulant of choice for the osmotic fragility test because it does not affect the size of red cells. Films made from heparinized blood have a light bluish background when stained with Wright-Giemsa stain.

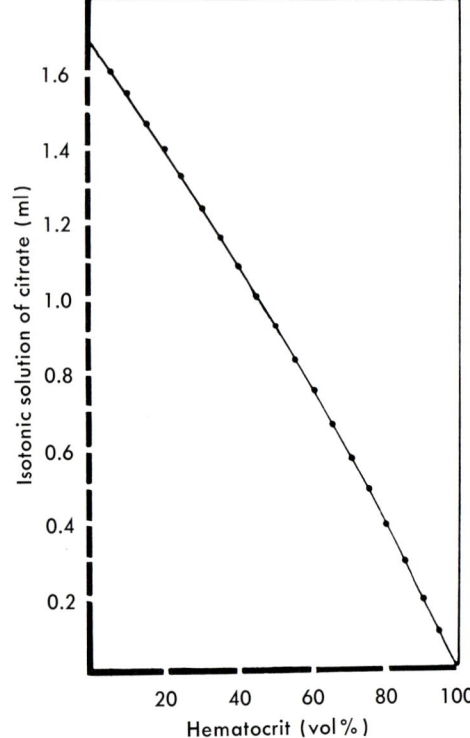

Fig. 3-6. Nomogram based on hematocrit and amount of anticoagulant to use in order to keep constant 1:10 ratio of anticoagulant in total volume of 10 ml blood. Citrate/plasma ratio is 1:4.95 at any hematocrit value shown in graph. (From Hellem, A.J.: Scand. J. Clin. Lab. Invest. **51**[suppl.]:1, 1960.)

Defibrination

1. Add 25 ml venous blood to a 125 ml Erlenmeyer flask containing 20 glass beads 3-4 mm in diameter.
2. Rotate the flask until the beads are covered with fibrin and cease to make a rattling noise.
3. Continue for another 2 min and decant the defibrinated blood.
4. The liquid portion of this blood is serum and not plasma, since fibrinogen has been removed.

STORAGE OF SPECIMENS

If a specimen cannot be handled immediately, the test tube should be stoppered and placed in a refrigerator. For some tests (e.g., plasma hemoglobin level) it is necessary to separate plasma from the red cells immediately after the specimen is obtained and before it is stored in a refrigerator. Blood specimens for platelet counts, sedimentation rate determinations, and prothrombin time should not be stored longer than 2 hr. Before any examination is undertaken, stored anticoagulated blood must be thoroughly mixed on blood rotators for at least 2 min after it has reached room temperature. Serum to be tested for cold agglutinins should be separated as soon as possible and should not be stored in the refrigerator in contact with the red cells.

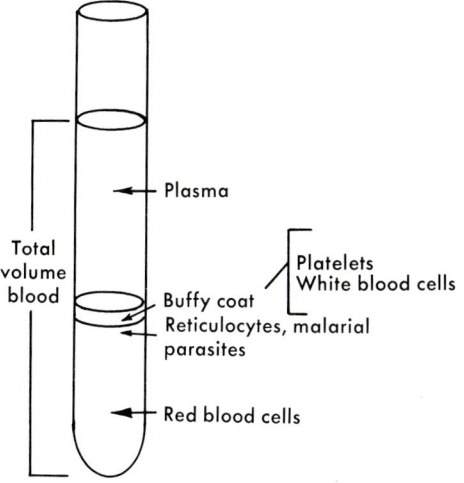

Fig. 3-7. Different layers of venous hematocrit.

SEPARATION METHODS
Serum and plasma

Serum: Clotted blood, when allowed to stand, separates into (1) a red cell–fibrin mass that collects at the bottom of the tube and (2) an overlying liquid, the serum. The separation of serum can be accelerated by centrifuging the blood after clotting has taken place. Serum differs from plasma primarily in its lack of coagulation factors I (fibrinogen), II (prothrombin), V (labile factor), and VIII (antihemophilic factor). Blood clotting can be accelerated by the use of thrombin tubes, and serum separation is aided by SST tubes (both available from Becton-Dickinson & Co., Rutherford, N.J.).

Plasma: If anticoagulated blood is centrifuged, it separates into three main layers: the red cell mass at the bottom of the liquid column, the plasma on top, and the buffy coat at the interface. Reticulocytes concentrate on top of the red cell column. The buffy coat consists of platelets and white blood cells, the former closest to the plasma column (Fig. 3-7).

Buffy coat preparations: Buffy coat preparations are well suited for the study of the morphology of platelets and white cells in cases of thrombocytopenia, leukopenia, lymphoma, and the aleukemic phase of acute leukemia. They aid in the discovery of abnormal circulating elements such as cancer cells, lymphosarcoma cells, Reed-Sternberg cells, fragments of megakaryocytes, and erythrophagocytic cells.

Because the height of the buffy coat column depends on the number of platelets and white cells, it reflects the presence of thrombocythemia and leukocytosis if of sufficient magnitude.

Procedure: Anticoagulated blood is centrifuged at low speed and the buffy coat thus formed is aspirated by means of a disposable Pasteur pipet inserted directly into the white buffy coat ring. Neither plasma nor red cells should be allowed to contaminate the specimen. The buffy coat is collected on a watch glass (see bone marrow aspiration method, Chapter 5) and is gently mixed before one small drop is transferred by means of a white cell counting pipet to a clean slide. It is then smeared, air dried, and stained like a blood smear.

The buffy coat may also be transferred into a Wintrobe hematocrit tube and spun again at low speed to

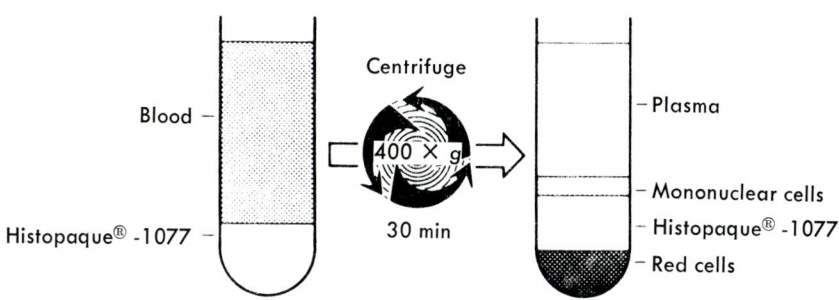

Fig. 3-8. Lymphocytes isolated by centrifuging anticoagulated blood with Histopaque-1077. (Courtesy Sigma Chemical Co., St. Louis.)

separate platelets and various white cells according to their specific gravity. (Platelets, lymphocytes, and monocytes are lighter than granulocytes.)

Cell preparation: The most widely used separation method depends on density gradients. The density stratification can be rendered more precise by centrifugation and by the addition of one or several solutions of differing specific gravity. The heaviest cells collect at the bottom of the centrifuge tube, whereas the other cell groups form layers at the interfaces of the various media in which they are suspended. Histopaque (Sigma Chemical Co., St. Louis) in conjunction with centrifugation is used to separate mononuclear cells (mainly lymphocytes) from anticoagulated blood (Fig. 3-8).

PREPARATION OF THE SPECIMEN
Unstained hematologic preparations

Wet preparation: Staining of tissues renders certain structures visible by differential adsorption of dyes but produces some undesirable side effects, such as coagulation of proteins and solubilization of carbohydrates and fats. If unstained preparations are examined, their physical properties are unchanged, and structures can be made visible that cannot be detected in stained preparations.

Procedure: Place one small drop of blood on a coverslip, immediately invert coverslip over slide, and allow the blood to spread evenly to form a thin film. Repeat with larger drop to form a thick film. Secure the corners of the coverslip with minute drops of nail polish or of 60° C liquid paraffin and use the same material to rim the preparation.

Interpretation: Microscopic examination of the preparation allows the recognition (1) of morphologic red cell changes (e.g., sickling, acanthoctosis,[2] and rouleaux formation), (2) of abnormal pigment (e.g., malaria pigment), and (3) of living parasites (e.g., trypanosomes, microfilaria, and spirochetes of relapsing fever). To exclude the erroneous diagnosis of crenated red cells on the basis of a stained smear, examine fresh blood immediately between two coverslips.

Imprints: Imprints are prepared by gently and swiftly touching a microscope slide with fresh unfixed tissue. The material is not smeared on the slide surface like a blood film. Imprints should be prepared from lymph nodes, spleen, and bone marrow biopsies. The imprints are air dried and then stained like a bone marrow smear (Fig. 3-9).

Blood smears: For best results use fresh capillary or venous blood and stain films as soon as they have dried. Fresh EDTA-anticoagulated venous blood may also be utilized. Only new precleaned microscopic slides with frosted ends and precleaned new coverslips should be employed. To prevent artifacts, dry slides rapidly in moving air.

Slide wedge procedure: Place one small drop of capillary or fresh venous blood near one end of a clean slide that is supported by a flat, firm, horizontal surface. (For best results, apply one small drop of venous blood using a microhematocrit tube.) Place spreader slide in front of the drop at an angle of about 30 degrees and allow the blood to spread in the angle between the slides (Fig. 3-10). Then, just before the blood has spread to the edges, push spreader slide ahead of the drop of blood so that a blood smear is produced. Label slide, allow it to air dry, stain it, then place a coverslip over it (if indicated) using Permount (Fisher Scientific Co., Pittsburgh).

Blood films of the proper thickness will dry quickly and will appear yellow when placed on white paper. The more acute the angle between the slides and the more slowly the blood is spread, the thinner will be the film. A well-made blood film consists of a thick band (at the application point) that is drawn out into a thin feathery portion. In the thick portion the cells are too closely placed and overlapping to be studied, while in the thin portion they exhibit artifacts because of their wide separation. Thus cell morphology is best in the intermediate zone where the cells just touch each other. The blood smear should be about 2 cm wide and 3 cm long, and its sides should not extend to the edges of the glass slide.

Defects of manual smears: Manual wedge smears are inherently variable, lack uniformity, and are affected by the hematocrit and the distribution of white cells. Increased blood volume and viscosity negatively influence the quality of manual smears; small white cells have a tendency to concentrate in the center of the

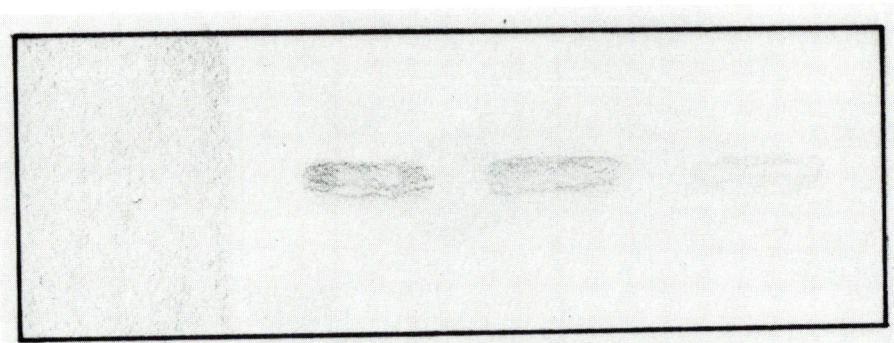

Fig. 3-9. Imprints of bone marrow biopsy.

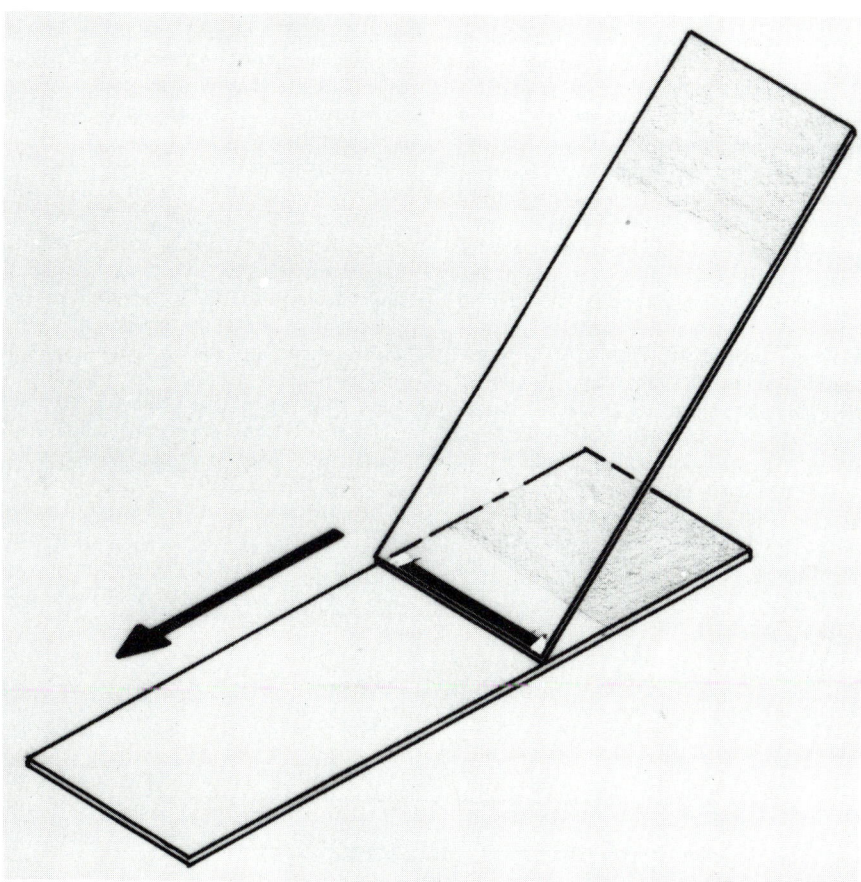

Fig. 3-10. Wedge procedure.

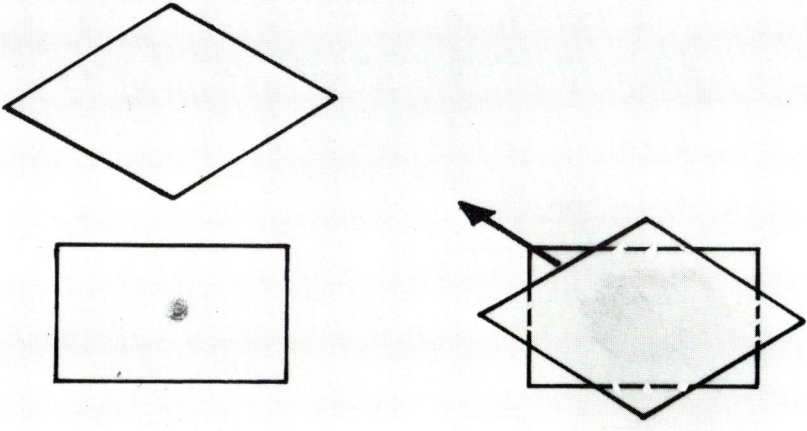

Fig. 3-11. Coverslip procedure.

smear, whereas larger cells are moved toward the periphery. White cells appear smaller if found in the body of the smear and larger if located in the periphery.

Coverslip procedure: The coverslip procedure is preferred to obtain the best possible cell definition and distribution. Place a small drop of blood (or bone marrow) in the middle of a coverslip held between thumb and forefinger by adjacent corners. Place a second coverslip over the first so that the second cover glass is rotated 45 degrees on the first. The slides can now be handled by their free corners and can be pulled apart immediately after the drop of blood has spread between them (Fig. 3-11). Air dry both slides; stain. Use rubber stoppers to support the coverslips during the staining procedure.

Automated smear procedure: The basis for reproducible manual or automated white cell differential counts is a well-prepared smear that provides a monolayer of cells that are well separated, not overlapping, and not distorted.[3] The cell distribution should reflect the volume distribution in the whole blood.

Minniprep: The Minniprep (Geometric Data Corporation, Wayne, Pa.) is an instrument that utilizes the wedge procedure to obtain reproducible blood smears. A precision blood spreader prepares dual smears simultaneously by spreading one small drop of blood at a constant angle and speed. This leads to consistent cell distribution and eliminates cell distortion, though it shares some of the other disadvantages of the manual wedge procedure.

Cytocentrifuge: The Cytocentrifuge (Shandon Scientific Co., Sewichley, Pa.) is a device that allows concentration and spreading of cells in one operation. While its primary use is in the preparation of body fluids for cytology,[4,5] it may also be used for bone marrow smears (Fig. 3-12). The specimen is placed into a centrifuge chamber, the exit port of which is in contact with a microscope slide. A filter paper strip with a 7 mm perforation separates the centrifuge chamber and glass slide but allows contact at the perforation site. Cells are collected by sedimentation on the slide in a small circle, and any fluid is absorbed by the filter paper. The small amount of specimen and the small area to be examined are advantages of this procedure.

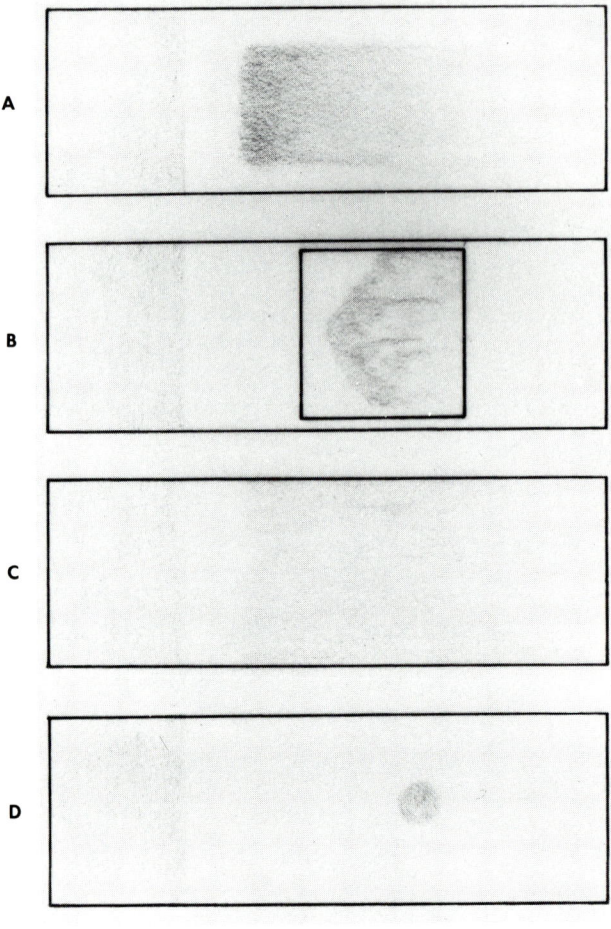

Fig. 3-12. Blood film procedures. **A,** Wedge procedure; **B,** coverslip procedure; **C,** spin procedure; and **D,** cytocentrifuge procedure.

METHODS OF MICROSCOPY
Compound light microscopy

In a compound light microscope, the objective forms an enlarged inverted image of the object, which the ocular (eyepiece) reverses and brings closer to the eye (Fig. 3-13). A third optical system, the condenser, controls the transillumination. The objective magnifies the object from 2 times to 100 times. The product of the magnification of the objective multiplied by the magnification of the ocular represents the total magnification. The light microscope usually magnifies up to 1000 times.

Phase-contrast microscopy

Phase-contrast microscopy allows observation of living cells without any prior treatment or staining by transforming slight differences in the refractive index or thickness of the various cell structures into degrees of brightness and contrast. Such small differences in the refractive index are not visible in stained preparations but require darkfield or phase-contrast microscopy. The physical principles of phase-contrast microscopy are well described by Benneth et al.[6] Two sets of light waves are used, one incident to the object and one diffracted by the object. These two sets are recombined

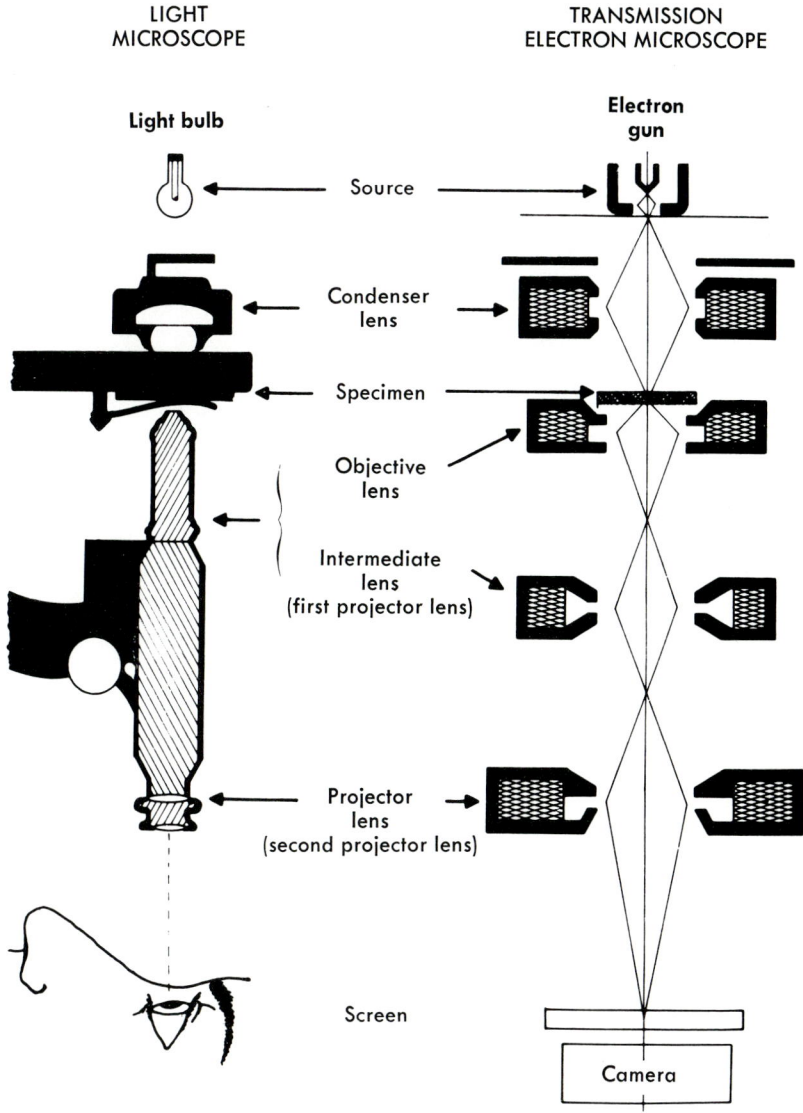

LIGHT
MICROSCOPE

TRANSMISSION
ELECTRON MICROSCOPE

Light bulb

Electron
gun

Source

Condenser
lens

Specimen

Objective
lens

Intermediate
lens
(first projector lens)

Projector
lens
(second projector lens)

Screen

Camera

Fig. 3-13. Schematic drawing comparing the essentials of the electron microscope with those of the light microscope. (Reproduced with permission from Transmission electron microscopy in medicine, Skokie, Ill., 1973, College of American Pathologists.)

in the objective. The object affects the amplitude of each wave and the relationship of the two wave sets to each other so that darker and lighter areas are visualized within the object. Phase contrast permits the observation of living cells containing nuclei, nucleoli, organelles (e.g., mitochondria, centrosomes, microtubules, lysosomes, granules, and ergastoplasm), and nonorganelle structures (e.g., glycogen).

To obtain an adequate phase-contrast preparation, the cell suspension must form a thin film between microscope slide and cover slip so that the cells are well separated from each other and do not assume a spherical shape.

Darkfield microscopy

If objects are illuminated by a beam of light directed onto their surfaces and no light is allowed to transilluminate them, they appear self-luminous against a dark background.

Interference microscopy

Whereas the phase-contrast microscope reveals refractive index gradients within tissue, the interference microscope evaluates the magnitude of these gradients. Unstained tissues, transparent preparations, and living cells can be examined.[7] In the split beam system utilized by interference microscopy, one beam of light is divided into two or more beams; one beam traverses the specimen, whereas the other passes around it. After the two beams are recombined, the path difference determines the thickness of the specimen. When monochromatic light is used, changes in brightness correspond to the path differences; white light indicates path differences by the production of variable colors. The thickness of the cell suspension between coverslip and microscope slide is not as critical as it is for phase-contrast microscopy.

Electron microscopy

In principle the electron microscope is similar to the light microscope, though its appearance is quite different. A large vacuum tube contains the electron beam. A high voltage power supply is used to produce electrons by heating a tungsten filament (cathode) in an electron gun. An electromagnetic condenser is used to "illuminate" the specimen. The electron microscope is focused by varying the focal length of another electromagnetic field (Fig. 3-13). The range of magnification is determined by the projector electromagnetic lens. The invisible electronic image is made visible by a fluorescent screen and can be photographed.[8] The most commonly used magnification is 20,000 times, though magnifications up to 1,000,000 times may be achieved. The specimen must be thin enough so as not to impede the flow of electrons and cause loss of energy, and a rapid method of fixation must be used that produces the least alteration of its molecular arrangement. Glutaraldehyde (1%) stored at 4° C in the dark can be used as a fairly satisfactory fixative. Epoxy resins are utilized as embedding compounds. Special glass or diamond knives are required to cut the specimen.

Scanning electron microscopy

The scanning electron microscope allows three-dimensional study of the shape and surfaces of specimens at high resolution. Electrons scan the surface of the specimen, leading to the production of various forms of secondary radiation that are picked up by the oscilloscope on which the image of the cell surface is synthesized.[9]

REFERENCES

1. So you're going to collect a blood specimen, Chicago, Ill., 1974, College of American Pathologists.
2. Weed, R.I.: Semin. Hematol. **7:**249, 1970.
3. Megla, G.K.: Acta Cytol. (Baltimore) **17:**3, 1973.
4. Hansen, H.H., Bender, R.A., and Shelton, B.J.: Acta Cytol. (Baltimore) **18:**259, 1974.
5. Drewinko, B., Sullivan, M.P., and Martin, T.: Cancer **31:**1331, 1973.
6. Benneth, A.H., et al: Trans. Am. Microsc. Soc. **65:**99, 1946.
7. Evans, E.A., and Fung, Y.C.: Microvasc. Res. **4:**335, 1972.
8. Dickerson, L.G.: Transmission electron microscopy in medicine, Chicago, 1973, College of American Pathologists.
9. Hayes, T.L., and Pease, R.F.W.: Adv. Biol. Med. Phys. **12:**85, 1968.

Laboratory investigation of hemoglobin

Hemoglobin is a red conjugated protein (molecular weight, 64,458) present in the red cell. It occupies 28% of the red cell mass, the rest being mainly water (71%) and some lipids (7% cholesterol and lecithin). Each hemoglobin molecule consists of one globin molecule and four heme molecules. Heme, a ferroprotoporphyrin, is responsible for the color of the entire compound and consists of four protoporphyrin rings, each ring containing one iron (Fe) atom in the center (Fig. 4-1). The four heme groups are located on the surface of the almost globoid globin molecule

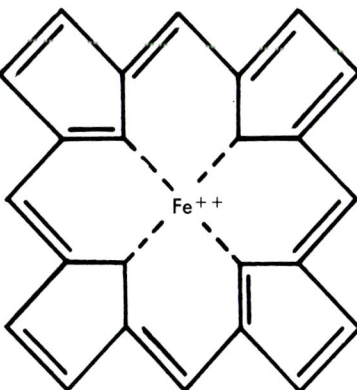

Fig. 4-1. Diagram of structure of heme. One iron atom is related to four pyrrole rings, which are joined to each other through methylene bridges.

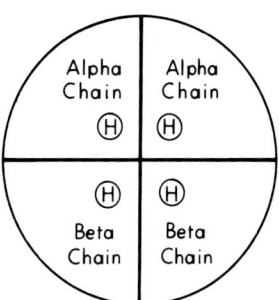

Fig. 4-2. Diagram of structure of Hb A molecule. Four heme groups are attached to one globin molecule, which consists of four polypeptide chains, two of which have an identical amino acid sequence of one type and the other two an identical amino acid sequence of another type. Each polypeptide chain is conjugated to one heme moiety. *H,* Heme.

(Fig. 4-2). The iron is present in the bivalent ferrous form, and, because of its unique association with globin, it is able to bind or give up oxygen without producing any changes in the heme group and with only minimal configurational changes in the globin molecule. Because of the close functional association of globin and heme, relatively minor changes in either one lead to physiochemical changes of the entire hemoglobin molecule, altering its oxygenation, solubility, and oxygen dissociation curve.

Heme is synthetized by nucleated red cells and reticulocytes, as outlined in the section on porphyrin metabolism (Chapter 27). The iron that is inserted into the protoporphyrin ring is derived from iron metabolism.

The globin fraction is synthetized by nucleated red cells and by reticulocytes from amino acids according to a genetically controlled sequence, which will be discussed further in the section dealing with normal and abnormal hemoglobins. Each globin molecule is a tetramere of four polypeptide chains, each combined with one heme group.

LABORATORY INVESTIGATION OF THE OXYGEN-BINDING CAPACITY OF HEMOGLOBIN

The reversible binding of oxygen and its transport are the main functions of hemoglobin. The oxygen-saturated hemoglobin is called **oxyhemoglobin,** while the nonoxygenated hemoglobin is termed **reduced hemoglobin,** or deoxyhemoglobin. Oxygen-saturated hemoglobin is bright red and easily soluble in water. Under normal circumstances the hemoglobin-oxygen union occurs extremely rapidly (within a fraction of a second). The maximal oxygen-binding capacity of blood parallels its hemoglobin contents, and for many years the oxygen consumption of blood has been accepted as a measure of its hemoglobin concentration, based on the formula that 1 g hemoglobin binds 1.34 ml oxygen and 1 g hemoglobin iron binds 401 ml oxygen. Under normal oxygen pressure (pulmonary alveolar pressure of 100 mm Hg P_{O_2}) the arterial blood is 95-98% saturated with oxygen and the venous blood is 67-75% saturated. Under conditions of decreased arterial oxygen tension an increased amount of reduced hemoglobin is responsible for the change in color of the blood from bright red to shades of dark red.

The oxygen dissociation curve

The physiologically advantageous low oxygen affinity of blood, which allows it to be an oxygen donor to fulfill its respiratory function, is dependent on the heterogenous tetrameric structure of hemoglobin, the binding of 2,3-diphosphoglycerates (2,3-DPG), and the heme-heme interaction. The combination of these factors is responsible for the sigmoid-shaped oxygen dissociation curve, which expresses the ability of hemoglobin to readily load or unload oxygen.[1] The oxygen dissociation curve is obtained when the percentage of oxygen saturation of hemoglobin is measured point by point and plotted against a range of discrete partial

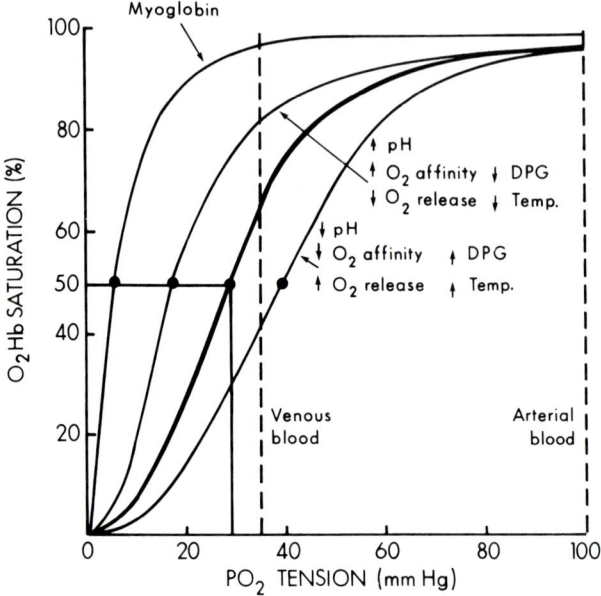

Fig. 4-3. Oxygen dissociation curves of normal human hemoglobin. Heavy middle line shows dissociation curve of normal adult blood (temperature 37° C, pH 7.4, P_{CO_2} 35 mm Hg). Dots represent P_{50} values, partial pressure of oxygen (27 mm Hg) at which hemoglobin solution is 50% oxyhemoglobin and 50% deoxyhemoglobin. If temperature increases, pH decreases, or P_{CO_2} increases, curve shifts to right. This shift increases release of oxygen from hemoglobin at given oxygen tension by decreasing its oxygen affinity. If temperature decreases, pH rises, or carbon dioxide tension decreases, oxygen dissociation curve moves to left. This shift increases oxygen-binding capacity of hemoglobin at given oxygen tension, thus decreasing oxygen release. (Modified from Oski, F.A., and Naiman, J.L.: Hematologic problems in the newborn, Philadelphia, 1972, W.B. Saunders Co.)

pressures of oxygen (Po_2) (Fig. 4-3). The steep slope of the central segment of the curve indicates that hemoglobin oxygen is released rapidly in response to relatively small changes in the oxygen pressure. The position of the curve along the Po_2 axis is determined by such characteristics of the blood as the pH, Pco_2, and temperature and by the intraerythrocytic 2,3-DPG concentration. An increase in any of these physical characteristics, except for the pH, moves the curve to the right, and a decrease moves it to the left. An increase in the pH value shifts the curve to the left, and a decrease shifts it to the right. The P_{50} value, the partial pressure of oxygen at which hemoglobin is half saturated, is generally accepted as an indicator of the position of the oxygen dissociation curve. If P_{50} is increased, the curve shifts to the right, indicating decreased oxygen affinity; a shift to the left is indicative of increased oxygen affinity.

Heme-heme interaction

The binding of oxygen to the heme iron leads to a number of structural changes in the hemoglobin molecule, which exists in two conformations: the T (taut), or deoxy, form and the R (relaxed), or oxy, form. The T form has a lower affinity for oxygen and a higher affinity for carbon dioxide than does the R form. The addition of oxygen to the T form changes its configuration to the R form. As soon as one oxygen molecule is bound by hemoglobin, the oxygen affinity of the partially oxygenated hemoglobin molecule is increased, a phenomenon referred to as the heme-heme interaction.

As stated, the position of the P_{50} of the oxygen dissociation curve is influenced by the concentration of the intraerythrocytic 2,3-DPG, the hemoglobin binding of which is related to the T-R configurational changes of the hemoglobin molecule. 2,3-DPG is located in the space between the β-chains, which are pulled apart when oxyhemoglobin releases oxygen and are pulled together when hemoglobin takes up oxygen and releases 2,3-DPG.[2,3]

Generation of the oxygen dissociation curve

The point-by-point measurement of fractional oxyhemoglobin levels over a range of partial oxygen pressures is a tedious and time-consuming procedure, outside the range of most clinical laboratories. The Hem-O-Scan (American Instrument Co., Silver Springs, Md.), an oxygen dissociation analyzer, eliminates the problems associated with the preparation of the oxygen dissociation curve. It requires 2 μl of undiluted blood in hemolysate to produce a complete continuous oxygen curve in approximately 20 min. The curve is generated using dual-wavelength spectrophotometry coupled with an oxygen monitoring electrode.

Because the temperature and the pH are controlled, the main variable is the 2,3-DPG.

Interpretation: The oxygen affinity of hemoglobin is inversely proportional to the intraerythrocytic 2,3-DPG concentration. The oxygen dissociation curve is shifted to the right (decreased oxygen affinity) by the following:
1. Increased intraerythrocytic 2,3-DPG levels as

seen in hypoxic conditions such as severe anemia and cardiac or pulmonary insufficiency
2. Functionally abnormal hemoglobin variants such as Hb Seattle,[4] Hb J Buda,[5] and a few others (Table 4-2)

The oxygen dissociation curve is shifted to the left (increased oxygen affinity) by the following:
1. Decreased intraerythrocytic 2,3-DPG concentration as seen in neonatal respiratory distress syndrome, following transfusion of stored blood, and in septic shock
2. Functionally abnormal hemoglobins such as Hb Chapel Hill,[6] Hb G Norfolk,[7] and many others (Table 4-2)
3. Methemoglobinemia
4. Carbon monoxide intoxication

Increased oxygen affinity of blood may result in tissue anoxia of clinical importance.

2,3-Diphosphoglycerate assay

The determination of 2,3-DPG may be made either enzymatically or colorimetrically. In the enzymatic method a series of coupled reactions is used with the final step involving the conversion of NADH to NAD^+ with the measurement of the change of absorbance at 340 nm. In the colorimetric method the amount of inorganic phosphate liberated in the reactions is measured by the usual colorimetric method for phosphorus. A correction is made for the inorganic phosphate originally present in the sample. The colorimetric test is available in kit form (Sigma Chemical Co., St. Louis, Bulletin no. 665) and utilizes the following reaction[8]:

$$2,3\text{-DPG} \rightarrow 3\text{-Phosphoglycerate} + \text{Inorganic phosphate}$$

This reaction is catalyzed by the enzyme 2,3-DPG phosphatase (phosphoglycerate mutase) when activated by the presence of 2-phosphoglycolate.

Normal values: The normal values when expressed as micromoles per milliliter are the same for males and females at 1.6 to 2.6 μmole/ml 2,3-DPG. Since males generally have higher hematocrits and hemoglobin levels than females, the normal levels for the sexes will differ when expressed in terms of hemoglobin or packed cells. The levels are then for males, 4.2-5.4 μmole/ml packed cells and 9.2-17.4 μmole/g hemoglobin; for females, 4.5-6.1 μmole/ml packed cells and 8.4-18.8 μmole/g hemoglobin. Levels of 2,3-DPG in newborns are similar to adult levels.[9]

Interpretation[10]: Red cell 2,3-DPG is increased in hypoxia[11] (high altitude, cardiac disease, anemia, and lung disease), in thyrotoxicosis, in pyruvate kinase deficiency, and in uremia.

2,3-DPG is lowered in acidosis and in stored blood bank blood.[12]

Oximeters

The I-L 282-Computerized CO-Oximeter (Instrumentation Laboratory, Lexington, Mass.) uses narrow-band interference filters to measure the absorption at three wavelengths (548, 568, and 578 nm) and calculates the total hemoglobin, percentages of oxyhemoglobin, carboxyhemoglobin, and methemoglobin; and oxygen content. At one wavelength, 548 nm, all compounds have the same molar absorption. The wavelength 568 nm is an isobestic point for reduced hemoglobin and carboxyhemoglobin. The dilution is accomplished anaerobically by introducing the sample and diluting fluid into a closed system by means of peristaltic pumps. Thus contact with air that causes consequent changes in the concentration of the various hemoglobins is avoided. The absorbances at the three wavelengths are fed to a small self-contained computer, and digital readouts are presented in grams per 100 ml for total hemoglobin and percentages for oxyhemoglobin and carboxyhemoglobin.

The American Optical Corp. (Buffalo, N.Y.) has the Unistat Oximeter in which the oxygen saturation is calculated from the reflected light measured at two wavelengths (660 and 805 nm) using nonhemolyzed heparinized whole blood. The percent saturation is read directly on a calibration scale. The micro model of this instrument requires only 0.2 ml blood.

Oxygen saturation may also be determined by measuring the Po_2 in a **blood gas apparatus.** The oxygen saturation is then calculated from the Po_2 by reference to curves or a slide rule obtained from the manufacturer. The measurements are made at 37° C, and the particular curve to be used depends on the pH of the blood, which also must be measured.

Spectrophotometric method: The spectrophotometric method, with some modifications, is also used to determine the concentrations of carboxyhemoglobin, methemoglobin, and sulfhemoglobin.

A discussion of the theoretical and experimental basis for this method is given in the monograph by van Assendelft,[13] which follows the earlier studies of van Kampen and Zijlstra.[14] Some of the methods use the technic of determining the two components in a binary mixture by measuring the absorbance at two different wavelengths. By the use of a calibration curve obtained from measurements with different known mixtures of the two compounds, their proportion in an unknown sample can be determined. If one of the wavelengths used is one at which the two compounds have the same absorbance (isobestic point), the calculations are simplified and the calibration curve is (theoretically) linear. Then only two calibration points obtained from separate solutions of the two components are needed. Preferably the spectrophotometer used should have a narrow band width, an accurately calibrated wavelength scale, and the capability of being read to 0.001 absorbance units.

To determine the absorbance of a blood sample accurately, it must be diluted somewhat and the cells completely lysed. In the determination of oxygen saturation this presents a difficulty because the dilution and lysing must be carried out anaerobically, for any contact with air (oxygen) may change the oxygen saturation of the sample. For this reason the dilution of the blood is kept to a minimum. The smaller the amount of solution added, which may not be completely oxygen free, the less the chance of error. A concentrated hemoglobin solution, however, requires a very short light path through the cuvet for measurement. Light paths that have been used are 0.1 and 1.0 mm. Since the measurements are made at two wavelengths on the

same solution in the same cuvet and only the ratio of the two absorbances is used in the calculations, the exact length of the light path is not important as long as it is constant during the measurements. If the measurements are made in the range of 500-600 nm, a 0.1 mm light path is required. If longer wavelengths are used (650-800 nm) where the hemoglobin absorbance is less, a 1.0 mm light path can be utilized.[15] Absorption cells with a 1 mm light path can be obtained from Pyrocell Manufacturing Co. (Westwood, N.J.) and other suppliers. These may require a special cuvet holder, but a simple U-shaped spacer can be made from plastic or 1 mm thick aluminum sheeting to hold the cells in the regular holder without obscuring the light path. To obtain a 0.1 mm light path, optically flat glass spacers having a thickness of slightly less than 0.9 mm are inserted in the 1 mm cell after some lysed blood has been added. This gives an effective light path of about 0.1 mm. If 1 mm cells alone are to be used, a holder containing four demountable cells that is of the same size as the cuvet carrier used in the Beckman DU spectrophotometer may be obtained. The assembly is made of metal and plastic. Although there is not the breakage problem associated with the fragile glass cuvets and spacers, care must be taken not to scratch the optical surfaces of the plastic cells.

Reagents:

1. Hemolyzing solution (15% Triton X-100 or 2% Sterox SE). Add 15 ml Triton X-100 to 85 ml 0.1% aqueous sodium carbonate solution or 2 ml Sterox SE to 98 ml water. Boil the solvent for a few minutes, cool somewhat, and add the surface-active agent. Then mix with a minimum of agitation and carefully transfer to a bottle that is kept tightly stoppered. The Sterox SE solution is recommended for use with the 0.1 mm cuvets[13] and the Triton X-100 solution for use with the 1 mm cuvets.[15]

2. Hemolyzing and reducing solution. In a small stoppered tube, dissolve 0.5 g sodium dithionite ($Na_2S_2O_4$, also known as sodium hydrosulfite) in 5 ml hemolyzing solution. If the solution is not perfectly clear when dissolved, it should be stoppered and centrifuged.

Procedure: Collect the blood samples (3-5 ml of arterial [preferable] or venous blood as required) in heparinized syringes, preferably of glass. Fill the dead space in the syringe and needle with heparin solution. If desired, to facilitate mixing after blood collection, inject a small amount of metallic mercury through the tip into the blood-filled syringe with another small syringe and needle. Eject any air bubbles and seal the syringe by replacing the needle and impaling a rubber stopper on the needle or preferably by using the B-D no. 3087 syringe adapter (Becton-Dickinson & Co., Rutherford, N.J.), which is actually a metal cap for the Luer tip. Keep the sample in ice and make the determination within a few hours. Just before sampling for the determination, mix the blood in the syringe thoroughly with the aid of the mercury drop.

For the determination, mix the blood anaerobically with a portion of the hemolyzing solution. With the Sterox SE solution and the 0.1 mm cuvets, the proportion of blood and solution is usually about 1:1; with Triton X-100 solution and the 1 mm cuvets, the proportion is about 1:5. There are two slightly different ways in which the solution can be added anaerobically to the blood and mixed:

1. The simplest method is to connect the two syringes via a short section of plastic tubing with their tips butting against each other. The tubing should make a tight fit on the tips and be of such a length that the two tips meet when inserted in the opposite ends of the tubing. Place the tubing on the syringe containing the hemolyzing solution, expel any air bubbles, and expel sufficient solution to fill the remainder of the tubing. Then uncap the blood syringe, expel a small amount of blood, and insert the tip into the open end of the tubing. The hemolyzing solution can be forced into the syringe containing the blood. If the latter contains a drop of mercury, it can be used to aid in mixing the two solutions. Otherwise mix by forcing the blood and solution back and forth between the two syringes. The syringes must have sufficient capacity to permit this.

2. A somewhat better method is to use an Ayer three-way stopcock (B-D no. MS02, Becton-Dickinson & Co., Rutherford, N.J.) instead of the tubing. The stopcock has two female sockets for the tips of the syringes and a tip to which a needle can be attached for filling the cuvet. If Luer-Lok syringes are used, fasten securely to the stopcock so that there will be no chance of leakage. Add and mix the solutions in the same way as when using the tubing.

For filling the cuvet, a long 23-gauge needle may be attached to the syringe or the three-way stopcock. After expelling any air bubbles and a small portion of the solution, insert the needle carefully into the cuvet for filling. To avoid trapping air bubbles in the cuvet, the needle must reach to the bottom of the cuvet. If the plastic cuvets are used, take care not to scratch the optical surfaces. With all cuvets, it is preferable to attach a 5 cm length of small polyethylene tubing to the needle. Fill the 1 mm cuvets completely and the 0.1 mm cuvets partially and carefully insert the spacers.

Then wipe the cuvets clean and insert in the spectrophotometer. Measure at 560 and 506 nm with the 0.1 cuvets and at 650 and 805 nm with the 1 mm light path, in each case using a blank of the hemolyzing solution. When measured at the shorter wavelengths, the ratio A560/A506 is calculated, where A560 represents the absorbance at 560 nm, etc. With the 1 mm light path the ratio A650/A805 is used. Then determine the percent saturation from the calibration curve.

Preparation of calibration curve: To obtain the calibration curve, measure in a similar manner on blood samples containing 100% and 0% oxyhemoglobin (O$_2$-Hb). The latter is obtained by using with the blood sample the reducing and hemolyzing solution containing the dithionite in the same proportion as used in the test. This reduces all the hemoglobin present. The 100% point is obtained by using a blood sample that has been fully saturated by equilibration with pure ox-

ygen. About 5 ml of blood is introduced into a 100 ml cylindric bottle, which is then rotated with its axis in a horizontal position while a slow stream of pure oxygen is passed in. It is preferable to obtain such a blood sample from an individual who has had as little exposure to carbon monoxide as possible. Since one of the wavelengths used is always an isobestic point, only the two calibration points are needed and a straight line drawn between them.

The following values of the ratios as found by the investigators cited are given as a guide. They should be checked with the instrument used, but values close to these should be obtained.

	100% Hb	100% O$_2$-Hb	Investigator
A560/A506	2.57	1.74	Ref. 16
A650/A805	4.0	0.5	Ref. 17

Measurements with the 1 mm cuvets with the longer wavelengths give a larger difference in the ratios between the two ends of the curve. Theoretically this should be more accurate, as well as somewhat simpler. It has been stated that the effect of turbidity and non-hemoglobin light absorption is much greater in the near infrared than in the visible portion (the greater errors being attributable to this) and that the isobestic point near 800 nm is rather elusive (in fact, van Assendelft[13] gives the wavelength as 815 nm, whereas Johnston[15] used 805 nm).

Normal values: With the method given, the oxygen saturation of normal arterial blood is 95-98%. The range of saturation of venous blood is from 67-75%.

False positive results: Since the absorption curve of carboxyhemoglobin (CO-Hb) is somewhat similar to that of O$_2$-Hb, an appreciable amount of CO-Hb in the blood will cause a spuriously high oxygen saturation with the spectrophotometric methods. The presence of 5% CO-Hb in the blood will cause an increase in the measured oxygen saturation by about 3-4%. Usually the oxygen saturation is measured in hospitalized patients who have not been recently subjected to carbon monoxide exposure, but if oxygen saturation must be measured by the method outlined in patients after recent exposure to carbon monoxide, this fact must be kept in mind. It is possible to simultaneously determine O$_2$-Hb, hemoglobin, and CO-Hb in one sample by making measurements at three wavelengths. This is not simple to do by ordinary methods, but it has been done with the I-L CO-Oximeter (see previous discussion), where the necessary dilution is made anaerobically and the results automatically calculated.

Interpretation: The following may cause decreased arterial oxygen tension (oxygen-binding capacity):
  Decreased atmospheric pressure (high altitude)[18]
  Impaired cardiopulmonary function[19]
  Congenital heart disease with right to left shunt[20]
  Hemoglobinopathies
  Chemical changes of the hemoglobin molecule
    Methemoglobinemia
    Sulfhemoglobinemia
    Carboxyhemoglobinemia

Carboxyhemoglobin (carbon monoxide)

Chemical changes of the hemoglobin molecule lead to the formation of CO-Hb methemoglobin, (Met-Hb), and sulfhemoglobin (S-Hb) and to alterations of the maximal oxygen-binding capacity of blood.

The affinity of carbon monoxide to hemoglobin is 210 times that of oxygen, so that inhalation of carbon monoxide–containing air readily leads to the formation of CO-Hb, which markedly reduces the oxygen-carrying capacity of blood. At a carbon monoxide concentration of 0.1% in the inhaled air, more than 50% of the hemoglobin is not available for oxygen transport. Carbon monoxide combines with hemoglobin more slowly than does oxygen, but the union is much firmer and the dissociation is 10,000 times slower than the release of oxygen from O_2-Hb. In the presence of carbon monoxide, even the O_2-Hb dissociates more slowly.

Tentative rapid tests

Dilution test:

Procedure: Dilute 1 ml blood with 50 ml water.

Results: CO-Hb is cherry red and a dilute solution appears pink or bluish red, whereas O_2-Hb solutions are yellowish red.

NaOH test:

Reagent: NaOH, 40% (40 g/dl).

Procedure: Add a few drops of NaOH to EDTA-anticoagulated blood and warm gently.

Results: If CO-Hb is present, a red color will appear, whereas in the presence of O_2-Hb a black-brown discoloration occurs.

Tannic acid test:

Reagent: Tannic acid, 1% (1 g/dl).

Procedure: Dilute blood four times with water, add 3 volumes of tannic acid solution, and mix.

Results: CO-Hb produces a red precipitate, whereas O_2-Hb produces a grayish brown precipitate.

Spectrophotometric method[13,14,21]

For determination of the abnormal hemoglobin pigments, CO-Hb Met-Hb, and S-Hb, a slight amount of contact with air is not harmful, and high dilutions can be used with ordinary cuvets that have a 10 mm light path.

Principle: Carbon monoxide may be determined by converting all the O_2-Hb present to reduced hemoglobin and then making measurements at two wavelengths in the two-component system hemoglobin–CO-Hb. The O_2-Hb is converted to reduced hemoglobin by the addition of a small amount of dithionite, which does not immediately affect the CO-Hb.

Reagents:

1. Ammonium hydroxide, 0.25M. Dilute 16 ml concentrated ammonium hydroxide to 1 L with water.
2. Sodium hydrosulfite (sodium dithionite). Weigh out portions of 35 mg fresh salt and place in small stoppered tubes for use as required.
3. Oxygen and carbon monoxide cylinders for preparation of standards if needed.
4. Sample. Collect venous blood in a heparinized Vacutainer; keep it stoppered and refrigerated until analyzed.

Procedure: Dilute 0.05 ml whole blood with 10 ml ammonium hydroxide solution. NOTE: Since only the ratio of absorbances is used, the volumes need not be accurately measured unless one wishes to also determine the total hemoglobin content. In this case, dilute accurately and then measure the absorbance of the dilution at 548 nm before the addition of dithionite. With a 1 cm light path, $A \times 26.5 =$ Total hemoglobin (g/dl). Mix by inversion and allow to stand for 2 min or until completely clear. Add 35 mg dithionite, mix by inversion, and start the stopwatch.

Exactly 5 min after the addition of dithionite, read the solution at 555 nm against a blank of the ammonium hydroxide solution; then read it also at 541 nm. NOTE: The wavelengths must be set very accurately on the wavelength scale. It is also advisable to check the cuvets to be used for samples by making a reading with the blank solution and making a correction for absorption by cuvets.

Calculations: Calculate R = A541/A555. Then calculate as follows:

$$\text{\% CO-Hb in sample} = \frac{R_S - R_0}{R_{100} - R_0} \times 100$$

R_S is the ratio for the sample; R_0 is the ratio for 0% CO-Hb; R_{100} is the ratio for 100% CO-Hb. R_0 and R_{100} should be determined as outlined below. For an occasional determination one can take R_0 as 0.830 and R_{100} as 1.220. NOTE: The values found by Tietz and Fiereck[22] are $R_0 = 0.825 \pm 0.005$, and $R_{100} = 1.225 \pm 0.005$.

Standardization: Obtain a quantity of heparinized blood from a nonsmoker. Place about 5 ml well-mixed blood in each of two 100 ml bottles. Pass in a slow stream of 100% oxygen from a small tank for about 15 min while rotating the bottle slowly in a horizontal position. Stopper and allow to stand for 15 min with occasional rotation. Repeat the flushing with oxygen and rotation several times to completely saturate the blood. Stopper tightly until ready for use.

Repeat the process with the other bottle using carbon monoxide instead of oxygen. CAUTION: This must be done in a good fume hood. Use the oxygenated sample to determine R_0 and the sample saturated with carbon monoxide to obtain R_{100}.

Normal values and interpretation[23]: The amount of CO-Hb in the blood depends on the recent exposure of the subject to carbon monoxide. Under the most favorable conditions the carbon monoxide content will be on the order of 1-2% (some carbon monoxide if formed by the metabolism of heme in the destruction of red cells, so that the level never falls to zero). In smokers (one to two packs of cigarettes per day) the level may vary from 4-6%, and in very heavy smokers the level may rise to 6-20%. Taxi drivers, traffic policemen, and garage workers, having a greater exposure to carbon monoxide, may have up to 10% in the blood. Mild symptoms such as slight headaches and slight dyspnea on exertion may occur at levels of 10-15% saturation. At levels of 20-30% there will be more severe headaches, ready fatigue, and impaired judgment. Levels of more than 50% cause increasingly severe symptoms, and 70% saturation is usually fatal, although death has occurred at levels as low as 40%. The actual fatal dose depends greatly on the general condition of the patient. The half-life for elimination of carbon monoxide is approximately 4 hr[24] for a person breathing atmospheric air,[25] although in smokers the level remains elevated.[26]

Methemoglobin

As mentioned in the discussion of O_2-Hb, hemoglobin is able to reversibly bind oxygen, a process called **oxygenation,** but this is not the only form of oxygen binding of which hemoglobin is capable. Under certain conditions the iron of the heme moiety binds oxygen so closely that it is unable to dissociate and is therefore not available for respiration. This process is called **oxidation of hemoglobin,** in which the iron of the heme moiety (which is bivalent) is oxidized to the trivalent ferric form and the reduced hemoglobin is transformed into a brown pigment, Met-Hb, that accumulates in the red cells. Methemoglobinemia refers to the clinical condition in which cyanosis is produced in proportion to the concentration of the abnormal Met-Hb (over 1%). Met-Hb is incapable of being oxygenated and is therefore devoid of any respiratory function. The ferric iron can be reduced to the original ferrous form by reducing agents and by certain enzymes. In vivo and in vitro, Met-Hb formation is therefore reversible.

Met-Hb produced by the addition of potassium ferricyanide to hemoglobin forms the basis of present-day hemoglobinometry.

Normally after prolonged standing, O_2-Hb is turned brown by Met-Hb formation. The brown color of blood in acid urine is also caused by Met-Hb formation.

Under physiologic conditions Met-Hb is continuously being formed within erythrocytes because of oxidation of hemoglobin, but it is prevented from accumulating within the red cell by a specific NADH diaphorase system called **Met-Hb reductase** that maintains a physiologic Met-Hb concentration of about 0.1 g/dl blood, or 0.1% saturation. Larger amounts than 0.1% are always pathologic and are found in the blood when (1) the rate of formation and the amount of Met-Hb overwhelm the physiologic reducing enzyme system; (2) there is a defect in the intraerythrocytic enzyme system that normally reduces Met-Hb, which, like all proteins, is genetically controlled; or (3) there is present a hereditary globin abnormality, as found in Hb M diseases and some non-M abnormal hemoglobins, e.g., Hb Freiburg (Tables 4-2 to 4-9).

Methemoglobinemia can thus be divided into one acquired and two congenital hereditary forms.

Acquired methemoglobinemia (toxic methemoglobinemia)

Acquired methemoglobinemia results from the action of oxidizing chemicals[27] and drugs such as nitrites, aniline derivatives, sulfonamides, acetanilid, nitroglycerin, and acetophenetidin, which accelerate the oxidation of hemoglobin. Toxic methemoglobinemia is characterized by elevated levels of Met-Hb in blood in the absence of any abnormality of the globin component of hemoglobin or any NADH diaphorase deficiency.

Newborn infants and those up to about 3 months of age have a tendency to form Met-Hb and are thus particularly sensitive to these oxidizing substances. The increased risk of Met-Hb formation in newborns is caused by (1) the increased speed with which Hb F (concentration at birth, 50-85%) can be oxidized and (2) the diminished or slowed activity of Met-Hb reductase. Nitrates, which may be found in high concentrations in spinach and in well water, can be converted into potentially dangerous nitrites by intestinal bacteria. Severe bacterial enteritis may also lead to the absorption of large amounts of nitrites. Met-Hb formation also accompanies some forms of hemolytic anemias, so that Met-Hb is found in the serum and urine, both of which turn brown.

Hereditary (congenital) methemoglobinemia

Hereditary methemoglobinemia can be divided into two groups. In group 1 there is a congenital intraerythrocytic deficiency of NADH diaphorase (Met-Hb reductase) and often also of glutathione. The reductase (diaphorase) is the enzyme that normally reduces the Met-Hb to hemoglobin. Two such enzymes have been described, one dependent on NADH and the other on NADPH.[28]

In group 2, Met-Hb formation is the result of a genetically abnormal hemoglobin molecule, the abnormality residing in the globin structure (amino acid sequence of the α- or β-chains). These abnormal hemoglobins are designated Hb M (Tables 4-2 to 4-9).

All congenital forms of methemoglobinemia are characterized by permanent cyanosis of long duration.

Enzyme-deficient methemoglobinemia

Enzyme-deficient methemoglobinemia may be manifest at birth and is associated with a deficiency in Met-Hb reductase activity. It is inherited as an autosomal recessive characteristic. Heterozygous subjects are not cyanotic and are therefore not usually investigated for Met-Hb, but their red cells are much more sensitive to oxidant stress than those of normal individuals.[29] In the homozygous form the red cells are severely deficient in Met-Hb reductase. A relatively high percentage of Alaskan Eskimos and Indians have been found to have hereditary enzyme-deficient methemoglobinemia. Mental retardation may result from diaphorase deficiency.[30] Methylene blue is not only used clinically to reverse acquired and congenital diaphorase-deficient methemoglobinemia but also serves as a rapid in vitro diagnostic test.

Screening tests:

1. A few drops of anticoagulated blood are aerated on a glass slide by blowing on it. In methemoglobinemia the blood is chocolate brown and retains its color, whereas hypoxic blood will brighten. A modification of this test consists of placing 1 drop of blood on a piece of filter paper, which is oxygenated by moving it slowly in the air for 30 sec. If Met-Hb is present, the color of the drop will not change.[31] The test serves to rapidly differentiate the cyanosis of methemoglobinemia from other forms of cyanosis, e.g., of heart and lung disease.

2. If the methemoglobinemia is caused by a reductase deficiency, the addition of 1% solution of methylene blue changes the chocolate brown color of the blood to red.

Spectroscopic method[13,14,32]: The most widely

used method is based on the work of Evelyn and Malloy.[32] In this method the blood is diluted with phosphate buffer and the absorbance of an aliquot of the diluted blood is measured at 630 nm before and after the addition of a few milligrams of potassium cyanide. The cyanide converts any Met-Hb present into cyanmethemoglobin and abolishes the absorption peak of the former compounds at 630 nm. In another aliquot all the hemoglobin is converted to Met-Hb by the addition of potassium ferricyanide. The absorbance of this solution is also measured at 630 nm before and after the addition of cyanide as a measure of the total amount of hemoglobin present. The difference in absorbance for the untreated sample divided by that for the sample that has been first treated with potassium ferricyanide will give the proportion of Met-Hb in the sample.

Reagents:
1. Stock phosphate buffer. Dissolve 34.6 g KH_2PO_4 and 36.1 g anhydrous Na_2HPO_4 in water to make 250 ml. Adjust the pH so that a 1:20 dilution will have a pH of 6.8.
2. Sterox SE, 5%. Dilute 5 ml Sterox SE to 1 dl with water.
3. Working solution. Dilute 1 ml stock buffer and 6 ml 5% Sterox to 50 ml with water.
4. Potassium ferricyanide, fine crystals.
5. Potassium cyanide, fine crystals.

Procedure: Dilute 0.2 ml well-mixed blood with 10 ml working solution. Mix and allow to stand for a few minutes for complete hemolysis. If the solution is not completely clear, centrifuge and use the supernatant. If only the percent of Met-Hb is required, the blood need not be measured too accurately, but if one wishes to measure the absolute amount as mentioned below, the working solution and blood should be accurately measured.

Divide the hemolyzed solution into two equal parts. Add a portion of one aliquot to a cuvet and read against a blank of the working buffer at 630 nm (A_1). Then add a few milligrams of potassium cyanide, mix to dissolve, and read again at the same wavelength (A_2). If the two readings are exactly the same, no Met-Hb is present and the rest of the procedure need not be done.

To the other aliquot, add a few milligrams of solid potassium ferricyanide and mix well. Then transfer to a cuvet and read, as with the first aliquot, before and after the addition of cyanide (A_3 and A_4). If the same cuvet is used for reading the two aliquots, be sure that it is completely rinsed before transferring the second aliquot.

The percent of Met-Hb is then given by:

$$Met\text{-}Hb\ (\%) = (A_1 - A_2) \times 100/(A_3 - A_4)$$

If the total hemoglobin content of the blood is known, then the amount of Met-Hb present may be calculated from the percentage and the total hemoglobin concentration. If the original dilution was exact, then the solution remaining after reading A_4 may be accurately diluted 1:5 with the usual Drabkin solution (Sigma Chemical Co., St. Louis) and the hemoglobin read at 540 nm. The result from the usual hemoglobin calibration curve is multiplied by 1.02 to take into account the fact that the dilution used here is 1:255 instead of the usual 1:251 for hemoglobin determination.

Range of values and interpretation: As already stated, small amounts of Met-Hb may be found in the blood of normal subjects. Values up to 0.1 g/dl blood have been found in hospitalized patients who have not been receiving any recognized Met-Hb–producing drugs. In methemoglobinemia, cyanosis becomes apparent when the saturation reaches levels of about 15%, but levels even up to 30% may not produce any obvious symptoms other than cyanosis. At levels of 35-45%, symptoms such as dyspnea may be observed. Lethargy and semistupor may not occur until levels of about 60% have been reached; the lethal level is generally above 70% saturation.

The test cannot be used to assay methemoglobinemia caused by Hb M variants because they react anomalously with cyanide.

Determination of NADH diaphorase activity: A screening method is presented in detail, but the quantitative method is only referenced.

Screening method:

Principle: This enzyme catalyzes the reduction of methemoglobin to hemoglobin by NADH.

$$Met\ Hb^{+++} + NADH \longrightarrow Hb^{++} + NAD^+$$

In vitro this reaction proceeds rather slowly and is difficult to measure. For the actual determinations different substrates are used. The screening method uses a substrate of the dye dichlorophenolindophenol, which is reduced to the leuko form by NADH as catalyzed by the enzyme. In this procedure the hemoglobin present is first changed to Met-Hb by the action of nitrite, since the hemoglobin would otherwise reduce the dye noncatalytically. The rate of reaction is observed as in the other screening methods by noting the change in the NADH fluorescence.

If the hemoglobin used to prepare the substrate is obtained from red cells, it is treated with DEAE cellulose to remove the NADH diaphorase present so that any enzyme present is from the sample itself and not from the substrate.

Reagents:
1. Tris buffer, 0.06M, pH 7.5, containing 0.027M EDTA. Dissolve 7.2 g tris(hydroxymethyl)aminomethane and 1 g disodium ethylenediamine tetraacetic acid (EDTA) in about 9 dl water. Add about 40 ml 1M HCl (83 ml concentrated acid to 1 L), check the pH, and add more HCl to bring the pH to 7.6.
2. Dichlorophenolindophenol, 19 mmole. Dissolve in water in a concentration of 6.25 mg/ml.
3. Saponin, 1 g/dl. Dissolve 1 g saponin (Sigma Chemical Co., St. Louis) in water to make 1 dl.
4. Sodium nitrite, 0.18M. Prepare fresh as required by dissolving 125 mg sodium nitrite in 10 ml water.

Procedure: Add 0.6 ml sodium nitrite solution to 100 μl whole blood sample (heparin or acid-citrate-dextrose [ACD], and allow to stand at room temperature for 30 min. (Prepare a normal control as well as a sample.) Mix together 1.0 ml tris buffer, 10 μl dye solution, and 200 μl saponin solution. Transfer 0.4 ml portions of this to small test tubes. Add 20 μl nitrite-treated sample or control to 0.4 ml reagent mixture. Spot on paper at once and at 15 min intervals for 1 hr, incubating at room temperature.

Dry the paper and observe the spots under ultraviolet light. The first spot should fluoresce brightly in all cases. With normal blood the fluorescence should disappear within 30 min, while with an enzyme-deficient sample the fluorescence will still be detected after 45 min or even 1 hr.

Quantitative method[35,36]:

Principle: In the quantitative method the substrate used is the Met-Hb–ferrocyanide complex, which gives a fairly rapid reduction with NADH; the change in absorbance at 475 nm is noted.

Methemoglobinemia caused by Hb M

Methemoglobinemia caused by Hb M is rare and occurs only in the heterozygous form. The homozygous form is probably not compatible with life. Several variants of Hb M have been described, not all of which are associated with Met-Hb formation but rather depress the oxygen affinity (Tables 4-2 to 4-9). Hb M variants show a dominant inheritance pattern and, unlike many other hemoglobinopathies, are usually not responsible for the production of hemolytic anemias. Cyanosis may be present at birth, or it may appear in the first few weeks of life. It does not respond to intravenous methylene blue, in contrast to other forms of methemoglobinemia, which readily improve under such treatment. The differentiation of Hb M methemoglobinemia from the other forms of methemoglobinemia is of some importance since it does not require treatment.

Diagnosis of Hb M: The diagnosis can be suspected clinically, and some variants can be confirmed by the analysis of the absorption spectrum of hemolysates oxidized to the Fe^{+++} state with ferricyanide. The abnormal spectral pattern is compared with that of normal Met–Hb A.[33] The technic of Evelyn and Malloy mentioned above is not applicable to Hb M variants because they react abnormally with cyanide. Other diagnostic methods include hemoglobin electrophoresis on agar gel at pH 7.1 and gel electrofocusing after treatment with ferricyanide. Both technics reveal a brown band of Hb M on the anodal side of the red Hb A band.[34]

Sulfhemoglobin

S-Hb is an intraerythrocytic hemoglobin derivative resulting from a stable linkage of hemoglobin and sulfur. The toxic effect of certain drugs on hemoglobin not only leads to the formation of Met-Hb but also to concomitant S-Hb production. S-Hb formation is the result of an irreversible (thus differing from the reversible Met-Hb formation) structural change within the protoporphyrin portion of the heme moiety produced by such substances as aniline dyes, acetanalid, acetophenetidin, sulfonamides, and sulfur-containing cathartics. Since the formation of the sulfur-linked pigment is irreversible, the compound does not disappear from the circulation until the involved red cells complete their life cycle. The cyanosis resulting from sulfhemoglobinemia resists treatment.

Spectrophotometric methods for sulfhemoglobin detection[13,14,37]

The determination of S-Hb presents difficulties not found in the other methods. It is difficult to prepare pure S-Hb, which creates uncertainty about its exact millimolar extinction coefficient, and it is not practical to prepare standards in the laboratory as was done, for example, with CO-Hb. We present two methods for its determination. The first, a simple screening method, is satisfactory for most clinical purposes.

Screening method

This method is based on the studies of van Kampen and Zijlstra.[14] The details of the derivation of the formula used will not be given here, and those interested should refer to the publications cited. The method is based on the fact that although the addition of cyanide will abolish the absorption of Met-Hb at 620 nm, it will not affect S-Hb, which has an absorption peak at this wavelength. The measurement of the absorption of 620 nm is corrected for the absorption of other hemoglobin compounds by an experimentally determined factor.

Reagents:
1. Sterox SE, 2%. Dilute 2 ml Sterox SE to 1 dl with distilled water.
2. Potassium cyanide crystals.

Procedure: To 10 ml 2% Sterox solution, add 0.1 ml blood. Allow to stand for a few minutes until hemolysis is complete. If the solution is not perfectly clear, centrifuge it and use the clear supernatant. Transfer about 3 ml of the solution to a cuvet, add about 3 mg potassium cyanide, and mix. Read the solution in a spectrophotometer at 577 and 620 nm against a blank of the Sterox solution. The percentage of S-Hb is then given by:

$$\text{S-Hb (\%)} = 1.3\left[F\frac{A620}{A577} - 1 \right]$$

A620 and A577 are the measured absorbances at the two wavelengths, and F is the ratio of the absorbance of pure O_2-Hb at 577 nm to that at 620 nm. This was found to be about 35 using the Beckman DU spectrophotometer, but it should be determined experimentally with the spectrophotometer used by diluting a sample of normal oxygenated blood 1:100 with 2% Sterox and measuring the absorbance at the two wavelengths. The equation given is slightly different from that given in the references cited, since we have used the later value for the extinction coefficient of S-Hb given by Nichol and Morell.[37]

Method of Nichol and Morell[37]

The method of Nichol and Morell is somewhat more elaborate and requires the use of a good spectrophotometer with a very narrow band and accurate wavelength calibration and cuvets with a 1 cm light path. Both S-Hb and Met-Hb may be determined.

Reagents:
1. Phosphate buffer 0.1M, pH 6.0. Dissolve 11.8 g K_2HPO_4 and 1.9 g Na_2HPO_4 in water and dilute to 1 L. Check the pH and adjust to 6.0 if necessary.

2. Sodium dithionite, fresh crystals.
3. Carbon monoxide from small lecture-type tank.

Procedure: Dilute 1 ml blood (oxalated or citrated) with water to make 10 ml. After hemolysis is complete, centrifuge strongly to remove stroma. Dilute 1 ml of the clear supernatant to 10 ml with the phosphate buffer. Pass a moderate stream of carbon monoxide in the form of large bubbles through the solution for 3 min. CAUTION: Use a fume hood with a good exhaust. Using cuvets with a 1 cm light path, measure the absorption at once against a blank of the phosphate buffer at 569 and 638 nm. Add a few crystals of fresh dithionite to the solution in the cuvet, mix by gentle inversion, and read again at 569, 614, and 638 nm. The percent of Met-Hb is then calculated from the formula:

$$\text{Met-Hb (\%)} = (\Delta A569 + \Delta A638) \times 10.4$$

The percent S-Hb is calculated from the formula:

$$[A614 - (A569 \times 0.036)] \times 6.4 = \%\text{S-Hb}$$

In the first formula, $\Delta A569$ is the change in the absorbance at 569 nm, and $\Delta A638$ is the change in absorbance at 638 nm before and after the addition of dithionite to the solution containing the carbon monoxide derivatives. Both the differences are taken as positive in this formula. In the second formula, $A614$ and $A569$ are the absorbances at these wavelengths after the addition of dithionite.

If the absolute amounts of Met-Hb or S-Hb must be determined, the total amount of hemoglobin compounds present must be known. If the total hemoglobin is determined by the cyanmethemoglobin method, remember that S-Hb is only very slowly converted into cyanmethemoglobin, so that in the presence of appreciable amounts of S-Hb the solution for hemoglobin measurement must be allowed to stand for at least 30 min after blood is added before the measurement is made.

Range of values and interpretation: Normally only very small amounts of S-Hb are found in the blood. It is usually formed after ingestion of the previously mentioned drugs, which may lead to S-Hb production that rarely exceeds 10%.

CLINICAL HEMOGLOBINOMETRY

The traditional manual procedures for the determination of hemoglobin concentration are adequately described in earlier editions of this book. In most laboratories they have been replaced by automated technics that have several advantages, e.g., greater reproducibility, accuracy coupled with greater speed, lower cost per test, less technician fatigue, and savings in glassware. The automated equipment requires careful standardization and accurate calibration. All dilutions must be prepared by carefully standardized automatic diluters.

The clinical hemoglobinometers measure hemoglobin spectrophotometrically either as cyanmethemoglobin or as O_2-Hb. The majority employ the cyanmethemoglobin method in which the ferrous iron in the heme molecule is oxidized to ferric iron to produce Met-Hb, which is then converted to cyanmethemoglobin by the potassium cyanide in the modified Drabkin reagent.

Use of the cyanmethemoglobin method is preferred primarily because a stable (1 year) cyanmethemoglobin standard is commercially available (Hycel, Houston) and because the method measures all hemoglobin derivatives, irrespective of their ability to carry oxygen, and the values obtained provide an acceptable basis for the calculation of the hematologic constants.

The O_2-Hb method measures only hemoglobin capable of being oxygenated and excludes abnormal non-oxygen-carrying pigments such as Met-Hb and CO-Hb, which lack respiratory function.

Coulter hemoglobinometer

Whole blood is diluted 1:501 with a modified isotonic electrolyte diluent (Isoton) to which 3 drops of a lysing and cyanmethemoglobin reagent (Zapoglobin) are added. An aliquot of the 1:501 Isoton dilution may also be used for the automated leukocyte count on Coulter Models S and S_{SR}. The Coulter hemoglobinometer (Coulter Electronics, Hialeah, Fla.) is equipped with a flow-through cuvet that is automatically rinsed after each determination with a blended neutral nonhemolytic detergent (Isoterge), which also serves as a reference blank. The cyanmethemoglobin concentration (grams per deciliter) is instantly computed and shown on a digital readout. It is based on the comparison of the optical density of the blank with the lysed, diluted hemoglobin sample. The entire operation requires less than 1 min.

IL hemoglobinometer

The IL hemoglobinometer (Instrumentation Laboratory, Andover, Mass.) does not utilize the cyanmethemoglobin method and therefore requires a special artificial standard for calibration. Its operation is based on the fact that at wavelength 548.5 nm identical concentrations of reduced hemoglobin, O_2-Hb, Met-Hb, and CO-Hb have the same optical density. The blood sample is automatically aspirated and diluted, and the concentration of hemoglobin appears on a digital readout. After completion of the test the instrument is automatically flushed.

Normal values:
Men: 14.0-16.0, mean 15.0 g/dl
Women: 12.0-15.0, mean 13.5 g/dl
Children at different ages: see Table 7-2
If values are expressed in molar concentration, multiply the values given here by 0.6206 to convert them to millimoles per liter.

Standardization of hemoglobin determination by measurement of total iron content[38]

Principle: The iron is split off from the hemoglobin with hypochlorite and determined directly with a sensitive-color reagent. Only a small blood sample is used, and a surfactant is added to eliminate any turbidity caused by the small amounts of protein present.

Reagents:
1. Sodium hypochlorite. Any commercial liquid bleach containing 5% available chlorine can be used.
2. Brij-35 solution (Technicon Instruments Corp., Tarrytown, N.Y.). Dilute the 25% solution of

polyethylene lauryl ether as purchased 1:5 with deionized water.

3. Ferrozine color reagent. Dissolve 150 mg ferrozine (Hack Chemical Co., Ames, Iowa) in 10 ml deionized water.

4. Acetate–ascorbic acid buffer. Dissolve 41.0 g sodium acetate (trihydrate) in water, add 30.3 ml glacial acetic acid, and dilute to 500 ml with deionized water. Just before use, dissolve 1 g ascorbic acid in 30 ml buffer.

5. Iron standard, 50 mg/dl iron. Dissolve 100 mg pure iron wire in 2 ml concentrated hydrochloric acid, 5 ml water, and 3 ml 70% perichloric acid by gentle warming in a small beaker. (NOTE: It is difficult to weigh out exactly 100 mg iron wire. Any amount between 90 and 110 mg may be weighed out exactly and the equivalent hemoglobin concentration calculated as given above.) When all the iron is dissolved, transfer solution to a 200 ml volumetric flask and dilute to volume with deionized water. This solution has an iron content of 50 mg/dl or, since hemoglobin is assumed to contain 0.347% iron, the solution is equivalent to 0.050/0.00347, or 14.4 g/dl hemoglobin.

Procedure: In a series of test tubes (preferably disposable plastic tubes) place 1 ml hypochlorite solution and 1 ml diluted Brij-35 solution. Add to the tubes 20 μl samples of well-mixed whole blood, reserving one tube as reagent blank. NOTE: Sahli pipets are not accurate enough for the calibration unless they have been individually calibrated. More accurate micropipets such as Accupettes with bulb (Scientific Products Co., McGaw Park, Ill.) are used. To eliminate the difficulties in pipetting duplicate samples of whole blood the following method may be used. Collect about 5 ml normal anticoagulated blood. Centrifuge it and remove the plasma. Wash once with saline. To the packed washed cells add 1.5 volumes water and 0.5 volume carbon tetrachloride. Shake vigorously, then centrifuge strongly. Remove a portion of the supernatant and use it for determination of hemoglobin by the above method and by the method being calibrated.

Allow the tubes to stand for 10 min, then add 3 ml buffer and 1 ml ferrozine color reagent to each tube. Mix and allow to stand for 20 min, then read standard and samples against blank at 568 nm.
Calculation:

$$\frac{\text{Absorbance sample}}{\text{Absorbance standard}} \times \text{Conc. standard} =$$
$$\text{g/dl Hemoglobin in sample}$$

The concentration of the standard is given above as 14.4 g/dl hemoglobin, but see note above. The hemoglobin content of the blood samples is determined by the cyanmethemoglobin or O_2-Hb method used routinely, and the results are compared with the iron determination.

LABORATORY INVESTIGATION OF NORMAL HEMOGLOBINS: QUALITATIVE AND QUANTITATIVE ASSAYS

Each hemoglobin molecule consists of four polypeptide chains to each of which one heme group is attached. Greek letters are used to designate the polypeptide chains: α (alpha), β (beta), γ (gamma), δ (delta), ε (epsilon), and ζ (zeta). The normal hemoglobins differ according to the developmental age of the individual.[39] There are three embryonic hemoglobins (Table 4-1)—Hb Portland $(\zeta_2\gamma_2)$,[40] Hb Gower 1 $(\zeta_2\varepsilon_2)$, and Hb Gower 2 $(\alpha_2\varepsilon_2)$; two fetal hemoglobins—Hb F $(\alpha_2\gamma_2)$ and Hb F_1 $(\alpha_2[\gamma\text{-}N\text{-acetyl}]_2)$; and several adult hemoglobins—Hb A $(\alpha_2\beta_2)$, Hb A_2 $(\alpha_2\delta_2)$, and Hb A_{1a}, A_{1b}, and A_{1c} $(\alpha_2[\beta\text{-}N\text{-glucose}]_2)$. The α-chain, which takes part in the formation of A_1, A_2, F, and Gower 2, consists of 141 amino acids; the β-, γ-, δ-, and ζ-chains consist of 146 amino acids each.

The laboratory approach to the identification or normal hemoglobins is the same as that used for the diagnosis of hemoglobinopathies.

Hemoglobin A

Hb A $(\alpha_2\beta_2)$ makes up the major portion (95-98%) of the adult hemolysates. Small amounts of Hb A form during intrauterine life, so that at birth cord blood contains about 10-30% Hb A, the remainder being Hb F.

Table 4-1. Normal hemoglobins

Hemoglobin	Peptide structure	Alkali resistant	Adult hemolysate (%)
Adult hemoglobins			
Hb A	$\alpha_2\beta_2$	No	95-98
Hb A_2	$\alpha_2\delta_2$	No	2-3
Hb A_{1a}		No	
Hb A_{1b}		No	
Hb A_{1c}	$\alpha_2(\beta\text{-}N\text{-glucose})_2$	No	1-5
Fetal hemoglobins			
Hb F	$\alpha_2\gamma_2$	Yes	<1
Hb F_1	$\alpha_2(\gamma\text{-}N\text{-acetyl})_2$	Yes	<1
Embryonic hemoglobins			
Hb Gower 1	$\zeta_2\varepsilon_2$	Yes	0
Hb Gower 2	$\alpha_2\varepsilon_2$	Yes	0
Hb Portland	$\zeta_2\gamma_2$	Yes	0

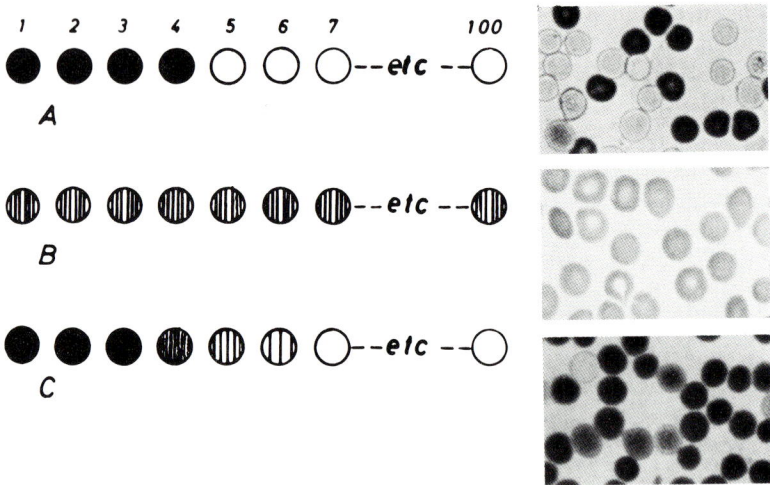

Fig. 4-4. Distribution patterns of Hb F and Hb A in red cells. **A,** Two separate cell populations, Hb F–containing cells and Hb A–containing cells **B,** Even distribution of Hb A and Hb F within cells. **C,** Irregular distribution of Hb A and Hb F within cells, some cells containing more Hb F than others and some containing none. (From Kleihauer, E.: Beihefte Arch. Kinderheilkd. **53**[suppl.], 1966.)

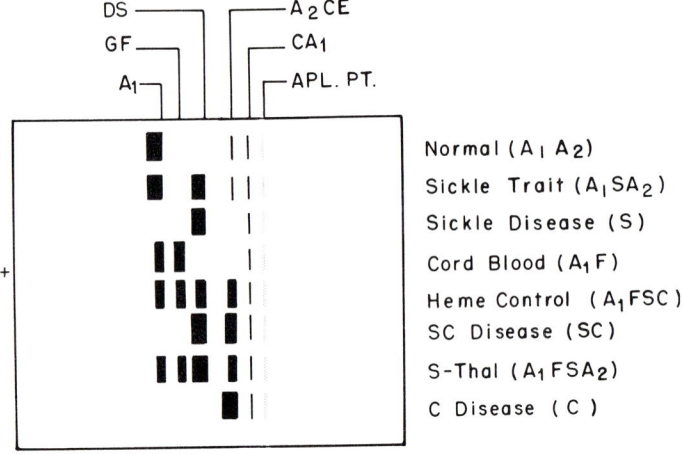

Fig. 4-5. Cellulose acetate electrophoretic patterns of normal and abnormal hemoglobins at pH 8.6. *Apl. pt.,* Application point; *CA₁,* carbonic anhydrase; + indicates anode. Heme Control is manufactured by Helena Laboratories, Beaumont, Tex.

During the ensuing 6-12 months Hb A reaches adult concentrations and is accompanied by only traces of Hb F and A₂ (Table 4-1 and Fig. 4-4). On the cellulose acetate electrophoretogram Hb A is closest to the anode and furthest from the application point (Fig. 4-5) except for the fast abnormal hemoglobins H and Bart's, small amounts of which may be present in normal cord blood. The citrate agar gel pattern also reveals Hb A (together with Hb G, D, and E) in the most anodal position furthest from the application point except for the Hb F band, which, if Hb F is present in high concentrations, is further anodal than the Hb A band (Fig. 4-6).

Stain for hemoglobin A

Principle: Selective staining of Hb A leaves Hb F unstained, representing a reversed Kleihauer stain. Hb A is less soluble in concentrated salt solution than is Hb F.[41]

Reagents:
1. Potassium phosphate buffer, pH 7.2
   K₂HPO₄, 24.1 g
   KH₂PO₄, 18.8 g
   Water, 100 ml
   Mix and confirm the pH.
2. Ethanol, 95%

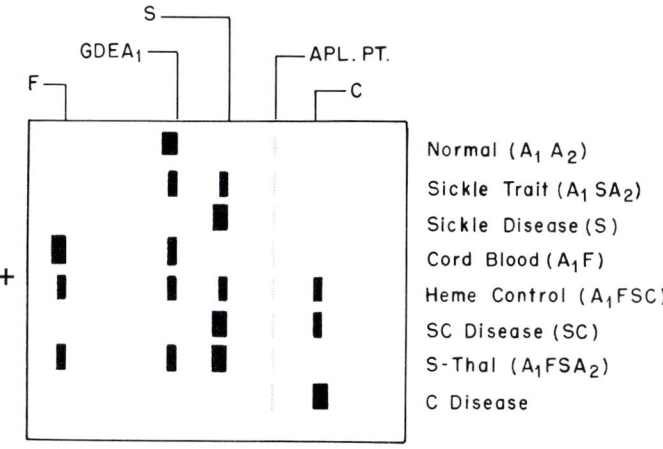

Fig. 4-6. Citrate agar electrophoretic patterns of normal and abnormal hemoglobins. Note separation of Hb D and Hb S and of Hb E and Hb C. *Apl. pt.,* Application point; + indicates anode. Heme Control is manufactured by Helena Laboratories, Beaumont, Tex.

3. Methanol, absolute
4. Erythrosin B, aqueous 0.1%

Procedure: Prepare thin direct or anticoagulated blood smears and allow them to dry for 30 min at room temperature. Insert them into the buffer for 2-3 min at 25° C and agitate gently. Transfer the slides rapidly into ethanol for 10 min. Then wash them in water for 5 sec and methanol for 5 min. Rinse the slides in water and stain them with erythrosin B for 4 min.

Result: Cells containing Hb A stain red; cells containing Hb F appear as ghost cells.

Hemoglobins A$_{Ia}$, A$_{Ib}$, and A$_{Ic}$ (glycosylated hemoglobins)

Using cation exchange resin chromatography Allen et al.[42] demonstrated the heterogeneous nature of Hb A, 90% of which is made of the main heme protein Hb A; the remainder is composed of the minor heme proteins Hb A$_1$ and A$_2$. Hb A$_1$ can be rechromatographed and split into Hb A$_{Ia}$, A$_{Ib}$, and A$_{Ic}$.[42] These components, which have faster chromatographic mobilities than the main band of Hb A, are collectively referred to as fast hemoglobins or as glycosylated hemoglobins, as they have a carbohydrate attached to the β-chain.[43] Hb A$_{Ic}$ has glucose attached, Hb A$_{Ia}$ forms a complex with fructose, and Hb A$_{Ib}$ may have G-6-PD attached. Hb A$_{Ic}$ has been found to be increased twofold in patients with insulin-dependent diabetes mellitus.[44,45] Because acute elevations of the blood sugar level encountered during intravenous glucose therapy do not affect the Hb A$_{Ic}$ level and because the highest levels are demonstrated in diabetics with hyperglycemia of several weeks' duration, it appears that the Hb A$_{Ic}$ elevation in diabetics is truly an expression of the diabetic state.[46] The formation of Hb A$_{Ic}$ represents a postsynthetic nonenzymatic glycosylation of red cells early in their development and remains constant until their

death.[47,48] Each generation of red cells thus reflects the glucose concentration at the time of their hemoglobinization.[49] The concentration of Hb A$_{Ic}$ can thus be used as an index of the adequacy of the long-term control of blood glucose concentration in diabetic patients.[49] A single Hb A$_{Ic}$ determination reflects the duration as well as the level of hyperglycemia[50] in diabetics during the previous 1-2 months, thus providing information not obtainable by single or serial blood sugar determinations, which reflect only moments in time. Raised concentrations of Hb A$_{Ic}$ indicate poor diabetic control.[51]

Clinical studies have reported glycosylated hemoglobins separately as Hb A$_{Ia + Ib}$ and Hb A$_{Ic}$ or collectively as the total "fast hemoglobins" Hb A$_{Ia + Ib + Ic}$. In diabetics the Hb A$_{Ic}$ values correlate well with the values for total glycosylated hemoblobins, and the latter appear to be as informative as Hb A$_{Ic}$ values alone for the assessment of long-term glucose control.[49] Glycosylated hemoglobins are measured by elution from cation-exchange resin columns. The commercially available columns measure total glycosylated hemoglobins rather than Hb A$_{Ic}$ alone. The high-performance liquid chromatography technic[52] for Hb A$_{Ic}$ alone offers optimal sensitivity for Hb A$_{Ic}$ and may ultimately prove to have an advantage over the total fast hemoglobins, but it requires special equipment and the advantage of Hb A$_{Ic}$ over the total fast hemoglobins has not been definitely established.[53]

Glycosylated (fast fraction) hemoglobin Quick column technic

Principle: The Quick column technic utilizes commercially available microcolumns containing negatively charged carboxymethyl cellulose resin (*Helena Laboratories, Beaumont, Tex.), which exhibits an affinity for positively charged molecules.[54] At selected ionic strength and pH the glycosylated hemoglobins are less positively charged than Hb A. Therefore the former components bind to the negatively charged resin less tightly than Hb A. With the application of the first developing buffer the glycosylated hemoglobins are eluted while the other hemoglobin components are retained. With the application of the second developing buffer, the remaining hemoglobins, the majority of which are Hb A, are eluted. Following elution the absorbance of each fraction is read on a spectrophotometer and the glycosylated hemoglobin percentage is calculated.

Results[54]:
Normal fast hemoglobins (Hb A_{1a} + Hb A_{1b} + Hb A_{1c}), 6.9 ± 1.7% of total hemoglobin
Range, 6-8.6% of total hemoglobin
Interpretation: For interpretation see introduction. Diabetic fast hemoglobin values are 8-14% of total hemoglobin.

There are a few conditions that cause falsely elevated or lowered glycosylated hemoglobin levels.[55] Elevated levels have been reported in postsplenectomy patients, in renal dialysis patients, and in individuals with high Hb F values, since Hb F elutes with the fast hemoglobins. The latter group includes neonates and women in the last trimester of pregnancy. Lowered values are found in hemolytic anemias because of the shortened life span of the red cells and in chronic renal failure.

Hemoglobin A_2[34]

Hb A_2 ($\alpha_2\delta_2$) is a minor component of hemoglobin that makes its first appearance close to term and remains at a low concentration (2.5% of total adult hemolysate) throughout adult life. Its exact function is unknown, but it is probably similar to that of Hb A.[56] Its rise and fall in a number of hematologic disorders give its concentration some importance in differential diagnosis.

Methods of quantitation

Quantitation by cellulose acetate electrophoresis followed by densitometry has proved to be inaccurate, since it does not allow clear separation of normal and abnormal values, apparently because of the relatively low concentrations of Hb A_2 and the variable concentration of the hemolysate.[57] Quantitation by electrophoresis[58] followed by elution[59] and quantitative spectrophotometric analysis of the eluate is a satisfactory procedure but requires a fresh sample, consistency in cutting fractions, and adequate time for elution.[60] Column chromatographic technics are preferred at the present time because of their precision[61] and the commerical availability of the equipment and reagents.

Hb A_2 Quick column chromatography utilizing a simplified fast micromethod*

Principle[62]: Hb A_2 is separated by chromatography on a small anion-exchange cellulose column, and the percentage of Hb A_2 is calculated from the absorbance of the eluate at 415 nm. At the pH of the first eluting fluid Hb A_2 is not bound to the cellulose microgranules, in contrast to the other normal and most abnormal he-

moglobins, which are bound and retained and are eluted by the second eluting fluid. The method requires only 1 drop (20 μl) of whole blood collected in EDTA. Hb C, E, and O may be partially eluted with the first eluting fluid and give rise to erroneous Hb A_2 results. The presence of these abnormal hemoglobins should be ascertained by prior hemoglobin electrophoresis.

Technic: The technic is adequately described in the product information.

Rapid batch fractionation method for Hb A_2

Principle: Hb A_2[63] may be determined in the presence of Hb F and Hb S by a batch absorption method on DEAE gel A without electrophoresis or column chromatography. With use of a buffer of carefully controlled pH and chloride content, Hb A_1 and F are absorbed on the gel, but Hb A_2 is not. After separation of the gel the Hb A_2 in the supernatant is measured in a spectrophotometer at 414 nm. The absorbance is compared with that obtained from a dilution of the total hemolysate representing the total hemoglobin present. If Hb S is present, the conditions can be adjusted so that it is absorbed and Hb A_2 can be measured. The method requires careful control of the pH and chloride content of the buffer and special preparation of the hemolysate, but otherwise it is not technically difficult, is accurate, and requires only 5 min.

Quantitation of Hb A_2 by immunodiffusion[64,65]

There is the promise that immunologic tests such as radial immunodiffusion will provide specific assays for a variety of normal and variant hemoglobins as soon as specific antihemoglobin antibiotics are commerically available. In the experimental laboratory, anti-Hb A_2, F, and S antibodies have proved their value in identifying the corresponding antigens in whole blood specimens.

Normal values:
Adult: 1.5-3.5% of total hemoglobin
Cord blood: Less than 1% of total hemoglobin
Interpretation: Increased Hb A_2 values[66] are encountered in β-thalassemia trait, homozygous thalassemia, megaloblastic anemias,[67] unstable hemoglobin variants,[68] malaria, viral hepatitis, Down's syndrome, and rheumatic heart disease. The elevated Hb A_2 concentration of β-thalassemia trait is only one of its diagnostic criteria and should be supported by detailed hematologic and biochemical investigations as outlined in the thalassemia section. The combination of iron deficiency and β-thalassemia trait may depress the Hb A_2 concentration to normal levels. If Hb A_2 is calculated in milligrams per deciliter of whole blood and plotted against MCV values of the peripheral blood, β-thalassemia trait can usually be clearly separated from iron deficiency.[69] The formula for converting percent Hb A_2 into milligrams per deciliter is as follows:

$$\% \text{ (decimal)} \times \text{Hb (g/dl)} \times 1000 = \text{mg/dl}$$

For example, if Hb A_2 is 4% of the total hemoglobin and the total hemoglobin is 16.0 g/dl:

$$0.04 \times 16 \times 1000 = 640 \text{ mg/dl Hb } A_2$$

---

*Helena Laboratories, Beaumont, Tex.

In homozygous β-thalassemia the concentration of Hb A_2 varies from 0-5%, the mean being only slightly higher than the upper limit of normal; it is always lower than the mean Hb A_2 concentration of the β-thalassemia carrier with normal serum iron.[70]

Hb A_2 levels are decreased in cord blood[66]; adult values are not reached until the fifth or sixth month after birth. They are also diminished in severe iron deficiency anemia,[71] sideroblastic anemia,[72] trisomy D, and in α-, δ-, or δ-β-thalassemia.

Hemoglobin F (fetal hemoglobin)

Hb F[73,74] has a globin formula $\alpha_2\gamma_2$ and has been shown to consist of two almost identical fractions, F_1 and F_2.[42,74-76] It is the predominant hemoglobin during fetal life (90-95%, 20% of which is F_1). After about the sixth month of pregnancy the Hb F values slowly decrease to about 80% (60-97%), so that at the time of birth the cord blood contains 70-80% Hb F, 10-15% Hb A, and less than 0.5% Hb A_2. Hb F_1 contains acetylated amino groups on the *N*-terminals of the γ-chains.[77] After birth, Hb F decreases fairly rapidly to about 70% of the total hemoglobin at about 1 month of age, to about 50% at 2 months, and to 25% at 3 months. After 6 months and in the first year of life the blood contains an average value of 2.9% Hb F, in the second year it falls to 1.8%, in the third year it falls to 1.0%, and it finally levels off to the adult level of 0.8% (Fig. 4-7).

Characteristics of hemoglobin F

1. Electrophoretically it is slower than Hb A.
2. It is resistant to alkali denaturation. This feature is the basis of the Singer test for Hb F.[78]
3. It is twice as resistant to acid elution as Hb A. This characteristic behavior of Hb F is the basis of the Kleihauer elution technic.[73]
4. Hb F is oxidized into Met-Hb twice as fast as Hb

A. This fact partially explains the tendency of newborns to form Met-Hb rather readily.
5. Hb F has a relatively high oxygen affinity and a decreased affinity to bind 2,3-DPG.

Demonstration of hemoglobin F

By the commonly used cellulose acetate electrophoretic methods employing alkaline buffer systems, Hb F is difficult to separate from Hb A and thus difficult to quantitate. Furthermore, the densitometric quantitation of large amounts of Hb F as seen in hereditary persistence of Hb F is considered to be inaccurate.[79] A number of specific characteristics of Hb F are used for its detection and quantitation.

Alkali-denaturation procedures
Method of Singer, Chernoff, and Singer[78,80]

Principle: Fetal hemoglobin is more resistant to denaturation by potassium hydroxide than other adult hemoglobins. Under the conditions of the test, potassium hydroxide converts adult hemoglobin to alkaline hematin within a period of 1 min. The denaturation is stopped by the addition of half-saturated ammonium sulfate, which lowers the pH and precipitates the denatured hemoglobin. The method of Singer et al. is adequately described in previous editions of this book, but it is not as accurate as the method of Pembrey over a wide range of values.

Method of Pembrey[81]

Although the determination of fetal hemoglobins by the alkali denaturation method of Singer et al. has been widely used, it is inaccurate for levels of fetal hemoglobin below about 5% and thus is not suitable for the determination of small amounts of Hb F in adults. The following method is also an alkali denaturation method but differs in that the hemolysate is first diluted and the hemoglobin converted to cyanmethemoglobin. The

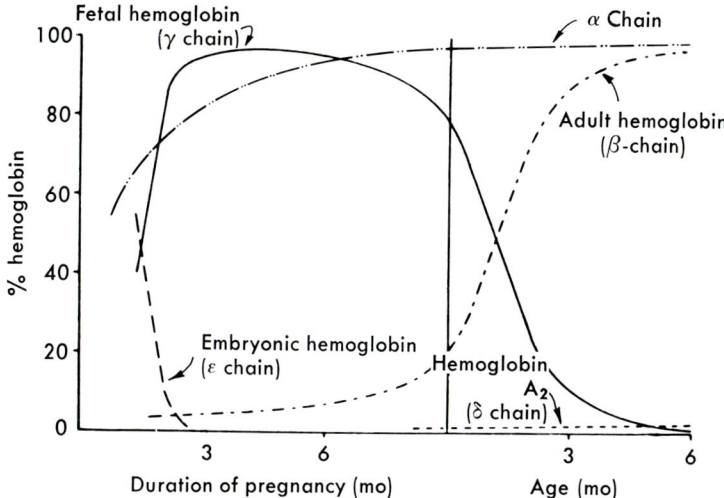

Fig. 4-7. Developmental changes in human hemoglobins. α-Chain synthesis begins well before third month of fetal life and continues into adult life. γ-Chain synthesis replaces embryonic ε-chain at about third month, and at about same time β-chain synthesis begins. (Modified from Huehns, E.R., and Shooter, E.M.: J. Med. Genet. **2:**48, 1965.)

method is accurate for very low levels of Hb F but may also be used for levels up to 50%.

Reagents:

1. Sodium hydroxide, 1.2M. Prepare solution fresh each time by dissolving 4.8 g sodium hydroxide in water to make 1dl, or a 6M solution may be prepared by dissolving 24 g in water to make 1dl. This is stable if kept in a tightly stoppered bottle in the refrigerator. As required, dilute 1 ml of this with 4 ml of water.
2. Drabkin solution. Dissolve 50 mg potassium cyanide and 200 mg potassium ferricyanide in water to make 1 L.
3. Saturated ammonium sulfate. Mix 100 g ammonium sulfate and 1 dl water. Allow to stand for some time with occasional vigorous shaking to saturate the solution. The saturated solution may then be decanted.

Procedure: Prepare a quantity of hemolysate by one of the methods given in the section on abnormal hemoglobins. The hemolysate should contain between 8 and 10 g/dl hemoglobin for accurate results. Dilute 0.6 ml hemolysate with 10 ml Drabkin solution and mix well.

Pipet 5.6 ml diluted hemolysate into a test tube. Rapidly add 0.4 ml 1.2M sodium hydroxide solution, start a stopwatch, and mix at once. Exactly 2 min after the addition of the sodium hydroxide, rapidly pipet in 4.0 ml saturated ammonium sulfate and mix well. Allow the solution to stand for about 15 min and then filter it through a retentive paper (Whatman no. 6 or equivalent). If the first filtrate comes through cloudy, pour it back into the filter. The final filtrate should be perfectly clear.

Also mix 1.4 ml diluted hemolysate, 1.6 ml water, and 2 ml saturated ammonium sulfate. Make a further 1:10 dilution of an aliquot of this mixture. Label this dilution "total hemoglobin."

Calculation: Read the filtrate and total hemoglobin tubes against a water blank at 415 nm. Then calculate as follows:

$$\frac{\text{Absorbance of filtrate}}{\text{Absorbance of total Hb}} \times 5 = \text{Fetal hemoglobin (\%)}$$

The factor of 5 arises as follows: In the fetal hemoglobin filtrate the original diluted hemolysate is diluted 5.6 ml to 10 (5.6 + 0.4 + 4.0) or 1.4 to 2.5. The tube marked "total hemoglobin" is diluted 1.4 to 5 (1.4 + 1.6 + 2) multiplied by an additional 1:10 dilution of 1.4 to 50. The ratio of these dilutions is 2.5:50 or 1:20. Thus 100 (to convert to percent) divided by 20 = 5.

If in the measurement the filtrate reading is too high (as it may be for higher levels of Hb F), make a further dilution of the filtrate and multiply the result obtained by the dilution factor.

Normal values[82]:

Adult: 0.9%
Newborn at birth: 70-90%
1 month: 50-75%
2 months: 25-60%
3 months: 10-35%

6 months: 8%
1 year: 2%

In adult life a few red cell clones continue to produce Hb F, so that occasional red cells contain small quantities of Hb F mixed with Hb A, giving an average ratio of Hb F–containing cells to pure Hb A cells of 1:5000. Pregnancy stimulates the synthesis of maternal Hb F so that the number of Hb F–containing cells increases about 5 times and the maternal Hb F level is raised to about 10-15% of total hemoglobin.[83,84]

Conditions associated with high or low values: There are a great number of neoplastic and nonneoplastic conditions in which Hb F is increased[74,85,86] and only a few in which Hb F is decreased:

1. Conditions associated with high Hb F concentrations
   a. Anemias: Almost all acquired or congenital anemias raise the Hb F production 2-5%. Higher levels (up to 25%) are seen in myelofibrosis (primary or secondary), aplastic anemias (primary or secondary), and paroxysmal nocturnal hemoglobinuria.
   b. Thalassemias: High Hb F values (up to 50% or over) are encountered in β-thalassemia (homozygous) and in hemoglobinopathy-thalassemia interactions. Lesser values (up to 20%) are seen in δ-β-thalassemia.
   c. Hereditary persistence of fetal hemoglobin (HPFH): HPFH is responsible for 100% Hb F in the homozygous form and up to 40% in the heterozygous form.
   d. Hemoglobinopathies: Homozygous Hb S disease and unstable hemoglobins are accompanied by Hb F values up to 20% and 10%, respectively.
   e. Leukemias: The highest values (up to 50%) are encountered in Philadelphia chromosome (Ph[1])–negative juvenile myelocytic leukemia,[87] but any type of leukemia may be responsible for raised concentrations of Hb F.
   f. Endocrinopathies: Endocrinopathies include tumor-induced ectopic secretions[88] and thyrotoxicosis.[89]
   g. Chromosomal abnormalities: trisomy D_1.
2. Conditions associated with relatively low Hb F concentrations
   a. Heterozygous α-thalassemia
   b. Heterozygous β-thalassemia
   c. Down's syndrome (trisomy G_1)[90]

Acid elution technic of Kleihauer for determination of hemoglobin F within red blood cells[73]

Principle: Hemoglobin is precipitated within the red cells by drying and fixation with alcohol. The air-dried and fixed blood films are treated with a citric acid–phosphate buffer of low pH in which adult hemoglobins are soluble. Thus Hb A is dissolved out of the red cells, but Hb F remains precipitated and is stained with eosin or erythrosin.

Reagents:

1. Ethyl alcohol, 80%
2. Citric acid–phosphate buffer, pH 3.2
   a. Stock solution 1 (0.2M Na_2HPO_4). Dissolve

36.5 g disodium phosphate ($Na_2HPO_4 \cdot 2H_2O$) in distilled water and dilute to 1 L.
  b. Stock solution 2 (0.1M citric acid). Dissolve 21.0 g citric acid ($C_6H_8O_7 \cdot H_2O$) in distilled water and dilute to 1 L.
  c. Working solution
    Stock solution 1, 24.7 ml
    Stock solution 2, 75.3 ml
    Measure the pH on a meter and adjust to pH 3.2 if necessary. Before use, warm in a 37° C water bath for 15 min.
3. Alum hematoxylin
4. Erythrosin B or eosin, 0.1% aqueous

All the reagents for the Kleihauer method are commercially available (Simmler & Son, St. Louis).

Procedure: Prepare thin (1-cell–thick) blood films of capillary or fresh (less than 6 hr) EDTA-anticoagulated blood of the patient, of Hb F–negative (adult blood specimen) and Hb F–positive (cord blood specimen) controls, each blood sample diluted 1:1 with saline. If the hematocrit is low, the saline dilution is not necessary.

Air dry the slides and fix them in 80% ethyl alcohol for 5 min. Wash them well in water, the pH of which should be 6.6-7.1. It must not be acid. Immerse the slides in prewarmed working buffer in a Coplin jar in a 37° C water bath for 6 min; during this period move the slides up and down a few times. After elution, wash the slides in water and stain them in hematoxylin for 3 min. Wash and stain them in erythrosin B or eosin B for 3 min. Wash the slides, air dry them, mount them in Permount, and apply a coverslip.

Interpretation: Hb A–containing cells appear as un-

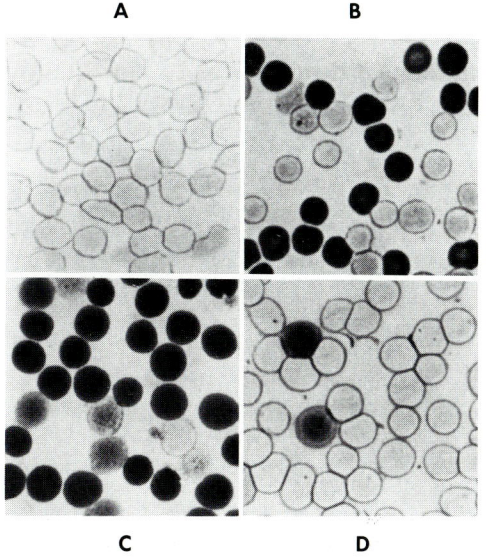

Fig. 4-8. Differentiation of fetal and adult hemoglobin by acid elution method. **A,** Empty "shadows" of adult cells from which hemoglobin has been eluted. **B,** Mixture of adult and fetal cells. Fetal cells are dark because of their acid-resistant Hb F content. **C,** Cord blood (Hb F, 85%). **D,** Blood of 5-month-old infant (Hb F, 25%). (From Kleihauer, E.: Beihefte Arch. Kinderheilkd. 53[suppl.], 1966.)

stained "ghosts," empty shells of red cells, while Hb F–containing cells stain red, the shade and distribution of the pigment depending on the concentration and pattern of distribution of Hb F (Fig. 4-8).

Examine the slides under high dry magnification, counting 500 red cells and expressing the number of Hb F–containing cells as a percent of the total red cell count. It may be necessary to count multiples of 500 cells.

Sensitivity of Kleihauer method[91]: The Kleihauer method is exquisitely sensitive, being able to identify 1 Hb F–containing cell per 1 million adult cells, or about 0.47% Hb F.

4 Hb F–containing cells/1 million adult cells = 1% Hb F
8 Hb F–containing cells/1 million adult cells = 2% Hb F
100 Hb F cells/100 adult cells = 10% Hb F

Difficulties with the Kleihauer stain: Smears obtained from fresh blood give best results; anticoagulated blood allowed to stand overnight may give false positive results. If the hematocrit is high, dilute the blood with normal saline solution in a ratio of 1:2.

As a fixative, 80% alcohol tends to render Hb A and Hb F more resistant to lysis; this effect increases with the fixation time, which should not exceed 5 min.

The pH of the buffer depends on the method of fixation. This interdependence of buffer and fixation is important. If 80% alcohol is used, the pH of the buffer should be 3.1-3.3.

Distribution of hemoglobin F within red cells (Fig. 4-4)

Hb F shows three distribution patterns: both Hb A and Hb F are present in strictly separated cell populations; both hemoglobins are present in equal concentrations in all cells; and both hemoglobins are irregularly distributed within the cells, some cells containing only Hb A, some only Hb F, and some varying amounts of both.

1. Hb A and F present in **strictly separate cell populations:** This distribution pattern is seen in fetal-maternal hemorrhage if the mother's blood is examined or in maternal-fetal hemorrhage if the infant's blood is examined.

In cases of anemia of the newborn or when an Rh-negative or Du-negative women delivers or miscarries (aborts), the mother's blood should be collected immediately after delivery and examined for fetal cells by the Kleihauer method (see discussion of RhoGam, Chapter 18). One vial of RhoGam neutralizes about 30-35 ml Rh-positive blood. The amount of fetal blood that has escaped into the maternal circulation can be roughly calculated using the following formula:

$$\text{ml fetal blood} = \%\text{Hg F cells} \times 50$$

If the fetal blood loss into the maternal circulation exceeds 35 ml blood, more than one vial of RhoGam is required. The efficiency of RhoGam can also be judged by the disappearance of Hb F–containing cells following its administration. If the fetal cells have not disappeared 12-24 hr after the administration of the first dose, more RhoGam is required.

2. **Even distribution** of Hb F and A within red cells:

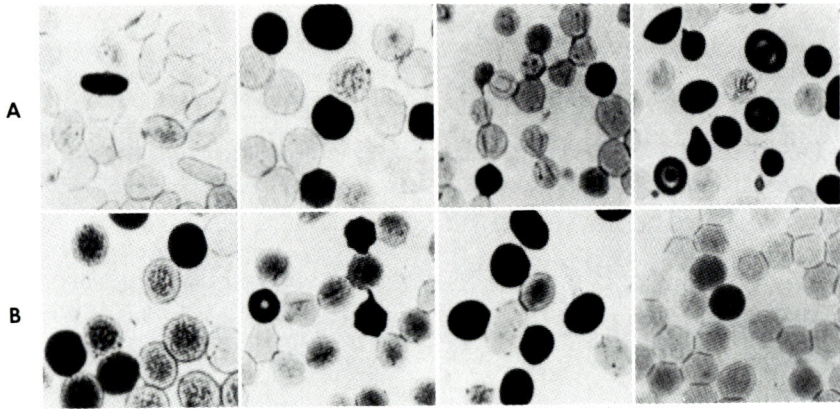

Fig. 4-9. Fetal hemoglobin in various hematologic disorders. **A** (from left to right), Elliptocytosis (Hb F, 1.2%), Fanconi anemia (Hb F, 12.4%), hereditary spherocytosis (Hb F, 0.9%), thalassemia major—after transfusion (Hb F, 30.5%). **B** (from left to right), Paroxysmal nocturnal hemoglobinuria (Hb F, 5.1%), erythroleukemia (Hb F, 2.28%), acute myelocytic leukemia in Down's syndrome in 9-month-old infant (Hb F, 46.6%), and thalassemia minor (Hb F, 1.9%). (From Kleihauer, E.: Beihefte Arch. Kinderheilkd. **53**[suppl.], 1966.)

This picture is seen in hereditary persistence of Hb F (see Chapter 8).

3. **Uneven distribution** of Hb A and Hb F in the red cells: This pattern is seen in thalassemia (minor and major), S-S disease, Fanconi anemias, and hereditary spherocytosis (Fig. 4-9).

The acid elution technic of Kleihauer can be utilized not only for the demonstration of Hb F in red cells but also for the detection of red cell inclusions such as Heinz bodies, which are indicative of unstable hemoglobin variants.[92] The inclusions appear as compact, densely stained structures within ghost cells. Kleihauer considers this method of detection of unstable hemoglobin variants superior to the brilliant cresyl blue technic (which also stains reticulocytes) and to the heat stability and isopropanol tests, the results of which may be equivocal. Small inclusion bodies are also seen in Hb S-S and in G-6-PD deficiency.

Embryonal hemoglobins

Embryonal hemoglobin occurs only in the 1- to 2-month-old embryo and is divided into two components, Gower 1 ($\delta_2\epsilon_2$) and Gower 2 ($\alpha_2\epsilon_2$). It can be demonstrated in blood smears of embryos by the Kleihauer acid elution method by lowering the pH of the buffer to 2.8-2.9 (Fig. 4-10).

LABORATORY DIAGNOSIS OF HEMOGLOBIN VARIANTS (HEMOGLOBINOPATHIES)

Hemoglobinopathies can be defined as congenital (genetic) hereditary disorders of hemoglobin synthesis in which there is a defect in the quality or quantity of the normal polypeptide chains of hemoglobin. They can be divided into two groups: the structural variants of hemoglobin and the thalassemia syndromes.

A current list of hemoglobin variants contains more than 400 entries (Tables 4-2 to 4-9). The molecular abnormalities responsible for the formation of mutant hemoglobins may affect any of the adult hemoglobin

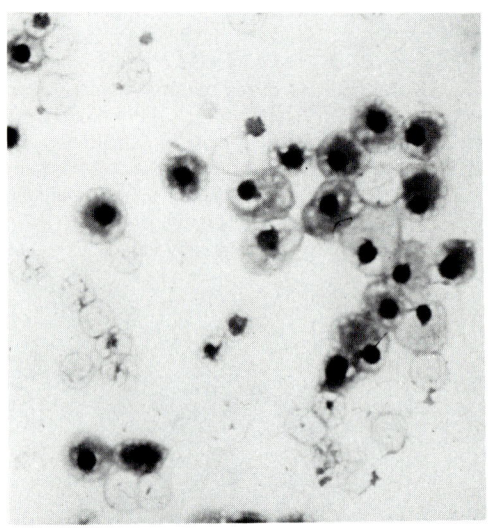

Fig. 4-10. Demonstration of embryonal hemoglobin in embryonal megalocytes and megaloblasts (nucleated cells) by modified (pH 2.8) Kleihauer method. (Courtesy Prof. Dr. E. Kleihauer.)

chains (α, β, γ, and δ) and are classified as follows:

1. The most common mutation is the substitution of one amino acid for another as in Hb S (glu → val) (Fig. 4-11).
2. Rarely there is more than one substitution in the same polypeptide chain as in Hb C Harlem (glu → val and asp → asn).
3. More common is the deletion of one or more amino acids as in Hb Leider (glu is deleted).
4. Other changes include the fusion of hemoglobins as in Hb Lepore (δ-β).
5. The extension of chains occurs, as in Hb Constant Spring (31 additional residues).

Text continued on p. 66.

Table 4-2. Variants of the α-chain

Residue	Substitution	Name	Major abnormal property	Reference no.*
1(NA1)	Val			
2(NA2)	Leu			
3(A1)	Ser			
4(A2)	Pro			
5(A3)	Ala→Asp	Hb J Toronto		1
6(A4)	Asp→Ala	Hb Sawara	↑ O₂ affinity	2,3
	Asp→Asn	Hb Dunn		418
7(A5)	Lys			
8(A6)	Thr			
9(A7)	Asn			
10(A8)	Val			
11(A9)	Lys→Glu	Hb Anantharaj		4
12(A10)	Ala→Asp	Hb J Paris-I		5
		J Aljezur		6
13(A11)	Ala			
14(A12)	Trp			
15(A13)	Gly→Asp	Hb I Interlaken		7
		J Oxford		8
		N Cosenza		9
	Gly→Arg	Hb Ottawa		10
		Siam		11
16(A14)	Lys→Glu	Hb I,		12
		I Philadelphia		13
		I Texas		14
		I Burlington		15
		I Skamania		16
17(A15)	Val			
18(A16)	Gly→Arg	Hb Handsworth		17
19(AB1)	Ala→Asp	Hb J Kurosh		18
20(B1)	His			
21(B2)	Ala→Asp	Hb J Nyanza		19
22(B3)	Gly→Asp	Hb J Medellin		20
23(B4)	Glu→Gln	Hb Memphis		21
	Glu→Lys	Hb Chad		22
	Glu→Val	Hb G Audhali		23
24(B5)	Tyr			
25(B6)	Gly			
26(B7)	Ala			
27(B8)	Glu→Gly	Hb Fort Worth		24
27(B8)	Glu→Val	Hb Spanish Town		25
28(B9)	Ala			
29(B10)	Leu			
30(B11)	Glu→Lys	Hb O Padova		26
	Glu→Gln	Hb G Honolulu		27
		G Singapore		28
		G Chinese		29
		G Hong Kong		29
31(B12)	Arg→Ser	Hb Prato		412
32(B13)	Met			
33(B14)	Phe			
34(B15)	Leu			
35(B16)	Ser			
36(C1)	Phe			
37(C2)	Pro			
38(C3)	Thr			
39(C4)	Thr			
40(C5)	Lys			
41(C6)	Thr			

Courtesy Ruth N. Wrightstone, International Hemoglobin Information Center, Medical College of Georgia, Augusta, Ga., 1979.
*See original list for references.

Continued.

Table 4-2. Variants of the α-chain—cont'd

Residue	Substitution	Name	Major abnormal property	Reference no.*
42(C7)	Tyr			
43(CE1)	Phe→Val	Hb Torino	Unstable, ↓ O₂ affinity	30
	Phe→Leu	Hb Hirosaki		31
44(CE2)	Pro			
45(CE3)	His→Arg	Hb Fort de France	↑ O₂ affinity	32
46(CE4)	Phe			
47(CE5)	Asp→Gly	Hb Umi		33
		Kokura,		33
		Michigan-I		
		Michigan-II		
		Yukuhashi-II		33
		L Gaslini		
		Tagawa-II		33,34
		Beilinson		35
		Mugino		33
	Asp→His	Hb Hasharon	Unstable	36
		Sinai		37
		Sealy		38
		L Ferrara		39,40
	Asp→Asn	Hb Arya	Sl. unstable	41
48(CE6)	Leu→Arg	Hb Montgomery		42
49(CE7)	Ser			
50(CE8)	His→Asp	Hb J Sardegna		43
51(CE9)	Gly→Asp	Hb J Abidjan		44
	Gly→Arg	Hb Russ		45
52(E1)	Ser			
53(E2)	Ala→Asp	Hb J Rovigo	Unstable	46
54(E3)	Gln→Arg	Hb Shimonoseki		47
		Hikoshima		
	Gln→Glu	Hb Mexico		48
		Hb J		48
		J Paris-II		49
		Uppsala		50
55(E4)	Val			
56(E5)	Lys→Thr	Hb Thailand		51
57(E6)	Gly→Arg	Hb L Persian Gulf		52
	Gly→Asp	Hb J Norfolk		53
		Kagoshima		54
		Nishik-I, II, III		55
58(E7)	His→Tyr	Hb M Boston	↓ O₂ affinity	56
		M Osaka		57
		Gothenburg		58
		M Kiskunhalas		59
59(E8)	Gly			
60(E9)	Lys→Asn	Hb Zambia		60
61(E10)	Lys→Asn	Hb J Buda		61
62(E11)	Val			
63(E12)	Ala→Asp	Hb Pontoise		62
64(E13)	Asp→Asn	Hb G Waimanalo		63
		Aida		64
	Asp→His	Hb Q India		65
	Asp→Tyr	Hb Perspolis		18
65(E14)	Ala			
66(E15)	Leu			
67(E16)	Thr			
68(E17)	Asn→Asp	Hb Ube-2		66
	Asn→Lys	Hb G-Philadelphia		67
		G Knoxville-1		68
		Stanleyville-I		69
		D Washington		68
		D St. Louis		70
		G Bristol		71
		G Azakuoli		68
		D Baltimore		68

Table 4-2. Variants of the α-chain—cont'd

Residue	Substitution	Name	Major abnormal property	Reference no.*
69(E18)	Ala			
70(E19)	Val			
71(E20)	Ala→Glu	Hb J Habana		72
72(EF1)	His→Arg	Hb Daneskgah-Tehran		73
73(EF2)	Val			
74(EF3)	Asp→His	Hb Mahidol		74
		G Taichung		75
		Q Thailand		76
	Asp→Asn	Hb G Pest		61
	Asp→Gly	Hb Chapel Hill		77
75(EF4)	Asp→His	Hb Q Iran		76
	Asp→Tyr	Hb Winnipeg		78
	Asp→Asn	Hb Matsue-Oki		79
76(EF5)	Met			
77(EF6)	Pro			
78(EF7)	Asn→Lys	Hb Stanleyville-II		80
79(EF8)	Ala			
80(F1)	Leu→Arg	Hb Ann Arbor	Unstable	81,82
81(F2)	Ser→Cys	Hb Nigeria		413
82(F3)	Ala→Asp	Hb Garden State		83
83(F4)	Leu			
84(F5)	Ser→Arg	Hb Etobicoke	↑ O_2 affinity	84,85
85(F6)	Asp→Asn	Hb G Norfolk	(?) ↑ O_2 affinity	86,87
	Asp→Tyr	Hb Atago		88
	Asp→Val	Hb Inkster		89
86(F7)	Leu→Arg	Hb Moabit	Unstable, ↓ O_2 affinity	416
87(F8)	His→Tyr	Hb M Iwate	Ferri-Hb, ↓ O_2 affinity	90
		M Kankakee		91
		M Oldenburg		92
88(F9)	Ala			
89(FG1)	His			
90(FG2)	Lys→Asn	Hb J Broussais		93,94,95
		Tagawa-I		55
	Lys→Thr	Hb J Rajappen		96
91(FG3)	Leu→Pro	Hb Port Phillip	Unstable	97
92(FG4)	Arg→Gln	Hb J Cape Town	↑ O_2 affinity	98,99
	Arg→Leu	Hb Chesapeake	↑ O_2 affinity	100,101
93(FG5)	Val			
94(G1)	Asp→Tyr	Hb Setif	Unstable	102
	Asp→Asn	Hb Titusville	↓ O_2 affinity, ↑ dissociation	103
95(G2)	Pro→Leu	Hb G Georgia	↑ dissociation, ↑ O_2 affinity	104
	Asp→His	Hb Sunshine Seth		419
	Pro→Ser	Hb Rampa	↑ dissociation, ↑ O_2 affinity	105,106
	Pro→Ala	Hb Denmark Hill	↑ O_2 affinity	107
	Pro→Arg	Hb St. Lukes	↑ dissociation	108
96(G3)	Val			
97(G4)	Asn			
98(G5)	Phe			
99(G6)	Lys			
100(G7)	Leu			
101(G8)	Leu			
102(G9)	Ser→Arg	Hb Manitoba	Sl. unstable	109
103(G10)	His			
104(G11)	Cys			
105(G12)	Leu			
106(G13)	Leu			
107(G14)	Val			
108(G15)	Thr			
109(G16)	Leu			
110(G17)	Ala			

Continued.

Table 4-2. Variants of the α-chain—cont'd

Residue	Substitution	Name	Major abnormal property	Reference no.*
111(G18)	Ala			
112(G19)	His→Asp	Hb Hopkins-II	Unstable, ↑ O_2 affinity	110,118
	His→Arg	Hb Strumica		111
		Serbia		112
113(GH1)	Leu			
114(GH2)	Pro→Arg	Hb Chiapas		48
115(GH3)	Ala→Asp	Hb J Tongariki		113
116(GH4)	Glu→Lys	Hb O Indonesia		114
		Buginese-X		115
		Oliviere		116
	Glu→Ala	Hb Ube-4		117
117(GH5)	Phe			
118(H1)	Thr			
119(H2)	Pro			
120(H3)	Ala→Glu	Hb J Meerut		119
		J Birmingham		120
121(H4)	Val			
122(H5)	His			
123(H6)	Ala			
124(H7)	Ser			
125(H8)	Leu			
126(H9)	Asp→Asn	Hb Tarrant	↑ O_2 affinity	121
127(H10)	Lys→Thr	Hb St. Claude		122
	Lys→Asn	Hb Jackson		123
128(H11)	Phe			
129(H12)	Leu			
130(H13)	Ala			
131(H14)	Ser			
132(H15)	Val			
133(H16)	Ser			
134(H17)	Thr			
135(H18)	Val			
136(H19)	Leu→Pro	Hb Bibba	Unstable, ↑ dissociation	124
137(H20)	Thr			
138(H21)	Ser			
139(HC1)	Lys			
140(HC2)	Tyr			
141(HC3)	Arg→Pro	Hb Singapore		125
	Arg→His	Hb Suresnes	↑ O_2 affinity	126
	Arg→Ser	Hb J Cubujuqui		127
	Arg→Leu	Hb Legnano	↑ O_2 affinity	128
	Arg→Gly	Hb J Camagüey		129

Table 4-3. Variants of the β-chain

Residue	Substitution	Name	Major abnormal property	Reference no.*
1(NA1)	Val→Ac-Ala	Hb Raleigh	↓ O$_2$ affinity, ↓ dissociation	130
2(NA2)	His→Arg	Hb Deer Lodge		131
3(NA3)	Leu			
4(A1)	Thr			
5(A2)	Pro			
6(A3)	Glu→Val	Hb S	Sickling	132
	Glu→Lys	Hb C		133
	Glu→Ala	Hb G Makassar		134
7(A4)	Glu→Gly	Hb G San José		135
	Glu→Lys	Hb Siriraj		136
8(A5)	Lys			
9(A6)	Ser→Cys	Hb Pôrto Alegre	Polymerization, ↑ O$_2$ affinity, ↓ heme-heme	137
10(A7)	Ala→Asp	Hb Ankara		138
11(A8)	Val			
12(A9)	Thr			
13(A10)	Ala			
14(A11)	Leu→Arg	Hb Sögn		139
	Leu→Pro	Hb Saki	Unstable	140,141
15(A12)	Trp→Arg	Hb Belfast	Unstable, ↑ O$_2$ affinity	142,143
16(A13)	Gly→Asp	Hb J Baltimore		144
		J Trinidad		145
		J Ireland		145
		N New Haven		146
		J Georgia		147
	Gly→Arg	Hb D Buchman		148
17(A14)	Lys→Glu	Hb Nagasaki		149
18(A15)	Val			
19(B1)	Asn→Lys	Hb D Ouled Rabah		150
	Asn→Asp	Hb Alamo		151
20(B2)	Val→Met	Hb Olympia	↑ O$_2$ affinity	152
21(B3)	Asp			
22(B4)	Glu→Lys	Hb E Saskatoon		153
	Glu→Gly	Hb G Taipei		154
	Glu→Ala	Hb G Saskatoon		155
		Hsin Chu		156
		G Coushatta		157
		G Taegu		158
	Glu→Gln	Hb D Iran		159
23(B5)	Val→Asp	Hb Strasbourg		160,161
24(B6)	Gly→Arg	Hb Riverdale-Bronx	Unstable	162
	Gly→Val	Hb Savannah	Unstable	163
	Gly→Asp	Hb Moscva	Unstable, ↓ O$_2$ affinity	164
25(B7)	Gly→Arg	Hb G Taiwan Ami		165
26(B8)	Glu→Lys	Hb E		166
	Glu→Val	Hb Henri Mondor	Unstable (slight)	167
27(B9)	Ala→Asp	Hb Volga	Unstable	168
		Drenthe		169
28(B10)	Leu→Gln	Hb St. Louis	Unstable, ferri-Hb, ↑ O$_2$ affinity	170,171
	Leu→Pro	Hb Genova	Unstable, ↑ O$_2$ affinity	172

Courtesy Ruth N. Wrightstone, International Hemoglobin Information Center, Medical College of Georgia, Augusta, Ga., 1979.
*See original list for references.

Continued.

Table 4-3. Variants of the β-chain—cont'd

Residue	Substitution	Name	Major abnormal property	Reference no.*
29(B11)	Gly→Asp	Hb Lufkin		
30(B12)	Arg→Ser	Hb Tacoma	Unstable, ↓ Bohr and heme-heme, normal O₂ affinity	174
31(B13)	Leu			
32(B14)	Leu→Pro	Hb Perth	Unstable	175
		Abraham Lincoln		176
	Leu→Arg	Hb Castilla	Unstable	177
33(B15)	Val			
34(B16)	Val			
35(C1)	Tyr→Phe	Hb Philly	Unstable, ↑ O₂ affinity	178
36(C2)	Pro			
37(C3)	Trp→Ser	Hb Hirose	↑ O₂ affinity	179
	Trp→Arg	Hb Rothchild		180
38(C4)	Thr			
39(C5)	Gln→Lys	Hb Alabama		181
	Gln→Glu	Hb Vaasa		182
40(C6)	Arg→Lys	Hb Athens-Ga	↑ O₂ affinity	183
		Waco		184
	Arg→Ser	Hb Austin	↑ O₂ affinity, ↑ dissociation	184
41(C7)	Phe→Tyr	Hb Mequon		185
42(CD1)	Phe→Ser	Hb Hammersmith	Unstable,	186
		Chiba	↓ O₂ affinity	187
	Phe→Leu	Hb Louisville	Unstable,	188
		Bucuresti	↓ O₂ affinity	189
43(CD2)	Glu→Ala	Hb G Galveston		190
		G Port Arthur		190
		G Texas		190
	Glu→Gln	Hb Hoshida		420
44(CD3)	Ser			
45(CD4)	Phe			
46(CD5)	Gly→Glu	Hb K Ibadan		191
47(CD6)	Asp→Asn	Hb G Copenhagen		192
	Asp→Gly	Hb Gavello		193
	Asp→Ala	Hb Avicenna		421
48(CD7)	Leu→Arg	Hb Okaloosa	Unstable, ↓ O₂ affinity	194
49(CD8)	Ser			
50(D1)	Thr→Lys	Hb Edmonton		195
51(D2)	Pro→Arg	Hb Willamette	↑ O₂ affinity	196
52(D3)	Asp→Asn	Hb Osu Christiansborg		197
	Asp→Ala	Hb Ocho Rios		198
53(D4)	Ala			
54(D5)	Val			
55(D6)	Met			
56(D7)	Gly→Asp	Hb J Bangkok		199
		J Meinung		200
		J Korat		200
		J Manado		201
	Gly→Arg	Hb Hamadan		202
57(E1)	Asn→Lys	Hb G Ferrara	Unstable	203
58(E2)	Pro→Arg	Hb Yukuhashi		55
		Dhofar		204
59(E3)	Lys→Glu	Hb I High Wycombe		205
	Lys→Thr	Hb J Kaohsiung,		206
		J Honolulu		207
	Lys→Asn	Hb J Lome		208
60(E4)	Val→Leu	Hb Yatsushiro		209
61(E5)	Lys→Glu	Hb N Seattle		210
	Lys→Asn	Hb Hikari		211

Table 4-3. Variants of the β-chain—cont'd

Residue	Substitution	Name	Major abnormal property	Reference no.*
62(E6)	Ala→Pro	Hb Duarte	Unstable, ↑ O₂ affinity	212
63(E7)	His→Arg	Hb Zürich	Unstable, ↑ O₂ affinity	213
63(E7)	His→Tyr	Hb M Saskatoon	Ferri-Hb, ↑ O₂ affinity	214
		M Emory		214
		M Kurume		215
		M Hida		
		M Radom		216
		M Arhus		217
		M Chicago		218
		Leipzig		219
		Hörlein-Weber		220
		Novi Sad		221
		M Erlangen		222
	His→Pro	Hb Bicêtre	Unstable, autoxidizing	223
64(E8)	Gly→Asp	Hb J Calabria	Unstable	224
		J Bari		
		J Cosenza		
65(E9)	Lys→Asn	Hb J Sicilia		225
	Lys→Gln	Hb J Cairo		226
66(E10)	Lys→Glu	Hb I Toulouse	Unstable, ferri-Hb	227
67(E11)	Val→Asp	Hb Bristol	Unstable	228
	Val→Glu	Hb M Milwaukee-I	Ferri-Hb, ↓ O₂ affinity	214
	Val→Ala	Hb Sydney	Unstable	229
68(E12)	Leu→Pro	Hb Mizuho	Unstable	230
69(E13)	Gly→Asp	Hb J Cambridge		192
		J Rambam		231
70(E14)	Ala→Asp	Hb Seattle	↓ O₂ affinity	232
71(E15)	Phe→Ser	Hb Christchurch	Unstable	233
72(E16)	Ser			
73(E17)	Asp→Tyr	Hb Vancouver	↓ O₂ affinity	234
	Asp→Asn	Hb Korle Bu		235
		G Accra		236
	Asp→Val	Hb Mobile	↓ O₂ affinity	237
74(E18)	Gly→Val	Hb Bushwich		238
	Gly→Asp	Hb Shepherds Bush	Unstable, ↑ O₂ affinity	239
75(E19)	Leu→Pro	Hb Atlanta	Unstable	240
76(E20)	Ala→Asp	Hb J Chicago		241
77(EF1)	His→Asp	Hb J Iran		242
78(EF2)	Leu			
79(EF3)	Asp→Gly	Hb G Hsi-Tsou	↑ O₂ affinity	243,244
80(EF4)	Asn→Lys	Hb G Szuhu		245
		Gifu		246
81(EF5)	Leu→Arg	Hb Baylor	↑ O₂ affinity, unstable	247
82(EF6)	Lys→Asn→Asp	Hb Providence	↓ O₂ affinity	248,249
	Lys→Thr	Hb Rahere	↑ O₂ affinity	250
	Lys→Met	Hb Helsinki	↑ O₂ affinity	251
83(EF7)	Gly→Cys	Hb Ta-li		252
	Gly→Asp	Hb Pyrogos		253,254
84(EF8)	Thr			
85(F1)	Phe→Ser	Hb Bryn Mawr	Unstable, ↑ O₂ affinity	255
		Buenos Aires		256
86(F2)	Ala			
87(F3)	Thr→Lys	Hb D Ibadan		257
88(F4)	Leu→Arg	Hb Böras	Unstable	258
	Leu→Pro	Hb Santa Ana	Unstable	259
89(F5)	Ser→Asn	Hb Creteil	↑ O₂ affinity	260
	Ser→Arg	Hb Vanderbilt		261

Continued.

Table 4-3. Variants of the β-chain—cont'd

Residue	Substitution	Name	Major abnormal property	Reference no.*
90(F6)	Glu→Lys	Hb Agenogi	↓ O₂ affinity	262
91(F7)	Leu→Pro	Hb Sabine	Unstable	263
	Leu→Arg	Hb Carribean	Unstable, ↓ O₂ affinity	264
92(F8)	His→Tyr	Hb M Hyde Park M Akita	Normal O₂ affinity, ferri-Hb	265 266
	His→Gln	Hb St. Etienne Istanbul	Unstable, ↑ O₂ affinity, ↑ dissociation	267 268
	His→Asp	Hb J Altgeld Gardens	Normal O₂ affinity	269
	His→Pro	Hb Newcastle		270
93(F9)	Cys			
94(FG1)	Asp			
95(FG2)	Lys→Glu	Hb N Baltimore Hopkins-I Jenkins, N Memphis Kenwood		271 272 273 274 275
	Lys→Asn	Hb Detroit		415
96(FG3)	Leu			
97(FG4)	His→Gln	Hb Malmö	↑ O₂ affinity	276
	His→Leu	Hb Wood	↑ O₂ affinity	277,278
98(FG5)	Val→Met	Hb Köln, San Francisco (Pacific) Ube I	Unstable, ↑ O₂ affinity	279 280 281
	Val→Gly	Hb Nottingham	Unstable, ↑ O₂ affinity	282
	Val→Ala	Hb Djelfa	Unstable, ↑ O₂ affinity	283
99(G1)	Asp→Asn	Hb Kempsey	↑ O₂ affinity	284
	Asp→His	Hb Yakima	↑ O₂ affinity	285
	Asp→Ala	Hb Radcliffe	↑ O₂ affinity	286
	Asp→Tyr	Hb Ypsilanti	↑ O₂ affinity	287
100(G2)	Pro→Leu	Hb Brigham	↑ O₂ affinity	288
101(G3)	Glu→Lys	Hb British Columbia	↑ O₂ affinity	289
	Glu→Gln	Hb Rush	Unstable	290
	Glu→Gly	Hb Alberta	↑ O₂ affinity	291
	Glu→Asp	Hb Potomac	↑ O₂ affinity	292
102(G4)	Asn→Lys	Hb Richmond	Asymmetric hybrids	293
	Asn→Thr	Hb Kansas	↓ O₂ affinity, ↑ dissociation	294
	Asn→Ser	Hb Beth Israel	↓ O₂ affinity	295
103(G3)	Phe→Leu	Hb Heathrow	↑ O₂ affinity	296
104(G6)	Arg→Ser	Hb Camperdown	Slightly unstable	297
	Arg→Thr	Hb Sherwood Forest		298
105(G7)	Leu			
106(G8)	Leu→Pro	Hb Southampton Hb Casper	↑ O₂ affinity Unstable	299 300
	Leu→Gln	Hb Tübingen	Unstable, ↑ O₂ affinity	301,302
107(G9)	Gly→Arg	Hb Burke	↓ O₂ affinity	303
108(G10)	Asn→Asp	Hb Yoshizuka	↓ O₂ affinity	304
108(G10)	Asn→Lys	Hb Presbyterian	↓ O₂ affinity	350
109(G11)	Val→Met	Hb San Diego	↑ O₂ affinity	305
110(G12)	Leu			
111(G13)	Val→Phe	Hb Peterborough	Unstable, ↓ O₂ affinity	306

Table 4-3. Variants of the β-chain—cont'd

Residue	Substitution	Name	Major abnormal property	Reference no.*
112(G14)	Cys→Arg	Hb Indianapolis	Very unstable	307
113(G15)	Val→Glu	Hb New York		308
114(G16)	Leu			
115(G17)	Ala→Pro	Hb Madrid	Unstable	309
116(G18)	His			
117(G19)	His→Arg	Hb P Galveston		310
118(GH1)	Phe			
119(GH2)	Gly→Asp	Hb Fannin-Lubbock	Unstable (slightly)	311,312
120(GH3)	Lys→Glu	Hb Hijiyama		313
	Lys→Asn	Hb Riyadh		314
		Karatsu		315
121(GH4)	Glu→Gln	Hb D Los Angeles	↑ O$_2$ affinity	316
		D Punjab		317,318
		D North Carolina		319
		D Portugal		320
		Oak Ridge		321
		D Chicago		322
	Glu→Lys	Hb O Arab		323
		Egypt		324
	Glu→Val	Hb Beograd		325
122(GH5)	Phe			
123(H1)	Thr			
124(H2)	Pro→Arg	Hb Khartoum	Unstable	326
	Pro→Gln	Hb Ty Gard	↑ O$_2$ affinity	414
125(H3)	Pro			
126(H4)	Val→Glu	Hb Hofu		327
127(H5)	Gln→Glu	Hb Hacettepe		328
128(H6)	Ala→Asp	Hb J Guantanamo	Unstable	329
129(H7)	Ala→Asp	Hb J Taichung		330
	Ala→Glu or Asp	Hb K Cameroon		191
	Ala→Pro	Hb Crete		424
130(H8)	Tyr→Asp	Hb Wien	Unstable	331
131(H9)	Gln→Glu	Hb Camden		332
		Tokuchi		333
132(H10)	Lys→Gln	Hb K Woolwich		191
133(H11)	Val			
134(H12)	Val→Glu	Hb North Shore	Unstable	334,335
135(H13)	Ala→Pro	Hb Altdorf	Unstable, ↑ O$_2$ affinity	336
136(H14)	Gly→Asp	Hb Hope	Unstable	337
137(H15)	Val			
138(H16)	Ala			
139(H17)	Asn			
140(H18)	Ala			
141(H19)	Leu→Arg	Hb Olmsted		276
142(H20)	Ala			
143(H21)	His→Arg	Hb Abruzzo	↑ O$_2$ affinity	338
	His→Gln	Hb Little Rock	↑ O$_2$ affinity	339
	His→Pro	Hb Syracuse	↑ O$_2$ affinity	340
144(HC1)	Lys→Asn	Hb Andrew-Minneapolis	↑ O$_2$ affinity	341
145(HC2)	Tyr→His	Hb Bethesda	↑ O$_2$ affinity	342
	Tyr→Cys	Hb Rainier	↑ O$_2$ affinity, alkali resistant	342
	Tyr→Asp	Hb Fort Gordon	↑ O$_2$ affinity	343
		Osler		344
		Nancy		345
	Tyr→Term	Hb Mckees Rocks	↑ ↑ O$_2$ affinity	346
146(HC3)	His→Asp	Hb Hiroshima	↑ O$_2$ affinity	347
	His→Pro	Hb York	↑ O$_2$ affinity	348
	His→Arg	Hb Cochin-Port	Normal oxygen	349
		Royal	affinity	

Table 4-4. Variants of the δ-chain

Residue	Substitution	Name	Reference no.*
2(NA2)	His→Arg	Hb A₂ Sphakiá	351
12(A9)	Asn→Lys	Hb A₂ NYU	352
16(A13)	Gly→Arg	Hb A₂' (B₂)	353
20(B2)	Val→Glu	Hb A₂ Roosevelt	354
22(B4)	Ala→Glu	Hb A₂ Flatbush	355
43(CD2)	Glu→Lys	Hb A₂ Melbourne	356
51(D2)	Pro→Arg	Hb A₂ Adria	357
69(E13)	Gly→Arg	Hb A₂ Indonesia	358
116(G18)	Arg→His	Hb A₂ Coburg	359
136(H14)	Gly→Asp	Hb A₂ Babinga	360

Courtesy Ruth N. Wrightstone, International Hemoglobin Information Center, Medical College of Georgia, Augusta, Ga., 1979.
*See original list for references.

Table 4-5. Variants of the γ-chain

Residue	Substitution	Name	Reference no.*
1(NA1)	Gly→Cys (136gly)	Hb F Malaysia	361
5(A2)	Glu→Lys (136ala)	Hb F Texas-I	362,363
6(A3)	Glu→Lys	Hb F Texas-II	364
7(A4)	Asp→Asn (136gly)	Hb F Auckland	365
12(A9)	Thr→Lys	Hb Alexandra	366
16(A13)	Gly→Arg (136gly)	Hb F Melbourne	367
22(B4)	Asp→Gly (136ala)	Hb F Kuala Lumpur	368
61(E5)	Lys→Glu (136ala)	Hb F Jamaica	369
80(EF4)	Asp→Tyr (136ala)	Hb F Victoria Jubilee	370
7(FG4)	His→Arg (136ala)	Hb F Dickinson	371
108(G10)	Asn→Lys	Hb F Ube	423
117(G19)	His→Arg (136gly)	Hb F Malta-I	372
121(GH4)	Glu→Lys (136ala)	Hb F Hull	373
121(GH4)	Glu→Lys (136gly)	Hb F Carlton	367
125(H3)	Glu→Ala (136gly)	Hb F Port Royal	374
130(H8)	Trp→Gly (136gly)	Hb F Poole	375

Courtesy Ruth N. Wrightstone, International Hemoglobin Information Center, Medical College of Georgia, Augusta, Ga., 1979.
*See original list for references.

Table 4-6. Fusion hemoglobins

	A6 9	A9 12	B4 22	D1 50	F2 86	F3 87	G18 116	G19 117	H2 124	H4 126	
δ-Chain:	Thr	Asn	Ala	Ser	Ser	Gln	Arg	Asn	Gln	Met	
β-Chain:	Ser	Thr	Glu	Thr	Ala	Thr	His	His	Pro	Val	Reference no.*
Lepore-Hollandia			δ	β							376
Lepore-Baltimore				δ	β						377
Lepore-Washington-Boston					δ	β					378
Miyada		β	δ								399
P Congo			β				δ				379
P Nilotic			β	δ							380

	NA1 1	EF4 80	EF5 81	F2 86	F3 87	HC3 146	
γ-Chain:	Gly	Asp	Leu	Ala	Gln	His	
β-Chain:	Val	Asn	Leu	Ala	Thr	His	Reference no.*
Kenya			γ	β			381

Courtesy Ruth N. Wrightstone, International Hemoglobin Information Center, Medical College of Georgia, Augusta, Ga., 1979.
*See original list for references.

Table 4-7. Deleted residues

Residue	Substitution	Name	Major abnormal property	Reference no.*
β6 or 7	Glu → O	Hb Leiden	Unstable, sl. ↑ O_2 affinity	393
β17-18	(Lys-Val)→O	Hb Lyon	↑ O_2 affinity	394
β23	Val → O	Hb Freiburg	↑ O_2 affinity	395
β42-44 or 43-45	(Phe-Glu-Ser)→O or (Glu-Ser-Phe)→O	Hb Niteroi	↓ O_2 affinity, unstable	396
β56-59	(Gly-Asn-Pro-Lys)→O	Hb Tochigi	Unstable, O_2 affinity not known	397
β74-75	(Gly-Leu)→O	Hb St. Antoine	Unstable, normal O_2 affinity	398
β87	Thr → O	Hb Tours	↑ O_2 affinity, unstable	398
β91-95	(Leu-His-Cys Asp-Lys)→O	Hb Gun Hill	Unstable, ↑ O_2 affinity	400
β131	Gln → O	Hb Leslie, Deaconess	Unstable, normal O_2 affinity	401,402,403
β141	Leu → O	Hb Coventry		404

Courtesy Ruth N. Wrightstone, International Hemoglobin Information Center, Medical College of Georgia, Augusta, Ga., 1979.
*See original list for references.

Table 4-8. Extended chains

Residue	Name	Major abnormal property	Reference no.*
α141 — 31 additional residues: Tyr-Arg-Gln-Ala-Gly-Ala-Ser-Val-Ala- [140] Val-Pro-Pro-Ala-Arg-Trp-Ala-Ser-Gln-Arg-Ala-Leu-Leu-Pro- [150,160] Ser-Leu-His-Arg-Pro-Phe-Leu-Val-Phe-Glu [170]	Hb Constant Spring		382,411
α141 — 31 additional residues: identical to Hb Constant Spring except for residue 142, which is lysine instead of glutamine	Hb Icaria		383
α141 — 16 or 17 additional residues: Tyr-Arg (Ser,Ala,Gly,Ala,Ser, [140] Val,Ala,Val,Pro,Pro,Ala)-Arg(?,Ala,Ser,Gln)-Arg-COOH [150]	Hb Koya Dora		384
β146 — 11 additional residues: Thr-Lys-Leu-Ala-Phe-Leu-Leu-Ser-Asn- [150] Phe-Tyr	Hb Tak	↑ O_2 affinity	385,386,387
α139-141 — Thr-Ser-Asn-Thr-Val-Lys-Leu-Glu-Pro-Arg (Frameshift) [140]	Hb Wayne		388
β145 — Lys-Ser-Ile-Thr-Lys-Leu-Ala-Phe-Leu-Leu-Ser-Asn-Phe-Tyr- [144,150,155] COOH	Hb Cranston	Unstable	389
α115-118 — Ala-Glu-Phe-Thr-*Glu-Phe-Thr*-Pro (insertion) [115 116 117 118 119]	Hb Grady, Dakar		390,391,392

Courtesy Ruth N. Wrightstone, International Hemoglobin Information Center, Medicine College of Georgia, Augusta, Ga., 1979.
*See original list for references.

Table 4-9. More than one point mutation in the same polypeptide chain

Residue	Substitution	Name	Major abnormal property	Reference no.*
β6(A3)	Glu → Val	Hb C Harlem	Normal O_2 affinity	405
	73Asp → Asn	G Georgetown		406
	Glu → Lys	Hb Arlington Park	Not done	407
	95Lys → Glu			
α78-79	Asn → Asp	Hb J Singapore	Not done	408
	Ala → Gly			
β(A3)	Glu → Val	Hb C Ziguinchor		409
	58Pro → Arg			
β6(A3)	Glu → Val	Hb S Travis	↑ O_2 affinity	410
	142Ala → Val			

Courtesy Ruth N. Wrightstone, International Hemoglobin Information Center, Medical College of Georgia, Augusta, Ga., 1979.
*See original list for references.

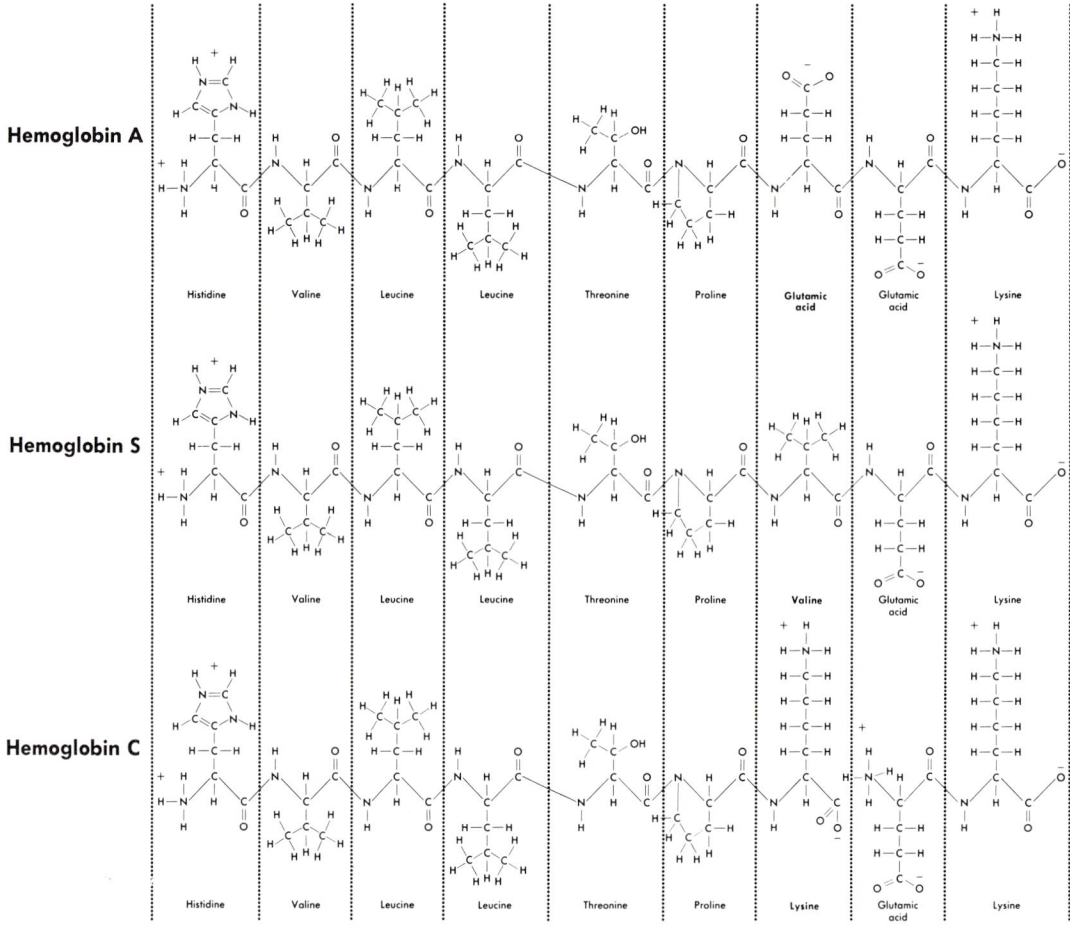

Fig. 4-11. Diagram of sections of globin amino acid patterns of Hb A, S, and C to show substitution of amino acids in sixth position of β-chain of globin. For each hemoglobin, amino acid that changes is underlined. (From Ingram, V.M.: Br. Med. Bull. **15:**27, 1959.)

The effect of these substitutions depends on the type of amino acid changed and on its position in the molecule. In most cases no clinical effects are produced, but in some patients severe clinical, physical, and chemical changes may include hemoglobin instability, methemoglobin formation, increased or decreased oxygen affinity, erythrocytosis, various types of anemia, shortened red cell survival, altered hemoglobin solubility, and red cell membrane changes.

Hemoglobins are analyzed by a number of electrophoretic, chromatographic, and unrelated methods. The methodology is divided into (1) presumptive electrophoretic identification of hemoglobins by cellulose acetate electrophoresis, (2) confirmatory hemoglobin identification by a second electrophoretic method with a buffer of different pH such as citrate agar electrophoresis and/or by electrophoresis of component globin chains, and (3) methods that do not depend on electrophoretic changes.

Cellulose acetate electrophoresis: presumptive identification of hemoglobins

Principle: Cellulose acetate electrophoresis provides a rapid, inexpensive, reproducible, semiquantitative hemoglobin screening method for Hb A, A_2 (F), S, G, C, E, O, and D. In alkaline tris-EDTA-borate buffer, pH 8.4, most hemoglobins have a negative charge and migrate from the cathodic application point toward the positive pole (anode). The ionic strength of the buffer is usually 0.05, the lower ionic strengths favoring wider separation of the hemoglobin bands. To prevent an increase in the ionic strength of the buffer during electrophoresis, evaporation should be kept to a minimum by controlling heat production and length of procedure. Electrophoresis is accomplished at 450 V for 15 min. The height of the voltage is directly proportional to the speed of the protein migration but has the disadvantage of greater heat production. The plates that accommodate 8 samples may be examined unstained or are stained with a protein stain, e.g., 0.5% Ponceau S in 7.5% trichloroacetic acid, or with a hemoglobin stain, e.g., *o*-tolidine, which differentiates the red-brown–staining heme from the red counterstained nonheme proteins such as carbonic anhydrase and also allows visualization of hemoglobin variants of very low concentration. A visual comparison of unknowns and controls is usually adequate for interpretation of the pattern. For quantitation the strips may be stained, cleared, and scanned with a densitometer, or the individual fractions may be eluted and measured in a spectrophotometer. Densitometry should not be used to quantitate Hb A_2 or F.

The following control hemolysates must be used with each "run": Hb A, F, S, and C.

Preparation of hemolysate

Principle: Quantitation and differentiation of various hemoglobins require a blood hemolysate. In most methods anticoagulated blood is concentrated by centrifugation and is hemolyzed by the addition of water and toluene or of saponin. White cells, platelets, stroma, and plasma proteins are removed by centrifugation because they interfere with staining. The hemoglobin concentration is adjusted to about 10 g/dl by the addition of water. If the blood is markedly anemic, a larger volume of packed cells and less water are used in the preparation of the initial hemolysate. For procedures that require larger amounts of blood, the macromethod is suggested; if only small amounts of blood are required or obtainable, the micromethod suffices. Potassium cyanide (KCN; extremely poisonous) may be added to convert Met-Hb to cyamethemoglobin if the specimen is old or is to be stored for any length of time.

Macromethod

Anticoagulated red blood cells are centrifuged, washed three times in saline, and concentrated after the last wash. Unwashed packed cells may be substituted for the washed cells but may lead to trailing and poorly defined bands. The hemoglobin solution should be clear and may be frozen or kept in the refrigerator for several weeks.

Reagent: Toluene.

Procedure: Centrifuge 5 ml anticoagulated blood at 3000 rpm for 20 min in a graduated conical centrifuge tube. Remove the plasma and wash three times in saline. After the last centrifugation remove the supernatant and measure the volume of packed cells. To each 1 ml cells add 1.4 ml distilled water and 0.4 ml toluene. Shake for 5 min and centrifuge at 3000 rpm for 20 min (preferably at 4° C).

Use a cotton-tipped swab to absorb the toluene, and with a Pasteur pipet inserted below the stromal ring remove the hemoglobin solution, which should be spun once more before use (3000 rpm for 20 min, preferably at 4° C). If the hemoglobin solution is not clear, repeat this step. NOTE: One drop of an 8-12 g/dl hemolysate from a disposable Pasteur pipet has a volume of about 0.04 ml and contains 3-6 mg hemoglobin.

A few difficulties may arise in the preparation of the hemolysate:

1. Target cells are somewhat resistant to lysis and the saponin lysing reagent may have to be added (see below).
2. Met-Hb production should be reduced to a minimum by shortening the contact of plasma and red cells. Electrophoretically Met-Hb at alkaline pH moves with Hb H.
3. The nonhemoglobin carbonic anhydrase, an intraerythrocytic carbon dioxide–binding enzyme, contaminates most hemolysates and at alkaline pH is seen close to the application point (Fig. 4-5). It gives a positive protein stain but is negative with the peroxidase stain for hemoglobin.

Micromethod

Reagent: Saponin lysing reagent:
1. Stock solution
   Saponin powder, 1 g
   Water in 100 ml volumetric flask, 50 ml
   Dissolve the powder in the water to make 1 dl.
2. Working solution
   Stock solution, 10 ml
   Water, 90 ml
   3% KCN, 2 ml

Procedure: Fill two heparinized microhematocrit tubes with finger-stick blood. Seal off one end with plastic seal and centrifuge both in a microhematocrit centrifuge for 5 min. The specimen is stable for 1 week in the refrigerator. With a sharp file score each hematocrit tube 1.6 cm above the upper level of the plastic sealing compound and break the tube. Drop the packed cell column into a test tube containing 6 drops saponin hemolyzing reagent. Shake well for 15 min to remove blood from the microhematocrit tube and to hemolyze it. NOTE: Half a microhematocrit tube of whole blood has a volume of about 0.04 ml and contains 3-6 mg hemoglobin.

Filter paper method

Procedure: Cut 1 × 3 in. filter paper strips (Whatman no. 3) and draw two 12 mm circles, one behind the other at one end. The opposite end is used for identification. Completely fill the circles with finger- or heel-stick blood by bringing the drop of blood in contact with the undersurface of the filter paper. Allow the blood filling the circles to dry completely. With a hole punch, punch out two bloody filter paper disks, each 1 cm in diameter. Place the filter paper disks into two separate test tubes, each containing 3 drops saponin hemolyzing reagent, mix, and allow to stand for 45 min at room temperature. Remove filter paper by pressing it against the wall of the tube with applicator stick or glass rod. Use specimen immediately or freeze. NOTE: One falling drop of blood collected on Whatman no. 3 filter paper contains 3-6 mg hemoglobin.

Electrophoresis of hemolysate

The method uses Mylar-backed cellulose acetate plates (sheets).

Reagents (Helena Laboratories, Beaumont, Tex.):
1. Hemolysate
2. Supre-Heme buffer diluted to 1000 ml, pH 8.4,

ionic strength 0.02, or the following buffer:
> Tris-EDTA-boric acid (TEB) buffer, pH 8.4
> Tris(hydroxymethyl)aminomethane, 10.2 g
> EDTA, 0.6 g
> Boric acid, 3.2 g
> Water to make 10 dl

3. Titan III plates, Mylar backed
4. Stains
   a. Protein stain
      > Ponceau S, 0.5 g
      > Trichloroacetic acid, 5%, to make 1 dl
   b. Hemoglobin-specific stain
      > Stock dye
      > *o*-Tolidine, 4 g
      > Glacial acetic acid, 1 dl
   c. Working dye: Immediately before use dilute the stock dye 1:4 with water and for each 1 dl add 2-3 drops fresh 30% H_2O_2.
5. Trichloroacetic acid
6. Acetic acid, 5%

Procedure: The method presented is essentially that of Helena Laboratories, Beaumont, Tex. Prepare the hemolysate with the hemolysate reagent by adding 1 part packed red cells to 6 parts hemolysate reagent, mix, let stand for 1 min, and mix again. Pour the buffer into the outer compartments of the electrophoresis chamber, soak the wicks, and position them. Identify the strips on the Mylar side, lower the rack of plates slowly into the buffer, and soak them ($2^3/_8 \times 3$ in.) in buffer for at least 5 min before use. Blot the plates between two pieces of absorbent paper quickly and evenly to remove excess moisture.

Apply the samples to the cellulose acetate side of the plate at a point approximately 3 cm from the cathode using a microdispenser. Place the plate, cellulose acetate side down, into the chamber with the application site near the cathode (black lead), and place a glass slide on the plate to establish good contact. Cover the chamber and apply 350 V for 15 min at room temperature. Remove the plates from the chamber and stain for 3 min with the Ponceau S stain. Remove the plates from the stain and place in three consecutive 2 min washes of 5% acetic acid until the background is white. Fix the plate in absolute methanol for 3-5 min. Clear the plate in 20% glacial acetic acid in absolute methanol for 10 min. Air dry the plate for 2 min with the strip placed on a blotter sheet. Place the blotter and strip in an 80° C oven for 3-4 min.

• • •

A simplified micromethod suitable for mass screening using 10 μl blood and the reagents and equipment mentioned above has been described by Rosenberg et al.[92a] and Barnes et al.[92b]

Hemoglobin-specific staining method

Principle: This method stains hemoglobin bands blue (see Chapter 5), thus differentiating them from non-heme proteins and aiding in the visualization of weak hemoglobin bands.

Procedure: After removing the strip from the electrophoresis chamber, fix it in 7.5% trichloroacetic acid for 3 min. Wash the strip in 5% acetic acid for 2-3 min. Stain the strip in working *o*-tolidine solution that has been prepared fresh and must be used immediately.

General remarks pertaining to all cellulose acetate procedures:

1. Cellulose acetate strips should be held by their edges only.
2. Air should not be trapped between the buffer and plates during the soaking period.
3. The blotting before the sample application should be adequate to remove excessive wetness but should not dry the plates.
4. The sample should be applied quickly after blotting and the plate should be placed into the chamber immediately.
5. The volume of the suggested hemolysate sample should not be exceeded so as not to impair the resolution.
6. The applicator should be washed with distilled water between applications.
7. Before densitometer screening is attempted, the strips must be adequately cleared. The densitometer should not be used to quantitate Hb A_2 and Hb F since the results do not conform to those of other quantitative methods.

Interpretation and limitations of alkaline cellulose acetate electrophoresis

All hemoglobins (Figs. 4-5 and 4-12) move from the area of the cathodic ($-$) application point to the anode ($+$). The application point may be faintly visible and there may be at the same level an equally faint non-hemoglobin band of carbonic anhydrase. According to their mobility, the hemoglobin variants can be classified into three groups: (1) the slow hemoglobins (Hb A_2, C, C Harlem, E, and O) are clustered near the cathode; (2) the "halfway" group is located between Hb C and A and includes Hb S, Lepore, D (G), and F; and (3) the faster (more anodal) than Hb A group includes the following variants: Hb K Woolwich, J, N, I, Bart's, and H. The hemoglobins with identical electrophoretic mobility can be differentiated by such methods as sickling and solubility tests, alkali denaturation tests, and citrate agar electrophoresis. They can also be differentiated by quantitative considerations. In the homozygous state of a hemoglobin variant (e.g., sickle cell disease) the variant hemoglobin is the major component and Hb A is absent, but there may be a small amount of Hb F. In the heterozygous state (trait) of a hemoglobin variant (e.g., sickle cell trait Hb A-S) there is usually more Hb A than variant hemoglobin present, although in some instances they are equal. The combination of a β-variant and β-thalassemia, (e.g., Hb S-thalassemia), characteristically exhibits a broad variant band and a small amount of Hb A, but in some cases of β-thalassemia in combination with a β-variant (e.g., Hb S–β-thalassemia or Hb C–β-thalassemia) Hb A is completely suppressed and the electrophoretic picture cannot be differentiated from the pattern of the homozygous state of the variant hemoglobin, e.g., Hb S-S or Hb C-C, which contain no Hb A but varying amounts of Hb F. In heterozygous thalassemia Hb A_2 is usually increased, but electrophoretically it is in-

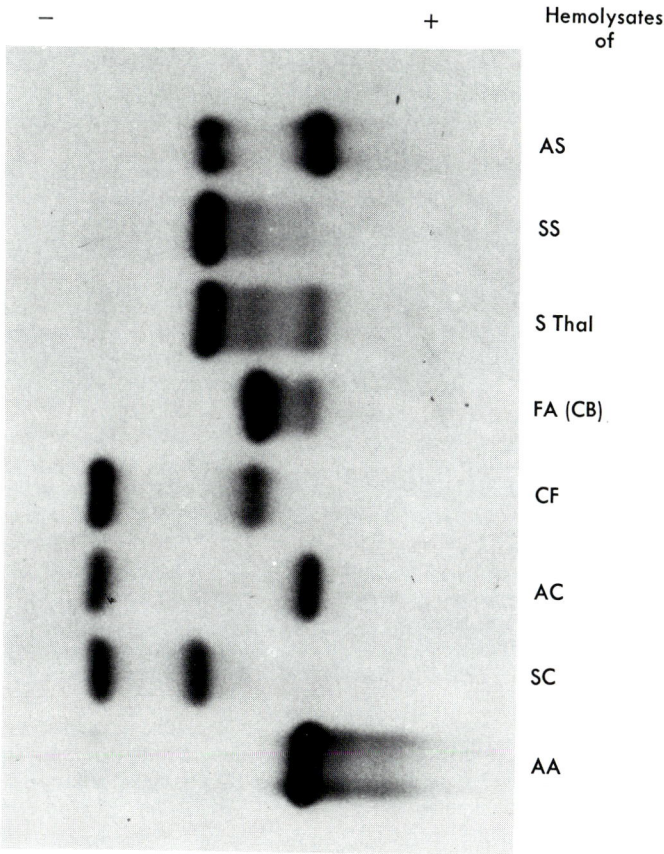

Fig. 4-12. Cellulose acetate hemoglobin electrophoresis, pH 8.5. (Courtesy R.G. Schneider.)

separable from Hb C. A heavy band in the A_2 position usually indicates Hb C, which pathologically may occupy 20-90% of the total hemoglobin mass, while Hb A_2 normally or pathologically does not exceed about 8%.

Hb A and F may not be separated adequately if the hemolysate contains normal amounts of Hb F or if it contains large amounts of one and small amounts of the other, as these two hemoglobins move close together. Hemoglobinopathies in the newborn cannot be detected by cellulose acetate electrophoresis but require isoelectric focusing (see below). Large amounts of Hb F can be diagnosed on cellulose acetate so that the association of Hb S and C with hereditary persistence of Hb F can be documented. The distribution of Hb F throughout the red cells should be confirmed by the Kleihauer staining method.

Citrate agar electrophoresis: confirmatory identification of hemoglobins

Principle: Citrate agar electrophoresis at pH 6.0-6.5 is essentially a chromatographic procedure depending on adsorption of the hemoglobin to the citrate agar rather than on the electric charge. The adsorption appears to be a function of the solubility of hemoglobin.

The method published by Schneider et al.[92c] uses Mylar-backed cellulose acetate plates impregnated with citrate agar that are stable for at least 6 months.

Reagents: All reagents are commercially available (Helena Laboratories, Beaumont, Tex.). Use deionized water for all procedures.

1. Stock citrate buffer, 0.5M
   Sodium citrate, 147 g
   Water, about 8 dl
   Citric acid solution (30 g/dl), about 80 ml
   Adjust the pH to 6.0. Add water to make 1 L. Mix well and store at 4° C.
2. Working citrate buffer
   Stock citrate buffer, 1 dl
   Add water to make 1 L. Adjust the pH to 6.0 if necessary with a small amount of citric acid solution. Mix well and store at 4° C.
3. Agar gel
   Bacto-agar, 10 g
   Working buffer, 1 L
   Dissolve the agar by placing the agar mixture into a boiling water bath. After the agar has dissolved, cool it to 65° C, add 1 ml potassium cyanide (50 g/L) as a preservative, and mix.
4. Staining solutions as described for cellulose acetate electrophoresis

Preparation of citrate agar plates: Holding the cellulose acetate plates vertical in a plate holder, soak them in the working buffer for 30 min. Slowly lower the sheets into the buffer to avoid the entrapment of air bubbles. Heat the agar solution to the melting point in a boiling water bath and then cool to 65° C. Remove rack of cellulose acetate plates from buffer, allow to drain, and slowly lower into melted agar, which should cover the plates. Keep in agar for 30 min at 65° C. Remove each plate separately, allow it to drain, and insert it into a sealable plastic bag containing 1 ml working buffer; seal and store at 4° C in a vertical position. The plates are stable for 6-8 months.

Procedure: Prepare the hemolysate by one of the methods given earlier. Hemolysates of adults are diluted with working buffer to a hemoglobin concentration of 0.5 gm/dl hemolysate; umbilical cord hemolysates are diluted to 5 g/dl hemolysate to allow the detection of small amounts of Hb A, S, and C.

Arrange the hemolysates (unknowns and Hb controls A-S, A-C, F-A-S) on a sample well plate (Helena Laboratories, Beaumont, Tex.) using the applicator supplied by the manufacturer. Because the system does not tolerate large hemolysate amounts, not more than 3 μl can be transferred. It is therefore suggested that prior to the performance of the test the technologist should practice the transfer of small amounts of hemolysate onto paper towels.

Remove the plate from the plastic bag and blot lightly; it must not be allowed to dry out at any time during the procedure. Depress the applicator once into the wells and apply hemolysate lightly to the plate,

holding it down for 10 sec. The application point should be about 3 cm from the cathodal end of the plate. Immediately invert the plate and place it agar side down into the electrophoresis chamber so that the agar touches the wicks. Weigh the plate down with a glass plate of suitable size to ensure proper contact with the wicks, and surround the electrophoresis chamber with crushed ice. Perform electrophoresis at about 100 V (5 mA/plate) for 15-30 min. Stain with O-tolidine stain for about 5 min until bands are clearly visible and wash well in water to which a few drops of 3% acetic acid have been added.

Discussion: Citrate agar electrophoresis is not a good screening method because many adult hemoglobin variants have the same mobility as Hb A. It does, however, distinguish Hb S from Hb D and Hb A from Hb F, even in small amounts. The wide separation of Hb A, F, S, and C makes it a good method for confirmation of these hemoglobins, for screening newborns for sickle cell trait or anemia, and for dectecting small amounts of Hb F and A in Hb S−β-thalassemia and Hb C−β-thalassemia to differentiate them from the homozygous variant forms (Figs. 4-6 and 4-13).

The hemoglobins move from the anode to the cathode, Hb F moving fastest and furthest to the cathode while Hb C stays closest to the anode. On cellulose acetate, Hb E, O, and C Harlem move with the Hb C. On citrate agar Hb E moves with Hb A, whereas Hb O migrates to a position between Hb A and S so that both can be separated from Hb C. Hb C Harlem moves with Hb S. On cellulose acetate, Hb D or G resembles Hb

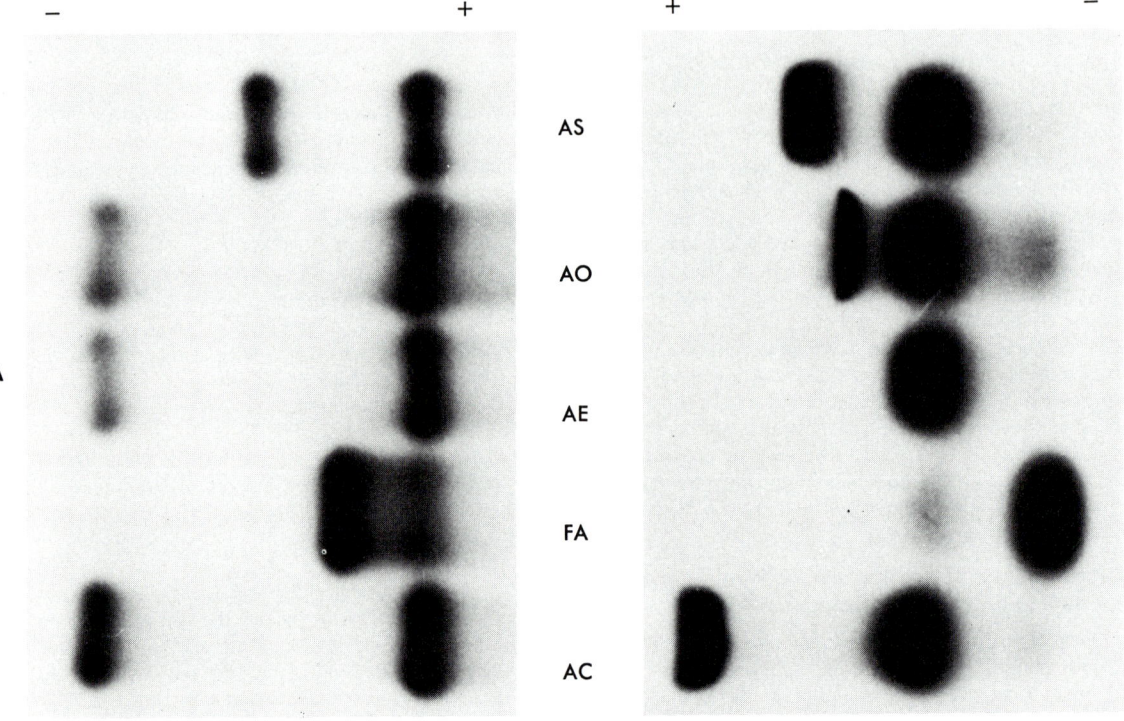

Fig. 4-13. Comparison of cellulose acetate hemoglobin electrophoresis, **A,** with citrate agar hemoglobin electrophoresis, **B.** (Courtesy R.G. Schneider.)

S, so that Hb SD disease produces the electrophoretic picture of homozygous Hb S. On citrate agar, Hb D moves with Hb A, producing the picture of sickle cell trait. The other nonsickling Hb S–like hemoglobins, e.g., Hb P and G, also migrate with Hb A. Hb A_2 also adheres to Hb A, so that citrate agar electrophoresis cannot be used to demonstrate Hb A_2.

Electrophoresis of globin chains

The net charge of a given hemoglobin is determined by the sum of the charges of its polypeptide chains. Electrophoresis of the globin chains separates the α-chains from the non-α-chains (β, δ, and γ). Chains with amino acid substitutions or with other amino acid changes (variant chains) exhibit a characteristic mobility that differs from the mobility of the normal chain at a given buffer pH. Electrophoresis of the globin chains determines which chain of a hemoglobin variant carries the abnormality and thus allows separation of hemoglobins that move at a similar rate on cellulose acetate or citrate agar because their total charge is similar. For instance, Hb N and Hb I move similarly on cellulose acetate at pH 8.6, but by globin chain electrophoresis they can be separated because Hb N is a β-chain variant and Hb I is an α-chain variant.

Principle: Electrophoresis of the hemolysate is done on cellulose acetate in urea-2-mercaptoethanol buffer in the presence of additional 2-mercaptoethanol. The latter cleaves heme from globin and allows it to leave the electrophoretic field during the procedure. Urea serves to separate the α- and non-α-chains. Each globin chain has a characteristic mobility at alkaline as well as acid pH so that the position of the normal α- and normal non-α-chain can be compared with the position of the variant chain.

Reagents: The reagents are commercially available (Mallinckrodt Chemical Works, St. Louis). Use only deionized distilled water.
1. Alkaline-urea-mercaptoethanol buffer
   a. Stock buffer
      Acid barbital, 11.2 g
      Water, boiling, 1 L
      Stir with glass rod until dissolved. Then add 82.4 g sodium barbital powder. Rinse the beakers with water and collect the solution in 4 L flasks; allow to cool. Add water to make 4 L. The pH should be 8.6-8.7. Refrigerate.
   b. Working buffer
      Stock buffer, 50%
      Water, 50%
2. Urea
3. 2-Mercaptoethanol (Eastman Kodak Co., Rochester, N.Y.). Store in a brown bottle in a refrigerator and remove only as needed. Do not allow it to become oxidized.
4. Titan II cellulose acetate strips (Helena Laboratories, Beaumont, Tex.)
5. Hemolysates prepared by methods described before
6. Ponceau S solution, 0.5%, as described before
7. Acetic acid, 5%

Procedure: Add 180 g urea to 3 dl working buffer. Use a glass rod only to handle the urea. Mix until dissolved, cover, and leave at room temperature. In a small test tube place 50 μl of the urea-buffer mixture, 40 μl 2-mercaptoethanol, and 50 μl hemolysate. Stopper the tube and refrigerate for $2^1/_2$ hr. Using the remaining urea-buffer mixture, add 2.5 ml 2-mercaptoethanol, mix, and soak Titan II cellulose acetate strips (4.5 × 6 in.) for 2 hr. Remove the strips and blot them lightly with paper towels. Mark the center of each strip with a dull pencil and draw six 2 cm lines, one for each sample. Place 3 μl hemolysate-urea-buffer mixture in sample wells (unknowns and at least one Hb A-S and one Hb A-C control). Position the strip on a filter paper wick in the chamber, the buffer wells of which contain equal volumes of urea-2-mercaptoethanol-buffer mixture. With a microliter pipet apply 3 μl hemolysate onto the pencilled lines. Move back and forth just once. Cover the strip with a glass plate to ensure contact and then surround chamber with ice water. Electrophorese at about 200 V for 1-$1^1/_2$ hr (2 mA/strip). Remove strip, stain in fresh 0.5% Ponceau S stain for 2 min, and rinse in 5% acetic acid to remove excess stain. Compare migration patterns of globin chains of normal hemoglobins with those of variant hemoglobins.

Result: The aberrant globin chain moves anodally or cathodally in relation to the normal chain of which it is a variant (Fig. 4-14).

The method can be refined by repeating the globin electrophoresis in acid-urea-mercaptoethanol buffer, pH 6.0-6.5. In the acid medium α- and β-chains move at the same rate and in the same direction as in the alkaline buffer, but γ- and β-chains can be separated and several other mutant globin chains move differently in the acid medium than in the alkaline medium.

Isoelectric focusing

Electrofocusing has the highest resolution of any technic for protein analysis. The method mentioned uses the LKB Multiphor system (LKB, Washington, D.C.) using thin-layer polyacrylamide gel slabs and high voltage.

Principle: The sample is applied to the surface of a thin layer of polyacrylamide gel containing carrier ampholytes. When a current is applied, a linear pH gradient results and the hemoglobins move toward the electrode of the opposite charge. As each molecule moves through the pH gradient it gradually loses its charge, until at a pH equal to the isoelectric point the charge is zero and the movement stops. Each hemoglobin is concentrated or focused at its isoelectric position into a narrow band. The method is sensitive enough to evaluate hemoglobins of neonates, fetuses, and embryos.

Nonelectrophoretic methods

The nonelectrophoretic methods of identification of hemoglobin variants include sickling, stability tests, and identification of morphologic red cell changes. The red cell changes include hypochromic microcytes (suggesting anemia), target cells (suggesting thalassemia), spherocytes and polychromatic cells (suggesting hemolysis), sickle cells (suggesting Hb S), red cell inclusions (suggesting Hb C and H) and Heinz bodies (suggesting unstable hemoglobin).

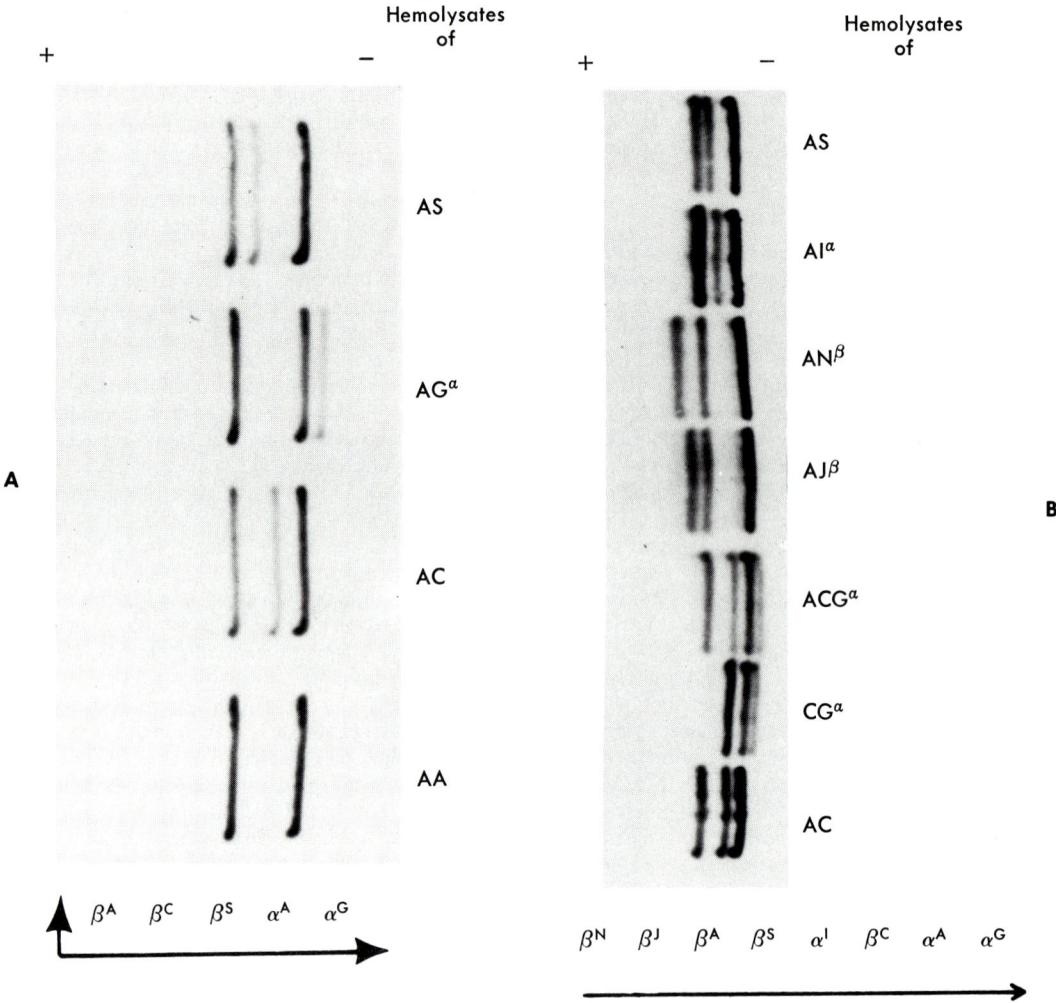

Fig. 4-14. **A,** Globin chain electrophoresis, alkaline pH 8.9. See text for explanation. **B,** Globin chain electrophoresis, alkaline pH. See text for explanation. (Courtesy R.G. Schneider.)

Hemoglobin S

The structural formula of Hb S, $\alpha_2\beta_2^{6val}$, indicates a substitution of valine for glutamic acid in the sixth position of the β-chain (Fig 4-11). In the United States Hb S is the most common hemoglobin variant, as it is found in 8-9% of American blacks. Higher concentrations are found in Africa and lower concentrations in the Middle East, Greece, and India. Very rarely is it found in Caucasians.[93] Deoxygenation of Hb S produces sickling of the red cells because of the intracellular polymerization of the deoxygenated Hb S into aligned elongated fibers that distort the cell membrane into the classic sickle shape, a process reversible on reoxygenation of the red cell. The intraerythrocytic crystallization is responsible for (1) the birefringence of sickled cells in wet preparations, (2) the low solubility of the reduced Hb S, (3) the condensation of hemoglobin in the center of the sickled cell in stained smears, (4) the rapid destruction of these cells by the reticu-

loendothelial system, and (5) the plugging of the smallest vessels by sickled cells causing painful infarcts. The increased viscosity of reduced Hb S in solution renders it about 50 times less soluble than reduced Hb A. A number of laboratory tests are based on the low solubility of Hb S, e.g., the original Itano solubility test,[41] the ferrohemoglobin solubility test,[94] the dithionite tube test,[95] the Sickledex test (Ortho Diagnostic Div., Raritan, N.J.),[96] and the Sickle-ID test (Hyland Diagnostics Div., Travenol Laboratories, Costa Mesa, Calif.).

The sickling phenomenon and the speed with which it occurs are influenced by the concentration of Hb S in the red cell and by the presence of other hemoglobins. Sickling is much more rapid in S-S cells (homozygous S) than in A-S cells (heterozygous S). Red cells containing Hb S and F are resistant to sickling. The protective influence of Hb F is seen in newborns with sickle cell anemia and in cases of hereditary persistence of Hb F associated with Hb S. The effect of Hb C and

D on Hb S is opposite to that of Hb F. S-C and S-D cells sickle more rapidly than do A-S cells with a similar Hb S concentration.

Laboratory diagnosis of Hb S is made by the following methods:

1. Tests based on the insolubility of reduced Hb S, such as turbidity or solubility tests, e.g., the dithionite tube test
2. Hemoglobin electrophoresis
3. Examination of the blood smear for sickled erythrocytes

Dithionite tube test for detection of Hb S and other sickling hemoglobins[95]

Principle: Red blood cells are lysed by saponin, and hemoglobin is reduced by dithionite in a phosphate buffer. Reduced Hb S is characterized by its very low solubility and by the formation of nematic insoluble liquid crystals, so that in the presence of Hb S or of non-S sickling hemoglobins the system becomes turbid.

Equipment:
1. Test tubes (12 × 75 mm)
2. Lined "reader"

Reagents: (Commerical kits are available from many laboratory supply houses.)
1. Stock buffer
   KH_2PO_4, 160.48 g
   K_2HPO_4, 281.88 g
   Add distilled water to make 1 L. The buffer is stable for 1 month if it is refrigerated.
   Working solution:
   Stock buffer, 8 dl
   $Na_2S_2O_4$, 20 g
   Mix until dissolved. Then add 60 ml saponin (Fisher Scientific Co., Pittsburgh) and distilled water to make 1 L. The solution is stable for 1 month under refrigeration.
2. EDTA-anticoagulated blood (patient's blood and positive and negative controls), 1 ml

Procedure: To 2 ml working solution in a 12 × 75 mm test tube (the test tube size is critical) add 20 μl well-mixed EDTA-anticoagulated blood and cover the tube with paraffin. Mix by inverting and allow the tube to stand at room temperature for 5 min. Read the test by holding the tube 3 cm from the lined reader scale.

Normal values: The solution is clear, and the reader lines are clearly seen.

Interpretation[97]: If no sickling hemoglobin is present in the specimen, the clear solution permits the lines to be seen through the test tube, and the test is recorded as negative for sickling hemoglobin. If the hemoglobin concentration of the blood specimen is below 8 g/dl, the volume of the specimen used in the test should be doubled[97]; false negative results may be caused by a low concentration of the abnormal hemoglobin. False negative results may also be encountered in infants with Hb S during the first 2 months of life, as the β-chains take several weeks to fully develop (Fig. 4-7). If Hb S or any other sickling hemoglobin is present, the solution is turbid and the lines behind the tube are not visible (Fig 4-15). A positive test means the specimen contains one of the following hemoglobins: Hb S, Hb C Harlan (synonymous with Hb C Georgetown), Hb S Travis, or Hb Bart's. The last is

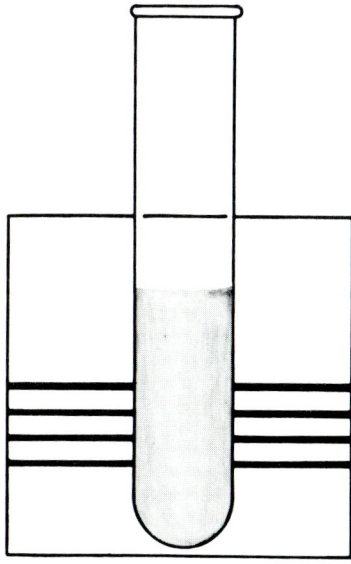

Fig. 4-15. Dithionite tube test for detection of Hb S. Reduced Hb S obscures black lines behind tube.

found only in fetuses dying from α-thalassemia. False positive results are encountered in hyperglobulinemia,[97] in which the globulin rather than the sickling hemoglobin is precipitated.

Electrophoresis: Cellulose acetate electrophoresis (pH 8.6) must be carried out on the specimen responsible for a positive turbidity test. On cellulose acetate Hb S moves roughly halfway between the application point and the Hb A band. It shares this position with Hb D Punjab, a nonsickling hemoglobin that can be separated from Hb S by citrate agar electrophoresis. Hb Lepore also has the mobility of Hb S and does not sickle. Electrofocusing in agarose or polyacrylamide gel may be used to demonstrate Hb S in cord blood in association with large amounts of Hb F and small amounts of Hb A.

Examination of the blood smear: Repeated sickling leads to persistent red cell membrane damage so that sickled cells remain in the circulation even after reoxygenation. They are readily found in sickle cell crisis and after prolonged stasis.

Sickle cell trait

In sickle cell trait the patient inherits one gene for Hb S from one parent and one gene for the normal Hb A from the other. The deoxyhemoglobin solubility test for Hb S is positive, and electrophoresis reveals 20-40% Hb S accompanied by 60% or more Hb A. Hb A_2 and F are within normal limits. The hemogram is entirely normal, and unless the patient is exposed to a severely hypoxic environment (anesthesia, diving, etc.), the demonstration of Hb S is of no clinical consequence, but it should suggest genetic counseling. There are reports of spontaneous hematuria and of impairment of the ability of the kidney to concentrate urine in individuals with sickle cell trait.[98]

Sickle cell anemia

In sickle cell anemia the gene for Hb S is inherited from both parents, and this fact may have to be ascertained to differentiate sickle cell–thalassemia from sickle cell anemia. In the steady state there is a normocytic hemolytic anemia with a pronounced reticulocytosis (usually over 10%) and a hemoglobin value of 5-10 g/dl. In the aplastic crisis both values fall dramatically. The solubility test and the electrophoresis are positive for Hb S, which makes up 80-95% of the total hemoglobin. The remainder is composed of Hb A_2 (2-4%) and of Hb F (2-20%). There is no Hb A since there are no normal β-chains. It is important to remember that solubility tests may be falsely negative because of the low hemoglobin concentration. Hematocrit must be raised prior to the test by removing some or all of the plasma. Citrate agar gel electrophoresis serves to identify the Hb S-D variant, which cannot be diagnosed by alkaline cellulose acetate electrophoresis. Severe sickle cell–β-thalassemia can be differentiated on the basis of red cell morphology. In sickle cell anemia and Hb S-D disease the peripheral smear shows target cells and various sickled forms, but in Hb S–β-thalassemia microcytic hypochromic cells alternate with numerous target cells and rare sickle cells. Careful quantitation of Hb A_2 by column chromatography may also aid in differentiating sickle cell–β-thalassemia from sickle cell anemia, as in the first the level of Hb A_2 is raised (4-6%). The bone marrow responds to the chronic hemolytic anemia by advanced erythroid hyperplasia. Hematuria, urine concentration[99] defects, and abnormal liver function tests are frequently encountered in sickle cell anemia.

Hemoglobin S-C disease

There is a moderate to mild hemolytic anemia with hemoglobin levels of 11-12 g/dl and 3-5% reticulocytes.[100] Cellulose acetate electrophoresis expresses the genetic defect of lack of normal β-chain synthesis. The pattern shows only Hb C and S bands. Hb A_2 is normal but its band is hidden by the Hb C band, and Hb F is normal or only minimally elevated (1-2%). Hb A is absent. At alkaline pH Hb O has the same mobility as Hb C, so that Hb S-O disease must be kept in mind whenever Hb S-C disease is diagnosed by alkaline electrophoresis. Citrate agar electrophoresis separates Hb O from Hb C. Hb O is located between Hb A and S, closer to the latter, and separated from Hb C. Family studies may be required to confirm the diagnosis of Hb S-O disease. In Hb S-C disease the blood smear shows target cells, swollen sickled cells, and often intraerythrocytic as well as free crystalline structures[101] (see Fig. 6-28).

Hemoglobin S-D disease[102]

Hb S-D disease produces a mild hemolytic anemia, the laboratory diagnosis of which is rendered difficult by the fact that the electrophoretograms appear to be misleading. The alkaline acetate electrophoretogram shows a pattern that cannot be distinguished from that of homozygous sickle cell anemia, and the citrate agar electrophoretogram shows the bands of Hb S trait, Hb D migrating as does Hb A distinct from Hb S (see discussion of sickle cell anemia).

Sickle cell–β-thalassemia

Double heterozygosity for β-thalassemia and for Hb S results in a hemolytic anemia, the severity of which depends on the degree of suppression of the β-chain synthesis, i.e., on the amount of Hb A synthesized.[103,104] In the most severe form no Hb A is demonstrable (S/β^0 thal), so that the electrophoretic pattern and the clinical picture suggest homozygous Hb S disease, but the anemia is hypochromic microcytic (low MCV and MCHC), and the Hb A_2 concentration is elevated (3-6%). The Hb F concentration is high (15%), and the reticulocyte count elevation reflects the degree of hemolysis. The electrophoretic pattern of patients with 10-30% Hb A (S/β$^+$ thal) resembles that of sickle cell trait except that in the latter there is always more Hb A than Hb S, while in S/β$^+$ thal there is more Hb S (55-75%) than Hb A (10-30%). Hb A_2 (3-6%) and Hb F (5-20%) are elevated. In S/β$^+$ thal the red cells are microcytic (the MCHC is less than normal), and on the blood smear they alternate with target cells and occasional sickled cells. If the Hb A_2 concentration is normal, family studies may be necessary to establish the diagnosis of S/β thal.

Sickle cell–α-thalassemia

The interaction of the Hb S (a β-chain variant) with an α-chain abnormality is rare and found only in Saudi Arabia. Homozygous sickle cell disease associated with thalassemia is responsible for a relatively mild hemolytic anemia, the hemoglobin pattern of which consists of Hb S, F, and Bart's.[105] The heterozygous form of sickle cell disease in combination with α-thalassemia leads to no clinical abnormality, and the electrophoretogram reveals a relatively small amount of Hb S.

Hemoglobin C

Hb C ($\alpha_2\beta_2^{6\ glu\rightarrow lys}$) has an incidence of 2-3% among American blacks. This formula indicates a β-chain variant with lysine replacing glutamic acid in the sixth position. Hb C occurs in the heterozygous and homozygous forms and in association with Hb S and β-thalassemia and is the second most common hemoglobin variant. The laboratory diagnosis involves hemoglobin electrophoresis and the demonstration of intraerythrocytic crystals and of abnormal red cells. Hb C, E, A_2, and O cannot be separated by alkaline electrophoresis because they have identical mobilities. Citrate agar electrophoresis separates Hb C from Hb A, A_2, E, and O. Hb A_2 and C can also be separated by column chromatography[106] and by quantitative consideration, as the concentration of Hb A_2 normally does not exceed 4% and even pathologically in β-thalassemia rarely reaches 8%, but Hb C concentrations vary from 30% (heterozygous form) to 90% (homozygous form). The ethnic background of the patient may also be helpful in the differential diagnosis; Hb C is relatively common in individuals of West African extraction, while Hb E occurs in Southeast Asia (and does not lead to intraerythrocytic crystals). The hemolytic anemia and the concomitant reticulocytosis are the result of Hb C–produced red cell changes, which include target cells, poikilocytes, crystal formation,[101] and folding of cells (Fig. 6-27). The crystals are best seen when the peripheral smear is allowed to deoxygenate and to dry slowly. They are intraerythrocytic and extraerythrocytic, reddish to brown (Wright-Giemsa stain), opaque, rodlike structures of varying length with rigid parallel sides and rounded or angular ends. Originally they were demonstrated following splenectomy, but they can also be discovered prior to splenectomy.[101] They are not seen in Hb A-C disease (Hb C trait) but are seen in other heterozygous forms of Hb C, such as Hb S-C and Hb C–thalassemia, and in association with hereditary persistence of Hb F. In Hb S-C disease some crystals show one half of the rod to be straight and the other half bent or curved (see Fig. 6-28).

Hemoglobin A-C disease

About 2% of American blacks are Hb A-C heterozygous. Hemoglobin electrophoresis reveals 30-40% Hb C, about 50-60% Hb A, 3-4% Hb A_2, and 1% Hb F. The stained blood film may show target cells but usually no other hematologic abnormality.

Hemoglobin C disease

Homozygous Hb C disease occurs in one out of 10,000 American blacks and leads to mild to moderate congenital hemolytic anemia with a hemoglobin level of about 8-12 g/dl and a moderate reticulocytosis (4-8%).[107,108] The stained blood smear reveals anisocytosis, the presence of numerous target cells accompanied by red cells containing Hb C crystalline inclusions. The target cells are responsible for increased osmotic fragility and a shortened red cell survival time. Quantitative electrophoresis reveals 95% Hb C, absence of Hb A, 3% Hb A_2, and 1-2% Hb F.

Hemoglobin E

Hb E ($\alpha_2\beta_2^{26\ glu\rightarrow lys}$) occurs in individuals of Southeast Asian extraction and is the third most common hemoglobin variant. It occurs in the heterozygous and homozygous forms and in association with β-thalassemia.

Hemoglobin A-E disease (heterozygous hemoglobin E disease)

The cellulose acetate electrophoretogram at pH 8.6 reveals about 25-30% Hb E; the remainder is Hb A. On cellulose acetate at pH 8.6, Hb A_2, E, and C have identical mobility, but Hb C and E can be separated on citrate agar. There are no hematologic abnormalities encountered in Hb E trait.

Hemoglobin E disease (homozygous hemoglobin E disease)

Cellulose acetate electrophoresis at pH 8.6 reveals about 95% Hb E and absence of Hb A. Hb A_2 and F as measured by nonelectrophoretic methods are within normal limits. There is a mild anemia associated with a slight erythrocytosis and microcytosis.[109]

Diagnosis of unstable hemoglobins

Approximately 200 unstable hemoglobins have been identified, most of which are of no clinical significance,[110-112] even though the majority show some abnormality of oxygen affinity. About one fourth are responsible for hemolytic anemias varying from well-compensated mild forms to severe hemolytic episodes. The anemia used to be referred to as **congenital nonspherocytic hemolytic anemia** or as **congenital Heinz**

body anemia. It appears at birth or after birth depending on whether α- or β-chains are involved. The urine may be dark, and the intensity of the color increases on standing. The cause of the pigment is unknown, but it is probably related to an abnormality of the heme metabolism leading to the excretion of **dipyrrole** or **mesobilifuscin.**

A number of structural changes of the hemoglobin molecule are responsible for the instability of the hemoglobin.[113-115] They include substitution in the α- and β-chains, heme loss, or dissociation of α- and β-chains. The unstable hemoglobins are precipitated in vivo and in vitro by insults that do not affect normal hemoglobins, e.g., drug ingestion and exposure to heat and cold. Unstable hemoglobins with α-chain abnormalities, such as Hb Torino, Constant Spring, and Ann Arbor, produce hemolytic anemias of varying intensity. β-Chain unstable hemoglobins are Hb Köln, Zurich, and H (β_4).[116,117]

The diagnosis of unstable hemoglobins is aided by the following:

1. Laboratory evidence of hemolytic anemia (see Chapter 8)
2. Pigmenturia (see Chapter 27)
3. Red cell morphology
4. Heat denaturation
5. Isopropyl alcohol precipitation
6. Heinz body formation
7. Hemoglobin electrophoresis
8. Globin chain electrophoresis
9. Oxygen affinity

Because of the instability of the hemoglobin, all testing should be done within 72 hr and the blood should be stored in the refrigerator.

Hemoglobin electrophoresis

Hemoglobin electrophoresis is not a sensitive method to differentiate the various unstable hemoglobins. The amino acid substitution may not change the electrophoretic charge of the unstable hemoglobin variant, so that Hb Torino, Hammersmith, Petersborough, and others move like Hb A. A number of variants move anodal to Hb A, e.g., Hb Tacoma, H, and I; others move cathodal to Hb A, e.g., Hb Freiburg; and others, such as Hb Köln, Sogn, and Sabine, move like Hb S. Hb E and Gun Hill accompany Hb A_2. Some hemoglobins separate only in the Met-Hb form, which should be electrophoresed at several pH levels. The electrophoretogram may reveal hemoglobin aggregates associated with free heme or free α- and β-chains. The precipitation of hemoglobin is caused by the heat generated during the electrophoresis.

Globin chain electrophoresis

Globin chain electrophoresis may demonstrate in which chain (α or β) the substitution responsible for the unstable hemoglobin has occurred.

Oxygen affinity

The molecular changes described above result in a poorly functioning hemoglobin with abnormal oxygen affinity and therefore abnormal oxygen dissociation curves. The previously described continuous method of plotting the oxygen dissociation curve distinguishes some unstable hemoglobins with low oxygen affinity, e.g., Hb S Seattle, Kansas, Hammersmith, Torino, and E, from unstable hemoglobins with high oxygen affinity, e.g., Hb Köln, Freiburg, Zurich, Hopkins-2, and H. The shift of the oxygen dissociation curve to the right or left is not accompanied by changes in the 2,3-DPG.

Heat denaturation test

Principle: Hb A, F, S, C, and D in solution are not precipitated when heated to 50° C for 1 hr or to 60° C for $^1/_2$ hr. Hemoglobins that are naturally partially and easily denatured precipitate at these temperatures[118-120] and render the solution turbid.

Reagents:
1. Buffer A
   Disodium phosphate (Na_2HPO_4), 0.1M, anhydrous, 14.2 g
   Water to make 1 L
2. Buffer B
   Monosodium phosphate ($NaH_2PO_4 \cdot 2H_2O$), 0.1M, 13.8 g
   Water to make 1 L
3. Working phosphate buffer
   Buffer A, 80.8 ml
   Buffer B, 19.2 ml
   Mix and adjust the pH to 7.4.
4. Normal and abnormal controls. For the normal control any fresh blood specimen suffices; for the abnormal control a 4-week-old specimen serves the purpose.

Procedure: Wash 1 ml fresh anticoagulated blood of the patient and a normal control in saline four times. Each time centrifuge at 3000 rpm for 5 min. After the last wash decant the supernatant and lyse the cells by the addition of 5 ml water to the packed cell button. Transfer the hemolysate to a prewarmed (60° C) thin-walled test tube and add 5 ml of working phosphate buffer at pH 7.4, mix, and centrifuge at 3000 rpm for 10 min. Transfer 2 ml of clear supernatant to a second set of prewarmed test tubes and place them in a 60° C water bath for 30 min. Prior to incubation determine the hemoglobin value by the cyanmethemoglobin method. Examine the tubes for precipitate at 1, 2, or 3 hr.

Result: Denatured hemoglobins (e.g., Hb H, Zurich, and Köln) precipitate and can be visualized grossly or centrifuged and filtered out. The remaining unprecipitated hemoglobin can be measured by the cyanmethemoglobin method to determine the amount of hemoglobin lost.

Isopropanol precipitation[121]

Principle: The addition of 17% buffered isopropyl alcohol to the hemolysate weakens the internal bonds of the hemoglobin molecule. In this solution normal hemoglobin is just stable and will precipitate after 40 min. Unstable hemoglobins precipitate rapidly and almost quantitatively.

Reagents:
1. Hemolysate. Wash fresh anticoagulated unknown and control red cells in saline three times; centrifuge at 3000 rpm for 5 min after each wash. After

the last wash add an equal volume of water and half the volume of carbon tetrachloride to the packed cells. Centrifuge for 10 min at 1500 *g*. Separate the clear supernatant.
2. Isopropyl alcohol 17% in 0.1 M tris-HC1 buffer, pH 7.4
   Tris (hydroxymethyl) aminomethane, 12.11 g
   Water, 7 dl
   Dissolve in 1 L volumetric flask. Then add 170 ml 100% isopropyl alcohol. Adjust the pH to 7.4 with HC1 and add water to make 1 L. Keep in a tightly closed container at room temperature.
3. Controls. See heat denaturation test above.

Procedure: Place 2 ml buffered isopropanol into two small test tubes labeled "unknown" and "control" and prewarm in a 37° C water bath for 10 min. Add 0.2 ml unknown clear hemolysate to one tube and the control hemolysate to the other. Stopper the tubes, mix, and incubate in a 37° C water bath. After 5 min examine the tubes for precipitated unstable hemoglobin, which renders the solution turbid; continue if necessary at 5 min intervals for 20 min.

Normal values: The normal control tube remains clear for 30-40 min.

Interpretation: The 17% isopropanol solution and the 37° C temperature are critical. The hemolysate should contain about 10 g hemoglobin per deciliter and no increased amounts of Hb F or Met-Hb, as they give false positive results. Met-Hb formation results from allowing the specimen to remain unrefrigerated for several days and can be prevented by the addition of 2% KCN to the specimen. Increased levels of Hb F, while interfering with the isopropanol test, do not interfere with the heat precipitation test. The presence of an unstable hemoglobin results in the formation of a fine turbidity after 5 min and after 20 min gives way to a flocculent precipitate.

Heinz body formation: acetylphenylhydrazine test

Heinz bodies are small, round, intraerythrocytic inclusions caused by oxidative denaturation of hemoglobin. They can be demonstrated in the susceptible red blood cell in a number of conditions such as drug-induced hemolytic anemias, defects in the intraerythrocytic reducing system (e.g., G-6-PD deficiency), unstable hemoglobins, excess α- and β-chains in homozygous α- and β-thalassemias, Hb Bart's (γ_4) disease, and Hb H (β_4) disease. Red cells of the hemolytic disorders mentioned form Heinz bodies more readily and in greater numbers than do normal cells (see Figs. 6-31 and 6-32).

Principle[121,122]: Because of the defect in the amino acid composition of the labile hemoglobins, globin is irreversibly denatured to Heinz bodies at the time the heme moiety is oxidized to the Met-Hb form (ferrous Fe^{++} to ferric Fe^{+++} state). Red cells containing unstable hemoglobins develop numerous small intraerythrocytic inclusions in mature red cells when exposed to acetylphenylhydrazine. They are stained with crystal violet.

Reagents:
1. Heparinized blood, 3-5 ml. Use within 1 hr of the time the sample is drawn.

2. Phosphate buffer, 0.067M, pH 7.6
   Solution A. KH_2PO_4, 0.067M
      KH_2PO_4, 9.08 g
      Distilled water to make 1 L
   Solution B. Na_2HPO_4, 0.067M
      Na_2HPO_4, anhydrous, 9.47 g
      Distilled water to make 1 L
   Mix 1.3 parts solution A and 8.7 parts solution B to obtain 1 dl or multiples of it. Immediately before use, add 200 mg glucose to 1 dl buffer.
3. Acetylphenylhydrazine solution
      Acetylphenylhydrazine powder, 100 mg
      Phosphate buffer, 1 dl
   This solution must be prepared fresh and used within 1 hr.
4. Crystal violet solution
      Crystal violet, 2 g
      NaCl solution, 0.73%, 10 ml
   Shake the solution for 5 min and filter it. Mix the filtrate with an equal quantity of 0.73% NaCl solution.

Procedure: Suspend 0.1 ml whole blood in 2 ml acetylphenylhydrazine solution in a 12 mm (inner diameter) test tube. The pipet used is a 0.1 ml "blowout" pipet that is left in the test tube. Mix the suspension immediately and aerate it two or three times by drawing it up into the pipet and blowing it out together with a small quantity of air. Incubate the material at 37° C for 4 hr. After completion of 2 hr incubation, aerate the mixture again briefly. After 4 hr, aerate again and place a small drop of the mixture on a coverslip. Invert the coverslip onto a microscope slide on which there is a slightly larger drop of crystal violet solution. Allow the mixture to stand for 5-10 min and then examine the wet preparation with the oil-immersion objective.

Result: Nonsensitive erythrocytes generally form one large, well-rounded Heinz body, 1-2 μm in diameter, situated at the margin of the cell. Seldom does the number of Heinz bodies within a cell exceed four. Sensitive erythrocytes usually contain many small Heinz bodies and very seldom the above-mentioned solitary, marginal, well-rounded body (see Figs. 6-31 and 6-32).

Interpretation: See introduction.

Heinz bodies inclusion test

Principle[123,124]: Unstable hemoglobin is denatured within the red cells by the use of a redux dye, such as brilliant cresyl blue, and shows up as intraerythrocytic stained bodies.

Reagents:
1. Brilliant cresyl blue, 1% in normal saline
2. Anticoagulated patient's blood
3. Normal and unstable controls, anticoagulated blood

Procedure: Mix the stain before use and filter a small amount through Whatman no. 42 filter paper. In a test tube mix one part stain and two parts fresh anticoagulated blood. Incubate in a 37° C water bath and prepare blood smears at 20 min, 1 hr and 2 hr intervals. Examine the unstained slides for intracytoplasmic blue inclusions with the oil-immersion lens.

Result: Normal red cells do not form Heinz bodies under the conditions of the test.

Interpretation: The test detects in vivo preformed Heinz bodies. Much longer incubation periods are required to stimulate de novo Heinz body inclusions. Heinz bodies are mostly single but also multiple, pale blue intraerythrocytic inclusions that differ from the dark blue filaments of reticulocytes. They are evidence of an unstable hemoglobin, the presence of which should be confirmed by the isopropranol and heat stability tests or by the acid dilution technic of Kleihauer.[125,126] As the normal spleen selectively removes Heinz bodies from the red cells, they are undetectable before splenectomy and a negative test in the nonsplenectomized patient is of no significance.

Red cell morphology

The precipitation of the unstable hemoglobin within the red cell renders the cell subject to premature splenic destruction, producing a chronic hemolytic anemia that exhibits the stigmata of most hemolytic anemias, such as reticulocytosis, increased serum bilirubin levels (indirect), and decreased haptoglobin concentration.[111] The peripheral smear reveals a somewhat unexpected anisocytosis because of the presence of macrocytes (reticulocytes) and hypochromic microcytes. The latter cells are an expression of the reduction of Hb A synthesis, although—as Weatherall[127] has pointed out many times—a patient with a congenital hemolytic anemia may also be iron deficient. The red cells may show a peripheral "bitten out" defect, the result of splenic pitting of the Heinz bodies.[128]

Hemoglobin H

Hb H (β_4) is an unstable tetramer of four normal β-chains formed in excess as the result of α-chain supression in α-thalassemia 2. In the α-thalassemic newborn there appears a fast hemoglobin called Hb Bart's (γ_4); it is the fetal precursor of Hb H, which replaces it as the infant matures. Hb H is easily precipitated in vivo (and in vitro) and is therefore responsible for the chronic hemolytic anemia described in the discussion of Heinz bodies. The reduction in Hb A is responsible for the hypochromia and microcytosis of the red cells. Peculiar to Hb H are the red cell inclusions that form as the red cell ages.[129-132] In the nonsplenectomized patient the inclusion-bearing cells are pitted or destroyed by the spleen, but Hb H can be precipitated and visualized in the red cells in vitro by incubating the blood in brilliant cresyl blue solution. In the splenectomized patient preformed Hb H inclusions can be demonstrated by in vitro exposure of the red cells to new methylene blue, the reticulocyte stain (see Fig. 6-30).

On cellulose acetate electrophoresis at pH 8.6 Hb H and Bart's move more rapidly than Hb A. The reduction in α-chain synthesis in Hb H disease is responsible for a reduction in Hb A_2 to about 1-1.5%.[133] In myeloproliferative disorders a similar but acquired depression of α-chain synthesis has been reported and may lead to the formation of Hb H.[134] Hb H has a high oxygen affinity, which is demonstrated by the pronounced displacement of the oxygen dissociation curve to the left.

In Southeast Asia about 50% of individuals with apparent Hb H disease have Hb H associated with Hb

Constant Spring,[135] which is responsible for a slow-moving hemoglobin band and consists of two normal β-chains and two abnormal α-chains, to each of which 31 amino acids are added.

Stain for hemoglobin H inclusions

Principle: If red cells containing Hb H are exposed to brilliant cresyl blue, the denatured Hb H precipitates in the red cells in the form of stained inclusions.[129,131,132]

Reagents:
1. Citrate saline
   a. Sodium citrate, 1.5 g
      Water, 50 ml
   b. Citrate solution, 10 ml
      Saline, 40 ml
2. Brilliant cresyl blue, 0.5 g
   Citrate saline, 50 ml
   Refrigerate; before use filter the solution through Whatman no. 42 or 44 filter paper.

Procedure: In two small test tubes (one for the unknown and one for the control) mix 2 drops of fresh anticoagulated blood and 2 drops of filtered stain. Incubate in a 37° C water bath for 20 min. Prepare smears and examine the wet preparations under oil immersion.

Result: Hb H precipitates in most erythrocytes as single or multiple pale bluish green, rounded bodies (see Fig. 6-30).

LABORATORY DIAGNOSIS OF THE THALASSEMIAS

The thalassemias are a heterogeneous group of inherited disorders of hemoglobin synthesis in which there is a defect in the synthesis of one or more of the normal polypeptide chains[136-140] that leads to a decrease in or complete absence of the affected chain (or chains). The disease is inherited as an autosomal dominant trait and has the highest incidence in people of Mediterranean, African, and Asian origin. If there is not total suppression of the affected chain, the fraction of the affected chain that is synthesized is structurally normal, unlike hemoglobin variants, in which the affected chain is always structurally abnormal. The decreased synthesis of one chain is responsible for (1) the reduction of the intracellular hemoglobin and for the hypochromic microcytic anemia and (2) the unbalanced production of the unaffected chain, which forms intracellular aggregates that are responsible for the accelerated destruction of the red cells and thus for the hemolytic anemia of the thalassemias. Thalassemias are defined according to the chain that is quantitatively reduced. In α-thalassemia the synthesis of α-chains is reduced and in β-thalassemia the β-chain synthesis is reduced. If the fetal hemoglobin chains (γ, ε, ζ) are involved, fetal or embryonic death results.

Genetically thalassemia may be caused by the following:
1. A defect in the messenger RNA, which contains instructions for amino acid polymerization, so that a certain globin chain is not produced
2. Deletion of all or part of the genes controlling the amino acid sequence of a given chain

The polypeptide sequence of the α-, β-, δ-, and γ-chains is controlled by separated allelic pairs of genes per individual, and in the case of the α- and γ-globin chains there is evidence of gene duplication.[141] In homozygous thalassemia both or all genes for the synthesis of a particular chain are affected, while in heterozygous thalassemia only one or two of the genes is mutant. Both α- and β-thalassemias may exist in association with structural hemoglobin variants and with other types of thalassemias.

The classification of thalassemia into major, intermediate, and minor forms describes the clinical severity of the disorder irrespective of the type of globin chain synthesis involved. Thalassemia major is a life-threatening congenital anemia, whereas thalassemia minor is a mild, asymptomatic disease.

The laboratory study of thalassemias requires the investigation of the following parameters:

Red cells: morphology, indices, osmotic fragility, intraerythrocytic inclusions, and red cell survival studies
Hemoglobin electrophoresis or chromatography
Quantitation of Hb F and A_2
Serum iron and total iron-binding capacity assays
Family studies
Study of the rate of chain synthesis in reticulocytes with ^{14}C leucine (a radioactive amino acid precursor)[142]

α-Thalassemia

There are four varieties of α-thalassemia, as there may be loss of function of one to four α-genes. The α-thalassemia genotypes are designated as α^1 or α^0, indicating the loss of two α-loci on the same chromosome, or as α^2 or α^+, indicating the loss of only one of four α-loci.[143] In Hb Constant Spring an abnormally long α-chain is synthesized, leading to an overall chain deficit.

Classification of α-thalassemias[144,145]

α-Thalassemia 1 (α^0 thal, α thal 1), heterozygous, homozygous
α-Thalassemia 2 (α^+ thal, α thal 2), heterozygous, homozygous, Hb Bart's (hydrops fetalis)
Hb H disease
Hb Constant Spring, heterozygous, homozygous
α-Thalassemia in association with α-chain hemoglobin variants (Hb Q, I, or Constant Spring)
α-Thalassemia with β-chain variants (HbS, C, or E) or β-chain thalassemia

Heterozygous α-thalassemia (thalassemia trait)

α-Thalassemia trait (α thal 1, α^0 thal) is the result of deletion or absent function of two of four α-genes. The patients are asymptomatic, and the disorder is usually discovered on routine laboratory examination. In the adult there may be no anemia at all or only a mild hypochromic anemia with a hemoglobin concentration of 10-12 g/dl and a reduction in the MCV, MCH, and MCHC levels. The red cell count may be normal or increased to about 5 million/mm³. The discriminant function of England and Fraser[146] derived from indices obtained on a Coulter S counter can be used to diagnose or suspect heterozygosity for α-thalassemia[147] (see Chapter 8). The blood film reflects the hypochromic microcytic nature of the anemia and shows slight anisocytosis, poikilocytosis, and very rare Hb H inclusions if suitably stained. The osmotic fragility is decreased and the serum iron level is normal. Hemoglobin electrophoresis reveals normal levels of Hb A and F and slightly decreased or normal Hb A_2 levels,[148] which distinguish it from β thal trait ($β^+$ thal or $β^0$ thal). The loss of three or four gene loci leads to the formation of Hb H ($β_4$). The diagnosis of heterozygous α-thalassemia may be difficult at times, and family studies may be necessary to find members with a mild hypochromic microcytic anemia that is not caused by iron deficiency.

In the newborn the diagnosis of α-thalassemia trait is easier because of the presence of Hb Bart's[148] ($γ_4$), which in the case of α-thalassemia 2 trait amounts to 1-2% at birth and in α-thalassemia 1 trait, 5-6%.[148] Within the first few months of life Hb Bart's disappears and no abnormal hemoglobins can be demonstrated, but after the first year of life a microcytic hypochromic anemia may develop.

Heterozygous α-thalassemia 2 (α thal 2, $α^+$ thal) is caused by deletion of one α-gene and is not accompanied by any abnormal hemotologic findings.

Homozygous α-thalassemia (Hb Bart's hydrops fetalis syndrome)

The homozygosity of α-thalassemia 1 ($α^0$ thal),[149] the complete suppression of all α-chains, is incompatible with life because the α-chains are essential for normal oxygen transport and release. The afflicted infants die in utero or shortly after birth of hydrops fetalis, a generalized form of anasarca and edema resulting from anoxic heart failure. The blood picture is that of severe thalassemia: small, deformed, and distorted hypochromic microcytic cells alternating with macrocytes that reflect the reticulocytosis and with a few Hb H–bearing cells. Hemoglobin electrophoresis reveals 80-100% Hb Bart's ($γ_4$), low concentrations of Hb H ($β_4$), and no Hb A, F, or A_2. The hemoglobin electrophoretogram reflects the formation of tetramers by the unmated (no α-chains) β- and γ-chains.[150]

Homozygosity of α-thalassemia 2 ($α^+$ thal), caused by deletion of one α-gene, leads to a mild anemia or is free of any abnormal hematologic findings.

Hemoglobin H (β₄) disease

Hb H disease is the result of the combination of α-thalassemia 1 and α-thalassemia 2. There is therefore complete suppression of one α-chain and partial suppression of the other, leading to various combinations of Hb A, H, Bart's, and A_2.[132] There is a mild hemolytic anemia from a slight to moderate reduction in the concentration of hemoglobin (7-10 g/dl) in the MCV, in the MCH, and in the MCHC, but the red cell count may be high. The blood film reflects the hypochromic microcytic nature of the anemia and shows the picture of a moderate homozygous α-thalassemia including fragmented cells, poikilocytosis, anisocytosis, basophilic stippling, and target cells. Reticulocytosis is moderate (10%) and reflects the bone marrow erythroid

hyperplasia. The bone marrow iron is usually normal. On the hemoglobin electrophoretogram the average concentration of Hb H varies from 8-10%, but it may reach values up to 40%. Hb Bart's is present in much lower concentrations than Hb H. Hb F, A_2, and A are present in low concentrations. In newborns and infants Hb Bart's ($γ_4$) is found in concentrations up to 40%. It is the precursor of Hb H. The latter is an unstable hemoglobin that precipitates in the majority of red cells and bone marrow normoblasts if they are incubated with brilliant cresyl blue or new methylene blue (see Chapter 8).

α-Thalassemia associated with α-chain hemoglobin variants, hemoglobin Constant Spring[151-154]

In a small percentage of patients with Hb H disease, cellulose acetate electrophoresis at pH 8.6 shows a slow-moving band between the origin and Hb A_2, which represents a hemoglobin variant with an abnormal elongated α-chain called Hb Constant Spring. The heterozygous form shows no hematologic abnormalities, and the homozygous form produces a picture similar to moderate Hb H disease. The hemoglobins are those of α-thalassemia 2 (Hb A and A_2) except for 3-5% Hb Constant Spring and Hb H in 50% of Oriental patients and Hb Bart's in infants.

β-Thalassemia

There are two main genetic variations of β-thalassemia, the $β^+$-thalassemia and the $β^0$-thalassemia, depending on the degree (partial or complete) of depression of the β-chain synthesis.[155] Clinically the two types are not distinguishable and can only be differentiated by hemoglobin electrophoresis. β-Thalassemia occurs in the heterozygous and homozygous forms as well as in association with β- and α-chain variants and with α-thalassemia. There is also a linkage between the β-thalassemia gene and the δ structural gene,[156] so that in the δ-β-thalassemias there is an absence of synthesis of both δ- and β-chains.

Classification of β-thalassemia

$β^+$-Thalassemia ($β^+$ thal), heterozygous, homozygous

$β^0$-Thalassemia ($β^0$ thal), heterozygous, homozygous

δ-$β^0$-Thalassemia (δ-$β^0$ thal), heterozygous, homozygous

δ-$β^+$-Thalassemia (δ-$β^+$ thal), heterozygous, homozygous

δ-β-Lepore, heterozygous, homozygous

Hereditary persistence of fetal hemoglobin (HPFH) heterozygous, homozygous

Heterozygous β-thalassemia

Weatherall considers the heterozygous β-thalassemia to be a homogeneous disorder characterized by a mild anemia (hemoglobin level of 9-11 g/dl) or by no anemia at all depending on the completeness of the suppression of the β-chain synthesis. The severity of the anemia and of the red cell changes is similar in heterozygous $β^+$- and $β^0$-thalassemia. The red cell count may be slightly lowered, normal, or increased (up to 7 million/dl). The MCV and MCH are strikingly low (MCH of 20 pg) even in the face of erythrocytosis. The MCV is usually between 55 and 56 fl; values greater than 75 fl rule out thalassemia.[140] The MCHC may be normal, slightly increased, or slightly lowered. The reticulocyte count is normal. The blood smear may reveal a normal picture but usually shows a moderate number of abnormal red cells, even if the hemoglobin level is almost normal. The red cell morphology may actually resemble that seen in the homozygous form—microcytic hypochromic cells mixed with target cells, poikilocytes, schistocytes, teardrop cells, and cells showing basophilic stippling and anisocytosis. Basophilic stippling is commonly seen in β-thalassemia trait but is distinctly uncommon in iron deficiency, which may be responsible for an otherwise very similar hematologic picture. Screening cellulose acetate electrophoresis at an alkaline pH reveals Hb A, F, and A₂. Hb A₂ is elevated and should be carefully quantitated by column chromatography. In β-thalassemia trait the amount of Hb A₂ is 5.1 ± 1.35%[110] (normal value: 1.5-3.5%). By depressing the Hb A₂ values iron deficiency may mask β-thalassemia trait,[111] but adequate treatment of the iron deficiency should restore the elevated Hb A₂ level. Family studies such as studies of Hb A₂ levels in first-degree relatives are also indicated. If iron deficiency is excluded, normal Hb A₂ levels in β-thalassemia trait are unusual, except in δ-β-thalassemia trait where the δ-chain of Hb A₂ is suppressed. Even though Hb A₂ elevation is the diagnostic criterion of heterozygous β-thalassemia, it must be noted that Hb A₂ may also be elevated when unstable hemoglobins are present. Hb F is slightly increased (2-7%) in about 50% of cases, a feature that is not characteristic, as Hb F is elevated in many blood diseases.[148] Hb F is normal in less than 1% of patients. The acid elution technic of Kleihauer reveals the heterogeneous distribution of Hb F within a few of the red cells. In heterozygous β-thalassemia it is the elevated Hb A₂ level that aids in the diagnosis; the Hb F level is helpful only in the diagnosis of homozygous thalassemia, in which its concentration may vary from 20-100%. The osmotic fragility is decreased, but such decreased values are also observed in iron deficiency. The serum iron and bone marrow iron are normal or slightly increased, just the opposite of what is found in iron deficiency anemia. The elevated erythrocyte protoporphyrin level of iron deficiency anemia may also be used to exclude thalassemia trait in which it is normal.

Differentiation from iron deficiency anemia

There are a number of considerations and calculations that aid in the differentiation of iron deficiency anemia from β-thalassemia trait in the absence of biochemical or electrophoretic tests.[157]

Blood smear: In iron deficiency at a hemoglobin level of 10-14 g/dl, the morphologic red cell changes are minimal, whereas in β-thalassemia they are quite striking. In iron deficiency the hemoglobin value must fall about 50% before severe morphologic red cell changes occur.

Gross inspection of serum: In iron deficiency anemia the serum is colorless; in β-thalassemia it has the normal yellowish tinge.

Calculations: Some cases of iron deficiency and heterozygous β-thalassemia can be differentiated on the basis of the preceding considerations alone, but the use of a mathematical formula called discriminant function (DF) identified 99% of these anemias correctly.[146] The formula is based on the MCV (fl), the red cell count $\times 10^6/\mu l$, and the hemoglobin concentration (g/dl):

$$DF = MCV - RBC - (5 \times Hb) - 3.4$$

Result: A positive value (over 0) indicates iron deficiency and a negative value (below 0) indicates thalassemia trait. The formula is not applicable in pregnancy and in iron deficiency superimposed on thalassemia.

A somewhat simpler formula was devised by Mentzer[158]:

$$DF = \frac{MCV\ (fl)}{RBC \times 10^6/\mu l}$$

Values below 13 indicate β-thalassemia trait; values over 13 are usually found in iron deficiency anemia.

Homozygous β-thalassemia (β⁺ and β⁰ thal, β-thalassemia major, Cooley's anemia)

Red cell pathology: The homozygous complete or incomplete suppression of β-chain production leads to a severe hypochromic microcytic hemolytic anemia with hemoglobin levels of 2-3 g/dl or less that is noted in the first year of life. In utero and during the first months of life the affected children fail to show evidence of an anemia because of the protection afforded by Hb F, but after the disappearance of Hb F the blood film shows striking variation in size and shape of red cells and the presence of target cells, basophilic stippling, normoblasts, polychromatic macrocytes, and teardrop cells (see Fig. 6-6). The reticulocyte count is elevated to about 10%. Staining of bone marrow and peripheral blood smears with methyl violet reveals α-**chain excess inclusions (Heinz bodies)** in polychromatophilic and orthochromatic normoblasts and in erythrocytes. Their size and number are a reflection of the overall deficiency of their partner β-chains.[159] This phenomenon of α-chain excess inclusions is not seen in heterozygotes[159] and is diagnostic of homozygous β-thalassemia. The **bone marrow** shows marked erythroid hyperplasia, mostly ineffective, with increased iron deposits in macrophages and in sideroblasts that also show increased glycogen deposits[159] as demonstrated by the PAS reaction.

Osmotic fragility: The red cell membranes show increased rigidity, and the flat, thin cells are responsible for a decreased osmotic fragility.

Hemoglobin electrophoresis[159]: The Hb F concentration may vary from 10-90%, and the distribution in the red cells as determined by the Kleihauer technic is heterogeneous in type. The Hb A₂ concentration may vary from 1.4-20%, embracing low, normal, elevated, and very high values. In homozygous β-thalassemia, even if the Hb A₂ value is low or normal in the patient, it will be high in both parents. If the Hb A₂ level in the patient is expressed as a percentage of the total hemoglobin, it spans the previously mentioned spectrum from low to high, but if it is expressed in relation to the Hb A value only, it is increased in all cases of β-thalassemia, e.g., an A/A_2 ratio of about 10:1 as compared to the normal A/A_2 ratio of about 40:1. If the Hb A_2 level is markedly increased Hb F is normal or only slightly elevated, and vice versa. In β^0-thalassemia there is a total absence of Hb A, so that the patient's hemoglobin consists only of Hb F and A_2, while in β^+ thalassemia diminished amounts of Hb A are found (5-20%). In both thalassemias free α-chains may be seen close to the application point of the electrophoretogram at alkaline pH.[160]

Iron metabolism: The serum iron and the bone marrow iron deposits are increased. The iron is seen not only in an increased number of sideroblasts and reticuloendothelial macrophages but also in the form of ring sideroblasts.[159] The total iron-binding capacity is completely saturated.

Other related biochemical findings: Because of the hemolytic component of the anemia, serum unconjugated bilirubin levels are elevated and haptoglobin is absent. Serum glutamic oxaloacetic transaminase (SGOT), lactic dehydrogenase (LDH), and erythropoietin concentrations are raised. The erythropoietin elevation is responsible for the 20-30% increase in erythropoietic marrow and is a result of the anemia and the high oxygen affinity of Hb F, which further increases the tissue anoxia. The liver involvement (hemosiderosis) may lead to a bleeding tendency. Gross examination of the urine may show the brown color of dipyrroles, which is probably caused by the excessive intramedullary hemolysis of normoblasts.

δ-β-*Thalassemia (F-thalassemia)*

The depression of β- and δ-chain synthesis leads to a variable anemia, depending on whether the condition is homozygous or heterozygous.

Heterozygous δ-β-*thalassemia*[161]

Red cell pathology: There is a mild anemia with red cell counts of 5-6 million/mm³ and with hemoglobin levels ranging from 11-12 g/dl. The blood film reveals abnormal red cell morphology classified as 1+ to 2+, similar to that seen in β-thalassemia trait. Despite this low-grade anemia, the MCV and MCH values are low, the latter ranging from 19-24 pg.

Hemoglobin electrophoresis and the Kleihauer stain: Hb F is increased to about 5-20%, or it may be normal. The remaining hemoglobin is made up of Hb A and normal levels of Hb A_2. The Kleihauer stain reveals heterogenous distribution of Hb F.

Family studies: It is clear from the preceding description that the relatively low F-variant of heterogenous δ-β thalassemia is difficult to diagnose, as it resembles iron deficiency anemia or α-thalassemia trait; family studies are necessary to arrive at a diagnosis.

Homozygous δ-β-*thalassemia*[162]

Red cell pathology: The hemoglobin values range from 4-10 g/dl. The hemolytic anemia is microcytic hypochromic and morphologically resembles homozygous β-thalassemia. Excess α-chain inclusions have been demonstrated both in the bone marrow and in the peripheral blood.

Hemoglobin electrophoresis[159]: Hb F completely replaces all other hemoglobins, so that Hb A and A_2 are absent.

Hemoglobin Lepore thalassemia[163]

Hb Lepore (named after the individual in whom it was first discovered) is a structurally abnormal hemoglobin in which the α-chain is normal and the non-α-chain is made up of one section of the δ-chain and one section of the β-chain. Hb Lepore is considered part of the δ-β-thalassemia syndrome because its concentration appears to be fixed at a low level[165] and there is absence of normal β- and δ-chain synthesis. Hb Lepore occurs in homozygous and heterozygous forms and in association with β-thalassemia and β-hemoglobin variants (Hb S and C).

Heterozygous Hb Lepore thalassemia

Red cell pathology: The hematologic findings are similar to those of heterozygous β-thalassemia.

Hemoglobin electrophoresis: Hb F is increased, while the concentration of Hb A_2 is slightly reduced (1.9-2.3%). Hb Lepore concentration varies from 10-15% and has the **electrophoretic mobility of Hb S**[164] at alkaline pH but does not sickle. The remaining hemoglobin consists of Hb A.

Homozygous Hb Lepore thalassemia

Red cell pathology: The hematologic findings are similar to those of homozygous β-thalassemia.

Hemoglobin electrophoresis: Hb F is about 80% of the total hemoglobin. The concentration of Hb Lepore amounts to about 30%, and Hb A and A_2 are absent.

Hereditary persistence of fetal hemoglobin

Hereditary persistence of fetal hemoglobin (HPFH) is considered to be a form of thalassemia, since the persistence of Hb F (γ-chain synthesis) into adult life can be regarded as a compensation for deficient δ- and β-chain synthesis and may thus represent a form of δ-β-thalassemia. HPFH may occur in the homozygous and heterozygous forms and in association with Hb S and C or with β-thalassemia.

Heterozygous hereditary persistence of fetal hemoglobin

Red cell pathology: There is no anemia and no morphologic red cell change.

Hemoglobin electrophoresis and Kleihauer stain: Hb F attains concentrations up to 15-35% and is evenly distributed throughout the red cells as demonstrated by the Kleihauer technic. The concentration of Hb A_2 is somewhat diminished to about 1.5%, and the remaining hemoglobin mass consists of Hb A.

Heterozygous hereditary persistence of fetal hemoglobin with hemoglobin S

Red cell pathology: There is no anemia and no morphologic red cell changes.

Hemoglobin electrophoresis and Kleihauer stain: The average concentration of Hb F is about 35%, and the hemoglobin is homogeneously distributed throughout all red cells. This distribution pattern is quite different from the heterogeneous distribution pattern seen in β-thalassemia with Hb S. The hemoglobin electrophoretograms of both conditions may be identical. The Hb A_2 concentration is increased. The remaining hemoglobin mass consists of Hb S, as Hb A is absent.

Homozygous hereditary persistence of fetal hemoglobin[166]

Red cell pathology: There is usually an erthrocytosis in response to the 100% Hb F level with its high oxygen affinity and the resulting relative oxygen starvation of the tissues.

Hemoglobin electrophoresis and Kleihauer stain: The total hemoglobin mass consists of Hb F. The outstanding feature of all forms of HPFH is the homozygous distribution of Hb F throughout the red cells as demonstrated by the Kleihauer technic. Hb A and A_2 are absent.

LABORATORY INVESTIGATION OF IRON

Iron in the form of iron-complexed proteins is widely distributed in the body. Some of these iron proteins are oxygen carriers, such as hemoglobin and myoglobin; others have to do with iron transport (**transferrin**) and storage (**ferritin**) and with electron transport (cytochromes). Aberrations in the iron metabolism affect the iron proteins directly and all other body systems and organs indirectly.

The biosynthesis of hemoglobin requires that its three components—iron, protoporphyrin, and globin—are available in optimal amounts.[167] About 70% of the body iron is locked in hemoglobin, 3% in myoglobin, 0.5% in heme enzymes, and 0.1% in transferrin.

Iron absorption and transport (Fig. 4-16)

The food iron in its bivalent form is taken up by the mucosa of the duodenum and by other segments of the small bowel. Within the mucosal cell it is oxidized to the trivalent form by ferroxidases[168] and ceruloplasmin.[169] The rate of iron absorption is a mucosal function influenced by the level of the body's iron stores. The iron traverses the mucosal cell and is taken up by the transferrin of the plasma within the rich capillary network of the intestinal mucosa. Iron that is not absorbed is bound by ferritin, an intracellular protein (iron plus aproferritin), some of which the mucosal cell excretes into the bloodstream.[170] In the bloodstream the transferrin-bound iron is carried to the bone marrow and offered to the normoblasts for hemoglobin synthesis, which takes place in their mitochondria. An enzyme, the heme synthetase (ferrochelatase), complexes the iron with protoporphyrin to form heme (Chapter 27). The iron-laden normoblasts (sideroblasts) can be visualized with the Prussian blue reaction, and under normal conditions the blue-stained granules are minute and not in the area of the mitochondria. If the heme synthesis is interfered with, mitochondrial iron can be visualized surrounding the nucleus, producing the picture of **ring sideroblasts**.[171]

Iron excretion

Iron is almost totally retained once it is incorporated into the body either through intestinal absorption or by means of parenteral administration (blood transfusions). The body is able to excrete or lose only minimal amounts of iron in the urine (0.1 mg/day), in feces (shed cells and microscopic amounts of blood, 0.6 mg/day), in shed cutaneous cells, and in perspiration (0.1 mg/day). Menstruation represents a large physiologic iron loss (25-30 mg/day).

Assessment of the iron status

Various routes and approaches are available to test the adequacy of iron:
1. The blood picture (see discussion of iron deficiency anemia in Chapter 8)

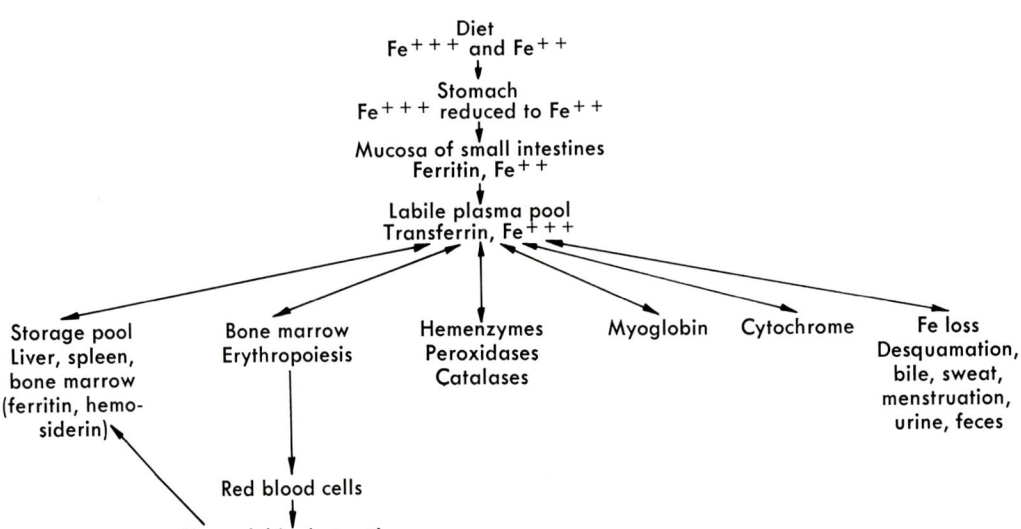

Fig. 4-16. Outline of iron metabolism.

2. Serum ferritin assay
3. Sideroblasts and siderocytes
4. Serum iron, total iron-binding capacity, and transferrin saturation
5. Ferrokinetics
6. Free erythrocyte porphyrin assay

Serum ferritin

Serum ferritin is a water-soluble storage protein for iron and is present in large amounts in the spleen, liver, and bone marrow. Its apo- form is produced intracellularly in response to the presence of iron, and when combined with the iron it becomes ferritin.[172] The relationship of ferritin to hemosiderin is not quite clear; both are increased when the iron stores increase, and both decrease in iron deficiency. Under normal conditions half the stored iron is in the form of ferritin. How ferritin reaches the circulating plasma is not known, as it reflects both parenchymal and reticuloendothelial iron. Ferritins of different organs reveal differences in electrophoretic mobility, and these differing proteins are called **isoferritins.**[173]

Serum ferritin assay

The small amounts of plasma needed for the assay make it ideal for the investigation of the iron status in infants and children.

The Corning Immo Phase ferritin (^{125}I) radioimmunoassay is supplied in kit form (Corning Medical and Scientific, Medfield, Mass.).

Principle: The Corning Immo Phase assay provides a sensitive and precise test utilizing a solid-phase antibody, which is covalently coupled to microscopic glass particles, and a second highly purified radioactive (^{125}I) ferritin antibody. The assay is quantitated in terms of radioactive ferritin antibody bound to solid-phase antibody-ferritin complexes. A test of this kind is known as a "sandwich assay," or a two-site immunoradiometric assay.

This ferritin sandwich assay employs constant amounts of two antibodies, one covalently bonded to glass particles and the other radioiodinated and free in solution. A variable amount of antigen is provided by the patient samples and the standards. The ferritin antibody bonded to the glass particles will bind to any ferritin present and form a solid-phase complex. After a short equilibration period a second ferritin antibody that has been iodinated is added to the reaction mixture. This serves to label the solid-phase complex formed in the first step. The solid-phase complex is separated by centrifugation and is counted for (^{125}I) radioactivity. A standard curve is constructed in which radioactivity is plotted against known ferritin concentrations (standards). The ferritin concentration of patient samples is determined by interpolation from the standard curve. Sandwich assays have a direct relationship between the amount of ferritin present and counts bound. The more ferritin present, the more counts will be bound.

Normal mean values[174]:
Adult men: 25-125 ng/ml
Adult women: 10-100 ng/ml
Newborns: 101 ng/ml
Infants (first month): 350 ng/ml

Infants (up to 6 months): 30 ng/ml
Children up to 15 years: 70 ng/ml

These values confirm the physiologically low iron stores of women and the high iron stores at birth, which then rapidly decrease.

Interpretation: Serum ferritin levels parallel the size of iron stores. In iron deficiency the serum ferritin level is consistently low (below 10 ng/ml) and appears to be a more reliable diagnostic criterion than serum iron or iron-binding capacity and bone marrow iron stains. A serum ferritin level below 10 ng/ml corresponds to a transferrin saturation of less than 16%. In the anemia of infection serum ferritin is normal or elevated. In addition to an iron deficiency, decreased levels are found in pregnant women, in hemodialysis patients, in patients with inflammatory bowel disease, and in patients who have had gastric surgery.[172]

Increased levels of ferritin are associated with a number of conditions. In acute myelogenous leukemia[175] and multiple myeloma[176] the increased synthesis of ferritin by the tumor cells can be used as an indicator of neoplastic activity, and the return to normal ferritin levels speaks for successful therapy.

Iron overload as seen in primary refractory anemia or following transfusion therapy raises the ferritin concentration to 1790 ± 266 ng/ml. In hemochromatosis markedly increased levels up to 4000 ng/ml may be obtained. Similar high levels are seen in hepatitis. In the precirrhotic stage of hemochromatosis the serum ferritin values are unexpectedly low, showing no correlation with serum iron, total iron-building capacity (TIBC), and transferrin saturation.[177,178]

In inflammatory and necrotizing disorders the elevated ferritin level reflects increased apoferritin synthesis, not increases in total body iron storage. Despite this disadvantage, the test is a valuable adjunct in the investigation of disorders of iron metabolism.

Sideroblasts and siderocytes
Bone marrow sideroblasts

Bone marrow smears and clot sections should routinely by stained with Prussian blue stain, and under certain circumstances peripheral smears should also be included.

Sideroblasts[171,179] are normoblasts that contain Prussian blue-positive granules within the cytoplasm, which can be visualized by light microscopy (oil-immersion lens). The granules vary from fine dustlike particles that are difficult to see to coarser masses that are evenly distributed and do not usually exceed four in number. By electron microscopy the iron granules are seen as aggregates of ferritin, free within the cytoplasm, not within mitochondria or associated with other cytoplasmic organelles.[180] The number of these granules as seen by light microscopy correlates well with the percent saturation of transferrin (see 1 and 2 in Plate 3, p. 147).

Normal values: The values for bone marrow are 30-50%.

Interpretation: In iron deficiency anemia and in anemia of infection when serum iron and percent saturation of transferrin values are low, sideroblasts are decreased or absent. Increased numbers of sideroblasts,[181] which contain an increased number of coarse iron granules evenly distributed, are found in hemolytic and megaloblastic anemias, siderosis, and hemochromatosis. In these conditions the serum iron level and the transferrin percent saturation are increased.[182]

Reticulated siderocytes

Reticulated siderocytes (R-S cells) are reticulocytes that not only contain a new methylene blue–positive reticulum but also Prussian blue–positive siderocytic granules. Two staining procedures are therefore necessary to distinguish R-S cells from reticulocytes (which are iron negative) and from siderocytes (which are new methylene blue negative). The R-S cells are young reticulocytes released into the peripheral blood from the bone marrow sideroblasts. They contain evenly distributed ferritin granules not associated with mitochondria or other organelles. The iron pattern is that of their precursor cells.

Normal value: The value for peripheral blood is 0.03%.

Interpretation: R-S cells are rarely found in normal peripheral blood. They are increased in the peripheral circulation whenever there is rapid blood regeneration, as in hemolytic anemias, which lead to a premature release of young reticulocytes into the circulation.

Siderocytes

Siderocytes (S cells) are mature red cells (thus devoid of mitochondria or ribosomes) that contain siderotic granules within the cytoplasm (see Fig. 6-33).

Normal value: The value for peripheral blood is 0.01%.

Interpretation: S cells are rarely found in the normal peripheral blood. They are increased after splenectomy and in hemolytic anemias.

Abnormal sideroblasts

There are two abnormal types of sideroblasts. One form as described above is associated with hemolytic anemias and contains an increased number of **coarse siderotic granules** in the cytoplasm. These granules are not related to mitochondria or to other organelles.

The second form has large amounts of iron deposited in perinuclear mitochondria. These cells are called **ring sideroblasts** and are always abnormal and associated with hereditary and acquired sideroblastic anemias, the prototype of which is pyridoxine deficiency, a disorder of heme synthesis. They have also been described in idiopathic and secondary aplastic anemias and in chronic alcoholism.[183] Light microscopy (Prussian blue stain) shows a ring of fine to coarse sideritic granules surrounding the nucleus. By electron microscopy the iron is seen not to be associated with ferritin but to lie between the cristae of distorted mitochondria. Normally ring sideroblasts are not found in the bone marrow, but in sideroblastic anemias 40-70% of normoblasts are ring sideroblasts. Maturation of ring sideroblasts leads to R-S cells with mitochondrial nonferritin iron deposits. However, by light microscopy with new methylene blue–Prussian blue stain these cells cannot be differentiated from normal R-S cells. Similarly their product of maturation, the S cell, cannot be differentiated from a normal S cell. The fact that the erythrocyte copropor-phyrin and protoporphyrin are elevated in ring sideroblastic erythropoiesis offers biochemical proof that ring sideroblasts are the result of a disturbance of the mitochondrial iron metabolism and of the heme synthesis pathway.[184]

Serum iron assay

Two chemical methods are described in Chapter 22. One recent radioactive method is outlined here.

Iron-binding capacity by radioassay kit

The test is marketed in kit form (Iron Binding Capacity Radioassay Kit [^{59}Fe]) by Becton-Dickinson & Co., Rutherford, N.J.[185]

Principle: The principle of isotope dilution is followed in the determination of total iron-binding capacity. Iron is dissociated from transferrin by lowering the pH of the serum below pH 5, and a known amount of iron, which includes radioiron, is added. The added iron mixes with the comparatively small amount of released endogenous iron, which causes a slight dilution of the specific activity of the radioiron. The reaction mixture is then neutralized, and binding of iron to transferrin takes place. Because there is a large excess of iron present, all of the binding sites become occupied. The unbound or free iron, both cold and radioactive, is removed by an ion-exchange resin (supplied in tablet form). After centrifugation the supernatants containing the bound iron are decanted and counted in a solid crystal scintillation counter.

The unsaturated iron-binding capacity (UIBC) is determined simply by adding a known amount of radioiron to serum at an alkaline pH. Radioiron saturates the unoccupied sites on the transferrin, and free iron is removed in the same way as in the TIBC procedure. The supernatants containing the bound radioiron are decanted and counted in a γ-counter.

The UIBC and TIBC are calculated from the recorded counts using formulas that take into account the amount of iron added and a dilution factor.

It should be reemphasized that this method, by focusing on transferrin, measures only the serum iron bound to it and does not give falsely elevated results because of hemolyzed blood.

Iron concentration is calculated as follows:

$$\text{Iron } (\mu g/dl) = \text{TIBC} - \text{UIBC}$$

Normal values: The normal range of serum iron is 80-150 µg/dl plasma in men and 70-130 µg/dl in women. If expressed in molar concentration, a factor of 0.179 converts these figures to micromoles per liter. The iron level in children below the age of 2 years is physiologically below 100 µg/dl. After the age of 2 years it rises, reaching the adult level at about adolescence. There is a distinct diurnal variation, the highest serum iron value occurring in the morning and the level gradually falling to the lowest value late in the evening. The variation may be as much as 40-100 µg/dl.[186] All blood specimens for serum iron determination should therefore be obtained in the morning in the fasting state, and repeat examinations performed on specimens drawn at identical times. The diurnal variation disappears in hematologic disorders and is reversed in persons who work at night and sleep in the day.[187-189]

Interpretation[190-192]: **Low values** are found in iron deficiency anemia, in chronic infections, in rheumatoid arthritis, in malignant tumors, after gastrectomy, and after surgical operations. Serum iron is also decreased during the period of recovery from hemorrhage and hemolytic anemias (e.g., pernicious anemia responding to treatment) when the stimulated erythropoiesis demands increased supplies of iron.

Increased serum iron levels are found (1) in anemias characterized by decreased hemoglobin formation not caused by iron deficiency, e.g., aplastic and sideroachrestic anemias, (2) in hemolytic anemias, e.g., pernicious anemia and thalassemias, characterized by ineffective erythropoiesis, (3) in acute hepatitis, and (4) after the administration of iron and blood.

Serum iron analysis is a measure of iron in transit, a measure of iron at a specific moment in time. Its level is the result of many interacting forces, e.g., hemoglobin destruction, iron absorption, and release of iron from iron stores. A single serum iron determination may be difficult to interpret and should be confirmed by repetition and by evaluation of the other parameters of the iron metabolism.[193]

Ladenson[194] discusses in detail the many nonanalytic sources of variation in the iron and iron-binding assays.

Total iron-binding capacity

The TIBC measures the maximal saturation of **transferrin** with iron, and it is thus a measure of the total amount of transferrin available for iron binding.[195]

Procedure: The method is described in Chapter 22.

Normal values: Normal values are 280-300 µg/dl serum.

Interpretation: Transferrin is quantitated in terms of the amount of iron it is able to bind. The fluctuations of transferrin concentration from birth to adolescence parallel the increase and decrease of the serum iron concentration just described.

Elevation of total iron-binding capacity: The TIBC is elevated in iron deficiency anemia and by the use of oral contraceptives. Physiologically it is elevated in pregnancy (Fig. 4-17).

Depression of total iron-binding capacity: Decreased levels are found (1) in chronic and acute infections, (2) in debilitating diseases characterized by protein loss or poor protein synthesis (e.g., nephrosis, malignancy, and liver disease), (3) in iron overload, as seen in hemochromatosis and siderosis, (4) in decompensated chronic hemolytic anemias (e.g., pernicious anemia and thalassemia), and (5) in sideroblastic anemia. Physiologically it is reduced in newborns (Fig. 4-17).

Unsaturated iron-binding capacity

The UIBC is a measure of the concentration of transferrin not bound to iron and is arrived at by subtracting the serum iron level from the maximal level of iron-saturated transferrin.

Normal values: Normal values are 200-220 mg/dl.

Interpretation: The UIBC is increased in iron deficiency and pregnancy and is decreased in infections, hemochromatosis, protein deficiencies, and hemolytic anemias (Fig. 4-17).

Laboratory evaluation of transferrin
Percent saturation of transferrin

The percent saturation of transferrin represents the proportion of iron-binding protein that is saturated with

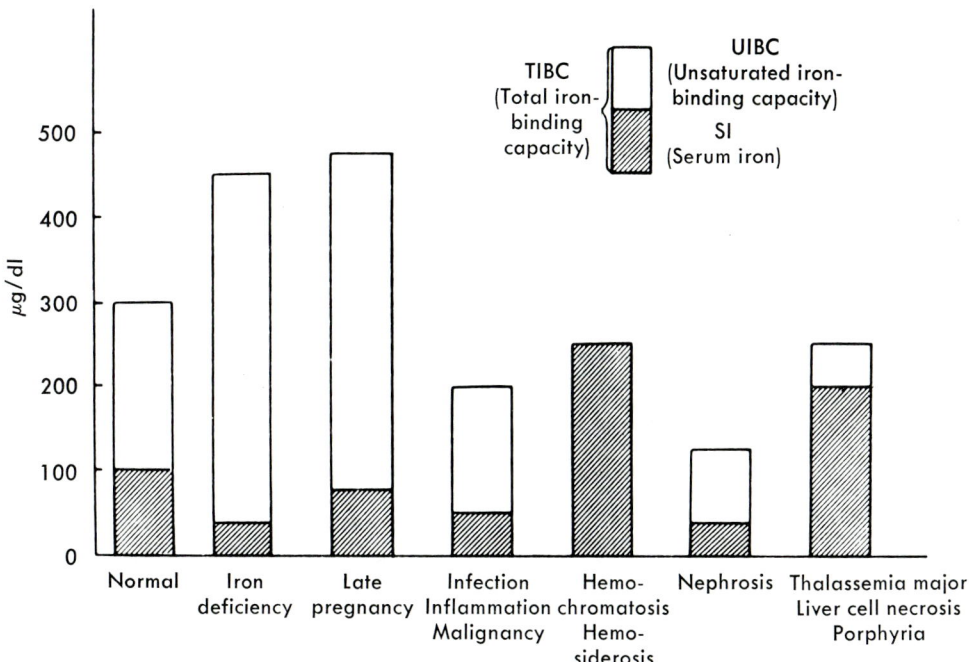

Fig. 4-17. Relationships of serum iron, unsaturated iron-binding capacity, and total iron-binding capacity in various clinical conditions. (From Brown, E.B.: Semin. Hematol. **3**:314, 1966.)

iron. This value is of physiologic importance, for if the degree of saturation is low, iron is mainly utilized for hemoglobinization in the bone marrow, whereas if the degree of saturation is high, the iron is deposited in the reticuloendothelial system and in various organs (liver, kidney, etc.).

$$\text{Saturation of transferrin (\%)} = \frac{\text{Serum iron conc.}}{\text{TIBC}} \times 100$$

Normal range: The normal range is 35-40%.

Interpretation: In iron deficiency anemia the percent saturation is very low—less than 15%.

Ferrokinetics—the path of radioiron[195,196]

Information about the dynamics of iron metabolism and utilization may be obtained by injecting plasma-bound radioiron ^{59}Fe intravenously, followed by activity measurements of appropriate samples of plasma and red cells, and by localization of radioiron in the liver, spleen, and bone marrow by surface counting. The radioiron technic is based on the fact that normally 75-80% of the plasma iron is assimilated by the bone marrow for hemoglobin formation and thus appears in the red cells. Myoglobin and cytochrome synthesis can be ignored as well as the small amount (10%) of feedback of radioactive iron from storage organs and lymphatics. A variety of studies can be undertaken with ^{59}Fe-tagged plasma, e.g., plasma iron clearance, plasma iron turnover rate, and iron utilization.

Technic of tagging plasma with ^{59}Fe

Venous blood is defibrinated with depyrogenized glass beads, and the serum is incubated with ^{59}Fe ferric citrate or ^{59}Fe transferrin.

Plasma iron disappearance time—radioiron plasma clearance

Definition: The plasma iron disappearance time (PIDT) refers to the length of time required for one half of the intravenously injected iron to disappear from the circulation.

Principle: Tagged plasma iron is injected intravenously, and 10, 20, 40, 60, and 120 min after the injection heparinized blood samples are obtained. The plasma radioiron is rapidly diluted in the labile plasma pool and is carried to the bone marrow to aid in hemoglobin synthesis (Fig. 4-18).

Normal values: The value is expressed as PIDT $^1/_2$ and represents the plasma iron disappearance half-time,

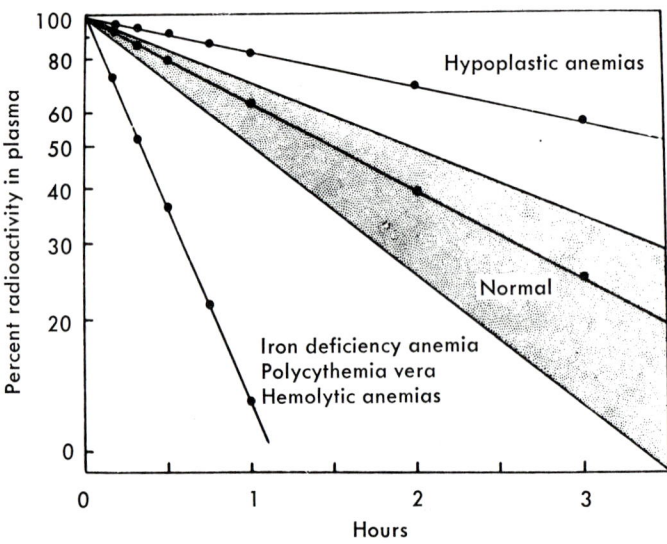

Fig. 4-18. Plasma radioiron clearance curves for normal subjects and patients with increased and decreased erythropoiesis. (From Brown, E.B.: Semin. Hematol. **3**:314, 1966.)

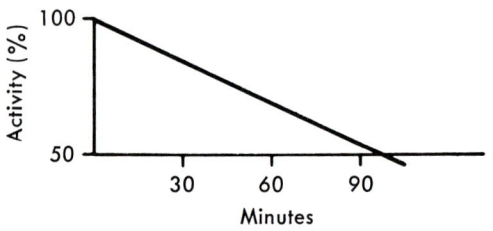

Fig. 4-19. Plasma iron turnover rate. (From Finch, C.A., et al.: Ser. Haematol. **6**:30, 1965.)

the time required for the activity of the plasma to reach half that of time zero, i.e., 50% activity. The normal PIDT $\frac{1}{2}$ is 60-120 min.

Interpretation: The clearance is more rapid when erythropoiesis is increased, as seen in iron deficiency anemia, polycythemia vera, hemolytic anemias, infections, and sideroachrestic anemias. The PIDT $\frac{1}{2}$ is delayed in bone marrow hypoplasia and in hemochromatosis.

The plasma radioiron curve can also be used to obtain the plasma volume and then, on the basis of the hematocrit, the total blood volume.

Plasma iron turnover rate

Definition: The plasma iron turnover rate (PITR) is the amount of iron leaving the plasma per unit time and is expressed as milligrams of iron per day or as milligrams per deciliter of whole blood per day (Fig. 4-19).

Normal values: The normal PITR ranges from 25-40 mg/day and 0.70 mg/dl of whole blood per day. It is assumed that 80% of the iron is taken up by the bone marrow. Uptake by the liver can be excluded by external counting over the liver area.

Interpretation: The PITR is elevated in polycythemia, hemolytic states, and ineffective erythropoiesis, conditions in which the plasma iron clearance is accelerated and the plasma iron is normal or high. The PITR is decreased in hypoplastic anemias, uremia, infections, and radiation exposure, conditions in which the plasma iron clearance is slow and the plasma iron level is low.

The PITR may be used to measure total **effective** and **ineffective erythropoietic** bone marrow **activity** (see below).

Iron utilization by red cells

Definition: Iron utilization by red cells is the percent of injected iron utilized in the production of red cells and is a measure of effective erythropoiesis, giving the amount of bone marrow iron appearing in the peripheral red cell mass (Fig. 4-20). This is in contrast to the PITR, which reflects the total erythropoiesis and thus also includes the ineffective erythropoiesis.

Effective erythropoiesis represents the number of red cells physiologically produced in the bone marrow and released into the circulation. **Ineffective erythropoiesis** represents the number of red cells produced in the bone marrow that are viable but are never released into the circulation.

Normal values: Normally approximately 80% of the administered ^{59}Fe is incorporated into hemoglobin by 14 days.

Interpretation: **Decreased** utilization is found when erythropoiesis is depressed, e.g., in aplastic anemia and in hemolytic anemias associated with ineffective erythropoiesis, such as pernicious anemia and thalassemia in which the maximal incorporation is less than 50%. **Increased** utilization, if erythropoiesis is effective, raises the normal figures only insignificantly and is therefore difficult to diagnose by iron utilization technics, but usually a plateau is reached earlier than is normally seen, i.e., on the fifth and sixth day versus the ninth and tenth day of the normal curve. The level of utilization may climb to 90-98%.

Measurement of radioactivity of various organs— in vivo iron storage

This method is used to investigate the iron deposits in various organs 24 hr after the injection of radioiron. Surface counts are obtained from over the sacrum (bone marrow), liver, spleen, and sternum (bone marrow). For each organ a radioactivity time curve is obtained by plotting against time the surface activity as a percent of the activity found immediately after injection of radioiron. The main areas of storage are the hepatic parenchymal cells and the reticuloendothelial cells of bone marrow, spleen, and liver.

Bone marrow: Normally radioactivity will be found localized in the bone marrow by 24 hr and is greater than the hepatic or splenic activity. The localization of the radioactivity is temporary, disappearing as the iron

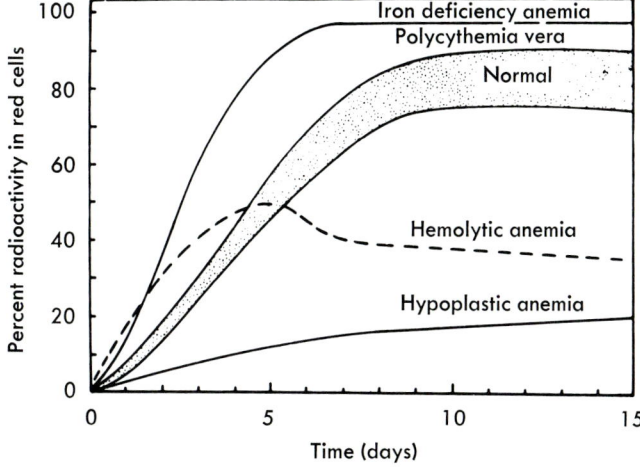

Fig. 4-20. Patterns of utilization of radioiron by peripheral red cells of normal subjects and of patients with hemolytic, hypoplastic, and iron deficiency anemias and polycythemia vera. (From Brown, E.B.: Semin. Hematol. **3:**314, 1966.)

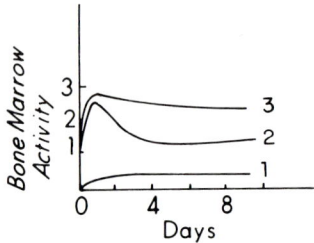

Fig. 4-21. Uptake of radioiron by bone marrow under three conditions. *1*, No radioiron acceptance, as in aplastic anemia; *2*, normal pattern—rapid radioiron incorporation, then slow release into peripheral circulation; *3*, rapid acceptance of radioiron but only minimal release, as seen in sideroachrestic anemia.

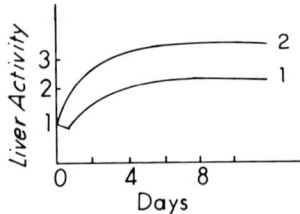

Fig. 4-22. Uptake of radioiron by liver. *1*, Normal pattern—fall of radioactivity in liver during first 24 hr, then slow return to initial level; *2*, radioiron in increased iron storage—initial fall is absent; hepatic iron concentration gradually increases.

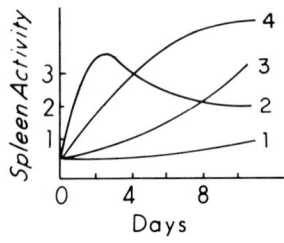

Fig. 4-23. Uptake of radioiron by spleen under four conditions. *1*, Normal gradual rise; *2*, characteristic pattern of extramedullary hematopoiesis; *3*, result of intravascular hemolysis; *4*, pattern of progressive iron storage.

moves into the peripheral circulation. The curve obtained over the bone marrow is thus complementary to the peripheral blood utilization curve of ^{59}Fe. In pathologic conditions the distribution of the radioactivity is altered. In bone marrow aplasia the characteristic steep incorporation phase of the normal curve is absent. In sideroachrestic anemia the marrow uptake is rapid, but the iron is not incorporated into the red cells and stays in the bone marrow (Fig. 4-21).

Liver: Under normal circumstances the liver activity curve falls slightly during the first 24 hr and then slowly increases, as it reflects the activity curve of the peripheral blood. As the radioactivity of the peripheral blood diminishes, it increases in the liver. If there is excessive iron storage in the liver, the initial fall of the

curve is absent and is replaced by a more or less steep initial phase. The ^{59}Fe activity curve of the liver and the ^{59}Fe utilization curve of the peripheral blood reflect only the relative distribution of ^{59}Fe. In bone marrow failure, for instance, the ^{59}Fe will concentrate in the liver since it is not utilized in the bone marrow, but this concentration in the liver does not imply pathologic hepatic iron concentration (Fig. 4-22).

Spleen: The normal splenic uptake of ^{59}Fe shows a gradual slow rise. In iron storage the uptake is rapid and the curve is steep. In extramedullary erythropoiesis the uptake is rapid at first, and then as the red cells are released into the circulation, the curve falls (Fig. 4-23).

Evaluation of porphyrins
Heme synthesis[198,199]

Heme is a tetrapyrrole ring structure composed of four pyrrole rings joined to each other through methane bridges (Fig. 4-1). One iron atom is bound to each pyrrole ring. Heme synthesis occurs in the mitochondria of erythroblasts and reticulocytes. The first heme precursor substance is δ-aminolevulinic acid (ALA), the result of the condensation of glycine and syccinyl coenzyme A from the citric acid cycle by the enzyme δ-aminolevulinic acid synthetase. Two molecules of ALA are combined by the enzyme ALA dehydrase to form porphobilinogen (PBG). Four molecules of PBG are polymerized to form uroporhyrinogen III and I by the enzymes PBG deaminase and PBG isomerase. Uroporphyrinogen III is autooxidated to uroporphyrin III. (Uroporphyrinogen I and its derivatives are not utilized for heme production.) Coproporphyrinogen III is formed by enzymatic decarboxylation of uroporphyrinogen III and is then autooxidated to coproporphyrin III. With the aid of carboxylases and dehydrogenases, coproporphyrinogen III is converted to protoporphyrin IX. Fe^{++} is inserted into the protoporphyrin ring with the aid of heme synthetase to form heme. Hemoglobin is formed by the combination of heme and protein (Fig. 4-2).

Porphyrins form complexes with metal ions to produce various compounds such as hemoglobin, an iron protoporphyrin attached to globin; myoglobin, an iron protoporphyrin occurring in muscle; and cytochrome, an iron-containing transfer agent. Porphyrins consist of four pyrrole rings joined by methane bridges to which various side chains are attached. Porphyrin synthesis occurs in all tissue cells but most richly in the bone marrow and the liver. The physiologic porphyrin levels are dependent on the adequacy of various enzyme systems and can be quantitated in urine, feces, and red cells. The overproduction of prophyrins, **porphyria,** is probably related to the absolute or relative overactivity of some of the various enzymes involved in porphyrin synthesis (see Chapter 27).

All technics mentioned are described in detail in Bauer.[200]

Total free erythrocyte porphyrin assay[201,202]

Principle: The porphyrins are extracted from the red cells with ethyl acetate–acetic acid and reextracted into hydrochloric acid solution in which they are determined fluorometrically. Normally the greater part of the por-

Table 4-10. Assay for porphyrins, ALA dehydratase, and porphyrinogen synthetase in blood: possible applications to detection of some disease states*

Assay	Finding	Disease	µg/dl Erythrocytes†	Confirmatory test
Porphyrins	Protoporphyrin			
	Normal	Normal	20-50	
	Decreased	Megaloblastic anemia	15-30	Low serum vitamin B_{12}
	Increased	Infection	50-300	
		Increased erythropoiesis (hemolytic anemias)	40-150	Decreased erythrocyte survival and bone marrow M/E
		Thalassemia		Target cell, no abnormal Hb
		Sideroachrestic anemia (acquired)	50-700	Siderocytes, increased tissue iron
		Iron deficiency anemia	200-800	Low serum Fe, increased Fe-binding capacity, decreased tissue Fe
		Lead poisoning	200-2000	Lead determination, low dehydratase, decreased osmotic fragility
		Erythropoietic protoporphyria	2200-4400	Photosensitivity, inheritance (dominant)
	Coproporphyrin			
	Normal	Normal	0.5-2.3	
	Increased	Sideroachrestic anemia	0-70	Siderocytes, increased tissue iron
		Congenital erythropoietic porphyria	90-125	Type I porphyrins
		Erythropoietic protoporphyria	135-938	Type III porphyrins
		Erythropoietic coproporphyria		Type III porphyrins
	Uroporphyrin			
	Normal	Normal	Trace	
	Increased	Congenital erythropoietic porphyria	280-420	Type I porphyrins
		Erythropoietic protoporphyria		
ALA dehydratase activity	Normal	Normal	33.8 ± 4.8 µmole/min/L RBCs	
	Decreased	Lead poisoning		Lead determination
	Increased	Increased erythropoiesis		Increased ferrokinetics and reticulocytes
		Iron deficiency		Low serum Fe, increased Fe-binding capacity Decreased tissue iron
Porphyrinogen (uroporphyrinogen and coproporphyrinogen) synthetase activity	Normal	Normal	nmole/ml erythrocytes/hr 35-50	
	Decreased	Acute intermittent porphyria		Neurologic symptoms, ALA, PBG in urine (dark urine particularly on standing)
	Increased	Hemolytic disorders		Decreased erythrocyte survival, increased osmotic fragility

*For details and references, consult original article. Modified from Granick, S., et al.: Proc. Natl. Acad. Sci. U.S.A. **69:**2381, 1972.
†Except when stated.

phyrins in red cells is protoporphyrin IX. In abnormal conditions much larger amounts of coproporphyrins or uroporphyrins may be found. If the increase in total porphyrins is not sufficient for diagnostic purposes, additional tests can be made to aid in distinguishing between abnormal amounts of coproporphyrins and uroporphyrins. Since coproporphyrin I is relatively stable in hydrochloric acid solution and is more readily available, it is often used as a standard, and the results are expressed in terms of equivalents of this porphyrin. Since the amount of porphyrins in the red cells is much

greater than that in the plasma, little error is made by using the much more convenient whole blood sample instead of washed cells.

Normal values: The normal levels of erythrocyte porphyrins as determined by this method are 20-50 µg/dl red cells. Some workers express the results as micrograms per liter of red cells, thus giving values 10 times as great, or 200-500 µg/L red cells.

Interpretation (Table 4-10): Erythrocyte protoporphyrin and coproporphyrin levels parallel the reticulocyte level except in iron deficiency anemia and dyserythropoietic anemias, e.g., lead poisoning. The most important clinical application of the test for free erythrocyte porphyrin (FEP) is to aid in the discrimination between two microcytic anemias: **iron deficiency anemia** and **β-thalassemia trait.** In the former the FEP is increased, while in the latter it is within the normal range.[203,204] In iron deficiency, as the transferrin saturation falls, the FEP increases. The FEP assay can also be employed for the detection of lead poisoning[205] and of other disturbances of **heme synthesis**, such as chronic infections, abnormalities of porphyrin metabolism, acquired sideroblastic anemias, and chronic alcoholism,[184] in which FEP elevations occur.

Erythrocyte aminolevulinic acid dehydratase assay[202,205]

Aminolevulinic acid dehydratase, now preferably termed **porphobilinogen synthetase** (E.C. 4.2.1.24), catalyzes the condensation of two molecules of ALA to form PBG with the elimination of two molecules of water. In many of the earlier methods[207,208] for its determination the rate of formation of PBG was measured by means of the reaction with Ehrlich's reagent. However, in the determination of the enzyme in blood samples and other biologic materials, other enzymes may be present that convert some of the PBG formed into porphyrins; thus the amount of PBG at the end of the reaction time may not be a true measure of the enzyme activity.

Principle: In the present method the rate of decrease in ALA is measured. The ALA remaining is separated from the PBG formed by extraction with ethyl acetate and condensed with acetoacetate to give a product reacting with a modified Ehrlich reagent.

Normal values: The normal range by this method is 33.8 ± 4.8 μmole/min/L red cells. The other methods mentioned have somewhat different units and thus different normal values. Values lower than normal are of greatest interest, and any method must be checked in the laboratory by determining the levels of a number of normal individuals.

Interpretation (Table 4-3): The assay of δ-ALA dehydratase allows the discrimination between iron deficiency anemia and lead poisoning, two conditions in which protoporphyrin levels are increased. In the first the ALA dehydratase activity is increased; in the latter it is decreased.

Erythrocyte uroporphyrinogen and coproporphyrinogen I synthetase (E.C. 4.3.1.8) assay[209]

Principle: A red cell hemolysate is incubated with PBG at pH 8.2. The enzyme present in the red cells catalyzes the condensation of the PBG to uroporphyrinogen I. This latter is spontaneously oxidized by the air to uroporphyrin I. The resulting porphyrin is measured fluorometrically after the heme and other proteins are precipitated with trichloroacetic acid. Since a coproporphyrin I standard is readily available, the results are expressed in terms of nanomoles coproporphyrin I equivalent produced per milliliter packed cells per hour.

Normal values: For normal individuals the values by

this method from 35-50 nmole/ml/hr packed cells (average 41).

Interpretation (Table 4-10): In conditions of accelerated erythropoiesis (e.g., hemolytic anemias) porphyrinogen synthetase activity is increased, but in acute intermittent porphyria, a hereditary porphyrin disorder, it is decreased.

LABORATORY INVESTIGATION OF VITAMIN B₁₂ CONCENTRATION

For effective erythropoiesis and hematopoiesis, factors other than proteins and iron are required. They are mainly vitamin B_{12}, intrinsic factor, and folic acid.

Vitamin B_{12}, the **anti–pernicious anemia factor** or **extrinsic factor of Castle,** is a red crystalline compound containing cobalt. Structurally it is a cyanocobalamin consisting of four substituted pyrrole rings surrounding a single central cobalt atom. The structure resembles the porphyrin ring of hemoglobin. The central structure of this ring is referred to as a "corrin" system, which like porphyrin is synthesized from δ-ALA. Methyl groups on the vitamin B_{12} molecule are derived from methionine. The basic compound is called cobalamin. The attachment of a cyanide group creates cyanocobalamin, which is vitamin B_{12}. The substitution of the cyanide group with a hydroxy group gives rise to a vitamin B_{12} analog, hydroxocobalamin. Vitamin B_{12} functions as a coenzyme in metabolism by means of two vitamin B_{12}–containing coenzymes, the cobamides; these have an adenine nucleoside or a methyl group, not a cyano group, attached to cobalt, creating the coenzymes adenosyl cobamide and methyl cobamide.[210]

Functions of vitamin B₁₂

The vitamin B_{12} coenzymes take part in a number of reactions in bacteria, but in humans there are only two reactions that require their participation[210]:

1. The conversion of methylmalonyl CoA to succinyl CoA,[211] which is part of the citric acid cycle, the major pathway of carbohydrate, protein, and lipid catabolism
2. The methylation of homocysteine to methionine,[212] the principle source of methyl groups in the body

Together with folic acid derivatives, vitamin B_{12} is required for DNA synthesis, as demonstrated by the morphologic changes of all cells of the body in vitamin B_{12} deficiency.

Absorption, transport, and excretion of vitamin B₁₂

Vitamin B_{12} is synthesized exclusively by microorganisms in soil, water, and animal intestines. Animal products are the principle source of dietary vitamin B_{12}.

In food the vitamin is protein bound. Its absorption in the ileum depends on the gastric factor designated **instrinsic factor** by Castle. This factor is a glycoprotein secreted by the parietal cells of the fundus and body of the stomach, which also secrete the gastric hydrochloric acid.[213] Gastric acid splits the protein–vitamin B_{12} linkage so that vitamin B_{12} is free to be bound by the intrinsic factor. The vitamin B_{12}–intrinsic factor complex is absorbed by the mucosa of the ileum, and vitamin B_{12} is freed and escapes into the portal circulation where it is bound to the **transcobalamins** I, II, and III[214-216] and carried to the tissues. Transcobalamin I is secreted by granulocytes and their precursor cells,[217] but its level is also influenced by other factors.[218] Transcobalamin II is synthesized in the liver,[219] and transcobalamin III is also of leukocytic origin.[216] Only a small amount of endogenous vitamin B_{12} is excreted into the urine and feces. In the latter it is contained within sloughed mucosal cells. Larger amounts are excreted into the bile and reabsorbed via the enterohepatic circulation. Exogenous vitamin B_{12}, manufactured by intestinal bacteria, is not absorbed by the body.

Vitamin B_{12} assay by competitive protein-binding radioimmunoassay

Recently introduced isotope methods have largely replaced the microbiologic assays using such microorganisms as *Euglena gracilis*,[219,220] *Lactobacillus leichmannii*, and *Escherichia coli*, which give somewhat lower values than the radioimmunoassay methods. It now appears that the extraction methods used for the microbiologic methods do not extract the vitamin as completely as the extraction methods used for radioimmunoassay. This accounts for many of the discrepancies between the two methods.[221]

The principles involved in this type of assay are explained very briefly. The essential materials and equipment required are given below. The first necessary component is radioactively labeled vitamin B_{12}, the substance being assayed. Since vitamin B_{12} contains cobalt, it is readily labeled with [57]Co. A second requirement is some protein substance that will bind or combine with the substance being assayed. Vitamin B_{12} combines readily either with a purified reference sample of intrinsic factor or with a sterile solution of human serum protein. The poor quality of the intrinsic factor used in earlier kits was responsible for erroneous assay results. A third requirement is some method of separating the vitamin B_{12} combined with the binding protein from that which is not bound (free). One substance that has been used is charcoal coated with an absorbed layer of large molecules such as hemoglobin or dextran. Charcoal by itself will absorb molecules of many different types. When first treated with hemoglobin or dextran, the charcoal particles are coated with an absorbed layer of these large molecules and will no longer absorb other large molecules such as vitamin B_{12} combined with serum protein. However, the free (nonprotein-combined) vitamin B_{12} molecules are relatively small enough to penetrate between the spaces of the large coating molecules and reach the charcoal surface to be absorbed. Therefore the free vitamin B_{12} will be absorbed by the charcoal, but that bound to the binding protein will not, thus separating the two fractions. One can also use DEAE cellulose, a cellulose derivative that will absorb the large serum-binding molecules but not the free vitamin B_{12}. Thus when cellulose is used, the bound form is in the precipitate (cellulose), whereas when coated charcoal is used, the free form is in the precipitate (charcoal). A counter is also required for

measuring the radioactivity. Some of the simpler instruments used for determinations are not suitable for counting [57]Co or other radioisotopes. The more sophisticated instruments can be adjusted to count a number of different isotopes such as ^{125}I, ^{59}Fe, [57]Co, and others.

Principle: The essential principle of the test is that when a definite amount of radioactively labeled vitamin B_{12} (the same holds for other molecules, but the mechanism is discussed in terms of vitamin B_{12}) and an amount of unlabeled vitamin B_{12} (from standards or sample) are added to an amount of binding protein not sufficient to bind all the vitamin B_{12} present, the amount of radioactivity bound by protein will vary with the amount of added unlabeled vitamin B_{12}. Thus by measuring either the amount of bound or the amount of unbound radioactivity (depending on the method used) and plotting the percent bound (or unbound) or some fraction of these against the amount of added standard, one can construct a standard curve from which can be determined the amount of vitamin B_{12} in the added sample. A number of different plotting methods have been used, depending on the procedure and type of material being assayed.

Commercially available radioassay kits allow the simultaneous determination of vitamin B_{12} and folate levels in a single serum sample and may also be used to measure red cell folate (Simultrac, Schwarz/Mann Div., Becton-Dickinson and Co., Orangeburg, N.Y.). The simultaneous assay is based on the differences in the counting spectrum of [57]Co and ^{125}I and on the radioisotope dilution procedure described by Lau et al.[221-223] In the vitamin B_{12} assay the standard or the endogenous unlabeled vitamin B_{12} in the patient's serum competes with the radioactive tracer ([57]Co) for binding sites on the intrinsic factor, while in the folate assay the standard or the endogenous unlabeled folate in the patient's serum competes with radioactive folate (^{125}I) for specific binding sites on milk derivatives.

Normal values: Normal values of serum B_{12} are 200-1000 pg/ml.[223]

Interpretation: Markedly elevated levels (1000-10,000 pg/ml) are found in myeloproliferative disorders (chronic and acute granulocytic leukemia, polycythemia vera, and myelosclerosis), in qualitative changes of the binding proteins (greater affinity for vitamin B_{12}), and in quantitative protein changes (increased protein mass). Increased transcobalamin levels have been reported in acute liver damage, in malignant hepatomas,[225] and in tumors metastatic to liver.[216] A significant percentage of vitamin B_{12}–binding protein appears to be derived from neutrophils, so its level can be used to measure the total granulocyte pool[226] (see discussion of neutropenia).

Decreased serum vitamin B_{12} values are found in a great number of conditions (as shown in the outline below and Table 4-11). In vitamin B_{12} deficiency the vitamin B_{12} level in serum falls below 100 pg/ml. Since vitamin B_{12} stores are adequate for 3-10 years, in acquired vitamin B_{12} deficiency it takes several years for anemia to develop.[227] Vitamin B_{12} (and folate) deficiency leads to a megaloblastic anemia characterized by ineffective erythropoiesis and reduced red cell survival.

Table 4-11. Laboratory diagnosis of vitamin B_{12} and folate deficiencies*

Deficiencies	IF	Serum		
		Anti-IF	Folate	Antibody B_{12}
Pernicious anemia[229]	−	+	+	+
Congenital intrinsic factor deficiency[230]	−	−	+	+
Juvenile autoimmune pernicious anemia[230]	−	+	+	−
Fish tapeworm infestation[231]	+	−	+	+
Stagnant loop syndrome[232]	+	−	+	+
Imerslund disease[233]	+	−	+	+
Tropical sprue[234]	+	−	−	−

*IF, Intrinsic factor; +, present; −, diminished.

The following outline gives the etiology of decreased B_{12} serum levels.
1. Abnormal absorption of vitamin B_{12}
   a. Gastric lesions: pernicious anemia (intrinsic factor deficiency), gastric resection, gastric carcinoma
   b. Intestinal lesions: some forms of sprue and celiac disease, blind loop syndrome, diverticulosis
2. Increased utilization of vitamin B_{12}
   a. *Diphyllobothrium latum* infection, diverticula, small-bowel stricture, blind loop syndrome
3. Diminished supply of vitamin B_{12}
   a. Nutritional deficiency: kwashiorkor, veganism
   b. Transcobalamin deficiency: cirrhosis, hepatitis
4. Chronic neutropenic states[228]

Test of vitamin B_{12} absorption: Schilling test

The Schilling test measures the absorption of ^{57}Co-B_{12} and is thus an indicator of **intrinsic factor activity.**[235] If radioactive vitamin B_{12} is administered orally to a normal individual and at the same time the blood is saturated with a "flushing" dose of nonradioactive vitamin B_{12} administered intramuscularly to saturate the body binding sites, the radioactive vitamin B_{12} is not utilized by the body and about 18% of it is excreted in the urine. Patients with pernicious anemia, who lack the intrinsic factor, are unable to absorb ^{57}Co-B_{12}, which is excreted in the feces and not in the urine (Fig. 4-24). If the test is repeated with ^{57}Co-B_{12} plus intrinsic factor, vitamin B_{12} will be absorbed from the bowel and excreted in the urine.

Determination of urinary ^{57}Co-B_{12} excretion is indicated in the investigation of macrocytic anemias and gastrointestinal malabsorption syndromes.

Procedure: The patient must be in the fasting state, and the urinary bladder must be emptied. Give 0.5 μCi ^{57}Co as radioactive cyanocobalamin orally. Herbert[236] suggests a dose of 2 μCi ^{57}Co, believing it challenges the absorptive ability of the ileum better. One hour after the oral dose administer 1000 μg crystalline vitamin B_{12} intramuscularly. Collect all urine for the next 24 hr, during which time the patient is allowed to eat and drink. Measure the total volume of urine. If it is less than 1 L, dilute it with water to 1 L. Prepare the standard by diluting 0.5 μCi ^{57}Co-B_{12} to 1 L. Count 3 ml urine and 3 ml standard.

Calculation:

$$\% \ ^{57}\text{Co-}B_{12} \text{ excreted} = \frac{\text{cpm 3 ml urine} \times \text{urine vol} \times 100}{\text{cpm 3 ml standard} \times \text{Dilution}}$$

Normal values: Of the administered dose of radioactive vitamin B_{12} 9-36% (average 18%) is excreted in the urine in 24 hr.

Interpretation: Low values are found in pernicious anemia (0.5%, range 0-2%) and in nontropical sprue (3.6%, range 0-19%). An abnormally low result allows two interpretations: absence of intrinsic factor and defective absorption in the ileum. The test is therefore repeated and 0.5 μCi ^{57}Co-B_{12} is given orally with 60 μg intrinsic factor. If the excretion of ^{57}Co-B_{12} rises to normal levels, the diagnosis is pernicious anemia, since in the latter the average excretion is 0-2% of the injected dose of ^{57}Co-B_{12} before the administration of intrinsic factor and about 15% after its administration. If the excretion of ^{57}Co-B_{12} does not rise, malabsorption may be the cause of the patient's anemia.

Sources of error: Incomplete urine collection is the greatest source of error. Since renal disease suppresses vitamin B_{12} excretion, the renal status should be ascertained before the test is started by noting the urinary specific gravity, total creatinine content, and the 24 hr volume. Urinary excretion of vitamin B_{12} is also depressed in diabetes, hypothyroidism, old age, and enteritis.

Quantitation of methylmalonic acid in urine: colorimetric technic[237]

The metabolism of proprionate to succinate, an energy-producing reaction, requires a vitamin B_{12} coenzyme,[211] which is necessary for the conversion of methylmalonyl CoA to succinyl CoA.

Principle: The methylmalonic acid is extracted from the urine with ether-ethanol and purified by the use of Permutit. The purified extract is then coupled with diazotized *p*-nitroaniline and determined colorimetrically. A more sensitive gas or thin-layer[237a] chromatographic method can be used.[238]

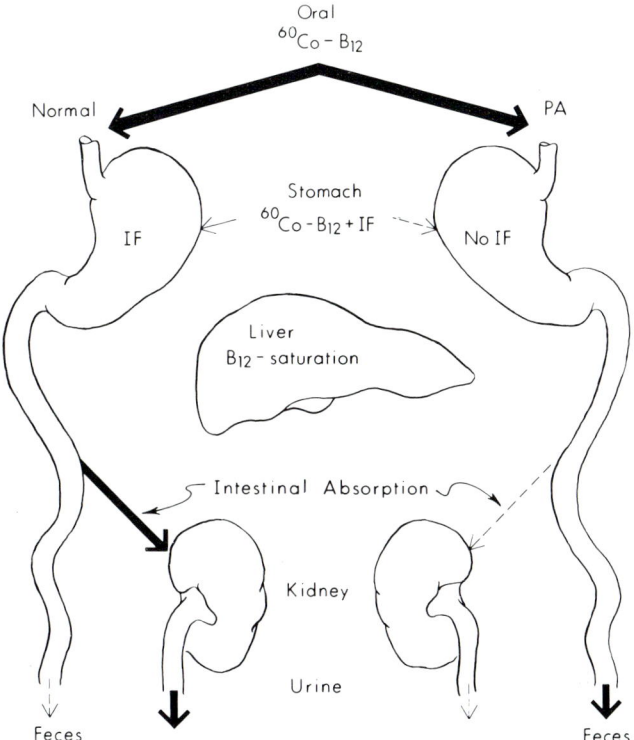

Fig. 4-24. Principle of Schilling test for measuring urinary excretion of ^{57}Co-B$_{12}$. See text.

Reagents:
1. Concentrated HCl used as preservative for urine.
2. HCl, 0.1N. Dilute 8.3 ml concentrated HCl to 1 L with water.
3. Deacidite FF (IP), <200 mesh, chloride form (Permutit Co., Paramus, N.J.).
4. Ethanol-ether mixture. Mix together 3 volumes diethyl ether and 1 volume 95% ethanol as needed.
5. Ammonium sulfate crystals.
6. Sodium acetate solution, 0.2M. Dissolve 27.2 g sodium acetate trihydrate in water to make 1 L.
7. Sodium acetate buffer, 1M, pH 4.3.
   a. Sodium acetate, 1M. Dissolve 136.1 g sodium acetate trihydrate in water to make 1 L.
   b. Acetic acid, 1M. Dilute 57.5 ml glacial acetic water to make 1 L.
   Mix 16.3 volumes sodium acetate solution and 33.9 volumes acetic acid solution. Check the pH and adjust by addition of more acid or salt as required.
8. Sodium hydroxide, 3M. Dissolve 12 g NaOH in water to make 1 dl.
9. Stock standard methylmalonic acid. Dissolve 100 mg pure methylmalonic acid (Calbiochem, La Jolla, Calif.) in water to make 1 dl. Store in a refrigerator.
10. Working standard. Dilute the stock 1:20 with 0.1N HCl as required, making a solution containing 0.05 mg/ml.
11. Diazo reagent. Prepare just before use as needed:

a. Sodium nitrite, 0.072M. Dissolve 0.5 g sodium nitrite in 1 dl water. Solution is not stable and is best prepared as needed.
b. *p*-Nitroaniline solution, 5.5 mM. Dissolve 75 mg *p*-nitroaniline in 1 dl 0.2N HCl (1.6 ml concentrated HCl to 1 dl).
c. Mix 4 ml sodium nitrite solution with 15 ml *p*-nitroaniline solution and cool in an ice bath. Add 4 ml 0.2M sodium acetate solution.
12. Valine, 10 g.

Procedure: Urine is collected for 24 hr after an oral dose of 10 g valine; 10 ml concentrated HCl may be added to the collection bottle as a preservative. The specimen should be well mixed and the total volume measured.

Adjust a portion of the total urine to pH 2 (narrow-range paper) by adding HCl as needed.

Transfer a 10 ml aliquot to a 50 ml separatory funnel, and add about 6 g ammonium sulfate crystals. Mix the solution well to dissolve the salt. Add additional ammonium sulfate if necessary so that the solution is saturated with salt; there should be a few crystals remaining undissolved, but a large excess should be avoided.

Then extract the urine three times with 15 ml aliquots of ether-alcohol (3:1) and combine the extracts.

Prepare the column of Permutit resin. Make a slurry of resin in water and pour it into a column 1-1.5 cm in diameter to give a column of resin about 5 cm high. After all excess water has drained from the column, pass the combined extract through the column, followed by wash of 50 ml water. Light suction may be used to increase flow through column. Discard the eluates. Now elute methylmalonic acid with 20 ml 0.1N HCl. Collect the eluate in a suitable flask or tube and mix well.

For development of color add 2 ml eluate to one tube. To the other tubes add 2 ml 0.1N HCl as a blank and 2 ml working standard for a standard. To each tube add 3 ml acetate buffer, then 3 ml diazo reagent. After mixing heat the tubes in a water bath at 95° C for 3 min. Then add 2 ml 3M NaOH to each tube and mix. Immediately stopper the tubes, avoiding contact with air. After cooling the tubes read the sample and standards against a blank at 620 nm.

Calculation:

$$\frac{A_x}{A_s} \times C_s \times \frac{V_1}{V_2} = \text{mg/ml MMA}$$

A_x is the absorbance of the sample, A_s is the absorbance of the standard, C_s is the concentration of the standard in milligrams per milliliter V_1 is the volume of eluate, and V_2 is the volume of urine used. With the volume given in the procedure, this reduces to:

$$\text{mg/ml} = \frac{A_x}{A_s} \times 0.1$$

Then

$$\text{mg/ml} \times \text{Total urine volume in ml} = 24 \text{ hr excretion}$$

If the reading of the sample is too high to read accurately, repeat the color reaction with an aliquot of eluate diluted 1:5 or greater with 0.1N HCl and make appropriate corrections in the calculations. Since other substances in urine will develop a slight amount of color, values under 15 mg/L are not reliable and are preferably reported as under 15 mg/L.

Normal values: Normal values are up to 9 mg/24 hr.

Interpretation: The normal excretion of methylmalonic acid is not increased following administration of valine (10 g), a methylmalonate precursor.[239] In vitamin B_{12} deficiency methylmalonic acid excretion is markedly raised, a phenomenon that appears to be specific,[240,241] as it is not seen in folic acid deficiency or in liver disease. In vitamin B_{12} deficiency methylmalonic acid excretion may reach values of 300 mg/24 hr[236] In folic acid deficiency accompanied by vitamin B_{12} deficiency methylmalonic acid excretion may initially be normal[242] but will show abnormally high values following valine administration.[243]

Methylmalonic aciduria also occurs as a congenital error of metabolism of vitamin B_{12} in infants but is not accompanied by a megaloblastic anemia.

Immunoassay of autoantibodies to intrinsic factor in serum and gastric juice[243]

Serum from patients with pernicious anemia may contain anti–intrinsic factor (anti-IF) and anti–parietal cell autoantibodies.[245] There are two types of anti-IF autoantibodies; the more common blocking antibody (type I) prevents the complexing of vitamin B_{12} to IF but fails to react with the IF-B_{12} complex.[246] The less common binding anti-IF antibody (type II) combines with either free IF or bound IF as in the IF-B_{12} complex.[246] The serum of 74% of patients with pernicious anemia contains blocking antibodies, and 48% of patients have binding antibodies in their sera, leaving about 25% of patients with pernicious anemia who show neither type of anti-IF antibody. The anti–parietal cell antibody is found in the serum of 95% of patients with pernicious anemia and can be detected by an immunofluorescent technic using parietal cells from a number of animals and humans.[247] The antibodies found in the gastric juice are secretory IgA antibodies, while the serum antibodies are IgG antibodies. The value of the detection of anti–parietal cell antibodies is somewhat lessened by the fact that they can be detected in the serum of about 10% of normal individuals in the pernicious anemia age group and also in patients with hepatic and thyroid disease and with chronic iron deficiency.[245,248] In 57% of patients with pernicious anemia, blocking anti-IF antibodies (IgA) but no binding antibodies are found in the gastric juice. There is no relationship between the serum and the gastric juice antibodies. Anti-IF antibodies are most commonly found in patients with pernicious anemia, but they have been demonstrated in other autoimmune disorders,[249] in thyrotoxicosis, and in atrophic gastritis.

No antibody is detected in folate-deficient megaloblastic anemia.

Principle: A modification of the vitamin B_{12} assay presented can be used as an immunoassay for gastric IF concentration.

The tests for blocking and binding antibodies as shown in the protocol are based on the following considerations. For blocking antibodies the test serum is incubated with diluted normal human gastric juice before the addition of the tracer vitamin B_{12}. If the serum does not contain blocking antibody, most of the added tracer vitamin B_{12} complexes with the IF rather than with the serum proteins because of the greater binding affinity of the former. If the serum does contain blocking antibody, the tracer vitamin B_{12} complexes with the unsaturated binding protein sites in the serum rather than with IF. To determine the binding, serum containing binding-type anti-IF antibody in excess of that needed to bind all the IF-bound tracer vitamin B_{12} is added. After incubation the immunoglobulins are precipitated by the addition of sodium sulfate solution. This precipitates all the IF bound to the antibody (along with the complexed vitamin B_{12}). If the serum does not contain blocking antibody, the tracer vitamin B_{12} precipitates bound to the IF. If the serum does contain blocking antibody, most of the tracer vitamin B_{12} remains in the supernatant (not precipitated bound to IF), and a higher radioactivity count is obtained in the supernatant.

A serum containing a very high level of cobalamin (as after a recent injection of cobalamin) will give false positive test results because the excess vitamin B_{12} competes with the tracer vitamin B_{12} for the binding sites. In such cases the excess vitamin B_{12} may be removed from the serum by treating it with 50-100 mg charcoal and centrifuging. The supernatant is used for the test.

The test for binding antibody is similar except that

the tracer vitamin B_{12} is added before the test serum. If the test serum contains binding antibody, it complexes with the tracer B_{12}-IF and precipitates on the addition of sodium sulfate solution. If no antibody is present, most of the added tracer vitamin B_{12} remains in the supernatant and gives a higher radioactivity count.

Reagents and technic: Details are found in Bauer.[200]

Folic acid assay

The term *folic acid* refers to a synthetic substance, pteroylglutamic acid (PGA), and several naturally occurring folates (substances with folic acid–like activity) that are widely distributed in various foods of plant and animal origin. Dietary folates are readily absorbed in the small intestine without the aid of IF. The biologically active forms of folic acid are conjugates of glutamic acid such as N-5-methyl tetrahydrofolic acid and N-5-formyl tetrahydrofolic acid (folinic acid, or citrovorum factor) These substances act as coenzymes in a variety of metabolic systems such as the conversion of ATP to ADP and NADP to NADPH. Folates are single-carbon donors to the purine nucleus, to serine, and to methionine and are needed for the catabolism of histidine to glutamic acid. An intermediate product of this reaction is formiminoglutamic acid (FIGLU), which is found in increased amounts in the urine in folic acid deficiency. Its assay is omitted in this edition.

In the serum about 90% of folates are carried unbound or loosely bound to albumin and 10% are bound to specific folate-binding proteins (FABP).[250] In folate-deficient serum, amounts of FABP present are eight times greater than in normal serum. Following treatment with folic acid the binding fraction falls to normal levels. Normal bound folate levels are also found in vitamin B_{12} deficiency and may aid in distinguishing vitamin B_{12} deficiency from folate deficiency.

Serum folate and folate-binding protein by radioassay with tritium-labeled pteroylglutamic acid[251]

The term *folic acid* as used here refers to the specific compound pteroylglutamic acid (PGA). The following is a radioassay method using PGA labeled with tritium. The radioactive counting must be done with a liquid scintillation counter. For details of the counting procedure and for corrections for quenching, reference must be made to the manual accompanying the particular instrument used. If more than a few assays are done at once, it is preferable to have an automatic counter.

Principle: The serum containing the unknown amount of folate is added to a definite amount of a folate-binding substance (lactoglobulin) along with a standard amount of tritium-labeled folate. The two folates, that from the serum and the added labeled material, compete for the binding sites of the lactoglobulin. The more folate present in the added serum sample, the smaller the amount of labeled folate that will be bound by the lactoglobulin. The free and bound folate are then separated by absorption of the former (but not the latter) on hemoglobin-coated charcoal. By themselves the charcoal particles would absorb all the folate. When the particles are first covered with an absorbed layer of hemoglobin molecules, the larger molecules of lactoglobulin with absorbed folate are not bound by the hemoglobin, but the smaller free folate molecules can still be absorbed by the charcoal, reaching the charcoal-binding sites between the hemoglobin molecules. After separation of the charcoal-absorbed free folate from the bound folate in solution, the radioactivity of the solution is measured. The radioactivity of the solution is calculated as the percent of the original radioactivity. A standard curve is prepared by treating a series of standards similarly to the serum. On the basis of this standard curve the percent of the radioactivity of the solution is used to determine the amount of folate in the original sample.

A radioassay kit is commercially available (Simultrac, Schwarz/Mann Div., Becton-Dickinson & Co., Orangeburg, N.Y.) in which levels of vitamin B_{12} and folate are determined simultaneously in a single tube.

Normal values: The normal range for serum folate by this method is 4-20 ng/ml.

Interpretation: See Table 4-11.

Contrary to serum vitamin B_{12} levels, which are stable, serum folate levels are labile, easily influenced by dietary factors.[252] Folate-containing foods may raise the value, and low folate intake may lower it. The level of the tissue folate stores more closely parallels the erythrocyte folate level than the serum folate level.

Elevated serum folate levels: Elevated values are seen in some patients with vitamin B_{12} deficiency[253]; others have normal values provided there is no concomitant folic acid deficiency. Elevated values may also be seen in the blind loop syndrome, in liver disease, in kidney failure,[253] and after oral administration of folic acid.[254]

Low serum folate values: Low serum values are rapidly produced (within a few weeks) by a folate-free diet,[253] and they do not allow any conclusion as to the bone marrow picture,[253] which may be normoblastic or megaloblastic. The folate level must remain low for about 20 weeks or more before anemia develops.[253] Folate stores are adequate for 4-6 months[253] and are depleted by the following conditions:

1. Abnormal absorption of folic acid
   a. Celiac disease
   b. Sprue
   c. Dermatitis herpetiformis
2. Increased utilization of folic acid
   a. Pregnancy
   b. Hemolytic anemias
   c. Myelosclerosis
   d. Acute leukemias (acute myelomonocytic)
   e. Chemotherapy with folic acid antagonists
   f. Administration of anticonvulsant drugs
3. Inadequate diet
   a. Iron deficiency
   b. Alcoholism

Red cell folate assay[255]

The erythrocyte folate level more closely reflects the tissue folate stores than does the serum folate level. In folate deficiency serum and erythrocyte folates are low, but the serum vitamin B_{12} level may be slightly increased. In vitamin B_{12} deficiency the serum folate level may be slightly increased, but the red cell folate

Table 4-12. Vitamin B_{12} and folate values in vitamin B_{12} and folate deficiencies*

	Vitamin B_{12} deficiency	Folate deficiency
Serum folate	N or ± or −	−
Red cell folate	−	−
Serum vitamin B_{12}	−	±

*N, Normal; −, low; ±, slightly increased; +, increased.

level is low (Table 4-12). Because of the areas of overlap, it is suggested that all three values (serum and erythrocyte folate and serum vitamin B_{12} levels) be determined at the same time.

Reagents and technic: Reagents and technic are discussed in detail in Bauer.[200]

Normal values: Individuals with normal serum folate levels show red cell levels above 200 ng/ml cells.

Interpretation: Individuals with lowered serum folate levels may have red cell levels of 25-275 ng/ml cells. Patients with folate deficiency and megaloblastic anemia usually have red cell folate levels below 100 ng/ml cells.

ENZYMES OF THE ERYTHROCYTE AND THEIR LABORATORY INVESTIGATION

The functional and physical integrity of hemoglobin and thus of the mature red cell is dependent on energy derived from the conversion of glucose to lactose either by the **oxidative (aerobic) hexose monophosphate shunt** or **pathway (HMP)** (also called the pentose-phosphate pathway) or by the **anaerobic Embden-Meyerhof pathway.** A number of enzymes are required to maintain the pathways on which glycosis depends. Congenital (or rarely acquired) severe deficiencies of these enzymes lead to functional changes in hemoglobin and to hemolysis, producing the picture of **hereditary nonspherocytic hemolytic anemias.**

Anaerobic glycolysis (Embden-Meyerhof pathway)

Aided by diffusion, glucose easily traverses the red cell membrane to enter the red cell. Glycolysis is initiated by phosphorylation of glucose to glucose-6-phosphate (G-6-P) and ultimately leads to the production of lactic acid, which leaves the red cell. More than 90% of the intraerythrocytic glucose is metabolized through this pathway.[256] The various intermediate enzymatic steps are noted in Fig. 4-25.

Aerobic glycolysis (pentose phosphate pathway)

The pentose phosphate pathway (PPP) involves less than 10% of the glucose flow but is nevertheless an important glycolytic process. The initial reactions (Fig. 4-26) involve the conversion of G-6-P to ribulose-5-phosphate with the aid of glucose-6-phosphate dehydrogenase (G-6-PD) and the conversion of NADP to NADPH. The latter acts as a coenzyme for the reduction of oxidized glutathione (GSSG) to reduced glutathione (GSH), which protects hemoglobin against oxidation (Fig. 4-27). As the anucleated red cell lacks any other mechanism of reduction of NADP to NADPH, it is very sensitive to enzymatic deficiencies involving the HMP.[257]

Laboratory detection of hereditary red cell enzymopathies

The most common enzymatic glycolytic defect is G-6-PD deficiency, which involves the HMP. Next in frequency, also involving the HMP, is glutathione reductase deficiency. In the Embden-Meyerhof pathway the most commonly deficient glycolytic enzymes are glucose phosphate isomerase, triosephosphate isomerase, and pyruvate kinase.[257]

For all enzyme determinations the use of Sigma kits (Sigma Chemical Co., St. Louis) is suggested. The details of the methods are not reiterated, but the specimen collection is given in detail, since in all cases the properly collected specimen can be stored in the refrigerator until a kit is obtained.

Glucose-6-phosphate dehydrogenase assay
(D-glucose-6-phosphate: NADP oxidoreductase, E.C. 1.1.1.49)

G-6-PD catalyzes the first step in the pentose phosphate shunt (Fig. 4-26), oxidizing G-6-P to 6-phosphogluconate (6-PG) and reducing NADP to NADPH.

In most biologic samples there will also be present some of the enzyme 6-phosphogluconate dehydrogenase (6-PGD), so that the following additional reaction occurs:

$$6\text{-PG} + NADP^+ \longrightarrow$$
$$\text{Ribulose-5-phosphate} + CO_2 + NADPH + H^+$$

Thus when G-6-PD is determined in red cell hemolysates using G-6-P as a substrate, the 6-PGD is also determined. The enzymes may be determined separately by making assays with G-6-P and 6-PG separately and with the two together as substrates. This requires several extra steps, and the G-6-PD activity is obtained as the difference between the total activity and that of the 6-PGD alone.

Quantitative ultraviolet kinetic determination of glucose-6-phosphate dehydrogenase in blood

The procedure presented avoids the interference from 6-PGD.

Principle: As mentioned above, NADP is reduced by G-6-PD in the presence of G-6-P as follows:

$$G\text{-6-P} + NADP \rightarrow 6\text{-PG} + NADPH + H^+$$

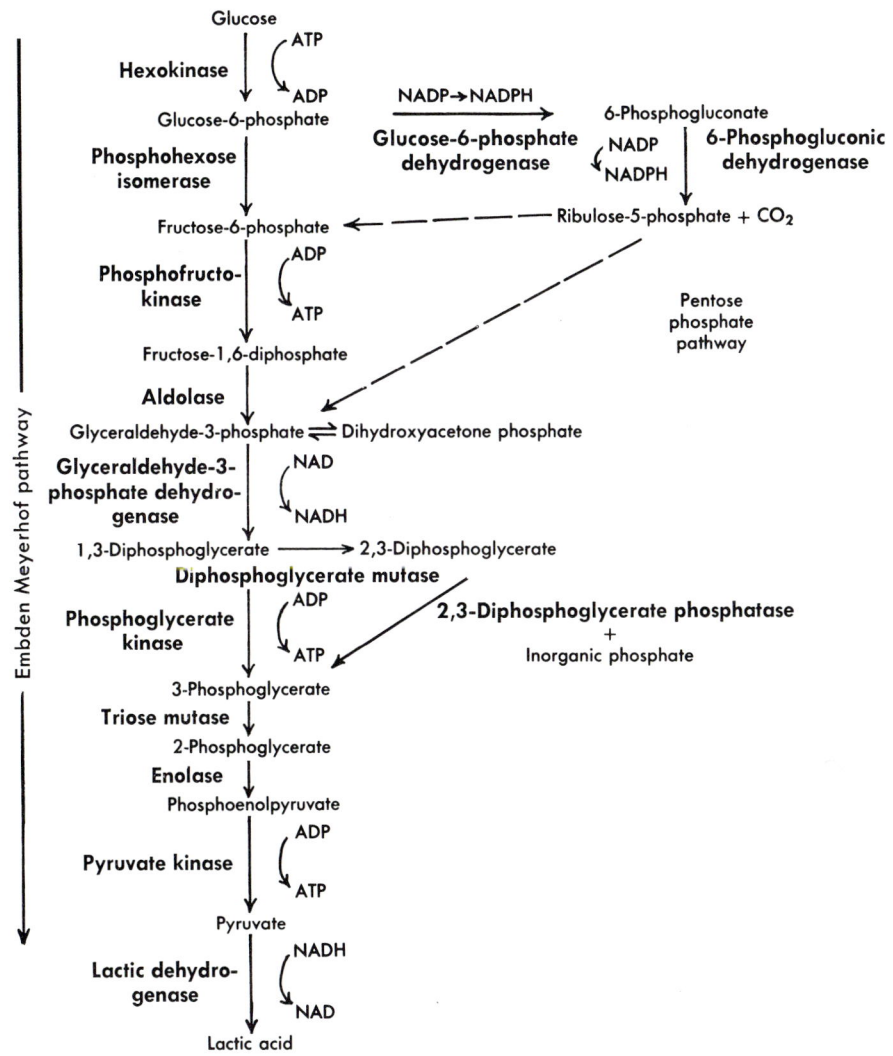

Fig. 4-25. Embden-Meyerhof pathway of glucose metabolism (anaerobic cycle). *ATP,* Adenosine triphosphate; *ADP,* adenosine diphosphate; *NADPH,* reduced nicotinamide adenine dinucleotide phosphate, formerly termed TPNH; *NAD,* nicotinamide adenine dinucleotide, formerly termed DPN, diphosphopyridine nucleotide; *NADP,* nicotinamide adenine dinucleotide phosphate, formerly termed TPN, triphosphopyridine nucleotide. (From Oski, F.A., and Naiman, J.L.: Major problems in clinical pediatrics, vol. 4. Hematologic problems in the newborn, Philadelphia, 1966, W.B. Saunders Co.)

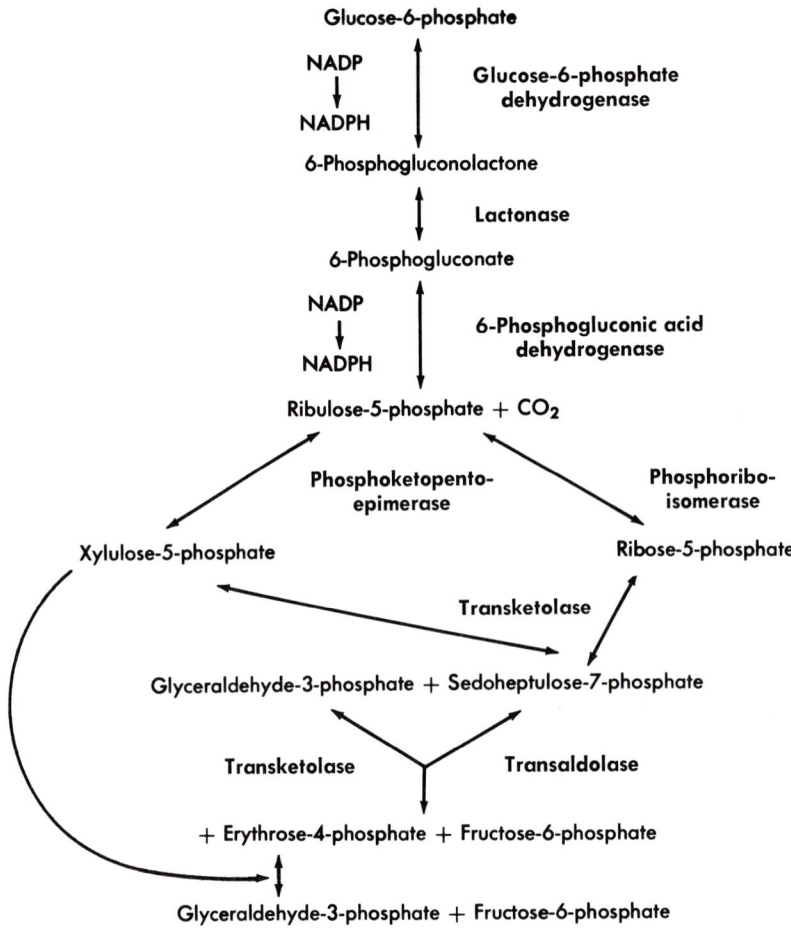

Fig. 4-26. Pentose-phosphate pathway. *NADP,* Nicotinamide adenine dinucleotide phosphate, formerly termed TPN; *NADPH,* reduced nicotinamide adenine dinucleotide phosphate. (From Oski, F.A., and Naiman, J.L.: Major problems in clinical pediatrics, vol. 4. Hematologic problems in the newborn, Philadelphia, 1966, W.B. Saunders Co.)

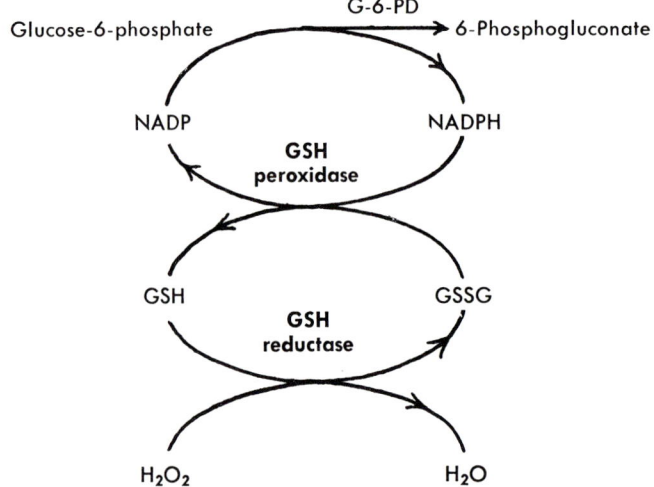

Fig. 4-27. Reduced glutathione, *GSH,* in presence of glutathione peroxidase, converts hydrogen peroxide to water. Oxidized glutathione, *GSSG,* is reduced again by $NADPH_2$ generated by the pentose pathway. (From Oski, F.A., and Naiman, J.L.: Major problems in clinical pediatrics, vol. 4. Hematologic problems in the newborn, Philadelphia, 1966, W.B. Saunders Co.)

The rate of the formation of NADPH is proportional to the G-6-PD activity and is determined spectrophotometrically as an increase in absorbance at 340 nm. The production of a second molar equivalent of NADPH by 6-PGD, an enzyme also present in the erythrocytes, is prevented by the addition of maleimide, which inhibits 6-PGDH.

Reagents: Reagents are supplied in Sigma kit no. 345.

Specimen collection:
Reagents:
1. ACD formula B
   Citric acid monophosphate, 0.48 g
   Trisodium citrate dihydrate, 1.32 g
   Dextrose, 1.47 g
   Water to make 1 dl
   Use 1 ml/4 ml whole blood.
2. EDTA
3. Heparin

Procedure for specimen collection: Collect the blood in ACD, although heparin and EDTA are also satisfactory. G-6PD is stable in heparinized blood for 7 days in the refrigerator and for several weeks in ACD. The enzyme is not stable in a hemolysate, and therefore freezing must be avoided. Determine the hemoglobin concentration, hematocrit, and red cell count.

Procedure for assay: See Sigma technical bulletin no. 345-UV, June 1980.

Qualitative screening procedures for glucose-6-phosphate dehydrogenase using spots prepared on paper

Principle: G-6-PD catalyzes the following reaction:

$$G\text{-}6\text{-}P + NADP \xrightarrow{\text{G-6-PD}} 6\text{-}PG + NADPH$$

(Not fluorescent) (Fluorescent)

The reaction mixture containing G-6-P, NADP, and a small amount of blood is incubated for 2 min. Drops of this mixture are spotted onto filter paper at zero time and at 5 min intervals. The spots are then visually inspected under long-wave ultraviolet light. Fluorescence is observed with normal blood, but there is no fluorescence when the blood is deficient in G-6-PD.

Specimen collection: Anticoagulated (heparin, EDTA, or ACD) venous blood is satisfactory (see above).

Procedure for assay: Follow the instructions in Sigma technical bulletin no. 202, March 1979.

Preparation of heaviest (oldest) erythrocytes for glucose-6-phosphate dehydrogenase assay[259]

The distribution of G-6-PD in blacks is dependent on red cell age: the younger cells contain normal levels of G-6-PD, and the older cells are enzyme poor. In a hemolytic episode the older cells are preferentially lysed, while the younger cells remain intact. Measuring the activity in the older cells allows the recognition of the enzymatic defect during the acute episode without resorting to family studies or without waiting several weeks for the acute hemolytic episode to subside.

Procedure: As they age, normal cells become in-creasingly dense and can be separated from young cells by high-speed centrifugation or by the use of density gradients.[200,260,261]

Genetics of glucose-6-phosphate dehydrogenase deficiency

G-6-PD deficiency is the most common type of hereditary red cell enzymopathy. It is transmitted by an X chromosome–linked gene ($\bar{X}$), so that the hereditary pattern is similar to that seen in hemophilia. It is fully expressed in affected males and is transmitted from mother to son.

Males have only one X chromosome and therefore are either G-6-PD deficient ($\bar{X}Y$ hemizygous) or nondeficient (XY). Females may be either homozygous for the deficient gene ($\bar{X}\bar{X}$—same deficient gene on each X chromosome) or heterozygous for it ($\bar{X}X$—one abnormal or one normal gene on each X chromosome). The heterozygous group has two populations of red cells, deficient cells and normal cells, since only one of the two chromosomes is active.[262] The variability of expression of the heterozygous form is explained by the Lyon hypothesis dealing with the variability of the process of inactivation.[263] In the heterozygous female ($\bar{X}X$) in whom the abnormal gene is only on one X chromosome, the effect of the defect varies widely from nearly normal to almost full expression. Since there are two cell populations, the final expression of the trait depends on the concentration of each cell population.[264]

Variants: Numerous mutants or variants have been described in G-6-PD deficiency that exhibit quantitative and qualitative changes, usually the result of a single amino acid substitution, as in hemoglobin variants. As in hemoglobinopathies, the diagnosis of variants is established by electrophoretic[265] and fingerprinting[266] methods. The normal enzyme is designated B+ (or B) and represents the standard of G-6-PD activity (the plus sign indicates activity) in all population groups. The most common variant found in **blacks** is **A+**, which travels faster than B+ on electrophoresis and is associated with some decreased activity compared to B+. The most common G-6-PD deficiency in **blacks** is **A−**. Other common variants are designated by geographic or other names.[257] The most common variants with fast electrophoretic mobility are Gd Debrousse[267] in North Africa and Gd Canton[268] in southern Asia (Gd, phenotypic or genotypic symbol). To date approximately 50 G-6-PD variants have been described. The quantitative methods for G-6-PD do not take into account variant forms.

Electrophoretic demonstration of variants: Quantitative and qualitative variations of G-6-PD can be demonstrated by electrophoresis employing a variety of media such as agar gel,[269] starch block,[270] and cellulose acetate.[270] The latter method lends itself to mass screening, a procedure that is probably seldom justified.[272] G-6-PD types A and B can readily be demonstrated by electrophoresis. The hemoglobin cellulose acetate electrophoresis method described can be modified to include G-6-PD types by means of a commercially available kit (Helena Laboratories, Beaumont, Tex.). The method is based on the reduction of the

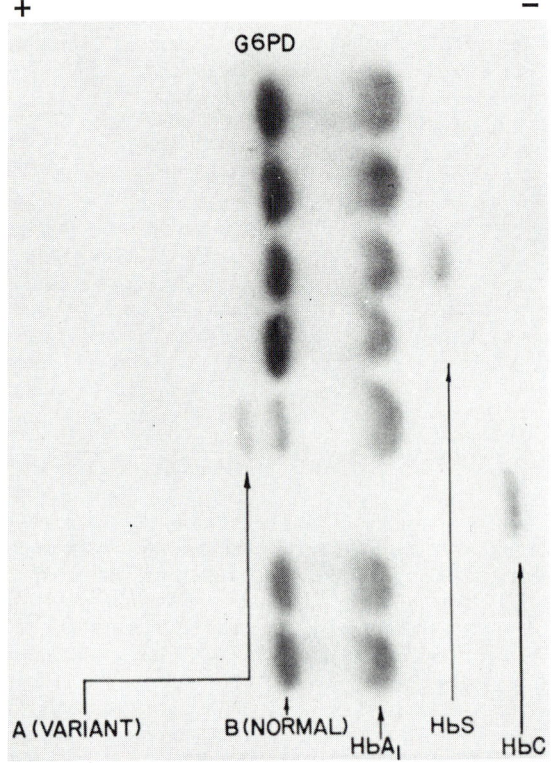

Fig. 4-28. Separation of G-6-PD (normal and variant) and simultaneous hemoglobin screening. (Courtesy Helena Laboratories, Beaumont, Tex.)

coenzyme NADP to NADPH in the presence of G-6-PD and G-6-P as substrate. The reduced NADPH is then oxidized by diaphorase, and the freed hydrogen reduces the colorless tetrazolium salt to form light blue bands in the G-6-PD areas. During electrophoresis normal type B G-6-PD migrates just ahead of Hb A. The deficient enzyme type A is faster than type B (Fig. 4-28).

Glutathione reductase (GR) assay *(NADPH: oxidized glutathione oxidoredctase, E.C. 1.6.4.2)*

Principle: Glutathione reductase catalyzes the reduction of oxidized glutathione (GSSG) to reduced glutathione (GSH) by NADPH or NADH. Glutathione reductase is a flavin enzyme and is activated by flavin adenosine dinucleotide (FAD). There may not be sufficient FAD in the red cell hemolysate to completely activate the enzyme, and in the quantitative method the test is run with and without added FAD. The degree of activation by the FAD may be used as an index of the nutritional state of the patient in regard to riboflavin. The addition of FAD is not needed for the screening test. The measurements are made in the usual way, noting the change in fluorescence of the spots for the screening procedure and the change in absorbance at 340 nm for the quantitative method.[200]

Screening procedure: See Sigma kit no. 205-2.

Specimen collection: Venous blood anticoagulated in

EDTA, heparin, or ACD is used. The enzyme is stable for about 20 days if the specimen is refrigerated.

Procedure for assay: See Sigma technical bulletin no. 205, Jan. 1980.

Glucose phosphate isomerase assay *(glucose-6-phosphate ketol isomerase, E.C. 5.3.9.1)*

Principle: Glucose phosphate isomerase enzyme catalyzes the following reaction:

$$\text{G-6-P} \longrightarrow \text{Fructose-6-phosphate}$$

A simple screening test and a quantitative method are given for this enzyme. In both, the reaction is run in the reverse direction with fructose-6-phosphate as substrate, and in both there is an additional step:

$$\text{G-6-P} + \text{NADP} \longrightarrow \text{6-PG} + \text{NADPH} + \text{H}^+$$

This reaction is catalyzed by added G-6-PD. In the **screening method** the amount of NADPH formed is estimated by noting the fluorescence of this compound in aliquots of the reaction mixture spotted on paper at timed intervals. In the **quantitative method** the additional enzyme 6-PGD is added so that the further reaction occurs:

$$\text{6-PG} + \text{NADP}^+ \longrightarrow$$
$$\text{Ribulose-5-phosphate} + \text{CO}_2 + \text{NADPH} + \text{H}^+$$

Two molecules NADPH are formed for each molecule G-6-P decomposed. The reaction rate is followed by measuring the absorbance of NADPH at 340 nm.

Screening and quantitative methods: See Bauer.[200]

Specimen collection: See glutathione reductase assay above.

Triosephosphate isomerase assay
(D-glyceraldehyde-3-phosphate ketol isomerase, E.C. 5.3.1.1)

Principle: Triosephosphate isomerase (TPI) catalyzes the introconversion of glyceraldehyde-3-phosphate (GAP) to dihydroxyacetone phosphate (DHAP):

Glyceraldehyde-3-phosphate → Dihydroxyacetone phosphate

In the methods presented here GAP is used as the substrate, and the dihydroxyacetone phosphate formed is measured by means of a coupled reaction with NADH catalyzed by the added enzyme α-glycerophosphate dehydrogenase:

$$NADH + H^+ + \text{Dihydroxyacetone phosphate} \rightarrow$$
$$NAD^+ + \alpha\text{-Glycerophosphate}$$

As in the other tests presented, the **screening procedure** uses the change in fluorescence of spots on paper as indicator of the extent of the reaction, and the **quantitive method** uses the measurement of the change in absorbance at 340 nm corresponding to the change in the amount of NADH present. For accurate quantitative measurements the concentration of the substrate is critical and must be accurately adjusted, and the added enzyme glycerophosphate dehydrogenase must be checked to be free of TPI.

Screening and quantitative methods: See Bauer.[200]

Specimen collection: See glutathione reductase assay above.

Pyruvate kinase assay *(ATP: pyruvate phosphotransferase, E.C. 2.7.1.40)*

Principle[273]: Pyruvate kinase catalyzes the phosphorylation of adenosine diphosphate (ADP) to adenosine triphosphate (ATP) by phospho(enol)-pyruvate (PEP):

$$PEP + ADP \rightarrow ATP + \text{Pyruvate}$$

The rate of formation of pyruvate is usually measured by means of the coupled reaction:

$$\text{Pyruvate} + NADH + H^+ \rightarrow \text{Lactate} + NAD^+$$

This reaction is catalyzed by added lactate dehydrogenase (LDH).

As in the other methods involving NADH, the change in absorbance at 340 nm is measured in the quantitative methods, and the change in fluorescence of spotted aliquots is noted in the **screening method.**

Leukocytes contain relatively large amounts of pyruvate kinase, and it is essential, particularly in cases of suspected enzyme deficiency in red cells, that the leukocytes be separated as completely as possible from the red cells. In removing the plasma and washing the red cells, one should remove the buffy coat as com-

pletely as possible. Thus it is helpful to have sufficient blood samples so that after centrifugation a little of the red cells can be removed from the top to aid in the complete removal of leukocytes. For the **quantitative method** the hemolysate can then be made in the usual manner. For the **screening test** a hemolysate is not made, but a suspension of the washed cells in the proportion of 1 volume cells to 4 volumes saline is made, and an aliquot of this is used in the test.

Screening and quantitative tests: See Bauer.[200]

Specimen collection: See glutathione reductase assay above.

LABORATORY INVESTIGATION OF HEMOLYSIS (DESTRUCTION OF ERYTHROCYTES)
Measurement of red cell survival time with ^{51}Cr (Na$_2$ ^{51}CrO$_4$)

The average life span of the normal red cell is 120 ± 5 days. The physiologic destruction of red cells does not occur at random but is a function of age, affecting only the senescent cells, which become more rigid and less pliable with advancing age. Because of increasing rigidity, these cells are destroyed in the reticuloendothelial system of the bone marrow and spleen.[274,275] If red cells are tagged with ^{51}Cr and their destruction is a function of age, the relationship between the radioactive remaining cells and time is essentially linear (Fig. 4-29). On the other hand, if red cell destruction is random and involves cells of all ages, the disappearance curve is exponential, indicating a certain constant loss affecting all cells.

Indications: A hemolytic disorder is characterized by a shorter than normal red cell life span. In chronic hemolysis the reticulocyte count is roughly inversely proportional to the erythrocyte life span; in these circumstances the reticulocyte count adequately reflects the bone marrow erythroid hyperplasia, rendering red cell survival studies unnecessary in most instances. On

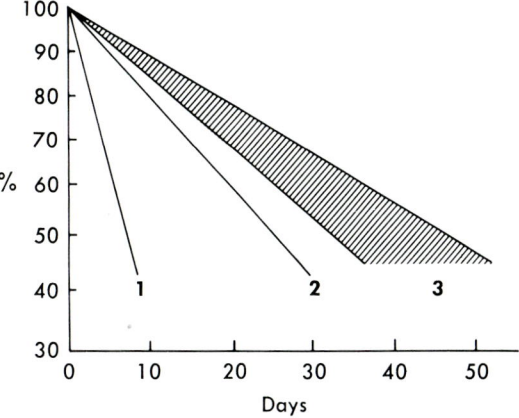

Fig. 4-29. Red cell survival time by ^{51}Cr method. Shaded area is normal range. *1,* Markedly shortened life span of red cells, as seen in severe hemolytic anemias; *2,* slightly shortened life span of red cells.

the other hand, in acute hemolytic episodes there may not be enough time for the reticulocyte response to occur,[276] and red cell survival studies may be indicated. Even if there is an increased reticulocyte response, its cause may be in doubt (since it may be caused by hemorrhage or by hemolysis), and red cell survival studies may be in order.[276]

Principle: Radioactive sodium chromate in the hexavalent form is able to tag about 90% of intraerythrocytic hemoglobin of an ACD-anticoagulated blood sample within 10 min at 37-39° C. After the incubation period ascorbic acid is added so that ^{51}Cr is reduced to the trivalent form, in which it is unable to penetrate red cells in vitro or in vivo. The tagged blood is then injected into the patient, and at suitable intervals blood samples are obtained and their radioactivity is determined. The half disappearance time of ^{51}Cr from the peripheral blood is used as an index of red cell survival. ^{51}Cr tags primarily the β-chains of hemoglobin, and after the destruction of the red cells it is not reutilized. The elution rate may vary from 0.6-1.4% under physiologic conditions and may reach 5% under pathologic conditions. In general a correction is made for a 1% elution rate per day.

Procedure: See Bauer.[200]

Normal values: The half-life ($T^{1/2}$) varies from 35-39 days and should be established for each technic and laboratory because the elution of ^{51}Cr is influenced by the method of tagging and by the type of hemoglobin.[277]

Interpretation: Values shorter than normal indicate decreased survival time. Not until the survival time falls to a $T^{1/2}$ of less than 20 days can the clinical signs of a hemolytic anemia be detected. Normal bone marrow and liver functions are able to compensate for lesser degrees of hemolysis.

Measurement of splenic and hepatic ^{51}Cr sites of red cell destruction

During the ^{51}Cr survival study, measurements are made over the sites of red cell destruction, the spleen and liver. The splenic activity consists of two components: the radioactivity derived from the circulating red cells and the activity caused by sequestration of red cells in the reticuloendothelial component. To eliminate the former as a factor contributing to the splenic activity, the latter is divided by the liver activity, which is assumed to have minimal hemolysis and to represent mainly the radioactive circulation and elution and decay of the label. It is preferable to use ^{59}Fe as a red cell label, thus eliminating the problem of elution and of measurement of liver activity. This method is mentioned in the discussion of ferrokinetics.

Normal values: At the half time in a normal individual splenic activity increases by about 35-50%.

Cross-transfusion studies using ^{51}Cr-tagged cells

To determine whether a hemolytic anemia is primarily caused by an intrinsic defect of the patient's cells or by an extrinsic factor, the patient's tagged red cells may be transfused into a compatible recipient and the recipient's tagged cells may be transfused into the patient (Fig. 4-30).

In intrinsic hemolytic disease there is a shortening of the survival time of the patient's cells in the normal recipient, but normal cells survive for a normal period of time in the patient's circulation. In extrinsic hemolytic disease normal cells exhibit accelerated destruction in the patient's circulation, whereas patient's cells survive for a normal length of time in a normal recipient.

Intravascular hemolysis

There are two principal mechanisms of red cell destruction: **intravascular** and **extravascular.** Severe hemolytic anemias may show evidence of both mechanisms, but usually one or the other predominates. The laboratory methods used in the investigation of these two processes differ.

A number of substances and conditions may lead to intravascular destruction of red cells and thus to escape of hemoglobin into the plasma (e.g., bacterial and

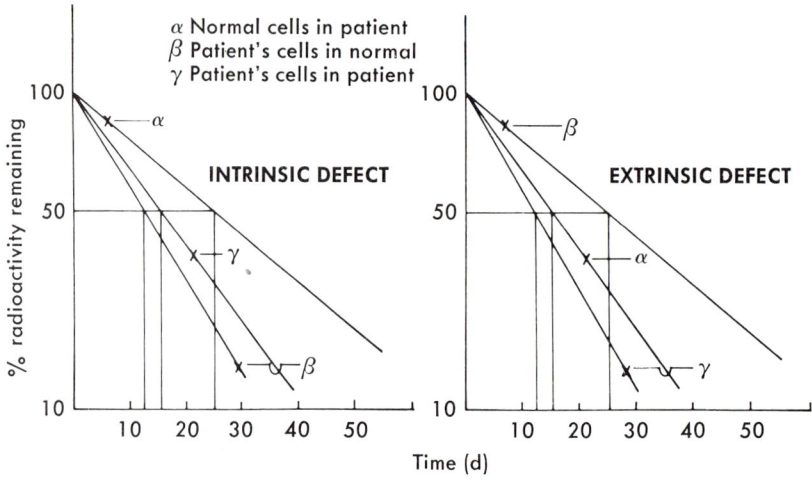

Fig. 4-30. Survival of red cells labeled with ^{51}Cr in transfusion studies. Normal half-life is about 25 days.

chemical lysins, immune antibodies, and osmotic and mechanical forces). After its release into the circulation, free hemoglobin is rapidly bound to **haptoglobin,** an α_2-glycoprotein, and the resulting hemoglobin-haptoglobin complex is cleared from the circulation by the liver. If the haptoglobin binding capacity is exceeded, the remaining **free hemoglobin** is excreted by the kidneys and any excess is oxidized to the trivalent **methemoglobin,** which is dissociated into the globin and the trivalent **hematin** (ferriheme) components.[275,278] Hematin is bound to albumin to form **methemalbumin** and to **hemopexin**[279] to form a hematin-hemopexin complex. Methemoglobin, methemalbumin, and hematin are not normally found in serum, and their presence is indicative of hemolysis.[280]

Plasma hemoglobin assay

Normal plasma contains a minute amount of free hemoglobin (0.3 mg/dl) that cannot be discerned on gross inspection, but intravascular hemolysis may raise this level to several hundred milligrams per deciliter, in which case the plasma appears grossly pink (**hemoglobinemia**).

The method presented is that of Blakney and Dinwoodie[281] as evaluated by Kahn et al.[282,283] It does not require the use of carcinogenic reagents (benzidine) or special equipment and is not affected by the presence of bilirubin or sample turbidity.

Principle: The fractional absorption of a portion of the 578 nm band of oxyhemoglobin (O_2-Hb) is used in conjunction with the absorption coefficient of O_2-Hb to relate absorption to hemoglobin concentration. The fractional absorbance of O_2-Hb at 578 nm is proportional to the hemoglobin concentration.

Reagents and equipment:
1. 18-gauge needle with attached tubing from infusion set
2. Heparinized and nonheparinized test tubes
3. Zeiss PMQ II spectrophotometer (bandpass width equal to 0.9-1.0 nm) or equivalent spectrophotometer
4. Two quartz microcuvets (type 9 Q, 10 mm, Precision Cells, Hicksville, N.Y.)

Sample collection: Sample collection is a critical part of the determination, since any hemolysis during collection or preparation of sample will give erroneously high results. The following procedure is suggested:
1. Remove the tops of a 3 ml red-top Vacutainer tube containing no anticoagulant and of a 5 ml green-top heparinized Vacutainer tube.
2. Place a tourniquet lightly around the upper arm.
3. Puncture the antecubital vein with an 18-gauge needle with attached tubing from an infusion set, and clamp the tubing with a hemostat as soon as blood is observed within the lumen.
4. Ready the tubes of step no. 1, open the hemostat, and allow blood to fill the red-top tube first and then direct the flow into the anticoagulated tube.
5. Clamp the tubing, withdraw the needle, and stop the bleeding.
6. Recap the heparinized tube and gently mix the contents by tipping the tube three or four times.

7. Discard the red-top tube or use the serum for other laboratory tests.
8. Centrifuge the heparinized blood for 10 min at 1000 *g*.
9. Draw off the plasma with a Pasteur pipet without disturbing the buffy layer and deliver it into a second tube.
10. Recentrifuge the plasma for 20 min at 1600 *g* and transfer the supernatant into a third tube.

Procedure: Place the plasma in one microcuvet and deionized water in the other. Adjust the wavelength to 520 nm and the slit width to 0.015 mm and set the absorbance to zero with a water blank. Read the sample absorbance, and record the result. Set the wavelength to 578 nm and the absorbance to zero with a water blank, read the sample absorbance, and record the result. Set the wavelength to 598 nm and the absorbance to zero with a water blank, read the sample, and record the result.

Calculation: The fractional absorption of O_2-Hb at 578 nm (A578) is calculated from the total absorption at 578 nm by substracting the tangential baseline absorption at 578 nm, which is determined by assuming a linear tangent between 562 and 598 nm. A calibration factor of 155 mg/dl is determined experimentally.

$$\frac{A562 - A598}{2.25} = X$$

$$A562 - X = Y$$

(A578 − Y) × 155 = Plasma hemoglobin (mg/dl)
Y = Calculated tangential baseline at 578 nm
(A578 − Y) = Fractional absorption of O_2-Hb

Interpretation: Elevated plasma hemoglobin levels are associated with intravascular hemolysis as seen in blood transfusion reactions, idiopathic and drug-induced autoimmune hemolytic anemia, lupus erythematosus, uremia, thrombotic thrombocytopenic purpura, disseminated intravascular coagulation, prosthetic heart valve, paroxysmal nocturnal hemoglobinuria, and malaria. The presence of hemoglobin in plasma aids in the differentiation between intravascular and extravascular hemolysis because extravascular hemolysis does not raise the plasma hemoglobin level. Determination of the serum haptoglobin level serves a similar discriminatory purpose (see below).

Plasma methemalbumin assay

Methemalbumin is the result of oxidation of free plasma hemoglobin to methemoglobin (trivalent iron), which is then dissociated into hematin and globin. **Hematin** complexes with **hemopexin** and also with albumin to form methemalbumin. The latter is not normally present in plasma (see the discussion of intravascular hemolysis) but may be detected in the plasma as an aftermath of a hemolytic episode when hemoglobinemia and hemoglobinuria have long disappeared. Methemalbumin imparts a brown color to the serum and can be identified by spectroscopic examination and by the **Schumm test.** Its presence is diagnostic of hemolysis.

Schumm test

The Schumm test[284] is based on the fact, discovered many years ago by **Schumm,**[285] that the addition of ammonium sulfide to a methemalbumin solution results in the formation of a compound with a strong absorption band at 558 nm. The interference of free hemoglobin is corrected by also making a reading at 576 nm, since the change in absorbance of a hemoglobin solution on the addition of ammonium sulfide is equal and opposite at wavelengths 558 and 576 nm.

Reagents:
1. Sodium sulfide solution, 1M. Dissolve 58.5 g NaCl in water and dilute to 1 L.
2. Ammonium sulfide, about 20%. This is purchased as a solution containing a minimum of 20% ammonium sulfide.
3. Hematin standard. Obtain unhemolyzed (CPDA-1) plasma from the blood bank. Dissolve 10 mg hematin in 1 ml of 1M sodium hydroxide and immediately dilute to 1 dl with blood bank plasma. Divide into small aliquots and store in freezer. As required, dilute stock standard to 1, 2, and 4 mg/dl hematin.

Procedure: Add a 1 ml sample to each of two tubes, to another pair add 1 ml standard, and to third pair add 1 ml water (as a blank). To one tube of each pair add 1 ml 1M NaCl solution and to the other add 1 ml ammonium sulfide solution. Mix and allow the tubes to stand for 15 min. Centrifuge if not clear and read each tube against the corresponding NaCl or sulfide blank at 558 and 576 nm.

Calculations: Calculate for each sample or standard:

$$A = (S_{558} - O_{558}) + (S_{576} - O_{576})$$

S_{558} is the absorbance of the sulfide solution at 558 nm, O_{558} is the absorbance of the NaCl solution at this wavelength, and corresponding symbols are used for the readings at 576 nm. Then:

$$\frac{A_{sample}}{A_{standard}} \times \text{Conc. of standard} =$$

Methemalbumin (mg/dl as hematin)

To obtain the result in terms of hemoglobin multiply the result by 25.

Normal values: Normal values are 0-8 mg/dl (as hemoglobin).

Interpretation: See introduction.

Plasma hemopexin assay

Hemopexin is a plasma β-glycoprotein that binds dissociated hematin (ferriheme) moieties forming complexes, which are removed from the circulation by the liver.[286] Its plasma concentration varies from 50-100 mg/dl[279] (see discussion of intravascular hemolysis). Following severe intravascular hemolysis, hemopexin is depleted as is haptoglobin, although its depletion is less complete.[287]

Plasma haptoglobin assay

Haptoglobins are glycoproteins that have an average plasma concentration of about 99 mg/dl (average range, 41-246 mg/dl). The haptoglobin level tends to remain stable in a given individual but varies from person to person depending on the phenotype. The latter can be demonstrated by starch gel[288] or polyacrylamide gel electrophoresis.[289] The highest values are found in phenotype Hp 1-1, with lower concentrations in phenotype Hp 2-2 and Hp 2-1.[290]

When hemoglobin escapes into the circulation, within minutes it complexes with haptoglobin, the binding capacity of which is 30-200 mg free hemoglobin. Not until the haptoglobin binding capacity is exceeded can free hemoglobin be detected in plasma (and in urine), as the hemoglobin-haptoglobin complex is too large to be excreted by the kidneys, but within hours it is cleared from the circulation by the liver at a rate of about 13 mg/dl/hr.[291]

Hb Bart's, Hb H, and myoglobin are not bound by haptoglobin. The haptoglobin level thus aids in the differentiation of **myoglobin** and hemoglobin.

Quantitation of haptoglobin serves a number of purposes: haptoglobin is a genetic marker,[290] it is an index of hemolysis, and it allows differentiation of hemoglobinemia from myoglobinemia. Several methods of haptoglobin quantitation are available. In the previous edition of this book the cellulose acetate electrophoresis method was described. Another method employs the principle of immunodiffusion.[292] The agarose–monospecific antiserum mixture is commercially available (Quantiplate, Kallestad Laboratories, Chaska, Minn.).

Manual nephelometric method using a laser light source[293]

Reagents and equipment:
1. Hyland Laser Nephelometer PDQ (Hyland Diagnostics, Div. Travenol Laboratories, Costa Mesa, Calif.)
2. Haptoglobin antiserum
3. Antiserum diluen
4. Sample blank solution

Principle: Unknown serum and reference sera are added to antiserum to human haptoglobin. The quantity of haptoglobin in each reaction mixture is determined using the nephelometer. A beam of collimated, monochromatic light is passed through the solutions, and the antigen-antibody complexes produce light scatter. The concentration of antigen is proportional to the amount of forward light scatter that is displayed by the instrument in relative light scatter (percent RLS) units. The percent RLS of the test specimen is compared to a reference curve constructed from the percent RLS of the reference sera, which have assigned haptoglobin values. The value of the test specimen is expressed in milligrams per deciliter.

Normal values: The normal value is 99 mg/dl; the range is 41-246 mg/dl.

Phenotypes:
1-1, 19% of population, 132 mg/dl; range, 67-261 mg/dl
2-1, 49% of population, 111 mg/dl; range, 49-252 mg/dl
2-2, 32% of population, 69 mg/dl; range, 19-247 mg/dl

Interpretation: Haptoglobin levels are physiologically low in newborn infants up to the age of 1 month, at which time adult levels are reached. Acquired haptoglobin **depletion** occurs in acute and chronic hepatocellular disease, rare cases of congenital ahaptoglobinemia, acute and chronic intravascular hemolysis, hemolytic blood transfusion reaction, tissue hemorrhage, and megaloblastic and hemolytic anemias and in Hp 0-0 individuals (4-6% of American blacks). Haptoglobin is rapidly diminished in response to even small amounts of intravascular lysis (e.g., lysis of 10 ml red cells decreases the level about 100 mg/dl,[294] thus depressing it to almost zero concentration). Following a hemolytic episode the lowest haptoglobin level is reached after about 8 hr.[291] Even if no further hemolysis occurs, the haptoglobin level remains depressed for several days, as long as 2 weeks may be required before hepatic synthesis restores prehemolytic levels.

Haptoglobin concentration is increased to six to eight times the normal value in pregnancy, following steroid and androgen administration (oral contraceptives), in conditions associated with tissue necrosis (myocardial infarct, inflammation), in malignancies, in rheumatoid arthritis, in ulcerative colitis, and after surgery. Increased haptoglobin synthesis may mask hemolytic haptoglobin depression,[295] so that haptoglobin values obtained in the above conditions should be compared with levels of other **acute-phase reactants** (e.g., α_1-antitrypsin or α_1-antichymotrypsin). The comparison of prehemolytic and posthemolytic haptoglobin levels is also helpful.[294]

Extravascular hemolysis

Extravascular hemolysis is the process of destruction of normal aged red cells and pathologic red cells of any age. The cells destined for destruction are phagocytosed by the reticuloendothelial cells of the spleen, liver, and bone marrow. In the process of red cell disintegration the cell membrane is broken down and hemoglobin is released and is split into the globin and heme moieties; the latter are further degraded into iron and protoporphyrins. The iron is carried to the bone marrow by transferrin, while the porphyrin ring is enzymatically converted into biliverdin and finally into bilirubin.[296] The common denominator of the destruction of aged normal erythrocytes or of pathologic red cells of any age is the **loss** of or **alteration** in the **red cell deformability**[297] caused by changes in the red cell membrane.[298]

Red cell deformability and membrane disorders

The extraordinary plasticity that characterizes the normal biconcave red cell allows it to survive in a microcapillary system with lumina measuring 3 μm in diameter and with pores of 0.5 μm in diameter. Impaired deformability of the red cell membrane and accompanying changes in the ratio of the erythrocyte surface to volume render the red cells subject to increased hemolysis and sequestration in the spleen. The membrane changes may be temporary, congenital, or acquired and follow intrinsic and extrinsic insults that include primary or secondary changes in the membrane chemistry, disorders of the hemoglobin structure and synthesis, metabolic red cell abnormalities, and trauma.[297,298]

There are a number of clinical laboratory procedures to test membrane disorders, such as osmotic

fragility determination, mechanical fragility determination, Heinz body formation test, cation concentration measurement, membrane lipid assay, and acetylcholinesterase assay.

Tests of osmotic fragility

The normal biconcave disk shape of the red cell is linked to an excess surface area in relation to its volume. This characteristic shape in conjunction with the fluid nature of the red cell is thought to be responsible for the **normal deformability** of the erythrocyte. If the red cell surface area decreases in relation to its volume, the red cell tends to assume a spheric shape, which imparts to the cell a certain degree of **rigidity** that interferes with the passage of the cell through small openings.

The osmotic fragility test roughly evaluates the relationship of surface area to volume of normal and abnormal cells.[298] Under conditions of the test spherocytes show decreased resistance to lysis in hypotonic saline solutions, allowing water to enter the cell at saline concentrations (e.g., 0.65%) that do not deform normal red cells. The entering water stretches the membrane, and hemoglobin escapes. **Increased osmotic fragility** is thus indicative of red cell sphere formation, i.e., of a decrease in surface area–to–volume ratio.[297] Increased resistance to hypotonic saline solutions, i.e., **decreased osmotic fragility,** is the result of an increase in surface area or a decrease in volume or biochemical contents of red cells. Under these conditions the cells assume the shape of target cells and fail to lyse completely in low saline concentrations (e.g., 0.3%) that completely lyse normal red cells.

Much of the information provided by osmotic and mechanical fragility tests can be obtained by careful scrutiny of a well-stained and well-prepared peripheral blood smear, rendering the performance of the fragility tests unnecessary.

Screening test: Perform the following test using only two Unopette reservoirs, one containing 0.85% saline and one containing 0.55% saline. Observe grossly for hemolysis in the 0.55% reservoir.

Result: Normal red cells do not hemolyze in 0.55% saline.

Dacie's technic:

Principle: The test is based on Dacie's method[299] and utilizes disposable blood-diluting pipets (Unopette, Becton-Dickinson & Co., Rutherford, N.J.). Unopette reservoirs contain 3.98 ml buffered sodium chloride solutions (pH 7.4) equivalent to percent sodium chloride concentrations of 0.85, 0.65, 0.60, 0.55, 0.50, 0.45, 0.40, 0.35, 0.30, and 0.0 (water). As the saline concentration decreases, the erythrocytes swell and finally rupture. The percent liberated hemoglobin is measured spectrophotometrically and is plotted on graph paper against the sodium chloride concentration.

Procedure: Dilute 20 μl free-flowing capillary or well-mixed venous blood in each of 10 reservoirs. Invert and allow to stand at room temperature for 20 min. Transfer each to a cuvet and centrifuge at 2000 rpm for 5 min. Measure the absorbance of the supernatant in each tube at 540 nm. Use the 0.85% tube to set the instrument at zero.

Calculation:

$$\text{Hemolysis } (\%) = \frac{A_x}{A_0} \times 100$$

A_x is the absorbance of the tubes with sodium chloride solutions (0.85, 0.65, 0.60, 0.55, 0.50, 0.45, 0.40, 0.35, and 0.30%) and A_0 is the absorbance of water.

A normal control specimen should be run with each test.

Normal values: Hemolysis begins at 0.50% or at 0.45% saline and is complete at 0.30% saline (Table 4-13 and Fig. 4-31).

Interpretation:

Increased fragility: Hemolysis begins at 0.65% saline and is complete at 0.35% saline. It occurs in all hemolytic disorders characterized by spherocytosis such as congenital spherocytosis, acquired immune hemolytic anemias, ABO hemolytic disease, anti-human globulin–positive anemias, and Zieve's syndrome (cirrhosis, hyperlipidemia, jaundice).[300] The spherocyte is characterized by the smallest surface area in relation to the greatest volume.

Decreased fragility: Hemolysis begins at 0.40% saline, and some nonhemolyzed cells may still be present at 0.30% saline. Decreased fragility occurs in all conditions characterized by target cell formation, such as hemoglobinopathies (Hb S, C, and E), severe hypochromic anemias (iron deficiency, thalassemia major, and sideroblastic anemias), and liver diseases (obstructive jaundice, cirrhosis, and Gilbert's disease). The increased osmotic resistance of the target cells is caused by the lack of thickness of the cells (decreased cation content and volume) in relation to the increased surface area resulting from the accumulation of cholesterol.

Table 4-13. Normal range of hemolysis

Saline (%)	Hemoglobin (%)
0.55	0
0.50	0-6
0.45	5-45
0.40	50-95
0.35	90-99
0.30	97-100

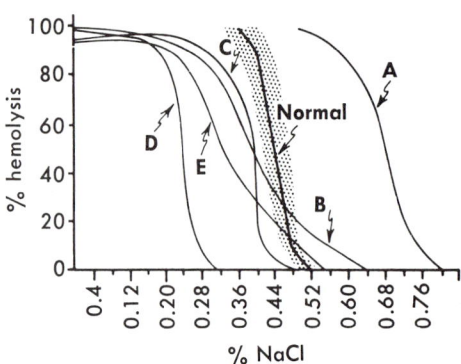

Fig. 4-31. Osmotic fragility of erythrocytes (method of Dacie). **A,** Hereditary spherocytosis. **B,** Thalassemia major. **C,** Thalassemia minor. **D,** Hb E disease. **E,** Thalassemia.

REFERENCES

1. Benesch, R., and Benesch, R.E.: Science **185:**905, 1974.
2. Winterhalter, K.M.: N. Engl. J. Med. **289:**41, 1973.
3. Edelstein, S.J.: Nature **230:**224, 1971.
4. Kurachi, S., et al.: Nature (New Biol.) **243:**275, 1973.
5. Brimhall, B., et al.: Biochim. Biophys. Acta **336:**344, 1974.
6. Orringer, E.P., Wilson, J.B., and Huisman, T.H.J.: FEBS Lett. **65:**297, 1976.
7. Cohen-Solal, M., et al.: FEBS Lett. **50:**163, 1975.
8. Nygaard, S.F., and Rorth, M.: Scand. J. Clin. Lab. Invest. **24:**399, 1969.
9. Greenwalt, T.J., and Ayers, V.E.: Blood **15:**698, 1960.
10. Bellingham, A.J., and Grimes, A.J.: Br. J. Haematol. **25:**555, 1973.
11. Hamasaki, N., et al.: Clin. Chim. Acta **50:**385, 1974.
12. Bunn, H.F., et al.: J. Clin. Invest. **48:**311, 1969.
13. van Assendelft, O.W.: Spectrophotometry of hemoglobin derivatives, Springfield, Ill., 1970, Charles C Thomas, Publisher.
14. van Kampen, E.J., and Zijlstra, W.G.: Adv. Clin. Chem. **8:**141, 1965.
15. Johnston, G.W.: In Seligson, D., editor: Standard methods of clinical chemistry, New York, 1963, Academic Press, Inc., vol. 4.
16. Perutz, M.F., et al.: Nature **185:**416, 1960.
17. De la Huerga, J., and Sherrick, J.C.: Ann. Clin. Lab. Sci. **1:**261, 1971.
18. Faura, J., et al.: Blood **33:**668, 1969.
19. Oski, F.A., et al.: N. Engl. J. Med. **280:**1165, 1969.
20. Valeri, C.R., and Fortier, N.L.: N. Engl. J. Med. **281:**1452, 1969.
21. Klendshoj, N.C., Feldstein, M., and Sprague, A.L.: J. Biol. Chem. **183:**297, 1950.
22. Tietz, N.W., and Fiereck, E.A.: Ann. Clin. Lab. Sci. **3:**36, 1973.
23. Davis, G.L., and Gartner, G.E.: J.A.M.A. **230:**996, 1974.
24. Godin, G., and Shephard, R.J.: Respiration **29:**317, 1972.
25. Astrup, P.: J.A.M.A. **230:**1064, 1974.
26. Castleden, C.M., and Cole, P.V.: Br. Med. J. **4:**736, 1974.
27. Bodansky, O.: Pharmacol. Rev. **18:**1091, 1951.
28. Kitao, T., et al.: Blood **44:**879, 1974.
29. Cohen, R.J., et al.: N. Engl. J. Med. **279:**1127, 1968.
30. Fialkow, P.J., et al.: N. Engl. J. Med. **273:**840, 1965.
31. Harley, J.D., and Lelermajer, J.M.: Lancet **2:**1223, 1970.
32. Evelyn, K.A., and Malloy, H.T.: J. Biol. Chem. **126:**655, 1938.
33. Shibata, S., et al.: Bull. Yamaguchi Med. Sch. **14:**141, 1967.
34. Bunn, F.H., Forget, B.G., and Ranney, H.M.: In Smith, L.M., editor: Hemoglobinopathies, Philadelphia, 1977, W.B. Saunders Co.
35. Hegesh, E., Calmenovici, N., and Avron, M.: J. Lab. Clin. Med. **72:**339, 1968.
36. Scott, E.M.: J. Clin. Invest. **39:**1176, 1960.
37. Nichol, A.W., and Morell, D.B.: Clin. Chim. Acta **22:**157, 1968.
38. Manasterski, A., et al.: Z. Klin. Chem. Klin. Biochem. **11:**335, 1973.
39. Stamatoyannopoulos, G.: Rev. Genet. **6:**47, 1972.

40. Capp, G.L., Rigas, D.A., and Jones, R.T.: Nature **228**:278, 1970.
41. Itano, H.A.: Arch. Biochem. Biophys. **47**:148, 1953.
42. Allen, D.W., Schroeder, W.A., and Balog, J.: J. Am. Chem. Soc. **80**:1628, 1958.
43. Bookchin, R.M., and Gallop, P.M.: Biochem. Biophys. Res. Commun. **32**:86, 1968.
44. Rahbar, S.: Clin. Chim. Acta **22**:296, 1968.
45. Paulson, E.P.: Metabolism **22**:269, 1973.
46. Schwartz, H.C., et al.: Diabetes **25**:1118, 1976.
47. Koenig, R.J., et al.: N. Engl. J. Med. **295**:417, 1976.
48. Bunn, H.F., et al.: J. Clin. Invest. **57**:1652, 1976.
49. Gabbay, K.H., et al.: J. Clin. Endocrinol. Metab. **44**:859, 1977.
50. Fraser, D.M., et al.: Br. Med. J. **1**:979, 1979.
51. Gonen, B., and Rubenstein, A.H.: Diabetologia **15**:1, 1978.
52. Davis, J.E., McDonald, J.M., and Jarett, L.: Diabetes **27**:102, 1978.
53. McDonald, J.M., and Davis, J.E.: Hum. Pathol. **10**:279, 1979.
54. Glycosylated (fast fraction) hemoglobin quick column technic, product insert, Beaumont, Tex., 1978, Helena Laboratories.
55. Dandona, P., Freedman, D., and Moorhead, J.F.: Br. Med. J. **1**:1183, 1979.
56. Bunn, H.F., and Briehl, R.W.: J. Clin. Invest. **49**:1088, 1970.
57. Schmidt, R.M., Rucknagel, D.L., and Necheler, T.F.: J. Lab. Clin. Med. **86**:873, 1975.
58. Marengo-Rowe, A.J.: J. Clin. Pathol. **18**:790, 1965.
59. Schneider, R.G.: In Schmidt, R.M., Moo-Penn, W., and Brosius, E.M., editors: Advanced laboratory methods of hemoglobinopathy detection, Atlanta, 1975, U.S. Department of Health and Human Services, Centers for Disease Control.
60. Schmidt, R.M., and Brosius, E.M.: Basic Laboratory Methods of hemoglobinopathy detection, Atlanta, 1976, U.S. Department of Health and Human Services, Centers for Disease Control.
61. Huisman, T.M.J., et al.: J. Lab. Clin. Med. **86**:700, 1975.
62. HbA$_2$ quick column, Product insert, Beaumont, Tex., 1980, Helena Laboratories.
63. Morin, L.G.: Clin. Chem. **21**:1490, 1975.
64. Chudewin, D.S., and Rucknagel, D.L.: Clin. Chim. Acta **50**:413, 1974.
65. Shukla, S.B., and Headings, U.E.: Immunochemistry **11**:741, 1974.
66. Huisman, T.M.J.: In Yunis, J.J., editor: Biochemical methods in red cell genetics, New York, 1969, Academic Press, Inc.
67. Josephson, A.M., et al.: Blood **13**:543, 1958.
68. White, J.M., and Dacie, J.V.: Prog. Hematol. **7**:69, 1971.
69. Ali, M.A.M., and Schwertner, E.: Am. J. Clin. Pathol. **63**:549, 1975.
70. Kattamis, C., Ladis, V., and Metaxotou-Maorometi, A.: In Schmidt, R.M., editor: Abnormal hemoglobins and thalassemia diagnostic experts, New York, 1975, Academic Press, Inc.
71. Chernoff, A.I.: Ann. N.Y. Acad. Sci. **119**:557, 1964.
72. Reed, L.J., and Mollin, D.W.: Synthesis of hemoglobin A$_2$ in sideroblastic and megaloblastic anemias, Abstracts, Twelfth Congress of International Society of Hematology, New York, 1968, The Society.
73. Kleihauer, E.: Beihefte Arch. Kinderheilkd. **53**(suppl.), 1966.
74. Cooper, M.A., and Hoagland, H.C.: Mayo Clin. Proc. **47**:402, 1972.
75. Naiman, J.L., and Gerald, P.S.: J. Lab. Clin. Med. **61**:508, 1963.
76. Newman, D.R., Pierre, R.V., and Linman, J.W.: Mayo Clin. Proc. **48**:199, 1973.
77. Minnich, V., et al.: Blood **19**:137, 1962.
78. Singer, K., Chernoff, A.J., and Singer, L.: Blood **6**:413, 1951.
79. Schmidt, R.M., Brosious, E.M., and Holland, S.: J. Lab. Clin. Med. **84**:720, 1974.
80. Singer, K., Chernoff, A.I., and Singer, L.: Blood **6**:429, 1951.
81. Pembrey, M.E., McWade, P., and Weatherall, D.J.: J. Clin. Pathol. **25**:738, 1972.
82. Schroeder, W.A., et al.: Anal. Biochem. **35**:235, 1970.
83. Pembrey, M.E., and Weatherall, D.J.: Br. J. Haematol. **21**:355, 1971.
84. Bromberg, T.M., Salzberger, M.M., and Abrahamov, A.: Blood **12**:1122, 1957.
85. Bertles, J.F.: Ann. N.Y. Acad. Sci. **241**:638, 1974.
86. Weatherall, D.J., Pembrey, M.E., and Pritchard, J.: Clin. Haematol. **3**:467, 1974.
87. Hardisty, R.M., Speed, D.E., and Till, M.: Br. J. Haematol. **10**:551, 1964.
88. Alexander, P.: Nature **235**:137, 1972.
89. Lie-Injo, L.E., Hollander, L., and Fudenberg, M.H.: Blood **30**:442, 1967.
90. Wilson, M.G., Schroeder, W.A., and Graves, D.A.: Pediatrics **42**:349, 1968.
91. Kiossoglow, K., Wolman, I.J., and Garrison, M.: Blood **21**:553, 1963.
92. Kleihauer, E., and Kohne, E.: In Schmidt, R.M., editor: Abnormal hemoglobins and thalassemia diagnostic aspects, New York, 1975, Academic Press, Inc.
92a. Rosenberg, A.P., Byrnes, N., and Sexton, L.: Clin. Chem. **5**:489, 1972.
92b. Barnes, M.G., Komarmy, L., and Novack, A.H.: J.A.M.A. **219**:701, 1972.
92c. Schneider, R.G., et al.: Clin. Chem. **20**:74, 1974.
93. Dunston, T., et al.: S. Afr. Med. J. **46**:1423, 1972.
94. Goldberg, C.A.J.: Clin. Chem. **3**:1, 1957.
95. Nalbandian, R.M., et al.: Clin. Chem. **17**:1033, 1971.
96. Diggs, L.W.: Postgrad. Med. **51**:277, 1972.
97. Hemoglobinopathies and thalassemias, Laboratory workshop, Rochester, Minn., 1979, Mayo Medical Laboratories, Mayo Clinic.
98. Statius van Eps, L. W., et al.: Lancet **1**:450, 1970.
99. Hatch, F.E., Culbertson, J.W., and Diggs, L.W.: J. Clin. Invest. **46**:336, 1967.
100. Tuttle, A.H., and Koch, B.: J. Paediatr. **56**:331, 1960.
101. Diggs, L.W., and Bell, A.: Blood **25**:218, 1965.
102. Stewart, J.W., and MacIver, J.E.: Lancet **1**:23, 1956.
103. Monti, A., Feldhake, C., and Schwartz, S.O.: Ann. N.Y. Acad. Sci. **119**:474, 1964.
104. Serjeant, G.R., et al.: Br. J. Haematol. **24**:19, 1973.
105. Weatherall, D.J., et al.: Br. J. Haematol. **17**:517, 1969.
106. Huisman, T.H.J.: Clin. Chim. Acta **40**:159, 1972.
107. Spaet, T.H., Alway, R.H., and Ward, G.: Pediatrics **12**:483, 1953.
108. Smith, E.W., and Krevans, J.R.: Johns Hopkins Med. J. **104**:17, 1959.
109. Chernoff, A.I., et al.: J. Lab. Clin. Med. **47**:455, 1956.
110. White, J.M.: Clin. Haematol. **3**:333, 1974.
111. Fairbanks, V.: In Schmidt, R.M., Moo-Penn, W., and Brosius, E.M., editors: Advanced laboratory methods of hemoglobinopathy detection, Atlanta, 1975, U.S. Department of Health and Human Services, Centers for Disease Control.
112. Necheles, T.F.: In Schmidt, R.M., Moo-Penn, W., and Brosius, E.M., editors: Advanced laboratory methods of hemoglobinopathy detection, Atlanta, 1975, U.S. De-

partment of Health and Human Services, Centers for Disease Control.

113. Jacob, H.S., and Winterhalter, K.H.: J. Clin. Invest. **49:**2008, 1970.

114. Huehns, E.R., and Shooter, E.M.: Biochem. J. **101:**843, 1966.

115. Rieder, R.F.: J. Clin. Invest. **49:**2369, 1970.

116. Morimoto, H., Lehmann, H., and Perutz, M.F.: Nature **232:**408, 1971.

117. Perutz, M.F., and Lehmann, H.: Nature **219:**902, 1968.

118. Betke, K., et al.: Klin. Wochenschr. **38:**529, 1960.

119. Huehns, E.R.: Annu. Rev. Med. **21:**157, 1970.

120. Motulsky, A.G., and Stamatoyannopoulos, G.: Ann. N.Y. Acad. Sci. **151:**807, 1968.

121. Carrell, R.W., and Kay, R.: Br. J. Haematol. **23:**615, 1972.

122. Beutler, E., Dern, R.J., and Alving, A.S.: J. Lab. Clin. Med. **45:**40, 1955.

123. Papayannopoulou, T., and Stamatoyannopoulos, G.: In Schmidt, R.M., Huisman, T.H.J., and Lehman, H., editors: The detection of hemoglobinopathies, Cleveland, 1974, CRC Press.

124. Schmidt, R.M., Moo-Penn, W., and Brocious, E.M.: Advanced laboratory methods of hemoglobinopathy detection, ed. 2, HEW Pub. (CDC) 75-8296, Atlanta, 1975, U.S. Department of Health and Centers for Disease Control.

125. Jacobi, H., H., et al.: Dtsch. Med. Wochenschr. **92:**98, 1967.

126. Schneider, R.G., et al.: N. Engl. J. Med. **280:**739, 1969.

127. Weatherall, D.J., and Clegg, J.B.: The thalassemia syndromes, ed. 2, Oxford, England, 1972, Blackwell Scientific Publications, Ltd.

128. Bunn, H.F., Forget, B.G., and Ranney, H.M.: Hemoglobinopathies, Philadelphia, 1977, W.B. Saunders Co., vol. 12.

129. Rigas, D.A., Koler, R.D., and Osgood, E.E.: Science **121:**372, 1966.

130. Todd, D., Lai, M., and Braga, C.A.: Br. Med. J. **3:**347, 1967.

131. Rigas, D.A., and Koler, R.D.: Blood **18:**1, 1961.

132. Lehmann, H., and Huntsman, R.G.: Man's hemoglobins, Amsterdam, 1968, North-Holland Publishing Co.

133. Kan, Y.W., Achwartz, E., and Nathan, D.G.: J. Clin. Invest. **47:**2515, 1968.

134. Hamilton, R.W., et al.: N. Engl. Med. J. **285:**1217, 1971.

135. Milner, P.F., Clegg, J.B., and Weatherall, D.J.: Lancet **1:**729, 1971.

136. Kan, Y.W., et al.: Blood **43:**411, 1974.

137. Kan, Y.W., et al.: N. Engl. J. Med. **287:**1, 1972.

138. Rowley, P.T., et al.: Blood **43:**607, 1974.

139. Headings, V., et al.: Blood **45:**263, 1975.

140. Hunt, J.A., and Ingram, V.M.: Nature **184:**640, 1959.

141. Wasi, P.: Br. J. Haematol. **24:**267, 1973.

142. Bank, A., and Marks, P.A.: J. Clin. Invest. **45:**330, 1966.

143. Wasi, P.: J. Med. Assoc. Thai. **53:**677, 1970.

144. Bank, A.: Blood **51:**369, 1978.

145. Weatherall, D.J.: In Hoffbrand, A.V., Brain, M.C., and Hirsh, J., editors: Recent advances in haematology, New York, 1977, Churchill-Livingstone.

146. England, J.M., and Fraser, P.M.: Lancet **1:**449, 1973.

147. Hodge, U.M., et al.: J. Clin. Pathol. **30:**884, 1977.

148. Wasi, P., Pootrakal, S., and Winichagoon, P.: In Schmidt, R.M., editor: Abnormal haemoglobins and thalassemia, New York, 1975, Academic Press, Inc.

149. Weatherall, D.J., Clegg, J.B., and Wong Hock Boon, Br. J. Haematol. **18:**357, 1970.

150. Boer, H.R., and Anida, G.: South. Med. J. **72:**1623, 1979.

151. Barrow, D.H.E., and Kohler, H.G.: Arch. Dis. Child. **35:**360, 1960.

152. Jacobs, P., Bothwell, T., and Charlton, R.W.: J. Appl. Physiol. **19:**187, 1964.

153. Worwood, M., Edwards, A., and Jacobs, A.: Nature **229:**409, 1971.

154. Charlton, R.W., et al.: J. Clin. Invest. **44:**543, 1965.

155. Ferras, P.H.: Heterogeneity of thalassemia. In Plenary Session Papers, Twelfth Congress, International Society of Hematology, New York, 1968, Cornell University.

156. Weatherall, D.J.: Br. Med. Bull. **25:**24, 1969.

157. Forget, B.G.: editor: In Stiene, E.A., editor: Hematology laboratory medicine: current aspects, New York, 1974, Intercontinental Medical Book Corp.

158. Mentzer, W.C., Jr.: Lancet **1:**882, 1973.

159. Fessas, P., and Loukopoulos, D.: Clin. Haematol. **3:**411, 1974.

160. Fessas, P., and Loukopoulos, D.: Science **143:**590, 1964.

161. Stamatoyannopoulos, G., Fessas, P., and Papayannopoulou, T.: Am. J. Med. **47:**194, 1969.

162. Brancati, C., and Baglioni, C.: Nature **212:**262, 1966.

163. Need, H., et al.: Trop. Geogr. Med. **13:**207, 1961.

164. Baglioni, C.: Proc. Natl. Acad. Sci. U.S.A. **48:**1880, 1962.

165. White, J.M., et al.: Nature (New Biol.) **235:**208, 1972.

166. Charache, S., and Conley, C.L.: Ann. N.Y. Acad. Sci. **165:**37, 1969.

167. Herbert, V.: Hosp. Pract. **15:**65, 1980.

168. Frieden, E.: Nutr. Rev. **31:**41, 1973.

169. Osaki, S., Johnson, D.A., and Frieden, H.: J. Biol. Chem. **241:**2746, 1966.

170. Halliday, J.W., Mack, V., and Powell, L.W.: Br. J. Haematol. **42:**535, 1979.

171. Cartwright, G.E., and Deiss, A.: N. Engl. J. Med. **292:**185, 1975.

172. Halliday, J.W., and Powell, L.W.: In Brown, E.G., editors: Progress in hematology, New York, 1979, Grune & Stratton, Inc., vol. 11.

173. Crichten, R.R., et al.: Biochem. J. **131:**51, 1973.

174. Siimes, M.A., Addiego, J.E., and Dallman, P.R.: Blood **43:**581, 1974.

175. Perry, D.H., Worwood, M., and Jacobs, A.: Br. Med. J. **1:**245, 1975.

176. Niitsu, Y., et al.: Ann. N.Y. Acad. Sci. **259:**450, 1975.

177. Wands, J.R., et al.: N. Engl. J. Med. **294:**302, 1976.

178. Crosby, W.H.: N. Engl. J. Med. **294:**333, 1976.

179. Cartwright, G.E.: Flow of iron, its diagnostic significance, Seventh Annual Sellman-Straus Memorial Seminar on Concology and Hematology, Kansas City, Mo., 1973, Menorah Medical Center.

180. Wintraub, L.R.: N. Engl. J. Med. **283:** 486, 1970.

181. Hines, J.D., and Grasso, J.A.: Semin. Hematol. **7:**86, 1970.

182. Bainton, D.F., and Finch, C.A.: Am. J. Med. **37:**62, 1964.

183. Pierce, H.I., McGuffin, R.G., and Hillman, R.S.: Arch. Intern. Med. **136:**283, 1976.

184. Ali, M.A.M., and Sweeney, G.: Blood **43:**291, 1974.

185. Unpublished data, Orangeburg, N.Y., 1977, Becton-Dickinson Immunodiagnostics.

186. Hamilton, L.D., et al.: Proc. Soc. Exp. Biol. Med. **75:**65, 1960.

187. Paterson, J.C.S., Marrach, D., and Wiggins, H.S.: J. Clin. Pathol. **6:**105, 1953.

188. Bowie, E.J.W., et al.: Am. J. Clin. Pathol. **40:**491, 1963.

189. Speck, B.: Helv. Med. Acta **34:**231, 1968.

190. Sinniah, R., and Neill, D.W.: J. Clin. Pathol. **21:**603, 1968.
191. Ramsay, W.N.M.: Adv. Clin. Chem. **1:**1, 1958.
192. Baird, I.M., and Padmone, D.A.: Clin. Sci. Mol. Med. **25:**323, 1963.
193. Beutler, E., Robson, M.J., and Buttonwieser, E.: Ann. Intern. Med. **48:**60, 1958.
194. Ladenson, J.H.: In Sonnenwirth, A.C., and Jarett, L., editors: Gradwohl's clinical laboratory methods and diagnosis, ed. 8, St. Louis, 1980, The C.V. Mosby Co.
195. Seltzer, C.C., Wenzel, B.J., and Mayer, J.: Am. J. Clin. Nutr. **13:**343, 1963.
196. Wasserman, L.R., J. Mt. Sinai Hosp. **32:**262, 1965.
197. Masouredis, S.P.: CRC Crit. Rev. Clin. Lab. Sci. **2:**139, 1971.
198. Burnham, B.F.: Semin. Hematol. **5:**296, 1968.
199. Kappas, A., Levere, R.S., and Granich, S.: Semin. Hematol. **5:**323, 1968.
200. Bauer, J.D.: Laboratory investigation of hemoglobin. In Sonnenwirth, A.C., and Jarett, L., editors: Gradwohl's clinical laboratory methods an diagnosis, ed. 8, St. Louis, 1980, The C.V. Mosby Co.
201. Chisolm, J.J., Jr., and Brown, D.H.: Clin. Chem. **21:**1669, 1975.
202. Granick, S., et al.: Proc. Natl. Acad. Sci. U.S.A. **69:**2381, 1972.
203. Stockman, J.A., III, et al.: J. Lab. Clin. Med. **85:**113, 1975.
204. McLaren, G.D., Carpenter, J.T., Jr., and Nino, H.V.: Clin. Chem. **21:**1121, 1975.
205. Piomelli, S., Young, D., and Gay, G.: J. Lab. Clin. Med. **81:**932, 1973.
206. Tomokuni, K.: Clin. Chem. **20:**1287, 1974.
207. Weissberg, J.B., Lipshutz, F., and Oski, F.A.: N. Engl. J. Med. **284:**565, 1971.
208. Bonsignore, D., Calissenmo, P., and Cortasangna, C.: Med. Lav. **56:**199, 1965.
209. Magnussen, C.R., et al.: Blood **44:**857, 1974.
210. Harper, H.A., Rodwell, V.W., and Mayes, P.A.: In Review of physiological chemistry, Los Altos, Calif., 1979, Lange Medical Publications.
211. Mahoney, M.J., and Rosenberg, L.E.: Am. J. Med. **48:**584, 1970.
212. Burton, E., and Sakami, W.: Eur. J. Biochem. **7:**1, 1968.
213. Hoedemacher, P.J., et al.: Lab. Invest. **15:**1163, 1966.
214. Hall, C.A.: Br. J. Haematol. **16:**429, 1969.
215. Bloomfield, F.J., and Scott, J.M.: Br. J. Haematol. **22:**33, 1972.
216. Carmal, R.: Br. J. Haematol. **22:**53, 1972.
217. Corcino, J.J., et al.: J. Clin. Invest. **49:**2250, 1970.
218. Carmel, R.: N. Engl. J. Med. **292:**282, 1975.
219. Pletsch, G.A., and Coffey, J.W.: J. Biol. Chem. **246:**4619, 1971.
220. Anderson, B.B.: J. Clin. Pathol. **17:**14, 1964.
221. Raven, J.L., and Robson, M.B.: J. Clin. Pathol. **28:**531, 1975.
222. Lau, K.S., et al.: Blood **26:**202, 1965.
223. Herbert, V., Gottlieb, C.W., and Lau, K.S.: Blood **28:**130, 1966.
224. Raven, J.L., et al.: Br. J. Haematol. **22:**21, 1972.
225. Waxman, S., and Gilbert, H.S.: N. Engl. J. Med. **289:**1053, 1973.
226. Chikkappa, G., et al.: Blood **34:**828, 1969.
227. Deller, D.J., and Witts, L.J.: Q. J. Med. **31:**71, 1962.
228. Carmal, R., and Coltman, C.A., Jr.: Clin. Res. **17:**531, 1969.
229. Chanarin, I.: The megaloblastic anemias, Oxford, England, 1969, Blackwell Scientific Publications, Ltd.
230. McIntyre, O.R., et al.: N. Engl. J. Med. **272:**981, 1965.
231. Nyberg, W., Grasbeck, R., and Sippola, V.: N. Engl. J. Med. **259:**216, 1958.
232. Gianella, R.A., Broitman, S.A., and Zamcheck, N.: Adv. Intern. Med. **16:**191, 1972.
233. Imerslund, O.: Acta Pediatr. Scand. Suppl. **49:**119, 1960.
234. O'Brien, W., and England, N.W.J.: Br. Med. J. **11:**1573, 1964.
235. Workman, J.B., and Rusche, E.: J. Nucl. Med. **7:**583, 1966.
236. Herbert, V.: Ann. Clin. Lab. Sci. **1:**193, 1971.
237. Green, A.: J. Clin. Pathol. **21:**221, 1968.
237a. Bashir, H.V., Hinterberger, H., and Jones, B.P.: Br. J. Haematol. **12:**704, 1966.
238. Frenkel, E.P., and Kitchens, R.L.: J. Lab. Clin. Med. **85:**487, 1975.
239. Gompertz, D.: Clin. Chim. Acta **19:**477, 1968.
240. Cox, E.V., and White, A.M.: Lancet **2:**853, 1962.
241. White, A.M., and Cox, E.V.: Ann. N.Y. Acad. Sci. **112:**915, 1964.
242. van de Weyden, M.B., Rother, M., and Firkin, B.G.: Blood **40:**23, 1972.
243. Giorgio, A.A., and Plant, G.W.E.: J. Lab. Clin. Med. **66:**667, 1965.
244. Rothenberg, S.P., Kantha, K.R.K., and Ficarra, A.: J. Lab. Clin. Med. **77:**476, 1971.
245. Irvine, W.J., et al.: Ann. N.Y. Acad. Sci. **124:**657, 1965.
246. Schade, S.G., Abels, J., and Schilling, R.F.: J. Clin. Invest. **46:**615, 1967.
247. Fisher, J.M., Dees, C., and Taylor, K.B.: Science **150:**1467, 1965.
248. Doniach, D., and Roitti, I.M.: Ser. Haematol. **1:**313, 1964.
249. Rose, M.S., et al.: Lancet **2:**9, 1970.
250. Waxman, S.: Br. J. Haematol. **29:**23, 1975.
251. Waxman, S., and Schreiber, C.: Blood **42:**281, 1973.
252. Chanarin, I.: The megaloblastic anemias, Philadelphia, 1969, F.A. Davis Co.
253. Herbert, V.; Trans. Assoc. Am. Physicians **75:**307, 1962.
254. Ratanasthien, K., et al.: J. Clin. Pathol. **27:**875, 1974.
255. Schreiber, C., and Waxman, S.: Br. J. Haematol. **27:**551, 1974.
256. Valentine, W.N.: Semin. Hematol. **8:**307, 1971.
257. Beutler, E.: Semin. Hematol. **8:**311, 1971.
258. Valentine, W.N.: Semin. Hematol. **8:**348, 1971.
259. Herz, F., Kaplan, E., and Scheye, E.S.: Blood **35:**90, 1970.
260. Borun, E.R., Figueroa, W.G., and Perry, S.M.: J. Clin. Invest. **36:**676, 1957.
261. Canon, D., and Marikovsky, Y.: J. Lab. Clin. Med. **64:**668, 1964.
262. Grumbach, M., Marks, P.A., and Morishima, A.: Lancet **1:**1330, 1962.
263. Lyon, M.F.: Nature **170:**372, 1961.
264. Kattamis, C.A.: Acta Paediatr. Scand. Suppl. **172:**103, 1967.
265. World Health Organization Scientific Group: WHO Tech. Rep. Ser. **366:**39, 1967.
266. Yoshida, A., Beutler, E., and Motulsky, A.G.: Bull. WHO **45:**243, 1971.
267. Kissin, C., and Dorche, C.: Bull. Soc. Chim. Biol. **52:**1233, 1970.
268. McCurdy, P.R., et al.: J. Lab. Clin. Med. **67:**374, 1966.
269. Haywood, B.J., et al.: J. Lab. Clin. Med. **71:**324, 1968.
270. Kirkman, H.N., and Henderickson, E.M.: Am. J. Hum. Genet. **15:**241, 1963.

271. Sparkes, R.S., and Baluda, M.C.: J. Lab. Clin. Med. **73:**531, 1969.
272. Conrad, M.E.: N. Engl. J. Med. **286:**1418, 1972.
273. Beutler, E.: Blood **28:**553, 1966.
274. Weed, R.I., LaCette, P.L., and Merill, E.W.: J. Clin. Invest. **48:**795, 1969.
275. Bunn, H.F.: Semin. Hematol. **9:**3, 1972.
276. Pollycove, M., and Tono, M.: Semin. Nucl. Med. **5:**11, 1975.
277. Pearson, H.A.: Blood **28:**563, 1966.
278. Pimstone, N.R.: Semin. Hematol. **9:**31, 1972.
279. Muller-Eberhard, U.: N. Engl. J. Med. **283:**1090, 1970.
280. Hershko, C.: Br. J. Haematol. **29:**199, 1975.
281. Blakney, G.B., and Dinwoodie, A.J.: Clin. Biochem. **8:**96, 1975.
282. Watkins, B.F., and Bermes, E.W.: In Sunderman, F.W., editor: Seminars on biochemical hematology, Philadelphia, 1979, Institute for Clinical Science, Inc.
283. Kahn, S.E., Watkins, B.F., and Bermes, E.W.: Ann. Clin. Lab. Sci. **2:**126, 1981.
284. Furlan, M. and Bucher, U.: Schweiz. Med. Wochenschr. **104:**124, 1974.
285. Schum, O.: Hoppe Seylers Z. Physiol. Chem. **80:**1, 1912.
286. Sears, D.A.: J. Clin. Invest. **49:**5, 1970.
287. Fertakis, A., Panitsas, G., and Angelopoulos, B.: Acta Haematol. **50:**149, 1973.
288. Smithies, O.: Biochem. J. **71:**585, 1959.
289. Hanks, G.E., et al.: J. Lab. Clin. Med. **56:**486, 1960.
290. Epstein, E., and Zach, B.: Ann. Clin. Lab. Sci. **2:**191, 1972.
291. Laurell, C.B., and Nyman, M.: Blood **12:**493, 1957.
292. Wert, E.B.: In Sunderman, F.W., editor: Seminars on biochemical hematology, Philadelphia, 1979, Institute for Clinical Science, Inc.
293. Lizana, J., and Helling, K.: Clin. Chem. **18:**335, 1972.
294. Fink, D.J., Petz, L.D., and Black, M.B.: J.A.M.A. **199:**615, 1967.
295. Whitten, C.F.: N. Engl. J. Med. **266:**529, 1962.
296. Tenhunun, R.: Semin. Hematol. **9:**19, 1972.
297. Weed, R.I.: Semin. Hematol. **7:**249, 1970.
298. Weed, R.I.: Clin. Haematol. **4:**3, 1975.
299. Dacie, J.V.: The haemolytic anemias, congenital and acquired. Part 1. The congenital anemias, London, 1960, J. & A. Churchill.
300. Zieve, L.: Ann. Intern. Med. **48:**471, 1958.

CHAPTER 5

Staining methods of blood and bone marrow preparations including cytochemistry

ROMANOWSKY STAINS

All Romanowsky stains use methylene blue and its oxidation products in combination with eosin and its derivatives. They are widely used as stains for blood and bone marrow smears and parasites and include Leishman stain, Giemsa stain, Wright stain, and many others. The Wright-Giemsa stain is explained in detail.

Wright-Giemsa stain

The Wright-Giemsa stain is a combination of acidic and basic components that allows the use of a single stain (polychrome stain) to produce a variety of predictable color reactions that are used to identify the cells of the peripheral blood, the bone marrow, and the biologic fluids described in Chapter 29.

Principle: The Wright-Giemsa stain uses methylene blue and variants of eosin. Methylene blue on standing at alkaline pH forms a complex dye (polychrome methylene blue) consisting of methyl violet, methylene blue, and several azures. The methylene azures are basic blue dyes that cause acidic tissue components such as nuclear DNA and cytoplasmic RNA to turn blue, while the acid esoins stain hemoglobin and eosinophilic granules pink. Other cellular structures show an affinity for the neutral dye component.[1] Methyl alcohol is the solvent for the dyes and the fixative for the material to be stained.

Reagents:
1. Stain
     Powdered commercial Wright stain, 9 g
     Powdered commercial Giemsa stain, 1.0 g
     Glycerin, 90 ml
     Absolute anhydrous methyl alcohol, 2910 ml
   Mix the ingredients in a brown bottle and allow to stand for 1 month before using. The bottle should be thoroughly shaken once daily for the first 3-4 days. Before using, filter into a small dropping bottle.
2. Phosphate buffer, 15M, pH 6.4 (Certified buffer tablets are commercially available from Coleman Instruments Corp., Maywood, Ill.)

Procedure: Use a horizontal staining rack for the slides and rubber stoppers for the coverslips. Arrange the air-dried blood films on the rack and the tops of the rubber stoppers so that the smears face upward. Apply the stain for 3 min (fixation), covering the slides completely. Gently add buffer (with a dropping bottle) of the same quantity as the stain and mix by blowing gently on the surface. Do not allow the dye-buffer mixture to spill off the slides or to dry out. Leave for 3-6 min. Some experimentation may be required to arrive at the best staining time for each lot of stain.

Wash the stain off with neutral distilled water until the stained area appears pink. Remove the stain on the back of the slide with alcohol-moistened gauze. Allow the slide to air dry by resting it on a blotter. The slide may be mounted under a coverslip using Permount (Fisher Scientific Co., Pittsburgh).

Results: A well-stained blood film appears pink macroscopically. Microscopically, erythrocytes are orange-pink to rose. Granules of neutrophils stain purple to lilac; granules of eosinophils, orange to pink; granules of basophils, deep blue to violet. The cytoplasm of neutrophils stains pale pink; the cytoplasm of lymphocytes, light blue; the cytoplasm of monocytes, pale gray-blue. Nuclei of neutrophils and lymphocytes stain deep blue-violet; of monocytes, light bluish purple. Platelets contain a central red-purple granule surrounded by a light blue halo.

Unsatisfactory staining results:

1. Causes of bluish red cells and dark blue structure-less nuclei: insufficient washing; pH of water, buffer, or stain too alkaline; prolonged staining; an overly thick film.
2. Causes of red cells staining too red and of pale gray-blue nuclei; inadequate staining; prolonged washing; pH of water, buffer, or stain too acidic.
3. Causes of a precipitate; insufficient washing; allowing stain to dry on slide; dirty slide. Use only new, precleaned slides and coverslips to make blood smears.
4. If slide is poorly stained or shows a precipitate, destain with absolute methyl alcohol and follow with rapid rinsing with water until all precipitate or stain has been removed. Control procedure under the microscope. The preparation can then be restained provided the cause of the initial failure has been removed.

Bone marrow: The timing of bone marrow smears is as follows: undiluted stain, 5 min; buffered diluted stain, 10 min.

Automated staining

Thin blood films may be prepared manually or by one of the automated smear technics discussed in Chapter 3 and then transferred into the automated slide stainer such as the Hema-Tek (Ames Co., Elkhart, Ind.) or the Hemastainer (Geometric Data Corp., Wayne, Pa.).

SUPRAVITAL (VITAL) STAINS

Vital dyes stain blood cells in vitro while they are still alive. A number of these stains are employed in hematology: tetrazolium salts, basic dyes such as Janus green, and fluorochromes. The use of colorless, soluble tetrazolium salts that are reduced into black formazan is mentioned in Chapter 6 in the discussion of the nitro blue tetrazolium (NBT) test, a leukocyte function test.

Fluorochromes are basic or acidic dyes that fluoresce when excited by ultraviolet light. The stained living cells are examined by a combination of fluorescence and phase microscopy. Ideal fluorochromes are acridine orange and neutral red, the latter having the advantage of also being a nonfluorescent dye. Fluorochromes can be used to identify cytoplasmic inclusions such as mitochondria, the Golgi apparatus, granules, and phagocytosed material.

The main advantage of supravital technics is the elimination of staining artifacts, since living, undamaged cells are examined. The main disadvantages are that (1) the preparations are not permanent and must be examined fresh before they dry out; (2) the living cells are extremely fragile and do not forgive any error in technic; and (3) the stain fades after a short time.

Janus green and neutral red stain[2]

Principle: Saturated stable solutions of the dyes are prepared in absolute alcohol. The working solution of the dye is spread evenly on clean slides that are allowed to dry and are then stable if stored at 4° C and protected from dust and moisture. At room temperature they deteriorate after 1 hr. The selective staining of mitochondria and of intracytoplasmic granules is probably the result of their enzymatic activity.[1]

Slides and coverslips must be washed in alcohol and dried with gauze.

Reagents:

1. Stock solution
   Neutral red, 0.2 g, in 50 ml absolute ethyl alcohol
   Janus green, 0.25 g, in 50 ml absolute ethyl alcohol
2. Working solution
   Janus green solution 0.25 ml
   Neutral red solution, 0.8 ml
   Absolute ethyl alcohol, 5 ml

Procedure: Flame the alcohol-washed clean microscopic slides, flood with stain, wipe off the edges, and dry in a horizontal position. Use only the slides with a uniform layer of dye, and mark the dye side with a wax pencil. Place 1 small drop of fresh (not anticoagulated) blood or bone marrow on the coverslip and invert it onto the dye side of the slide. Allow the specimen to spread between the coverslip and slide to produce a thin and even preparation. Seal with nail polish and allow to stain for 20 min. Examine under oil immersion using phase microscopy.

Results: Intracytoplasmic granules and vacuoles stain deep purple to orange; the mitochondria, green; the cytoplasm, pale yellow to pale green-blue or colorless; and the nuclei remain unstained.

Pinacyanol and neutral red stain

Pinacyanol, which stains the mitochondria deep blue, has the advantage over Janus green that it does not fade for many hours and can successfully be combined with neutral red.[3,4]

Reagents:

1. Pinacyanol, 0.03% in absolute alcohol
2. Neutral red, 0.4% in absolute alcohol
3. Stain: 1 ml of each solution added to 5 ml absolute alcohol

Procedure: Prepare slides and blood spreads as described in discussion of Janus green and neutral red stain.

Interpretation: The mitochondria stain deep blue.

Acridine orange supravital stain[5]

Principle: Living cells are stained with acridine orange and are examined under the fluorescence microscope.

Reagent: Acridine orange, 0.001% in saline, pH 6-8.

Procedure: Suspend 1 drop of fresh blood or bone marrow in several drops of stain on a slide, apply coverslip, allow to incubate at room temperature for 3 min, and examine with fluorescence microscope.

Results: Living nuclei (DNA) fluoresce yellow-green, while nucleolar and cytoplasmic RNA fluoresce orange-red; granules of polymorphonuclear cells light up bright red; eosinophilic granules fluoresce orange; mast cells fluoresce red; and dead nuclei exhibit red fluorescence.

CYTOCHEMICAL STAINS

In general about 90% of all normal and abnormal peripheral blood and bone marrow elements can be correctly identified by the use of one of the Romanowsky stains. In the past decade hematologic morphology has been expanded by the use of cytochemical investigations.[6,7] A variety of intracellular substances and metals can be demonstrated qualitatively by histochemistry, exactly localized within cytoplasmic organelles by electron microscopy, and quantitated by autoradiography. Cytochemistry aids in defining cellular differentiation, maturation, and function and in establishing internationally accepted reproducible standards for the diagnosis of leukemic cells and the evaluation of antileukemic therapy.

Gomori Prussian blue stain[8]

Principle: The Prussian blue reaction employs a fresh solution of acid ferrocyanide to demonstrate nonheme iron as it occurs in the iron storage compounds ferritin and hemosiderin. Ferritin is a relatively homogeneous substance composed of a protein shell (apoferritin) surrounding a ferric hydroxide core.[9] In the past ferritin has been described as Prussian blue negative, but more recent investigations have shown it to be Prussian blue positive, similar to hemosiderin, which is its polymer. The composition of hemosiderin is variable, depending on the incorporation of lipids, calcium, saccharides, and copper.[10] Compared to ferritin it contains about double the amount of iron (40%). Ferritin is a mobile storage form of iron, whereas hemosiderin's iron is slow to mobilize. The iron in both compounds is loosely bound and is easily unmasked by dilute acid to give the reactions of ionic iron. One of these reactions is the formation of a blue pigment, Prussian blue, a ferric ferrocyanide, the result of the combination of ferric ions with ferrocyanide.

Reagents:
1. Fixative: methyl alcohol or formol-ethanol (10 ml 40% formaldehyde in 90 ml 95% ethanol)
2. Hydrochloric acid, 10%
3. Potassium ferrocyanide, 5% (Stored in a dark bottle, it is stable for 3 weeks.)
4. Safranin, 0.05%, or 1% neutral red or nuclear fast red
   Nuclear fast red, 1 g
   Aluminum sulfate, 5% aqueous, 100 ml
   Heat, cool, filter, and add grain of thymol.
5. Stain: Just before use mix equal parts (25 ml) of solutions of hydrochloric acid and potassium ferrocyanide and filter the mixture into a Coplin jar.
   NOTE: (1) All glassware and reagents used must be free of iron. (2) Safranin, if too old, forms needle-shaped crystalline precipitates.

Procedure: Fix air-dried peripheral blood or bone marrow smears in absolute methyl alcohol or in formol-ethanol for 1 min. Rinse in deionized water. Stain in potassium ferrocyanide mixture for 30-60 min at room temperature or at 37° C. Rinse in distilled water (deionized). Counterstain in safranin for 5 min and rinse in distilled water. Apply coverslip with Permount.

Results: Hemosiderin and ferritin iron stain blue; nuclei stain red; cytoplasm stains pink (Figs. 5-1 to 5-3 and Plate 3 [p. 148]).

Leukocyte cytochemistry

The commercial availability of the Histozyme System (Sigma Chemical Co., St. Louis) for histochemical staining of white cells is of enormous benefit to the already burdened clinical laboratory because it provides dependable reagents, buffers, substrates, and coupling

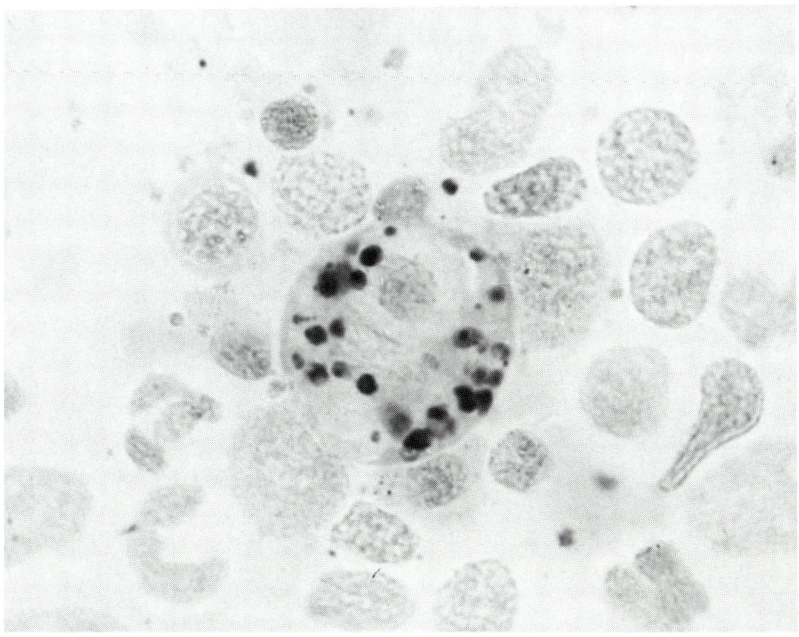

Fig. 5-1. Macrophage (bone marrow) containing iron-positive granules. (Gomori Prussian blue stain.)

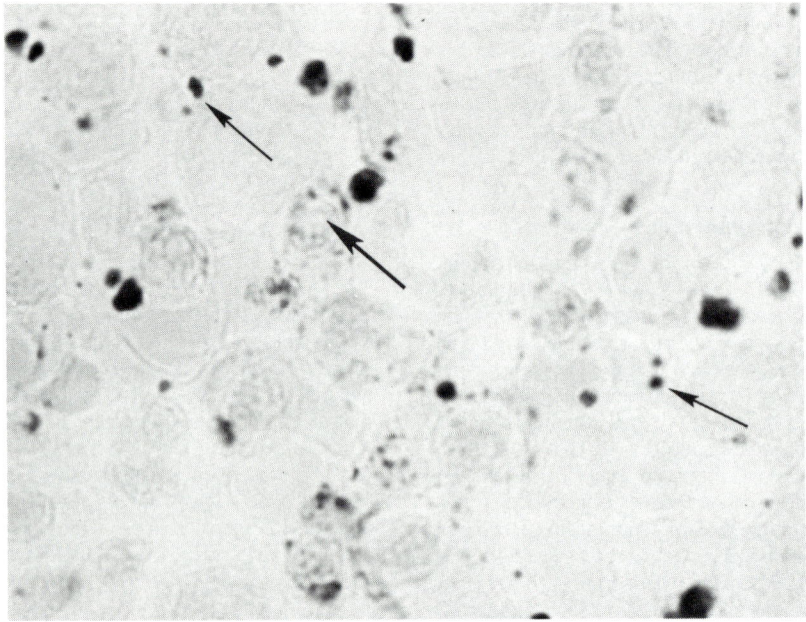

Fig. 5-2. Sideroblasts in bone marrow (thin arrows); ring sideroblast (heavy arrow). (Gomori Prussian blue stain.)

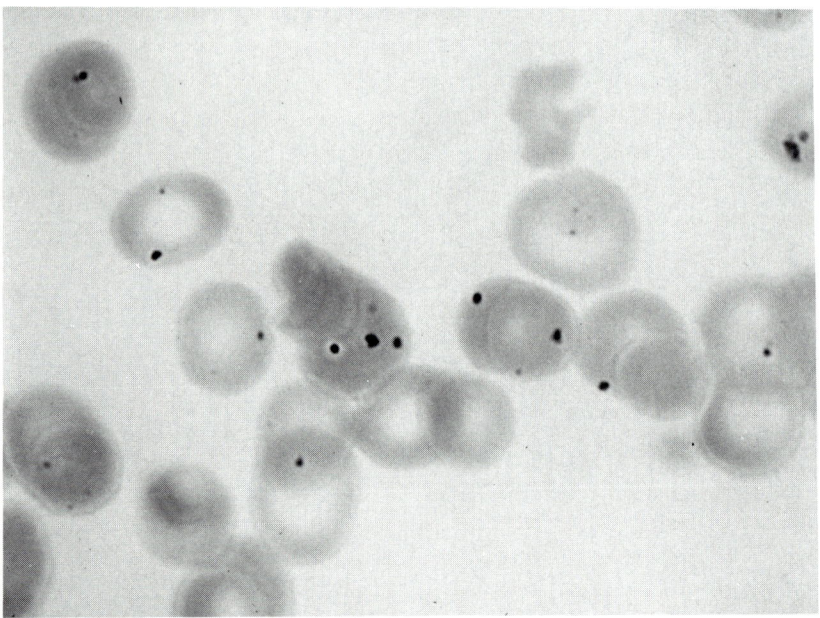

Fig. 5-3. Siderocytes in peripheral blood. (Gomori Prussian blue stain.)

agents optimized to ensure consistent results. The cytochemically stained slides can be scanned by automated light-sensing differential counters. Previous editions of this book contain detailed "recipes" for the various cytochemical stains, but because of the time- and effort-saving hematology kits offered by Sigma Chemical Co., these instructions are not repeated. Some of the less frequently used or modified histochemical reactions are described in detail elsewhere.[11]

Quality control

All histochemical stains must be run with positive and negative controls.

Leukocyte peroxidase stain

Principle: The intracellular peroxidase activity of neutrophils and their precursors transfers hydrogen from the colorless substrate (phenylenediamine) to hydrogen peroxide, thus oxidizing the substrate to a colored product, the location of which indicates the sites of peroxidase activity. The classic method utilizes benzidine or its derivatives,[12] the use of which is discouraged because of benzidine's carcinogenic properties. The Histozyme method uses *p*-phenylenediamine and catechol to detect peroxidase (POD) activity.[13]

Reaction:

p-Phenylenediamine + Catechol + H_2O_2

$$\xrightarrow{POD} \text{Brown-black insoluble product}$$

Specimen handling: Smears are prepared freshly from capillary or venous blood, heparin-anticoagulated specimen, or bone marrow. Allow smears to dry for 10 min prior to fixation and minimize exposure to light because peroxidase is photolabile. Samples are stable in the dark for 3 weeks.[12]

Fixation:
1. Formaldehyde, 37%, 5 ml
2. Ethanol, 95%, 45 ml

Prepare solution fresh daily and keep it tightly stoppered.

Procedure: Fix the slides for 30 sec. Wash in running water for 2 min and allow to dry for 10 min.

Reagents: Reagents are supplied in Sigma kit no. 390-A.

Staining procedure: Follow instructions of Sigma technical bulletin no. 390.

Result: Peroxidase activity is indicated by brown-black granular deposits (Figs. 5-4 and 5-5).

Interpretation: Cells of the lymphocytic, megakaryocytic, and erythroid series are peroxidase negative. Monocytes and monoblasts are usually negative, though they may exhibit weak activity. All cells of the myeloid series are peroxidase positive (primary azurophilic granules), including some of the myeloblasts. The peroxidase reaction is useful in the investigations of acute leukemias. In acute myelogenous leukemia at least 5%, and usually well over 50%, of the blast cells are positive. In acute myelomonocytic leukemia the monocytic elements are usually negative or only weakly positive. In acute lymphocytic leukemia the blast cells are negative. Auer bodies, which are derivatives of azurophilic granules, are peroxidase positive. The peroxidase reaction of mature neutrophils may be negative in severe infections (toxic granulation), in acute myeloid leukemia, in chronic granulocytic leukemia and other myeloproliferative disorders, and in hemophilia.[14]

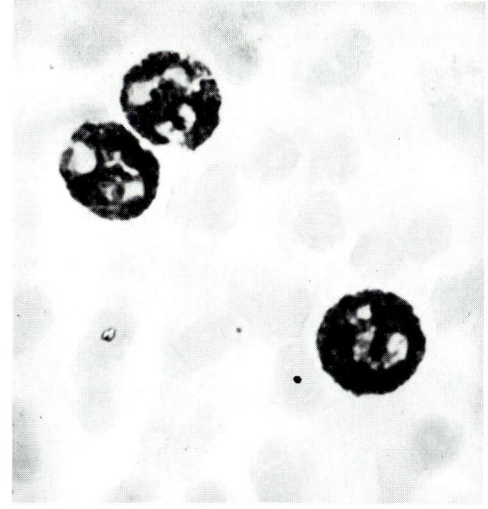

Fig. 5-4. Peroxidase-positive neutrophils.

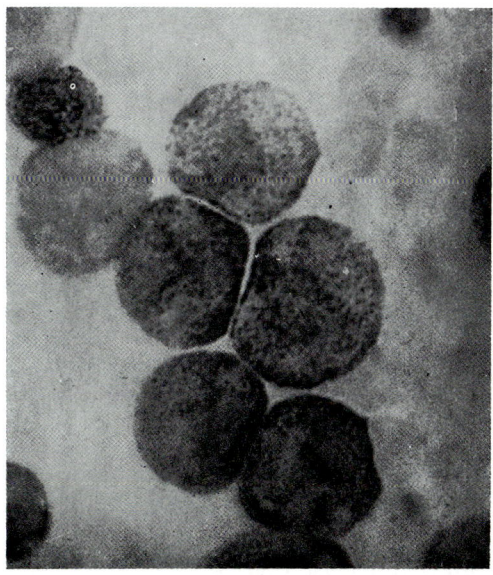

Fig. 5-5. Myelocytic leukemia. Blood spread per oxidase stain, showing selective staining of granules. ($\times 950$.)

Leukocyte alkaline phosphatase stain

Principle: Leukocyte alkaline phosphatase (LAP) is the enzyme present in the secondary granules of polymorphonuclear leukocytes and is identified by allowing it to act on a substrate containing naphthol AS-MX phosphate in an alkaline solution. As a result of the

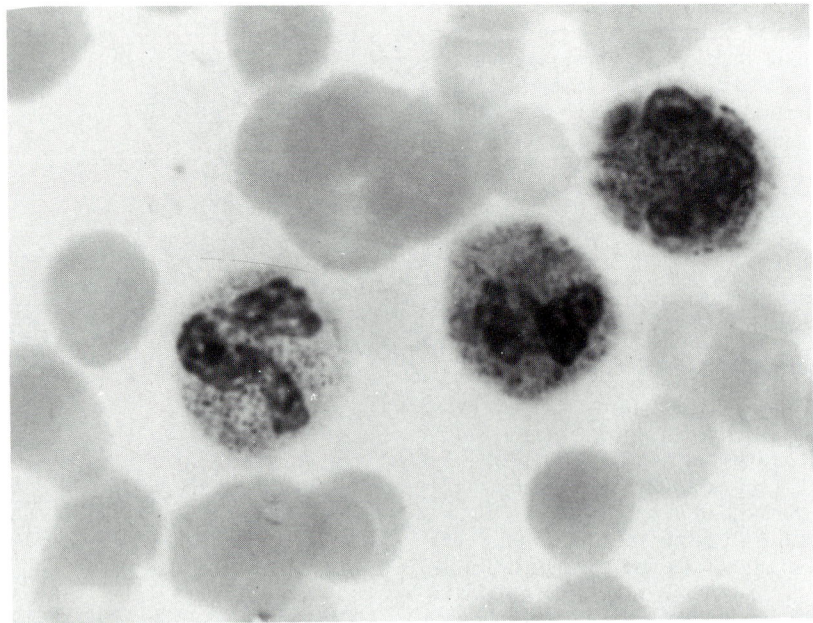

Fig. 5-6. Three alkaline phosphatase–positive neutrophils; from left to right, one rated grade 2, one rated grade 3, and one rated grade 4.

phosphatase activity, naphthol AS-MX is liberated and immediately coupled with the diazonium salt fast blue RR, forming an insoluble dark blue pigment at the site of phosphatase activity.

Specimen handling: Smears should be prepared from capillary or fresh venous blood or from heparin-anticoagulated specimen or bone marrow and should be allowed to dry at room temperature. The smears are fixed for 30 min in 60% citrate-buffered acetone at room temperature. Though immediate staining is the preferred approach, the fixed slides may be kept in the freezer for 1-3 weeks without loss of enzymatic activity.[15]

Fixation:
1. Acetone, 3 dl
2. Citrate buffer (supplied in kit), 2 dl
Add the acetone to the buffer and stir.

Procedure: Immerse the slides for 30 sec. Rinse them in tap water for 30 sec and air dry.

Reagents: Reagents are supplied in Sigma kit no. 85L-2.

Quality control: Positive and negative controls must be run with each unknown slide. Blood smears from women in their third trimester of pregnancy or their first few postpartum days serve as adequate positive controls, whereas negative controls are prepared by immersing an air-dried fixed smear in boiling water for 1 min to destroy the enzyme activity.

Staining procedure: Follow instructions of Sigma technical bulletin no. 85.

Results: Blue deposits are formed at the sites of LAP activity.

Interpretation[16,17]: Only mature polymorphonuclear cells and band or stab cells are scored. Physiologically 50% of these cells are LAP positive (Fig. 5-6). All other peripheral blood or bone marrow cells are LAP negative except reticulum cells, osteoblasts, and endothelial cells. There is no relationship between leukocyte alkaline phosphatase and serum alkaline phosphatase.

For the purpose of clinical evaluation it is adequate to divide band and polymorphonuclear cells into three groups of LAP activity: normal, low, and high. A rough scoring technic is based on the assignment of 0-4+ values to each of 100 consecutively examined band and polymorphonuclear neutrophils. The sum of the ratings is referred to as the score and may vary from a minimal value of 0 to a maximal value of 400. The normal score is 10-100 with an average of 60. Newborns have scores of up to 200 or over. Reactions are graded as follows (Fig. 5-6):

Grade 0	Colorless cytoplasm
Grade 1+	Pale blue cytoplasm, no granules
Grade 2+	Purple cytoplasm, occasional blue granules
Grade 3+	Moderate blue granules
Grade 4+	Many coarse blue granules

Since LAP levels are influenced by many factors, they fluctuate and lack diagnostic consistency and specificity. Nevertheless, LAP levels in the conditions mentioned are seen frequently enough to attain diagnostic significance.

1. Elevated LAP values
   a. Tissue necrosis
   b. Acute bacterial infections (granulocytic leukemoid reactions)
   c. Trauma and burns
   d. Immediate postoperative period
   e. Pregnancy and lactation

f. Stress

g. Oral contraceptives

h. Lymphomas: Hodgkin's disease, multiple myeloma, acute and chronic lymphatic leukemia, acute myelomonocytic leukemia

i. Myeloproliferative disorders: polycythemia vera, myelofibrosis, agnogenic myeloid metaplasia, myelosclerosis

j. Newborn period (up to 2 weeks)

k. Administration of adrenocortical steroids

2. Decreased values

a. Infectious mononucleosis (early)

b. Collagen diseases

c. Paroxysmal nocturnal hemoglobinuria

d. Chronic granulocytic leukemia (Ph[1] positive or Ph[1] negative)

e. Acute granulocytic leukemia (50%)

f. Erythroleukemia

g. Aplastic anemia

h. Acute myelogenous leukemia

3. Normal LAP values

a. Secondary polycythemia (erythrocytosis)

b. Chronic lymphatic leukemia

c. Acute myelogenous leukemia

d. Viral infections

In chronic granulocytic leukemia (CGL) the LAP score is not always characteristically low, since there may be a dual population of polymorphonuclear cells—some leukemic and some normal. Similar considerations apply to the LAP score in acute granulocytic leukemia. In CGL the score is also influenced and increased by bacterial infection, remission, and blast crisis. The low score in CGL aids in differentiating this form of leukemia from blood diseases that may mimic CGL, such as polycythemia vera, granulocytic leukemoid reactions, myelosclerosis, and myeloid metaplasia, in which the LAP levels are raised. In acute lymphatic leukemia and in acute myelomonocytic leukemia the LAP score is usually elevated, whereas in acute myelogenous leukemia the score is normal or low. The decreased level in infectious mononucleosis aids in its differentiation from acute lymphatic leukemia, and the lowered level in erythrocytosis distinguishes it from polycythemia vera. In paroxysmal nocturnal hemoglobinuria the LAP score is very low.

Sudan black B stain

Principle: Sudan black B stains phospholipids and some nonlipid cellular components, such as the azurophilic and specific granules of neutrophils. The staining pattern parallels that of peroxidase.

Specimen collection: Capillary, fresh or heparin-anticoagulated venous blood or bone marrow is used to prepare the film preparations, which should be fixed as soon as possible.

Fixation: Place several pieces of filter paper in the bottom of a Coplin jar with a screw-top lid. Moisten the paper with 3-4 drops of 37% formaldehyde. Place the air-dried smears in the Coplin jar and cap tightly. Fix for 10 min and wash in running water for 2 min.

Staining reagents: Reagents are supplied in Sigma kit no. 360-A.

Staining procedure[18]: Follow instructions of Sigma technical bulletin no. 380.

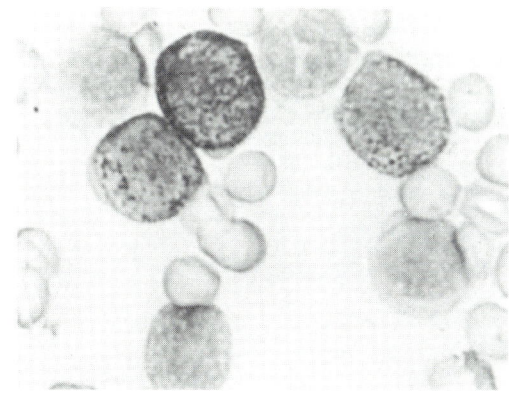

Fig. 5-7. Sudan black B stain of blast cells. Three are negative, two show discrete scattered granules, and one shows a granulocytic pattern of overall positivity. Negative granulocyte is present. (From Hayhoe, F. G. J., Quaglino, D., and Doll, R.: The cytology and cytochemistry of acute leukaemias, M.R.C. special report series, no. 304, London, 1964, Her Majesty's Stationery Office. By permission of the Controller.)

Results: Sudan-positive material stains blue-black (Fig. 5-7).

Interpretation: Members of the granulocytic series show increasing sudanophilia as they mature (Fig. 5-7). Normal myeloblasts are generally Sudan black B negative but may show a few fine perinuclear granules. Beginning with the promyelocytes, in which the positive granules are localized in one area, neutrophilic myelocytes, metamyelocytes, band cells, and segmented neutrophils become progressively more positive because of dense, coarse, closely placed granules that in the most mature cells partially cover the nucleus, fill the cytoplasm, and correspond to the specific neutrophilic granules. Eosinophilic granules show peripheral staining, while basophilic granules exhibit a variable reaction, some being negative and some positive. Lymphocytes are Sudan black B negative, whereas most monocytes show discrete scattered black granules. A small percentage are completely negative. Megakaryocytes, erythroblasts, normoblasts, and platelets are negative.

Leukocyte acid phosphatase stain

Acid phosphatase is a lysosomal enzyme that by disk electrophoresis can be demonstrated to consist of a number of isoenzymes.[19] L(+) Tartaric acid inhibits acid phosphatase isoenzymes 1-4, but isoenzyme 5 is resistant.[19]

Principle: The sites of acid phosphatase activity are discovered by incubating the specimen in a solution containing naphthol AS-BI phosphoric acid and fast garnet GBC. The acid phosphatase activity liberates naphthol AS-BI, which immediately couples with fast garnet GBC, forming insoluble maroon dye deposits at sites of enzyme activity. Duplicate samples are allowed to act on the same substrate to which L(+) tartaric acid has been added.

Specimen: Prepare smears of fresh capillary or venous blood or tissue imprints. Smears of heparinized blood specimens are also acceptable.

Fixation:
1. Acetone, 30 ml
2. Citrate buffer (dilute), 20 ml (citrate buffer concentrate supplied in kit)

Add the acetone to the buffer.

Procedure: Fix the slide for 30 sec. Wash it in deionized water and air dry.

Reagents: Reagents are supplied in Sigma kit no. 386-A.

Procedure: Follow instructions of Sigma technical bulletin no. 386, March 1980.

Result: Acid phosphatase activity is indicated by maroon-colored deposits.

Interpretation[19,20]: The acid phosphatase stain has a somewhat limited usefulness in diagnostic hematology, because most cells of the hematopoietic system are acid phosphatase positive in varying degrees. The least activity is seen in normoblasts and lymphocytes, and maximal expression is seen in osteoclasts and macrophages. Moderate activity is characteristic for monocytes, plasma cells, and megakaryocytes, whereas weaker reactions are encountered in neutrophils and their precursors. The acid phosphatase in all of these cells is not tartrate resistant. Increased acid phosphatase[21,22] levels are seen in hairy cell leukemia, infectious mononucleosis, macroglobulinemia, and T-cell leukemia.[23] Tartrate-resistant acid phosphatase is characteristic of the hairy cells of leukemic reticuloendotheliosis (hairy cell leukemia); however, rarely are the atypical lymphocytes of infectious mononucleosis also tartrate resistant.[24] It is the characteristic of tartrate resistance that differentiates the cells of hairy cell leukemia from the cells of chronic lymphocytic leukemia and leukosarcoma, which have low non-tartrate-resistant acid phosphatase.

Leukocyte esterase stains

Esterases are enzymes that hydrolyze short-chain esters of fatty acids. The differences between these enzymes include substrate specificity and optimal pH levels. The enzyme is classified as a nonspecific esterase if the substrate is a simple ester, such as α-naphthyl acetate or α-naphthyl butyrate. Specific chloroacetate esterase is best demonstrated by using naphthol AS-D chloroacetate as the substrate. Aminocaproate esterase is demonstrated in mast cells by using ε-aminocaproic acid as substrate, and acetylcholinesterase is demonstrated in megakaryocytes by using acetylthiocholine as substrate.

By most technics the cytochemical demonstration of esterases is based on the hydrolysis of naphtholic substrates and on the splitting off of the specific substituent, which leaves the naphthol free to couple with a diazonium salt to form insoluble azo-dye precipitates.

The pattern of esterase distribution in the various cell types varies according to the choice of substrate.

Naphthol AS-D chloroacetate esterase (specific esterase) stain

Principle: Specific chloroacetate esterase, a lysosomal enzyme, is demonstrated by using naphthol AS-D chloroacetate as substrate at pH 7.0-7.6 and is insensitive to fluoride inhibition.[25] The enzyme splits off naphthol AS-D, which forms a red diazo dye with Fast Corinth V salt.[26]

Specimen: Smears are prepared from capillary or venous blood or from heparinized specimens. They are allowed to dry and then fixed in citrate-acetone-methanol fixative.

Fixation:

Reagents:
1. Methanol, absolute
2. Acetone
3. Citrate concentrate solution (Sigma)
   Dilute 1 part citrate concentrate solution with 9 parts deionized water.

Fixative:
1. Acetone, 60 parts
2. Citrate dilute solution, 40 parts

Discard 10 parts this mixture and replace with 10 parts absolute methanol. Store solution at room temperature, tightly stopped red. Discard after 24 hr.

Procedure: Fix the slides in citrate-acetone-methanol fixative for 30 sec. Wash them well in deionized water and allow to dry. The fixed slides may be stored at room temperature without loss of enzymatic activity.

Reagents: Reagents are supplied in Sigma kit no. 90-C1.

Procedure: Follow instructions of Sigma technical bulletin no. 90, May 1980.

Results: Red deposits indicate sites of enzymatic activity.

Interpretation: The specific naphthol AS-D chloroacetate esterase staining pattern and distribution are essentially those of peroxidase and of Sudan black B (Tables 5-1 and 5-2). Their main contribution to the armamentarium of the hematologist is that monocytes are consistently chloroacetate esterase negative.

Mast cells and granulocytes and their precursors (band and juvenile cells, myelocytes, and promyelocytes) are chloroacetate positive. Normal myeloblasts are negative, but leukemic myeloblasts may be positive. Lymphocytes, normoblasts, eosinophils, megakaryocytes, plasma cells, and monocytes are chloroacetate negative.

α-Naphthyl acetate esterase[26] (nonspecific esterase) stain

Principle: The principle is similar to that of the stain for naphthol AS-D chloroacetate esterase except that α-naphthyl acetate is used as a substrate and fast blue RR salt as a coupling azo dye, the optimal pH is 6.0-6.3, and the esterase is inhibited by fluorides.[25]

Specimen: The specimen is the same as that for naphthol AS-D chloroacetate esterase.

Fixation: Fixation is the same as for naphthol AS-D chloroacetate esterase.

Reagents: Reagents are supplied in Sigma kit no. 90-A1.

Procedure: Follow instructions of Sigma technical bulletin no. 90, March 1980.

Result: Black granulation indicates enzymatic activity.

Interpretation: The nonspecific α-naphthyl esterase

Table 5-1. Characteristics of leukemic blast cells

Type	Romanowsky features*	Cytochemical features*
Acute lymphoblastic leukemia (ALL)	Nuclear cytoplasmic ratio high Nuclei not indented or twisted Erythroblasts not present in peripheral blood Erythroblasts not predominant in bone marrow	5% or less of cells Sudan positive 5% or less of cells peroxidase positive Neutrophil alkaline phosphatase (LAP) score normal or high PAS score in erythroblasts, polychromatophilic and oxyphilic, low
Acute granulocytic (myeloblastic) leukemia (AGL)	Cell outlines not irregular Nuclear cytoplasmic ratio not high Monocytes form less than 1% of nucleated cells of peripheral blood Erythroblasts not predominant in marrow	Neutrophil alkaline phosphatase (LAP) score low Invariably more than 5% and usually more than 85% of cells Sudan black positive of strong local or heavy overall type More than 5% of cells peroxidase positive
Myelomonocytic leukemia	Nuclei indented and twisted Monocytes form more than 1% of nucleated cells of peripheral blood Nuclear cytoplasmic ratio not high Erythroblasts not present in peripheral blood Erythroblasts not predominant in marrow	More than 5% and less than 85% of cells Sudan black positive of more finely granular type than in myeloblastic leukemia
Erythremic myelosis	Cell outlines irregular Nuclear cytoplasmic ratio not high Erythroblasts present in peripheral blood Erythroblasts predominant in marrow	PAS score high More than 5% of cells Sudan black positive More than 5% of cells peroxidase positive

From Hayhoe, F.G.J., and Cawley, J.C.: Clin. Haematol. **1**:49, 1972.
*The features listed for each group are its "group discriminating features."

Table 5-2. Cytochemical reactions in normal blood cells and blasts of acute leukemias

	Peroxidase Sudan black B	Esterases			PAS	Acid phosphatase
		α-Naphthyl acetate	α-Naphthyl butyrate	Naphthol-ASD chloroacetate		
Promyelocyte	+/+ +	−/±	−	+/+ +	±/+	+/+ +
Neutrophil	+ +	−/±	−	+/+ +	+ + +	+
Monocyte	−/±	+ + +	+ +/+ + +	−/±	±	+ +
Lymphocyte	−	−/± *	−/± *	−	−/+	−/+ +
Normoblast	−	−/± †	−	−	−‡	±/−
Megakaryocyte	−	+ + +	±	−	+ +	+ +
ALL	−	−/+ §	−	−	+/+ +‖	−/+
AGL	+/+ +	−	−	+/+ +	−/±	+
APL	+ + +	±	−	+ + +	±/+	+ +
AMML	−/+ +	+/+ + +	+/+ + +	±/+ +	−/+ +	+/+ +
AUL	−	−	−	−	−	−

From Nelson, D.A., and Davey, F.R.: In Williams, W.J., et al., editors: Hematology, ed. 2. Copyright © 1977 by McGraw-Hill Book Co. Used with permission of McGraw-Hill Book Co.
Key:
    − Negative   ALL = Acute lymphocytic leukemia
    ± Weak or few positive cells   AGL = Acute granulocytic leukemia
    + Moderate   APL = Acute promyelocytic leukemia
   + + Moderately strong   AMML = Acute myelomonocytic leukemia
  + + + Strongly positive (most cells)   AUL = Acute undifferentiated leukemia
*Positivity is focal, not diffuse.
†In erythroleukemia and in some erythroid maturation defects, positivity is strong.
‡Positive in erythroleukemia and to a lesser degree in iron deficiency and thalassemia.
§Focal cytoplasmic positivity in a small proportion of ALLs.
‖Coarse blocks are typical.

is strongest in monocytes, monoblasts, megakaryocytes, and platelets and is inhibited by sodium fluoride. Strong activity is also seen in basophils and plasma cells, whereas the activity in lymphocytes and neutrophils is absent, very weak, or only sporadic. A second nonspecific esterase stain, the α-naphthyl butyrate esterase stain is not available in kit form and is described elsewhere.[11,25] Both nonspecific esterases react strongly with myelomonoblasts and monocytes in acute myelomonocytic leukemia (Tables 5-1 and 5-2) and fail to react with myeloblasts and promyelocytes of acute granulocytic leukemia. On the basis of the Wright-Giemsa stain, without the aid of esterase stains, the distinction between promonocyte and promyelocyte may be inaccurate and difficult.[27]

A double staining technic for both specific and nonspecific esterases is also available and colors the granules of granulocytes and their precursor cells red and the monocytic granules black (Sigma technical bulletin no. 90, May 1980).

Periodic acid–Schiff (PAS) stain

Principle: In hemic cells glycogen is the most important polysaccharide that reacts positively with the Schiff reagent. Other polysaccharides that give a positive PAS reaction are starch, chitin, cellulose, and glycoproteins (mucoproteins). The initial phase of the PAS stain[14,28-32] is the oxidation of polysaccharides, which are polyhydric alcohols, by periodic acid to aldehydes. The latter are detected by the addition of colorless pararosaniline plus sodium metabisulfite (Schiff reagent), which is transformed into a red compound. Excess Schiff reagent is then removed by sulfurous rinses.

To distinguish the reaction given by glycogen from that given by other PAS-positive polysaccharides, duplicate slides are treated with diastase and then stained with PAS stain.

Specimen: Smears prepared from capillary, fresh venous, or heparinized blood or from bone marrow are allowed to dry and should be fixed as soon as possible.

Fixation:
Reagents:
1. Formaldehyde, 37%
2. Ethanol, 95%
Fixative:
1. Formaldehyde, 5 ml
2. Ethanol, 95 ml
Prepare solution fresh daily, and keep it tightly stoppered.
Procedure: Fix the air-dried smears for 10 min at room temperature. Rinse them in slowly running tap water for 5-10 min.
Reagents: Reagents are supplied in Sigma kit no. 395-A.
Procedure: Follow instructions of Sigma technical bulletin no. 395, March 1980.
Result: PAS-positive material is colored pink to pale violet-red.
Controls:
Positive control: Normal polymorphonuclear leukocytes are used as a positive control.
Cytochemical control: Pretreat smear with diastase

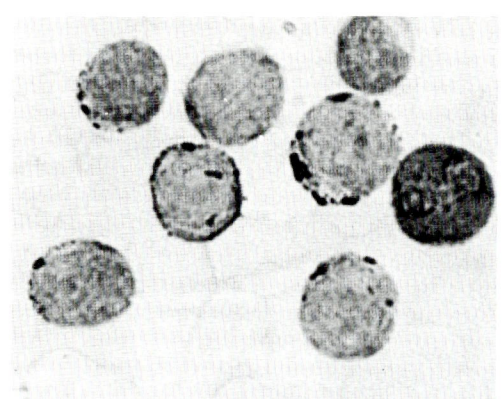

Fig. 5-8. PAS reaction of blast cells. One cell is negative and the remainder are all strongly positive with coarse granules and blocks. A granulocyte shows normal positivity and a mature lymphocyte is negative. (From Hayhoe, F. G. J., Quaglino, D., and Doll, R.: The cytology and cytochemistry of acute leukaemias, M.R.C. special report series, no. 304, London, 1964, Her Majesty's Stationery Office. By permission of the Controller.)

solution, which hydrolyzes positive-reacting glycogen. A blood smear prepared from the same specimen as the PAS-positive smear will react negatively after diastase treatment when stained with PAS stain if the PAS-positive material is glycogen.

Diastase control: The reagent is diastase solution: 0.5 g diastase and 1 dl water. Stored in a refrigerator, the solution remains good for 1 week. The technic involves treating control and duplicate films with diastase solution for 30 min and staining with PAS stain.

Interpretation: Cells of the granulocytic series beginning with the myelocytes show increasing granular cytoplasmic PAS positivity reminiscent of their reaction pattern with Sudan black B. Myeloblasts are normally PAS negative, although they may show a faint diffuse cytoplasmic pink tinge, while in promyelocytes and myelocytes a pink halo may surround the nucleus. Later stages of the maturing granulocytic cells, such as juvenile and stab cells, show increasing numbers of PAS-positive intracytoplasmic granules, until finally the segmented polymorphonuclear leukocyte is densely packed with granules that spare the nucleus but hide the cytoplasm (Fig. 5-8).

Eosinophils contain finely granular PAS-positive material that does not involve the specific granules.

Basophils at times contain coarsely granular PAS-positive deposits.

Twenty percent or fewer lymphocytes and their precursors show delicate, discrete, somewhat coarse PAS-positive granules arranged in rings parallel to the periphery of the cytoplasm. The granules vary in number from 2-4 to about 30-40. Pale pink staining of the perinuclear area is commonly seen and is not interpreted as PAS positivity. Slight elevation of the number of PAS-positive lymphocytes is seen in viral lymphocytosis.

Monocytes vary in their PAS response from com-

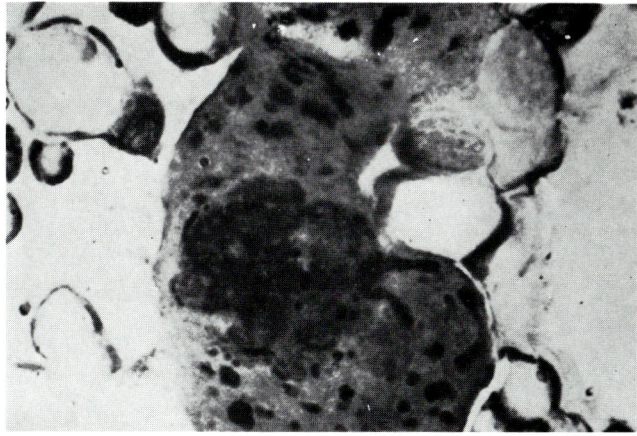

Fig. 5-9. PAS-positive clumps in cytoplasm of megakaryocyte. (From Bauer-Sic, P., and Lambers, K.: In Merher, H., editor: Zyto- und Histochemie in der Hämatologie, Berlin, 1963, Springer-Verlag.)

pletely negative to a pink hue to fine or coarse red granules.

Plasma cells also vary from negative to weakly positive, with occasional granules against a light pink background, but plasmacytoid cells of Waldenström's macroglobulinemia and the myeloma cells of IgA multiple myeloma contain intracytoplasmic and intranuclear glycogen deposits.

Megakaryocytes are PAS positive, showing a diffuse cytoplasmic positivity with occasional large PAS-positive glycogen blocks (Fig. 5-9). Newly formed platelets are also PAS positive and adorn the periphery of the platelet-forming megakaryocyte with a red rim. The **Reed-Sternberg** cells of Hodgkin's disease, which may be confused with megakaryoblasts, are PAS negative.

The lymphoblasts of about 80% of patients with acute lymphatic leukemia contain fine to coarse PAS-positive granules and at times even large blocks of positively reacting glycogen (Fig. 5-8). In acute myelocytic leukemia the myeloblasts and promyelocytes may be completely PAS negative or may show diffuse positivity. In acute monocytic or myelomonocytic leukemia the cells may be negative or show diffuse positivity with fine to coarse granules. In acute erythroleukemia (Di Guglielmo syndrome) normoblasts and erythroblasts that are normally PAS negative may show a strong PAS-positive reaction that may involve all erythrocytic precursors or only a few. A positive reaction of normoblasts may also be seen in thalassemia, in some cases of iron deficiency anemia, and in idiopathic sideroblastic anemia.

In chronic lymphocytic leukemia a greater number of lymphocytes and prolymphocytes show heavier PAS granular deposits than are seen in normal lymphocytes. This finding contrasts with the PAS staining in chronic granulocytic leukemia, in which the PAS positivity of the white cells is somewhat reduced compared to the nonleukemic cells.

Sézary cells and the cells of hairy cell leukemia are positive (diffuse or granular), but PAS positiveness is not a constant finding.

Demonstration of lysozyme using lysozyme substrate (lyophilized *Micrococcus lysodeikticus*)

Principle: Lysozyme activity can be demonstrated by lysis of *Micrococcus lysodeikticus*[33] and can be used to separate monocytes from lymphocytes. The technic is a modification of the cytochemical method of Briggs.[34]

Reagents:
1. Fixative
   Neutral formalin, 10%, 1 vol
   Ethanol, 96%, 3 vol
2. Substrate
   Lysozyme substrate (Difco Laboratories, Detroit), 60 mg
   Saline, 1 ml
   Prepare substrate fresh, mixing gently but well.
3. Phosphate buffer, 0.01 M, pH 7.0
   KH_2PO_4, 0.70g
   Na_2HPO_4, 0.65 g
   Water, 9 dl
   Adjust pH and dilute to make to 1 L.

Procedure: Perform the test within 1 hr of collecting EDTA-anticoagulated bone marrow or peripheral blood buffy coat. Mix in a test tube equal volumes of buffy coat or bone marrow and *M. lysodeikticus* suspension (0.25-0.5 ml each) and shake gently for 5-10 sec. Prepare the smear from the mixture, allow it to dry, and fix it in fixative for 1 min. Rinse in buffer and incubate in buffer at 37° C for 10 min. Air dry the smear and stain with Wright-Giemsa stain.

Result: Lysozyme activity is indicated by a variably sized zone of lysed bacteria surrounding the appropriate leukocytes. Some bacteria are completely lysed, whereas others stain weaker than the surrounding unaffected bacteria.

Interpretation: Normal monocytes, neutrophils, and their precursor cells back to myelocytes show strong lysozyme activity, whereas lymphocytes, leukemic lymphoblasts, and myeloblasts are lysozyme negative. Leukemic monoblasts, promonocytes, and myelomonoblasts are lysozyme positive in more than 50% of patients.[35]

Quantitative determination of lysozyme activity in serum and urine

In the above mentioned acute leukemias the stimulated production of lysozymes is responsible for high lysozyme blood levels and for spillover into the urine. Lysozyme concentration is also elevated in renal homograft rejection and in Crohn's disease.[36]

Principle: The rate of lysis of *M. lysodeikticus* in a suspension is a measure of lysozyme concentration.

Reagents: The test is available in kit form from Worthington Diagnostics, Millipore Corp., Freehold, N.J.

REFERENCES

1. Sheehan, D.C., and Hrapchak, B.B.: Theory and practice of histotechnology, ed. 2, St. Louis, 1980, The C.V. Mosby Co.
2. Gurr, E.: A practical manual of medical and biological staining techniques, ed. 2, New York, 1956, Interscience Publishers, Inc.
3. Rosse, C.: Blood **34:**72, 1969.
4. Schwind, J.L.: Blood **5:**597, 1950.
5. Kosenow, W.: Acta Haematol. **7:**217, 1952.
6. Pearse, E.A.G.: Histochemistry theoretical and applied, vol. 2, Edinburgh, 1972, Churchill Livingstone.
7. Kaplow, L.S.: Special stains for blood cells, methods and applications. Medcom famous teachings in modern medicine, New York, 1975, Medcom, Inc.
8. Gomori, G.: Am. J. Pathol. **12:**655, 1936.
9. Harrison, P.M.: J. Mol. Biol. **6:**404, 1963.
10. Richter, G.W., and Bessis, M.: Blood **25:**370, 1965.
11. Bauer, J.D.: In Sonnenwirth, A.C., and Jarett, L., editors: Gradwohl's clinical laboratory methods and diagnosis, ed. 8, St. Louis, 1980, The C.V. Mosby Co, vol. 1.
12. Kaplow, L.S.: Blood **26:**215, 1965.
13. Hanker, J.S., et al.: Histochem. J. **9:**789, 1977.
14. Hayhoe, F.G.J.: In Custer, R.P., editor: An atlas of the blood and bone marrow, Philadelphia, 1974, W.B. Saunders Co.
15. Beutler, E.: In Williams, W.J., et al., editors: Hematology, New York, 1977, McGraw-Hill Book Co.
16. Rosenblum, D., and Petzold, S.J.: Blood **45:**335, 1975.
17. Schmidt, D.Z.: Am. J. Med. Sci. **252:**465, 1966.
18. Sheehan, H.L., and Storey, G.W.: J. Pathol. **59:**336, 1947.
19. Li, C.Y., Yam, L.T., and Lam, K.W.: J. Histochem. Cytochem. **18:**473, 1970.
20. Kaplow, L.S., and Burstone, M.S.: J. Histochem. Cytochem. **12:**805, 1964.
21. Yam, L.T., Li, C.Y., and Finkel, H.E.: Arch. Intern. Med. **130:**248, 1972.
22. Yam, L.T., Li, C.Y., and Lam, K.W.: N. Engl. J. Med. **284:**357, 1972.
23. Davey, F.R., and Nelson, D.A.: In Williams, W.J., et al., editors: Hematology, ed. 2, New York, 1977, McGraw-Hill Book Co.
24. Katayama, I., Li, C.Y., and Yam, L.T.: Cancer **29:**157, 1972.
25. Li, C.Y., Lam, K.W., and Yam, L.T.: J. Histochem. Cytochem. **21:**1, 1973.
26. Yam, L.T., Li, C.Y., and Crosby, W.H.: Am. J. Clin. Pathol. **55:**283, 1971.
27. Glick, A.D., and Horn, R.G.: Br. J. Haematol. **26:**395, 1974.
28. Hayhoe, F.G.J., and Flemans, R.J.: An atlas of haematological cytology, New York, 1970, John Wiley & Sons, Inc.
29. Hayhoe, F.G.J., Quagline, D., and Doll, R.: The cytology and cytochemistry of acute leukemias, a study of 140 cases. Medical Research Council Special Report Series, no. 304, London, 1964, Her Majesty's Stationery Office.
30. Hayhoe, F.G.J., and Cawley, J.C.: Clin. Haematol. **1:**49, 1972.
31. Merher, H.: Zyto- und Histochemie in der Haematologie, Berlin, 1963, Springer-Verlag.
32. Brynes, R.K., and Vardiman, J.W.: Histologic techniques in hematopathology, Chicago, 1974, University of Chicago Hospitals and Clinics.
33. Syrén, E., and Raeste, A.M.: Acta Haematol. **45:**29, 1971.
34. Briggs, R.S., Perillie, P.E., and Finch, S.C.: J. Histochem. Cytochem. **14:**167, 1966.
35. Catovsky, D., and Galton, D.A.G.: J. Clin. Pathol. **26:**60, 1973.
36. Falchuk, D.R., Perrotto, J.L., and Isselbacher, K.J.: N. Engl. J. Med. **292:**395, 1975.

CHAPTER 6

Morphology of blood and bone marrow cells

MATURATION OF BLOOD CELLS

Maturation of blood cells is a continuous process, but certain forms are singled out as morphologic indicators of various stages in the development of a cell line. Of special importance is the morphologic differentiation of mature from immature cells. The immature nucleus is large, occupying almost the entire cell, the nuclear chromatin is delicate and fine, and the nucleoli are large in relation to the nuclear size. The cytoplasm is scanty and basophilic and contains no specific secretions. As the cell matures, it usually decreases in size (the megakaryocyte is the exception), the nucleus becomes smaller, the nucleoli disappear, and the nuclear chromatin becomes dense and deeply stained. The cytoplasm loses its basophilia, and secretory products appear in it. The nuclear cytoplasmic ratio of the immature cell is greater than that of the mature cell.

The suffix ''-blast'' indicates an immature cell, whereas the mature cell is indicated by the suffix ''-cyte'' (myelocyte is an exception). The intermediate cell forms are labeled ''pro-'' and ''meta-.''

Overview of the Wright-Giemsa–stained cell

In this chapter the cells are described as they appear when stained with Wright-Giemsa stain and viewed by light microscopy, but pertinent features seen in phase or electron microscopy are added. Staining procedures and cytochemical investigations are described in Chapter 5. Cell structures visualized by the Wright-Giemsa stain include the nucleus, which is surrounded by a nuclear membrane and contains particulate material called chromatin, the basophilia of which is caused by DNA. Dense portions of the chromatin are called chromocenters. The lighter stained areas between the reticular chromatin are called parachromatin or nuclear sap. The pattern and distribution of chromatin vary according to type, age, and activity of the cell. The interphase nucleus of female cells contains a condensed mass of chromatin that is triangular in shape and closely applied to the inner surface of the nuclear membrane: the **sex chromatin.** The **nucleolus** is a condensation of RNA within the nucleus, which appears dark to light blue

and is often surrounded by condensed chromatin. The cytoplasm is surrounded by a cell membrane. Adjacent to the nucleus is an area of pale cytoplasm called the centrosome or hof (the Golgi system).

Electron microscopic structure of "typical" white cell as related to cellular function and cytochemistry

Electron microscopy (Fig. 6-1) has added materially to our understanding of cell structure. Because some of the structures defined by electron microscopy are visualized by cytochemistry and are related to function, electron microscopic terminology is essential for the understanding of both.

The **nucleus** is characterized by the pattern of its chromatin, which contains most of the cell's deoxyribonucleic acid (DNA). The latter stains purple-blue with Romanowsky stains, fluoresces green with acridine orange, and is Feulgen positive. The nucleus is surrounded by a double-layered **nuclear membrane,** which is interrupted by openings called **nuclear pores** and which on the nuclear side is lined by condensations of chromatin that are also interrupted in the areas of the pores, thus allowing interchange between nucleus and cytoplasm, e.g., messenger RNA. The nuclear membranes are surrounded by a space, the perinuclear cistern.

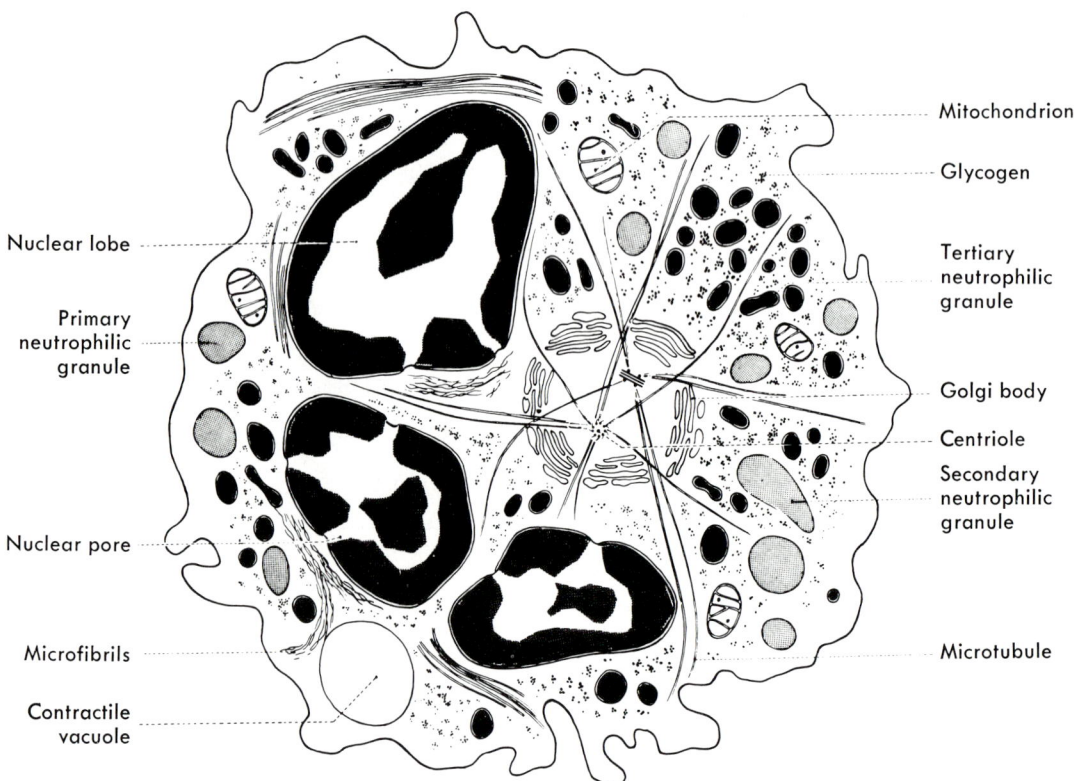

Fig. 6-1. Neutrophilic granulocyte as seen with electron microscope. (From Bessis, M.: Living blood cells and their ultrastructure, Heidelberg, West Germany, 1973, Springer-Verlag)

The **nucleolus** consists of RNA particles and/or protein particles or filaments and is surrounded by chromatin. It is pyronine positive, fluoresces red with acridine orange, and stains bluish with Romanowsky stains.

The **cytoplasm,** which is surrounded by a thin three-layer **membrane,** contains a number of **organelles,** a name given to different structures located within its matrix. A few organelles can be seen by light microscopy, some can be visualized by cytochemistry and phase microscopy, but most require electron microscopy for their detection. They are endoplasmic reticulum, Golgi body, centrioles, mitochondria, ribosomes, lysosomes, specific granulations, vacuoles, and storage granules.

The **endoplasmic reticulum** consists of linked saccular or tubular structures, which are called rough endoplasmic reticulum or ergastoplasm if ribosomes (RNA) are attached to the surface and smooth endoplasmic reticulum if ribosomes are not attached. The endoplasmic reticulum is in continuity with openings in the perinuclear cistern and in the cell membrane. The products produced by the ribosomes (amino acid units of proteins) enter the lumina of the endoplasmic reticulum and are ultimately transferred to the **Golgi apparatus,** a series of vesicles and sacs where enzymes are synthesized and can be demonstrated histochemically. The main functions of endoplasmic reticulum are protein synthesis and transport. Granulocytes that are not concerned with protein synthesis contain scant endoplasmic reticulum, whereas plasma cells, responsible for immunoglobulin production, are rich in ergastoplasm.

Mitochondria measure up to 4 μm in length and up to 0.8 μm in width and consist of a liquid matrix surrounded by two limiting membranes, the inner membrane of which is folded into cristae. Mitochondria can be visualized by phase microscopy. They form high-energy chemical bonds (ATP), contain enzymes of the citric acid cycle, and are involved in oxidation and phosphorylation in the respiratory chain. Mitochondria contain DNA, the structure of which may be different in leukemic and nonleukemic cells.[1] Plasma cells contain many large mitochondria, whereas lymphocytes contain only a few small mitochondria.

Ribosomes are minute accumulations of RNA and protein that occur singly (monoribosomes) or in groups (polyribosomes) and are responsible for protein synthesis within the cell. They are thus most highly developed in cells producing immunoglobulins, e.g., plasma cells. Immature cells are rich in RNA, so that the cytoplasm stains blue with Romanowsky stains. As the cells mature, the amount of RNA decreases and the cytoplasmic blue color disappears.

Lysosomes (granules) are collections of digestive acid proteolytic enzymes (acid hydrolases and oxidases) surrounded by a lipoprotein membrane. They are involved in the digestion of phagocytosed material and cell lysis; lysosomes are divided into primary and secondary. Acid phosphatase, ribonuclease, collagenase, and glucuronidase are their most important enzymes. The lysosomes of the various cell lines differ in their enzymatic composition; e.g., the lysosomes of lymphocytes do not contain peroxidase and are Sudan black B negative, whereas neutrophilic lysosomes are peroxidase and Sudan black B positive. The lysosomes of both cells are acid phosphatase and naphthol AS-D chloroacetate esterase positive. As long as the enzymes remain within the lipoprotein envelopes, the cell is protected and digestion of itself and of phagocytosed material within vacuoles does not take place. In the neutrophilic series of cells two types of granules are seen: **primary** or **azurophilic granules** and **secondary** or **specific granules.** Histochemically the azurophilic granules are peroxidase positive, whereas the neutrophilic granules are alkaline phosphatase positive (see Chapter 9 for a discussion of phagocytosis and leukocytic function tests).

The **Golgi apparatus** (also referred to as centrosome) is situated in the juxtanuclear area of the cell center and consists of a series of membranous sacs (tubules) and clusters of vesicles that are involved in synthesis of enzymes such as peroxidase and acid phosphatase and of mucopolysaccharides. In granulocytes the concave surface of the tubules gives rise to the large azurophilic granules, whereas the small specific neutrophilic granules arise from the convex surface of the Golgi apparatus (Fig. 6-1). The latter structure is thought to be the point of confluence of various cell products used for protein synthesis. The center of this apparatus is occupied by two **centrioles,** which appear as sheaves of small tubules to which satellites with their microtubules are attached. Functionally centrioles are involved in mitoses and cell movement.

Several types of **vacuoles** are seen within the cytoplasm, e.g., storage vacuoles and contractile vacuoles caused by pinocytosis and phagocytosis.

ORIGIN OF BLOOD CELLS
Stem cell

In the embryo and probably also in the adult one single fixed pluripotent stem cell gives rise to tissue and to blood cells. It has dual abilities to replicate itself and to differentiate into a multipotent cell that gives rise to a unipotent committed stem cell. The latter cell provides specific hematopoietic cell lines in response to various stimulating hormones, e.g., erythropoietin.

The Philadelphia chromosome found in chronic myeloid leukemia lends some credence to the above model. It is demonstrable in neutrophil and red cell precursors and in megakaryocytes.[2] The mature lymphocyte is probably its own and the plasma cell's stem cell. The morphologic identity of either the pluripotent or the unipotent stem cell is not well established, but based on the culture methods mentioned below and in the section on bone marrow culture, these cells probably resemble small circulating lymphocytes.

In the last decade experimental work has identified cells involved in the early stages of hematopoiesis.[3] In the spleen of irradiated mice Till and McCulloch demonstrated cells called CFUs (**colony-forming unit spleen**), which are pluripotent stem cells capable of forming erythroid, granulocytic, and thrombocytic colonies.[4] Bradley and Metcalf[5] grew a unipotent granu-

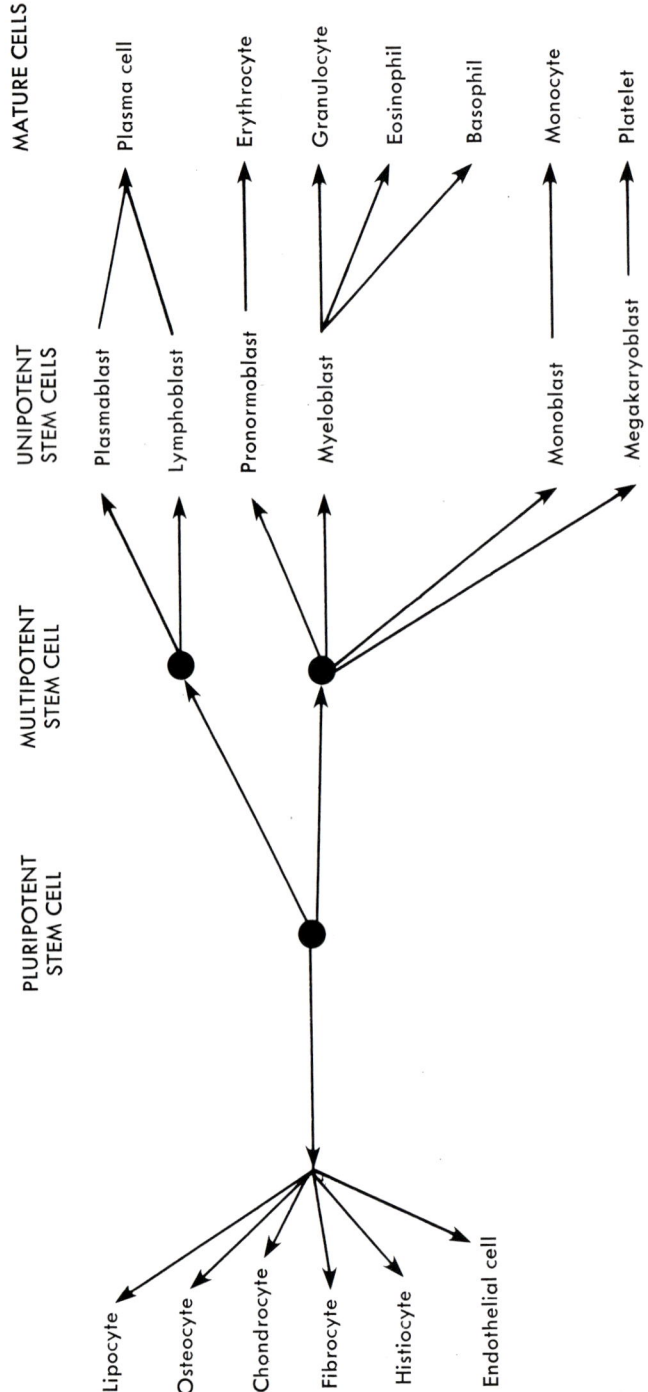

Fig. 6-2. Origin of blood and tissue cells.

locytic stem cell, the CFUc (colony-forming unit in culture), in semisolid agar medium with the aid of a colony-stimulating factor (Fig. 6-2).

Erythropoiesis

In the adult, normal erythropoiesis occurs in the bone marrow. In the embryo, erythropoiesis takes place in the liver, spleen, adrenal, pancreas, and other organs. In adult life, under pathologic conditions (bone marrow replacement by fibrous tissue), the call for blood is met by the reticuloendothelial organs that had hematopoietic function in fetal life, primarily the liver and the spleen where extramedullary hematopoiesis takes place. Erythropoiesis requires such building blocks as iron, folic acid, and vitamin B_{12}. If folic acid or vitamin B_{12} or both are missing, **megaloblastic erythropoiesis** supersedes or occurs simultaneously with physiologic **normoblastic erythropoiesis.** When there is a deficiency of iron, the cells mature but fail to acquire the normal amount of hemoglobin. Erythropoiesis follows the above outlined pattern of cell maturation. The pluripotent primitive stem cell destined to produce erythrocytes under the influence of erythropoietin differentiates into the multipotent cell, which in turn produces the pronormoblast. Within a period of 5 days each pronormoblast gives rise to four orthochromatic normoblasts. They extrude their nuclei and enter the bone marrow sinusoids as reticulocytes, which in 1 or 2 days become mature erythrocytes who spend their life of 120 days in the peripheral circulation.

Erythropoietin

Erythropoietin (EP) is a hormonelike substance that controls the red cell production and the red cell mass. It is a glycoprotein ($T^{1}/_{2} = 6$ hr) that causes the stem cell to metamorphose ultimately into the morphologically recognizable red cell precursor, the pronormoblast. Ninety percent of EP is produced in the kidney[6] in the juxtaglomerular areas,[7] whereas 10% is produced extrarenally, probably in the liver.[8] Since EP cannot be experimentally localized in the kidney and since nephrectomy does not completely suppress EP activity, it is assumed that the kidney produces an enzyme that acts on an inactive plasma factor (erythropoietinogen) to transform it into the biologically active EP. The renal EP is responsive to tissue hypoxia.[9] The urine concentration of EP reflects its plasma level, which in turn is inversely related to the hemoglobin concentration,[10] so that a feedback mechanism is established between kidney, oxygen, and EP.[11] EP increases the bone marrow pool of ''erythroid stem cells'' and shortens the red cell production and transit time,[12] so that ''stress'' reticulocytes appear in the peripheral blood (see discussion of reticulocytes, p. 128).

Erythropoietin assay: EP may be assayed by a number of different methods. An older method still in common use is a bioassay using hypoxia-induced polycythemic mice.[13] It is relatively insensitive in that it will barely detect the EP in the serum of normal individuals. Like all bioassays it is lengthy, requiring several days for completion. Agglutination inhibition studies and radioimmunoassay (RIA)[14,15] procedures depend for their success on the purity of the EP used for the production of the antibody.

MORPHOLOGY OF RED CELLS AND THEIR PRECURSORS

NORMOBLASTIC ERYTHROPOIESIS
(Plates 1 and 2, pp. 129 and 145)
Pronormoblast (rubriblast)

Size: The pronormoblast is 20-25 μm in diameter.

Nucleus: The nucleus is large, round to oval, and contains 0-2 light bluish, indistinct nucleoli. The chromatin forms a delicate network giving the nucleus a reticular appearance and allowing only tiny dots of pink parachromatin to shine through the interstices (Fig. 6-3).

Cytoplasm: There is a narrow (about 2 μm) rim of dark blue cytoplasm. It is more condensed and less in amount than that seen in the myeloblast or promyelocyte. There may be a perinuclear halo. The nuclear/cytoplasmic ratio is about 8:1.

Basophilic normoblast (basophilic rubricyte)

Size: The basophilic normoblast is 16-18 μm in diameter.

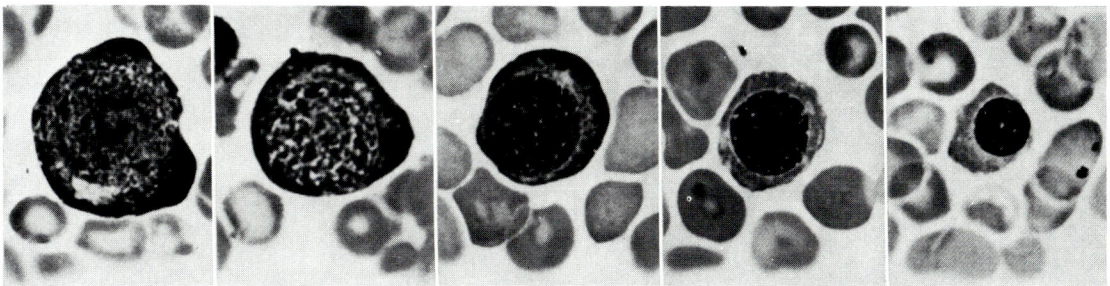

Fig. 6-3. Successive stages in normoblastic maturation of red cells as seen in bone marrow smear stained with Wright-Giemsa stain. Left to right: pronormoblast; basophilic normoblast; basophilic normoblast (later stage); polychromatophilic normoblast; orthochromatic normoblast. ($\times 2000$.) (From Bessis, M.: Life cycle of the erythrocyte, Basel, Switzerland, 1966, Sandoz.)

Nucleus: The nucleus is round or oval and smaller than in the previous stage. The chromatin forms delicate clumps so that its pattern appears to be denser and coarser than that seen in the pronormoblast. No nucleoli are seen. The parachromatin is arranged in irregular small pink dots.

Cytoplasm: There is a slightly wider ring of deep blue cytoplasm than in the pronormoblast, and there is a perinuclear halo. The nuclear/cytoplasmic ratio is about 6:1 (Fig. 6-3).

Vacuolated basophilic normoblast

Vacuolated basophilic normoblasts have been reported in a number of conditions: chloramphenicol administration,[16] acute alcoholism,[17] severe malnutrition,[18] leukemia, chemotherapy,[19] aplastic anemia,[20] phenylalanine deficiency,[21] riboflavin deficiency,[18] and episodes of hyperosmolarity.[22]

Polychromatophilic normoblast (polychromatophilic rubricyte)

Size: The polychromatophilic normoblast is 9-12 μm in diameter.

Nucleus: The nucleus is smaller than in the previous cell, has a thick membrane, and contains coarse chromatin masses. The parachromatin forms pink, small, irregular areas in the interstices.

Cytoplasm: As the nucleus is shrinking, the band of cytoplasm is widening. It has a lilac (polychromatic) tint because of beginning hemoglobinization. The nuclear/cytoplasmic ratio varies from 2:1 to 4:1 (Fig. 6-3).

Orthochromatic normoblast (metarubricyte)

Size: The orthochromatic normoblast is 7-10 μm in diameter.

Nucleus: The nucleus is small and central or eccentric with condensed homogeneous structureless chromatin.

Cytoplasm: A wide rim of pink cytoplasm surrounds the shrinking nucleus. The entire cell is somewhat smaller than the polychromatophilic normoblast. The nuclear/cytoplasmic ratio varies from 1:2 to 1:3.

Nuclear degeneration: When the nucleus disappears atypically or incompletely, as it often does in pernicious anemia, myelocytic leukemia, and very severe anemia, it may leave a remnant of the nuclear membrane or it may break up and leave small spheroid pyknotic portions known as **Howell-Jolly bodies** (Plate 1 [p. 129], *41* and *42*).

Variations in polychromatophilic normoblasts

Multinucleated normoblasts: Failure of cytoplasmic division leads to the formation of normoblasts with two to four or even more nuclei. Such cells may occur in pernicious anemia and in erythroleukemia. In erythroleukemia the nuclei contain nucleoli, and the cytoplasm may vary from deep blue to lavender because of beginning hemoglobinization.

Small normoblasts: Unusually small cells may occur in iron deficiency anemia and in erythroleukemia.

Vacuolated normoblasts: See previous discussion of vacuolated basophilic normoblasts.

Reticulocyte

After the expulsion of the nucleus a large somewhat basophilic anuclear cell remains, which, when stained with new methylene blue, a vital dye, is seen to contain a network of bluish granules. This network is responsible for the name of the cell and consists of precipitated ribosomes (Fig. 6-4). As the bone marrow reticulocyte matures, the network becomes smaller, finer, thinner, and finally within 3 days disappears. If the hematocrit is normal, about 1% of reticulocytes enter the

---

Plate 1. Blood cells (Giemsa stain; scale: 1 mm = 1 μm). (From Sonnenwirth, A.C., and Jarett, L., editors: Gradwohl's clinical laboratory methods and diagnosis, ed. 8, St. Louis, 1980, The C.V. Mosby Co., vol. 1.)

1 Myeloblast	**26** Irritation cell
2 Promyelocyte	**27** Rubricyte, pernicious anemia type
3 and **4** Neutrophilic myelocytes	**28** Metarubricyte, pernicious anemia type
5 Eosinophilic myelocyte	**29** and **30** Metarubricytes
6 Basophilic myelocyte	**31** Metarubricyte with nucleus showing karyorrhexis
7 Metamyelocyte	**32** Megalocyte
8 and **9** Band granulocytes	**33** Macrocyte
10 Degenerated band granulocyte	**34** Erythrocyte
11 Segmented neutrophil	**35** Microcyte
12 Eosinophil	**32-35** Example of anisocytosis
13 Basophil	**36** Erythroblast with mitotic nucleus
14 Lymphoblast	**37** Faintly polychromatophilic erythrocyte
15 Large lymphocyte	**38** Polychromatophilic erythrocyte
16 Small lymphocyte	**39** Basophilic punctation, fine
17 Reticuloendothelial cell	**40** Basophilic punctation, coarse
18-20 Monocytes	**41** Poikilocytes with Howell-Jolly bodies
21 Endothelial cell	**42** Howell-Jolly body
22 Atypical promyelocyte	**43** Ring form of malarial parasite
23 Micromyeloblast	**44** and **45** Cabot rings
24 Twin-nuclear cell	**46** Erythrocyte showing achromia
25 Plasma cell	**47** Hyperchromic erythrocyte
	48 Platelets

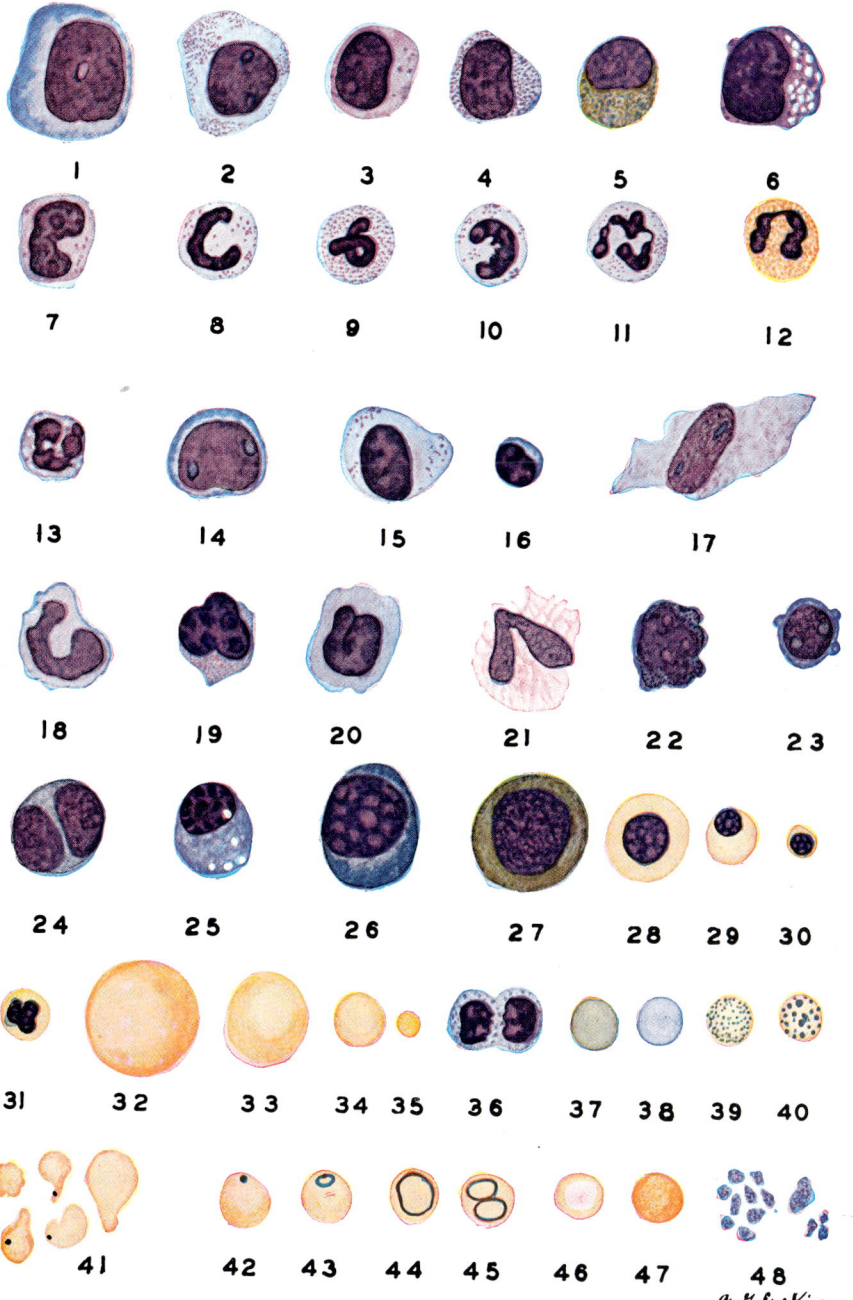

Plate 1. For legend see opposite page.

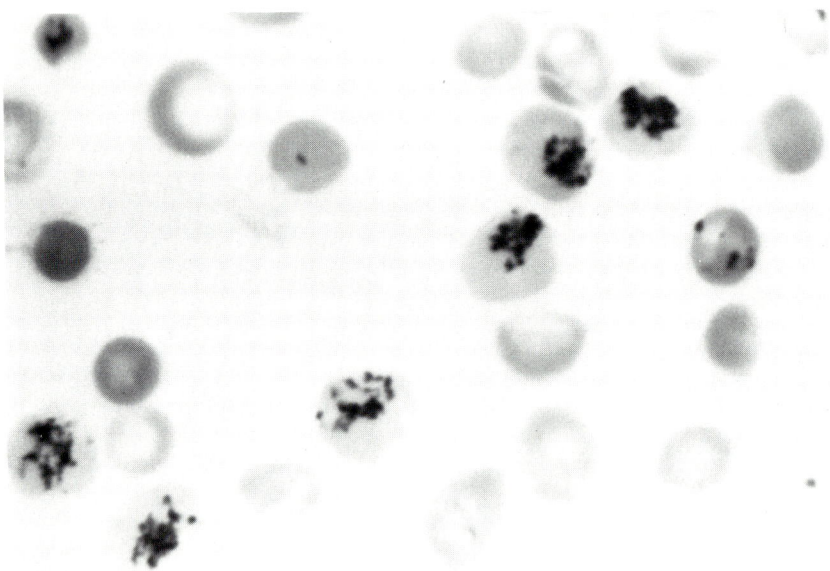

Fig. 6-4. Young reticulocytes stained with vital stain.

bone marrow sinusoids by way of diapedesis and thus enter the circulation. In the peripheral blood the remaining reticulum disappears within 24-48 hr.

In anemias associated with high erythropoietin levels, young large reticulocytes are swept into the peripheral blood, the so-called "shift cells." They are a measure of effective erythropoiesis and are further discussed in the section on reticulocyte count in Chapter 7.

Size: The reticulocyte is 8-10 μm in diameter. It is usually larger than the mature erythrocyte, and if it is harassed by accelerated erythropoiesis, it may reach almost twice the normal red cell size. The presence of these macrocytic cells, if in sufficient numbers (over 30%), shifts the size distribution curve of automated particle counters to the right and may increase the mean corpuscular volume (MCV).

Nucleus: The reticulocyte does not contain a nucleus.

Cytoplasm: The cell outline may be irregular because of shallow indentations. The cytoplasm is faintly polychromatophilic (basophilic).

Erythrocyte

Size: The erythrocyte is about 7.5-8.3 μm in diameter and 1.7 μm thick.[23]

Nucleus: There is no nucleus present in the erythrocyte.

Cytoplasm: The biconcave orange-pink cytoplasm has a paler staining center occupying one third of the cell area[24] (Fig. 6-5).

Variations of erythrocytes in stained smear

Method of reporting: The number (percentage) of abnormal cells per 100 normal red cells should be reported after counting several hundred cells.

Variations in size

Normal range: The normal range includes a few cells as small as 6 μm in diameter and a few as large as 9 μm in diameter.

Anisocytosis: Anisocytosis implies that the variation in size of erythrocytes is greater than normal (Fig. 6-6). If there is marked anisocytosis, the mean corpuscular hemoglobin concentration (MCHC) loses its significance because the individual cells differ too much in hemoglobin content. On the basis of their diameters, the cells are divided into gigantocytes, macrocytes, megalocytes, microcytes, and spherocytes (see discussion of variations in shape).

Gigantocytes: The cells are larger than 10 μm in diameter because of a failure of cell division (polyploidy).

Macrocytes: The cells are larger than 8 μm in diameter and may be caused by vitamin B_{12} or folic acid deficiency, or they may be young red cells that can be shown by supravital staining to be reticulocytes. Macrocytes are found in megaloblastic anemias, cirrhosis, and hemolytic anemias. The macrocytes of pernicious anemia are oval, whereas in liver disease they tend to be round and flat and are often target cells (Figs. 6-7 and 6-8).

Megalocytes: Megalocytes measure 9-12 μm in diameter and are usually caused by folic acid or vitamin B_{12} deficiency. The central depression may be absent or only minimal. The best way to decide whether macrocytic cells are caused by B_{12} or folic acid deficiency or both is to determine the serum B_{12} and the serum or red cell folate levels. The hemoglobin concentration within the cell is normal but tinctorially appears to be increased because of the increased thickness of the cell (hyperchromia).

Microcytes: Microcytes measure less than 6 μm in

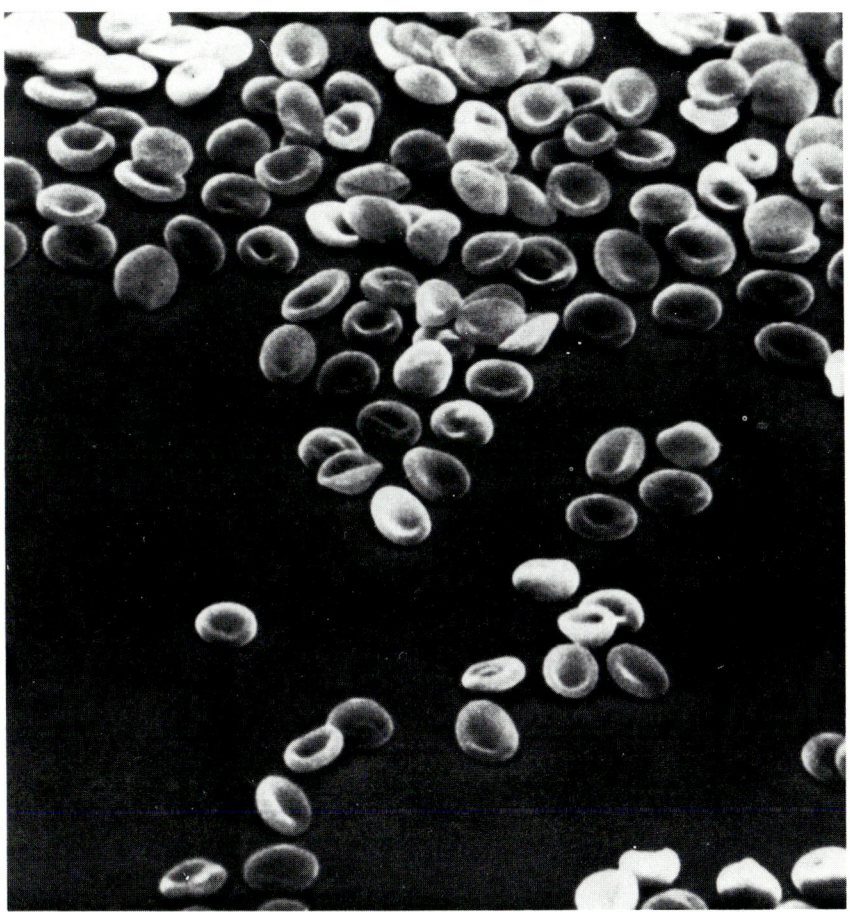

Fig. 6-5. Normal human red cells as seen with scanning electron microscopy. (From Salsbury, A.J., and Clarke, J.A.: Triangle **8**(7):261-263, 1968.)

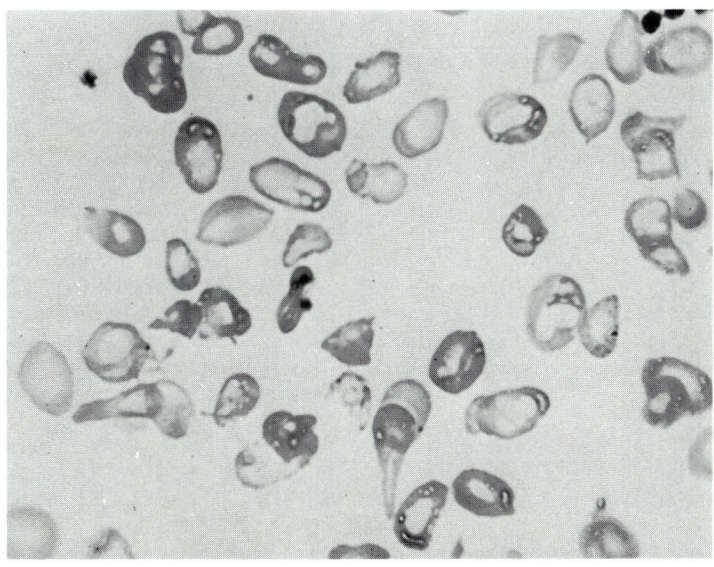

Fig. 6-6. Anisocytosis (thalassemia major).

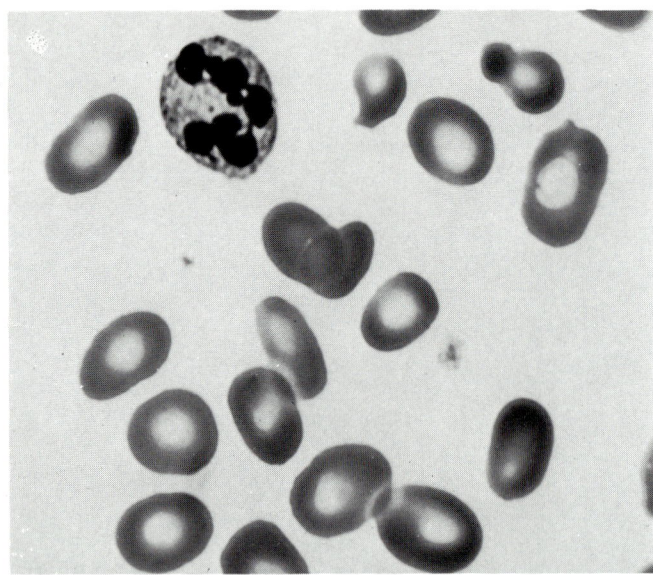

Fig. 6-7. Oval macrocytes (pernicious anemia); hypersegmented granulocyte.

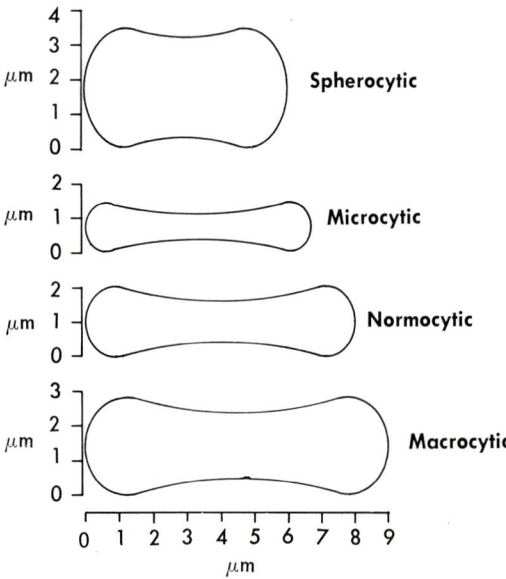

Fig. 6-8. Side views of various types of red cells.

diameter and are caused by iron deficiency. The presence of the normal or exaggerated central pallor differentiates these cells from spherocytes (see anulocytes).

Variations in staining (Plate 1, p. 129)

Anulocytes: Anulocytes are thin cells that are poorly hemoglobinized and exhibit a thin peripheral ring of stained hemoglobin surrounding a large central clear area (Fig. 6-9).

Hyperchromia: The hemoglobin content of the individual cell **appears** to be increased since the cell is thicker than normal. The entire cell stains deep pink, lacking the usual central pallor. Spherocytes and megalocytes are hyperchromatic cells (Fig. 6-10).

Hypochromia: When hemoglobin content is greatly decreased, the central pale area increases in size and becomes more prominent (see previous discussion of anulocytes). The cells are usually microcytes, although flattened macrocytic cells and target cells also appear to be hypochromic.

Polychromasia: Polychromasia (polychromatophilia) refers to diffuse, light blue coloration (diffuse basophilia) of Wright-Giemsa–stained young erythrocytes. The basophilic material represents nuclear substance remaining in an immature red cell after expulsion of the normoblastic nucleus. The normal blood smear may contain 1-2 polychromatic cells/500 normal orthochromatic erythrocytes. Polychromatic cells are usually larger than normal cells and frequently contain a reticulum that is only seen when the cells are stained with supravital dyes. Polychromatic cells have the same significance as reticulocytes, indicating rapid blood regeneration.

Target cells (leptocytes): The target cell (Figs. 6-11 and 6-12) is an abnormally thin red cell that tends to buckle and, in Wright-stained preparations, presents a bull's-eye appearance because of a central condensation of hemoglobin surrounded by a clear zone. This appearance is probably an artifact of unusually thin cells but may be due to an excessive ratio of membrane lipid (cholesterol and phospholipid lecithin)[25] to cell volume. Target cells are found in hemolytic anemias and are most numerous in thalassemia, Hb C disease, sickle cell disease, sickle cell–Hb C disease, sickle cell thalassemia, and obstructive liver disease. In contradistinction to the thick spherocyte, the target cells are unusually resistant to hypotonic solutions of sodium chloride. When these cells are present in any significant number (over 40%), they result in a shift of the osmotic fragility curve to the left.

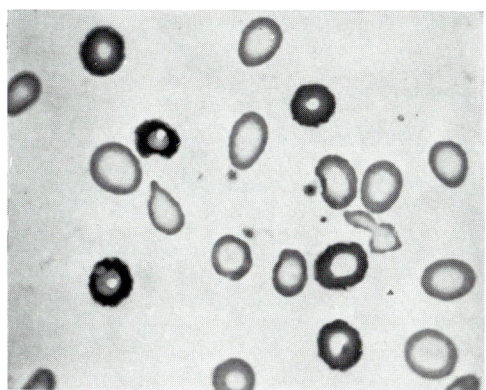

Fig. 6-9. Anulocytes, anisocytosis, and microcytes in iron deficiency anemia.

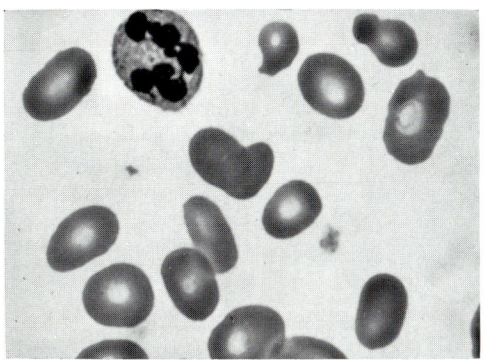

Fig. 6-10. Oval macrocytes and hypersegmented polymorph in pernicious anemia.

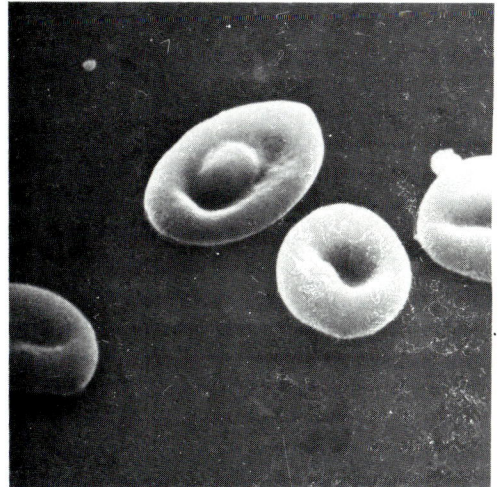

Fig. 6-11. Target cells from patient with hemolytic anemia as shown by scanning electron microscopy. (From Salsbury, A.J., and Clarke, J.A.: Triangle **8**(7):261-263, 1968.)

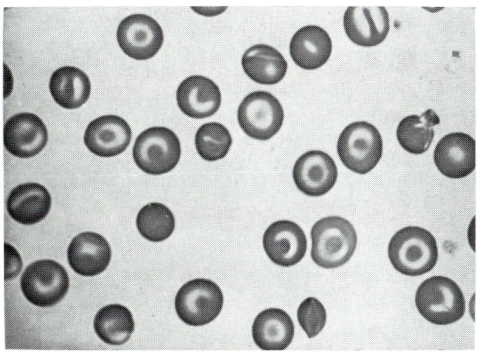

Fig. 6-12. Target cells in Hb C disease.

Table 6-1. Nomenclature of red cell shapes suggested by Bessis

Name	Meaning of greek prefix	Comments
Discocyte	Disc	Normal biconcave erythrocyte
Echinocyte (I, II, III)	Sea urchin	Different stages of crenation
Stomatocyte (I, II, III)	Mouth	Different stages of cup shapes
Acanthocyte	Spike	Abetalipoproteinemia
Codocyte	Bell	Thin, bell-shaped erythrocyte (target cell = codocyte flattened on a surface, or a cell with a single spicule in dimple)
Dacryocyte	Teardrop	Frequent in thalassemia
Drepanocyte	Sickle	Hemoglobin S
Elliptocyte	Oval	Congenital or acquired
Keratocyte	Horn	With one or more pointed projections
Leptocyte	Thin	Flattened cell
Megalocyte	Giant	Oval macrocyte in megaloblastic states
Schistocyte	Cut into pieces	Cut into pieces
Spherocyte	Sphere	Spheric shape without change in volume (macro = swollen sphere; micro = reduced volume)
Torocyte	Torus (doughnut)	Thinned dimple (center) with redistribution of hemoglobin to periphery

Modified from Bessis, M.: Living blood cells and their ultrastructure, New York, 1973, Springer-Verlag New York, Inc.

Table 6-2. Nomenclature of red cell shapes suggested by Bessis

Compound names	Comments
Sphero-echinocytes	Fine spicules
I, II	Few small spicules
Sphero-stomatocytes	Small hilum (concavity)
I, II	Irregularities at site of hilum (concavity)
Sphero-schistocyte	Sphering as result of fragmentation
Echino-schistocyte	Crenated schistocyte
Drepano-echinocyte	Echinocyte that undergoes sickling
Drepano-stomatocyte	Stomatocyte that undergoes sickling
Echino-acanthocyte	Echinocytic change in acanthocyte
Stomato-acanthocyte	Stomatocytic change in acanthocyte

Modified from Bessis, M.: Living blood cells and their ultrastructure, New York, 1973, Springer-Verlag New York, Inc.

Variations in shape (Plate 1, p. 129)

Acanthocytes: Acanthocytes[26] are irreversibly thorny, spheric erythrocytes (Fig. 6-13) with irregularly arranged spinous processes, some of which are bent at their tips. Their presence indicates permanent red cell damage. They are found in a rare hereditary disease, **abetalipoproteinemia**, that is characterized by pigmentary degeneration of the retina and by various metabolic defects, among which a low plasma β-lipoprotein level is outstanding, contributing to an imbalance between erythrocytic and plasmic lipids.[27] The occurrence of acanthocytes has also been reported in certain forms of cirrhosis associated with hemolytic anemia,[28] in hepatic hemangioma,[29] and in neonatal hepatitis.[30] The cells have normal osmotic and mechanical fragility. The cell shape is probably related to a membrane defect characterized by a progressive increase in the sphingomyelin/lecithin ratio.[31]

Blister cells: Blister cells[32] (Fig. 6-14) are red cells that contain single or multiple vacuoles or markedly thinned areas at the periphery. The vacuoles may rupture, leaving distorted and fragmented cells, which, according to their shape, are called helmet cells, burr cells, triangle cells, spherocytes, and schistocytes. The blister cell is the result of trauma to the cell occurring during its passage through injured and altered blood vessels. Blister cells and their derivatives are the hallmarks of **microangiopathic hemolytic anemias**, which result from the traumatic interaction of blood vessels and circulating blood. The injury may be due to intimal fibrin deposits, as seen in diffuse intravascular clotting, or it may be due to platelet thrombi, tumor or blood emboli, or passage of blood through the maze of angiomas. In sickle cell anemia the injury is indicative of pulmonary emboli.[33] Bessis coined the name **keratocyte** for the cell remaining after the rupture of the blister. It is half-moon shaped, the central depression flanked by two horns (see later discussion of helmet cells).[34]

Burr cells: Burr cells,[35,36] or echinocytes, are elongated or rounded, crenated erythrocytes. The normal biconcave disk shape of the red cell endows it with a certain amount of plasticity or deformability, which allows it to withstand the passage through the various microcirculations of the body. This deformability depends on a variety of factors, e.g., the relationship of surface area to volume, the type of hemoglobin, and membrane characteristics such as lipid contents. Loss of deformability leads to increased rigidity and to premature destruction of the red cell. Burr cells or spur cells are reversibly spiculated cells that are not synonymous with the nonreversible acanthocyte. Bessis designated these cells as echinocytes and described a four-stage sequence of discocyte-echinocyte transformation[37,38] (Fig. 6-15). The last stage may be induced by extrinsic factors, e.g., ionophose,[39] bile acids, fatty acids, and salicylates, and by intrinsic factors, e.g., ATP depletion.[31] The four stages of the transformation are echino-

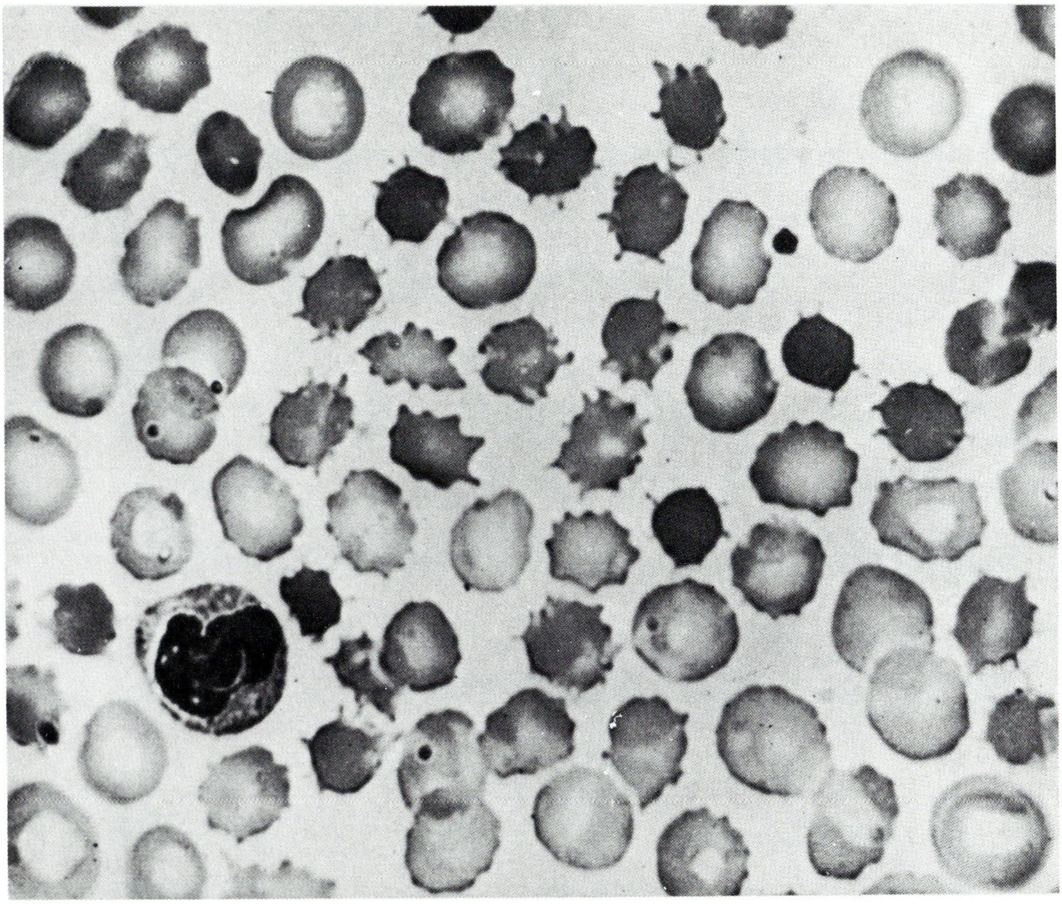

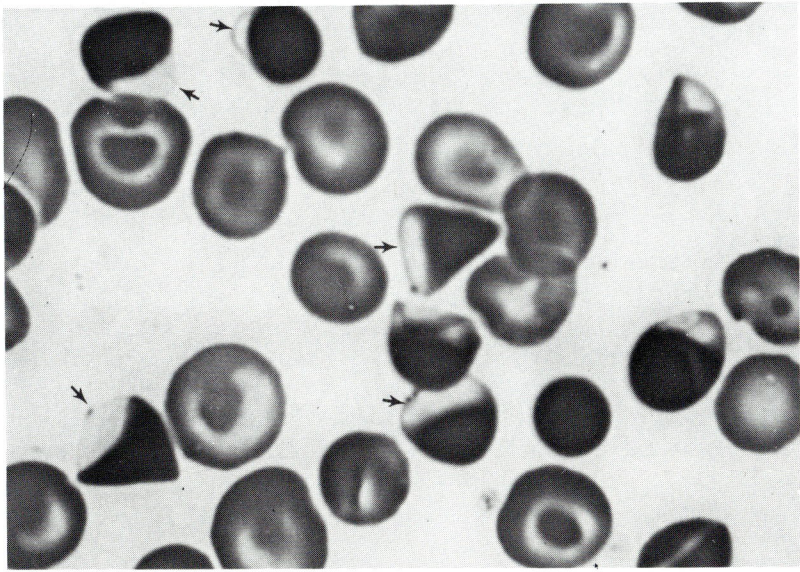

Fig. 6-13. Blood smear from child with acanthocytosis. Red cells are almost uniformly distorted. Many possess spiny projections; others have irregularly spaced protuberances. Note small and deeply stained red cells resembling spherocytes with irregularly spaced spines. (×500.) (From Smith, C.H.: Blood diseases of infancy and childhood, ed. 3, St. Louis, 1972, The C.V. Mosby Co.)

Fig. 6-14. Blister cells. If blisters burst, triangular cells are produced. (Courtesy Dr. L.W. Diggs.)

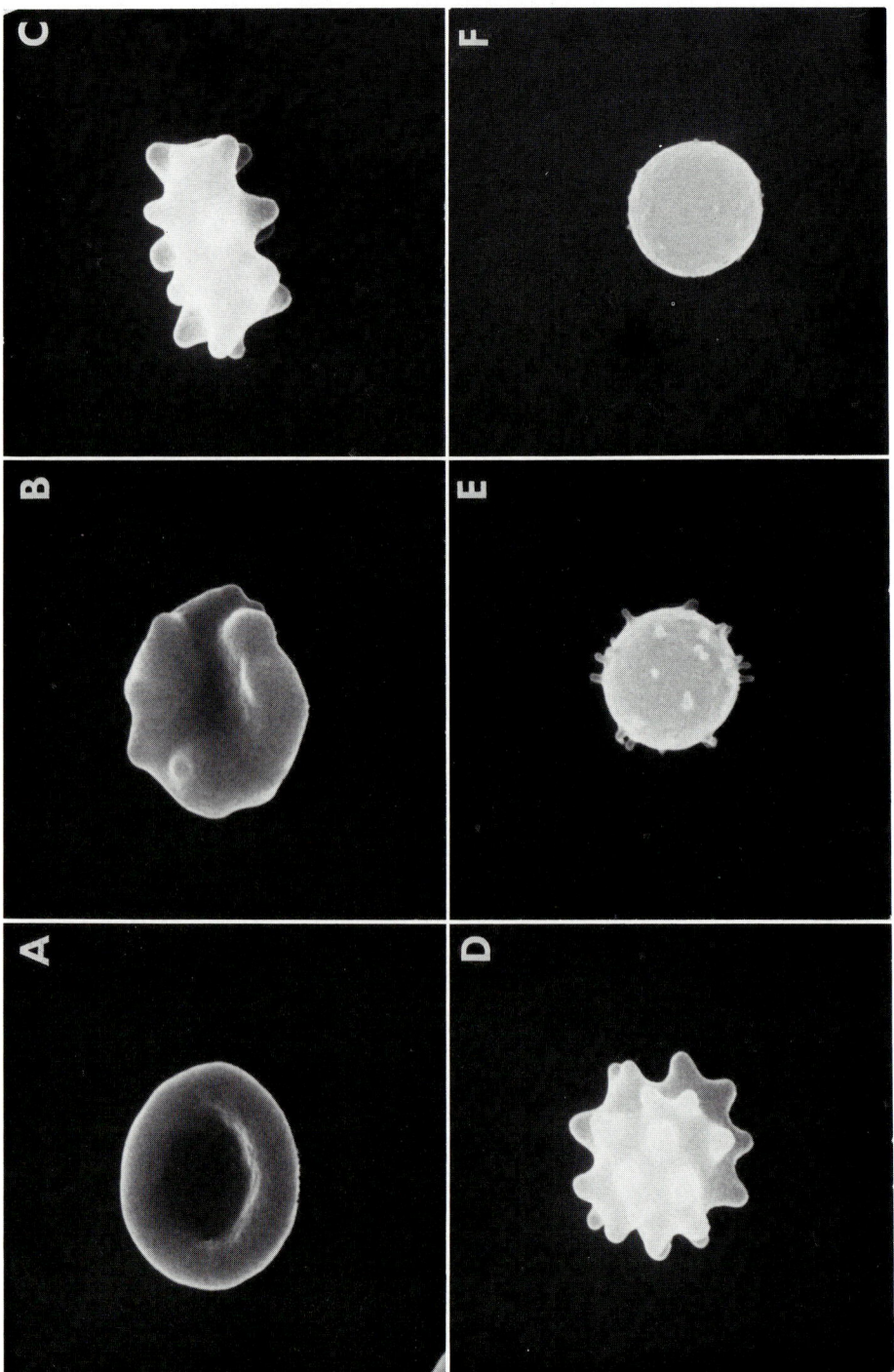

Fig. 6-15. Discocyte-echinocyte shape change as shown by scanning electron microscopy. **A,** Discocyte. **B,** Echinocyte I. **C,** Echinocyte II. **D,** Echinocyte III. **E** and **F,** Spheroechinocyte. (From Weed, R.I.: Clin. Haematol. **4:**3, 1975.)

cyte I (a flat cell), echinocyte II (a flat cell with spicules), echinocyte III (an ovoid cell with spicules), and the spheroechinocyte (a spheric cell with spicules).[38] In vivo burr cells occur in uremia, gastric carcinoma, peptic ulcer, pyruvate kinase deficiency, and other anemias. To establish the fact that crenated cells exist in vivo and are not artificially produced in vitro, one drop of fresh blood sandwiched between two coverslips should be examined for crenated cells immediately after the blood specimen has been obtained.

Echinocytes: See discussion of burr cells above.

Elliptocytes (ovalocytes)[40] (Fig. 6-16): Normally about 1% of all red cells are oval in shape. In severe anemias the number of ovalocytes may increase to 15%. They are frequently seen in pernicious anemia and in anemias associated with malignant lesions. Elliptocytes may also be due to a congenital anomaly of red cells, which is mendelian dominant and is not sex linked.[41] In the congenital form over 25% of red cells are oval. Ovalocytosis is confined to the mature red blood cells and does not involve the precursor forms. In most cases elliptocytosis is asymptomatic, but occasionally it is associated with a hemolytic anemia.

Helmet cells: Helmet cells (Fig. 6-17; keratocytes of Bessis)[42,43] are irregular, contracted, triangular cells. The intravascular obstructions enumerated earlier (see discussion of blister cells) may mechanically divide passing red cells so as to snare off small fragments, which become spherocytes, leaving larger scooped-out cells, helmet cells. The latter cells may also be caused by the rupture of a previously formed blister (blister cell).

Keratocytes: See previous discussion of helmet cells.

Ovalocytes: See previous discussion of elliptocytes.

Poikilocytes: Poikilocytes (Fig. 6-18) are cells that show marked variation not only in shape but also in size and hemoglobin content. The cells may be teardrop shaped, pear shaped, racket shaped, or pessary shaped. These changes are characteristically found in severe hemolytic anemias, including pernicious anemia, in myelofibrosis, in thalassemia, and in microangiopathic hemolytic anemias. Poikilocytosis refers to the presence of these cells and can be graded from 1-4 + .

Pyknocytes: Pyknocytes[44] (Fig. 6-19) are distorted, contracted erythrocytes similar to burr cells that in small numbers may normally be seen in the first 2-3 months of life. In a condition called **infantile pyknocytosis** they are present in increased numbers (up to 50%) and are associated with an acute, severe hemolytic anemia. Some of these cells are associated with G-6-PD deficiency, microangiopathic hemolytic anemia, and **hereditary lipoprotein deficiency.**

Schistocytes: Schistocytes are fragmented red cells frequently seen in hemolytic anemias that are burn or prosthesis related or microangiopathic in type. They are small, irregular, pointed segments of cells (Fig. 6-17). They have also been reported as a sign of renal homograft rejection.[45]

Sickle cells (depranocytes): Sickle cells (Figs. 6-20 and 6-21) are elongated, drawn out, slightly curved cells with pointed ends that resemble a sickle blade. The center of the cell contains a dense, almost crystal-

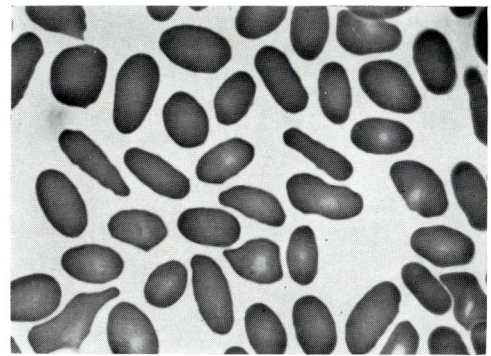

Fig. 6-16. Elliptocytes in congenital elliptocytosis.

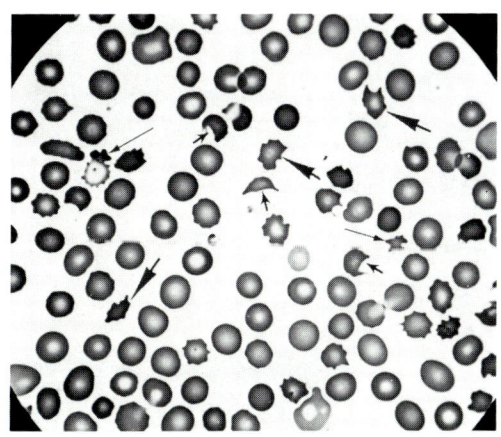

Fig. 6-17. Helmet cells (small arrows), pyknocytes (large arrows), and schistocytes (long thin arrows) in hemolytic uremic syndrome. (Courtesy Prof. Dr. J.V. Dacie.)

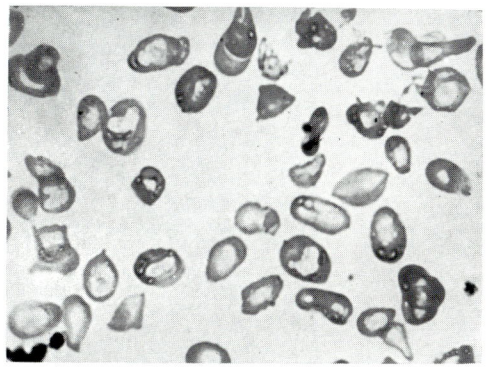

Fig. 6-18. Poikilocytes in thalassemia major.

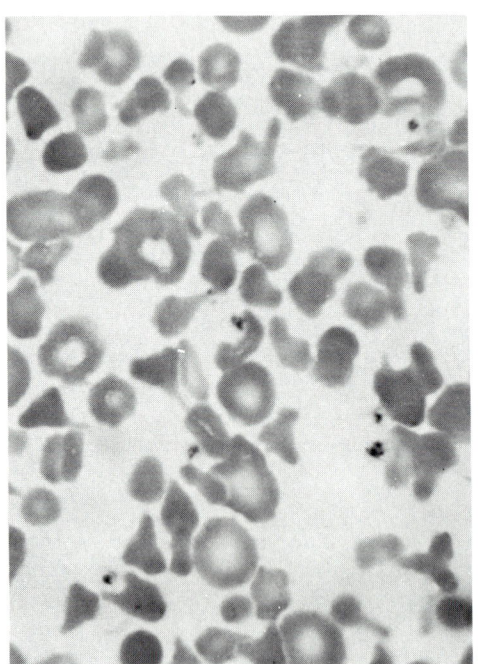

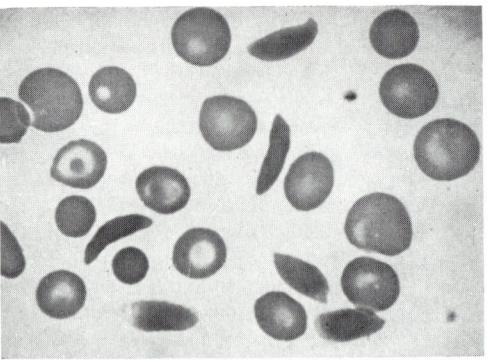

Fig. 6-20. Sickle cells, target cells, macrocytes, and spherocytes in sickle cell anemia.

Fig. 6-19. Pyknocytes in infantile pyknocytosis.

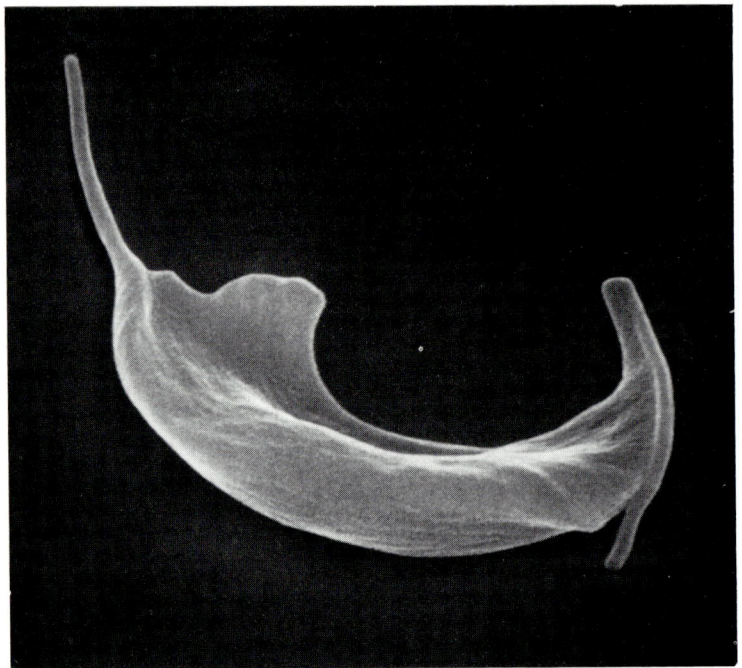

Fig. 6-21. Sickle cell as seen with scanning electron microscope. (×5000.) (From Weed, R.I.: Clin. Haematol. **4:**3, 1975.)

line area of hemoglobin that fades somewhat toward the periphery. A number of hemoglobins in the deoxygenated form sickle and thus induce the red cell to assume a sickle shape. The most important sickling hemoglobin is Hb S, although other hemoglobins also sickle, e.g., Hb Bart's, Hb C Harlem, Hb C Georgetown, and Hb I Memphis. In Hb S the sickle shape is produced by reversible molecular interaction (see p. 72). Electron microscopic studies of sickled cells show the aggregates of sickled hemoglobin to be arranged in parallel rodlike structures.[46]

Spherocytes: Spherocytes (Fig. 6-22) are spheric red cells that have a diminished diameter, at times reduced to 4 μm (microspherocytes), and a central thickened portion instead of the normal pallor. Compared to normal red cells their surface area is markedly reduced. In blood spreads they appear circular and have a dark-stained center. Spherocytes occur in a number of conditions of varied etiology, e.g., congenital spherocytosis, acquired hemolytic anemias, and diffuse intravascular coagulation. They are found in ABO hemolytic disease of the newborn, in transfusion reactions, and in hemolytic anemias associated with burns. In ABO erythroblastosis the spherocytes are a valuable clue to the diagnosis because they are absent in erythroblastosis caused by Rh incompatibility. Transfused cells (storage phenomenon) appear as microspherocytes in the recipient's blood.

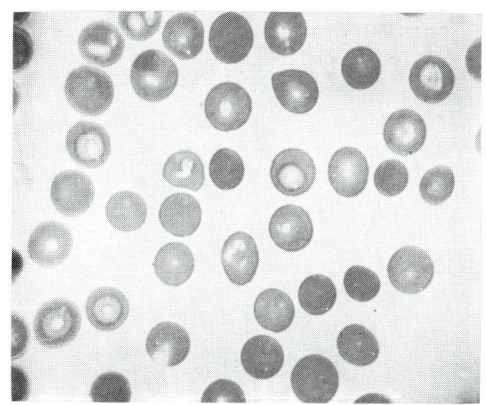

Fig. 6-22. Spherocytes in congenital spherocytosis.

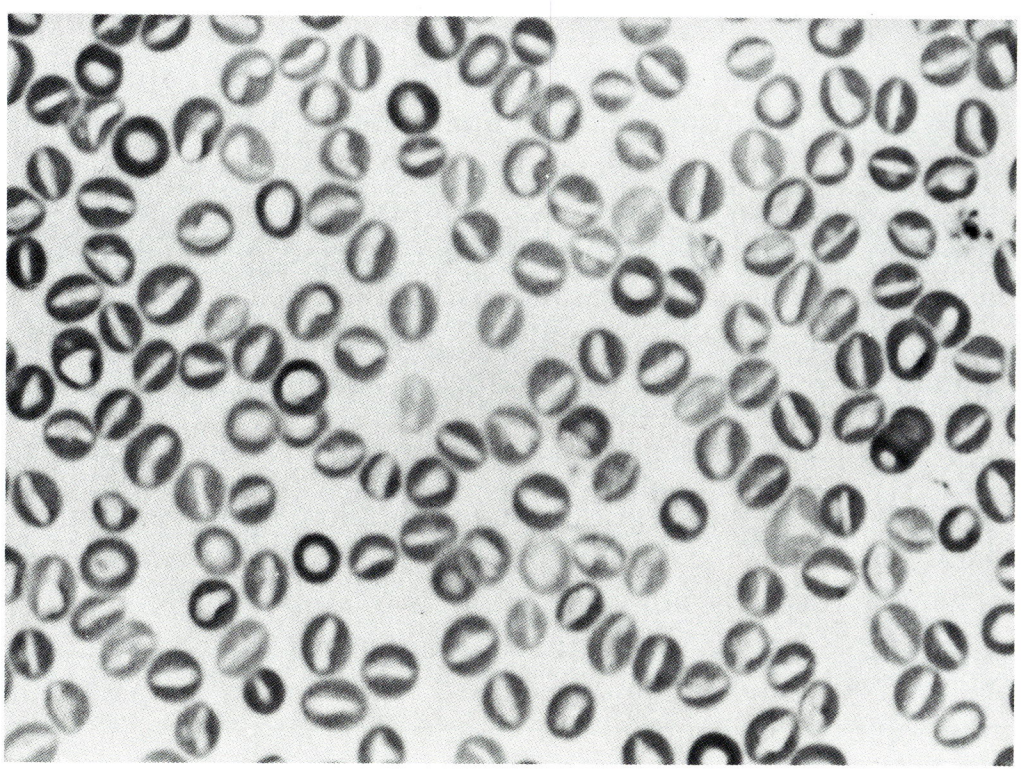

Fig. 6-23. Stomatocytes. (×5000.) Note mouthlike area in cell instead of normal circular area of central pallor. (From Oski, F.A., and Naiman, J.L.: Hematologic problems in the newborn, ed. 2, Philadelphia, 1972, W.B. Saunders Co.)

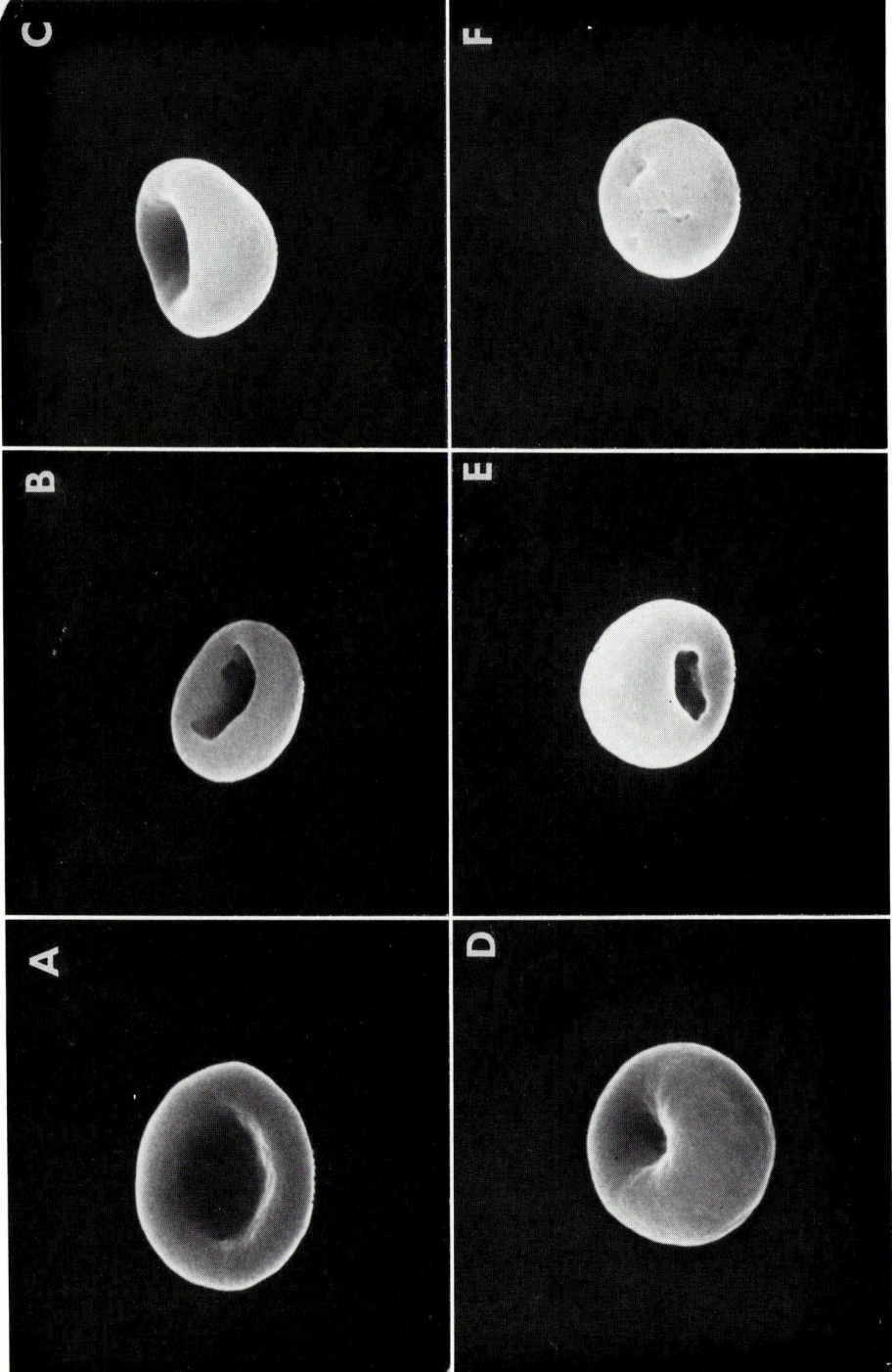

Fig. 6-24. Discocyte–stomatocyte shape change as shown by scanning electron microscopy. **A,** Discocyte. **B,** Stomatocyte I. **C,** Stomatocyte I. **C,** Stomatocyte II. **D,** Stomatocyte III. **E** and **F,** Spherostomatocyte. (From Weed, R.I.: Clin. Haematol. **4:**3, 1975.)

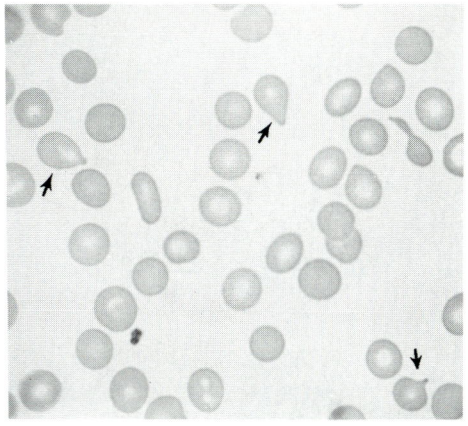

Fig. 6-25. Teardrop cells.

In vitro, spherocytes can be produced by the action of lytic agents on red cells. They may also result from fragmentation of normal erythrocytes. If the factors leading to echinocyte formation are strong, echinocytes III are transformed into spheroechinocytes. Spherocytes represent a prelytic state. They exhibit increased osmotic fragility when brought in contact with hypotonic solutions (see discussion of osmotic fragility test in Chapter 4).

Stomatocytes: Stomatocytes[47,48] are morphologically abnormal red cells in which the normally present rounded pale central area seen on Wright-Giemsa–stained films is rectangular or slitlike (stoma means mouthlike opening) (Fig. 6-23). In three-dimensional preparations the cells are cup shaped (Fig. 6-24). These cells exhibit an abnormally increased osmotic fragility and increased autohemolysis at 37°-40° C. Certain chemical agents (phenothiazine, chlorpromazine) produce a reversible cup-shaped deformity of red cells, which on dried smears produces the previously described appearance.[49] If the action of these chemicals continues, the cells become spherostomatocytes.[39] Stomatocytes with high sodium and low potassium contents have been found to be associated with a rare form of congenital hemolytic anemia.[50] Transient stomatocytosis accompanied by hemolysis has been observed in acute alcoholism,[51] alcoholic cirrhosis, glutathione deficiency, hereditary spherocytosis, infectious mononucleosis, lead poisoning, thalassemia minor, and malignant diseases.

Spur cells: See earlier discussion of burr cells.

Teardrop cells: Teardrop cells are pear-shaped cells seen in severe anemias, myelofibrosis, and homozygous β-thalassemia (Fig. 6-25).

Triangle cells: Triangle cells are seen in microangiopathic anemia and are thought to be remnants of ruptured blister cells (Fig. 6-15).

Red cell artifacts

A number of artifacts in the preparation of peripheral blood smears (see later discussion) may be responsible for the appearance of red-cell-variant-like cells in the preparation. It is very important that the true nature of

these red cell changes is recognized and is not mistaken for a pathologic red cell condition. Because the differentiation of red cell variants from red cell artifacts may be difficult at times, the latter must be prevented by perfect technic. Factors that aid in the recognition of artifacts are (1) the total hemogram, (2) clinical history, (3) repeat blood smear by skilled laboratory personnel, (4) the use of plastic coverslips to make the blood smear (to eliminate glass artifacts), and (5) immediate examination of a small drop of fresh blood by phase microscopy. If no abnormal cells are observed, the red cell alterations seen on the blood film are artifacts.

Red cell artifacts may be caused by the following factors:
1. Delay in making the smear
2. Abnormal temperatures (freezing or heating)
3. Drying (too slow)
4. Crowding of cells as in polycythemia
5. Increased viscosity
6. Presence of abnormal proteins
7. Glass effect
8 Abnormal pH (too acid or too alkaline)
9. Anionic or cationic changes of the red cell milieu
10. Pressure when making the smear
11. Errors in staining

Erythrocytic inclusions[52] (Plate 1, p. 129)

Method of reporting: It is probably best to report the percentage of affected cells, i.e., the number of cells with inclusions per 100 red cells.

Basophilic stippling: Basophilic stippling (Fig. 6-26) refers to the basophilic granules that appear in red cells in cases of disturbed erythropoiesis, as seen in lead poisoning and in severe anemias. The number of polychromatic and stippled cells parallels the number of reticulocytes seen by the supravital technic (the reverse is not true). Stippling appears as fine or coarse dots that stain blue or purple with Wright stain and are scattered either around the edge or throughout the entire red cell. Coarse stippling reflects increased erythropoietin stimulation. Agglutination of ribosomes accounts for the punctate pattern.

Cabot rings: Cabot rings (Fig. 6-26) are delicate, circular, figure eight or loop-shaped, threadlike bodies seen in polychromatic or stippled erythrocytes and at times in erythrocytes with Howell-Jolly bodies. They are sometimes seen in lead poisoning and in pernicious anemia. Cabot rings are neither nuclear remnants (they are Feulgen negative) nor remnants of the nuclear membrane, but are artifacts produced by denatured protein, persistent spindle fibers, or fused microtubules.

Congenital red cell inclusions: Lange and Akeroyd,[53] Scott et al.,[54] and Sansone and Pik[55] have described a congenital hemolytic anemia in which 14% of the red cells contained unusual inclusion bodies as seen with a Wright stain. The urine contained an abnormal dark brown pigment (dipyrroles).

Crystals: In Hb C disease, Wright-stained blood films are seen to contain rodlike, angular, opaque, and brown structures within some erythrocytes (Fig. 6-27). In Hb S-C disease they may be curved (Fig. 6-28).

Hemoglobin H inclusions: Hb H inclusions are not

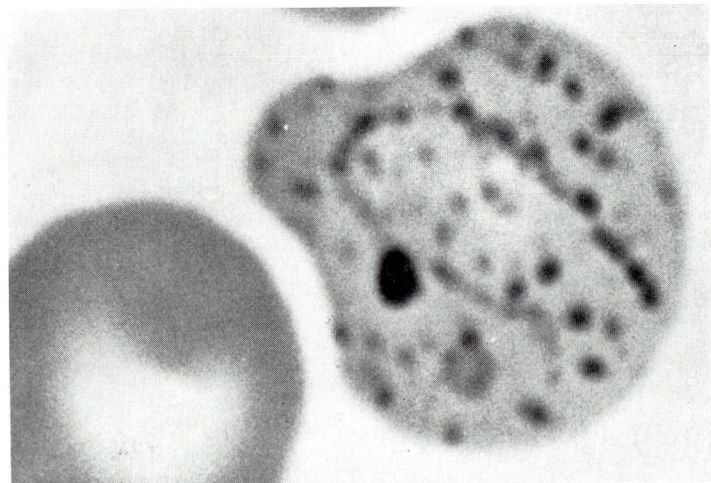

Fig. 6-26. Basophilic stippling, Cabot ring, diffuse basophilia, and Howell-Jolly body. (Courtesy Dr. L.W. Diggs.)

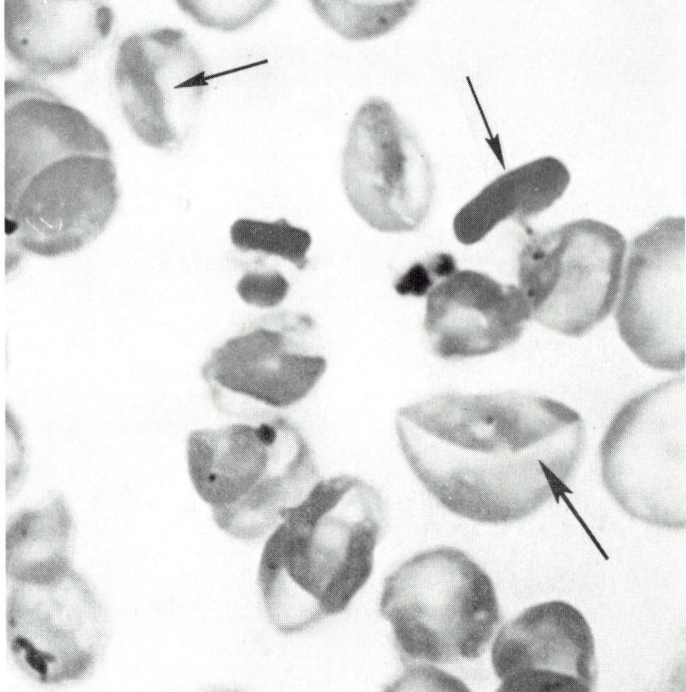

Fig. 6-27. Rodlike crystals in homozygous Hb C disease, intraerythrocytic and extraerythrocytic (thin arrows); folding of red cell (heavy arrow).

seen in unstained cells, but they can be visualized with supravital stains (Fig. 6-29). They are an expression of the instability of Hb H and consist of excess β-chain in α-thalassemia (see discussion of Heinz bodies).

Heinz bodies: Heinz bodies[56] are small, round, intraerythrocytic inclusions that result from precipitation of hemoglobin or globin. They are not seen in Wright-Giemsa–stained preparations but are easily visualized by supravital stains, e.g., methyl violet and brilliant cresyl blue, or by phase microscopy. They are Prussian blue negative. Usually they are attached to the cell membrane, but they may be free within the cell body. They are found in red cells after splenectomy in many hemolytic anemias of various etiology, e.g., G-6-PD deficiency, in hemoglobinopathies caused by unstable hemoglobins, and in thalassemia major. In the bone marrow of children they are diagnostic of homozygous β-thalassemia (excess α-chain inclusions). They are larger than the inclusions of Hb H and Zurich, which are unstable, easily precipitated hemoglobins. Heinz body formation can be induced in vitro by phenylhydrazine (Figs. 6-30 and 6-31).

Howell-Jolly bodies: Howell-Jolly bodies are small, spheric structures seen in erythrocytes (Fig. 6-27). In Wright-Giemsa–stained film they appear as single blue bodies about 1 μm in diameter within the red cells. They can also be seen in the unstained preparation by phase microscopy. They are methyl green–pyronine and Feulgen positive, indicating that they contain RNA and DNA. They may be nuclear remnants separated during the normal process of karyorrhexis or they may represent separated chromosomes. They are seen in hemolytic anemias, including pernicious anemia, and may be found after surgical or physiologic (atrophy) splenectomy.[57]

Maurer dots: Maurer dots are coarse dark violet

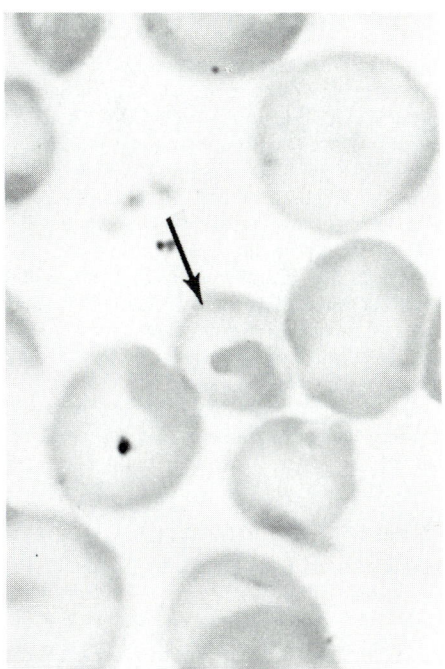

Fig. 6-28. Curved crystal in Hb S-C disease.

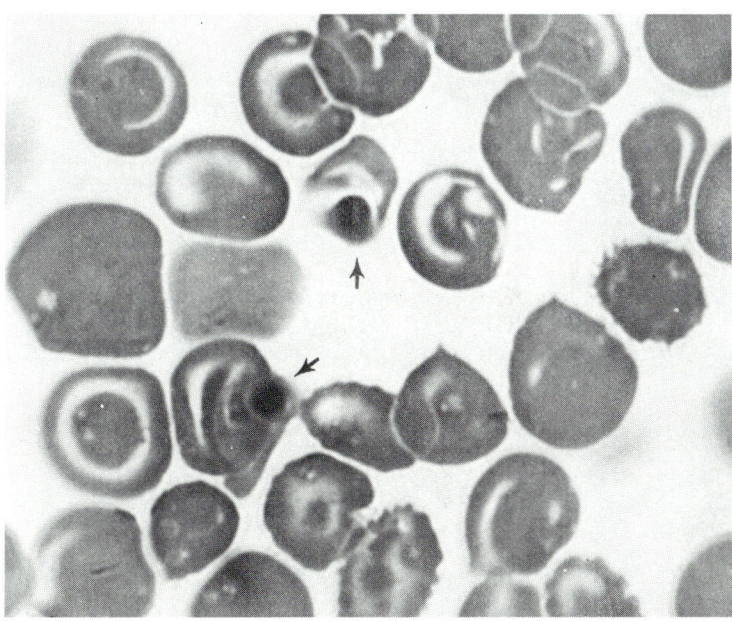

Fig. 6-29. Hb H intraerythrocytic inclusions. (From Rigas, D., and Kohler, R.D.: Blood **18:**1, 1961.)

pigment granules seen in *Plasmodium malariae* malaria.

Reticulocytes: Reticulocytes are young polychromatic erythrocytes that show a reticulum or net structure when stained by supravital methods (p. 195 and Figs. 7-13 and 7-14).

Schüffner dots: Schüffner dots are reddish violet granules occurring in *Plasmodium vivax* malaria. They are scattered over the entire erythrocyte.

Siderotic granules (Pappenheimer bodies): Siderotic granules (Figs. 6-32 and 6-33 and Plate 3 [p. 148]) are intraerythrocytic Prussian blue–positive aggregations of ferritin surrounded by a membrane (siderosomes). They may be single or multiple and probably represent iron not yet utilized in the hemoglobin synthesis. These aggregates stain a faint blue color with Wright-Giemsa stain. Erythrocytes containing these granules are called siderocytes (Fig. 6-33). Similar granules are seen in normoblasts (sideroblasts) in the bone marrow. In ringed sideroblasts the ferritin is present in the perinuclear mitochondria, in which physiologically the last step in hemoglobin synthesis occurs (see Chapter 4).

Megaloblastic erythropoiesis

Megaloblasts are pathologic cells that are not present in the normal adult bone marrow, their appearance being caused by a deficiency in vitamin B_{12} or folic acid or both, leading to defective DNA synthesis. Megaloblasts are characterized by nuclear/cytoplasmic dissociation, implying that the nucleus and the cytoplasm do not mature at the same rate, so that nuclear maturation lags behind cytoplasmic hemoglobinization. This nuclear lag appears to be caused by interference with DNA synthesis while RNA and protein synthesis continues at a near normal rate.[58] As the megaloblastic

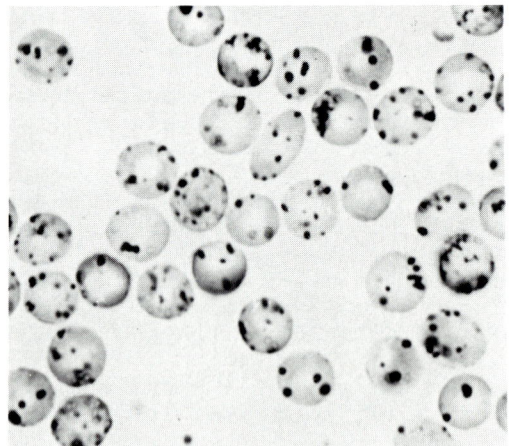

Fig. 6-30. Heinz body formation in drug-sensitive erythrocytes. Note multiple small bodies throughout cytoplasm. (From Beutler, E., Dein, R.J., and Alving, A.S.: J. Lab. Clin. Med. **45**:40, 1955.)

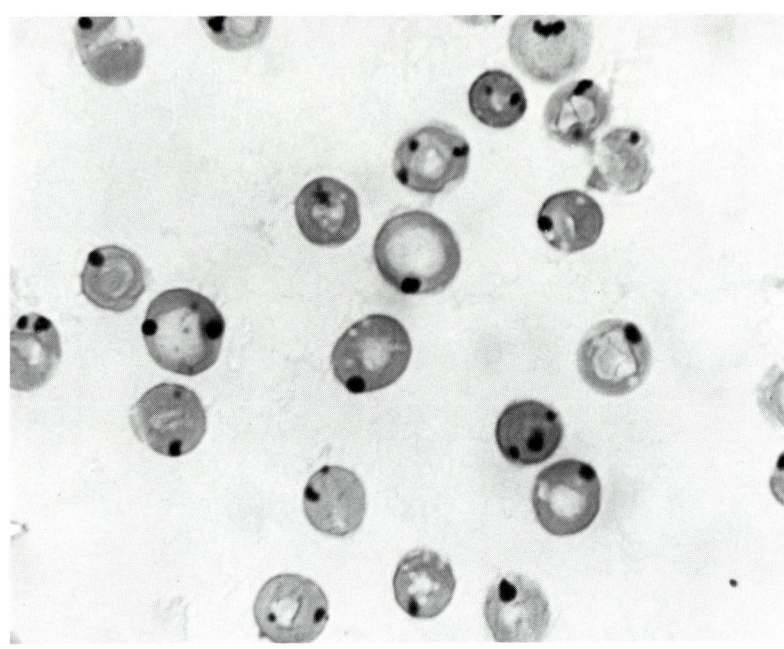

Fig. 6-31. Heinz body formation in normal nonsensitive erythrocytes. Note single marginal body in most red cells.

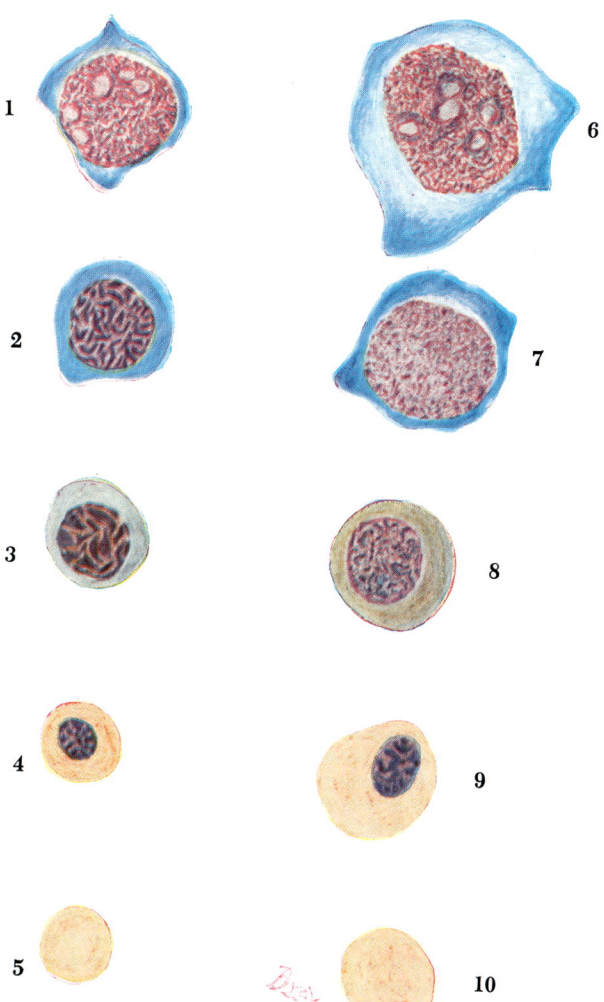

Plate 2. Red blood cell maturation (normoblastic and megaloblastic).

Normoblastic erythropoiesis
1 Pronormoblast
2 Basophilic normoblast
3 Polychromatophilic normoblast
4 Orthochromatic normoblast
5 Erythrocyte

Megaloblastic erythropoiesis
6 Promegaloblast
7 Basophilic megaloblast
8 Polychromatophilic megaloblast
9 Orthochromatic megaloblast
10 Macrocyte (megalocyte)

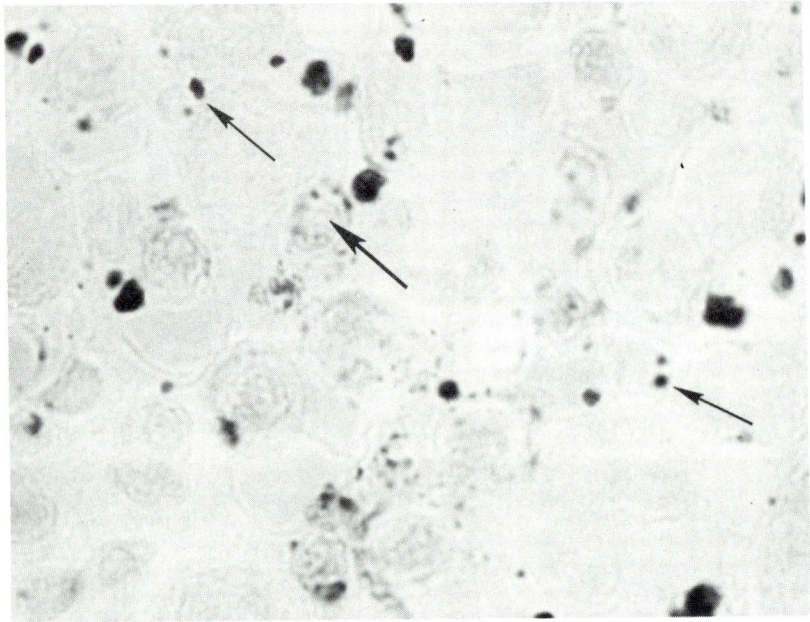

Fig. 6-32. Sideroblasts in bone marrow (thin arrows); ring sideroblast (heavy arrow).

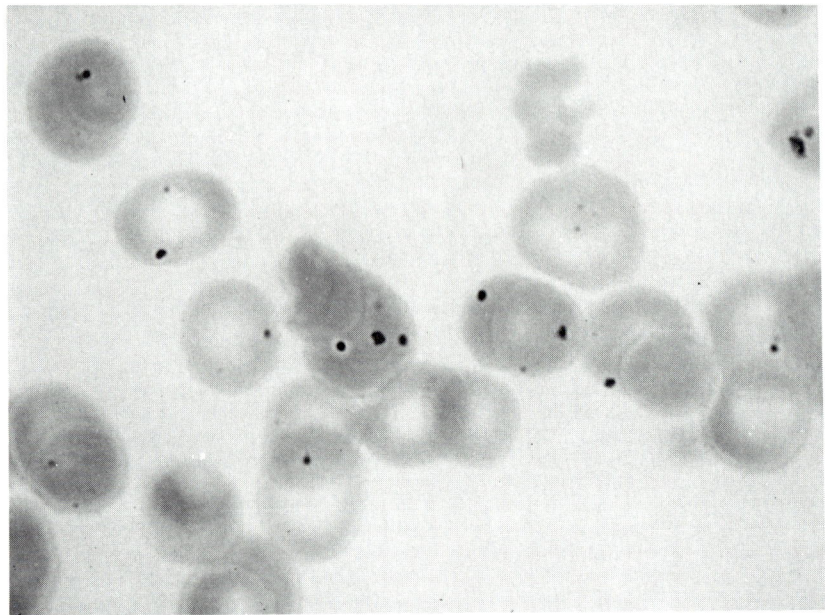

Fig. 6-33. Siderocytes in peripheral blood.

cells mature, the nuclear/cytoplasmic dissociation becomes more marked, so that the easiest way to make the diagnosis of megaloblastic erythropoiesis (Plates 1, 2, and 3, pp. 129, 145, and 148, respectively) is by recognizing the polychromatophilic megaloblast. The end stage of megaloblastic maturation is the megalocyte (Fig. 6-34). Megaloblastic erythropoiesis is a reversible process.

Megaloblastic erythropoiesis is only one expression of folic acid and vitamin B_{12} deficiency that involves all body cells, including leukocytes, megakaryocytes, epithelial cells, etc. Megaloblastic changes are also brought about by a number of chemotherapeutic agents, e.g., alkalizing agents,[59] and antimetabolites.[60]

Promegaloblast

Size: The promegaloblast is 25-30 μm in diameter.

Nucleus: The nucleus is round or oval and larger than that of the corresponding normoblastic cell. The chromatin is arranged in small delicate masses and bands that produce an open, somewhat stippled appearing network surrounding prominent areas of pinkparachromatin. One to four large pale nucleoli are seen surrounded by chromatin.

Cytoplasm: The nuclear/cytoplasmic ratio is greater than in the corresponding normoblast. The cytoplasm is basophilic and shows some purple mottling (Plate 2, p. 145).

Basophilic megaloblast

Size: The basophilic megaloblast is 18-25 μm in diameter.

Nucleus: The nucleus is round or oval in size, and the chromatin pattern is very similar to that of the promegaloblastic nucleus. Nucleoli are difficult to see or may be absent.

Cytoplasm: The cytoplasmic ring is wider than in the promegaloblast. It is basophilic and shows some purple mottling because of azurophilic granules (Plate 2, p. 145).

Polychromatophilic megaloblast

Size: The polychromatophilic megaloblast is 16-20 μm in diameter.

Nucleus: The nucleus is reduced in size and is usually eccentric. The chromatin network is coarse because of irregular pink chromatin masses.

Cytoplasm: There is a large ovoid area of lilac to greenish gray cytoplasm. The asynchronous precocious development (hemoglobinization) of the cytoplasm as compared to the nuclear development is characteristic (Plate 2, p. 145).

Orthochromatic megaloblast

Size: The orthochromatic megaloblast is 12-15 μm in diameter.

Nucleus: The nucleus is reduced in size and is usually eccentric. The chromatin is condensed and pyknotic.

Cytoplasm: The cytoplasm is orange-red because of hemoglobinization. The nuclear/cytoplasmic ratio greatly exceeds that of the orthochromatic normoblast. Howell-Jolly bodies that represent nuclear fragments may be seen in the cytoplasm (Plate 2, p. 145).

Megalocyte

Size: The megalocyte is 9-12 μm in diameter.

Nucleus: There are no nuclei present.

Cytoplasm: The cytoplasm is dark pink because it lacks the central area of clearing characteristic of the normal erythrocyte. Megalocytes of pernicious anemia are characteristically ovoid or pear shaped. Howell-Jolly bodies and azurophilic granules may be present (Plate 2, p. 145).

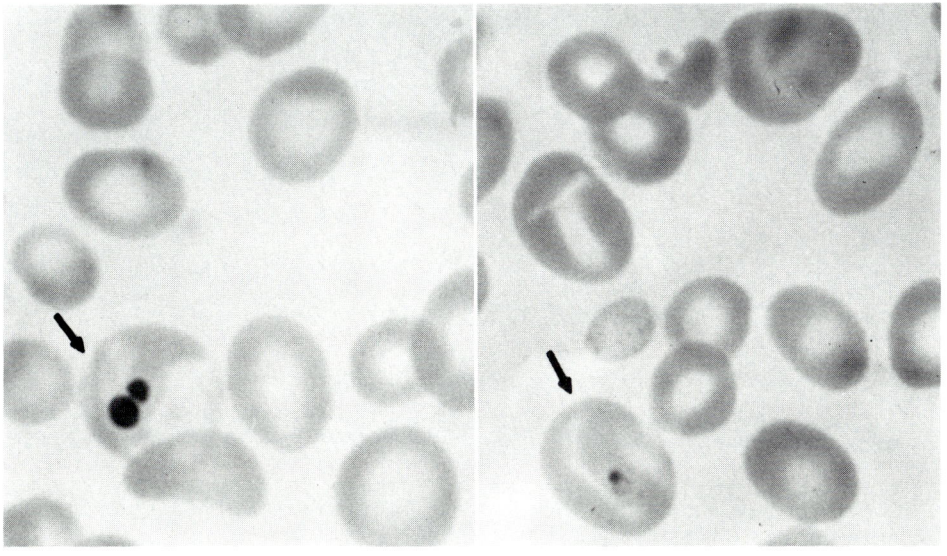

Fig. 6-34. Megalocytes with Howell-Jolly bodies *(arrows).*

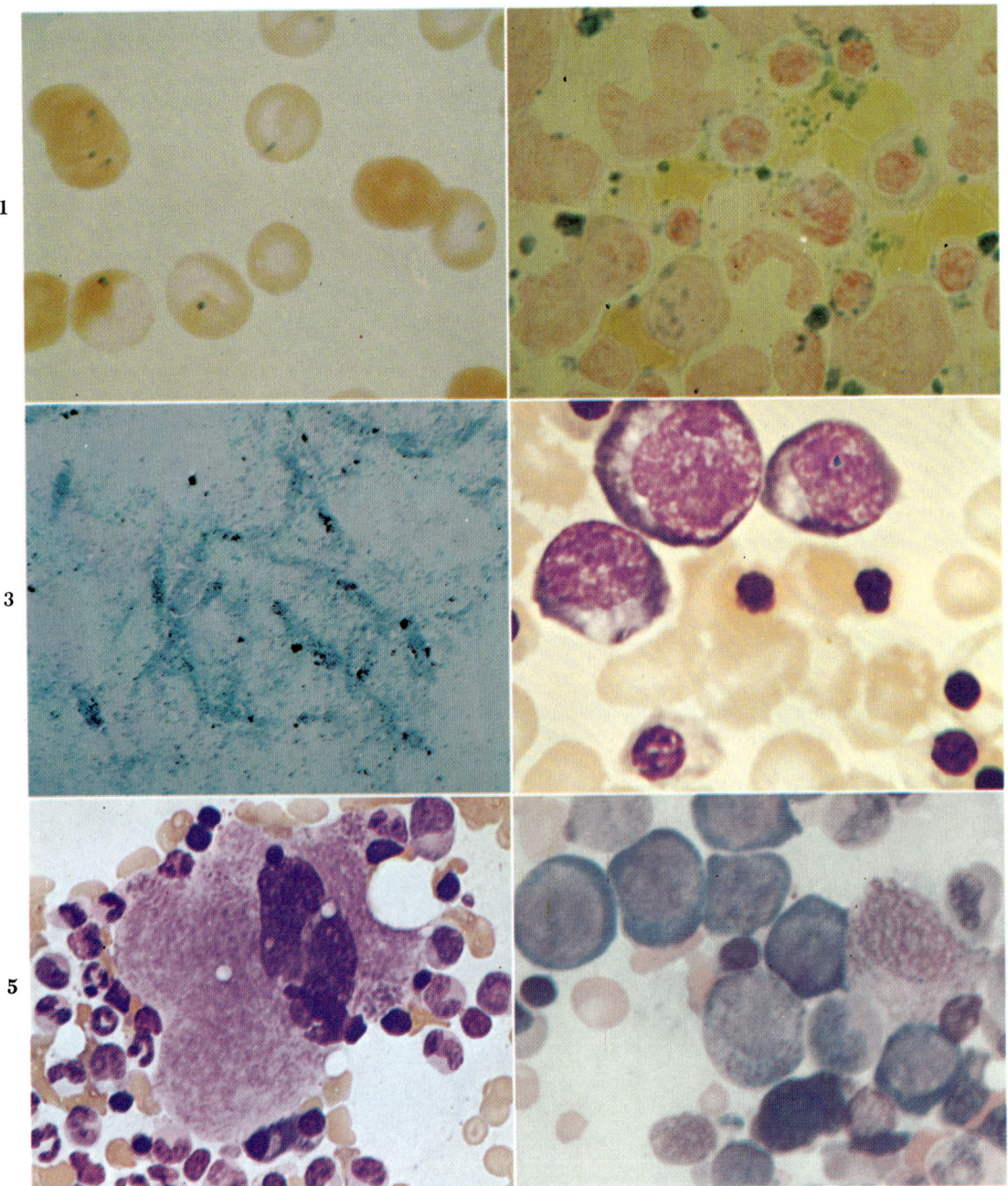

Plate 3. Peripheral blood, bone marrow, and urinary sediment in some anemias.

1 Siderocytes in peripheral blood in sideroachrestic anemia. (Prussian blue stain.) (Courtesy V. Minnich.)

2 Ring sideroblasts in bone marrow in sideroachrestic anemia. (Prussian blue stain.)

3 Hemosiderin casts in urinary sediment in paroxysmal nocturnal hemoglobinuria. (Prussian blue stain.) (Courtesy V. Minnich.)

4 Hemolytic disease of the newborn (erythroblastosis fetalis), normoblasts and erythroblasts in peripheral blood. (Wright stain.)

5 Platelet-producing megakaryocyte. (Wright stain.)

6 Megaloblasts in bone marrow in pernicious anemia. (Wright stain.)

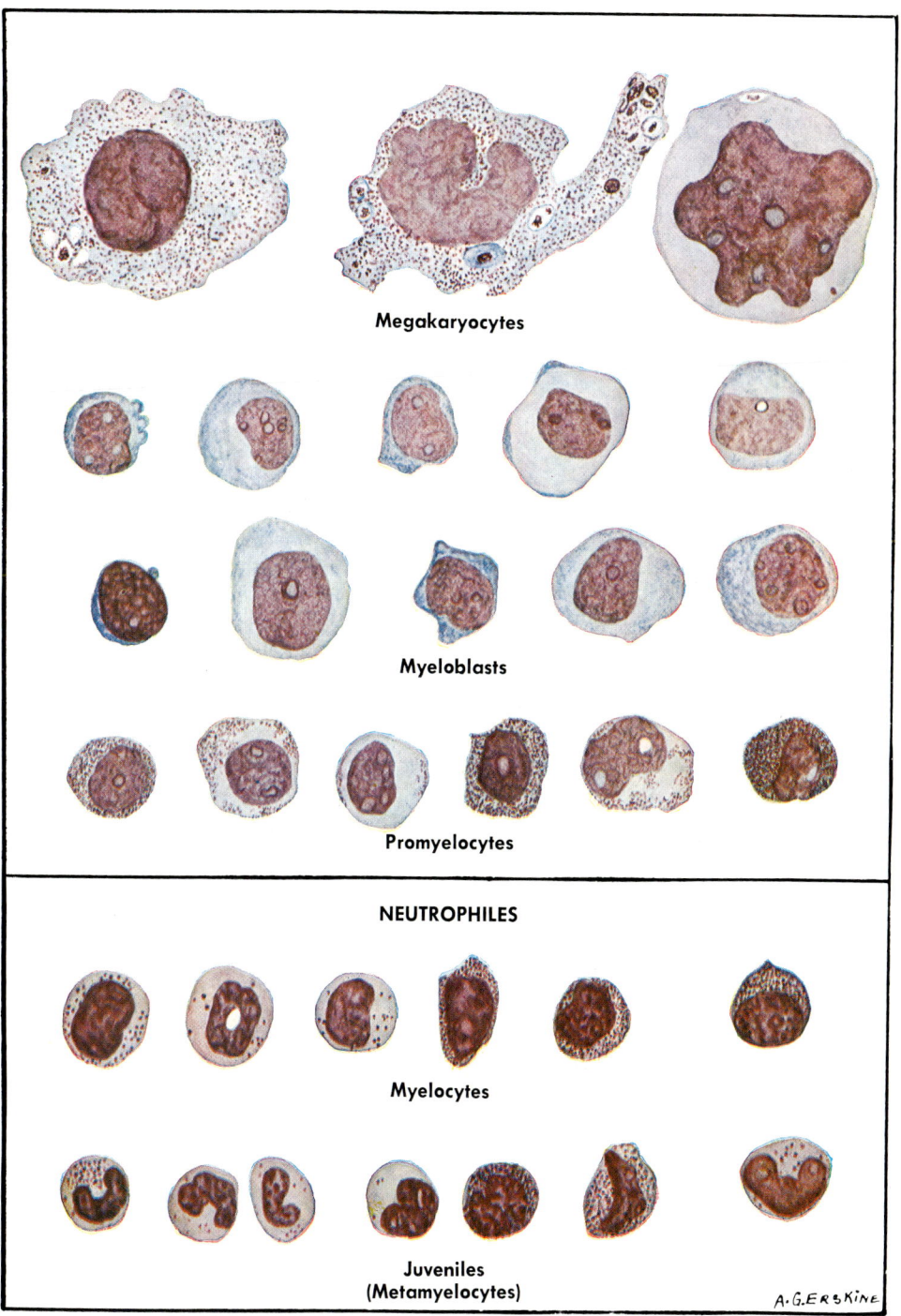

Plate 4. Leukocytes. (Wright-Giemsa stain; ×950.)

MORPHOLOGY AND FUNCTION OF WHITE CELLS

NEUTROPHILIC GRANULOCYTE AND PRECURSORS

Stem cell

In health, granulopoiesis occurs only in the bone marrow, which appears to provide the required hematopoietic inductive microenvironment (HIM) for the pluripotent stem cell, which by dividing replicates itself but at the same time produces a daughter cell that is sensitive to various "poietins," thus committing it to differentiate in one direction.

Myeloblast

Size and shape: The myeloblast is 20-25 μm in diameter depending on the cell's cycle, i.e., round or oval. In leukemia unusually large (macromyeloblasts) and very small (micromyeloblasts) cells may be found.

Nucleus: The nucleus is large, oval or round, and eccentric. It has a thin nuclear membrane and finely dispersed, granular, purplish, pale chromatin with well-demarcated, pink, evenly distributed parachromatin; two to five light blue-gray nucleoli surrounded by dense chromatin are seen (Plate 4 [p. 149] and Fig. 6-35).

Cytoplasm: The cytoplasmic mass is small in comparison to the nucleus, producing a nuclear/cytoplasmic ratio of about 7:1. It stains basophilic and shows a small, indistinct, paranuclear, lighter staining halo (Golgi apparatus). At the periphery, which stains somewhat darker, there are several blunt cytoplasmic projections. The cytoplasm lacks specific or nonspecific granules (see Chapter 5).

Cytochemistry: The peroxidase reaction may be positive.

Auer body

Auer bodies (Fig. 6-36) are elongated, rod-shaped structures that are not found in normal cells but may be seen in the myeloblasts, myelomonoblasts, and monoblasts of acute leukemias. They are not encountered in lymphoblasts. Tinctorially and histochemically they are large, tubercle bacilli–like rods that stain azurophilic with Wright-Giemsa stain and are peroxidase, naphthol AS-D chloracetate esterase, and acid phosphatase positive.[61-63] The histochemical reactions emphasize the Auer body's rich complement of lysosomal enzymes. By electron microscopy Auer bodies are surrounded by a double membrane and are either devoid of any internal structure or contain crystalline inclusions (see Chapter 5).

Promyelocyte

Size and shape: The promyelocyte is 14-20 μm in diameter and round or oval in shape (Plate 4, p. 149).

Nucleus: The nucleus is still large but is beginning to shrink. It is round or oval, eccentric, possibly slightly indented, and surrounded by a thin membrane. Within the finely granular purplish pale chromatin, chromatin condensations appear and one to three nucleoli may be faintly visible.

Cytoplasm: The cytoplasm is pale blue; it is somewhat larger in area than in myeloblasts, so that the nuclear/cytoplasmic ratio is 4:1 or 5:1. The basophilia is not quite as intense as in myeloblasts. The nonspecific, peroxide-containing azurophilic granules are characteristic of the promyelocytic stage of development. As the cell divides and slips into the myelocytic stage, the azurophilic granules diminish and brownish neutrophilic specific granules appear at the periphery of the centrosome. The specific granules are peroxidase negative and leukocyte alkaline phosphatase positive, and the maturing cells continue to produce them at the ex-

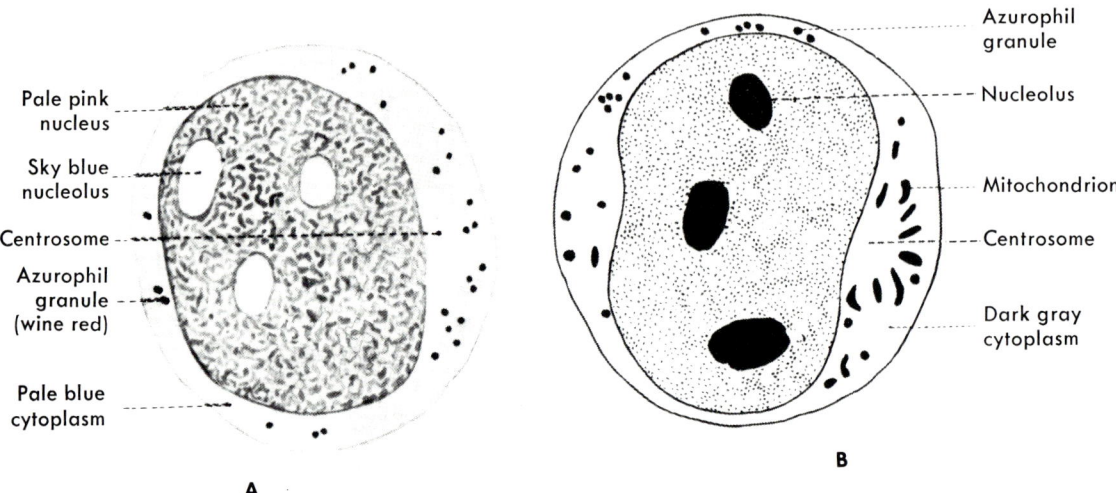

Pale pink nucleus

Sky blue nucleolus

Centrosome

Azurophil granule (wine red)

Pale blue cytoplasm

A

Azurophil granule

Nucleolus

Mitochondrion

Centrosome

Dark gray cytoplasm

B

Fig. 6-35. Myeloblasts. **A,** Wright-Giemsa stain. **B,** As seen in living state with phase microscopy. (From Bessis, M.: Living blood cells and their ultrastructure, Heidelberg, West Germany, 1973, Springer-Verlag.)

pense of the azurophilic granules. Close to the nuclear indentation there is an unstained zone devoid of granules, the hof or Golgi apparatus (Fig. 6-37).

Cytochemistry: The endoplasmic reticulum and the azurophilic granules are peroxidase, naphthol AS-D chloroacetate esterase, acid phosphatase, and Sudan black B positive. The neutrophilic granules are alkaline phosphatase positive. Leukemic promyelocytes contain a procoagulant that is related to brain tissue factor and that possesses potent clot-promoting activity.[64,65]

Myelocyte

Size and shape: The myelocyte is 15-18 μm in diameter and round.

Nucleus: The nucleus is condensed, oval, slightly indented, and eccentric. The chromatin is coarse. Nucleoli are absent.

Cytoplasm: The cytoplasm is light pink, acidophilic, and contains neutrophilic granules that may cover the nucleus and are coarse in the younger cells but become finer as the cell matures. A few azurophilic granules are also seen. The nuclear/cytoplasmic ratio is now about 2:1 or 1.5:1 (Plate 4, p. 149).

Cytochemistry: The cytochemical reactions are identical with those of granulocytes.

Metamyelocyte (juvenile cell)

The metamyelocyte is the last cell of the granulocytic series capable of mitotic division; further stages in the development are caused by maturation and nondivision.

Size and shape: The metamyelocyte is 12-18 μm in diameter and round.

Nucleus: The nucleus is eccentric, condensed, and

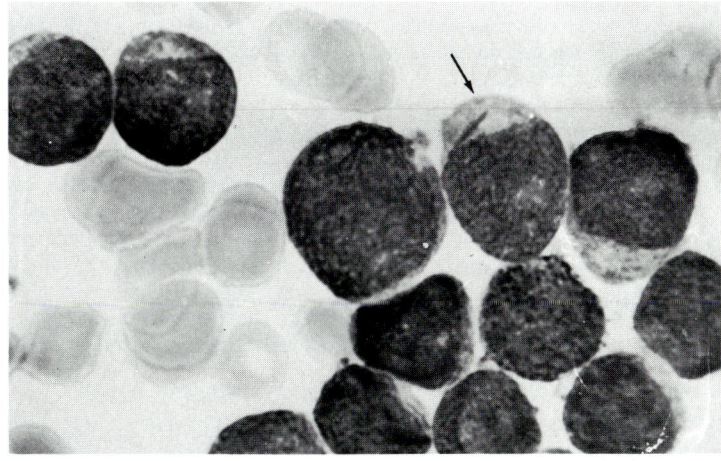

Fig. 6-36. Acute granulocytic leukemia, bone marrow smear. Auer body present in one myeloblast. (Wright-Giemsa stain.)

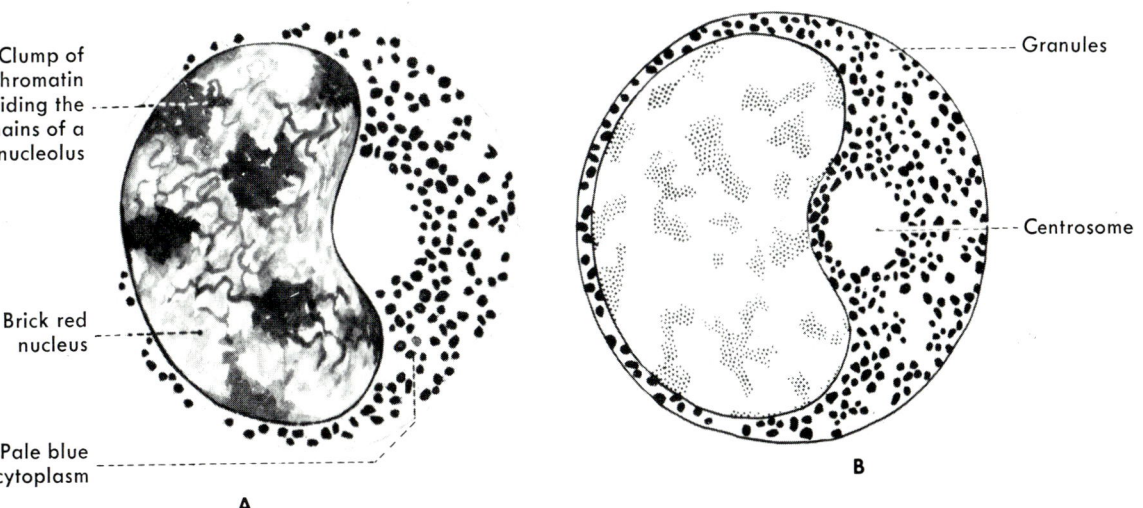

Fig. 6-37. Neutrophil promyelocytes. **A,** Wright-Giemsa stain. **B,** As seen in living state with phase microscopy. (From Bessis, M.: Living blood cells and their ultrastructure, Heidelberg, West Germany, 1973, Springer-Verlag.)

indented. The nuclear membrane is thick and heavy, and the chromatin is concentrated into irregular thick and thin areas.

Cytoplasm: The cytoplasm is abundant and pale or pink; it contains both nonspecific (a few) and specific granules that in the neutrophilic metamyelocytes vary somewhat in size, whereas the basophilic and eosinophilic granules are large and equal in size. The nuclear/cytoplasmic ratio is 1:1 (Plate 4, p. 149).

Cytochemistry: The cytochemical reactions are identical with those of granulocytes.

Band granulocyte (stab cell)

The juvenile cell and the band cell are the youngest granulocytes normally found in the peripheral blood.

Size: The band granulocyte is 10-15 μm in diameter.

Nucleus: The nucleus is elongated, curved, and usually U shaped, but it may be twisted. It is not segmented but may be slightly indented at one or two points. The chromatin is continuous, thick, and coarse, and the parachromatin is scanty. Some stab forms show a degree of nuclear constriction, which makes their differentiation from bilobed segmented polymorphonuclear cells difficult. If nuclear chromatin and parachromatin are still visible in the space between the nuclear membranes of the narrowest nuclear constriction, the cell is called a stab cell. If the bridge or filament between the two nuclear lobes consists of nuclear membranes only and measures less than 1.0 μm in thickness, the cell is a segmented polymorphonuclear leukocyte. If the nucleus is bent or folded on itself so that the fine nuclear bridge cannot be studied in detail, the cell is classified as a segmented leukocyte (Plate 5 [p. 153] and Fig. 6-38).

Cytoplasm: The cytoplasm contains specific and a few nonspecific granules and is pink or colorless. The nuclear/cytoplasmic ration is 1:2.

Cytochemistry: The cytochemical reactions are identical with those of granulocytes.

Segmented granulocyte

Size: The segmented granulocyte is 10-15 μm in diameter.

Nucleus: The nucleus is eccentric, with heavy, thick chromatin masses and a small amount of parachromatin. It is divided into two to five lobes (the three-lobed nucleus is the most common form) connected to each other by thin bridges of nuclear membrane. The nucleus usually surrounds the Golgi area and exhibits a variety of protrusions of nuclear material, e.g., spikes, sessile bodies, and drumsticks (see later discussion of drumsticks). The ratio of segmented to band forms is of clinical importance (shift to the left of the differential count) and is normally about 10:.1. It is therefore necessary to establish clear morphologic criteria for bilobed segmented granulocytes (see earlier description of band polymorphonuclear leukocyte). As the cell matures, the number of lobes increases from two to about five. If over 5% of the granulocytes have five or more lobes, this indicates B₁₂ or folic acid deficiency.

Cytoplasm: The cytoplasm is abundant and slightly eosinophilic or colorless and contains specific granules. The neutrophilic granules are very fine in texture and do not overlay the nucleus. The nuclear/cytoplasmic ratio is 1:2 (Plate 5, p. 153).

Cytochemistry: Granulocytes contain large amounts of glycogen, which render the cell periodic acid–Schiff (PAS) positive. The glycogen gradually accumulates as the cell matures, beginning with the myelocytic stages. In granulocytic leukemia the glycogen content is reduced. The leukocyte alkaline phosphatase (LAP) level parallels the glycogen contents. The specific or secondary granules are LAP and Sudan black B positive and peroxidase negative. LAP is a lysosomal enzyme that appears in the myelocytic stage and increases in amount as the cell matures. Its increased activity in infections is probably related to adrenal steroid activity, whereas its fall in chronic granulocytic leukemia, paroxysmal nocturnal hemoglobinuria, and many other hematologic

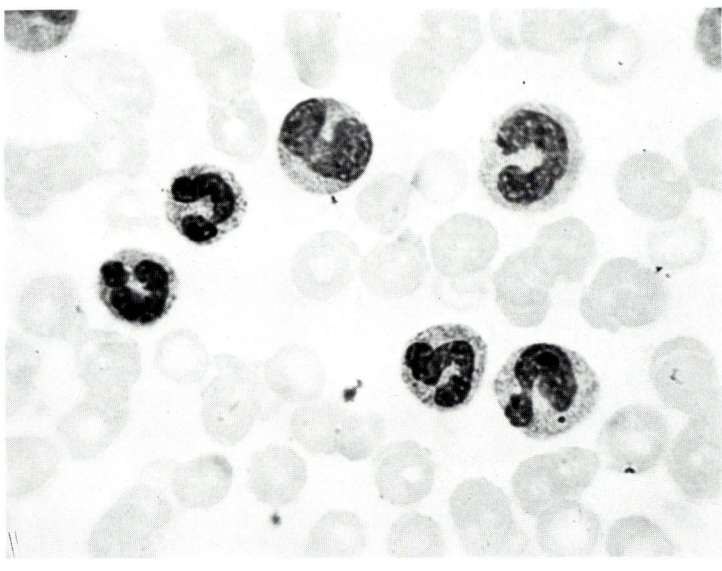

Fig. 6-38. Band granulocytes.

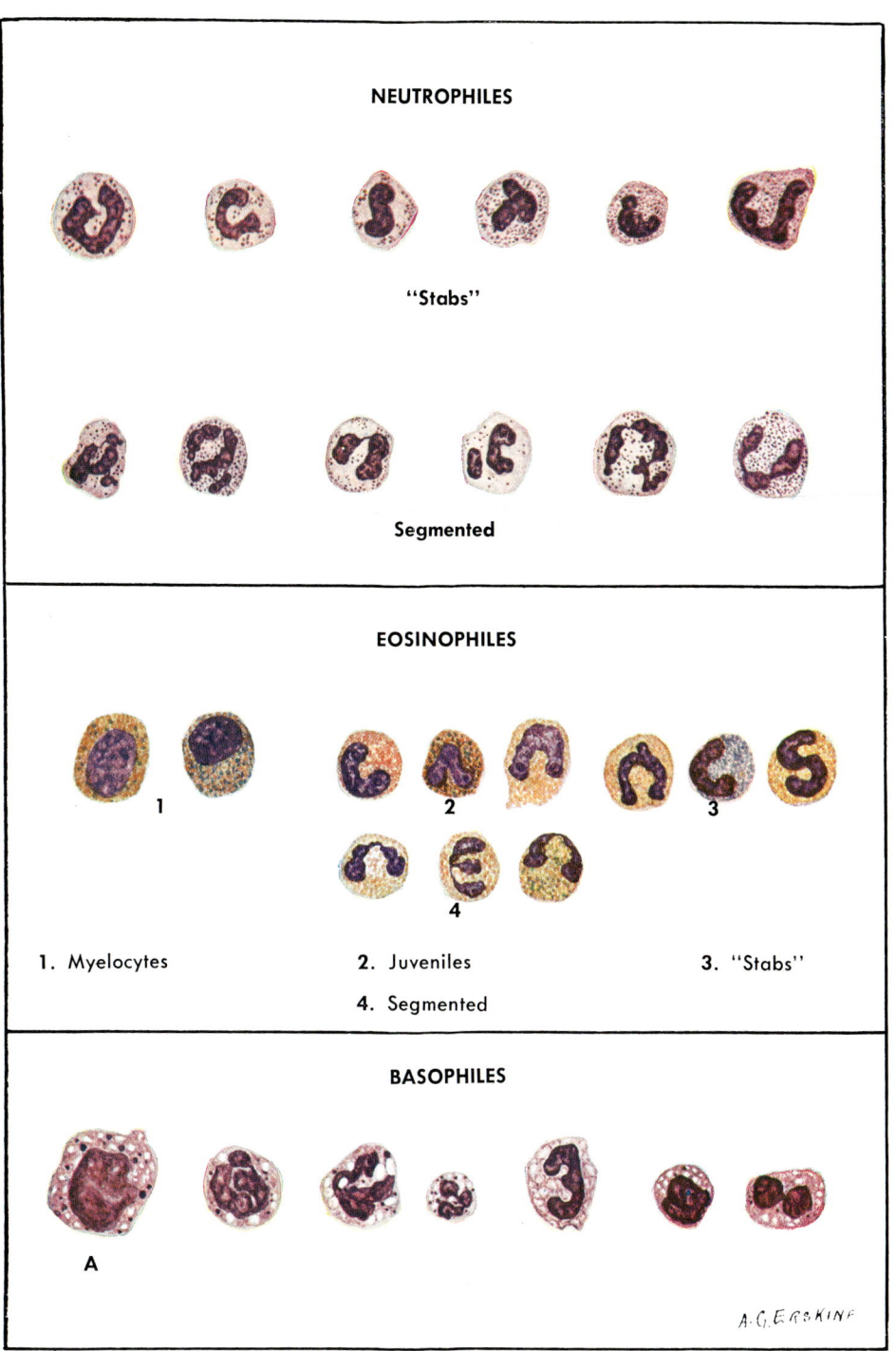

Plate 5. Leukocytes. *A*, Basophilic myelocyte. (Wright-Giemsa stain; ×950.)

conditions may be related to low zinc levels,[66] since normal granulocytes have high zinc levels. Whereas LAP is the enzyme of the mature cell, myeloperoxidase is the lysosomal enzyme of the immature cell, the myeloblast. The granulocytic lysosome (muramidase) content is responsible for the increase in serum and urinary lysosome in chronic granulocytic and in myelomonocytic leukemias (see Chapter 9). The mature granulocyte, like its precursors, has two types of granules; the smaller peroxidase-negative specific granules are twice as frequent as the peroxidase-positive nonspecific granules.

The function of neutrophils is described in the discussion of leukocytic function tests in Chapter 9.

NUCLEAR SEX DIMORPHISM IN SEGMENTED LEUKOCYTES, SEXING OF GRANULOCYTES[67]

Granulocytic nuclei may have many nuclear appendages, the best studied of which is the sex chromatin.

Drumsticks

In the female about one in 38-60 (1-8%) segmented neutrophils will have a solid nuclear appendage shaped like a drumstick attached by a narrow segment to one of the main lobes of the nucleus (Fig. 6-39). This structure can also be seen in eosinophils and basophils, although the granules of these cells may obscure it. The irregular tags, clubs, and pale racket bodies sometimes found extending from the nuclear lobes of polymorphonuclear cells in males must be distinguished from the typical drumstick appendage.

The peripheral blood film method of sexing uses a regular thin blood film stained with Wright stain. Because of the large number of polymorphonuclear cells that must be scanned, it is advisable to prepare a **buffy coat smear.** Five hundred leukocytes should be sexed and the percentage of drumsticks reported. The blood

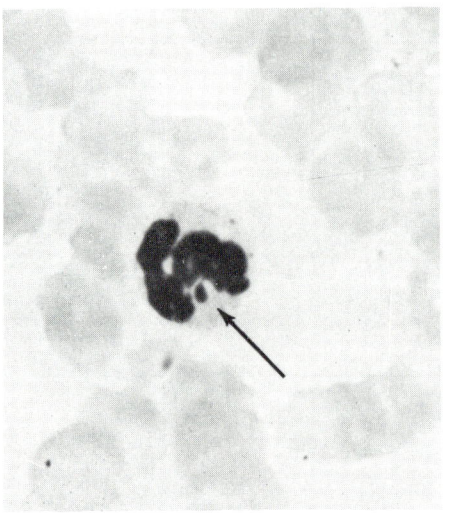

Fig. 6-39. "Drumstick" in polymorphonuclear leukocytes.

film findings should be confirmed by one or two additional methods of cellular sexing, e.g., the buccal smear method **(Barr body)** and chromosomal analysis by the leukocyte culture technic.

Interpretation: It is essential that in the differential count the strictest criteria for drumsticks be maintained and that other types of nuclear appendages not be mistaken for drumsticks (Fig. 6-40).

In females a minimum of seven drumsticks per 500 polymorphonuclear cells is found and reported as **sex-chromatin positive.** In female premature infants, up to 100 drumsticks per 500 polymorphonuclear cells may be found, and in female full-term newborns the average number is 13 drumsticks per 500 polymorphonuclear cells. After birth the number rapidly falls to the adult level.

In males, the usual finding is zero drumsticks per 500 polymorphonuclear cells; this finding is reported as **sex-chromatin negative.**

The correlation between the number and structure of X chromosomes and the number and morphology of drumsticks is not as good as it is between the number and structure of X chromosomes and Barr bodies (see later discussion).

Abnormally enlarged and numerically diminished drumsticks have been reported in the XXX syndrome.[68] In trisomy C[69] the frequency of drumsticks is increased (Fig. 6-41).

Sex chromatin in buccal smears

The buccal smear is described for two reasons: (1) it may be used to confirm nuclear sexing of leukocytes; and (2) it is usually handled by the routine laboratory rather than by the cytogenetic laboratory.

Barr bodies[70]

In females the nuclei of somatic cells contain a biconvex chromatin mass measuring about 1-1.5 μm in width and 1.5-2 μm in length (Fig. 6-42). It is called the **sex-chromatin Barr body** and is closely applied to the inside of the nuclear membrane, representing the condensed chromatin mass of the inactivated second X chromosome. In somatic cells only one X chromosome can be biologically active; the other is in some way inactivated (probably incompletely). It is therefore not seen in the somatic cells of males (Fig. 6-43).

Buccal smear technic of nuclear sexing

Reagents:

1. Fixative
   Ethyl alcohol, absolute ⎫
   Ether ⎭ Equal parts
2. Stain: cresyl violet, 1%

Procedure: Gently scrape the right and left buccal surfaces with tongue depressors and smear mucosal cells on separate slides. Immerse slides immediately in fixative for 30-60 min. After fixation, treat as follows:

Ethyl alcohol, 50%: 10 dips
Distilled water: 10 dips
Cresyl violet, 1%: 45 min
Ethyl alcohol, 95%: 3 dips
Ethyl alcohol, absolute: 3 dips
Xylene: 6 dips

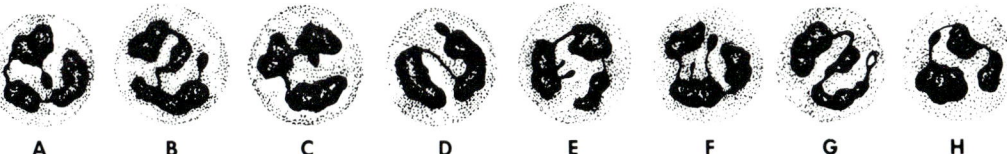

Fig. 6-40. Nuclear appendages of polymorphonuclear cells that may be mistaken for drumsticks. **A** and **B,** Typical drumsticks (the only diagnostic form). **C** and **D,** Sessile nodules. **E** and **F,** Small tags (**F** also shows a drumstick). **G,** Racket appendage. **H,** Small lobe. (From Hienz, H.A.: Chromosomen Fibel, Stuttgart, West Germany, 1971, Georg Thieme Verlag.)

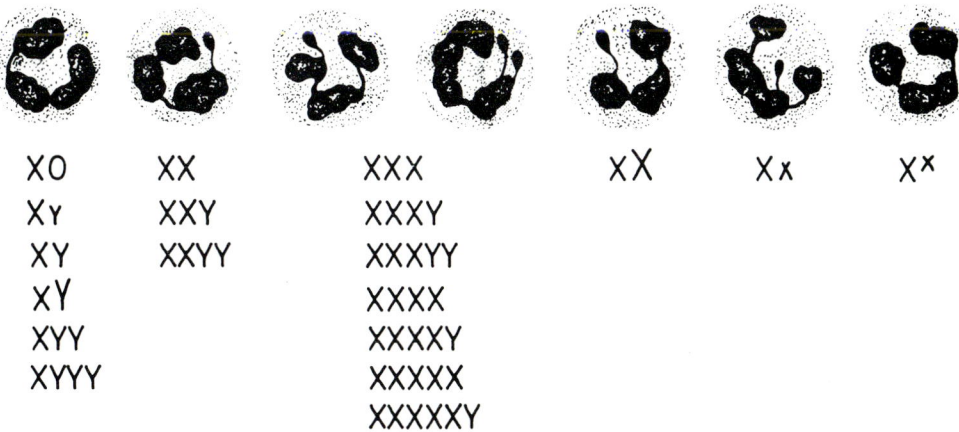

XO	XX	XXX		XX	Xx	Xx
XY	XXY	XXXY				
XY	XXYY	XXXYY				
XY		XXXX				
XYY		XXXXY				
XYYY		XXXXX				
		XXXXXY				

Fig. 6-41. Relationship between size and number of drumsticks and sex chromosome pattern. (From Hienz, H.A.: Chromosomen Fibel, Stuttgart, West Germany, 1971, Georg Thieme Verlag.)

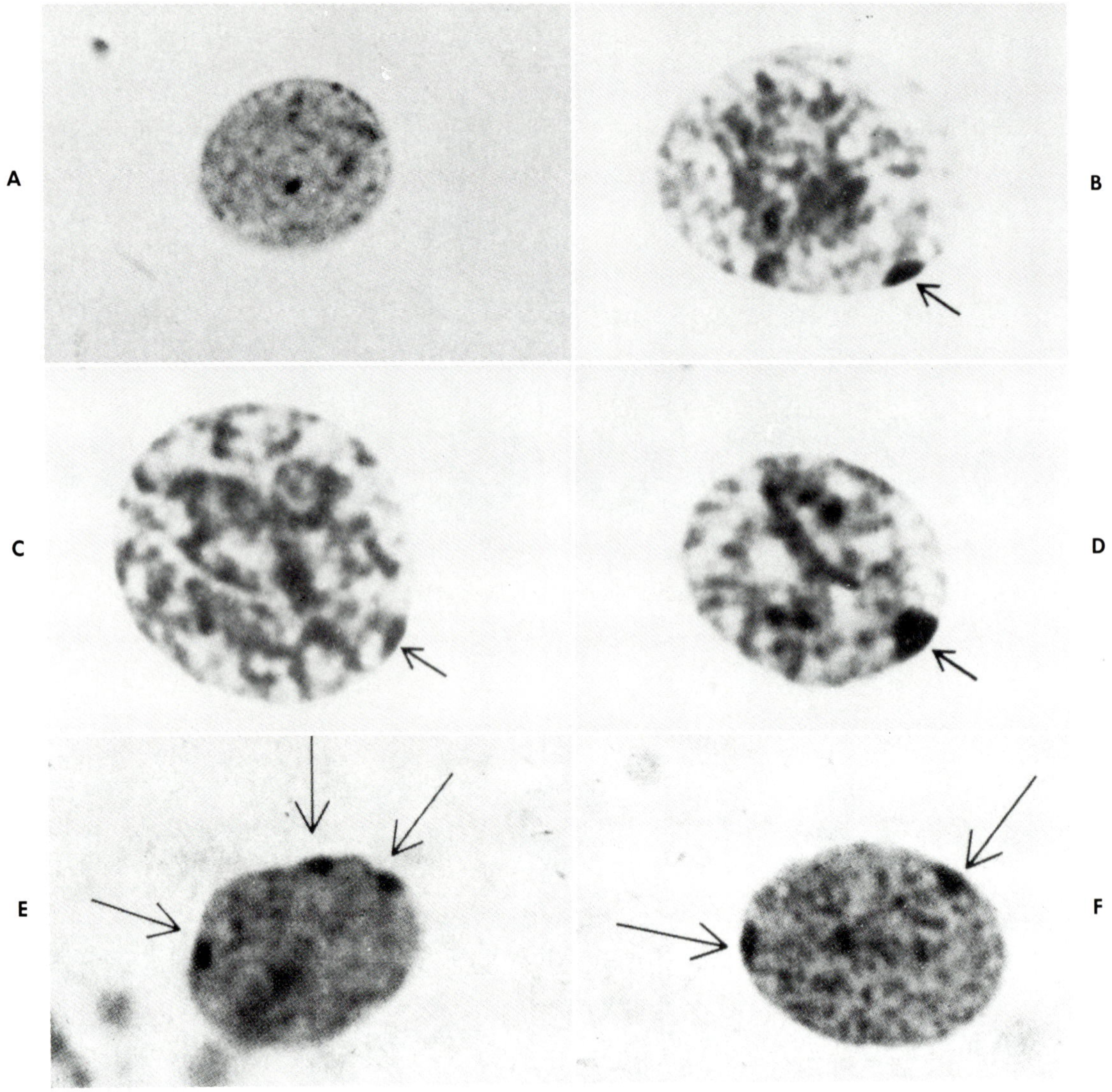

Fig. 6-42. Cells from buccal smears used for counting of X chromosomes. **A,** Chromatin-negative cell from normal male (XY). Cell has no Barr body, as male sex chromosome complement includes only one X chromosome. **B,** Normal typical single Barr body. **C,** Single Barr body, small size of which suggests partial deletion (loss of material) of one X chromosome. **D,** Barr body of large size, suggesting added material in long arm, isochromosome. **E,** Three Barr bodies in cell of anatomically normal male patient of inferred genotype *XXXY*. **F,** Two Barr bodies in anatomically normal female of genotype *XXX*. (From Ferguson-Smith, M.A.: Hosp. Pract. **5:**88, 1970.)

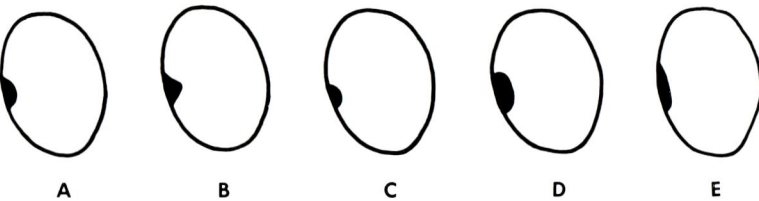

A   B   C   D   E

Fig. 6-43. Morphologic variation of Barr body. **A,** Classic form. **B,** Triangle. **C,** Microform. **D,** Macroform. **E,** Elongated form. (From Hienz, H.A.: Chromosomen Fibel, Stuttgart, West Germany, 1971, Georg Thieme Verlag.)

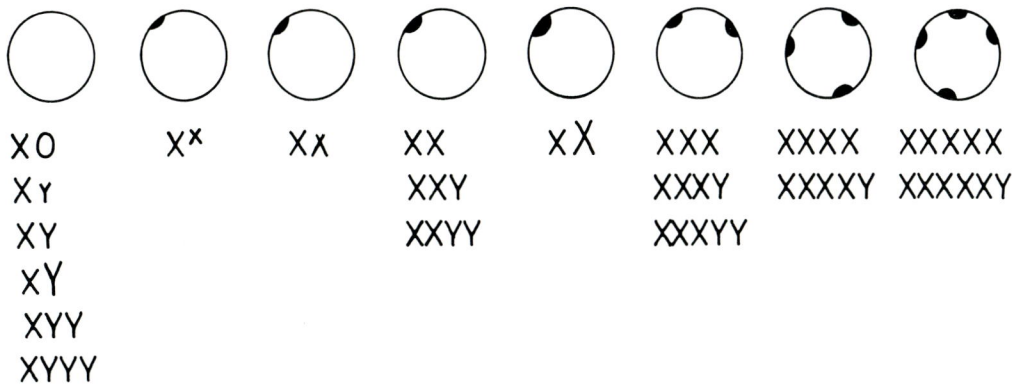

Fig. 6-44. Relationship between size and number of Barr bodies and sex chromatin patterns. (From Hienz, H.A.: Chromosomen Fibel, Stuttgart, West Germany, 1971, Georg Thieme Verlag.)

Mount in Permount (Fisher Scientific Co., Pittsburgh) under coverslip. Do not allow slides to dry during procedure.

Results: Under oil immersion examine 100-300 well-preserved flat cells free of bacteria with open-faced, chromatin-poor nuclei for Barr bodies. Use strictest criteria and accept only typical, well-preserved forms situated on the inside of the nuclear membrane.

Interpretation: Barr body frequency in women is 8-61%; in men, 0-1%.

The **X chromosome complement** of an individual can be determined by counting the maximal number of Barr bodies per cell and then adding 1. No Barr bodies indicate an XY sex chromosomal pattern (normal male) or XO pattern's (Turner's syndrome); one Barr body means an XX (normal female) or XXY pattern (Klinefelter's syndrome); two Barr bodies mean an XXX or XXXX pattern, etc.

There is not only a correlation between the number of X chromosomes and the number of Barr bodies but also between the size of Barr bodies and structural X chromosomal changes (Fig. 6-44) such as deletion of the short arm or long arm of the X chromosome or additional chromosome material added to the long arm (isochromosome formation). Combinations of numeric and structural aberrations of the X chromosome can also be evaluated.

Quinacrine fluorescence method of Y chromosome identification[71,72]

Well-preserved male cells contain a single, intranuclear, brightly fluorescent spot that represents the Y chromosome (Fig. 6-45).

Reagents:
1. Quinacrine chloride, aqueous, 0.5%
2. Citric acid phosphate buffer (McIlvaine), 0.01M, pH 5.5:
   2.84 g/dl: Na_2HPO_4, aqueous, 12.9 ml
   2.1 g/dl: Citric acid, aqueous, 8.6 ml
3. Phosphate buffer, 0.01M, pH 7.4:
   Na_2HPO_4, 15M, 12 ml
   KH_2PO_4, 15M, 3 ml

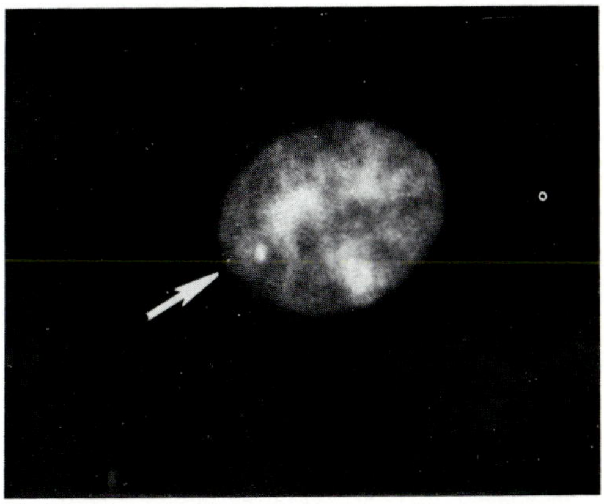

Fig. 6-45. Quinacrine fluorescence method of Y chromosome identification. Note bright spot in nucleus near eight o'clock position (arrow). (From Hollander, D.H.: Acta Cytol. [Baltimore] **15:**453, 1971.)

Add distilled water to 1 dl. Check pH and adjust with 0.1N HCl or 0.1N NaOH as needed.

Procedure: The buccal smear is obtained and prepared as in the Barr body method. Fix smear, without drying, in 95% ethyl alcohol 1 hr or longer and then treat as follows:
Methyl alcohol, absolute: 3 min
Graded ethyl alcohol to water: 3 min
Quinacrine chloride, aqueous, 0.5%: 5 min (or longer)
Citric acid–phosphate buffer, 0.01M: 3 min
Phosphate buffer, 0.01M, 2 changes: 3 min
Mount with 0.01M phosphate buffer (pH 7.4) and seal with clear nail polish. Examine with fluorescence microscope and darkfield illumination.

Interpretation: About 40% of the nuclei of males contain a discernible fluorescent Y body. A similar structure is seen in less than 2% of females. The described method should be useful in rapidly identifying Y polysomy, e.g., XYY.

Fluorescent male sex chromatin in hair root cells

Engel et al.[73,74] applied the "buccal smear" method to the identification of Y chromosomes in cells of the external root sheath of plucked hairs. According to their method, the cells are spread, flattened, and stained.

Interpretation: The results and interpretation of the hair root method are similar to those of the buccal smear method.

PATHOLOGIC FORMS OF POLYMORPHONUCLEAR LEUKOCYTES[75]
Cytoplasmic changes

Alder-Reilly granulation[76]: Alder's anomaly (Fig. 6-46) is a rare hereditary anomaly characterized by

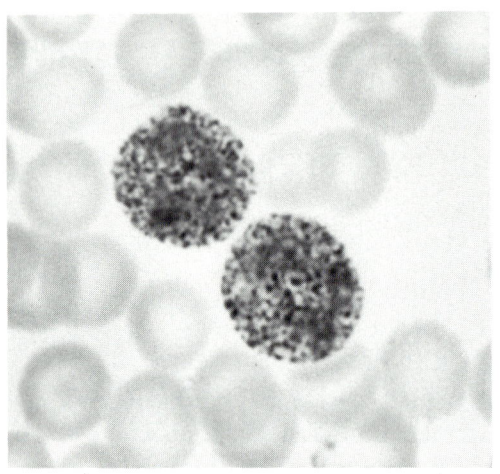

Fig. 6-46. Alder's anomaly in gargoylism.

coarse, dark, azurophilic granules in the cytoplasm of polymorphonuclear cells that cover the nucleus. They also occur in monocytes, lymphocytes, and the bone marrow precursor cells. Eosinophilic and basophilic granules are abnormally dark. Alder's anomaly occurs in white cells of patients with genetic mucopolysaccharidoses (e.g., gargoylism) but may also occur as a hereditary abnormality in healthy patients. The granules contain acid polysaccharides and glycogen and are similar to Reilly bodies.[77] They are larger than toxic granulation seen in infections.

Amato bodies: See later discussion of Döhle bodies.

Chédiak-Higashi syndrome: In Chédiak-Higashi syndrome[78,79] (Fig. 6-47) the neutrophils show large, azurophilic inclusions that vary in size and color. The giant granules alternate with normal granules. Cytochemically they resemble primary azurophilic granules (lysosomes) and are Sudan black B, peroxidase, and acid phosphatase positive.[80] Electron microscopy[81] supports the concept that these giant granules are the result of fusion of normal azurophilic granules.[82] The granules in the eosinophils and basophils are also abnormally large as are the azurophilic granules in lymphocytes, monocytes, and plasma cells. The anomaly of the white cells is part of a hereditary autosomal recessive syndrome that includes albinism, abnormal skin pigmentation, and repeated infections, ultimately leading to anemia, neutropenia, thrombocytopenia, and death. A Chédiak-Higashi anomaly–like aberration has recently been reported in acute myelomonocytic leukemia.[83] The Chédiak-Higashi syndrome represents one of the few instances of a familial leukotactic defect, although a cause-and-effect relationship between the large lysosomal granules and the bactericidal defect has not been established (see Chapter 9).[84,85] The polymorphonuclear cells show not only a chemotactic defect but also impaired adhesion to artificial surfaces[86] and delayed killing of intracellular bacteria because of defective lysosomal emptying into phagocytic vacu-

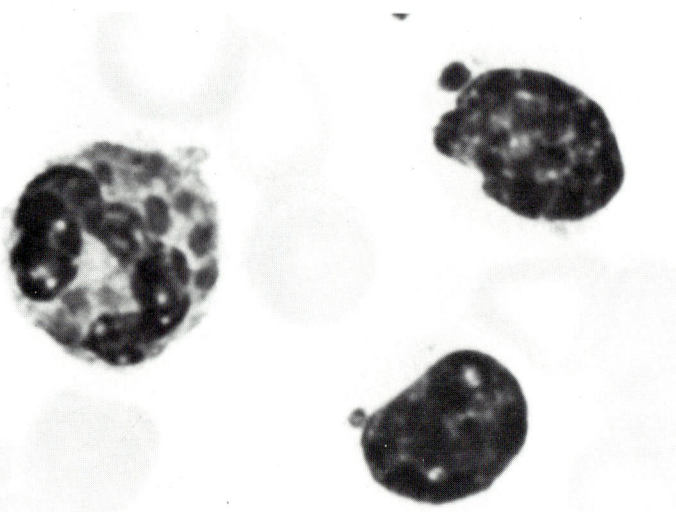

Fig. 6-47. Abnormal granulation of lymphocytes and granulocytes in Chédiak-Higashi syndrome. (Courtesy Dr. L.W. Diggs.)

oles.[87] Recent investigations have focused on a defect in the membrane-associated microtubules as the cause of the functional defect of the polymorphonuclear cells in Chédiak-Higashi syndrome.[88,89] A platelet storage-pool defect is responsible for the bleeding tendency of the affected patients.[90]

Döhle (Amato) bodies: Döhle bodies[91] are irregular, blue-staining cytoplasmic inclusions that vary from the size of cocci to about 2 μm in diameter (Fig. 6-48). They are found in severe infections and disappear as the infection subsides. They are found after chemotherapy,[92] in severe burns,[93] and in May-Hegglin anomaly, in which they persist for life. By electron microscopy Döhle bodies are sacs of ergastoplasm. It must be noted

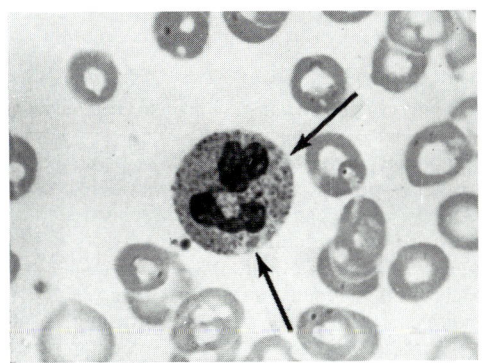

Fig. 6-48. Döhle bodies.

that the structures that appear in May-Hegglin anomaly and that in Wright-Giemsa–stained preparations resemble Döhle bodies by electron microscopy[94] are seen to be made of granules that contain rodlike structures and thus differ from the usual Döhle bodies.

Giant neutrophils: See later discussion of hypersegmented forms.

Granulocytic anomaly in Down's syndrome[95]: Down's syndrome (trisomy 21) is characterized by a series of abnormalities involving the heart, soft tissues, and the nervous system. Hematologic findings may include a raised level of fetal hemoglobin and morphologic changes of neutrophils consisting of clumping of nuclear chromatin, hypersegmentation, and hooklike appendages. The changes are not unlike those described in the later discussion of malignancy-associated changes (MAC).

Hurler's disease (gargoylism): Hurler's disease is an autosomal recessive inborn error of the metabolism of mucopolysaccharides, which are important normal molecular constituents of connective tissue and of granulocytes. It is one of 12 forms of polysaccharides characterized by the gargoyl-like appearance of the patient and by increased excretion of mucopolysaccharides in the urine.[96] In Hurler's disease, Alder's anomaly–like granules may appear in granulocytes, lymphocytes, and monocytes in the peripheral blood and bone marrow.[97,98] In the bone marrow they are also seen in histiocytes.

Jordans' anomaly: Jordans[99] described vacuoles in granulocytes and monocytes in two brothers who had progressive muscular dystrophy. Similar changes were

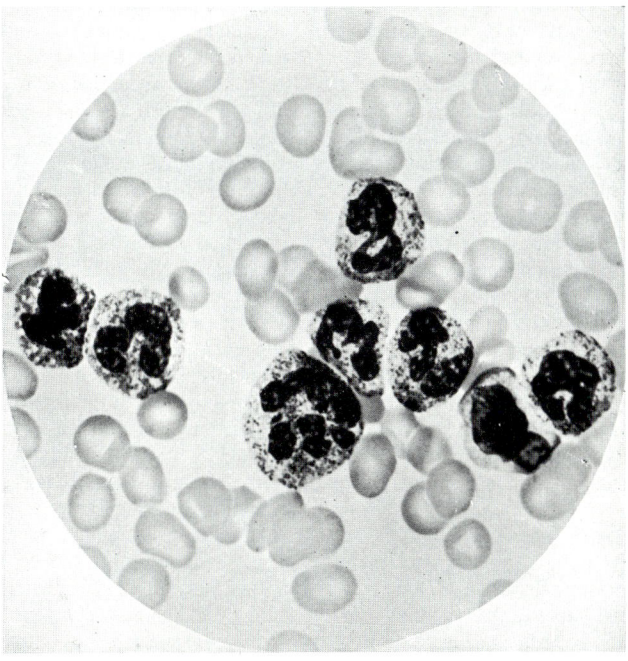

Fig. 6-49. Acute lobar pneumonia. Toxic granules in all segmented and nonsegmented polymorphonuclear neutrophils. Note anisocytosis of leukocytes and also large polymorphonuclear neutrophils. (Jenner-Giemsa stain.) (From Kugel, M.A., and Rosenthal, N.: Am. J. Med. Sci. **183:**657, 1932.)

seen in two sisters with ichthyosis.[100] The vacuoles may represent fatty degeneration or glycogen, or they may be due to autophagosomes because they are frequently observed in septicemia, in association with toxic granulation, and in immune complex disorders. In some patients vacuoles appear only in the lymphocytes and monocytes and have proved to be associated with mucopolysaccharidosis, although the majority of patients with gargoylism show no vacuoles in any of their white cells.

May-Hegglin anomaly[101,102]: Hegglin described an autosomal dominant disorder characterized by irregularly sized, 2-5 μm, multiple or single inclusions in the polymorphonuclear cells; these inclusions are similar to Döhle bodies, are also found in monocytes, basophils, eosinophils, and rarely in lymphocytes, and are related to infections. They are associated with abnormal giant platelets and thrombocytopenia. May-Hegglin anomaly is of no clinical significance except for a bleeding tendency, reported in 50% of cases, that is related to the abnormal platelets. By electron microscopy the May-Hegglin inclusions differ from the usual Döhle bodies because they contain glycogen and RNA, the latter being methyl green pyronine positive.

Reilly bodies: In the leukocytes of patients with gargoylism there are darkly stained granules that vary in size and shape and are referred to as Reilly bodies[103] (Fig. 6-49). They may alternate with vacuoles. Reilly bodies are an expression of an inherited disorder of mucopolysaccharide metabolism and are similar to the granules seen in Alder's anomaly (see earlier discussion). These granules stain metachromatically with toluidine blue O stain but fail to stain with PAS stain because they contain acid mucopolysaccharides.

Toxic granulation: In severe infection, in chemical poisoning, and in toxic states, the cytoplasm may contain large, dark-staining granules (toxic granules; Fig. 6-49). Toxic granulation must be differentiated from the abnormal granules of Alder's anomaly and Chédiak-Higashi syndrome and from artifacts produced by poor staining. The latter can be excluded by examination of a control slide stained at the same time as the original slide or by examination of other cells on the same slide. Toxic granules may be larger than normal neutrophilic granules and may thus represent a kind of granular/cellular dissociation, i.e., a mature cell with large immature granules. On the other hand, some toxic granules (as proven by electron microscopy) may represent secondary lysosomes or autophagosomes that contain immune complexes. Autophagosomes[104] are lysosomes that have fused with a phagocytic vacuole and have discharged their enzymatic contents into it.

Vacuoles: See discussions of Jordans' anomaly and vacuolated lymphocytes.

Nuclear changes

Basket cells: See later discussion of smudge cells.

Hypersegmented forms: Large forms with many (6-10) nuclear lobes and large reddish granules are often found in pernicious anemia (Fig. 6-50). Similar cells may also occur as a congenital abnormality,[105,106] in chronic anemia, and in Down's syndrome. In pernicious anemia the cell outline is oval instead of round,

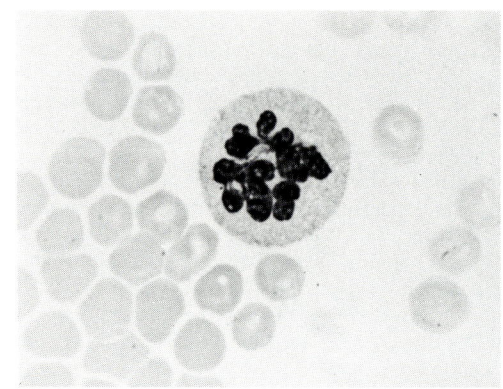

Fig. 6-50. Hypersegmented polymorphonuclear cell in pernicious anemia.

and the hypersegmentation may involve eosinophils and basophils.

Malignancy-associated changes: In about 88% of all patients with cancer, malignancy-associated changes (MAC) can be recognized in polymorphonuclear cells and monocytes. According to Johnston and Brady[107] these changes consist of thin, threadlike, pointed, small (about 1 μm) inclusions surrounded by halos within the cytoplasm of monocytes. The entire structure is about the size of a Döhle body (2-3 μm). Nieburgs et al.[108] described nuclear chromatin changes that can be seen under oil immersion and that in the granulocyte consist of the absence of the normal chromocenter in several or all lobes. In place of the usually single prominent chromocenter there are numerous clear spheric areas surrounded by a rim of chromatin, or there may be enlarged chromocenters that vary in size and shape.

In Down's syndrome delicate hooked nuclear appendages are noted, somewhat similar to the changes seen associated with malignancy.

Pelger-Huët anomaly: Pelger-Huët anomaly[109,110] (Fig. 6-51) is characterized by marked condensation of nuclear chromatin in all white cells and by decreased lobulation of the neutrophils, so that most polymorphonuclear cells are bilobed or band forms. Completely round nuclei with coarse, clumped chromatin are also seen in some neutrophils. The abnormality is either congenital (true Pelger-Huët anomaly) or acquired (pseudo Pelger-Huët anomaly).[111] The congenital form is asymptomatic in the heterozygous state, although its association with muscular dystrophy has been reported.[112] It is apparently lethal in the homozygous form. The acquired form is seen in such blood diseases as chronic myelocytic leukemia, acute leukemia, myeloid metaplasia, agranulocytosis, infectious mononucleosis, following myelotoxic therapy, and in Fanconi's anemia; it can be differentiated from the congenital disease by examination of other members of the family and by evidence of the primary disease. A functional defect in mature leukocytes exhibiting Pelger-Huët–like chromatin clumping has been described.[113]

Pyknotic cells: In pyknotic cells the nucleus becomes smaller and denser and the chromatin bridges

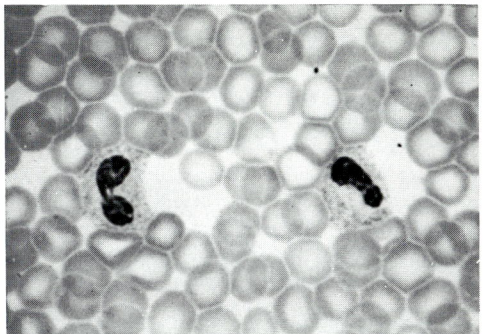

Fig. 6-51. Pelger-Huët anomaly, congenital. (Courtesy V. Minnich.)

between the nuclear segments disappear, leaving several small balls of dense chromatin. This phenomenon is seen in infections and in aging cells.

Twinning deformity (tetraploid neutrophils with diploid nuclei): Segmented neutrophils that exhibit twinning deformity are twice the size of normal neutrophils and are round, whereas the hypersegmented polymorphs of pernicious anemia are oval. The apparent hypersegmentation of the twinning deformity is due to the presence of two nuclei in one cell and occurs in pernicious anemia and in myeloproliferative states.

Smudge cells: Smudge (basket) cells represent the squashed, degenerative nuclei of cells that defy identification. Nevertheless, the percent distribution of these structures should be ascertained at the time of the differential count. Less than 5% smudge cells per 100 white cells is of no significance. Over 5% smudge cells is indicative of poor technic in preparing the blood smear, which should therefore by repeated. There is one exception to this statement: In chronic lymphatic leukemia the cells characteristically smudge easily despite the use of good technic because they are dead or degenerated and fragile.

Lysosomes and functional defects in polymorphonuclear leukocytes

For a discussion of lysosomes and functional defects in polymorphonuclear leukocytes, see Chapter 9.

EOSINOPHILIC GRANULOCYTE AND PRECURSORS

Eosinophils[114,115] mature in the same manner as neutrophils. The eosinophilic myeloblast is not recognizable as such, since it apparently contains only azurophilic granules. In the eosinophilic promyelocyte in the Wright-Giemsa−stained preparation the granules are at first bluish and later mature into orange granules, which are larger than neutrophilic granules, are round or ovoid, and are prominent in the eosinophilic myelocyte.

Mature eosinophil

Size and shape: The mature eosinophil is 12-17 μm in diameter, slightly larger than a segmented polymorphonuclear granulocyte (Plate 5, p. 153).

Nucleus: The nucleus is usually bilobed, rarely single or trilobed, and contains dense chromatin masses. Eosinophils with more than two nuclear lobes are seen in vitamin B_{12} and folic acid deficiency and in allergic disorders.

Cytoplasm: The cytoplasm is densely filled with granules, so that its pale blue color can be appreciated only if the granules escape. The granules are uniform in size, large, and usually spheric and do not cover the nucleus. They show highlights when the micrometer adjustment is moved up and down.

In the differential count all the eosinophils are placed in one group, except the eosinophilic myelocytes and promyelocytes, which are counted separately.

Cytochemistry: Eosinophils are alkaline phosphatase and naphthol AS-D chloroacetate esterase negative; they contain a peroxidase that differs from the myeloperoxidase found in other leukocytes.[116] Acid phosphatase is localized in the small granules, which on electron microscopy do not contain a crystalline core[117]; alkaline phosphatase activity is restricted to nuclear and mitochondrial membranes.[118]

Function: Eosinophils are phagocytic and bactericidal, similar to neutrophils.[119] Eosinophilia is frequently associated with allergic and parasitic disorders,[120] since eosinophils selectively respond to a number of eosinophil chemotactic factors, e.g., immune complexes after activation of the complement system,[121] sensitized lymphocytes,[122] the eosinophil chemotactic factor of anaphylaxis (ECF-A),[123] and lymphokine-immune complex (IgE), and the eosinophil stimulation promoter (ESP)[124] released by a number of parasites, e.g., schistosomes and *Trichinella* organisms. Other eosinophil chemotactic factors are complement complexes and histamine. Once the eosinophil has been attracted to an area of activity it is called upon to phagocytose a number of materials, e.g., immune complexes, mast cell granules, monocytes, bacteria, and inert particles.[115] The mechanism of bacterial killing in the eosinophil differs from that in the polymorphonuclear leukocytes since the peroxidase enzymes of these cells are not the same.[115]

Damaged and degenerated eosinophils give rise to **Charcot-Leyden** crystals (see Fig. 29-17), which can be found in sputum, exudates, and stool specimens in conditions characterized by a large number of eosinophils, e.g., asthma, granulocytic leukemia, and amebiasis.

BASOPHILIC GRANULOCYTE AND PRECURSORS

The early maturation of the basophilic granulocyte[125] is similar to that of the neutrophilic granulocyte. The specific granules appear in the promyelocytic and myelocytic stages and arise like all secretory granules from the Golgi apparatus.

Mature basophil[126]

Size: Basophils are somewhat smaller than eosinophils, measuring 10-14 μm in diameter (Plate 5, p. 153).

Nucleus: The nucleus is indented, giving rise to an S pattern. It is difficult to see because it contains less chromatin and is masked by the cytoplasmic granules.

Cytoplasm: The cytoplasm is pale blue to pale pink and contains basophilic granules that often overlie the nucleus but do not fill the cytoplasm as completely as the eosinophilic granules do. The granules are dark purple to blue-black, vary in size, and are water soluble. They may therefore dissolve during the staining process, leaving clear cytoplasmic vacuoles.[127]

Cytochemistry: The granules are alkaline and acid phosphatase, nonspecific esterase, and phosphorylase negative but peroxidase positive.[128] A minority of special small granules are peroxidase negative.[129] Specific cytoplasmic granules contain histamine, which is released in response to antigen-antibody reactions. This phenomenon forms the basis for the basophil degranulation test.[130] The granules are also rich in acid mucopolysaccharides, probably heparin, which stains metachromatically at low pH with certain basic dyes.[127] Basophils also contain a platelet activating factor (PAF), which stimulates platelets to release serotonin.[131] The cytoplasm contains glycogen[130] and several dehydrogenases and diaphorases.[132]

Function[133]: Basophils contain large amounts of histamine, which is released in response to IgE-mediated antigen-antibody reactions and leads to degranulation. Wolf-Jürgensen,[134] using Rebuck's skin window technic, demonstrated that basophils are part of the delayed hypersensitivity reaction as seen in patients with ulcerative colitis and Henoch's ulcer of the urinary bladder.

MAST CELL AND PRECURSORS

Mast cells,[135] which are essentially tissue basophils, are not found in the peripheral blood but sparsely populate the bone marrow. They appear to arise from basophils by a process of differentiation and replication.[136]

Mastoblast

In systemic mastocytosis and in tissue mast cell leukemia immature mast cells (mastoblasts) are seen in the peripheral blood and bone marrow.

Size and shape: The mastoblasts is 25-30 μm in diameter and round.

Nucleus: The nucleus is round and has the fine chromatin pattern of all blast nuclei.

Cytoplasm: The cytoplasm contains azurophilic granules and some metachromatic granules, which do not completely cover the nucleus or fill the entire cell body.

Mast cell

Size and shape: The mast cell is 5-25 μm in diameter and irregular in outline or elongated.

Nucleus: The nucleus is usually oval or round and almost completely covered by granules.

Cytoplasm: The cytoplasm can hardly be seen because of numerous, small, closely packed, deep blue–staining spheric granules of uniform size, which are water soluble and stain metachromatically with toluidine blue.

LYMPHOCYTE AND PRECURSORS

The ontogeny of lymphocytes follows the pattern of erythrocytic and granulocytic development. In response to an increased demand for lymphocytes the totipoten-

tial bone marrow stem cell pool develops pluripotential cells, which generate lymphoblasts. Morphologically the pluripotential cell is a small lymphocyte or a reticulum cell that is poietin sensitive. In the central lymphoid organs the immature lymphocytes develop into either B or T cells.[137] In humans these organs are the thymus for T cells and the bursa equivalent for B cells. These cells are discussed in detail in Chapter 36. T cells perform functions of cell-mediated immunity, and B cells differentiate into plasma cells, the secretors of antibodies, responsible for humoral immunity.

Lymphoblast

Size: The lymphoblast is 15-20 μm in diameter.

Nucleus: The nucleus is central, round, or oval, and the magenta chromatin has a delicate stippled pattern. The nuclear membrane is distinct, and one or two pink nucleoli are present and are usually well outlined (Plate 6, p. 164).

Cytoplasm: The cytoplasm is nongranular and sky blue and may have a darker blue border. It forms a thin perinuclear ring.

Histochemistry: The T cell lineage leukemic stem cell contains terminal deoxynucleotidyl transferase and stains weakly positive for acid phosphatase and acid α-naphthol acetate esterase, whereas the B cell lineage stem cell lacks all histochemical markers,[138] except that of acid phosphatase.

Prolymphocyte

Size: The prolymphocyte is 15-18 μm in diameter.

Nucleus: The nucleus is oval but slightly indented and may show a faint nucleolus. The chromatin is slightly condensed into a mosaic pattern; the denser chromatin is not sharply demarcated from the light-staining, pale blue parachromatin.

Cytoplasm: There is a thin rim of basophilic, homogeneous cytoplasm that may show a few azurophilic granules and vacuoles.

Cytochemistry: The cytochemistry of the prolymphocyte is identical with that of the mature lymphocytes.

Lymphocytes

Lymphocytes that are larger than polymorphonuclear cells are classified as large lymphocytes and the smaller cells as small lymphocytes. The morphologic difference lies mainly in the amount of cytoplasm, but functionally most small lymphocytes are T cells and most large lymphocytes are B cells.

Small lymphocyte

The small (T-) lymphocyte survives for several months or years and has a number of receptors, e.g., for sheep red blood cells (SRBC) and for Fc fragments, which are discussed in Chapter 36.

Size: The small lymphocyte is 6-9 μm in diameter.

Nucleus: The nucleus of the small lymphocyte is round or oval to kidney shaped and occupies nine tenths of the cell diameter. The chromatin is dense and clumped and not sharply delineated from the small amount of bluish parachromatin. A poorly defined nucleolus may be seen depending on the pressure used in the preparation of the smear.

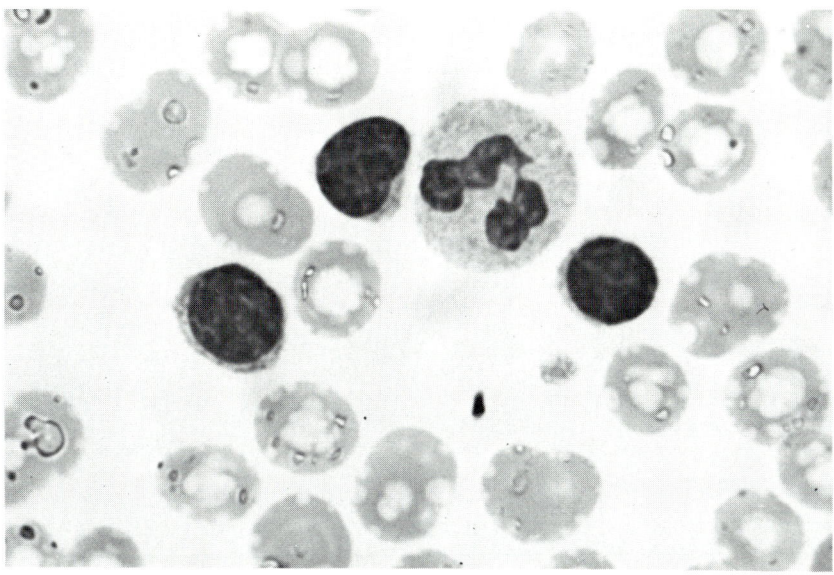

Fig. 6-52. Three small lymphocytes and one segmented neutrophil.

Cytoplasm: The cytoplasm is basophilic and forms a narrow rim around the nucleus or at times a thin blue line only (Fig. 6-52). Leukemic lymphocytes are fragile, so that the cytoplasm elongates and projects with tapering ends beyond either pole of the oval nucleus in response to the pressure used in making the smear. The long nuclear axis overlies the long cell axis, a pattern not seen in any other cell. The cytoplasm contains a few azurophilic granules and occasional vacuoles.

Cytochemistry: The nucleolus and the basophilic cytoplasm contain RNA, which can be demonstrated by the methyl green pyronine stain. The periodic acid–Schiff stain reveals variable amounts of intracytoplasmic glycogen. A number of enzyme reactions are positive, e.g., non-tartrate-resistant acid phosphatase and α-naphthol butyrase in T cell lymphoma and leukemia only, whereas peroxidase and nonspecific esterase are negative.

Scanning electron microscopy: For a discussion of scanning electron microscopy as applied to the samll lymphocyte, see the following discussion of large lymphocytes.

Large lymphocyte

The large (B-) lymphocyte's life span is short lived (days). Its surface immunoglobulins and various receptors are discussed in Chapter 36.

Size: The large lymphocyte is 17-30 μm in diameter.

Nucleus: The dense, oval, or slightly indented nucleus is centrally or eccentrically located. Its chromatin is dense and clumped, fusing imperceptibly without sharp demarcation with the samll amount of pale blue parachromatin. Depending on the pressure with which the smear has been made a nucleolus may be visible.

Cytoplasm: The cytoplasm is abundant, gray to pale blue, unevenly stained, and streaked at times. A few azurophilic granules are contained in 30-60% of the cells. Leukemic cells do not contain these granules. In addition to granules, the cytoplasm contains one or two vacuoles (Gall bodies).[139] The cell margins are indented by surrounding cells so that the cell outline, often accentuated by a darker blue thin streak, is irregular.

Cytochemistry: The B cell is acid phosphatase and α-naphthol butyrase negative.

Scanning electron microscopy: The surface topography of T- and B-lymphocytes as seen in the scanning electron micrograph allows the differentiation of the villous bone marrow–derived lymphocytes from the smooth thymus-derived cells.[140]

Variations in lymphocytes

Atypical lymphocytes: Atypical lymphocytes have been described under a variety of names and occur in a great number of conditions. They are called **immunocytes**[141] because they are involved in humoral immunity and serve as the memory bank of previous immunologic experience. On the basis of morphology they are called blastoid lymphocytes, **plasmacytoid lymphocytes** and lymphocytoid plasma cells, Türk cells, or hyperbasophilic lymphocytes. They are also called Downey cells and transformed, stimulated, or **atypical lymphocytes.**[142] Since their cytoplasm stains heavily red with pyronine, a red basic dye staining RNA, they are called **pyroninophilic cells.** Because of their occurrence in viral diseases, they are referred to as virocytes. A number of agents called mitogens or plant lectins, e.g., pokeweed mitogen or bacterial products, stimulate lymphocytes in vitro to change from small lymphocytes into plasmacytoid and plasma cells, a metamorphosis that carries with it morphologic and biochemical changes. Clinically, atypical lymphocytes are seen primarily in viral diseases, e.g., infectious mononucleosis, viral hepatitis, viral pneumonias, herpes zoster and simplex, and cytomegalic inclusion

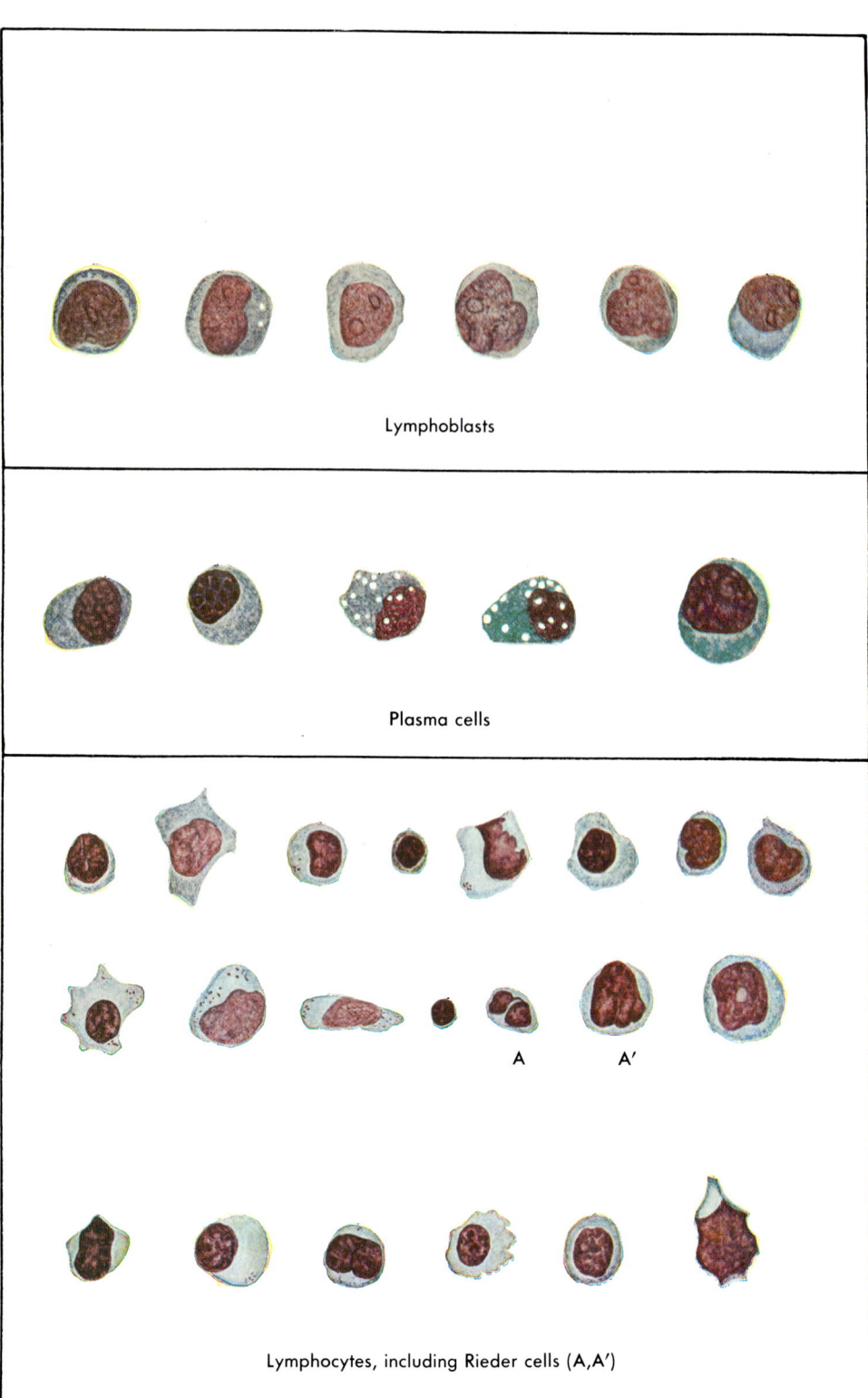

Lymphoblasts

Plasma cells

Lymphocytes, including Rieder cells (A,A')

A.G.Erskine

Plate 6. Leukocytes. (Wright-Giemsa stain; ×950.)

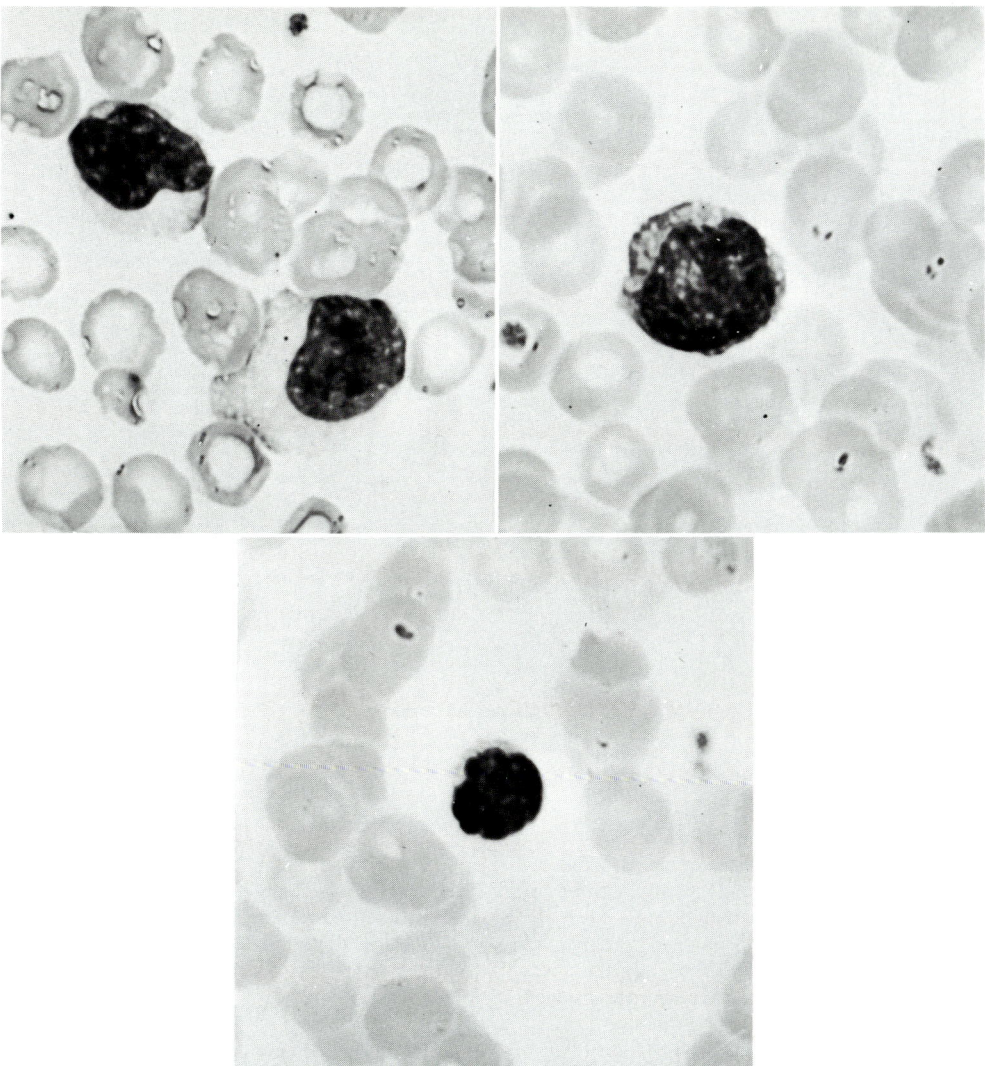

Fig. 6-53. Reactive lymphocytes in infectious mononucleosis cells, blood film.

disease, and in allergic autoimmune reactions (Fig. 6-53). Up to 10% atypical lymphocytes may be found in the differential count of normal individuals, representing morphologic evidence of a normal immune mechanism. Very rare mitotic figures seen in the peripheral blood smear usually belong to reactive lymphocytes.

The percentage of atypical lymphocytes in the peripheral blood smear should be recorded, even though morphologic description of these cells is complicated by the fact that they embrace all transition changes from mature unstimulated lymphocytes to immunoblasts and plasma cells. Reactive lymphocytes represent stimulated B-lymphocytes showing increased DNA and RNA activity. The activated nucleus becomes larger and its chromatin masses smaller and less dense, while the increasing cytoplasmic RNA is responsible for the deepening basophilia of the augmented, at times vacu-

olated, foamy cytoplasm. The formation of clearly discernible nucleoli characterizes the immunoblast, the further transformation of which produces plasma cells or small sensitized committed lymphocytes called memory cells.[143]

Size: The atypical lymphocyte is 16-30 μm in diameter.

Nucleus: The nucleus is usually indented, irregular in outline, and often cleaved and eccentric. The shape varies from cell to cell. The nuclear membrane is thick; the chromatin pattern is coarse and lymphocytic or at times lighter and more delicate, resembling the blast nucleus. One to three nucleoli, often irregular in shape, may be present.

Cytoplasm: The cytoplasm is usually increased in amount and basophilic (increased RNA), at times deep blue and represented only by a rim. It may or may not contain azurophilic granules and vacuoles. There is of-

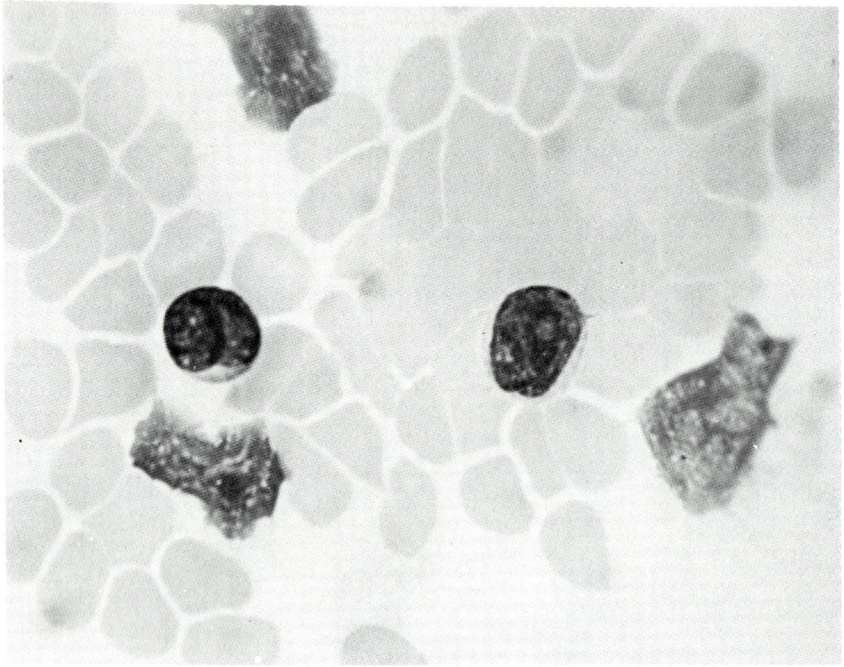

Fig. 6-54. Two Rieder cells and three smudge cells. (×1250.)

ten a perinuclear halo. The hyperplastic Golgi apparatus pushes the nucleus toward the periphery. The cell
margins may be irregular and indented by surrounding
cells.

Cytochemistry: The already mentioned pyroninophilia results from formation of new nuclear and cytoplasmic RNA. The normal small lymphocyte produces
only traces of RNA.

Rieder cell: The Rieder cell (Fig. 6-54) is similar to
a lymphocyte except that it has a notched, indented,
lobulated, cloverleaf-like nucleus. These cells occur in
chronic lymphatic leukemia. Bizarre leukemic myeloblasts with pseudolobulations are also often called
Rieder cells. Bessis and Breton-Gorius[144] consider
Rieder cells to be nonspecific, often artificially produced in the preparation of the smear.

Vacuolated lymphocyte: Vacuolated lymphocytes
have been described in Niemann-Pick disease,[145] amau-
rotic familial idiocy,[146] Tay-Sachs disease,[147] Hurler's
syndrome, and in type II glycogen storage disease.
Vacuoles are also seen in the cytoplasm of atypical
lymphocytes and in lymphocytes reacting to radiation
and chemotherapy.

Crystalline inclusions: IgG, rod-shaped deposits
may be seen as negative images in the dark blue cytoplasm. **Dutcher bodies** are IgM intramuscular inclusions that stain pale with Wright-Giemsa stain and histochemically are diastase-resistant PAS positive. They
are encountered in macroglobulinemia.

Lymphocytic mitoses or binucleated lymphocytes:
In general, mitotic figures or binucleated cells are seldom found in the peripheral blood smear but may

be encountered in viral infections, e.g., infectious
mononucleosis. An increased number of binucleated
cells (over 5%) suggests lymphocytic leukemia or leukosarcoma (hematologic spread of lymphosarcoma).

Smudge cells: Smudge cells frequently occur in
chronic lymphocytic leukemia (Fig. 6-54).

PLASMA CELLS AND PRECURSORS

Plasma cells are not normally found in the peripheral
blood, and even in the normal bone marrow their concentration does not usually exceed 4-5%.

There are two experimentally well-established pathways of plasma cell development and maturation. Some
plasma cells arise from stimulated small lymphocytes
via intermediate cells and plasmablasts,[148] whereas others may arise from an immature plasma cell.[149]

Plasmablast

Size: The plasmablast is 8-20 μm in diameter.

Nucleus: The nucleus is round or oval and eccentric.
The chromatin is bluish purple and arranged in a fine
chromatin network with some clumping. The nucleus
resembles the reticulum cell nucleus. The blue nucleoli
are difficult to see, although several may be present.

Cytoplasm: The nongranular cytoplasm is moderate
in amount and blue and may be mottled.

Proplasmacyte

Size: The proplasmacyte is 15-25 μm in diameter.

Nucleus: The round or oval nucleus is eccentric and
contains a coarse chromatin network. Parachromatin
spaces are irregular, and nucleoli may be visible.

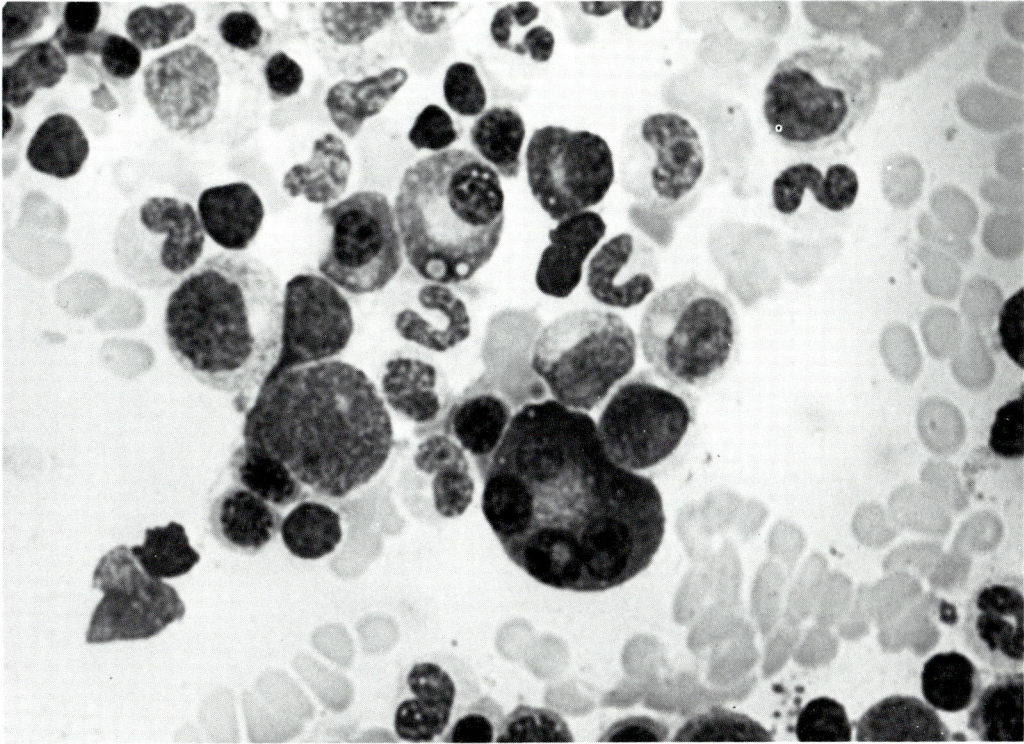

Fig. 6-55. Plasma cells; one has four nuclei. (Bone marrow; Wright-Giemsa stain.)

Cytoplasm: An abundant, deep blue, nongranular cytoplasm shows a clear perinuclear zone.

Plasmacyte

The plasmacyte (plasma cell) is not normally found in the peripheral blood, although about 1-2% of plasma cell–like transformed lymphocytes may be encountered under physiologic conditions.

Size: The plasmacyte is 14-20 μm in diameter.

Nucleus: The nucleus is small, eccentric, and oval. Its long axis is at a right angle to the long axis of the cell. The condensed chromatin forms large angular clumps that may be concentrated in the periphery and center of the nucleus, creating the so-called cartwheel pattern, which is best seen in tissue sections. The parachromatin is pale pink. In the bone marrow a few plasma cells may normally be binucleated or trinucleated (Plate 6, p. 164).

Cytoplasm: The cytoplasm is dark blue, ovoid, and somewhat fibrillar (Fig. 6-55). There is a clear zone (centrosome) between the nucleus at one end and the dark blue marginal cytoplasm at the other end. The cytoplasm is nongranular but may contain secretory globules that represent protein secretion and are called **Russell bodies** (Fig. 6-56). These globules vary in size, are usually colorless but may be pink, red, or blue, and are prominent in hyperglobulinemic states. If the cytoplasm is completely filled with secretory globoid structures, the cell is called a **grape cell** or Mott cell. Russell bodies are contained within endoplasmic sacs[150] filled with

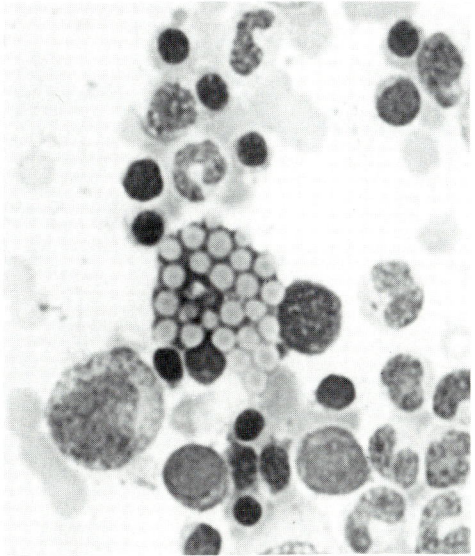

Fig. 6-56. "Grape" cell with Russell bodies.

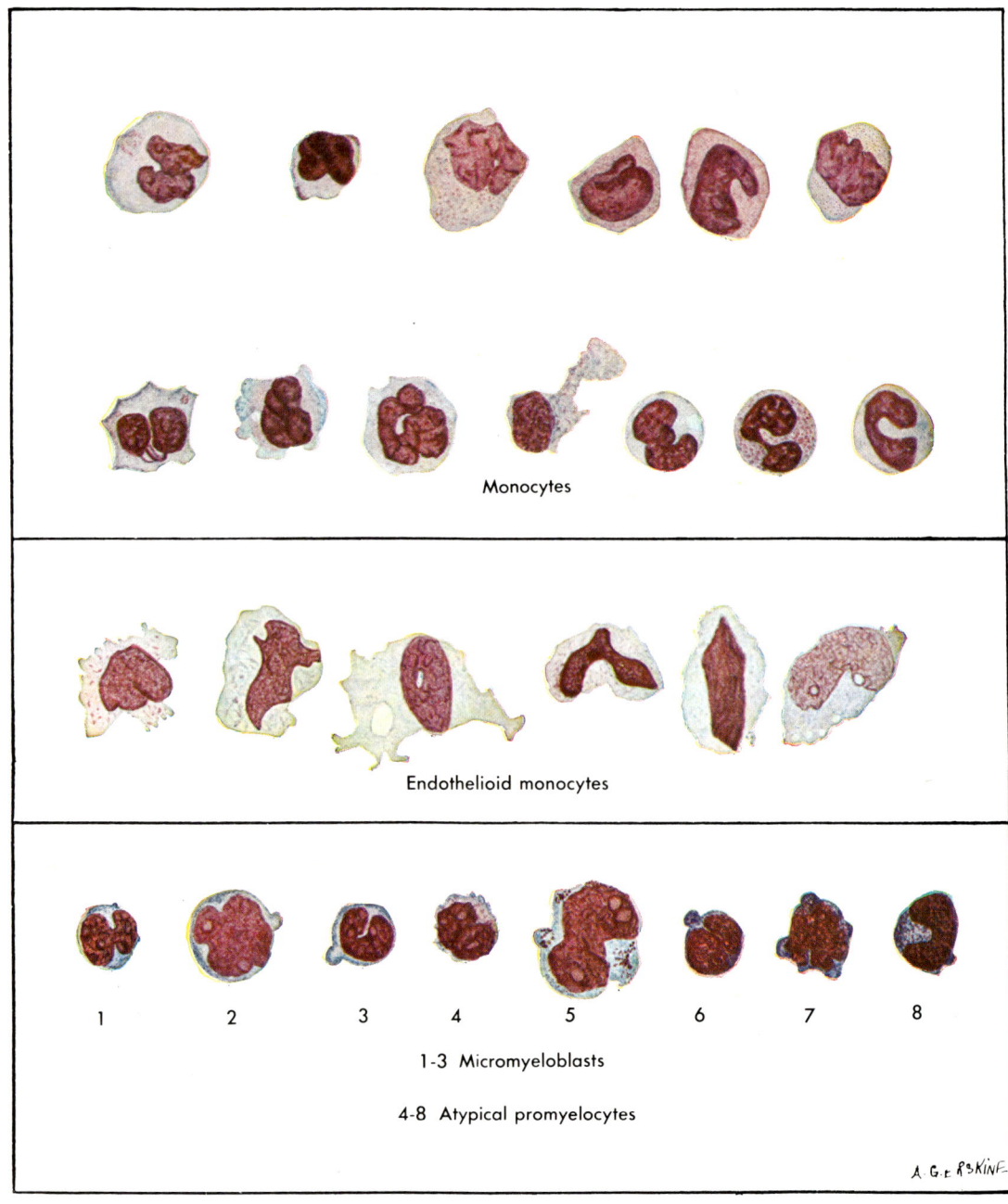

Monocytes

Endothelioid monocytes

| 1 | 2 | 3 | 4 | 5 | 6 | 7 | 8 |

1-3 Micromyeloblasts

4-8 Atypical promyelocytes

A. G. ERSKINE

Plate 7. Monocytes. (Wright-Giemsa stain).

γ-globulins[151] and are PAS positive by virtue of their glycoprotein contents. Protein may also be seen in the form of crystals in the cytoplasm. The intracytoplasmic deposition of amorphous material may give rise to **flame cells** with pink cytoplasm.

Pathologic conditions associated with hypergammaglobulinemia usually show an increase in bone marrow plasma cells, whereas hypogammaglobulinemia states are related to a diminution or absence of these cells.

Function: Plasma cells synthesize and excrete immunoglobulins (antibodies). They are able to assemble all known classes of antibody molecules: IgG, IgA, IgD, IgM, and IgE (see Chapter 36).

MONONUCLEAR PHAGOCYTE AND PRECURSORS

The mononuclear phagocyte system[152] is the modern successor to the reticuloendothelial system of phagocytic cells of several decades ago. It is found throughout the body and includes the circulating blood monocytes, their bone marrow precursors, and fixed tissue macrophages, e.g., pulmonary alveolar macrophages, hepatic Kupffer cells, splenic littoral cells, and the sinusoidal cells of lymph nodes. The fixed tissue macrophages contrast with the ubiquitous free histiocytes that are encountered at sites of inflammation and in serous cavities of the body. The fixed and free macrophages are derived from blood monocytes and from local macrophage proliferation.[153,154] The peripheral blood monocytes trace their origin to bone marrow monoblasts[152] and promonocytes.

Monoblast

Since the monoblast cannot be differentiated from the myeloblast on morphologic or histochemical criteria, one may assume that our criteria for recognizing the monoblast are either inadequate or that the myeloblast can give rise to myeloid and monocytic cells. Cytogenetic,[155] cytochemical,[156] and tissue culture studies of acute myelomonocytic leukemia favor this concept.

Size: The monoblast is 15-20 μm in diameter.

Nucleus: The nucleus is round or oval and at times notched and indented. The chromatin pattern may resemble that of a myeloblast (**Naegeli type**), i.e., delicate blue to purple stippling with small, regular, pale pink or blue parachromatin areas. On the other hand, the chromatin pattern may resemble that of a reticulum cell (**Schilling type**), i.e., irregular network of strands and granules with irregular masses of parachromatin. The nucleoli (three to five in number) are pale blue, large, and round.

Cytoplasm: The cytoplasm is often relatively large in amount, contains a few azurophilic granules, and stains pale blue or gray. The cell border is irregular with pseudopods and indentations. The cytoplasm filling the nuclear indentation is lighter in color than the surrounding cytoplasm. The surrounding cytoplasm may contain Auer bodies.

Promonocyte

The earliest monocytic cell recognizable as belonging to the monocytic series is the promonocyte, which is capable of mitotic division. Its product, the mature

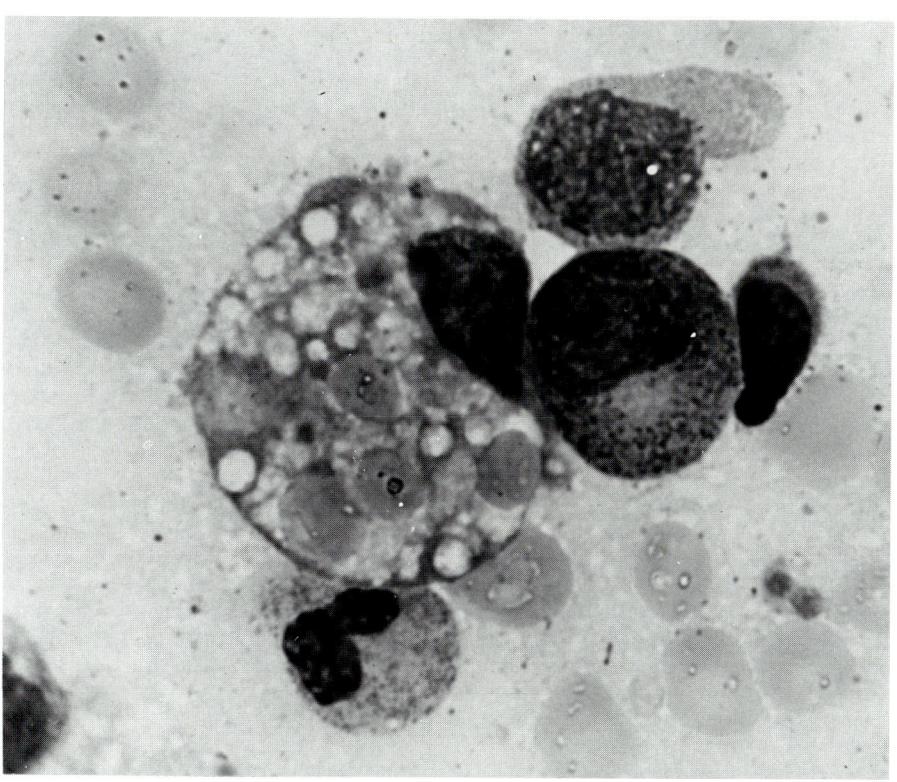

Fig. 6-57. Bone marrow macrophage showing erythrophagocytosis.

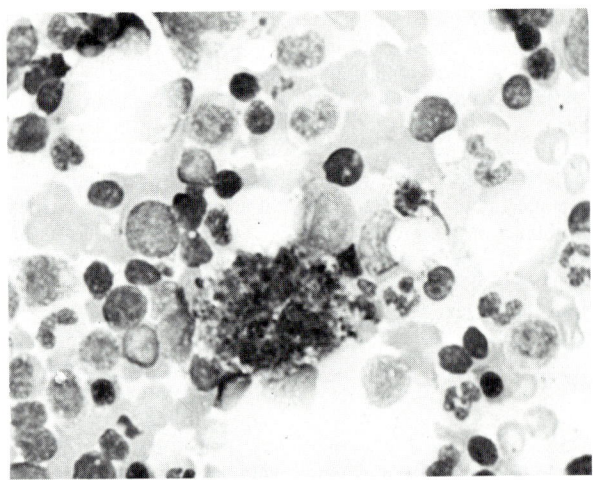

Fig. 6-58. Sea-blue histiocyte. (×600.)

monocyte, is only capable of maturation into a macrophage.[157]

Size: The promonocyte is 15-25 μm in diameter.

Nucleus: The nucleus is large, ovoid to round, convoluted, grooved, and indented. The chromatin forms a loose open network containing a few larger clumps. There may be two or more nucleoli.[158]

Cytoplasm: The sparse gray-blue cytoplasm contains fine azurophilic granules. The nuclear/cytoplasmic ratio is about 7:1.

Monocyte

Size: The monocyte is 14-20 μm to 30-40 μm in diameter.

Nucleus: The nucleus may be eccentric or central, is kidney shaped and often lobulated (with two or more lobes), and at times is folded at the periphery with brainlike convolutions. The chromatin network consists of fine, pale, loose, linear threads producing small areas of thickening at their junctions. No nucleolus is seen. The overall impression is that of a pale nucleus quite variable in shape (Plate 7, p. 168).

Cytoplasm: The cytoplasm is abundant, opaque, gray-blue, and unevenly stained and may be vacuolated. It contains azurophilic dust and often phagocytosed material and vacuoles; it is often described as having a ground-glass appearance.

Cytochemistry: Monocytes, unlike myelocytes and promyelocytes, are positive for nonspecific esterases, but the monocytic esterase is inhibited by sodium fluoride.[159]

Function of monocyte-macrophage group: The cell's phagocytic function is related to its immunologic activity. The phagocytosed material includes bacteria, dying and damaged cells, erythrocytes (Fig. 6-57), debris, hemosiderin, and metals. The monocyte's immunologic function consists of two phases: (1) the induction of immunity, when antigenic information is transferred to lymphocytes[160,161] and (2) expression of cellular immune response and the development of delayed hypersensitivity.[160]

Pathologic macrophages: In a number of congenital and acquired disorders large tissue macrophages are found, which store glycolipids (Gaucher's disease), sphingomyelin (Niemann-Pick disease), and granulocytic debris (sea-blue histiocyte as seen in the syndrome of the sea-blue histiocyte[162,163] [Fig. 6-58] and in chronic granulocytic leukemia).[164]

LEUKOCYTE FUNCTION TESTS

The time-honored methods of evaluating white cell changes include white cell and differential counts. The first method discovers numeric fluctuations, whereas the second sheds light on the type and degree of maturity of the cells involved. In recent years a third dimension has been added to the investigation of leukocytes, i.e., the evaluation of their function in host defense reactions. Two groups of leukocytes are involved in the defense of the body against infection: lymphocytes (T and B cells) and macrophages (neutrophils and monocytes). They are joined by serum proteins called complement. The function of lymphocytes and complement is discussed in detail in Chapter 36.

The main purpose of polymorphonuclear leukocytes is the localization, eradication, and destruction of microorganisms, a goal achieved by a number of synchronized steps, which can be broken down into four components[165] (Fig. 6-59):

1. Chemotaxis,[166] the initial phase of the chemotactic response, is the margination of the circulating neutrophils. They adhere to the endothelial lining of the vessel wall, penetrate it, leave the bloodstream, and proceed toward the focus of infection, guided by chemotactic forces. The chemotaxins are a cocktail of complement components, kinins, bacterial products, damaged tissue,[154] and the contact factors of the intrinsic pathway of coagulation plus platelet components.

2. In opsonization[167] opsonins, components of fresh serum, coat the foreign particles, thus making them more acceptable to phagocytic cells. The chief compo-

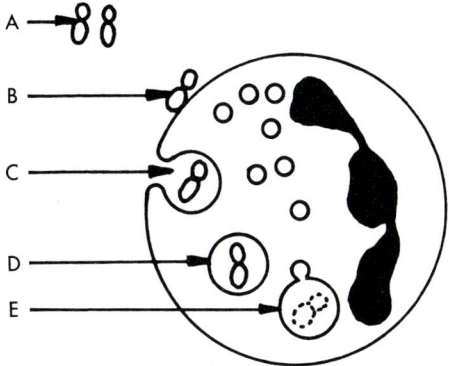

Fig. 6-59. Schema of phagocytosis by polymorphonuclear leukocyte. **A,** Bacteria. **B,** Contact of cell surface with bacterium. **C** and **D,** Formation of phagosome. **E,** Lysosomal enzymes are discharged into phagosome, destroying bacterium. Small circles are lysosomes.

nents of opsonins are complement, mainly C3, and IgG. Opsonization increases the speed with which foreign substances are phagocytosed.

Deficiencies in immunoglobulins (agammaglobulinemia) and/or complement interfere with opsonization, a step that allows the neutrophil to recognize phagocytizable microorganisms or particles. It attaches itself by means of membrane receptors to the opsonized organisms and to portions of the IgG molecule (Fc portion).[166]

3. Ingestion[168] or phagocytosis involves invagination of the cell membrane so that the foreign particulate substance adherent to the surface of the phagocytic cell is encircled by cytoplasmic arms and thus carried into an intracytoplasmic vacuole, the phagosome.

4. Degranulation, killing, digestion, and the destruction of the ingested bacteria or fungi trapped within the phagosome are caused by the lytic action of lysozymes.[169] Primary and secondary granules of the polymorphonuclear cell fuse with the phagosome, discharge their enzymatic content into the vacuole, and thus kill the organisms found within it. This process leads to disappearance of the granules from the cytoplasm and hence to degranulation.

The killing of the engulfed organism is enhanced by the presence of oxygen. All phagocytic cells employ a hydrogen peroxide generating system as a bactericidal mechanism[170] supported by myeloperoxidase activity.

SELECTED LABORATORY TESTS FOR NEUTROPHIL FUNCTION[171-174]

1. White cell count (neutropenia)
2. Nylon fiber adherence (to study adherence or stickiness of neutrophils)
3. Boyden chamber (to study chemotaxis)
4. Oil red O (paraffin oil injection to study degranulation of lysosomal enzymes into phagolysosomes)
5. Nitro blue tetrazolium (NBT) reduction tests (to study oxygen generation by neutrophils)
6. Bactericidal assay (to study bacterial killing by neutrophils)

Details of the technics of all tests mentioned (except no. 2) are discussed in the reference by Bauer.[175]

White cell count (neutropenia)

A minimal number of polymorphonuclear cells in the peripheral blood are essential to allow adequate phagocytic function. A fall of the absolute neutrophil count to neutropenic levels below 1500/mm^3 carries with it the danger of increased susceptibility to infection, especially with gram-negative organisms.[176]

Nylon fiber adherence[177]

Principle: A white cell and differential count is performed on heparinized blood. Aliquots, 1 ml, of the blood specimen are added to the top of three Pasteur pipets packed with nylon fiber columns. The blood is allowed to filter through the columns for 5-10 min. The granulocytes in the effluent are counted, and the percentage of granulocyte adherence is calculated as follows:

$$100\% - \dfrac{\dfrac{\text{PMNs/ml in effluent sample}}{\text{PMNs/ml in original sample}}}{} \times 100 =$$

$$\text{PMN adherence (\%)}$$

The results of the three columns are averaged.

Normal values:
Men: 76% ± 12%
Women: 91.1% ± 7%

Interpretation: The blood of patients receiving alcohol, salicylates, and glucocorticoids inhibits granulocyte adherence. Neutrophils of some patients with diabetes mellitus, acute leukemia, and Chédiak-Higashi disease also fail to adhere to nylon fibers.[178]

Polymorphonuclear leukocyte chemotaxis, Boyden technic

Principle: Leukocytes move toward (or away from) certain chemical substances. The technic described quantitates the chemotactic effect of various sera and additives utilizing a plastic chamber separated into two compartments by a filter membrane, the pore size of which is such that leukocytes cannot pass through it except by active migration. The leukocytes are concentrated on one side of the membrane, while the diluted serum is placed on the other side. After incubation the membrane is fixed, stained, and cleared, and the number of cells that have migrated to the other side are counted microscopically.

Normal range: The normal range is 20-275 cells/hpf.

Normal value: The average normal value is 133 cells per high-power field.

Interpretation: Defective chemotaxis has been described in a variety of conditions (e.g., diabetes, rheumatoid arthritis, lupus erythematosus)[179] and in newborns.[180] In all these conditions it appears to be related to deficiencies of C3 and C5 components of the serum complement system.[181,182]

Limitations: The original technic and its modifications are difficult to standardize since they are subject to observer errors and depend on a number of variables, e.g., filter variability[183] and standardization of cell numbers.[184]

Serum-dependent phagocytosis of paraffin oil emulsified with bacterial lipopolysaccharide (method of Stossel[185,186])

Principle: Phagocytic cells are isolated from peripheral blood and brought in contact with *E. coli* lipopolysaccharide-coated paraffin oil droplets containing oil red O. The droplets are first opsonized with fresh human serum (see p. 170) and are then phagocytosed by normal phagocytic cells. The rate of ingestion of opsonized particles by the cells is constant for 5 min, the period during which cells and oil droplets are incubated. The uningested oil droplets are then separated by centrifugation from the cells containing ingested particles. The cells are heavier and thus sediment, while the lighter oil particles float. The sedimented cells are then washed, and oil red O is extracted with dioxane and measured spectrophotometrically.

Normal value: The normal value for paraffin oil is 0.138 (0.121-0.175) mg/10^7 phagocytes/min.

Comment: The method allows (1) comparison of different sera against a set of control cells and the same serum against different cells and (2) a screening procedure. The above method can also be combined with the quantitative NBT reduction technic.[187,188]

Interpretation: Defects of phagocytosis are found in congenital disorders (e.g., chronic granulomatous disease, myeloperoxidase deficiency, Chédiak-Higashi disease, G-6-PD–deficient polymorphonuclear cells) and in acquired defects (e.g., related to the administration of certain drugs).

Tests of ingestion and opsonization: nitro blue tetrazolium reduction tests

The soluble yellow oxidized nitro blue tetrazolium (NBT) salt is reduced to a dark blue insoluble formazan when normal phagocytic cells (granulocytes and monocytes) are incubated with NBT.[189,190] In healthy individuals less than 10% of phagocytic cells are NBT positive (spontaneous NBT reduction test). A much higher percentage of positive cells results if the cells are stimulated in vitro or in vivo by bacteria and are then incubated with NBT (stimulated NBT reduction test), since granulocytes exposed to bacteria have a markedly stimulated metabolic activity.[191]

Spontaneous nitro blue tetrazolium reduction test

Principle: The percentage of NBT-positive neutrophils increases markedly in bacterial infections but remains normal or near normal in nonbacterial diseases. The spontaneous NBT test may thus aid in the differentiation of bacterial from nonbacterial conditions.[192-194] The mechanism of the formazan production is poorly understood but is related to the fact that if active phagocytes are brought in contact with the soluble, oxidized, yellow NBT dye, the latter enters the phagocytic vacuoles with the ingested bacteria and is reduced by the hydrogen peroxide formed within the cell as a result of its phagocytic activity to an insoluble blue-black pigment. The proportion of neutrophils containing formazan inclusions is calculated.

Reagents and equipment: All reagents are marketed by Sigma Chemical Co. (St. Louis) in kit form (Sigma technical bulletin no. 840) and allow a degree of standardization that cannot be achieved by use of any of numerous modifications of the test.

1. NBT vial (Sigma no. 840-10) containing nitro blue tetrazolium, sodium chloride, and phosphate buffer
2. Siliconized glass vials (Sigma no. 840-50)
3. Heparin vial (Sigma no. 840-20), siliconized, containing 20 USP units heparin
4. Wright stain (Sigma no. 840-100)
5. Stimulant solution (Sigma no. 840-15), a soluble bacterial extract used only in the stimulated NBT test

Procedure:

1. Use a plastic syringe to obtain 1 ml fresh venous blood; remove needle and place blood in siliconized collection vial containing 20 units heparin. Mix gently.
2. Add 1 ml water to NBT vial; agitate intermittently to dissolve.
3. Transfer 0.1 ml clear yellow solution from step 2 to siliconized vial.
4. Add 0.1 ml heparinized blood; mix gently and cover vial.
5. Incubate for 15 min at 37° C and for additional 15 min at room temperature.
6. Mix and transfer 1 small drop with capillary pipet from incubated vial onto clean microscope slide and gently (without pressure) prepare blood smear. Avoid too thin a smear to prevent damage to fragile positive cells.[187,188]
7. Air dry smear, stain with Wright-Giemsa stain, and apply coverslip.
8. Examine stained smear under oil immersion lens and determine number (percent) of positive neutrophils in 100 consecutive polymorphonuclear leukocytes. Count only intact neutrophils (not band or juvenile cells) that contain large irregularly shaped black masses (positive cells) (Fig. 6-60).

Controls: Blood from healthy adults should be used for controls.

Normal values: The mean normal value is 5-10% positive cells, although the figure may reach 17%.[187]

Interpretation: Normal values are found in viral diseases,[187,188] postpartum and postoperative patients,[195] febrile conditions not of bacterial origin,[195] and localized infections.[195] Low values are seen in response to effective antibiotic therapy,[196] in the course of immu-

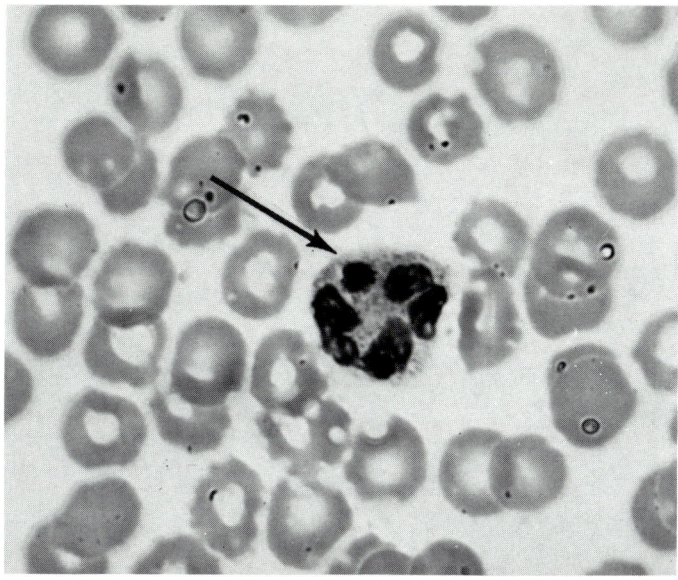

Fig. 6-60. NBT-positive polymorphonuclear leukocyte. NBT inclusion (arrow).

nosuppressive therapy, during administration of corti-sone[196] and oral contraceptives,[197] and in diseases associated with phagocytic dysfunction, e.g., chronic granulomatous disease (CGD),[198] myeloperoxidase[199] and G-6-PD deficiencies,[200] lupus erythematosus,[201] nephrosis,[195] and sickle cell disease.[195]

Elevated values are reported in bacterial disease,[187,188] including miliary tuberculosis,[195] and in some parasitic,[202] fungal,[193] and protozoal infections.[203]

There is some doubt as to the clinical value of the spontaneous NBT reduction test in the differential diagnosis of bacterial vs. nonbacterial[190,204,205] and noninfectious diseases, although Feigin and Pickering consider the test to be an aid in the differential diagnosis of febrile disorders.[206] Numerous false positive and false negative results require the consideration of additional laboratory and clinical parameters to aid in the above differential diagnosis. It appears that the test is best suited to study the clinical course of a patient with initially positive values.[194]

Stimulated nitro blue tetrazolium reduction test

Principle: Phagocytosis is stimulated in vitro by the addition of stimulant (Sigma no. 840-15), a soluble bacterial extract, to step 3 of the preceding procedure.

Procedure:

1 and 2. Follow steps 1 and 2 for spontaneous NBT reduction test.

3. To siliconized vial (Sigma no. 840-50) add 0.05 ml stimulant solution and 0.05 ml heparinized blood (step 1).

4. Cover vial, mix gently, and incubate for 30 min at 37° C.

5. Add 0.1 ml NBT solution (step 2).

6 and 7. Follow steps 6 and 7 for spontaneous NBT reduction test.

Normal values: The stimulant should cause formazan deposits in 10-50% of neutrophils of healthy individuals.

Interpretation: Failure to exhibit a positive response to in vitro stimulation is seen in diseases associated with phagocytic dysfunction, including defects in chemotaxis, opsonization, and intracellular killing of bacteria. (See interpretation of skin window technic and of spontaneous NBT test.) In patients with chronic granulomatous disease (CGD) fewer than 10% of polymorphonuclear leukocytes reduce the dye. CGD is an X-chromosome–linked defect in leukocyte function[198,207] in which the neutrophilic leukocytes ingest bacteria normally but the intracellular killing of the organisms is delayed because of dihydronicotinamide adenine dinucleotide (NADH) oxidase deficiency.[198,207]

Quantitative nitro blue tetrazolium test

Quantitation of the NBT test has been proposed to detect not only patients with CGD but also the female carriers. Two technics are available,[198,208] one of which is described in detail in Bauer.[175]

Tests of fungicidal and bactericidal mechanisms
Candidacidal (fungicidal) activity assay

Principle: Leukocytes are concentrated by dextran sedimentation and are incubated with yeast and fresh serum (opsonins) to maximally stimulate phagocytosis. Fungicidal activity is determined by a differential count technic employing methylene blue to distinguish between viable and nonviable organisms.[209,210] Viable yeast cells remain unstained while nonviable organisms take a deep blue stain.

Normal values: Normal neutrophils kill 29.0% ± 7.4% of ingested *Candida albicans* in 1 hr.

Interpretation: Leukocytes of patients with heredi-

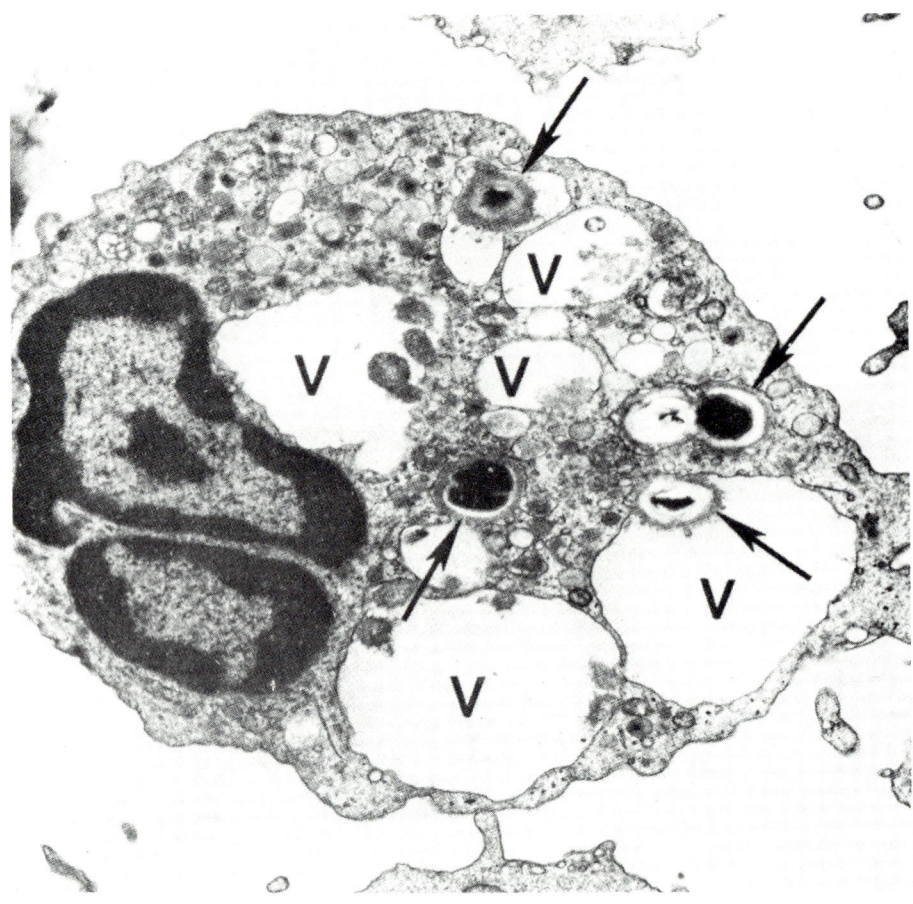

Fig. 6-61. Polymorphonuclear leukocyte from normal control patient incubated with staphylococci for 30 min. Electron micrograph. Many bacteria (arrows) in various stages of destruction are evident within cell. Note cytoplasmic vacuoles *(V)* around and adjacent to degenerating bacteria. (From Quie, P.G., et al.: J. Clin. Invest. **46:**668, 1967.)

tary myeloperoxidase deficiency or with chronic granulomatous disease (CGD) phagocytose *C. albicans* normally but fail to kill the yeast.[201]

Bactericidal activity assay

*Principle***:** See principle of candidacidal assay above. The bactericidal activity is evaluated by incubating leukocytes with bacteria *(Staphylococcus aureus),* and phagocytosis is estimated by the disappearance of viable bacteria as determined by culture.[209,211,212]

*Normal values***:** After 45 min of incubation of test mixture there is a reduction of viable organisms of $91.8\% \pm 2.2\%$[186] (Fig. 6-61).

*Interpretation***:** Myeloperoxidase-deficient leukocytes produce a reduction of viable organisms of only $36.0\% \pm 9.1\%$.[186]

REFERENCES

1. Clayton, D.A., and Vinograd, J.: Nature **216:**652, 1967.
2. Whang, J., et al.: Blood **22:**664, 1963.
3. Lajtha, L.G.: Br. J. Haematol. **29:**529, 1975.
4. Till, J.E., and McCulloch, E.A.: Radiat. Res. **14:**213, 1961.
5. Bradley, T.R., and Metcalf, D.: Aust. J. Exp. Biol. Med. Sci. **44:**287, 1966.
6. Brown, R.: Br. Med. J. **2:**1036, 1965.
7. Mitus, W.J., Toyama, K., and Brauner, M.J.: Ann. N.Y. Acad. Sci. **149:**107, 1968.
8. Fried, W.: Blood **40:**671, 1972.
9. Nathan, D.G., et al.: J. Clin. Invest. **43:**2158, 1964.
10. Movassaghi, N., Shore, N.A., and Hammond, D.: Proc. Soc. Exp. Biol. Med. **126:**615, 1967.
11. Thorling, E.B., and Erslev, A.J.: Blood **31:**332, 1968.
12. Fogh, J.: Radiat. Res. **45:**563, 1971.
13. Kazal, I.A., and Erslev, A.J.: Ann. Clin. Lab. Sci. **5:**91, 1975.
14. Fisher, J.W., Thompson, J.F., and Espada, J.: Isr. J. Med. Sci. **7:**873, 1971.
15. Lertora, J.L., et al.: J. Lab. Clin. Med. **86:**140, 1975.
16. Saidi, P., Wallerstein, R.O., and Aggeler, P.M.: J. Lab. Clin. Med. **57:**247, 1961.
17. McCurdy, P.R., Pierce, L.E., and Rath, C.E.: N. Engl. J. Med. **266:**505, 1962.
18. Kondi, A., and Foy, H.: Lancet **2:**1157, 1964.
19. Kundel, D.W., and Nies, B.A.: Am. J. Clin. Pathol. **44:**146, 1965.
20. Powars, D.: N. Engl. J. Med. **273:**700, 1965.

21. Sherman, J.D., Greenfield, J.B., and Ingall, D.: N. Engl. J. Med. **270:**810, 1964.
22. Lehane, D.E.: Arch. Intern. Med. **134:**763, 1974.
23. Evans, E., and Fung, Y.C.: Microvasc. Res. **4:**335, 1972.
24. Bull, B.S., and Brailsford, J.D.: Blood **41:**833, 1973.
25. Cooper, R.A., et al.: J. Clin. Invest. **51:**3182, 1972.
26. Florman, A.L., and Wintrobe, M.M.: Johns Hopkins Med. J. **63:**209, 1938.
27. Salt, H.B., et al.: Lancet **2:**325, 1960.
28. Douglass, C.C., McCall, M.S., and Frenkel, E.P.: Ann. Intern. Med. **68:**390, 1968.
29. Gingold, N., Gherman, I., and Comanescu, N.: Folia Haematol. (Leipz.) **86:**436, 1966.
30. Tchernia, G., et al.: Arch. Fr. Pediatr. **25:**729, 1968, cit. no. 3247220.
31. Weed, R.I.: Clin. Haematol. **4:**3, 1975.
32. Barreras, L., Diggs, L.W., and Bell, A.: J.A.M.A. **203:**569, 1968.
33. N. Engl. J. Med. **271:**898, 1964.
34. Bessis, M., and Boisfleury, A.: Nouv. Rev. Fr. Hematol. Blood Cells **10:**223, 1970.
35. Schwartz, S.O., and Moto, S.A.: Am. J. Med. Sci. **218:**563, 1949.
36. Bell, R.E.: Br. J. Haematol. **9:**552, 1963.
37. Bessis, M., and Lessin, L.S.: Blood **36:**399, 1970.
38. Brechner, G., and Bessis, M.: Blood **40:**333, 1972.
39. White, J.G.: Am. J. Pathol. **77:**507, 1974.
40. Pryor, D.S., and Pitney, W.R.: Br. J. Haematol. **13:**126, 1967.
41. Scholnik, A.P., Van Tilburg, C.P., and Hoffman, G.C.: Cleve. Clin. Q. **41:**23, 1974.
42. Brain, M.C., Dacie, J.V., and Hourihane, D.O.: Br. J. Haematol. **8:**358, 1962.
43. Propp, R.P., and Scharfman, W.B.: Blood **28:**623, 1966.
44. Tuffy, P., Brown, A.K., and Zuelzer, W.W.: Am. J. Dis. Child. **98:**227, 1959.
45. Guevarra, A.K., Morita, Y., and Reyman, T.A.: Transplantation **14:**683, 1972.
46. White, J.G.: Arch. Intern. Med. **133:**545, 1974.
47. Lock, S.P., Smith, S., and Hardisty, R.: Br. J. Haematol. **7:**303, 1961.
48. Miller, G., Townes, P.L., and MacWhinney, J.B.: Pediatrics **35:**906, 1965.
49. Weed, R.I., and Bessis, M.: Blood **41:**471, 1973.
50. Oski, F.A., et al.: N. Engl. J. Med. **280:**909, 1969.
51. Douglass, C.C., and Twomey, J.J.: Ann. Intern. Med. **72:**159, 1970.
52. Barnes, A.: J.A.M.A. **198:**151, 1966.
53. Lange, R.D., and Akeroyd, J.H.: Blood **13:**950, 1958.
54. Scott, J.L., et al.: Blood **16:**1239, 1960.
55. Sansone, G., and Pik, C.: Br. J. Haematol. **11:**511, 1965.
56. Beutler, E., Dern, R.J., and Alving, A.S.: J. Lab. Clin. Med. **45:**40, 1955.
57. Larrimer, J.H., Mendelson, D.S., and Metz, E.N.: Arch. Intern. Med. **135:**857, 1975.
58. Wickramasinghe, S.N.: Br. J. Haematol. **22:**111, 1972.
59. Galton, D.A.G.: Semin. Hematol. **6:**323, 1969.
60. Elion, G.B., and Hitchings, G.M.: Adv. Chemother. **2:**91, 1965.
61. Bessis, M.: Living blood cells and their ultrastructure, New York, 1973, Springer-Verlag New York, Inc.
62. Breton-Gorius, J., and Houssay, D.: Lab. Invest. **28:**135, 1973.
63. Hayhoe, F.G.J., and Cowley, J.C.: Clin. Haematol. **1:**49, 1972.
64. Gralnick, H.R., and Tan, H.K.: Hum. Pathol. **5:**661, 1974.

65. Gouault-Heilmann, M., et al.: Br. J. Haematol. **30:**151, 1975.
66. Prasad, A.S., et al.: Clin. Chem. **21:**582, 1975.
67. Overzier, C.: Triangle **8:**32, 1967.
68. Mittwoch, U.: Cytogenetic. Cell Genet. **2:**24, 1963.
69. Lawler, S.D., Kay, H.E.M., and Birbeck, M.S.C.: J. Clin. Pathol. **19:**214, 1966.
70. Ferguson-Smith, M.A.: Hosp. Pract. **5:**88, 1970.
71. Hollander, D.H., and Borgaonkar, D.S.: Acta Cytol. (Baltimore) **15:**452, 1971.
72. Borgaonkar, D.S., and Hollander, D.H.: Nature **230:**52, 1971.
73. Engel, E., et al.: South. Med. J. **64:**161, 1971.
74. Engel, E., et al.: Lancet **1:**789, 1970.
75. Brunning, R.D.: Hum. Pathol. **1:**99, 1970.
76. Alder, A.: Dtsch. Arch. Klin. Med. **183:**372, 1938.
77. Reilly, W.A.: Am. J. Dis. Child. **62:**489, 1941.
78. Chediak, M.: Rev. Haematol. **7:**362, 1952.
79. White, J.G.: Blood **28:**143, 1966.
80. Mauri, C., and Silingardi, V.: Acta Haematol. (Basel) **32:**114, 1964.
81. Efrati, P., and Danon, D.: Br. J. Haematol. **15:**173, 1968.
82. Bessis, M., Bernerd, J., and Seligmann, M.: Nouv. Rev. Fr. Hematol. Blood Cells **1:**422, 1961.
83. Van Slyck, E.J., and Rebuck, J.W.: Am. J. Clin. Pathol. **62:**673, 1974.
84. Ward, P.A.: Am. J. Pathol. **77:**520, 1974.
85. Clark, R.A., and Kimball, H.R.: J. Clin. Invest. **50:**2645, 1971.
86. Provisor, D., et al.: Clin. Res. **25:**382A, 1977.
87. Stossel, T.P., Root, R.K., and Vaughan, M.: N. Engl. J. Med. **282:**120, 1972.
88. Haak, R.A., et al.: J. Cell. Biol. **75:**582, 1977.
89. Hoffstein, S., Goldstein, I.M., and Weissmann, G.: J. Cell. Biol. **73:**242, 1977.
90. Boxer, G.J., et al.: Br. J. Haematol. **35:**521, 1977.
91. Döhle, V.: Central blatt fur Bakt. **61:**63, 1911.
92. Itoga, T., and Laszlo, J.: Blood **20:**668, 1962.
93. Weiner, W., and Topley, E.: J. Clin. Pathol. **8:**324, 1955.
94. Jenis, E.H., et al.: Am. J. Clin. Pathol. **55:**187, 1971.
95. Powars, D., Rohde, R., and Graves, D.: Lancet **1:**1363, 1964.
96. Dorfman, A., and Matalon, R.: Am. J. Med. **47:**691, 1969.
97. Griffiths, S.B., and Findlay, M.: Arch. Dis. Child. **33:**229, 1958.
98. Lagunoff, D., Ross, R., and Benditt, E.P.: Am. J. Pathol. **41:**273, 1962.
99. Jordans, G.H.W.: Acta Med. Scand. **145:**419, 1953.
100. Rozenszajn, L., Klajman, A., and Efrati, P.: Blood **28:**258, 1966.
101. Hegglin, R.: Arch. Julius Klaus Stift. Vererbungsforschg. **20:**1, 1945.
102. Jordan, S.W., and Larsen, W.E.: Blood **25:**921, 1965.
103. Mittwoch, U.: Br. J. Haematol. **5:**365, 1959.
104. Zucker-Franklin, D.: Arthritis Rheum. **9:**24, 1966.
105. Undritz, E.: Schweiz. Med. Wochenschr. **88:**996, 1958.
106. Davidson, W.M., Milner, R.D.G., and Lawler, S.D.: Br. J. Haematol. **6:**339, 1960.
107. Johnston, B., and Brady, J.M.: Acta Cytol. (Baltimore) **14:**399, 1970.
108. Nieburgs, H.E., et al.: Acta Cytol. (Baltimore) **11:**415, 1967.
109. Undritz, E.: Rev. Hematol. **5:**644, 1950.
110. Huet, G.J.: Maandschr. Kindergeneeskd. **1:**4, 1932.
111. Dorr, A.D., and Moloney, W.C.: N. Engl. J. Med. **261:**742, 1959.
112. Schneiderman, L.J., et al.: Am. J. Med. **46:**380, 1969.

113. Gustke, S.S., et al.: Blood **35**:637, 1970.
114. Donohugh, D.L.: Calif. Med. **104**:421, 1966.
115. Clark, R.A., and Kaplan, A.P.: Clin. Haematol. **4**:635, 1975.
116. Bujak, J.S., and Root, R.K.: Blood **43**:727, 1974.
117. Parmley, R.T., and Spicer, S.S.: Lab. Invest. **30**:557, 1974.
118. Makita, T., and Sandborn, E.B.: Histochemistry **24**:8, 1970.
119. Sullivan, T.J.: The role of eosinophils in inflammatory reactions. In Brown, E.B., editor: Progress in hematology, New York, 1979, Grune & Stratton, Inc., vol. 11.
120. Goetzl, E.J., Wasserman, S.I., and Austen, K.F.: Arch. Pathol. **99**:1, 1975.
121. Laster, C.E., and Gleich, G.J.: J. Allergy Clin. Immunol. **48**:297, 1971.
122. Cohen, S., and Ward, P.A.: J. Exp. Med. **133**:133, 1971.
123. Wasserman, S.I., Goetzl, E.J., and Austen, K.F.: J. Immunol. **112**:351, 1974.
124. Greene, B.M., and Colley, D.G.: J. Immunol. **113**:910, 1974.
125. Padawer, J.: Ann. N.Y. Acad. Sci. **103**:87, 1963.
126. Dvorak, H.F., and Dvorak, A.M.: Clin. Haematol. **4**:651, 1975.
127. Ackerman, G.A.: Ann. N.Y. Acad. Sci. **103**:376, 1963.
128. Ackerman, G.A., and Clark, M.A.: Acta Haematol. (Basel) **45**:280, 1971.
129. Nichols, B.A., and Bainton, D.F.: Lab. Invest. **29**:27, 1973.
130. Lindell, S.E., Rorsman, H., and Westling, H.: Acta Allergol. (Kbh.) **16**:216, 1961.
131. Benveniste, J.: Nature **249**:581, 1974.
132. Balogh, K., Jr., and Cohen, R.B.: Blood **17**:491, 1961.
133. Ishizaka, T., Soto, C.S., and Ishizaka, K.: J. Immunol. **111**:500, 1973.
134. Wolf-Jürgensen, P.: Ser. Haematol. **1**:45, 1968.
135. Code, C.F., Hurn, M.M., and Mitchell, R.G.: Mayo Clin. Proc. **39**:715, 1964.
136. Dvorak, H.F., and Dvorak, A.M.: Hum. Pathol. **3**:454, 1972.
137. Kay, N.E., Ackerman, S.K., and Douglas, S.D.: Semin. Hematol. **16**:252, 1979.
138. Gupta, S., and Good, R.A.: Henry Ford Hosp. Med. J. **27**:224, 1979.
139. Hemplemann, L.H., and Knowlton, N.P., Jr.: Blood **8**:524, 1953.
140. Lin, P.S., Cooper, A.G., and Wortis, H.H.: N. Engl. J. Med. **289**:548, 1973.
141. Dameslich, W.: Blood **21**:243, 1963.
142. Yoffey, J.M., et al.: Br. J. Haematol. **11**:488, 1965.
143. Dutton, R.W.: Adv. Immunol. **6**:253, 1967.
144. Bessis, M., and Breton-Gorius, J.: C.R. Acad. Sci. **261**:1392, 1965.
145. Rossier, A., Caldera, R., and Sarraut, S.: Nouv. Presse Med. **66**:535, 1958.
146. Bagh, K., and Hortling, H.: Nord. Med. **38**:1072, 1948.
147. Sjövall-Lund, E.: Verh. Dtsch. Ges. Pathol. **27**:185, 1934.
148. Murphy, M.J., et al.: Am. J. Pathol. **66**:25, 1972.
149. Nossal, G.J.V., and Mäkela, O.: J. Exp. Med. **115**:209, 1962.
150. Movat, H.Z., and Frenando, N.V.P.: Exp. Mol. Pathol. **1**:535, 1962.
151. Bangle, R., Jr.: Am. J. Pathol. **43**:437, 1963.
152. van Furth, R., et al.: Bull. W.H.O. **46**:845, 1972.
153. Lessin, L.S., Bessis, M., and Douglas, S.D.: Morphology of monocytes and macrophages. In Williams, W.J., et al., editors: Hematology, ed. 2, New York, 1977, McGraw-Hill Book Co.
154. Cline, M.J., and Golde, D.W.: Granulocytes and monocytes, function and functional disorders. In Hoffbrand, A.V., Brain, M.C., and Hush, J., editors: Recent advances in hematology, New York, 1977, Churchill Livingstone, no. 2.
155. Brandt, L., et al.: Scand. J. Haematol. **12**:117, 1974.
156. Leder, L.D.: Blut **16**:86, 1967.
157. van Furth, R.: Semin. Hematol. **7**:125, 1970.
158. Fedorko, M.E., and Hirsch, J.G.: Semin. Hematol. **7**:109, 1970.
159. Shnitka, T.K., and Seligman, A.M.: J. Histochem. Cytochem. **9**:504, 1961.
160. Mackaness, G.B.: Semin. Hematol. **7**:172, 1970.
161. Unanue, E.R., and Cerottini, J.C.: Semin. Hematol. **7**:225, 1970.
162. Sawitsky, A., Rosner, F., and Chodsky, S.: Semin. Hematol. **9**:285, 1972.
163. Silverstein, M.N., and Ellefson, R.D.: Semin. Hematol. **9**:299, 1972.
164. Dosik, H., Rosner, F., and Sawitsky, A.: Semin. Hematol. **9**:309, 1972.
165. Graham, R.C., Jr.: Cleve. Clin. Q. **42**:33, 1975.
166. Stossel, T.P.: N. Engl. J. Med. **290**:717, 1974.
167. Winkelstein, J.A.: J. Pediatr. **82**:747, 1973.
168. Stossel, T.P.: N. Engl. J. Med. **290**:774, 1974.
169. Hansen, N.E.: Ser. Haematol. **7**:1, 1974.
170. Territo, M.C., and Cline, M.J.: Clin. Haematol. **4**:685, 1975.
171. Bachner, R.L., and Boxer, L.A.: Semin. Hematol. **16**:158, 1979.
172. Harvath, L., and Anderson, B.R.: N. Engl. J. Med. **300**:1130, 1979.
173. Gallin, J.I., and Wolf, S.M.: Clin. Haematol. **4**:567, 1975.
174. Klebanoff, S.J., and Clark, R.A.: The neutrophil: function and clinical disorders, Amsterdam, 1978, North-Holland Publishing Co.
175. Bauer, J.D.: Leukocyte function tests. In Sonnenwirth, A.C., and Jarett, L., editors: Gradwohl's clinical laboratory methods and diagnosis, ed. 8, St. Louis, 1980, The C.V. Mosby Co.
176. Br. Med. J. **281**:1091, 1980.
177. MacGregor, R.R., Spagmualo, P.J., and Lenlnek, A.L.: N. Engl. J. Med. **291**:642, 1974.
178. Bachner, R.L.: Neutrophil dysfunction syndromes. In Granulocytes, normal and dysplastic, morphology and function, clinical and laboratory review, Milwaukee, 1979, School of Allied Health Professions, Continuing Education, University of Wisconsin.
179. Baum, J., Mowet, A., and Kirk, J.: Clin. Res. **18**:422, 1970.
180. Miller, M.E.: Pediatr. Res. **3**:497, 1969.
181. Ward, P.A., et al.: J. Immunol. **110**:1003, 1973.
182. Alper, C.A., et al.: J. Clin. Invest. **49**:1975, 1970.
183. Gallin, J.I., Clark, R.A., and Kimball, H.R.: J. Immunol. **110**:233, 1973.
184. Miller, M.E.: Assays of phagocytic function. In Vyas, G.N., Stites, D.P., and Brecher, G., editors: Laboratory diagnosis of immunologic disorders, New York, 1975, Grune & Stratton, Inc.
185. Stossel, T.P.: Blood **42**:121, 1973.
186. Stossel, T.P.: J. Exp. Med. **137**:690, 1973.
187. Feigin, R.D., et al.: J. Pediatr. **78**:230, 1971.
188. Feigin, R.D., Shakelford, P.G., and Choi, S.C.: J. Pediatr. **79**:943, 1971.
189. Farnes, P.: NBT. In Stiene, E.A., editor: Hematology laboratory medicine: current aspects, New York, 1974, IMBC.
190. Nathan, D.G.: N. Engl. J. Med. **290**:280, 1974.
191. Quie, P.G., and Hill, H.R.: DM **1**:32, Aug. 1973.

192. Park, B.H., and Good, R.A.: Lancet **2:**616, 1970.
193. Park, B.H., Fibrig, S.M., and Smithwick, E.M.: Lancet **2:**532, 1968.
194. Lace, J.K., Tann, J.S., and Watanakunakorn, C.: Am. J. Med. **58:**685, 1975.
195. Park, B.H.: J. Pediatr. **78:**376, 1971.
196. Miller, D.R., and Kaplan, H.G.: Pediatrics **45:**861, 1970.
197. Norden, C.W., and Reese, R.: N. Engl. J. Med. **287:**254, 1972.
198. Baehner, R.L., and Nathan, D.G.: N. Engl. J. Med. **278:**971, 1968.
199. Lehrer, R.I.: Clin. Res. **18:**443, 1970.
200. Cooper, M.R., et al.: J. Clin. Invest. **49:**21, 1970.
201. Douwes, F.R.: N. Engl. J. Med. **287:**822, 1972.
202. Chretien, J.H., and Garagusi, V.F.: Lancet **2:**549, 1971.
203. Anderson, B.R.: Lancet **2:**317, 1971.
204. Steigbigel, R.T., and Johnson, P.K.: N. Engl. J. Med. **290:**235, 1974.
205. Ashburn, P., et al.: Blood **41:**921, 1973.
206. Feigin, R.D., and Pickering, L.K.: South. Med. J. **68:**237, 1975.
207. Newsome, J.: Nature **214:**1092, 1967.
208. Stossel, T.P.: Personal communication.
209. Lehrer, R.I., and Cline, M.J.: J. Clin. Invest. **48:**1478, 1969.
210. Lehrer, R.I., and Cline, M.J.: J. Bacteriol. **98:**996, 1969.
211. Klebanoff, S.J.: Annu. Rev. Med. **22:**39, 1971.
212. Hirsch, J.G., and Strauss, B.: J. Immunol. **92:**145, 1964.

CHAPTER 7

Numeric evaluation of formed elements of blood

AUTOMATED TECHNICS

The cellular components of blood should be counted by automated instruments and not by manual technics, which are reserved for counting cells in biologic fluids (synovial, pleural, cerebrospinal, etc.) that cannot be handled by automated equipment. Manual methods are tedious and time consuming and have a coefficient of variation ranging from 8-20%, whereas the coefficient of variation[1] of the Coulter method (Coulter, Model S[+], Coulter Electronics, Hialeah, Fla.) is 2-4%.[2] All counting procedures (manual or automated) share three basic steps: (1) dilution of blood, (2) sampling of a measured amount, and (3) enumeration of particles.

The advantages of the electronic methods for particle counting over the manual methods are well accepted: (1) speed, (2) precision, (3) automated calculation of hematocrit and hematologic constants, and (4) printouts, which eliminate errors of transcription and calculation.

The automated counters operate on one of two general principles: (1) electronic counting and sizing and (2) optical detection of particles.

The first method is based on the fact that cells passing through a small aperture change the electrical resistance, because the resistance of the intact cell is much greater than that of the conducting suspension fluid. As the cell passes through the aperture of the Coulter S[+], there is a momentary increase in resistance that creates a voltage impulse proportional in height to the volume of the cells counted. If two or more cells enter the aperture at the same time, they are counted as one, creating a coincidence error for which a correction must be made.

The optical counting method allows the cell suspension to flow through a small rectangular cell, which is illuminated by a narrow beam of light at right angles to the direction of the flow. As each cell enters the beam it reflects a small flash of light, which is converted to electric pulses by a photomultiplier tube. The light scattering method is used in the Technicon 8/90 system (Technicon Instruments Corp., Tarrytown, N.Y.) and in the ELT-8 Hematology analyzer (Ortho Instruments, Westwood, Mass.).

Electronic particle counters
Coulter Model S[+]

The Coulter Model S[+],[1,3,4-6] the latest Coulter S model, provides not only the already mentioned hematologic data but also two additional parameters: platelet count and red cell size distribution widths (RDW).

At a maximal rate of 3 samples per minute the Coulter Models S[+] and S[SR] (Coulter Electronics, Hialeah, Fla.) measure directly the concentration of white cells, red cells, mean corpuscular volume (MCV), and hemoglobin concentration. They calculate electronically packed cell volume (hematocrit), mean corpuscular hemoglobin (MCH), and mean corpuscular hemoglobin concentration (MCHC). Anticoagulated whole blood or prediluted capillary specimens are aspirated and diluted 1:224 with an isotonic particle-free fluid. The white cell count and the hemoglobin determination are performed on this dilution. The red cell count and the MCV determination are performed on the second dilution of 1:50,000. There are six apertures, three for red cells and three for white cells. The result from each aperture is recorded separately and corrected for coincidence. The values are averaged and printed on special cards or sent to a computer. The instrument is programmed to reject data from any channel if unacceptable variations occur. The MCV is calculated on the basis of the summation of the height of the red cell impulses divided by the red cell count and is measured in duplicate, and the mean value is recorded on the printout. Hemoglobin is measured as cyanmethemoglobin. An aliquot of the red cell–containing sample is mixed with a lysing agent, which converts hemoglobin into cyanmethemoglobin and at the same time lyses the red cells but leaves the white cells intact. The hemoglobin concentration is measured photometrically, and the white cells of the lysed sample are counted simultaneously with the red cell sample in triplicate. The packed cell volume is calculated from the MCV multiplied by the red cell count. The MCH is computed from the hemoglobin value and the red cell count. The MCHC is calculated from the hemoglobin value and the packed cell volume. A special system is used to count platelets. It uses a smaller aperture to increase sensitivity, a sweep-flow to remove potentially interfering particles, and a concentrated solution to increase the number of platelets. The Coulter S^+ determines the actual cell wall volume as a true measurement of size and computes the red cell size distribution and spread of the erythrocytes counted. (See discussion of Price-Jones curve.)

Sources of error: The Coulter S^+ has eliminated most of the problems of previous models. It still requires the attention of a full-time operator, but the carry-over problem is solved. However, very low white and red cell counts should be repeated at least once and the second values reported. The turbidity produced by a high white cell count may be responsible for erroneous values of hemoglobin, MCV, and hematocrit. Errors in the MCV can be eliminated by using normocytic and microcytic cells for standardization.[7] In chronic lymphocytic leukemia and in other leukemias the cells are easily damaged by the aperture, so that spuriously low white cell counts may appear on the printout, the values of which should be confirmed by manual counts. The mentioned inaccuracies of manual counts are of little clinical significance in leukemias with high white cell counts. Falsely low counts may also be expected in uremia and immunosuppression.[8] High-titered cold agglutinins, which clump the red cells at room temperature, are responsible for spurious macrocytosis and very high MCHC values.[9]

Optical particle counters
Hemac 4000-Laser Hematology Counter

The Hemac 4000-Laser Hematology Counter (Ortho Instruments, Westwood, Mass.) counts red and white cells as they pass through a laser beam, measures the hemoglobin concentration by a modified cyanmethemoglobin method, and determines the hematocrit by summing the pulse amplitudes produced by narrow-angle diffraction measurements. MCV, MCH, and MCHC levels are derived from measured values. All the results appear on a digital printout.[10]

The heart of the instrument is the flow chamber, a microcuvet with a diameter of 250 μm. Within the flow chamber the diluted blood sample is constrained to flow in the exact center of a laminar flow of sheath fluid. As the sample stream and the sheath fluid flow upward, the diameter of the fluid sheath progressively diminishes, constricting the central core of the specimen to an aperture of 18 μm. At the center of the flow channel the sample cells maintained in "single-file" configuration by the lamina flow conditions pass through the 20 μm thickness of the focused laser beam at the approximate rate of 2500 cells/sec. As each cell passes through the beam, the light is interrupted, deflected, or scattered, and the detector and associated electronics generate a pulse. The pulses appear on the oscilloscope and are accumulated for printout of the red cell count and hematocrit. A second aliquot of specimen enters the flow chamber for the white cell count.

ELT-8

The ELT-8 (Ortho Instruments, Westwood, Mass.) provides the traditional seven parameters of multichannel instruments plus a platelet count. The instrument uses the above described laser counting mechanisms and the laminar flow technic called hydrodynamic focusing, rendering the unit unsusceptible to aperture clogging. Counts are performed on separate channels.

Electronic counting of leukocytes

The previously described systems for counting red cells are used to enumerate white cells, provided the red cells are lysed before the white cell counting phase. The error of the method comes close to ±2 SD or to 5% if two counts are made. This figure represents a vast improvement over the coefficient of variation of manual counts, which varies from 12-20%.[11]

Electronic platelet counts

Automated platelet counts use the electronic (platelet phase of Coulter S^+) or the optical counting systems (Technicon AutoCounter, Technicon Instruments Corp., Tarrytown, N.Y.) described for the enumeration of red and white cells. The great variation in platelet size poses a technical problem, because some platelets are as small as debris and others as large as red cells. The counts may be performed on diluted whole blood or on platelet-rich plasma prepared by centrifugation (Thrombocounter, Coulter Electronics, Hialeah, Fla.).

Thrombocounter

With the Thrombocounter platelet-rich plasma is prepared by slow centrifugation (750 rpm) of EDTA-anticoagulated blood. This method of preparation of the platelet suspension is fast, accurate, and reproducible. It is superior to the separation of red cells from platelets by sedimentation, because the latter method requires transfer of EDTA blood to plastic sedimentation tubes and a sedimentation period of 1 hr. The platelet-rich plasma is diluted in plastic-capped glass vials containing 15 ml Isoton II (Coulter Electronics, Hialeah, Fla.). The platelet count is performed by using the electronic particle counter technic. To arrive at a whole blood platelet count the raw count must be corrected for coincidence effect, dilution, actual volume aspirated through the aperture, and hematocrit. A circular slide rule supplied by the manufacturer allows the completion of the calculation in one operation.[12,13]

Standardized glutaraldehyde- and osmium tetroxide–fixed platelets, postfixed with uranyl acetate, may be used as control and standard for the Coulter counter.[14] A suspension of fixed human platelets is also supplied by Technicon Instruments Corp., Tarrytown, N.Y.

Sources of error: There are innate inaccuracies associated with the preparation of platelet-rich plasma by sedimentation or centrifugation. The counting procedure is the only automated step; all other steps are manual and relatively time consuming. Platelet carry-over assumes importance in the counting of thrombocytopenic blood samples[13,15] that may follow high platelet counts. Capillary blood samples require special handling, e.g., anticoagulation in glass capillary tubes and subsequent transfer to sedimentation tubes.[12,16] Finally the raw plasma platelet count must be corrected for coincidence error and hematocrit level. Also, abnormal plasma proteins and extremes of platelet size affect the method.[17] If there is much platelet clumping, severe thrombocytopenia, or numerous giant platelets, the electronic counting results may be inaccurate.

AutoCounter system

The AutoCounter system uses anticoagulated whole blood samples in macro quantities (0.6 ml) or micro quantities $(44.7 \mu l)$[15] and performs a completely automated optical platelet count in about 3 min. The blood samples are aspirated at the rate of 40/h and automatically diluted 1:1500 with 2M urea. The urea lyses the red cells, leaving the platelets and white cells in suspension; they are counted by a darkfield microscope optical system that detects light diffracted by them. The scatter light is transformed into electronic pulses, which are amplified and converted into voltage signals that are automatically compared to a standard voltage equivalent to a particular number of platelets. The compared voltage value is recorded on a strip chart as a specific number of platelets per cubic millimeter.

When finger-stick blood is used, it is immediately diluted 1:200 with specially prepared Unopettes (Becton-Dickinson & Co., Rutherford, N.J.) having a 20 μl capillary and containing 3.98 ml 0.1% K_3-EDTA in saline. The proportioning pump of the AutoCounter is adjusted to give a final dilution of 1:1500 with 2M urea.

If the expected platelet count is less than 50,000, an initial dilution of 1:40 is suggested using Unopettes with a 40 μl capillary and 1.56 ml saline per diluent.

A standardized suspension of fixed platelets is available to serve as reference material and standard.

Sources of error: As both platelets and white cells are enumerated by the optical method, an independent total white cell count should be performed and subtracted from the total platelet count. Inconsistent counting results are obtained when much platelet clumping

occurs.[18] To exclude carry-over of thrombocytopenic counts following thrombocythemic samples, the thrombocytopenic counts must be repeated at least once. The calibration of the optical count method is more cumbersome and must be performed more frequently than that of the electronic particle counter.

Automated differential counts

The manual differential count is subject to many errors, including errors in preparation and staining of the slides, cell distribution, cell interpretation, and number of cells counted. A successfully automated differential system should eliminate most of these errors, and (1) it should be able to identify normal and abnormal cells; (2) the results should be reproducible in repetitive counts; (3) the total number of leukocytes identified and counted should exceed the manually counted 100-200 cells to provide greater precision; (4) the count should be performed in a minimal amount of time; and (5) provision must be made for documentation and storage of results. The classification of white cells should include segmented neutrophils, band or juvenile neutrophils, lymphocytes, monocytes, eosinophils, basophils, and other "cells."

Conceptual approaches to automatic white cell counts fall into three groups.

1. Cells are classified by selective cytochemical stains in a liquid milieu and are pumped through transparent capillary columns passing a light source and a sensing device that measures light scatter and light absorption caused by specific stains.[19] (See discussions of Technicon D/90 and H6000 systems.)

2. Cells are classified on the basis of stained blood smears using an automated microscope and morphologic and tinctorial criteria for cell identification. (See discussions of Hematrak automatic white cell analyzers and differential counters.)

3. Unstained cells are classified by phase microscopy on the basis of size and refractive index in a liquid milieu as they are pumped through transparent columns, or they are classified on the basis of size and density by using a Coulter transducer (Coulter Electronics, Hialeah, Fla.) in conjunction with a multichannel analyzer.

Technicon D/90 and H6000 systems

The Technicon D/90 is an automated leukocyte differential analyzer, which is also incorporated in the H6000 hematology system (Technicon Instruments Corp., Tarrytown, N.Y.). It classifies 30,000 white cells per sample in less than 1 min using an automated continuous-flow cytochemical staining technic.[20,21] Eosinophils and neutrophils are identified by their peroxidase contents. A mixture of hydrogen peroxide and 4-chloro-1-naphthol is added to stain the peroxidase-positive granules. Neutrophils are stained various shades of gray, and eosinophils are stained black. Neutrophils with high peroxidase activity are identified as juvenile population. Lymphocytes remain unstained and are measured by electronic sizing. The monocytic esterase is reacted with α-naphthyl butyrate, so that α-naphthol is released to combine with diazotized basic fuchsin in the mixture to form a red intracellular precipitate. The heparin of the granules of basophils reacts with alcian

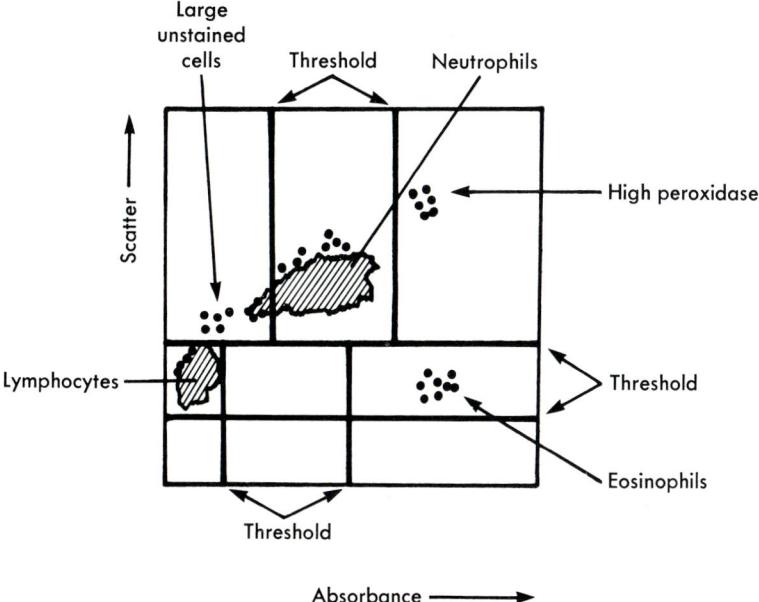

Fig. 7-1. Sketch of *X-Y* display of peroxidase channel of normal blood.

blue, a stain used for the demonstration of acid muco-polysaccharides. The remaining group of "large, un-stained cells" includes large lymphocytes, atypical lymphocytes, and blast cells. Results are reported as percentages and as absolute values (number of white cells per cubic millimeter). The Technicon D/90 system also provides a two-dimensional *X-Y* display of 10,000 cells for each channel from each sample. The *X* axis shows the absorbance, and the *Y* axis displays the scatter (Fig. 7-1). Each dot represents a single cell passing through the flow cell. The display thus provides a graphic presentation of the distribution of the various white cell types of the sample being processed in the channel selected. The instrument identifies and sorts leukocyte types by their respective scatter and absorbance characteristics on staining. In selected white cell disorders the distribution pattern of the *X-Y* presentation displays diagnostic features.

The H6000 combines the white cell differential count with an automated platelet count and a red cell size histogram. A stained monolayer slide is also prepared automatically.

Hematrak Automated Differential Counter

Hematrak (Geometric Data Corp., Wayne, Pa.) is a computerized electro-optical system to scan Wright-stained blood smears. The number of leukocytes counted may vary from 50-800 cells. A high-speed morphologic analysis is made of nuclear shape, chromatin pattern, nuclear/cytoplasmic ratio, and color of granules.[22] These recognition factors determine the differentiation criteria of normal cells. When abnormal white cells or nucleated red cells are detected, the scanning stops and the cell's image is displayed. The technologist then views the cell through the microscope and enters its classification on the keyboard. Blood films are prepared by manual or automated wedge technic,

so that finger-stick and bedside preparations may be used. The counter is trained to recognize Wright-stained smears and adjusts to some variations in their color and intensity, so that manually prepared and stained slides may be scanned. One hundred white cells can be analyzed in about 40 sec.

Rapid automated differential counts using dilute leukocyte suspensions[23,24]

Leukocytes in dilute suspensions may be classified according to size with a Coulter Model TPS Cell Sorter (Coulter Electronics, Hialeah, Fla.) in conjunction with a multichannel analyzer. Two peaks can be distinguished on an oscilloscope screen if leukocyte-rich plasma is analyzed: a lymphocytic peak and a granulocytic and monocytic peak. Heparinized venous blood is obtained, the red cells are sedimented by the addition of Plasmagel (Laboratoire Roger Bellon, Neuilly-sur-Seine, France), and leukocyte-rich plasma is aspirated and centrifuged. The leukocyte pellet is dispersed in Hank's balanced salt solution (HBSS), and the size distribution of 100,000 cells is obtained.

The main advantage of this method is the rapid counting of a large number of cells, so that the purity of a representative population of leukocytes can be established in a short period of time. The major disadvantage is that granulocytes and monocytes overlap in size and are therefore indistinguishable. One area of clinical application is the rapid enumeration of blast cells in the peripheral blood of leukemic patients to monitor their response to treatment.

Pulse cytophotometry (PCP) and flow microfluorometry (FMF)

Cell flow analysis is an extension of the electronic cell counting and sizing systems. The Cytofluorograf System 50 (Ortho Instruments, Westwood, Mass.) is a

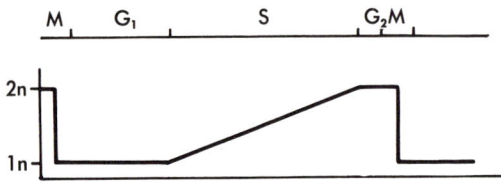

Fig. 7-2. Division of intermitotic time span into postmitotic resting phase *(G₁)*, DNA synthesis time *(S),* and premitotic resting phase *(G₂). M* = mitosis; *n* = haploid number of chromosomes; *2n* = diploid number of chromosomes.

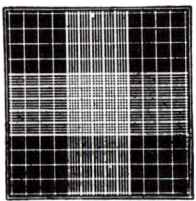

Fig. 7-3. Improved Neubauer hemocytometer counting chamber ruling. (Courtesy E.H. Sargent Co., Chicago.)

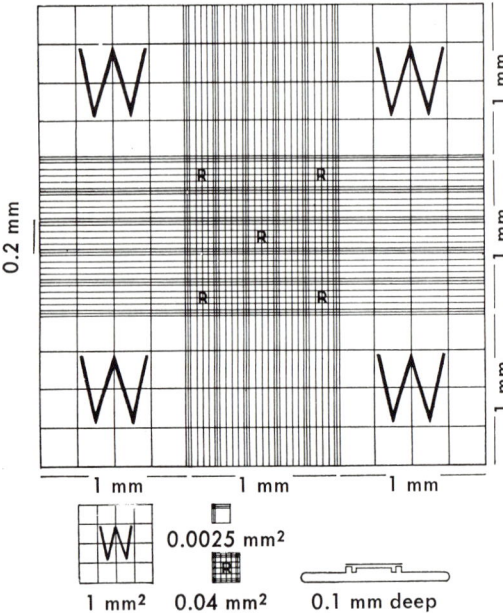

Fig. 7-4. Counting chamber rulings and dimensions. Hemocytometer of counting chamber has two ruled areas etched on its surface, each consisting of a 3 mm square divided into nine large squares *(W),* each measuring 1 mm². Center square, which is used for red cell counting, is subdivided into 25 smaller squares *(R),* each occupying an area of 0.04 mm². Red cells in five *R* squares are enumerated. Depth of the chamber is 0.1 mm. The four large corner squares, each 1 mm² in area, are subdivided into 16 smaller squares and are used for leukocyte counting.

refinement of the laser optical cell counter. The instrument enumerates and sizes the cells and after the addition of different fluorochromes allows quantitation of the most important intracellular components, e.g., DNA,[25] RNA, proteins, lipids, and enzymes.[26]

The cytofluorographic method can be used for fluorescent antibody studies,[27] histocompatibility testing,[28] lymphocyte cultures,[26] and cancer cell identification.[29] The great advantage of pulse cytophotometry is that a large number of cells can be examined in a short time, 1000 cells/sec, to obtain a statistically significant histogram. The disadvantage is that cell morphology cannot be appreciated.

PCP also provides insight into the DNA and the mitotic division pattern of cells. Since different phases of the mitotic cell cycle contain different amounts of DNA, the percentage of cells in the G_1, S, G_2, and M phases can be calculated[29a] (Fig. 7-2).

MANUAL TECHNICS

Manual counting technics are still used for cell counts on body fluids (cerebrospinal paracentesis, synovial, pericardial, and thoracocentesis fluids) and are also employed for high leukemic white cell counts, for eosinophil, basophil, and platelet counts, and when the electronic particle counters break down.

Manual erythrocyte count
Unopette technic

Equipment:
1. Unopette (Becton-Dickinson & Co., Rutherford, N.J.) reservoir no. 5851 containing 1.99 ml diluting fluid made up of 8.5 g sodium chloride, 0.1 g sodium azide, and 1 L water.
2. Capillary pipet, 10 μl. The desired dilution ratio of 1:200 is obtained when the volume of blood sample in the capillary pipet is mixed with the diluent in the reservoir.
3. Hemocytometer (improved Neubauer chamber) and coverslip (Figs. 7-3 and 7-4).

Procedure: Fill capillary with sample (EDTA-anticoagulated venous blood or capillary blood) and allow negative pressure of reservoir to draw it into the diluent. Mix well. Convert to dropper assembly and fill the hemocytometer.

Red cell diluting pipet technic

Equipment:
1. The red cell diluting pipet contains a red bead in the bulb and has 10 divisions on the capillary end, with

points 0.5 and 1 numbered. If blood is drawn to the 0.5 mark and the pipet filled with diluting fluid, the resultant dilution is 0.5:100 or 1:200, the dilution used in routine counting. One volume of diluting fluid remains in the stem, does not enter the bulb, is blown out first before the counting chamber is filled, and therefore does not dilute the blood. Various dilutions may be obtained by using different divisions on the capillary or stem for measuring the amount of blood used. (See below and Fig. 7-5.)

2. Hemocytometer. The most commonly used method employs the Neubauer counting chamber (Fig. 7-6 and Table 7-1). A single chamber (of which there are two per hemocytometer) consists of nine large

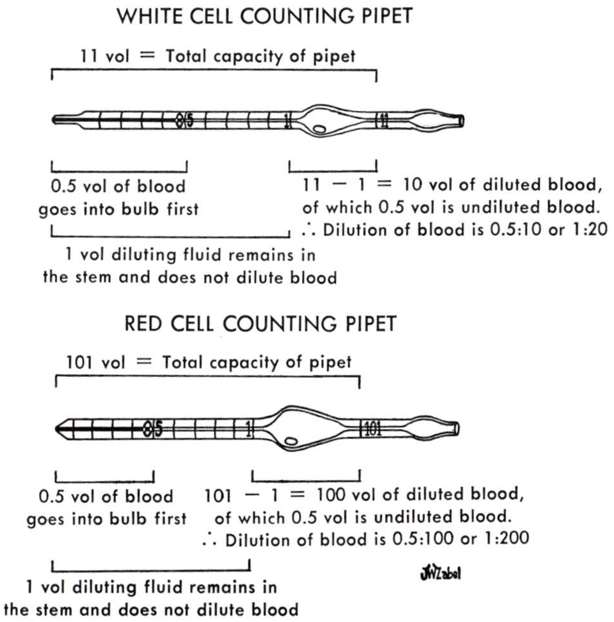

WHITE CELL COUNTING PIPET

11 vol = Total capacity of pipet

0.5 vol of blood
goes into bulb first

11 − 1 = 10 vol of diluted blood,
of which 0.5 vol is undiluted blood.
∴ Dilution of blood is 0.5:10 or 1:20

1 vol diluting fluid remains in
the stem and does not dilute blood

RED CELL COUNTING PIPET

101 vol = Total capacity of pipet

0.5 vol of blood
goes into bulb first

101 − 1 = 100 vol of diluted blood,
of which 0.5 vol is undiluted blood.
∴ Dilution of blood is 0.5:100 or 1:200

JWZabel

1 vol diluting fluid remains in
the stem and does not dilute blood

Fig. 7-5. Explanation of dilution of blood in red and white cell counting pipets. (From Bauer, J.D.: In Frankel, S., Reitman, S., and Sonnenwirth, A.C., editors: Gradwohl's clinical laboratory methods and diagnosis, ed. 7, St. Louis, 1970, The C.V. Mosby Co., vol. 1.)

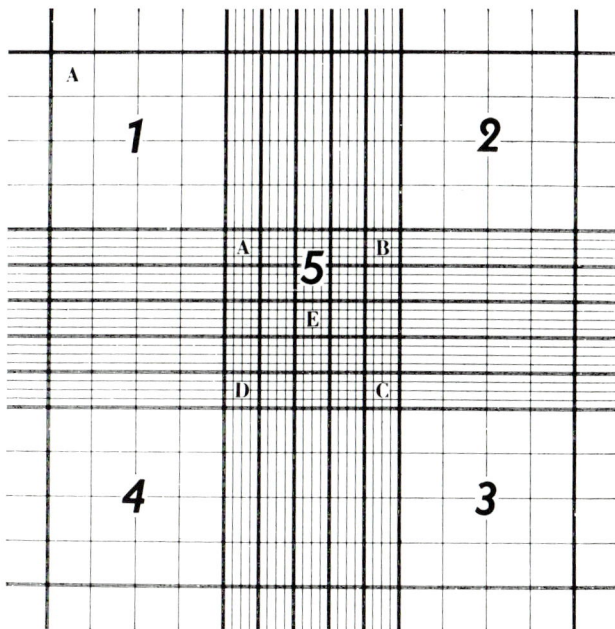

Fig. 7-6. Improved Neubauer ruling for one counting chamber. White cell count is done on the four large corner squares *(1, 2, 3,* and *4)* of each of two counting chambers. Red cell count is done on square *5 (A, B, C, D,* and *E)* of each of two counting chambers. Platelet count is done on two large corner squares *(1 and 3)* of each of two counting chambers. (From Page, L.B., and Culver, P.J.: A syllabus of laboratory examination in clinical diagnosis, Cambridge, Mass., 1960, Harvard University Press.)

Table 7-1. Dimensions of counting chamber and subdivisions

Square	Length (mm)	Area (mm²)	Depth (mm)	Volume (mm³)
Chamber	3	9	0.10	0.90
1	1	1	0.10	0.10
1A	0.25	0.0625	0.10	0.00625
5A	0.20	0.040	0.10	0.0040

From Page, L.B., and Culver, P.J.: The successor to Thomas Hale Ham's syllabus of laboratory examinations in clinical diagnosis. Cambridge, Mass., 1956. Harvard University Press.

squares, each measuring 1 mm². In Fig. 7-6 these squares are labeled 1, 2, 3, 4, and 5. The central square of the chamber (5) is subdivided into 25 smaller squares, each $^1/_{25}$ mm². Five of these squares in Fig. 7-6 are marked A, B, C, D, and E. Each of these 25 squares is further divided into 16 squares of $^1/_{400}$ mm² each. The five squares marked A, B, C, D, and E are used for erythrocyte counting.

Diluting fluid:

Hayem red cell counting solution:
  Mercuric chloride, 0.5 g
  Sodium sulfate, 5.0 g
  Sodium chloride, 1.0 g
  Distilled water, 2 dl

Dissolve all the chemicals in the distilled water and filter. Hayem solution is fairly stable. If a precipitate forms, discard the solution. This solution must be used at room temperature, because cold causes clumping of the erythrocytes; clumping may also occur in diseases associated with hyperglobulinemia, e.g., multiple myeloma and lymphomas.

Procedure: Draw the EDTA-anticoagulated blood to exactly the 0.5 mark of the counting pipet. Capillary blood may also be used. Wipe the tip of the pipet clean with a piece of dry gauze without touching the opening of the capillary. Then immerse the pipet in the freshly filtered diluting fluid, which should be in a small tube. Do not insert the pipet in a bottle of counting solution. By gentle mouth suctioning, draw the diluting fluid steadily into the pipet to exactly the 101 mark past the bulb. Rotate the pipet on its long axis to ensure thorough mixing of blood and diluent. Gradually bring the pipet to a vertical position, so that the measurement at the top of the pipet is accurate. Do not permit the capillary tip of the pipet to come out of the diluting fluid while drawing up the solution, and do not permit any of the blood to run out of the capillary while filling the pipet.

If the diluting fluid has been permitted to go beyond the 101 mark or if air bubbles are present in the pipet, discard the mixture and begin again with a clean, dry pipet. Immediately mix the contents of the pipet thoroughly by placing the thumb over one end and the first finger over the other end and shaking the pipet for about 1 min.

Diluted samples must be examined within 2 hr. They must be thoroughly mixed just before their admission into the hemocytometer, preferably on a pipet rotator for 2-3 min.

Filling the counting chamber: Place the special coverslip in its proper position over the ruled areas of the hemocytometer. Shake the pipet, discard the first 3 or 4 drops of diluted blood from the pipet, and then carefully and exactly fill the counting chamber via capillary attraction by placing the tip of the pipet at one of the open ends of the chamber. Overfilling can be readily observed by the presence of fluid in the moat surrounding each ruled area. If this occurs, clean and refill the counting chamber. An insufficient amount of fluid may be noted by the failure of fluid to cover a ruled area. Rectify by adding more fluid to the chamber. If air bubbles are present in the chamber, they usually indicate moisture or a dirty hemocytometer or coverslip. Clean again and refill both ruled areas of the chamber.

Allow the mixture to settle in the chamber. Locate the ruled area for erythrocyte counting under low magnification and then change to the high dry objective for actual counting of the cells.

Making the count: All counts should be made in duplicate. Watch the correction factor on the pipet or make two counts with balanced pipets (e.g., correction factors of $+2$ and -2).

For a routine erythrocyte count, enumerate the cells in the five squares labeled A, B, C, D, and E (Fig. 7-6). Since Hayem solution does not dissolve leukocytes, do not count such cells in the red cell count. Leukocytes are larger than erythrocytes, appear grayish, and are usually granular. Only one such cell is seen in approximately 750-1000 erythrocytes; therefore leukocytes do not present a problem in routine red cell counting. When the white cell count is very high, as in leukemias, it is important to make this differentiation.

A standardized pattern of counting should be adopted. It is recommended that counting begin in the left upper corner of each A, B, C, D, and E square and proceed as follows: Count the first row of small subdivisions to the right, drop down to the second row and

No. of cells/mm³ undiluted blood = Counted cells × 10,000

This formula is based on the following:

$$\text{No. of cells/mm}^3 \text{ undiluted blood} = \frac{\text{Total no. of counted cells in 5 squares}}{\text{Surface area counted} \times \text{Height of counting chamber} \times \text{Dilution of blood}}$$

which equals:

$$\frac{\text{Counted cells}}{^1/_5 \times {}^1/_{10} \times {}^1/_{200}}$$

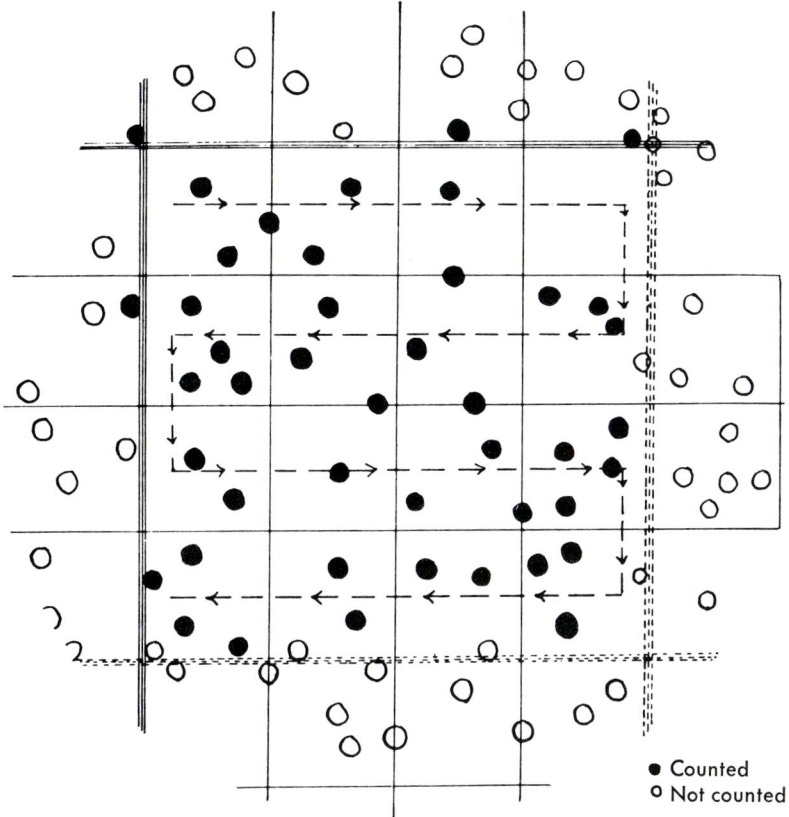

● Counted
○ Not counted

Fig. 7-7. Diagrammatic representation of red cell count. Square shown, comparable to square *5A* in Fig. 7-6, is magnified 400 times, using high-power dry objective of microscope. Order of counting of the small squares is indicated by the arrows. A red cell is counted only once by counting those within small square and those touching any line at left or top but not counting those touching any line at right or bottom of small square. By this procedure, all cells touching triple lines shown as solid lines will be included and all cells touching triple lines shown as broken lines will be excluded. (From Page, L.B., and Culver, P.J.: A syllabus of laboratory examinations in clinical diagnosis, Cambridge, Mass., 1960, Harvard University Press.)

count to the left, drop down to the third row and count across to the right, and then finish the fourth row counting to the left. In the enumeration include all cells touching or half in and half out of the upper line and the line to the left, excluding those half in and half out of the lower and right-hand lines. Take care not to count any cell twice, and do not omit any cells. Remember that the boundary line is the center line of the triple ruling. Count the first square at the upper left of the ruling (A square), the second at the upper right (B square), the third at the lower right (C square), the fourth at the lower left (D square), and the fifth in the center (E square) (Fig. 7-7).

Record the counts in each of the A, B, C, D, and E squares and add them together.

Calculation: The basic formula for the calculation of the number of blood cells per cubic millimeter undiluted blood is as shown at the bottom of p.184.

Variations in procedure in polycythemia and severe anemias: If the red cells are markedly increased in number (polycythemia), increase the dilution by drawing blood to the 0.3 mark on the red cell pipet and

dilute to mark 101. Count and calculate as before but multiply the result by $^5/_3$, since only 3 volumes of blood were counted instead of 5 volumes. If the number of red cells is markedly diminished (anemia), decrease the dilution by drawing blood up to the 1 mark in the red cell pipet and dilute to mark 101. The dilution is then 1:100. On the basis of the previous formula, the counted erythrocytes have to be multiplied by 5000 instead of 10,000.

Normal values: Normal values of the erythrocyte count are as follows (Tables 7-2 to 7-4):

Men: 4.2-5.4 million/mm^3

Women: 3.8-5.2 million/mm^3

Infants and children: See Fig. 7-8 and Tables 7-2 and 7-4.

Variations in number of red cells

Increase (polycythemia): Polycythemia (see Chapter 8) may be secondary (erythrocytosis) or primary (erythremia, polycythemia vera). Secondary polycythemia results from factors that do not change the red cell mass, e.g., dehydration or anoxia. A physiologic form

Table 7-2. Erythrocyte and hemoglobin values from birth to maturity

Age	Erythrocyte count (million/mm³ blood)	Erythrocyte packed volume (hematocrit) (ml/dl blood)	Erythrocyte volume (mean corpuscular) (μm³)	Hemoglobin concentration		Erythrocyte hemoglobin content (pg)
				g/dl blood	g/dl erythrocytes	
At birth*	5.7 (4.8-7.1)	56.6	106	21.5 (18.0-27.0)	38.0	38
1 d	5.6 (4.7-7.0)	56.1	106	21.2 (17.7-26.5)	37.8	38
1 wk	5.3 (4.5-6.4)	52.7	101	19.6 (16.2-25.5)	37.2	37
2 wk	5.1 (4.3-6.0)	49.6	96	18.0 (14.5-24.2)	36.3	35
3 wk	4.9 (4.1-6.0)	46.6	93	16.6 (13.2-23.0)	35.6	34
4 wk	4.7 (3.9-5.9)	44.6	91	15.6 (12.0-21.8)	35.0	33
2 mo	4.5 (3.8-5.8)	38.9	85	13.3 (10.8-18.0)	34.2	30
4 mo	4.5 (3.8-5.3)	36.5	79	12.4 (10.2-15.0)	34.0	27
6 mo	4.6 (3.9-5.3)	36.2	78	12.3 (10.0-15.0)	34.0	27
8 mo	4.6 (4.0-5.4)	35.8	77	12.1 (9.8-15.0)	33.8	26
10 mo	4.6 (4.0-5.5)	35.5	77	11.9 (8.4-14.9)	33.5	26
12 mo	4.6 (4.0-5.5)	35.2	77	11.6 (9.0-14.6)	33.0	25
2 yr	4.7 (3.8-5.4)	35.5	78	11.7 (9.2-15.5)	33.0	25
4 yr	4.7 (3.8-5.4)	37.1	80	12.6 (9.6-15.5)	34.0	27
6 yr	4.7 (3.8-5.4)	37.9	80	12.7 (10.0-15.5)	33.5	27
8 yr	4.7 (3.8-5.4)	38.9	80	12.9 (10.3-15.5)	33.2	27
10 yr	4.8 (3.8-5.4)	39.0	80	13.0 (10.7-15.5)	33.3	27
12 yr	4.8 (3.8-5.4)	39.6	81	13.4 (11.0-16.5)	33.8	28
14 yr and over						
Males	5.4 (4.6-6.2)	47	87	15.8 (14.0-18.0)	33.5	29
Females	4.8 (4.2-5.4)	42	87	13.9 (11.5-16.0)	33.5	29

From Altman, P.L., and Dittmer, D.S., editors: Blood and other body fluids, Bethesda, Md., 1961, Federation of American Societies for Experimental Biology.

*When cord was clamped after placental separation rather than immediately after birth, erythrocyte count was 560,000/mm³ greater and hemoglobin 2.6 g/dl greater during first week of life. Erythrocyte and hemoglobin values were higher for heel blood (capillary) than for blood from superior sagittal sinus.

Table 7-3. Erythrocyte and hemoglobin values in nonpregnant, pregnant, and postpartum females

Condition	No. of observations	Erythrocyte count (million/mm³ blood)	Erythrocyte packed volume (hematocrit) (ml/dl blood)	Hemoglobin concentration (g/dl blood)
Nonpregnant	42	4.44 (3.68-5.20)	41.5 (37.5-45.0)	13.4 (11.7-15.1)
Pregnant				
3 mo	7	4.49 (4.00-4.98)	40.6 (35.0-46.2)	13.2 (11.4-15.0)
4 mo	9	3.83 (3.43-4.23)	37.0 (32.0-42.0)	12.0 (10.8-13.2)
5 mo	9	3.98 (3.50-4.46)	34.8 (31.0-38.6)	12.1 (10.1-14.1)
6 mo	20	3.85 (3.19-4.51)	36.0 (30.0-42.0)	12.2 (10.1-14.3)
7 mo	24	3.90 (3.25-4.65)	36.0 (31.0-41.0)	12.1 (10.4-13.8)
8 mo	34	3.89 (3.20-4.58)	36.4 (31.5-41.3)	11.9 (10.1-13.7)
9 mo	38	3.97 (3.02-4.92)	37.5 (31.5-43.5)	12.3 (10.2-14.4)
Postpartum	16	4.14 (3.23-5.05)	38.7 (33.5-43.9)	12.7 (10.4-15.0)

From Altman, P.L., and Dittmer, D.S., editors: Blood and other body fluids, Bethesda, Md., 1961, Federation of American Societies for Experimental Biology.

Table 7-4. Average normal blood values at different age levels

	At birth	At 2 d	At 14 d	At 3 mo	At 6 mo	At 1 yr	At 2 yr	At 4 yr	At 8-21 yr
Red cells/mm³ (in millions)	5.1	5.3	5.0	4.3	4.6	4.7	4.8	4.8	5.1
Hemoglobin									
g/dl	17.6	18.0	17.0	11.4	11.5	12.2	12.9	13.1	14.1
Percentage of normal	113	115	109	73	74	78	83	84	90
White cells/mm³ (in thousands)	15.0	21.0	11.0	9.5	9.2	9.0	8.5	8.0	8.0
Platelets/mm³ (in thousands)	350.0	400.0	300.0	260.0	250.0	250.0	250.0	250.0	250.0
Differential smears (percentages)									
Polymorphonuclear neutrophils	45	55	36	35	40	40	40	50	60
Eosinophils and basophils	3	5	3	3	3	2	2	2	2
Lymphocytes	30	20	53	55	51	53	50	40	30
Monocytes	12	15	8	7	6	5	8	8	8
Immature white cells	10	5	—	—	—	—	—	—	—
Percentage of nucleated red cells in total nucleated cells	1-5	2	—	—	—	—	—	—	—
Percentage of reticulocytes in total red cells	2	3	1	0.5	0.8	1	1	1	1

From Blackfan, K.D., et al.: Atlas of the blood in children, Cambridge, Mass., 1944, Harvard University Press.

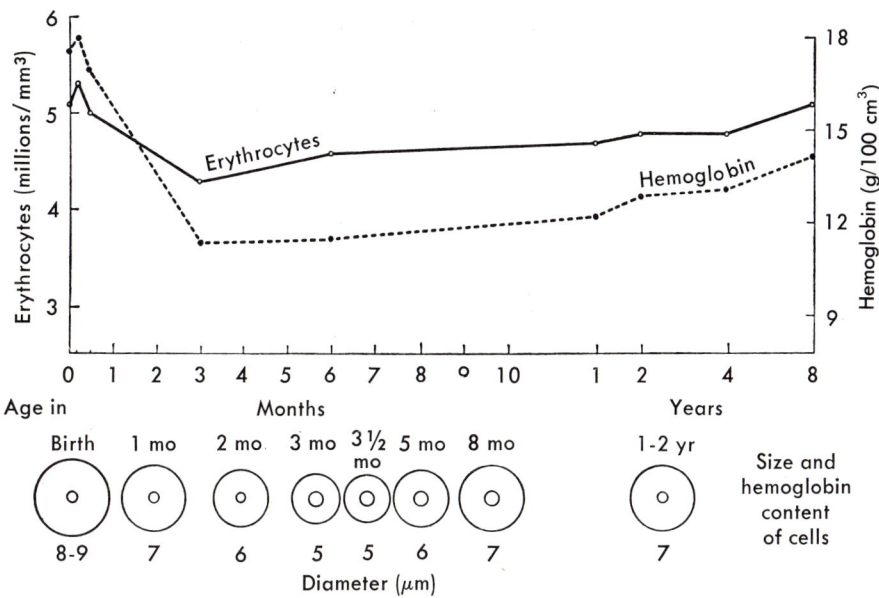

Fig. 7-8. Normal values of erythrocytes and hemoglobin at different age levels. (From Blackfan, K.D., et al.: Atlas of the blood in children, Cambridge, Mass., 1944, Harvard University Press.)

of erythrocytosis occurs in newborns. Polycythemia vera is a purposeless, idiopathic pancytosis leading to a progressive increase in the red cell mass.

Decrease (anemia): Anemia (see Chapter 8) may also be secondary or primary. Secondary anemia follows dilution of blood by an increase in plasma volume, as seen in pregnancy, whereas primary anemia results from a decreased red cell mass.

Errors in manual red cell counts

Red cell counts are subject to many errors involving the equipment, performance of the test, and sampling of the blood. The errors concerning blood sampling, pipetting, and unclean glassware are the same as those in hemoglobin determination. Restricted to counting procedures are such defects as inadequate filling of the counting chamber or drying of the specimen in the chamber, dirt or debris in the counting fluid, incorrect enumeration of cells, air bubbles and fat droplets in the counting area, and inadequate mixing of the specimen in the counting pipet.

Cleaning of pipets

Immerse stained pipets in 2.5% aqueous sodium hypochlorite solution. Attach the pipet to a suction pump and clean by siphoning through in this order: fresh water, 95% alcohol, acetone, and air. The counting chamber must be gently cleaned after each use.

HEMATOCRIT (PACKED RED CELL VOLUME)

The venous hematocrit measures the percent of the total volume of a venous blood sample that is occupied by red cells or, stated slightly differently, it is the ratio of the volume of erythrocytes to that of the whole blood. It is expressed as a percentage or as a decimal fraction.

Procedures: The hematocrit (Hct) can be determined by several methods: the manual macromethod and micromethod and the automated methods.

Principle: The hematocrit is determined by centrifuging an anticoagulated blood sample under standardized conditions. The anticoagulant may be dried heparin, EDTA, or balanced oxalate. The result is calculated from the following formula:

$$Hct = \frac{\text{Height of red cell column}}{\text{Height of plasma column (red cells + plasma)}}$$

Manual methods

Macromethod: Wintrobe's macromethod for hematocrit determination is replaced by the speedier, cheaper, and equally accurate microhematocrit method but can be used to obtain the buffy coat. The technic is described in previous editions of this book.

Buffy coat: If anticoagulated blood is centrifuged, several layers separate. Red cells occupy the bottom part of the test tube and plasma fills the upper portion. Between the plasma and the red cells is a thin, yellowish white layer called the buffy coat, which consists of white cells and other nucleated cells and platelets. The platelets are closest to the red cell mass; the white cells and nucleated cells face the plasma. The uppermost

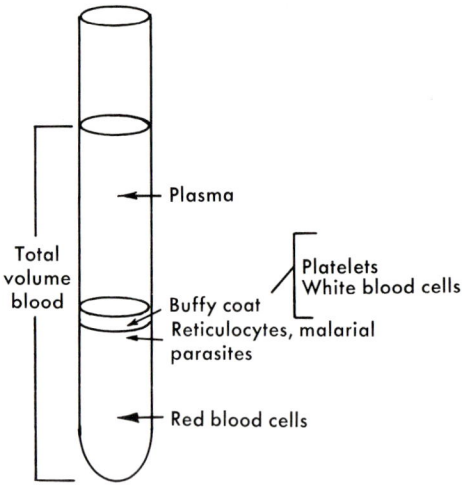

Fig. 7-9. Different layers of venous hematocrit.

layer of the red cell column contains the reticulocytes (Fig. 7-9).

The degree of red cell packing depends on the speed and time of centrifugation, the radius of the centrifuge, and the height of the blood column. Even under standardized conditions the amount of plasma trapped between red cells will vary with the height of the cell column and with the shape of the cells. An increased amount of plasma is trapped in thalassemia, sickle cell anemia, and hereditary spherocytosis.

Microhematocrit method

Principle: Blood in capillary tubes is centrifuged at a relative centrifugal force of 14,490 *g* for 4 min.

Equipment:
1. Capillary tubes (heparinized for blood taken without an anticoagulant; plain for anticoagulated blood)
2. Standardized high-speed centrifuge
3. Hematocrit linear scale for direct reading

Procedure: Fill the heparinized capillary tube with the blood sample. If the blood is anticoagulated, use a plain capillary tube. Seal one end of the tube with special sealing clay. Place the capillary tube in the centrifuge with the sealed end toward the outside, balancing it against another tube of the same size on the opposite side of the centrifuge head. Place the cover on the centrifuge and begin centrifugation, setting the automatic timer at 4 min or according to the manufacturer's directions.

Read percent blood cell volume directly from the graphic reader. Hold the tube against the linear chart so that the top of the blood column is exactly at the top line and the bottom of the column is against the bottom line. Move the tube until it reaches this position and then read volume of packed cells directly from the reader. The seal at the bottom of the tube must be flat.

Normal values: Normal values of the microhematocrit determination are as follows:

Men: 47 ± 7 vol%
Women: 42 ± 5 vol%
At birth: 56 ± 10 vol%
First year: 35 ± 5 vol%

Duplicate determinations decrease the chance of error. The coefficient of variation is 1-2%.

Interpretation: At the time of the hematocrit determination the plasma should be examined for evidence of jaundice (yellow color) or hemolysis (red color). The thickness of the buffy coat should also be judged.

Increased hematocrit: The hematocrit is increased in hemoconcentration, as seen in shock associated with surgery, trauma, and burns and in polycythemia.

Decreased hematocrit: The hematocrit is decreased in anemias and in conditions associated with hydremia, e.g., cardiac decompensation, pregnancy, and excessive administration of fluids. In the recovery phase after blood loss the blood volume is being restored by an increase in plasma volume, so that the hematocrit may be depressed in the initial phase of transfusion therapy.

Sources of error:

1. The centrifugal force must be strictly standardized so that maximal packing is achieved. The speed of the centrifuge and the accuracy of the timer must be checked and recorded at least once a week.
2. If the red cells are normal in size and shape, the trapped plasma, platelets, and white cells amount to about 3% of the microhematocrit red cell column. If the cells are pathologic in size and shape (sickle cells, macrocytes, microcytes, spherocytes, schistocytes, etc.), the amount of trapped plasma increases to 6% or over.[30]
3. Nelson[31] mentions that the hematocrit is an unreliable indicator of anemia immediately following blood loss or transfusions.

Automated methods

The automated methods are based on sizing of red cells in an electronic particle counter, on the conductivity of blood, or on automated centrifugation. The automated hematocrit values are lower than those obtained by the micromethod and the macromethod because plasma trapping is eliminated, and therefore they show excellent reproducibility.

ERYTHROCYTE CORPUSCULAR INDICES OR CONSTANT

On the basis of the erythrocyte count and hemoglobin and hematocrit values, characteristics of individual red cells (i.e., the red cell indices) can be formulated, which aid in the diagnosis of anemias. Electronically obtained values of red cell indices reproduce within ± 2% limits 95% of the time, but they apply only to relatively homogeneous cell populations. In cases of mixed cell populations, e.g., in sideroblastic anemias, in which a mixture of hypochromic and normochromic cells is encountered, the red cell constants may not convey the true red cell picture, so that the red cell indices must always be confirmed by examination of the peripheral blood smear.[32]

Mean corpuscular volume

The MCV is the volume of the average red cell in a given sample of blood. It is calculated as follows:

$$\frac{\text{Hct (\%)} \times 10}{\text{RBCs (million/mm}^3)} = \text{MCV } (\mu m^3 \text{ or femtoliters [fl])}^{33}$$

The normal value is 90 ± 8 μm^3 or fl.

MCV values below 82 μm^3 are indicative of microcytosis, whereas values higher than 100 μm^3 indicate macrocytosis. The hematocrit value obtained by centrifugation differs from the Coulter S hematocrit, because the first contains significant amounts of trapped plasma and thus leads to falsely elevated MCV (hematocrit per red cells) and falsely low MCHC (hemoglobin per hematocrit) values. Electronically obtained hematocrit values are independent of the amounts of trapped plasma and of the concentration of anticoagulants and thus favor accurate MCV and MCHC values.[30] The modulation of the electric current by nonconductive red cells as they pass through the aperture of electronic particle counters is determined mainly by the cell membrane. The magnitude of the modulation is proportional to the cellular volume. Some evidence indicates that injury to the cell membrane may lead to errors in the electronic volume measurements.[34] The electronic measurement of the erythrocyte volume makes it possible to detect microcytosis and macrocytosis[35] before anemia develops and before these changes can be detected by visual examination of the blood smear, since the automated equipment is more sensitive to size changes than is the human eye.[9,36] The MCV may be spuriously high in the presence of high-titer cold agglutinins because of clumping of the red cells. This error can be prevented by using a diluent warmed to 37° C, a procedure that requires recalibration of the Coulter Model S.[37]

Automatic erythrocyte volume distribution pattern by electronic cell counters

The cell size distribution pattern formerly was determined by the tedious, slow, and inaccurate Price-Jones method, which produced a symmetric, bell-shaped distribution curve of the normal red cells. The erythrocyte volume distribution curve as measured by an aperture counter is skewed to the right,[38] a phenomenon that may result from a preponderance of young red cells or from an artifact directly related to the aperture counting device. The pulse height depends not only on the cell volume but also on the orientation of the cell in the electric field, its shape, and its location in the aperture. In the center of the electric field the particle path is shorter than in the periphery of the field along the wall of the aperture. Despite these drawbacks the electronically measured volume distribution pattern is far superior and faster than the manual methods used in the past. The introduction of a long-pulse rejector (LPR), an electronic module that eliminates all signals except the ones originating from the erythrocytes flowing in the aperture core, reduces the artifacts related to the flow dynamics of the electronic field.[39] The Coulter Model S⁺ uses the Price-Jones principle to create a red cell distribution width (RCDW) parameter, but instead

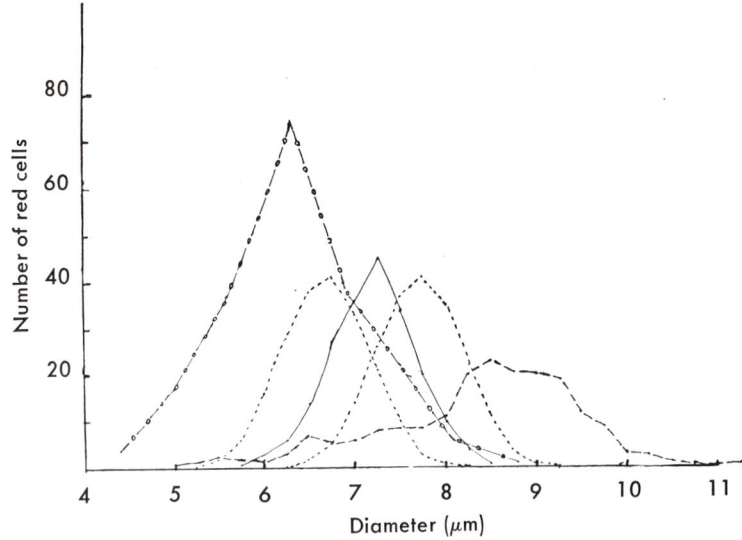

Fig. 7-10. Price-Jones curves. Red cell diameters. o-o-o, Chronic hemolytic jaundice curve superimposed on Price-Jones curves modified by plotting 200 cells. Solid line, the normal mean; dotted lines, the normal range; broken line, a case of pernicious anemia. (Chronic hemolytic jaundice curve from Cheney, W.F., and Cheney, G.: Am. J. Med. Sci. **187:**191, 1934; remaining curves from Price-Jones: Red blood cell diameters, London, 1933, Oxford University Press, Inc.)

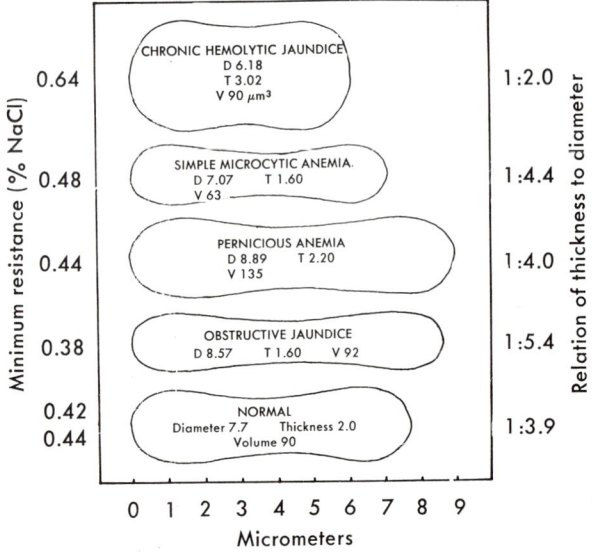

Fig. 7-11. Cross section and measurements of mean erythrocyte in different clinical conditions. (From Haden, R.L.: Am. J. Med. Sci. **188:**441, 1934.)

of measuring the erythrocytic diameter, which is only an indicator of cell size and volume (and not a good one), it records the mean erythrocyte volume and supplies a red cell size distribution curve. Normal red cells produce a gaussian bell-shaped distribution curve, with the peak at 7-7.5 μm. Hemolytic anemias and severe iron deficiency anemias produce a shift to the left of the Price-Jones curve, whereas pernicious anemia produces a shift to the right (Fig. 7-10).

An impression of the mean diameter of red cells can be obtained by careful examination of the peripheral blood smear and is indeed an important part of the smear evaluation.

Mean corpuscular hemoglobin

The MCH is the amount of hemoglobin by weight in the average red cell of the sample of blood. Its value is based on the following formula:

$$\frac{\text{Hb (g/dl)} \times 10}{\text{RBCs (million/mm}^3)} = \text{MCH (pg)}$$

The normal value is 30 ± 4 pg. A factor of 0.0155 converts this figure to femtomoles.

The formulas for MCV and MCH have the same denominator (RBC) and are thus essentially expressing a relationship between hematocrit and hemoglobin. MCV (based on the hematocrit) is normally three times the MCH (based on hemoglobin).[32]

Mean corpuscular hemoglobin concentration

The MCHC is the concentration of hemoglobin (weight per volume) in the average red cell of the sample of blood. It is calculated as follows:

$$\frac{\text{Hb (g/dl)} \times 100}{\text{Hct (\%)}} = \text{MCHC (\% or g/dl)}$$

The normal value is 34% ± 3%. A factor of 0.01 converts this figure to SI units.

In hypochromia the MCHC is lower than normal. "Hyperchromia" of a normal sized erythrocyte is not possible, because the normal red cell contains the maximal amount of hemoglobin.

Value of blood indices

Differences in size of erythrocytes and in the concentration and amount of hemoglobin in each erythrocyte form the basis of a clinically useful and widely accepted morphologic classification of anemias[40] (Fig. 7-11). Blood indices may be chosen as parameters of a quality control system in hematology (see Chapter 1).

BLOOD VOLUME

The measurement of total circulating blood volume is of clinical value in selected surgical and medical patients to determine the type of therapy for blood or plasma loss or overload. The indications include preoperative and postoperative patient evaluation, trauma, chronic or acute blood loss, shock, burns, polycythemia, and anemia. Despite some clear indications blood volume determinations have fallen into disuse because the results are difficult to interpret and technical errors and poor technic may lead to inconsistent results.[41] The

total blood volume is the sum of the red cell volume plus the plasma volume.

Total red cell volume

The total red cell volume (TRCV) may be measured by using ^{51}Cr as an isotope label for the patient's own (autologous) cells. An aliquot of the patient's red cells is incubated with ^{51}Cr for a short period, and a measured amount is injected into the patient's bloodstream after the excess (not-bound-to-red-cells) isotope has been removed by washing of the cells. Since mixing is complete after about 3 min, the first patient sample is obtained 15 min after injection and the amount of isotope in the red cells is measured. As the red cells pool in an enlarged spleen and delay adequate mixing, several samples must be obtained 10 min apart from patients with splenomegaly to ensure complete mixing.[42] The difference between the 3 min and 30 min volume is a measure of the blood trapped and pooled in the spleen.

The TRCV is calculated as follows:

$$\text{TRCV} = \frac{\text{Vd}}{\text{C}}$$

where Vd = measured dose of isotope injected, and C = concentration of dose measured after dilution by unknown volume.

Normal values: The average normal values for TRCV are as follows:

Men: 29 ml/kg
Women: 25 ml/kg

Physiologic variations: The red cell volume is increased in newborns, during pregnancy, and in high altitudes.

Plasma volume

The plasma volume is measured with ^{125}I-labeled albumin.[43]

Normal values: The average plasma volume in men and women is 35-45 ml/kg.

Physiologic variations: The plasma volume is increased in newborns and during pregnancy and is decreased after prolonged bed rest and in high altitudes.

Total blood volume

The total blood volume is the sum of the red cell and plasma volumes, which may be measured simultaneously by tagging the red cells with ^{51}Cr and the plasma with ^{125}I-labeled albumin.

Method of simultaneous red cell mass and plasma volume determination using ^{51}Cr-tagged red cells and ^{125}I-labeled albumin[44]

Principle: If ^{125}I-labeled albumin is used as the plasma tag together with ^{51}Cr as the red cell tag, the two isotopes can be quantitated satisfactorily in the same specimen by simultaneously measuring the radioactivity of plasma and the red cells in a well counter with two pulse-height analyzers.

The method is based on the dilution principle, which was utilized prior to the advent of radioindicators in the Evans blue dye test for estimating blood volume. If a known quantity of material (activity of injected material) is added to an unknown volume, the amount of material in a given volume after dilution (activity of diluted sample) is directly proportional to the unknown volume. Therefore the unknown volume may be calculated by the following formula:

$$\frac{\text{Activity of diluted sample}}{\text{Activity of injected material}} = \frac{\text{Volume of diluted sample}}{\text{Unknown total volume}}$$

or:

Unknown total volume = Volume of diluted sample ×

$$\frac{\text{Activity of injected material}}{\text{Activity of diluted sample}}$$

Procedure: Obtain 15 ml venous blood. Inject 10 ml into a sterile siliconized collecting bottle containing modified ACD solution (Mallinckrodt Chemical Works, St. Louis). Inject 5 ml into an EDTA solution to obtain a background sample. Add 45 μCi sodium chromate ^{51}Cr to ACD bottle. (The average concentration is 3 μCi/ml.) Incubate the solution at room temperature for 15 min, and add 50 mg ascorbic acid to stop further tagging.

Dilute 5 ml ^{125}I-labeled albumin in sterile normal saline solution to 2 μCi/ml. Inject intravenously into the patient 10 ml tagged red cell mixture and, through the same needle, the diluted tagged albumin. Wait 15 min and collect 7 ml venous blood in EDTA solution from the opposite arm. Dilute 1 ml of this blood in 1 dl normal saline solution to obtain the whole blood ^{51}Cr standard. Centrifuge 3 ml EDTA blood. Dilute 1 ml plasma in 1 dl normal saline solution to provide the plasma ^{125}I standard. Determine the hematocrit of the EDTA blood. One milliliter EDTA blood serves as the whole blood sample. Mix 5 ml albumin solution with 1 dl normal saline solution to provide the albumin standard. Centrifuge 3 ml premixed EDTA blood to obtain 1 ml plasma sample and also the patient's hematocrit. Use 1 ml background blood as the whole blood background sample; 1 ml background plasma also serves as the plasma background sample. Count all samples under the above conditions and correct to net counts per minute per milliliter.

Calculation: The final formula for arriving at the red cell and plasma volumes is based on the following formula:

$$V = \frac{N}{n} \times v$$

where V = total unknown volume, N = activity of injected material, n = activity of sample, and v = volume of sample.

Normal values: The normal values for total blood volume are as follows:

Men: 61.5 ± 8.5 ml/kg
Women: 59.0 ± 5 ml/kg
Infants: 77.0 ml/kg

Physiologic variations: The blood volume is elevated in infancy and in pregnancy.

Interpretation (Fig 7-12):

Hypervolemia: Excessive volume occurs in congestive heart failure, overtransfusion, primary aldosteronism, polycythemia vera, and Cushing's syndrome.

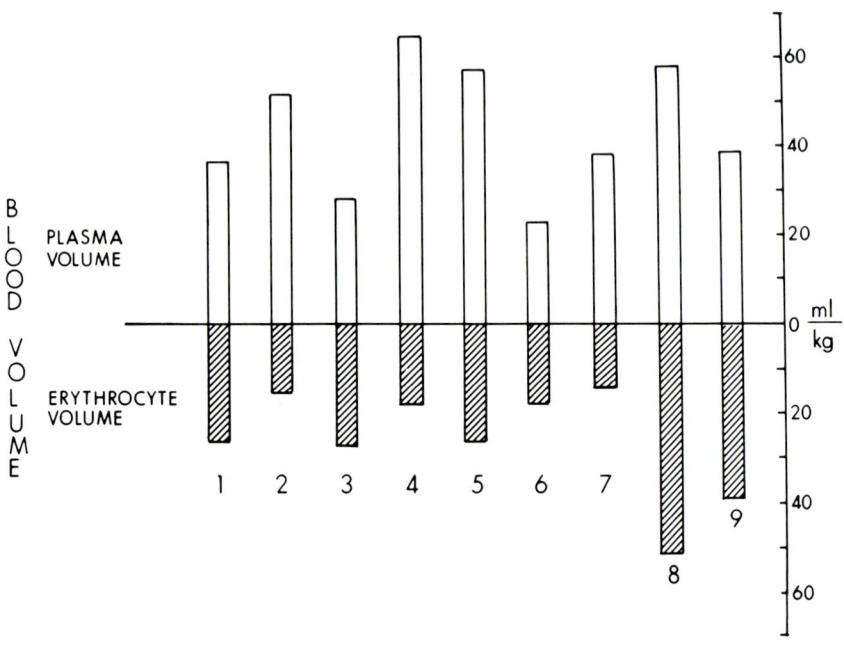

Fig. 7-12. Blood volume determination under normal and abnormal conditions.

1 Normal values
2 Anemia
3 Hemoconcentration
4 Anemia plus increased plasma volume
5 Anemia caused by increased plasma volume
6 Acute blood loss (hypovolemia)
7 Anemia with normal plasma volume
8 Polycythemia vera
9 Erythrocytosis

Hypovolemia: An abnormally decreased volume appears in severe hemorrhage, severe burns, severe diarrhea, nephrotic syndrome, peritoneal dialysis, and surgical shock.

• • •

Blood volume determinations are of value in the following situations:
1. To evaluate blood and fluid losses during major surgical procedures and following trauma (burns)
2. To serve as a guide in preoperative and postoperative transfusion therapy
3. To evaluate gastrointestinal and uterine bleeding
4. To aid in the diagnosis of hypovolemic shock
5. To aid in the diagnosis of polycythemia vera

Discussion[45]: The isotope tracer–dilution technics make several assumptions: (1) that the blood volume remains relatively steady during measurement, (2) that the mixing time is shorter than the clearance time of the isotope from the bloodstream, (3) that uniform mixing and distribution are achieved before blood samples are obtained, and (4) that blood volume correlates with the lean body mass.

Autologous red cells tagged with ^{51}Cr are well confined to the vascular system, show little loss of label during the first 30-60 min, and therefore represent a suitable system for the measurement of red cell volume. The same considerations do not apply to ^{131}I-labeled albumin used to measure the plasma volume, because it is subject to rapid loss from the bloodstream through diffusion from the capillaries into interstitial spaces. To prevent this loss, labeling of larger protein molecules, e.g., fibrinogen, paraproteins, and most recently ^{113m}In-labeled transferrin, has been suggested.[46]

In normal individuals the mixing time of labeled erythrocytes and albumin is about 3-5 min, and there is an insignificant loss of the isotope label of red cells or of albumin, but under pathologic conditions the mixing time may be prolonged, the albumin loss rapid, and the distribution of tagged red cells variable and erratic.[47]

In healthy individuals of ideal weight the blood volume correlates fairly well with the lean tissue mass, which is approximately 75% of the actual weight of women and 80% of the weight of men,[47] but even under physiologic conditions, blood volume is affected by plasma volume determinants, e.g., capillary permeability, plasma proteins, and hormones (aldosterone and antidiuretic hormone), and by red cell volume determinants, e.g., rate and adequacy of erythropoiesis, red cell life span,[45] and hormones (testosterone).

Errors in blood volume determinations[48]
1. Single tag methods measure dilutions and must be corrected for blood volume. The calculated values of red cell and plasma volumes represent approximations only.
2. Blood volume is not a constant but a dynamic equilibrium that may be difficult to correctly interpret.
3. Inadequate mixing time leads to erroneous results.
4. Mistakes in the administration of the tracer, spill-

age of the tracer, and incorrect sampling are responsible for most technical errors.

HEMATOLOGIC VALUES IN INFANTS AND CHILDREN

The red cell count at birth has a mean value of 5.7 million/mm^3 blood (hematocrit, 56.6 vol%). The count drops progressively within the first 4 months to about 4.5 million/mm^3 (hematocrit, 36.5 vol%) and then gradually rises to about 4.6 million/mm^3 (hematocrit, 35.2 vol%) the first year and to 4.7 million/mm^3 (hematocrit, 35.5 vol%) the second year. By the tenth year the average value is 4.8 million/mm^3 (hematocrit, 39.0 vol%) (Table 7-4 and Fig. 7-8).

The average hemoglobin value of 21.5 g/dl blood at birth falls rapidly to 13.3 g/dl at the end of the second month. It then hovers around 12 g/dl until the end of the first year and may drop even lower in the second and third year (11.5 g/dl). After the fourth year it begins to rise, reaching 13.0 g/dl at the end of the tenth year.

The MCV is highest at birth, 106 μm^3, at which time the red cells have the greatest diameter (8.6 μm). In the first year of life the MCV drops to the lowest level of 77 μm^3 and gradually rises to the adult level of 87 μm^3 at age 14 years or older.

The MCH drops from 38 pg to its lowest value of 25 pg in the first or second years, reaching normal levels of 29 pg at puberty.

The MCHC drops from an initial 38% to the adult level of approximately 34% at about 4 months of age.

The white cell count (Table 7-6) is high at birth, about 18,000/mm^3. It rises to about 22,000/mm^3 during the first 12 hr and drops to about the original level after 24 hr. It then falls rapidly during the first week to about 12,000/mm^3. At age 1 year the count is approximately 11,500/mm^3. Adult values are reached between the ages of 4 and 10 years.

The differential count shows a neutrophilic leukocytosis at birth of about 61% and at age 12 hr of 68%. Having reached this height, the percentage of granulocytes continues to drop, reaching a low level of 30% at about 10 months of age, after which it slowly rises to adult levels. The drop in granulocytes is accompanied by a progressive lymphocytosis, which gradually increases from a birth level of 31% (falling after 12 hr to 24%) to about 63% at 10 months of age. The number of monocytes is also increased in the early weeks of life.

At birth the reticulocyte count is about 4.5%; this rapidly falls to below 1% within 1-2 weeks. After about 3 weeks, reticulocyte counts show a slow rise to the adult level of just over 1%.

The platelet count in the first few days of life reveals about 100,000-300,000 platelets/mm^3 (although marked variations may occur). After 1 week, the number of platelets reaches the adult range.

The average blood volume at birth is 88 ml/kg body weight. The volume is somewhat higher if cord clamping is delayed. Within 1 month the blood volume adjusts itself to the adult level.

The bone marrow in the first day of life shows marked normoblastic hyperplasia (predominantly with orthochromatic normoblasts), so that the erythroid/myeloid ratio is about 1:1.5. After about 1 week, the erythroid/myeloid ratio becomes 1:6.5, and after 2 months, the adult ratio of 1:3.5 is established. Plasma cells are scarce in the marrow of newborns.

ERYTHROCYTE SEDIMENTATION RATE

The erythrocyte sedimentation rate (ESR) measures the rate of settling of erythrocytes in their native anticoagulated plasma. Sedimentation occurs in three stages[49]: (1) rouleaux formation, (2) sinking of rouleaux at a constant speed, and (3) slowing of sedimentation as the cells begin to pack.

The length of the fall of the meniscus of the red cell column (measured from the plasma meniscus) in a unit time is the ESR.

Mechanism of erythrocyte sedimentation rate

The erythrocytes in suspension repel each other because of their negatively charged surface sialic acid[50] (the ζ-potential), but increasing amounts of asymmetric macroglobulins, mainly fibrinogen and to a lesser extent gammaglobulins,[51] weaken the repellent forces between adjacent erythrocytes, so that rouleaux and aggregate formation take places. Since the red cell rouleaux and aggregates have a relatively large volume, they sediment faster than single cells.

The ESR depends on several factors[52]:

1. Plasma factors: Proteins other than fibrinogen and γ-globulins also influence the ESR; some like albumin retard it, whereas others like α- and β-globulins increase it. The fact that fibrinogen is one of the **acute-phase reactants** (the other elements being haptoglobin, transferrin, ceruloplasmin, C-reactive protein, α_1-antitrypsin, α_1-acid glycoprotein, and α_2-macroglobulin) robs the test of its diagnostic specificity and renders it responsive and sensitive to a wide variety of abnormal states. Increasing IgM levels in macroglobulinemia are responsible for maximal rouleaux formation and, at the same time, for increasing plasma viscosity. The latter tends to retard the ESR and may eventually reach a point where the viscosity exceeds the accelerating protein effect, so that a normal or near normal ESR results. The occurrence of rouleaux formation associated with normal or near normal ESR suggests the **hyperviscosity syndrome**.[52,53] Monoclonal gammopathy as seen in plasma cell–lymphoproliferative disorders stimulates rouleaux formation, thus accelerating the ESR.

2. Red cell factors: The size and number of erythrocytes play a minor role in the ESR. When normal cells sediment, the downward force is almost counterbalanced by the upward forces[54] generated by the plasma and the confines of the sedimentation tube. Changes in the shape and size of red cells, e.g., in microcytosis, anisocytosis, poikilocytosis, sickling, and acanthocytosis, interfere with their ability to form rouleaux and aggregates and thus slow the sedimentation rate.[55] Macrocytosis[56,57] and anemia[58] accelerate the ESR, whereas polycythemia causes it to slow down

considerably. Heparin accelerates the rate of the fall of the erythrocytes.[59]

3. Physical factors: The temperature, size, and bore of tube and the angle of the tube during the test influence the ESR.

Measurement of erythrocyte sedimentation rate

The International Committee for Standardization in Hematology (ICSH) has standardized the Westergren method,[60] because the Wintrobe method has major drawbacks, e.g., the 100 mm tube length and the narrow bore, which limit readings in excess of 60 mm/hr because of packing of red cells.

Reagent and equipment:
1. Sodium citrate solution
2. Westergren tube (disposable, glass)
3. Tube-holding device

Procedure: Collect venous blood in a sodium citrate tube and mix it well. Perform the test within 2 hr, or within 6 hr if the blood is kept at 4° C. Draw the blood to the 200 mm level in the Westergren tube, place it in a strictly vertical rack, and leave it undisturbed. At the end of 1 hr measure the height of the clear plasma above the red cell column. The height is an expression of the rate of the fall of the red cells and is expressed as millimeters in the first hour.[60]

Normal values[49]: The normal values for men given in Westergren units per millimeter per hour are as follows:

17-50 yr: 4 ± 3
51-60 yr: 6 ± 3
> 60 yr: 6 ± 4

The normal values for women are as follows:

17-50 yr: 6 ± 3
51-60 yr: 9 ± 5
> 60 yr: 10 ± 5

Interpretation: Physiologically the ESR is elevated in pregnancy, in the puerperium, and in 10% of apparently normal children.[49]

The test is nonspecific but sensitive to inflammation, tissue injury, and lymphoproliferative disorders. It has been labeled outdated because of its lack of specificity, but clinically a normal ESR gives the assurance that the conditions detected by an abnormal ESR are not present,[61] though there are reasons to prefer the C-reactive protein test[62] over the ESR.

The ESR is increased in the following conditions:

1. Infections, e.g., tuberculosis, pelvic inflammatory disease, systemic lupus erythematosus, and rheumatoid and pyogenic arthritis, because of the increase in immunoglobulins and acute-phase reactants (fibrinogen, haptoglobins, transferrin, ceruloplasmin, and α_2-macroglobulins)

2. Relative increase of globulins: conditions that lead to loss of albumin and thus to a relative increase of globulins, e.g., kidney disease, chronic liver disease, and enteritis

3. Absolute increase of globulins, e.g., multiple myeloma, cryoglobulinemia, macroglobulinemia, and lymphomas

4. Extensive tissue necrosis, as seen in malignant tumors and in myocardial infarction

5. Other conditions, e.g., pregnancy (increase in fi-

brinogen), menstruation, lead poisoning (anemia?), and cirrhosis (In cirrhosis, depression of albumin production is associated with a polyclonal globulin increase. Severe hypofibrinogenemia may counteract the accelerated ESR.)

6. Coombs'-positive hemolytic anemia (The globulin-coated cells exhibit an increased tendency to agglomerate.)

7. Unexplained causes (On rare occasions, especially in elderly patients, elevated levels may be found.[63])

The ESR is normal or near normal in the following conditions:

1. Hematologic disorders, e.g., infectious mononucleosis
2. Localized infection
3. Benign neoplasms

The ESR is decreased in the following conditions:

1. Polycythemia vera (may even be zero)
2. Sickle cell anemia
3. Some forms of macroglobulinemia, e.g., hyperviscosity syndrome

ζ-Sedimentation rate

The ζ-sedimentation rate (ZSR) is a measure of the degree of packing of the erythrocytes of a blood sample contained in a vertically oriented, special, quantitated pipet subjected to four 45 sec cycles of dispersion and compaction.[51] The hematocrit of the red cells, representing the standardized, modified sedimentation rate, is expressed as vol% (milliliters per deciliter). The method requires a special instrument, the Zetafuge (Coulter Electronics, Hialeah, Fla.), but has several advantages over the Westergren method: (1) it is unaffected by anemia; (2) it is linearly related to increases in fibrinogen and/or γ-globulin; (3) the normal range is the same for men and women; (4) the test is performed in micro quantities; (5) 6 samples can be handled in 3 min; and (6) temperature and age of sample do not affect the test.

The normal range is 40-51 ml/dl.

RETICULOCYTE COUNT

The extrusion of the nucleus of the orthochromatic normoblast transforms it into the reticulocyte, which through its motility spills by diapedesis into the bone marrow sinusoids and into the circulation. It owes its name to a tinctorial artifact, because the vital dyes used for its demonstration kill it and precipitate the intracytoplasmic organelles, e.g., mitrochondria and ribosomal and residual RNA, and conjure up a filamentous intercytoplasmic reticulum.

Manual method
Unopette technic

Principle: Equal volumes of blood and stain are incubated, and smears are made of the mixture. For mode of action of dye see above.

Reagent and equipment:

1. Stain (Unopette dropper bottle containing 7 ml diluent mixture, 5 g new methylene blue N, 16 g potassium oxalate, and distilled water to make 1 L)
2. Unopette capillary pipet, 25 μl

Dilution ratio of blood-dye mixture is 1:1.

Procedure: Mix 1 drop fresh capillary or anticoagulated venous blood with equal amounts of stain on microscope slide. Aspirate the blood-dye mixture into the capillary pipet and cover the pipet with a shield. Allow the mixture to stand at room temperature for 10 min.

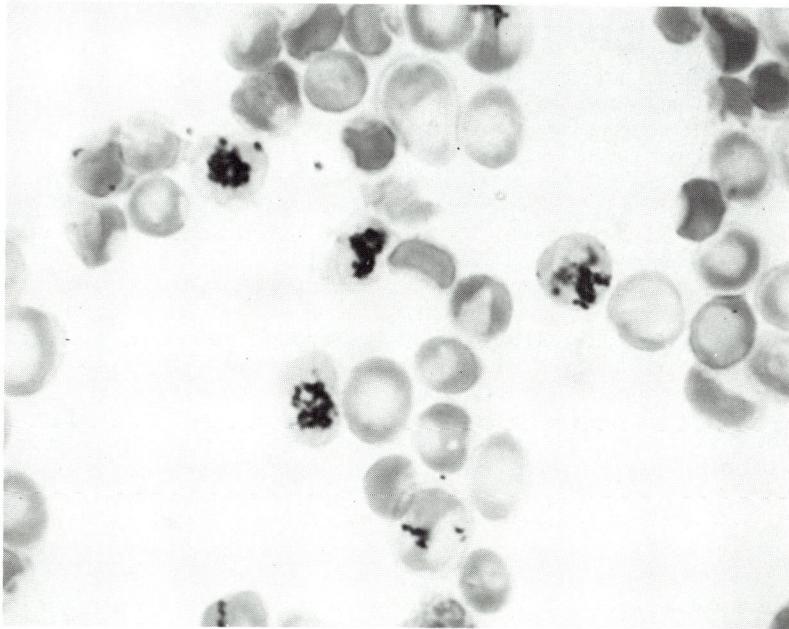

Fig. 7-13. Reticulocytes stained with methylene blue.

Prepare thin coverslip preparations of blood-dye mixture using 1 small drop of mixture and allowing it to air dry after spreading. Count 1000 red cells in consecutive oil immersion fields and record the number of cells that contain dark blue material in granules or strands (Fig. 7-13). The enumeration of reticulocytes in 1000 erythrocytes is adequate for high reticulocyte counts, but for low counts 2000 or more cells must be examined.

Calculations:
1. Determine percent of reticulocytes by using the following formula:

$$\text{Reticulocytes (\%)} = \frac{\text{Reticulocytes counted in 1000 RBCs}}{10}$$

The normal values are as follows:
Adult: 0.5-1.5%
At birth: 2.5-6.0%

2. Determine absolute reticulocyte count by using the following formula:

Absolute reticulocyte count =

$$\frac{\text{Reticulocytes (\%)}}{100} \times \text{Red cell count (cells/mm}^3)$$

The normal value is 60,000 mm³. The absolute count expresses the number of reticulocytes present in 1 mm³ blood rather than the number as a percentage of red cells, which is subject to change.

Automated reticulocyte counting method

Because of the inaccuracy of the blood film method, flow microfluorometry has been adapted to count several thousand reticulocytes in seconds. The method is based on the selective staining of the RNA reticulum with acridine orange, which fluoresces when exposed to ultraviolet light.[64]

The Hematrak Automated Differential system has an automated reticulocyte identification feature incorporated.

Discussion[65,66]: Reticulocytes are young, newly produced polychromatic, macrocytic red cells that contain residual cytoplasmic RNA and organelles that fail to stain with Wright-Giemsa stain but are visualized when treated with vital dyes, e.g., new methylene blue. The reticulocyte count loosely reflects the erythropoietic activity of the bone marrow. Stimulated effective erythropoiesis as seen in some hemolytic anemias and in erythropoietin stimulation leads to an elevated reticulocyte count, whereas ineffective erythropoiesis, as seen in pernicious anemia, thalassemia, and sideroblastic anemia, is responsible for a decreased, normal, or only slightly raised reticulocyte count. The latter is in sharp contrast to the erythroid hyperplasia of the bone marrow.

Reticulocyte index

The reticulocyte-erythropoiesis relationship is not absolute, because probably some of the young, too-soon-released bone marrow reticulocytes are destroyed by the spleen when they enter the circulation.[67] The younger the reticulocyte, the more filamentous and plentiful is the reticulum, whereas in the older reticulocyte a single small dot represents a reticular remnant.

According to the degree of maturation and the pattern of the reticulum, reticulocytes can be divided into four groups, group I being the youngest and group IV the most mature (Fig. 7-14).

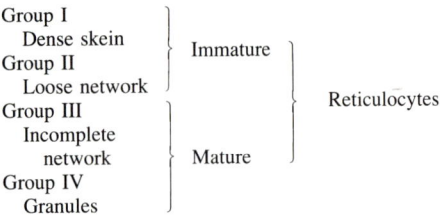

The prematurely released reticulocytes are called **stress or shift reticulocytes**. The reticulum normally disappears after the cells have spent their first day in the peripheral circulation. If there is increased erythropoietin stimulation, the residual RNA is increased and requires 2 or 2½ days to disappear. If the reticulocyte count is used to evaluate the erythropoiesis, it must be corrected for the red cell count and the reticulocyte maturation time.[68]

The first correction for the patient's red cell count is arrived at as follows:

Corrected reticulocyte count =

$$\text{Reticulocytes (\%)} \times \frac{\text{Patient's Hct}}{45 \text{ (normal Hct)}}$$

To arrive at the **reticulocyte index** the second correction makes allowance for the erythropoietin-induced shortened bone marrow maturation time and the lengthened peripheral blood maturation time of the reticulocytes (Table 7-5). This is accomplished by dividing the result of the first correction by an empiric figure arrived at experimentally or by multiplying the hematocrit by a factor derived from a nomogram (Fig. 7-15).

The formula is as follows:

Reticulocyte index =

$$\frac{\text{Reticulocyte count (\%)} \times \dfrac{\text{Patient's Hct}}{45 \text{ (normal Hct)}}}{2 \text{ (reticulocyte maturation time)}}$$

Interpretation: The reticulocyte index gives a numeric value to the hematopoietic stimulation over and above normal baseline activity, e.g., two times basal activity.

Elaborate corrections do not alter the fact that considerable error (±2% in low counts and up to ±7% in high counts) and lack of reproducibility are inherent in the reticulocyte count.

Variations in number:

Increased count: The reticulocyte count is increased in response to (1) hemorrhage (acute and chronic), (2) treatment of iron deficiency and of vitamin B_{12} and folic acid deficiency anemias (Figs. 7-16 and 7-17), and (3) chronic and acute hemolysis. In hemolytic crises of hemolytic anemias the reticulocyte count may reach 40% or higher.

Decreased count: The diminished reticulocyte count indicates a decreased rate of red cell production as seen in aplastic anemias and in aplastic crises of hemolytic anemias. In general a low peripheral reticulocyte count

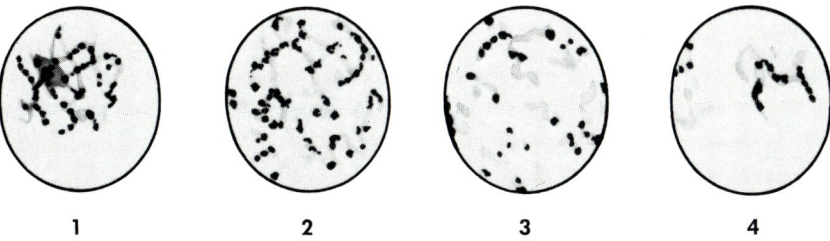

Fig. 7-14. Classification of reticulocytes according to density of reticulum. **1,** Youngest cell. **4,** Oldest cell.

Table 7-5. Maturation correction

Hematocrit (%)	Maturation time (d)
45	1.0
35	1.5
25	2.0
15	2.5

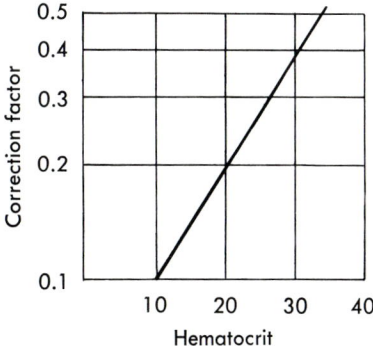

Fig. 7-15. Nomogram showing relationship of hematocrit to reticulocyte index correction factor.

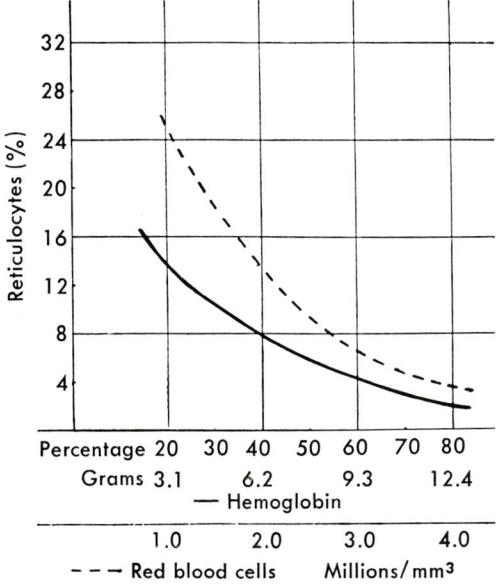

Fig. 7-16. Expected reticulocyte rise on iron deficiency anemia after administration of iron, showing relation of response to hemoglobin and red cell levels. (From Heath, C.W.: Arch. Intern. Med. **51:**459, 1933.)

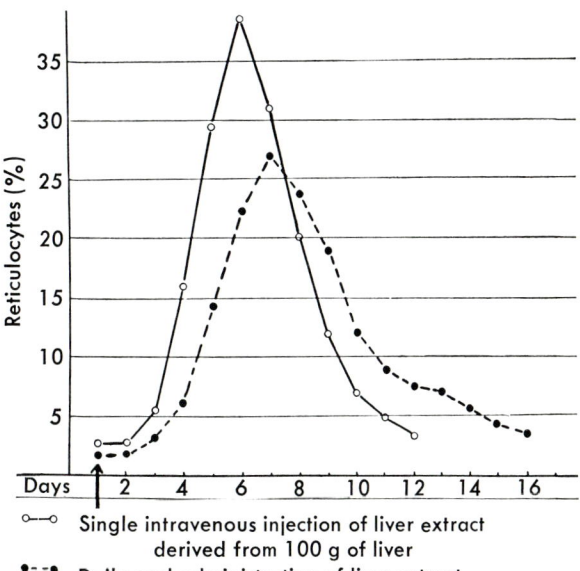

Fig. 7-17. Average reticulocyte response in pernicious anemia to liver extract by single injection (13 cases) and by uniform oral daily doses (20 cases). Average red cell count 1.2 million/mm^3. (From Minot, G.R.: Trans. Assoc. Am. Physicians **49:**287, 1934.)

carries a greater degree of inaccuracy than does a high count. A low count may therefore be misleading, suggesting an unfounded diagnosis of erythroid hypoplasia or aplasia.

LEUKOCYTE COUNTS

The total leukocyte count enumerates all types of nucleated cells in the peripheral blood, the white cells and the nucleated red cells.

Manual counts

The manual method is not suggested for everyday white cell counts, but it must be available (1) for confirmation of severely leukopenic and leukemic counts performed by multichannel analyzers, (2) as a backup method in an emergency, and (3) as a poor (and not recommended) quality control procedure for automated counts.

Unopette technic

Equipment:
1. Unopette reservoir no. 5856 containing 0.475 ml diluent mixture—28.6 ml glacial acetic acid in water to make 1 L. The acetic acid hemolyzes red cells but does not affect white cells and nucleated red cells, which are thus counted together with white cells.
2. Capillary pipet, 25 μl. A 1:20 dilution ratio is obtained when volume of sample drawn into capillary pipet is mixed with diluting fluid in reservoir.
3. Hemocytometer (Neubauer) and coverslip.

Procedure: Fill the capillary pipet with capillary or EDTA-anticoagulated venous blood. Dilute the specimen with reservoir fluid and allow to stand 10 min to hemolyze the erythrocytes. Convert to dropper assembly and fill both sides of the hemocytometer. Focus under low-power magnification with the condenser lowered. Adjust the light so that the leukocytes appear as round, slightly iridescent bodies with a definite outline. If there is doubt as to whether an object is a leukocyte or an artifact, examine it under high magnification. Leukocytes have definite cell outlines and well-defined nuclei. Platelets appear as very small refractive bodies about one fifth to one seventh the size of leukocytes, have no nuclei, and exhibit slight Brownian movement. Occasionally ghost outlines of red cells may be seen.

Enumerate cells in four large corner 1 mm squares (W), each of which is divided into 16 smaller squares for convenience in counting. Enumeration should follow the pattern described for erythrocyte counting. Include in the count those leukocytes that are half in and half out of the upper and left-hand lines but not those half in and half out of the lower and right-hand lines. Enumerate cells in four corner squares of ruled area (Fig. 7-18).

Calculation: Calculate the number of leukocytes per cubic millimeter undiluted blood by multiplying the to-

tal number of leukocytes in four corner squares by 50. The factor 50 is based on the formula shown at the bottom of the page.

Normal values: The normal value is 4000-11,000 WBCs/mm^3. A factor of 10^6 converts these figures to cells per liter. For normal range of leukocyte count at different ages, during pregnancy, and in children see Tables 7-6 and 7-7 and Fig. 7-19. Also consult the following interpretation.

Interpretation: Because the main white cell groups, e.g., neutrophils, eosinophils, basophils, monocytes, and lymphocytes, represent physiologically independent systems under varying controls, it is difficult to define a normal white cell count. The lower limits of the leukocyte count may be depressed to 2000 cells/mm^3 in white individuals and to 1500 cells/mm^3 in blacks[69,70] and still be within physiologic limits. The count is not only influenced by race but also by age and somewhat by sex. As neutrophils make up a major sector of the total white cell count, their fluctuations materially affect the result of the total count. The neutrophilic peripheral blood pool is visualized as having two compartments, the **circulating** and the **marginal pools**. The first is evaluated by the peripheral blood count and represents about 50% of the available peripheral white cells. It is in constant flux, because a rapid exchange occurs from one pool to the other. Demargination of neutrophils is encouraged by epinephrine, stress, exercise, time of day, exposure to light, postprandial state, lithium, and inflammation, whereas margination is favored by anesthetics, barbiturates, and tranquilizers. White cell counts should be repeated at the same time with the patient in basal condition.

Procedure for very low counts: For leukopenia use twice the amount of blood for the leukocyte count. Draw blood up to the 1 mark, dilute to the 11 mark, thus diluting 1:10, and multiply by 12.5.

Procedure for very high counts: For very high leukocyte counts, as in leukemia, make the blood dilution in the red cell pipet. If diluted 1:100, multiply by 125; if the dilution is 1:200, multiply by 250.

If eight large squares are counted, multiply the sum of cells as follows:

If dilution is 1:10:
  Cells counted × 12.5 = Leukocytes/mm^3 blood
If dilution is 1:20:
  Cells counted × 25 = Leukocytes/mm^3 blood
If dilution is 1:100:
  Cells counted × 125 = Leukocytes/mm^3 blood
If dilution is 1:200:
  Cells counted × 250 = Leukocytes/mm^3 blood

Errors in white cell counting procedure

Errors in white cell counts are similar to the errors in red cell counts, although since the dilution used is not as great as in the red cell count, they are not magnified to the same extent.

$$\text{Leukocytes/mm}^3 \text{ blood} = \frac{\text{Cells counted in 4 large squares}}{\text{Area counted} \times \text{Height of chamber} \times \text{Dilution}} = \frac{\text{Counted cells}}{4 \times \frac{1}{10} \times \frac{1}{20}} = \text{Counted cells} \times 50$$

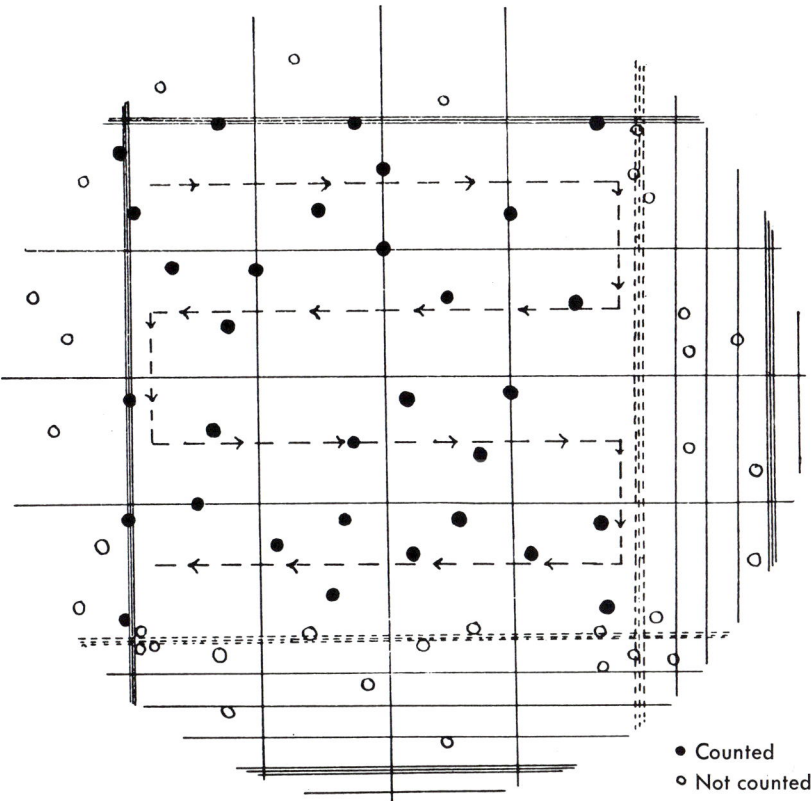

Fig. 7-18. Diagram of white cell count. Square shown, comparable to square 1 shown in Fig. 7-6, is magnified 100 times, using low-power objective of microscope. Order of counting of medium-sized squares is the same as that shown in Fig. 7-7. A white cell is counted only once by counting those within medium-sized square and those touching any line at left and top but not counting those touching any line at right and bottom of medium-sized square. By this procedure, all cells touching triple lines shown as broken lines will be excluded. (From Page, L.B., and Culver, P.J.: A syllabus of laboratory examinations in clinical diagnosis, Cambridge, Mass., 1960, Harvard University Press.)

Table 7-6. Leukocyte values from birth to maturity

Age	Leukocytes (total) (in thousands)	Neutrophils			Eosinophils	Basophils	Lymphocytes	Monocytes
		Total	Band	Segmented				
At birth	18.1 (0.0-30.0)	11.0 (6.0-26.0) 61%	1.65 9.1%	9.4 52%	0.40 (0.02-85) 2.2%	0.10 (0-0.64) 0.6%	5.5 (2.0-11.0) 31%	1.05 (0.40-3.1) 5.8%
12 hr	22.8 (13.0-38.0)	15.5 (6.0-28.0) 68%	2.33 10.2%	13.2 58%	0.45 (0.02-0.95) 2.0%	0.10 (0-0.50) 0.4%	5.5 (2.0-11.0) 24%	1.20 (0.40-3.6) 5.3%
24 hr	18.9 (9.4-34.0)	11.5 (5.0-21.0) 61%	1.75 9.2%	9.8 52%	0.45 (0.05-1.00) 2.4%	0.10 (0-0.30) 0.5%	5.8 (2.0-11.5) 31%	1.10 (0.20-3.1) 5.8%
1 wk	12.2 (5.0-21.0)	5.5 (1.5-10.0) 45%	0.83 6.8%	4.7 39%	0.50 (0.07-1.10) 4.1%	0.05 (0-0.25) 0.4%	5.0 (2.0-17.0) 41%	1.10 (0.30-2.7) 9.1%
2 wk	11.4 (5.0-20.0)	4.5 (1.0-9.5) 40%	0.63 5.5%	3.9 34%	0.35 (0.07-1.00) 3.1%	0.05 (0-0.23) 0.4%	5.5 (2.0-17.0) 48%	1.00 (0.20-2.4) 8.8%
4 wk	10.8 (5.0-19.5)	3.8 (1.0-9.0) 35%	0.49 4.5%	3.3 30%	0.30 (0.07-0.90) 2.8%	0.05 (0-0.20) 0.5%	6.0 (2.5-16.5) 56%	0.70 (0.15-2.0) 6.5%
2 mo	11.0 (5.5-18.0)	3.8 (1.0-9.0) 34%	0.49 4.4%	3.3 30%	0.30 (0.07-0.85) 2.7%	0.05 (0-0.20) 0.5%	6.3 (3.0-16.0) 57%	0.65 (0.13-1.8) 5.9%
4 mo	11.5 (6.0-17.5)	3.8 (1.0-9.0) 33%	0.45 3.9%	3.3 29%	0.30 (0.70-0.80) 2.6%	0.05 (0-0.20) 0.4%	6.8 (3.5-14.5) 59%	0.60 (0.10-1.5) 5.2%
6 mo	11.9 (6.0-17.5)	3.8 (1.0-8.5) 32%	0.45 3.8%	3.3 28%	0.30 (0.07-0.75) 2.5%	0.05 (0-0.20) 0.4%	7.3 (4.0-13.5) 61%	0.58 (0.10-1.3) 4.8%
8 mo	12.2 (6.0-17.5)	3.7 (1.0-8.5) 30%	0.41 3.3%	3.3 27%	0.30 (0.07-0.70) 2.5%	0.05 (0-0.20) 0.4%	7.6 (4.5-12.5) 62%	0.58 (0.08-1.2) 4.7%
10 mo	12.0 (6.0-17.5)	3.6 (1.0-8.5) 30%	0.40 3.3%	3.2 27%	0.30 (0.06-0.70) 2.5%	0.05 (0-0.20) 0.4%	7.5 (4.5-11.5) 63%	0.55 (0.05-1.2) 4.6%

12 mo	11.4 (6.0-17.5)	3.5 (1.5-8.5) 31%	0.35 3.1%	3.2 28%	0.30 (0.05-0.70) 2.6%	0.05 (0-0.20) 0.4%	7.0 (4.0-10.5) 61%	0.55 (0.05-1.1) 4.8%
2 yr	10.6 (6.0-17.0)	3.5 (1.5-8.5) 33%	0.32 3.0%	3.2 30%	0.28 (0.04-0.65) 2.6%	0.05 (0-0.20) 0.5%	6.3 (3.0-9.5) 59%	0.53 (0.05-1.0) 5.0%
4 yr	9.1 (5.5-15.5)	3.8 (1.5-8.5) 42%	0.27 (0-1.0) 3.0%	3.5 (1.5-7.5) 39%	0.25 (0.02-0.65) 2.8%	0.05 (0-0.20) 0.6%	4.5 (2.0-8.0) 50%	0.45 (0-0.8) 5.0%
6 yr	8.5 (5.0-14.5)	4.3 (1.5-8.0) 51%	0.25 (0-1.0) 3.0%	4.0 (1.5-7.0) 48%	0.23 (0-0.65) 2.7%	0.05 (0-0.20) 0.6%	3.5 (1.5-7.0) 42%	0.40 (0-0.8) 4.7%
8 yr	8.3 (4.5-13.5)	4.4 (1.5-8.0) 53%	0.25 (0-1.0) 3.0%	4.1 (1.5-7.0) 50%	0.20 (0-0.50) 2.4%	0.05 (0-0.20) 0.6%	3.3 (1.5-6.8) 39%	0.35 (0-0.8) 4.2%
10 yr	8.1 (4.5-13.5)	4.4 (1.8-8.0) 54%	0.24 (0-1.0) 3.0%	4.2 (1.8-7.0) 51%	0.20 (0-0.60) 2.4%	0.04 (0-0.20) 0.5%	3.1 (1.5-6.5) 38%	0.35 (0-0.8) 4.3%
12 yr	8.0 (4.5-13.5)	4.4 (1.8-80) 55%	0.25 (0-1.0) 3.0%	4.2 (1.8-7.0) 52%	0.20 (0-0.55) 2.5%	0.04 (0-0.20) 0.5%	3.0 (1.2-6.0) 38%	0.35 (0-0.8) 4.4%
14 yr	7.9 (4.5-13.0)	4.4 (1.8-8.0) 56%	0.24 (0-1.0) 3.0%	4.2 (1.8-7.0) 53%	0.20 (0-0.50) 2.5%	0.04 (0-0.20) 0.5%	2.9 (1.2-5.8) 37%	0.38 (0-0.8) 4.7%
16 yr	7.8 (4.5-13.0)	4.4 (1.8-8.0) 57%	0.23 3.0%	4.2 54%	0.20 (0-0.50) 2.6%	0.04 (0-0.20) 0.5%	2.8 (1.2-5.2) 35%	0.40 (0-0.8) 5.1%
18 yr	7.7 (4.5-12.5)	4.4 (1.8-7.7) 57%	0.23 3.0%	4.2 54%	0.20 (0-0.45) 2.6%	0.04 (0-0.20) 0.5%	2.7 (1.0-5.0) 35%	0.40 (0-0.8) 5.2%
20 yr	7.5 (4.5-11.5)	4.4 (1.8-7.7) 59%	0.23 (0-0.7) 3.0%	4.2 (1.8-7.0) 56%	0.20 (0-0.45) 2.7%	0.04 (0-0.20) 0.5%	2.5 (1.0-4.8) 33%	0.38 (0-0.8) 5.0%
21 yr	7.4 (4.5-11.0)	4.4 (1.8-7.7) 59%	0.22 (0-0.7) 3.0%	4.2 (1.8-7.0) 56%	0.20 (0-0.45) 2.7%	0.04 (0-0.20) 0.5%	2.5 (1.0-4.8) 34%	0.30 (0-0.8) 4.0%

From Altman, P.L., and Dittmer, D.S., editors: Blood and other body fluids, Bethesda, Md., 1961, Federation of American Societies for Experimental Biology.

Table 7-7. Leukocyte values in pregnant and postpartum females

Condition	No. of subjects	Leukocytes (total) (thousands/mm³)	Polymorphonuclear cells (%)	Eosinophils (%)	Lymphocytes (%)	Monocytes (%)
Pregnant						
2 mo	12	9.5 (6.8-15.0)	68 (56-71)	1.7 (0.6-7.8)	28 (23-39)	2.0 (0-6)
3 mo	13	10.5 (6.6-14.1)	71 (57-76)	1.5 (0.6-4.8)	23 (17-33)	4.0 (1-8)
4 mo	9	10.3 (7.5-14.6)	71 (65-76)	1.3 (0.2-2.5)	23 (17-30)	2.5 (0-4)
5 mo	16	10.6 (8.9-14.8)	76 (67-88)	1.1 (0.2-2.8)	18 (8-26)	3.0 (1-7)
6 mo	15	11.1 (6.9-17.1)	73 (67-81)	1.3 (0.3-2.9)	21 (10-23)	3.5 (0.8)
7 mo	18	10.5 (6.8-20.3)	77 (69-92)	1.3 (0.3-4.1)	18 (3-25)	2.3 (0-8)
8 mo	17	10.1 (7.5-15.3)	76 (61-88)	1.3 (0.06-3.80)	19 (9-28)	3.0 (0-8)
9 mo	9	10.8 (5.9-14.7)	75 (68-81)	1.2 (0.2-2.2)	18 (12-24)	3.5 (0-8)
Labor	11	12.7 (9.8-17.8)	82 (72-88)	0.21 (0.01-0.60)	14 (8-20)	2.5
Postpartum						
1 wk	7	16.4 (9.7-25.7)	83 (70-94)	0.35 (0-1.5)	13 (5-30)	2.0
1-2 mo	12	8.5 (6.4-11.8)	63 (52-79)	2.42 (0.9-7.3)	29 (17-44)	4.0

From Altman, P.L., and Dittmer, D.S., editors: Blood and other body fluids, Bethesda, Md., 1961, Federation of American Societies for Experimental Biology.

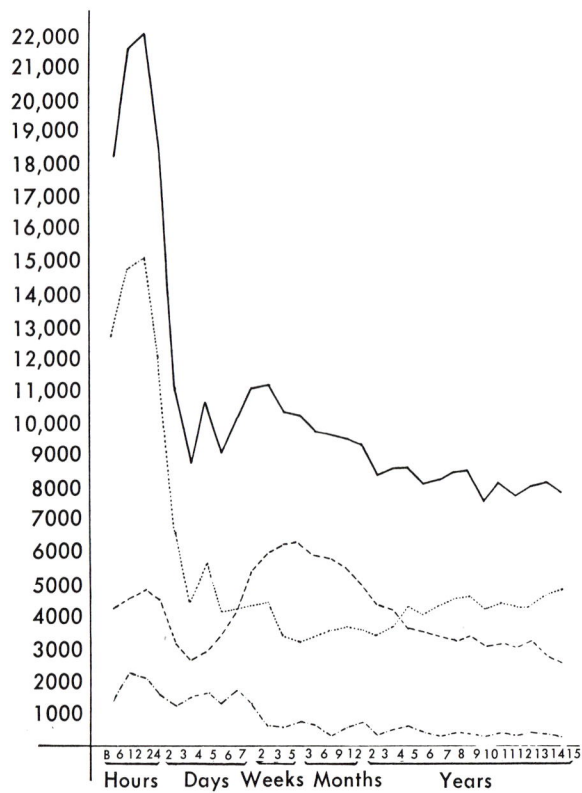

Fig. 7-19. Leukocytes in infancy and childhood. (From Kato, K.: J. Pediatr. **7:**7, 1935.)

Correction of white cell count for nucleated red cells

If nucleated red cells are present, the white cell count has to be corrected because nucleated red cells are counted along with the white cells. Use the following formula:

Corrected WBC count =

$$\frac{\text{No. of uncorrected WBCs} \times 100}{100 + (\text{No. of nucleated RBCs}/100 \text{ WBCs})}$$

The number of nucleated red cells per 100 white cells is obtained from the differential count.

Automated white cell count

All automated hematology counters include in their profile the white cell count. The Coulter S (Coulter Electronics, Hialeah, Fla.) measures the white cell count in duplicate. Each count is based on the displacement of an amount of diluent proportional to the volume of each cell. The volume of each cell is also recorded on a size distribution graph or on a screen display.

Absolute white cell count

The absolute white cell count expresses the numbers of the various cell types present in 1 mm³ blood.

The relative and the absolute numbers of a given cell type do not express the same information. The leukocyte differential count establishes the relative number of the various cell types in the peripheral blood. If the percentage of one cell type is increased, it implies that this cell type is more numerous than normal, but it does not explain whether the number of these cells is actually increased or whether there is a decrease in the other types of cells. If the percent distribution of white cells and the total leukocyte count are known, the absolute white cell values can be calculated as follows:

Absolute value (leukocytes/mm³) =
Total leukocyte count (cells/mm³) × Relative value (%)

Example:

Total leukocyte count = 6000
Segmented forms (relative no.) = 50%

Segmented forms (absolute no.) = $6000 \times \frac{50}{100} = 3000/\text{mm}^3$

Table 7-8. Relative and absolute leukocyte values (adult)

	Relative values (%)	Absolute values (no./mm³)
Total leukocytes		5000-11,000
Myelocytes	0	0
Metamyelocytes	0-1	30-110
Band granulocytes	2-5	100-550
Segmented granulocytes	36-66	1800-7260
Eosinophils	1-4	50-440
Basophils	0-1	0-110
Lymphocytes	22-40	1100-4400
Monocytes	4-8	200-880

Normal values: Normal absolute values are given in Table 7-8. The absolute value establishes the actual number of the various types of leukocytes and their relationship to each other as demonstrated by the examples that follow.

Example 1: WBCs = 22,000/mm³

Differential count	%	Absolute values (cells/mm³)
Segmented neutrophils	19	4180
Band neutrophils	1	220
Lymphocytes	75	16,500
Eosinophils	2	440
Basophils	0	0
Monocytes	3	660

The percentage of neutrophils is decreased, but the absolute number is within normal limits. The percentage and the absolute number of lymphocytes are increased and are responsible for the high white cell count.

Example 2: WBCs = 3000/mm³

Differential count	%	Absolute values (cells/mm³)
Segmented neutrophils	19	570
Band neutrophils	1	30
Lymphocytes	75	2250
Eosinophils	1	30
Basophils	1	30
Monocytes	3	90

There is a relative and an absolute decrease in neutrophils. The percentage of lymphocytes is increased, but the absolute value is within normal limits. The increased percentage of lymphocytes is the result of the decrease in neutrophils. Although the differential counts of examples 1 and 2 are almost identical, the basic processes are not.

Manual absolute eosinophil count
Unopette technic

The inaccuracy of the leukocyte differential count performed on a limited number of cells is discussed in the sections on automated and manual differential counts. When dealing with leukocytes of low frequency this counting error is much increased, so that direct counting methods based on selective staining have been developed for eosinophils and basophils. They allow the counting of about 2500 leukocytes in the Fuchs-Rosenthal chamber (Fig. 7-20) (as compared to about 100

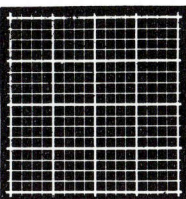

Fig. 7-20. Fuchs-Rosenthal hemocytometer counting chamber ruling. (Courtesy E.H. Sargent Co., Chicago.)

cells in the Neubauer chamber), so that increases or decreases in the number of these cells in physiologic and pathologic states can be recognized.[71]

Principle: The red cells are lysed, and eosinophils only stain bright orange-red with Phloxin B.

Equipment:
1. Unopette no. 5877. Reservoir with 0.775 ml diluent mixture containing 1 g Phloxin B, 5 dl propylene glycol, and water to make 1 L.
2. Capillary pipet, 25 μl. Dilution of 1:32 is obtained if blood sample drawn into capillary is mixed with diluent in reservoir.
3. Fuchs-Rosenthal hemocytometer (Fig. 7-20). The ruled area has the following measurements: area = 16 mm², depth = 0.2 mm, and volume = 3.2 μl.

Procedure: Dilute the blood and mix it using the Unopette system technic. Mix it thoroughly by inversion, convert to dropper assembly, fill the hemocytometer, and place it on moistened filter paper in a Petri dish. Cover the Petri dish and allow it to stand 10 min to permit cells to settle. Count all eosinophils in one ruled area using a high-power lens (×100). Eosinophils appear bright orange-red and are clearly distinguishable from all other leukocytes. Calculate the absolute number of eosinophils per cubic millimeter by multiplying the total number of cells by 10. The calculation is based on the formula mentioned in the discussion of manual counts.

$$\text{Eosinophils/mm}^3 = \frac{\text{Cells counted}}{16 \times 0.2 \times \frac{1}{32}} = \text{Cells counted} \times 10$$

Results: Normal absolute range is 0-450 eosinophils/mm³ blood. A factor of 10⁶ converts this figure to eosinophils per liter.

$$\text{Eosinophils (\%)} = \frac{\text{Eosinophils counted}}{\text{WBCs counted} \times 100}$$

Manual absolute basophil count
Toluidine blue method of Cooper and Cruickshank[72]

Principle: The staining method is based on the fact that basophilic granules contain heparin, which stains metachromatically with toluidine blue, leaving other leukocytes unstained. Cetylpyridinium chloride is used to lyse the erythrocytes and to complex with the mucopolysaccharides, thus rendering the basophilic granules insoluble. Aluminum sulfate is used as a mordant to improve the staining qualities of the toluidine blue. EDTA prevents platelet agglutination.

Reagents:
1. Solution 1
   EDTA (disodium salt), 0.1% in saline
2. Solution 2
   Cetylpyridinium chloride, 0.5%, 25 ml
   Distilled water, 25 ml
   Toluidine blue, 0.8%, in aluminum sulfate, 5%, 20 ml
   Filter before use.

Procedure: Place 0.08 ml solution 1 in a 75 × 10 mm test tube. Add 0.02 ml blood from free-flowing skin puncture and mix. Add 0.1 ml solution 2, mix,

and stopper. Fill two Fuchs-Rosenthal chambers (see discussion of eosinophil counting technic) using a Pasteur pipet. Keep the chamber in a moist atmosphere (Petri dish and moist filter paper), and allow 5 min for cells to settle. Count the basophils in both chambers and average the results. Dilution of whole blood is 1:10.

Results: Basophils are seen as purple-red metachromatically stained cells. Other leukocytes, platelets, and red cells do not stain.

Calculation:

$$\text{Basophils/mm}^3 \text{ blood} = \frac{\text{Total count} \times 10}{3.2}$$

Normal values: Counts range from 0-200 basophils/mm³, the average value being 40 basophils/mm³ blood. A factor of 10⁶ converts these figures to basophils per liter.

Interpretation: See function of basophils, p. 162.

SOURCES OF ERROR IN HEMOCYTOMETER COUNTING PROCEDURES

1. Errors in equipment
   a. Moist syringes
   b. Incorrectly calibrated equipment
2. Errors in blood sampling
   a. Finger-stick blood not freely flowing
   b. Anticoagulated blood contains clots
   c. Incorrect ratio of blood to anticoagulant or diluent
3. Errors in performance of test
   a. Inadequate filling of micropipet
   b. Inadequate mixing of blood sample in reservoir before filling counting chamber
   c. Failure to discard first 4 drops before applying sample to counting chamber
   d. Errors in counting and in arithmetic[73] (In general, manual counts are higher than counts performed by electronic particle counters.)

Manual differential count and its sources of error

The manual differential count technic is adequately discussed in previous editions of this book, but its accuracy deserves reassessment in view of the advent of automated differential counters. The purpose of the differential count is to evaluate the distribution of various formed elements in the bloodstream by identifying a limited number of these cells in the blood smear and by reporting their percentage distribution. The examination of the blood smear is one of the most important hematologic procedures allowing the morphologic study of red and white cells and of platelets, but as a quantitative method it is most unreliable. The assessment of the frequency of each leukocyte type on the basis of manually counting a very limited number of cells is an inaccurate and nonreproducible procedure because the method is burdened by a number of errors that cannot be eliminated. The sampling error for each cell type is determined by the frequency of the cell type in the total leukocyte population and by the number of cells counted, usually 100-200 cells. In leukopenic bloods it may not be possible to count more than 50 cells. For cell populations of low frequency, e.g., eosinophils and basophils, the sampling error is significant.[71] Additional sources of error are the location of the cell on the slide and the error of interpretation, or the human error, which is most significant in the differentiation of bands and bilobed neutrophilic granulocytes and in the identification of blast cells.[74-76]

In the age of automatic particle counters the manual differential count technic is the weakest link in the hematologic workup. The more cells that are classified and the more frequently a given leukocytic cell type is present in the smear, the greater will be the accuracy of the differential count. The absolute concentration of each leukocyte type is based on the percent differential count and on the total white cell count. (See discussion of absolute white cell count.) In doing the differential count, one should pay attention to the percent distribution of normally found leukocytes, of young or abnormal forms, and of shifts to the right or left and to morphologic changes such as nuclear/cytoplasmic abnormalities, e.g., twinning deformity, increased lobulation, toxic granulation, cytoplasmic inclusions, abnormal size and shape of cells. In addition, consideration is given to platelet and red cell morphology, including nucleated red cells. Red cell abnormalities should be quantitated, although the presence of a few abnormal red cells is difficult to interpret.

Automated differential count

Completely automated differential counters are available that combine a 10-cell white cell count, evaluation of red cell size, shape, and color, and estimation of platelets.

REFERENCES

1. Pinkerton, P.H., et al.: J. Clin. Pathol. **23**:68, 1970.
2. Brittin, G.M., and Brecher, G.: Prog. Hematol. **7**:299, 1971.
3. Sharp, A.A., and Ballard, B.C.D.: J. Clin. Pathol. **23**:327, 1970.
4. Brittin, G.M., Brecher, G., and Johnson, C.A.: Am. J. Clin. Pathol. **52**:679, 1969.
5. Hamilton, P.J., and Davidson, R.L.: J. Clin. Pathol. **26**:700, 1973.
6. Alpert, N.L.: Lab. World **26**:16, 1975.
7. England, J.M., and Down, M.C.: Br. J. Haematol. **32**:403, 1976.
8. Luke, R.G., Koepke, J.A., and Siegel, R.R.: Am. J. Clin. Pathol. **56**:503, 1971.
9. Hattersley, P.G., et al.: Am. J. Clin. Pathol. **55**:442, 1971.
10. Cytographic analysis prepared by staff of Bio/Physics Systems, 1973, Mahopac, N.Y.
11. Eilers, R.J.: Br. J. Haematol. **13**(suppl.):32, 1967.
12. Bull, B.S., Schneiderman, M.A., and Brecher, G.: Am. J. Clin. Pathol. **44**:678, 1965.
13. Bull, B.S.: Am. J. Clin. Pathol. **54**:707, 1970.
14. Nakatsui, T., et al.: Am. J. Clin. Pathol. **53**:659, 1970.
15. Brittin, G.M., Dew, S.A., and Fewell, E.K.: Blood **38**:422, 1971.
16. Hart, J.E., Hogue, K.A., and Hartmann, J.R.: Am. J. Clin. Pathol. **53**:914, 1970.
17. Weisbrot, I.M., and Ewing, N.S.: Am. J. Clin. Pathol. **62**:693, 1974.
18. Watkins, S.P., Jr., and Shulman, N.R.: Blood **36**:153, 1970.
19. Megla, G.K.: Acta Cytol. (Baltimore) **17**:3, 1973.
20. Mansberg, H.P., Saunders, A.M., and Groner, W.: J. Histochem. Cytochem. **22**:711, 1974.
21. The Announcer Newsletter, Tarrytown, N.Y., July 1975, Technicon Instruments Corp.
22. Clinical evaluation report, Wayne, Pa., 1973, Geometric Data Corp.
23. Oberjat, T.E., Zucker, R.M., and Cassen, B.: J. Lab. Clin. Med. **76**:518, 1970.
24. Zucker, R.M., and Casse, A.B.: Blood **34**:591, 1969.
25. Hillen, H., Wessels, J., and Haanen, C.: Lancet **1**:609, 1975.
26. Editorial: Lancet **1**:435, 1975.
27. Julius, M.H., Massuda, T., and Herzenberg, L.A.: Proc. Natl. Acad. Sci. U.S.A. **69**:1934, 1972.
28. Drake, W.P., Ungaro, P.C., and Mardiney, M.R., Jr.: Transplantation **14**:127, 1972.
29. Horan, P.K., et al.: J. Natl. Cancer Inst. **52**:843, 1974.
29a. Patrick, J., and Linstrom, J.: Science **180**:871, 1973.
30. England, J.M., Walford, D.M., and Waters, D.A.W.: Br. J. Haematol. **23**:247, 1972.
31. Nelson, D.A.: In Henry, J.B., editor: Basis methodology in clinical diagnosis and management by laboratory methods, Philadelphia, 1979, W.B. Saunders Co.
32. Rutzsky, J.: An orientation to the CBC: technical improvement service no. 18, Chicago, 1974, American Society of Clinical Pathologists.
33. Dutcher, T.F.: Lab. Med. **2**:32, 1971.
34. Penttila, A., and Trump, B.F.: Am. J. Clin. Pathol. **63**:581, 1975.
35. McPhedran, P., et al.: Ann. Intern. Med. **78**:677, 1973.
36. Petrucci, J.V., Dunne, P.A., and Chapman, C.C.: Am. J. Clin. Pathol. **56**:500, 1971.
37. Komarmy, L., and Barnes, M.G.: Med. Lab. Sci. **29**:293, 1972.
38. Winter, H., and Sheard, R.P.: Aust. J. Exp. Biol. Med. Sci. **43**:687, 1965.
39. Waterman, C.S., et al.: Clin. Chem. **21**:1201, 1975.
40. Wintrobe, M.M.: Arch. Intern. Med. **54**:256, 1934.
41. Ihnen, M., and Kelsey, D.: J. Nucl. Med. **4**:211, 1963.
42. Tizianello, A., and Pannaciulli, I.: Acta Haematol. **21**:346, 1959.
43. International Committee for Standardization in Hematology (ICSH): Br. J. Haematol. **25**:801, 1973.
44. Wood, G.A., and Levitt, S.H.: J. Nucl. Med. **6**:433, 1965.
45. Besa, E.C.: C.R.C. Crit. Rev. Clin. Lab. Sci. **6**:67, 1975.
46. Wochner, R.D., et al.: J. Lab. Clin. Med. **75**:711, 1970.
47. Wright, R.R., Tono, M., and Pollycove, M.: Semin. Nucl. Med. **5**:63, 1975.
48. Sodee, D.B., and Early, P.J.: Mosby's manual of nuclear medicine procedures, ed. 3, St. Louis, 1981, The C.V. Mosby Co.
49. Lewis, S.M.: ACP Broadsheet 94, June 1980.
50. Touster, O.: Annu. Rev. Biochem. **31**:407, 1962.
51. Bull, B.S., and Brailsford, J.D.: Blood **40**:550, 1972.
52. Ballas, S.K.: Am. J. Clin. Pathol. **63**:45, 1975.
53. Benninger, G.W., and Kreps, S.I.: Am. J. Med. **51**:287, 1971.
54. Weicker, H., and Kuhn, D.: German Med. Monthly **12**:37, 1967.
55. Bunting, H.: Am. J. Med. Sci. **198**:191, 1939.
56. Phear, D.: J. Clin. Pathol. **10**:357, 1957.
57. Rogers, K.B.: Br. Med. J. **1**:1109, 1952.
58. Lascari, A.D.: Pediatr. Clin. North Am. **19**:1113, 1972.
59. Penchas, S., Stern, Z., and Bar-Or, D.: Arch. Intern. Med. **138**:1864, 1978.

60. International Committee for Standardization in Hematology (ICSH): Am. J. Clin. Pathol. **68:**505, 1977.
61. Hutchinson, R.M., and Eastham, R.D.: J. Clin. Pathol. **30:**345, 1977.
62. Editorial: Lancet **2:**1166, 1977.
63. Boyd, R.V., and Hoffbrand, B.I.: Br. Med. J. **1:**901, 1966.
64. Vander, J.B.: J. Lab. Clin. Med. **62:**132, 1963.
65. Hillman, R.S., and Finch, C.A.: Red cell manual, Philadelphia, 1974, F.A. Davis Co.
66. Hillman, R.S.: Hematology laboratory manual, Seattle, 1970, University of Washington Medical School.
67. Jandl, J.H.: J. Lab. Clin. Med. **55:**663, 1960.
68. Hillman, R.S.: J. Clin. Invest. **48:**443, 1969.
69. Broun, G.O., Herbig, F.K., and Hamilton, J.R.: N. Engl. J. Med. **275:**1410, 1966.
70. Karayalcin, G., Rosner, F., and Sawitsky, A.: N.Y. State J. Med. **72:**1815, 1972.
71. Gilbert, H.S.: Advances in automated analysis, Tarrytown, N.Y., 1972, Technicon International Congress, Mediad, vol. 3.
72. Cooper, J.R., and Cruickshank, C.N.D.: J. Clin. Pathol. **19:**402, 1966.
73. Mattern, C.F.T., Brackett, F.S., and Olson, B.J.: J. Appl. Physiol. **10:**56, 1957.
74. Bacus, J.W.: Am. J. Clin. Pathol. **59:**223, 1973.
75. Simmons, A., and Elbert, G.: Am. J. Clin. Pathol. **64:**512, 1975.
76. Barnett, C.W.: J. Clin. Invest. **12:**77, 1933.

CHAPTER 8

Laboratory investigation of red cell disorders

ANEMIAS

Pathophysiologically, **anemia** is defined as a condition in which the circulating hemoglobin is reduced to levels that are inadequate to oxygenate the peripheral tissues, but in the laboratory it is defined by hemoglobin or hematocrit levels more than 2 SD below normal values. In men, hemoglobin and hematocrit levels of 13 g/dl and 41 vol%, respectively, are considered to be in the anemic range; the corresponding values for women are 11 g/dl and 36 vol%.

CLASSIFICATION

The morphologic classification of anemias is based on the **Wintrobe blood indices** (the average size and hemoglobin content of red cells) and is of practical importance in the investigation of the anemic patient, since accurate red cell characteristics are not only readily available but also furnish information as to the most likely cause of the anemia.

The anemias are divided into three groups:

1. **Macrocytic anemias,** characterized by erythrocytes with mean corpuscular volume (MCV) and mean corpuscular hemoglobin (MCH) greater than normal but with normal mean corpuscular hemoglobin concentration (MCHC)
2. **Normocytic anemias,** characterized by erythrocytes with normal MCV, MCH, and MCHC
3. **Microcytic hypochromic anemias,** characterized by erythrocytes with lower than normal MCV, MCH, and MCHC (Table 8-1)

The Wintrobe indices are most meaningful when obtained by automated technics, but they must still be corroborated by a careful evaluation of the red cell

Table 8-1. Morphologic classification of anemias

	MCV (μm^3)	MCH (pg)	MCHC (g/dl)
Anemia			
Macrocytic normochromic	95-160	32-50	32-36
Normocytic normochromic	80-94	27-31	32-36
Microcytic hypochromic	50-79	19-29	24-30
Normal values			
Men	80-94	27-31	32-36
Women	81-99	27-31	32-36

morphology of a well-stained blood smear. The indices are least reliable in diphasic anemias.

Etiologic and morphologic classification

I. Microcytic hypochromic anemias: iron deficiency
   A. Inadequate iron intake
   B. Inadequate iron absorption
      1. Achlorhydria, gastric resection
      2. Chronic diarrhea
         a. Celiac disease
         b. Sprue
         c. Small bowel resection
      3. Absence or suppression of factors necessary for iron absorption
   C. Increased demand for iron
      1. Pregnancy
      2. Growth periods
      3. Blood regeneration
   D. Excessive iron loss
      1. Hemorrhage
         a. Acute
         b. Chronic
      2. Hemosiderin loss: pulmonary siderosis
   E. Disturbance of iron utilization
      1. Sideroblastic anemias
         a. Hereditary
         b. Acquired
      2. Thalassemia
   F. Selected hemoglobinopathies
      1. Hb Lepore
      2. Hb Köln
      3. Hb H
   G. Anemia of chronic disorders
   H. Transferrin deficiency
II. Macrocytic normochromic anemias
   A. Vitamin B_{12} deficiency
      1. Pernicious anemia
      2. Malabsorption
         a. Gastric resection
         b. Gastric carcinoma
         c. Some forms of sprue and celiac disease
      3. Increased utilization
         a. *Diphyllobothrium latum* infection
         b. Pathologic intestinal flora in small bowel stricture, blind loop operations, diverticula
         c. Pregnancy
      4. Diminished supply: nutritional deficiency (kwashiorkor)
   B. Folic acid deficiency
      1. Abnormal absorption
         a. Sprue
         b. Celiac disease
      2. Increased utilization
         a. Pregnancy
         b. Some acute leukemias
      3. Treatment with folic acid antagonists
   C. Several causative factors involved
      1. Severe liver disease
      2. Hypothyroidism
      3. Administration of antimetabolic drugs and anticonvulsants

III. Normocytic normochromic anemias
   A. Acute blood loss
   B. Hemolytic anemias
      1. Intrinsic erythrocytic defects
         a. Abnormal red cell morphology
            (1) Hereditary spherocytosis
            (2) Hereditary elliptocytosis
            (3) Infantile pyknocytosis
            (4) Hereditary stomatocytosis
         b. Enzymatic deficiencies of red cells
            (1) Glycolytic enzymes
               (a) Glucose-6-phosphate dehydrogenase (G-6-PD) deficiency
               (b) Pyruvate kinase deficiency
               (c) Triosephosphate insomerase deficiency
               (d) Galactose-1-phosphate uridyl transferase deficiency (galactosemia)
               (e) 2,3-Diphosphoglycerate mutase deficiency
            (2) Nonglycolytic enzymes
               (a) Hereditary glutathione absence
               (b) Glutathione reductase deficiency
               (c) ATPase deficiency
         c. Hemoglobinopathies
         d. Paroxysmal nocturnal hemoglobinuria
         e. Pernicious anemia
         f. Erythropoietic porphyria
      2. Extrinsic factors leading to hemolytic anemias: antibodies
         a. Acquired isoimmune hemolytic anemias
         b. Acquired autoimmune hemolytic anemias
         c. Infections
            (1) Bacterial
            (2) Viral
            (3) Parasitic
         d. Hypersplenism
         e. Drugs and toxins: Heinz body anemia
         f. Physical agents: burns
         g. Micronangiopathic hemolytic anemias
            (1) Intracardiac prosthesis
            (2) Intravascular clotting
            (3) Vasculitis
            (4) Sickle cell anemia
IV. Aplastic (aregenerative) anemias
   A. Pure red cell anemia
      1. Thymic tumors
      2. Myasthenia gravis
   B. Hypoplastic anemia of Diamond and Blackfan
   C. Anemia associated with pancytopenia
      1. Congenital
         a. Fanconi's
         b. Estren and Dameshek
      2. Acquired
         a. Chemical agents and drugs
         b. Radiation
         c. Myelophthisic anemias
         d. Idiopathic anemias

Classification based on activity of erythroid marrow units

Anemias can be classified according to the activity of the erythroid marrow units.

1. **Hypoproliferative anemias:** anemias caused by lack of iron (cytoplasmic maturation defect), depression of erythropoietin (renal disease), marrow damage (myelofibrosis)
2. **Dyserythropoietic anemias:** anemias caused by deficiency of B_{12} or of folic acid or both (nuclear maturation defect)
3. **Hyperproliferative (hemolytic) anemias:** autoimmune anemias, hemoglobinopathies, enzyme-deficient anemias, microangiopathic anemias

MICROCYTIC HYPOCHROMIC ANEMIAS
IRON DEFICIENCY ANEMIA

Iron deficiency leads to a reduced rate of erythropoiesis and to the production of morphologically and structurally altered erythrocytes with a shortened life span (apparently caused by decreased glutathione peroxidase activity).[1-3]

Erythrocyte count: The erythrocyte count may be normal at the beginning but decreases as the iron deficiency continues. Unless there is severe iron deprivation, the erythrocyte count is usually affected less than the hemoglobin level.

Hemoglobin concentration: Hemoglobin concentration is decreased (usually to a greater degree than the red cell count) and is considered to be in the anemic range if it falls below the following values[4]:

Children (6 months-6 years): 11 g/dl
Children (6-14 years): 12 g/dl
Adult men: 13 g/dl
Adult women: 12 g/dl
Pregnant women: 11 g/dl

Red cell indices: Red cells will have an MCV less than 80 μm^3, an MCH less than 27 pg, and an MCHC less than 32%. The Coulter S$^+$ (Coulter Electronics, Hialeah, Fla.) measures hypochromia and microcytosis of red cells so accurately that mildly lowered MCH and MCV values may be obtained at a time when the peripheral smear and the total red cell count are well within normal limits.

Blood film: In the early stages the red cell morphology is normal, since the initial anemia is normocytic and normochromic, but as it progresses, the peripheral smear reveals hypochromia, microcytosis, anulocytosis, occasional target cells, some anisocytosis, and poikilocytosis.

Reticulocytes: Reticulocytes are decreased or normal.

Osmotic fragility: Osmotic fragility is normal, although it may be decreased (target cells).

White cell count and differential count: The white cell and differential counts are usually normal, although neutropenia and leukocytosis after acute blood loss have been reported.[5]

Platelets: Acute blood loss is one of the long-accepted causes of thrombocytosis,[6] but recent work has revealed that it is the iron deficiency that is responsible for the increase in megakaryocytes and platelets.[7]

However, normal platelet levels and thrombocytopenic levels have been documented, especially in children.[6,8,9]

Serum iron: In states of iron depletion the serum iron level is low (below 30 $\mu g/dl$), but the iron-binding capacity (i.e., the iron-binding protein, transferrin) is increased. This combination of low serum iron and increased iron-binding capacity is responsible for a fall in transferrin saturation.[10] If transferrin saturation falls below 16%, iron-deficient erythropoiesis and depletion of iron stores result. In anemia caused by chronic infection and chronic disease, the serum iron and iron-binding capacity both decrease, but the transferrin saturation usually remains close to the normal range (20-25%).

Bone marrow examination: Bone marrow examination is indicated for the evaluation of tissue-storage iron, sideroblasts, and defective erythropoiesis. The latter condition is evidenced by small normoblasts with pyknotic nuclei surrounded by a thin rim of irregular, ragged basophilic cytoplasm lacking hemoglobinization. The cytoplasm appears to be mechanically weak so that the edges are irregular, and often naked nuclei appear (ineffective erythropoiesis). There is usually an increase in basophilic and polychromatic normoblasts **(normoblastic hyperplasia)** with a marked decrease in orthochromic normoblasts. In established iron deficiency there is complete **absence of stainable iron** in bone marrow reticulum cells and normoblasts.

Erythrocyte protoporphyrin (EP): The last step in the biosynthesis of heme in the normoblast is the incorporation of iron into the protoporphyrin molecule. If iron is not available in adequate amounts, unused protoporphyrin accumulates in the normoblasts and in the erythrocytes into which they develop. The level of free EP is thus increased whenever adequate amounts of iron are not available for heme synthesis or when, because of enzymatic defects, iron cannot be incorporated into the protoporphyrin molecule, even if present in adequate amounts. EP level is thus elevated in iron deficiency anemia, in chronic anemia caused by infection, and in sideroblastic anemias. It remains elevated in the iron-deficient erythrocytes until they are destroyed, even if the hemoglobin level has returned to normal after treatment. The normal EP level is 15.5 ± 8.3 $\mu g/dl$ erythrocytes, whereas in iron deficiency anemia the value is 159.2 ± 96.5 $\mu g/dl$ erythrocytes.[10]

Serum ferritin: The serum ferritin level reflects the magnitude of the iron stores. Normal values are 39 ng/ml for women and 140 ng/ml for men. The serum ferritin level is low (about 9 ng/ml) in patients with an iron deficiency and high in patients with excessive iron storage. Elevated values up to 850 ng/ml have been seen in patients with chronic hemolytic anemias such as β-thalassemia.[11]

Selected iron deficiency states
Iron deficiency in infants and children

Iron deficiency is a common cause of anemia in infants and children.[12] Physiologically the hemoglobin level and number of red cells fall rapidly between birth and the age of 3 months, so that the storage depots become filled with iron from the breakdown of red cells. After the age of 3 months, the depots become gradually depleted if the infant is on a pure milk diet, since milk alone does not supply enough iron to restore the depleted iron reserves. This physiologic (?) iron deficiency is even more marked if (1) the child was premature or is a twin, (2) the placental blood was not allowed to drain into the infant at the time of birth (cesarean section), or (3) the infant bled into the maternal circulation[13] or was born after placental hemorrhage had occurred. Iron deficiency anemia is common at the end of the first year or in the second year of life. Frequent infections may well be a contributing factor. A second peak of iron deficiency may accompany the beginning of menstruation and the increased growth rate of adolescence.

Chronic blood loss

The hemorrhage causing chronic blood loss[14] (and subsequent iron loss) may be intermittent. It may be so small in amount as to be difficult to detect and may come from hidden lesions (e.g., diverticula, hiatus hernia, peptic ulcers, and gastrointestinal tumors) that are difficult to diagnose. Excessive menstrual loss, frequent pregnancies, and frequent blood donations to blood banks may also lead to iron loss. At first the bone marrow is able to maintain the equilibrium between blood loss and production and there is no manifest anemia. Later, however, a normocytic normochromic anemia develops. If the blood loss continues, the marrow production is unable to counterbalance the blood loss, and a hypochromic anemia results.

The first response to iron loss is depletion of the iron stores, followed by an increase in plasma transferrin. The increase may represent an attempt to augment iron absorption. The serum iron level falls because of the rapid removal of iron to cover the increasing compensatory erythroid hyperplasia.

The most frequent site of occult chronic blood loss is the gastrointestinal tract. Repeated stool specimens should be examined for occult blood. If the results are doubtful, the patient's red cells can be labeled with ^{51}Cr and the feces examined for radioactivity.

Hookworm anemia

The anemia caused by hookworm disease[4] is a typical iron deficiency anemia. Its severity depends on the severity of the infection, the nutritional state of the patient, and coexisting iron (blood) losses (e.g., menses). It is reported that each worm consumes 0.67 g hemoglobin daily. Additional factors are nutritional hypoproteinemia and malabsorption related to the hyperperistalsis of the diarrhea.

Acute blood loss

In general, the blood count after acute hemorrhage will not immediately reflect the blood loss. After 24 hours, however, as the body attempts to compensate for the blood loss by mobilizing interstitial fluid (which is poor in protein), the blood count, hemoglobin level, and hematocrit will decrease in proportion to the plasma dilution and the blood loss (roughly 50 mg iron is lost per 100 ml blood). This fall may continue for several days even though the hemorrhage has ceased. Bone marrow erythroid hyperplasia will follow within a matter of days, leading to temporary serum iron depletion and defective erythropoiesis. If the blood loss is sudden and of any magnitude, young marrow reticulocytes together with nucleated red cells are released into the circulation.

HYPOCHROMIC ANEMIA NOT CAUSED BY IRON DEFICIENCY

There are a number of anemias that must be differentiated from iron deficiency anemia. They are **sideroblastic anemias, anemia caused by chronic disorders,** and **thalassemia.** Differentiating laboratory findings are discussed briefly; thalassemia is discussed under congenital hemoglobinopathies.

Sideroblastic anemias

By definition sideroblastic anemias are associated with the presence of **ringed sideroblasts** in the bone marrow. They are a result of interference with hemoglobin synthesis so that iron, although present in adequate amount, cannot be used.

Idiopathic refractory sideroblastic anemia

Idiopathic refractory sideroblastic anemia (IRSA)[15,16] varies in intensity from moderate to marked and is normocytic or slightly macrocytic. The MCHC is normal or slightly reduced. The peripheral blood smear shows a **mixed field** of microcytic hypochromic cells alternating with normal or slightly macrocytic cells. This **dimorphism** (or *partial hypochromia*) is characteristic and is almost always associated with some degree of anisocytosis and poikilocytosis and with heavily stippled hypochromic cells. The reticulocytes may be normal in number, decreased, or even slightly increased. The bone marrow exhibits erythroid hyperplasia, which may be megaloblastic. The normoblasts are PAS negative, a feature that distinguishes IRSA from erythroleukemia. The sideroblasts may be normal in number, increased, or even decreased, but the pathologic **ringed sideroblasts** (Fig. 8-1) are always increased, as is the reticuloendothelial iron. The leukocytes and platelets are usually normal, but the neutrophilic alkaline phosphatase level may be reduced.

In most cases serum iron and percent saturation of transferrin are increased. Kinetic studies show very poor iron utilization by red cells (less than 35%, compared to the normal 90%). The red cells are only reluctantly released into the circulation, so that **ineffective erythropoiesis** and an **increase in free EP** are common.

Lead poisoning

The hematologic changes produced by lead intoxication are most pronounced in children. They are essentially similar to those seen in other sideroblastic anemias, with some exceptions (e.g., increased Hb F and A_2 levels,[17] masking of the usual serum iron increase by a concomitant iron deficiency,[18] and increased plasma and urine lead levels). If the lead levels are borderline (just below 80 μg/dl), lead deposits in the bone may be mobilized by injection of calcium

EDTA, and the plasma and urine lead levels can be reassayed.[17] Large-scale screening programs for lead poisoning have made use of lead-induced abnormalities in porphyrin metabolism.[19] Urinary δ-aminolevulinic acid (ALA) is greatly increased and is accompanied by increased urinary porphobilinogen (PBG) and coproporphyrin levels. Free EP is also greatly increased, so that the red cells may **fluoresce** when examined under the fluorescent microscope. The basic defect is probably related to the toxic action of lead on the enzymes heme synthetase, coproporphyrinogen oxidase, ALA synthetase, and ALA dehydrase.[20]

Blood picture[21,22]: Acute and chronic forms of lead poisoning are associated with a variable anemia that is usually hypochromic microcytic but may be normochromic normocytic. Hematocrit, hemoglobin, MCV, and MCHC are about 30% reduced. The Wright-Giemsa–stained film shows a moderate increase in polychromatic and basophilic stippled red cells. By supravital staining technic, the polychromatic cells are recognized as increased numbers of reticulocytes. **Basophilic stippling** (see Fig. 6-26) is characteristic of lead poisoning but is not diagnostic, and its absence does not exclude this diagnosis. Normally a stippled cell may occasionally (less than 0.3% of the time) be found, but in lead poisoning the percentage may vary from 1-10%. Stippling may also be seen in thalassemia and pernicious anemia and is caused by ribosomal aggregates. Lead also affects the erythrocytic surface, so that the affected erythrocytes show increased resistance to hypotonic saline solution.[23] The damaged erythrocytes have a shortened life span and are selectively destroyed in the spleen so that a toxic **hemolytic component** may be partly responsible for anemia caused by lead poisoning. In the bone marrow, **ringed sideroblasts** (Fig. 8-1) have been observed that are the result of interference with normal heme synthesis (thus the inclusion of lead poisoning anemia in the group of sideroblastic anemias). Moderate erythroid hyperplasia may also be seen.

Anemia of chronic disorders

A great number of systemic diseases (e.g., infections, collagen diseases, and malignancies) produce varying degrees of chronic refractory anemias that are of variable cause but have one common denominator: the interference with iron metabolism. Cartwright collectively calls these rather common anemias **anemias of chronic disorders.**[24,25]

The anemia is usually of moderate degree (with hematocrit levels ranging from 30-40 vol%), normocytic, and normochromic, although considerably more than 50% are mildly hypochromic; some of the latter may also be microcytic. The hypochromia and the microcytosis do not reach the degree associated with iron deficiency anemia. The MCV and the MCHC are often within normal limits or only slightly decreased. The blood film may show moderate anisocytosis, but poikilocytosis and polychromatic regenerative cells are absent. The reticulocyte count is normal, reduced, or slightly increased. Prussian blue–stained preparations of bone marrow show a reduced number of sideroblasts and iron retained within macrophages.

The serum iron level and the TIBC are reduced (serum iron, 10-70 μg/dl, and TIBC, 100-300 μg/dl), so that the percent saturation is low normal or only slightly reduced (25% or lower).[25] Plasma copper levels[24] and concentrations of free EP[25] are increased.

MACROCYTIC NORMOCHROMIC ANEMIAS

Macrocytic anemias are characterized by erythrocytes that exceed normal red cells in size and that usually contain a hemoglobin complement proportional to their size. The presence of these cells leads to increased

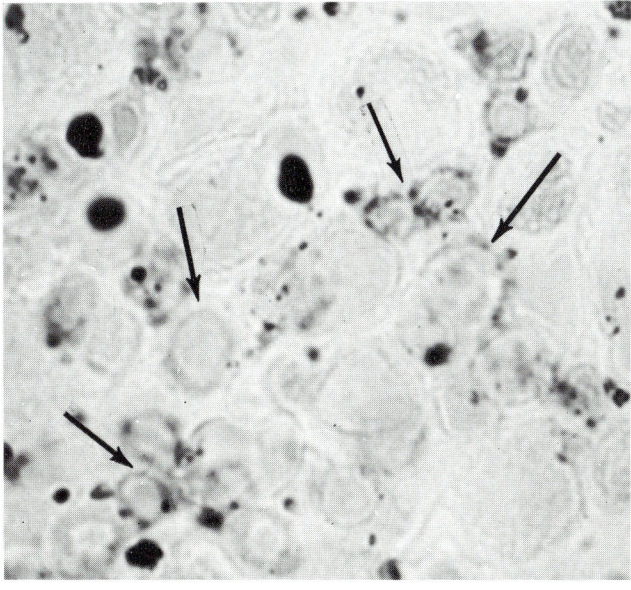

Fig. 8-1. Ringed sideroblasts in sideroblastic anemia (Prussian blue stain.)

MCV and MCH values, but the MCHC remains within normal limits.

Peripheral macrocytosis occurs in a large number of conditions that, when the bone marrow is examined, show megaloblastic or normoblastic erythroid hyperplasia or a mixture of both.

There are thus two main groups of macrocytic anemias: the **nonmegaloblastic form** and the **megaloblastic form.** The first group includes a variety of anemias that are primarily normocytic or even microcytic in type but may on occasion contain large numbers of macrocytes, which are an expression of the intense **reticulocytosis** (about 30%). Anemias characterized by large, thin target cells also fall into this group. The laboratory diagnosis of the nonmegaloblastic macrocytic anemias is discussed under the heading of normocytic normochromic anemias. The megaloblastic form, on the other hand, is always caused by defective DNA synthesis resulting from a deficiency of **vitamin B₁₂, folic acid,** or both. For classification, see etiologic and morphologic classification of anemias.

Vitamin B₁₂ deficiency

Vitamin B₁₂ deficiency[26] (as well as folic acid deficiency) leads to (1) disturbed nucleic acid metabolism, (2) megaloblastic maturation of the erythroid elements, and (3) a disturbance of most tissue cells, both hematopoietic and somatic. Miale calls this involvement of the body's cells **megaloblastic dyspoiesis.** Megaloblastic dyspoiesis is characterized by abnormal nuclear maturation and configuration as well as by nuclear/cytoplasmic dissociation. In the erythroid elements, nuclear/cytoplasmic dissociation is expressed by unimpaired hemoglobinization (in the absence of iron deficiency) in a cell with an immature nucleus. The abnormal nuclear maturation caused by vitamin B₁₂ deficiency (or folic acid deficiency) leads to an abnormal chromatin pattern and impairs the cell's ability to divide; so a result, not only is the production of mature cells markedly delayed but the individual cell components—both nucleus and cytoplasm—are unusually large. Impaired maturation and delayed aging are also seen in the myeloid series and in megakaryocytes and lead to leukopenia, thrombocytopenia, and the formation of giant metamyelocytes, hypersegmented and giant polymorphonuclear cells, and giant platelets. Thus there is ineffective erythropoiesis, granulocytopoiesis, and thrombocytopoiesis. Pernicious anemia[27] is the most common megaloblastic anemia and serves as a prototype of the entire group, since the blood picture is the same whether the anemia is caused by the lack of vitamin B₁₂ or of folic acid.

Hematologic findings

Red cell count: The red cell count varies from almost normal to levels below 1 million/mm³.

Hemoglobin concentration: Hemoglobin concentration is markedly reduced, often as low as 7-8 g/dl.

Blood indices: The MCV is greater than normal, but the degree of difference depends on the degree of anemia. The MCV may vary from values just above normal (95 μm³) to high values (130 μm³ or higher). The MCH also depends on the degree of anemia, varying

from slightly raised values (33 pg) to high values (up to 56 pg). The MCHC is within normal limits (34 g/dl) because the anemia is normochromic (although macrocytic). The hematocrit may vary from 5-25 vol% (with an average of 20 vol%).

White cell count: There is usually a slight-to-moderate leukopenia, with the white cell count varying from 1000-6000/mm³, the result of an absolute neutropenia and a relative lymphocytosis (greater than 50%).

Platelet count: The platelet count is moderately decreased, but it seldom drops below 80,000-90,000/mm³ (although platelet-related bleeding episodes have been reported).[28]

Blood film: The characteristic cell of the blood film (Fig. 6-7) is the somewhat oval, hemoglobin-filled macroovalocyte, the longest axis of which varies from 10-15 μm. Because the cell is filled with hemoglobin, the normal central pallor is not seen. The oval shape of the macrocyte is characteristic of megaloblastic anemias, since nonmegaloblastic macrocytes are round. There is a pronounced anisocytosis and poikilocytosis because of the presence of pear-shaped, comma-shaped, and racquet-shaped erythrocytes alternating with some normal red cells, microcytes, and the oval macrocytes. Polychromatic young cells are absent, but the red cells may show basophilic stippling, Howell-Jolly bodies, and Cabot rings (Plate 8, p. 214), as well as occasional nucleated forms with characteristics of megaloblastic maturation.

The white cells show neutropenia and lymphocytosis as already mentioned. The nuclei of the neutrophils are hypersegmented. There are sometimes 6-8 nuclear segments united to each other by fine stringlike connections. **Hypersegmentation** of neutrophils is one of the first manifestations of vitamin B₁₂ deficiency or folic acid deficiency and is one of the last to disappear after successful treatment (see Fig. 6-50).[29] The cells may also be larger than normal and, at times, oval; they are then called **macropolycytes.**

The platelets are decreased, irregular in form and size, and often of giant dimensions.

Red cell survival time: Red cell survival is shortened to one half to one fourth the normal time. Pernicious anemia has a hemolytic component because of intraerythrocytic and extraerythrocytic defects.[30,31]

Reticulocytes: In untreated pernicious anemia the reticulocyte count is below 1%. The level of the reticulocyte count is helpful in differentiating vitamin B₁₂ deficiency from folic acid deficiency. In vitamin B₁₂ deficiency the reticulocyte count is below 1%, whereas in folic acid deficiency it varies from 1.5-8.0%.[32] Following treatment it shows a characteristic response that is delayed for 2-3 days (the period during which the megaloblasts develop into erythroblasts). After the third day there is a rapid increase in the number of reticulocytes, reaching a maximal level of 25% or more in 5-8 days (Plate 9, p. 214). The degree of anemia in part determines the extent of the reticulocytosis; the more anemic the patient, the greater the reticulocyte response.

Bone marrow: There is a marked (as much as 10-30 times normal) erythroid hyperplasia (most of the cells belonging to the megaloblactic series) that can be ob-

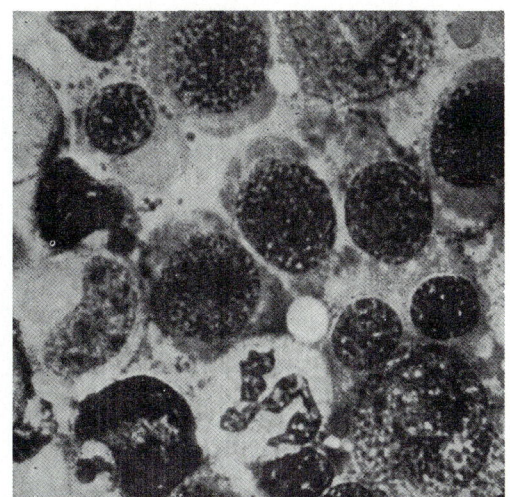

Fig. 8-2. Bone marrow smear in pernicious anemia showing abnormal number of megaloblasts. ($\times 950$.)

served from the youngest promegaloblast to the orthochromatic megaloblast (Fig. 8-2). These cells show nuclear/cytoplasmic asynchronism as well as disturbance of the normal nuclear/cytoplasmic ratio. The cells crowd out most of the normal erythropoietic elements. The diagnosis of megaloblastic maturation is facilitated by identification of the orthochromatic megaloblast, which differs in size and nucleus from its normocytic counterpart, the orthochromatic normoblast.

The myelocytic elements are also abnormal; large myelocytes, giant metamyelocytes, and hypersegmented granulocytes appear. Not only are the giant metamyelocytes large in size but their nuclei are also distorted and bizarre in shape and size and exhibit an abnormal chromatin pattern (Plate 10, p. 215). Some abnormal leukocytic forms persist even after the erythroid series has returned to normal after therapy.

Abnormal non-platelet-producing megakaryocytes with irregular nuclei (see Fig. 12-7) and abnormal reticulum cells are also noted. Some of the latter cells show erythrophagocytosis (see Fig. 6-57).

The bone marrow iron stores are increased; sideroblasts and reticuloendothelial iron are prominent.

Nonhematologic findings

Examination of gastric juice: Examination of the gastric juice[33] shows **histamine-fast achlorhydria** associated with achylia, a diminution of the total volume of gastric juice, and the absence or reduction of pepsin and rennin, which Wenger et al. call **total gastric failure.**[34] However, the aspiration of gastric juice, an unpleasant procedure at best, should not be necessary for the diagnosis of pernicious anemia.

Serum vitamin B₁₂ level

In pernicious anemia the serum B_{12} level (as determined by radioimmunoassay) is consistently low. This finding can be confirmed by the Schilling test or by the

increased urinary excretion of methylmalonic acid after ingestion of valine.[35] In about 30% of patients with folate deficiency the serum vitamin B_{12} concentration is also lowered; it returns to normal levels after treatment with pteroylglutamic acid, since these patients are able to normally absorb vitamin B_{12}. Patients with true vitamin B_{12} deficiency are unable to absorb the vitamin. In megaloblastic anemias both the vitamin B_{12} and folate levels should be assayed using the same specimen.[36]

Deoxyuridine suppression test

If a small amount of peripheral blood (0.1 ml) is incubated with deoxyuridine,[37,38] the deoxyuridine is converted into thymidine and incorporated into newly synthesized DNA. ^{3}H-thymidine is handled by the peripheral lymphocytes in a similar way. If the blood specimen is preincubated with deoxyuridine in the presence of normal folate coenzyme function (indicating normal folate and vitamin B_{12} functions), the deoxyuridine is converted to thymidine, and very little of the added radioactive thymidine is incorporated into the DNA. Thus the amount of radioactivity incorporated into the DNA is suppressed. With lymphocytes (and bone marrow cells) from patients with megaloblastic anemia, deoxyuridine is not converted into thymidine because of the lack of normal folate coenzyme function. Under these conditions the uridine is not used for thymidine synthesis, and a larger amount of radioactive thymidine is utilized. The test can be used to differentiate folic acid deficiency from B_{12} deficiency by determining which compound, when added, normalizes the suppression test.

Urine examination: Vitamin B_{12} deficiency leads to increased excretion of methylmalonic acid.[39] which is normal in folate deficiency and in liver disease. Physiologically, methylmalonic acid is converted into succinic acid by the methylmalonyl CoA, which contains cobamide coenzymes. In vitamin B_{12} deficiency the coenzyme is not available, and methylmalonate is excreted in greater quantities than normal, providing a reliable index of B_{12} deficiency.

Serum iron level: The serum iron level is increased, the TIBC is normal or decreased, and the percent saturation of transferrin is increased.

Haptoglobin: In all intravascular hemolytic anemias, haptoglobins are diminished or absent, and methemalbumin may be present. If, in a patient with a megaloblastic bone marrow picture, the serum iron is normal, the TIBC is increased, and stainable bone marrow iron is readily discovered, then iron deficiency complicating a megaloblastic process should be suspected.[32]

Pigment metabolism: The serum bilirubin may be increased, with the major component being the unconjugated (indirect) bilirubin. Urobilinogen excretion is greatly increased.[30]

Lactic acid dehydrogenase: Marked increases of up to 26,000 units in serum lactic acid dehydrogenase (LDH)[40] have been reported in pernicious anemia. With histochemical technics, megaloblastic bone marrow cells can be shown to contain increased amounts of LDH.[41] The increased intramedullary destruction of these cells is probably responsible for the elevated

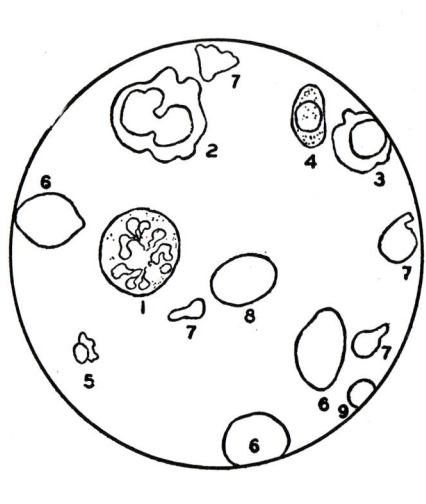
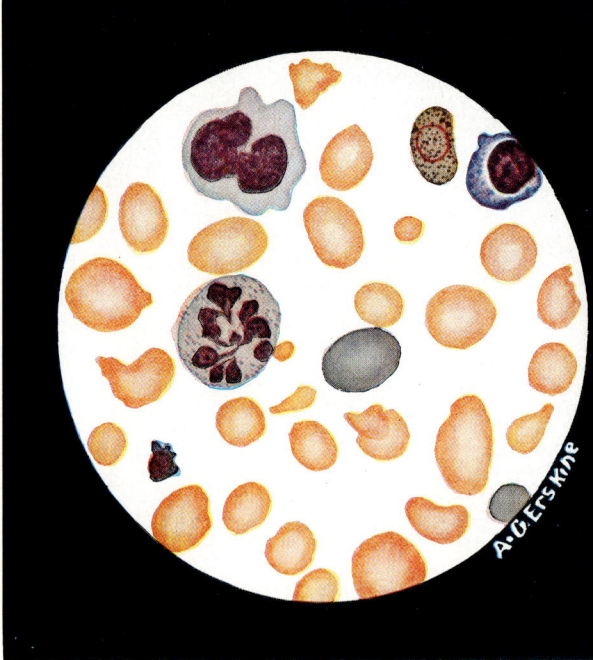

Plate 8. Peripheral blood smear in pernicious anemia. Note anisocytosis, poikilocytosis, polychromasia, and basophilic punctation in **9**; erythrocytes are macrocytic. (Wright-Giemsa stain; ×950.)

1 Giant hypersegmented neutrophil
2 Monocyte
3 Lymphocyte
4 Cabot ring body and basophilic punctation in macrocyte
5 Large blood platelet

6 Megalocyte
7 Poikilocyte
8 Polychromatic megalocyte
9 Polychromatic erythrocyte

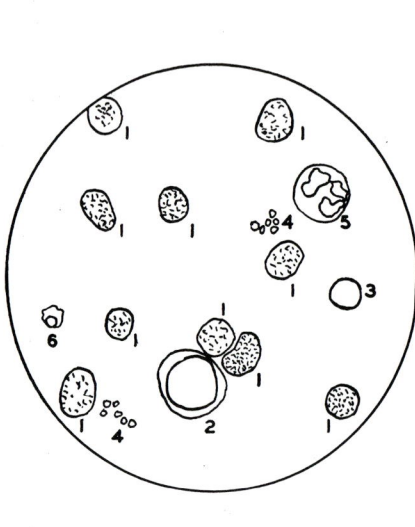
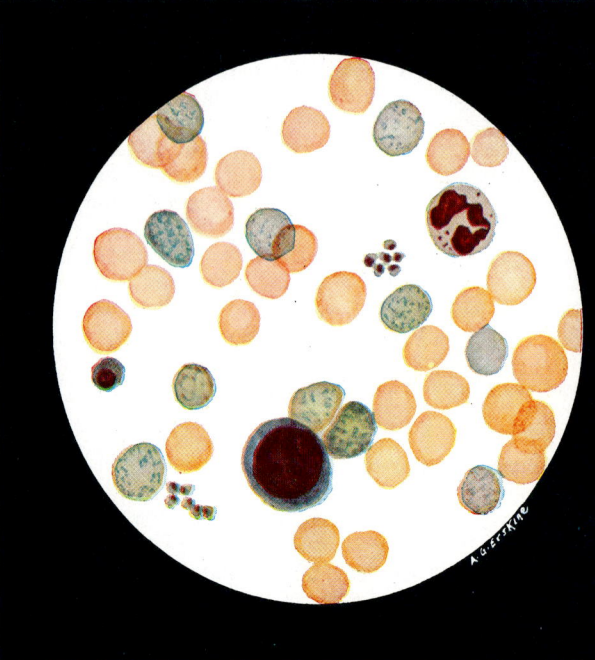

Plate 9. Peripheral blood smear in pernicious anemia responding to treatment. (Brilliant cresyl blue; Wright-Giemsa stain; ×950.)

1 Reticulocytes
2 Megaloblast
3 Polychromatic erythrocyte showing no reticulum

4 Blood platelets
5 Segmented neutrophil
6 Polychromatic micronormoblast

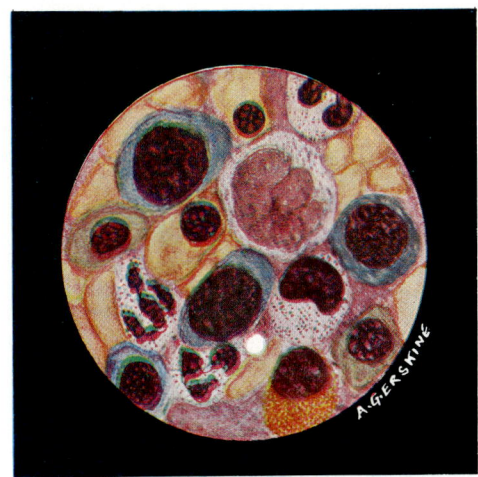

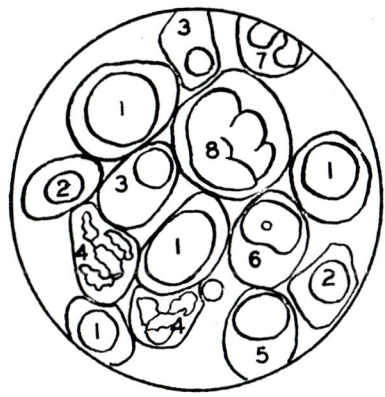

Plate 10. Giant metamyelocyte and megaloblasts in bone marrow smear in pernicious anemia. (Wright-Giemsa stain; ×950.)
1 Basophilic megaloblast
2 Polychromatic macrocyte
3 Orthochromatic macrocyte
4 Segmented granulocyte
5 Eosinophilic myelocyte
6 Neutrophilic myelocyte
7 Band granulocyte
8 Atypical young giant metamyelocyte

serum levels. The isoenzymes primarily affected are the fast LDH_1 and LDH_2. In megaloblastic anemias LDH_1 exceeds LDH_2, whereas in other hemolytic anemias that usually show a moderate LDH rise, isoenzyme LDH_2 activity exceeds LDH_1 activity.

Autoantibodies: Three types of antibodies have been demonstrated in the serum of patients with pernicious anemia: antiparietal cell antibodies and two types—blocking and binding—of anti-intrinsic-factor antibodies.

Folate deficiency

For causes of folate deficiency see classification of macrocytic normochromic anemias (p. 208).

Hematologic picture

The changes in the peripheral blood and bone marrow brought about by folic acid deficiency are similar to those found in vitamin B_{12} deficiency. Thus both serum folate and vitamin B_{12} levels must be assayed to substantiate the diagnosis. The degree of pancytopenia usually parallels the degree of folic acid deficiency, although in some instances the severity of the thrombocytopenia and leukopenia outweighs that of the anemia. In folate deficiency caused by erythroid (e.g., hemolytic anemias) and neoplastic diseases (leukemias), the primary blood disease influences the blood picture.

Assay of serum and red cell folates

The stability of the serum vitamin B_{12} level contrasts with the lability of the serum folate level, which is somewhat influenced by dietary intake or absence of folates.[29] Serum folate levels below 3.0 ng/ml are considered significantly low, but a dietary cause cannot be excluded. The erythrocyte folate levels closely mirror the tissue folate stores.[42,43] In severe folic acid deficiency, the excretion of **formimino-L-glytamic acid** (Figlu) is increased 8 hr after the oral administration of a loading dose of histidine. Since this test is neither specific nor sensitive,[44] it has been replaced by the radioimmunoassay of serum folates.

NORMOCYTIC NORMOCHROMIC ANEMIAS
ACUTE POSTHEMORRHAGIC ANEMIA

When dealing with a normocytic normochromic anemia of acute onset, an acute posthemorrhagic anemia should be differentiated from an acute hemolytic episode. Because acute blood loss leads to loss of both red cells and plasma, the hematocrit does not reflect the red cell mass loss until several days have passed and the blood volume has been normalized by the influx of water, electrolytes, and albumin. At that time the bone marrow, responding to erythropoietin stimulation, will show erythroid hyperplasia; after about 6-10 days, the marrow will release an increased number of reticulocytes[45] into the peripheral blood that are responsible for the polychromasia seen in the blood smear. Since the initial hematologic workup of posthemorrhagic and posthemolytic patients may produce an identical picture, specific laboratory tests must be used to differentiate these two anemias and identify the hemolytic episode. A haptoglobin assay and an assay for unconjugated bilirubin are suggested as discriminatory procedures to identify intravascular and extravascular hemolysis and separate it from acute blood loss anemia. The former process leads to a fall in **haptoglobin,** and the latter process leads to an increase in **unconjugated bilirubin.** Neither is found in acute blood loss.

HEMOLYTIC ANEMIAS

The common denominator of all hemolytic anemias is the increased rate of red cell destruction and the shortened life span of the average red cell. Hemolytic anemias may be classified as acute or chronic, as congenital (hereditary) or acquired, and as resulting from intracorpuscular or extracorpuscular defects. **Four groups of laboratory tests** may be employed to establish the hemolytic nature of the anemia.

Group I

Group I tests measure the product of inappropriate red cell destruction (intravascular or extravascular) to determine whether there is excessive hemolysis.

Tests for intravascular hemolysis

1. *Haptoglobins:* If there is intravascular hemolysis, the concentration of haptoglobin is markedly diminished or no haptoglobin is identified.

2. *Free hemoglobin in plasma:* The depletion of haptoglobin allows free hemoglobin to accumulate in the plasma (hemoglobinemia).[46] Free hemoglobin is a small molecule that escapes into the glomerular filtrate and (once the tubular reabsorptive capacity of the proximal convoluted tubules is exceeded) can be demonstrated in the urine (**hemoglobinuria**). If hemolysis is chronic, iron from the absorbed and catabolized hemoglobin is stored in the form of hemosiderin in the tubular cells, which, when desquamated into the urine, can be demonstrated in the urinary sediment as cells with granular, brown, Prussian blue–positive pigment (**hemosiderinuria**). Pronounced hemoglobinemia leads to some breakdown of the hemoglobin in the plasma and to the formation of hematin, which binds to albumin to form **methamalbumin**,[47] the presence of which is always indicative of past hemolysis.

Tests for extravascular hemolysis

Bilirubin formation: Reticuloendothelial cells phagocytose dying, senescent normal red cells, pathologic red cells of any age, and the previously mentioned haptoglobin and hemopexin-hemoglobin complexes. Hemoglobin is catabolized to globin and heme, and the heme is converted to biliverdin. Biliverdin reductase is responsible for the conversion of biliverdin to bilirubin.[48] The latter substance is released into the plasma in its water-insoluble, albumin-bound form and is conjugated in the liver with the aid of glucuronyl transferase. The conjugated form is excreted into the bile and discharged into the small bowel. The system just described is able to handle markedly increased amounts of nonconjugated bilirubin resulting from excessive hemolysis because of the phenomenon of enzyme induction. Bacterial action in the bowel converts the water-soluble, conjugated bilirubin to urobilinogen, which is then partly reabsorbed into the plasma and excreted in the urine. Excessive hemolysis leads to increased production of nonconjugated bilirubin and, ultimately, of **urobilinogen.** Urobilinogen is a colorless pigment that is oxidized on standing to form a brown pigment, urobilin.

Group II

Group II tests evaluate changes in peripheral blood and bone marrow in response to hemolysis.

Red cell count: The red cell count usually shows an anemia, although there may be none. The degree of anemia depends on the rate of hemolysis and on the ability of the bone marrow to compensate for the red cell loss. If the bone marrow is adequately supplied with the essential elements for normal erythropoiesis, it can increase its erythroid output six to eight times that of normal; this compensates for the reduction in the red cell life span (to about 20 days) so that no anemia develops, even in the face of hemolysis. The anemia may vary from mild to severe and is usually normochromic and normocytic, but it may be microcytic and megaloblastic depending on associated iron, vitamin B_{12}, or folate deficiencies. If the reticulocytes are markedly increased in number, the anemia will appear to be macrocytic. A very severe anemia may be indicative of an aplastic or hemolytic crisis.

Blood film: Films from even moderate hemolytic anemias usually show pronounced anisocytosis, which in severe anemias is associated with poikilocytosis and basophilic stippling. An increase in polychromatic macrocytes is indicative of an increase in reticulocytes, an impression that may be confirmed by supravital staining. This reticulocytosis is a valuable indicator of erythroid marrow hyperplasia. A reticulocyte response of 30% or more may be responsible for macrocytic red cell indices, for polychromatic cells, and for "shift" reticulocytes. The peripheral blood smear also shows morphologic evidence (e.g., fragmented cells, schistocytes, blister cells, spherocytes, and echinocytes) of destruction of red cells within the circulation. Special stains may reveal Heinz bodies and siderocytes. Pitted red cells or "bite" cells without the help of special stains suggest the negative image of Heinz bodies that have been removed by the spleen. Other indicators of hemolysis are Hb C and Hb S-C crystals, autoagglutination of red cells, and the presence of parasites. In severe anemias, nucleated red cells are released into the circulation, and Howell-Jolly bodies can be seen.

Osmotic fragility testing: Osmotic fragility is increased in hemolytic anemias caused by membrane defects (congenital spherocytosis and elliptocytosis), normal in enzymopathies, and decreased in hemoglobinopathies and thalassemias.

White cells: In hemolytic anemias there is usually a moderate leukocytosis with a shift to the left. Leukopenia may be seen in acquired hemolytic anemias.

Platelets: The number of platelets is often increased but may be normal; in paroxysmal nocturnal hemoglobinuria and in some acquired hemolytic anemias the number is decreased.

Bone marrow findings: The physiologic bone marrow response to hemolysis is erythroid hyperplasia, which can be evaluated by examination of the aspirated bone marrow and by the number of reticulocytes in the peripheral blood. The myeloid/erythroid ratio is reduced or reversed; compared to normal erythropoiesis, there is usually a more pronounced increase in basophilic and polychromatic normoblasts, so that they are about equal in number to the orthochromatic normoblasts. Erythroid hyperplasia is not diagnostic of hemolysis, since it simply indicates a response to blood loss.

Erythropoiesis has been classified into effective and ineffective erythropoiesis. **Effective erythropoiesis** can be measured by (1) the reticulocyte count, which should be corrected for the red cell count and for shift reticulocytes, and by (2) the red cell iron utilization assayed after the injection of radioactive iron compounds. **Ineffective erythropoiesis** can be estimated by measuring the **early-labeled bilirubin fraction** following injection of ^{15}N-glycine.[49,50]

• • •

Crises

In all hemolytic anemias periods of acute exacerbations occur called **crises.** They are of two types: hemolytic and aplastic.

In a **hemolytic crisis** there is a sudden increase in the hemolytic process, often associated with further reduction of red cell life span. This crisis is frequently precipitated by an infection.

In the **aplastic** (or **aregenerative**) **crisis,** despite continuing hemolysis, the bone marrow suddenly (but only temporarily) ceases to produce mature erythroid elements. The cause for this failure is unknown, but clinically it is often related to infections or immune processes. The laboratory expression is a precipitous drop in the hemoglobin level and exacerbation of the anemia, which lacks the usual reticulocytosis and marrow erythroid hyperplasia. The nonerythroid marrow elements are not affected.

Group III

Group III tests evaluate erythrocyte survival.

Red cell survival time: It is seldom necessary to employ the lengthy and expensive methods of erythrocyte tagging to determine erythrocyte survival time. The half disappearance time of ^{51}Cr is always reduced in hemolytic anemias, usually to about half normal value.

Cross-transfusion studies using ^{51}Cr-tagged cells: To determine whether a hemolytic anemia is primarily caused by an intrinsic defect in the patient's cells or by an extrinsic factor, the patient's tagged red cells may be transfused into a compatible recipient, and the recipient's tagged cells may be transfused into the patient (see Fig. 4-30). In intrinsic hemolytic disease there is a shortening of the survival time of the patient's cells in both the normal recipient and the patient, but normal cells survive normally in the patient's circulation. In extrinsic hemolytic disease, normal cells exhibit accelerated destruction in the patient's circulation, whereas the patient's cells survive normally in a normal recipient.

Group IV

Group IV tests focus on the cause and mechanism of the hemolytic process by concentrating on four main components of the red cell: the **membrane,** the **glycolytic enzyme activity,** the **hemoglobins,** and the presence or absence of specific **immune mechanisms.**

Hemolytic anemias caused by membrane defects

The red cell membrane defect is either congenital or acquired.

Congenital membrane defects

Hereditary spherocytosis: Hereditary spherocytosis[51] is transmitted as an autosomal dominant characteristic. In its clinical expression it varies from an almost normal carrier state to a severe hemolytic anemia and from a disease appearing in early infancy and childhood to a condition that may manifest itself for the first time

in the later years of life. It is accentuated by acute episodes of varying frequency. The outstanding clinical findings are anemia, jaundice, splenomegaly, skeletal changes, and gallbladder calculi; however, the exact nature of the membrane defect is not known. The increased permeability to sodium appears to be only a manifestation of the basic membrane defect, which may lie in an abnormal contractile membrane protein.[52]

Red cell count and hemoglobin: The hematologic picture varies among patients. In the asymptomatic phase the red cell count and the hemoglobin value may be normal. In the neonatal period and in early infancy the anemia is usually slight to moderate. However, because of the inability of the liver in the newborn to handle even small excesses of bilirubin, hereditary spherocytosis is one of the causes of hemolytic anemia and jaundice in the newborn. There is usually a mild hemolytic anemia with a hemoglobin value of 8-12 g/dl and a corresponding reduction in the number of red cells. Automated particle counters reveal a red cell population with lowered MCV but normal to slightly raised MCHC.

Blood film: The characteristic cell is the **microspherocyte** (see Fig. 6-24), an abnormally shaped cell that does not develop until after the reticulocyte stage. The spherocytes may not always be readily apparent (e.g., only after an exchange transfusion in a newborn or after a hemolytic episode when large numbers of reticulocytes and macrocytes appear in the blood). Because most of the red cells in the newborn are macrocytic, spherocytosis may not be recognizable until 8 days after birth.

Reticulocytosis: Depending on the degree of anemia, reticulocytosis may be minimal or as much as 20% or more. In aplastic crises and after splenectomy the number of reticulocytes decreases markedly.

Osmotic fragility: Characteristically the resistance to hypotonic saline is reduced (see Fig. 4-31).

Pigment metabolism: Unconjugated bilirubin is increased and may, in the newborn, suggest ABO incompatibility.

Hereditary elliptocytosis: Hereditary elliptocytosis (ovalocytosis) is a rare cause of congenital hemolytic anemia. The abnormality is inherited as an autosomal dominant characteristic and may be linked to the Rh gene. The homozygous form may lead to a severe hemolytic anemia in infancy[53] whereas the heterozygous form may or may not show evidence of hemolysis. The cause of elliptocytosis is not known but may be related to location of cholesterol in the erythrocyte membrane.[54]

Hereditary stomatocytosis: Stomatocytes are red cells in which the normally present round, pale, central depressed area is replaced by a linear, "fishmouth-line," pale, depressed zone (see Fig. 6-24).[55] Three-dimensional views show the cell to be cup shaped. Stomatocytes can be observed in a number of anemias, mostly hemolytic (e.g., thalassemia minor, lead poisoning, and hereditary spherocytosis[56]) and in alcoholic cirrhosis, but their role in these anemias is not established. There are a number of reports of hereditary hemolytic anemias associated with about 20-40% stomatocytes. The cause of the defect is not known, but it involves a cation abnormality inasmuch as the red cells contain increased sodium and decreased potassium concentrations.[57]

Infantile pyknocytosis: Pyknocytes are irregularly contracted, small, densely staining red cells with multiple spiny processes. Some pyknocytes (0.5-2.0%) may be normally found in infants up to 3 months of age and are three times more common in premature than in full-term infants. Infantile pyknocytosis[58-60] (see Fig. 6-20) is characterized by 4-20% pyknocytes, a transitory hemolytic anemia, jaundice, reticulocytosis, and often splenomegaly, thus mimicking the clinical picture of erythroblastosis fetalis.

Acanthocytosis (abetalipoproteinemia): Acanthocytes are found in a very rare condition called *Bassen-Kornzweig syndrome*,[61] (or *abetalipoproteinemia*),[62] in which the plasma has decreased levels of lipids, cholesterol, lecithin, and lecithin cholesterol transferase.[63] The lowered lecithin and cholesterol levels and the increased sphingomyelin levels in the red cell membrane may be responsible for the red cell abnormality, which affects mainly aged cells. Abetalipoproteinemia is inherited as an autosomal recessive trait and is associated with a number of pigmentary and neurologic abnormalities and with vitamin E deficiency.

Acquired membrane defects

Paroxysmal nocturnal hemoglobinuria: Paroxysmal nocturnal hemoglobinuria (PNH) is a rare acquired chronic hemolytic anemia accentuated by paroxysms of acute intravascular hemolysis occurring when the patient is asleep.[64] It is characterized by a red cell membrane defect that renders one population of red cells markedly sensitive to lysis by normal complement (C'), while another population is less sensitive.[65]

Red cell pathology: The red cell count may vary from $1\text{-}3 \times 10^6$ μl so that the hematocrit value is usually below 30%. In the majority of patients, the MCV and MCH are increased because of the macrocytosis resulting from the reticulocytosis. The MCHC is usually reduced, a sign of the iron deficiency brought about by renal siderosis and loss of iron in the urine.[66]

White cells and platelets: More than 50% of patients exhibit thrombocytopenia[67] and leukopenia (the latter primarily caused by neutropenia[67]) so that the total hematologic picture is suggestive of the pancytopenia of aplastic anemia. The leukocyte alkaline phosphatase (LAP) score is low.[68]

Bone marrow: The bone marrow picture not only varies among different patients but also in an individual patient at different times. There may be erythroid hyperplasia characteristic of most hemolytic processes or the marrow may be hypoplastic or aplastic, thus mimicking aplastic anemia. Paroxysmal nocturnal hemoglobinuria may also appear in the course of myelosclerosis[69] and leukemia.[70]

Nonhematologic findings: The plasma may be pink as the result of free hemoglobin, or it may be brown because of the presence of methemoglobin. Chronic hemolysis is responsible for depression of haptoglobin levels and for elevation of nonconjugated bilirubin and LDH levels. Hemoglobinuria is found after sleep, although much longer periods of acute hemolysis may be observed. **Hemosiderinuria** is one of the diagnostically more important laboratory findings in PNH.

Serologic investigation: The diagnosis of PNH depends on the in vitro demonstration of the lysis of PNH red cells by complement (e.g., in the sucrose hemolysis test).

Sugar water screening test: The sugar water screening test[71] is a valid screening procedure only if the sucrose solution is freshly prepared, specific anticoagulants are used, and the hematocrit is not too low. The hemolysis should be read spectrophotometrically, since hemolysis values below 5% are not diagnostic.

Principle: PNH red cells lyse when exposed to serum solutions of low ionic strength containing complement; this is a result of the sensitivity of these cells to this protein. Normal red cells under similar circumstances do not lyse.

Reagent: Prepare fresh sugar water as follows:
Sucrose, 92.4 g
Distilled water, 1 L
Mix well.

Procedure: Add 1 volume citrated or oxalated blood (do not use any other form of anticoagulant) to 9 volumes sugar water. Mix ingredients and incubate at room temperature for 3 min. Centrifuge and examine supernatant grossly and spectrophotometrically for hemolysis. Always run a normal and positive control (see Ham test).

Interpretation: If hemolysis exceeds 5%, the specific acid hemolysin test or the sucrose hemolysis test must be performed. A negative test result renders the diagnosis of PNH unlikely.

Sucrose hemolysis test[72]:

Principle: See discussion of sugar water screening test.

Reagents:
1. Aqueous sucrose, 92.4 g/L
2. Serum ABO compatible with patient's red cells
3. Saline suspension (50%) of patient's washed (three times) oxalated or citrated red cells

Procedure: Set up two small tubes and label them "1" (test) and "2" (control). Follow tabulated outline in Table 8-2. Mix reagents and incubate at 37° C for 30 min. Centrifuge tubes and examine for lysis grossly and, if indicated, examine spectrophotometrically as follows:
1. Zero blank: Add 0.05 ml ABO compatible serum to 0.85 ml saline.
2. Hemolysis (100%): Add 0.1 ml red cell suspension to 0.9 ml Drabkin's solution.
3. Patient's hemolysis: Add 0.5 ml supernatant of tube 1 to 5 ml Drabkin's solution.

Table 8-2. Sucrose hemolysis test

Reagents	Test tubes	
	1	2
Fresh serum	0.05 ml	0.05 ml
Sucrose solution	0.85 ml	—
Saline	—	0.85 ml
50% patient's red cell suspension	0.1 ml	0.1 ml

Read absorption *(A)* on spectrophotometer at 540 nm using microcuvets.

Result:

$$\frac{\text{Patient's hemolysis}}{100\% \text{ hemolysis}} \times 100 = \text{Sucrose hemolysis (\%)}$$

Interpretation: Less than 10% lysis should be considered negative, because red cells from some patients with leukemia[73,74] or myelosclerosis[68,75] may give small amounts of lysis. PNH lysis varies from 10-80%. Red cells of congenital dyserythropoietic anemia (hereditary erythrocytic multinuclearity associated with a positive acidified serum test, or HEMPAS) give a negative sucrose lysis test (see discussion of acidified serum lysis test).

Acidified serum lysis test (Ham test):

Principle: PNH cells are lysed in acidified (pH 6.5-7.0) ABO campatible normal or patient's serum at 37° C.

Reagents:

1. HCl, 0.2N (17 ml/L).
2. Defibrinate 10 ml patient's blood in an Erlenmeyer flask containing ten 3-4 mm glass beads. Centrifuge the defibrinated specimen to separate the serum, and wash the red cells twice in saline before preparing a 50% red cell suspension in saline.
3. Defibrinate normal donor blood (ABO compatible with the patient's blood) and handle as previously instructed to prepare 50% red cell suspension in saline.
4. Inactivate complement in 3 ml normal donor's serum and in 3 ml patient's serum by placing test tubes in 56° C water bath for 30 min to destroy the lytic action of the serum samples on PNH cells.

Procedure: Label six 75 × 12 mm test tubes and proceed as outlined in Table 8-3. Mix contents of tubes and incubate at 37° C for 1 hr. Centrifuge and observe for lysis.

The amount of hemolysis may also be measured spectrophotometrically as free hemoglobin as follows:

1. Zero blank: Add 0.5 ml patient's serum to 0.85 ml saline.
2. 100% hemolysis: Add 0.05 ml 50% patient's red cell suspension to 0.9 ml Drabkin's solution.
3. Add 0.5 ml supernatant from tubes 1 and 3 to 5 ml Drabkin's solution each.

4. Read absorbance *(A)* on spectrophotometer at 540 nm using microcuvets.

Result:

$$\frac{\text{Patient's hemolysis (tube 1)}}{100\% \text{ hemolysis}} \times 100 = \text{Hemolysis (\%)}$$

Repeat same calculation for tube 3.

Interpretation: If the cells are from a patient with PNH, lysis should occur in tubes 1 and 3 in the acidified serum. No lysis or much less lysis should occur in tubes 2 and 4. No lysis should be observed in tube 5, which contains the normal control red cells, or in tube 6, which contains inactivated acidified serum. In PNH the lysis usually amounts to 10-50%; rarely does it fall to 5% or reach 80%. A **positive acidified serum test** is **essential** for the diagnosis of PNH, provided the following controls are included in the test protocol. The normal serum must be ABO compatible with the patient's red cells, pH 5.6 must be maintained in the acidified mixtures, and tube 6 must be negative. The most important variable is the PNH hemolytic activity of the normal serum, which, when severely impaired, leads to false negative results.[76] The potency of the donor's serum can be evaluated by testing it with known PNH cells or with **AET cells.** The latter are normal red cells rendered PNH-like by treatment with S-2-aminoethyl isothiuronium bromide (AET).[77]

Acid hemolysis (tube 3) is also positive in **congenital dyserythropoietic anemia** (HEMPAS).[78] Tube 1, however, is negative, since the HEMPAS cells give a negative test with the patient's own serum but a positive test with a number of normal sera that contain an appropriate antibody.

According to Sirchia and Lewis,[66] both the acid hemolysis and the sucrose hemolysis tests should be utilized to diagnose PNH. The former test is more specific and less sensitive, while the latter one is more sensitive and less specific.

Spur cell anemia of severe liver disease (acanthocytosis): The disturbed lipid metabolism encountered in severe liver disease is responsible for an imbalanced accumulation of cholesterol and phospholipids in the red cell membrane.[79]

Congenital red cell enzymopathies

About 35% of patients with **congenital nonspherocytic hemolytic anemias** have red cell enzymopathies, a diagnosis suspected if the previously mentioned tests establish the congenital, hemolytic, and nonspherocytic

Table 8-3. Acidified serum test*

Reagents	Test (ml)			Control (ml)		
	1	2	3	4	5	6
Patient's fresh serum	0.5	0.5	—	—	0.5	—
Heat-inactivated patient's serum	—	—	—	—	—	0.5
Fresh normal serum	—	—	0.5	0.5	—	—
HCl, 0.2N	0.05	—	0.05	—	0.05	0.05
50% patient's red cells	0.05	0.05	0.05	0.05	—	0.05
50% normal red cells	—	—	—	—	0.05	—

*The pH of acidified mixtures must be 5.6 (pH electrode).

nature of the anemia but establish no extrinsic cause (except, in some cases, an apparent drug sensitivity). Enzyme deficiencies of the **Embden-Meyerhof pathway** are rare and are not drug sensitive, whereas the hemolytic anemias associated with the **pentose phosphate pathway** are relatively common and are drug related.

Glucose-6-phosphate dehydrogenase deficiency

G-6-phosphate dehydrogenase (G-6-PD) deficiency[80] is the most common enzymopathy, but in the majority of individuals it is asymptomatic unless the individual is exposed to certain drugs.

Hematologic findings: The blood picture is normal unless the patient is exposed to oxidant drugs, infections, or acidosis, all of which may cause hemolysis in sensitive individuals. The severity of the self-limiting hemolytic episode (excessive destruction of older cells) depends on the G-6-PD variant enzyme, which is transmitted by a sex-linked gene ($\overline{X}$) of intermediate dominance. G-6-PD deficiency is red cell age dependent, so that older cells show an increased rate of destruction, whereas younger cells with higher G-6-PD activity resist hemolysis. In blacks (G-6-PD variant A$^-$) the hemolytic episode following drug exposure is self limiting and biphasic, even if the drug administration is continued. The hemolytic episode is followed by a recovery period (young cells) that in turn is terminated by a second hemolytic episode (excessive destruction of the by now aging "young" cells) (Fig. 8-3). Mediterranean deficiency, found in persons who live near the Mediterranean Sea, is much more severe, so that even the young red cells are enzyme deficient and the hemolytic episode is not self limiting.

The hematologic findings in sensitive individuals following drug exposure are similar to those found in other enzymopathies. Full exposure of the trait is seen in hemizygous males ($\overline{X}$Y) and in homozygous females ($\overline{X}\overline{X}$), whereas intermediate expression is found in heterozygous females ($\overline{X}X$). G-6-PD deficiency produces variable degrees of anemia and morphologic red cell changes. The deficiency may not produce any clinical manifestations, or it may lead to a severe hemolytic anemia when challenged by drugs. On the other hand, the deficiency may be so severe that the survival time of red cells is shortened even if not challenged by drugs. During a hemolytic episode the hemoglobin may fall to 8-9 g/dl, and the red cell count will be correspondingly reduced. In general the reticulocyte count is elevated, and the supravital stain, in addition to showing the reticulocytes, may also reveal Heinz bodies.

The blood film often reveals anisocytosis and poikilocytosis produced by pyknocytes (Fig. 8-4); however, morphologic changes may be absent. The presence of Heinz bodies may be responsible for "bitten" cells.

Pigment metabolism: The plasma bilirubin level may be increased, depending on the degree of hemolysis and on the ability of the liver to use the unconjugated bilirubin. In the newborn the excretory ability of the liver is physiologically impaired, so that the liver is unable to handle even moderate increases in indirect-reacting bilirubin. G-6-PD deficiency is one of the causes of hemolytic jaundice in the newborn.

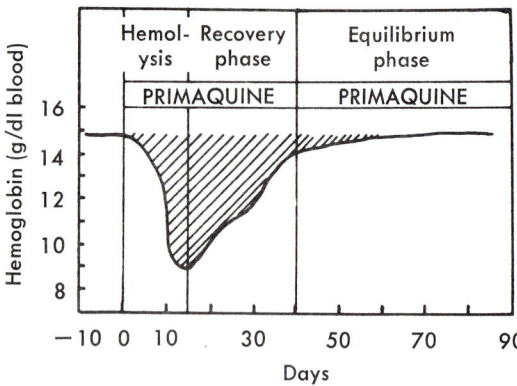

Fig. 8-3. Transient hemolysis caused by G-6-PD deficiency in response to continuous administration of primaquine.

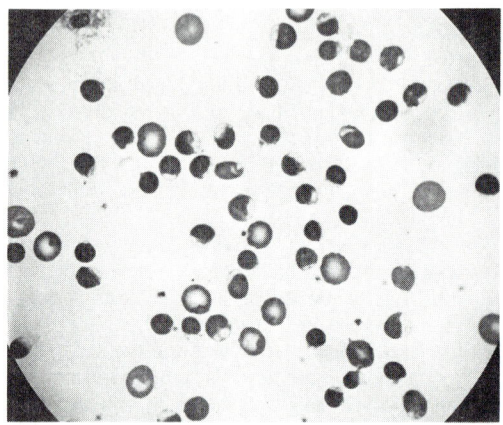

Fig. 8-4. Blood film in severe hemolytic anemia showing numerous blister cells. Child had demonstrated G-6-PD deficiency after exposure to fava beans. (Courtesy Prof. Dr. J. V. Dacie.)

G-6-PD assay: It is clear from the preceding discussion that in the severe Mediterranean form the G-6-PD assay during the hemolytic episode is always meaningful (0-7% activity). On the other hand, in the A$^-$ variant (and in heterozygotes) the presence of young cells may obscure a G-6-PD deficiency; therefore the assay should be repeated 2-3 months after the hemolytic episode.[81] G-6-PD values in hemizygous males and in homozygous females vary from 0-20% activity, whereas heterozygous females exhibit variations from 8-20% activity.

Congenital hemoglobinopathies

Hemoglobinopathies are diseases produced by molecular abnormalities of hemoglobin. Structural alterations of the hemoglobin molecule may be responsible for a wide spectrum of clinical changes varying from no effect at all to profound, often lethal, consequences. Hemoglobinopathies are divided into three large groups: (1) hemoglobinopathies caused by qualitative defects, (2) hemoglobinopathies caused by quantitative

Table 8-4. Incidence of common hemoglobinopathies in blacks in the United States[82]

Condition	Hb	Percentage
Sickle cell trait	AS	8-14
Sickle cell anemia	SS	0.3-1.3
Hb C trait	AC	2-3
Hb C disease	CC	Rare
Hb S-C disease	SC	0.1-0.25
Hemoglobin D trait	AD	0.08-0.4
Hemoglobin D disease	DD	Very rare
Hemoglobin E trait	AE	Occasional
Sickle cell–thalassemia	S-thal	0.04
β-Thalassemia trait	Thal-minor	1

defects, and (3) hemoglobinopathies caused by a combination of the two.

Like all genetic abnormalities, hemoglobinopathies occur in heterozygous and homozygous forms. In the heterozygous state, in combination with Hb A, most hemoglobin variants are asymptomatic, whereas in the homozygous state they produce clinical disease. About 35% of all congenital nonspherocytic hemolytic anemias are a result of enzyme deficiencies, and another 35% are caused by hemoglobin variants (Table 8-4).

The **hematologic findings** are essentially those described for enzymopathies. Once the presence of a **congenital nonspherocytic hemolytic anemia** has been established, the phenylhydrazine test for Heinz bodies should be performed. If the result is positive, it should be followed by a screening test for G-6-PD (the most common enzymopathy) and by the isopropanol or heat stability tests for unstable hemoglobins. If both tests are negative, screening tests for other enzymopathies should be performed. If the Heinz body test is negative, screening for hemoglobinopathies should be undertaken using alkaline cellulose acetate and citrate agar electrophoresis supported by assays of Hb F and A_2 and the dithionite test for Hb S.

Pyruvate kinase deficiency

Pyruvate kinase (PK) deficiency[83] is the most common defect of the Embden-Meyerhof pathway. This hemolytic anemia is usually quite severe and may appear in the neonatal period or be delayed until early adult life. The blood film shows the pattern of all anemias associated with enzymopathies.

Pyruvate kinase assay: Patients homozygous for PK deficiency may show enzyme values 5-20% lower than normal controls. The values are red cell age dependent, since reticulocytes are rich in PK. Heterozygotes for PK deficiency also demonstrate decreased PK activity.

Hemolytic anemias caused by extracorpuscular defects
Classification

I. Acquired autoimmune hemolytic anemias: warm or cold antibodies
   A. Idiopathic
   B. Secondary: lymphoproliferative disorders
      1. Lymphatic leukemia, chronic and acute
      2. Macroglobulinemia

3. Multiple myeloma
4. Lymphoma
5. Hodgkin's disease
   C. Viral infections
      1. Epstein-Barr (EB) virus (infectious mononucleosis)
      2. Cytomegalovirus
      3. Bacterial infections—syphilis: paroxysmal cold hemoglobinuria
      4. Drugs
         a. α-Methyldopa
         b. Penicillin
      5. Disorders with known autoimmune aspects
         a. Collagen diseases
            (1) Periarteritis nodosa
            (2) Systemic lupus erythematosus
            (3) Rheumatoid arthritis
         b. Immunodeficiency states
         c. Thyroiditis (Hashimoto's disease)
         d. Ulcerative colitis
         e. Hepatitis
         f. Thrombocytopenic purpura
         g. Thrombotic thrombocytopenic purpura
         h. Neoplasms
         i. Glomerulonephritis
         j. Myeloproliferative syndromes
II. Acquired isoimmune hemolytic anemias
   A. Hemolytic disease of the newborn
   B. Transfusion incompatibility
III. Acquired nonimmune hemolytic anemias: infections
   A. Bacterial
      1. *Treponema pallidum:* paroxysmal cold hemoglobinuria
      2. *Mycoplasma pneumoniae,* meningococci, gram-negative enteric bacteria, clostridia, streptococci, staphylococci
   B. Parasitic
      1. Malaria
      2. *Leishmania*
      3. *Bartonella*
   C. Viral
      1. EB virus, infectious mononucleosis
      2. Cytomegalovirus
   D. Drugs and chemical agents
   E. Paroxysmal nocturnal hemoglobinuria
   F. Mechanical
      1. Burns
      2. March hemoglobinuria
      3. Intracardiac prosthesis, chronic valvular disease
      4. Diffuse intravascular coagulation (DIC)
         a. Thrombotic thrombocytopenic purpura
         b. Uremia

Autoimmune hemolytic anemias

Autoimmune hemolytic anemias (AIHA) are acquired hemolytic anemias, the hemolytic component of which is the result of the action of autoantibodies directed against antigens on the individual's own red cell membranes. In about 50% of cases the cause of these anemias is unknown (**idiopathic AIHA**), while the other 50% occur in association with well-defined disease entities, primarily lymphomas or diseases of known autoimmune etiology (see classification).[84] It is convenient to divide the AIHAs according to the in vitro behavior of the antibodies involved.

1. Warm antibodies that bind the corresponding antigen best at 37° C are usually IgG.
2. Cold antibodies that bind the corresponding antigen at temperatures below 31° C are usually IgM.
3. The Donath-Landsteiner antibody, which is an IgG, is the cause of paroxysmal cold hemoglobinuria.

Antibodies may also be divided according to whether they react with the patient's own cells (autoantibodies) or with all human red cells (isoantibodies).

Serologic investigation of autoimmune hemolytic anemias

Serologic investigation of AIHA[85-87] should include the following steps.

1. The first test to be performed is the **direct antiglobulin test** (DAT) to determine whether the patient's red cells are coated with immunoglobulin or complement or both. In the case of warm AIHA the red cells are usually strongly agglutinated by wide-spectrum antiglobulin sera reacting with IgG and complement absorbed onto the patient's red cells. In the case of cold autoagglutinins the DAT is also positive, despite the fact that in the course of the procedure the cold autoagglutinins are eluted from the red cells as the wide-spectrum antiglobulin serum reacts with the complement (C), which resists elution at 37° C. If the DAT is negative, the diagnosis of AIHA is doubtful.

2. The patient's ABO blood group, other blood groups, and the Rh genotype should be determined as completely as possible to later confirm the autoantibody nature of the warm agglutinin/hemolysin identified in the serum or the eluate or both.

3. If the DAT is positive, it should be determined whether the coating antibody is an immunoglobulin or complement by repeating the DAT, using serial four-fold saline dilutions[86] of a broad-spectrum antiglobulin serum and of monospecific anti-IgG and anti-C sera. IgG-coated cells are best agglutinated by dilute antisera (1:64 to 1:256), whereas complement-coated cells are best agglutinated by concentrated broad-spectrum antiglobulin and anti-C sera (1:1 to 1:4). Warm antibodies are usually of IgG and IgG + C type, whereas in the presence of cold autoantibodies, the complement is responsible for the positive DAT.

4. To determine the specificity of the autoantibody (step 5) it must be eluted from the red cells by the heat elution method. If cold agglutinins are to be removed, special technics must be used to first absorb the cold autoantibodies onto the patient's red cells at 4° C and then to elute them by the preceding technic.

5. Cold or warm autoantibodies are almost always present in the serum of patients with AIHA, although there are times when they cannot be detected (e.g., after a hemolytic episode). Their presence can be detected by testing the patient's serum with enzyme-treated and non-enzyme-treated pooled adult group O

cells of known antigenic composition. The patient's own enzyme-treated and non-enzyme-treated red cells must also be included. the serum is screened for agglutinins/hemolysins by saline, albumin, and antiglobulin methods. The first two procedures are performed at 4° C, 20° C, and 37° C. The purpose is to determine at what temperature and in what medium (saline, albumin, or enzymes) the antibodies react best. The use of enzyme-treated cells is important, because it increases the sensitivity of the DAT by about 50%.

If the serum reacts with the test cells, three possibilities exist.[88,89] These possibilities are (1) that an isoantibody is present that does not react with the patient's own cells as seen in a delayed transfusion reaction, (2) that an autoantibody is present that reacts with the patient's own cells and is similar in specificity to the antibody found in the eluate of the patient's cells, and (3) that a combination of (1) and (2) is present that requires complicated cross-absorption and elution studies.

Warm agglutinins/hemolysins are always incomplete antibodies (usually IgG), acting best in albumin at 37° C with enzyme-treated red cells and are detected by the indirect globulin technic. Cold agglutinins/hemolysins (usually IgM) are saline agglutinins, acting best on non-enzyme-treated cells at temperatures lower than 31° C (usually 4-20° C). IgG and IgM antibodies may also be differentiated by the treatment of the serum with 2-mercaptoethanol.

6. If the serum antibody is incomplete (warm), determine the specificity of the antibody in the serum and the eluate by using the indirect globulin technic with commercially available enzyme-treated "panels" of red cells of known antigenic composition and ABO compatibility. Also include the patient's own cells, enzyme and nonenzyme treated.

7. The antibody titer may be established by using the most appropriate enzyme-treated test cells (i.e., those that gave the strongest reactions in step 5).

8. If the antibody is complete (cold), its specificity is determined by using the panel of enzyme-treated and non-enzyme-treated cells from step 6 suspended in saline at 4° C. It should be expanded by adding the patient's own enzyme-treated and non-enzyme-treated cells and cord blood (i) cells.

9. Titration of cold antibodies usually reveals very high titers (greater than 1:1000), especially if enzyme-treated cells are used.

10. In rare instances the test for Donath-Landsteiner antibody is indicated.

11. If the hemolytic anemia is thought to be **drug induced**, two types of procedures must be used.
    a. If α-methyldopa (Aldomet) is the cause of the hemolytic anemia, the antiglobulin test system does not need to include the responsible drug, since the IgG responsible for the anemia reacts with normal red cells.[90]
    b. In hemolytic anemias caused by other drugs, even if the direct antiglobulin test is positive the antibody cannot be identified unless the drug is included in the test system[91] or, as in the case of antipenicillin antibodies, penicillin-pretreated compatible test cells are used.

12. The C3 concentration may be estimated in fresh

serum by immunodiffusion or by laser nephelometry. The serum of patients with AIHA is frequently complement deficient, so that tests for hemolysins require the addition of fresh human serum complement to show hemolytic antibodies.

13. Other serologic tests may be indicated (e.g., tests for antinuclear and antimitochondrial antibodies and for heterophil antibodies).

Autoimmune hemolytic anemia caused by warm antibodies

The investigation of AIHA involves (1) the demonstration of an anemia characterized by a shortened life span of the erythrocytes, (2) the detection of immune antibodies coating the patient's red cells, and (3) the bone marrow response to the hemolytic process.

Serologic investigation: In 86% of AIHA cases, the antibody coating the red cells is a warm incomplete autoantibody, IgG, which in about 50% of the cases is associated with complement.[85] The coated red cells are therefore agglutinated by wide-spectrum antiglobulin sera and by monospecific anti-IgG; about 50% of the cells are also agglutinated by monospecific anticomplement sera. When the IgG antibodies are eluted from the red cells, about 90% can be shown to have Rh specificity,[86] but a few have anti-U specificity.[85] Eight percent of the warm AIHA cases are associated with IgM autoantibodies, which appear to be difficult to elute[86] and lack any detectable specificity. They are always combined with complement.[85] Six percent of warm AIHA cases are associated with IgA autoantibodies that are often combined with IgG[86] and always with complement. In vitro at 37° C, warm autoantibodies combined with complement reacting with enzyme-treated red cells may be agglutinating and hemolytic.

Hemolytic disease of newborn

Hemolytic disease of the newborn (HDN, or erythroblastosis fetalis) is a hemolytic anemia of the fetus and newborn that is caused by the transplacental transfer of maternal antierythrocytic isoantibodies into the fetal circulation where they destroy the appropriate red cells, producing variable degrees of anemia. Three mechanisms may be involved.

1. Within the ABO blood group system, the transplacental transfer of immune IgG anti-A or anti-B antibodies may be responsible for lysis of the fetal red cells (**ABO hemolytic disease**).
2. Within the Rh system, Rh-negative women are stimulated by Rh-positive cells to form immune anti-D antibodies (IgG) that are transferred through the placenta and lyse the Rh-positive fetal cells (**Rh hemolytic disease**).
3. IgG antibodies against other blood group systems (e.g., anti-Kell) are rarely involved in the production of HDN.

ABO hemolytic disease: IgG anti-A and anti-B antibodies are most likely to be formed in group O individuals and although both types of antibodies are able to pass through the placenta, group A infants of group O mothers are more frequently affected by HDN than group B infants. The physiologic anti-B or anti-A is IgM that does not pass through the placenta.

Red cell pathology: The red cell count may be normal or reveal only slight to moderate anemia. A severe hemolytic process is quite unusual and should stimulate a search for a different cause. The mildness of the hemolytic process is related to the weak isoimmunizing stimulus provided by the undeveloped fetal A and B red cell antigens and by the absorption of the maternal IgG anti-A and anti-B antibodies by the infant's tissue cells or plasma proteins. The hemoglobin level may be normal or fall to 10 g/dl. The blood film should be searched for characteristic **microspherocytes** that contrast with the physiologic macrocytes of the newborn. The picture may suggest **congenital spherocytosis,** an impression reinforced by the increased osmotic fragility of the red cells. Family studies may be required to differentiate hereditary spherocytosis from ABO HDN.

Related biochemical findings: Hyperbilirubinemia is quite rare. Low haptoglobin levels are a sensitive indicator of intravascular hemolysis.

Serologic investigations: High titers of IgG anti-A or anti-B antibodies can be demonstrated in the mother's blood after neutralization of the maternal IgM antibodies with the appropriate A or B substances or after treatment of the serum with 2-mercaptoethanol. The immune anti-A or anti-B antibodies are able to react with the appropriate enzyme-treated or non-enzyme-treated red cells when the antiglobulin technic is used.

The infant's blood group will be either A or B. The direct antiglobulin test is frequently negative or only slightly positive—a remarkable phenomenon, since the immune anti-A or anti-B antibodies can often be eluted from the infant's red cells and can then be demonstrated in the eluate by the indirect antiglobulin technic using appropriate enzyme-treated or non-enzyme-treated cells. The latter method can also be used to demonstrate relatively high titers of IgG anti-A or anti-B antibodies in the cord blood. Low titers of IgG antibodies may be found in normal infants.

Rh hemolytic disease: Virtually all (99%) cases of Rh HDN are caused by the lysis of the infant's Rh-positive cells by IgG anti-D antibodies produced by an Rh-negative mother and transmitted transplacentally. Rh HDN has been conquered by the preventive program of intramuscular injection of IgG anti-D antibodies into unimmunized Rh-negative women immediately after the delivery of an Rh-positive fetus or infant.

Hematologic findings: To evaluate the degree of the infant's anemia, it is essential that the hemoglobin level be determined from cord blood rather than from the infant's venous or capillary blood, both of which give values from 3-6 g/dl higher than cord blood.[92] A cord hemoglobin value of 14 g/dl is in the anemic range, and values below 12 g/dl require exchange transfusion. Peripheral blood smears reveal macrocytosis, polychromatophilia, anisocytosis, and normoblastosis. Spherocytes characteristic of ABO HDN are not seen. More than six normoblasts per 100 white cells indicates increased hemolysis. Reticulocytosis exceeds 6%. The white cells reveal neutrophilic leukocytosis with a shift to the left. The platelet count is normal or decreased.

Related biochemical findings: The cord blood unconjugated bilirubin level is closely related to the severity of the disease, so that values of 5 mg/dl or higher demand treatment by exchange transfusion. Additional indications for this form of treatment are (1) an increase in bilirubin level of 1 mg/dl/hr, (2) a bilirubin level of 20 mg/dl, or (3) a bilirubin level that remains at 5 mg/dl for an extended period of time.[93] **Hypoglycemia** may be present at birth and is frequently discovered 1-2 hr after exchange transfusion.[94]

Serologic investigation: In Rh HDN, the direct antiglobulin test on the cord blood is always positive (unless intrauterine transfusion therapy has been used) and is of prognostic significance; a strong reaction indicates a more severe form of HDN. The mother's blood group and Rh type should be confirmed and her serum tested for IgG anti-D. The infant's blood should be similarly tested and the Rh type established by using a saline-acting anti-D, since albumin-acting anti-D may agglutinate the sensitized red cells whether they are Rh positive or negative. If there is reason to believe that the infant's cells reacted falsely negatively with saline anti-D because of the blocking activity of the immune anti-D coating, the infant's red cells must be eluted by the heat elution technic and retyped with saline anti-D serum.

Autoimmune hemolytic anemias caused by cold antibodies

Cold agglutinin disease: Cold agglutinin disease (CAD),[86,95] like AIHA (p. 221), may be an idiopathic disorder or may be caused by lymphomas, *Mycoplasma pneumoniae* infections, or some viral infections (e.g., **Epstein-Barr** virus and cytomegalovirus).

Red cell pathology: Gross examination of anticoagulated blood in a test tube or on a slide usually reveals clumping of the red cells, which at room temperature are collected into small irregular aggregates. The red cell clumps may deceive some automated particle counters into recording falsely elevated MCV values. There is usually a moderate normocytic normochromic anemia, with the red cell count varying from 2-4 million/mm^3. The peripheral smear prepared at 37° C shows polychromatophilic macrocytes, an expression of the moderate reticulocytosis, and occasional spherocytes.

Sedimentation rate: At room temperature the sedimentation rate is markedly increased because of the autoagglutinated red cells. Determination of the sedimentation rate at 37° C reflects its true value.

Serologic investigation: The majority of cold agglutinins are IgM antibodies that are capable of agglutinating and lysing non-enzyme-treated red cells in saline at lower temperatures than 35° C. Complement is always involved in this reaction, which nearly always has anti-I specificity, although other specificities such as anti-M and anti-N have also been identified. Some of the anti-I antibodies also have anti-A, anti-B, anti-H, and anti-P specificity.[96] Depending on their cause, the cold antibodies occur in **transient episodes** or in **chronic form.** The cold IgM antibodies have a **wide temperature range** and are of **high titer** (greater than 1:1000). Cold agglutinins of low titer and with a narrow temperature range may be found in normal individuals.

Paroxysmal cold hemoglobinuria: Paroxysmal cold hemoglobinuria (PCH) is the rarest form of AIHA (p. 221), since it is usually associated with **congenital syphilis** and seldom with the acquired form. The control of syphilis is responsible for the disappearance of PCH, which is now seen only occasionally in association with the same viral diseases as cold agglutinin disease (e.g., infectious mononucleosis).[97] The antibody responsible for PCH is a **biphasic anti–red cell autoantibody** described by **Donath** and **Landsteiner** (the D-L type of cold hemolysin).[98]

Serologic investigation: The D-L cold hemolysin of PCH is a biphasic autoantibody capable of lysing non-enzyme-treated red cells in vitro. It differs from the high-titer, monothermal, thermolabile cold hemolysin of cold agglutinin disease in that it is a biphasic and thermostable IgG antibody of low titer that acts in non-acidified serum (pH 7.4) and often has anti-P specificity.[99] The D-L cold hemolysin attaches itself to the red cells at 0-10° C, but hemolysis does not occur until the temperature increases to 15-37° C. The hemolysis fails to take place in the cold, because the complement is not completely activated at this low temperature.

Immediately following or during an attack, the direct antiglobulin test (DAT) is positive, since the red cells coated with D-L hemolysin (IgG) are agglutinated by wide-spectrum antiglobulin serum because of its reaction with the complement attached to the red cell membranes. Between attacks, however, the DAT is negative.

Donath-Landsteiner antibody qualitative screening test

Principle: The D-L reaction requires complement and a cold and warm phase to achieve lysis of red cells.

Equipment:
1. Prewarmed syringe
2. Test tubes
3. Water bath

Procedure:
1. Obtain 10 ml patient's EDTA-anticoagulated blood, using a syringe warmed to 37° C
2. Place 5 ml into each of two test tubes prewarmed to 37° C
3. Allow one sample to clot at 37° C (control)
4. Place the other sample immediately into crushed ice and leave undisturbed for 1 hr
5. Return tube (step 4) to 37° C water bath and leave for about 30 min
6. Examine sera of steps 3 and 5 after clots have retracted

Result: In PCH the serum of the blood that was chilled and then warmed shows hemolysis, which is absent from the control blood.

Drug-induced immune hemolytic anemias

Drug-induced immune hemolytic anemias can be classified into several groups according to the pathways of red cell sensitization and laboratory methods of diagnosis.[88,100]

Group 1

Group 1 hemolytic anemias[101] are induced by a number of drugs (**quinindine,** stibophen, and quinine) that first combine with their respective antibodies to form immune complexes, which are then absorbed onto the red cell membranes, carrying complement with them.

Red cell pathology: There is often a rapidly developing severe anemia with the characteristics of intravascular hemolysis (e.g., hemoglobinemia, ahaptoglobinemia, and hemoglobinuria). The blood smear may show spherocytes and polychromatophilic macrocytes that reflect the reticulocytosis.

Serologic investigation: The DAT is positive. If monospecific antiglobulin sera are used, the cells react best with anticomplement and less with anti-G or anti-G + complement sera. The antidrug antibody in the serum is an IgM that activates complement and does not react with normal enzyme-treated or non-enzyme-treated cells unless the drug is included in the test system.

Group 2

Group 2 hemolytic anemias closely resemble warm AIHAs. The most important drug inducing this group is **penicillin,**[102] but **cephalothin**[103] and possibly carbromal[104] are also included. Penicillin is absorbed onto the cells, and the antipenicillin antibody (IgG) present in the serum of most patients receiving penicillin therapy acts on the penicillin-coated erythrocytes. Since complement is not involved in this reaction (although there are exceptions[105]), intravascular lysis does not occur and the coated red cells are destroyed by the reticuloendothelial system.[91,102]

Red cell pathology: The anemia is slow in developing but progresses rapidly if the administration of penicillin is continued. It is characterized by a rising reticulocyte count in the face of falling hemoglobin levels.

Serologic investigation: The DAT is strongly positive with wide-spectrum antiglobulin and monospecific anti-G sera because of the IgG coating of the patient's red cells. The attachment of complement to the red cells can seldom be demonstrated by the use of monospecific anti-C antiserum. The antibody in the serum and in the eluate obtained from the Coombs-positive red cells reacts only with penicillin-treated red cells. Because of the chemical similarity between penicillin and cephalothin, antipenicillin antibodies may also react with cephalothin-coated red cells[103,106] and produce a hemolytic anemia in patients who have had penicillin contact but are presently on cephalothin therapy. In other patients cephalothin acts similar to penicillin. It attaches itself to the red cells and stimulates the production of specific anticephalothin antibodies that then react with the cephalothin-coated cells.

Group 3

In group 3 anemias, cephalothin may be responsible for a positive DAT not accompanied by a hemolytic anemia by modifying the red cell membranes so that they nonimmunologically absorb a variety of globulins and proteins that react with wide-spectrum and nonspecific antiglobulin sera. The eluate of these cells is usually nonreactive.[88]

NOTE: If the DAT is positive, and the serum and eluate contain isoantibodies or autoantibodies reacting with normal red cells, a drug-induced hemolytic anemia can be excluded.

Mechanical hemolytic anemias

There are groups of hemolytic anemias in which the red cells are destroyed mechanically within the vascular system by (1) an impediment to the blood flow in a high-pressure system causing turbulence (as in **cardiac hemolytic anemias)** or (2) incompletely obstructing lesions located in the smallest blood vessels (as in **microangiopathic hemolytic anemias**).

Cardiac hemolytic anemias

The laboratory diagnosis of cardiac hemolytic anemias is aided by the clinical history, which may include chronic valvulitis with stenosis or insufficiency, coarctation of the aorta, valve replacement by prosthetic devices, repair of congenital cardiac anomalies, or any combination of these. In about 5% of patients with chronic valvulitis the red cell survival time is significantly shortened,[107] but a much higher percentage of hemolytic anemias (up to 12%) occurs following the insertion of an incorrectly functioning valve prosthesis.[108]

Red cell pathology: The degree of the anemia varies from a mild compensated hemolysis to a severe, rapidly progressing intravascular lysis.[109] The hemoglobin and hematocrit values reflect the red cell loss. The blood film is fairly characteristic, showing contracted, fragmented cells (helmet cells, triangle cells, and schistocytes) and spherocytes alternating with macrocytes and polychromatophilic cells resulting from the increased reticulocytosis. Hypochromic cells express the iron deficiency following hemosiderinuria and renal siderosis.

Microangiopathic hemolytic anemia

The term *microangiopathic hemolytic anemia*[110,111] embraces a number of anemias of varying cause that are characterized by intravascular fragmentation and destruction of red cells as a result of diseased or abnormal microvasculature. The changes in the smallest blood vessels are produced by a number of pathologic processes, e.g., (1) thrombi **(hemolytic-uremic syndrome, diffuse intravascular coagulation (DIC), thrombotic thrombocytopenic purpura, homograft rejection, purpura fulminans),** (2) emboli (carcinomatosis), (3) fibrinoid necrosis (polyarteritis nodosa, Wegener's granulomatosis, lupus erythematosus, acute glomerular nephritis, renal cortical necrosis, eclampsia), and (4) vascular and cardiac valvular abnormalities (cavernous hemangioma and valve prostheses).

Hematologic findings: The red cell destruction leads to hemolysis, decreased hemoglobin and hematocrit values, and to a fall in red cell concentration. The peripheral blood film reveals the characteristic contracted and fragmented cells (e.g., helmet cells, spherocytes, schistocytes, and occasional polychromatophilic macrocytes), acanthocytes, and hypochromic microcytes resulting from iron deficiency (Figs. 6-18 and 8-5). The reticulocyte count is increased. The osmotic fragility is influenced by the number of spherocytes. Leukocytes are commonly increased, often exhibiting a shift to the left. The platelets are usually decreased. (In cardiac hemolytic anemias they are usually normal.)

The bone marrow shows the expected erythroid hyperplasia. The histologic sections of bone marrow biopsies or of bone marrow clots may reflect the etiologi-

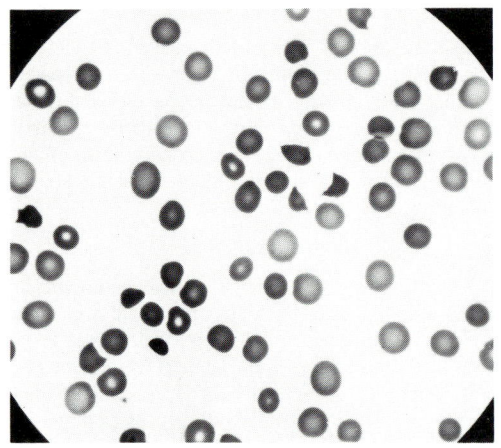

Fig. 8-5. Blood film of patient with thrombotic thrombocytopenic purpura. Note anisocytosis caused by pyknocytes, helmet cells, schistocytes, and triangle cells. (From Dacie, J.V.: The haemolytic anaemias, Edinburgh, 1967, Churchill Livingstone.)

cally important microvascular changes (e.g., intravascular thrombi and fibrinoid degeneration[112] of the blood vessel walls).

Hemolytic anemias caused by foreign substances or conditions

Parasitic and bacterial infections

The anemias accompanying bacterial and parasitic infections[113] are usually multifactorial in origin with the hemolytic phase only a minor component, but there are circumstances in which the hemolysis dominates the clinical and laboratory picture. A variety of mechanisms may be responsible for the hemolysis, including (1) direct parasitic invasion of the red cells (malaria, bartonellosis) followed by intravascular rupture of the parasitized cells or by their accelerated extravascular removal by the stimulated reticuloendothelial system.[114] (2) direct action of bacterial toxins on red cells[115] *(Clostridium perfringens),* (3) immune reactions between antibacterial, antiparasitic, and antidrug antibodies and parasitized or nonparasitized red cells (malaria),[116] and (4) DIC (gram-negative and meningococcal septicemia).[117]

Laboratory findings: The hemolytic anemia is often quite overwhelming and fulminating (as in **blackwater fever** [in *Plasmodium falciparum* malaria] and **Clostridium perfringens infections**), with intense hemoglobinemia and hemoglobinuria. The peripheral blood smear may show spherocytes and polychromatophilic macrocytes. Leukopenia is slightly less common than leukocytosis; both are usually accompanied by thrombocytopenia.

Viral infections

Complete (IgM)[118] or incomplete (IgG)[119] anti-I antibodies are present in the serum of 70-90% of patients with **infectious mononucleosis.** They are usually of low titer and only rarely produce a hemolytic anemia[120] but may result in a positive direct antiglobulin test.

Cold agglutinins and a positive direct antiglobulin test may develop in the course of **cytomegalovirus (CMV) infections** and may lead to acute and chronic hemolysis.[121] Hemolytic anemia may develop in conjunction with acquired CMV infection in the adult, in CMV infectious mononucleosis, and in postperfusion syndrome associated with CMV.[122]

Venoms

Snake, spider, and bee venoms contain components that may trigger hemolytic anemias in the victims. The anemias are caused by intravascular lysis of red cells, the membrane phospholipids of which are damaged by the various lytic enzymes present in the venoms.[123]

Thermal injury

Extensive cutaneous burns may be followed by severe hemolytic anemias bearing all the stigmata of fulminant intravascular hemolysis. Red cells exposed to heat in vivo and in vitro develop membrane changes that result in fragmentation of the cells and in the production of small bubbly projections; these projections ultimately separate from the parent cell and can be seen in the blood film as **blood dust** mixed with microspherocytes and schistocytes.[124,125]

APLASTIC (REFRACTORY) AND PURE RED CELL ANEMIAS

Aplastic anemia is a pancytopenia resulting from failure of the hematopoietic bone marrow. Theoretically this failure is explained in three ways.[126]
1. Reduction of stem cells to levels that fail to support adequate erythropoiesis (The etiology may be intrinsic to the stem cells or extrinsic.)
2. Failure of the totipotential precursor cells to develop into their mature forms because of lack of some poietic factors
3. A T cell–dependent autoimmune process

Classification

I. Aplastic anemias
   A. Congenital (Fanconi's anemia)
   B. Acquired chronic
      1. Idiopathic
      2. Secondary
         a. Chemical and physical agents (radiation)
         b. Drugs
         c. Infections (viral hepatitis)
         d. Infiltrating bone marrow lesions (myelophthisic anemia); metastatic tumors, miliary tuberculosis, multiple myeloma
         e. Paroxysmal nocturnal hemoglobinuria (PNH)-aplastic crisis
         f. Preleukemic states
II. Pure red cell anemia (aplasia): acute, transient
   A. Crises of hemolytic anemia
   B. Congenital (Diamond-Blackfan)
   C. Acquired, chronic: secondary
      1. Thymoma
      2. Metabolic (erythropoietin deficiency of renal disease)
      3. Drugs

Hematologic findings in aplastic anemia

Irrespective of their cause, the hematologic manifestations of aplastic anemia are similar. There is usually a severe normocytic normochromic anemia with normal MCV and MCHC, or it may be macrocytic with a high MCV, in which case the blood film shows some poikilocytosis and anisocytosis caused by the presence of macrocytes.[127]

The reticulocyte count is always subnormal and may even drop to zero. The blood film is devoid of the morphologic stigmata of blood regeneration, e.g., basophilic stippling, nucleated red cells, and polychromatophilic macrocytes.

The leukopenia associated with granulocytopenia (and often with lymphopenia) significantly influences the clinical course of the disease (infection). The segmented forms present may show high alkaline phosphatase levels[128] that contrast with the low LAP level in the aplastic crisis of PNH.

Thrombocytopenia is essential for the diagnosis of aplastic anemia, but the platelet level only infrequently falls below 10,000/mm³ to become clinically significant and responsible for petechial hemorrhages.

Bone marrow aspiration and biopsy are important steps in the diagnosis of aplastic anemia. The Jamshidi needle technic, which allows aspiration and biopsy in one procedure should be used on both posterior iliac crests.[129] The **aspirated material** contains only sparse marrow particles that, when smeared, are almost acellular, consisting mainly of adipose and fibrous tissue containing scattered lymphocytes, plasma cells, plasmacytoid cells, reticulum cells, and mast cells. These cells appear to be increased because of the almost complete absence of granulocytes, stab cells, and juvenile cells and the marked diminution of myelocytes and promyelocytes. Megakaryocytes may be conspicuous by their complete absence, or there may be so few that they are difficult to find. Erythroblasts are also depressed, but groups of normoblasts, although absolutely diminished, may attract the attention of the examiner (Figs. 8-6 and 8-7). Rarely do the erythroblastic elements show dyserythropoietic features, e.g., asynchronism of nuclear and cytoplasmic maturation, and mitotic abnormalities, e.g., nuclear gigantism, lobulations, and megaloblastic features. If the dyserythropoiesis is part of dyshematopoiesis, the myelocytes and promyelocytes may show granulation abnormalities and cytoplasmic vacuoles. Similar vacuoles may also appear in normoblasts (chloramphenicol-induced asplastic anemia; Fig. 8-8). The stainable iron is increased and is primarily located in the phagocytic reticulum cells, since sideroblasts are absent or difficult to locate.[130] Excessive iron deposits in the mitochondria lead to the formation of **ring sideroblasts.** Small islands of normal or even hyperplastic marrow may be encountered, but although it can be argued that they are either remnants of a vanishing marrow or foci of its reappearance, they may instead be indicative of a different disease process, e.g., the **aplastic phase** of **PNH** or of **aleukemic acute leukemia.**[131] The **bone marrow biopsy** either confirms the aspiration findings or explains the "dry tap" by revealing myelosclerosis (Fig. 8-9), tuberculosis, or metastatic tumor.

As indicated previously, aplastic bone marrow aspirates may be encountered in the preleukemic phase of acute leukemia and in PNH. The differential diagnosis may require repeated bone marrow examinations using different sites, prolonged periods of observation, and ferrokinetic studies.

Drugs are the most frequent agents associated with hypoplastic or aplastic marrow.[132] They can be divided into two large groups: (1) drugs that have a predictable dose-related bone marrow depressant effect (e.g., nitrogen mustard and 6-mercaptopurine) and (2) drugs that cause an unpredictable, idiosyncratic, non-dose-dependent, and often delayed bone marrow–damaging reaction.

Pure red cell aplasia

Pure red cell aplasia[133] implies a selective suppression of the bone marrow erythroid elements. It is classified into three types: (1) acute (transient), (2) chronic, and (3) congenital.

Acute pure red cell aplasia

The term *acute pure red cell aplasia* is synonymous with an *acute aplastic crisis,* which is a self-limiting episode that occurs in hemolytic anemias but is not confined to them. It has been observed in patients with acute infectious processes either of bacterial or viral etiology and in patients with drug toxicity, mainly during phenytoin (Dilantin) therapy. As a complication of hemolytic anemias it is seen in thalassemia major, sickle cell anemia, paroxysmal nocturnal hemoglobinuria, and hemolytic disease of the newborn.

Laboratory findings: The hematologic picture is indicative of the underlying disease or, if the crisis occurs in a previously hematologically normal patient, of a severe anemia with normal or slightly depressed white cells and platelets. The reticulocytes are absent. Bone marrow examination reveals a striking, almost complete absence of the red cell precursors so that the overall cellularity of the marrow and the erythroid/myeloid ratio are decreased. Megaloblastic dyserythropoiesis of the remaining nucleated red cells is seldom encountered. The nonerythroid bone marrow elements are quantitatively and qualitatively within normal limits (Fig. 8-10). Stainable iron is usually increased. The recovery phase of the aplastic crisis is usually initiated by the appearance of large numbers of reticulocytes and, at times, normoblasts in the peripheral blood.

Chronic pure red cell aplasia

A chronic acquired red cell aplasia is seen in 50% of patients with thymomas[134] and in patients following the administration of drugs such as chloramphenicol, phenytoin, and others.[135]

The anemia is normocytic, normochromic, or at times macrocytic. Characteristically the reticulocytes are decreased or absent. The white cells and the platelets are normal. The bone marrow findings are identical to those found in acute red cell aplasia.

Congenital pure red cell aplasia

The congenital form of red cell aplasia is exceedingly rare and is associated with other congenital deformities.

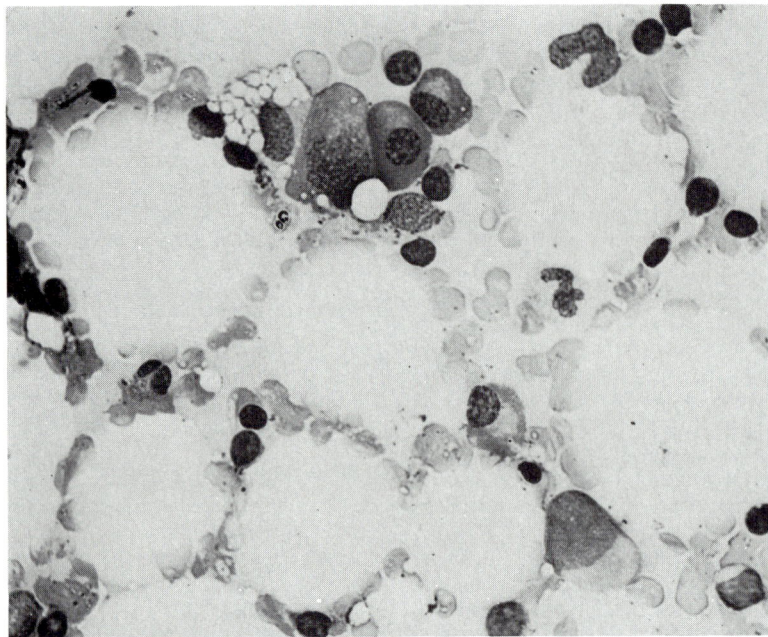

Fig 8-6. Bone marrow smear in drug-induced aplastic anemia. Sparse cell population consists mainly of plasma cells, reticulum cells, and lymphocytes.

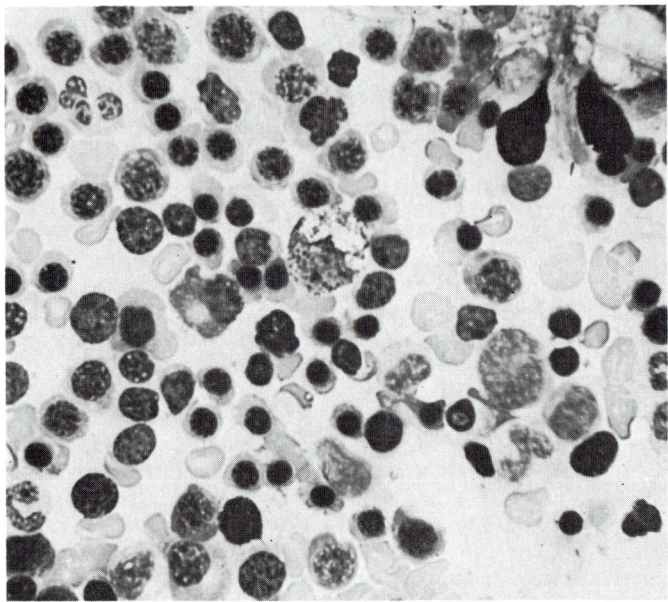

Fig. 8-7. Bone marrow smear in Fanconi's anemia showing erythroid hyperplasia associated with myeloid hypoplasia and increase in plasma cells. Peripheral blood film shows pancytopenia.

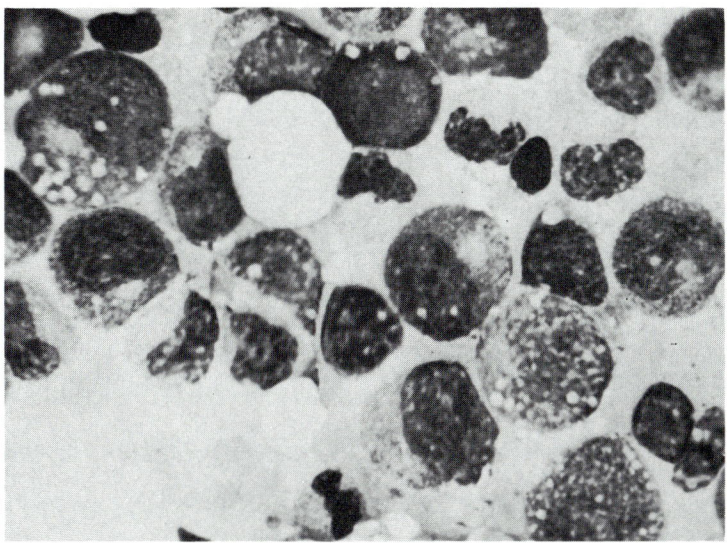

Fig. 8-8. Bone marrow smear in chloramphenicol toxicity showing vacuoles in basophilic normoblasts, progranulocytes, and myelocytes.

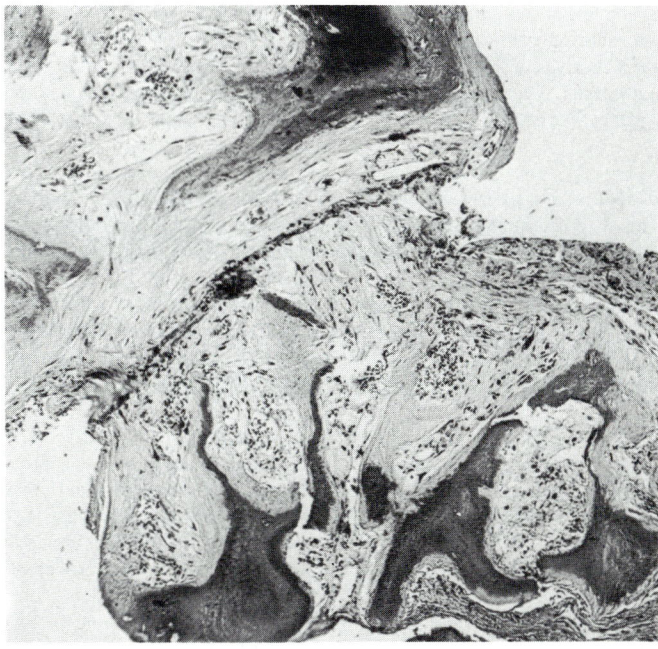

Fig. 8-9. Histologic section of bone marrow needle biopsy in myelosclerosis. Bone marrow spaces are replaced by fibrous tissue and by mature and young bone.

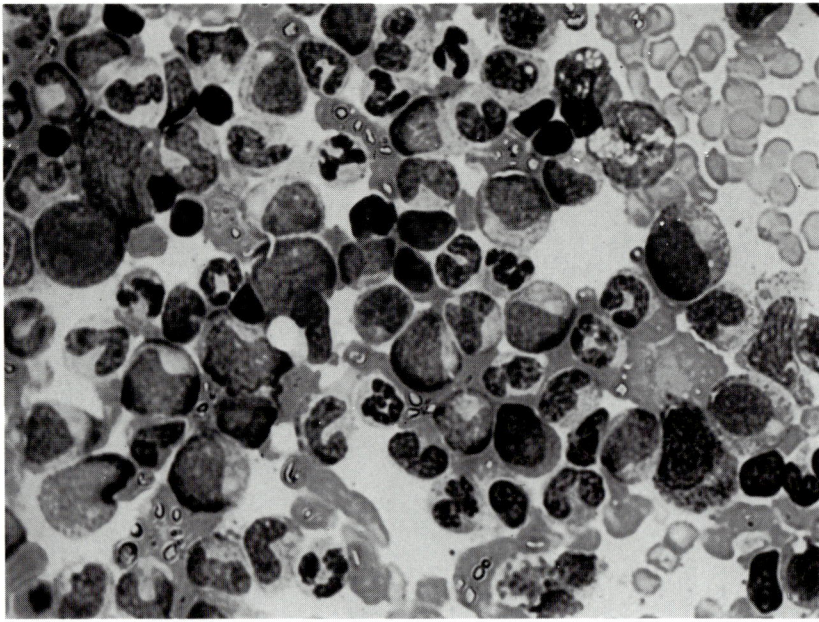

Fig. 8-10. Bone marrow smear in pure red cell anemia. Note cellular marrow but absence of erythroid elements.

POLYCYTHEMIAS

A number of hematologic conditions are characterized by increased levels of red cell concentration, hemoglobin, and hematocrit; these conditions are collectively called the *polycythemias* and can be classified as follows: (1) polycythemia vera, (2) secondary polycythemia, and (3) relative polycythemia.[136]

CLASSIFICATION

I. Increased red cell volume
  A. Primary polycythemia: polycythemia vera (erythremia)
  B. Secondary polycythemia
    1. Hypoxic (physiologic increase in erythropoietin)
      a. High altitude
      b. Chronic obstructive lung disease
      c. Congenital heart disease (right-to-left shunt)
      d. High–oxygen affinity hemoglobinopathies
      e. Congenital methemoglobinemia
      f. Pickwickian syndrome
      g. Congenital decreased red cell 2,3-diphosphoglycerate
    2. Nonhypoxic (inappropriate increase in erythropoietin)
      a. Tumors of kidney, liver, brain, uterus, adrenal, and lung
      b. Kidney disease, ischemia
      c. Kidney cysts and hydronephrosis
      d. Kidney transplant
    3. Benign familial polycythemia

II. Normal red cell volume: relative polycythemia (erythrocytosis)
  A. Hemoconcentration: dehydration, burns
  B. Gaisböck's (stress) syndrome

POLYCYTHEMIA VERA

Polycythemia vera is a myeloproliferative disorder characterized by an idiopathic (primary) absolute increase in the red cell mass associated with a panmyelosis.

Hematologic findings: The red cell count ranges from 7-12 million/mm^3, and the hematocrit varies from 50-80%.[137] The hemoglobin concentration is also increased (18-24 g/dl) but often to a lesser degree than the red cell count because of the frequent concomitant iron deficiency that renders the cells microcytic.

A technically good peripheral blood smear is difficult to obtain because of the high blood viscosity. The morphologic red cell picture varies with the developmental stage of the disease. A normocytic normochromic pattern prevails in the early stages until iron deficiency reduces the cells to hypochromic microcytes. As the disease progresses, anisocytosis, poikilocytosis, and occasional normoblasts and teardrop cells make their appearance. In the later stages of the disease the blood smear reflects the development of myelofibrosis, myeloid metaplasia, and acute leukemia.

The reticulocyte count is normal or only slightly increased (1.5-6.0%); greater increases follow hemorrhages. The sedimentation rate is greatly reduced because of the hyperviscosity of the blood and may not exceed 1 mm/hr.

The **white cell count** is moderately increased, varying from 10,000-20,000/mm^3, although much higher values may be encountered in a small percentage of

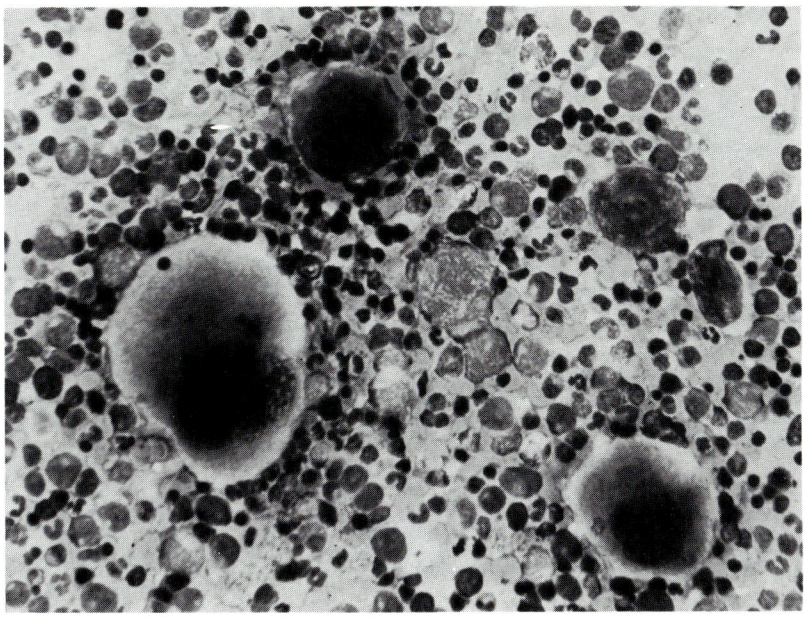

Fig. 8-11. Bone marrow smear in polycythemia vera. Hyperplasia of megakaryocytic, myeloid, and erythroid elements.

patients. The leukocytosis is caused by an absolute granulocytosis that often shows a shift to the left evidenced by increased numbers of band granulocytes and by the appearance of occasional metamyelocytes and even promyelocytes and blast cells. The presence of these cells in the peripheral blood may be caused by myeloid metaplasia and myelofibrosis but may also presage the development of acute myelogenous leukemia.[138] The differential count may also show a slight increase in basophils[139] and eosinophils. The LAP content of the mature polymorphonuclear cells is increased to above the upper limits of normal[140] in almost 90% of the patients with polycythemia vera and fails to return to normal even after apparently successful therapy. However, a normal LAP score does not exclude the diagnosis of polycythemia vera. The correct interpretation of the LAP score is also influenced by the presence or absence of clinical infection at the time the blood specimen is obtained.

The **platelet count** is usually moderately increased from 400,000 to 1 million/mm^3, but in about 20% of patients with polycythemia vera, it is below 400,000/mm^3. High platelet and white cell values are reflected in the height of the buffy coat layer of the hematocrit specimen.

The peripheral blood smear may reveal megakaryocytic fragments and bizarre and giant platelets, a picture very similar to that seen in myelofibrosis and thrombocythemia.

Platelet function tests reveal a variety of defects related to faults in platelet factor 3, in adenosine diphosphate (ADP) release, and in aggregation.[141] Coagulation studies may show a slightly increased fibrinolytic activity, normal to slightly depressed fibrinogen levels, and clot retraction with increased "fallout" of free red cells.[141]

Bone marrow examination: Bone marrow examination does not establish the diagnosis of polycythemia vera, but in untreated patients it adds information of diagnostic significance, e.g., (1) increased cellularity, (2) hyperplasia of all marrow elements but especially of megakaryocytes, (3) eosinophilia, (4) increases in reticulin or collagen fibers or both, and (5) iron deficiency[142-144] (Fig. 8-11). The differential count is usually within normal limits, but the normoblastic hyperplasia is responsible for the increase in the erythroid/myeloid ratio. The frayed, thin, blue cytoplasmic rim of the normoblasts reflects the iron deficiency. The bone marrow biopsy aids in the evaluation of the hypercellularity of the hematopoietic marrow as it replaces the adipose tissue and in the study of reticulin and collagen production. It also confirms the megakaryocytic hyperplasia seen in 95% of patients with polycythemia vera. The megakaryocytes are mature and appear in large clumps.

Procedures for investigation of the polycythemic patient

If the hematologic investigation suggests the diagnosis of polycythemia, a number of diagnostic procedures must be carried out to accurately classify the disease (Table 8-5).[136] The list includes tests for total red cell volume, arterial oxygen saturation, clinical search for tumors, and erythropoietin assay of urine or serum.

Red cell volume determination is a critical procedure, since it separates patients with absolute polycythemia from those with relative polycythemia. A red cell volume greater than 36 ml/kg in men and 32 ml/kg in women is considered to be in the polycythemic range.

The normal **arterial blood oxygen** saturation (92%

Table 8-5. Laboratory tests in the differential diagnosis of polycythemias in order of suggested protocol

Laboratory test	Polycythemia vera	Secondary polycythemia	Relative polycythemia
Hemoglobin	Increased	Increased	Increased
Hematocrit	Increased 60-80%	Increased 60-80%	Increased up to 60%
No. of WBCs	Normal or slightly increased	Normal	Normal
Immature RBCs	Occasional	None	None
No. of platelets	Increased	Normal	Normal
Bone marrow	Hyperplasia of all hematopoietic elements	Erythroid hyperplasia	Normal
LAP	Increased	Normal	Normal
Sedimentation rate	Decreased, 1 mm	Normal	Normal
Red cell volume	Increased	Increased	Normal
Plasma volume	Normal or decreased	Normal	Decreased
Arterial O_2 saturation	Normal	Decreased	Normal
Serum iron	Decreased	Increased	Normal
Plasma iron clearance and turnover	Accelerated	Normal	Normal
Uric acid	Increased	May be increased	Normal
Erythropoietin	Normal or decreased	Increased	Normal
Blood histamine	Increased	Normal	Normal
Unsaturated vitamin B_{12}– binding capacity	Increased	Normal	Normal
Serum vitamin B_{12}	Increased	Normal	Normal
Basophil count	Increased	Normal	Normal
Absolute reticulocyte count	Slightly increased	Increased	Normal

or more) of patients with polycythemia vera separates this group of patients from the hypoxic secondary group of polycythemias with values below 92%. Patients with nonhypoxic secondary polycythemias have a normal arterial blood oxygen saturation,[145] and 10% of patients with polycythemia vera have arterial oxygen values between 88-92%.[136] In patients with secondary polycythemia and normal oxygen saturation, a clinical search for **tumors** should be undertaken, and if the oxygen saturation is diminished, the $p_{50}O_2$ may be determined, since it is reduced in **abnormal hemoglobins with high oxygen affinity.**

Urinary **erythropoietin** is low or absent in polycythemia vera and is increased in secondary polycythemia vera, particularly if the erythropoietin is inappropriately produced by tumors.

SECONDARY POLYCYTHEMIA

Secondary polycythemia is characterized by erythrocytosis resulting from an absolute increase in the red cell mass consequent to some underlying condition that stimulates increased erythropoietin production (Table 8-5). If this condition is removed, the erythrocytosis disappears.[146]

RELATIVE POLYCYTHEMIA

The term *relative polycythemia* or *pseudopolycythemia* refers to conditions in which the hematocrit is raised following stress and fluid loss (e.g., in burns and severe gastroenteritis).[147] According to Weinreb et al. there may also be some patients with pseudopolycythemia who have an unusually high normal red cell volume associated with an unusually low but normal plasma volume.[148]

REFERENCES

1. Bainton, D.F., and Finch, C.A.: Am. J. Med. **37:**62, 1964.
2. Brown, E.B.: Semin. Hematol. **3:**314, 1966.
3. Rodvien, R., Gillum, A., and Weintraub, L.R.: Blood **43:**281, 1974.
4. Cowan, B., and Bharucha, C.: Clin. Haematol. **2:**353, 1973.
5. Voigt, D., et al.: Blut **14:**267, 1967.
6. Dincol, K., and Aksoy, M.: Acta Haematol. **41:**135, 1969.
7. Karpatkin, S., Garg, S.K., and Freedman, M.L.: Am. J. Med. **57:**521, 1974.
8. Gross, S., Keefer, V., and Newman, A.J.: Pediatrics **34:**315, 1964.
9. Lopas, H., and Rabiner, S.F.: Clin. Pediatr. **5:**609, 1966.
10. Dagg, J.H., and Goldberg, A.: Clin. Haematol. **2:**365, 1973.
11. Siimes, M.A., Addiego, J.E., and Dallman, P.R.: Blood **43:**581, 1974.
12. Burman, D.: Clin. Haematol. **2:**257, 1973.
13. Woodrow, J.C., and Finn, R.: Br. J. Haematol. **12:**297, 1966.
14. Baird, I.M.: Clin. Haematol. **2:**291, 1973.
15. Petz, L.D., et al.:Am. J. Clin. Pathol. **45:**581, 1966.
16. Verloop, M.C., et al.: Ser. Haematol. **5:**76, 1965.
17. Albahary, C.: Am. J. Med. **52:**367, 1972.
18. Watson, R.J., Decker, E., and Lichtman, H.C.: Pediatrics **21:**40, 1958.
19. Goldberg, A.: Semin. Hematol. **5:**424, 1968.
20. Chisolm, J.J., Jr.: J. Pediatr. **64:**174, 1964.
21. Hutchinson, H.E., and Stark, J.M.: J. Clin. Pathol. **14:**548, 1961.
22. Waldron, H.A.: J. Clin. Pathol. **17:**405, 1964.
23. Melamed, M.R., et al.: Am. J. Med. Sci. **252:**301, 1966.

24. Cartwright, G.E.: Semin. Hematol. **3**:351, 1966.
25. Cartwright, G.E., and Lee, G.R.: Br. J. Haematol. **21**:147, 1971.
26. Björkman, S.E., editor: Vitamin B$_{12}$ and folic acid, Ser. Haematol., vol. 3, 1965.
27. Heinrich, H.C.: Semin. Hematol. **1**:199, 1964.
28. Smith, M.D., Smith, D.A., and Fletcher, M.: Br. Med. J. **1**:982, 1962.
29. Herbert, V.: Trans. Assoc. Am. Physicians **75**:307, 1962.
30. Finch C.A., et al.: Blood **11**:807, 1956.
31. Owen, J.A., et al.: Br. J. Haematol. **6**:242, 1960.
32. Herbert, V.: Hosp. Pract. **15**:65, 1980.
33. Kay, A.W.: Br. Med. J. **2**:77, 1953.
34. Wenger, J., et al.: Am. J. Med. Sci. **253**:539, 1967.
35. Kahn, S.B., et al.: J. Lab. Clin. Med. **66**:75, 1965.
36. Chanarin, I.: The megaloblastic anaemias, Philadelphia, 1969, F.A. Davis Co.
37. Das, K.C., Manusselis, C., and Herbert, V.: Clin. Chem. **26**:72, 1980.
38. Das, K.C., and Herbert, V.: Br. J. Haematol. **38**:219, 1978.
39. White, A.M., and Cox, E.V.: Ann. N.Y. Acad. Sci. **112**:915, 1964.
40. Goldfarb, T.G., and Papp, B.J.: Am. J. Med. **34**:578, 1963.
41. Libnoch, J.A., Yakulis, V.J., and Heller, P.: Am. J. Clin. Pathol. **45**:302, 1966.
42. Tisman, G., and Herbert, V.: Blood **41**:465, 1973.
43. Hoffbrand, A.V., Newcombe, B.F.A., and Mollin, D.L.: J. Clin. Pathol. **19**:17, 1966.
44. Zalusky, R., and Herbert, V.: J. Clin. Invest. **40**:1091, 1961.
45. Hillman, R.S.: J. Clin. Invest. **48**:443, 1969.
46. Müller-Eberhard, U., et al.: Blood **32**:811, 1968.
47. Gartner, L.M., and Arias, I.M.: N. Engl. J. Med. **280**:1339, 1969.
48. Tenhunen, R., Marver, H.S., and Schmid, R.: Proc. Natl. Acad. Sci. U.S.A. **61**:748, 1968.
49. Israels, L.G., et al.: Science **139**:1054, 1963.
50. Schmid, R., Marver, H.S., and Hammaker, L.: Biochem. Biophys. Res. Commun. **24**:319, 1966.
51. Jacob, H.S.: Semin. Hematol. **2**:139, 1965.
52. Jacob, H.S., et al.: J. Clin. Invest. **50**:1800, 1971.
53. Nielsen, J.A., and Strunk, K.W.: Scand. J. Haematol. **5**:486, 1968.
54. Murphy, J.R.: J. Lab. Clin. Med. **65**:756, 1965.
55. Miller, G., Townes, P.L., and MacWhinney, J.B.: Pediatrics **35**:906, 1965.
56. Ducrou, W., and Kimber, R.J.: Med. J. Aust. **2**:1087, 1969.
57. Miller, D.R., et al.: Blood **38**:184, 1971.
58. Keimowitz, R., and Desforges, J.F.: N. Engl. J. Med. **273**:1152, 1965.
59. Zannos-Mariolea, L., Kattamis, C., and Paidoucis, M.: Br. J. Haematol. **8**:258, 1962.
60. Ackerman, B.D.: Am. J. Dis. Child. **117**:417, 1969.
61. Bassen, F.A., and Kornzweig, A.L.: Blood **5**:381, 1950.
62. Ways, P., Reed, C.F., and Hanahan, D.J.: J. Clin. Invest. **42**:1248, 1963.
63. Cooper, R.A., and Gulbrandsen, C.L.: J. Lab. Clin. Med. **78**:323, 1971.
64. Crosby, W.H.: Blood **8**:769, 1953.
65. Rosse, W.F.: Br. J. Haematol. **24**:327, 1973.
66. Sirchia, G., and Lewis, S.M.: Clin. Haematol. **4**:199, 1975.
67. Dacie, J.V., and Lewis, S.M.: Ser. Haematol. **5**:3, 1972.
68. Lewis, S.M., and Dacie, J.V.: Br. J. Haematol. **11**:549, 1965.
69. Lewis, S.M., et al.: Scand. J. Haematol. **8**:451, 1971.
70. Holden, D., and Lichtman, H.: Blood **33**:283, 1969.
71. Hartmann, R.C., and Jenkins, D.E., Jr.: N. Engl. J. Med. **275**:155, 1966.
72. Hartmann, R.C., Jenkins, D.E., Jr., and Arnold, A.B.: Blood **35**:462, 1970.
73. Gardner, F.H., and Blum, S.F.: Semin. Hematol. **4**:250, 1967.
74. Catowsky, D., Lewis, S.M., and Sherman, D.: Br. J. Haematol. **21**:541, 1971.
75. Stratton, F., and Evans, D.I.K.: Br. J. Haematol. **13**:862, 1967.
76. Sirchia, G., Ferrone, S., and Mercuriali, F.: Br. J. Haematol. **16**:269, 1969.
77. Sirchia, G., et al.: Br. J. Haematol. **24**:751, 1973.
78. Crookston, J.H., et al.: Br. J. Haematol. **17**:11, 1969.
79. Forget, B.G.: Hosp. Pract. **15**:67, 1980.
80. Carson, P.E., and Frischer, H.: Am. J. Med. **41**:744, 1966.
81. Herz, F., Kaplan, E., and Scheye, E.S.: Blood **35**:90, 1970.
82. Schmidt, R.M., and Brosious, E.M.: Basic laboratory methods, Atlanta, 1974, Centers for Disease Control, U.S. Department of Health & Human Services.
83. Tanaka, K.R., Valentine, W.N., and Miwa, S.: Blood **19**:267, 1962.
84. Weens, J.H., and Schwartz, R.S.: Ser. Haematol. **7**:303, 1974.
85. Engelfriet, C.P., et al.: Ser. Haematol. **7**:328, 1974.
86. Worlledge, S.M., and Dacie, J.V.: In Dacie, J.V., and Lewis, S.M., editors: Practical haematology, Edinburgh, 1975, Churchill Livingstone.
87. Worlledge, S.M.: In Hardisty, R.M., and Weatherall, D.J., editors: Blood and its disorders, Oxford, England, 1974, Blackwell Scientific Publications, Ltd.
88. Petz, L.D., and Garratty, G.: Clin. Haematol. **4**:181, 1975.
89. Vos, G.H., Petz, L.D., and Fudenberg, H.H.: J. Immunol. **106**:1172, 1971.
90. Worlledge, S.M., Carstairs, K.C., and Dacie, J.V.: Lancet **2**:135, 1966.
91. Petz, L.D., and Fudenberg, H.H.: N. Engl. J. Med. **274**:171, 1966.
92. Moe, P.J.: Acta Paediatr. Scand. **56**:391, 1967.
93. Odell, G.B., Storey, G.N.B., and Rosenberg, L.A.: J. Pediatr. **76**:12, 1970.
94. Barrett, C.T., and Oliver, T.K., Jr.: N. Engl. J. Med. **278**:1260, 1968.
95. Schubothe, H.: Semin. Hematol. **3**:27, 1966.
96. Feizi, T., et al.: J. Immunol. **106**:1578, 1971.
97. Worlledge, S.M., and Rousso, C.: Vox Sang. **10**:293, 1965.
98. Donath, J., and Landsteiner, K.: Munch. Med. Wochenschr. **51**:1590, 1904.
99. Lay, W.H., and Nussenzweig, V.: J. Exp. Med. **128**:991, 1968.
100. Worlledge, S.M.: Semin. Hematol. **10**:327, 1973.
101. Harris, J.W.: J. Lab. Clin. Med. **44**:809, 1954.
102. Levine, B., and Redmond, A.: Int. Arch. Allergy Appl. Immunol. **31**:594, 1967.
103. Gralnick, H.R., Wright, L.D., Jr., and McGinniss, M.H.: J.A.M.A. **199**:725, 1967.
104. Stefanini, M., and Johnson, N.L.: Am. J. Med. Sci. **259**:49, 1970.
105. Ries, C.A., et al.: J.A.M.A. **233**:432, 1975.
106. Gralnick, H.R., et al.: J.A.M.A. **217**:1193, 1971.
107. Forshaw, J., and Harwood, L.: J. Clin. Pathol. **20**:848, 1967.

108. Kloster, F.E., Bristow, J.D., and Griswold, H.E.: Prog. Cardiovasc. Dis. **7:**504, 1965.
109. Yacoub, M.H., Roger, K., and Tayler, P.C.: Thorax **20:**367, 1965.
110. Symmers, W.S.C.: Br. Med. J. **2:**897, 1952.
111. Brain, M.C., Dacie, J.V., and Hourihane, D.O.: Br. J. Haematol. **8:**358, 1962.
112. Burkhardt, R.: Semin. Hematol. **2:**29, 1965.
113. Conrad, M.E.: Semin. Hematol. **8:**267, 1971.
114. Esan, G.J.F.: Clin. Haematol. **4:**247, 1975.
115. Dacie, J.V.: The hemolytic anaemias, III: congenital and acquired, New York, 1967, Grune & Stratton, Inc.
116. Gilliland, B.C., Baxter, E., and Evans, R.S.: N. Engl. J. Med. **285:**252, 1971.
117. Corrigan, J.J., Jr., Ray, W.L., and May, N.: N. Engl. J. Med. **279:**851, 1968.
118. Hossaini, A.A.: Am. J. Clin. Pathol. **53:**198, 1970.
119. Capra, J.D., et al.: Vox Sang. **16:**10, 1969.
120. Stites, D.P., and Leikola, J.: Semin. Hematol. **8:**243, 1971.
121. Zuelzer, W.W., et al.: Transfusion **6:**438, 1966.
122. Kantor, G.L., and Goldberg, L.S.: Semin. Hematol. **8:**261, 1971.
123. Condrea, E., et al.: Biochim. Biophys. Acta **84:**365, 1964.
124. Ham, T.H., et al.: Blood **3:**373, 1948.
125. Karle, H.: Br. J. Haematol. **16:**409, 1969.
126. Goldstein, M.: Hosp. Pract. **15:**85, 1980.
127. Lewis, S.M.: Nouv. Rev. Fr. Hematol. **9:**49, 1969.
128. Lewis, S.M.: Br. J. Haematol. **8:**322, 1962.
129. Jamshidi, K., and Swaim, W.R.: J. Lab. Clin. Med. **77:**335, 1971.
130. Nixon, R.K., and Olson, J.P.: Ann. Intern. Med. **69:**1249, 1968.
131. Melhorn, D.K., Gross, S., and Newman, A.J.: J. Pediatr. **77:**647, 1970.
132. Kelton, J.G.: N. Engl. J. Med. **301:**621, 1979.
133. Yune-Gill, J., Jung, Y., and River, G.L.: J.A.M.A. **229:**314, 1974.
134. Hirst, E., and Robertson, T.I.: Medicine **46:**225, 1967.
135. Bithell, T.C., and Wintrobe, M.M.: Semin. Hematol. **4:**194, 1967.
136. Berlin, N.I.: Semin. Hematol. **12:**339, 1975.
137. Wasserman, L.R., and Gilbert, H.S.: Semin. Hematol. **3:**199, 1966.
138. Laudaw, S.A.: Semin. Hematol. **13:**33, 1976.
139. Gilbert, H.S., Warner, R.R.P., and Wasserman, L.R.: Blood **28:**795, 1966.
140. Meislin, A.G., Lee, S.L., and Wasserman, L.R.: Cancer **12:**760, 1959.
141. Glass, J.L., and Wasserman, L.R.: In Williams, W.J., et al., editors: Hematology, New York, 1972, McGraw-Hill Book Co.
142. Ellis, J.T., et al.: Semin. Hematol. **12:**433, 1975.
143. Kurnick, J.E., Ward, H.P., and Block, M.H.: Arch. Pathol. **94:**489, 1972.
144. Lundin, P.M., Ridell, B., and Weinfeld, A.: Scand. J. Haematol. **9:**271, 1972.
145. Donati, R.M., et al.: Ann. Intern. Med. **58:**47, 1963.
146. Balcerzak, S.P., and Bromberg, P.A.: Semin. Hematol. **12:**353, 1975.
147. Frankerd, T.A.J.: Proc. R. Soc. Med. **59:**1089, 1966.
148. Weinreb, J.J., and Shih, C.F.: Semin. Hematol. **12:**397, 1975.

CHAPTER 9

Laboratory investigation of white cell disorders

LABORATORY EVALUATION OF LEUKOCYTOSIS AND LEUKEMOID REACTIONS

The benign, self-limiting absolute increase in circulating leukocytes is termed *leukocytosis,* a term that does not take into account the degree of maturity of the cells involved or the predominant cell type. It usually results from an increase of only one cell type and should be designated by the name of the principal cell involved, e.g., neutrophilic (granulocytic), eosinophilic, basophilic, lymphocytic, or monocytic leukocytosis. The term *granulocytosis* refers to the increase of leukocytes containing granules, e.g., neutrophils, eosinophils, and basophils. Leukocytosis refers to absolute leukocyte counts above 12,000/mm³ in adults and above 6000/mm³ in children below the age of 10. Leukocytosis may be acute or chronic and may represent a physiologic reaction or a pathologic phenomenon.

In certain diseases the increase in leukocytes is so great and the shift to immature forms so marked that the blood picture may suggest leukemia. The leukemoid reaction should be defined as to the cell type primarily involved. The lymphocytosis seen in measles, chickenpox, infectious lymphocytosis, infectious mononucleosis, and pertussis may suggest chronic lymphatic leukemia, and the granulocytosis coupled with a shift to the left seen in septicemic states, miliary tuberculosis, and myelophthisic anemias may mimic chronic granulocytic leukemia.

Careful evaluation of the clinical history and of the complete hematologic investigation usually allows the differentiation of chronic leukemia from leukemoid reactions.

Granulocytic leukocytosis

Granulocytic leukocytosis may be acute or chronic and is defined as the absolute increase in circulating neutrophils (>8000/mm³). In the acute phase stress and a number of other stimuli rapidly lead to the mobilization of pooled granulocytes, whereas in the chronic form the increased production of precursor and mature cells is responsible for the granulocytosis. The stimuli for the chronic form are many and varied.

The causes of neutrophilic leukocytosis (granulocytosis) are as follows:

1. Physiologic conditions: newborns, pregnancy, delivery, ovulation, lactation, menstruation, emotional disturbances, nausea and vomiting, strenuous physical and mental exercise, and exposure to ultraviolet light, cold, and severe stress
2. Pathologic conditions
   a. Infections: bacterial and parasitic
   b. Inflammatory disorders: rheumatoid arthritis and rheumatic fever
   c. Metabolic disturbances: uremia, diabetic acidosis, and eclampsia
   d. Hematologic disorders: after hemorrhage, hemolytic anemias, leukemias, and myeloproliferative disorders
   e. Tissue breakdown: burns, myocardial infarction, gangrene, carcinoma, and lymphoma
   f. Brain lesions: tumors
   g. Drugs and toxins: heparin, digitalis, epinephrine, and venoms
   h. Stress: allergies

In leukemoid reactions the differential count may show a marked shift to the left characterized by the appearance of myelocytes, promyelocytes, and very occasional myeloblasts. The number of lymphocytes, monocytes, and eosinophils is reduced. Basophils are usually absent, although in polycythemia vera and in myelosclerosis they may be prominent. Auer bodies and granular abnormalities are absent, but toxic granulation and Döhle bodies are frequently encountered. The leukemoid reaction is usually not accompanied by severe anemia (although the latter is commonly seen in myelosclerosis) or by thrombocytopenia. Thrombocytosis, on the other hand, is of no differential diagnostic importance, since it may be present in chronic granulocytic leukemia and in granulocytic leukemoid reactions. Nucleated red cells are found in highest percentage in myelosclerosis and only occasionally in other leukemoid reactions. The **leukocyte alkaline phosphatase score** is usually high, and the Philadelphia (Ph[1]) chromosome is absent. Examination of the bone marrow smears often allows clear delineation of the leukemoid blood picture by absence of significant numbers of myeloblasts and absence of suppression of erythroid elements. The bone biopsy section aids in the diagnosis of myelosclerosis.

Eosinophilic leukocytosis

The variety of diseases responsible for eosinophilia (>450 cells/mm[3]) are as follows:
1. Diseases of blood-forming organs: chronic granulocytic leukemia (eosinophilic leukemia), polycythemia vera, Hodgkin's disease (at times), multiple myeloma (at times), heavy-chain disease, and after splenectomy
2. Allergic conditions: asthma, hay fever, urticaria, eczema, Henoch's purpura, favism, arachnidism, insect bites and wasp stings, reactions to foreign proteins, and angioneurotic edema
3. Parasitic diseases: trichinosis, visceral larva migrans *(Toxocara canis* or *T. cati),* and strongyloidiasis
4. Skin diseases: dermatitis, psoriasis, eczema, pemphigus, scabies, and erythema multiforme
5. Certain infectious diseases: scarlet fever and pyogenic infections during convalescence
6. Familial eosinophilia
7. Collagen diseases: polyarteritis (periarteritis nodosa) and lupus erythematosus
8. Lung diseases: Löffler's syndrome and tropical eosinophilia
9. Tumors: metastasizing carcinoma
10. Hormonal changes: hyperthyroidism and hypofunction of adrenal, thyroid, and pituitary glands

Recent literature uses the term *hypereosinophilic syndrome* to embrace what had been called eosinophilic leukemia, idiopathic eosinophilia, and Löffler's endocarditis and pneumonia. Three criteria delineate the hypereosinophilic syndrome[1,2]: (1) presistent eosinophilia exceeding 1500/mm[3], (2) tissue dysfunction because of infiltration with mature eosinophils, and (3) absence of known etiology of eosinophilia and tissue dysfunction.

Basophilic leukocytosis

The conditions associated with basophilic leukocytosis (>50 cells/mm[3]) are as follows:
1. Myeloproliferative disorders: polycythemia vera, chronic granulocytic leukemia, and basophilic leukemia
2. Hypersensitivity states: drugs
3. Urticaria pigmentosa (mast cell disease)
4. Chronic hemolytic anemias
5. Ulcerative colitis
6. Myxedema

Of clinical importance are (1) the basophilia heralding sensitization to an allergen and its regression as the antigenic stimulation ceases and (2) the association of basophilia with myeloproliferative disorders.

Basophils and eosinophils should be counted by special technics (see Chapter 7), because the usual differential count evaluates too few cells to arrive at a meaningful figure.

Lymphocytic leukocytosis

Lymphocytosis[3] is defined as an absolute increase in circulating lymphocytes exceeding 4000/mm[3] in adults, 9000/mm[3] in infants, and 7200/mm[3] in children.[4] The etiology, which varies from viruses to tumors, is as follows:
1. Physiologic conditions: newborns and children up to 4 years
2. Pathologic conditions
   a. Viral infections: infectious mononucleosis, infectious lymphocytosis, cytomegalovirus infection, hepatitis, whooping cough, mumps, herpes zoster and herpes simplex, chickenpox, viral pneumonia, and measles
   b. Bacterial infections: typhoid and paratyphoid, tuberculosis, brucellosis, syphilis, and healing infections
   c. Postperfusion syndrome
   d. Chronic exposure to radiation
   e. Blood diseases: lymphatic leukemia (chronic and acute), Felty's syndrome, Banti's syndrome, aplastic anemia, agranulocytosis, heavy-chain disease, and multiple myeloma
   f. Dysproteinemia: hypogammaglobulinemia and agammaglobulinemia
   g. Endocrine disorders: thyrotoxicosis

Because of the multifaceted etiology of lymphocytic leukocytosis careful morphologic evaluation of the lymphocytes is essential. Many of the viral diseases are responsible for the appearance of stimulated (atypical) lymphocytes in the peripheral blood, which exceeds the upper limit of their normal concentration of 10-11%.

Monocytic leukocytosis

Monocytosis is defined as an increase in monocytes exceeding 750/mm[3] in children[5] and 500-700/mm[3] in adults.[4,6] The varied diseases that cause a monocytic reaction are as follows:
1. Hematologic disorders
   a. Leukemia: chronic myelomonocytic leukemia and acute monocytic leukemia
   b. Lymphomas: Hodgkin's disease and non-Hodgkin's lymphomas
   c. Histiocytic medullary reticulosis
   d. Myeloproliferative disorders: myelosclerosis, agnogenic myeloid metaplasia, and polycythemia vera
   e. Hemolytic anemias
   f. Preleukemic states
2. Bacterial infections: tuberculosis, subacute bacterial endocarditis, syphilis, and brucellosis
3. Storage diseases: Hand-Schüller-Christian disease
4. Viral diseases: hepatitis and mumps
5. Rickettsial infections
6. Collagen diseases: periarteritis nodosa, lupus erythematosus, and rheumatoid arthritis
7. Ulcerative colitis
8. Regional ileitis

9. Cirrhosis
10. Malignancies
11. Parasitic diseases: malaria and kala-azar

From the clinical point of view the association of monocytosis and malignant tumors should be emphasized.

Plasmacytic leukocytosis

The causes of plasmacytosis are plasma-lymphoproliferative disorders, e.g., macroglobulinemia, multiple myeloma, and lymphocytic leukemia.

Plasma cells are not usually found in the peripheral blood. Plasmacytoid lymphocytes may be found in viral diseases such as measles and infectious mononucleosis and in hypersensitivity states.

LABORATORY INVESTIGATION OF LEUKOPENIA: NEUTROPENIA (GRANULOCYTOPENIA)

Leukopenia is a reduction in the number of granulocytes in the circulating blood to below 1000/mm[3]. The term *leukopenia* includes eosinophils, basophils, monocytes, and granulocytes, but in practice it denotes a reduced number of granulocytes only. Eosinopenia, monocytopenia, and basopenia cannot be clearly associated with clinical disorders, since the normally low blood concentration of these cells leads to a considerable counting error. Automated differential counters, some of which identify several thousands of white cells, will in the near future shed some light on the clinical interpretation of abnormally low concentrations of monocytes, eosinophils, and basophils.

Finch[7] classifies the **mechanism responsible for neutropenia** as follows:
1. Diminished production of peripheral blood granulocytes
   a. Depression of bone marrow synthesis of precursor cells
   b. Ineffective granulocytopoiesis despite the presence of morphologically adequate granulocytopoiesis
   c. Impaired release from bone marrow
2. Accelerated utilization or loss of granulocytes
   a. Accelerated egress into tissues (infection, inflammation)
   b. Reduced survival because of maturation defect, contact with leukotoxic factors, or hyperactive reticuloendothelial system (hypersplenism)

A functional classification into drug-induced and non-drug-induced granulocytopenia follows the classification of aplastic anemias (see p. 227) and recognizes the predictable as well as the nonpredictable, idiosyncratic, drug-induced forms.

The absolute granulocyte count in the peripheral blood falls to about 1000 cells/mm[3] or less. The blood film may show complete disappearance of the mature neutrophilic granulocytes, or they may constitute not more than 5-10% of the total white cell mass, which consists mainly of lymphocytes, reduced numbers of monocytes and basophils, and the usual complement of eosinophils. Younger granulocytic forms, e.g., stab granulocytes, metamyelocytes, or even myelocytes,

may make their appearance. These cells may show morphologic changes, e.g., nuclear clumping, cytoplasmic vacuolization, and toxic granulation. The **leukocyte alkaline phosphatase** score is increased. Red cells and platelets are characteristically within normal limits, unless the neutropenia is part of a pancytopenic process or is associated with some forms of leukemia, in which case the leukemic cells reflect the primary disease. To correctly interpret the neutropenia, serial hematologic profiles on the patient and on his closest relatives may be necessary at times to establish patterns such as fluctuations, chronicity, or cycles and to discover a possible familial etiology. The causes of neutropenia are as follows:
1. Infections
   a. Bacterial: typhoid fever, brucellosis, and septicemia (mainly gram negative)
   b. Viral: hepatitis, infectious mononucleosis, measles, rubella, and influenza
2. Myeloid hypoplasia: aplastic anemia, vitamin B_{12} and folic acid deficiency, agranulocytosis, and space-occupying bone marrow lesions (lymphoma, leukemia, myelofibrosis, and metastatic carcinoma)
3. Toxic agents: radiation, drugs, e.g., chloramphenicol, phenothiazine, anticonvulsants, antibiotics, antihistaminics, and alkalytic agents
4. Familial: hereditary neutropenia
5. Cyclic neutropenia[8]
6. Chronic infantile agranulocytosis[9]
7. Chronic benign granulocytopenia of childhood[10]
8. X-linked agammaglobulinemia
9. Increased destruction (immune mechanisms)
   a. Drugs: drug-hapten antibody[11]
   b. Autoantibodies: lupus erythematosus, lymphomas, rheumatoid arthritis, and infectious mononucleosis
   c. Isoantibodies: neonatal neutropenia
10. Hypersplenism[12]
11. Mechanical: hemodialysis

The peripheral blood count establishes the diagnosis of neutropenia, but bone marrow aspiration and biopsy relate it to decreased production or increased destruction of granulocytes. The **marrow** is almost always hypocellular, showing complete disappearance of segmented and band forms, leaving the myeloid elements represented by increased numbers of juvenile cells, myelocytes, and promyelocytes (Fig. 9-1). If the marrow is severely damaged, the promyelocytes dominate the picture. Further damage leads to almost complete aplasia of the granulopoietic elements, so that the white cell mass of the marrow consists only of lymphocytes, plasma cells, atypical myelocytes, and promyelocytes with giant polyploid deformities and vacuolated cytoplasm. The bone marrow aspirate and biopsy section may reveal a primary disease such as multiple myeloma, leukemia, or metastatic tumor. The total granulopoietic activity of the bone marrow can be gauged by the **mitotic index.**[13,14] In the normal bone marrow there are about 20 dividing granulocyte precursor cells (myelocytes and promyelocytes) per 1000 nucleated cells. A decrease in cell production reduces this figure to well below 10% of normal (e.g., 2 per 1000).

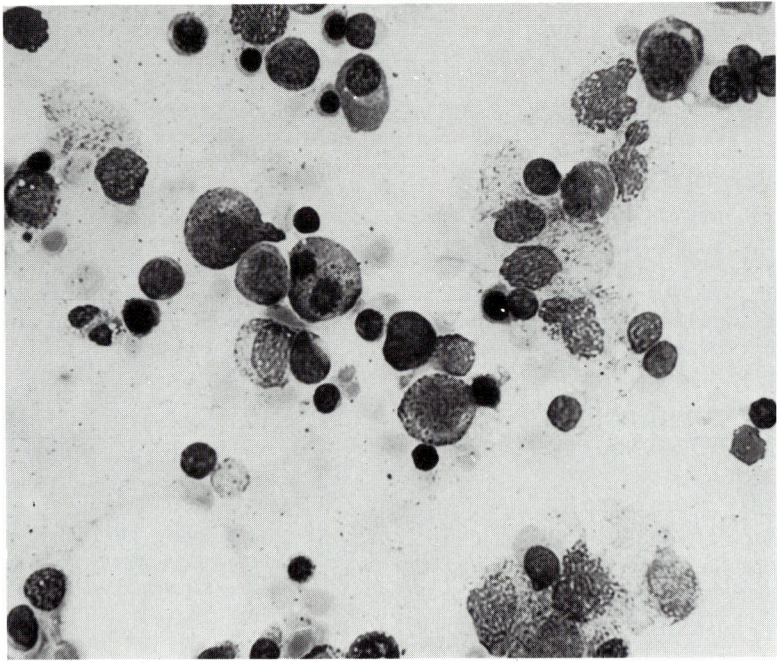

Fig. 9-1. Drug-induced agranulocytosis, bone marrow film. Absence of metamyelocytes, band granulocytes, and segmented granulocytes. Increase in lymphocytes; red cell precursors are not involved.

Tests to evaluate the granulocyte pool

Neither the absolute differential count nor the bone marrow examination provides a picture of the total granulocyte pool or of any abnormality in the disappearance rate or kinetics of granulocytes. Labeling of granulocytes with **diisopropyl fluorophosphate** (DFP) supplies a measure of their distribution in the peripheral blood and of their disappearance rate. The latter ($t_{1/2}$) averages 6.7 hr (range: 4-10 hr).[15,16]

The size of the circulating granulocyte pool may also be gauged by assaying the **total vitamin B$_{12}$ binding capacity** (BBC), the plasma **muramidase level,** or both.[17] The BBC varies directly with the granulocyte count and parallels it more closely than does the muramidase level, since it is derived in large measure from intact intravascular granulocytes rather than from dying extravascular cells.[18]

Muramidase is a hydrolytic enzyme with significant activity in granulocytes and monocytes and in the precursors of both.[19] Increased muramidase activity appears to be associated with increased granulocyte destruction and increased turnover rate.[20] Low muramidase levels have been reported in the neutropenia of acute lymphatic leukemia.[19]

CLASSIFICATION OF LYMPHOPENIA

Lymphopenia (congenital and acquired) can be caused by the following conditions or disorders:
1. Congenital: agammaglobulinemia (Swiss type)
2. Acquired: toxic agents (drugs, radiation, and antilymphocytic serum), leukemias, and stress (ACTH, cortisone, and epinephrine)

LABORATORY INVESTIGATION OF LEUKEMIAS

Leukemia is a purposeless, malignant, neoplastic proliferation of abnormal leukocytes in hematopoietic tissues. Based on the degree of differentiation of the leukemic cell line, leukemias are divided into acute and chronic forms. Undifferentiated hematopoietic cells are responsible for the acute leukemias, whereas differentiated cells are associated with chronic leukemias.

All classifications are a mixture of morphologic, immunologic, cytochemical, and clinical observations, but all suffer from the lack of insight into the true nature of leukemic cells.

Laboratory investigation of acute leukemias

All types of **acute** leukemias are sufficiently similar in some of their hematologic and other laboratory findings that they can first be discussed as a group and then analyzed as individual forms.

The hematologic findings are related to the leukemic infiltration of the bone marrow, leading to anemia, leukopenia, and thrombocytopenia and to the release of leukemic cells into the peripheral blood.

All forms of acute leukemia are accompanied by an **anemia** that is normocytic normochromic and that even in the early stages depresses the hemoglobin concentration to 6-10 g/dl. There are no characteristic morphologic red cell changes. The reticulocyte level may be normal, depressed, or minimally elevated in response to hemorrhage.

In about one third of patients the initial **white cell count** is within normal limits or leukopenic, but in

Table 9-1. Cytochemical reactions in leukemias

	Leukemias						
Cytochemistry	Acute granulocytic leukemia	Acute lymphocytic leukemia	Acute myelomonocytic leukemia	Chronic granulocytic leukemia	Chronic lymphocytic leukemia	Di Guglielmo syndrome (erythroblasts)	Monocytic and myelomonocytic leukemia
Peroxidase	+ to ++	−	− to ++	+++	−	− to +	− to ±
Periodic acid–Schiff (PAS)	+ to ++	− to +	− to +	± to ++	− to +	+ to ++*	− to ±
Sudan black B	+ to ++	−	− to ±	+ to ++	−	− to +	¬ to ±
Acid phosphatase	+	−†	+ to ++	+ to ++	−	+ to ++	+++‡
Naphthol AS-D acetate esterase	++§	−	++‖		±	+++	++‖
Naphthol AS-D chloro-acetate esterase	+ to ++	−	−	+ to +++	−	−	−
Lysozyme	−	−	++ to +++	−	−	++ to +++	++ to +++
Iron	+	+	+	+	+	+¶	+
Leukocyte alkaline phosphatase (LAP)	−	+ to ++	−	−	+ to ++	+ to ++	+ to ++

NOTE: −, Diminished or absent; ±, +, ++, +++, degrees of positivity.
*Positive in all stages of red cell maturation and in leukemic myeloblasts.
†Negative in B cell leukemia, positive in T cell leukemia.
‡Tartrate resistant in hairy cell leukemia, sensitive in Sézary syndrome.
§Not inhibited by sodium fluoride.
‖Inhibited by sodium fluoride.
¶Ringed sideroblasts.

most patients it is somewhere between 10,000-50,000/mm^3 and seldom exceeds the latter figure. As the disease progresses the initial leukopenia gives way to leukocytosis, but the level of the white cell count is of no diagnostic significance. The presence of immature and undifferentiated cells in the peripheral blood is the decisive diagnostic feature.

Thrombocytopenia is common to all acute leukemias, and if not present in the initial phase it usually results from chemotherapy or is related to diffuse intravascular coagulation (DIC). Bleeding episodes can be expected if the level falls below 10,000 platelets/mm^3. In acute myeloblastic leukemia the bleeding episodes are more closely related to the high white cell count than to the concentration of the platelets.[21] and in **acute promyelocytic leukemia** (a form of acute myeloblastic leukemia)[22] they are related to hypofibrinogenemia.

The **bone marrow** is usually hypercellular because of the apparently unrestricted proliferation of the same immature white cells that are seen in the peripheral blood. In the early stages of acute leukemia the marrow may be **hypoplastic** or even aplastic, so that it may be difficult to decide whether the disease is an acute leukemia, aplastic anemia, or agranulocytosis. Repeated examinations of marrow obtained from several sites may be necessary to arrive at a correct diagnosis. In the acute leukemias of adults depression of the erythroid precursors seen in acute childhood leukemia may not be present in the early stages of the disease. Frequently there is megaloblastic erythroid hyperplasia, producing the picture of **erythroleukemia.**

Cytochemical investigations: Acute lymphocytic leukemia can be separated from the "myeloid" group of acute leukemias by cytochemical technics, provided cells show some degree of cytoplasmic or granular differentiation and are not uniformly immature. However, a considerable overlap occurs in the myeloid group, so that myeloblastic, myelomonocytic, and erythroblastic leukemias cannot be differentiated adequately (Table 9-1).

Chromosomal abnormalities: No marker chromosome similar to the Ph^1 chromosome in chronic granulocytic leukemia has been demonstrated in acute leukemias, but the relationship of acute leukemias and preleukemic states[23] to chromosomal abnormalities,[24] e.g., trisomy 21 syndrome, Bloom's syndrome,[25] and Fanconi's anemia,[26] is well established. In acute leukemias not related to preexisting chromosomal abnormalities additional chromosomes of the D or E groups or the loss of G group chromosomes has been reported.[24,25]

Related laboratory findings: The markedly elevated serum and urine **lysozyme** levels in acute myelomonocytic and acute monocytic leukemias contrast with the normal or reduced serum lysozyme level and the absence of urinary lysozyme activity in acute lymphocytic leukemia.[27] High uric acid levels in serum and urine are frequently found in patients with acute leukemias[28] and rarely are responsible for the presenting symptoms.[29]

Meningeal involvement of acute leukemia in children is responsible for pleocytosis of the spinal fluid.[30]

Acute lymphocytic leukemia

Classification: Three classifications of acute lymphocytic leukemia (ALL) are presented in the following outline:

A. ALL (acute nongranulocytic leukemia)
  1. ALL
    a. With T cell markers
    b. With B cell markers (Burkitt's type)
    c. Non–T and non–B cell markers
  2. Acute undifferentiated leukemia (stem cell leukemia, non-Burkitt's type)
B. European classification of Mathé[31]
  1. Microlymphoblastic leukemia
  2. Prolymphocytic leukemia
  3. Macrolymphoblastic leukemia
  4. Prolymphoblastic leukemia
  5. Immunoblastic leukemia
C. French, American, and British cooperative working group (FAB)[32]
  1. L1: small blast cells with scanty cytoplasm, regular nuclei, and indistinct or no nucleoli
  2. L2: larger blast cells with more cytoplasm, irregular nuclei, and one or more distinct nucleoli
  3. L3: vacuolated blast cells with deep blue cytoplasm similar to Burkitt's lymphoma cells or the immunoblasts of Mathé

According to Mathé the first two types in his classification have a better prognosis, but American workers have not been able to duplicate the classification or the results.[33]

Laboratory investigation: The accurate diagnosis of ALL is important, since present-day therapy produces complete remission in about 94% of previously untreated patients below the age of 30 years. In fact, lack of response to treatment is an indication for review of the diagnosis.[34]

In about 40% of ALL the total white cell count is below 5000/mm³, whereas in 10% it is over 100,000/mm³ (Table 9-2). In about 50% there is an initial leukopenia (<500/mm³). The predominant cell in the **peripheral blood** and in the **bone marrow** is the lymphoblast, which has a thin rim of blue cytoplasm, a high nuclear/cytoplasmic ratio, and 1-2 nucleoli (Fig. 9-2). Auer bodies are not identified. **Rieder's cells** are frequent but not diagnostic (see Fig. 6-54). The lymphoblasts are accompanied by mature-appearing lymphocytes that cytochemically can be shown to have been derived from the leukemic blast cells.[35] The blast cells are essentially lysozyme, Sudan black B, peroxidase, and naphthol AS-D chloroacetate esterase negative.[35] The latter three reactions are strongly positive in acute granulocytic and acute myelomonocytic leukemias and are therefore of differential diagnostic significance. The blast cells usually show diagnostically important coarse granules or blocks of PAS-positive material against a negative cytoplasmic background.[35] The leukocyte alkaline phosphatase level of the diminished number of normal granulocytes is normal or high.[35] The erythroblasts surviving in the bone marrow are PAS negative and are not involved in the leukemic process. Fewer than 5% of lymphoblasts are T or B cells. The majority are non–B and non–T cells.

Subacute lymphocytic leukemia

In subacute lymphocytic leukemia (SLL) (Fig. 9-3) the majority of leukemic cells in the peripheral blood and bone marrow are prolymphocytes. The bone mar-

Table 9-2. Peripheral blood presenting features in two series of consecutive cases of acute leukemias

		Percent of cases	
		Acute lymphocytic leukemia	**Acute granulocytic leukemia**
Hemoglobin (g/dl)	>12	5.5	6
	8-12	27.5	56
	4-8	52.5	37
	<4	11.5	1
Platelets/μl	>50,000	34	42
	<50,000	66	58
Total leukocytes/μl	>100,000	10.5	9
	20-100,000	19	33.5
	5-20,000	33	20
	<5,000	37.5	29.5
Blasts	Present	82	92
	Absent	18	8
Neutrophils/μl	>2,000	19	32
	500-2,000	32	28
	<500	49	40

From Kay, H.E.M.: In Hardisty, R.M., and Weatherall, D.J., editors: Blood and its disorders, Oxford, England, 1974, Blackwell Scientific Publications, Ltd.

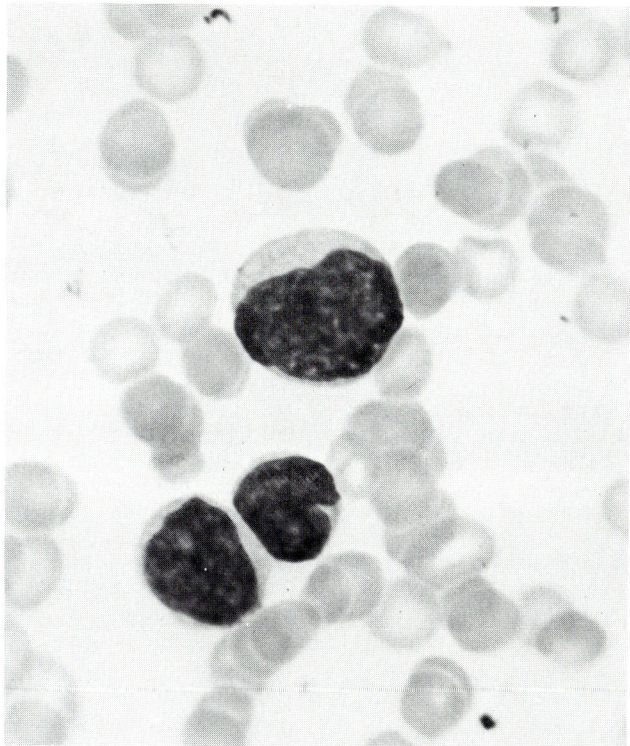

Fig. 9-2. Peripheral blood film in acute lymphocytic leukemia.

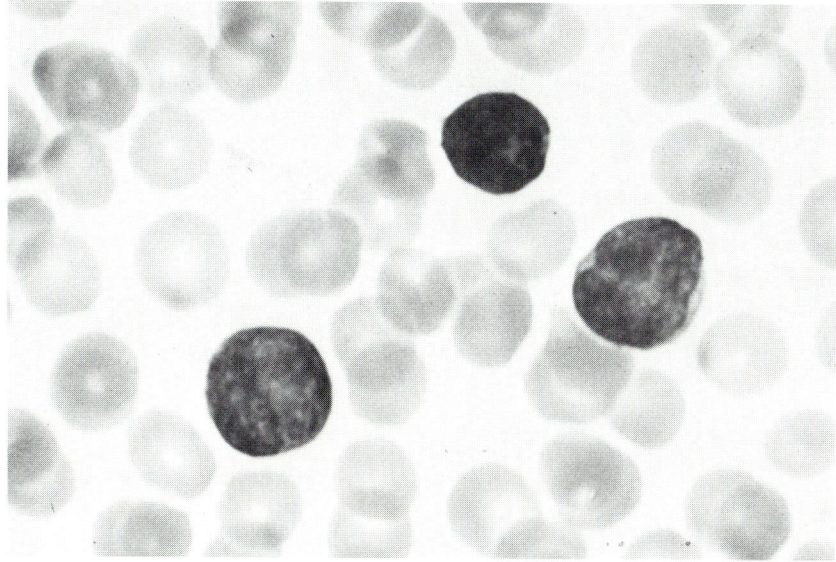

Fig. 9-3. Subacute lymphocytic leukemia.

row lymphoblastic concentration is reduced to less than 30%. The cytochemistry of lymphoblasts is mentioned in the discussion of acute lymphocytic leukemia. The majority of acute lymphocytic leukemias in childhood and half of the acute lymphocytic leukemias in adults are SLL. Cells of SLL and of acute lymphocytic leukemia when tested for surface markers include both non–T and non–B cells and T cells (see ALL above). T cells are strongly focally acid phosphatase positive, whereas non–T and non–B cells are weakly and diffusely positive.[36] Anti–lymphoblastic sera react with most non-T and non-B lymphoblasts, so that the reacting form of leukemia is designated as ''common'' lymphoblastic leukemia. The sera fail to react with leukemic cells of the T cell and B cell types, so that this form of leukemia is referred to as null type.[37]

A number of enzymes appear to be restricted to lymphoblasts and to the cells of the blast crisis of chronic granulocytic leukemia because they are not found in other blast cells. These enzymes are terminal deoxynucleotidyl transferase,[38] adenosine deaminase,[39] and lysosomal hydrolase hexosaminidase.[40]

Stem cell (undifferentiated) leukemia (Burkitt's type)

The Burkitt type of leukemia (Fig. 9-4) is characterized by monoclonal proliferation of large blast cells that contain punched-out vacuoles in the cytoplasm that stain with oil red O. The nuclear chromatin is more coarse than that in the lymphoblasts. This leukemia is frequently associated with a lymphoma, often in the ileocecal area. The Burkitt cells are methyl green–pyronine positive, peroxidase and PAS negative, and immunoglobulin surface marker positive and are therefore of B cell origin.

Stem cell (undifferentiated) leukemia (non-Burkitt's type)

The non-Burkitt type of acute lymphocytic leukemia (Fig. 9-5) is characterized by undifferentiated blast cells that lack the cytoplasmic vacuoles of the Burkitt cells but are still surface immunoglobulin positive. Both types of stem cell leukemia are quite rare.

Acute myeloid (myelogenous granulocytic) leukemia

Classification: Three classifications of acute myeloid leukemia (AML) are presented in the following outline:
A. AML[41]
 1. Myeloblastic leukemia
 2. Myelomonocytic leukemia
 3. Promyelocytic leukemia
 4. Erythroleukemia
 5. Blast cell crisis of chronic granulocytic leukemia
  a. Acute myeloid leukemia
  b. Acute lymphoid leukemia
B. French, American, and British cooperative working group (FAB)[33]
 1. M1: myeloblastic leukemia without maturation
 2. M2: myeloblastic leukemia with maturation
 3. M3: hypergranular promyelocytic leukemia

4. M4: myelomonocytic leukemia
5. M5: monocytic leukemia, differentiated
6. M5: monocytic leukemia, poorly differentiated
7. M6: erythroleukemia
C. Classification of AML that corresponds to FAB classification[42]
 1. M1: acute myelogenous leukemia
 2. M2: subacute myelogenous leukemia
 3. M3: acute promyelocytic leukemia
 4. M4: acute myelomonocytic leukemia (Naegeli type)
 5. M5: acute monocytic leukemia
 6. M5: acute monoblastic leukemia (Schilling type)
 7. M6: erythroleukemia

Laboratory investigation: The peripheral blood shows well over 60% myeloblasts with fairly regular cell outlines and fairly uniform cell shape (see Fig. 6-36). The cytoplasmic ring is wider than that in the lymphoblast, so that the nuclear/cytoplasmic ratio is decreased. The cytoplasm may contain scattered azurophilic granules that increase in number as the cells mature to the promyelocytic stage. **Auer bodies** can frequently be discovered if searched for diligently and are of great value in differentiating acute lymphocytic leukemia from acute granulocytic leukemia (see Fig. 6-36). About 5% of the blast cells react positively with myeloperoxidase, Sudan black B, and chloroacetate esterase stains. The erythroid and megakaryocytic elements are severely depressed.

The peripheral blood smear shows evidence of a normocytic normochromic anemia and thrombocytopenia. If the patient is leukopenic, the myeloblasts may be difficult to find and buffy coat preparations should be examined. If there is a leukocytosis, 100% of white cells may be myeloblasts.

Subacute myeloid leukemia

In subacute myeloid leukemia (Fig. 9-6) fewer bone marrow myeloblasts are seen, and they are accompanied by promyelocytes, myelocytes, and even more mature cells that show the stigmata of dysgranulopoiesis. The nuclei may exhibit Pelger-Huët nuclear anomaly and nuclear cytoplasmic dissociation is evident. The cytoplasmic granules are diminished and often replaced by vacuoles. The observer may still be able to discover Auer bodies. The dyserythropoiesis is expressed in megaloblastoid changes of the red cell precursor forms. These changes, which are an expression of the leukemia rather than of folic acid deficiency, also involve the megakaryocytes. The cytochemical reactions are as in AML.

Myelomonocytic leukemia

In the peripheral blood and the bone marrow over 20% monocytoid blast cells, promonocytes, and/or monocytes are seen, an impression that can be confirmed by the nonspecific esterase stain. The monocytic leukemic cells have indented, folded, irregularly shaped nuclei with fine chromatin and 3-5 nucleoli (Fig. 9-7). The fairly wide cytoplasmic rim contains vacuoles and azurophilic granules that may be fused into **Auer bodies.** The peroxidase, Sudan black B, and

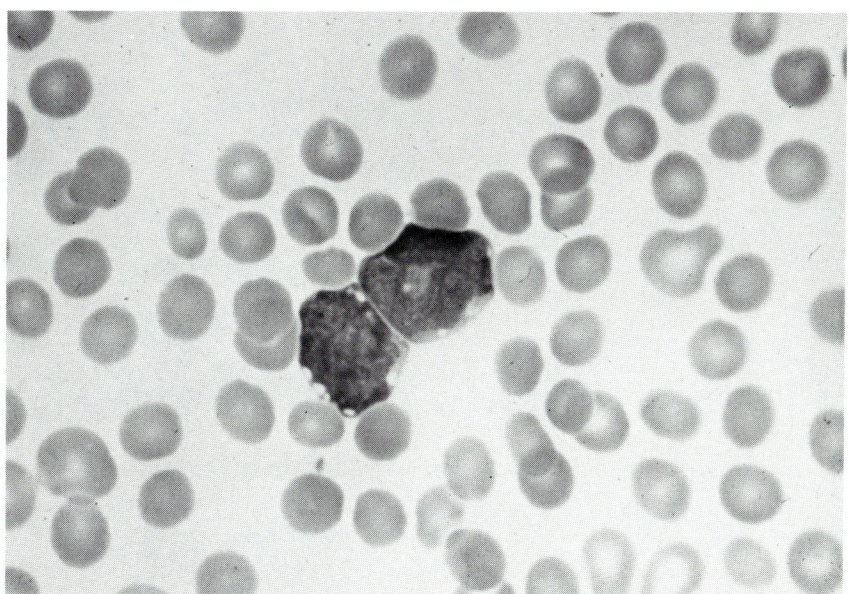

Fig. 9-4. Stem cell leukemia (Burkitt's type).

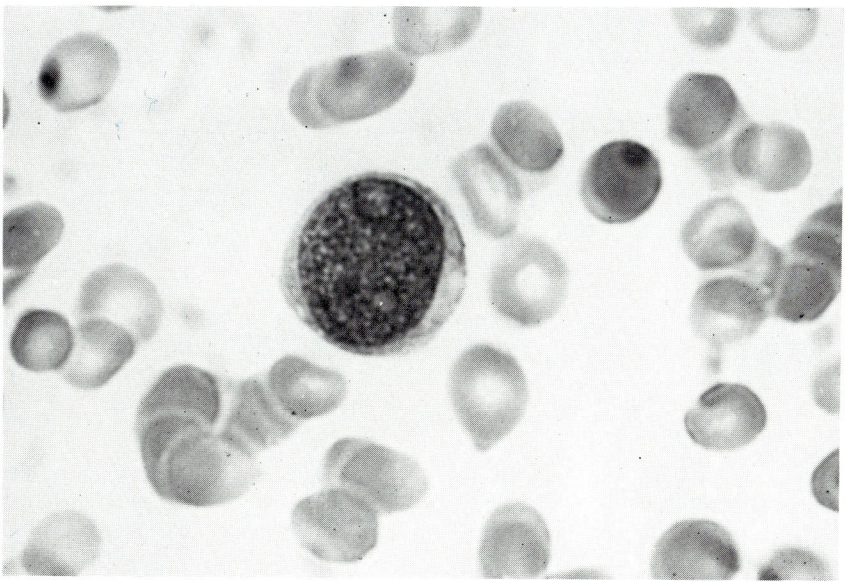

Fig. 9-5. Stem cell leukemia (non-Burkitt's type).

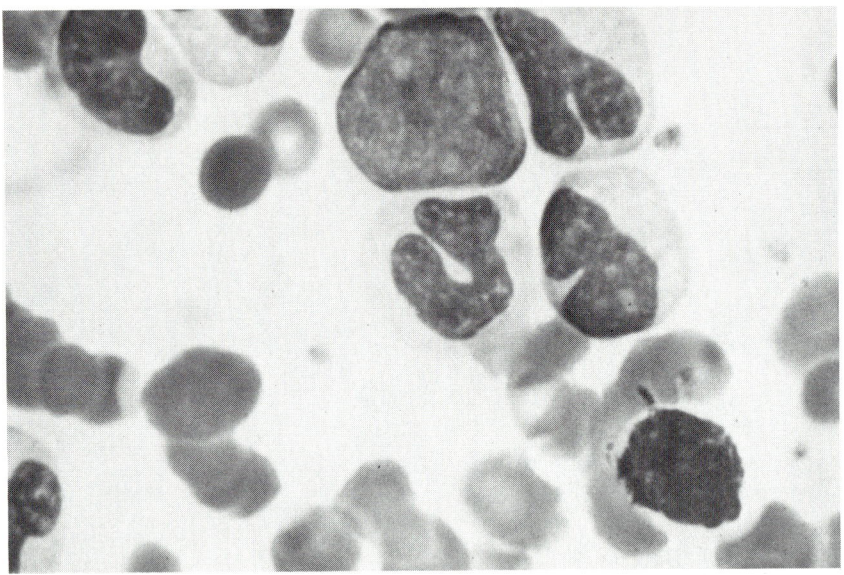

Fig. 9-6. Subacute myeloid leukemia.

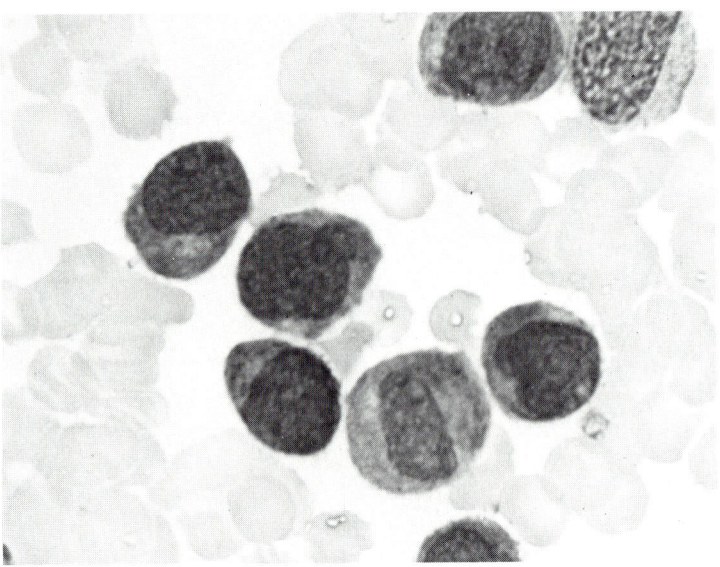

Fig. 9-7. Blood film in acute myelomonocytic leukemia.

naphthol AS-D chloroacetate esterase reactions are negative, and the α-naphthol AS-D acetate esterase activity is strongly positive but inhibited by sodium fluoride,[43] a reaction that is diagnostic of monocytes, since granulocytic α-naphthol AS-D acetate esterase is not inhibited by sodium fluoride. Consistently elevated values of lysozyme have been found in the sera and urine of patients with acute myelomonocytic (and monocytic) leukemia,[44] whereas in acute lymphocytic leukemia these values are normal or decreased. The elevated urinary lysozyme is responsible for a positive urinary protein reaction and for a peculiar glomerular-tubular dysfunction.[45] The elevated serum lysozyme gives rise to a monoclonal γ-peak in the serum electrophoretogram. The dyserythropoietic megaloblastoid red cell precursor cells and the depressed and abnormal megakaryocytes bear evidence that the leukemic process has spread to a second and third cell line. The peripheral blood shows monocytoid blast cells, monocytes, and abnormal segmented cells. Morphologic evidence of severe thrombocytopenia and of normocytic normochromic anemia is present.

Acute monocytic leukemia (Schilling type)

Schilling believed that the malignant cells of acute monocytic leukemia (Fig. 9-8) were of reticuloendo-

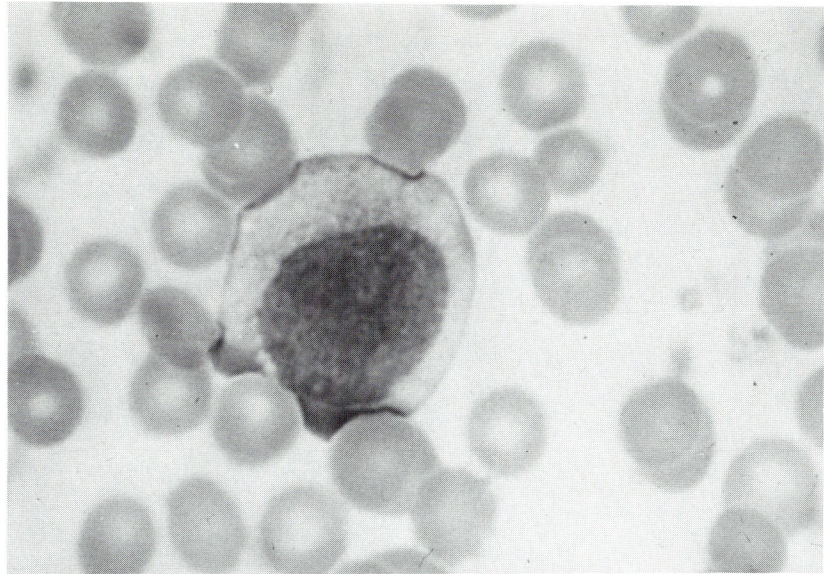

Fig. 9-8. Acute monocytic leukemia (Schilling type).

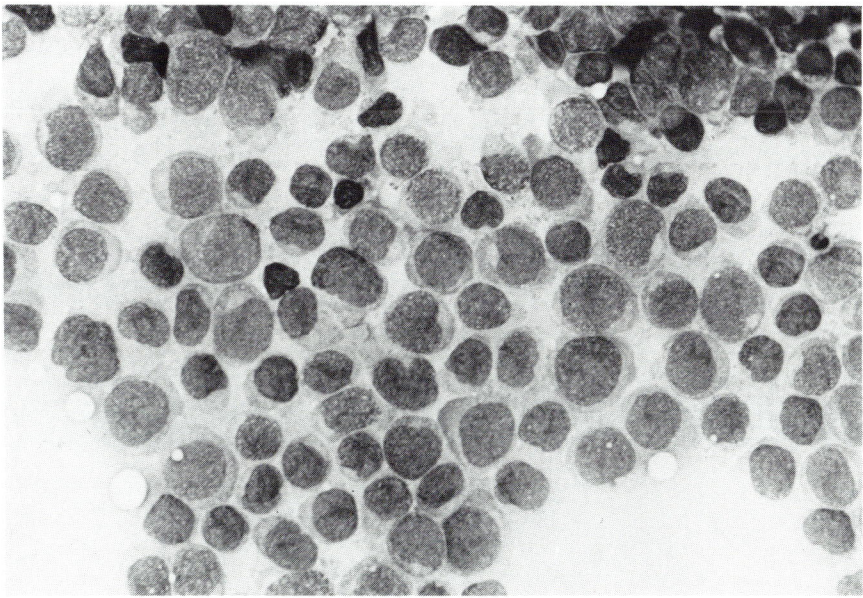

Fig. 9-9. Acute monoblastic leukemia.

thelial origin, whereas Naegeli considered all monocytic leukemias to originate from myeloblastic precursors. The peripheral blood and bone marrow contain monoblasts that are seen to mature into promonocytes and monocytes that stain positively with α-naphthol acetate esterase and do not react with myeloperoxidase stain.

Acute monoblastic leukemia

Acute monoblastic leukemia (Fig. 9-9) is a rare form of acute leukemia that is still subject to dispute.[46] Cultures of leukemic bone marrows have settled the Schilling-Naegeli dispute. The monoblasts do not show evidence of maturation but cytochemically can be unmasked as monoblasts by their strong positivity when stained with α-naphthol esterase, a positivity inhibited by sodium fluoride.[47]

Acute promyelocytic leukemia

In acute promyelocytic leukemia (Fig. 9-10) the predominant cell in the bone marrow and peripheral blood is an abnormal promyelocyte with heavy granules and frequently with numerous Auer bodies. These inclu-

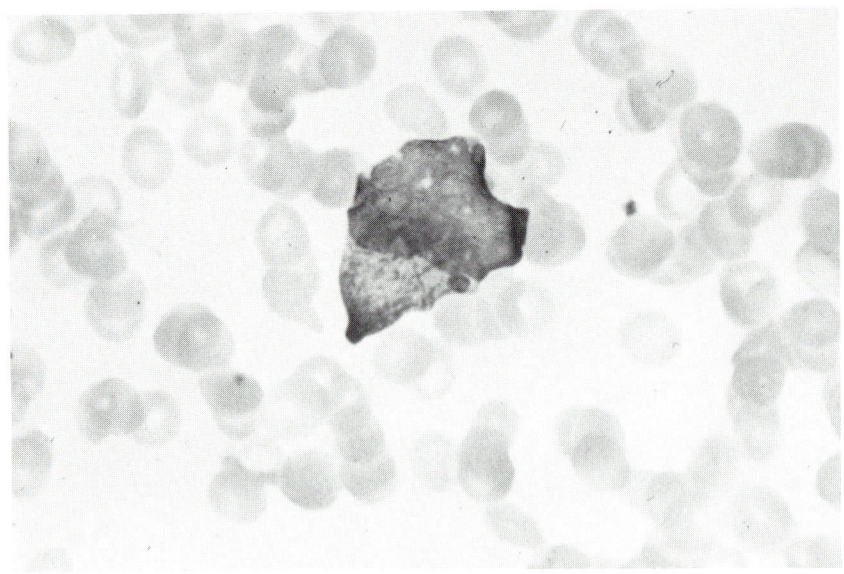

Fig. 9-10. Acute promyelocytic leukemia.

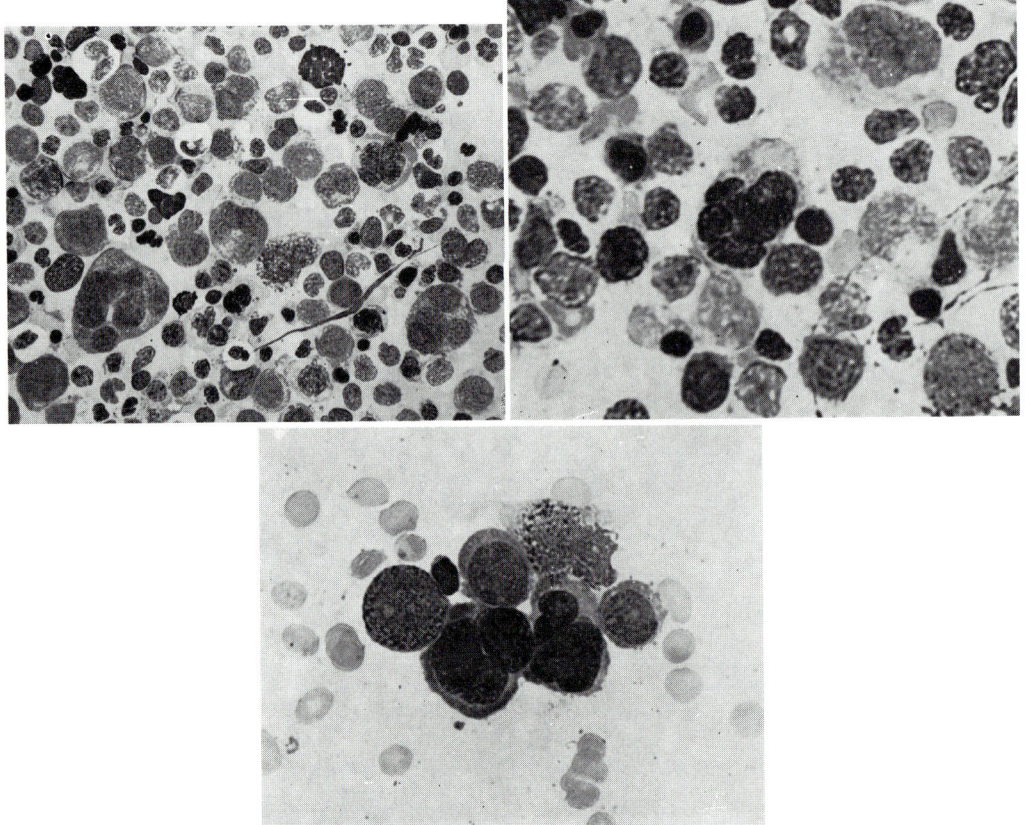

Fig. 9-11. Bone marrow in erythroleukemia. Giant multinucleated bizarre pathologic normoblasts.

sions are intensely myeloperoxidase positive. In many blast cells are globoid inclusions that stain similar to Auer bodies. In the peripheral blood the myeloblasts and promyelocytes are difficult to find. Acute promyelocytic leukemia is characterized by a strong bleeding tendency, since almost all patients develop diffuse intravascular coagulation. The disintegrating leukemic cells release activators of plasminogen and factor VII. The activated factor VII acts on the common pathway coagulation factors, and thrombin and fibrin are produced. Thrombin activates factor's VIII, V, and XIII. The activated plasminogen is responsible for the production of plasmin, a proteolytic enzyme, which attacks fibrinogen, fibrin, and factors VIII and V.

Acute red cell leukemia (erythroleukemia; Di Guglielmo syndrome)

In erythroleukemia (Fig. 9-11) the leukemic process not only involves the myeloid series but also spreads to the megakaryocytic and erythroid elements. The erythroid involvement is evidenced by erythroid hyperplasia, nuclear malformations, and pathologic multinucleation of normoblasts.

The peripheral blood reveals a striking erythroblastemia. The myeloid cells are strongly α-naphthol AS-D acetate esterase and acid phosphatase positive and show the already described variable positive reaction with peroxidase and Sudan black B. The leukemic erythroblasts are strongly PAS positive, thus differing from normal erythroblasts, which are PAS negative. Other conditions in which the erythroblasts are PAS positive are thalassemia, refractory sideroblastic anemia, and at times iron deficiency anemia. If these conditions can be excluded, the PAS positivity of the erythroblasts is diagnostic for erythroleukemia.

The ineffective erythropoiesis is responsible for a marked elevation of serum lactic dehydrogenase (LDH).

Preleukemia syndromes

Preleukemic manifestations of acute nonlymphocytic leukemia have been recognized for a number of years.[48,49] They may vary in duration from several months to years, or the acute phase of the disease may never surface. The hematologic manifestations may vary from leukocytosis to neutropenia and from moderate anemia to severe hemolytic episodes. The neutrophils may be hypersegmented, and Pelger-Huët nuclear anomaly may be evident. A Coombs-negative hemolytic anemia may arise, which is responsible for abnormally shaped and sized red cells, reticulocytosis, and erythroblastosis. The platelets show anisocytosis and abnormal shapes and are usually decreased in number. Bone marrow chromosomal abnormalities are found in 50-60% of patients with preleukemia.[50]

Laboratory investigation of chronic leukemias

Each type of chronic leukemia has its own characteristics because of the involvement of well-differentiated cells. The classification is as follows:

1. Chronic granulocytic leukemia (CGL)
2. Chronic myelomonocytic leukemia (CML)

3. Chronic lymphocytic leukemia (CLL)
   a. B cell CLL
   b. T cell CLL

Myeloproliferative disorders

Chronic granulocytic leukemia is one member of a group of closely related diseases embraced by the unifying concept of **myeloproliferative disorders.**[51] This designation is based on the well-supported evidence of a single multipotential hematopoietic stem cell (see Chapter 6) that in response to an unknown stimulus is responsible for an abnormal proliferation of mature progeny. Based on the cell type primarily involved in the myeloproliferative process, the following variants can be distinguished[52]: (1) polycythemia vera and erythroleukemia—disorders of the red cell series, (2) essential thrombocythemia and megakaryocytic leukemia—disorders of the megakaryocytes, (3) chronic granulocytic leukemia—disorder of the granulocytic series, (4) myelofibrosis (myelosclerosis)—disorder of fibroblasts, and (5) osteosclerosis—disorder of osteoblasts. **Agnogenic myeloid metaplasia** resulting from extramedullary hematopoiesis has also been included in the scheme of myeloproliferative disorders.[53] Chronic granulocytic leukemia has some distinctive features, e.g., Ph[1] chromosome, so that its relationship to the other members of the group has been questioned.[51]

Laboratory investigation of chronic granulocytic leukemia

In the early stages of chronic granulocytic leukemia (CGL) the red cell count and the hemoglobin level are normal, and a slight polycythemia may actually be present, which in the later stages of the disease gives way to a moderate normocytic normochromic anemia with hemoglobin values ranging from 8-12 g/dl.[54] The anemia is aggravated by hypersplenism or by myelosclerosis and is independent of the concentration of platelets or white cells. When the hematocrit tube is examined, the increased number of leukocytes and platelets forms a creamy layer that is almost equal in length to the underlying red cell column (Fig. 9-12). When the disease is fully developed, there is a marked leukocytosis with levels from 100,000-350,000 cells/mm³ or even higher. In the early stages the increase in cells is only moderate, varying from 20,000-50,000 cells/mm³. The number of platelets is usually greatly increased, from 350,000/mm³ to several million. The number of reticulocytes is normal.

The **peripheral blood smear** reveals normocytic normochromic red cells that show only slight variation in shape and size. The differential count is suggestive of the myelogram of normal bone marrow: 20-35% of the white cells are mature polymorphonuclear leukocytes, 25-30% are band forms, and the remainder of the cells (immature myeloid cells) in order of decreasing percentage are 12-18%, metamyelocytes; 6-10%, myelocytes; 2-4%, promyelocytes; and 1-3%, myeloblasts (Fig. 9-13). Lymphocytes and monocytes each represent less than 5%,[55] but usually basophilia and eosinophilia are present. In certain forms of CGL the numbers of eosinophils and basophils are strikingly in-

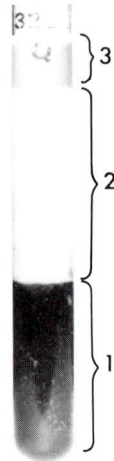

Fig. 9-12. Hematocrit in chronic granulocytic leukemia. *1*, Red cell column; *2*, white cell column; *3*, serum.

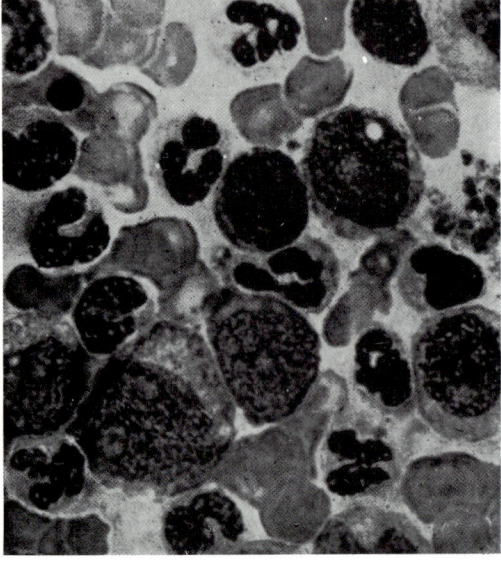

Fig. 9-13. Chronic granulocytic leukemia, blood film, showing crowding of cells, myelocytes, and promyelocytes. ($\times$950.)

creased (up to 20%). There are about 1-3 nucleated red cells per 100 leukocytes. Normally the platelets are increased in number, show variation in size and shape, and may be seen attached to megakaryocytic fragments.

The **bone marrow** is hypercellular and hyperplastic at the expense of the fatty marrow and contains a higher percentage of immature myeloid cells (myeloblasts, promyelocytes, and myelocytes) than does the peripheral blood.[56] The increase in peripheral eosinophils and basophils is reflected in a corresponding increase of these cells in the marrow. They may show granulation abnormalities, e.g., incomplete granulation exposing degranulated areas and a mixture of baso-

philic and eosinophilic granules. The myeloid hyperplasia leads to a markedly decreased erythroid/myeloid ratio (1:30 compared to the normal 1:4) and, because of the ineffective leukopoiesis, to an increase in phagocytic cells, which engulf leukemic white cells, their lipid components forming **Gaucher-like** cells and **sea-blue histiocytes.**[57] The number of megakaryocytes, including their precursor cells (megakaryoblasts and promegakaryocytes), is characteristically increased in the earliest stages of the disease.

The erythroid elements may show a rarely seen initial hyperplasia corresponding to the initial polycythemic red cell count. In the course of the disease the erythropoiesis is always depressed and may terminate in aplasia. With time the myelogram changes as rapidly proliferating myeloblasts overtake the more mature marrow elements and initiate the **terminal blast cell phase** of CGL, which must not be confused with primary acute granulocytic leukemia. Some of the differentiating morphologic features that are **not** seen in de novo acute granulocytic leukemia are[58] (1) high percentage of morphologically normal neutrophils with low alkaline phosphatase score; (2) normal or high platelet counts; (3) basophilia, eosinophilia, or both; (4) raised vitamin B_{12} levels and B_{12}-binding proteins; (5) blast cells of transformed CGL that are often micromyeloblasts, resembling lymphoblasts rather than the myeloblasts of acute granulocytic leukemia, and have high terminal deoxynucleotidyl transferase levels[59,60]; and (6) karyotype of bone marrow cells that shows a number of cytogenetic changes added to the preexisting Ph^1 chromosome,[58] the most common of which is the appearance of a second Ph^1 chromosome.[61,62]

Cytochemical investigations: In most myeloproliferative disorders the leukocyte alkaline phosphatase activity is increased, but in CGL it is markedly reduced. This reduction is not diagnostic, because lowered levels are also found in some cases of paroxysmal nocturnal hemoglobinuria, infectious mononucleosis, pernicious anemia, myelosclerosis (variable), and aplastic anemia. An increase in the leukocyte alkaline phosphatase score may accompany a period of remission or the transformation into the acute blast cell phase.[58] The glycogen content of the mature neutrophils is also decreased in CGL.

Chromosomal abnormalities: In 85-95% of patients with CGL an acquired chromosomal abnormality, the **Philadelphia (Ph^1) chromosome,** is found[63] (Fig. 9-14). It is limited to megakaryocytic, erythroid, and myeloid precursor cells and persists during remissions and in the blast crisis.[62] The Ph^1 chromosome is caused by the loss of about half the greater arm of one member of the no. 22 chromosome pair. It is now known that variant translocations can occur, e.g., a simple translocation of no. 22.[64] Chromosomal abnormalities other than the Ph^1 chromosome are found in 30% of patients with CGL.[65] The Ph^1 chromosome is rare in acute leukemia but has been found in the blast cells of acute lymphocytic, myelocytic, and myelomonocytic leukemias.[66] The Ph^1 chromosome is not related to the leukocyte alkaline phosphatase level. **Ph^1-positive patients** usually have a better prognosis and form a more homogeneous group than Ph^1-negative patients.[63] **Ph^1-**

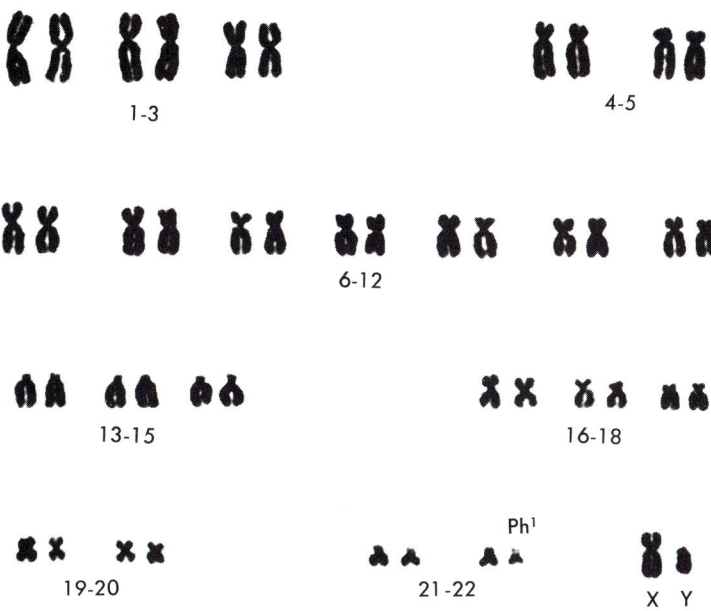

1-3
4-5
6-12
13-15
16-18
19-20
Ph¹
21-22
X Y

Fig. 9-14. Ph¹ chromosome–positive karyotype from a bone marrow sample of patient with chronic granulocytic leukemia. (Courtesy Dr. J.M. Trujillo.)

negative CGL is usually seen in children (juvenile form)[67] and in older individuals[68,69] who exhibit a less favorable response to therapy and have a shorter median survival and lower leukocyte and platelet counts.[70] The association of a missing Y chromosome ($-Y$) in male patients with CGL who are Ph¹ positive is reported as offering a better prognosis,[71] but evidence indicates that it is a mere expression of early aging of bone marrow cells.[64]

• • •

Other distinctive hematologic features in CGL are high levels of **Hb F** in the red cells of the juvenile type[72] and occasional **Hb H** in the red cells of the adult form.[58]

The accelerated breakdown of large numbers of granulocytes is responsible for the high **uric acid** levels in serum and urine that may damage the kidneys and lead to raised BUN levels.[73] Elevated potassium[74] and LDH levels[75] have also been reported. The serum vitamin B_{12} concentration is markedly increased to about 15 times the normal level, since the disintegration of the leukemic (and normal) leukocytes releases a transcobalamin I–like protein that delays the normal clearance of vitamin B_{12}.[76] The serum vitamin B_{12} level and the total vitamin B_{12}–binding capacity are increased in most myeloproliferative disorders.

The median survival of patients with CGL is about 3 years, death being caused by the upsurgence of blast cells, the blast crisis, or by relentlessly progressing myelofibrosis. The blast cells may be quite immature, so that they are myeloperoxidase negative, or they may be myeloblasts (part of a blast cell panmyelosis), or they may, as mentioned previously, have the characteristics of lymphoblasts.

The major differential diagnosis of CGL includes agnogenic myeloid metaplasia, myelofibrosis, and leukemoid reaction. In agnogenic myeloid metaplasia and in myelofibrosis the leukocyte alkaline phosphatase level is elevated, the Ph¹ chromosome is not seen, and teardrop cells appear in the peripheral blood. In leukemoid reactions the following features are not encountered: teardrop red cells, normoblasts, the Ph¹ chromosome, a depressed leukocyte alkaline phosphatase level, and an elevated vitamin B_{12} level.

Laboratory investigation of chronic myelomonocytic leukemia

In the elderly patient a form of chronic granulocytic leukemia, chronic myelomonocytic leukemia, occurs that is characterized by a predominantly monocytic pattern in the peripheral blood, a predominantly myelocytic pattern in the bone marrow,[77] and a relatively benign course if left untreated (Fig. 9-15).

The hemoglobin value may be slightly reduced, the average concentration being 11.7 g/dl, but about 40% of patients are not anemic when first investigated. The total white cell count varies from 3900-38,800 cells/mm³. About 60% of patients are thrombocytopenic, the remaining 40% having fairly normal platelet counts. The peripheral smear reveals a moderate macrocytosis and a monocytosis ranging from about 30-80%. Morphologically the monocytes are mature cells, although some may show coarse cytoplasmic granulation. The polymorphonuclear cells, on the other hand, may show no granulation.[77]

The **bone marrow** is cellular, the majority of the cells being myelocytes and promyelocytes mixed with a variable number of myeloblasts and myelomonoblasts. The more mature myeloid elements are also rep-

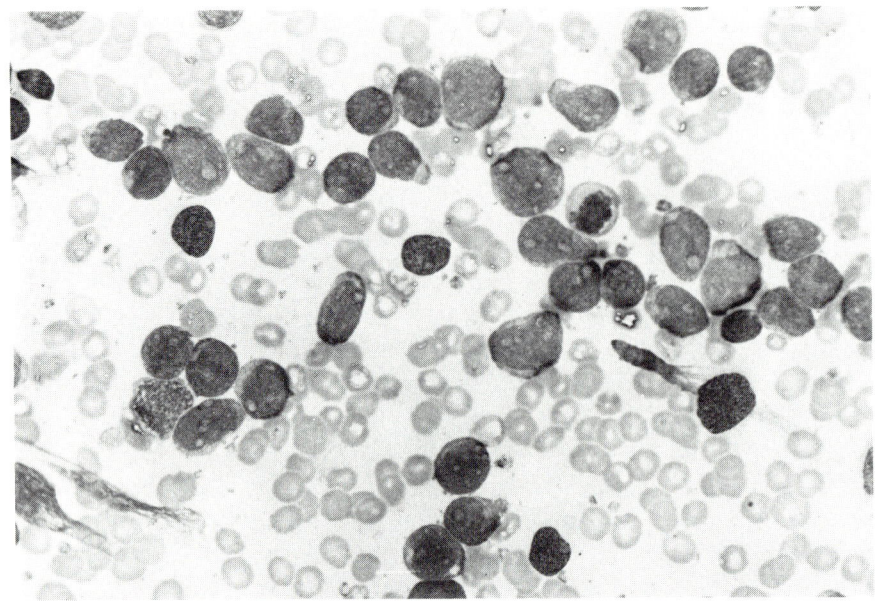

Fig. 9-15. Myelomonocytic leukemia.

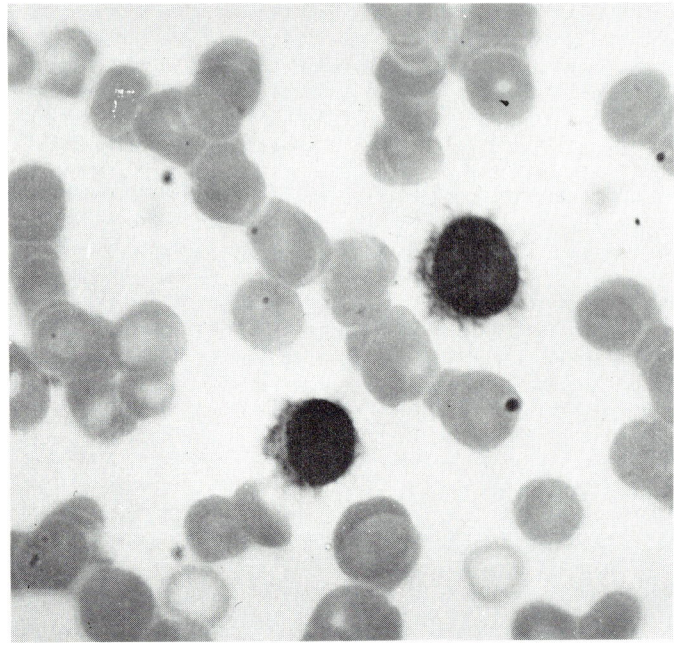

Fig. 9-16. Peripheral blood film in ''hairy cell'' leukemia.

resented, but there is only a sprinkling of the mature monocytes that are so readily seen in the peripheral blood. The erythoid elements may be hyperplastic in the early stages, and as the disease progresses they are decreased. The megakaryocytes, reticulum cells, and lymphocytes are not remarkable.

The leukocyte alkaline phosphatase level is normal. The monocytes are naphthol AS-D chloroacetate esterase positive, but not as sensitive to sodium fluoride as are normal monocytes.

Serum and urine lysozyme concentrations are greatly increased. Vitamin B_{12} levels are normal or moderately increased, whereas folate levels (serum and red cells) and serum LDH concentrations are normal.

Laboratory diagnosis of "hairy cell" leukemia (leukemic reticuloendotheliosis)

"Hairy cell" leukemia is a disease characterized by marked splenomegaly, a chronic course, hypersplenic pancytopenia, and "hairy cells" in the peripheral blood and bone marrow. The latter frequently resist aspiration, so that "dry" taps are obtained.[78] An accurate morphologic diagnosis is essential, since vigorous chemotherapy is contraindicated.

The anemia[78-80] is normocytic normochromic, the hemoglobin concentration varying from 6-12 g/dl and the white cell count ranging from 500-4800/mm³. The differential count reveals a relative lymphocytosis. Of these cells, 10% are **hairy cells,** which on Wright-Giemsa preparations measure 12-20 μm in diameter and contain a round-to-oval nucleus with delicate nuclear chromatin interrupted by nucleoli. The nucleus is often eccentric, indented, folded, and contained by a delicate membrane (Fig. 9-16). The cytoplasm is pale blue and exhibits fine filamentous projections arising from the cell membrane that are seen best by phase microscopy, using unstained fresh preparations, and can easily be demonstrated by electron microscopy.[81]

The average platelet count is 60,000/mm³ but may go as high as 150,000/mm³.

Bone marrow aspiration is unsuccessful in about 50% of patients. Bone marrow biopsy sections show diffuse infiltration of the marrow by hairy cells. **Cytochemically** these cells can be shown to contain **tartrate-resistant acid phosphatase,** a reaction considered specific for the disease.[82] **Immunologic investigations** of these cells in the peripheral blood reveal a significant number bearing surface immunoglobulins, a B-lymphocyte marker,[83] but, on the other hand, receptor sites for IgG complexes, a characteristic of monocytes, can be demonstrated.[84] The latter phenomenon favors a monocytic origin of hairy cells.[81,85] The hairy cell may be a hybrid of lymphocyte and monocyte.

Laboratory investigation of myelofibrosis (myelosclerosis)

Myelofibrosis (MF) is a syndrome that normally has the following characteristics: fibrosis of the bone marrow, a leukoerythroblastic peripheral blood picture, and splenomegaly as the result of agnogenic myeloid metaplasia. MF may arise de novo or in the course of other myeloproliferative disorders, e.g., polycythemia vera,

essential thrombocythemia, or chronic granulocytic leukemia.[51,86,87] The classification of MF is as follows:

1. Primary: idiopathic with agnogenic myeloid metaplasia
2. Secondary
   a. Chemicals and toxins: benzene
   b. Myelosuppressive drugs
   c. Radiation
   d. Infiltrative marrow diseases: metastatic tumors, multiple myeloma, leukemia, and lymphoma
   e. Other myeloproliferative disorders: polycythemia vera, essential thrombocythemia, and chronic granulocytic leukemia
   f. Granulomatous inflammation: tuberculosis
   g. Bone diseases: osteopetrosis

The **peripheral blood picture** is quite variable, but a moderate-to-severe normocytic normochromic anemia is present in about 75% of patients, although anemia may not be evident when a patient is first seen. Repeated hemorrhages may change the character of the anemia to hypochromic microcytic. The degree of anemia is also influenced by the large size of the spleen, which not only allows pooling of the blood—thus exacerbating the anemia—but also adds a hemolytic component.[53] Several other red cell anomalies have been described, e.g., Coombs' positivity,[88] enzyme anomalies,[89] and increased mechanical fragility,[90] which may be responsible for a mild hemolytic component leading to slight reticulocytosis, polychromatophilia, and basophilic stippling. Usually the number of reticulocytes is normal or only slightly increased (1.5%).

The white cell count is at the lower limit of normal or lower (leukopenic) in about 10% of patients in the late stage of the disease; it is normal (4000-10,000 cells/mm³) in about 40% and may reach 50,000 cells/mm³ in the remaining patients, but it does not attain the high levels often found in chronic granulocytic leukemia.

The **blood film** shows fairly characteristic but not diagnostic red cell changes, e.g., poikilocytosis, anisocytosis, and **teardrop** cells, that probably relate to the splenic pooling or to extramedullary hematopoiesis. The differential count reveals a leukoerythroblastic picture characterized by nucleated red cells, often up to 20 cells/100 WBCs, in association with immature granulocytes usually not younger than myelocytes, although myeloblasts occur in 5-13% of patients and are not indicative of a blast crisis. The leukocyte alkaline phosphatase level is usually high but not invariably so. Basophilia and eosinophilia are seen in one fourth of MF patients. Fragments of megakaryocytes alternate with morphologically abnormal and normal platelets.

The **platelet count** is as variable as the other hematologic parameters. In about one third of patients it is normal and reaches high levels (1 million/mm³ or over) in only a few cases. Thrombocytopenic levels are associated with the late stages of the disease, but whatever the level of the platelet count abnormally shaped platelets, e.g., giant platelets, are always seen. The platelets are functionally deficient and are responsible for some of the abnormalities of hemostasis that appear to be independent of the number of platelets and are expressed in such laboratory findings as inadequate clot retraction, prolonged bleeding time, abnormal prothrombin consumption, and poor platelet adhesiveness.[91,92]

Bone marrow examination: In about 10% of patients in the early stages of the disease the bone marrow aspirate may be normal or even hypercellular, but in the majority of patients the bone is difficult to penetrate because of cortical thickening, and the tap is dry or hypocellular because of marrow fibrosis. Bone marrow biopsy is necessary in all patients suspected of having MF. It may reveal complete fibrosis or a mixture of increased connective tissue with hypercellular areas consisting of increased numbers of megakaryocytes and varying admixtures of granulocytic and erythocytic precursor cells (see Fig. 8-9).

Cytochemical investigations: Some of the erythroblasts are PAS positive.[93] The erythrocytic reduced glutathione level, the leukocytic 6-phosphogluconic dehydrogenase activity (6-PG), and the glucose-6-phosphate dehydrogenase (G-6-PD) level are increased.[89] The latter is normal in chronic granulocytic leukemia and only slightly elevated in polycythemia vera.

Related biochemical findings: Serum vitamin B_{12} and unsaturated B_{12}–binding proteins are normal or may be elevated, thus contrasting with the high levels found in chronic granulocytic leukemia.[53] There may be a relationship between the increased serum alkaline phosphatase level,[86] the serum protein[86] and immunoglobulin fluctuation,[94] and the degree of hepatic extramedullary hematopoiesis. The serum LDH level[95] and the serum uric acid concentration[96] are increased.

Lymphoreticular disorders

The lymphoreticular system embraces the tissues that are intimately connected with the defense of the body but by common usage excludes the granulocytes. The discovery of lymphocytic subpopulations on the basis of the B and T cell markers has unified our concept of the disorders of B- and T-lymphocytes and plasma cells. They include quantitative variations such as lymphocytosis and lymphopenia (see pp. 236 and 238) and immunoproliferative disorders such as B and T cell malignancies, e.g., lymphocytic leukemia, Hodgkin's disease, non-Hodgkin's lymphoma, disorders of the plasma cells (multiple myeloma, macroglobulinemia, benign monoclonal gammopathy), and T cell malignancies such as Sézary syndrome (mycosis fungoides).

Laboratory investigation of chronic lymphocytic leukemia

Chronic lymphocytic leukemia (CLL)[97] is the commonest form of chronic leukemia. About 30% of CLL patients have a normal red cell count and hemoglobin level when first seen by the physician. The other 70% have a normocytic normochromic anemia with reduced numbers of reticulocytes. About one fourth of all patients develop a hemolytic anemia during the course of the disease. This anemia may be severe and show all the features of an **autoimmune hemolytic process** because of warm or cold antibodies, e.g., a positive direct antiglobulin test, spherocytosis, reticulocytosis, and

hyperbilirubinemia. On the other hand, it may show no more than a shortened red cell survival time and increased urobilinogen production. About 60% of patients develop progressive hypogammaglobulinemia that because of the high incidence of infections may lead to the development of a microcytic hypochromic anemia. The association of CLL with a severe pure red cell anemia with erythroblastopenia (0%) and reticulocytopenia (0%) has been reported as a rare cause of anemia in CLL.[98]

The leukocyte count may rise steadily or very slowly with long stationary periods of months or years to reach the highest level of about 200,000-500,000 cells/mm^3 in the late stages of the disease.

The **platelet count** is normal unless the megakaryocytes are replaced by lymphoid tissue or the platelets are destroyed by antiplatelet antibodies.

The peripheral blood differential count at first shows 60-80% mature lymphocytes, but as the disease progresses the lymphocytosis becomes 100% (Fig. 9-17). The lymphocytes are interrupted here and there by naked nuclei and smudge cells, and, depending on the pressure used in making the blood smear, they may show single nucleoli and trailing of the ctyoplasm. Azurophilic granules are absent. The leukemic lymphocytes are frequently larger than the nonleukemic lymphocytes, and their nuclei have a round contour. Prolymphocytes, which are rare (less than 10%), stand out because of the larger size, wider rim of cytoplasm, and conspicuous nucleolus. They are the characteristic cell[99] in the prolymphocytic form of CLL and are responsible for a less favorable response to treatment.[100]

Functional studies of T- and B-lymphocytes in patients with CLL show the leukemic cells to be predominantly of B cell origin[101] and rarely (5-10%) of T cell ancestry.[102] The depression of the T cell function may be a dilutional effect of the large numbers of neoplastic B cells.[103] The T-CLL differs from the B-CLL not only in lymphocytic surface markers but also in clinical behavior and manifestations.[104,105] The lymphocytes are

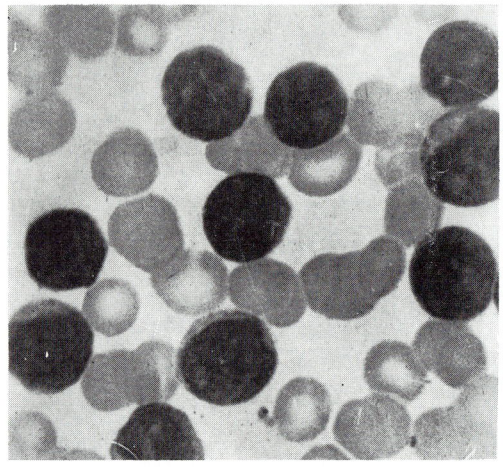

Fig. 9-17. Chronic lymphocytic leukemia, blood film, showing crowding of lymphocytes. ($\times 950$.)

small, and the slightly increased amount of cytoplasm contains azurophilic granules.

The **bone marrow** aspirate shows closely placed lymphocytes similar to the cells seen in the peripheral blood. The normal marrow elements are diminished in number, but their relative proportions to each other excluding the neoplastic cells are preserved. Bone marrow biopsy sections and several bone marrow smears should be examined to exclude the outside possibility that the original aspirate contained a lymph follicle, a normal bone marrow component. In CLL the lymphocytic aggregates are large, irregular, and numerous.

Related biochemical findings: The serum protein concentration is reduced, and in the course of the disease most patients develop a progressive **hypogammaglobulinemia** that in late stages of CLL is responsible for the occurrence of viral, bacterial, and fungal infections. In the late stages small monoclonal immunoglobulin elevations may occur, mainly of IgG or IgM, which are responsible for Coombs'-positive warm or cold hemolytic anemias in 5-10% of patients, but in general all immunoglobulins are reduced.

Differential diagnosis: The spectrum of CLL includes malignant lymphomas in the leukemic phase (lymphosarcoma cell leukemia) and Waldenström's macroglobulinemia, from which it can be differentiated by clinical, morphologic, and cytochemical criteria.

CLL can be distinguished from Waldenström's macroglobulinemia by the presence of plasmacytoid lymphocytes and PAS-positive intranuclear inclusions in some of the lymphocytes. The differentiation of CLL from hematogenous spread of diffuse, well-differentiated lymphocytic lymphosarcoma is a matter of semantics, because pathologically both diseases are the same. Bone marrow examination may at times be required to differentiate CLL from viral types of lymphocytosis. In the viral types the bone marrow only reflects the peripheral changes but does not show the infiltrative pattern of CLL.

Laboratory investigation of lymphosarcoma cell leukemia

Lymphosarcoma cell leukemia (LSCL) describes the leukemic phase of a **poorly differentiated** or **well-differentiated** lymphocytic lymphoma.[106] The peripheral blood smears mimic the picture of chronic lymphocytic leukemia.

There is a mild-to-moderate normocytic normochromic anemia with hematocrit values ranging from 22-47%. The majority of white cell counts range from 12,000-82,000/mm^3, although leukopenic levels may also be encountered. The concentration of platelets is not affected. The differential count of the peripheral blood and the bone marrow reveals 20-90% lymphosar-

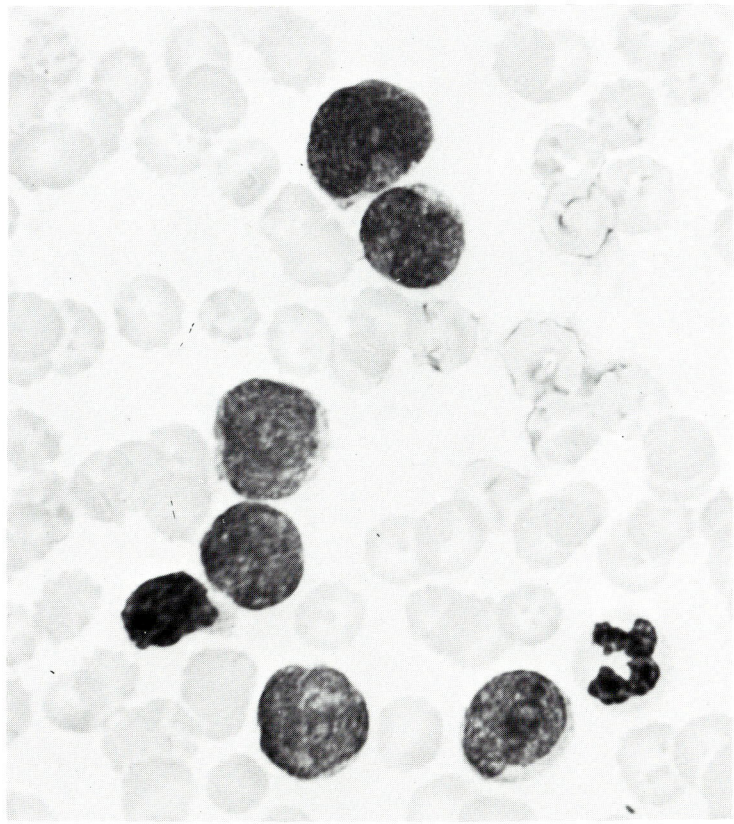

Fig. 9-18. Peripheral blood film in lymphosarcoma cell leukemia.

coma cells. The bone marrow sections show complete replacement of the marrow by lymphosarcoma or large irregular islands of the tumor. Lymphosarcoma cells are larger than normal lymphocytes and have irregular nuclei that are often indented, notched, and cleft. The moderately coarse chromatin is interrupted by one large, eccentric nucleolus. The cytoplasm forms a thin, gray-blue ring around the large, eccentric nucleus and may contain vacuoles and occasional azurophilic granules (Fig. 9-18).

Laboratory investigation of Sézary syndrome

The main clinical finding in Sézary syndrome is a pruritic, generalized exfoliative dermatitis, and the main laboratory findings are lymphocytosis and Sézary cells in the peripheral blood and usually not in the bone marrow.[107-109]

In most patients the red cell and platelet concentrations are normal and the hemoglobin concentration varies from 13-14 g/dl. In fewer than 1% of patients there is a moderate thrombocytopenia (40,000-50,000/mm^3), contrasting with the average platelet count of 200,000/mm^3 found in most patients. There is a leukocytosis of varying degree, averaging about 15,000 WBCs/mm^3, with the extremes spanning about 5000-72,000 WBCs/mm^3. The peripheral blood smear reveals a striking lymphocytosis consisting of 50-90% lymphoid cells, a designation used to include lymphocytes and Sézary cells at the expense of neutrophils. The average monocyte concentration is 6%. **Two types** of **Sézary cells** are seen in most patients, although one type usually predominates. The **large Sézary cell** measures 12-20 μm in diameter. The cytoplasm forms a thin, clear basophilic ring around the large, oval, or round nucleus, which is convoluted or cerebriform, folded and grooved, and devoid of nucleoli (Fig. 9-19). The **small Sézary cell** resembles a lymphocyte by light microscopy, and if it is the predominant cell it may be incorrectly diagnosed as a lymphocytic leukemic cell. It measures about 8-11 μm in diameter and has a delicate rim of blue cytoplasm surrounding a rather large nucleus that shares the grooved appearance of the large cell nucleus. By electron microscopy[108] the Sézary cells show the characteristic cerebriform nucleus, which has a large nucleolus. The cytoplasm contains a striking number of cytoplasmic fibrils, incomplete viruslike particles,[110] clusters of glycogen granules, a variable number of mitochondria, and a Golgi apparatus. By electron microscopy these cells are identical with the cells found in mycosis fungoides.[111]

The bone marrow is normally cellular and usually spared, but if a great number of Sézary cells are in the peripheral blood, they also invade the marrow.[104]

Cytochemical investigations[109]: The cells contain both diastase-resistant and diastase-sensitive PAS-positive granules and show a positive acid phosphatase re-

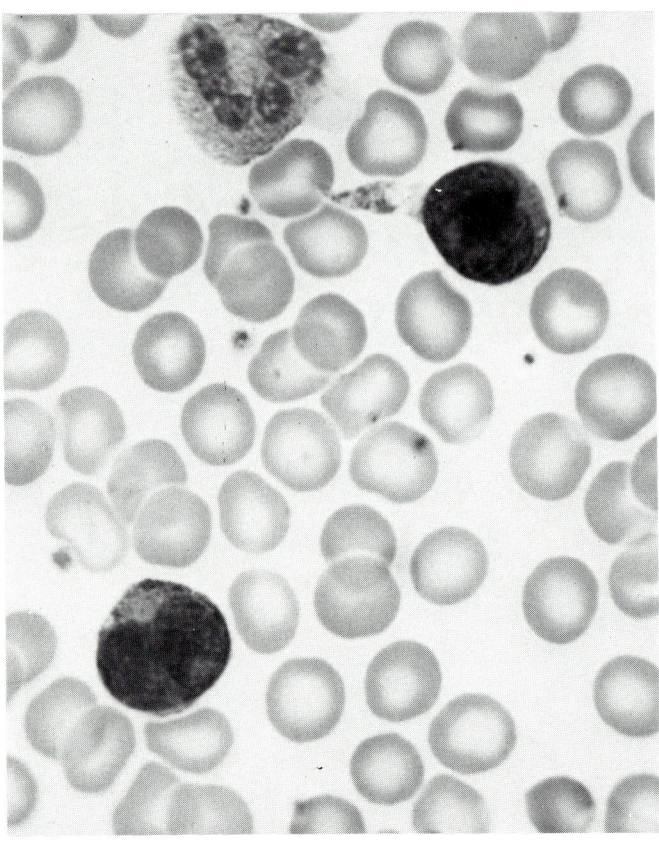

Fig. 9-19. Sézary cells in peripheral blood smear.

action that is inhibited by tartaric acid. The naphthol AS-D esterase activity is low, contrasting with the strong β-glucuronidase contents. Cytochemically the Sézary cell resembles lymphocytes more closely than monocytes or histiocytes.

Immunologic investigation: Evidence strongly indicates that the Sézary cell is of T-lymphocyte origin, since it reacts with anti–T cell sera, responds to phytohemagglutinin stimulation, and forms spontaneous rosettes with sheep erythrocytes.

LABORATORY INVESTIGATION OF M-COMPONENT (MONOCLONAL IMMUNOGLOBULIN) DISORDERS

M-component disorders deal with the hematologic features of plasma cell–lymphocyte disorders. The immunologic aspects and the protein abnormalities are discussed in Chapter 36. M-component disorders are classified as follows:

1. Multiple myeloma and light-chain disease
2. Heavy-chain diseases
3. Benign monoclonal gammopathy
4. Waldenström's macroglobulinemia

Laboratory investigation of multiple myeloma

Myeloma is a neoplastic proliferation of plasma cells of varying degrees of maturation and differentiation.

During the course of the disease almost all patients develop an **anemia** that is usually normocytic normo-chromic but because of its multifactorial etiology may be macrocytic, megaloblastic,[112] or (rarely) microcytic.[113] The factors that contribute to the development of the anemia are bone marrow replacement, kidney impairment or failure, hemolysis, blood loss, chemotherapy, infection, and hemodilution resulting from an increase in the plasma volume. The anemia is usually moderate with hemoglobin concentration varying from 9-10 g/dl, but as the disease progresses it increases in severity.

The **white cell count** is usually normal, although in about 35% of patients neutropenia forces it into the leukopenic range (2000-4000 cells/mm³). The differential counts shows a relative lymphocytosis, at times accompanied by eosinophilia.[114] The lymphocytosis, which rarely exceeds 60%, is the result of proliferation of stimulated and plasmacytoid lymphocytes that in about 70% of patients are mixed with occasional plasma cells. The yield of plasma cells is much richer if buffy coat preparations are examined. In the terminal stages of myeloma, plasmablasts and proplasmacytes amounting to about 50% of the white cells may be swept into the peripheral blood, creating the picture of a **plasma cell leukemia**[115] with total white cell counts rising to concentrations of 10,000-15,000 cells/mm³, although much higher values have been reported. In rare individuals with IgE[116] and IgD[117] myeloma the leukemic phase is the presenting symptom (Fig. 9-20).

Examination of the blood smear confirms the diag-

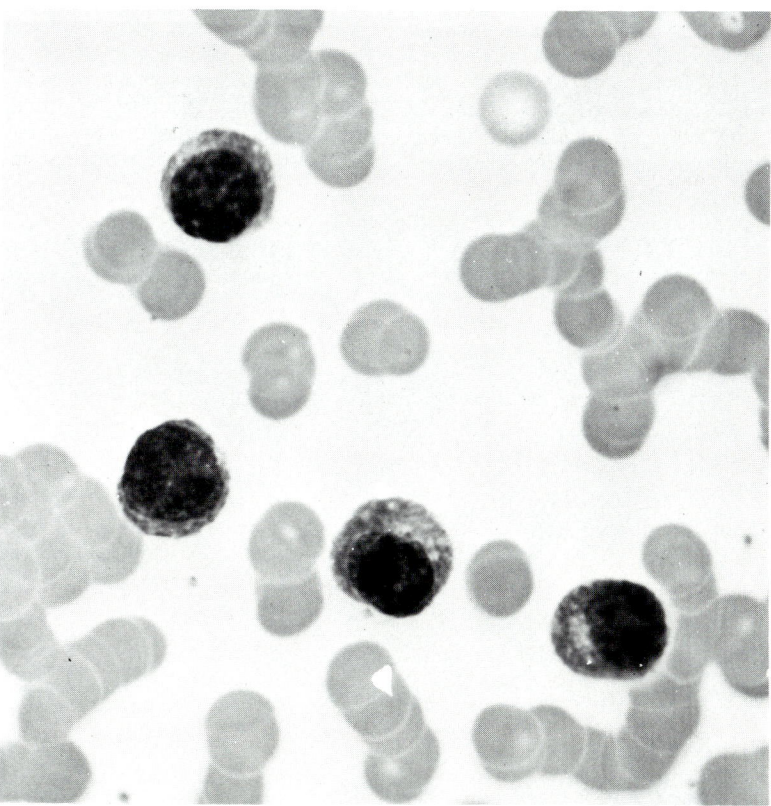

Fig. 9-20. Peripheral blood film in plasma cell leukemia.

nosis of **thrombocytopenia** found in about 50% of patients with myeloma.[118] In the initial stages the platelet count is normal.

The **M proteins** are responsible for a number of characteristic changes seen in the peripheral blood smear. The blood may not spread evenly, and the thin, feathery edge of the unstained blood film may show a play of colors. The red cells form short chains of 2-4 cells (rouleaux formation) against a bluish proteinaceous background that surrounds each erythrocyte with a bluish halo.

In the well-established plasmacytic neoplasia the **bone marrow** smear reveals proliferating plasma cells replacing most normal hematopoietic elements. The majority of cells may be mature-appearing plasma cells mixed with a small number of abnormal plasma cells, or the cells may be proplasmacytes, plasmablasts, or both, their concentration varying from 10-90% in different aspirates (Fig. 9-21; Plate 11, p. 257). Several aspirations and biopsies of different sites may be necessary to establish a definite diagnosis of myeloma and to distinguish it from reactive plasmacytosis. In myeloma the **biopsy** section reveals a lytic marrow space—occupying lesion consisting of homogeneous nodules and sheets of plasma cells with little intervening hematopoietic tissue or supportive reticular framework.[119] These nodules are not seen in **nonmyelomatous reactive plasmacytosis,** which exhibits a perivascular arrangement of the plasma cells without aggregation and demonstrates intermingling of predominantly single plasma cells with normal hematopoietic elements.[119] The diagnosis of reactive plasmacytosis, a common finding in bone marrow aspirates of inflammatory and neoplastic conditions, is further supported by the presence of plasmacytic satellitosis, lymphoid follicles, and lipid granulomas.[120] Plasmacytic satellitosis is a morphologic configuration consisting of a central histiocyte surrounded by three or more plasma cells.[120] The bone marrow smear allows not only quantitation of the plasma cells but also study of their morphology and cytochemistry. The percentage of plasma cells is an unreliable criterion of plasma cell neoplasia, since **reactive plasmacytosis** with up to 60% plasma cells has been observed in liver diseases, e.g., cirrhosis and hepatitis, in carcinomas, particularly of the gastrointestinal tract and breast metastasizing to the skeleton,[121] and in rheumatoid arthritis. The usual concentration of plasma cells in plasmacytosis ranges from 10-20%. In myeloma, on the other hand, the plasma cells are more numerous than 20%, the average being 32%.[122] **Morphologic criteria** allow the classification of myeloma into mature and less mature plasma cell types. The proteins secreted by the plasma cells are responsible for the **basophilia** and **pyroninophilia (RNA)** of the cytoplasm and, if produced in pathologic quantities, lead to the formation of spheroidal hyaline or crystalline inclusions. The first are called **Russell bodies** and consist of intracytoplasmic or intranuclear protein globules that stain various shades of blue with Wright-Giemsa stain and by immunofluorescence can be shown to contain light chains.[123] The crystals are precipitated cryoglobulins. If the Russell bodies are dissolved during the process of staining, vacuolated plasma cells remain that have been called grape cells, Mott cells, or morular cells (Fig. 9-22). Soluble M proteins are responsible for red-staining "**flame**" **cells** and for **thesaurocytes,** cells distended with stored proteins frequently but not exclusively found in the IgA type of myeloma.[124] Except for the latter, attempts to correlate plasma cell morphology and clinical behavior have not been successful.[125] The fate of the erythroid precursor cells is quite variable. They may be partially replaced by the proliferating neoplastic cells, or they may show normoblastic hyperplasia in response to a hemolytic com-

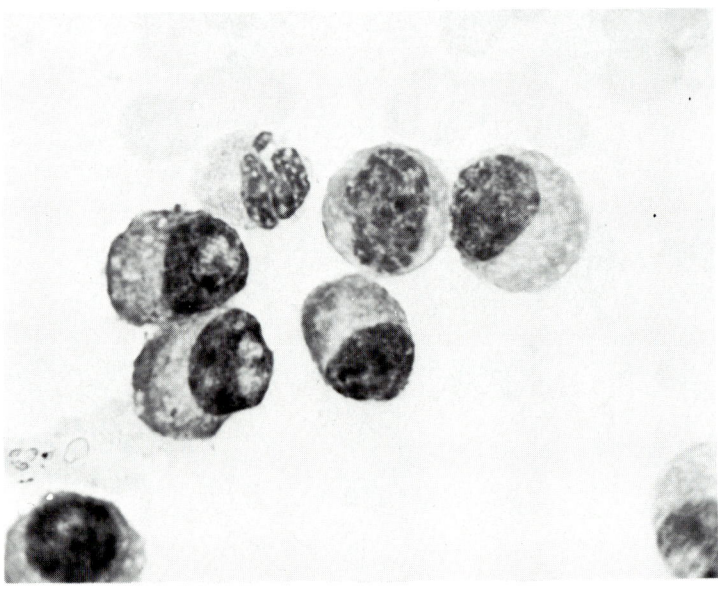

Fig. 9-21. Myeloma cells, bone marrow smear.

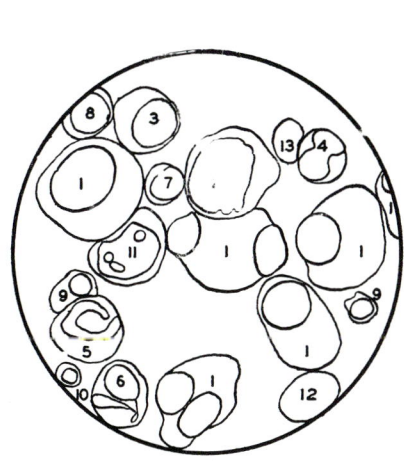

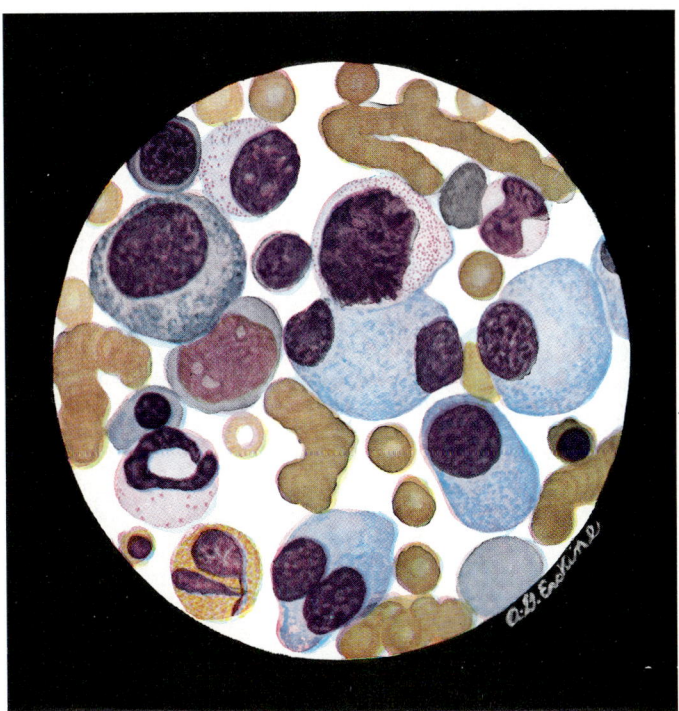

Plate 11. Multiple myeloma. (Bone marrow smear; Wright-Giemsa stain; ×1000.)
 1 Large plasma cells, two with double nuclei
 2 Degenerated promyelocyte
 3 Neutrophilic myelocyte
 4 Neutrophilic metamyelocyte
 5 Neutrophilic band granulocyte
 6 Eosinophil
 7 Small lymphocyte
 8 Polychromatic macroblast
 9 Polychromatic normoblast
10 Orthochromatic normoblast
11 Myeloblast
12 Polychromatic macrocyte
13 Polychromatic red cell

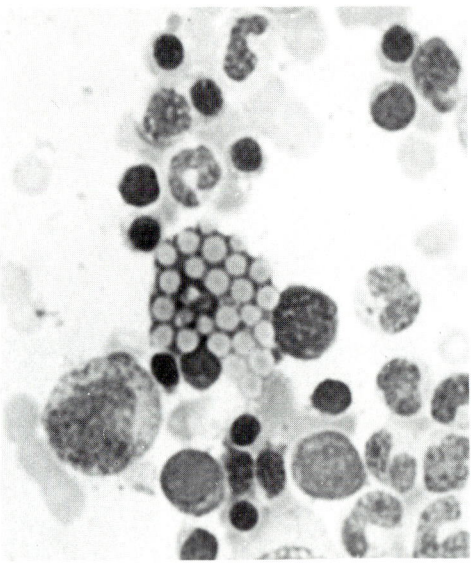

Fig. 9-22. Russell bodies.

ponent or to blood loss. Megaloblastic erythropoiesis associated with myeloma has been known to occur for many years,[112] but **sideroblastic** marrow changes in response to therapy have only recently been reported.[126] They herald a rapidly progressive **acute myelomonocytic leukemia.**[127] In the rare nonsecretory myeloma it may be necessary to utilize immunofluorescence to demonstrate the intracellular synthesis of monoclonal M proteins in the bone marrow or peripheral blood B cells that are unable to release their products.

Cytochemical investigations: The cytoplasm of myeloma cells contains PAS-positive secretory protein granules that are responsible for the PAS-positive reaction of the Russell bodies. The ATPase activity is decreased,[128] contrasting with the increased acid phosphatase.[129]

Sedimentation rate: The sedimentation rate is greatly increased because of rouleaux formation and abnormal fibrin aggregation found in 75% of patients. The increased rate may be held in check by the high viscosity of some of the serum M proteins, which may even reduce it to zero.

Hemostatic abnormalities: Bleeding tendencies occur in 15% of patients with IgG myeloma and in double that number of patients with IgA myeloma and macroglobulinemia.[126,130] The hemostatic defects are related to the dysproteinemia and may be aggravated by such complications as uremia, liver involvement, and sepsis. The already mentioned thrombocytopenia that by itself is not of sufficient magnitude to cause bleeding is augmented by impaired platelet function, resulting in a prolonged bleeding time.[131] The often noted abnormal clot retraction is caused not only by platelet dysfunction but also by complexing of fibrin monomers with M proteins, so that the formation of normal fibrin is inhibited and the clot fails to retract spontaneously (**"gelation"** of the clot).[131] Prolongation of many of the clotting tests may result from interference with fibrin for-

mation and depression of clotting factors complexed with the abnormal proteins.[130]

Serum and urine abnormalities are described in Unit Six.

Nonhematologic findings: Hypercalcemia and hyperuricemia occur frequently and damage kidneys already compromised by nephrotoxic paraproteins, or amyloid, or both. Hyperviscosity and cryoprecipitates, although infrequent, increase the renal damage, so that urea and creatinine concentrations climb. Even in the face of extensive bone destruction the alkaline phosphatase level remains normal.

Laboratory investigation of light-chain disease

Light-chain disease (LCD) is a variant of multiple myeloma in which the monoclonal gammopathy consists of an excess production of light chains, either κ− or λ−Bence Jones proteins that because of their low molecular weight are cleared by the glomeruli and accumulate in abnormal concentration in the urine. They are not detected in the serum until the kidneys fail. LCD accounts for less than 15% of myeloma cases[132] and is characterized as follows[133]: (1) the usual marker of multiple myeloma, the monoclonal M spike in the serum electrophoretogram, is absent and is replaced by hypogammaglobulinemia and hypoimmunoglobulinemia (Fig. 9-23); (2) because of the absence of hypergammaglobulinemia the peripheral blood smear fails to show rouleaux formation; (3) unless special tests are used the Bence Jones proteinuria may not be discovered since it may not be sought; (4) elevated BUN and creatinine levels may be the initial laboratory findings; (5) 2.5% of cases are associated with amyloidosis; and (6) thrombocytopenia, anemia, and leukopenia are absent. LCD shares hyperuricemia, hypercalcemia, and bone marrow plasmacytosis with myeloma.

Laboratory investigation of heavy-chain diseases

Heavy-chain diseases (HCDs) are uncommon forms of monoclonal gammopathies associated with serum proteins composed of heavy-chain fragments without L chains.[134] The three recognized forms correspond to the H chains of the major immunoglobulins: α-,[135] γ-,[136] and μ-[137]HCD. The diagnosis rests on the identification of the H chains in serum and urine that react with one of the monospecific anti−H chain antisera and fail to react with both anti−L chain antisera.[138]

Hematologic findings in γ-HCD[134]: All patients are anemic, and about 50% show leukopenia and thrombocytopenia. The peripheral smear reveals a relative lymphocytosis resulting from a mixture of lymphocytes, plasmacytoid lymphocytes, and plasma cells. The lymphocyte−plasma cell lines also infiltrate the bone marrow. Agammaglobulinemia associated with a monoclonal γ-chain spike and proteinuria without Bence Jones protein are present in 75% of patients.

Laboratory findings in α-HCD: The laboratory diagnosis is rendered difficult by the small amount of α-chains found in the sera of most cases and by the small or nonexistent amount excreted into the urine.

Laboratory findings in μ-HCD[137]: The rarest form of HCD, μ-HCD is recognized as an unusual complication of long-standing chronic lymphocytic leukemia. The

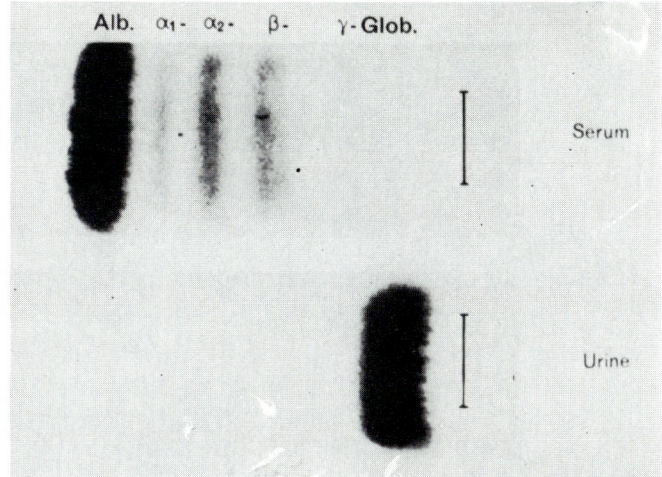

Fig. 9-23. Serum: aclonal (agammaglobulinemia) serum electrophoretic pattern in multiple myeloma. Urine: Bence Jones protein band in urine electrophoretogram of above case. (From Phlippen, R.: Triangle **6:**111, 1963.)

serum shows hypogammaglobulinemia with an abnormal monoclonal component that migrates more rapidly than normal or monoclonal IgM. The bone marrow smear reveals vacuolated plasma cells. Urine immunoelectrophoresis may demonstrate small amounts of μ-chains and Bence Jones protein.

Laboratory investigation of benign monoclonal gammopathy

In recent years a number of patients have been described who have a monoclonal protein in the serum but no clinical evidence of multiple myeloma, macroglobulinemia, amyloidosis, or lymphoma.[139,140] Kyle refers to this benign form of monoclonal gammopathy as the **monoclonal gammopathy of undetermined significance,** because reviews and subsequent studies reveal myeloma in 10% of patients 5-15 years later. In the remaining 90% of patients no disease process can ever be demonstrated. This benign form is probably the most common type of monoclonal gammopathy and it has certain characteristic features: (1) the level of the γ-protein remains the same through the years; (2) the serum α-protein level usually does not exceed 2 g/dl; (3) the bone marrow contains fewer than 5% plasma cells; (4) no monoclonal proteins appear in the urine; and (5) in the 70 years and over age group benign M protein elevation is seen in about 3% of patients.[141]

Laboratory investigation of Waldenström's (primary) macroglobulinemia

Waldenström's macroglobulinemia (WM) is the result of the neoplastic proliferation of the lymphocyte–plasma cell system, which under physiologic conditions is responsible for the normal IgM level but under pathologic conditions synthesizes excessive quantities of monoclonal IgM macroglobulins that are directly responsible for the salient features of this disease: the **hy-**perviscosity syndrome and the **hemorrhagic diathesis.**

Hematologic findings[142]: Of patients with this disease, 90% show a normocytic normochromic anemia with hemoglobin values ranging from 6-10 g/dl. Many factors are involved in the production of the anemia, e.g., marrow infiltration by normal and atypical lymphocytes and plasma cells, hemorrhage, hemolysis resulting from shortened red cell survival, erythroid depression,[143] and an increased plasma volume that may amount to more than twice the normal value of 41 ml/kg. The reticulocyte and white cell counts are usually normal, but moderate leukocytosis and leukopenia have been reported. The differential count reveals rouleaux formation and an absolute lymphocytosis or monocytosis, the first caused by atypical plasmacytoid lymphocytes. The platelet count is slightly to moderately depressed to levels that by themselves cannot account for the bleeding tendency of patients with WM. The effect of the mild thrombocytopenia is augmented by a functional platelet defect that is apparently related to the interference of the macroglobulins with the release of platelet factors and is responsible for the prolonged bleeding time. The macroglobulins may also interfere with hemostasis by complexing with clotting factors or by having anti–clotting factor activity. Prolonged prothrombin times have been reported.

The **sedimentation rate** varies from 1 mm/hr to increased levels.

The **bone marrow** smear reveals infiltration and replacement of the normal marrow by an infiltrate consisting of small lymphocytes, lymphocytoid cells, and plasma cells (Fig. 9-24). If most of the normal marrow cells are replaced, the differentiation from chronic lymphocytic leukemia may be difficult, but the differentiation from multiple myeloma is usually self-evident. Dutcher and Fahey[144] have drawn attention to the characteristic PAS-positive intranuclear inclusions in the

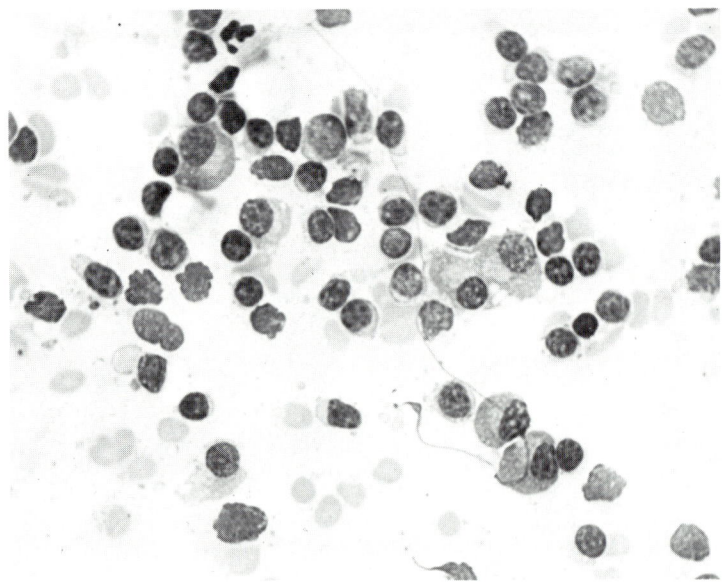

Fig. 9-24. Bone marrow smear in macroglobulinemia. Increased number of plasma cells, lymphocytes, and lymphocytoid cells; absence of other marrow elements.

plasmacytoid lymphocytes of WM, which may appear as vacuoles in Wright-Giemsa stain preparations. The megakaryocytes are not reduced in number, whereas the other normal marrow elements are more or less replaced by the infiltrate.

Serum protein studies reveal a monoclonal M protein that by immunoelectrophoresis can be proven to be IgM. In one third of patients it is associated with Bence Jones protein, since apparently the macroglobulins interfere with the formation of complete immunoglobulins. One third of the macroglobulins are thermoproteins, usually **cryoglobulins,** but the presence of pyroglobulins has been demonstrated in about 7% of cases. The macroglobulins are responsible for a positive **Sia test,** for the markedly increased **serum viscosity,** for false-positive serologic tests for syphilis, and for rheumatoid factor activity.[138] Despite the monoclonal M protein, the levels of the other immunoglobulins are not significantly reduced.

Nonhematologic findings: Many of the nonhematologic laboratory findings encountered in multiple myeloma are absent in WM, e.g., hyperuricemia, and elevated creatinine and urea nitrogen levels, since bone destruction, tumor necrosis, and renal infiltration by myeloma cells are not seen in WM. Macroglobulins are devoid of renal toxicity.

LABORATORY INVESTIGATION OF INFECTIOUS MONONUCLEOSIS

Infectious mononucleosis (IM) is an acute or subacute sporadic, benign, infectious, self-limiting lymphoproliferative disorder predominantly of young adults that is responsible for a persistent antibody titer against the viral capsid antigen of the herpeslike Epstein-Barr virus (EBV).[145] A heterophil antibody may or may not be demonstrable.[146] Variants of IM that are heterophil

antibody negative are caused by the cytomegalovirus[152] or by *Toxoplasma.*[152]

Hematologic findings

The red cells are usually normal in number and morphology, so that anemia is a rare occurrence, but in about 3% of patients a Coombs-positive, mild-to-moderate hemolytic anemia is encountered.[153] In such cases spherocytes are seen in the peripheral blood smear, and cold agglutinins with anti-I activity are found in the serum.[154]

There is usually a moderate to sometimes pronounced **leukocytosis** (10,000-20,000 WBCs/mm^3) that is well established by the second week of the disease, reaches maximal levels during the third week, and subsides during the fourth and following weeks (Fig. 9-25). Much higher lymphocytic leukemoid reactions do not exclude the diagnosis of IM, especially in young children. Initially normal or leukopenic white cell concentrations may be seen in about 20% of patients,[155] or there may be a transient **leukopenic** (agranulocytic) episode during the course of IM.[156] The **differential count** reveals an absolute and relative lymphocytosis (20-90%) because of elevated numbers of normal and atypical lymphocytes (Fig. 9-26). Their various stages of development, originally classified by Downey into three types, are seen in the blood smear of almost every patient with IM. The atypical lymphocytes are not diagnostic of IM, because they are also seen in viral infections such as hepatitis, mumps, rubella, rubeola, varicella, herpes simplex, herpes zoster, and cytomegalovirus infections, in drug-induced hepatitis, and in toxoplasmosis. The atypical lymphocytes in IM are **T cells** stimulated by lymphocytes containing the EBV.[152,153] The **leukocyte alkaline phosphatase** level is decreased. The **platelet** concentration is slightly dimin-

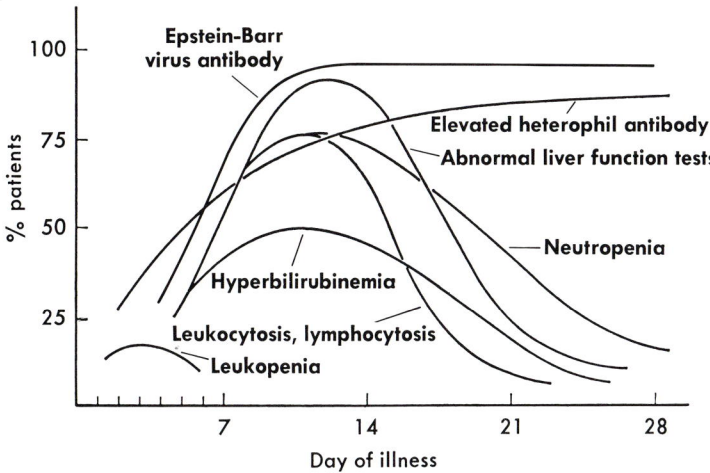

Fig. 9-25. Major laboratory changes in adults with uncomplicated infectious mononucleosis. (Modified from Finch, S.C.: In Carter, R.L., and Penman, H.G., editors: Infectious mononucleosis, Oxford, England, 1969, Blackwell Scientific Publications, Ltd.)

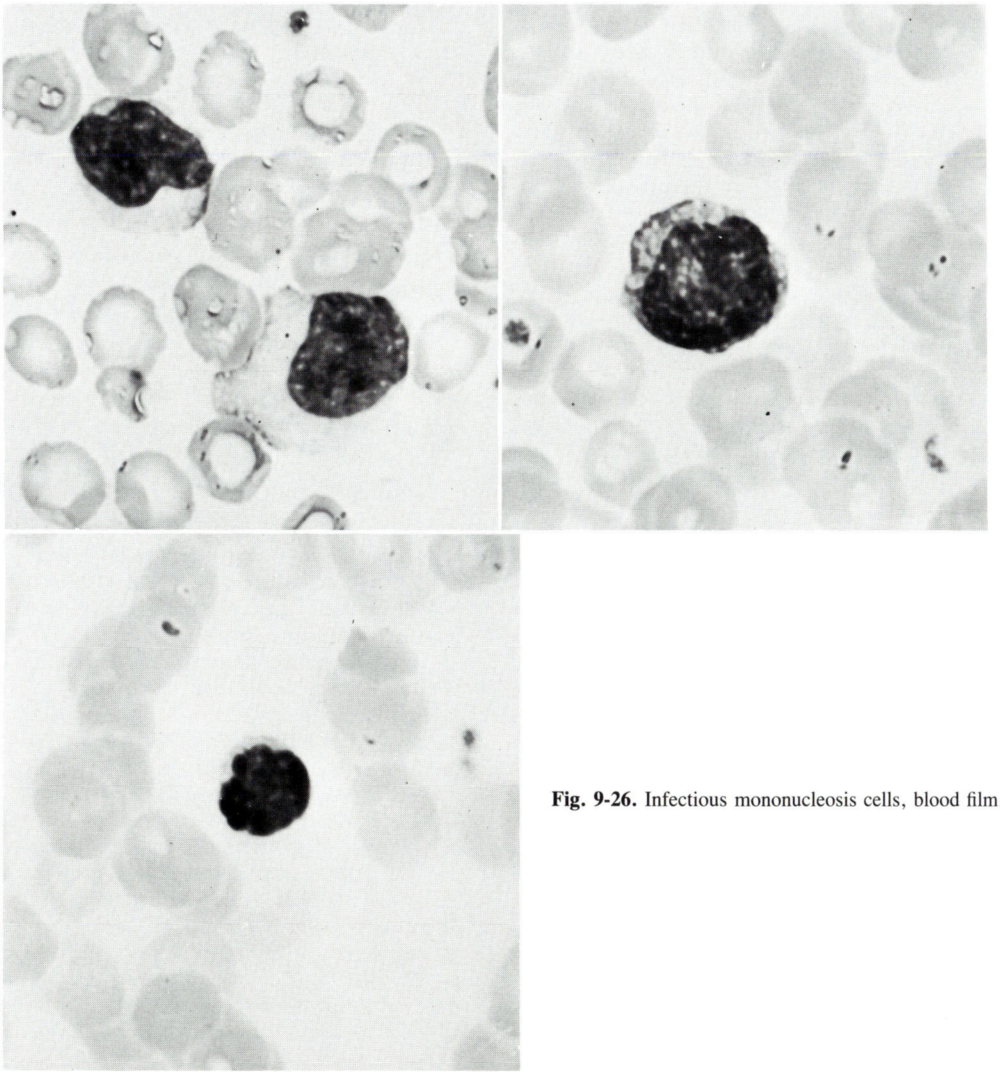

Fig. 9-26. Infectious mononucleosis cells, blood film.

ished in about 50% of patients[154] but may be so severely depressed as to be responsible for petechiae.

Serologic findings

Heterophil antibodies: The most widely used serologic test for IM was first described more than 40 years ago[155] and is based on the presence of IgM **heterophil antibodies** that agglutinate sheep red cells. Davidsohn[156] modified the test to differentiate normally occurring heterophil antibodies (Forssman antibodies) from the agglutinins found in IM by treating the serum with guinea pig kidneys, which are rich in the Forssman antigen and absorb the normally occurring heterophil antibodies but fail to absorb the heterophil antibodies of IM. On the other hand, beef erythrocytes completely absorb the IM heterophil antibodies. In recent years a number of slide tests have been developed that simplify and accelerate the original Davidsohn test. All appear to be satisfactory in terms of specificity and sensitivity,[157] but only the Monospot test[158] (Ortho Diagnostics, Raritan, N.J.) is described below.

Monospot test:

Principle: The test uses formalized horse erythrocytes as indicator cells, because they are more sensitive than sheep erythrocytes and allow the demonstration of low titers of IM heterophil antibodies. The Forssman antibodies are absorbed by ground guinea pig kidney that does not absorb the heterophil antibodies of IM, which are, however, absorbed by ox erythrocytes. Horse red cells are added to each system as indicator cells. If IM heterophil antibodies are present in the patient's serum or plasma,[159] the horse erythrocytes will be agglutinated by the guinea pig kidney–absorbed serum or plasma within 2 min.

Procedure: See manufacturer's instructions.

Discussion[157]: A positive **heterophil antibody test** is specific for IM and EBV infection. False positive results are very rare,[160] and only five such cases have been reported in 33 years of experience with this test.[161] In about 75% of patients heterophil antibodies are present in the first week of illness. During the following 2-3 weeks the titers rise in about 90% of patients and decline gradually to disappear completely after about 12 weeks (see Fig. 9-25). On the other hand, they may persist for 6-12 months or longer and may be anamnestically recalled during subsequent viral illnesses[148,162] that clinically and hematologically are not IM. Apparently no relationship exists between heterophil antibody titer and severity of the disease.

In about 10% of adults with clinical and hematologic manifestations of IM the heterophil antibody test is persistently negative or the titer never exceeds 1:16. **Negative heterophil responses** are found more frequently in children and uniformly in infants with EBV infections.[163] These patients present a diagnostic challenge to the clinical pathologist. In some patients the disease may be an expression of **cytomegalovirus** (CMV) infections, which can be confirmed by growing the virus from urine or throat washings on **human fetal fibroblast cultures** or by demonstrating anti-CMV IgM in the serum by using immunofluorescence. In other patients dye or hemagglutination tests may point to *Toxoplasma* as the responsible agent. Even if these two

groups of patients are excluded, a significant number remain that are **heterophil antibody negative** but clinically have evidence of IM. Recent investigations demonstrate IgM antibodies specific for EBV in almost all of these patients (45 of 46).[146] It is possible that very rarely other viruses, e.g., hepatitis or adenoviruses, may be responsible for heterophil-negative IM.

Other antibodies: In addition to the heterophil antibodies, other heteroantibodies and autoantibodies appear during the course of IM, e.g., antinuclear, anti-smooth muscle and antithyroid antibodies. Abnormal globulins may be responsible for rheumatoid factor, cryoglobulins.[164] and hemolysins of Donath-Landsteiner.[165] During the course of IM, IgM antibodies (heterophil and anti-I) increase to a greater extent than do anti-IgG or anti-IgA[166] antibodies. **Anti-I antibodies** can be demonstrated in about 70% of patients,[150] but rarely are they responsible for an autoimmune hemolytic anemia or an associated thrombocytopenia.

Antibodies to Epstein-Barr virus: A number of **antibodies** to **EBV** appear at different times during the course of IM and are directed against virus-related cell-associated antigens. The demonstration of these antibodies is of diagnostic importance in the seronegative and the chronic or recurring IM and in the determination of susceptibility or immunity to IM.[168]

Other laboratory findings

A mild-to-moderate form of **hepatitis** is always associated with IM.[167] If it is absent, the diagnosis of IM should be questioned.

LABORATORY INVESTIGATION OF SYSTEMIC LUPUS ERYTHEMATOSUS

Systemic lupus erythematosus (SLE) is a diffuse connective tissue disorder that has many features of a complement-dependent autoimmune disease, characterized by a variety of antibodies, e.g., antinuclear, anticytoplasmic, anti-IgG, and antierythrocytic, and by such plasma proteins as lymphocytotoxins and circulating anticoagulants.[168]

Hematologic findings

A mild-to-moderate hypochromic microcytic anemia is seen in almost every patient with SLE. It can be classified as an **anemia of chronic** disorders, since both the serum iron concentration and the total iron binding capacity are low. The anemia is multifactorial in origin. There may be some difficulty in iron absorption, a mild degree of hemolysis, some blood loss because of hemorrhages, and bone marrow depression resulting from kidney involvement. A frank autoimmune hemolytic anemia is found in about 5% of patients and is often combined with an immune thrombocytopenia. The autoimmune anemia is Coombs positive, reacting best with broad-spectrum anticomplement–anti-γ-globulin antisera, and may precede by weeks and months the development of SLE. The erythrocyte **sedimentation rate** is elevated mainly because of the dysproteinemia and can therefore be used as a rough indicator of disease activity. If the hemolysis is a significant factor, it may be responsible for a mild leukocytosis (less than 40,000 cells/mm³), which contrasts with the moderate leukopenia seen in about 80% of patients with SLE.[169] The **differential** count may be normal but frequently shows an absolute lymphopenia, and fewer than 5% of patients have a moderate eosinophilia.[169] **Thrombocytopenia** (less than 100,000/mm^3) is seen in about 25% of patients and is thought to result from an immune mechanism, even though antiplatelet antibodies cannot be demonstrated in all cases,[169] but the giant young platelets found in the peripheral smear and the megakaryocytic hyperplasia of the bone marrow are reminiscent of idiopathic thrombocytopenic purpura. The thrombocytopenia like the AIHA may precede by months or years the onset of SLE.

The **bleeding tendency** in SLE results from a number of factors, thrombocytopenia being one of the least important contributors. The development of lupoid hepatitis is responsible for hypofibrinogenemia and depression of the vitamin K–depending factors. Lupoid nephritis adds a vascular component, and dysproteinemia is responsible for the development of circulating anticoagulants that may be antithrombins or specifically directed against factor X[170] and against activation of factors VIII and IX.[171]

The fractionation of ANA antibodies is discussed in Chapter 36.

REFERENCES

1. Churid, M.J., et al.: Medicine **54:**1, 1975.
2. Sullivan, T.J.: In Brown, E.B., editor: Progress in hematology, New York, 1979, Grune & Stratton, Inc.
3. Murdoch, J.M., and Smith, C.C.: Clin. Haematol. **1:**619, 1972.
4. Miale, J.B.: Laboratory medicine, ed. 5, St. Louis, 1977, The C.V. Mosby Co.
5. Oski, F.A., and Naiman, J.L.: Hematologic problems in the newborn, Philadelphia, 1966, W.B. Saunders Co.
6. Linman, J.W.: Principles of hematology, New York, 1966, Macmillan Publishing Co., Inc.
7. Finch, S.C.: In Williams, W.J., et al., editors: Hematology, ed. 2, New York, 1977, McGraw-Hill Book Co.
8. Page, A.R., and Good, R.A.: Arch. Dis. Child. **94:**623, 1957.
9. Barak, Y., et al.: Blood **38:**74, 1971.
10. Zuelzer, W.W., and Bajoghli, M.: Blood **23:**359, 1964.
11. Huguley, C.M., Jr.: J.A.M.A. **118:**817, 1964.
12. Crosby, W.H.: Annu. Rev. Med. **13:**127, 1962.
13. Japa, J.: Br. J. Exp. Pathol. **23:**272, 1942.
14. Fliedner, T.M., et al.: Acta Haematol. **22:**65, 1959.
15. Mauer, A.M., et al.: J. Clin. Invest. **39:**1481, 1960.
16. Boggs, D.R.: Clin. Haematol. **4:**535, 1975.
17. Carmel, R., and Coltman, C.A., Jr.: Clin. Res. **17:**531, 1969.
18. Chikkappa, G., et al.: Blood **34:**828, 1969.
19. Zucker, S., et al.: J. Lab. Clin. Med. **75:**83, 1970.
20. Fink, M.E., and Finch, S.C.: Proc. Soc. Exp. Biol. Med. **127:**365, 1968.
21. Gaydos, L.A., Freireich, E.J., and Mantel, N.: N. Engl. J. Med. **266:**905, 1962.
22. Didisheim, P., et al.: Blood **23:**717, 1964.
23. Nowell, P.C.: Cancer **28:**513, 1971.
24. Hart, J.S., et al.: Ann. Intern. Med. **75:**353, 1971.
25. Bloom, G.E., et al.: N. Engl. J. Med. **274:**8, 1966.
26. Silver, H.K., Blair, W.C., and Kempe, C.H.: Am. J. Dis. Child. **83:**14, 1952.
27. Perillie, P.E., and Finch, S.C.: Med. Clin. North Am. **57:**395, 1973.
28. Sandberg, A.A., Cartwright, G.E., and Wintrobe, M.M.: Blood **11:**154, 1956.
29. Boggs, D.R., Wintrobe, M.M., and Cartwright, G.E.: Medicine **41:**163, 1962.
30. Evans, A.E., Gilbert, E.S., and Zandstra, R.: Cancer **26:**404, 1970.
31. Mathé, G., et al.: Eur. J. Clin. Biol. Res. **16:**554, 1971.
33. Bennett, J.M., Klemperer, M., and Segel, J.B.: Recent Results Cancer Res. **43:**23, 1973.
32. Bennett, J.M., et al.: Br. J. Haematol. **33:**451, 1976.
34. Spiers, A.S.D.: Clin. Haematol. **1:**127, 1972.
35. Hayhoe, F.G.J., and Cawley, J.C.: Clin. Haematol. **1:**49, 1972.
36. Catovsky, D., et al.: Lancet **1:**749, 1978.
37. Belpomme, D., et al.: Br. J. Haematol. **38:**85, 1978.
38. McCoffrey, R., et al.: N. Engl. J. Med. **292:**775, 1975.
39. Smyth, J.F., and Harrop, K.R.: Br. J. Cancer **31:**544, 1975.
40. McKenna, R.W.: In Recent advances in laboratory hematology and hematopathology, Minneapolis, 1978, University of Minnesota Press.
41. Beard, M.E.J., and Whitehouse, J.M.A.: In Hoffbrand, A.V., Brain, M.C., and Hirsh, J., editors: Recent advances in haematology, New York, 1977, Churchill Livingstone, Inc.
42. Brunning, R.: In Recent advances in laboratory hematology and hematopathology, Minneapolis, 1978, University of Minnesota Press.
43. Daniel, M.-Th., et al.: Nouv. Rev. Fr. Hematol. Blood Cells **11:**233, 1971.
44. Kiossoglou, K.A., Mitus, W.J., and Dameshek, W.: Blood **26:**610, 1965.
45. Pruzanski, W., and Platts, M.E.: J. Clin. Invest. **49:**1694, 1970.
46. Schiffer, C.H., et al.: Blood **46:**17, 1975.
47. McKenna, R.W., et al.: Blood **46:**481, 1975.
48. Gralnick, H.R., et al.: Ann. Intern. Med. **87:**740, 1977.
49. Pierre, R.V.: Blood Cells **1:**163, 1975.
50. Sokal, G., Michaux, J.L., and Van den Berghe, H.: Clin. Haematol. **9:**129, 1980.
51. Gilbert, H.S.: Med. Clin. North Am. **57:**355, 1973.
52. Gilbert, H.S.: Mt. Sinai J. Med. (N.Y.) **37:**426, 1970.
53. Ward, H.P., and Block, M.H.: Medicine **50:**357, 1971.
54. Medical Research Council's Working Party for Therapeutic Trials in Leukaemia: Br. Med. J. **1:**201, 1968.
55. Rundles, W.R.: In Williams, W.J., et al., editors: Hematology, New York, 1972, McGraw-Hill Book Co.
56. Athens, J.W.: Clin. Haematol. **4:**553, 1975.
57. Sawitsky, A., Rosner, F., and Chodsky, S.: Semin. Hematol. **9:**285, 1972.
58. Galton, D.A.G.: In Hardisty, R.M., and Weatherall, D.J., editors; Blood and its disorders, Oxford, England, 1974, Blackwell Scientific Publications, Ltd.
59. Marks, S.M., Baltimore, D., and McCaffrey, R.: N. Engl. J. Med. **298:**812, 1978.
60. Sarin, P.S., Anderson, P.N., and Gallo, R.C.: Blood **47:**11, 1976.
61. Nowell, P.C., and Hungerford, D.A.: J. Natl. Cancer Inst. **27:**1013, 1961.
62. Tjio, J.H., et al.: J. Natl. Cancer Inst. **36:**567, 1966.
63. Kardinal, C.G., Bateman, J.R., and Weiner, J.: Arch. Intern. Med. **136:**305, 1976.
64. Rowley, J.D.: Clin. Haematol. **9:**55, 1980.
65. Mitelman, F., and Levan, G.: Hereditas **89:**207, 1978.
66. Bloomfield, C.D., et al.: Br. J. Haematol. **36:**347, 1977.
67. Hardisty, R.M., Speed, D.E., and Till, M.: Br. J. Haematol. **10;**551, 1964.
68. Ezdinli, E.Z., et al.: Ann. Intern. Med. **72:**175, 1970.
69. Whang-Peng, J., et al.: Blood **23:**755, 1968.

70. Strykmans, P.A.: Semin. Hematol. **11:**101, 1974.
71. Sakurai, M., and Sandberg, A.A.: Cancer **38:**762, 1976.
72. Weatherall, D.J., Edwards, J.A., and Donahue, W.T.A.: Br. Med. J. **1:**679, 1968.
73. Yu, T.-F.: Arthritis Rheum. **8:**765, 1965.
74. Bronson, W.R., et al.: N. Engl. J. Med. **274:**369, 1966.
75. Magill, G.B., Wroblewski, F., and LaDue, J.E.: Blood **14:**870, 1959.
76. Gilbert, H.S., et al.: Ann. Intern. Med. **71:**719, 1969.
77. Miescher, P.A., and Farguet, J.J.: Semin. Hematol. **11:**129, 1974.
78. Burke, J.S., Byrne, G.E., Jr., and Rappaport, H.: Cancer **33:**1399, 1974.
79. Scully, R.E., and McNelly, B.U.: N. Engl. J. Med. **292:**689, 1975.
80. Lee, S.L., et al.: N.Y. State J. Med. **69:**422, 1969.
81. Rozenszajn, L.A., et al.: Am. J. Clin. Pathol. **66:**432, 1976.
82. Yam, L.T., Li, C.-Y., and Finkel, H.E.: Arch. Intern. Med. **130:**248, 1972.
83. Catovsky, D., et al.: Br. J. Haematol. **26:**29, 1974.
84. Huber, H., et al.: Science **162:**1281, 1968.
85. Scheinberg, M., et al.: Cancer **37:**1302, 1976.
86. Takácsi-Nagy, L., and Gráf, F.: Clin. Haematol. **4:**291, 1975.
87. Rosenthal, D.S., and Moloney, W.C.: Postgrad. Med. **45:**136, 1969.
88. Khumbananda, M., Horowitz, H.I., and Eyster, M.E.: Am. J. Med. Sci. **258:**89, 1969.
89. Goswitz, F., et al.: J. Lab. Clin. Med. **67:**615, 1966.
90. Lind, I.: Acta Haematol. **23:**247, 1960.
91. Lakatos, E.K., and Hadnagy, Cs.: Folia Haematol. (Leipz) **96:**365, 1971.
92. Didisheim, P., and Bunting, D.: Am. J. Clin. Pathol. **45:**566, 1966.
93. Müller, D., and Haberlandt, W.: Blut **20:**205, 1970.
94. Boivin, P., et al.: Acta Haematol. **51:**91, 1974.
95. Hoffbrand, A.V., et al.: Br. Med. J. **1:**577, 1966.
96. Hickling, R.A.: Lancet **1:**175, 1958.
97. Catovsky, D., et al.: Br. J. Haematol. **33:**173, 1976.
98. Lewis, S.M., and Szur, L.: Br. Med. J. **2:**472, 1963.
99. Catovsky, D., et al.: Lancet **2:**232, 1973.
100. Galton, D.A.G., et al.: Br. J. Haematol. **27:**7, 1974.
101. Aisenberg, A.C., and Bloch, K.J.: N. Engl. J. Med. **287:**272, 1972.
102. Brouet, J.-C., et al.: Lancet **2:**890, 1975.
103. Thong, Y.H., et al.: South. Med. J. **67:**138, 1974.
104. Dickler, H.B., et al.: Clin. Exp. Immunol. **14:**97, 1973.
105. Bronet, J.C., et al.: Lancet **2:**390, 1975.
106. Schnitzer, B., and Lass, L.: Cancer **31:**547, 1973.
107. Editorial: Br. Med. J. **1:**590, 1975.
108. Labaze, J.J., et al.: J. Clin. Pathol. **25:**312, 1972.
109. Flandrin, G., and Brouet, J.-C.: Mayo Clin. Proc. **49:**575, 1974.
110. Zucker-Franklin, D.: Mayo Clin. Proc. **49:**567, 1974.
111. Robinowtiz, B.N., Noguchi, S., and Roenigk, H.H., Jr.: Cancer **37:**1747, 1976.
112. Hoffbrand, A.V., et al.: J. Clin. Pathol. **20:**699, 1967.
113. Cline, M.J., and Berlin, N.I.: Am. J. Med. **33:**510, 1962.
114. Osserman, E.F.: N. Engl. J. Med. **261:**952, 1959.
115. Pruzanski, W., Platts, M.E., and Ogryzlo, M.A.: Am. J. Med. **47:**60, 1969.
116. Ogawa, M., et al.: N. Engl. J. Med. **281:**1217, 1969.
117. Ben-Bassat, I., et al.: Arch. Intern. Med. **121:**361, 1968.
118. Lackner, J.: Semin. Hematol. **10:**125, 1973.
119. Canale, D.D., Jr., and Collins, R.D.: Am. J. Clin. Pathol. **61:**382, 1974.
120. Hyun, B.H., et al.: Am. J. Clin. Pathol. **65:**921, 1976.
121. Isobe, T., and Osserman, E.F.: Ann. N.Y. Acad. Sci. **190:**507, 1971.
122. Zawadski, Z.A., and Edwards, G.A.: Prog. Clin. Immunol. **1:**105, 1972.
123. Blom, J., Mansa, B., and Wilk, A.: Acta Pathol. Microbiol. Scand. **84:**335, 1976.
124. Paraskevas, F., Heremans, J., and Waldenström, J.: Acta Med. Scand. **170:**575, 1961.
125. Drivsholm, Aa., and Clausen, J.: Acta Med. Scand. **175:**609, 1964.
126. Khaleeli, M., Keane, W.M., and Lee, G.R.: Blood **41:**17, 1973.
127. Kyle, R.A., Pierre, R.V., and Bayrd, E.D.: N. Engl. J. Med. **283:**1121, 1970.
128. Lejeune, F., et al.: Pathol. Biol. **20:**486, 1972.
129. Kaplow, L.S., and Burstone, M.S.: J. Histochem. Cytochem. **12:**805, 1964.
130. Perkins, H.A., MacKenzie, M.R., and Fudenberg, H.H.: Blood **35:**695, 1970.
131. Cohen, I., et al.: Am. J. Med. **48:**766, 1970.
132. Williams, R.C., Jr., Brunning, R.D., and Wollheim, F.A.: Ann. Intern. Med. **65:**471, 1966.
133. Stone, M.J., and Frenkel, E.P.: Am. J. Med. **58:**601, 1975.
134. Frangione, B., and Franklin, E.C.: Semin. Hematol. **10:**53, 1973.
135. Seligmann, M., et al.: Science **162:**1396, 1968.
136. Seligmann, M.: Rev. Eur. Etudes Clin. Biol. Res. **17:**349, 1972.
137. Bonhomme, J., et al.: Blood **43:**485, 1974.
138. Wells, J.V., and Fudenberg, H.H.: DM, February 1974.
139. Kyle, R.A.: Am. J. Med. **64:**814, 1978.
140. Kyle, R.A.: Arch. Intern. Med. **125:**20, 1975.
141. Axelsson, U., Bachman, R., and Hallén, J.: Acta Med. Scand. **179:**235, 1966.
142. McCallister, B.D., et al.: Am. J. Med. **43:**394, 1967.
143. MacKenzie, M.R., and Fudenberg, H.H.: Blood **39:**874, 1972.
144. Dutcher, T.F., and Fahey, J.L.: J. Natl. Cancer Inst. **22:**887, 1959.
145. Greaves, F.M., Brown, G., and Rickinson, A.B.: Clin. Immunol. Immunopathol. **3:**514, 1975.
146. Nikoskelainen, J., Leikola, J., and Klemola, E.: Br. Med. J. **4:**72, 1974.
147. Jordan, M.C.: J.A.M.A. **234:**45, 1975.
148. Hoagland, R.J.: Infectious mononucleosis, New York, 1967, Grune & Stratton, Inc.
149. Hossaini, A.A.: Am. J. Clin. Pathol. **53:**198, 1970.
150. Chervenick, P.A.: DM, December 1974.
151. Koziner, B., et al.: J.A.M.A. **225:**1235, 1973.
152. Sheldon, P.J., et al.: Lancet **1:**1153, 1973.
153. Steel, C.M., and Ling, N.R.: Lancet **2:**861, 1973.
154. Carter, R.L.: Blood **25:**817, 1965.
155. Paul, J.R., and Bunnell, W.W.: Am. J. Med. Sci. **183:**90, 1932.
156. Davidsohn, I.: J.A.M.A. **108:**289, 1937.
157. Goldin, M.: Am. J. Med. Technol. **40:**317, 1974.
158. Lee, C.L., Davidsohn, I., and Panczyszyn, O.: Am. J. Clin. Pathol. **49:**12, 1968.
159. Davidson, R.J.L., and Main, S.R.: J. Clin. Pathol. **24:**259, 1971.
160. Davidsohn, I., and Lee, C.L.: In Carter, R.L., and Penman, H.G., editors: Infectious mononucleosis, Oxford, England, 1969, Blackwell Scientific Publications, Ltd.
161. Davidsohn, H.: Clinical diagnosis by laboratory methods, Philadelphia, 1969, W.B. Saunders Co.
162. Finch, S.C.: In Carter, R.L., and Penman H.G., editors: Infectious mononucleosis, Oxford, England, 1969, Blackwell Scientific Publications, Ltd.

163. Henle, W., Henle, G.E., and Howitz, C.A.: Hum. Pathol. **5:**551, 1974.

164. Carter, R.L.: Br. J. Haematol. **12:**268, 1966.

165. Wishart, M.M., and Davey, M.G.: J. Clin. Pathol. **26:**332, 1973.

166. Stites, D.P., and Leikola, J.: Semin. Hematol. **8:**243, 1971.

167. Chang, M.Y., and Campbell, W.G.: Arch. Pathol. Lab. Med. **99:**185, 1975.

168. Hughes, G.R.V.: Br. J. Haematol. **25:**409, 1973.

169. Harvey, A.M., et al.: Medicine **33:**291, 1954.

170. Wall, R.L., Haq, A., and Moore, D.: J. Lab. Clin. Med. **70:**861, 1967.

171. Bithell, T.C., and Bunting, D.L.: Clin. Res. **15:**103, 1967.

Examination of bone marrow

The bone marrow is a large hematopoietic and lymphoreticular organ housed in the marrow spaces of the skeleton. It consists of a system of sinusoids lined by phagocytic endothelial cells supported by a framework of fibrofatty tissue. The fibrofatty framework contains the precursors of hematopoietic cells, mature blood elements, localized aggregates of lymphoreticular cells, and a number of large phagocytic cells called *reticulum cells*. The marrow can be divided into a hematopoietic and a nonhematopoetic component. In response to disease one component may expand at the expense of the other.

In the newborn and infant all bones contain hematopoietic marrow, whereas in adults it is restricted to the axial skeleton (vertebrae and flat bones).

The examination of the bone marrow is an essential diagnostic and prognostic step in the evaluation of patients with a wide variety of hematologic and neoplastic disorders. The absolute indications for bone marrow examination include the following conditions:

1. Anemia of unknown etiology
2. Megaloblastic anemia
3. Myelosclerosis and other leukoerythroblastic anemias
4. Metastatic tumor and other bone marrow invasive diseases
5. Staging of Hodgkin's disease[1] and other lymphomas[2]
6. Hypersplenism
7. Thrombocytopenia
8. Pancytopenia, assessment of hypocellularity[3]
9. Leukopenia (agranulocytosis)
10. Myeloproliferative disorders (polycythemia vera, leukemia)
11. Lymphoproliferative disorders
12. Refractory (aplastic) anemia
13. Malignant reticuloendothelioses and histiocytoses (storage diseases)
14. Management of patients undergoing chemotherapy
15. Plasma cell and immunoglobulin disorders

The relative indications are as follows:

1. Iron deficiency anemia
2. Macrocytic anemia
3. Follow-up of certain hematologic disorders
4. Granulomatous diseases (sarcoidosis, tuberculosis)
5. Fungal and parasitic diseases (histoplasmosis, malaria)
6. Bone marrow culture
7. Cytogenetic studies

The only contraindication is hemophilia.

EQUIPMENT FOR BONE MARROW PUNCTURE

The following equipment is used for bone marrow punctures:

1. Skin antiseptic and sterile drape material
2. Local anesthetic
3. Sterile needles (25 g 5/8 in and 21 g 1½ in) and syringes
4. Sterile scalpel with no. 11 blade
5. Sterile biopsy and aspiration needle (Jamshidi needle, Kormed, St. Paul)
6. Gauze, small dressing (adhesive strip)
7. B5 fixative, glass slides, watch glasses, coverslips, pipets
8. Sterile surgical gloves

The Jamshidi needle[4-6] is the instrument of choice for the bone marrow biopsy and aspiration of the posterior superior iliac spine. The needle is available in various sizes so that aspirations and biopsies can be obtained from children as well as adults with minimal discomfort. The specimen is adequate in size and shows little or no distortion. The needle has a tapered distal cutting tip that allows the specimen to enter the lumen without distortion and prevents it from escaping after completion of the biopsy procedure. The marrow aspiration must precede the biopsy. The Jamshidi needle is not suitable for sternal marrow aspiration, which should be performed with the University of Illinois needle.

ASPIRATION SITES

The following are recommended bone marrow aspiration sites.

1. The posterior superior iliac spine is the ideal site for bone marrow aspiration and biopsy in children and adults alike.

2. The manubrium just above the angle of Lewis or the body of the sernum just below the angle of Lewis is a suitable site for bone marrow aspiration in adults. This approach should not be used for biopsies or in children.

3. The anterior aspect of the tibia just below the tibial tubercle is a suitable site in infants under $1^1/_2$ years of age. Biopsy should not be attempted.

4. The spinous process of the third lumbar vertebra is suitable for aspiration only.

5. The anterior superior iliac spine can be utilized for aspiration and biopsy. The biopsy specimen is usually shorter than that obtained from the posterior iliac crest.

Procedure for posterior iliac crest aspiration[7,8]

1. The patient is placed in a right or left lateral decubitus position with the lower leg extended and the upper leg flexed toward the chest. The back is curved so that the position is similar to the ''spinal puncture position'' (Fig. 10-1).

2. After the posterior superior iliac spine is located and outlined with a methyl blue pencil, the area is disinfected with an iodine preparation and draped.

3. Skin, subcutaneous tissue, and underlying periosteum are infiltrated with a local anesthetic (1% lidocaine).

4. A no. 11 Bard-Parker blade is used to make a 3 mm skin incision through which the needle, with the stylet locked in place, is inserted and allowed to penetrate to the underlying bone. The direction of the needle is parallel to the bed, pointing toward the anterior superior iliac spine.

5. With one hand use firm pressure to rotate the needle in an alternating clockwise-counterclockwise motion to penetrate the outer cortex of the bone while the other hand identifies the anterior superior spine and at the same time steadies the patient by applying counter pressure.

6. After the marrow cavity is entered, remove stylet and aspirate about 0.5 ml bone marrow into a 20 ml syringe attached to the hub of the Jamshidi needle. The aspiration of a larger specimen only dilutes the marrow with peripheral blood.

7. The aspirated blood and marrow mixture is ejected into a 10 cm diameter watch glass, which is handed to the technologist to judge the adequacy of the aspirated bone marrow and to prepare the smears.

8. If the marrow aspirate is adequate, obtain the core biopsy specimen by advancing the needle into the marrow cavity for a distance up to 3 cm by gently clockwise-counterclockwise motion.

9. Break off the marrow biopsy specimen caught within the needle by rotating the hub of the needle in a wide circle, thus displacing the cutting edge from its original position.

10. Withdraw the needle with alternating rotating movements and expel the biopsy specimen into a watch glass by means of the probe supplied by the manufacturer and introduced through the narrow cutting end of the needle.

11. Use sterile gauze to apply pressure until bleeding has stopped.

12. Handle marrow as described below.

Procedure for sternal marrow aspiration

1. With the patient in a supine position locate (a) the midline sternal notch, (b) the angle of Lewis at the level of the second rib attachment, (c) the lateral borders of the body of the sternum, and (d) the puncture site above or below the angle of Lewis in the midline (Fig. 10-2).

2. Shave the area if necessary, paint with iodine disinfectant, and drape.

3. Infiltrate the future puncture site, including skin, subcutaneous tissue, and periosteum, with 1-2% local anesthetic.

4. Employing sterile technic and using a bone marrow aspiration needle with the stylet in place, holding it at a 60-90 degree angle, puncture skin and underlying tissue until the outer table of the sternum is reached.

5. Using straight downward pressure, penetrate the anterior bony plate. When the marrow cavity is entered, the operator experiences a ''give.''

6. Remove the stylet from the aspiration needle and with a dry plastic 20 ml syringe aspirate about 0.5 ml marrow.

7. Apply sterile gauze and pressure until bleeding has stopped.

8. Handle marrow specimen as described below.

Procedure for tibial aspiration in infants

The following method is only used in infants under $1^1/_2$ years of age. In older children the cortex is too firm and the cellularity of the hematopoietic marrow varies.

1. The proximal half of the tibia is surgically prepared and draped as for iliac crest aspiration.

2. Locate the puncture site in the upper third of the tibia medially and below the tibial tubercle (Fig. 10-3).

3. Infiltrate the area with local anesthetic and direct the needle posteriorly and laterally.

4. When needle ''sits tight'' (no ''give'' is felt), remove stylet and aspirate.

5. Apply gauze and pressure until bleeding has stopped.

6. Handle aspirate as described below.

HANDLING OF MARROW SPECIMEN

The laboratory technologist's duties begin as soon as the marrow specimen is obtained. They include the preparation of the bone marrow smears and imprints and the fixation of the bone marrow biopsy specimen and clot.

The marrow aspirate is quickly deposited in a watch glass and the excess blood is drained into a second watch glass, leaving the yellowish white bone marrow particles adherent to the glass surface. One or two bone marrow particles are aspirated into the tip of a white cell diluting pipet attached to suction tubing and are transferred onto the center of a 22 × 40 mm coverslip.

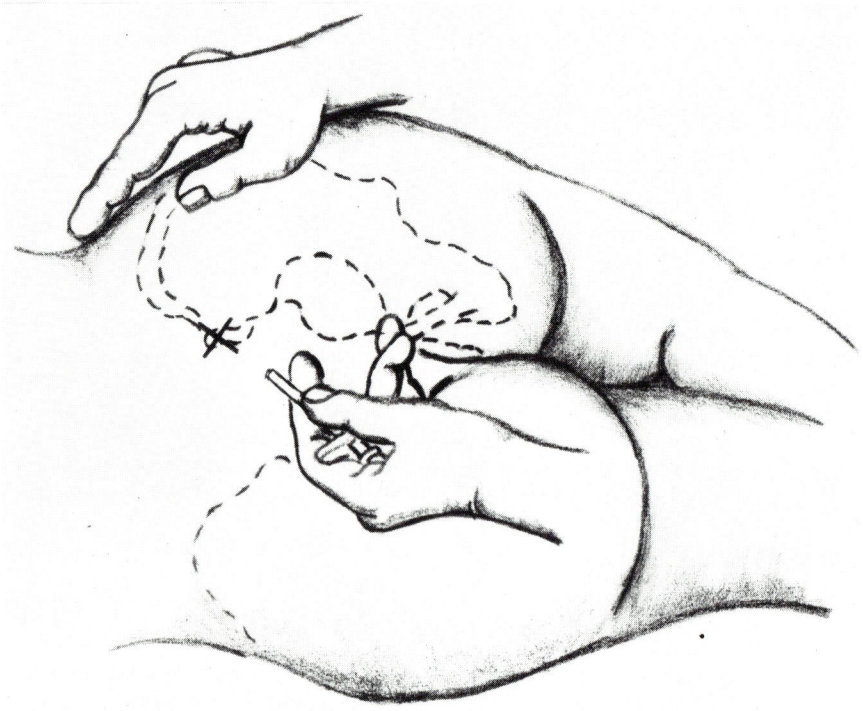

Fig. 10-1. Bone marrow posterior iliac crest aspiration site (*x*).

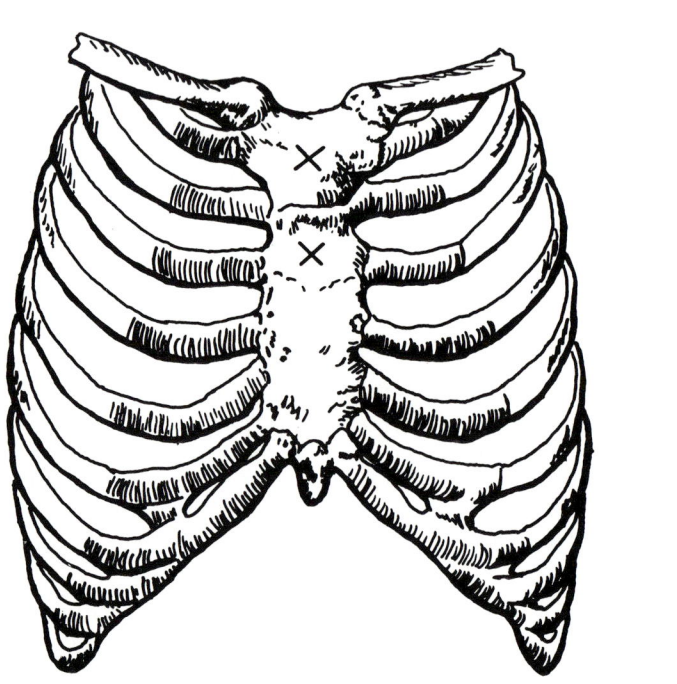

Fig. 10-2. Bone marrow sternal aspiration sites (*x*).

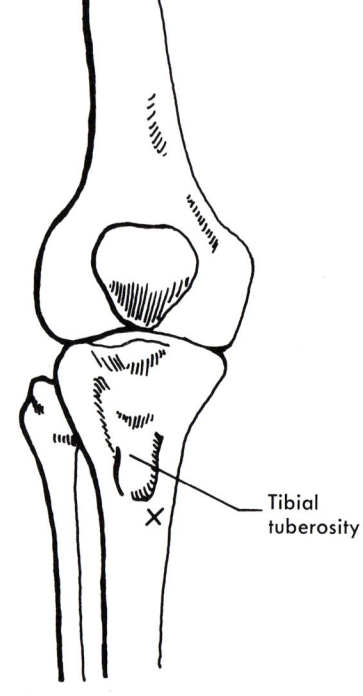

Fig. 10-3. Bone marrow tibial aspiration site (*x*).

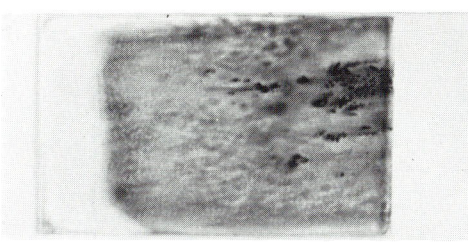

Fig. 10-4. Bone marrow smear.

Table 10-1. Cytochemical fixatives

Leukocyte studies	Fixatives
Peroxidase	Formaldehyde, 37%, 10 ml Absolute ethyl alcohol, 90 ml
Alkaline phosphatase	Citrate buffered acetone (Sigma Chemical Co., St. Louis)
PAS	AS peroxidase
Acid phosphatase	Citric acid–sodium citrate buffer (Sigma Chemical Co.)
Esterases	Citrate-acetone-methanol (Sigma Chemical Co.)

A second coverslip is placed over the bone marrow particles, which spread between the coverslips under very gentle pressure. The coverslips are quickly pulled apart and allowed to air dry. A satisfactory preparation shows a central streak of white greasy marrow flanked by a delicate pink halo of blood (Fig. 10-4). As many smears as possible are made before the marrow coagulates. No anticoagulant should be used unless buffy coat preparations, bone marrow culture, or Cytocentrifuge (Shandon Southern Instruments, Sewickley, Pa.) preparations are contemplated. In the case of a Cytocentrifuge preparation a second bone marrow sample should be aspirated into a sterile heparinized syringe. Send bone marrow smears to the laboratory for staining.

Special procedures

Special investigations require modification of the usual method of handling of bone marrow particles.

Cytochemical staining procedures are preceded by immersing the air-dried smears in special fixatives. See discussion of cytochemistry (p. 113) and Table 10-1.

Phase microscopy and vital staining require unfixed, unstained marrow preparations.

For electron microscopic examination place one or two bone marrow particles into glutaraldehyde (Glutaraldehyde, practical, Eastman Kodak Co., Rochester, N.Y.) and store in refrigerator.

Immunopathologic studies require the following technic:

1. Slides must be cleaned in 95% alcohol and wiped dry before making smears.
2. Prepare six smears and air dry.
3. Fix in acetone for 10 min as soon as dry.
4. Air dry and place in slide box kept in refrigerator.

For cytogenetic investigations the bone marrow aspirate is immediately deposited in 5 ml chromosome culture medium or into 5 ml sterile Hanks salt solution containing 2 drops of sodium heparin.

Points to remember in preparation of bone marrow slides

1. The technologist must work rapidly so that the marrow does not clot. All necessary supplies must be laid out before the procedure is begun. There is no time to look for equipment. Speed is preferable to heparin, which may produce artifacts.
2. In preparing the slides, excessive pressure must be avoided to prevent distortion and destruction of marrow cells.

3. A good bone marrow preparation consists of an evenly spread thin film.
4. If in leukemia the cells are so tightly packed as to make routine aspiration impossible, a 50 ml syringe may produce enough suction to dislodge bone marrow particles.
5. A "dry" tap (i.e., a tap devoid of bone marrow particles) may be caused by (a) faulty positioning of the needle, (b) tightly packed leukemic cells, or (c) myelofibrosis. Items b and c are indications for needle bone biopsies, and item a is an indication for repeating the biopsy with a new needle (tissue thromboplastin may clot the marrow) at a different site.
6. Normal or leukemic marrow of young patients and metastatic tumors may yield only minute, hardly visible particles.

Handling of bone marrow clot

When the marrow clots in the watch glass, no further marrow smears can be prepared and the clotted tissue is transferred to B-5 fixative for $1\frac{1}{2}$ hr, washed in 70% alcohol, and transferred to the 10% formalin beaker of the tissue processor.

B-5 fixative:
1. Mercuric chloride, 6 g
2. Sodium acetate (anhydrous), 1.25 g
3. Distilled water, hot, 90 ml

At the time of use, add 1.0 ml 37-40% formaldehyde to 9 ml B-5 fixative.

Handling of bone marrow biopsy specimen: preparation of imprints

As soon as the biopsy specimen is removed from the needle it is quickly and without smearing brought into contact with different areas of a slide. The imprints (Fig. 10-5) may reveal cells and groups of cells not seen in smears. They are air dried and stained in the same manner as the bone marrow smear. After completion of the imprints, the biopsy specimen is fixed in B-5 for $1\frac{1}{2}$ hr, transferred to decalcifying solution for $1\frac{1}{2}$ hr, washed in 90% alcohol, and added to the surgical specimens in the formalin beaker of the tissue processor.

Staining of bone marrow smears and imprints

Bone marrow smears and imprints are stained with Wright-Giemsa stain (see p. 111) using the following staining times: 6 min undiluted stain and 8 min buffered stain.

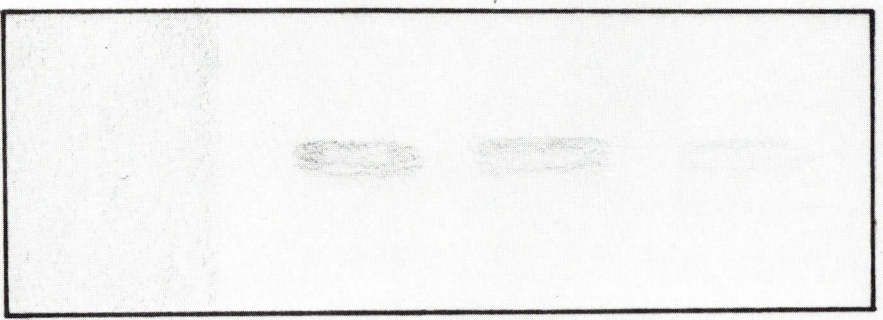

Fig. 10-5. Imprints of bone marrow biopsy specimen.

Staining of sections of bone marrow clot and biopsy

The sections of the bone marrow clot and biopsy are stained with hematoxylin-eosin (H and E) after treatment with iodine to remove the mercuric chloride crystals.

Removal of mercuric chloride crystals

Reagents:
1. Alcoholic iodine solution, 0.5%
   Iodine, 1.0 g
   Absolute alcohol, 160.0 ml
   After iodine has dissolved, add 40.0 ml distilled water.
2. Sodium thiosulfate (Hypo), 5%

Procedure: Deparaffinize slides using xylene and alcohol. Leave in iodine solution for 5-10 min. Wash in water. Bleach in Hypo solution for 1-5 min (to remove iodine). Wash in running water. Proceed with H and E staining procedure.

Additional staining procedures

Bone marrow smears and sections of clot and biopsy must be stained for iron (see p. 113). Cytochemical stains and stains for tubercle bacilli, fungi, amyloid, and reticulum fibers, etc. are added as indicated.

GUIDELINES TO MICROSCOPIC EXAMINATION OF BONE MARROW SMEARS AND IMPRINTS

Detailed bone marrow findings are mentioned wherever they contribute to the laboratory diagnosis of hematologic disorders, but a few general guidelines to the microscopic evaluation of bone marrow smears apply to all bone marrow preparations.[10-13] Smears are screened under low power to discover areas that are thin and well stained and allow recognition of individual cells. The differential count of the bone marrow smear (myelogram) is seldom worth the effort even if 200-500 cells are counted (a count of 100 cells is always inadequate) since a number of factors render standardization of bone marrow aspiration impossible. The most important one is the fact that most bone marrow cells represent stages in a continuous growth process, so that it may be difficult or impossible to correctly categorize each cell. Furthermore, the adequacy of the

Table 10-2. Myelogram of normal adult

Cell type	Range (%)
Stem cells	0.0
Myeloblasts	0.3-5.5
Progranulocytes	1.3-8.3
Myelocytes	7.0-20.0
Neutrophilic	4.5-18.5
Eosinophilic	0.0-3.0
Basophilic	0.0-0.5
Metamyelocytes	4.0-30.0
Neutrophilic	12.5-42.0
Eosinophilic	0.3-3.6
Basophilic	0.0-0.1
Band granulocytes	10.0-35.0
Neutrophilic	15.0-33.0
Eosinophilic	0.0-1.5
Basophilic	0.0-0.5
Segmented granulocytes	8.0-27.0
Neutrophilic	14.5-35.0
Eosinophilic	0.0-0.5
Lymphocytes	7.0-38.0
Monocytes	0.0-5.0
Megakaryocytes	0.0-1.0
	(1-2/lpf)
Reticulum cells	0.0-2.0
Plasma cells	0.0-3.0
Pronormoblasts	0.0-6.0
Basophilic normoblasts	1.0-6.0
Polychromatophilic normoblasts	5.0-26.0
Orthochromatic normoblasts	1.5-21.0
Erythroid/myeloid ratio	1:3-1:6

From Miale, J.B.: Laboratory medicine: hematology, ed. 4, St. Louis, 1972, The C.V. Mosby Co.

aspiration depends on such variables as the angle of the needle and puncture site. Several fields of multiple bone marrow smears should be screened and examined to evaluate the interplay of peripheral blood, hematopoietic marrow, and fat (Table 10-2). Counting of marrow cells is indicated only when preleukemic marrow pictures are encountered or when chemotherapeutic results are to be appraised.[14] For chemotherapeutic purposes the bone marrow in acute leukemias is graded as follows: category 1 contains 0-5% blast cells, category 2 contains 6-25%, and category 3 contains over 25%.

The marrow smears should be examined for quanti-

Table 10-3. Myelogram of children

	Control figures for various age groups									
	1-2 mo	3-12 mo	1-2 yr	3-4 yr	5-6 yr	7-8 yr	9-10 yr	11-12 yr	13-14 yr	15-16 yr
Myeloblasts	1.6	1.9	0.7	1.4	1.8	1.0	1.4	1.1	1.2	1.3
Progranulocytes	5.6	1.8	3.4	3.2	3.2	1.8	2.0	1.7	1.1	1.9
Myelocytes	18.1	16.7	13.3	15.9	17.2	17.4	16.5	15.31	16.4	16.8
Metamyelocytes	25.6	23.9	21.8	22.0	22.9	23.4	26.1	22.2	21.6	23.2
Band and segmented cells	9.3	7.2	14.1	16.4	12.6	12.3	10.9	12.2	12.2	13.3
Pronormoblasts	0.8	0.6	0.8	0.4	0.5	0.4	0.3	0.2	0.4	0.5
Basophilic normoblasts	1.9	2.1	1.2	1.0	1.2	1.7	1.6	1.8	1.3	2.2
Polychromatophilic normoblasts	12.6	14.5	19.5	16.4	17.3	19.4	19.1	21.8	18.3	15.1
Orthochromatic normoblasts	1.6	2.5	2.1	1.2	3.6	3.4	2.4	2.7	3.1	2.5
Lymphocytes	19.7	25.4	19.3	18.6	17.5	13.6	13.6	16.0	18.0	17.4
Myeloid/erythroid ratio	5.5	3.5	2.5	3.4	2.8	2.6	2.9	2.3	2.7	3.3

From Miale, J.B.: Laboratory medicine: hematology, ed. 4, St. Louis, 1972, The C.V. Mosby Co.

tative and qualitative changes of the cellular elements. Hyperplasia and/or hypoplasia of one or the other cell line as well as normal or abnormal maturation is noted. Under low power the adequacy of megakaryocytes is determined. Three to four such cells should be present per low power field and about 40% of these cells should be platelet producing as seen under high power. The pale granulocytic elements are differentiated from the darker staining erythroid elements to arrive at a rough mycloid/crythroid (M/E) ratio. The normal M/E ratio varies from 3:1 to 4:1. Lastly, tumor cells, fungi, granulomas, and evidence of storage diseases and of aminoaciduria may be discovered. The evaluation of stainable iron (hemosiderin) is discussed under the heading of iron metabolism.

Physiologic variations of bone marrow picture

The age of the patient and the aspiration site must be known to allow correct evaluation of the marrow preparation.

Premature infants: Premature infants at birth show erythroid hyperplasia that may be megaloblastic.

Infants and children: In the first year all marrow is hematopoietic and shows lymphocytosis (Table 10-3).

Adults: In the adult[15] the sternal marrow is the most cellular; then follow in order of decreasing cellularity the marrow of vertebrae and of the iliac bone. In the first decade the cellularity of the iliac marrow falls to 75% and during the ensuing 40 years to 50%, the level at which it remains for two to three decades to fall to 30% during the eighth decade. The hematopoietic marrow is thus gradually replaced by fatty tissue.

Pregnant women: In the last trimester the marrow becomes unusually cellular as a result of erythroid hyperplasia of predominantly the younger forms, plasmacytosis, and shift to the left of the myeloid series.

Bone marrow biopsy

Sections of bone marrow biopsy specimens provide information that imprints or smears fail to reveal, since ground substance, blood vessels, and stroma are usually not seen in bone marrow smears and seldom in sections of bone marrow clots. Histologic sections of

the bone marrow biopsy specimen[16-20] allow the evaluation of the following parameters of marrow activity, although decalcification may produce some artifacts.

1. Hematopoietic cellularity: Hematopoietic cellularity is best evaluated in tissue sections, whereas cytomorphologic evaluation is best accomplished by smear examination. The diagnosis of myelophthisic, aplastic, or hypoplastic anemia should never be made without tissue examination.

2. Hemosiderin deposits. Hemosiderin deposits are best evaluated in biopsy sections that are of uniform thickness and lack the thin and thick areas of bone marrow smears.

3. Tumor cells, storage diseases, and granulomas: The presence of tumor cells, storage diseases, and granulomas should be confirmed by examination of tissue sections that also lend themselves to evaluation by histochemical and ''special'' stains.

4. Localization of foci of erythropoiesis and leukopoiesis: Normal leukopoiesis is found close to the endosteum, whereas pathologic leukopoiesis follows capillaries in addition to maintaining the endosteal site. Normal erythropoiesis occurs in perisinusoidal foci, and in erythroid hyperplasia there is a marked increase in the activity and the number of erythropoietic units.

5. Ground substance: Changes in the ground substance include the presence of lipogranulomas, deposits of fibrin, fibrinoid, amyloid,[21] delicate argentophile fibrils, and fibrous tissue. Ground substance changes are important in the diagnosis of immune diseases, plasma cell proliferative disorder, myelofibrosis, and sclerosis.

6. Nuclear necrosis, necrobiosis, and phagocytosis: Necrobiosis is the term used for an LE cell type of nuclear homogenization and swelling occurring in immune reactions. The other type of necrosis, also seen in immune processes, is karyorrhexis. True necrosis and lysis of nuclei producing nuclear shadows are seen in infarcts (sickle cell anemia).

7. Blood vessels: The smallest arterioles may show fibrinoid degeneration or amyloid deposits. There may be perivascular fibrosis, edema, platelet or fibrin thrombi, or plasmacytosis.

8. Cellular patterns: The fixation described gives

such excellent results that bone marrow cells can be identified and evaluated accurately in the section. Protein lakes may be seen around plasma cells, which may contain Russell bodies. It has been pointed out that the perivascular arrangement of mature plasma cells differentiates plasmacytosis from plasma cell myeloma that replaces marrow areas.

9. Changes in the sinusoids: There may be endothelial swelling or sclerosis. The sinuses may be dilated, thrombosed, or atrophied.

Bone marrow culture

The purpose of bone marrow culture is the evaluation of the number and function of hematopoietic cells. In days to come, in vitro hematopoietic cell culture technics will be part of the study of patients with malignant or immunologic hematologic diseases.[22] Semisolid agar media support the growth of neutrophils, macrophages, eosinophils, megakaryocytes, T- and B-lymphocytes, multipotent stem cells,[23] and leukemic cells. When human bone marrow is cultured, the mature cells die rapidly and only a few morphologically undefinable mononuclear cells survive and proliferate. They are called colony-forming cells (CFC) or progenitor cells, and in the process of hematopoiesis they are thought to be interpolated between the multipotent stem cells and the morphologically identifiable blast cells, e.g., erythroblasts, myeloblasts, and myelomonoblasts,[24] which are the parent cells of the mature elements of the peripheral blood. In order for the cells to grow in a semisolid agar medium, for each type of cell specific colony-stimulating factors (CSF) must be added. The CSF for the granulocyte-macrophage stimulation (GM-CSF), for instance, is a glycoprotein supplied by human white cells suspended in an underlayer of agar gel.[25] This socalled feeder layer is covered by the bone marrow aspirate suspended in a similar agar gel overlay (Fig. 10-6). In a successful culture the CFC progenitor cells enlarge and proliferate to form tight aggregates (clusters of fewer than 50 cells) at first, which are followed by the development of colonies containing over 50 cells each. After about 2 weeks the cells die. Normally clusters outnumber colonies 5:1 to 10:1. This ratio is often important, since in acute leukemia it is distorted by the absence of CFC.[26] The aggregates and colonies are a clone of a single progenitor cell and therefore lend themselves to the investigation of certain aspects of preleukemia and acute and chronic leukemia and of immunologic hematologic disorders. In immunologic hematologic disorders, bone marrow cultures serve to demonstrate the immunologic cell injury[22] whereas in preleukemia and acute and chronic leukemia there are important correlations between growth patterns of cultured cells and clinical behavior, e.g., remission rate, survival, and response to treatment. On the basis of the growth pattern, acute myeloid leukemia can be divided into a good prognosis group with a remission rate of about 52% and a poor prognosis group with a 10% remission rate.[27] The leukemic cells of the first group form small clusters only, which, for reasons unknown, indicate a better response to chemotherapy.[27,28] In acute myeloid leukemia and in preleukemia the leukemic

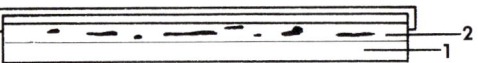

Fig. 10-6. Sketch of semisolid agar gel bone marrow culture. *1*, Underlay; *2*, overlay with colonies.

cells in bone marrow culture form clusters only and suppress the colony formation of normal CFC.[29] According to Metcalf[24] the clinical uses of the agar culture technic in the diagnosis and management of leukemia include (1) the diagnosis of acute nonlymphocytic leukemia, which can clearly be differentiated from acute lymphocytic leukemia; (2) the assessment of likely responses to chemotherapy based on the cluster/colony ratio; (3) confirmation of remission based on the development of normal cluster/colony ratio; (4) early warning of blast transformation in chronic myelogenous leukemia based on a rising cluster/colony ratio associated with a progressive increase in morphologic abnormalities; and (5) the observation of transition of myeloproliferative states to acute nonlymphocytic leukemia or the absence and nonoccurrence of such a transition.

CYTOGENETIC STUDIES OF BONE MARROW

Chromosomal studies can be performed on fresh bone marrow aspirates or on cultured bone marrow. The first approach is preferred because it eliminates possible culture-induced artifacts, although Moore and Metcalf[30] show that the clones of cultured leukemic bone marrow cells exhibit the same karyotypic markers as the original cells. Cytogenetic studies are useful in the evaluation of acute nonlymphocytic leukemia since they shed light on the patients' therapeutic response and thus on their survival, prognosis, and remission rate. The prognosis is poor in patients with acute nonlymphocytic leukemia who have no normal metaphases or in patients who have a mixture of normal and abnormal metaphases but are over 70 years of age,[31-33] Cytogenetically normal patients with acute leukemia have a better survival rate than those with chromosomal abnormalities. The most frequent abnormalities involve chromosomes 8 and 21,[34] which can be used as markers in a number of clonal hematologic disorders in which the neoplastic cells arise from a single abnormal progenitor, which, as in acute leukemia of adults,[35] is often pluripotential; as the clonal diseases progress, additional karyotypic abnormalities are superimposed on the original changes.

There are a number of hematologic illnesses that are classified as preleukemic disorders and that are associated with a high frequency of chromosomal abnormalities. They include the very early stages of acute nonlymphocytic leukemia[36] and potentially leukemic disorders such as Fanconi's and Bloom's syndromes.[9] Progression of the karyotypic abnormality almost always heralds the development of acute leukemia.[37]

One of the best-studied chromosomal abnormalities is the Ph[1] chromosome in chronic myelogenous leukemia (CML); this chromosome is the result of a trans-

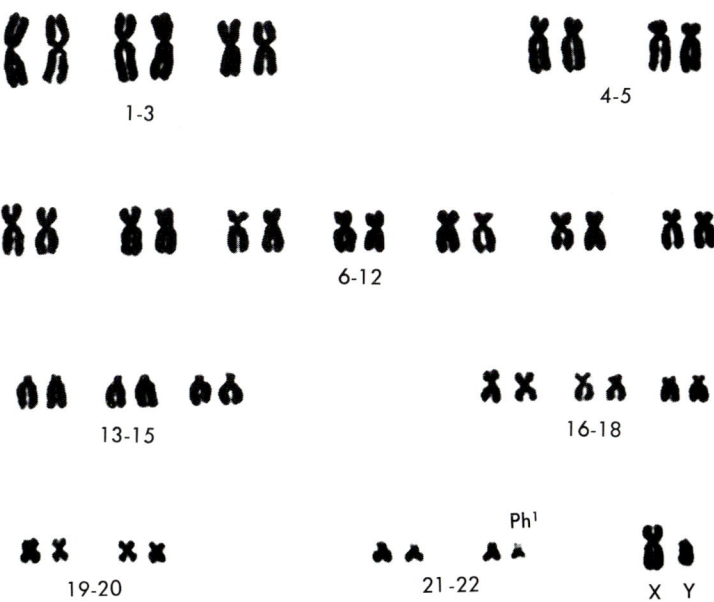

Fig. 10-7. Ph[1] chromosome–positive karyotype from bone marrow sample of patient with chronic granulocytic leukemia. (Courtesy Dr. J.M. Trujillo.)

location of material from the long arm of the G22 chromosome to the long arm of the C9 chromosome. It occurs in about 85% of patients with CML and when present is diagnostic (Fig. 10-7). It remains during remission, is clinically associated with longer survival, is not related to leukocyte alkaline phosphatase levels, and can be detected in myeloid-erythroid cell lines and in megakaryocytes. It remains demonstrable during clinical remission. In blast transformation of CML two Ph[1] chromosomes may be found, often associated with abnormalities in the E and D groups. CML without the Ph[1] chromosome may be seen in older patients and usually implies a poorer prognosis.

Procedures for bone marrow chromosome studies

One of the earliest methods for bone marrow chromosome study is described by Lam-Po-Tang[38]; in this method demecolcine (Colcemid) solution is added directly to the bone marrow specimen and allowed to incubate for 60 min to stop mitotic activity. The cells are harvested in warm hypotonic KCl solution, fixed in Carney's fixative, and finally allowed to spread on a slide.

Banding procedures

Since the introduction of the chromosome banding technic in 1966,[39,40] new approaches are responsible for the recognition of the C,[41] G,[42] R,[43] T,[44] and N[45] bands. The choice of the banding method depends on the information being sought.[46] Q banding identifies the individual chromosomes and their abnormalities using fluorescent technic, which is responsible for its lack of permanence. C banding selectively stains the centro-

meric heterochromatin and identifies characteristic features on the chromosomes by selective staining.

G banding and Q banding produce essentially the same pattern. The trypsin Giemsa technic is the most widely used method because of its relative ease.

The R bands are the reverse of G bands and are induced by heat treatment of chromosome slides.

The T bands are confined on the terminal ends (telomeres)—hence the name of one or both arms of each chromosome.

The N bands are confined to the nucleolus organizer regions (NOR).

Fixed tissue cells of bone marrow

The cellular supporting framework of the bone marrow is part of the granular cell macrophage system consisting of cells that have been described under a variety of names, e.g., reticulum cells (large and small), histiocytes, and phagocytes. These cells are phagocytic and are able to produce reticulin. Sinusoidal lining cells are sometimes included in the classification because of their phagocytic activity, although they do not produce reticulin.

Sinusoidal lining cell (endothelial cell): The lining cells of sinusoids and of blood and lymph vessels resemble phagocytic monocytes. In smears of bone marrow and of peripheral blood they usually appear in clumps, resembling syncytial masses (Fig. 10-8).

Size: The sinusoidal lining cell is 20-30 μm in length.

Nucleus: The nucleus is round or oval, it is eccentric, and it contains fine chromatin arranged in delicate threads. There is a single blue nucleolus.

Cytoplasm: The cytoplasm is bluish gray, surrounds

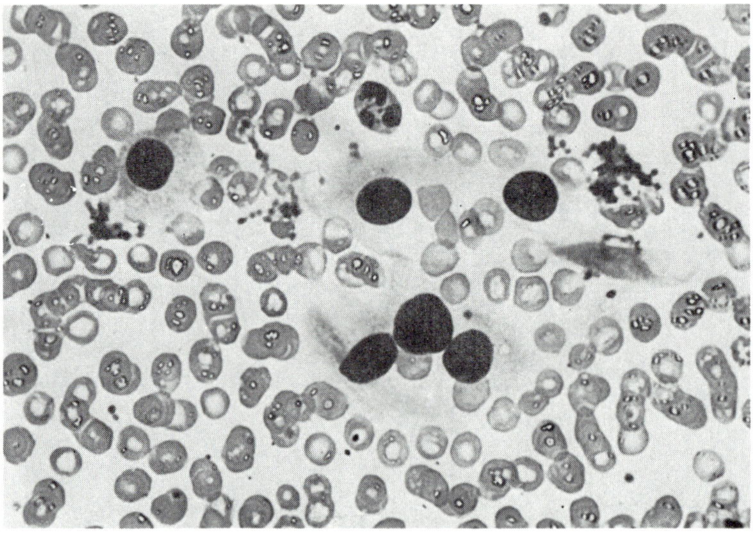

Fig. 10-8. Endothelial cells, peripheral blood.

the nucleus, and extends into drawn-out, elongated, and at times irregular and indistinct shapes. It often contains phagocytosed material.

REFERENCES

1. Rosenberg, S.A., and Kaplan, H.S.: Cancer Res. **26:**1225, 1966.
2. Vinciguerra, V., and Silver, R.T.: Blood **41:**913, 1973.
3. Morley, A., and Blake, J.: J. Clin. Pathol. **28:**104, 1975.
4. Jamshidi, K., and Swaim, W.R.: J. Lab. Clin. Med. **77:**335, 1971.
5. Buskard, N.A., and Gray, G.R.: Abstract no. 183. Sixteenth Annual Meeting of the American Society of Hematology, Chicago, Dec. 1973.
6. Roeckel, I.E.: Ann. Clin. Lab. Sci. **4:**193, 1974.
7. Instrument manual for Jamshidi needle.
8. Dutcher, T.F.: In Morphologic haematology, ASCP Educational Center Program, Chicago, 1974, American Society of Clinical Pathologists.
9. Lillie, R.D.: Histopathologic technic and practical histochemistry, ed. 3, New York, 1965, McGraw-Hill Book Co.
10. Custer, R.P.: An atlas of the blood and bone marrow, ed. 2, Philadelphia, 1974, W.B. Saunders Co.
11. Hyun, B.H., Blank, M., and Custer, R.P.: Filmstrip presentations in hematology—a morphologic study, Philadelphia, 1970, W.B. Saunders Co.
12. Hyun, B.H., and Ashton, J.K.: Filmstrip presentations in hematology—a morphologic study, Philadelphia, 1972, W.B. Saunders Co.
13. Schleicher, E.M.: Bone marrow morphology and mechanics of biopsy, Springfield, Ill., 1973, Charles C Thomas, Publisher.
14. Hewlett, J.S., et al.: Cancer Chemother. Rep. **42:**25, 1964.
15. Hartsock, R.J., Smith, E.B., and Petty, C.S.: Am. J. Clin. Pathol. **43:**326, 1965.
16. Ellis, L.D., Jensen, W.N., and Westerman, M.P.: Arch. Intern. Med. **114:**213, 1964.
17. Conrad, M.E., and Crosby, W.H.: J. Lab. Clin. Med. **57:**642, 1961.
18. Burkhardt, R.: Clin. Wochenschr. **43:**1300, 1965.
19. Burkhardt, V.R.: Folia Haematol. (Leipz.) **9:**353, 1964.
20. Rywlin, A.M.: Hum. Pathol. **6:**523, 1975.
21. Kyle, R.A., et al.: Am. J. Clin. Pathol. **45:**252, 1966.
22. Cline, M.J.: N. Engl. J. Med. **301:**658, 1979.
23. Fauser, A.A., and Messner, H.A.: Blood **52:**1243, 1978.
24. Metcalf, D.: In Recent results in cancer research, New York, 1977, Springer-Verlag New York, Inc.
25. Metcalf, D., et al.: Blood **43:**847, 1974.
26. Senn, J.S., McCulloch, E.A., and Till, J.E.: Lancet **2:**597, 1967.
27. Moore, M.A.S., et al.: Blood **44:**1, 1974.
28. Spitzer, G., et al.: Blood Cells **2:**139, 1976.
29. Chiyoda, S., et al.: Br. J. Cancer **31:**355, 1975.
30. Moore, M.A.S., and Metcalf, D.: Int. J. Cancer **11:**143, 1973.
31. Mitelman, F., et al.: Int. J. Cancer **18:**31, 1976.
32. Sakurai, M., and Sandberg, A.A.: Cancer **37:**285, 1976.
33. Sakurai, M., and Sandberg, A.A.: Cancer **33:**1548, 1974.
34. Yamada, K., and Furusawa, S.: Blood **47:**679, 1976.
35. Blackstock, A.M., and Garson, O.M.: Lancet **2:**1178, 1974.
36. Cline, M.J., et al.: Ann. Intern. Med. **81:**801, 1974.
37. Lawler, S.D., Millard, R.E., and Kay, H.E.M.: Eur. J. Cancer **6:**223, 1970.
38. Lam-Po-Tang, P.R.L.C.: Scand. J. Haematol. **5:**158, 1968.
39. Caspersson, T., et al.: Exp. Cell Res. **58:**141, 1969.
40. Yoshida, M.C., Ikeuchi, T., and Sasaki, M.: Proc. Jpn. Acad. **51:**184, 1975.
41. Pardue, M.L., and Gall, J.G.: Science **168:**1356, 1970.
42. Kato, H., and Yosida, T.H.: Chromosoma **36:**272, 1972.
43. Dutrillaux, B.: Nobel Symposium **23:**38, 1973.
44. Dutrillaux, B.: Chromosoma **41:**395, 1973.
45. Funaki, K., Matsui, S-I., and Sasaki, M.: Chromosoma **49:**357, 1975.
46. Sandberg, A.A., and Abe, S.: Clin. Haematol. **9:**19, 1980.

CHAPTER 11

Laboratory investigation of hemostasis

Hemostasis is concerned with the maintenance of the liquid state of the circulating blood. Imbalance in the hemostatic mechanism may lead to hemorrhage or thrombosis. Thrombosis is the localized transformation of the liquid blood into a gel that may completely occlude the blood vessel. The laboratory investigation of hypercoagulability that may lead to thrombosis is discussed on p. 348. Hemorrhage follows a vascular injury and allows plasma and cellular components of the blood to escape. The effectiveness or the failure of hemostasis to control bleeding depends on the type of injury (bruise, clean cut, or laceration), the size and the ability of the injured vessel to contract, the pressure within the vessel and in the surrounding tissues, the availability of platelets, fibrinogen, and other clotting factors, and the presence of inhibitors and fibrinolysis.[1,2]

BLOOD VESSELS IN HEMOSTASIS

Although a transected large or medium-sized artery or vein requires rapid surgical intervention to prevent exsanguination, small arteries or veins are able to control bleeding by vasoconstriction and fibrin plug formation. When arterioles and venules are injured, they control bleeding by means of platelet plugs, and injured capillaries reduce blood loss by constriction and apposition of endothelial surfaces. Vasoconstriction, a reflex action of the smooth muscle of the blood vessel wall, narrows the vascular lumen and reduces the blood flow not only in the injured vessel but also in the surrounding vascular bed, allowing increased contact time of the injured vessel wall with platelets and coagulation proteins. The short-lived immediate reflex vasoconstriction is sustained and maintained by the subsequent release of serotonin from platelets[1-3] and the formation of thromboxane A_2 (see later discussion).

Blood vessels are lined by an intimal monolayer of flat endothelial cells that is supported by the subendothelium. Normal endothelium does not interact with platelets or with plasma procoagulants[3] but is involved in the clotting process by producing (or storing) antigenically active factor VIII,[4] platelet thrombosthenin,[5] tissue thromboplastin,[6] and a plasminogen activator.[7]

PLATELETS IN HEMOSTASIS

Platelets have a unique and vital function in the various stages of hemostasis at the site of a blood vessel injury.[8] They are metabolically active sol-gel structures that are capable of rapid morphologic changes and of synthesis of proteins such as fibrinogen, of enzymes such as glucuronidase, cathepsin, of amines such as serotonin, catecholamines, and histamine, and of nucleotides such as adenosine diphosphate (ADP) and adenosine triphosphate (ATP) (Chapter 12 deals with platelets). The delicate endothelial monolayer of blood vessels is easily damaged and in response to such an injury platelets adhere immediately and selectively to the exposed subendothelial collagen fibers (**platelet adhesion**) and spread pseudopods along the fiber surfaces[9] (**platelet spreading**). The intensity of the interaction of platelets with collagen and their adherence to it depend on the degree of polymerization of the collagen and are best if the collagen has a quaternary structure with microfibrils 60 nm in diameter.[2,10] The spreading phenomenon is the result of a change in the platelet morphology: The smooth circulating platelet disk is transformed into a sphere with projecting pseudopods, the center of which collects the organelles.[11] This transformation leads to a surface membrane reorganization resulting in the production of a procoagulant phospholipoprotein called platelet factor 3, which takes part in the formation of complexes with calcium and coagulation factors (V, VIII, and IXa) that accelerate and potentiate some phases of the clotting cascade.[12] The platelet membrane enzyme glucosyltransferase[13] interacts specifically with collagen and may be responsible for the platelet adhesion to collagen that triggers the platelet shape change, and the concomitant release of ADP. ADP causes other platelets to metamorphose into globoid structures with pseudopods that interact with each other and with the adherent platelets to form a rather loose clump, the **platelet plug of primary hemostasis**.[1] The ADP-induced aggregation is accompanied by the **platelet release reaction (degranulation),** which discharges the contents of the platelet granules onto the platelet surface. The electron-dense granules release ADP, ATP, platelet factor 4, and vasoactive amines serotonin and catecholamines (release I),[14] and the α-granules liberate lysosomal enzymes,[15] chemotactic factors,[16] and platelet fibrinogen[17] (release II). The platelet release reaction potentiates the early ADP-induced aggregation and is responsible for further ADP release, thus initiating a self-perpetuating ADP release. Platelet fibrinogen under the influence of small amounts of thrombin precipitates as polymerized fibrin surrounding each platelet with a fibrin network, thus stabilizing and consolidating the now irreversibly fused hemostatic plug (**secondary hemostasis**). Thrombin has a collagen-like effect on platelets causing them to release further ADP, to aggregate, and to discharge the α-granules[18] and thrombosthenin. Platelet aggregation is also sustained and promoted by a secondary mechanism that involves arachidonic acid transformation products, cyclic endoperoxides,[19] and thromboxane A_2,[20] a potent vasoconstrictor and releasing agent. Aggregation of platelets by ADP, thrombin, and collagen is accompanied by hydrolysis of the platelet membrane phospholipids, which releases arachidonic acid. The latter substance is converted to cyclic endoperoxides (prostaglandins), which are transformed to thromboxane A_2, a potent platelet-aggregating and vessel-constricting agent.[21] Aspirin interferes with the production of thromboxane A_2 and thus with the release II reaction. The aspirin effect is important to patients with a preexisting factor deficiency (e.g., von Willebrand's disease) since they may bleed after aspirin administration.[22]

Collagen not only interacts with platelets but also activates the Hageman factor,[23] a plasma procoagulant that initiates the **intrinsic clotting** sequence while at the same time the **extrinsic clotting** sequence is called into action by the activation of factor VII by tissue thromboplastin[24] exposed by the vascular injury.

The role of platelets in hemostasis is not confined to their participation in primary and secondary hemostasis or to the release of platelet factor 3 with its procoagulant activity. Platelet factor 4, a lipoprotein, has antiheparin activity[23] and is stored in the α-granules.[25] It is discharged during the release reaction[26,27] to neutralize heparin, thus preventing the inhibition of thrombin in the area of the hemostatic platelet plug.[28] As in patients with diffuse intravascular coagulation[29] or after myocardial infarction,[28] the platelet factor 4 level is raised; its concentration may be a marker of in vivo platelet activation and utilization[30] (see also discussion of laboratory tests in the investigation of diffuse intravascular coagulation). Platelet factor 4 may also play a role in clinical heparin sensitivity or resistance.

Some coagulation factors are adsorbed to the surfaces of platelets, e.g., factors V, XI, and XIII. Other coagulation-related factors, e.g., fibrinogen, plasminogen, factor VIII, and thrombosthenin, reside within the platelet substance. The platelet surface may well be the stage on which clotting takes place.[31]

Platelets are also involved in the maintenance of the normal endothelial integrity by somehow ''nurturing'' the endothelial cells with some platelet secretion[32,33] or by insinuating themselves into gaps between the endothelial lining cells.[34]

CLOTTING FACTORS (PLASMA PROCOAGULANTS)

The coagulation of blood is the end result of a series of enzymatic processes involving plasma proteins

Table 11-1. Nomenclature of clotting factors

Factor	Synonyms*
I	Fibrinogen
II	Prothrombin
III	Tissue thromboplastin, tissue factor
IV	Calcium
V	Proaccelerin, labile factor, AC globulin
VI	Not assigned
VII	Proconvertin, stable factor, autoprothrombin I
VIII	Antihemophilic factor A (AHF), antihemophilic globulin (AHG)
IX	Christmas factor, plasma thromboplastin component (PTC), antihemophilic factor B, autoprothrombin II
X	Stuart-Prower factor, autoprothrombin II
XI	Plasma thromboplastin antecedent (PTA), antihemophilic factor C
XII	Hageman factor
XIII	Fibrin stabilizing factor, Laki-Lorand factor
—	Fletcher factor (prekallikrein)
—	Fitzgerald factor (high-molecular-weight kininogen)

*List of synonyms is not complete.

called procoagulants or clotting factors, which are supported by phospholipids and calcium in some of their reactions. A protein is designated as a clotting factor if (1) its deficiency leads to a clinical disorder usually characterized by a bleeding tendency (deficiencies of factor XII and of Fletcher and Fitzgerald factors are the exceptions); (2) it can be assayed; (3) its physical and chemical characteristics are known,[2] e.g., polypeptide composition, half-life, and adsorbability; and (4) it is synthesized independently from other proteins. In the International Nomenclature the clotting factors are assigned Roman numerals in order of their discovery (Table 11-1). The enzymatically active forms of the factors that are enzymes (factors XII, XI, X, IX, VII, and II) are designated by a lowercase "a" following the Ro-

man numeral. Since factors III, IV, V, and VIII are nonenzymatic, they do not qualify for the "a" designation, although factors V and VIII form complexes with calcium and platelet phospholipids that have enzymatic activity.

COAGULATION PATHWAY OR CASCADE

The ultimate aim of blood clotting is the transformation of fibrinogen to a fibrin clot with the aid of thrombin, a proteolytic enzyme (Fig. 11-1). Thrombin is not normally present in the plasma and is the result of the activation of prothrombin by a complex of factor Xa, factor V, calcium, and phospholipids: the **prothrombin-converting complex** (thrombokinase, prothrombinase). The formation of this complex depends

EXTRINSIC PATHWAY OF
FACTOR X ACTIVATION

INTRINSIC PATHWAY OF
FACTOR X ACTIVATION

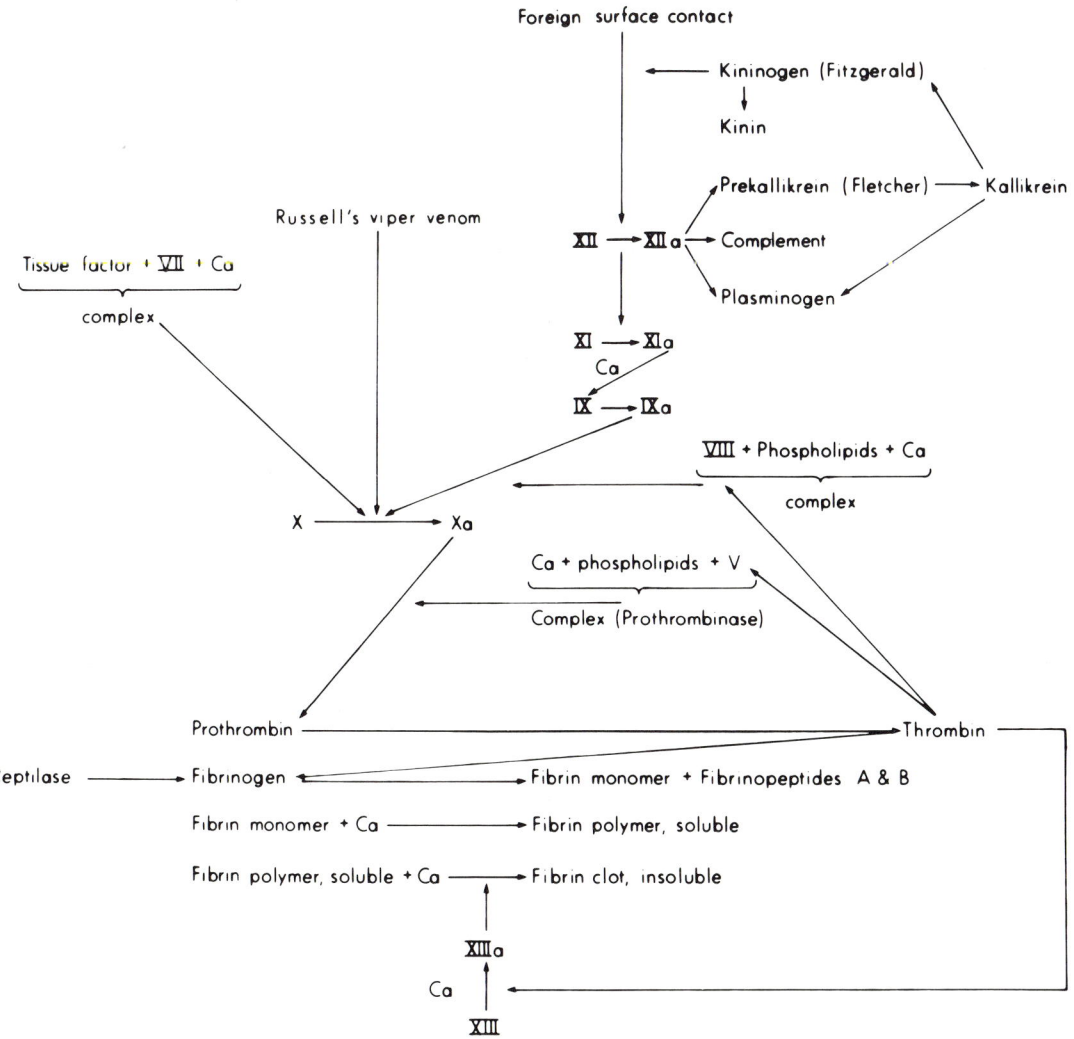

COMMON PATHWAY

Fig. 11-1. Scheme of blood coagulation.

on the activation of factor X. This activation is the pivotal reaction of the clotting scheme and can be achieved in three ways: (1) by the extrinsic pathway when blood is exposed to collagen at the site of tissue injury, (2) by the intrinsic pathway when blood comes in contact with an abnormal or foreign negatively charged surface, and (3) by the addition of Russell's viper venom or trypsin. After the activation of factor X the clotting process follows a single common pathway to the formation of fibrin.

Extrinsic activation of factor X

The extrinsic pathway is activated by exposure of blood (plasma) to a lipoprotein complex released by injured tissue called the **tissue factor,** which is not normally present in the blood. If plasma comes in contact with the tissue factor, it binds with factor VII and calcium to form an enzymatically active high-molecular-weight complex[8] that activates factors X (X to Xa). Factor VII takes part only in the extrinsic pathway, and factors XII, XI, IX, and VIII do not participate. The activation of factor X is followed by thrombin formation as outlined in the common pathway. Platelet phospholipids are not required to initiate the extrinsic pathway, since tissue factor supplies its own phospholipids.

Intrinsic activation of factor X

Recent investigations into the biochemistry of blood coagulation have led to changes in the classic waterfall or cascade concept of factor X activation.[35,36] According to the cascade hypothesis, each clotting factor circulates in the plasma in an inactive zymogen or precursor form and during blood clotting is converted to its biologically active enzymatic form by the activated, mildly proteolytic preceding factor. The activated forms are proteases that carry the amino acid serine on their enzymatically active sites and are therefore called serine proteases. Activation is caused by the splitting of some peptide groups off the original precursor protein, which is then restructured to become enzymatically active. The following factors, when activated, are serine proteases: XII, XI, X, IX, VII, and II.[37] Exceptions to the cascade concept may be factor XII, which is not inhibited by conventional serine esterase inhibitors,[38] factor XIII, which is a transglutaminase,[39] and factors V and VIII, which are nonenzymatic and form complexes with activated coagulation proteins, calcium ions, and platelet-derived phospholipids.[37] These complexes then activate the next factor in the clotting sequence to convert it to an active enzyme. The intrinsic pathway is initiated by the activation of factor XII by contact with foreign surfaces that are strongly negatively charged solids, e.g., glass and kaolin.[39] It is also activated by collagen, elastin, platelet surfaces, injured intima of bood vesslels, trypsin, kallikrein, plasmin, and high-molecular-weight kininogen.[39,40] When Hageman factor becomes activated, molecular surface alterations expose the enzymatically active esterolytic sites,[41] which function as arginine aminopeptidases[2] and are not inhibited by serine esterase inhibitors.[39] Activation of the Hageman factor is a two-step procedure leading first to an initial cleavage without fragmentation followed by a second cleavage which liberates Hageman factor fragments that have a dimininshed procoagulant activity but are able to activate **Fletcher factor**. The activated Hageman factor converts factor XI to its activated form (XIa), a reaction that is accelerated by the activation of an additional plasma protein, the Fletcher factor, a prekallikrein.[42] The Fletcher factor is activated by activated factor XII (XIIa), a proteolytic enzyme that results in the formation of kallikrein (activated Fletcher factor), an enzyme that releases kinins from high-molecular-weight kininogen.[43] Kinins are small, biologically active peptides, e.g., bradykinin, which activate Hageman factor and are involved in the vascular and leukotactic response to inflammation, thus establishing a bridge between inflammation, a defense mechanism, and coagulation. The high-molecular-weight kininogen acts as a cofactor in the surface activation of factor XII, its concentration being directly related to the concentration of activated factor XII.[44] The high-molecular-weight kininogen cofactor has received various labels, e.g., **Fitzgerald,** Flaujeac, and Williams factor.[39] Kininogen can also be activated to release kinin by endotoxins and by immune complexes, thus establishing a link between inflammation and coagulation.

The activated factor XII (XIIa) is not only necessary for the activation of factor XI and of the kallikrein-kinin system,[43] but it is also capable of activating the complement[45] and the plasminogen-plasmin systems.[46] The activated factor XI (XIa) is a serine protease that in the presence of calcium converts factor IX to its active form (IXa). The latter complexes with factor VIII, calcium, and phospholipids to activate factor X, which as factor Xa enters the common pathway of prothrombin conversion to thrombin, which hydrolyzes fibrinogen to form fibrin.

There are some links between the intrinsic and extrinsic pathways of factor X activation. Cold (4° C) activation of plasma depends on the activation of factor VII of the extrinsic pathway by factor XII[47] and kallikreins[48] of the intrinsic pathway. The factor VII activation is expressed in a markedly shortened thrombotest time. A further link is established by factor VIII of the intrinsic pathway, which, to complete its physiologic role, requires a small amount of thrombin and/or factor Xa, both proteases originating in the extrinsic pathway.

Common pathway

The common pathway (the road to fibrin formation) is shared by both extrinsic and intrinsic systems of coagulation. Irrespective of the method or agent of activation, the activated factor X (Xa), a serine protease, rapidly converts prothrombin in the presence of calcium, phospholipids, and factor V to thrombin, a proteolytic enzyme. The final phase of the clotting sequence is initiated by the hydrolysis of fibrinogen by thrombin, a step that leads to the formation of fibrin monomers and fibrinopeptides. The fibrin monomers polymerize to fibrin polymers, the fibrin clot, which, in the presence of calcium, is rendered insoluble by the action of a plasma transamidase, factor XIII.

CHARACTERISTICS OF COAGULATION FACTORS

The clotting factors can be collected into three groups, each containing factors with somewhat similar characteristics.[2]

The **fibrinogen group** embraces high-molecular-weight factors I, V, VIII, and XIII. They are consumed during coagulation and are therefore present in plasma and lacking in serum. They are produced in the liver without the aid of vitamin K, are not adsorbed by $BaSO_4$, and are destroyed by thrombin and plasmin. They are increased in inflammatory conditions, pregnancy, fear, and stress and after the administration of oral contraceptives. Three factors (I, V, and VIII) are nonenzymatic, and factors V and VIII are unstable in stored plasma and are therefore absent in blood bank blood.

The **prothrombin,** or **vitamin K–dependent, group** consists of the relatively low-molecular-weight factors II, VII, IX, and X. The zymogen form of these factors is synthesized in the liver and requires vitamin K to render it physiologically active. The enzymatic forms are serine proteases, the activity of which is depressed by oral anticoagulants, e.g., sodium warfarin (Coumadin). Factors VII, IX, and X are not consumed during clotting and are therefore of equal activity in serum and plasma. They are heat stable and are adsorbed by $BaSO_4$.

The **contact group** includes factors XI, XII, Fletcher, and Fitzgerald. They are not consumed during clotting and are not (or only partially) adsorbed by $BaSO_4$. They are stable, do not require vitamin K for their synthesis, and are found in serum and plasma.

Fibrinogen group
Fibrinogen (factor I)

Fibrinogen is a large (molecular weight 340,000) nonenzymatic glycoprotein with a half-life of 3-6 days; it may be rod shaped or pentagonal and is synthesized in the liver. Its plasma concentration of 200-400 mg/dl exceeds that of all other clotting factors. The molecule consists of three pairs of dissimilar polypeptide chains, $A\alpha$, $B\beta$, and γ, linked by disulfide bonds (Fig. 11-2).[49,50] The conversion of fibrinogen to fibrin occurs in several steps.[51]

1. Thrombin, a protease, splits 3% off the fibrinogen molecule in the form of two pairs of **fibrinopeptides**. Fibrinopeptides A are removed first and rapidly from the amino (N) terminal portions of the $A\alpha$ chains, followed by the release of the B fibrinopeptides from the $B\beta$ chains[52] (Fig 11-2). Reptilase, a snake venom, also activates fibrinogen but releases only fibrinopeptides A.[53]

2. After the release of the fibrinopeptides, the remaining fibrin monomers spontaneously polymerize to form fibrin polymer, a loose fibrin gel (fibrin$_s$), the "s" signifying solubility in 5M (30%) urea and in 2% acetic acid.

3. The fibrin polymers in the presence of calcium aggregate to form insoluble fibrin$_i$, which is reinforced by factor XIII, a transpeptidase, which by the introduction of peptide bonds[54] renders the fibrin clot insoluble in 30% urea or in 2% acetic acid solutions and less subject to lysis by fibrinolytic agents, e.g., plasmin.

Labile factor (factor V)

Factor V is an unstable, nonenzymatic plasma protein[39] with a half-life of 15 hr and a concentration of 50-150% of normal,[31] the biologic activity of which in plasma is labile at room and higher temperatures.[55] It is not adsorbed onto $BaSO_4$. During clotting it acts as a catalyst and forms a complex (**prothrombin-converting complex** or **prothrombinase**) with calcium and phospholipids to accelerate the activation of prothrombin by factor Xa in the presence of small amounts of thrombin.[56] Thrombin is not the only factor V–activat-

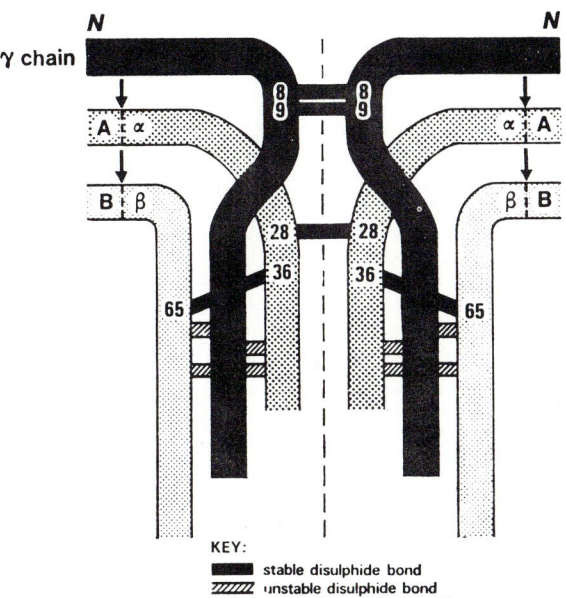

Fig. 11-2. Schematic model of N-terminal disulfide knot (N-DSK) portion of dimeric fibrinogen molecule. Shown are the two γ-chains forming a stable covalently bonded structure onto which the other chains seem to be tied. (From Gaffney, P.J.: Br. Med. Bull. **33:**245, 1977.)

N
γ chain

N
γ chain

A $\pm$ α

α $\pm$ A

B $\vdots$ β

β $\vdots$ B

8 9

8 9

28

28

36

36

65

65

KEY:
▬ stable disulphide bond
▨ unstable disulphide bond
↓ site of cleavage by thrombin

ing enzyme,[57] since it shares this activity with plasmin, papain, and Russell's viper venom.[58] Factor V is thought to be synthesized in the liver because its plasma concentration is markedly reduced in patients with severe liver disease.

Antihemophilic factor (AHF, factor VIII)

The exact nature of factor VIII is unknown, but it may be visualized as a complex of two molecules with separate activities and properties[59-61] (Fig 11-3). The smaller molecule has factor VIII clotting activity (F VIII C), while the larger molecule is responsible for the factor VIII–related antigen (F VIII RAG), which controls the bleeding time, glass-bead retention of platelets, and ristocetin platelet aggregation. Normal fresh plasma contains all factor VIII activities. Unless it is specified differently, when factor VIII is mentioned it refers to its procoagulant activity.

Factor VIII procoagulant

Factor VIII procoagulant is a labile glycoprotein with a half-life of 12-18 hr; it is present in normal fresh plasma and is diminished or almost absent in plasma of patients with hemophilia A[62] or von Willebrand's disease. It is an essential link in the intrinsic pathway of clotting in which it complexes with phospholipids, calcium, and activated factor IX (factor IXa) to activate factor X (factor Xa). Its procoagulant activity is demonstrated by a clotting test, the partial thromboplastin time, which is prolonged in significant factor VIII deficiency. The normal factor VIII concentration may vary from 45-180% of the average normal plasma level. The level not only varies in normal individuals (hence normal reference control plasmas must be pooled), but it increases in pregnancy, fear, exercise, and stress and after administration of birth control pills. It decreases in old age and is rapidly degraded in stored plasma or in crude as well as purified preparations. Factor VIII is activated by thrombin and other proteolytic enzymes, e.g., plasmin. The reaction with thrombin may be an essential step in the activation of factor X. Factor VIII procoagulant activity is inherited by an X-linked recessive mechanism. Its site of synthesis is unknown, and in acute yellow atrophy of the liver it is not reduced. It is not adsorbed by $BaSO_4$.

The physiologic role of factor VIII in the coagulation scheme is not well defined. Esnouf believes that factor VIII is a regulatory protein enhancing the rate of factor X activation similar to the rate controlling action of factor V on the prothrombin activation.[56] Factor VIII, factor IXa, phospholipids, and calcium react together to activate factor X.[56] For the physiologic activity of factor VIII, thrombin must be available, the origin of which may be traced to activation of the extrinsic pathway, thus establishing a link between the two major forms of activation of factor X[63] and continuous minimal activation of prothrombin.

Factor VIII–related antigen

The factor VIII–related antigen (factor VIII RAG) is measured by an antigen-antibody reaction as it precipitates with heterologous (rabbit) antiserum to factor VIII cryoprecipitates, a high-molecular-weight, factor VIII–

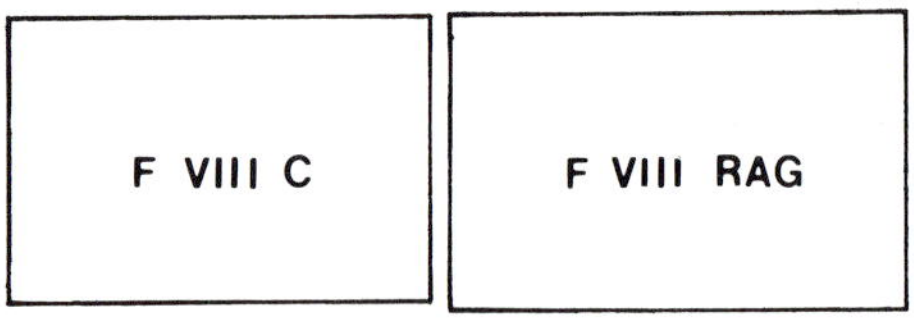

Fig. 11-3. Scheme of two molecular configuration of Factor VIII. *F VIII C,* procoagulant factor VIII; *F VIII RAG,* factor VIII–related antigen with determinants that control bleeding time, glass-bead retention of platelets, and ristocetin platelet aggregation.

rich plasma fraction. Factor VIII RAG is present in normal fresh plasma and in the plasma of hemophilia A patients, where it may actually be increased. In the plasma of von Willebrand's disease patients, it is reduced to the same extent as the procoagulant factor VIII activity.[62,64] Factor VIII lacks procoagulant activity, and together with the ristocetin cofactor it is probably synthesized in endothelial cells but can also be demonstrated in platelets and in megakaryocytes. Together with ristocetin cofactor it is inherited as an autosomal dominant trait.

Factor VIII–related von Willebrand factor*

Both ristocetin cofactor and factor VIII RAG are produced by endothelial cells and are probably present on the same molecule, which has a dual function. Factor VIII procoagulant activity, on the other hand, resides on a separate molecule closely linked to the factor VIII RAG molecule from which it can be separated by a variety of methods (gel filtration; ion exchange chromatography).

The von Willebrand factor is reduced in patients with von Willebrand's disease. It is demonstrated and identified by a number of abnormal platelet function tests, e.g., platelet aggregation with ristocetin, diminished platelet retention in glass-bead columns, and a prolonged bleeding time. When added to platelet-rich plasma of normal individuals, ristocetin, an antibiotic now discontinued, causes platelet aggregation, but it fails to do so when added to platelet-rich plasma of patients with von Willebrand's disease.[65,66] Since this apparent platelet defect can be corrected by the addition of normal plasma, it is assumed that the platelets themselves are not abnormal but that a plasma factor is missing in patients with von Willebrand's disease, namely, the von Willebrand factor. The latter also expresses itself by inhibiting platelet retention in glass-bead columns[67] and by prolonging the bleeding time. A fourth determinant of the von Willebrand factor is the characteristic response of the von Willebrand patient to factor VIII transfusion (Fig. 11-4). In hemophilia, factor VIII transfusion leads to a short-lived rise in the factor VIII concentration in the patient's plasma, while in von Willebrand's disease such a transfusion is followed by a sustained rise of factor VIII concentration, exceeding the level of the transfused factor VIII,[68] proving that in von Willebrand's disease the patient has

---

*Synonyms: von Willebrand factor, vWF, factor VIII R vWF, ristocetin cofactor, RiCoF.

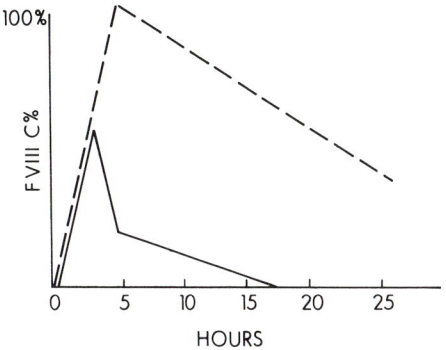

Fig. 11-4. Scheme of response of factor VIII concentration in plasma of patients with hemophilia (———) or von Willebrand's disease (— — —) in response to factor VIII transfusions.

the potential to synthesize factor VIII. Prior to the transfusion the von Willebrand patient does not show any evidence of factor VIII synthesis.

Fibrin stabilizing factor (factor XIII, Laki-Lorand factor)

Activated factor XIII is the last enzyme to form in the clotting cascade and is the last step in the formation of a firm fibrin clot. The factor circulates in the plasma as an inactive 2-chain proenzyme that is activated by thrombin to form an enzyme with transamidase activity (XIIIa, fibrinase, fibrinoligase). This activation is a two-step procedure in which thrombin in the presence of calcium first releases peptides from each α-chain leaving the β-chain pair intact.[69] The second phase consists of the formation of an enzymatically active α-2 dimer and an enzymatically inactive β-2 dimer. Factor XIII can also be activated by trypsin, papain, and reptilase, a commercially available snake venom (Abbott Diagnostic Products, North Chicago, Ill.). The activated factor XIII catalyzes the production of intermolecular γ-γ chain links of the fibrin$_s$ gel molecules to cross-linked fibrin$_i$, which is not soluble in 5M (30%) urea or in 2% acetic acid and which is more resistant to the digestive action of fibrinolytic enzymes, e.g., plasmin. The plasma concentration of factor XIII is about 20 units/ml with a half-life of 90 hr.[2] Since severe liver disease does not lead to a reduction in the concentration of factor XIII, it is assumed that it is not produced by hepatocytes.[70] It has been isolated from platelets and megakaryocytes[71,72] and from the placenta.[68]

Prothrombin group (vitamin K–dependent clotting factors)

The vitamin K–dependent clotting factors embrace the prothrombin group, which includes prothrombin (factor II), stable factor (factor VII), Christmas factor (factor IX), and Stuart-Prower factor (factor X). These factors share a number of characteristics[68,73]:

1. They are single-chain glycoproteins.
2. They show significant homology of their polypeptide chains.
3. They are serine protease precursors and are activated by limited proteolysis to serine proteases with trypsinlike activity.
4. They are adsorbed by $BaSO_4$.
5. With the exception of factor II they are not consumed during clotting.
6. They require vitamin K for their coagulant activity.
7. They are depressed by coumarin derivatives.
8. They are produced in the liver as inactive precursors.
9. They are activated by the vitamin K–dependent introduction of an extra carboxyl group at the γ-position of some of the glutamic acid residues.[74]
10. They are elevated during pregnancy and in patients on oral contraceptives.
11. In the fetus and newborn their concentration is low.[75]
12. Acquired deficiencies occur if vitamin K is not absorbed.
13. Activated factors II, IX, and X are inhibited by heparin and antithrombin III.

Vitamin K is supplied in the diet as vitamin K_1, and as vitamin K_2 it is synthesized by bacteria in the intestinal tract, from where, with the aid of bile salts, it is absorbed to be utilized by the liver. If vitamin K absorption is interfered with or inhibited, or a coumarin-type drug has been administered, the clotting activity of all four prothrombin group factors is reduced or absent, but the liver continues to produce the biologically inactive precursor forms, which immunochemically are similar to the functioning proteins.[76] These "pre-forms" have been called PIVKA-II, -VII, -IX, and -X, PIVKA being the acronym for protein-induced by vitamin K absence or antagonists.[77] A newer nomenclature suggests the names acarboxy-II, -VII, etc. for the "pre-forms."[73] The precursor forms have certain features in common:

1. In the absence of vitamin K they cannot be activated to physiologically active forms and therefore do not promote clotting.
2. Their calcium-binding ability and adsorption to $BaSO_4$ are reduced.[68]
3. They contain glutamic acid residues in the N-terminal region of the peptide chains. In order for the proteins to be biologically active after completion of their synthesis, the glutamic acid residues must be carboxylated; i.e., a carboxyl group is inserted into the γ-carbon of some glutamic acid residues to form the amino acid γ-carboxy glutamic acid.[68] This amino acid is found in all vitamin K–dependent physiologically active clotting factors and is responsible for their calcium-binding ability.[68] The carboxylation requires a vitamin K–dependent carboxylase system.[78]
4. They act as specific inhibitors of the vitamin K–dependent clotting factors (II, VII, IX, and X): the **PIVKA effect**.[79]

Prothrombin (factor II) and thrombin

Prothrombin is one of the vitamin K–dependent glycoproteins with a half-life of 5 hr and a concentration of 83-110%; it is degraded by the vitamin K–dependent enzyme factor Xa, a serine protease (see p. 278) to form thrombin, a proteolytic enzyme that almost specifically catalyzes the hydrolysis of the arginyl bonds of fibrinogen. The prothrombin peptide is produced in the liver, and its glutamic acid residues are carboxylated with the aid of vitamin K. The degradation of prothrombin to thrombin requires factor Xa, which forms a complex with factor V, platelet phospholipids, and calcium,[80] a mixture that has enzymatic activity (**prothrombinase**) and increases the rate of thrombin generation.[56] The cleavage of prothrombin by factor Xa produces two enzymes in sequence, prothrombin E with esterase activity and thrombin with esterase and proteolytic activity.[81] Further degradation by autolysis results in a peptide with esterase activity only (thrombin E).[82] **Thrombin** cleaves **fibrinopeptides A** and **B** off the fibrinogen molecule to form fibrin monomers, which initiate the final phase of fibrin formation. According to Seegers et al.,[80] small amounts of prothrombin are continuously degraded in the circulation to produce small amounts of thrombin, which are required to activate factors VIII and XIII and platelet fibrinogen. Thrombic activity can also be generated by snake venom (Russell's viper venom) and by trypsin, which are able to activate factor X.

Stable factor (factor VII)

Factor VII is a liver-synthesized, single-chain glycoprotein[68] with a half-life of 5 hr; it participates in the extrinsic pathway and, when activated, is a serine protease that requires vitamin K for the formation of its calcium-binding site, an activity that is rapidly lost during treatment with vitamin K antagonists.[56] After oral anticoagulant therapy the prothrombin group factors disappear in order of their half-life, factor VII ($t^1/_2$ 5 hr) first, followed by factor IX ($t^1/_2$ 25 hr), factor X ($t^1/_2$ 40 hr), and factor II ($t^1/_2$ 60 hr). In the extrinsic pathway of factor X activation, tissue phospholipids, calcium, and factor VII form a complex that has enzymatic activity and becomes the factor X activator.[83,84] According to Laake and Ellingsen[85] as quoted by Stormorken,[83] factor VII can also be activated by contact with glass, kaolin, and the intrinsic pathway factors XII, XI, and IX, by cold storage (0-4° C),[86] by thrombin,[87] and by factor Xa,[87] thus establishing connecting bridges between extrinsic and intrinsic pathways of coagulation.

Christmas factor (factor IX)

Factor IX is a vitamin K–dependent, liver-synthesized, single-chain glycoprotein with a half-life of 25 hr; it participates in the intrinsic pathway. It is activated by factor XIa, a serine protease, to form factor IXa, also a serine protease. The activation is a two-step process that cleaves two peptide bonds off the precursor protein, the first step leading to a factor devoid of coagulant activity, while the second step leads to the formation of the activated enzyme.[88] The activation process involves the conversion of the single-chain peptide into a smaller two-chain structure (one heavy and one light chain), the reactive serine residue being located on the heavy chain[63] while the vitamin K–dependent calcium-binding site is located on the light chain.[68] Factor IX is adsorbed from normal plasma with $BaSO_4$,

one of several characteristics that distinguish it from factor VIII. Factor IXa joins factor VIII, phospholipids, and calcium to form a complex that has enzymatic activity and activates factor X (factor X → factor Xa), which by cleavage becomes a serine protease. The complex is called **factor X–converting principle** in which factor VIII is the rate-controlling constituent.

Stuart-Prower factor (factor X)

Factor X is a vitamin K–dependent, liver-synthesized, single-chain glycoprotein with a half-life of 40 hr; it consists of one heavy and one light chain linked by disulfide bonds. The inactive plasma form is activated to the proteolytic enzyme form (Xa) by the extrinsic and/or intrinsic pathways, by Russell's viper venom, and by trypsin. The activation is a two-step procedure, both steps involving the cleavage of the heavy chain.[89-91] The intermediate product (α-Xa) as well as the final product (β-Xa) are serine proteases with coagulant activity able to slowly convert prothrombin to thrombin. This conversion is accelerated by the **prothrombin-converting complex** consisting of factor V, phospholipids, and calcium. Like most activated vitamin K–dependent factors (factor VIIa is the exception), factor Xa is inhibited by heparin and by antithrombin III[92] except when it is locked in the prothrombin-converting complex.[93] Factor X is found in serum and plasma.

Contact group
Plasma thromboplastin antecedent (factor XI)

Factor XI is a plasma glycoprotein with a half-life of 48 hr; it consists of two polypeptide chains and is involved in the intrinsic activation of factor X. Upon glass contact the activated factor XII (factor XIIa), a serine protease, activates prefactor XI by limited proteolytic digestion to form factor XIa, also a serine protease.[94] The latter reaction does not require calcium. Factor XIa is inhibited by heparin in the presence of antithrombin III. The prefactor is synthesized in the liver, and, in contradistinction to the factors of the prothrombin group, it is decreased in pregnancy and in patients on oral contraceptives.[95]

Hageman factor (factor XII), Fletcher factor, and Fitzgerald factor

The inactive factor XII is a biologically inert plasma protein with a half-life of 48 hr; it is synthesized in the liver without the aid of vitamin K and consists of three polypeptide chains held together by disulfide bonds. Increased levels are encountered during pregnancy.[96] Upon contact with foreign surfaces, e.g., glass, kaolin, elastin, collagen, cartilage, trypsin, plasmin, platelet surfaces, and kallikreins, and with endotoxins, the factor XII zymogen is converted to an active clot-promoting coagulation factor (XIIa) that initiates the intrinsic pathway of factor X activation by activating the inactive prefactor XI to the active factor XIa. The latter step requires two additional clotting factors, the Fletcher factor[97] and the Fitzgerald factor.[98] The first one has been identified as prekallikrein, and the second one is a high-molecular-weight kininogen; both are plasma factors involved in the kinin-generating system, and both appear to be necessary for the optimal activation of factor XII (see p. 278). All three factors are not adsorbed by $BaSO_4$ and are found in serum and plasma, since they are not consumed during clotting. The half life of the Fletcher factor is not known, and that of the Fitzgerald factor is 5-6 days.

Tissue factor (factor III)

Tissue factor is a lipoprotein complex[99] that initiates the extrinsic pathway of factor X activation but is not a plasma-derived component. It is found in many organs,[100] e.g., brain, lung, kiney, liver, and aorta, which influence its protein component rather than the lipid portion. Injury to the vascular endothelium, which is rich in tissue factor,[101] exposes plasma to its procoagulant activity. The tissue factor in the presence of calcium interacts with factor VII to form a complex that activates factor X.

Calcium (factor IV)

Ionized plasma calcium is needed for a number of reactions of the coagulation cascade (Fig. 11-1), e.g., in the formation of the various complexes, and for the synthesis of the vitamin K–dependent procoagulants. Despite the fact that when calcium is removed in vitro with citrates or oxalates to form nonionized salts or with ethylenediamine tetraacetate (EDTA) to form complexes clotting is inhibited and is reestablished when calcium is added, the exact role of calcium in coagulation has not been established.[102] Even severe hypocalcemia or hypercalcemia fails to produce appreciable changes in the clotting mechanism, although exceptions have been reported.[103]

FIBRINOLYSIS

Fibrinolysis (the plasminogen-plasmin fibrinolytic system) is the progressive physiologic enzymatic process that removes fibrin[50] and is responsible for the ultimate dissolution of blood clots in test tubes, blood vessels, soft tissues, and body cavities. Fibrinolysis is caused by the activation of a normally present inactive plasma protein, a proenzyme called **plasminogen,**[104] to **plasmin,** a trypsinlike proteolytic enzyme capable of cleaving not only insoluble fibrin and soluble fibrinogen but also fibrin monomers, factors V and VIII,[105] and plasma proteins such as complement.

Plasminogen is a single-chain plasma polypeptide that occurs in two major forms. One has glutamic acid

in the NH_2-terminal (gluplasminogen), and the other has lysine in the same position (lysplasminogen).[105] The site of production of plasminogen is unknown, but bone marrow eosinophils, endothelium, liver, kidney, and platelets appear to be involved in its metabolism.[106-108] Increased plasminogen concentrations are found in conditions that call forth **acute phase reactants,**[107] e.g., inflammatory and neoplastic diseases, trauma, surgery, and myocardial infarction.[108] Increased levels of plasminogen are found in infants[108] and in advanced liver disease and diffuse intravascular coagulation.

Plasminogen activation to plasmin is the result of the activity of a number of proteolytic enzymes (kinases), the **plasminogen activators,**[105] which specifically cleave susceptible bonds of the plasminogen molecule (Fig. 11-5). Plasminogen activators are found in various sites and biologic fluids.[105] Tissue activators originate from vascular endothelial cells[109] and from lysosomal granules,[110] while other plasminogen activators are found in biologic fluids, e.g., plasma,[106] saliva, urine, and semen. In urine a kidney-derived activator, urokinase,[111] is of therapeutic significance. Other activators are enzymes such as trypsin and thrombin, bacterial products such as streptokinase[112] from β-hemolytic streptococci, and staphylokinase. Plasminogen activators are also produced by leukocytes[113] and malignant tumors.[114]

The plasminogen-plasmin system in some ways resembles the coagulation system with which it interacts. Tissue activators of the plasminogen-plasmin system represent the extrinsic system of plasminogen activation, whereas the intrinsic system is represented by the activated factor XII (XIIa)[105] supported by activated Fletcher and Fitzgerald factors. The intrinsic activation of plasminogen is not only interwoven wih the kininogen, kallikrein, and complement systems,[108] but also interacts with platelets, which it causes to aggregate and degranulate (release reaction).[115]

Raised concentrations of plasminogen activators are found in many conditions, e.g., exercise, mental stress, cirrhosis,[116] venous occlusion, infections, and malignancies, and after surgery, shock, and administration of insulin and vasoconstrictive drugs, e.g., catecholamines, adrenalin, vasopressin, and nicotinic acid.[106]

Plasmin specifically cleaves fibrin and fibrinogen by peptide hydrolysis of susceptible bonds to produce progressively smaller fragments (**split products**) accom-

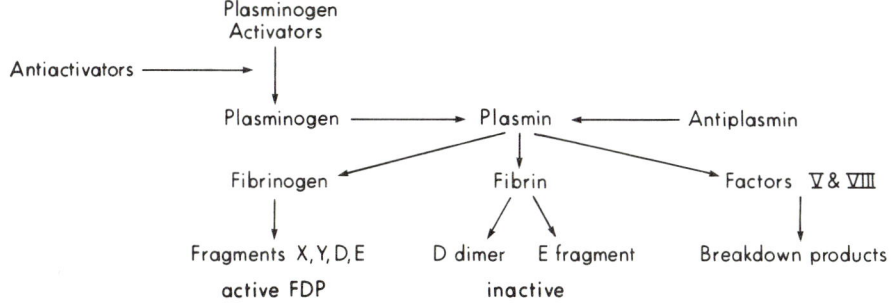

Fig. 11-5. Fibrinolytic system of blood and inhibitors.

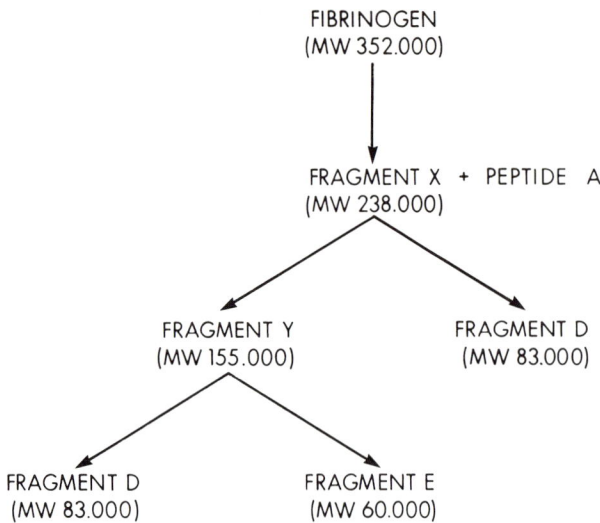

Fig. 11-6. Summary of action of plasmin on fibrinogen. Similar fragments are produced by the action of plasmin on non-cross-linked fibrin (fibrin$_s$), but fibrin$_s$ does not contain fibrinopeptide A. Action of plasmin on cross-linked fibrin (fibrin$_i$) produces D dimer and fragment E.

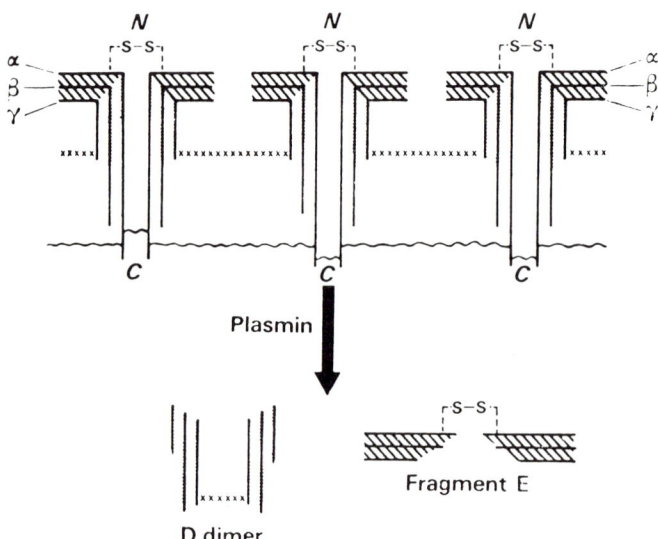

The cross-linked γ-chain dimers (γ–γ cross-links shown by xxxxx), the cross-linked α-chain polymers (α$_p$ cross-links shown by ∿∿∿), and the non-cross-linked β chains, are here related to each other schematically. All the cross-links are shown for convenience as being close to the carboxyl (C) ends of the chains; while this localization is true for the γ-chain cross-links, the α-chain cross-links are at least 20 000 molecular-weight distance from the C-terminal end. Disulphide (S—S) bonds (not shown here except for one S—S bond joining the two N-terminal ends of each fibrin molecule) link the individual polypeptide chains (α, β and γ) of each fibrin molecule. Non-covalent bonds also hold the units of the fibrin polymer together but are omitted for the sake of simplicity. The location of the antigenically distinct sections of fibrin, D and E, are shown in each of three fibrin molecules of the fibrin polymer. Digestion by plasmin yields a fragment, D, which is cross-linked to another D fragment from an adjacent fibrin molecule; this is called "D dimer". Fragment E and a variety of cross-linked and non-cross-linked peptides (not shown) are also released during the lysis of cross-linked fibrin.

Fig. 11-7. Schematic representation of polypeptide chains of cross-linked human fibrin and its plasmin-mediated degredation products D dimer and fragment E. (From Gaffney, P.J.: Br. Med. Bull. **33**:245, 1977.)

panied by small-molecular-weight peptides. In the course of digestion a large number of fragments are produced, which are collected into groups of structurally similar polypeptides to indicate stages and progression of degradation.[117]

The first fragment to result from fibrinogen degradation by plasmin is fragment X and smaller peptides. As the degradation proceeds, fragment Y appears followed by fragments D and E. According to Marder and Budzynski, the molecular weights of the structures involved are as follows: fibrinogen, 352,000; fragment X, 238,000; fragment Y, 155,000; fragment D, 83,000; and fragment E, 60,000.[118] Asymmetric degradation of fibrinogen gives rise to one X molecule, which is unequally split into one Y and one D fragment (Fig. 11-6). Fragment Y then yields a second fragment D and one fragment E.[118,119] The fibrinogen (or fibrin) split or degradation products (FDPs or fdp) are anticoagulants. Fragments X and Y have stronger anticoagulant activity than fragments D and E by interfering with fibrin monomer polymerization, despite the fact that fragment X is clottable with thrombin. The interference with fibrin monomer polymerization leads to the appearance of excess soluble fibrin monomers in the plasma and to slowly and poorly formed fibrin clots. Fibrin monomers form complexes with fibrinogen and fibrin, which precipitate in the cold (4° C) (**cryofibrinogen**) and are evidence of fibrinolysis.[120]

The degradation products derived from fibrinogen and from fibrin are dissimilar, but the fragments released from non-cross-linked fibrin (fibrin$_s$: absence of factor XIIIa) are similar to those produced by the plasmin-fibrinogen interaction.[50]

Digestion of cross-linked fibrin (fibrin$_i$) by plasmin yields unique fragments that differ from the fibrinogen and the non-cross-linked fibrin degradation products.[50] Although lysis of fibrinogen rapidly leads to polypeptide fragments, the digestion of cross-linked fibrin slowly yields a D fragment, which is cross-linked to another D fragment from an adjacent fibrin molecule forming a D dimer[50] accompanied by an E fragment. The D dimer has double the molecular weight of the fragment D derived from fibrinogen and contains the cross-linked γ-chain remants of the original fibrin molecule[121] (Fig. 11-7).

The fragments resulting from the cleavage of fibrinogen also differ from the fibrin degradation products by the fact that fibrinogen cleavage products contain fibrinopeptides A and B, which are absent in the fibrin digest because in the production of fibrin, fibrinopeptides A and B are split off the fibrinogen molecule.[108]

The fibrinolytic system is held in check by a number of naturally occurring inhibitors, some of which prevent activation of plasminogen while others are antiplasmins (see following discussion). The end result is the prevention of uncontrolled fibrinolysis.

Naturally occurring inhibitors of the fibrinolytic system and of the coagulation sequence

Plasma contains a number of natural inhibitors that limit intravascular clotting and fibrinolysis by inactivation of activated clotting factors such as the proteases XIa, IXa, Xa, or IIa (thrombin) and/or interference with the plasminogen-plasmin system. Four of these factors are well documented: antithrombin III, CI inactivator, α_2-macroglobulin inhibitor, and α_1-antitrypsin. These natural inhibitors are very similar in their action, and although their excess does not appear to be responsible for a hemorrhagic diathesis their decrease may be responsible for thrombosis.

Antithrombin III and heparin

Antithrombin III is an α_2-globulin synthesized in the liver and circulating in the plasma; it progressively and irreversibly but slowly inhibits thrombin by forming a 1:1 stable complex with it that is devoid of any thrombic or antithrombic activity. The complex formation occurs by the interaction of the active serine site of thrombin with the reactive arginine site of the antithrombin.[122] Since the inhibition of thrombin by antithrombin III is markedly accelerated by heparin, antithrombin III is considered to be identical with the heparin cofactor, which in combination with heparin effectively and rapidly inhibits thrombin.[122] Heparin is a sulfated mucopolysaccharide prepared from liver (hence the name) that by itself is an ineffective antithrombin or anticoagulant, but when complexed with antithrombin III heparin is transformed into a potent inhibitor of coagulation. The inhibition of thrombin is thought to be accomplished (1) by heparin binding the lysine sites on the antithrombin III molecule, which then undergoes conformational changes to expose reactive arginine residues (the arginine residues then neutralize the serine sites of thrombin causing its inhibition [Fig 11-8])[123]

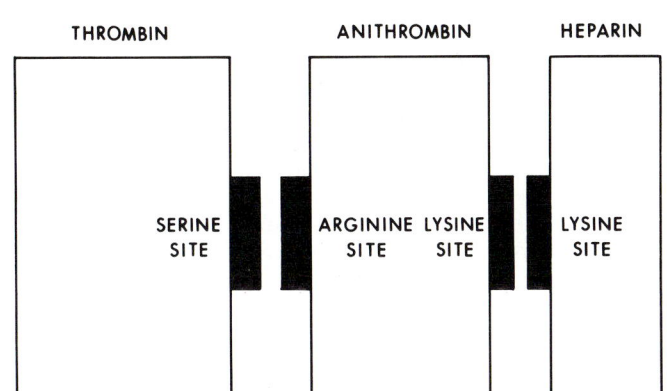

Fig. 11-8. Scheme of inhibition of thrombin by heparin.

and (2) by accelerating the adsorption of thrombin onto fibrinogen.[124] The antithrombin-heparin complex inhibits not only thrombin but also the serine proteases Xa,[125] IXa,[126] XIa,[92] and XIIa[127] of the clotting cascade, plasmin,[128] kallikrein,[37] fibrinogen,[124] platelets,[129] Cl$_s$ subunit of complement,[130] factor VII,[131] and tissue factor.[132] Some of these reactions do not require heparin.

Cl inactivator (or inhibitor)

A normal serum protein–labeled Cl esterase inhibitor[133] is capable not only of inhibiting the enzymatic activity of the Cl component of complement but also of inhibiting the fibrinolytic activity of plasmin,[133,134] factors XIIa and XIa,[135] and kallikrein.[136] The Cl inhibitor is precipitated with the euglobulin fraction of serum.

α_2-Macroglobulin inhibitor

α_2-Macroglobulin is a high-molecular-weight glycoprotein of hepatic origin that complexes with some serine proteases, e.g., kallikrein,[137] thrombin,[138] and plasmin,[139] of which it is the main inhibitor.

α_1-Antitrypsin

α_1-Antitrypsin is a plasma glycoprotein that is capable of inhibiting a number of proteases, including trypsin,[140] plasmin,[141] and factor XIa.[142] Its antithrombic activity is probably limited.[143]

Acquired coagulation inhibitors

Acquired coagulation inhibitors are abnormal (pathologic) acquired endogenous plasma proteins that inhibit clotting.[144,145] They thus differ from the naturally occurring inhibitors (antithrombin III, α_2-macroglobulin, Cl esterase inhibitor, and α_1-antitrypsin) and are delineated from therapeutically administered anticoagulants, e.g., heparin and coumarin derivatives. Most of these pathologic proteins are autoantibodies of the IgG immunoglobulin class directed against certain clotting factors, e.g., factor VIII. Acquired inhibitors with unusual features are encountered in disseminated intravascular coagulation (fibrin degradation products),[146] in lupus erythematosus, the lupus anticoagulant,[147] and in macroglobulinemia and other plasma cell dyscrasias.[148]

Acquired inhibitor of factor VIII

The acquired inhibitor of factor VIII is the most common specific inhibitor of a coagulation factor. It has been demonstrated not only in patients with hemophilia A treated with factor VIII but also in nonhemophilic individuals, e.g., in the postpartum period,[149] following abortions,[145] in immunologic disorders[150] such as rheumatoid arthritis[151] and cutaneous penicillin allergy,[152] in lupus erythematosus,[153] and in older individuals.[144] About 7-10% of transfused hemophilia A patients develop anti–factor VIII antibodies,[154] but according to Biggs they do not fare worse than those who do not develop this complication.[155]

The cause of anti–factor VIII antibodies in hemophilic and nonhemophilic patients is unknown, but in the first group the development of antibodies is clearly related to transfusions of factor VIII. Since the majority of treated hemophilic patients fail to develop inhibitors,

it has been postulated that immunologic differences in the hemophilic population explain the response to factor VIII transfusion.[147] Tolerant individuals contain in their plasma a factor VIII procoagulant that experimentally cross reacts with heterologous anti–factor VIII antibodies but is biologically inactive.[144] This immunologically recognizable but coagulatively inactive material is called **cross-reacting material** (CRM).[156] CRM-positive hemophiliacs who have CRM in their blood fail to recognize exogenous factor VIII as foreign antigen, whereas CRM-negative hemophiliacs produce antibodies to exogenous factor VIII. This hypothesis fails to explain the occurrence of antibodies in mild hemophiliacs[144] and the low percentage of CRM-negative patients who develop antibodies.[157] Antibodies to factor VIII may also be found in patients with severe von Willebrand's disease who have complete absence of factor VIII.[158] It should be noted that in testing for an inhibitor of factor VIII, the mixture of normal and test plasmas must be allowed to incubate for 30-120 min at room temperature to allow full development of the inhibitor's activity. All other inhibitors act immediately.

Antibodies to other coagulation factors

Antibodies to factor IX rarely occur in hemophilia B patients[144] (factor IX deficiency) and are hardly ever encountered in normal individuals.[144] Most of the inhibitors of factor IX are IgG antibodies. In hemophilia B patients[144] the incidence of inhibitors is about half (3%) that reported in hemophilia A patients. In a number of hemophilia B patients CRM capable of neutralizing factor IX has been demonstrated and has been found to be absent (CRM−) in patients who develop antibodies,[159] but the presence or absence of CRM does not adequately explain the occurrence of anti–factor IX antibodies in some cases of hemophilia B in the same way that it does not solve all problems of anti–factor VIII antibodies in hemophilia A patients.

The development of anti–factor V antibodies is unusual, and the majority of cases reported do not occur in factor V–deficient individuals[144] but rather following transfusions, major surgery with or without transfusions, and streptomycin therapy.[144] In patients with congenital factor V deficiency who develop inhibitors, CRM is absent.[160]

Acquired inhibitors have also been reported to factors XI, I, and XIII. The majority of inhibitors to factor XI occur in lupus erythematosus patients[161] and not in congenitally deficient individuals, although one such case has been recorded.[161] The incidence of inhibitors to fibrinogen is very low even in multitransfused patients with congenital afibrinogenemia.[144] Of the few inhibitors of fibrin stabilizing factor reported, most are encountered in previously normal individuals[144] and only one patient with congenital factor XIII deficiency[162] is recorded as having developed acquired inhibitors to it. Long-term treatment with isoniazid[144] is in some way responsible for the development of anti–factor XIII antibodies.

Inhibitors associated with lupus erythematosus

About 6% of patients with lupus erythematosus (LE) develop a circulating anticoagulant that lengthens both the prothrombin time and the partial thromboplastin time.[147] The LE inhibitor is specific for phospholipids and interferes with phospholipid-dependent complexes involving factors VIII and V.[145] This inhibitor may also be responsible for the high incidence of false reactive serologic tests for syphilis in LE.[147] As mentioned above, inhibitors to factors VIII and XI have also been reported.

Inhibitors associated with plasma cell dyscrasias

Multifaceted coagulation inhibitors have been reported in plasma cell dyscrasias, e.g., multiple myeloma and macroglobulinemia; in these conditions the autoantibodies are either specific or nonspecific protein-binding IgG or IgM antibodies.[144]

LABORATORY DIAGNOSIS OF THE BLEEDING PATIENT

The laboratory diagnosis of the bleeding patient has three phases to allow meaningful interpretation of the laboratory results. These phases are (1) a detailed history, (2) an adequate physical examination, and finally (3) a well-chosen battery of laboratory tests. The history should cover the following points: hematuria, gastrointestinal bleeding, easy bruising following minimal or apparently absent trauma, bleeding from nose and gums or following circumcision, tonsillectomy, surgery, tooth extraction, or heavy menses. The history of recent blood loss should be evaluated in the light of the hematologic findings and any treatment for anemia the patient may have received. A careful drug review should include the use of aspirin in all its many forms and preparations, of anticoagulants, and of birth control pills. The examiner must delve into the possibility of any underlying blood, liver, or kidney disease and determine the patient's age at the time of the first bleeding episode. The patient's age together with a careful family history aids in the separation of acquired from congenital bleeding disorders, since the latter usually begin early in life while the former make their appearance in adult life. The family history should include the sex of the member affected.

The clinical examiner should note superficial capillary and petechial bleeding into skin and mucous membrane (nose, gums), which suggests platelet defects, as well as hemorrhages (ecchymoses) into muscle, joints, and deep tissues, which suggests coagulation factor defects. Biggs points out that deep hemorrhages do not cause blue discoloration but rather pain in joints and muscles.[163]

The third phase of the investigation of the bleeding patient includes the laboratory studies.

Laboratory tests

Two groups of laboratory tests are performed on the blood of patients suspected of having a bleeding disorder. The first series of tests represents the minimum of "screening" tests, which are designed to prove or disprove the existence of a hemorrhagic diathesis. The second group consists of specific investigations designed to identify and pinpoint the coagulation disorder discovered by the screening tests.

The screening panel consists of the following tests:
1. Tests of platelet evaluation
   a. Bleeding time
   b. Whole blood clotting time, primarily for the observation of clot retraction and clot lysis
   c. Platelet count or scrutiny of blood smears for numeric and morphologic adequacy of platelets
   d. Platelet aggregation using epinephrine and ristocetin
2. Tests of coagulation factor disorders
   a. One-stage prothrombin time
   b. Activated partial thromboplastin time
   c. Thrombin time
   d. Screening tests for inhibitors
   e. Fibrinogen level
   f. Fibrin degradation products
   g. Clot solubility in 5M urea
3. Tests to discover etiology of hemorrhagic diathesis
   a. Complete blood count
   b. Examination of blood film with evaluation of red and white cells and platelet morphology
   c. Chemical screening, e.g., blood urea concentration, LDH level, globulin concentration

It is essential that the *entire* group of tests be performed at the time of the initial investigation. Even so, not all coagulation defects will be discovered since some of the tests employed are too insensitive and some require additional specific studies to aid in their correct interpretation. The screening panel may miss a mild deficiency (e.g., mild hemophilia A or von Willebrand's syndrome) that nevertheless may be of clinical significance in periods of stress, e.g., during surgery. When confronted with a suggestive history and negative screening tests, a number of special tests, e.g., factor level determinations, may be necessary to arrive at a diagnosis since the heterozygous carrier of a congenital defect may have a low enough concentration of a given factor to produce clinical symptoms but not low enough to affect screening tests. By increasing the concentration of some clotting factors (I, V, VIII, and XIII) pregnancy, oral contraceptives, and stress may temporarily mask minor deficiencies, which will then not be discovered by screening tests. In some instances laboratory tests may suggest a bleeding disorder (factor XII and Fletcher factor deficiencies) but the patient will be asymptomatic, whereas in other instances (factor XIII deficiency) the patient is symptomatic but the screening tests are normal.

Reagents used in coagulation procedures

The following are general guidelines for reagents used in coagulation procedures:
1. Reagents not in use should be tightly capped and stored at 4° C.
2. Incubate only enough reagent required for testing and refrigerate the balance.
3. Lyophilized reagents must be fully dissolved before use.
4. Water used in reconstitution must have a pH of 6.8-7.2.

Adsorbed plasma: The reagents used as adsorbents

Table 11-2. Coagulation factors present in fresh and aged plasma, in serum, and in BaSO₄-adsorbed plasma

Factor	Fresh normal plasma*	Aged normal plasma*	Normal serum*	Adsorbed normal plasma†	BaSO₄ eluate*‡	Adsorbed serum†
Fibrinogen (I)	+	+	0	+	0	0
Prothrombin (II)	+	+	0	0	+	0
Factor V	+	0	0	+	0	0
Factor VII	+	+	+	0	+	0
Factor VIII	+	0	0	+	0	0
Factor IX	+	+	+	0	+	0
Factor X	+	+	+	0	+	0
Factor XI	+	+	+	±	+	+
Factor XII	+	+	+	±	+	+
Factor XIII	+	+	+	+	+	0

* +, Factor present; 0, factor absent.
† +, Factor not adsorbed (present in plasma or serum); 0, factor adsorbed (not present in plasma or serum); ±, factor slightly adsorbed.
‡Or BaCO₃, Al(OH)₃, and Ca₃(PO₄) eluate.

are barium sulfate for oxalated plasma and aluminum hydroxide for citrated plasma. In the process of adsorption both remove the vitamin K–dependent factors (II, VII, IX, and X) from the plasma so that after adsorption it contains factors I, V, VIII, XI, XII, and XIII (Table 11-2).

Aged plasma: Using sterile equipment, transfer oxalated plasma into sterile test tube and incubate for 24-48 hr at 37° C. The prothrombin time on the plasma should be over 60 sec. All clotting factors are present in the plasma except the labile factors V and VIII.

Aged serum: Allow blood to clot in a glass tube at room temperature for 24 hr. Rim the clot, centrifuge, and harvest the serum. It contains factors VII, IX, X, XI, XII, and XIII (Table 11-2).

Aluminum hydroxide–adsorbed plasma: Add 10 volumes fresh oxalated or citrated plasma to 1 volume aluminum hydroxide gel. Mix, allow to incubate for 1 hr at room temperature, separate plasma by centrifugation for 15 min at 2000 *g* at 4° C, and refrigerate. Refrigerated plasma should be used within 2 hr to prevent loss of factor V, or it may be distributed into small aliquots and frozen. See discussion of adsorbed plasma above and Table 11-2.

Aluminum hydroxide gel: Prepare 4% suspension of Amphogel (Wyeth Laboratories, Philadelphia) (without flavor).

Anticoagulants: Sodium oxalate or citrate functions as an anticoagulant by binding ionized calcium. Nine volumes freshly drawn blood is added to 1 volume anticoagulant. This ratio is correct for blood with relatively normal hematocrit. Severely anemic blood, because of its large plasma volume, requires more anticoagulant, and severely polycythemic blood requires less. The latter fact must be considered when tests are performed on the blood of newborns. Fig. 11-9 correlates hematocrit values with amounts of anticoagulant. Oxalates in the plasma suppress platelets and labile factors V and VIII.

Barium sulfate–adsorbed plasma: Add 50 mg barium sulfate to 1.0 ml oxalated (not citrated) plasma and allow to stand for 1 min. Centrifuge suspension for 15 min at 2000 *g*. The prothrombin time of the supernatant will be infinite.

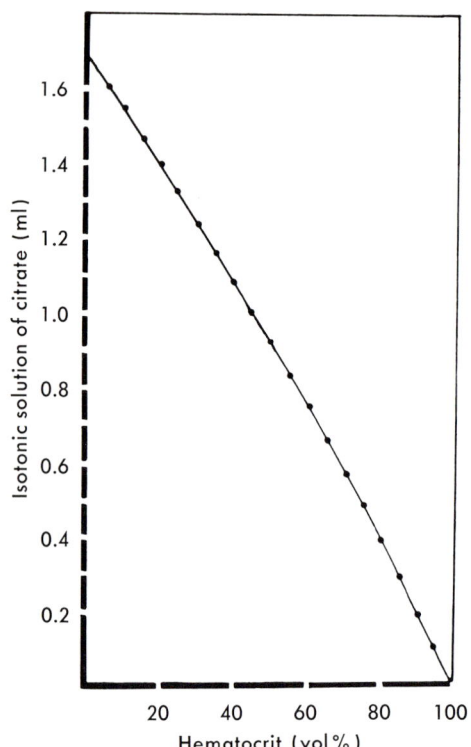

Fig. 11-9. Nomogram based on hematocrit and amount of anticoagulant to use in order to keep constant 1:10 ratio of anticoagulant in blood. Correct amount of citrate is pipetted into siliconized tube and blood is drawn to a final volume of 10 ml. (From Hellem, A.J.: Scand. J. Clin. Lab. Invest. [Suppl.] **51:**1, 1960.)

Calcium chloride: A 0.02M (2.2 g/L) solution is commercially available from Bio/Data Corp., Willow Grove, Pa.

Citrated plasma: Add 9 volumes freshly drawn blood to 1 volume 3.8% sodium citrate. Centrifuge to obtain plasma.

EACA (ε-aminocaproic acid) in buffered saline: Dissolve 1.31 g ε-aminocaproic acid (Amicar, Lederle Laboratories, Pearl River, N.Y.) in 1 L imidazole buffered saline.

EDTA (2%): A 2% solution of dipotassium ethylenediamine tetraacetate is used.

Factor-deficient plasmas: Factor-deficient plasmas are deficient in a specific factor but have normal levels of all other factors. They are commercially available, e.g., from Dade Diagnostics, Miami, or they may be prepared in the laboratory according to the following instructions.

Factor II–deficient plasma: Mix equal parts adsorbed plasma and serum.

Factor V–deficient plasma:

1. Age sterile oxalated plasma for 48 hr at 37° C and store in aliquots at −20° C. The prothrombin time should be greater than 45 sec.
2. Or adsorb factor V by adding 100 mg Celite powder (Filter-Cel, Johns-Manville, Denver) to each milliliter of plasma and stir magnetically for 4-6 hr until the prothrombin time of the plasma is greater than 45 sec.
3. Centrifuge and store plasma in aliquots at −20° C.

Factors VII– and X–deficient plasma:

1. Filter 1 dl bovine plasma (Colorado Serum Co., Denver) through a Seitz filter and 30% asbestos filter pad by gentle suction. Change pad after every 100 dl plasma.
2. Discard first 20 ml of plasma.
3. Store remaining 80 ml aliquots at −20° C.
4. Use prothrombin time test to check on adequacy of asbestos absorption of factors VII and X.

Factor XI–deficient plasma:

1. Adsorb citrated, fresh, platelet-poor plasma with 15 mg/ml of Filter-Cel with constant mixing for 10 min.
2. Centrifuge for 30 min at 3000 rpm at 4° C.
3. Using a plastic pipet, aspirate the supernatant and transfer to plastic tube.
4. Adjust to pH 7.0 using 0.1N HCl or NaOH.
5. Incubate plasma for 5 hr at 37° C with frequent mixing.
6. Store aliquots in plastic tubes at −20° C.
7. The activated partial thromboplastin time should be 80-120 sec.

Factors XI– and XII–deficient plasma: Prepare as described for factor XI–deficient plasma but use Filter-Cel, 50 mg/ml of plasma.

Heparin: Use sodium heparin for injection. (Abbott Laboratories, North Chicago, Ill.).

Imidazole buffer: Commercially available from Bio/Data Corp., Willow Grove, Pa.

Imidazole buffered saline: Use 1 volume buffer, pH 7.4, to 2 volumes 0.9% NaCl. Imidazole buffered saline is commercially available from Bio/Data Corp., Willow Grove, Pa.

Kaolin suspension: Use a 0.5% suspension of kaolin in saline.

Normal saline: Normal saline is commercially available from Bio/Data Corp., Willow Grove, Pa.

Oxalated plasma: See citrated plasma, except that 1 volume 0.1M (1.34%) sodium oxalate is used. Oxa-lates in the plasma suppress platelets and labile factors V and VIII.

Owren veronal buffer: Owren veronal buffer is commercially available from Dade Diagnostics, Miami, Fla.

Partial thromboplastin: A platelet substitute is commercially available, e.g., from Dade Diagnostics, Miami.

Platelet-poor plasma: Centrifuge citrated plasma at room temperature for 30 min at 2500 g. Most clotting tests employ platelet-poor plasma to eliminate platelet variability.

Platelet-rich plasma: Centrifuge citrated blood at room temperature for exactly 3 min at 1500 rpm (250 g) and separate plasma. The number of platelets suspended in the plasma cannot be adequately controlled by this method. Since platelet factor 3 influences the various plasma clotting time tests, platelet-poor plasma should be used for these tests.

Protamine sulfate reagent: Protamine sulfate reagent is commercially available from Dade Diagnostics, Miami, Fla.

Sodium citrate: Sodium citrate is commercially available from Bio/Data Corp., Willow Grove, Pa.

Synthetic chromogenic substances: Synthetic chromogenic substances are commercially available from Abbott Laboratories, North Chicago, Ill.

Synthetic fluorescent substances: Synthetic fluorescent substances are commercially available from Dade Diagnostics, Miami, Fla.

Thromboplastin: Thromboplastin, usually an acetone-dried rabbit brain preparation, is commercially available, e.g., from Dade Diagnostics, Miami, Fla.

Tris buffer: Tris buffer is commercially available from Bio/Data Corp., Willow Grove, Pa.

Thrombin: Thrombin reagent is available from Dade Diagnostics, Miami, Fla., or from Parke, Davis & Co., Detroit. The Parke Davis 5000 unit desiccated thrombin is dissolved in 2.5 ml glycerol and 2.5 ml veronal buffered saline and the 1000 units/ml solution is stored at −20° C. It is rediluted when needed with veronal buffer to give a thrombin time of 10-15 sec (usually about 5 units/ml) with normal plasma. Thrombin is also supplied by Ortho Diagnostics, Raritan, N.J., as Fibrindex.

Veronal buffer: See Owren veronal buffer.

Equipment in the coagulation laboratory

Minimal equipment includes automated clot timers, temperature-controlled water baths, refrigerator, −70° C deep freeze, disposable plastic and glass test tubes, and plastic transfer and automatic pipets.

Collection of blood for coagulation procedures

The two-syringe method: A clean, rapid venipuncture is required to prevent tissue thromboplastin or air from entering the blood sample. Tissue thromboplastin activates the extrinsic pathway of clotting and air renders the sample frothy and unsuitable. For all clotting tests except the one-stage prothrombin time test, the two-syringe method for obtaining the blood sample should be used.

Procedure: Apply the tourniquet and, using sterile

technic (sponge with alcohol first and then blot dry with sterile gauze), enter vein with disposable needle and release tourniquet. The size of the needle used is determined by the amount of blood to be withdrawn. A 20-gauge needle is satisfactory for the average 10 ml sample. Large amounts of blood require needles with larger bores.

Place sterile gauze below the hub of the needle to absorb any blood that may escape in switching syringes.

Withdraw 1-2 ml of blood into the first syringe, detach it but leave needle in place, and attach a second plastic syringe in which the test sample is collected.

After the collection withdraw the needle and apply a small sterile pressure dressing since patients with a hemorrhagic tendency may bleed. Do not leave the patient until the bleeding has stopped.

Transfer the specimen into a plastic tube by allowing it to run down the side of the tube after the needle has been removed from the syringe. If the specimen is unsatisfactory for any reason, discard it and do not use it for coagulation tests.

Two-Vacutainer method:

Procedure: Draw 1-2 ml venous blood into vacuum tube. Leave needle in place, remove tourniquet, and replace initial tube with second Vacutainer tube. Care of the puncture site before and after the proce-

dure is similar to that described for the two-syringe method.

Precautions: Blood samples from patients suspected of having hepatitis or other infectious diseases should be specially tagged to demand extreme caution when handling.

Bleeding time

Principle: The bleeding time measures the time required for bleeding from a small superficial cutaneous cut that injures only capillaries to cease. It tests platelet plug formation in injured capillaries. Since the test is sensitive to the ingestion of aspirin, it should be delayed for 1-2 weeks if the patient has taken as little as 10 grains (2 tablets) of aspirin during the past 2 weeks.[164]

Several modifications of the basic tests have been proposed.[165] The Duke method, which employs a puncture wound of the earlobe, is not described in detail since it is difficult to standardize and appears to be less sensitive than the Ivy method. If bleeding is excessive, it is not easily controlled and repeat tests may run out of testing area.

Ivy bleeding time using a commercial template

The Ivy method using a commercial template[166] (Simplate, General Diagnostics, Morris Plains, N.J.) is the method of choice because the capillary pressure and

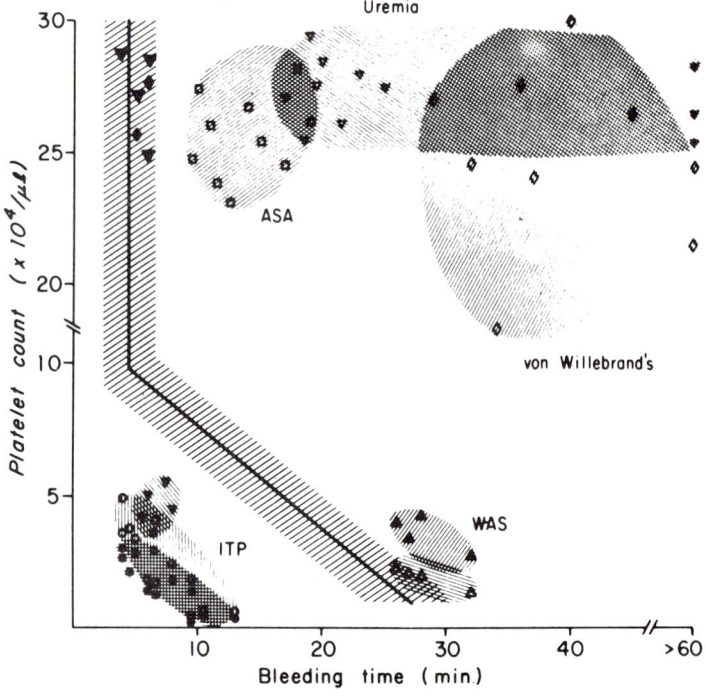

Fig. 11-10. More than predictable shortening of bleeding time for normal platelets by young platelets, as found in patients with ITP (solid circle) or rapidly returning bone-marrow function after chemotherapy (inverted solid triangle). Bleeding times remain short even after adjustment for increase in platelet volume (open circle). Impaired platelet plug formation is reflected as bleeding times longer than predicted by platelet count as shown by 3 g of ASA daily (open square) and von Willebrand's disease (open diamond), which corrects with cryoprecipitate infusion (diamond with cross in it). In uremia platelets have marked dysfunction in untreated state (inverted solid triangle), which improves after hemodialysis (inverted open triangle) and reverses to normal with peritoneal dialysis (inverted solid triangle). Modestly disparate bleeding times in Wiskott-Aldrich syndrome (WAS) (solid triangle) become appropriate after adjustment for small platelet volume (open triangle). (Reprinted, by permission, from The New England Journal of Medicine **287:**155, 1972.)

the incision can be standardized; the area allows multiple testing and easier control of the bleeding should it become excessive.

Procedure: Apply a sphygmomanometer cuff to the patient's upper arm and inflate it to 40 mm Hg. Maintain this pressure, clean the volar surface of one forearm with an alcohol swab, and dry with sterile gauze.

Using the template, make one or two small incisions (9 mm long, 1 mm deep) in the skin of the volar aspect of the forearm avoiding superficial veins and scars.

Start a stopwatch at the time of the incision and blot the bleeding point or points with filter paper disks at 30 sec intervals by just touching the tip of each drop.

The timing ends with the cessation of bleeding, and the stopwatch is stopped.

Quantitation of the blood loss has been suggested, because even though the bleeding time may be normal, the actual volume of blood lost may be excessive,[165,167] as in von Willebrand's disease.

Normal values: Normal values are 1-6 min.

Interpretation: The test measures the formation of the hemostatic platelet plug in injured capillaries (see p. 276). Prolonged values are seen in quantitative and qualitative platelet disorders, in von Willebrand's disease, in congenital deficiencies of factors I and V, in fibrinolytic states in the presence of inhibitors, and in heparin therapy. If the platelet count is below 100,000/mm[3], the bleeding time progressively increases (Fig. 11-10). In hemophilia A and B the bleeding time is normal, but bleeding may occur from the wound 24 hr after the test procedure. The presence of an anti–factor VIII antibody may lead to an abnormal bleeding time if the bleeding disorder is severe. Quick[164] noted that the ingestion of 10 grains of aspirin 2 hr before the Ivy test prolongs the bleeding time. Since this prolongation is most marked in patients with von Willebrand's disease, the "aspirin tolerance test" has been suggested as a means of diagnosing von Willebrand's disease.

Capillary fragility test (tourniquet test, Rumpel-Leede test)

Principle: Temporarily increased intracapillary pressure tests the fragility of the capillary walls and, if positive, leads to petechial rhexis bleeding into the skin. Since the test is positive in a number of apparently healthy individuals, especially women over 40 years of age, and in a great variety of metabolic, immunologic, and hematologic disorders,[168] it is difficult to interpret and is of little value in the investigation of the bleeding patient. The technic is described in previous editions of this book. If petechiae are present prior to the performance of the test, there is no need to proceed.

• • •

The above two tests are the only in vivo tests employed in the investigation of clotting defects.

Whole blood clotting time (Lee-White clotting time)

All coagulation tests must be run in duplicate and parallel with appropriate high, low, and normal controls as indicated, which should also be run in duplicate. See section on quality control in coagulation (p. 13).

The whole blood clotting time[169] measures the intrinsic pathway of coagulation of blood that is unadulterated except for the venous stick and glass contact. The test is poorly reproducible and is so insensitive to even significant intrinsic coagulation factor deficiencies that it should not be used as a test for coagulation factor defects but may be utilized as an indicator of clot formation, retraction, and lysis. It is useful for following patients on heparin therapy and is the first step in the preparation of serum for the serum prothrombin time (prothrombin consumption test). The three-tube method is described, but several one- to two-tube modifications exist, which may or may not require water baths and which are equally satisfactory for the stated purposes of the test.[170] The two-syringe method of obtaining blood reduces the amount of tissue thromboplastin entering the system and the use of three tubes further diminishes the tissue thromboplastin effect, since the effect is most likely to be present in the first milliliter of aspirated blood, which according to the test protocol is deposited in the third tube, which is tilted first. Precalibrated (2 or 3 ml marks) Vacutainers may be used. For heparin therapy control the test must be strictly standardized as to volume of blood tested, frequency of tilting, caliber and type of test tube, temperature, etc.

Equipment:
1. Water bath
2. Three glass test tubes, 10 × 75 ml, edged at 1 ml mark
3. Stopwatch

Procedure: Label three edged glass test tubes nos. 1, 2, and 3. Place tubes in 37° C water bath.

Obtain 5 ml blood by the two-syringe method and start stopwatch. Place 1 ml blood in each tube, starting with tube no. 1, by removing the needle and allowing the blood to run down the sides of the tubes.

Gently tilt tube no. 3 (the last tube to receive blood) every 30 sec until the blood clots solidly. Tubes no. 2 and 1 are then treated in the same manner until no flow of blood is observed on tilting.

The clotting time is the time required for the blood to clot in tube no. 1.

Normal values: Normal values for the whole blood clotting time are 5-15 min.

Interpretation: Clotting time is prolonged when circulating anticoagulants or heparin is present and in severe deficiencies of clotting factors of the intrinsic and common pathways (less than 3% concentration). The clotting time is unaffected by deficiencies of factor VII (extrinsic pathway), factor XIII, and platelets. If the blood fails to clot, the diagnosis of afibrinogenemia or hyperheparinemia should be considered. If the clotting time is markedly prolonged, severe hemophilia is the most likely cause.

Clot retraction phase of whole blood clotting time

Principle: Normal clot retraction requires quantitatively and qualitatively adequate platelets[171] and is influenced by the contractile platelet protein, thrombosthenin.

Equipment: See discussion of whole blood clotting time.

Procedure: The tubes used for the whole blood clot-

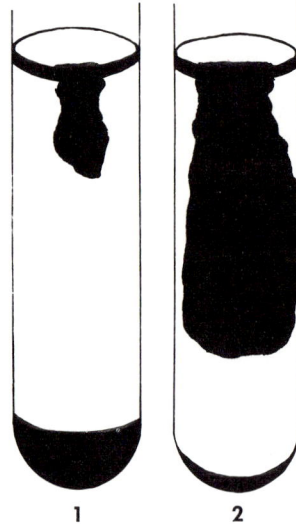

Fig. 11-11. Concept of clot retraction. **1,** Abnormal clot retraction. During retraction, large amount of free blood ("fallout") collects at bottom of tube, leaving small irregular clot attached to tube. **2,** Normal clot retraction. Large clot is adhering to one side of tube. Fallout is minimal.

ting time are allowed to remain in the 37° C water bath and are examined 1-2 hr after clotting has taken place, for adequacy of clot retraction.

Normal values: Clot retraction begins 30-60 min after the blood has clotted and is complete in 2 hr, at which time the clot should be retracted from at least three sides of the test tube. In the process of shrinking the clot decreases in size to about half of its original volume and expresses 40-60% of its volume as serum. This process is accompanied by a minimal amount of "fallout," the escape of unclotted red cells that collect at the bottom of the test tube (Fig. 11-11).

Clot retraction is reported as normal, impaired, or indeterminate.

Interpretation: Clot retraction is impaired in severe thrombocytopenia, Glanzmann's thrombasthenia, polycythemia, hypofibrinogenemia, and fibrinolysis. Impaired clot retraction implies a clot that is fragile, soft, and irregular and is accompanied by an increased fallout of red cells. The correlation of the clot retraction with the platelet count is poor, since significant thrombocytopenia may fail to affect the test result. The whole blood clot retraction is inversely proportional to the hematocrit, anemia accelerating it and erythrocytosis delaying it. The hematocrit variable can be circumvented and at the same time the method can be semiquantitated by the use of the red cell–free, platelet-rich plasma clot retraction,[172] which represents a refinement of the method that is usually not indicated.

Lysis phase of the whole blood clotting time

Principle: Hyperplasminemia (excessive fibrinolysis) leads to rapid dissolution of the clot once formed or to the formation of a small, shaggy, inadequate clot right from the beginning (Fig. 11-11).

Equipment: See discussion of whole blood clotting time.

Procedure: The clot is allowed to remain in the water bath for 12-24 hr and is inspected for lysis at 2, 12, and 24 hr.

Interpretation: Under the conditions of the test, the normal solid clot does not dissolve for 48 hr. Excessive fibrinolysis may lead to rapid lysis of the clot within a few minutes or hours. It is important to ascertain that initially a clot had actually formed, however small or fleeting. Since a small clot may hide at the bottom of the tube, its contents should be poured into a Petri dish for examination. If, because of circulating anticoagulants or hyperheparinemia, no clot forms at all, the test cannot be interpreted. Fragmentation of a clot because of dysfibrinogenemia or hypofibrinogenemia must not be mistaken for lysis. The test is insensitive to mild forms of fibrinolysis and may be falsely normal because of the inactivation of plasmin by antiplasmin or the depletion of plasminogen. It should be replaced by the euglobulin lysis time. If the fibrinogen level is severely reduced, the addition of compatible blood allows a clot to form, which can then be observed for lysis.

Activated coagulation time (ACT) of whole blood

Principle: The coagulation time of whole blood is an insensitive test for the detection of hemorrhagic diatheses. Its sensitivity can be increased by drawing the blood directly into a contact activant (Celite, an inert diatomite) that provides maximal activation.[173]

Equipment:
1. Evacuated Celite tubes
2. Heat block
3. Shaker
4. Timer

The reagents, tubes, and equipment for the ACT are marketed under the name of Hemochron by the International Technidyne Corp., Metuchen, N.Y.

Procedure: Use the two evacuated tubes method to obtain the specimen. Draw at least 1 ml blood into vacuum tube and discard blood. With the needle still in place, remove tourniquet and replace the initial tube with a vacuum Celite tube, prewarmed to 37° C. Start timer when blood appears in tube. Allow tube to fill, mix, and place in heat block. Allow 1 min to pass and then tilt tube every 5 sec until a clot appears and stop timer.

Normal values: Normal values are 1 min 45 sec ± 25 sec.

Discussion: Clotting times of 2 min 10 sec or less are considered normal; clotting times of 2 min 15 sec are borderline; and clotting times of 2 min 20 sec are abnormal. The test closely parallels the activated partial thromboplastin time in its sensitivity to factor VIII deficiency and to heparin. Adequate heparin therapy prolongs the ACT to 8 min.[174,175] The ACT offers the advantage of immediate bedside information. See discussion of monitoring of heparin therapy.

Plasma recalcification time

Principle: Like the whole blood clotting time, the plasma recalcification time (plasma clotting time) measures the intrinsic clotting potential of plasma. Plasma

Table 11-3. Shortened outline of protocol of differential plasma clotting time*

Patient's plasma	Effect of the addition of mixing reagents			
	Adsorbed plasma	Aged serum	Factor VIII–deficient plasma	Factor IX–deficient plasma
Deficient in:				
Factor VIII	+	0	0	+
Factor IX	0	+	+	0
Contains a circulating anticoagulant	0	0	0	0

* +, Prolongation of clotting time normalized or nearly normalized; 0, prolongation of clotting time not normalized.

contains all the clotting factors necessary for clot formation except calcium. When calcium is replaced, the clotting is initiated by the glass contact factors and proceeds as outlined according to the intrinsic and common pathways. The test is sensitive to severe (10% or less) clotting factor defects primarily of the intrinsic system (factors XII, XI, IX, and VIII) and is also influenced by the quality of platelets and the presence of inhibitors. If performed on platelet-rich plasma (PRP) and platelet-poor plasma (PPP) of the same individual, the test can be used as an indicator of platelet procoagulant activity since it is inversely proportional to the concentration of platelet factor 3.

Reagents:
1. CaCl$_2$, 0.025M
2. Citrated platelet-rich plasma

The method described uses the Bio/Data Coagulation Profiler (Bio/Data Corp., Willow Grove, Pa.).

Procedure[176]: Place the CaCl$_2$ in the vial test well. Add 0.2 ml plasma to 7 × 70 mm tube and incubate for 2 min. Place the sample in the test well of the Analyzer and add 0.1 ml of prewarmed CaCl$_2$. The digital timer will stop at the first detection of a fibrin clot.

Normal values: Normal values for PRP clotting time are 90-120 sec. For PPP, clotting time exceeds 130 sec.

Interpretation: The clotting time is prolonged in severe deficiencies (less than 10%) of one or more plasma procoagulants, but mainly of the contact factors XI and XII and of factors VIII, IX, and X. It is not affected by deficient factors VII and XIII. The clotting time is also influenced by the quality and concentration of platelets. If the PRP clotting time is equal to the PPP clotting time, a platelet defect may be present since normally the PRP clotting time is at least 20 sec shorter than the PPP clotting time. The plasma clotting time is also abnormally long when a circulating anticoagulant is present or the patient is on heparin therapy. The clot once formed may be observed for lysis.

Differential recalcification time (mixing or substitution test) to differentiate inhibitors from factor deficiency

If the recalcification time is prolonged, mixing tests are indicated to determine (1) whether the prolongation is caused by circulating inhibitors, or heparin, or a factor deficiency and (2) if the prolongation is caused by a factor deficiency, which factor is responsible.

Reagents:
1. Fresh normal platelet-rich plasma

2. Fresh platelet-rich patient's plasma

Procedure: Prepare 1:10 mixture of normal plasma (0.1 ml) and patient's plasma (0.9 ml). Repeat recalcification time.

Interpretation: If the addition of 10% normal plasma corrects or almost corrects the prolonged clotting time, a coagulation factor deficiency is probably responsible for the prolongation of the clotting time. If the prolongation is not corrected, a circulating anticoagulant or heparin is probably present.

Mixing (differential) tests to qualitatively identify a single factor deficiency

Principle: Mixing tests using adsorbed plasma reagent containing factors I, V, VIII, XI, and XII and aged serum reagent containing factors VII, IX, X, XI, and XII aid in the qualitative identification of a single coagulation factor defect, but the use of specific, known factor–deficient plasmas is preferred to pinpoint the factor responsible for the prolongation of the recalcification time. Cephalin (Ortho Pharmaceutical Corp., Raritan, N.J.), a platelet substitute, corrects the defect produced by inadequate platelets. The final diagnosis of a specific factor defect should be confirmed by a factor assay.

Reagents:
1. Platelet-rich patient's plasma
2. Adsorbed plasma
3. Aged serum
4. Known deficient plasmas (commercially available)
5. Cephalin (platelet substitute)

Procedure: Repeat recalcification time using a 1:10 mixture of adsorbed plasma and patient's plasma and a 1:10 mixture of aged serum and patient's plasma.

Interpretation: If adsorbed plasma (and not serum) corrects the recalcification time to normal or near normal, this indicates that adsorbed plasma has supplied the most likely missing factor, which in 85% of cases is factor VIII. If aged serum (and not adsorbed plasma) corrects the recalcification time to normal or near normal, this indicates that it has supplied the most likely missing factors, namely, factor IX or X. Mixing tests with known deficient plasmas are necessary to identify the factor IX or X deficiency. If a specific factor-deficient plasma fails to correct the recalcification time, this indicates that the patient has the same deficiency as the plasma used (Table 11-3).

Activated partial thromboplastin time

Principle: The activated partial thromboplastin time (aPTT), a modification of the plasma clot time, measures the intrinsic pathway of clotting. Two variables of the plasma recalcification time are removed by two modifications that shorten the testing time and provide a crisper end result. The addition of a partial thromboplastin, a platelet factor 3 substitute, eliminates the test's sensitivity to the quantity and quality of platelets. The addition of kaolin eliminates the variability of the glass contact activation. **Partial thromboplastin** is a petroleum ether soluble extract of acetone-dried brain that is called "partial" because it requires the assistance of the plasma procoagulants (except factor VII) to induce clotting and because it does not clot hemophilic plasma as rapidly as normal plasma. It is used as a platelet phospholipoprotein substitute in various clotting tests. **Complete thromboplastin,** on the other hand, is a whole brain dried acetone extract that has tissue factor activity in the prothrombin time test and clots hemophilic plasma as rapidly as normal plasma. Plasma contains all the procoagulants necessary for the intrinsic pathway of clotting except calcium. If calcium is added to the system, the clotting time becomes a measure of the intrinsic procoagulant activity of the plasma since the intrinsic prothrombinase that is formed acts on prothrombin to release thrombin, which converts fibrinogen to fibrin.

Reagents and equipment:
1. Bio/Data Coagulation Profiler (Bio/Data Corp., Willow Grove, Pa.)
2. Citrated normal plasma control
   For the sake of reproducibility use a lyophilized plasma control and reconstitute according to the manufacturer's instructions. Store at 2-8° C.
3. Platelet-poor citrated patient's plasma
   Remove from cells within 30 min and store at 2-8° C. Prewarm just prior to use. Plasma must be tested within 2 hr after collection.
4. Partial thromboplastin reagent containing kaolin (usually 2% in 0.45% saline)
   Reconstitute according to manufacturer's instructions, store at 2-8° C, and prewarm just before use.
5. CaCl$_2$, 0.025 M
   Prewarm to 37° C.
6. Glass test tubes, 7 × 70 mm

Procedure: Place 0.1 ml control plasma into test tube and place in the 37° C incubation block. Incubate for 2 min. Add 0.1 ml partial thromboplastin reagent to the plasma, mix well, and incubate mixture for 3 min (not longer). For the sake of reproducibility the incubation time must be kept constant.

Place the mixture into the test well, aspirate 0.1 ml prewarmed CaCl$_2$ and discharge into thromboplastin-plasma mixture. The timer will record the clotting time.

Repeat test with patient's plasma.

Perform all tests in duplicate, calculate the mean values, and report results as aPTT in seconds.

Normal value: Normal values are 35-45 sec.

Critical areas: The type of thromboplastin and the incubation time of the plasma and thromboplastin are critical areas in the performance of the aPTT.

Table 11-4. Differentiation of hemorrhagic disorders using aPTT and prothrombin time (PT)

aPTT	PT	Factor deficiency
Prolonged	Normal	Factors VIII, IX, XI, and XII
Prolonged	Prolonged	Factors II , V, and X (circulating anticoagulant)
Normal	Prolonged	Factor VII

Interpretation: The test is sensitive to severe to moderate (10-20% factor concentration) deficiencies of the intrinsic pathway factors XII, XI, IX, and VIII, to inhibitors (fibrin degradation products, etc.), and to heparin. It is slightly sensitive to deficiencies of the common pathway factors V, X, II, and I, but it is not sensitive to deficiencies of platelets and factors VII and XIII. Fibrinogen levels below 100 mg/dl prolong the aPTT. The test can be used to observe patients on heparin therapy.

The aPTT should always be performed in conjunction with the one-stage prothrombin time because the combination of these two tests allows the evaluation of the intrinsic, extrinsic, and common pathways of coagulation (Tables 11-4 and 11-5).

Differential partial thromboplastin time (mixing or substitution test)

Principle: The principle of the differential test is discussed under the heading of recalcified plasma clotting time (p. 292). If a 10% dilution of the patient's plasma with normal plasma corrects the prolonged aPTT, this indicates that normal plasma has supplied the missing factor. If the prolonged aPTT is not corrected, a circulating anticoagulant, e.g., fibrin degradation products or heparin, may be present in the patient's plasma. If the screening test suggests a missing factor, known factor−deficient plasma is used to identify the specific factor deficiency. If heparin is thought to be responsible for the prolongation of the aPTT, it should be neutralized by one of the methods discussed in the section on monitoring of heparin therapy. If known factor−deficient plasmas are not available, the aPTT is set up with a 10% or 50% dilution of the patient's plasma with adsorbed plasma and a 10% or 50% dilution of the patient's plasma with aged serum. If the adsorbed plasma corrects the prolonged aPTT, this suggests factor V, VIII, XI, or XII deficiencies. If factor V is abnormal, the prothrombin time will also be abnormal. If aged serum corrects the prolonged aPTT, this suggests factor IX or X deficiency (Table 11-5). If factor X is deficient, the prothrombin time and the Russell viper venom time will also be prolonged (Table 11-5). If both adsorbed plasma and aged serum correct the prolonged aPTT, a deficiency of factor XI or XII should be considered. Factor XII deficiency can be distinguished from factor XI deficiency by the relatively normal glass clotting time of the latter deficiency. If neither adsorbed plasma nor aged serum correct the aPTT, a factor II deficiency should be considered.

Table 11-5. Combined use of aPTT and prothrombin time (PT) differential studies*

Results of original tests		Correction studies					Probable factor deficiency
		aPTT		PT			
aPTT	PT	Adsorbed plasma	Serum	Adsorbed plasma	Serum		
P	N	C	NC	—	—		VIII
P	N	C	C	—	—		XI, XII†
P	N	NC	C	—	—		IX
P	P	C	NC	C	NC		V
P	P	NC	C	NC	C		X‡
P	P	NC	NC	NC	NC		II
N	P	—	—	NC	C		VII

*P, Prolonged; C, clotting time corrected; —, does not apply; NC, clotting time not corrected.
†Suggested additional test is Lee-White clotting time.
‡Suggested additional test is Russell's viper venom time.

One-stage prothrombin time

Principle: The one-stage prothrombin time is the clotting time obtained when an excess of tissue (complete) thromboplastin (tissue phospholipid) and optimal calcium are added to citrated plasma. The test evaluates the extrinsic and common pathways of clotting, which involve factors I, II, V, VII, and X, and bypass the intrinsic factors XII, XI, IX, and VIII. The tissue extract activates factor VII, which in turn activates factor X. Factor Xa interacts with factor V, calcium, and phospholipids to form prothrombinase, which activates prothrombin. The thrombin thus formed converts fibrinogen to fibrin. The test is sensitive to the vitamin K−dependent factors II, VII, and X. Factor IX, which is also vitamin K dependent, is evaluated by the aPTT.

Reagents and equipment:
1. Bio/Data Coagulation Profiler
2. Citrated normal plasma control
3. Platelet-rich citrated patient's plasma
4. Thromboplastin-calcium reagent

Procedure: Reconstitute thromboplastin-calcium reagent and citrated normal plasma control. Pipet 0.1 ml control plasma and patient plasma into each of two 7 × 70 mm test tubes.

Place plasma samples in the incubation block. Allow the samples to incubate for a minimum of 5 min but not longer than 10 min. Insert a control plasma tube into the test well.

Resuspend the thromboplastin-calcium reagent by gently swirling the vial. Aspirate 0.2 ml and discharge the thromboplastin-calcium reagent into the plasma tube. Note and record results shown on the digital timer. Run control and patient plasma samples twice and calculate the mean values.

Normal values: Normal values are 12-14 sec.

Controls: Two controls should be run in duplicate with each test (or series of tests): a normal plasma control and a therapeutic control of about 20 sec. The duplicate normal results should fall within ±0.5 sec of each other and the therapeutic control should fall within ±1 sec of each other.

Methods of reporting: The preferred method is to record the patient's plasma clotting time in seconds and to compare it with the normal control time also reported in seconds.

The prothrombin time may be reported as a percentage concentration by referring to a hyperbolic calibration curve (Fig. 11-12) that expresses the relationship of prothrombin concentration to clotting time. This method of reporting should be discouraged since it is based on the incorrect assumption that the prothrombin time measures the concentration of prothrombin.

Interpretation: The prothrombin time is prolonged if there is a deficiency of one or more of the following plasma procoagulants: factors I, II, V, VII, and X, or if circulating inhibitors, e.g., fibrin degradation products or heparin, are present. The factor deficiency may involve only one factor, as in congenital deficiencies, or it may involve several, as in acquired deficiencies. The latter deficiencies may be an expression of liver disease, of exposure to coumarin drugs, or of vitamin K deficiency.

Liver disease: If the liver parenchyma is severely damaged, the liver is unable to synthesize factors I and V and the vitamin K−dependent factors (VII, IX, X, and II) even if adequate amounts of the vitamin are available (see p. 281).

Coumarin drugs: The administration of bishydroxycoumarin or other coumarin derivatives interferes with the production of the vitamin K−dependent factors: prothrombin and factors VII, IX, and X. The coumarin drugs are therefore used to lower the coagulability of blood in patients with thromboembolic phenomena. After the administration of bishydroxycoumarin, factor VII is suppressed first, followed by factors IX and X and prothrombin. After cessation of treatment, the procoagulants recover in the same order (see discussion of vitamin K on p. 281).

Prothrombin time in newborn infants: In newborn infants the maternal supply of vitamin K is largely used up in 3-5 days and a decrease of prothrombin (hypoprothrombinemia) occurs before the intestinal flora necessary for the production of vitamin K is established. The prothrombin time is variable, tending to be within the normal adult range (method of Quick) on the first day, rising to a peak that is definitely higher than the normal adult range between the second and fifth days (usually the third day), and falling within the normal adult range after the fifth day (Fig. 11-13).

Vitamin K deficiency: Failure to absorb the fat-soluble vitamin occurs in external biliary fistula and in obstructive jaundice because of the absence of bile from the intestinal tract and in sprue and related diseases because of the inability to absorb fat. Sterilization of the intestinal flora by **antibiotics** leads to diminished vitamin K supply because of the disappearance of the normal flora. As already stated, severe liver disease interferes with the utilization of vitamin K (See discussion of PIVKA on p. 281).

Influence of drugs on prothrombin time[177]: Apart

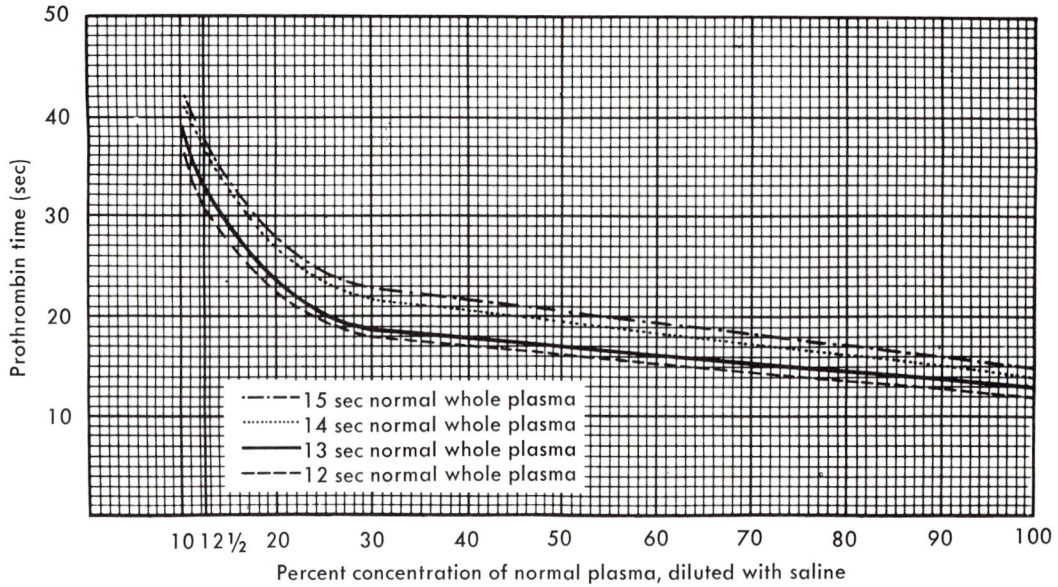

Fig. 11-12. Typical prothrombin activity curves. (Courtesy Warner-Chilcott Laboratories, Morris Plains, N.J.)

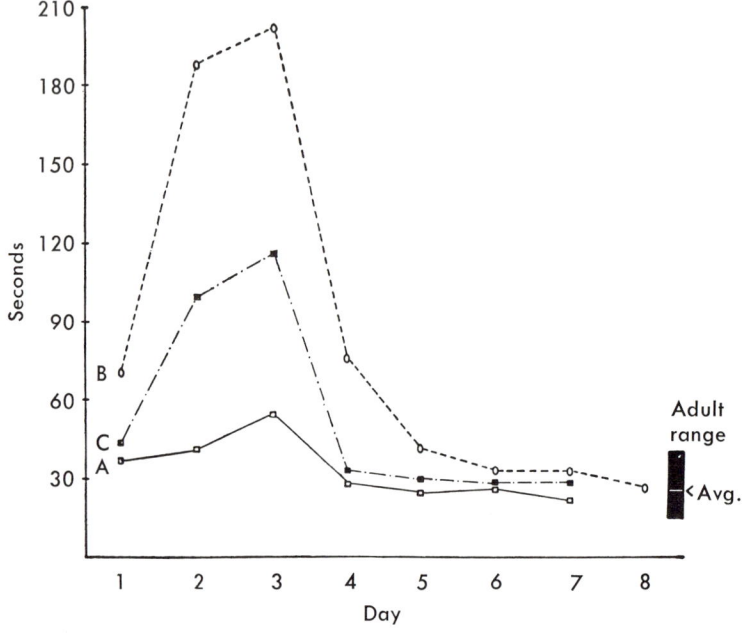

Fig. 11-13. Average prothrombin time (Quick) in newborn infant. **A,** Fourteen cases with clotting time not over 5 min; **B,** nine cases with clotting time over 5 min; **C,** average of all cases. (From Bray, W.E., and Kelley, O.R.: Am. J. Clin. Pathol. **10:**154, 1940.)

from the coumarin derivatives previously mentioned, there are many drugs that **lengthen** the prothrombin time by (1) suppressing vitamin K–synthesizing bacteria in the intestinal tract, e.g., antibiotics; (2) preventing the absorption of fat-soluble vitamin K, e.g., mineral oil; or (3) interacting with coumarin anticoagulants, e.g., salicylates.

Drugs may **shorten** the prothrombin time by interacting with anticoagulants. Many frequently used drugs belong to this group, e.g., barbiturates, digitalis, diuretics, vitamin K, and oral contraceptives.

Preparation of calibration curve

Principle: Various dilutions of normal citrated plasma are made with adsorbed plasma. The prothrombin time of each of these dilutions is determined so that a prothrombin activity curve can be constructed. If the patient's prothrombin time in seconds is known, the corresponding prothrombin concentration can then be read off the curve. The clotting time of the normal control plasma determines which curve is used (Fig. 11-12).

Dilution of normal plasma with saline solution decreases the concentration of factor V, fibrinogen, prothrombin, factor X, and factor VII. If prothrombin-free plasma (BaSO$_4$-adsorbed plasma) is used as the diluent, a curve having a slightly different slope is obtained, since BaSO$_4$-adsorbed plasma contains factor V and fibrinogen, and these factors therefore remain constant in the various dilutions. Because the concentrations of prothrombin and factors VII and X are the only variables in these dilutions, the BaSO$_4$-adsorbed plasma method more closely reflects the changes occurring in the plasma in coumarin therapy.

Table 11-6. Outline of preparation of prothrombin calibration curve

Tube	1	2	3	4	5	6	7	8
Normal plasma (ml)	1.0	0.8	0.6	0.5	0.4	0.3	0.2	0.1
Adsorbed plasma (ml)	0	0.2	0.4	0.5	0.6	0.7	0.8	0.9
Prothrombin (%)	100	80	60	50	40	30	20	10

Reagents:
1. Lyophilized normal control plasma with prothrombin time of 12-13 sec
2. BaSO$_4$-adsorbed normal citrated plasma
3. Commercial thromboplastin–calcium chloride mixture

Procedure: Label eight tubes as follows: 100%, 80%, 60%, 50%, 40%, 30%, 20%, and 10%. Prepare the dilutions shown in Table 11-6 and mix. Determine the prothrombin time of each tube in triplicate and take average values. Using lined graph paper, plot clotting time in seconds on the ordinate versus prothrombin concentration in percent on the abscissa (Fig. 11-12).

Differential prothrombin time test (mixing or substitution test)

The one-stage prothrombin time is prolonged if (1) there is an acquired or congenital deficiency of the procoagulants of the extrinsic and common pathways or (2) the patient is on heparin therapy or circulating anticoagulants are present. A deficiency of the following factors leads to a prolongation of the one-stage prothrombin time: factors I, V, VII, X, and II. Of these procoagulants, factors VII, X, and II are vitamin K dependent. The circulating anticoagulants that prolong the prothrombin time include heparin, the LE inhibitors, fibrin degradation products, and plasmin. The identification of the deficiency responsible for the prolongation of the one-stage prothrombin time is accomplished by the use of mixing tests employing normal plasma, absorbed plasma, serum, and factor-deficient plasmas.

Reagents: Reagents are the same as those used in the differential plasma clotting time (p. 293) plus plasmas deficient in factors II, V, VII, and X.

Procedure: Add 0.1 ml normal plasma to 0.9 ml patient's plasma and repeat the prothrombin time.

Interpretation (Table 11-7): If the originally prolonged clotting time is corrected or nearly corrected by the use of the mixture, a factor deficiency is responsible for the original prolongation. If the clotting time is not corrected, a circulating anticoagulant is present in the patient's plasma. If the screening test indicates a factor deficiency, proceed as follows to identify the factor.

Prepare a 10% mixture of adsorbed plasma (0.1 ml) and of the patient's plasma (0.9 ml). If the fibrinogen level is normal (established by the thrombin time), the adsorbed plasma supplies factor V. If the patient's

Table 11-7. Shortened outline of protocol of differential prothrombin time test*

Patient's plasma	Effect of the addition of mixing reagents				
	Adsorbed plasma	Aged serum	Factor V–deficient plasma	Factor VII–deficient plasma	Factor X–deficient plasma
Deficient in:					
Factor V	+	0	0	+	+
Factor VII	0	+	+	0	+
Factor X	0	+	+	+	0
Contains circulating anticoagulant	0	0	0	0	0

*+, Prolongation of prothrombin time normalized or nearly normalized; 0, prolongation of prothrombin time not normalized.

plasma lacks factor V, the activated partial thromboplastin time should also be prolonged (Table 11-5).

Prepare a 10% mixture of serum (0.1) containing factors VII and X and of patient's plasma (0.9 ml). If the addition of serum corrects the prothrombin time, the patient's plasma lacks factor VII or X. If factor VII is decreased, the activated partial thromboplastin time is normal; if factor X is diminished, the activated partial thromboplastin time and the Russell viper venom time will be prolonged (Table 11-5).

If neither the addition of adsorbed plasma nor of serum corrects the prothrombin time, factor II is deficient. This fact may be confirmed by the use of factor II–deficient plasma.

Confirmation of the factor deficiency can be obtained by using factor-deficient plasmas, which, if they fail to correct the prolonged prothrombin time, indicate that the patient has the same deficiency as the plasma reagent used (Table 11-7).

Russell's viper venom time test (Stypven time test)

Principle: The venom of the Russell viper has procoagulant activity and can be substituted for tissue thromboplastin in the one-stage prothrombin time. Contrary to tissue thromboplastin the snake venom does not require factor VII for its activity since it interacts directly with factors V and X and platelet phospholipids.[178,179] The principal area of application of this test lies in assessing factor X deficiency if the one-stage prothrombin time is prolonged and corrected by the addition of serum.

Reagents and equipment:
1. Bio/Data Coagulation Profiler
2. Platelet-poor citrated plasma (control and unknown)
3. Russell's viper venom with calcium (General Diagnostics, Morris Plains, N.J.)
4. Platelin (platelet factor 3) (General Diagnostics, Morris Plains, N.J.)

Procedure: Combine equal parts of reconstituted viper venom reagent and Platelin. Place 0.2 ml combined reagent into 7 × 70 mm test tube and incubate at 37° C for at least 2 min. Transfer tube into test well and add 0.1 ml control plasma and time clot formation. Repeat procedure with unknown plasma.

Normal values: Normal values are 8-10 sec.

Interpretation: The clotting time is considered prolonged if it exceeds the control time by 3 sec. If the prolonged one-stage prothrombin time is corrected by the addition of aged serum, the correction may be caused by the aged serum's factor VII or factor X contents. Stypven time, by circumventing factor VII, differentiates factor VII deficiency from factor X deficiency. The test is also sensitive to deficiencies of factors I, II, and V. The use of platelet-rich plasma renders the test sensitive to qualitative and quantitative platelet deficiencies.

Thrombin time

Principle: The thrombin time is the time required for a standardized thrombin solution to clot plasma by converting plasma fibrinogen into the insoluble fibrin gel.

No other clotting factors are involved in this reaction.

Reagents and equipment:
1. Bio/Data Coagulation Profiler
2. Platelet-poor citrated plasma (unknown and control)
3. Fibrindex (Ortho Pharmaceutical Corp., Raritan, N.J.), source of thrombin (50 NIH units)
4. Imidazole buffered saline (Bio/Data Corp., Horsham, Pa.)

Thrombin solution: Reconstitute 1 vial Fibrindex with 1 ml imidazole buffered saline and dilute the solution with imidazole buffer so that the addition of 0.1 ml solution to 0.1 ml normal plasma results in a normal clotting time of 13-18 sec.

Procedure: Add 0.1 ml control plasma to a 7 × 70 mm test tube and allow to equilibrate at 37° C for 5 min. Place tube into test well, add 0.1 ml thrombin solution, and measure clotting time.

Normal values: Normal values are 13-18 sec.

Interpretation: The thrombin time is abnormally prolonged (over 20 sec) in hypofibrinogenemia (fibrinogen level below 90 mg/dl), dysfibrinogenemia, and paraproteinemia[148] and in the presence of circulating anticoagulants (antithrombin), e.g., heparin, fibrin degradation products, and plasmin. The presence of circulating anticoagulants can be confirmed by mixing tests.

Differential thrombin time (mixing test)

Repeat thrombin time using a 1:9 mixture of normal citrated plasma (0.1 ml) and of unknown citrated plasma (0.9 ml). If normal plasma fails to correct the prolonged thrombin time, a circulating anticoagulant is most likely responsible for the prolongation of the thrombin time.

The thrombin time is very sensitive to heparin, the presence of which can be documented in a number of ways. See discussion of monitoring of heparin therapy on p. 343.

Reptilase time test

Principle: Reptilase (Eli Lilly & Co., Indianapolis), a thrombinlike snake venom enzyme, acts directly on fibrinogen, but unlike thrombin it is not inhibited by heparin. The addition of reptilase to plasma results in a clot that is more fragile than the normal fibrin gel, since reptilase splits off fibrinopeptide A only from the fibrinogen molecule while thrombin splits off fibrinopeptides A and B.[180]

Reagents and equipment:
1. Bio/Data Coagulation Profiler
2. Platelet-poor citrated plasma (unknown and control)
3. Reptilase, reconstituted

Procedure: Add reconstituted reptilase to 7 × 70 mm test tube and allow it to equilibrate at 37° C for 5 min. Add 0.1 ml patient's plasma to test tube and warm at 37° C for 2 min. Add 0.1 ml reptilase to plasma and determine clotting time.

Normal values: Normal values are 18-22 sec.

Interpretation: The reptilase clotting time is unaffected by heparin, moderately prolonged by fibrin degradation products, and markedly prolonged by dysfibrinogenemia.[181]

Prothrombin consumption time (serum prothrombin time)

Principle: During normal clotting intrinsic prothrombinase (the activity of all intrinsic factors that activate factor X) continues to be formed and continues to convert prothrombin to thrombin after the blood has clotted. If serum is tested for prothrombin 1 hr after coagulation has occurred, practically all prothrombin has been consumed. If there is a deficiency in any of the factors required for the formation of the intrinsic prothrombinase, not all prothrombin will be consumed, leaving residual prothrombin in the serum 1 hr after clotting. The prothrombin consumption time[182] measures the residual prothrombin in the serum by a modified Quick one-stage method. The concentration of prothrombin in the serum is inversely proportional to the prothrombinase concentration generated during coagulation. The prothrombinase concentration depends primarily on the adequacy of platelets and the concentration of the hemophilic factors VIII and IX. In the test system, serum supplies factors VII and X, and Simplastin A (Warner-Chilcott Laboratories, Morris Plains, N.J.) supplies fibrinogen, factor V, calcium, and thromboplastin, the materials needed for the prothrombin time.

Reagents and equipment:
1. Bio/Data Coagulation Profiler
2. Simplastin A
3. Unknown and control sera

Procedure: Allow 1 ml venous blood obtained by the two-syringe method to clot in the test tube undisturbed and separate serum exactly 1 hr after coagulation has taken place by centrifuging the clot at 3000 rpm for 1 min. Remove serum and return to water bath.

Reconstitute Simplastin A and allow to equilibrate at 37° C for 2 min. To 0.2 ml reconstituted Simplastin A add 0.1 ml serum and record clotting time.

Run test in duplicate parallel with a normal control.

Normal values: Normal values are over 30 sec.

Interpretation: The serum prothrombin time evaluates the intrinsic thromboplastin (prothrombinase) formation. Since normal serum is essentially free of prothrombin, the normal serum prothrombin time is prolonged. A defect in the intrinsic thromboplastin formation leads to an abnormally short serum prothrombin time because of the increased prothrombin concentration in the serum. The serum prothrombin time is shortened in deficiencies of factors VIII and IX, in qualitative and quantitative platelet abnormalities, and in the presence of circulating anticoagulants, but it must be recognized that the serum prothrombin time is an indicator of the entire intrinsic clotting system, platelets, and factors XII, XI, X, and IX. If the serum lacks factors VII, X, and II, the prothrombin time will be prolonged because of inadequacy of the "prothrombin" factors and the prothrombin consumption time will be normal (prolonged), masking any deficiencies in the intrinsic pathway factors.

Differential prothrombin consumption test (mixing test)

If the serum prothrombin time is shortened, the defect can be pinpointed by substituting the following reagents and repeating the test to see whether the subtitution corrects the shortened time. Platelin (General Diagnostics, Morris Plains, N.J.) corrects the platelet deficiency, adsorbed plasma supplies factor VIII, and serum supplies factor IX. Factor-deficient plasmas may also be used.

Thromboplastin generation test

The thromboplastin generation test (TGT) is more time consuming and more difficult to perform than the other tests described that evaluate deficiencies in the intrinsic pathway of clotting, but it pinpoints the nature of the clotting defect by the use of the following "reagents": diluted aged serum, adsorbed plasma, platelets, substrate plasma, and calcium chloride. The dilution of the "reagents" results in increased sensitivity of the test system to coagulation factor defects.

Principle: The TGT is a two-stage procedure. In the first stage the intrinsic thromboplastin reaction mixture (intrinsic prothrombinase) is formed by using the three "reagents" of the patient's blood and of the control blood. The "reagents" are platelets or a platelet substitute, adsorbed fresh plasma supplying factors V, VIII, XI, and XII, aged serum supplying factors VII, IX, X, XI, and XII, and $CaCl_2$. In the first phase of the TGT the mixture of the above reagents generates prothrombinase, which cannot express iteslf since the mixture lacks prothrombin and fibrinogen. In the second phase small amounts of the thromboplastin reaction mixture are added to a substrate plasma that is platelet poor but supplies prothrombin and fibrinogen and thus allows a clot to form. The normal control "reagents" and the substrate plasma are commercially available (TGT reagents [TGTR], General Diagnostics, Morris Plains, N.J.).

Reagents and equipment[183]:
1. Bio/Data Coagulation Profiler
2. Electric timer and stopwatches
3. Plastic test tubes for preparation of platelets
4. Platelet substitute: Platelin or Inosithin (Associated Concentrates, Woodside, Long Island, N.Y.)
5. $CaCl_2$, 0.25M
6. Adsorbed plasma (patient's and controls)
   Maintain in ice water, and prior to use dilute 1:5 in saline.
7. Aged serum (patient's and controls)
   Prior to test dilute 1:10 in saline and keep in ice water for 1 hr before use.
8. Platelets (patient's and controls)
   Use platelet substitute unless patient's platelets are suspect.

Plan of test: The various reaction mixtures are prepared as stated below and $CaCl_2$ is added. At 2 min intervals (1, 3, 5, 7, 9, 11, etc.), aliquots of the reaction mixture are transferred to six tubes of substrate plasma and the clot formation is timed. The procedure is performed with the following reaction mixtures:
1. Normal serum, normal plasma, platelet substitute
2. Patient's serum, patient's plasma, platelet substitute
3. Patient's serum, normal plasma, platelet substitute
4. Normal serum, patient's plasma, platelet substitute

5. Repeat of no. 1 to check on degree of deterioration of reagents

***Procedure*:**

1. Add 4.0 ml $CaCl_2$ to a vial and place in the incubation block.

2. Add 0.1 ml normal substrate plasma to each of six 7 × 70 mm test tubes and place in the incubation block.

3. To a test tube labeled ''reaction mixture'' add the following:

    a. 0.3 ml normal 1:10 diluted serum

    b. 0.3 ml normal 1:5 diluted adsorbed plasma

    c. 0.3 ml normal platelet suspension

4. Place the reaction mixture in the incubation block. Incubate for 2 min.

5. Add 0.3 ml $CaCl_2$ to the mixture and immediately start the stopwatch. Mix the contents of the tube by gentle agitation.

6. At 45 sec, transfer 0.1 ml reaction mixture to the first tube of substrate and immediately place the tube into the test well of the Analyzer. Aspirate 0.1 ml $CaCl_2$ with the Bio/Ette.

7. At 60 sec, add the $CaCl_2$. Note the clotting time.

8. Repeat steps 6 and 7 for each of the remaining tubes of substrate plasma at successive 60 and 120 sec intervals. After the second or third minute a clot usually forms in the incubation mixture because of traces of thrombin. This will not interfere with the test and should be removed by winding the clot around a wooden applicator stick.

9. Using the patient's reagents, repeat steps 2-8.

10. Combinations of normal and patient's serum, and patient's plasma and normal serum should be assayed in a similar manner.

***Interpretation and normal values*:** The reaction of normal reagents produces the shortest clotting time (7-12 sec) in about 3-5 min. If the amount of thromboplastin generated in the reaction mixture is deficient, a long clotting time will be obtained in about 3-5 min when it should be shortest. If the rate of thromboplastin formation is deficient, the rate of shortening of the clotting time is abnormal, so that the shortest clotting time is obtained after 7 or 9 min.

ASSAYS OF CLOTTING FACTORS

Newer assay methods of coagulation factors and of activation products employ a combination of functional clotting techniques, immunologic methods, and the use of synthetic chromogenic or fluorescent substrates. A short introduction to the latter three technics follows.

Immunologic diagnosis of coagulation defects

The immunologic methods[184] depend on the availability of specific antisera to specific factors and can be used for qualitative and quantitative analyses. They include the double diffusion technic of Ouchterlony, radial immunodiffusion, counterimmunoelectrophoresis, latex agglutination, rocket electroimmunodiffusion technic of Laurell, hemagglutination inhibition, and radioimmunoassay. The decision of which method to use depends on its sensitivity, precision, reproducibility, and the time required to complete the procedure (Tables 11-8 and 11-9). Because the antigen-antibody interaction is highly specific and involves only certain antigenic determinants of the antigen molecule, immunologic methods are ideal for the demonstration of fibrin-fibrinogen degradation products and are essential in the differential diagnosis of fibrinolysis. In the diagnosis of hemophilia A, von Willebrand's disease, the hemophilia A carrier, and hypercoagulability, quantitative immunologic methods are combined with functional assays.

Use of chromogenic substrates in the coagulation laboratory

Chromogenic substrates are synthetic peptides that are used as substrates in the assay of clotting enzymes such as thrombin, plasmin, and serine proteases; they consist of two parts, an amino acid sequence and an organic chromophore, paranitroaniline.[185,186] On enzymatic hydrolysis free paranitroaniline is liberated. This is measured by its absorbance at 415 nm. As with other enzyme assays, either an end point or a kinetic assay method may be used. Differences in the peptide chain result in differences in the sensitivity and specificity for the different coagulation factors. By the use of the proper concentration of the correct substrate in a buffer (pH 8.3), the absorbance changes produced by the aliquots of the sample plasma are compared with the changes produced by different dilutions of the standard (a purified solution of the proper factor, or more simply, pooled normal plasma), and the activity of the factor in the sample can be calculated. The procedure is very similar to that given in Chapter 24 for the determination of the activity of trypsin and α_1-antitrypsin in which a similar substrate, benzoyl-arginine-paranitroaniline, is used.

Chromogenic substrate S2222 is used for the assay of factor X, factor Xa, heparin, factor VIII, factor IX, antithrombin III, and platelet factor 4. Substrate S2160 is used for the determination of thrombin, prothrombin, and antithrombin III, and substrate S2251 is available for the analysis of plasmin, plaminogen, antiplasmin, and plasminogen activators.

There are a number of advantages to the use of these substrates. The analysis requires only 5-20 μl of plasma, it can be automated, and it is easier to standardize than the clotting procedures. The reactions are specific and of high sensitivity,[187] and factor-deficient plasmas are not required. The substrates are commercially available (Ortho Diagnostics, Raritan, N.J.) but at present are expensive. Substrates for factors XIIa, XIa, and IXa are in the research state. The results of these methods are expressed in microkatals, units of enzyme activity.

Use of fluorescent synthetic substrates

The Dade (Dade Diagnostics, Miami, Fla.) Protopath Synthetic Substrate Assays[188] are based on the assays of proteolytic coagulation enzymes by the use of synthetic substrates, but the colorimetric determination is replaced by a fluorometric method. The synthetic substrate consists of a special sequence of amino acids and a fluorometric tag. When the reaction between the synthetic substrate and a particular proteolytic enzyme occurs, the tag, which in its free state fluoresces, is lib-

Table 11-8. Immunologic methods for determination of individual coagulation factors (Normal ranges of values for these factors are shown.)*

Protein	Methods	Normal range (% of norm)	Remarks
F I, fibrinogen	RID, EID, RIA	59-141	
FDP	RID, EID, CIEP, TRCHII, LAT, RIA		EID with anti-D serum: normal value in fibrinogen equivalents = 0-5 μg/ml
Fibrinopeptide A	RIA		
F II, prothrombin	RID, EID	67-133	
F VIII, antihemophilic globulin A	EID	47-185	High voltage and buffers of high ionic strength are unsuitable
F IX, antihemophilic globulin B	RID, EID	ca. 70-130	
F XII, Hageman factor	RID, EID	48-151	
F XIII, fibrin stabilizing factor	EID, ANT	50-140	
Antithrombin III	RID, EID	72-128	Determination in serum with EID only as heparin complex
α₂-Macroglobulin	RID, EID	62-145	
Plasminogen	RID, EID	75-125	

From Heimburger, N., and Karges, H.E.: Med. Lab. **5:**1, 1978.
*RID, Radial immunodiffusion; EID, electroimmunodiffusion (Laurell method); RIA, radioimmunoassay; CIEP, counterimmunoelectrophoresis; TRCHII, tanned red cell hemagglutination inhibition immunoassay; LAT, latex agglutination test; ANT, antibody neutralization test.

Table 11-9. Sensitivities of immunologic methods

Method	Sensitivity (μg/ml)	Application	Time needed for evaluation
Double diffusion (Ouchterlony)	10-40	Semiquantitative	24 hr
Precipitation analysis (Heidelberger)	12.5-20	Quantitative	24 hr
Radial immunodiffusion (Mancini)	10-20	Quantitative	24 hr
Counterimmunoelectrophoresis	1-5	Semiquantitative	1-2 hr
Latex agglutination	0.5-5	Semiquantitative	10 min
Electroimmunodiffusion (Laurell)	0.5-2	Quantitative	12 hr
Complement fixation test	0.05-0.2	Semiquantitative	4 hr
Indirect hemagglutination	0.02-0.04	Semiquantitative	4 hr
Hemagglutination inhibition test	0.006-0.01	Semiquantitative	4 hr
Radioimmunoassay, enzyme-linked immunosorbent assay	0.00004-0.005	Quantitative	2-3 hr

Modified from Heimburger, N., and Karges, H.E.: Med. Lab. **5:**1, 1978.

erated. The total fluorescence is a direct measure of the amount of enzyme in the sample.

Fibrinogen assay

The available technics can be grouped into three main categories: clotting methods, physicochemical determinations, and immunologic measurements.[189]

Clotting method

The measurement of fibrinogen as clottable protein is based on two reactions that are intrinsic to fibrinogen: (1) fibrinogen, when exposed to thrombin, a proteolytic enzyme, is degraded into smaller fragments, the soluble fibrin monomers, and (2) the smaller fragments polymerize to form a fibrin clot. Conversion of fibrinogen to fibrin is accomplished by adding thrombin to plasma. The protein content of the fibrin clot is determined by the biuret reaction[190] or by the addition of the Folin-Ciocalteau reagent[191] and the determination of the ty-

rosine concentration. Details of the first method are described in the previous edition of this book and are not repeated since the test, although precise and accurate, takes 1-2 hr to perform. The method described is the Data-Fi fibrinogen determination, which utilizes a commercially available kit (Data-Fi reagents, Dade Diagnostics, Miami, Fla.) and an automated clot timer.

Data-Fi fibrinogen determination

Principle: Plasma is diluted so that when excess thrombin is added, the rate of fibrin formation is a function of the concentration of firbinogen only.[192,193]
Reagents and equipment:
1. Data-Fi thrombin reagent
2. Data-Fi fibrinogen calibration reference
3. Owren's veronal buffer
4. Ci-Trol normal citrated plasma control
5. Fibrometer (Becton-Dickinson & Co., Rutherford, N.J.)

6. Graph paper (supplied by Dade Diagnostics, Miami, Fla.)

Procedure:

1. Prepare 1:5, 1:15, and 1:40 dilutions of Data-Fi fibrinogen calibration reference in Owren's veronal buffer according to Table 11-10. Mix gently.

2. Incubate 0.2 ml fibrinogen calibration reference dilution at 37° C for 2 min and add 0.1 ml thrombin reagent, which must be at room temperature, and determine clotting time. Run duplicate determinations on each dilution and average clotting time.

3. Prepare calibration curve by plotting the three average clotting times on furnished graph paper using the three vertical lines marked 1:5, 1:15, and 1:40. The calibration curve may be extended beyond the 1:5 and 1:40 values to a maximum of 800 mg/dl and a minimum of 50 mg/dl (Fig. 11-14).

4. Dilute unknown and control plasma samples 1:10 with Owren's veronal buffer (0.1 ml plasma plus 0.9 ml buffer) and test specimens in duplicate as outlined in step 2. Read results of fibrinogen concentration from the calibration curve and report in milligrams per deciliter.

5. The calibration curve is set up for a 1:10 dilution of the plasma. If the dilution exceeds 1:10, multiply results by the dilution factor (e.g., multiply by 2 for a dilution of 1:20; if the plasma dilution is less than 1:10, divide by the dilution factor (e.g., divide by 2 for a dilution of 1:5).

Normal range: Normal range is 200-400 mg/dl.

Discussion: Falsely low fibrinogen levels may be caused by antithrombins such as heparin concentrations exceeding 0.6 units/ml or fibrin degradation products exceeding 100 μg/ml. Lesser concentrations of antithrombins do not interfere with the fibrinogen quantitation because the dilution of the test plasma and the use of excess thrombin overcome the inhibitory effect of heparin or fibrin degradation products. If heparin is present, it may be neutralized by protamine sulfate (see discussion of laboratory control of heparin therapy, p. 343).

Elevated fibrinogen levels (**hyperfibrinogenemia**) are encountered in some obese individuals, in pregnancy (up to 700 mg/dl), and in women on oral contraceptives. They are also encountered in conditions that call forth an acute phase protein (reactant) response, e.g., stress, infection, neoplasms, collagen diseases, and defibrination. Decreased levels (**hypofibrinogenemia**) are found in infants and children and in congenital afibrinogenemia or hypofibrinogenemia. Acquired deficiencies accompany severe liver disease, diffuse intravascular coagulation, fibrinolysis, and glomerulonephritis and other immune complex diseases.

Laboratory diagnosis of dysfibrinogenemias

Dysfibrinogenemias are qualitative abnormalities of the fibrinogen molecule. Immunologic or chemical fibrinogen assays are usually normal, but since the abnormal fibrinogen reacts abnormally to thrombin and other enzymes, the thrombin and reptilase time tests are prolonged. The prolongation may be reduced by the addition of excess thrombin. The commonly performed screening tests, e.g., prothrombin time and activated partial thromboplastin time, may be normal or may be prolonged. The **thrombokinetogram** may be abnormal.

Fibrinogen titer

Fibrinogen titer is a rapid semiquantitative method that has been used in the past to assess the defibrination syndrome in pregnant women,[195] but it is too crude a test to be recommended. Plasma is diluted until fibrinogen can no longer be demonstrated by the addition of thrombin.

Immunologic methods

The immunologic methods for measuring fibrinogen include radial immunodiffusion, rocket electroimmunodiffusion (Fig. 11-15), and radioimmunoassay. They lack specificity since they are unable to distinguish clottable normal fibrinogen from abnormal fibrinogen or from fibrinogen degradation products. As a matter of fact, it is in the demonstration of fibrinogen degradation products that immunologic methods are most useful.

Assay procedures for extrinsic factors
One-stage assay of factor V

If the one-stage prothrombin time is prolonged, it may be necessary to assay the activity of the individual factors that are responsible for the test.

Principle[196-198]: The degree that a prolonged one-stage prothrombin time of factor V–deficient plasma is shortened (corrected) by the addition of normal or unknown plasma is proportional to the amount of factor V present in the normal or unknown plasmas. The factor V–deficient substrate supplies factors II, VII, X, and I, rendering the assay sensitive to factor V only. The prothrombin time correcting action of the patient's plasma is compared to that of a normal control plasma and the activity of factor V is expressed as a percent of normal plasma.

Reagents and equipment:

1. Thromboplastin-calcium reagent, dried
2. Owren's veronal buffer (diluting fluid)
3. Normal platelet-poor control plasma, citrated
4. Patient's platelet-poor plasma, citrated
5. Factor V–deficient substrate plasma, dried (Dade Diagnostics, Miami, Fla.)
6. Bio/Data Profiler (Bio/Data Corp., Willow Grove, Pa.).

Procedure: Maintain all plasma samples and reconstituted factor V–deficient plasma in ice water.

Table 11-10. Outline of preparation of Data-Fi fibrinogen calibration

Dilution	1:5	1:15	1:40
Buffer (ml)	1.6	0.8	2.8
Fibrinogen calibration reference (ml)	0.4	—	—
Mix and transfer (ml)		0.4	0.4

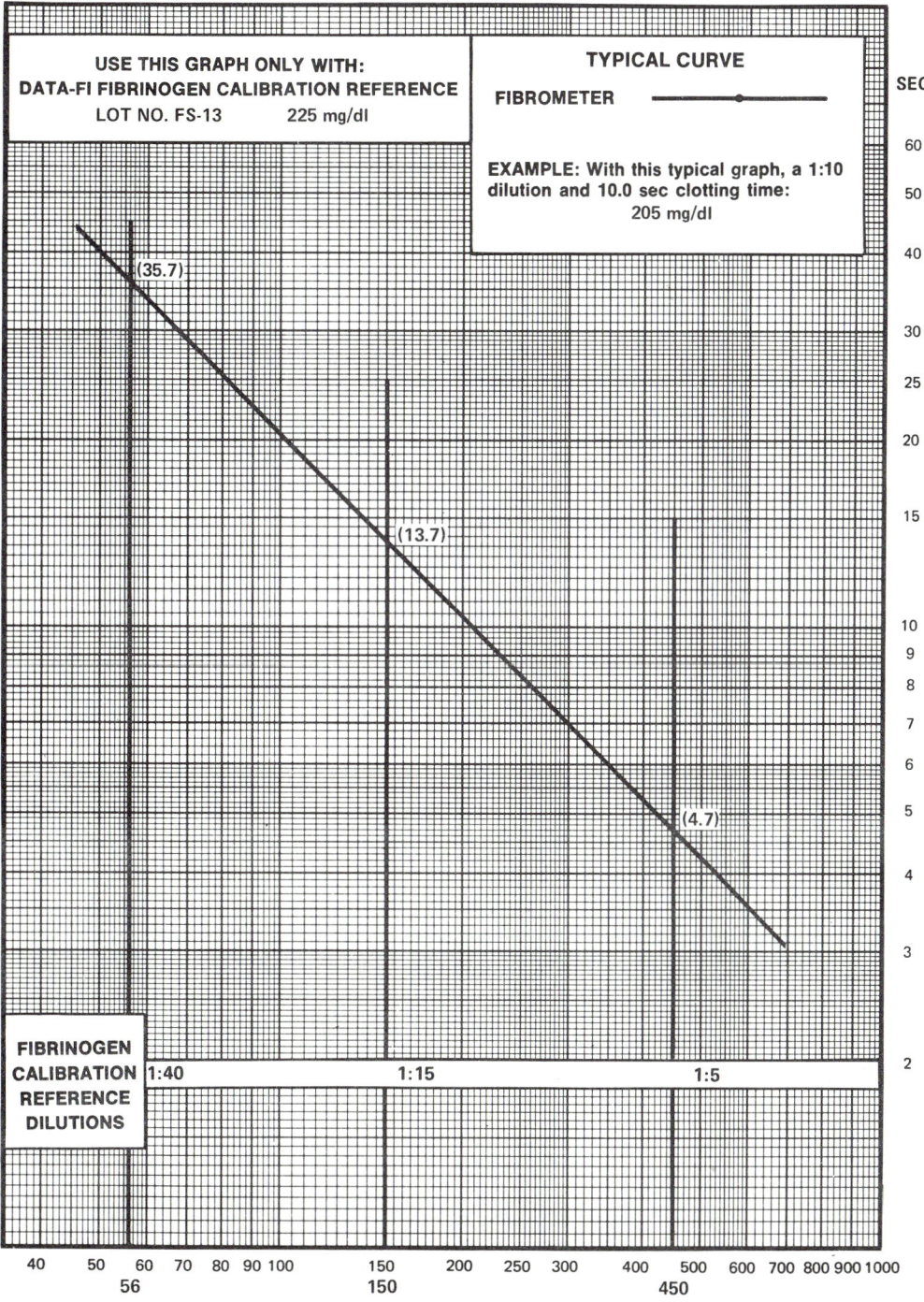

USE THIS GRAPH ONLY WITH:
DATA-FI FIBRINOGEN CALIBRATION REFERENCE
LOT NO. FS-13   225 mg/dl

TYPICAL CURVE
FIBROMETER

EXAMPLE: With this typical graph, a 1:10
dilution and 10.0 sec clotting time:
205 mg/dl

(35.7)

(13.7)

(4.7)

FIBRINOGEN
CALIBRATION
REFERENCE
DILUTIONS

1:40   1:15   1:5

SEC
60
50
40
30
25
20
15
10
9
8
7
6
5
4
3
2

40   50   60   70   80   90 100   150   200   250   300   400   500   600   700 800 900 1000
56   150   450

FIBRINOGEN IN mg/dl

Fig. 11-14. Typical fibrinogen calibration curve. NOTE: Calibration curve is valid as long as the Data-Fi thrombin reagent used in test has same lot number as that used in making curve. (Produced with permission of author and publisher. © American Hospital Supply Corp.)

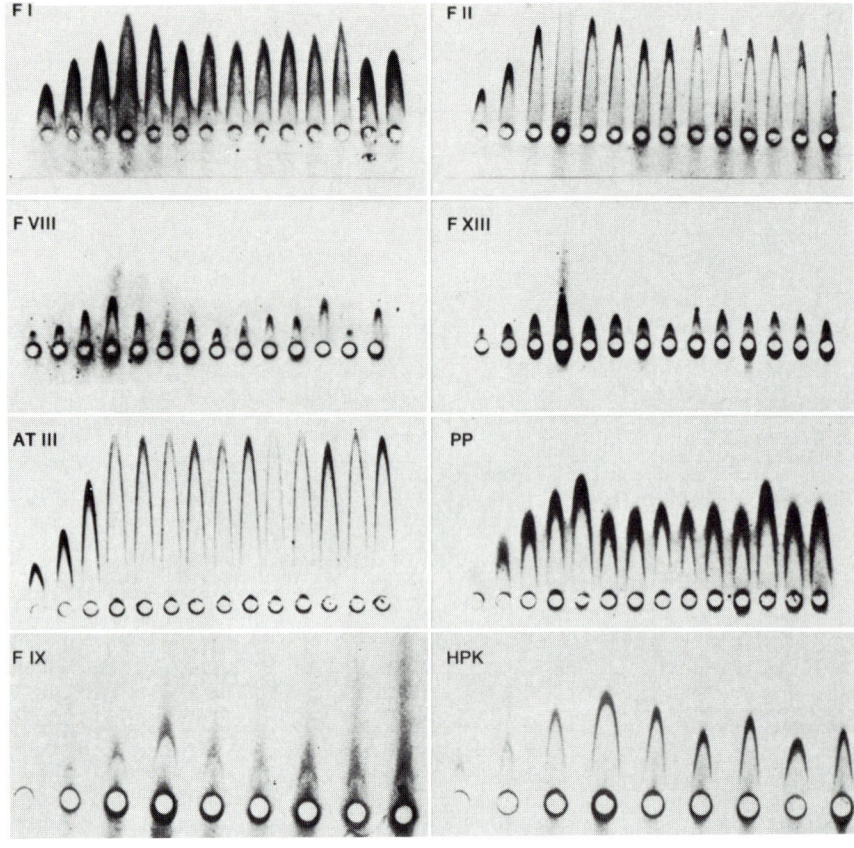

Fig. 11-15. Determination of fibrinogen *(F I)*, prothrombin *(F II)*, antihemophilic globulin A *(F VIII)*, fibrin stabilizing factor *(F XIII)*, antithrombin III *(AT III)*, plasminogen *(PP)*, antihemophilic globulin B *(F IX)*, and human plasma kallikrein *(HPK)* by electroimmunoassay. First four samples on left of each plate are dilutions of standard human plasma (for construction of calibration curve), and these are followed by 5 or 10 samples of plasma from normal individuals. (From Heimburger, N., and Karges, H.E.: Med. Lab. **5:**1, 1978.)

Table 11-11. Outline of preparation of normal factor activity (dilution) curve

Tube	1	2	3	4	5	6	7
Buffer (ml)	0.9	0.5	0.5	0.5	0.5	0.5	0.5
Normal plasma control (ml)	0.1	—	—	—	—	—	—
Mix and transfer (ml)	0.5	0.5	0.5	0.5	0.5	0.5	0.5
Dilution	1:10	1:20	1:40	1:80	1:160	1:320	1:640
Factor V activity (%)	100	50	25	12.5	6.25	3.1	1.5

1. Prepare reference curve.
   a. Prepare seven dilutions (1:10, 1:20, 1:40, 1:80, 1:160, 1:320, and 1:640) of normal control plasma by dilution with buffer (Table 11-11). The dilutions represent 100%, 50%, 25% 12.5%, 6.25%, 3.1%, and 1.5% of factor V activity.
   b. In a glass tube add 0.1 ml factor V–deficient substrate plasma to 0.1 ml 1:10 normal diluted plasma from tube 1, mix well, and incubate in heating block for 3 min.
   c. Place tube in test well and add 0.2 ml thromboplastin-calcium reagent and record clotting

time. Repeat test and record average time, which should be 18-28 sec.
   d. Repeat steps b and c using each normal plasma dilution and perform duplicate determinations, which should agree within 5%.
   e. Plot result on two cycle log-log paper with percent of dilution on the abscissa and the time in seconds on the ordinate. Connected points should produce a straight line.
2. Perform assay of patient's plasma.
   a. Dilute patient's plasma 1:10 in buffer (0.1 ml plasma plus 0.9 ml buffer)
   b. Test plasma as outlined in steps b and c

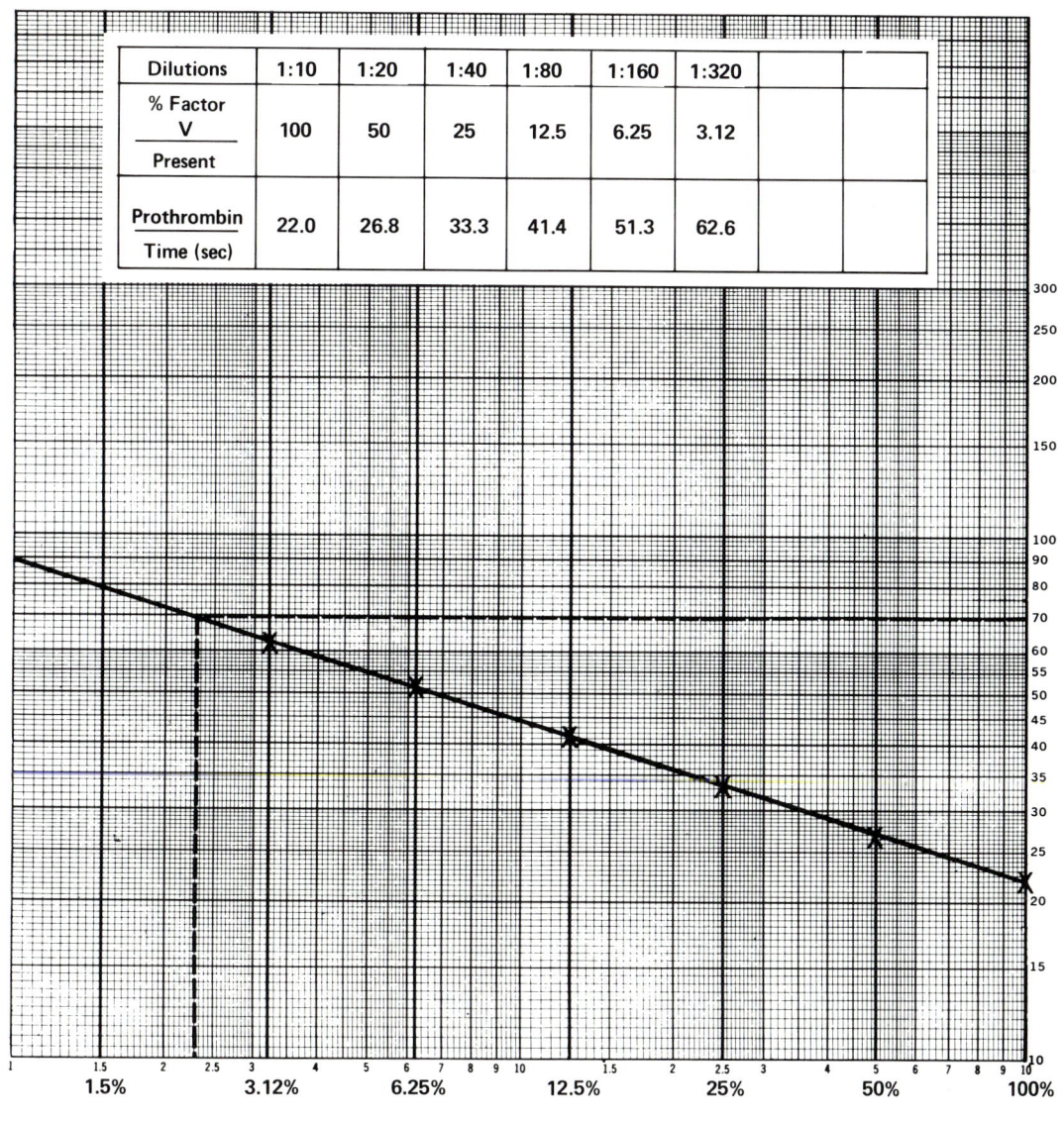

Dilutions	1:10	1:20	1:40	1:80	1:160	1:320		
% Factor V Present	100	50	25	12.5	6.25	3.12		
Prothrombin Time (sec)	22.0	26.8	33.3	41.4	51.3	62.6		

Plasma Dilutions in Percent

Fig. 11-16. Typical normal factor V assay curve. (Produced with permission of author and publisher. © American Hospital Supply Corp.)

c. The time in seconds is related to percent activity by reading the latter value off the normal control activity curve (Fig. 11-16).

One-stage assay of factors II, VII, and X

The theory and technic of the assays of factors II, VII and X are the same as described earlier for factor V, except that factor II–, VII–, and X–deficient substrate plasmas are used (Dade Diagnostics, Miami, Fla.).

Assay procedures for intrinsic factors
One-stage assay of factor VIII

Principle[196-198]: The prolonged partial thromboplastin time of a substrate plasma deficient in factor VIII is shortened by the addition of normal (control) or patient's plasma. The degree of correction is proportional to the amount of factor VIII in the normal or unknown plasma.

Reagents and equipment:
1. Activated partial thromboplastin reagent (Actin, Dade Diagnostics, Miami, Fla.)
2. CaCl$_2$, 0.02M
3. Owren's veronal buffer, pH 7.35
4. Fresh citrated normal control plasma pool
5. Factor VIII–deficient substrate plasma (Dade Diagnostics, Miami, Fla.)
6. Patient's plasma, citrated
7. Ice bath
8. Coagulation Profiler (Bio/Data Corp., Willow Grove, Pa.)

Table 11-12. Serial dilution of normal plasma

Tube	1	2	3	4	5	6	7
Buffer (ml)	0.9	0.5	0.5	0.5	0.5	0.5	0.5
Normal plasma (ml)	0.1	—	—	—	—	—	—
Mix and transfer (ml)	0.5	0.5	0.5	0.5	0.5	0.5	0.5
Dilution	1:10	1:20	1:40	1:80	1:160	1:320	1:640
Factor VIII activity (%)	100	50	25	12.5	6.25	3.1	1.5

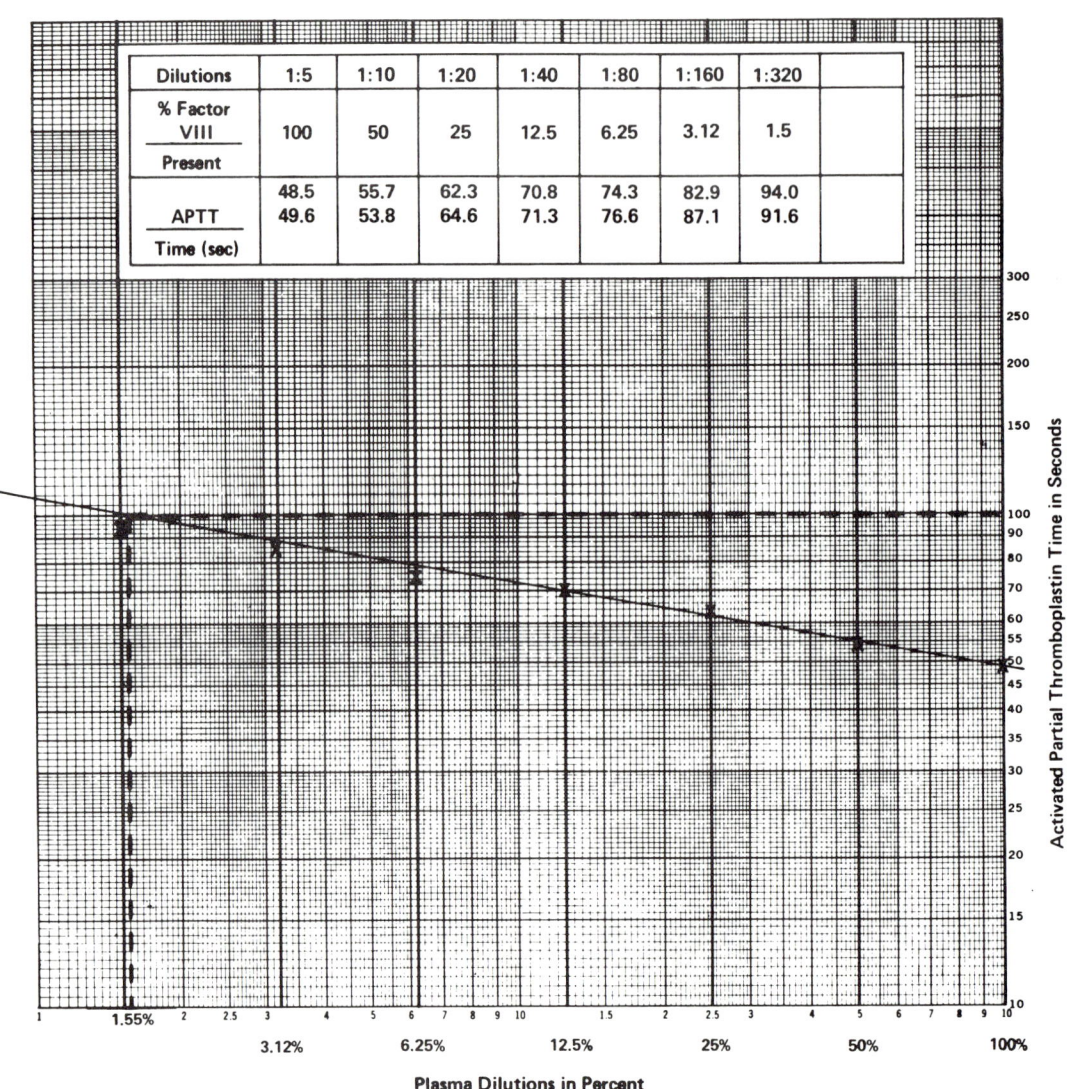

Dilutions	1:5	1:10	1:20	1:40	1:80	1:160	1:320	
% Factor VIII Present	100	50	25	12.5	6.25	3.12	1.5	
APTT Time (sec)	48.5 49.6	55.7 53.8	62.3 64.6	70.8 71.3	74.3 76.6	82.9 87.1	94.0 91.6	

Plasma Dilutions in Percent

Fig. 11-17. Typical normal factor VIII assay curve. (Produced with permission of author and publisher. © American Hospital Supply Corp.)

Procedure: Keep all plasma samples in ice water until just prior to use. Keep partial thromboplastin reagent at room temperature. Keep $CaCl_2$ at 37° C.

Preparation of normal factor activity dilution curve:
1. Prepare serial dilution of normal plasma in buffer as shown in Table 11-12.
2. To 0.1 ml partial thromboplastin reagent add 0.1 ml factor VIII–deficient substrate and 0.1 ml 1:10 diluted normal plasma.
3. Mix well and incubate for exactly 3 min.
4. Add prewarmed $CaCl_2$ and record clotting time.
5. Run duplicate determination of 1:10 dilution and repeat steps 2, 3, and 4 in duplicate for each plasma dilution. Duplicates should agree within 5%.
6. Plot results on two-cycle log-log paper with percent dilution on the abscissa and the time in seconds on the ordinate. Connected points should produce a straight line (Fig. 11-17).

Assay of patient's plasma:
1. Dilute patient's plasma 1:10 in buffer.
2. Test plasma as outlined in steps 2, 3, and 4.
3. The time in seconds is related to percent activity by reading off the normal control activity curve (Fig. 11-17).

NOTE: The activity curve need not be prepared each time a factor VIII assay is performed if the same lot of control plasma, partial thromboplastin reagent, and factor-deficient substrate is used. On a daily basis a 1:10 dilution of the control plasma should be run and the resulting clotting time should closely approximate the times obtained when the original curve was derived.

One-stage assay of factors IX, XI, and XII

The procedure for assay of factors IX, XI, and XII is the same as that for factor VIII except that commercially available factor IX–, XI–, and XII–deficient substrate plasmas are used.

Immunologic diagnosis of factor VIII activity

Laurell rocket electrophoresis and **cross immunoelectrophoresis** share certain reagents and pieces of equipment, which are discussed below.

Reagents:
1. Barbital buffer, 0.075 mole/L, pH 8.6
   Dissolve 2.76 g barbital and 14.5 g barbital sodium in about 950 ml water in a 1 L volumetric flask. Gentle heating may be needed in dissolving the barbital. Cool, dilute to 1 L, and mix well. Check the pH and adjust to 8.60 ± 0.05 with a few drops of 0.5 mole/L NaOH (NaOH, 200 g/L) or HC1 (concentrated, 42 ml/L) as required.
2. Coomassie blue stain
   Dissolve 1.25 g Coomassie brilliant blue R (C.I. 42660) in a mixture of 225 ml methanol, 240 ml water, and 45 ml glacial acetic acid. When all the dye has dissolved, filter once.
3. Barbital-buffered saline for sample dilution
   Dissolve 2.06 g barbital sodium, 2.76 g barbital, and 7.31 g sodium chloride in water to make 1 L. Check the pH and, if necessary, adjust to 7.5 ± 0.1.
4. Acetic acid destaining solution, 1.3 moles/L
   Dilute 75 ml glacial acetic acid to 1 L with water.

5. Agarose (Sea-Kem, Marine Colloids, Rockland, Me.) for the preparation of the slides
   Agarose is made into a gel for coating the slides in which the electrophoresis takes place. A convenient size for the slides is 8 × 10 cm (3¼ × 4 in). Other sizes can be used if they are better adapted to the particular electrophoresis chamber used. The one suggested is the Gelman Deluxe (Gelman Instrument Co., Ann Arbor, Mich.) with the Gelman power supply.

Before the slides are used in the electrophoresis with agarose containing the appropriate antibody, they are first precoated with a thin layer of plain agarose. For this purpose prepare a solution of 3.0 g agarose in 2 dl water. Heat the water to boiling and add the agarose. Stir until dissolved. Cook somewhat and place the solution in a water bath at 54° C. With a prewarmed pipet add 2 ml agarose solution to a prewarmed slide. Spread the agarose evenly over the slide with an applicator stick. Allow to dry overnight at room temperature and then store at 4° C.

Equipment:
1. Electrophoresis chamber and power supply
2. Glass slides, 3¼ × 4 in (Kodak, Rochester, N.Y.)
3. Water bath, boiling and 54° C
4. Well cutter, 4 mm (BioRad Laboratories, Richmond Calif.)
5. Wicks, 8 × 10 cm (Schleicher & Schuell, Keene, N.H.)
6. Bibulous paper (Scientific Products, McGaw Park, Ill.)
7. Pipets, 25 ml, 0-20 μl, and 0-200 μl (adjustable)
8. Magnifying loop (Bausch & Lomb, Rochester, N.Y.)
9. Two-cycle semi-log paper

Quantitation of factor VIII–associated antigen

Principle: The high-molecular-weight antigenic portion of the factor VIII molecule is measured by means of the Laurell "rocket" electrophoresis. The factor VIII antigen is electrophoresed through an agar gel containing antiserum to factor VIII. The length of the rocket-shaped immunoprecipitate formed is a measure of the amount of the antigen present. The results obtained with various dilutions of the sample plasma are compared with the results obtained with dilutions of pooled normal plasma. Except for the dilutions and the antisera used, the procedure as given is the same for a number of other specific proteins and can be used for them with obvious modifications. After electrophoresis the slide may be stained to enhance the visibility of the precipitate.

Reagent: Use antiserum to human factor VIII–associated protein (Calbiochem-Behring Corp., San Diego, Calif.).

Procedure: Dilute a portion of the 0.075 mole/L barbital buffer given earlier 1:3 with water. Heat 5 dl diluted buffer to boiling, add 4.5 g agarose, and continue heating with constant stirring until a clear solution is obtained. Then cool the solution somewhat and place in a water bath at 54° C.

When the solution has cooled to 54° C, add the appropriate amount of the antiserum to an aliquot of the agarose solution to give a 1:100 concentration of the antiserum. The actual amount of the antiserum used will depend on the particular lot used; the package insert should give information in this regard. Mix well by gentle stirring and avoid the formation of air bubbles in the agarose.

Using a prewarmed 25 ml Mohr pipet, slowly deliver 15 ml agarose-antibody mixture onto a precoated glass slide. The slide should be on a perfectly level surface, and the solution on the slide should be level and run up to the corners of the slide. When the agarose has solidified, store in a container with moist gauze (to prevent drying out) at 4° C for up to 2-3 weeks.

For use, dilute aliquots of the control plasma 1:2, 1:4, and 1:8 and dilute the sample plasma 1:2 and 1:4. Just before use mark the starting positions on a prepared slide as indicated in Fig. 11-18. The positions are in a row 6 mm apart and 2 cm from the long edge of the slide. Then punch 14 wells about 2.5 mm in diameter following the hole punch guide (Figs. 11-15 and 11-18), removing the agar by suction.

Place 15 μl undiluted control plasma and the three dilutions at various positions in the row and the undiluted sample and its two dilutions at other positions. Positions 1 and 2 should contain the same plasma or dilutions as should positions 13 and 14. This is to compensate for the fact that sometimes the migration from the two end positions is not as uniform as from the other positions.

Fill the electrophoresis chambers with the undiluted buffer. Place the slides in the chamber with the wells toward the cathode and establish good wick contact with the agarose surface as outlined in the procedure manual for the instrument.

Place the cover on the chamber, set the power source to 10 mA per slide at constant current and electrophorese for 18 hr (overnight).

After electrophoresis, turn off the current and remove the slide from the chamber. Press the slide using filter paper and paper towels covered by a glass plate and additional weight of several kilograms. This should be done with care to prevent wrinkling or cracking of the agarose. Press for 15 min, change the paper, and press for another 15 min.

Rinse the slides twice for 15 min each in normal saline, then rinse the slides once in distilled water for 15 min. Next cover the slide with a wet bibulous paper and allow to dry at room temperature or in an oven at 60-70° C.

After drying, place the slides in the Coomassie blue stain for 15 min, and then rinse the slides briefly in the acetic acid solution. Remove the excess stain from the back of the slides and allow them to dry at room temperature.

Measure the lengths of the rockets obtained in nanometers using a measuring magnifier. Plot the standards (pooled normal plasma dilutions) against the rocket height on semi-log paper with the heights on the linear scale, or plot the logarithms of the standard concentrations against the rocket height on regular linear graph paper (Fig. 11-19). Note that the undiluted normal plasma and the 1:2, 1:4, and 1:8 dilutions correspond to 100%, 50%, 25%, and 12.5% of normal activity. In the example that follows, the calculations are given for plotting the logarithm using the same type of calculations; an example is given using semi-log paper. The values for the sample dilutions are read off the curve and multiplied by the appropriate dilution factor (see following example).

Example: Suppose that the values obtained with the dilutions of the normal plasma were as follows:

Activity (%)	Rocket height	Log (% of activity)
100	15.4	2.000
50	11.5	1.699
25	7.6	1.398
12.5	3.5	1.097

These values are plotted as the small dots in Fig. 11-19.

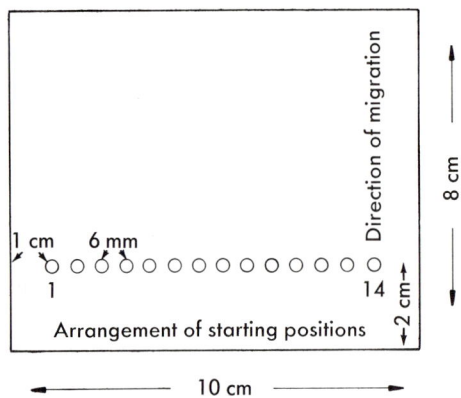

Fig. 11-18. Agarose antiserum plate.

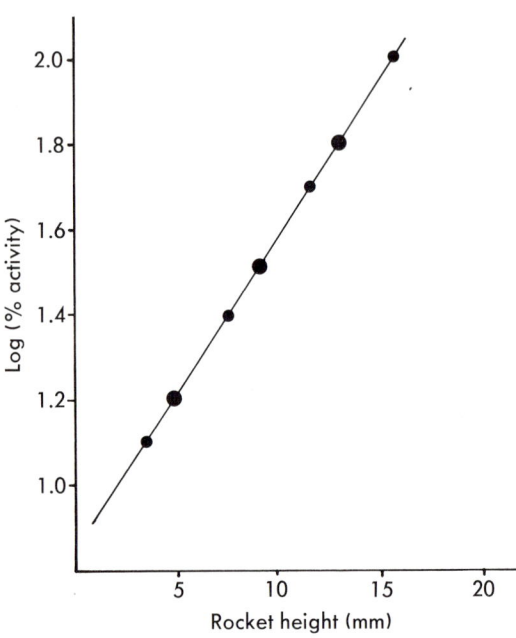

Fig. 11-19. Linear graph showing relationship of rocket height to log percent activity.

Example: Suppose also that the following values were obtained for the dilutions of the sample:

Dilution	Rocket height (mm)	Log (% of activity) read from curve	Activity (%) of dilution	Total activity
1:4	5.0	1.200	15.9 × 4 =	63.6
1:2	9.0	1.500	31.6 × 2 =	63.2
1	12.0	1.800	63.1	63.1

These points are plotted on the curve as the large dots.

NOTES: Each laboratory must experiment with the details of the electrophoresis, e.g., amperage and time, to get the optimal results. The dilutions of the sample plasma to be used will depend on the activity expected. As noted below, some patients may have greater than normal activity in the plasma, whereas other patients may have very low values, in which case the undiluted serum should be run.

Interpretation: Patients with hemophilia A have normal levels of factor VIII–related antigen, and female carriers of hemophilia A may show levels that are normal or above normal. On the other hand, patients with von Willebrand's disease lack factor VIII–related antigen (Fig. 11-20).

Factor VIII crossed immunoelectrophoresis

The molecular weight structure of the high-molecular weight, antigenically active portion of the factor VIII molecule (factor VIII–associated antigen) may be estimated by two-dimensional crossed immunoelectrophoresis.

A linear distribution of the different subunits making up the factor VIII–related antigen is obtained by electrophoresis in agarose gel. The distribution of these components is then characterized by electrophoresis a second time at right angles through a gel containing antiserum to the factor VIII–related antigen. Immunoprecipitate arcs are formed, the shape and position of which are then compared with those obtained from normal pooled plasma (Figs. 11-21 and 11-22).

Factor XIII deficiency screening test

Principle[199]: The normal cross-linked fibrin clot is the result of the action of the thrombin activated factor XIII on the polymerized fibrin monomers (fibrin$_s$) in the presence of calcium. The polymerized fibrin monomer clot is soluble in 5M (30%) urea and in 2% acetic acid but the cross-linked fibrin clot (fibrin$_i$) is produced by the action of factor XIII. The screening test for factor XIII is based on the differential clot solubility.

Reagents:
1. 30% urea solution (aqueous)
2. 2% acetic acid
3. $CaCl_2$, 0.025M (37° C)
4. Citrated plasma (patient and control, platelet poor)
5. Glass tubes, 12 × 75 mm
6. Water bath, 37° C

Procedure: Place 0.2 ml plasma into each of two glass tubes in 37° C heating block. To each tube add

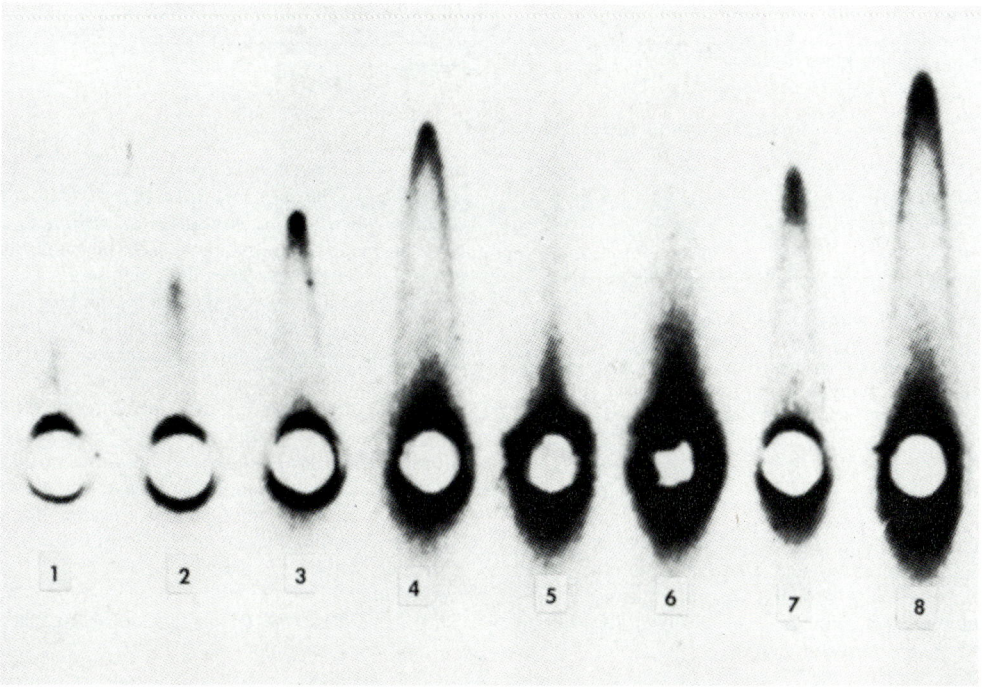

Fig. 11-20. Electroimmunodiffusion (Laurell method) in agarose with antiserum against factor VIII–associated antigen. Standard human plasma in dilutions of 1:8, 1:4, 1:2, and 1:1 (in wells 1- 4); von Willebrand's plasma (in wells 5 and 6); hemophilia A plasma in dilutions of 1:2 and 1:1 (in wells 7 and 8). (From Heimburger, N., and Karges, H.E.: Med. Lab. **5:**1, 1978.)

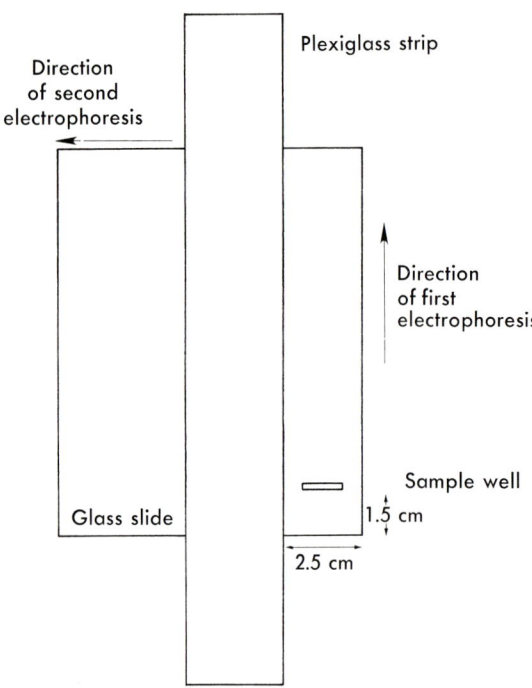

Fig. 11-21. Factor VIII crossed immunoelectrophoresis in agarose gel.

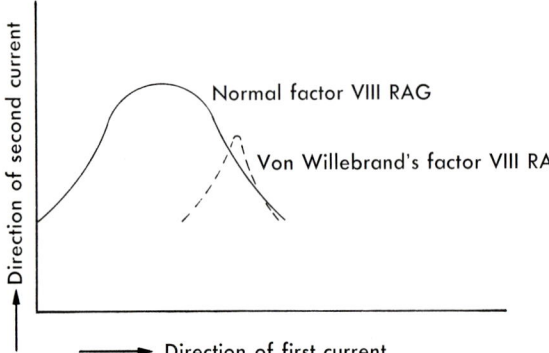

Fig. 11-22. Sketch of qualitative evaluation of factor VIII RAG by crossed immunoelectrophoresis, allowing differentiation between normal and von Willebrand's disease.

0.2 ml prewarmed CaCl$_2$. Allow clot to stand for 10 min after which time add 2.5 ml urea solution to one tube and 2.5 ml acetic acid solution to the other. Free clot from sides with glass rod without injuring it. Observe clot every 15 min for 1 hr and then allow to sit overnight and observe in morning.

Result: Normal clots (over 2% factor XIII) do not dissolve in either solution.

Interpretation: Disappearance of the clot is evidence of inadequate factor XIII levels.

TESTS OF FIBRINOLYSIS AND INTRAVASCULAR COAGULATION

The fibrinolytic system is made up of a number of components, which can be assayed individually or their combined activity can be measured.

The tests can be grouped as follows:
1. Tests evaluating systemic fibrinolysis
    a. Whole blood or plasma clot lysis time (p. 292)
    b. Fibrinogen assay (see p. 301)
    c. Euglobulin lysis time
    d. Plasminogen assays
2. Tests for fibrin (fibrinogen) degradation products (FDPs)
    a. Thrombo-Wellco test (direct latex agglutination test)
3. Estimation of circulating soluble fibrin monomers
    a. Ethanol gelation test
    b. Protamine sulfate test
    c. Cryofibrinogen determination
4. Assays of inhibitors of the fibrinolytic system

Tests evaluating systemic fibrinolysis
Whole blood clot lysis time and plasma clot lysis time

Tests for whole blood clot lysis time and plasma clot lysis time are discussed under the heading of the Lee-White clotting time and the plasma clotting time.

Interpretation: The tests are too insensitive to discover low-grade fibrinolytic activity and should be replaced by the euglobulin lysis time and the thrombin time. The lack of sensitivity is a result of the presence of natural inhibitors of fibrinolysis, which rapidly neutralize plasmin as it forms and thus prevent fibrinolysis. The euglobulin lysis time test reduces the concentration of inhibitors by dilution and uses an inhibitor-free protein clot.

Euglobulin lysis time

The euglobulin lysis time[200-202] is a sensitive test for plasma plasminogen activators.

Principle: The euglobulin fraction of plasma is precipitated when plasma is diluted and acidified. It contains fibrinogen, plasminogen, and plasminogen activators and lacks the fibrinolytic inhibitors present in normal plasma. Very dilute acetic acid is added to plasma to precipitate the euglobulins, which are separated from the normal inhibitors present in plasma by differences in their solubility in water. After centrifugation the supernatant is discarded, the precipitate is dissolved in borate buffer, and the fibrinogen is clotted with thrombin. In the absence of plasmin or plasminogen inhibitors, plasminogen is activated to plasmin by the precipitated plasminogen activators, and the time it takes for plasmin to dissolve the fibrin clot completely is the euglobulin lysis time.

Reagents:
1. Citrated plasma (test and control) in plastic test tubes in ice water
2. Acetic acid, 1% aqueous
    The pH of the plasma acid mixture is a critical 6.2
3. Sodium borate buffer, pH 9.0:

a. NaCl, 9g

b. Sodium borate, 1 g

c. Distilled water to 1 L

4. Thrombin, bovine, 5 units/ml in normal saline solution in plastic test tubes at 37° C

Procedure: Perform test in duplicate within 20 min of obtaining the specimen. Most handling should be at 4° C. Add 0.5 ml plasma to 9.0 ml distilled water and mix by inversion against Parafilm. Add 0.1 acetic acid and mix as above (pH 6.2). Allow euglobulin to precipitate by incubating tubes at 4° C for 30 min. Centrifuge mixtures as above at 4° C. Invert tube and allow it to drain on filter paper for 2 min. Wipe walls of tube dry with cotton applicator to prevent antiplasmin from draining back onto the sediment. Do not disturb button of precipitate.

Insert tube in 37° C water bath. Add 0.5 ml sodium borate and stir with glass rod until euglobulin precipitate is dissolved. Clot euglobulin by adding 0.5 ml thrombin solution at 37 ° C, and mix thoroughly. Confirm clot formation by tilting.

Incubate at 37° C and observe for clot dissolution at 5 min intervals for $^1/_2$ hr and then at 10 min intervals for 2 hr or until clot has disappeared. The end point is complete dissolution of the clot.

Normal values: Normal euglobulin lysis takes longer than 120 min. There are marked variations from day to day.

Interpretation: If the plasminogen and fibrinogen levels are known to be normal, and since plasmin is usually not present in plasma because of the action of antiplasmin, an accelerated (below 2 hr) euglobulin lysis time is indicative of increased plasminogen activator activity as seen in disseminated intravascular coagulation, but it may also be caused by vascular irritation from failure to release the tourniquet rapidly, excessive pumping, or excessive rubbing with the alcohol swab. The plasma must be platelet poor since platelets contain plasmin and plasminogen inhibitors. The inhibitors of plasminogen activators are kept ineffective by handling the plasma in the cold and by diluting it. If the fibrinogen concentration is low, the test cannot be interpreted since small clots may lyse rapidly. The test should then be repeated after the addition of plasminogen and plasminogen activator–free fibrinogen, which is available commercially (Organon, West Orange, N.J.). Heparin does not interfere with the test since it is discarded with the inhibitors in the supernatant.[203]

Plasminogen assays

Two technics are presented, the time-honored caseolytic method and the more recent fluorometric assay.

Caseolytic method[204]

Principle: Plasma is treated with acid to inactivate the antiplasmins and is then restored to neutral pH. The plasminogen is then activated by the addition of streptokinase, and the plasmin thus produced is assayed by its ability to digest α-casein. After hydrolysis the undigested casein is precipitated with trichloroacetic acid and the tyrosine in the supernatant is measured at 275 nm. The amount is proportional to the original plasminogen concentration.

Reagents:

1. Hydrochloric acid, 0.17 mole/L
   Dilute 14 ml concentrated acid to 1 L with water.

2. Sodium hydroxide, 0.17 mole/L
   Dissolve 6.7 g NaOH in water to make 1 L. NOTE: The exact normality of these two solutions is not as important as the fact that they should be equivalent in strength. After preparation, one solution should be titrated against the other and the stronger solution diluted so that both are of the same concentration.

3. TES-NaCl (Calbiochem-Behring Corp., San Diego) buffer, pH 7.5
   Dissolve 13.75 g of *N*-tris(hydroxymethyl)methyl-2-aminoethane sulfonic acid and 5.26 g sodium chloride in about 9 dl water, adjust the pH to 7.5 with the addition of 1 mole/L NaOH, and then dilute to 1 L with water.

4. Gelatin buffer
   Dissolve 2 g purified calfskin gelatin in 2 dl buffer by heating in a boiling water bath until all the gelatin has dissolved. Then filter through Whatman no. 1 paper. Store frozen in 10 ml aliquots.

5. Streptokinase (20,000 units/ml)
   Dissolve the contents of a lyophilized vial (Sigma Chemical Co., St. Louis) in the gelatin buffer to give a concentration of 20,000 units/ml. Store frozen in small capped tubes.

6. Trichloroacetic acid, 0.6 mole/L
   Dissolve 10 g trichloroacetic acid in water to make 1 dl.

7. α-Casein (Sigma C-7891, Sigma Chemical Co., St Louis) 14 g/L
   Dissolve 1.4 g casein in 1 dl buffer. Store frozen in aliquots sufficient for 1 day's use.

8. Plasminogen standard*
   Dissolve lyophilized contents of a vial in buffer to give a concentration of 10.0 CTA units per ml. Store frozen in aliquots of 0.4 ml. Thaw just before use and add 3.6 ml buffer to give a concentration of 1.0 unit/ml.

Procedure: Obtain platelet-poor plasma by centrifuging citrated blood at 5° C in plastic tubes, carefully remove plasma, and store in refrigerator until used.

In a 13 × 100 mm test tube place 0.5 ml plasma, warmed to room temperature. Add 0.5 ml of 0.17 mole/L HC1 and mix on a vortex briefly. Allow to stand for 15 min.

Add 0.5 ml of 0.17 mole/L NaOH and mix. Transfer 0.5 ml of the mixture to each of two small test tubes (duplicate plasma samples), and add 1.9 ml buffer.

Add 0.1 ml streptokinase reagent to one tube and mix on a vortex briefly. Twenty seconds after the addition of the streptokinase, add 2.5 ml casein solution (previously warmed to 37° C) and mix.

Place in water bath at 37° C and at 2 min and 32 min after the addition of the casein, remove 2 ml aliquots

---

*This may be obtained from Dr. Alan J. Hohnson, American National Red Cross, New York University Medical Center, 550 First Avenue, New York, N.Y. 10016.

Table 11-13. Suggested schedule of operations

Time (min:sec)	Operation	Time (min:sec)	Operation	Time (min:sec)	Operation*
00:00	SK-10	12:00	SK-4	32:20	TCA-10
00:20	CA-10	12:20	CA-4	36:20	TCA-8
02:20	TCA-10	14:20	TCA-4	40:20	TCA-6
04:00	SK-8	16:00	SK-2	44:20	TCA-4
04:20	CA-8	16:20	CA-2	48:20	TCA-2
06:20	TCA-8	18:20	TCA-2	52:20	TCA-0
08:00	SK-6	20:00	SK-0		
08:20	CA-6	20:20	CA-0		
10:20	TCA-6	22:20	TCA-0		

*The second TCA precipitation must be distinguished from the first.

of the incubating mixture and add to 3.0 ml trichloroacetic acid solution. Mix and allow to stand for 30 min at room temperature. Treat other tube similarly.

Centrifuge the tubes at 2000 *g* at 5° C for 15 min or until a clear supernatant is obtained.

Transfer the supernatant to cuvets (preferably with a 1 cm light path) and read the 32 min sample against the 2 min sample as blank at 275 nm.

Obtain the activity of the sample from a standard curve prepared as given in the next discussion.

Standard curve: To a series of small test tubes add 1.0, 0.8, 0.6, 0.4, 0.2, and 0.0 ml plasminogen standard and buffer to bring the volume in each tube to 2.4 ml. Then, in a series of timed steps, add 0.1 ml streptokinase to the first tube; 20 sec later add 2.5 ml casein solution to this tube. Place tube in 37° C water bath, and at 120 min withdraw 2.0 ml of the incubating solution and add to a labeled tube containing 3.0 ml trichloroacetic acid solution and mix. Continue incubation of the remaining solution in the first tube and start the timed reactions in the second tube in a similar manner.

As an example of how the timing might be done, consider the following schedule where SK-10 means add the streptokinase (0.1 ml) to tube 10 (for convenience the tubes are labeled 10, 8, 6, 4, 2, and 0 in the order given above), CA-10 means add 2.5 ml of the casein solution to tube 10 and place in incubator, and TCA-10 means withdraw 2 ml of the mixture from tube 10 and add this to labeled tube containing 3 ml trichloroacetic acid solution and treat as mentioned above for sample. Then a schedule might be made up like the one given in Table 11-13.

After centrifugation, as for the samples, the clear supernatants are read at 275 nm. As with the sample, each supernatant obtained after 30 min incubation (TCA-10, etc. in schedule above) is read against the corresponding 2 min supernatant. Subtract the net reading for the 0 tubes from the net for the others and plot the resulting absorbances against the activity (1.0, 0.8, 0.6, 0.4, and 0.2 units/ml). Draw the best straight line through the points. For the sample absorbance (average of duplicates) read off activity from the curve and multiply by 6 to give the activity of the sample in units per milliliter (one third of a 0.5 ml sample is used in the final determination).

NOTE: If preliminary experiments indicate that the equipment available does not give a perfectly clear su-

pernatant for the absorbance readings, the supernatant may be filtered through a Millipore filter (Millipore Corp., Bedford, Mass.) (AAWP 01300, 0.8 using Swinnox filter units SX 0001300).

Normal values: The normal level by this method is 2.7-4.5 ±0.5 units/ml.

Interpretation: Since plasminogen is the precursor of plasmin, it may be reduced in clinical fibrinolytic states. Usually this reduction wil be secondary to disseminated intravascular coagulation, but it may also be primary as a result of cirrhosis or plasminogen activator–secreting tumors or as a result of treatment with streptokinase or urokinase infusions. A further reason for plasminogen reduction in disseminated intravascular coagulation is the fact that it is coprecipitated with fibrin.

Plasminogen is commonly elevated in the latter part of pregnancy and in inflammatory exudates.

Plasminogen assay (fluorometric method)

A synthetic substrate is hydrolyzed by plasmin produced by the conversion of plasminogen to plasmin by adding streptokinase. The rate of formation of the fluorescent hydrolysis product is observed with a recording spectrofluorometer. The activity is compared with that of a standard plasmin preparation. The actual plasmin concentration in the original sample may be measured by omitting the initial activation with streptokinase.

The fluorometric method[205] is somewhat more sensitive than the colorimetric methods, which yield paranitroaniline as the chromogen.[204] However, they do require a spectrofluorometer such as the Turner Model 430 (Turner Associates, Palo Alto, Calif.) with a good recorder or the special instrument produced by Dade Diagnostics, Miami, Fla., for this and similar assays.

The reagents and procedure outlined below are for use with a spectrofluorometer. When the Dade instrument is used, the reagents are supplied in kit form.

Collection of plasma sample: Blood is collected in a plastic syringe and immediately mixed with the anticoagulant: 9 volumes blood + 1 volume trisodium citrate solution (0.147 mole/L, 38 g/L) in a plastic tube. Contact with glass should be avoided for the undiluted plasma. The blood is centrifuged for 15 min at 2000 *g* and the plasma carefully removed. If the samples are not assayed at once, they should be stored at −20° C.

Reagents:

1. Assay buffer, 0.05 mole/L tris, 0.05 mole/L glycine, pH 8.0

   Dissolve 6.05 g tris (hydroxymethyl)aminomethane and 3.76 g glycine in about 9 dl distilled water in a 1 L volumetric flask. Adjust the pH to 8.0 by the addition of 1 mole/L HCl (83 ml concentrated acid diluted to 1 L). Add 0.3 ml Brij-35 (30% solution) and dilute to 1 L and mix well.

2. Activation buffer, 0.05 mole/L tris, 0.1 mol/L glycine

   Dissolve 6.05 g tris and 7.51 g glycine in about 9 dl water, adjust pH to 7.5 with 1 mole/L HCl, and then dilute to 1 L.

3. Bovine albumin, 12 g/dl

   A commercial 30% bovine albumin solution is diluted by adding 20 ml of the solution to 30 ml saline (8.8 g/L NaCl).

4. Streptokinase, 2000 units/ml

   A lyophilized vial containing 100,000 units (Lederle Laboratories, Pearl River, N.Y.) is diluted to 50 ml with the activation buffer. The mixture is then divided into small aliquots and stored at −20° C.

5. Plasminogen reference material (standard)

   A solution containing 9.7 CTA units per ml in 50% glycerol* is diluted 1:2 with 12 g/dl bovine albumin solution to give a solution containing 4.85 units/ml. Further dilutions with 6 g/dl may be made if it is desired to construct a calibration curve.

6. Substrate solution, 0.8 mmole/L

   Sixty-two milligrams H-D-valine-leucine-lysine-5-amidoisophthalic acid, dimethyl ester (Enzyme System Products, Indianapolis), is dissolved in 1 dl assay buffer. Portions are warmed to 37° C before use.

Procedure: Add 10 μl plasma or standard (4.85 units/ml) to 0.5 ml streptokinase solution. Mix on a vortex and incubate for 15 min at 37° C.

To 2.0 ml assay substrate solution warmed to 37° C add 200 μl of incubated mixture and follow the rate of change of fluorescence in the fluorometer for 4 min. The relative rate of change of the fluorescence is obtained from the recorder tracing. Then

$$\text{Plasmin (CTA units/ml)} = \frac{\text{Relative rate of sample}}{\text{Relative rate of standard}} \times 4.85$$

Normal range: The normal range by this method is 2.5-5.2 units/ml. (NOTE: A somewhat narrower range is given by the Dade instrument.)

Tests for fibrin (fibrinogen) degradation products

The Thrombo-Wellco test (direct latex agglutination test)†

Plasmin lyses fibrin/fibrinogen into progressively smaller fragments starting with the high-molecular-weight degradation products X and Y and ending with the completely degraded materials D and E. All fibrin/fibrinogen degradation products (FDPs) share antigenic determinants with fibrin/fibrinogen and can therefore be demonstrated immunologically by the use of antifibrinogen antiserum. In order to avoid interference by fibrinogen, thrombin is added to the test specimen to ensure complete clotting and complete removal of fibrinogen, a process that has the disadvantage of trapping some of the FDPs and falsely reducing the total FDP concentration in serum. A falsely elevated FDP level is guarded against by the addition of soybean trypsin inhibitor to the test system to avoid in vitro activation of fibrinolysis and in vitro production of FDPs. Other inhibitors of fibrinolysis may be added, e.g., ε-aminocaproic acid (EACA).

Principle: The Thrombo-Wellco test is a rapid, reliable, direct latex slide test for the semiquantitative assay of FDPs. Latex particles suspended in glycine saline buffer are coated with specific antifragment D and E globulins. In the presence of FDP in the serum or urine, the latex particles clump together producing macroscopic agglutination. By testing the unknown sample at different dilutions, the approximate concentration of FDPs can be determined. The sensitivity of the test is standardized at 1 μg FDPs/ml.

Reagents and equipment: Each kit contains the following:

1. Latex suspension
2. Positive and negative control sera
3. Sample collection vacuum tubes containing bovine thrombin and soybean trypsin inhibitor
4. Glycine saline buffer
5. Glass test slide with four rings for testing one or two samples and two controls
6. Disposable pipets, mixing rods, and rubber bulb Store kit at 4° C.

Procedure[206]: Collect 2 ml venous blood in special sample collecting tube and immediately mix by inverting tube several times. Ring clot and allow tube to stand at 37° C for 1/2 hr or centrifuge tube immediately after sample has clotted. If the patient is on heparin therapy, 0.2 ml of Reptilase R (Abbott Laboratories, North Chicago, Ill.) should be added to 2 ml blood to promote clotting in the presence of heparin. Reptilase treatment will lower the FDP concentration.

Mark two small test tubes 1 and 2 and mark two of the rings on the glass slide 1 and 2. Place 0.75 ml glycine saline buffer in each test tube.

Add 5 drops serum sample to test tube 1 (1:5 dilution of serum) and 1 drop to test tube 2 (1:20 dilution of serum) and mix. Transfer 1 drop from test tube 2 to position 2 of the reaction slide and 1 drop from test tube 1 to position 1.

Mix latex suspension vigorously and add 1 drop to each position on the glass slide. Stir serum/latex mixtures, starting with position 2 and spread mixtures to fill the circles. Rock slide gently for exactly 2 min and examine for macroscopic agglutination by viewing slide against a dark background.

Result: The agglutination in position 1 indicates an FDP concentration in the original serum in excess of 10 μg/ml. Agglutination in position in position 2 indi-

---

*May be obtained from Dr. David Aronson, National Institutes of Health, Bethesda, Md. 20014.

†Burroughs Wellcome & Co., Research Triangle Park, N.C.

cates an original FDP concentration greater than 40 μg/ml.

The Thrombo-Wellco test may be used to assay FDP in urine, but the method differs from that used for the demonstration of FDP in serum.[207]

Other methods for the demonstration of FDP

The rocket method of Laurell (see discussion of factor VIII–related antigen assay, p. 280) is time consuming, but it has the advantage of specifically identifying the various FDPs, e.g., fragment D or E by the use of specific anti-D or anti-E antisera. The method also allows the addition of fragments D or E to the fragments already present so that the height of the corresponding peaks will increase.

An indirect latex agglutination method has been reported in which the latex particles are coated with fibrinogen.[208] The FDPs in the patient's urine or serum are neutralized by antifibrinogen antiserum and the addition of the fibrinogen-coated latex particles does not lead to agglutination. This method is less sensitive to D and E fragments than to the high-molecular-weight FDPs.[208]

Radioimmunoassay for FDPs in urine and serum is so sensitive to changes in molecular configuration that it allows the differentiation of degradation products of fibrin from those of fibrinogen, so that primary fibrinolysis can be separated from secondary fibrinolysis as seen in disseminated intravascular coagulation (p. 310).[209]

Interpretation[209]: FDPs are increased in a number of conditions, which include malignant tumors with vascular spread,[210] acute and chronic renal failure,[210,211] the hemolytic-uremic syndrome,[212] renal transplant rejection,[213] and diffuse intravascular coagulation (p. 310).

Estimation of circulating soluble fibrin monomers

Soluble fibrin monomers are the result of systemic thrombic action on fibrinogen in diffuse intravascular coagulation. The excess soluble fibrin monomers fail to polymerize, so that they form soluble complexes with fibrinogen and with FDPs resulting from the activity of plasmin. The soluble fibrin monomer complexes can be detected by their **gelation** (paracoagulation), by ethanol, by protamine sulfate, and by cooling (cryofibrinogens). These tests are collectively called **paracoagulation tests.**

Ethanol gel test

Principle: Fibrin monomers are gelled by ethanol.[214]
Reagents:
1. Freshly prepared 50% ethanol
   Dilute 53 ml in 95% ethanol with 47 ml distilled water.
2. Platelet-poor citrated plasma obtained by the two-syringe method
Perform test within 1 hr of obtaining the blood.
Procedure: Add 0.5 ml plasma to 10 × 75 mm glass tube and add 0.15 ml ethanol. Mix gently and leave undisturbed for exactly 10 min. Tilt tube to inspect for gel formation. Run normal control.

Normal values: Normal values are indicated by no particulate matter visible in the test tube.

Interpretation: The presence of a fibrin gel indicates the presence of fibrin monomers in the plasma. Formation of discrete granules or of fibrin strands is considered negative or doubtful. Gelled fibrin monomers are pathognomonic of disseminated intravascular coagulation since they are not present in primary fibrinolytic states without disseminated intravascular coagulation. See interpretation of protamine sulfate test below. A falsely negative result may be encountered in severe hypofibrinogenemia,[215] and a falsely positive result may be caused by dysproteinemia or hyperfibrinogenemia.[215] There should, therefore, always be other supportive evidence for disseminated intravascular coagulation.

Protamine sulfate test[216]

Principle: The addition of protamine sulfate to soluble fibrin monomer complexes splits the XYD fragments off the complexes, allowing the fibrin monomers to polymerize into a visible gel.
Reagents and equipment:
1. Protamine sulfate, 1% solution (Eli Lilly & Co., Indianapolis)
2. Platelet-poor patient's and control plasmas
3. Incubator, 37° C
4. Micropipets, 50 μl
5. Glass test tubes, 13 × 75 mm

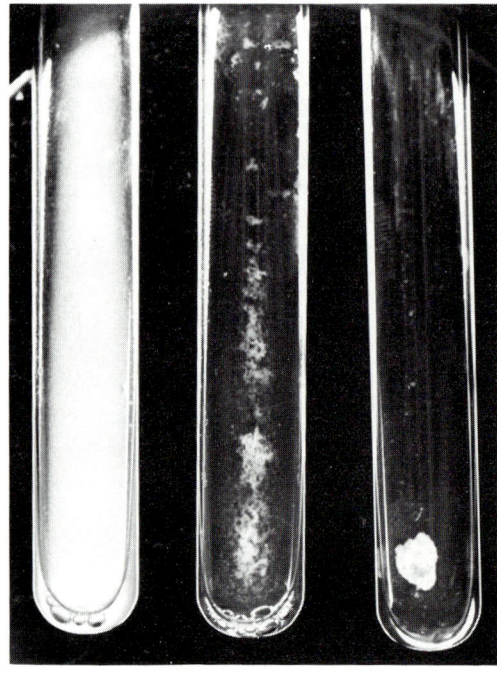

Fig 11-23. Interpretation of protamine sulfate serial dilution test. Left tube shows amorphous precipitate; middle tube shows fibrin strands; right tube shows gelation. Fibrin strands and gelation are positive reactions for fibrin monomer and fibrin degeneration products. (From Niewiarowski, S., and Gurewich, V.: J. Lab. Clin. Med. **77:**665, 1971.)

Procedure: Pipet 0.5 ml plasma into test tube and prewarm in water bath for 3 min. At end of this period make sure that no fibrin bands are present. Add 0.5 ml protamine sulfate and mix gently. Incubate at 37° C for 15 min. Remove tube and observe for clot formation.

Normal values: Normal values are indicated by no precipitated material within the test tube.

Interpretation: A white granular precipitate or fibrin web indicates the presence of fibrin monomers in the plasma. A positive test, therefore, suggests disseminated intravascular coagulation. The test is negative in primary fibrinolysis (Fig. 11-23).

NOTE: The request for the demonstration of excess soluble fibrin monomers should be supported by clinical and laboratory findings that suggest the possibility of disseminated intravascular coagulation, e.g., hypofibrinogenemia, thrombocytopenia, prolonged activated partial thromboplastin time, prothrombin time, and thrombin time. These safeguards are necessary since the paracoagulation may be caused by careless sampling of the blood specimen and fibrin monomer formation after the blood specimen has been obtained.[217]

Demonstration of cryofibrinogen

Principle: Cryofibrinogens are fibrinogen complexes that precipitate in plasma on cooling.

Procedure: Collect patient's blood in EDTA tube and separate plasma by centrifugation. Incubate plasma at 4° C for 24-48 hr. Examine for precipitate.

Normal values: Normal values are indicated by no precipitate in test tube.

Interpretation: A white precipitate indicates cryofibrinogens that redissolve at 37° C. McKee et al.[218] demonstrated the relationship of cryofibrinogens to hypercoagulability, but other investigators fail to agree.[219]

Assays of inhibitors of the fibrinolytic system

The natural inhibitors described on p. 285, e.g., antithrombin III, C1 inactivator, α_2-macroglobulin, and α_1-antitrypsin, have antiplasmin activity. The latter may be assayed by a number of methods. A modified caseinolytic method[220,221] (see discussion of plasminogen analysis) allows plasmin to be incubated with plasma containing the inhibitor for a given period at a given temperature. The residual plasmin activity is then assayed by allowing it to lyse casein.[222] Plasmin, a serine protease, may also be measured by its ability to hydrolyze synthetic substrates, e.g., S2251.[223] Plasmin and inhibitor are incubated together and at suitable intervals aliquots are transferred to a spectrophotometer cuvet containing dissolved S2251. The reaction is then observed over several minutes in a double-beam spectrophotometer that compares it with a blank free of enzymatic activity. The results are expressed in nanomoles or as a percentage of inhibition of plasmin activity.[224] Lastly, inhibitors may be assayed by radial immunodiffusion. The plates containing monospecific antisera are available from Calbiochem-Behring Corp., San Diego, Calif.

REFERENCES

1. Mustard, J.F., and Packham, M.A.: Br. Med. Bull. **33:**187, 1977.
2. Harker, L.A.: Hemostasis manual, ed. 2, Philadelphia, 1974, F.A. Davis Co.
3. Stemerman, M.B.: Prog. Hemost. Thromb. **2:**1, 1974.
4. de los Santos, R.P., and Hoyer, L.W.: Fed. Proc. **31:**262 (abstract), 1972.
5. Becker, C.G., and Nachman, R.L.: Am. J. Pathol. **71:**1, 1973.
6. Zeldis, S.M., et al.: Science **175:**766, 1972.
7. Todd, A.S.: J. Pathol. **78:**281, 1959.
8. Sixma, J.J., and Wester, J.: Semin. Hematol. **14:**265, 1977.
9. Erichson, R.B., and Cintron, J.R.: Thromb. Diathes. Haemorrh. **18:**80, 1967.
10. Jaffe, R., and Deykin, D.: J. Clin. Invest. **53:**875, 1974.
11. White, J.G.: Blood **31:**604, 1968.
12. Sixma, J.J., and Nijessen, J.G.: Thromb. Haemost. **24:**206, 1970.
13. Jamieson, G.A., Urban, C.L., and Barber, A.J.: Nature **234:**5, 1971.
14. Holmsen, H., Day, H.J., and Stormorken, H.: Scand. J. Haematol. **8**(suppl.):1, 1969.
15. Marcus, A.J., et al.: J. Clin. Invest. **45:**14, 1966.
16. Nachman, R.L., Weksler, B., and Ferris, B.: J. Clin. Invest. **49:**274, 1970.
17. Day, H.J., and Solum, N.O.: Scand. J. Haematol. **10:**136, 1973.
18. Holmsen, H., and Day, H.J.: J. Lab. Clin. Med. **75:**840, 1970.
19. Smith, J.B., et al.: J. Clin. Invest. **53:**1468, 1974.
20. Hamberg, M., Svensson, J., and Samuelsson, B.: Proc. Natl. Acad. Sci. U.S.A. **72:**2994, 1975.
21. Marx, J.L.: Science **196:**1072, 1977.
22. Williams, W.J., and Gottlieb, A.J.: Practical problems in hemostasis. Workshop no. 623, American College of Physicians, Audio Ed. Courses, 1976.
23. Walsh, P.N.: Blood **43:**597, 1974.
24. Nemerson, Y., and Esnouf, M.P.: Proc. Natl. Acad. Sci. U.S.A. **70:**310, 1973.
25. Niewiarowski, S., and Thomas, D.P.: Nature **222:**1269, 1969.
26. Kubisz, P., et al.: Rev. Eur. Etudes Clin. Biol. **15:**429, 1970.
27. Walsh, P.N., and Gagnatelli, G.: Blood **44:**157, 1974.
28. Caen, J.P., Cronberg, S., and Kubisz, P.: Platelets: physiology and pathology, New York, 1977, Stratton Intercontinental Medical Book Corporation.
29. O'Brien, J.R., et al.: Lancet **2:**656, 1974.
30. Fuster, V., et al.: Blood **40:**592, 1972.
31. Triplett, D.A.: Thrombosis and hemostasis, no. TH-1, Chicago, 1979, American Society of Clinical Pathologists.
32. D'Amore, P., and Shepro, D.: J. Cell Physiol. **92:**177, 1977.
33. Gingrich, R.D., and Hoak, J.C.: Semin. Hematol. **16:**208, 1979.
34. Tranzer, J.P., and Baumgartner, H.R.: Nature **216:**1126, 1967.
35. MacFarlane, R.G.: Nature **202:**498, 1964.
36. Davie, E.W., and Ratnoff, O.D.: Science **145:**1310, 1964.
37. Triplett, D.A.: Lab. Manage. **15:**40, 1977.
38. Bennett, B.: Semin. Hematol. **14:**301, 1977.
39. Folk, J.E., and Chung, S.I.: Adv. Enzymol. **38:**109, 1973.
40. Cochrane, C.G., et al.: In Lepow, I.H., and Wark,

P.A., editors: Inflammation mechanisms and control, New York, 1972, Academic Press, Inc.

41. Ulevitch, R.J., Letchford, D., and Cochrane, C.G.: Thromb. Haemost. **31**:30, 1974.
42. Zimmerman, T.S., Fierer, J., and Rothberger, H.: Semin. Hematol. **14**:391, 1977.
43. Wuepper, K.D.: In Lepow, I.H., and Ward, D.A., editors: Inflammation mechanisms and control, New York, 1972, Academic Press, Inc.
44. Liu, C.Y., et al.: Fed. Proc. **35**:692, 1976.
45. Muller-Eberhard, H.J., et al.: In Lepow, I.H., and Ward, P.A., editors: Inflammation mechanisms and control, New York, 1972, Academic Press, Inc.
46. Niewiarowski, S., and Prou-Wartelle, O.: Thromb. Diathes. Haemorrh. **3**:593, 1959.
47. Gjønnaess, H.: Thromb. Diathes. Haemorrh. **28**:194, 1972.
48. Gjønnaess, H.: Thromb. Diathes. Haemorrh. **28**:182, 1972.
49. Blomback, B., and Blomback, M.: Ann. N.Y. Acad. Sci. **202**:77, 1972.
50. Gaffney, P.J.: Br. Med. Bull. **33**:245, 1977.
51. Murano, G.: Semin. Thromb. Hemostas. **1**:1, 1974.
52. Blomback, B., et al.: Biochim. Biophys. Acta **115**:371, 1966.
53. Blomback, B.: Acta Physiol. Scand. [Suppl.] **43**(148):1, 1958.
54. Finlayson, J.S.: Semin. Thromb. Hemostas. **1**:33, 1974.
55. Colman, R.W.: Prog. Hemost. Thromb. **3**:109, 1976.
56. Esnouf, M.P.: Br. Med. Bull. **33**:213, 1977.
57. Kandall, C.L., Rosenberg, R., and Colman, R.W.: Eur. J. Biochem. **58**:203, 1975.
58. Prentice, C.R.M., and Ratnoff, O.D.: Br. J. Haematol. **16**:291, 1969.
59. Bloom, A.L., and Peake, I.R.: Br. Med. Bull. **33**:219, 1977.
60. Hougie, C., et al.: Proc. Soc. Exp. Biol. Med. **147**:58, 1974.
61. Ekert, H., et al.: Thromb. Haemost. **36**:78, 1976.
62. Bloom, A.L., and Peake, I.R.: Semin. Hematol. **14**:319, 1977.
63. Davie, E.W., and Fujikawa, K.: Annu. Rev. Biochem. **44**:799, 1975.
64. Bloom, A.L.: In Poller, L., editor: Recent advances in blood coagulation, no. 2, Edinburgh, 1977, Churchill Livingstone.
65. Hoyer, L.W.: Prog. Hemost. Thromb. **3**:231, 1976.
66. Howard, M.A., and Firkin, B.G.: Thromb. Haemost. **26**:362, 1971.
67. Meyer, D., et al.: Nature **243**:293, 1973.
68. Baugh, R.F., and Hougie, C.: In Poller, L., editor: Recent advances in blood no. 2, coagulation, Edinburgh, 1977, Churchill Livingstone.
69. Chung, S.I., Lewis, M.S., and Folk, J.E.: J. Biol. Chem. **249**:940, 1974.
70. Nachman, R.L., and Jaffe, E.A.: Thromb. Haemost. **35**:120, 1976.
71. Hoyer, L.M., de los Santos, R.P., and Hoyer, J.R.: J. Clin. Invest. **52**:2737, 1973.
72. Kiesselbach, T.H., and Wagner, R.H.: Ann. N.Y. Acad. Sci. **202**:318, 1972.
73. Prydz, H.: Semin. Thromb. Hemostas. **4**:1, 1977.
74. Prydz, H.: Thromb. Diathes. Haemorrh. (Stuttg.) **59**(suppl.):61, 1974.
75. Bonnar, J.: In Poller, L., editor: Recent advances in blood coagulation, no. 2, Edinburgh, 1977, Churchill Livingstone.
76. Shah, D.V., and Suttie, J.W.: Proc. Natl. Acad. Sci. U.S.A. **68**:1653, 1971.

77. Hemker, H.C., Muller, A.D., and Loeliger, E.A.: Thromb. Haemost. **23**:633, 1970.
78. Hauschka, P.V., et al.: Biochem. Biophys. Res. Commun. **71**:1207, 1976.
79. Lancet **1**:317, 1975.
80. Seegers, W.H., et al.: Semin. Thromb. Hemostas. **1**:211, 1975.
81. Landaburu, R.H., and Seegers, W.H.: Am. J. Physiol. **197**:1178, 1959.
82. Seegers, W.H., et al.: Thromb. Res. **4**:829, 1974.
83. Stormorken, H.: In Poller, L., editor: Recent advances in blood coagulation, no. 2, Edinburgh, 1977, Churchill Livingstone.
84. Osterud, B., et al.: Biochemistry **11**:2853, 1972.
85. Laake, K., and Ellingsen, R.: Thromb. Res. **5**:539, 1974.
86. Gjønnaess, H.: Thromb. Diathes. Haemorrh. **28**:155, 1972.
87. Radcliffe, R., and Nemerson, Y.: J. Biol. Chem. **250**:388, 1975.
88. Fujikawa, K., et al.: Biochemistry **13**:4508, 1974.
89. Henriksen, R.A., and Jackson, C.M.: Semin. Thromb. Hemost. **1**:284, 1975.
90. Jesty, J., Spencer, A.K., and Nemerson, Y.: J. Biol. Chem. **249**:5614, 1974.
91. Fujikawa, K., et al.: Biochemistry **13**:5290, 1974.
92. Damus, P.S., Hicks, M., and Rosenberg, R.D.: Nature **246**:355, 1973.
93. Marciniak, E.: Br. J. Haematol. **24**:391, 1973.
94. Kaplan, A.P., Meier, H.L., and Mandle, R., Jr.: Semin. Thromb. Hemost. **3**:1, 1976.
95. Nossel, H.L., et al.: Thromb. Diathes. Haemorrh. **16**:185, 1966.
96. Biland, L., and Duckert, F.: Thromb. Diathes. Haemorrh. **29**:644, 1973.
97. Wuepper, K.D.: J. Exp. Med. **138**:1345, 1973.
98. Wuepper, K.D., Miller, D.R., and Lacombe, M.J.: J. Clin. Invest. **56**:1663, 1975.
99. Hvatum, M., and Prydz, H.: Thromb. Diathes. Haemorrh. **21**:217, 1969.
100. Astrup, T.: Thromb. Diathes. Haemorrh. **14**:401, 1965.
101. Zeldis, S.M., et al.: Science **175**:766, 1972.
102. Lovelock, J.E., and Porterfield, B.M.: Biochem. J. **50**:415, 1952.
103. Aggeler, P.M., Perkins, H.A., and Watkins, H.B.: Transfusion **7**:35, 1967.
104. Sherry, S., Fletcher, A., and Alkjaersig, N.: Physiol. Rev. **39**:343, 1959.
105. Davidson, J.F.: In Poller, L., editor: Recent advances in blood coagulation, no. 2, Edinburgh, 1977, Churchill Livingstone.
106. Barnhart, M.I., and Riddle, J.M.: Blood **21**:306, 1963.
107. Lackner, H., and Javid, J.P.: Am. J. Clin. Pathol. **60**:175, 1973.
108. Kernoff, P.B.A., and McNicol, G.P.: Br. Med. Bull. **33**:239, 1977.
109. Warren, B.A.: Br. Med. Bull. **20**:213, 1964.
110. Lack, C.H.: Br. Med. Bull. **20**:217, 1964.
111. Lesuk, A., Terminiello, L., and Traver, J.: Science **147**:880, 1965.
112. Summaria, L., and Robbins, K.C.: J. Biol. Chem. **251**:5810, 1976.
113. Plow, E.F., and Edgington, T.S.: J. Clin. Invest. **56**:30, 1975.
114. Reich, E.: In Reich, E., Rifkin, D.B., and Shaw, E., editors: Proteases and biological control, Cold Spring Harbor, New York, 1975, Cold Spring Harbor Conferences on Cell Proliferation.
115. Stormorken, H.: Thromb. Diathes. Haemorrh. **34**:378, 1975.

116. Fletcher, A.P., et al.: J. Clin. Invest. **43**:681, 1964.
117. Marder, V.J., and Budzynski, A.Z.: Thromb. Diathes. Haemorrh. **51**(suppl.):267, 1972.
118. Marder, V.J., and Budzynski, A.Z.: Prog. Hemost. Thromb. **2**:141, 1974.
119. Marder, V.J., and Budzynski, A.Z.: Schweiz. Med. Wochenschr. **104**:1338, 1974.
120. Shainoff, J.R., and Page, I.H.: J. Exp. Med. **116**:687, 1962.
121. Gaffney, P.J., and Brasher, M.: Biochim. Biophys. Acta **295**:308, 1973.
122. Rosenberg, R., and Damus, P.: J. Biol. Chem. **248**:6490, 1973.
123. Damus, P.C., Hicks, M., and Rosenberg, R.D.: Nature **246**:356, 1973.
124. Klein, P.D., and Seegers, W.H.: Blood **5**:742, 1950.
125. Yin, E.T., Wessler, S., and Stoll, P.: J. Biol. Chem. **246**:3703, 1971.
126. Rosenberg, J.S., McKenna, P.W., and Rosenberg, R.D.: J. Biol. Chem. **250**:8883, 1975.
127. Stead, N., Kaplan, A.P., and Rosenberg, R.D.: J. Biol. Chem. **251**:6481, 1976.
128. Highsmith, R.F., and Rosenberg, R.D.: J. Biol. Chem. **249**:4335, 1974.
129. Lane, J.L., and Biggs, R.: In Poller, L., editor: Recent advances in blood coagulation, no. 2, Edinburgh, 1977, Churchill Livingstone.
130. Ogston, D., Murray, J., and Crawford, G.P.M.: Thromb. Res. **9**:217, 1976.
131. Marciniak, E., and Tsukamura, S.: Br. J. Haematol. **22**:341, 1972.
132. Egeberg, O.: Thromb. Diathes. Haemorrh. **14**:473, 1965.
133. Pensky, J., Levy, L., and Lepow, I.: J. Biol. Chem. **236**:1674, 1961.
134. Schreiber, A., Kaplan, A., and Austen, K.F.: J. Clin. Invest. **52**:1394, 1973.
135. Forbes, C.D., Pensky, J., and Ratnoff, O.D.: J. Lab. Clin. Med. **76**:809, 1970.
136. McConnell, D.J.: J. Clin. Invest. **51**:1611, 1972.
137. Harpel, P.C.: J. Exp. Med. **138**:508, 1973.
138. Lanchantin, G.F., et al.: Proc. Soc. Exp. Biol. Med. **121**:444, 1966.
139. Ganrot, P.O.: Clin. Chim. Acta **16**:328, 1967.
140. Bundy, H., and Mehl, J.: J. Biol. Chem. **234**:1124, 1959.
141. Shamash, Y., and Rimon, A.: Biochim. Biophys. Acta **121**:35, 1966.
142. Heck, L.W., and Kaplan, A.P.: J. Exp. Med. **140**:1615, 1974.
143. Learned, L.A., Bloom, J.W., and Hunter, M.J.: Thromb. Res. **8**:99, 1976.
144. Shapiro, S.S., and Hultin, M.: Semin. Thromb. Hemost. **1**:336, 1975.
145. Margolius, A., Jackson, D., and Ratnoff, O.: Medicine (Baltimore) **40**:145, 1961.
146. Kwaan, H.: Med. Clin. North Am. **56**:177, 1972.
147. Feinstein, D.I., and Rapaport, S.I.: Prog. Hemost. Thromb. **1**:75, 1972.
148. Lackner, H.: Semin. Haematol. **10**:125, 1973.
149. Greenwood, R., and Rabin, S.: Obstet. Gynecol. **30**:362, 1967.
150. Green, D.: Br. J. Haematol. **15**:57, 1968.
151. Sise, H., et al.: Am. J. Med. **32**:964, 1962.
152. Bowie, E.J.W., and Owen, C.A.: In Poller, L., editor: Recent advances in blood coagulation, no. 2, Edinburgh, 1977, Churchill Livingstone.
153. Gobbi, F., and Stefanini, M.: Acta Haematol. **28**:155, 1962.

154. Biggs, R., and Spooner, R.J.D.: Br. J. Haematol. **36**:447, 1977.
155. Biggs, R., editor: Complications of treatment. In Biggs, R., editor: The treatment of haemophilia A and B and von Willebrand's disease, Oxford, England, 1978, Blackwell Scientific Publications, Ltd.
156. Weigle, W.O.: J. Exp. Med. **114**:111, 1961.
157. Hougie, C.: In Ogston, D., and Bennett, B., editors: Haemostasis: biochemistry, physiology, and pathology, New York, 1977, John Wiley & Sons, Inc.
158. Mannucci, P.M., et al.: Nature **262**:141, 1976.
159. George, J.N., Miller, G.M., and Breckenridge, R.T.: Br. J. Haematol. **21**:333, 1971.
160. Feinstein, D.I., et al.: J. Clin. Invest. **49**:1578, 1970.
161. Castro, O., Farber, L., and Clyne, L.P.: Ann. Intern Med. **77**:543, 1972.
162. Lorand, L., et al.: J. Clin. Invest. **48**:1054, 1969.
163. Biggs, R.: In Biggs, R., editor: The treatment of haemophilia A and B and von Willebrand's disease, Oxford, England, 1978, Blackwell Scientific Publications, Ltd.
164. Quick, A.J.: Am. J. Med. Sci. **252**:265, 1966.
165. Bowie, E.J.W., and Owen, C.A.: Prog. Hemost. Thromb. **2**:249, 1974.
166. Mielke, C.H., et al.: Blood **34**:204, 1969.
167. Sutor, A.H., et al.: Am. J. Clin. Pathol. **55**:541, 1971.
168. Owen, C.A., Bowie, W.E.J., and Thompson, J.H.: The diagnosis of bleeding disorders, ed. 2, Boston, 1975, Little Brown & Co.
169. Lee, R.I., and White, P.D.: Am. J. Med. Sci. **145**:495, 1913.
170. Didisheim, P.: Am. J. Clin. Pathol. **47**:622, 1967.
171. Tocantins, L.M.: Am. J. Physiol. **110**:278, 1934.
172. Friedman, L.L., et al.: Mayo Clin. Proc. **39**:908, 1964.
173. Hattersley, P.G.: J.A.M.A. **196**:150, 1966.
174. Bull, B.S., et al.: J. Thorac. Cardiovasc. Surg. **69**:674, 1975.
175. Roth, J.A., Cukingnan, R.A., and Sott, CR.: Ann. Thorac. Surg. **28**:69, 1979.
176. Owen, C.A., et al.: Am. J. Clin. Pathol. **25**:1417, 1955.
177. Martin, E.W., et al.: Hazards of medication. A manual of drug interaction, incompatibilities, contraindications, and adverse effects, Philadelphia, 1978, J.B. Lippincott Co.
178. MacFarlane, R.G., and Barnett, B.: Lancet **2**:985, 1934.
179. Prentice, C.R.M., and Ratnoff, O.D.: Br. J. Haematol. **16**:291, 1969.
180. Holleman, W.H., and Weiss, L.J.: J. Biol. Chem. **251**:1663, 1976.
181. Latallo, Z., and Teisseyre, E.: Scand. J. Haematol. **13**(suppl.):261, 1971.
182. Quick, A.J.: Am. J. Clin. Pathol. **45**:105, 1966.
183. Biggs, R., and Douglas, A.S.: J. Clin. Pathol. **6**:23, 1953.
184. Heimburger, N., and Karger, H.E.: Med. Lab. **5**:1, 1978.
185. Triplett, D.A., Harms, C.S., and Smith, C.S.: The use of synthetic chromogenic substrates in the coagulation laboratory, Muncie, Ind., 1978, Department of Hematology, Ball Memorial Hospital.
186. Claeson, G., et al.: Haemostasis **7**:62, 1978.
187. Bang, N.U., and Mattler, L.E.: Haemostasis **7**:98, 1978.
188. Rasalhi, S.B., editor: New pathways in laboratory medicine. Transactions of the Merz and Dade exploratory seminar, Dudinger, 1977, Vienna, 1978, Hans Huber Publishers.
189. Deegan, M.J.: Clinical chemistry check sample, no. CC-89, Chicago, 1974, Commission on Continuing Education, American Society of Clinical Pathologists.

190. Ware, A.G., Guest, M.M., and Seegers, W.H.: Arch. Biochem. Biophys. **13**:231, 1947.

191. Ratnoff, O.D., and Menzie, C.: J. Lab. Clin. Med. **37**:316, 1951.

192. Morse, E.E., Panek, S., and Menga, R.: Am. J. Clin. Pathol. **55**:671, 1971.

193. Stevens, D.J., and Sanfelippo, M.J.: Am. J. Clin. Pathol. **60**:182, 1973.

194. Technical Information Bulletin, CO19-2152E, Miami, 1976, Dade Diagnostic Inc.

195. Schneider, C.L.: Am. J. Obstet. Gynecol. **64**:141, 1952.

196. Methods manual, Horsham, Pa., 1977, Bio/Data Corporation.

197. Vollmer, K.: Coagulation procedures, Miami, 1976, Dade Diagnostics Inc.

198. Fekete, L.F., and Bick, R.L.: In Recent concepts and developments in evaluating disorders of hemostasis and thrombosis, Chicago, 1976, American Society of Clinical Pathologists.

199. Alami, S.Y., et al.: Am. J. Med. **44**:1, 1968.

200. von Kaulla, K.N., and Schultz, R.L.: Am. J. Clin. Pathol. **29**:104, 1958.

201. Buckell, M.: J. Clin. Pathol. **11**:403, 1958.

202. Blix, S.: Scand. J. Clin. Lab. Invest. [Suppl.] **13**(58):3, 1961.

203. Blix, S.: Scand J. Clin. Lab. Invest. **14**:528, 1962.

204. Johnson, A.J., Kline, D.L., and Alkjaersig, N.: Thromb. Diathes. Haemorrh. **21**:259, 1969.

205. Pochron, S.P., et al.: Thromb. Res. **13**:733, 1978.

206. Detection of fibrinogen degradation products and fibrinogen, Research Triangle Park, N.C., 1977, Wellcome Reagents Division, Burroughs Wellcome Co.

207. Laurell, C.B.: Anal. Biochem. **15**:45, 1966.

208. Donati, M.B., Semeraro, N., and Vermylen, J.: J. Clin. Pathol. **26**:760, 1973.

209. Hedner, N.: In Davidson, J.F., Samoma, M.M., and Desmoyers, P.C., editors: Progress in chemical fibrinolysis and thrombolysis, vol. 2. Methodology, New York, 1976, Raven Press.

210. Hedner, U., and Nilsson, I.M.: Acta Med. Scand. **189**:471, 1971.

211. Briggs, J.D., Prentice, C.R.M., and Hutton, M.M.: Br. Med. J. **4**:82, 1972.

212. Ekberg, M., Nilsson, I.M., and Denneberg, T.: Acta Med. Scand. **196**:373, 1974.

213. Carlsson, S., et al.: Transplantation **10**:366, 1970.

214. Breen, F.A., and Tullis, J.L.: Ann. Intern. Med. **69**:1197, 1968.

215. Conard, J., Bogaty-Yver, J., and Samama, M.: Nouv. Presse Med. **3**:2639, 1974.

216. Latallo, Z.S., et al.: Scand. J. Haematol. [Suppl.] **13**:387, 1971.

217. Jacobsen, C.D., and Senthees, N.J.: Thromb. Diathes. Haemorrh. **29**:130, 1973.

218. McKee, P.A., Kalbfleisch, J.M., and Bird, R.M.: J. Lab. Clin. Med. **61**:203, 1963.

219. Mosesson, M.W., Colman, R.W., and Sherry, S.: N. Engl. J. Med. **278**:815, 1968.

220. Shamash, Y., and Rimon, A.: Thromb. Diathes. Haemorrh. **12**:119, 1964.

221. Sherry, S., et al.: J. Clin. Invest. **38**:810, 1959.

222. Remmer, L.F., and Cohen, P.P.: J. Biol. Chem. **181**:431, 1949.

223. Svendsen, L., et al.: Thromb. Res. **1**:267, 1972.

224. Crawford, G.P.M.: In Davidson, J.F., Samama, M.M., and Desmoyers, P.C., editors: Progress in chemical fibrinolysis and thrombolysis, vol. 2, New York, 1976, Raven Press.

CHAPTER 12

Laboratory investigation of platelets

PLATELETS AND THEIR PRECURSORS

Platelets (thrombocytes) are produced by megakaryocytes in the bone marrow (Fig. 12-1). The earliest recognizable cell of this series is the megakaryoblast. By nuclear replication it changes into the promegakaryocyte, which matures into the granular megakaryocyte that releases the platelets.[1] These steps of replication and maturation are also referred to as stages I, II, and III.[2] Multipotent cells preceding megakaryoblasts appear in agar culture systems of bone marrows but cannot be identified morphologically.[3]

Megakaryoblasts (stage I)

Size: The megakaryoblast ranges from 10-30 μm in diameter. The cell is smaller than its mature form but larger than all other blast cells (Fig. 12-2).

Nucleus: The single, large, oval or indented nucleus has a loose chromatin structure and a delicate nuclear membrane. Multilobulated nuclei also occur, representing a polyploid stage. Several pale blue nucleoli are difficult to see. The parachromatin is pink.

Cytoplasm: The cytoplasm forms a scanty, bluish,

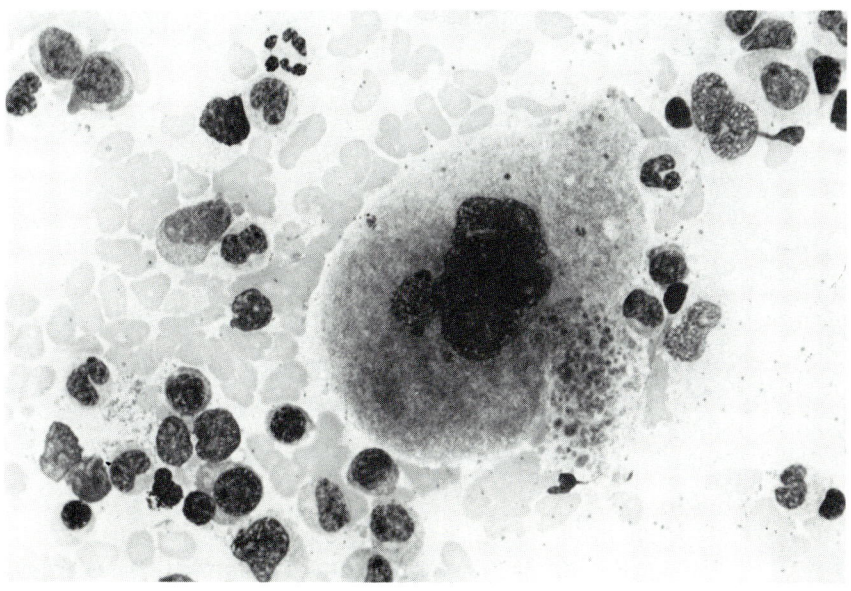

Fig. 12-1. Megakaryocyte functioning.

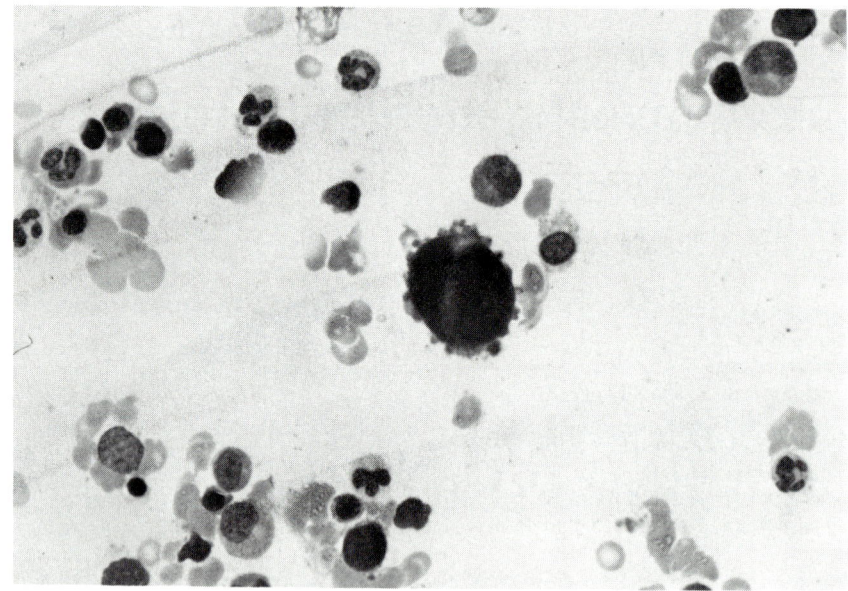

Fig. 12-2. Megakaryoblast.

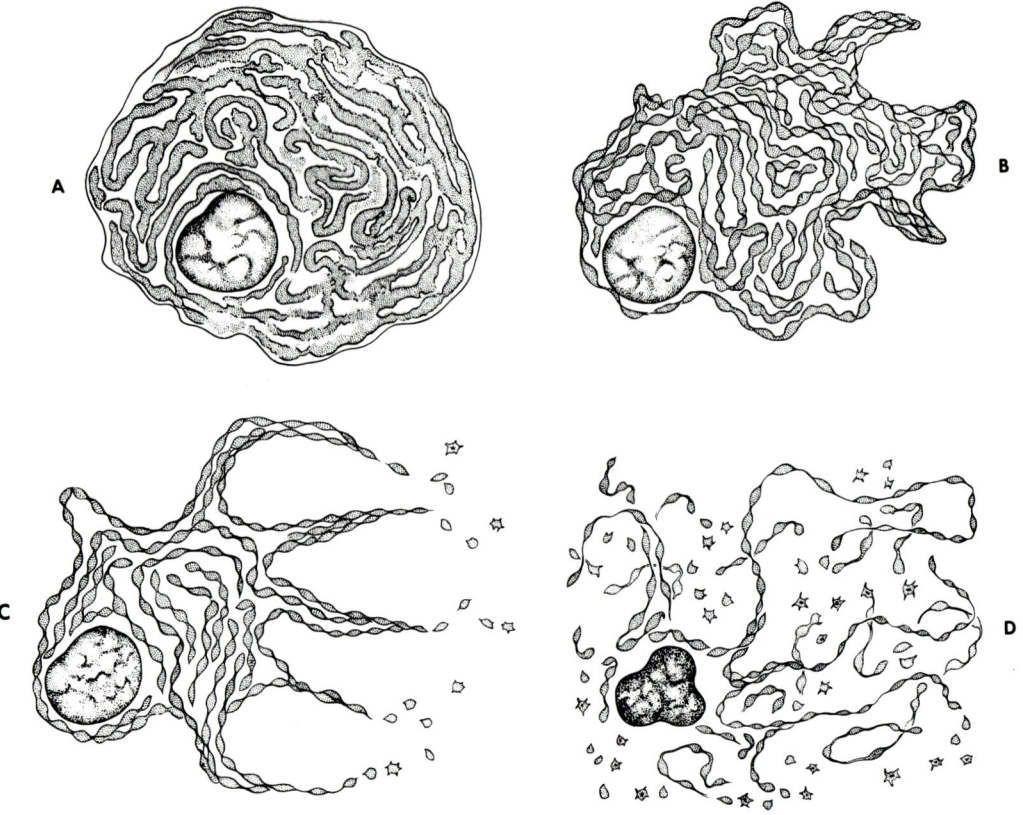

Fig. 12-3. Demarcation membrane system of megakaryocytes. Stages in platelet formation and liberation of platelets. (From Bessis, M.: Living blood cells and their ultrastructure, Heidelberg, 1973, Springer-Verlag.)

patchy, irregular ring around the nucleus. The periphery shows cytoplasmic projections and pseudopodia-like structures. The immediate perinuclear zone is lighter stained than the periphery.

Phase microscopy: According to Bessis,[4] the size of the cell is the most outstanding feature. The thin cytoplasmic rim contains numerous large mitochondria and a prominent Golgi apparatus.

Electron microscopy: The nucleus shows a fine chromatin pattern. The cytoplasm contains numerous prominent Golgi sets, peripheral immature granules, some endoplasmic reticulum,[5] ribosomes, glycogen, and numerous large mitochondria. Electron microscopy lends itself to follow the **demarcation membrane system** (DMS), which defines small cytoplasmic segments destined to become platelets. The DMS arises near the cell wall and extends toward the nucleus and Golgi apparatus (Fig. 12-3).

Promegakaryocytes (stage II)

Size: The promegakaryocyte (basophil megakaryocyte) ranges from 20-50 μm in diameter. It is larger than the megakaryoblast, and in the process of maturation it reaches the size of the stage III cell (Fig. 12-4).

Nucleus: The nucleus is large, indented, and polylobulated. The chromatin appears to have coarse, heavily stained strands and may show some clumping. The total number of nucleoli is decreased, and they are more difficult to see than in the blast cell. The nuclear membrane is thin and fine.

Cytoplasm: The characteristic feature is the intensely basophilic cytoplasm that is being filled with increasing numbers of azurophilic granules radiating from the Golgi apparatus toward the periphery, sparing a thin peripheral ring that remains blue in color.

Phase microscopy: The cell is large and contains a large nucleus, which may show nucleoli. The small amount of cytoplasm is dense and often darker around the nucleus.

Electron microscopy: The nucleus is lobulated and has a delicate chromatin structure. Nucleoli may be prominent. The cytoplasm may show blunt extensions and is packed with polyribosomes, rough endoplasmic reticulum, and granules. The Golgi apparatus is prominent. The DMS is convoluted and fills the entire cell, and small subdivisions appear in its cylindric, tubular structures.

Granular megakaryocytes (stage III)

The majority of megakaryocytes of a bone marrow aspirate are in stage III, which is characterized by progressive nuclear condensation and indentation and by the beginning of platelet formation within the cytoplasm (Fig. 12-5).

Size: The granular megakaryocyte ranges from 30-100 μm in diameter and is the largest cell found in the bone marrow.

Nucleus: The nucleus is plump, multilobulated, indented, and at times multinucleated. The nuclei are arranged in chains or rings and may partially cover each other. The chromatin is in heavy clumps, and nucleoli are not visible.

Cytoplasm: A large amount of polychromatic cytoplasm produces blunt, smooth, pseudopodia-like projections that contain aggregates of azurophilic granules surrounded by pale halos. These structures give rise to platelets at the periphery of the megakaryocytes. The line of cleavage goes through the hyaline cytoplasm of the ''halo'', so that the granular mass becomes the platelet center. Platelet formation requires about 9-11 days[6] and appears to be under the control of a thrombopoietic factor (thrombopoietin). A number of experimental methods of assay of thrombopoietin are avail-

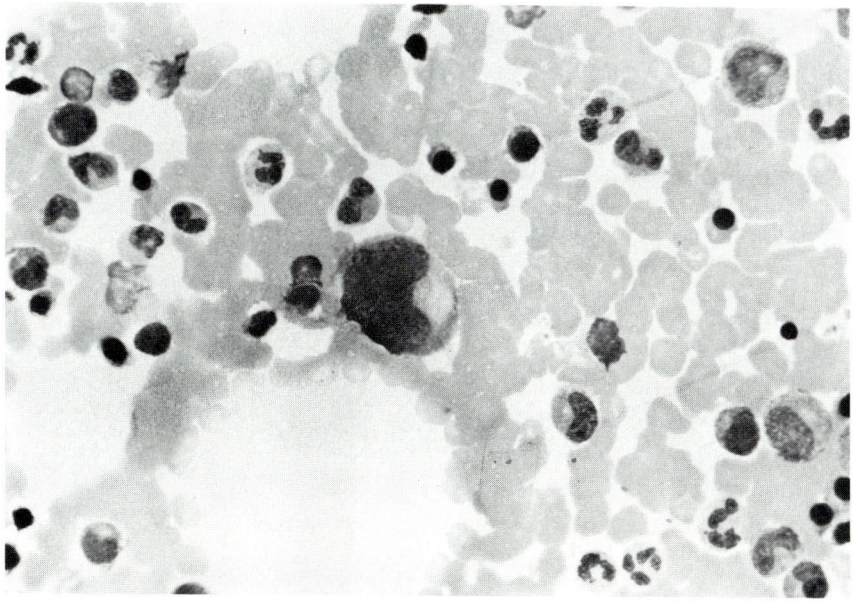

Fig. 12-4. Promegakaryocyte.

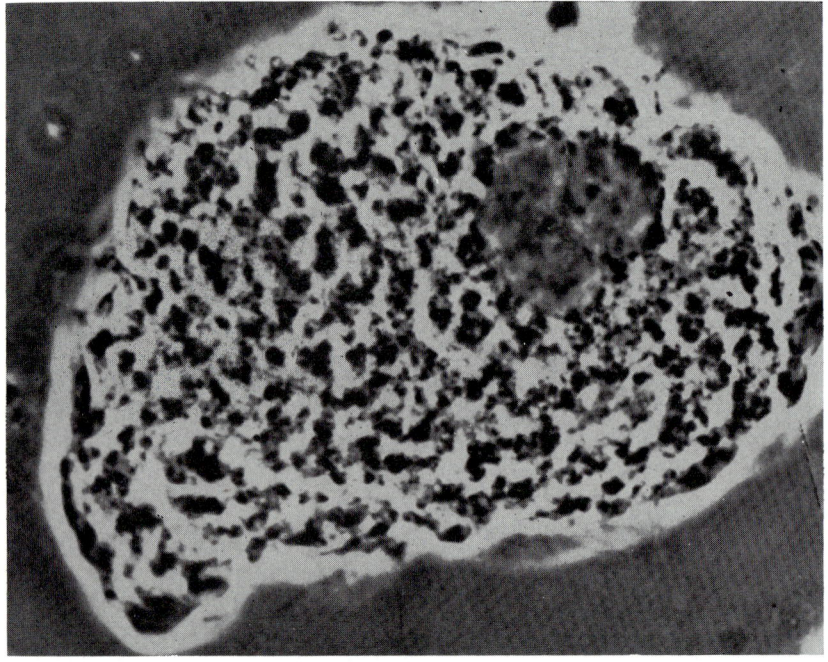

Fig. 12-5. Phase contrast photomicrograph of megakaryocyte showing division of cytoplasm in areas resulting from developing platelets. (From Bernard, J., and Bessis, M.: Hématologie clinique, Paris, 1958. Masson & Cie.)

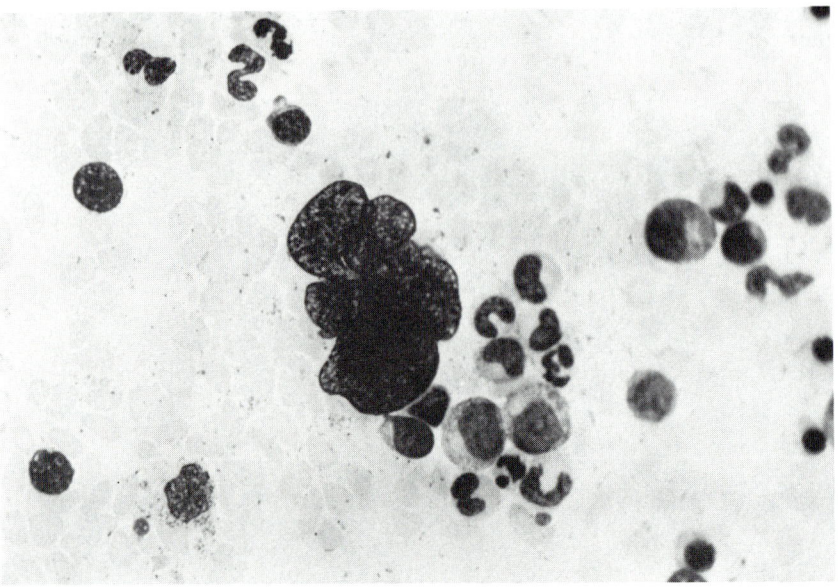

Fig. 12-6. Degenerating megakaryocyte.

able, two of which, an immunoassay and a bioassay method, hold some promise for the future development of an inexpensive, quick assay method.[7]

Phase microscopy: Small black dots in the cytoplasm represent the future platelets. The nucleus is difficult to see (Fig. 12-5).

Electron microscopy: The nucleus becomes progressively more condensed and indented and contains mainly membranous chromatin interrupted by many pores. The large mitochondria and the polyribosomes of the cytoplasm disappear, so that the picture is dominated by the DMS and granules. About 30% of megakaryocytes are in the inactive, non-platelet-producing phase.

Cytochemical investigations: Megakaryocytes and the precursor forms are PAS (glycogen), cholinesterase, and acid phosphatase positive.

Degenerating megakaryocytes

After platelets have been shed, only the perinuclear rim of cytoplasm remains, the nuclear chromatin condenses, the lobulation becomes more pronounced, and finally only the naked nucleus remains (Fig. 12-6).

Abnormal megakaryocytes

In vitamin B_{12} and folate deficiencies megakaryocytes are diminished in number (hypoplasia) and their nuclei may show hyperlobulation (hypersegmentation)[8] and multinucleation, whereas the cytoplasm retains the basophilia of immaturity and its inability to produce platelets[9] (Fig. 12-7). In immunologic thrombocytopenic purpura, either primary or secondary, megakaryocytes are increased in number (hyperplasia) but their thrombocytopoietic activity is diminished (Fig. 12-8). Secondary immunologic thrombocytopenic purpura may accompany hypersplenism of any etiology, lupus erythematosus, or drug reactions. The reduction

in platelet formation is apparently related to the vacuolation and hypogranularity of the megakaryocytic cytoplasm[8] and to hyperlobulation of the nuclei.[10] Neither the cytoplasmic nor the nuclear defects in immunologic thrombocytopenic purpura are confirmed.[11] Hypersegmentation of nuclei and lack of cytoplasmic granularity may be seen in Wiskott-Aldrich syndrome.[12] Hyperplasia of megakaryocytes in association with peripheral thrombocytopenia is also reported in thrombotic thrombocytopenic purpura,[8] Wiskott-Aldrich syndrome, and megakaryocytic leukemia. Atypical mononuclear and binuclear megakaryocytes can be found in a variety of disorders, e.g. hereditary macrothrombocytopathia associated with nephritis and deafness,[13] chronic granulocytic leukemia,[14] acute megakaryocytic leukemia,[8] acute myelogenous leukemia,[9] erythroleukemia, myelomonocytic leukemia, and preleukemia.[15] Atypical megakaryocytes have also been reported in a large number of nonleukemic conditions, e.g., radiation and folic acid antagonist therapy, heat stroke,[16] and May-Hegglin anomaly.[17]

Megakaryocytes in peripheral blood

Megakaryocytes or fragments of these cells normally appear in the peripheral blood,[18-20] but buffy coat preparations are usually required to discover them. Megakaryocyte counts reveal from 1-100 megakaryocytes/5 ml blood. They are found in increased numbers in the peripheral blood in chronic myelocytic leukemia, leukoerythroblastic anemias, extramedullary hematopoiesis, polycythemia vera, myelofibrosis, and acute megakaryocytic leukemia.

Platelets (thrombocytes)

Size: Platelets may vary from 1-4 μm in diameter. Young platelets may be two to three times as large.[21]

Nucleus: No nucleus is present.

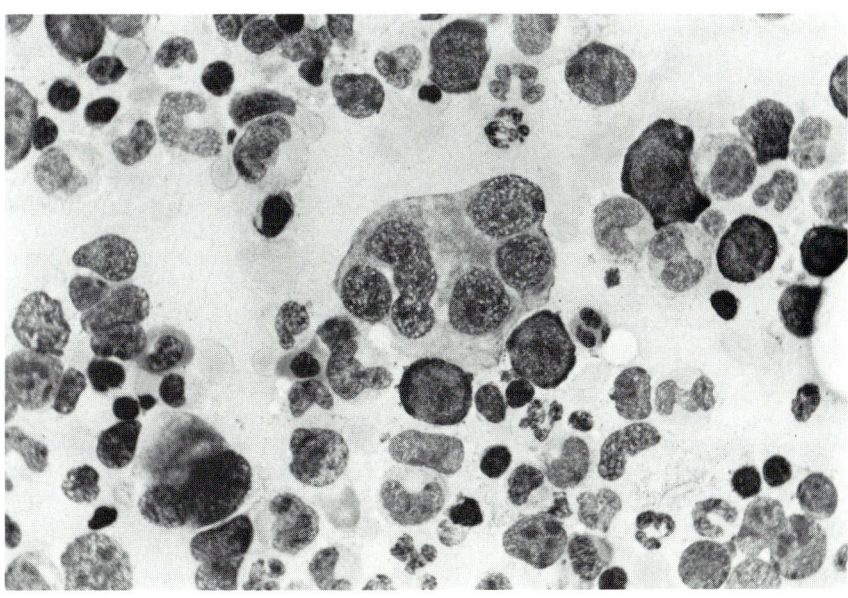

Fig. 12-7. Megakaryocyte in vitamin B_{12} deficiency.

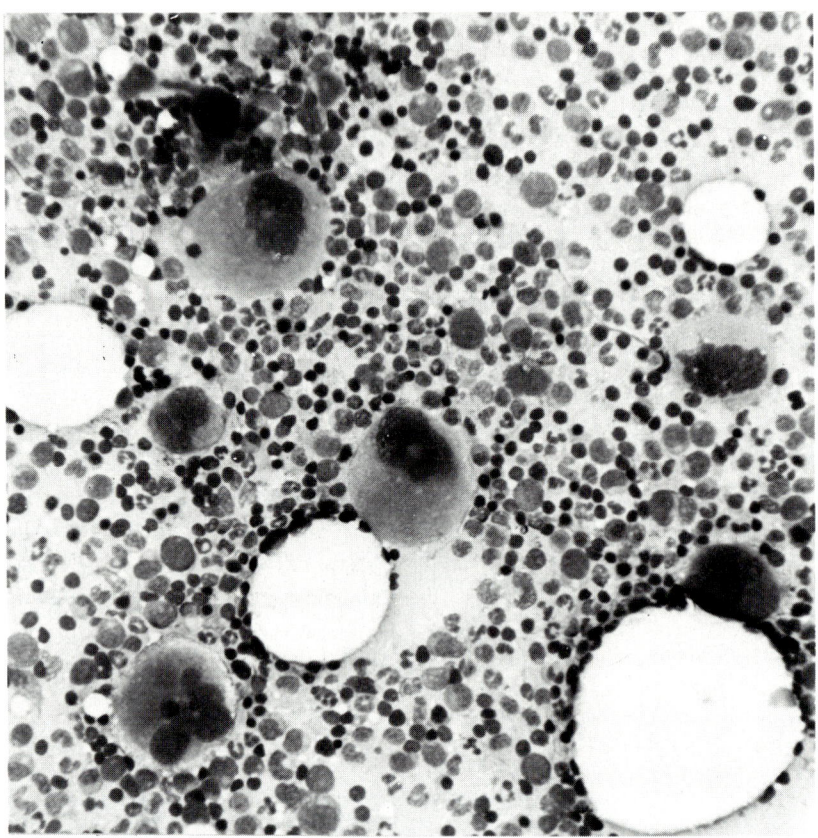

Fig. 12-8. Bone marrow in thrombocytopenia purpura.

In the Wright-Giemsa–stained film, platelets appear as small, bright, azure, rounded or elongated bodies with a delicately granular structure. Each platelet consists of a central group of azurophillic granules, **chromomere,** and a surrounding light blue **hyalomere.** Platelets have a tendency to agglutinate on contact with glass, so that if isolated platelets are to be studied, heparin or EDTA must be used as an anticoagulant. EDTA induces platelets to become round and globoid.

Phase microscopy: Circulating platelets are round or oval structures containing central granules. After contact with glass, slender protoplasmic projections appear that precede the "spread form," the large clear cell, the center of which contains the granules that are surrounded by a thin membrane (**viscous metamorphosis)** (Figs. 12-9 and 12-10).

Electron microscopy: By electron microscopy (Fig. 12-11) platelets are seen to be much more complicated than light and phase-contrast microscopy suggest. White proposes an electron microscopy nomenclature that combines morphologic-anatomic features with physical and functional considerations[22-24]: (1) the peripheral zone, which is the site of adhesion and aggregation, consists of a trilaminar membrane and submembranous microtubules; (2) the matrix inside platelets is a sol-gel containing an irregular network of fiber systems and microtubules that support the platelet discoid shape and contractile mechanism; (3) the organelle zone embedded in the sol-gel contains the dense bodies, the specific α-granules, a few round, small mitochondria, occasional vacuoles, and the elements of the dense tubular system, all structures related to metabolic processes and to storage and release of products. The fuzzy exterior coat, the glycocalyx, is rich in carbohydrates and is the site of adhesion and of nonspecific absorption of plasma constituents such as fibrinogen and factor VIII.[25] The trilaminar units membrane lies under the exterior coat and protects the intracellular organelles. The cytoplasmic aspect of the membrane includes a surface-connecting canalicular-vesicular system that supports the shape of the platelets.[26] The membrane is involved in the transformation of the platelets from the disk shape to the spined globe that occurs during adhesion and aggregation and may be responsible for the release of such membrane substances as ADP and platelet factor 3. The interior of the platelet, the sol-gel zone, is composed of microtubules and microfilaments. The microtubules form marginal bundles that maintain the platelet shape, whereas the smaller microfilaments are randomly distributed and have contractile properties. The sol-gel zone houses glycogen granules and the intracellular organelles, which include the mitochondria and two types of oval-to-round granules that have secretory and storage capabilities. The **α-granules** are of moderate electron density and contain hydrolytic enzymes such as acid phosphatases and fibrinogen, thrombasthenin, platelet factor 3, ATP, ADP, and serotonin.[27] The second type

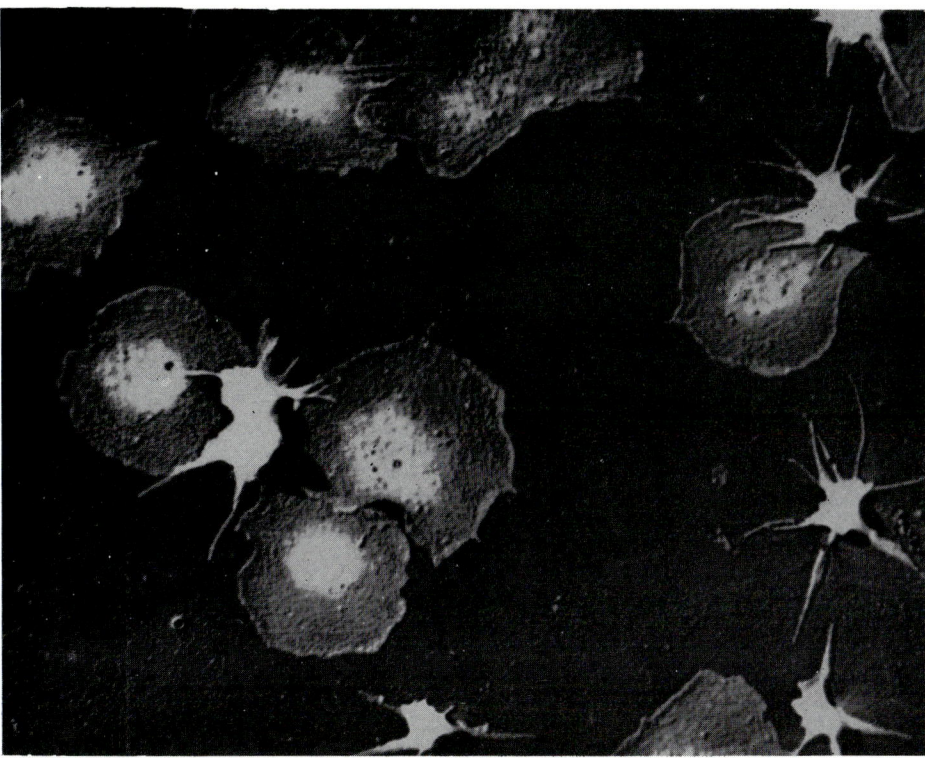

Fig. 12-9. Electron micrograph of normal platelets with pseudopods and spreading of hyaloplasm. (Courtesy Prof. H. Braunsteiner, Innsbruck, Austria.)

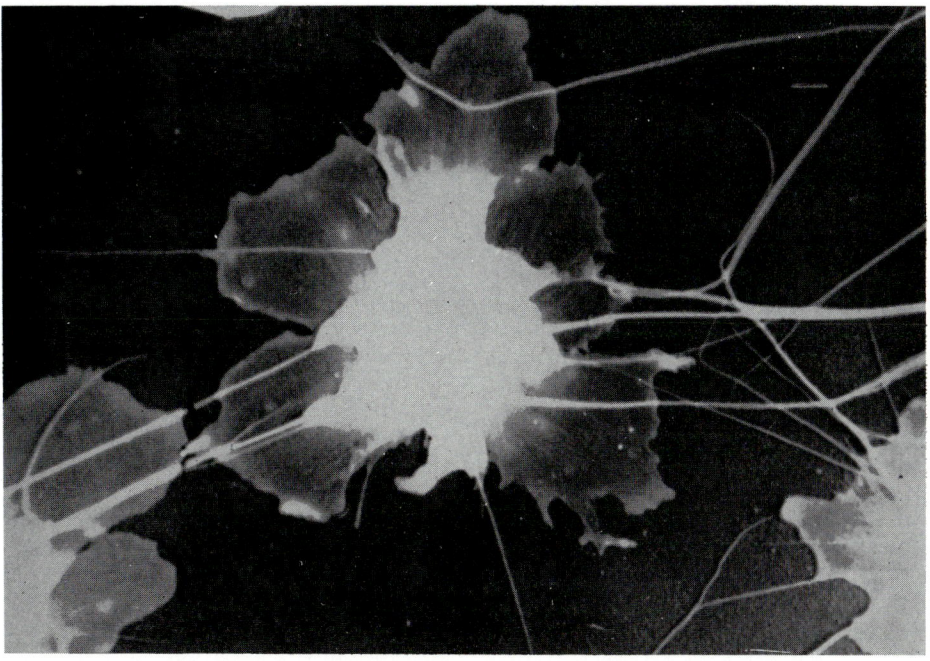

Fig. 12-10. Electron micrograph of platelets in early stages of coagulation, showing viscous metamorphosis. (Courtesy Prof. H. Braunsteiner, Innsbruck, Austria.)

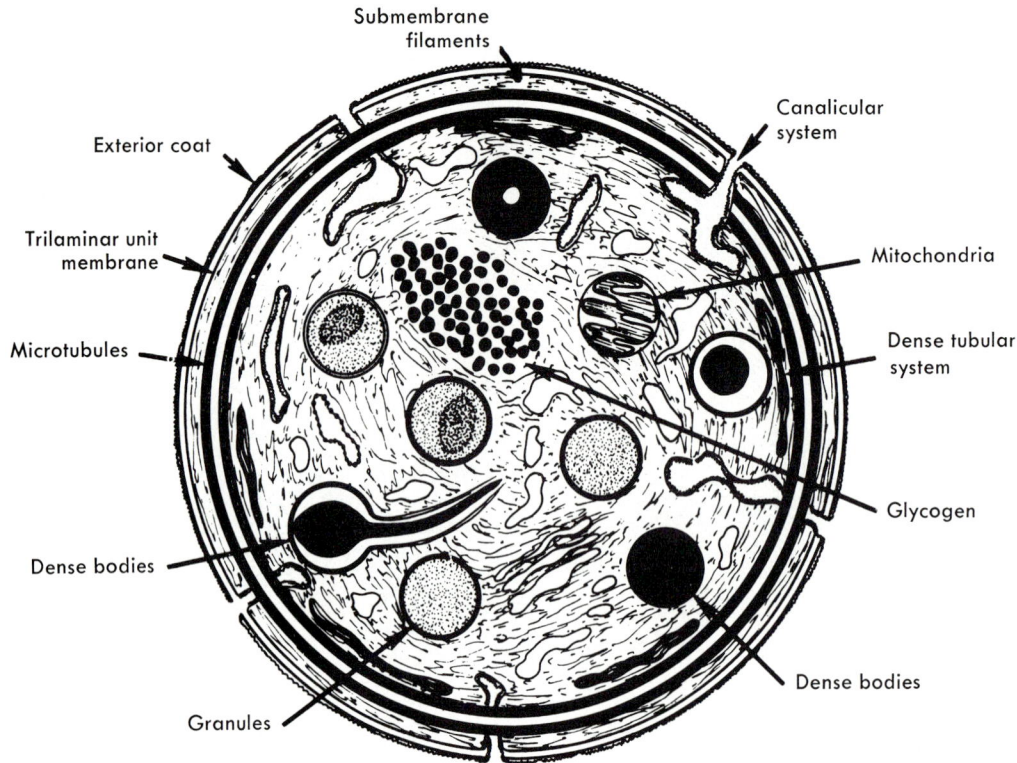

Fig. 12-11. Blood platelet as it appears in thin section by electron microscopy; platelet cut in equatorial plane. Components of peripheral zone include exterior coat, trilaminar unit membrane, and submembrane area, which form wall of platelet and line channels of open canalicular system. Matrix of platelet is sol-gel zone containing microfilaments. submembrane filaments, circumferential band of microtubules, and glycogen. Formed elements embedded in sol-gel zone include mitochondria, granules, dense bodies, and channels of dense tubular system. (From White, J.G.: Ann. N.Y. Acad. Sci. **201:**205, 1972.)

of granules, the **dense bodies,** are electron opaque because of their calcium content and are the primary secretory organelles of platelets. Moving toward the surface of the platelets as they transform into spiny spheres during the process of aggregation they secrete serotonin, platelet factor 4, and catecholamines.[28]

• • •

Metabolically, platelets are contractile, secretory cells that are able to store and/or synthesize glycogen, ATP, prostaglandin, and serotonin.

Functionally, platelets play a pivotal role in the various stages of primary hemostasis, e.g., platelet adhesion, aggregation, release reaction, and plug formation. Several steps of the coagulation cascade require platelet factor 3, a lipoprotein. Other hemostatic functions involve clot retraction, mediated by thrombasthenin and platelet-endothelial interaction. Evidence indicates that some of the substances within the platelets, e.g., ferritin, antigen-antibody complexes, viruses, and bacteria, are acquired by phagocytosis. Platelets are also capable of activating complement and are thus involved in the inflammatory response.

Immunologically, platelets possess weak A and B antigens, specific platelet antigens, and histocompatability antigens (HLA), which they share with many other tissues.

Cytochemically, acid mucopolysaccharides are the main component of the surface coat. The sol-gel zone does not reveal cytochemically significant localities except for its organelles, which contain a variety of substances as described above.

Variations in platelet morphology

Platelets are markedly heterogeneous in physical appearance; generally young platelets are large, whereas aged platelets are small. An increased number of large platelets (macrothrombocytes or megathrombocytes) in the peripheral circulation (Fig. 12-12) stems from two factors: (1) release of young platelets following hyperutilization or hyperdestruction of platelets[21] and (2) dysthrombocytopoiesis resulting from abnormal membrane demarcation within the megakaryocytes.[29] The first has been described in immunologic thrombocytopenic purpura, diffuse intravascular coagulation, posthemorrhagic thrombocytosis,[21] May-Hegglin anomaly,[8,30] and Alport's syndrome.[31] Increased platelet size has also been noted in malaria,[32] often with parasitic inclusions, von Willebrand's disease,[33] and Bernard-Soulier syndrome.[34,35] The second form of macrothrombocytosis, which results from **dysthrombocytopoiesis,** occurs in chronic myelogenous leukemia and other myeloproliferative disorders, refractory anemia, myelofibrosis, hereditary macrothrombocyto-

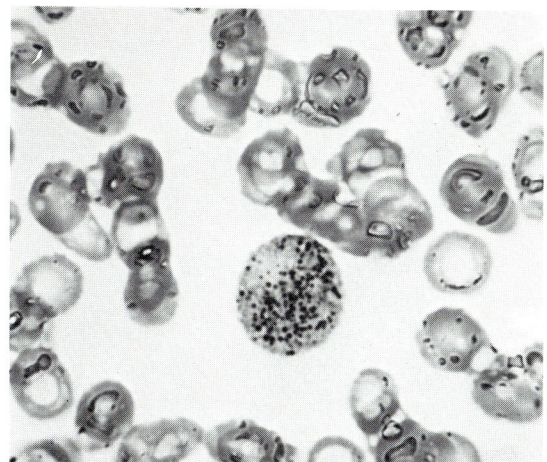

Fig. 12-12. Macrothrombocyte. (×1250.)

pathia, and the preleukemic phase of acute myeloid leukemia.[36]

Small platelets have been found following aspirin therapy[37] and in Wiskott-Aldrich syndrome.[38]

Platelet abnormalities detected by electron microscopy are described in Glanzmann's thrombasthenia,[39] **Hermansky-Pudlak syndrome,**[40] and **gray platelet syndrome.** In the latter condition, because of almost complete absence of granules, platelets reveal a gray color in Wright-Giemsa–stained blood smears.[41]

Tests of platelet function[42]

1. Platelet count and blood film examination
2. Bleeding time (a) before aspirin and (b) after aspirin
3. Clot retraction
4. Prothrombin consumption time
5. Tourniquet test
6. Platelet aggregation (with or without aggregating agents)
7. Platelet adhesion
8. Platelet factor 3 assay
9. Platelet factor 4 assay
10. Factor VIII evaluation, including factor VIII procoagulant activity, factor VIII antigen, and von Willebrand's factor (ristocetin cofactor activity)
11. Antiplatelet antibodies

Tests 2, 3, 4, and 5 are described in Chapter 11.

Platelet count:

Manual method: Platelets are characterized by a tendency to agglutinate and adhree to foreign surfaces. To obtain reproducible and representative results, the blood specimen should be collected in a plastic syringe and immediately mixed with EDTA.

Reagents and equipment:

1. Unopette reservoir no. 5855, containing 1.98 ml diluent mixture:
   Ammonium oxalate, 11.45 g
   Sörensen's phosphate buffer, 1.0 g
   Thimerosal, 0.1 g
   Dilute with water to make 1 L. Store in the refrigerator.

2. Micropipet, 20 μl
   A dilution ratio of 1:100 is obtained when the volume of sample drawn in the capillary is mixed with the diluent in the reservoir.
3. Hemocytometer (Neubauer) and coverslip

Procedure: Obtain capillary or venous blood in EDTA vacuum tube or in plastic syringe and transfer the latter to EDTA test tube. Fill the micropipet, mix with the diluent in the reservoir, and let it stand for 10 min to allow red cells to hemolyze. Convert to dropper assembly, mix well, discard 4 drops, and fill the hemocytometer. Deposit it in a Petri dish containing moist filter paper in the bottom half and wait 10 min for the platelets to settle. Count the platelets in the central 1 mm² "red cell counting area" at least twice using the high dry objective. Platelets are oval, round, or comma shaped, varying in size from 1-5 μm. Use light or phase microscopy (the latter adds a pink-purple hue to the platelets). Calculate the number of platelets per cubic millimeter of blood by multiplying the total number of platelets counted in 1 mm² by 1000. The calculation is based on the formula found in the discussion of manual red cell counts (see Chapter 7).

Normal values: The average value is 250,000 platelets/mm³ blood. Normal variations range from 175,000-350,000 platelets/mm³ blood. A factor of 10^6 converts these figures to platelets per liter.

Sources of error in hemocytometer counting procedure:

1. Errors in equipment
   a. Moist syringes
   b. Incorrectly calibrated equipment
2. Errors in blood sampling
   a. Fingerstick blood not freely flowing
   b. Clots in anticoagulated blood
   c. Incorrect ratio of blood to anticoagulant or diluent
3. Errors in performance of test
   a. Inadequate filling of micropipet
   b. Inadequate mixing of blood sample in reservoir before filling counting chamber
   c. Failure to discard first 4 drops before applying sample to counting chamber
   d. Errors in counting and arithmetic (In general, manual counts are higher than those performed by electronic particle counters.)[43]

Automated counts: The count may be performed on diluted whole blood or on platelet-rich plasma, and it may be accomplished by an electronic aperture counter or by an optical electronic counting system. The platelet-rich plasma may be prepared by centrifugation or by sedimentation of anticoagulated blood (see Chapter 7).

Confirmation of platelet count by examination of peripheral blood smear: The platelet count should be supplemented by examination of a Wright-Giemsa–stained blood smear to confirm the number of platelets counted and to study their morphology:

Less than 1 platelet per oil-immersion field = Decreased number of platelets
Several platelets with occasional clumps per oil-immersion field = Adequate supply of platelets
More than 25 platelets per oil-immersion field = Increased number of platelets

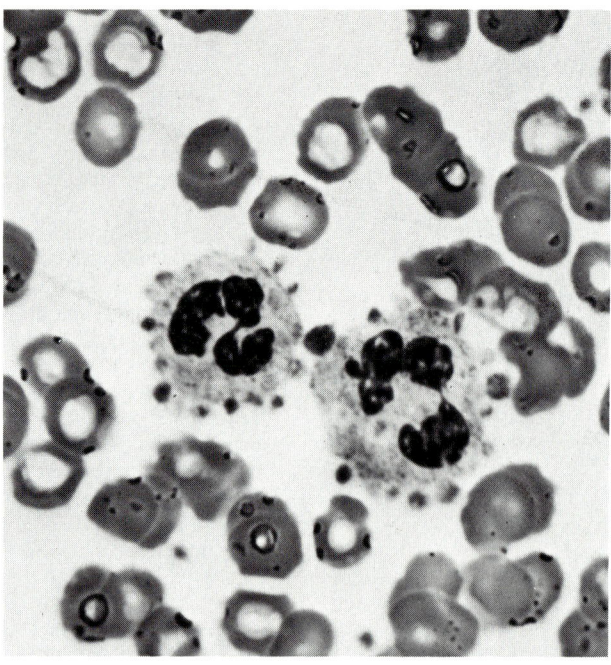

Fig. 12-13. Platelet satellitosis.

If the number of platelets are counted in 10 oil-immersion fields and the total figure multiplied by 2000, the result closely approximates the platelet count obtained by the manual method.

It is also important to note the platelet configuration and size (see previous discussion of variations in platelet morphology). Confirmation of the platelet count by examination of the peripheral blood smear is essential in cases of **pseudothrombocytopenia** in which the automated count is spuriously low because the platelets are arranged around and adhere to neutrophils, a phenomenon called **platelet satellitosis** or platelet rosette formation (Fig. 12-13).[44]

Platelet aggregation: Adequately functioning platelets are essential for hemostasis and for the formation of the intravascular platelet plug (see p. 276).[45] To fulfill their mission platelets must be able to adhere, aggregate, and secrete. Qualitatively inadequate platelets may lose these functions. Since acquired qualitative platelet deficiencies are the most frequent cause of bleeding disorders,[46] platelet aggregation with epinephrine and ristocetin is suggested as a screening test.[47] If the bleeding time is abnormal in the face of a normal platelet count or if all screening tests are normal in a bleeding patient, the platelet aggregation test[48, 49] becomes an essential step in the investigation of the bleeding disorder.

Principle: Platelet-rich citrated plasma is a turbid suspension that at a given wavelength transmits a certain amount of light relative to a platelet-poor citrated plasma blank. This light transmittance can be measured and recorded in a spectrophotometer (aggregometer). The addition of an aggregation-producing agent, e.g., ADP, thrombin, epinephrine, ristocetin, or collagen causes platelets to aggregate into large clumps, a phenomenon responsible for increased light transmittance. Platelet aggregation depends primarily on the quantity and quality of the platelets.[50] Patients must not have taken aspirin in any form during the 2 weeks preceding the test.

Reagents and equipment:
1. Platelet-rich citrated plasma (PRP) (The instrument determines the adequacy of the specimen.)
2. Platelet-poor citrated plasma (PPP)
3. Aggregating agents (Suggested agents are epinephrine and ristocetin, but ADP, collagen, and others may be used. They are commercially available.)
4. Aggregometer with recorder
5. Plastic pipets and test tubes (Do not use glass.)

Procedure: Follow the instructions that accompany the instrument. The critical areas are the concentration of the aggregating agent, the time it takes to complete the test (2-3 hr), the time the PRP is allowed to stand (30 min), the temperature at which the test is performed, and the speed of stirring the sample, The basic steps of the technic using a Bio/Data Platelet Aggregation Profiler (Bio/Data Corp., Willow Grove, Pa.) are as follows: The PRP and PPP samples are inserted into the labeled optical test wells and on the basis of their difference in optical density the instrument determines if the platelet count is sufficient for proper testing. The light that passes through both specimens is transformed into electronic signals that are continuously and differentially compared, amplified, and finally split into two parts. One part is converted to numeric values and on a continuous basis displays the percent aggregation, while the other part is fed into the galvanometer-ac-

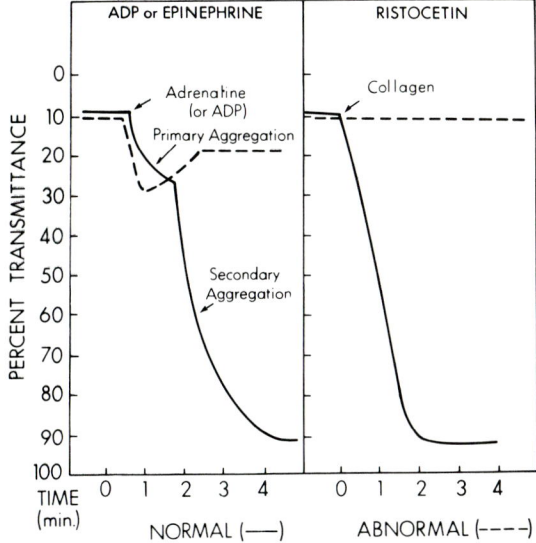

Fig. 12-14. Typical platelet aggregation curves following addition of ADP, epinephrine, and ristocetin.

tuated recorder from which the aggregation curve is generated. The latter reflects the changes in the optical density recorded on a moving paper strip.

Normal values: The patient's aggregation curve is compared with the normal control curve obtained at the same time. Attention is paid to the height and slope of the tracing and to the monophasic or diphasic response.

Interpretation: If epinephrine is used at 37° C as an aggregating agent, two waves of aggregation are produced in about 50% of normal individuals (Fig 12-14). An almost immediate small primary wave of aggregation results from the direct effect of the exogenous epinephrine on platelets and is followed by a secondary larger wave resulting from endogenous release of ADP from the granules. The secondary wave of aggregation is absent in the remaining 50% of normal individuals. Ristocetin aggregation is usually responsible for a single wave only, but at times a double wave response may be seen. If ADP is used at 37° C, a single wave is usually observed, although a double curve occasionally may be encountered. Collagen is usually responsible for a single wave of aggregation.

In congenital platelet abnormalities, e.g., Glanzmann's thrombasthenia, platelets fail to aggregate with any agent, and in Bernard-Soulier syndrome and in von Willebrand's disease they fail to do so with ristocetin. However, in the latter the apparent defect is corrected by the addition of normal plasma (von Willebrand's factor),[51] whereas in Bernard-Soulier disease the defect is not corrected by the addition of fresh plasma.[52] Acquired platelet defects have been described in some types of myeloproliferative disorders,[53] in acquired von Willebrand's disease, in uremia, in liver disease (often associated with thrombocytopenia), in macroglobulinemia and other plasma cell dyscrasias, and following or accompanying the use of a number of drugs. Medications that interfere with platelet aggregation include aspirin and the almost endless list of aspirin-containing

prescription and over-the-counter drugs, anticoagulants (heparin), anti-inflammatory drugs (clofibrate), psychotropic drugs,[49] antihistaminics, and analgesics.

Increased platelet aggregation has been described in thrombosing states (hypercoagulability), hyperlipidemia, diabetes mellitus, and atheromatosis.

Owen et al.[54] stress the fact that even if aggregation is carefully standardized, it may be difficult to interpret, because it may vary in the same control from day to day and is subject to interference by many commonly used drugs. It can be assumed that if epinephrine causes a well-demonstrated biphasic response the test result is normal. Abnormal results must always be confirmed by repeat tests.

Spontaneous platelet aggregation: Spontaneous aggregation of platelets in the optic chamber of the aggregometer may occur without the addition of any aggregating agent[55] in normal individuals[56] but more frequently in patients with arterial insufficiency [57] who are in the process of forming platelet thrombi. Circulating platelet aggregates may also be detected in formalized platelet preparations without the aid of the aggregometer. The increased aggregation may be a reflection of an accelerated turnover and of the appearance of increased numbers of metabolically hyperactive young platelets.

The technic of spontaneous aggregation is a modification of the standard aggregation method described above.[55]

Platelet adhesion:

Principle: The test measures primarily the adhesiveness of platelets to glass beads and, to a lesser extent, platelet aggregation to each other.[58, 59] Native blood is passed through a column of glass beads at a constant rate. A platelet count is performed on the untreated blood and on the blood passed through the glass bead column. The percentage of platelets retained by the glass beads is calculated. Variables that must be standardized are the flow rate, the length of the glass bead column, and the size, number, and material of the glass beads.

Reagents and equipment: The reagents and equipment necessary to perform Bowie and Owen's modification of the platelet adhesion method is marketed by Pacific Hemostasis Laboratories, Los Angeles.

Procedure: Draw 12 ml blood into a 20 ml plastic syringe. Immediately place 10 ml whole blood into the EDTA tube (marked "C" for control). Connect the syringe to the adhesion column and insert the syringe into the constant perfusion pump. Immediately start the pump at a rate of 5.82 ml/min. Collect the first 3 ml blood as 1.0 ml aliquots into EDTA tubes marked 1, 2, and 3. Discard the remainder of the blood, syringe, and column. Perform platelet counts on tubes 1, 2, 3, and control. Calculate the platelet retention as follows:

$$\text{Platelet retention} = \frac{\text{C tube count} - \text{Tube no. 3 count}}{\text{C tube count}} \times 100$$

Normal range: The normal range is 75-97% retention.

Interpretation: The test is difficult to interpret, because it measures two separate platelet functions (adhesiveness and aggregation), which may be independently abnormal.

Decrease retention is encountered in certain hereditary and acquired disorders. The most important hereditary conditions are von Willebrand's disease, Bernard-Soulier syndrome, and Chédiak-Higashi syndrome. The acquired disorders include myeloproliferative disorders, uremia, plasma cell dyscrasias, and disorders resulting from taking aspirin and other drugs.

Increased retention has been reported in hypercoagulability states, hyperlipedemia, carcinoma, and pregnancy and in patients taking oral contraceptives.

Platelet factor 3 availability test: kaolin clotting time: Platelet phospholipid (platelet factor 3) is required in the common pathway for the formation of prothrombinase and in the intrinsic pathway for the formation of factor VIII complex. It is released from stimulated platelets in the course of platelet aggregation induced by various agents or after traumatization of platelets by sonification or by freezing and thawing. The avilability of platelet factor 3 can be evaluated not only by the kaolin clotting time[60,61] but also by the recalcification time of platelet-rich plasma, the Stypven time,[62] the prothrombin consumption test,[54] and the thrombin time.

Principle: The normal recalcification time of PRP is based on a limited release of platelet factor 3. Clotting time can be signficantly shortened by releasing platelet factor 3 from platelets aggregated by kaolin. The PRP is incubated with kaolin before the addition of calcium.

Reagents and equipment:
1. Bio/Data Coagulation Profiler (Bio/Data Corp., Willow Grove, Pa.) (may be used)
2. Platelet-poor plasma (PPP), control and patient (p. 289)
3. Platelet-rich plasma (PRP), control and patient (p. 289) (Perform platelet count on each PRP sample and standardize both in the range of 200,000-600,000/mm^3.)
4. Calcium chloride, 0.035M (p. 288)
5. Kaolin suspension (p. 289)

Procedure: Perform the test according to the following chart:

| | Test tubes (glass) | | | |
	1	**2**	**3**	**4**
PRP, patient (ml)	0.1		0.1	
PRP, control (ml)		0.1		0.1
PPP, patient (ml)		0.1	0.1	
PPP, control (ml)	0.1			0.1
Warm to 37° C.				
Kaolin (ml), 37° C	0.2	0.2	0.2	0.2
Incubate at 37° C, agitating occasionally.				
Calcium chloride (ml), 37° C, added to each tube 1 min apart	0.2	0.2	0.2	0.2

Start timer as soon as calcium is added and record clotting time.

Result: The average clotting time is less than 60 sec.

Interpretation: Prolongation of the clotting times of tubes 1 and 3 (test platelets) compared to those of tubes 2 and 4 (normal platelets) points to reduced platelet factor 3 availability in the test platelets. Such a deficiency has been reported in G-6-PD deficiency.[63]

Platelet factor 4: Platelet factor 4 is an antiheparin capable of neutralizing the anticoagulant activity of heparin. It is released by platelets into the plasma during the platelet plug formation. Increased levels therefore indicate increased platelet utilization somewhere in the body. It is measured by a heparin thrombin method.[64,65]

Principle: The control plasma, rendered platelet poor by centrifugation, serves as the substrate plasma. The patient's plasma is also rendered platelet poor by centrifugation and is then heated in a water bath to destroy fibrinogen and antithrombin III. The mixture of substrate plasma, test plasma, and heparin is clotted by the addition of thrombin. The shorter the clotting time, the higher is the antiheparin activity released by platelets into the plasma. Elevated platelet factor 4 levels have been reported in myocardial infarction, thromboembolism, diffuse intravascular coagulation, and immune thrombocytopenia.[66]

LABORATORY INVESTIGATION OF DISEASES OF PLATELETS

Platelets may be numerically abnormal by being deficient or markedly increased in number, or they may be functionally deficient or overactive (see discussion of hypercoagulability).

The classification of numeric platelet abnormalities is as follows:

I. Thrombocytopenia
  A. Decreased production
    1. Acquired abnormalities
      a. Marrow depression: aplastic anemia, radiation, myelosuppressive drugs
      b. Marrow infiltration: acute leukemia, carcinoma, myelofibrosis, multiple myeloma
      c. Drugs[67,68]: alcohol, thiazide
      d. Severe iron deficiency anemia
      e. Megaloblastic anemias: vitamin B_{12} and/or folic acid deficiency
      f. Paroxysmal nocturnal hemoglobinuria
    2. Congenital abnormalities: Wiskott-Aldrich syndrome, immune deficiency states, Bernard-Soulier syndrome, thrombocytopenia with absent radius (TAR), May-Hegglin anomaly, hereditary thrombocytopenia resembling idiopathic thrombocytopenic purpura, rubella, maternal thiazide therapy, hereditary hypogranular thrombocytopenia, Alport's syndrome
  B. Increased destruction
    1. Immunologic abnormalities
      a. Isoimmune: erythroblastosis fetalis
      b. Autoimmune: idiopathic thrombocytopenic purpura (autoimmune thrombocytopenia), Evans' syndrome, infectious mononucleosis
      c. Antigen-antibody complexes: systemic lupus erythematosus, lymphoma, chronic lymphocytic leukemia
      d. Infections: bacterial, viral, etc.

2. Dilution: exchange transfusion, multiple transfusions
3. Coagulopathies: diffuse intravascular coagulation, septicemia, hemolytic-uremic syndrome, thrombotic thrombocytopenic purpura, large and/or multiple hemangiomas
4. Hypersplenism
5. Heparin
  C. Increased loss: severe hemorrhage
  D. Pseudothrombocytopenia: platelet satellitosis or platelet rosette formation
II. Thrombocytosis
  A. Reactive (secondary): infection, acute blood loss, disseminated carcinoma, splenectomy (e.g., in hereditary spherocytosis), surgery (stress), malignant lesions (e.g., in carcinoma)
  B. Primary: thrombocythemia (myeloproliferative disorders, polycythemia vera, chronic granulocytic leukemia, myelosclerosis, essential thrombocythemia)

Laboratory investigation of idiopathic thrombocytopenic purpura

In adults idiopathic thrombocytopenic purpura (ITP)[69,70] is usually a chronic process, whereas in children it is often acute. No diagnostic laboratory test is available that clearly differentiates ITP from ITP-like conditions as seen in systemic lupus erythematosus, lymphoma, chronic lymphocytic leukemia, drug reactions, and viral infections, e.g., infectious mononucleosis. From the point of view of the clinical pathologist, ITP is characterized by thrombocytopenia in the presence of megakaryocytic hyperplasia in the bone marrow. The platelet survival time is shortened, a phenomenon linked to the action of antiplatelet autoanti-bodies. The platelet destruction exceeds the capability of the bone marrow to replace them.

Hematologic findings: There may be a normocytic normochromic anemia that, depending on the duration of the disease, may give way to a hypochromic microcytic iron deficiency. The leukocyte count is normal or slightly increased, and the differential count may reveal stimulated lymphocytes and eosinophils. In the acute form the platelet count may be depressed below 10,000/mm^3, whereas in the chronic form it is usually below 50,000/mm^3. At levels exceeding 60,000-70,000/mm^3 petechiae are seldom seen. The peripheral blood smear supports the numeric findings in as much as the red and white cells are essentially normal and the number of platelets is severely reduced. Large platelets (megathrombocytes) are seen that alternate with microthrombocytes and with abnormal bizarre platelet forms. The sizes of platelets in thrombocytopenia help to differentiate ITP from two other thrombocytopenic syndromes. Predominantly large platelets are seen in **Bernard-Soulier syndrome,**[71] whereas predominantly small platelets are seen in **Wiskott-Aldrich syndrome.**[38] The bone marrow megakaryocytes are increased in number in ITP. They are large, bizarre, and non–platelet producing and alternate with small immature forms such as promegakaryocytes and megakaryoblasts (Fig. 12-8). However, in some cases of ITP the megakaryocytopoiesis is depressed, a phenomenon thought to be caused by the extension of the antiplatelet action of the autoantibodies to the marrow megakaryocytes. The cytoplasm is agranular and often peripherally vacuolated (Fig. 12-15). Eosinophilia may be noted.

Coagulation tests: The numeric lack of platelets markedly prolongs the bleeding time, shortens the prothrombin consumption time, and interferes with the clot retraction. The partial thromboplastin, prothrombin,

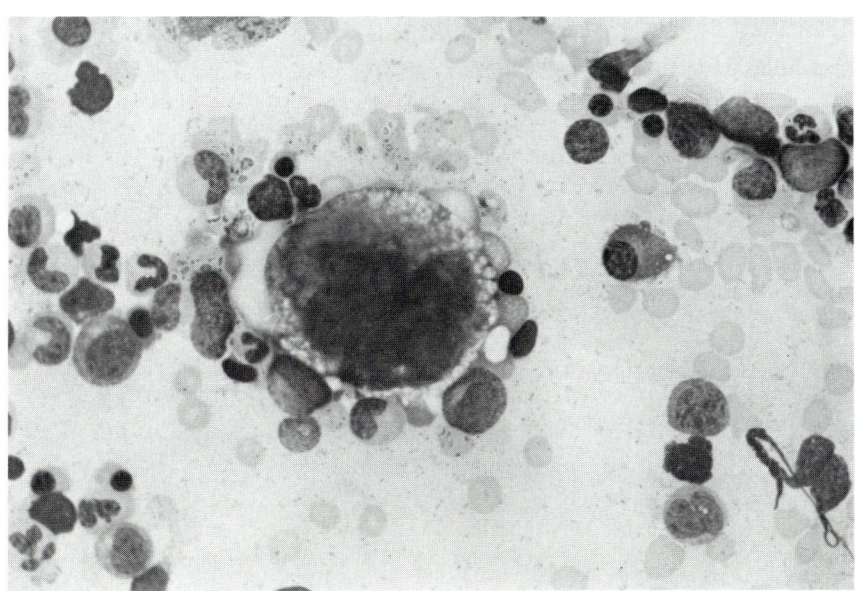

Fig. 12-15. Peripherally vacuolated megakaryocyte.

and clotting times are not affected. The capillary fragility is abnormal.

Platelet survival and determination of platelet sequestration site: In ITP radioactively labeled (^{51}Cr) autologous or compatible isologous platelets are rapidly removed from the circulation within a few hours[72] and are sequestrated in the spleen or the liver.[73]

Differential diagnosis: Additional laboratory tests designed to exclude ITP-like syndromes should include (1) screening for antinuclear antibodies to exclude systemic lupus erythematosus, (2) testing for red cell sensitization by the direct antiglobulin technic to exclude immune hemolytic syndromes, and (3) testing for infectious mononucleosis by the heterophil antibody test. Other ITP-like syndromes that must be considered in the differential diagnosis are included in the discussion of antiplatelet antibodies.

ANTIPLATELET ANTIBODIES

Antiplatelet antibodies may appear in the sera of patients in a number of clinical settings. Autoantibodies may be responsible for the production of thrombocytopenia secondary to lymphoproliferative disorders such as chronic lymphocytic leukemia, to collagen diseases such as systemic lupus erythematosus, and to viral diseases such as infectious mononucleosis. The development of isoantibodies may follow multiple transfusions and may occur during pregnancy if the mother is sensitized by fetal platelets.[74] Also, a number of drugs are known to lead to drug-dependent antiplatelet antibodies, e.g., quinine and digitoxin.[75] In ITP the autoantibodies appear for no known reason. The long list of laboratory methods available for the demonstration of antiplatelet antibodies speaks for the difficulty in demonstrating their existence in all cases of immune thrombocytopenia, especially in ITP. The available technics include the platelet factor 3 availability test,[76-78] complement fixation,[79] lysis of ^{51}Cr-labeled platelets,[80] and a number of recent competitive binding assays for quantitation of platelet-bound immunoglobulins.[81,82]

Antiplatelet antibody determination by platelet factor 3 assay[83]

Hirschman and Gralnick[84] modified the original platelet factor 3 assay of Horowitz et al.[85] and introduced a rapid test that is sensitive and reproducible and can be performed in most laboratories since it requires no specialized equipment.

Principle: Platelet factor 3 is released from platelets by immune injury, and its activity is measured by a clotting-time procedure. Increased antibody activity leads to a higher concentration of factor 3, which is responsible for a shortened clotting time.

Reagents:
1. Platelet-rich plasma (PRP: 350,000-700,000 platelets/mm^3)
   Anticoagulate 10 parts blood with 0.1 part 40% sodium citrate. Centrifuge immediately at 1200 g for 3^1/$_2$ min at room temperature. Decant 1-2 ml PRP and store at 22° C.
2. Platelet-poor plasma (PPP)
   Anticoagulate blood as above. Centrifuge at 1800 g for 10 min. Decant 1-2 ml PPP and store at 22° C.

3. Patient's serum and control sera
   Allow 10 ml blood to clot and incubate it for 4 hr at 37° C. Centrifuge at 1800 g for 10 min at 22° C.
4. CaCl$_2$, 0.025M, 2.75 g/L

Procedure:
The reaction is carried out in a Fibrometer (BioQuest, Cockeysville, Md.).
1. Add 0.1 ml test serum to 0.1 ml PRP.
2. Incubate the mixture at 37° C for 10 min.
3. Add 0.1 ml mixture to 0.1 ml PPP and incubate it for 30 sec at 37° C.
4. Add 0.2 ml CaCl$_2$ and record the clotting time.
5. Repeat the test with five control sera and perform all tests in duplicate.

Results: Results that deviate by more than 2 SD from the results of five control sera with each platelet suspension are considered positive.

Discussion: The higher the concentration of platelets in the PRP, the shorter is the clotting time for both controls and antibody serum samples. For 300,000 platelets/mm^3 the normal mean clotting time may be about 110 sec, whereas the isoantibody clotting time for the same platelet concentration may be 80 sec.[84] Karpatkin et al.,[86] who employed a modification of Horowitz's original platelet factor 3 assay, demonstrated antiplatelet antibodies in 65% of patients with autoimmune thrombocytopenic purpura and in 78% of patients with systemic lupus erythematosus.

Platelet factor 3 assay for antidrug antibodies[87]

Reagents:
1. For the preparation of PRP, PPP, and unknown and control sera see platelet factor 3 assay for antiplatelet antibodies above.
2. Saline solutions of drugs, e.g., the following:
   Quinidine sulfate, 0.005M, 1.85 g/L
   Hydrochlorothiazide, 1.2 mg/ml
   Digoxin, 0.02 mg/ml
3. For controls substitute saline for test serum.

Procedure: Inactivate the sera at 56° C for 30 min, and store at −40° C if not used immediately. Mix 0.1 ml test serum, 0.1 ml drug solution, and 0.1 ml PRP. Allow it to incubate at 37° C for 10 min. Continue with steps 3, 4, and 5 of procedure above.

Results: Results are considered positive when the clotting times deviate by more than 2 SD from the results of five control specimens. Results obtained by Okuno and Crockatt[83] are as follows:

Test serum + quinidine: 48.8 sec
Test serum + saline: 70.2 sec
Control sera + quinidine: 62.4 ± 4.8
Control sera + saline: 60.5 ± 5.4

Coombs' antiglobulin test to detect IgG and C$_3$ on platelets

The radiolabeled Coombs' antiglobulin test[88] substantiates the fact that the majority of patients with idiopathic thrombocytopenic purpura have increased levels of IgG on their platelets. Platelet-associated C$_3$ is elevated in some patients with idiopathic thrombocytopenic purpura even if the IgG is within normal limits, suggesting a role of C_3 in the pathogenesis of idiopathic thrombocytopenic purpura.

Procedure: PRP is obtained by centrifuging EDTA-anticoagulated blood at 170 g for 10 min. Wash platelets three times (2500 g for 10 min) with modified Tyrode's buffer and resuspend to 1 ml (10^8/ml). Incubate at 37° C for 30 min with an aliquot of ^{125}I anti-IgG or ^{125}I anti-C_3. Platelets are washed four times with Tyrode's buffer containing EDTA, resuspended to 1 ml, and the amount of platelet-associated radioactivity determined in a γ-scintillation counter. Results can be reported as platelet-associated radioactivity.

Pseudothrombocytopenia

Platelet adherence to the periphery of neutrophils is called platelet satellitosis or platelet rosette formation. Its importance lies in that it is a cause of spurious thrombocytopenia if EDTA blood samples are tested. It probably results from an IgG platelet satellitosis factor (Fig 12-13).[45,89,90]

Heparin-associated thrombocytopenia

Heparin administration in a dosage-dependent phenomenon may be responsible for complement-mediated platelet injury that may lead to at times severe thrombocytopenia.[91]

LABORATORY INVESTIGATION OF ESSENTIAL THROMBOCYTHEMIA

An increase in the platelet concentration to over 400,000/mm^3 is designated **thrombocytosis,** whereas an excess of platelets of 1 million or over is referred to as **thrombocythemia,**[92] which may fall into the group of myeloproliferative disorders such as polycythemia vera, chronic granulocytic leukemia, and myelofibrosis.

Hematologic findings: Patients with essential thrombocythemia suffer from a combination of thromboembolic and hemorrhagic episodes that influence the red cell picture. Because of the blood loss there is usually a hypochromic microcytic anemia with low mean corpuscular hemoglobin and low mean corpuscular hemoglobin concentration, but low-grade erythrocytosis and the occurrence of macrocytic anemia have been documented. There is usually a moderate leukocytosis. A platelet count of 1 million/mm^3 is not unusual and is often exceeded, values up to 10-14 million have been reported.[93] The blood film is quite characteristic, because it is flooded with platelets that vary in size and alternate with megakaryocytic fragments. The red cell morphology expresses the iron deficiency, and most of the erythrocytes are small and show ring staining. There is a neutrophilic shift to the left with myelocytes making their appearance. The **leukocyte alkaline phosphatase** level is normal or high. The **bone marrow** may show hyperplasia of all hematopoietic elements but predominantly of platelets and megakaryocytes, which form closely packed masses. The megakaryocytes are large with polylobulated nuclei and excessive platelet production. Some younger, smaller, immature forms are also observed. On the other hand, the aspirate may contain only sheets of platelets and fragments of megakaryocytic cytoplasm. The normal

erythroid/myeloid ratio is preserved. The erythropoiesis is normoblastic or shows features of megaloblastoid maturation. Stainable iron is absent except for a few ring sideroblasts. Bone marrow biopsy sections show a moderate increase in reticulin fibers.[94]

Other laboratory findings: The high levels of serum acid phosphatase, serum potassium, uric acid, and serum lactic dehydrogenase are probably related to the rapid platelet turnover rate. The bleeding tendency is an expression of intrinsic platelet deficiencies.[95]

FUNCTIONAL PLATELET DISORDERS

The functional (qualitative) platelet disorders are divided into the rare congenital disorders and the frequently encountered acquired forms that are secondary to some primary disease process[96] or to drugs.

Inherited platelet disorders

The hereditary congenital defects of platelet function can be classified as follows:

1. Defective adhesion to collagen: Bernard-Soulier (giant platelet) syndrome,[97] (a platelet membrane abnormality)
2. Defective release reaction: storage pool disease (defective storage and defective release,[98] aspirin-like defect (normal storage and defective release),[99] Hermansky-Pudlak syndrome,[100] and Wiskott-Aldrich syndrome[38]
3. Defects of primary aggregation: Glanzmann's thrombasthenia
4. Unclassified disorders (e.g., gray platelet syndrome.[41])

Laboratory features of the main congenital platelet disorders are given in Table 12-1.

Acquired platelet disorders

Clinically significant (bleeding) platelet abnormalities have been documented in chronic kidney disease (uremia), liver disease, and a number of hematologic malignancies, e.g., lymphoproliferative and myeloproliferative disorders, and monoclonal gammopathies. In uremia the bleeding time is prolonged in the face of a usually normal platelet count, although about 40% of patients develop thrombocytopenia. Platelet aggregation (secondary wave) and adhesion[101] are abnormal, and platelet factor 3 is not released when platelets are stimulated.[102,103] In coagulation disorders of chronic liver disease, the shortened half-life of the prothrombin factors and hypofibrinogenemia comes to mind first, but the uremic platelet defect has also been described in liver disease,[104,105] as well as the thrombocytopenia secondary to hypersplenism. Severe thrombocytopenia is frequently encountered in acute leukemia and multiple myeloma, whereas in macroglobulinemia[106] and myeloproliferative disorders (with the exception of chronic myelogenous leukemia) defective release of platelet factor 3 has been demonstrated coupled with abnormal aggregation response and morphologic changes (anisocytosis and giant forms) of platelets resulting from bone marrow dysthrombopoiesis.[107]

Of the drugs that affect platelet function, aspirin and phenylbutazone are the most important ones, because they produce the aspirin-like platelet defect character-

Table 12-1. Laboratory findings in some inherited platelet disorders

Disorder	Platelet count	Clot retraction	Bleeding time	Aggregation					Morphology			Platelet adhesion
				ADP (primary)	Epinephrine (secondary)	Ristocetin	Release of ADP		Light microscopy	Electron microscopy		
Glanzmann's thrombasthenia	Normal	Absent	Prolonged	Absent	Absent	Normal	Normal		Isolated platelets, not clumped	Normal		Decreased
Bernard-Soulier syndrome	Decreased	Normal	Prolonged	Normal	Normal	Absent (not normalized by normal plasma)	Normal		Giant platelets; anisocytosis	Swiss cheese pattern		Decreased
Storage pool disease	Normal	Normal	Prolonged	Normal	Absent	Normal	Decreased		Normal	Absent; dense bodies		Decreased
Aspirin-like defect	Normal	Normal	Prolonged	Normal	Absent	Normal	Decreased		Normal	Normal		Normal

ized by a prolonged bleeding time, inhibition of the second wave of aggregation, and decreased ADP release.[108]

REFERENCES

1. Penington, D.G., and Streatfield, K.: Ser. Haematol. **8:**22, 1975.
2. Breton-Gorius, J.: Nouv. Rev. Fr. Hematol. **13:**504, 1973.
3. Nakeff, A., Dicke, K.A., and van Noord, M.J.: Ser. Haematol. **8:**4, 1975.
4. Bessis, M.: Rev. d'Hematol. **4:**294, 1949.
5. Jones, O.P.: Anat. Rec. **138:**105, 1960.
6. Schulman, I., et al.: Blood **16:**943, 1960.
7. MacDonald, T.P.: In Baldini, M.G., and Ebbe, S., editors: Platelets: production, function, transfusion, and storage, New York, 1974, Grune & Stratton, Inc.
8. Rebuck, J.W., Boyd, C.B., and Monto, R.W.: In Brinkhous, K.M., Shermer, R.W., and Mostofi, F.K., editors: The platelet, Baltimore, 1971, The Williams & Wilkins Co.
9. Jones, O.P.: Proc. Soc. Exp. Biol. Med. **34:**694, 1936.
10. Harker, L.A., and Finch, C.A.: J. Clin. Invest. **48:**963, 1969.
11. Brecher, G.: In Baldini, M.G., and Ebbe, S., editors: Platelets: production, function, transfusion, and storage, New York, 1974, Grune & Stratton, Inc.
12. Pearson, H.A., et al.: J. Pediatr. **68:**754, 1966.
13. Epstein, C.J., et al.: Am. J. Med. **52:**299, 1972.
14. Franzen, S., Strenger, G., and Zajicek, J.: Acta Haematol. **26:**182, 1961.
15. Saarni, M.I., and Linman, J.W.: Am. J. Med. **55:**38, 1973.
16. Malamud, N., Haymaker, W., and Custer, R.P.: Milit. Med. **99:**397, 1946.
17. Kass, L.: Arch. Pathol. Lab. Med. **98:**112, 1974.
18. Melamed, M.R., et al.: Am. J. Med. Sci. **252:**301, 1966.
19. Maldonado, J.E., Pintado, T., and Pierre, R.V.: Blood **43:**797, 1974.
20. Maldonado, J.E.: Blood **43:**811, 1974.
21. Karpatkin, S., and Garg, S.: Br. J. Haematol. **26:**307, 1974.
22. White, J.G.: Ann. N.Y. Acad. Sci. **201:**205, 1972.
23. Hattori, A., et al.: Ser. Haematol. **8:**126, 1975.
24. White, J.G.: In Williams, W.J., et al., editors: Hematology, ed. 2, New York, 1977, McGraw-Hill Book Co.
25. Crawford, N., and Taylor, D.G.: Br. Med. Bull. **33:**199, 1977.
26. Caen, J.P., Cronberg, S., and Kubisz, P.: Platelets: physiology and pathology, New York, 1977, Stratton Intercontinental Medical Book Corp.
27. White, J.G.: In Brinkhous, K.M., Shermer, R.W., and Mostofi, F.K., editors: The platelet, Baltimore, 1971, The Williams & Wilkins Co.
28. Holmsen, H., Day, H.J., and Stormorken, H.: Scand. J. Haematol. **8**(suppl.):3, 1969.
29. Paulus, J., et al.: In Baldini, M.G., and Ebbe, S., editors: Platelets: production, function, transfusion, and storage, New York, 1974, Grune & Stratton, Inc.
30. Beck, E.A., and Baumgartner, H.R.: Schweiz. Med. Wochenschr. **100:**330, 1970.
31. Bernheim, J., et al.: Am. J. Med. **61:**145, 1976.
32. Fajardo, L.F., and Rao, S.: Milit. Med. **136:**463, 1971.
33. Marx, R., and Jean, G.: Klin. Wochenschr. **42:**491, 1964.
34. Bithell, T.C., Parekh, S.J., and Strong, R.R.: Ann. N.Y. Acad. Sci. **201:**145, 1972.
35. Maldonado, J.E., et al.: Mayo Clin. Proc. **50:**402, 1975.

36. Breton-Gorius, J.: Ser. Haematol. **8:**49, 1975.
37. Fajardo, L.F.: Am. J. Clin. Pathol. **63:**554, 1975.
38. Grottum, K.A., et al.: Br. J. Haematol. **17:**373, 1969.
39. Caen, J.P., et al.: Am. J. Med. **41:**4, 1966.
40. White, J.G., et al.: Am. J. Pathol. **63:**319, 1971.
41. Raccuglia, G.: Am. J. Med. **51:**818, 1971.
42. Henry, R.L.: Semin. Thromb. Hemostas. **4:**93, 1977.
43. Mattern, C.F.T., Brackett, F.S., and Olson, B.J.: J. Appl. Physiol. **10:**56, 1957.
44. Hyun, B.H., Gulliani, G.L., and Woodall, M.: Hematology "Check Sample" No. H-78, Chicago, 1976, Commission on Continuing Education, American Society of Clinical Pathologists.
45. Zeigler, Z.: Haemostasis **3:**282, 1974.
46. Kjeldsberg, C.R., and Hershgold, E.J.: J.A.M.A. **227:**628, 1974.
47. Packham, M.A., and Mustard, J.F.: Semin. Hematol. **8:**30, 1971.
48. Day, H.J., and Holmsen, H.: Ann. Clin. Lab. Sci. **2:**63, 1972.
49. Swatman, L.E.: Med. Lab. **12:**22, 1976.
50. O'Brien, J.R.: J. Clin. Pathol. **15:**446, 1962.
51. Weiss, H.J., Rogers, J., and Brand, H.: J. Clin. Invest. **52:**2697, 1973.
52. Howard, M.A., Hutton, R.A., and Hardisty, R.M.: Br. Med. J. **2:**586, 1973.
53. Neemeh, J.A., et al.: Am. J. Clin. Pathol. **57:**336, 1972.
54. Owen, C.A., Jr., Bowie, E.J.W., and Thompson, J.H.: The diagnosis of bleeding disorders, ed. 2, Boston, 1975, Little, Brown and Co.
55. Wu, K.K., and Hoak, J.C.: Thromb. Haemost. **35:**702, 1976.
56. Kardinal, C.G., Wegener, L.T., and Anderson, L.K.: Am. J. Clin. Pathol. **63:**559, 1975.
57. Wu, K.K., and Hoak, J.C.: Blood **44:**934, 1974.
58. Bowie, E.J.W., and Owen, C.A., Jr.: Am. J. Clin. Pathol. **56:**479, 1971.
59. Bowie, E.J.W., and Owen, C.A., Jr.: Am. J. Clin. Pathol. **60:**302, 1973.
60. Hardisty, R.M., and Hutton, R.A.: Br. J. Haematol. **11:**258, 1965.
61. Austen, D.E.G., and Rhymes, I.L.: A laboratory manual of blood coagulation, London, England, 1975, Blackwell Scientific Publications, Ltd.
62. Fekete, L.F.: In Recent concepts & developments in evaluating disorders of hemostasis and thrombosis, Chicago, 1976, Commission on Continuing Education, American Society of Clinical Pathologists.
63. Schartz, J.P., Cooperberg, A.A., and Rosenberg, A.: Br. J. Haematol. **27:**273, 1974.
64. Dana, B., Carvalho, A.C.A., and Ellman, L.: Am. J. Clin. Pathol. **65:**964, 1966.
65. Fuster, V., et al.: Mayo Clin. Proc. **48:**103, 1973.
66. Fabiszewski, R., et al.: Thromb. Haemost. **19:**578, 1968.
67. Mills, D.C.B.: Clin. Haematol. **1:**295, 1972.
68. Miescher, P.A.: Semin. Hematol. **10:**311, 1973.
69. Prankerd, T.A.J.: Clin. Haematol. **1:**327, 1972.
70. Mueller-Eckhardt, C.: Semin. Thromb. Hemostas. **3:**125, 1977.
71. Bernard, J., and Soulier, J.P.: Bull. Mem. Soc. Med. Hop. Paris **64:**969, 1948.
72. Ries, C.A., and Price, D.C.: Ann. Intern. Med. **80:**702, 1974.
73. Najean, Y., and Ardaillou, N.: Br. J. Haematol. **21:**153, 1971.
74. Pearson, H.A., et al.: Blood **23:**154, 1964.
75. Young, R.C., Nachman, R.L., and Horowitz, H.I.: Am. J. Med. **41:**605, 1966.
76. Karpatkin, S., and Siskind, G.W.: Blood **33:**795, 1969.
77. Spaet, T.H., and Cintron, J.: Br. J. Haematol. **11:**269, 1965.
78. Mueller-Eckhardt, C., and Mersch-Baumert, K.: Vox Sang. **33:**221, 1977.
79. Aster, R.H., Cooper, H.E., and Singer, D.L.: J. Lab. Clin. Med. **63:**161, 1964.
80. Aster, R.H., and Enright, S.E.: J. Clin. Invest. **48:**1199, 1969.
81. McMillan, R., et al.: Blood **37:**316, 1971.
82. Dixon, R., Rosse, W., and Ebbert, L.: N. Engl. J. Med. **292:**230, 1975.
83. Okuno, T., and Crockatt, D.: Am. J. Clin. Pathol. **66:**475, 1976.
84. Hirschman, R.J., and Gralnick, H.R.: J. Lab. Clin. Med. **84:**292, 1974.
85. Horowitz, H.I., et al.: Transfusion **5:**336, 1965.
86. Karpatkin, S., et al.: Am. J. Med. **52:**776, 1972.
87. Okuno, T., and Crockatt, D.: Am. J. Clin. Pathol. **65:**523, 1976.
88. Cines, D.B., and Schreiber, A.D.: N. Engl. J. Med. **300:**106, 1979.
89. Ravel, R., and Bassart, J.A.: Lab. Med. **5:**41, 1974.
90. Kjeldsberg, C.R., and Swanson, J.: Blood **43:**831, 1974.
91. Cines, D.B., et al.: N. Engl. J. Med. **303:**788, 1980.
92. Lewis, S.M., Szur, L., and Hoffbrand, A.V.: Clin. Haematol. **1:**339, 1972.
93. Fanger, H., Cella, L.J., and Litchman, H.: N. Engl. J. Med. **250:**456, 1954.
94. Horowitz, H.I., and Nachman, R.L.: Semin. Hematol. **2:**287, 1965.
95. Jellett, L.B., and Bonnin, J.A.: Aust. N.Z. J. Med. **15:**51, 1966.
96. Lusher, J.M., and Barnhart, M.I.: Semin. Thromb. Hemostas. **4:**123, 1977.
97. Bernard, J., and Soulier, J.P.: Sem. Hop. Paris **24:**3217, 1948.
98. Weiss, H.J., et al.: N. Engl. J. Med. **281:**1264, 1969.
99. Weiss, H.J.: Ann. N.Y. Acad. Sci. **201:**161, 1972.
100. Hermansky, F., and Pudlak, P.: Blood **14:**162, 1959.
101. Salzman, E.W., and Neri, L.L.: Thromb. Haemost. **15:**84, 1966.
102. Horowitz, H.I., et al.: Blood **30:**331, 1967.
103. Rabiner, S.F.: Prog. Hemost. Thromb. **1:**233, 1972.
104. Thomas, D.P., Ream, V.J., and Stuart, R.K.: N. Engl. J. Med. **276:**1344, 1967.
105. Weiss, H.J., and Eichelberger, J.W.: Arch. Intern. Med. **112:**827, 1963.
106. Pachter, M.R., et al.: Am. J. Clin. Pathol. **31:**467, 1959.
107. Lisiewicz, J.: Semin. Thromb. Hemostas. **4:**241, 1978.
108. Weiss, H.J., Aledort, L.M., and Kochwa, S.: J. Clin. Invest. **47:**2169, 1968.

CHAPTER 13

Laboratory investigation of hemorrhagic diseases and hypercoagulability

HEMORRHAGIC DISEASES

Hemorrhagic diseases are divided into congenital and acquired conditions. The congenital diseases usually result from a single coagulation defect, although multiple congenital deficiencies have been described. The acquired conditions often have more than one coagulation defect.

Hemorrhagic diseases may further be classified according to the nature of the main defect into (1) vascular defects, (2) coagulation factor defects, (3) coagulation defects resulting from circulating anticoagulants, and (4) platelet defects (see Chapter 12).

HEMORRHAGIC DISEASES RESULTING FROM VASCULAR DEFECTS: NONTHROMBOCYTOPENIC OR VASCULAR PURPURAS

The pathophysiology of vascular purpuras is complex, because it may involve platelets, connective tissue, capillaries, and clotting factors. The diagnosis is established by exclusion of the other hemorrhagic disorders and by an abnormal bleeding time in the absence of quantitative and qualitative platelet abnormalities.

Congenital vascular disorders (primary purpuras)
Hereditary hemorrhagic telangiectasia

Hereditary hemorrhagic telangiectasia is inherited as an autosomal dominant disorder of venules and capillaries that form thin-walled dilated masses of vessels that are unable to contract in response to an injury. These angiomas are widely distributed, but the nasal lesions are responsible for the most frequent presenting symptom of epistaxis.[1]

Purpuras resulting from mesenchymal dysplasias[2]

Ehlers-Danlos syndrome is an inherited autosomal dominant defect of elastic tissue fibers. The bleeding tendency may be caused by a collagen-platelet interaction defect.[3] **Marfan's syndrome** also falls into this group, because its bleeding tendency is based on the lack of adequate connective tissue support of the capillaries and smallest vessels.[4]

Acquired vascular disorders
Purpura simplex

Purpura simplex is manifested by cutaneous petechiae and includes "easy bruising," a common complaint of women over 40 years. Ecchymoses follow minimal trauma, which frequently cannot be recalled by the patient. Owen and Thompson[5] report evidence indicating that the loss of vascular integrity results from a platelet defect. A familial form of purpura simplex has been described.[6]

Senile purpura

Senile purpura is seen in older and debilitated individuals who develop petechiae and ecchymoses in the skin of the extremities, face, and back following minimal trauma, e.g., pressure of clothing. It is probably related to loss of perivascular supportive fibrous tissue.[7] The purpura seen in Cushing's disease, following the administration of ACTH, and in vitamin C deficiency (scurvy) also appears to be connected to changes in the connective tissue support framework.[8,9]

Stasis and mechanical purpura

Stasis purpura results from an acute or chronic increase in intraluminal capillary pressure and may follow interference with the venous return from the lower extremities or cutaneous pressure changes caused by paroxysmal coughing, weight lifting, or decompression sickness.

Dysproteinemic purpura[10]

Coating of platelets with abnormal globulins may explain the purpura seen in macroglobulinemia, multiple myeloma, chronic lymphatic leukemia, lupus erythematosus, cryoglobulinemia,[11] and amyloidosis. In amyloidosis absence of factor X has also been demonstrated.[12]

Autoerythrocyte and DNA sensitivity

Gardner and Diamond[13] describe painful cutaneous ecchymoses of women in whom intradermal testing with red cells, red cell stroma, and hemoglobin produces similar lesions at the injection site.[14]

Allergic purpura

Allergic purpura is primarily a vasculitis of children,[15] although cases in adults have been reported. The etiologically responsible antigen has not been isolated or identified, if indeed there is a single antigen responsible for all cases. The antigens that have been investigated include β-hemolytic streptococci,[16] immune complexes,[17] and the various causes of secondary purpuras, e.g., foods, drugs, and infections.[18] Schönlein associated the characteristic purpuric rash of the buttocks and lower extremities with rheumatic joint manifestations, and Henoch added gastrointestinal symptomatology (melena and pain) to the description of the disease now referred to as **Schönlein-Henoch purpura.** The disease may also give rise to hematuria caused by a focal acute glomerulonephritis. The **purpuras secondary to infection** may complicate meningococcal and streptococcal septicemias, viremias as seen in measles and infectious mononucleosis, and rickettsial infections, e.g., Rocky Mountain spotted fever. Purpura at times may be quite extensive as in **purpura fulminans.**

Congenital coagulation factor defects
Congenital factor I (fibrinogen) deficiency

Congenital abnormalities of fibrinogen may be quantitative, e.g., afibrinogenemia and hypofibrinogenemia, or qualitative, e.g., dysfibrinogenemia.

Afibrinogenemia and hypofibrinogenemia: Afibrinogenemia, or absence of fibrinogen, is very rare and is inherited through an autosomal recessive gene. It occurs with equal frequency in both sexes. In the homozygous patient no fibrinogen is demonstrable in the plasma. According to Bommer, Künzer, and Schröer[20,21] 50% of these infants bleed from the umbilical stump and in later life from cuts and injuries. Epistaxis and hemarthroses have also been reported.[19-21]

Laboratory diagnosis: No clot forms in clotting tests since the blood is incoagulable, and no fibrinogen can be demonstrated by any method. The tests can be normalized by the addition of fibrinogen or normal plasma. It should be noted that incoagulable blood is also encountered in hyperplasminemia and hyperheparinemia. Hyperplasminemia can be exluded by the repetition of the clotting test after the addition of ε-aminocaproic acid. Hyperheparinemia can be excluded by repetition of the clotting test after neutralization of heparin by protamine sulfate (see p. 347). The heterozygous (carrier) form of afibrinogenemia may be asymptomatic or show a mild bleeding tendency. Low levels of fibrinogen (below 100 mg/dl) can be demonstrated by all methods employed to demonstrate fibrinogen,

Table 13-1. Coagulation tests in hypofibrinogenemia

Test	Result
Whole blood clotting time	Prolonged
Ivy bleeding time	Normal
Platelet count	Normal
Clot retraction	Prolonged
Prothrombin time	Prolonged
Activated partial thromboplastin time	Prolonged
Prothrombin consumption	Normal
Fibrinogen	Below 100 mg/dl
Thrombin time	Prolonged
Reptilase time	Prolonged

Table 13-2. Clotting tests in dysfibrinogenemia

Test	Result
Whole blood clotting time	Normal
Ivy bleeding time	Normal
Platelet count	Normal
Prothrombin time	Normal
Activated partial thromboplastin time	Normal
Thrombin time	Prolonged
Reptilase time	Prolonged
Fibrinogen assay	
Clotting technic	Normal
Immunologic technic	Normal
Precipitation technic	Normal

e.g., clotting, precipitation, and immunologic technics.[22] Traces of fibrinogen may be demonstrable by immunologic technics even in homozygous afibrinogenemia, rendering the diagnosis of afibrinogenemia dependent on the sensitivity and specificity of the method employed. In hypofibrinogenemia the clotting times are prolonged (Table 13-1), depending on the fibrinogen concentration, and thrombokinetic instruments demonstrate abnormal clot formation.

Dysfibrinogenemia: Qualitative abnormalities of the fibrinogen molecule are called dysfibrinogenemias.[19] They are inherited in an autosomal dominant manner. Clinically the patient may be asymptomatic or show a mild bleeding tendency, abnormal wound healing, and even a tendency to develop thrombi. The structural change in the fibrinogen molecule is caused by an amino acid substitution in one of the polypeptide chains[23] and expresses itself in abnormal clot formation and dissolution. The fibrinogen concentration of the plasma is within normal limits. The abnormal fibrinogens are named according to the cities in which they were discovered, e.g., fibrinogen Detroit[23] and fibrinogen St. Louis.[24] More than two dozen abnormal fibrinogens are now recognized.

Laboratory diagnosis: Clotting tests in dysfibrinogenemia are given in Table 13-2.

Congenital factor II (prothrombin) deficiency (hypoprothrombinemia)

The rarely encountered congenital deficiency of factor II is inherited as an autosomal recessive trait.[25] The few cases reported present the clinical picture of umbilical and postcircumcision bleeding and subcutaneous and joint hemorrhages.[26] Some patients have an abnormally low concentration of functionally normal prothrombin, whereas others have a functionally defective but immunologically normal prothrombin.[27,28]

Laboratory diagnosis: Clotting tests in factor II deficiency are given in Table 13-3.

Congenital factor V (proaccelerin) deficiency (parahemophilia)

Factor V deficiency is inherited as an autosomal recessive trait and is clinically expressed by epistaxis and by posttraumatic and gingival bleedings[29,30] which may be severe in homozygous patients.

Table 13-3. Clotting tests in factor II deficiency (hypoprothrombinemia)

Test	Result
Whole blood clotting time	Normal
Prothrombin time	Prolonged, depending on prothrombin concentration
Stypven time	Normal
Factor II concentration	Diminished
Taipon time	Prolonged
Activated partial thromboplastin time	Normal to prolonged, depending on prothrombin concentration
Bleeding time	Normal
Platelet count	Normal
Factor II–deficient plasma	No correction

Table 13-4. Clotting tests in factor V deficiency

Test	Result
Whole blood clotting time	Prolonged
Ivy bleeding time	Prolonged
Clot retraction	Normal
Platelet count	Normal
Prothrombin time	Prolonged
Activated partial thromboplastin time	Prolonged
Prothrombin consumption	Shortened
Prothrombin consumption plus platelet substitute	Shortened
Fibrinogen	Normal
Factor V assay	Decreased

Table 13-5. Clotting tests in factor VII deficiency

Test	Result
Whole blood clotting time	Normal
Ivy bleeding time	Normal
Clot retraction	Normal
Prothrombin time	Prolonged
Activated partial thromboplastin time	Normal
Prothrombin consumption	Normal
Fibrinogen	Normal
Stypven time	Normal
Factor VII assay	Decreased

Laboratory diagnosis: Clotting tests in factor V deficiency are given in Table 13-4.

Congenital factor VII (proconvertin) deficiency

Factor VII deficiency is inherited as an autosomal recessive trait and is responsible for gingival and mucosal bleeds and posttraumatic hemorrhages,[31] although more severe hemophilia-like symptoms and thrombotic episodes have been reported.[32] There are two types of deficiencies—with or without cross-reacting material.[33]

Laboratory diagnosis: Clotting tests in factor VII deficiency are given in Table 13-5. Since factor VII is involved only in the extrinsic pathway, the prothrombin time is prolonged, whereas the activated partial thromboplastin time is unaffected. The Stypven time is normal, because it does not require factor VII, thus differentiating between factor VII and factor X deficiencies, provided factor I, factor V, and platelets are adequate. The Taipon time may be used to exclude prothrombin deficiency, and factor V deficiency is excluded by the lack of correction of the prolonged prothrombin time by adsorbed normal plasma. The use of commercially available factor VII–deficient plasma clinches the diagnosis.

Congenital factor VIII (antihemophilic factor) deficiency (hemophilia A)

Factor VIII deficiency is inherited as a sex-linked recessive trait in hemophilia A or as an autosomal dominant trait in von Willebrand's disease. A combined defect of factor V and factor VIII is also transmitted as an autosomal recessive trait.[34] In hemophilia A the defective gene is linked to the X chromosome ($\overline{X}$). (The term *hemophilia* generally refers to hemophilia A, the factor VIII deficiency.) If a hemophilic male ($\overline{X}Y$) marries a normal female (XX), the male children will be normal (XY), but all female children will be obligatory carriers (heterozygous $\overline{X}X$), the defective gene ($\overline{X}$) being counterbalanced by a normal X chromosome. If the latter marry normal males (XY), half of the female children will be carriers ($\overline{X}X$) and half will be normal females (XX), whereas half of the male children will be hemophiliacs ($\overline{X}Y$) and half will be normal males (XY). In the unlikely circumstance that a hemophilic male ($\overline{X}Y$) marries a heterozygous female ($\overline{X}X$), one of the children may be a hemophilic female ($\overline{X}\,\overline{X}$).

Hemophilia is a rare disease (about 6 per 100,000 population),[35] and the seriousness of the disease depends on the concentration of factor VIII, which forms the basis for its clinical classification into three groups: mild (6-30% factor VIII), moderate (1-5% factor VIII), and severe (less than 1% factor VIII). Although mild and moderate hemophiliacs may lead a relatively normal life and bleed only when challenged by experiences such as trauma, surgery, and childbirth, severe hemophiliacs are in continuous fear of hemarthroses, extensive bleeding, painful, deep hematomas, hematuria, and prolonged hemorrhages lasting for days and weeks following minimal injuries. Carriers have a factor VIII concentration varying from 25-75% (average 50%). By the use of a highly specific rabbit antiserum against factor VIII in a system of crossed immunoelectrophoresis of Laurell,[36] antigenically active but functionally ineffective cross-reacting material (CRM) can be demonstrated in all hemophilic plasmas,[37] thus eliminating the division of hemophilia into hemophilia A + (CRM +) or hemophilia A − (CRM −).

Laboratory diagnosis: Clotting tests in factor VIII deficiency are given in Table 13-6. Factor VIII is involved in the intrinsic pathway, and the results of tests of the intrinsic pathway are influenced by the concentration of factor VIII and their sensitivity to this concentration. In severe and moderate hemophilia all clotting tests are abnormal, whereas in mild hemophilia the activated partial thromboplastin time is prolonged and other forms of plasma recalcification time will be within the normal range. The abnormal activated partial thromboplastin time is corrected with fresh adsorbed plasma but not with factor VIII–deficient or aged plasma. The clot in hemophilia is poorly formed and is responsible for an abnormal thrombokinetogram,[38] which may be the only abnormality found in mild hemophilia. The bleeding time in hemophilia is normal, but 24 hr after the test, when the scab is removed, secondary bleeding may occur and may be persistent. In the diagnosis of hemophilia the family history is most important, but the possibility of spontaneous mutations must be kept in mind. The assay of factor VIII concentration is the final procedure.

Table 13-6. Clotting tests in factor VIII deficiency (hemophilia A)

Test	Result
Whole blood clotting time	Prolonged
Ivy bleeding time	Normal
Clot retraction	Normal
Platelet count	Normal
Prothrombin time	Normal
Activated partial thromboplastin time	Prolonged
Prothrombin consumption	Shortened
Prothrombin consumption plus platelet substitute	Shortened
Fibrinogen	Normal
Factor VIII assay	Decreased
Platelet aggregation with ristocetin	Normal

Laboratory diagnosis of the carrier of hemophilia: The plasma of the (female) carrier of hemophilia contains about 50% of the normal factor VIII concentration. Because of the wide spread of normal factor VIII concentration (55-145%), the rather large error in its assay methods, and its augmentation by many physical and psychologic factors, factor VIII assay cannot be used in the detection of the carrier. The ratio of factor VIII:C (procoagulant) to factor VIII:AG (related antigen) provides a means to detect carriers of hemophilia.[39] In the normal individual the factor VIII:C%/factor VIII:AG% ratio is 1 or over, because there is as much or more procoagulant activity as there is factor VIII–related antigen. Under conditions of stress both increase, so that the ratio remains unchanged. In carriers the procoagulant level falls to about 50% or lower of normal, but the factor VIII–related antigen concentration remains at its normal level. The factor VIII:C%/factor VIII:AG% ratio therefore falls to about 0.6% or lower, and under conditions of stress the ratio does not change. In most cases the carrier can thus be diagnosed by assaying the factor VIII:C%/factor VIII:AG% ratio.[40,41,41a]

Von Willebrand's disease

Von Willebrand's disease is a familial bleeding disorder that is inherited as an autosomal dominant trait, thus affecting males and females, and is clinically characterized by cutaneous and mucosal bleeds. The disease varies in severity from a mild form, which is asymptomatic until stressed by surgery and other forms of trauma, to a severe form, which may mimic hemophilia.

Laboratory diagnosis: In von Willebrand's disease all three components of the factor VIII complex are absent: factor VIII:C (procoagulant), factor VIII:AG (related antigen), and factor VIII R:WF (von Willebrand's factor). The absence of the latter is responsible for the prolonged bleeding time, the absence of retention of platelets to glass beads, and the absence of ristocetin-induced platelet aggregation. For differentiation of von Willebrand's disease from hemophilia A see Table 13-7.

In response to plasma transfusion (even the plasma of hemophiliacs), the factor VIII:C concentration in the plasma of von Willebrand's patients rises higher than expected from the amount of factor VIII transfused and remains elevated for 2 or more days.[42] It dissociates

Table 13-7. Differentiation of von Willebrand's disease and hemophilia A

	Von Willebrand's disease	Hemophilia A
Factor VIII:C (AHF)	Reduced (10-30%)	Reduced (2% or less)
Factor VIII:C response to transfusion of factor VIII	In excess of transfused factor VIII:C	Not in excess of transfused factor VIII:C
Factor VIII:AG	Reduced	Normal
Factor VIII R:WF	Reduced or absent	Normal
Bleeding time	Prolonged	Normal
Ristocetin-induced platelet aggregation	Reduced or absent	Normal
Inheritance	Autosomal dominant	Sex-linked recessive
Capillary bleeding	Common	Absent

Table 13-8. Clotting tests in von Willebrand's disease

Test	Result
Whole blood clotting time	Prolonged or normal
Ivy bleeding time	Prolonged
Clot retraction	Normal
Platelet count	Normal
Prothrombin time	Normal
Activated partial thromboplastin time	Prolonged
Prothrombin consumption	Shortened
Prothrombin consumption plus platelet substitute	Shortened
Fibrinogen	Normal
Platelet adhesion and ristocetin aggregation	Diminished
Factor VIII assay	Diminished

itself from factor VIII R:WF and from factor VIII:AG, the concentrations of which decrease at the same time as the factor VIII:C concentration increases.[43] The prolonged bleeding time response to the plasma transfusion in von Willebrand's disease is variable; it may remain prolonged or it may be corrected for only a few hours. In hemophilia A the transfusion response is directly proportional to the factor VIII concentration transfused, and the activity is lost in 12-14 hr.[44] The bleeding time remains normal (see Fig. 11-4).

Overwhelming evidence indicates that the apparently primary platelet abnormalities encountered in von Willebrand's disease are not the expression of an intrinsic platelet defect but rather the result of the absence of a plasma factor, because they are corrected by the administration of plasma and/or factor VIII.[45] The expressions of the platelet dysfunction include a prolonged bleeding time, lack of platelet adhesion to endothelium and glass beads, and lack of ristocetin-induced platelet aggregation. The prolonged bleeding time, an expression of the platelet disorder, is sensitive to the administration of aspirin, a fact that can be used in the diagnosis of mild cases of von Willebrand's disease in patients who have a normal bleeding time, but after the ingestion of 10 grains of aspirin the bleeding time is prolonged[46] in excess of the expected post-aspirin prolongation. The low platelet retention to glass beads is an indication of the abnormal platelet adhesion.[47] Ristocetin, an antibiotic that is not in clinical use, induces aggregation of normal platelets but not of platelets derived from patients with von Willebrand's disease,[48] whereas other aggregating agents, e.g., epinephrine and ADP, induce normal aggregation.[49]

Clotting tests in von Willebrand's disease are given in Table 13-8. The laboratory findings are influenced by the severity of the factor VIII deficiency, which may at times be masked by a number of conditions, e.g., birth control pills and pregnancy, that temporarily increase its concentration (see p. 280). The platelet-controlling factor of von Willebrand's disease is not subject to these fluctuations and aids in the diagnosis of mild von Willebrand's disease, which may require repeated coagulation workups before the diagnosis can be established.

Not all patients with von Willebrand's disease have the typical coagulation profile described above but deviate from it by demonstrating normal values for one or the other parameter that is usually abnormal in von Willebrand's disease; e.g., factor VIII:C, the bleeding time, or the platelet aggregation is normal. These forms of von Willebrand's disease are referred to as **variants** of the disease.[50]

Congenital factor IX (Christmas factor) deficiency (hemophilia B or Christmas disease)

Hemophilia B, a congenital factor IX deficiency, is clinically and genetically indistinguishable from hemophilia A but occurs less frequently. The asymptomatic female carriers have slightly depressed factor IX concentrations,[51] whereas the affected males show severe factor IX depression. Of all hemophiliacs 10-15% suffer from hemophilia B, which like hemophilia A shows a wide spectrum of clinical expression varying from an asymptomatic state to a severe bleeding tendency. Almost all patients with hemophilia B when tested with anti-factor IX antibody produced in rabbits have cross-reacting functionally abnormal but immunologically reactive material in their blood.[52] Most patients are therefore CRM+, leaving only a few who are CRM−. Almost all patients with Christmas disease have a normal prothrombin time when the test is performed with human brain thromboplastin, but in a variant of the disease the prothrombin time is prolonged if bovine brain thromboplastin is used. This variation in the prothrombin time is caused by a molecular abnormality of factor IX that inhibits the thromboplastin-factor VII reaction of the extrinsic pathway.[53] Other molecular varients have been investigated and named according to the location in which they were discovered, e.g., hemophilia B Leyden.[54]

Laboratory diagnosis: Clotting tests in factor IX deficiency are given in Table 13-9. Factor IX deficiency leads to a prolonged activated partial thromboplastin time, which can be corrected by the addition of normal serum and fails to be corrected by the addition of factor IX-deficient plasma. The diagnostic test is the factor IX assay.

Congenital factor X (Stuart-Prower factor) deficiency

Factor X deficiency is a rare disease that is inherited as an autosomal recessive characteristic[55] and, depending on the factor X concentration, may be responsible for easy bruising only or for severe posttraumatic hemorrhages.

Laboratory diagnosis: Clotting tests in factor X deficiency are given in Table 13-10. The one-stage prothrombin time is prolonged and is corrected by serum but not by factor X-deficient plasma nor by adsorbed plasma. The Stypven time is prolonged, ruling out factor VII deficiency. Of the other deficiencies responsible for a prolonged Stypven time, factor V deficiency is rules out by the lack of correction with adsorbed plasma, and neither serum nor adsorbed plasma correct a prothrombin deficiency. Factor X assay clinches the diagnosis.

Table 13-9. Clotting tests in factor IX deficiency (Christmas disease, hemophilia B)

Test	Result
Whole blood clotting time	Prolonged
Ivy bleeding time	Normal
Clot retraction	Normal
Platelet count	Normal
Prothrombin time	Normal
Activated partial thromboplastin time	Prolonged
Prothrombin consumption	Shortened
Prothrombin consumption plus platelet substitute	Shortened
Fibrinogen	Normal
Factor IX assay	Diminished

Table 13-12. Clotting tests in factor XII deficiency

Test	Result
Whole blood clotting time	Prolonged
Ivy bleeding time	Normal
Clot retraction	Normal
Platelet count	Normal
Prothrombin time	Normal
Activated partial thromboplastin time	Prolonged
Prothrombin consumption	Shortened
Prothrombin consumption plus platelet substitute	Shortened
Fibrinogen	Normal
Factor XII assay	Diminished

Table 13-10. Clotting tests in factor X deficiency

Test	Result
Whole blood clotting time	Normal
Ivy bleeding time	Normal
Clot retraction	Normal
Platelet count	Normal
Prothrombin time	Prolonged
Activated partial thromboplastin time	Prolonged
Prothrombin consumption	Normal
Fibrinogen	Normal
Stypven time	Prolonged
Factor X assay	Diminished

Table 13-11. Clotting tests in factor XI deficiency (hemophilia C)

Test	Result
Whole blood clotting time	Prolonged or normal
Ivy bleeding time	Normal
Clot retraction	Normal
Prothrombin time	Normal
Activated partial thromboplastin time	Prolonged
Prothrombin consumption	Shortened
Prothrombin consumption plus platelet substitute	Shortened
Fibrinogen	Normal
Factor XI assay	Diminished

Congenital factor XI (plasma thromboplastin antecedent) deficiency (hemophilia C)

Hemophilia C is inherited as an autosomal recessive trait[56] that occurs almost exclusively in Jews and usually leads to a mild bleeding disorder with easy bruising, epistaxis, and posttraumatic hemorrhage.

Laboratory diagnosis: Clotting tests in factor XI deficiency are given in Table 13-11. The activated partial thromboplastin time and the nonactivated partial thromboplastin time are equally prolonged (normally the activated time is shorter) and correction by serum and adsorbed plasma may be variable and the correction by adsorbed plasma is less than that achieved by the addition of serum. Factor XI–deficient plasma fails to correct the prolonged activated partial thromboplastin time. Factor XI assay clinches the diagnosis.

Congenital factor XII (Hageman factor) deficiency

Factor XII deficiency is not accompanied by any bleeding diathesis; in fact, some of the Hageman factor–deficient patients died of thromboembolic phenomena, including the first patient ever described.[57,58] The disease is inherited as an autosomal recessive or dominant trait.[59]

Laboratory diagnosis: Clotting tests in factor XII deficiency are given in Table 13-12. The prolongation of all clotting tests measuring the intrinsic pathway is in glaring contrast with the almost complete absence of clinical symptoms. The prothrombin time that measures the extrinsic pathway of clotting is normal. The partial thromboplastin time is not shortened by the addition of kaolin, since the contact factor is missing from the plasma (see discussion of factor XI deficiency). Factor XII–deficient plasma fails to correct the prolonged clotting time.

Congenital deficiency of Fletcher factor

Fletcher factor deficiency is clinically asymptomatic.[60] The defect is inherited as an autosomal recessive trait.

Laboratory diagnosis: The activated partial thromboplastin time is prolonged and is corrected by the addition of serum or adsorbed plasma. An important feature of the prolonged activated partial thromboplastin time is the fact that it shortens, even to normal, on incubation, because apparently extended activation of factors XII and XI corrects the plasma kallikrein deficiency.[61]

Congenital deficiency of Fitzgerald factor

Fitzgerald factor deficiency,[62] like Fletcher factor deficiency, is clinically asymptomatic and in the laboratory is characterized by a prolonged activated partial thromboplastin time and a normal prothrombin time.

The prolonged activated partial thromboplastin time is corrected by the addition of fresh plasma, including that from patients with Fletcher factor or factor XII deficiencies.[63] Williams and Flaujeac traits[64] appear to be identical to Fitzgerald trait.[63]

Congenital deficiency of Passovoy factor

Hougie et al.[65,66] report a coagulation abnormality of the extrinsic pathway of coagulation that clinically produces easy bruising and excessive hemorrhage after minor trauma. The activated partial thromboplastin time is markedly prolonged, whereas the prothrombin time, the intrinsic factor levels, platelets, prekallikrein, and high-molecular-weight kininogen are normal. The deficiency is inherited as an autosomal dominant trait.

Congenital factor XIII (fibrin stabilizing factor) deficiency

Congenital factor XIII deficiency is a rare disorder that must be considered if there is a history of neonatal umbilical cord bleeding of the patient and of his siblings, easy bruising, and prolonged bleeding from wounds that heal slowly and lead to keloid formation. Other manifestations of factor XIII deficiency are ecchymoses and slowly disappearing subcutaneous hematomas.[67-69] The disease is inherited as an autosomal recessive trait. Since only very small amounts of factor XIII (1% or less) are active in the coagulation sequence, heterozygous individuals are asymptomatic, and homozygous individuals show complete absence of factor XIII.

Laboratory diagnosis: All routine clotting tests are normal, except the clot is friable and the thrombokinetogram (Bio/Data Corp., Willow Grove, Pa.) is abnormal. If factor XIII is absent as in homozygous patients, the diagnosis is readily made, because the clot is abnormally soluble in 5M urea or in 2% acetic acid solution. The heterozygous patient is identified by immunologically measuring the subunits A (proenzyme) and S (carrier protein).[70,71]

Congenital combined coagulation factor deficiencies

Combined congenital factor deficiencies are rare, since the majority of combined deficiencies are acquired abnormalities. A number of cases with congenitally decreased factors V and VIII have been reported.[72] Other combined deficiencies include factors VIII and IX, VII and IX, and VII and VIII.[73]

Acquired coagulation disorders

Acquired deficiencies of coagulation factors result from nonavailability of vitamin K to the liver, severe liver disease, defibrination syndrome and DIC (p. 310), appearance of antibodies to coagulation factors (p. 286), and administration of oral anticoagulants and heparin.

Acquired coagulation abnormalities in liver disease

Severe hepatocellular damage leads to an acquired deficiency of the vitamin K–dependent factors (factors II, VII, IX, and X)[74] fibrinogen, and factor V. Fibrinogen and factor V are produced in the liver but do not require vitamin K for their synthesis. By the combined use of functional and immunologic assay methods it can be demonstrated that in liver disease there is loss of coagulation protein synthesis[75] that fails to respond to the parenteral injection of vitamin K. This lack of response aids in the diagnosis of hepatocellular jaundice.[76] The etiology of the coagulation factor depression in liver disease thus differs from that seen in vitamin K deficiency (see below). Hepatic depression leads to prolongation of the one-stage prothrombin time, which is paralleled by the depression of the plasma albumin.[77] Prolongation of the prothrombin time to twice its normal level is a poor prognostic sign[78] in liver disease. Impaired hepatic synthesis is also responsible for the depression of factors V and I. The contact factors (XI and XII) are not significantly affected by liver disease, whereas factor VIII may be strikingly elevated.[74,79] The mosaic of coagulation disorders in liver disease is modified by the frequent reduction of factor XIII,[80] thrombocytopenia secondary to hypersplenism or disseminated intravascular coagulation,[81] the appearance of increased fibrinolytic activity, increase in circulating fibrin degradation products,[81] and decrease in antithrombin III levels.[82]

Vitamin K deficiency: Vitamin K is essential for the hepatic synthesis of the vitamin K–dependent clotting factors (II, VII, IX, and X).[83] If the supply of vitamin K is inadequate, the activity of the coagulation factors decreases in the following order: factor VII first, followed by factors IX, X, and II.[84] In the absence of vitamin K the liver produces biologically abnormal, coagulationwise inactive proteins, which are called PIVKA[85] (see p. 281) and have a clotting inhibitory effect.

Vitamin K is derived from green leafy vegetables in the diet and from the activity of coliform intestinal bacteria. Since it is fat soluble, of bacterial origin, and requires bile for its absorption, a large number of conditions interfere with vitamin K availability and absorption, e.g., malabsorption syndromes, intestinal sterilization by antibiotics, obstructive jaundice, and oral anticoagulants.

HYPERCOAGULABILITY

LABORATORY CONTROL OF ANTICOAGULANT THERAPY

The purpose of anticoagulant therapy is to prevent intravascular fibrin formation. This goal is achieved by the use of two groups of drugs: heparin and warfarin sodium, (Coumadin) derivatives. Although their clinical anticlotting effect is similar, they achieve their therapeutic result by different routes and require different laboratory controls, dosages, and forms of administration. The prime indication for their use is the prevention and treatment of venous thrombosis. Their use in arterial thromboses is still controversial after 30 years of use.[86]

Oral anticoagulants

Oral anticoagulants prevent the hepatic synthesis of the biologically active vitamin K–dependent clotting factors (VII, IX, X, and II), reducing their concentration to such levels as to interfere with fibrin clot formation. Although oral anticoagulants lack fibrinolytic or thrombolytic activity, an already formed clot will fail to propagate if the blood is anticoagulated and, since it remains small, it is more likely to be digested by the physiologic fibrinolytic processes. Two groups of oral anticoagulants are available: coumarin derivatives and indanedione derivatives. The most commonly prescribed drugs, bishydroxycoumarin (Dicumarol) and warfarin sodium (Coumadin) belong to the first group. By inhibiting hepatic vitamin K reductase they render vitamin K ineffective in transforming the inactive precursor coagulation proteins (CRMs) into functional coagulation factors[87-89] (see PIVKA, p. 281), thus reducing the concentration of factors VII, IX, X, and II. While the effect of the anticoagulant on vitamin K is immediate, the disappearance rate of the factors in the plasma is a function of their half-life. The concentration of factor VII with a half-life of 5-6 hr decreases first, whereas the levels of factors IX, X, and II fall more slowly.[90] It takes about 1 week of treatment before all vitamin K–dependent factors are equally depressed.[91] A large number of variables influence the anticoagulant effect of warfarin sodium drugs.[89] Conditions and drugs that may potentiate the response to oral anticoagulants are liver disease,[92] vitamin K deficiency, fever,[89] thyrotoxicosis,[93] heart failure, and drugs[94] such as phenylbutazone, salicylates, and steroids. Conditions and drugs that may inhibit or increase the resistance to oral anticoagulants are hereditary resistance,[95] pregnancy,[96] and drugs[94] such as barbiturates, oral contraceptives, and griseofulvin. The drug-induced variations[97] are related to inhibition or acceleration of warfarin sodium metabolism, stimulation or depression of clotting factors, inference with vitamin K, or unknown factors. The one-stage prothrombin time is used to monitor patients on oral anticoagulant therapy, the aim of which is to provide adequate anticoagulation with minimal risk of hemorrhage, a goal that is usually achieved if the prothrombin time does not exceed the control level by twice the norm. In the first week of anticoagulant therapy the prothrombin time is not a good indicator of antithrombotic effect, because the prolongation of the prothrombin time depends largely on the depression of factor VII, whereas the antithrombotic effect of warfarin sodium is primarily related to the depression of factor IX (not measured by prothrombin time) and factor X.[89] During this period heparin should be administered concomitantly with warfarin sodium. When heparin therapy is discontinued and replaced by oral anticoagulants only about 6 hr need to be allowed to pass before the prothrombin time can be used to monitor the effect of oral anticoagulation.

Heparin

Heparin requires binding to antithrombin III for its anticoagulant activity, which depends on the neutralization of factors IXa, Xa, and XIa and thrombin.[98] In the prevention of venous thrombosis the pivotal reaction is the inhibition of the activated serine protease factor Xa.[99] Once a clot has formed, the emphasis shifts to the antithrombin activity[99] of heparin, which requires higher doses than does the prethrombic prophylaxis,[100] and even higher doses are required for the prevention of platelet-induced arterial thrombi.[100]

Administration and control

The aim of heparin therapy is identical with that of oral anticoagulants, i.e., to achieve adequate anticoagulation without the danger of hemorrhage. Since heparin cannot be administered orally, the most common methods of administration are by intermittent or continuous intravenous injection or by the subcutaneous route. The intravenous route provides immediate onset of action that can be adequately controlled by a number of laboratory tests. The low doses of prophylactic heparin therapy do not require laboratory monitoring.

Laboratory monitoring

A large number of coagulation tests can be employed to monitor heparin therapy. They include activated partial thromboplastin time, Lee-White clotting time, activated clotting time of whole blood, and thrombin time. If the expected prolongation of the clotting tests in response to heparin fails to occur, the antithrombin III level must be assayed. In general it can be stated that no laboratory test can predict bleeding caused by heparin therapy and that all the coagulation tests mentioned—if at least doubly prolonged in response to heparin—indicate adequate antithrombin III levels and an adequate heparin response. Linearity between activated partial thromboplastin time and heparin concentration has been reported[101] if a kaolin-activated partial thromboplastin reagent (Hyland Laboratories, Costa Mesa, Calif.) or an improved activated cephaloplastin (Dade Diagnostics, Miami, Fla.) is used, but the type of thromboplastin is only one of many variables that affect the clotting tests. The others are the type of heparin administered[102] (bovine, porcine, calcium, or sodium salt), the presence of kidney or liver disease, the antithrombin III level, and the platelet concentration (antiheparin activity of platelet factor 4). All the clotting tests mentioned are "global" tests and are influenced not only by heparin but also by factor deficiencies. If there is any doubt concerning the etiology of the prolongation, heparin must be neutralized (see below) and the clotting test repeated. Bick[103] suggests the following approach to the monitoring of heparin therapy. The activated partial thromboplastin time is obtained 60 min after infusion of heparin. If the result is prolonged to about twice the norm, no further testing is necessary, because this proves that the patient's antithrombin III level is adequate to respond to the dose of heparin administered. If the antithrombin III prolongation is unexpectedly inadequate, the antithrombin III level should be determined. Lastly, the plasma heparin level may be assayed, which should vary from 0.1-1 unit/ml plasma.

Colorimetric determination of heparin in plasma by use of synthetic substrate

Principle[104]: Heparin is determined in the plasma by a series of reactions. In the first step, heparin combines with antithrombin III to form heparin–antithrombin III complex:

Heparin + Antithrombin III $\longrightarrow$
$$\text{Heparin–antithrombin III complex}$$

Since the following step depends on the complete binding of all heparin present, normal plasma is added to the sample to ensure an adequate supply of anti-thrombin III. In the next step the heparin–antithrombin III complex combines with and inactivates added coagulation factor Xa. An excess of factor Xa is added so that some free factor Xa remains after all the heparin–antithrombin III complex has combined with and inactivated some of the factor Xa. The free factor Xa then enzymatically catalyzes the hydrolysis of an artificial peptide substrate containing p-nitroaniline as a terminal group. The free p-nitroaniline removed by the hydrolysis is then determined colorimetrically.

The amount of p-nitroaniline formed in a given time interval is proportional to the amount of free factor Xa present and thus is a measure of the amount of the heparin–antithrombin III complex and thus of the amount of heparin present in the sample. The more heparin present in the original sample, the smaller is the amount of free factor Xa present and the smaller the amount of p-nitroaniline formed. The method has some disadvantages. If the amount of heparin present in the sample is sufficient to inactivate all of the added factor Xa, there will be only a minimal amount of hydrolysis, and one will be unable to judge between samples containing just enough heparin to inactivate all of the added factor Xa and samples containing larger amounts of heparin. On the other hand, if one adds sufficient factor Xa to take care of all the expected levels of heparin, the accuracy at low levels of heparin will be small, since one will be measuring the small difference between two large numbers (hydrolysis with no heparin and hydrolysis with only a small amount of heparin). To reduce these errors, the procedure calls for two standard curves, one from 0.00-0.20 IU/ml for small amounts of heparin and one from 0.00-0.80 IU/ml when larger amounts are expected.

The procedure as outlined calls for cuvets having a working volume of 1 ml and, preferably, a light path of 1 cm. There is no theoretic reason why the procedure could not be scaled upward to use larger volumes, but this would require larger amounts of the reagents, some of which are expensive.

Reagents:
1. Substrate S-2222 (Ortho Diagnostics, Raritan, N.J.) (a polypeptide with p-nitroaniline as a terminal group), 1 mmole/L
   Prepare the substrate by adding 25 mg substrate to 34 ml water at 50° C, and stir to dissolve. If prepared under sterile conditions, this solution is stable for 6 months in the refrigerator.
2. Coagulation factor Xa, (Diagen[Diagnostic Reagents, Thame, Oxon, England])
   Dissolve one ampule in 0.8 ml distilled water. The solution is stable for about 10 hr at room temperature.
3. Tris buffer, 50 mmole/L, pH 8.4, with 7.5 mmole/L EDTA and 175 mmole/L NaCl
   Dissolve 6.1 g tris(hydroxymethyl)aminomethane, 2.6 g disodium ethylenediamine tetraacetate dihydrate, and 10.2 g NaCl in about 8 dl water. Adjust the pH to 8.4 by adding 1 mole/L HCl (83 ml concentrated acid per liter) (17-20 ml of the acid will generally be required), and dilute to 1 L. This buffer is stable for 2 months in the refrigerator.

4. Normal plasma
   Obtain blood samples from a number of normal donors. Collect the blood in sodium citrate, 1 volume of 0.1 mole/L sodium citrate (29 g/L) to 9 volumes of blood. Discard the first milliliter of blood, and keep the rest in an ice bath. Prepare the plasma by centrifuging at 2000 g for 20 min in a refrigerated centrifuge. Mix approximately equal volumes of plasma from a number of donors, and dispense into small tubes in volumes of 3-4 ml. Tightly stopper the tubes and store them at −20° C. For use thaw the tubes at 37° C, and then keep them on ice.
5. Acetic acid, 5.25 moles/L
   Dilute 30 ml glacial acetic acid with water to make 1 dl.

Procedure: Treat the test plasma samples the same way as the normal control plasma.

As mentioned above, standard curves in two different ranges are used; these will be the high (0-0.8 IU heparin/ml) and the low (0-0.2 IU/ml) ranges. The procedure is slightly different for the two ranges. Both are given below.

Just before analysis dilute the standard or sample plasma by adding 100 μl plasma to 100 μl normal plasma and 800 μl buffer solution. This will be referred to as the diluted plasma and should be used as soon as possible after preparation.

The protocol for the analysis is given below. The appropriate standards are used in the high and low ranges. Usually the sample is run in both ranges unless one has good reason to assume that the sample level is high or low.

	High range	Low range
1. Diluted sample or standard plasma	200 μl	200 μl
Incubate at 37° C for exactly:	4min	4 min
2. Coagulation factor Xa Add at room temperature.	100 μl	100 μl
Mix and incubate at 37° C for:	30 sec	180 sec
3. Substrate S-2222 Add at 37° C. Mix rapidly and start stopwatch.	200 μl	200 μl
Incubate at 37° C for exactly:	180 sec	180 sec
4. Acetic acid, 5.25 moles/L Add rapidly at end of incubation period.	500 μl	500 μl
Mix at once and allow to stand for:	20 min	20 min

Read standards and samples against blank (see below) at 405 nm. The blank is prepared from 200 μl diluted plasma, 500 μl acetic acid solution, and 300 μl water. With clear sample plasmas the samples and standards can be read against the same standard blank, but with icteric (total bilirubin over 6 mg/dl) or hyperlipemic samples the plasma sample should be read against its own blank.

Preparation of standard curves: The standards are prepared in pooled normal plasma.
1. To 1 dl normal saline add 300 μl heparin solution

containing 5000 units/ml to give a solution containing 15 units/ml. If possible, the same heparin as given to the patient should be used in preparing the standards.

2. To 1400 μl normal plasma add 100 μl of the above diluted heparin solution (15 units/ml) to give a solution containing 1 unit/ml. Prepare the high standards as follows:

Heparin solution (μl)	Normal plasma (μl)	Final concentration (unit/ml)
0	500	0.00
100	400	0.20
200	300	0.40
300	200	0.60
400	100	0.80

For the low standards dilute 100 μl of each of the above standards with 300 μl normal plasma or prepare as follows:

Heparin solution (μl)	Normal plasma (μl)	Final concentration (unit/ml)
0	1000	0.00
50	950	0.05
100	900	0.10
150	850	0.15
200	800	0.20

The standard curve is prepared by using the appropriate standards and the procedure as given above. The values for the samples are read from the appropriate curve.

Fluorometric determination

Principle: Heparin is determined by a series of reactions similar to those used for antithrombin III as follows[105-108]:

Heparin + Antithrombin III (excess) ⟶

Antithrombin III–heparin complex

Antithrombin III–heparin complex + Thrombin ⟶

Antithrombin III–heparin–thrombin complex +

Residual thrombin

Residual thrombin + Synthetic substrate–fluorescent

compound complex ⟶ Substrate + Fluorescent compound

The substrate is hydrolyzed by the residual thrombin, and the rate of the reaction is measured. The rate depends on the amount of residual thrombin present, which in turn depends on the amount of antithrombin III–heparin complex present to react with the added thrombin, and the amount of complex depends on the amount of heparin present, since the antithrombin III is added in excess. (In the antithrombin III assay the heparin is added in excess, and the final rate of reaction depends on the amount of antithrombin III originally present.) The residual thrombin is used to hydrolyze a substrate that will liberate a fluorescent compound, and the rate of formation of the fluorescence is measured. This procedure thus requires the use of a good spectrofluorometer with a thermostated cell compartment. The determination may also be run on a special fluorometer designed for such tests (Protopath [Dade Division, American Hospital Supply Corp., Miami, Fla.]).

Reagents:

1. Buffer A, 0.25 mole/L glycine, pH 8.3
   Dissolve 18.8 g glycine, 0.74 g dipotassium EDTA, and 1.8 g NaCl in water to make about 9 dl in a 1 L volumetric flask. Adjust the pH to 8.3 by adding 5 moles/L NaOH (200 g/L). Add 0.1 g thimerosol, dilute to 1 L, and mix well.

2. Buffer B, 0.25 mole/L glycine with 0.15 mole/L NaCl
   Dissolve 18.8 g glycine, 8.8 g NaCl, and 0.74 g dipotassium EDTA in about 9 dl water in a 1 L volumetric flask. Adjust the pH to 8.3 by adding 5 moles/L NaOH. Add 0.3 ml 30% bovine albumin solution, dilute to 1 L, and mix well.

3. Thrombin solution
   Dilute a lyophilized vial of human thrombin containing 2500 NIH units/mg (Calbiochem-Behring Corp., San Diego) with buffer B to make 10 units/ml. Store it in 1 ml aliquots at −20° C. Just before use thaw an aliquot, and dilute it to 2 units/ml with the same buffer.

4. Sodium heparin solution and standards
   Dilute one vial of sodium heparin U.S.P. (beef lung) (Upjohn Co., Kalamazoo, Mich.), 10,000 units/ml, to make 80 units/ml with buffer A (2-250 ml). A standard containing 0.8 unit/ml is prepared by diluting 100 μl of the 80 units/ml with 9.9 ml pooled normal plasma. Standards of 0.1, 0.2, and 0.4 unit/ml are prepared by diluting 1 ml of the 0.8 unit/ml standard with 7, 3, and 1 ml plasma, respectively.

5. Pooled normal plasma
   Obtain specimens from five normal individuals in plastic syringes, and mix 9 volumes of blood with 1 volume of 3.8% sodium citrate in plastic tubes. Separate the plasma by centrifugation at 1200 g for 15 min. Pool the samples, store them at 4° C, and use within 8 hr. Dilute one part of the plasma with buffer A 1:40 (1 ml plasma + 39 ml buffer), and use in all determinations as an equalizer of antithrombin III activity.

6. Substrate solution
   The substrate used is D-phenylalanine-proline-arginine-5-amidoisophthalic acid, dimethyl ester diacetate (Enzyme System Products, Indianapolis). Prepare a stock solution by dissolving 560 mg in 50 ml absolute ethanol. This is stored at 4° C. For use dilute the stock with buffer A 1:80 (0.5 ml stock + 39.5 ml buffer). Warm an aliquot to 37° C just before use.

Procedure: Set the spectrofluorometer for an excitation wavelength of 335 nm, with a slit width of 6 nm, and an emission wavelength of 430 nm with a slit width of 12 nm. Set the recorder speed to 25 mm (1 in)/min. Use rectangular cuvets with a capacity of 4 ml. Add 200 μl of the 1:40 diluted normal plasma and 5 μl of the test plasma or heparin standard in plasma to a cuvet and warm to 37° C. Add 50 μl thrombin solution (2 units/ml) and mix. Incubate for 60 sec at 37° C. (This preincubation time is fairly critical and should be kept constant for the samples and standards.) Add 2 ml diluted substrate, mix by inversion, and place it in a spectrofluorometer. The change in fluorescence is measured over a 4-5 min interval. A blank is run by using the normal plasma without heparin, and the heparin standards given above are also run. The result is calculated as follows:

Initial thrombin (%) =

$$\frac{\text{Rate of change of test or standard}}{\text{Rate of change of blank}} \times 100$$

The values obtained for the blank and the various heparin standards are plotted against the amounts of heparin in the standards, and the amount in the samples is read from the curve.

Antithrombin III

Determination by amidolytic colorimetric method by use of artificial substrate (Chromozym TH)

Principle: Thrombin hydrolyzes the artificial colorless substrate toluene-sulfonyl-glycyl-prolinyl-arginyl-p-nitroaniline (Tol-Gly-Pro-Arg-p-Na) to release the compound p-nitroaniline, which has a strong absorbance at 405 nm. Thus, as with other enzymatic reactions, the increase in absorbance per unit of time is a measure of the enzyme activity. Antithrombin III inhibits the action of thrombin, and thus in the presence of antithrombin III the absorbance change will be smaller. Thus by comparing the absorbance change with and without the presence of serum containing antithrombin the amount of the latter may be estimated.[109]

Reagents:
1. Triethanolamine buffer, pH 8.4, 0.1 mole/L
   Dissolve 18.57 g triethanolamine hydrochloride and 11.69 g NaCl in about 8 dl water. Adjust the pH to 8.4 by adding 2 moles/L NaOH. Add 300 units of heparin (0.6 ml from a vial containing 5000 units/ml) and dilute to 1 L. Dissolve the above substrate (as hydrochloride[Chromozym TH, Boehringer Mannheim Biochemicals, Indianapolis]) in water to make a concentration of 1 mg/ml. This solution is stable for about 6 months when kept in the refrigerator.
2. Thrombin solution, 10 units/ml
   Dissolve the contents of a vial containing 50 NIH units of thrombin (Fibrindex, Ortho Diagnostics, Raritan, N.J.) in isotonic saline to make 5 ml.
3. Albumin stock solution
   Dissolve 4 g bovine albumin in isotonic saline to make 1 dl.
4. Glacial acetic acid

Procedure: Dilute the plasma sample and the control (4 g/dl bovine albumin) to 1:100 with the buffer (0.1 ml plasma or albumin solution + 9.9 ml buffer). Place a tube containing 0.4 ml diluted test plasma or control in a water bath at 37° C. After warming to the temperature, add 0.1 ml thrombin solution, mix it rapidly, and start the stopwatch. After exactly 30 sec add 0.2 ml substrate solution previously warmed to 37° C. After exactly 30 sec more stop the reaction by adding 0.3 ml glacial acetic acid. Then read the sample against a blank consisting of 0.4 ml diluted plasma (or control), 0.3 ml water, and 0.3 ml acetic acid at 405 nm.

NOTE: The above procedure yields a total volume for absorbance measurement of 1 ml. If the cuvets used require larger volumes, the procedure can be scaled up, but in this case one must be certain that all the reagents

except the acetic acid are at 37° C before adding them to the reaction mixture.

• • •

The plasma antithrombin activity (PATA) is expressed as the amount of thrombin amidolytic activity inhibited as measured by the difference between the thrombin alone control and that of the thrombin plus test plasma using the following formula:

$$\text{PATA (μmole/min/ml)} = \frac{A \times V_1}{E \times V_2 \times t}$$

As is usual with enzyme reactions (see discussion of LDH determinations in enzyme section), A is the difference in absorbance between the control and test samples, E is 9.9 (the millimolar absorption coefficient for p-nitroaniline), V_1 is the assay volume in microliters, V_2 is the amount of sample used (4 μl [0.4 ml of a 1:100 dilution]), and t is the time of reaction in minutes (30 sec = 0.5 min). Thus the above reduces to the following:

$$\text{PATA} = A \times 50.5$$

Note that this assumes a light path of 1 cm. To correct for other light paths see the discussion of LDH determination. Also, if all the reagents are scaled up proportionately, the above factor remains the same.

Normal value: The normal value is 9.4 ± 1.6 μmole/min/ml.

Interpretation: The above procedure has several advantages. The antithrombin is expressed quantitatively rather than as a percentage of activity as in other similar methods.[110] It is not affected by fibrin degradation products that interfere with clotting procedures for antithrombin III.[111] Low levels of antithrombin III are associated with hypercoagulability and with recurrent thromboembolic disease. Rarely are they encountered as a congenital deficiency[112] but are more commonly secondary to liver disease, disseminated intravascular coagulation, and heparin therapy[113] or in women using oral contraceptives.[114]

Fluorometric determination

Principle[115]: Antithrombin III may be determined by using the following series of reactions:

Antithrombin III + Heparin (excess) ⟶

Antithrombin III–heparin complex

Antithrombin III–heparin complex + Thrombin (excess) ⟶

Antithrombin III–heparin–thrombin complex +

Residual thrombin

The residual thrombin may then be used to hydrolyze a colorimetric or fluorometric substrate. The greater the amount of antithrombin III originally present, the greater will be the amount of added thrombin complexed in an inactive form and the smaller will be the amount of hydrolysis of the substrate. In the procedure outlined a substrate is used that when hydrolyzed yields a fluorescent compound. The method thus requires a sensitive spectrofluorometer with thermostated sample cell. (The determination may also be made by using a specially designed fluorometer [Protopath] for this purpose, which along with the required lyophilized reagents may be obtained from the Dade Division, American Hospital Supply Corp., Miami, Fla.) The rate of change of fluorescence and hence of the reaction is an indication of the amount of residual thrombin present. The results are compared with those obtained with different dilutions of pooled normal plasma.

Reagents:
1. Buffer A, 0.25 mole/L glycine, pH 8.3
   Dissolve 18.8 g glycine, 1.8 g NaCl, and 0.74 g dipotassium salt of EDTA in about 9 dl water in a 1 L volumetric flask. Adjust the pH to 8.3 by adding 5 moles/L NaOH (200 g/L). Then add 0.1 g thimerosol and dilute to 1 L.
2. Buffer B, 0.25 mole/L glycine with 0.15 mole/L NaCl
   Dissolve 18.8 g glycine, 8.8 g NaCl, and 0.74 g dipotassium salt of EDTA in about 9 dl water in a 1 L volumetric flask. Adjust the pH to 8.3 by adding 5 moles/L NaOH, add 0.3 ml 30% solution of bovine albumin, and dilute to 1 L.
3. Thrombin, human, lyophilized, 100 units/vial (obtained from WHO International Laboratory for Biological Standards, London MW3 6RB, England)
   Each vial is reconstituted and diluted to 20 units/ml with buffer B. Place the solution in siliconized glass tubes, and store them at −20° C. Before use thaw the heparin and further dilute it with the buffer to a concentration of 1 unit/ml.
4. Heparin, bovine mucosal, lyophilized, 1250 units/vial (obtained from the same source as the thrombin)
   The vial is reconstituted and diluted to a concentration of 10 units/ml, and 0.2 ml aliquots are placed in siliconized glass tubes and stored at −20° C. For use thaw the aliquot and dilute it with the buffer to a working concentration of 2 units/ml.
5. Fluorometric substrate, CBZ-glycine-proline-arginine (HCl)-4-methoxy-β-naphthylamide (Enzyme System Products, Indianapolis)
   a. Stock solution, 18.3 mmole/L
      Dissolve 0.600 g of the salt in absolute ethanol to make 50 ml. Store it at 4° C.
   b. Working solution, 0.23 mmole/L
      Before use dilute 1.25 ml of the alcohol solution to 1 dl with buffer A. Warm aliquots of this to 37° C just before use.

Specimen collection: The blood is collected with a plastic syringe and 9 volumes of blood added to 1 volume 3.8% sodium citrate solution in a plastic tube. After mixing, the tubes are centrifuged for 15 min at 1000 g to obtain the plasma. The plasma is removed and stored at −20° C in plastic tubes. Before use, an aliquot of the plasma is diluted 1:400 with buffer A (0.25 ml plasma to 100 with buffer). (It is best to use a plastic-tipped syringe for this to prevent the undiluted plasma from coming into contact with glass.)

For the test a spectrofluorometer connected to a good recorder is used. The excitation wavelength is 345 nm, and the emission wavelength is 415 nm with slit widths of 6 nm and 12 nm, respectively. The recorder is run at 25 mm (1 in)/min.

Procedure: Of 100 µl diluted plasma and 100 µl working heparin solution, mix 2 units/ml in the fluorometer cuvet and warm to 37° C. Add and mix 100 µl working thrombin solution (1 unit/ml) previously warmed to 37° C. After incubation at 37° C for 1 min, add and mix 2 ml working substrate solution previously warmed to 37° C. Then place the cuvet in the spectrofluorometer, and note the change in fluorescence. A blank is run by using 100 µl buffer A instead of the diluted plasma. The rate of change for the sample and blank are calculated in any convenient unit. Then

$$\text{Inhibited thrombin (\%)} = \frac{(\text{Blank rate} - \text{Plasma rate})}{\text{Blank rate}} \times 100$$

Normal value: The normal value is 85-115%.

NOTE: The above formula does not give values over 100%. In the determination of the normal range, one may use plasma diluted an additional 1:2 and multiply the result by 2. In practice this is not necessary. Abnormal conditions result in low inhibition rates. If a value of close to 100% is obtained, the sample would be considered normal, and it is rarely necessary to run a dilution to see by how much the sample may have exceeded 100%.

Interpretation: See interpretation of amidolytic method of antithrombin III assay.

Neutralization of heparin in laboratory

A number of methods are available to neutralize heparin in a plasma sample, so that a given coagulation test can be repeated without heparin interference. The available methods include the use of protamine sulfate (Eli Lilly & Co., Indianapolis), Heparsorb (General Diagnostics, Morris Plains, N.J.), and Polybrene (Aldrich Chemical Co., Milwaukee).

Neutralization of heparin by protamine sulfate

Principle: Heparin is neutralized by protamine sulfate. A precise titration is usually not necessary. One milligram of protamine sulfate neutralizes 1 mg (100 units) of heparin.

Method 1:
Reagent: Protamine sulfate, 1% solution in normal saline, is available in 5 ml glass vials (50 mg/5 ml).

Procedure: Add 0.1 ml 1% protamine sulfate solution to 4 ml anticoagulated blood, mix, and separate plasma by centrifugation.

Method 2: If the exact neutralizing dose of protamine sulfate needs to be determined, the heparin titration is required.

Reagents:
1. Protamine sulfate solution, 10 mg/ml (see above)
2. Barbitol-buffered saline (see p. 289)
3. Thrombin solution (see p. 289)
4. Citrated plasma, patient's and control

Procedure[116]:
1. Dilute protamine sulfate as outlined on the following page:

A. 1 ml protamine + 99 ml buffered saline = 100 µg/ml
B. 0.5 ml A + 4.5 ml buffered saline = 10 µg/ml
C. 2.0 ml B + 2.0 ml buffered saline = µg/ml
D. 2.0 ml C + 2.0 ml buffered saline = 2.5 µg/ml
E. 2.0 ml D + 2.0 ml buffered saline = 1.25 µg/ml

2. To five test tubes add 0.1 ml patient's plasma and label A, B, C, D, and E. To each tube add 0.1 ml of the corresponding protamine solution.
3. To each tube add 0.1 ml thrombin and determine the clotting time.
4. Note the lowest concentration of protamine that gives a thrombin time equal to that of normal plasma (see p. 298).
5. The test determines the neutralizing protamine concentration per millimeter of plasma. The total dose of protamine (µg/ml) required to neutralize x millimeters of plasma is arrived at by multiplying the result of step 4 by the plasma volume. An excess of protamine sulfate prolongs the prothrombin time and the activated partial thromboplastin time but not the thrombin time.

Neutralization of heparin by Heparsorb tablets

Heparsorb is an ion exchange column in tablet form that removes 30 units of heparin from 1 ml plasma. The tablet contains 10 mg triethylaminoethyl cellulose plus a binder. The ion exchange procedure has the advantage over the protamine sulfate method in that it does not require titration and excess neutralizing material does not interfere with clotting tests.[117]

Reagent: Heparsorb tablets are the reagent used.

Procedure: Add 1 tablet of Heparsorb to 1 ml plasma in plastic 12 × 75 mm test tube. Incubate it at room temperature for 5 min to allow tablets to swell. Tap the tube vigorously for 5 sec to distribute the cellulose uniformly throughout the plasma sample. Mix the contents of the test tube slowly by using an Ames aliquot mixer (Ames Co., Elkart, Ind.) for 10 min at room temperature. Centrifuge for 5 min and remove the plasma slowly and carefully.

Neutralization of heparin by Polybrene

Hexadimethrine bromide (Polybrene) is a specific heparin-neutralizing agent. There is an almost direct proportionality between heparin and Polybrene, since about 0.08 mg/ml Polybrene neutralizes 1 unit/ml heparin.[118] The amount of 0.01 mg/ml Polybrene neutralizes a heparin concentration of 0.2 unit/ml, which prolongs the clotting time to two to three times normal.[118]

Reagents:
1. Stock Polybrene solution in 0.9% saline containing 1 mg/ml Polybrene
2. Working solution
   Dilute 1 ml stock with 1 dl saline to obtain 0.01 mg/ml Polybrene.

Procedure: Obtain citrated venous blood. Centrifuge to obtain plasma. Place 1 ml plasma into 10 × 75 mm test tube and add 0.1 ml Polybrene working solution. Mix it and perform clotting tests on the plasma.

LABORATORY TESTS IN HYPERCOAGULABILITY

Although deficiencies in the coagulation system usually lead to bleeding episodes of varying severity, the relationship of the overactivity of its components to thrombosis or to the hypercoagulable state is not well established. The hypercoagulable state indicates an abnormal tendency toward thrombotic vascular occlusion, either arterial or venous, and to embolic episodes. The thrombi may not only occlude blood vessels but also attach themselves to diseased or prosthetic heart valves. In clinical practice thrombotic episodes by far exceed hemorrhagic states in importance, because arterial thrombosis in myocardial infarction and venous thrombosis resulting in pulmonary embolism are frequently occurring maladies. The pathophysiologic mechanisms[119,120] underlying arterial and venous thromboses are not identical. The **arterial thrombus** builds up within a more or less freely flowing bloodstream and consists primarily of a large, white platelet plug to which a small amount of clotted blood is adherent. The **venous thrombus,** on the other hand, forms in a more or less static bloodstream and consists primarily of a fibrin and red cell coagulum with only a small number of platelets participating. The hypercoagulable state is related to a number of factors:

1. Increased levels of coagulation factors as seen in pregnancy and following the administration of oral contraceptives in which factors VII, VIII, IX, X, and I are increased[121]
2. The release of thromboplastic substances into the circulation as seen in some leukemias,[122] malignant tumors,[123] and disseminated intravascular coagulation
3. Stasis in the venous circulation as encountered in postsurgical states[124]
4. Antithrombin III deficiency as seen in liver disease or congenital deficiency[125]
5. Platelet hyperfunction[126] as seen in thrombocytosis, thrombocythemia, atherosclerosis, and diabetes mellitus (The metabolically stimulated platelets may have excessive procoagulant activity.)[127]
6. Increased levels of activated coagulation factors as encountered following the administration of commerical prothrombin complex to bleeding patients with liver disease[128]

A number of coagulation tests may draw attention to the existence of a hypercoagulable state:

1. Activated partial thromboplastin time (see p. 294)
2. Tests for thrombin for thrombic activity, e.g., radioimmunoassay for thrombin or fibrinopeptide A, paracoagulation tests (protamine sulfate test and ethanol gel test [see p. 314]) for fibrin monomers, and test for cryofibrinogen (see p. 315)
3. Thrombo-Wellco test for fibrin degradation products (see p. 313)
4. Tests for antithrombin III concentration (see p. 346)
5. Tests for platelet hyperactivity: spontaneous platelet aggregation (see p. 329), megathrombocyte index, and platelet factor 4 level (see p. 330)

Gallus, Hirsh, and Gent[129] reported shortening of the activated partial thromboplastin time in patients with deep vein thrombosis, probably resulting from circulating activated clotting factors. Since thrombin is essential for the generation of fibrin, radioimmunoassays have been developed that measure thrombin[120,130] itself or byproducts of its activity, e.g., fibrinopeptide A.[131,132] Fibrin monomers also result from thrombic activity, and fibrin monomer complexes are demonstrated by the paracoagulation tests that encompass the protamine sulfate and the ethanol gelation tests. Both have been reported positive in patients with deep vein thrombosis.[133,134] The appearance of cryofibrinogens is also associated with the hypercoagulable state.[135] As soon as fibrin is deposited within blood vessels, the plasmin-plasminogen system is activated, and fibrin degradation products are generated, which can be detected by the Thrombo-Wellco test (see p. 313). Above-normal concentrations of fibrin degradation products have been reported in deep vein thrombosis and pulmonary embolism.[136] There is a good relationship between anti-thrombin III deficiency and deep vein thrombosis.[137]

A number of investigators have used various parameters to measure platelet hyperfunction as evidence of rapid platelet turnover and/or increased concentration of metabolically activated young platelets following accelerated platelet consumption. The tests used include a modification of the standard platelet aggregation,[119] spontaneous platelet aggregation,[138] platelet factor 4 activity, and the sizing of platelets (see p. 326). Platelet sizing devices attached to automated platelet counters allow the calculation of the megathrombocyte index, which closely reflects the production of young platelets.[139]

REFERENCES

1. Bird, R.M., et al.: N. Engl. J. Med. **257:**105, 1957.
2. McKusick, V.A.: Heritable disorders of connective tissue, ed. 4, St. Louis, 1972, The C.V. Mosby Co.
3. Karaca, M., Cronberg, L., and Nilsson, I.M.: Scand. J. Haematol. **9:**465, 1972.
4. Estes, J.W., Carey, R.J., and Desai, R.G.: Arch. Intern. Med. **116:**889, 1965.
5. Owen, C.A., Jr., and Thompson, J.H.: Am. J. Clin. Pathol. **33:**197, 1960.
6. Davis, E.: Lancet **2:**160, 1943.
7. Tattersall, R.N., and Seville, R.: Q. J. Med. **19:**151, 1950.
8. Scarborough, H., and Shuster, S.: Lancet **1:**93, 1960.
9. Stolman, J.M., Goldman, H.M., and Gould, B.S.: Arch. Pathol. Lab. Med. **72:**535, 1961.
10. Perkins, H.A., et al.: Blood **35:**695, 1970.
11. Lerner, A.B., and Watson, C.J.: Am. J. Med. Sci. **214:**410, 1947.
12. Pechet, L., and Kastrul, J.J.: Ann. Intern. Med. **61:**315, 1964.
13. Gardner, F.H., and Diamond, L.K.: Blood **10:**675, 1955.
14. Kremer, W.B., et al.: Blood **30:**62, 1967.
15. Allen, D.M., Diamond, L.K., and Howell, D.A.: Am. J. Dis. Child. **99:**833, 1960.
16. Vernier, R.L., et al.: Pediatrics **27:**181, 1961.
17. Cochrane, C.G., and Weigle, W.O.: J. Exp. Med. **108:**591, 1958.
18. Ackroyd, J.F.: Am. J. Med. **14:**605, 1953.
19. Mammen, E.F.: Semin. Thromb. Hemostas. **1:**184, 1974.
20. Bommer, V.W., Künzer, W., and Schröer, H.: Ann. Paediat **200:**46, 1963.
21. Bommer, V.W., Künzer, W., and Schröer, H.: Ann. Paediat **200:**180, 1963.
22. Werder, E.: Helv. Paediatr. Acta **18:**208, 1963.
23. Blombäck, M., et al.: Nature **218:**134, 1968.
24. Sherman, L.A., Gaston, L.W., and Spivack, A.R.: J. Lab. Clin. Med. **72:**1017, 1968.
25. Borchgrevink, C.V., et al.: Br. J. Haematol. **5:**294, 1959.
26. de Bastos, O., Reno, R.S., and Correa, O.T.: Thrombos. Diathes. Haemorrh. **11:**467, 1964.
27. Josso, F., Lavergne, J.M., and Soulier, J.R.: Nouv. Rev. Fr. Hematol. **10:**633, 1970.
28. Kattlove, H.E., Shapiro, S.S., and Spivack, M.: N. Engl. J. Med. **282:**57, 1970.
29. Owren, P.A.: Lancet **1:**446, 1947.
30. Brink, A.J., Kingsley, C.S.: Q. J. Med. **21:**19, 1952.
31. Owen, C.A., Jr., et al.: Am. J. Med. **37:**71, 1964.
32. Hall, C.A., et al.: Am. J. Med. **37:**172, 1964.
33. Goodnight, S.H., Jr., et al.: Blood **38:**1, 1971.
34. Jones, J.H., et al.: Br. J. Haematol. **8:**120, 1962.
35. Biggs, R., and Spooner, R.J.D.: Br. J. Haematol. **36:**447, 1977.
36. Laurell, C.B.: Anal. Biochem. **15:**45, 1966.
37. Zimmerman, T.S., Ratnoff, O.D., and Powell, A.E.: J. Clin. Invest. **50:**244, 1971.
38. Eichelberger, J.W.: Fundamentals of thrombokinetics, Willow Grove, Pa., 1975, Bio/Data Corp.
39. Rizza, C.R., et al.: Br. J. Haematol. **30:**447, 1975.
40. Zimmerman, T.S., Ratnoff, O.D., and Littell, A.S.: J. Clin. Invest. **50:**255, 1971.
41. Meyer, D., et al.: Thromb. Res. **1:**183, 1972.
41a. Zimmerman, T.S., and Meyer, D.: Thrombosis and hemostasis, no. Th-4, Chicago, 1979, American Society of Clinical Pathologists.
42. Nilsson, I.M., Blomback, M., and Blomback, B.: Acta Med. Scand. **164:**263, 1959.
43. Bennett, B., Ratnoff, O.D., and Levin, J.: J. Clin. Invest. **51:**2597, 1972.
44. Biggs, R., and Densen, K.W.E.: Br. J. Haematol. **9:**532, 1963.
45. Perkins, H.A.: Blood **30:**375, 1967.
46. Quick, A.J.: Am. J. Med. Sci. **253:**520, 1967.
47. Weiss, H.J., Rogers, J., and Brand, H.: Blood **41:**809, 1973.
48. Weiss, H.J., Rogers, J., and Brand, H.: J. Clin. Invest. **52:**2697, 1973.
49. Sanderson, J.H., Burn, A.M., and Cooke, S.: Scand. J. Haematol. **12:**249, 1974.
50. Hoyer, L.W.: Prog. Hemost. Thromb. **3:**231, 1976.
51. Didisheim, P., and Vandervoort, R.L.E.: Blood **20:**150, 1962.
52. Meyer, D., Bidwell, E., and Larrieu, M.J.: J. Clin. Pathol. **25:**433, 1972.
53. Denson, K.W.E., Biggs, R., and Mannucci, P.M.: J. Clin. Pathol. **21:**160, 1968.
54. Veltkamp, J.J., et al.: Scand J. Haematol. **7:**82, 1970.
55. Girolami, A., et al.: Thrombos. Diathes. Haemorrh. **24:**175, 1970.
56. Rosenthal, R.L., Dreskin, O.H., and Rosenthal, N.: Blood **10:**120, 1955.
57. Ratnoff, O.D., and Colopy, J.E.: J. Clin. Invest. **34:**602, 1955.
58. Ratnoff, O.D., Busse, R.J., and Sheon, R.P.: N. Engl. J. Med. **279:**760, 1968.
59. Bennett, R., et al.: Blood **40:**412, 1972.

60. Abildgaard, C.F., and Harrison, J.: Blood **43**:641, 1974.
61. Hathaway, W.E., and Alsever, J.: Br. J. Haematol. **18**:161, 1970.
62. Saito, H., et al.: J. Clin. Invest. **55**:1082, 1975.
63. Bowie, E.J.W., and Owen, C.A., In Poller, L., editor: Recent advances in blood coagulation, New York, 1977, Churchill Livingstone.
64. Wuepper, K.D., Miller, D.R., and Lacombe, M.J.: J. Clin. Invest. **56**:1663, 1975.
65. Hougie, C., McPherson, R.A., and Aronson, L.: Lancet **2**:290, 1975.
66. Hougie, C., et al.: N. Engl. J. Med. **298**:1045, 1978.
67. Aziz, M.A., and Siddiqui, A.R.: Blood **40**:11, 1972.
68. Duckert, F.: Thrombos. Diathes. Haemorrh. **13**(suppl.):115, 1963.
69. Francis, J., and Todd, P.: Br. Med. J. **2**:1532, 1978.
70. Barbui, T., et al.: Br. J. Haematol. **38**:267, 1978.
71. Bohn, H.: Blut **28**:81, 1974.
72. Smit Sibinga, C.Th., Gokemeyer, J., and ten Kate, L.P.: Br. J. Haematol. **23**:467, 1972.
73. Owen, C.A., Bowie, E.J.W., and Thompson, J.H.: The diagnosis of bleeding disorders, Boston, 1975, Little, Brown & Co.
74. Lechner, K., Niessner, H., and Thaler, E.: Semin. Thromb. Hemostas. **4**:40, 1977.
75. Lechner, K.: Thrombos. Diathes. Haemorrh. **27**:19, 1972.
76. Lord, J.W., and Andrus, W.D.: Arch. Intern. Med. **68**:199, 1941.
77. Roberts, H.R., and Cederbaum, A.I.: Gastroenterology **63**:297, 1972.
78. Shapiro, S.S.: In Williams, W.J., et al., editors: Hematology, ed. 2, New York, 1977, McGraw-Hill Book Co.
79. Straub, P.W., Riedler, G., and Meili, E.O.: Schweiz. Med. Wochenschr. **96**:1199, 1966.
80. Nussbaum, M., and Morse, B.S.: Blood **23**:669, 1964.
81. Straub, P.W.: Semin. Thromb. Hemostas. **4**:29, 1977.
82. Workman, E.F., and Lundblad, R.L.: Semin. Thromb. Hemostas. **4**:15, 1977.
83. Prydz, H.: Semin. Thromb. Hemostas. **4**:1, 1977.
84. Kazmier, F.J., et al.: Arch. Intern. Med. **115**:667, 1965.
85. Hemker, H.C., Veltkamp, J.J., and Loeliger, E.A.: Thrombos. Diathes. Haemorrh. **19**:346, 1968.
86. Gurewich, V.: Semin. Thromb. Hemostas. **2**:176, 1976.
87. Mackie, M.J., and Douglas, A.S.: Br. Med. Bull. **34**:177, 1978.
88. Brozović, M.: Semin. Hematol. **15**:27, 1978.
89. Breckenridge, A.: Semin. Hematol. **15**:19, 1978.
90. Williams, W.J.: In Williams, W.J., et al., editors: Hematology, ed. 2, New York, 1977, McGraw-Hill Book Co.
91. Loeliger, E.A., et al.: Thrombos. Diathes. Haemorrh. **9**:74, 1963.
92. Kliesch, W.F., Young, P.C., and Davis, W.D.: J.A.M.A. **172**:223, 1960.
93. Owens, J.C., Neely, W.B., and Owen, W.R.: N. Engl. J. Med. **266**:76, 1962.
94. Kock-Weser, J., and Sellers, E.M.: N. Engl. J. Med. **285**:547, 1971.
95. O'Reilly, R.A., et al.: N. Engl. J. Med. **271**:809, 1964.
96. O'Reilly, R.A., and Aggeler, P.M.: Pharmacol. Rev. **22**:35, 1970.
97. Soloway, H.B.: Am. J. Clin. Pathol. **61**:622, 1974.
98. Barrowcliffe, T.W., Johnson, E.A., and Thomas, P.: Br. Med. Bull. **34**:143, 1978.
99. Thomas, D.P.: Semin. Hemat. **15**:1, 1978.
100. Gurewich, V.: Semin. Thromb. Hemostas. **2**:176, 1976.
101. Ts'ao, C.H., et al.: Am. J. Clin. Pathol. **71**:17, 1979.
102. Thomas, D.P., et al.: Thromb. Res. **9**:241, 1976.
103. Bick, R.L.: Diagnostic Dialog. **5**:4, 1979.
104. Teien, A.N., Lie, M., and Abildgaard, U.: Thromb. Res. **8**:413, 1976.
105. Mitchell, G.A., et al.: Thromb. Res. **13**:47, 1978.
106. Package insert instructions of heparin synthetic substrate assay, CO56-5365, Miami, Dade Diagnostics.
107. Teien, A.N., and Lie, M.: Thromb. Res. **10**:399, 1977.
108. Estes, J.W., and Poulin, P.F.: Thrombos. Diathes. Haemorrh. **33**:26, 1975.
109. Frigola, A., Angeloni, S., and Cerqueti, A.R.: J. Clin. Pathol. **32**:21, 1979.
110. Ødegård, O.R., Lie, M., and Abildgaard, U.: Thromb. Res. **6**:287, 1975.
111. Frigola, A.: J. Clin. Pathol. **30**:881, 1977.
112. Ødegård, O.R., and Abildgaard, U.: Scand. J. Haematol. **18**:86, 1977.
113. Collen, D., et al.: Eur. J. Clin. Invest. **7**:27, 1977.
114. Zuck, T.F., Bergin, J.J., and Raymond, J.M.: Surg. Gynecol. Obstet. **133**:609, 1971.
115. Mitchell, G.A., et al.: Thromb. Res. **12**:219, 1978.
116. Bowie, E.J.W., et al.: Mayo Clinic Laboratory Manual of Hemostasis, Philadelphia, 1971, W.B. Saunders Co.
117. LeRoy, G.V., Halpern, B., and Dolkart, R.E.: J. Lab. Clin. Med. **35**:446, 1950.
118. Grann, V.R., Homewood, K., and Golden, W.: Am. J. Clin. Pathol. **58**:26, 1972.
119. Arkin, C.F., and Hartman, A.S.: CRC Crit, Rev. Clin. Lab. Sci. **10**:397, 1979.
120. Davies, J.A., and McNicol, G.P.: Br. Med. Bull. **34**:113, 1978.
121. Bonnar, J., McNicol, G.P., and Douglas, A.S.: Br. Med. J. **2**:200, 1970.
122. Brodsky, I.: J. Med. **5**:38, 1974.
123. Sun, N.C.J., et al.: Mayo Clin. Proc. **49**:636, 1974.
124. Lipinska, I., et al.: Am. J. Clin. Pathol. **66**:958, 1976.
125. Shapiro, S.S., Prager, D., and Martinez, J.: Blood **42**:1001, 1973.
126. Yamazaki, H., Takahashi, T., and Sano, T.: Thrombos. Diathes. Haemorrh. **34**:94, 1975.
127. Hoak, J.C., Warner, E.D., and Connor, W.E.: Cir. Res. **20**:11, 1967.
128. Blatt, P.M., et al.: Ann. Intern. Med. **81**:766, 1974.
129. Gallus, A.S., Hirsh, J., and Gent, M.: Lancet **2**:805, 1973.
130. Shuman, M.A., and Majerus, P.W.: J. Clin. Invest. **58**:1249, 1976.
131. Kockum, C.: Thromb. Res. **8**:225, 1976.
132. Nossel, H.L.: N. Engl. J. Med. **295**:428, 1976.
133. Seaman, A.J.: Arch. Intern. Med. **125**:1016, 1970.
134. von Kaulla, E., and von Kaulla, K.N.: Am. J. Clin. Pathol. **61**:810, 1974.
135. Smith, S.B., and Arkin, C.: Am. J. Clin. Pathol. **58**:524, 1972.
136. Rickman, F.D., et al.: Ann. Intern. Med. **79**:664, 1973.
137. von Kaulla, E., and von Kaulla, K.N.: Am. J. Clin. Pathol. **48**:69, 1967.
138. Wu, K.K., and Hoak, J.C.: Thromb. Haemost. **35**:702, 1976.
139. Garg, S.K., Amorosi, E.L., and Karpatkin, S.: N. Engl. J. Med. **284**:11, 1971.

IMMUNOHEMATOLOGY

Blood group systems

There are hundreds of red cell antigens known today, many of which appear to be related to each other.* When one group of related antigens is shown to be inherited independently from any other group of related antigens, they are said to belong to a particular blood group system. Such related blood factors are usually inherited as allelomorphic genes at one genetic locus.

---

*Standard references are *Technical Manual of the American Association of Blood Banks*,[1a] Mollison's *Blood Transfusion in Clinical Medicine*,[2] Prokops and Uhlenbruck's *Human Blood and Serum Groups*,[3] Erskine's *Principles and Practice of Blood Grouping*,[4] and Barrett's *Textbook of Immunology*.[5]

Occasionally more than one locus is involved in the expression of a blood group system; in such an instance, the second locus involves modifying genes, which are also considered an integral part of that blood group system.

The antigen composition of all blood groups is written as the **phenotype,** i.e., all the antigens of that system known to be present on the basis of serologic typing. The **genotype** is the collection of all genes responsible for producing the phenotype. Most of the genes controlling erythrocyte antigens are located on autosomes and are dominant in effect; probably no blood group antigens result from recessive genes. When a gene produces no detectable product, it is termed a **silent gene** or an **amorph;** examples of amorph genes are found in many of the blood group systems, including ABO, rhesus, Duffy, P, Kell, Lutheran, Kidd, and Lewis. The only commonly occurring amorph gene occurs in the ABO system, all other such genes being very rare.

ABO BLOOD GROUP SYSTEM

The ABO blood group system is of great importance because A and B substances are strongly antigenic, because anti-A and anti-B occur naturally in the serum of persons lacking the corresponding antigen, and because these antibodies are capable of producing hemolysis in vivo.

General principles
Antigens and subgroups

There are two antigens, A and B, in the ABO blood group system that are controlled from one genetic locus. By serologic reactions each antigen has subtle divisions, often referred to as subgroups. Common to all these antigens and their subgroups is still another antigen, H; the H antigen is controlled from a separate and independent genetic locus. The H antigen is considered a basic substance from which the A and B antigens are made. Since group O cells have neither A nor B anti-

Table 14-1. Basic ABO phenotypes

Phenotype	Genotype	Antigens present on surface	Antibodies present in serum	Frequency (%) Whites	Frequency (%) Blacks
A	*AA, AO*	A, H	Anti-B	41	27
B	*BB, BO*	B, H	Anti-A	10	20
AB	*AB*	A, B, H	None	4	4
O	*OO*	H	Anti-A, anti-B	45	49

Table 14-2. ABO blood group system including subgroups*

Blood group	Phenotype	Genotype	Frequency	Reactions with:				
				Anti-A	Anti-A$_1$	Anti-A,B	Anti-B	Anti-H
A	A$_1$	A_1A_1, A_1A_2, A_1O	32%	4+	4+	4+	−	±
	A$_2$	A_2A_2, A_2O	9%	3-4+	−	3-4+	−	3+
	A$_3$	A_3A_3, A_3O	<1%	1+ MF	−	2-4+ MF	−	3+
	A$_x$		Rare	0-±	−	2-4+	−	4+
	A$_m$		Rare	0-±	−	0-2+	−	4+
	A$_{end}$		Rare	±	−	±	−	4+
	A$_{el}$		Rare	−	−	−	−	4+
B	B	BB, BO	10%	−	−	4+	4+	2-3+
AB	A$_1$B	A_1B	2.8%	+	+	+	+	±
	A$_2$B	A_2B	1.2%	+	−	+	+	±
O	O	OO	45%	−	−	−	−	4+
	O$_h$ (gene interaction)	ABO, hh	Rare	−	−	−	−	−

*+, Agglutination; −, no agglutination; MF, mixed field; Occ, occasional; Freq, frequent; Dec, decreased.

gen, they have the most H antigens on their surface; A and B cells have much less H antigen since H antigen has been largely converted into A and B antigen. Table 14-1 gives the characteristics of the four basic ABO phenotypes.

Soon after the discovery of the ABO blood group system[1] it was recognized that there were two types of anti-A in the serum of group B and group O persons; these two antibodies have been designated anti-A and anti-A$_1$. Their use has allowed the classification of group A red cells into A$_1$ and A$_2$ cells, based on the serologic reactions observed:

	Anti-A	Anti-A$_1$
A$_1$ cells	+	+
A$_2$ cells	+	−

In an identical manner, AB red cells can be classified as A$_1$B or A$_2$B. Most red cells that are group A or AB belong to the subgroup A$_1$ or A$_1$B, respectively; a smaller percentage belong to the subgroup A$_2$ or A$_2$B.

Rare subgroups of A are also known and have been designated A$_3$, A$_x$, A$_m$, A$_{el}$, and A$_{end}$. There is little uniformity of nomenclature with these rare subgroups, all of which are inherited as rare alleles at the ABO locus. These rare subgroups are all characterized serologically by a weak or absent agglutination with anti-A; hence they are often termed **weak** A subgroups. If there is no agglutination after exposure to anti-A, the cells can be shown to belong to the A blood group system if one or both of the following can be shown:

1. Presence of A substance in the saliva of secretors
2. Ability of the cell to absorb and elute anti-A

Table 14-2 summarizes the current knowledge of the ABO blood group system, including the A subgroups.

Genetics and biochemistry

Two independent genetic loci regulate the ABO phenotype of red cells: the ABO locus and the Hh locus. The ABO locus is located on chromosome 9; it has four principal alleles: A_1, A_2, B, and O. A_1 and B

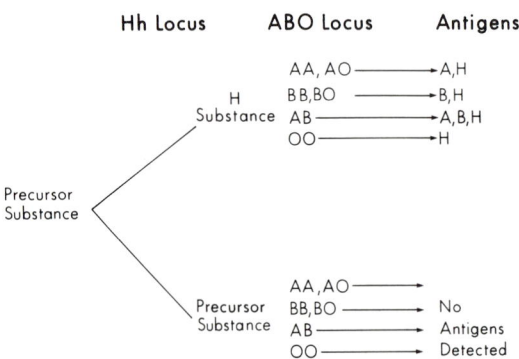

Fig. 14-1. Interaction between ABO and Hh genetic loci.

are codominant genes; O is an amorph gene; A_2 appears masked by A_1. Also present at this locus are the rare alleles that give rise to the weak A and B subgroups. The Hh locus is located on an unknown chromosome; the H gene is responsible for the production of H antigenic substance from a precursor substance. The A and B genes transform H substance into A and B antigenic substances; the O gene is unable to change H substance because it is an amorph gene.[6] The amorph gene h is very rare, and inheritance of its homozygous state prevents the transformation of precursor substance; as a result, normal genes at the ABO locus have no H substance to act on. The inheritance of the homozygous h gene is called the Bombay phenotype (O$_h$), named after its place of discovery, Bombay, India. Fig. 14-1 illustrates these gene interactions.

The biochemistry of ABH antigens was elucidated by analyzing these antigenic substances as they are found in body fluids. Purification of these blood group substances reveals glycoproteins containing a high percentage of carbohydrate, which consists predominantly of four sugars: D-galactose, L-fucose, N-acetyl-D-galactosamine, and N-acetyl-D-glucosamine.[7,8] These

Antibodies in serum				Secretor			Absorbs and elutes:		
Anti-A	Anti-A₁	Anti-B	Anti-H	A	B	H	Anti-A	Anti-B	Anti-H
−	−	+	0.6%	+	−	+	+	−	+
−	1 − 2%	+	−	+	−	+	+	−	+
−	Occ	+	−	+	−	+	+	−	+
−	Freq	+	−	Dec	−	+	+	−	+
−	−	+	−	+	−	+	+	−	+
−	Occ	+	−	−	−	+	+	−	+
−	−	+	−	−	−	+	+	−	+
+	+	−	−	−	+	+	−	+	+
−	−	−	3%	+	+	+	+	+	+
−	25%	−	−	+	+	+	+	+	+
+	+	+	−	−	−	+	−	−	+
+	+	+	+	−	−	−	−	−	−

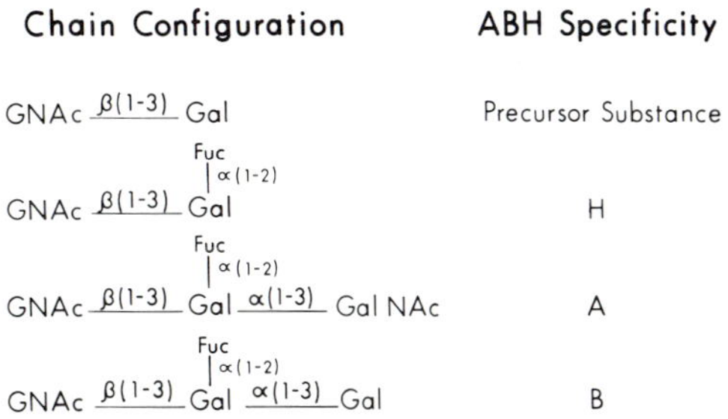

Chain Configuration — ABH Specificity

GNAc $\underline{\beta(1-3)}$ Gal — Precursor Substance

GNAc $\underline{\beta(1-3)}$ Gal, Fuc $|\alpha(1-2)$ — H

GNAc $\underline{\beta(1-3)}$ Gal $\underline{\alpha(1-3)}$ Gal NAc, Fuc $|\alpha(1-2)$ — A

GNAc $\underline{\beta(1-3)}$ Gal $\underline{\alpha(1-3)}$ Gal, Fuc $|\alpha(1-2)$ — B

Fig. 14-2. Terminal monosaccharides of ABH antigenic determinants. *Gal*, D-Galactose; *Gal NAc*, N-acetyl-D-galactosamine; *GNAc*, N-acetyl-D-glucosamine; *Fuc*, L-fucose.

Table 14-3. ABO genes and their enzymatic products

Gene	Enzyme
A	α-N-acetylgalactosaminyltransferase
B	α-Galactosyltransferase
O	None
H	L-Fucosyltransferase

sugars are linked together in a specific way and are attached to a protein backbone. The antigenic specificity of the structure is determined by the terminal nonreducing sugar that is under the direct control of the genes mentioned above (Table 14-3). Fig. 14-2 illustrates the configuration of the terminal monosaccharides given in Table 14-3 and indicates their antigenic specificity.

Distribution of ABH antigens

The antigens of the ABO system are present not only on erythrocytes, but on leukocytes, platelets, and tissue cells, as well as in most body fluids. The antigens are also widespread in nature. The appearance of these antigens in body fluids depends on the inheritance of genes at a locus independent of the ABO or Hh loci; these genes are designated *Se* and *se* (secretor). The *secretor* gene has no effect on the antigens as they appear on the red cells.

Differences between A₁ and A₂ red cells.

It is accepted that there are more A receptor sites on A₁ than A₂ red cells.[9] That the difference is more than just quantitative is suggested by the occurrence of an-ti-A₁ in the serum of some A₂ and A₂B persons. Further support for a qualitative difference is the observed kinetic differences of the A₁ and A₂ transferases.[10]

Atypical cold antibodies in the A₁ and A₂ subgroups

The sera of approximately 2% of A₂ individuals and 25% of A₂B individuals contain anti-A₁. Anti-A₁ may also be found in the sera of some of the weak A subgroups but not with any degree of regularity. Anti-H may be found in the sera of approximately 1% of A₁ and 3% of A₁B individuals; it also occurs regularly in the sera of Bombay individuals where it often is active at 37° C, although it is an IgM immunoglobulin. The anti-H in the sera of A₁ and A₁B individuals is a much weaker antibody than the anti-H of a Bombay individual and always reacts as a cold-reacting antibody.

ABO blood grouping

The antibodies of the ABO system are IgM immunoglobulins and agglutinate saline suspended red cells at or below room temperature. Heating to 37° C greatly weakens or eliminates the reaction. Because the antibodies occur naturally in the serum of persons lacking the corresponding antigen, the red cell phenotype is determined and confirmed by performing cell and serum groupings. The **cell grouping (forward typing)** is performed by testing unknown red cells with antisera of known type; the **serum grouping (reverse typing)** is performed by testing unknown serum with red cells of known type. Because commercial antisera are highly potent, the cell grouping can be performed either on a slide or in a test tube; because the naturally occurring antibodies in the unknown serum may be weak and of low titer, the serum grouping must be performed only in test tubes where centrifugation will intensify the reaction. The importance of correct ABO grouping cannot be overemphasized, and both cell and serum grouping must be performed on each specimen.

Cell grouping (forward typing)

Slide method: Specific manufacturer's instructions must always be followed. The following is one method that can be used.

Label slides with the patient's name or number. Draw three ceramic rings and label them A, B, and O.

Place 1 drop of anti-A serum in the circle marked A, 1 drop of anti-B serum in the circle marked B, and 1 drop of group O serum (anti-A,B) in the circle marked O.

Prepare a 10% saline suspension of unknown cells using freshly drawn, clotted, oxalate or citrate blood. With the aid of a wooden applicator stick, place a small amount of the cells (not greater than half the volume of serum used) next to each drop of antiserum within the circle.

Mix the cells and antisera with separate applicator sticks over an area about 1 in in diameter.

Tilt the slide backward and forward at room temperature continuously for a maximum of 2 min. Read macroscopically for agglutination.

Test tube method: The following method is preferred because of its increased sensitivity.

Use disposable 10 × 75 mm test tubes. Label each tube with the patient's name or number. For each specimen to be tested, mark two tubes A and B.

Prepare a 4% saline suspension of unknown cells using freshly drawn, clotted, oxalate or citrate blood after first washing the cells two times in saline.

Place 1 drop of anti-A serum in the tube labeled A and 1 drop of anti-B serum in the tube labeled B. Add 1 drop of 4% saline suspended patient cells to each tube. Mix the cells and antisera thoroughly. Centrifuge for 15 sec. Gently dislodge the sedimented cells and read for agglutination with an optical aid.

Serum grouping (reverse typing)

The cells used may be commercially prepared A_1 and B cells or a freshly prepared 2-5% saline suspension of washed A_1 and B cells.

For each specimen to be tested, label two 10 × 75 mm test tubes with the patient's name or number; mark one tube A and the other B.

Place 2 drops of unknown serum in each tube. Add 1 drop 5% saline suspended A_1 cells to the tube labeled A and 1 drop 5% saline suspended B cells to the tube labeled B. Mix thoroughly. Centrifuge for 15 sec. Gently dislodge the cells and read for agglutination with an optical aid.

Interpretation

Agglutination occurring in serum grouping tests may be very weak because of weak antibodies in the patient's serum. False negative readings may result unless very gentle resuspension of the cells is performed.

Hemolysis may occur with serum grouping tests because fresh serum contains complement and anti-A and anti-B are capable of acting as hemolysins. If hemolysis is observed, it indicates an antigen-antibody reaction has occurred and must be regarded as a positive reaction.

Agglutination results of cell and serum grouping tests are interpreted as outlined in Table 14-4.

Discrepancy between cell and serum grouping tests

When the results of cell and serum grouping tests do not agree as shown in Table 14-4, the discrepancy must be investigated and resolved. Such discrepancies may be the result of technical errors or an intrinsic property of the cells or serum.

Technical errors

The first step in resolving a discrepancy is a careful repeat of the entire test procedure, paying careful attention to details. Possible pitfalls are listed below:

1. Partial drying of the slide in cell groupings may be misinterpreted as agglutination.
2. Overcentrifugation or undercentrifugation may result in false positive or false negative readings, respectively.
3. Rough dislodgement of the centrifuged cell button may disrupt small agglutinates and result in a false negative reading.
4. The cell-serum mixture may be inadvertently heated, resulting in a false negative reading.
5. Use of improper concentration of cells or old cells may lead to a false negative reading.
6. Failure to observe hemolysis will result in false negative readings.

Table 14-4. Cell and serum grouping*

Cell grouping—unknown cells with:			Serum grouping—unknown serum with cells of group:		
Anti-A	Anti-B	Anti-A,B	A_1	B	Blood group
−	−	−	+	+	O
+	−	+	−	+	A
−	+	+	+	−	B
+	+	+	−	−	AB

*+, Agglutination; −, no agglutination.

7. Dirty glassware will simulate clumping and result in a false positive reading.
8. The specimen may be identified incorrectly.

Subgroups of Group A

Subgroups A_2 and A_2B: A_1 and A_2 cells are rapidly and strongly agglutinated by commercial anti-A; the distinction between these two subgroups will not be made unless the irregular cold agglutinin, anti-A_1, occurs in the serum of the A_2 individual. There is no need to distinguish between these two subgroups in routine blood bank work; but if anti-A_1 is present, a discrepancy in ABO cell-serum grouping will be detected and will need to be resolved. Table 14-5 illustrates the usual discrepancies detected.

The discrepancies are resolved by demonstrating that the unknown red cells are not A_1 and by showing that the irregular antibody has the specificity anti-A_1. The cell grouping is repeated, adding anti-A_1 serum; the serum grouping is repeated, adding known A_2 cells (Table 14-6).

There are two sources of anti-A_1:

1. Absorbed group B serum: When anti-A + anti-A_1 are absorbed with A_2 cells, the anti-A agglutinin fraction is removed, leaving the anti-A_1 fraction behind.
2. Anti-A_1 lectin: This extract of seeds from the plant *Dolichos biflorus* has specific anti-A_1 activity when properly diluted.

In addition to the above, anti-H lectin is also useful; this extract of seeds from the plant *Ulex europeus* reacts with H antigen on the surface of red cells. Because A_2 cells have more H antigen on their surface than A_1 cells, the former are more strongly agglutinated by anti-H lectin:

	Anti-H
A_1 cells	±
A_2 cells	3+

Anti-H lectin will show a similar strong agglutination with the weak A subgroups and therefore is only supportive evidence in identifying the specificity of such cells.

Although A_1 and A_2 cells cannot be distinguished on the basis of their reactivity with commercial anti-A, A_2B cells do react weaker than A_1B cells, allowing some distinction. This is caused by the greatly reduced number of A antigen sites on the surface of A_2B cells.[9]

Subgroup A_3: Cells belonging to subgroup A_3 react as if part of the cells have antigen A whereas the remainder lack the antigen, thus behaving like a mosaic (or chimera). If A_3 cells are acted on by anti-A serum, a mixed-field agglutination pattern results. A **mixed-field pattern** consists of small clumps of agglutinated cells surrounded by free nonagglutinated cells. Anti-H lectin, for reasons already given, reacts strongly with A_3 cells.

Subgroups of A weaker than A_3: A summary of the serologic reactions of cells of A subgroups weaker than A_3 is given in Table 14-2. Generally they all give weak reactions or no reaction with anti-A, strong reactions with anti-H lectin, and no reactions with anti-A_1 lectin. Of particular note is the strong reaction of some of these cells (A_x and A_m) with anti-A,B (group O serum), hence preventing their erroneous classification as group O cells.

Table 14-5. A_2 and A_2B subgroups with anti-A_1 in serum*

Unknown cell	Cell grouping—unknown cells with:		Serum grouping—unknown cells with:		Interpretation	
	Anti-A	Anti-B	A_1 cells	B cells	Cell grouping—belongs to group:	Serum grouping—belongs to group:
A_1	+	−	−	+	A	A
A_2	+	−	+	+	A	O
A_1B	+	+	−	−	AB	AB
A_2B	+, ±	+	+	−	AB	B

*+, Agglutination; −, no agglutination; ±, very weak agglutination.

Table 14-6. Expanded ABO grouping in A_2 and A_2B subgroups with anti-A_1*

Cell grouping—unknown cells with:				Serum grouping—unknown serum with:			
Anti-A	Anti-A_1	Anti-B	Anti-A,B	A_1 cells	A_2 cells	B cells	Blood group
+	+	−	+	−	−	+	A_1
+	−	−	+	+	−	+	A_2
+	+	+	+	−	−	−	A_1B
+, ±	−	+	+	+	−	−	A_2B

*+, Agglutination; −, no agglutination; ±, very weak agglutination.

Some of the weak subgroups only react very weakly or not at all with anti-A,B; their identification is aided by examination of their eluate after absorption of anti-A serum; if the eluate contains anti-A, it identifies the cell as belonging to group A. Identification of the group substance in the saliva of secretors may further aid in the identification of weak A subgroups.

Altered antigens

Disease: The subgroups described above refer to weak A antigens resulting from a rare allele at the ABO genetic locus. Weak A antigens may also result as an acquired characteristic in acute leukemia. Similar changes can occur to the B and H antigens, as well as antigens of other blood group systems.

Polyagglutinable cells: Red cells are said to be polyagglutinable if they are agglutinated by most normal human sera. Only three types of polyagglutination will be characterized.

T-activation:

Principle: All normal red cells possess antigens that are not demonstrable by ordinary technics; such antigens, called **hidden antigens,** can be exposed by the action of certain enzymes. One such antigen is the T antigen and cells with exposed T antigens are called **T activated.** Since all normal adult sera contain anti-T, T-activated cells are polyagglutinable. Cells become T activated by enzymes capable of removing sialic acid from the red cell membrane; such enzymes are produced by a variety of bacteria and viruses. Most clinical cases of polyagglutination caused by T-activation do show evidence of bacterial or viral infection; when the infection is treated, the cells are no longer T activated and no longer polyagglutinable. Polyagglutination caused by T-activation can be suggested in the following ways:

1. The cells are agglutinated by most adult sera, including ABO typing sera. Hence, the cells are agglutinated by anti-A, anti-B, anti-A,B, and group AB sera; those cells agglutinated on a T-anti-T basis show a mixed-field reaction.
2. The cells are not agglutinated by cord serum because cord serum lacks anti-T.
3. The cells are not agglutinated by the individual's own serum because the antibody is not an autoantibody.
4. The cells fail to be aggregated by Polybrene.

To diagnose T-activation, the red cells should be exposed to the peanut lectin *Arachis hypogea*, which has anti-T specificity. It is possible to obtain a correct ABO typing by preparing T-activated cells and using them to absorb the typing sera.

• • •

Three methods for determining T-activation are described in the following sections.

Polybrene aggregation: Hexadimethrine bromide (Polybrene) is a positively charged synthetic polymer (1,5-dimethyl-1,5 diazundecamethylene methobromide) capable of overcoming the negative charge present on normal red cells, thereby allowing nonspecific aggregation, which is easily reversed by hypertonic salt solution.

The procedure[11] is given below.

Stock Polybrene solution: Suspend Polybrene in physiologic saline at a concentration of 40 mg/ml (4 g/dl). Store the solution at room temperature in a plastic container.

Working Polybrene solution: Dilute the stock solution 1:40 in physiologic saline.

METHOD: Place 1 drop of Polybrene working solution into two 10×75 mm test tubes. Add 1 drop of a 5% suspension of the cells to be tested to one test tube and 1 drop of a 5% suspension of normal red cells to the other tube. Observe for aggregation.

INTERPRETATION: Red cells with a reduced negative surface charge are not aggregated by Polybrene; such cells include T-activated red cells, Tn-activated red cells, and En(a-) cells that are genetically deficient in sialic acid content.

If the degree of polyagglutination is only slight, the cells may show some aggregation by this method and thus lead to misinterpretation.

Arachis hypogea lectin[11]:

Preparation of lectin:

1. Grind 1 volume of raw peanuts with 4 volumes of physiologic saline in a blender.
2. Allow the emulsion to stand overnight.
3. Centrifuge and collect the supernatant.
4. Dilute the supernatant 1:10 to 1:100 depending on anti-T activity. Store at 4° C.

Procedure: Place 2 drops of undiluted anti-T extract in each of two 10×75 mm test tubes. To one tube add 1 drop of a 5% saline suspension of test cells; to the other tube add 1 drop of a 5% saline suspension of normal cells. Mix and centrifuge at 3000 rpm for 15 sec. Shake gently to resuspend the cell button and observe for agglutination. If no agglutination is seen, leave the tubes at room temperature or 4° C for 30-60 min. Spin and observe for agglutination.

Interpretation: Agglutination of the test cells by anti-T lectin indicates T-activation. No agglutination of the test cells by anti-T lectin excludes T-activation.

Absorption of anti-T from ABO typing sera[11]:

Preparation of T-activated red cells:

1. Mix 20 lambdas of neuraminidase (General Biochemical, Chagrin Falls, Ohio) with 12 ml of a 25% saline suspension of washed red cells.
2. Add enough $CaCl_2$ to give the final solution a strength of $10^{-3}M$ calcium.
3. Incubate 30 min at room temperature.
4. Wash the cells three times in saline.
5. Test with anti-T lectin to be certain of T-activation.

Absorption procedure: To 1 volume of packed, washed, T-activated cells, add 1 volume of the typing serum to be absorbed. Mix. Place in the refrigerator (4° C) for 60 min. Centrifuge. Collect absorbed serum.

Test the absorbed serum for anti-T by reacting with T-activated cells. If anti-T remains, a second absorption is required. Test the absorbed serum for anti-A and anti-B by reacting with normal A_1 and B cells, respectively.

Tn-activation:

Principle: The Tn antigen is also not demonstrable on red cells; all normal sera contain the corresponding antibody. Tn activation is a rather uncommon condition possibly resulting from insufficient amounts of sialic acid added to the cells during maturation. Tn-activated cells are similar to T-activated cells in the following ways:

1. They have reduced sialic acid levels.
2. They show no aggregation with Polybrene.
3. They show a mixed-field agglutination pattern.
4. They react with all normal adult sera (contain anti-Tn).
5. They fail to react with cord sera (lack anti-Tn).
6. They have reduced M and N surface antigens.

Tn-activation differs from T-activation in the following ways:

1. It is a permanent transformation.
2. It cannot be produced in vitro.
3. It is usually associated with hematologic abnormalities: hemolytic anemia, leukopenia, or thrombocytopenia.
4. The red cells are agglutinated by *Dolichos biflorus* extract.

Tn activation can be identified by using extracts from *Salvia sclarea* or *Salvia haematodes* seeds.[12] To obtain correct ABO grouping tests, treat the Tn-activated cells with 1% ficin or papain to destroy the Tn receptor sites.

Preparation of Salvia sclarea lectin[12]:

1. Grind the dry *Salvia sclarea* seeds in a mortar.
2. Add 3 volumes of physiologic saline and macerate thoroughly.
3. Centrifuge hard.
4. Remove the supernatant and filter. The raw extract has weak activity for T-activated and Cad cells, but this can be diluted out, leaving very specific and powerful anti-Tn activity. Test dilutions with known T-activated and Cad cells until negative.

Destruction of Tn-receptors with enzymes:

1. To 1 volume of washed, packed red cells, add 2 volumes of ficin or papain (See discussion of special test procedures); enzyme concentrations of 0.1-0.5% are suitable.
2. Mix. Incubate at 37° C for 10 min.
3. Wash the cells three times in saline.
4. Prepare the appropriate red cell suspension with saline.

Cad polyagglutinability: Cad cells appear polyagglutinable because they carry an extraordinary quantity of the antigen Sd[a], most red cells having a much smaller amount. Most sera contain a minute amount of anti-Sd[a]; the Cad cells are readily agglutinated by virtue of the large amount of antigen on their surface.[13] The name "Cad" is derived from the first recognized propositus, at a time when the explanation of the phenomenon was unclear.[14] Like Tn-activated cells, Cad cells are agglutinated by *Dolichos biflorus* extract: The Cad cells are even more strongly agglutinated by this extract than are A$_1$ cells. Unlike Tn-activated cells, the Cad receptor is not destroyed by enzyme treatment but may actually be enhanced.[15] The diagnosis of Cad polyagglutination is made by exclusion, aided by the reaction of the seed extract of *Salvia horminum*, which agglutinates both Tn and Cad polyagglutinable cells[12] (Table 14-7).

Table 14-7. Differentiation of T, Tn, and Cad polyagglutination*

Mode of treatment	Type of polyagglutination		
	T	Tn	Cad
Arachis hypognea	+	−	−
Salvia sclarea	−	+	−
Salvia haematodes	−	+	−
Salvia horminum	−	+	+
Dolichos biflorus	−	+	+
Ficin (1%)	NE	RD	RE

*+, Agglutination; −, no agglutination; NE, no effect; RD, receptor destroyed; RE, receptor enhanced.

Acquired B antigen: In this condition the red cells of some group A individuals have temporarily acquired a B-like antigen as the result of disease. These cells at first appear to be polyagglutinable because they react with most normal adult sera; however, they do not react with group AB serum. Most patients have a bacterial infection and on recovery lose their acquired antigen and revert to normal. Because the number of A receptor sites diminishes as the number of B receptor sites increases,[16] it is postulated that bacterial enzymes deacetylate the A antigen to form B antigen (*N*-acetyl-D-galactosamine ⟶ D-galactose).[17] This B-like antigen can be suspected by observing a very slow agglutination with anti-B antiserum and by the low agglutination scores.[16]

Altered antibodies

The absence of expected agglutinins may be seen in hypogammaglobulinemia and at both ends of the age spectrum. Infants do not develop recognizable anti-A and anti-B until 3-6 months of age; to avoid this problem, serum grouping is not attempted in an infant under 6 months old. In old age the isoagglutinin titers may become very low.

Cold alloantibodies and autoantibodies

Specific cold alloantibodies may be present in the serum being tested; if the reagent cells have the corresponding antigen, agglutination may occur at room temperature and may confuse the ABO grouping interpretation. Such antibodies are anti-Le[a], anti-Le[b], anti-M, anti-N, and anti-P$_1$. When such antibodies are suspected, test the serum against panel cells for identification.

More commonly, anti-I is the problem; this harmless cold autoantibody, if present in high titers or if active at room temperature, will agglutinate all test cells in the serum grouping procedure. The nature of the problem can be suspected by the following:

1. The autologous control is positive: Observe a reaction of the patient's serum with his own cells.
2. Repeat the ABO grouping tests and demonstrate increased agglutination at 4° C and absent agglutination at 37° C.

Although the auto−anti-I problem is more manifest in serum grouping tests, it is important to realize that the cell grouping tests may also be invalid if the antibody binds to the patient's cells at room temperature. Correct ABO grouping may be obtained by autoabsorbing the anti-I from the serum and repeating the grouping procedures.

Removal of autoantibody by autoabsorption[18]:

1. Prepare enzyme-treated patient cells (see discussion of special test procedures).
2. To 1 volume of enzyme-treated cells, add 1 volume of the patient's serum.
3. Mix. Incubate at 4° C for 30-60 min.
4. Centrifuge and remove the supernatant serum.
5. Test the autoabsorbed serum against patient's cells to ensure complete removal of the cold autoantibody. If cold autoagglutinin remains, repeat the above, using fresh cells.
6. If autoantibody has been completely removed, proceed with desired testing.

Pseudoagglutination

Pseudoagglutination is the nonspecific clumping of red cells, simulating true antigen-antibody–induced agglutination. Various agents can induce such an occurrence, some of which are described below.

Rouleaux formation: Rouleaux formation is the nonspecific clumping of red cells caused by a property of the serum in which they are suspended. Molecules producing rouleaux include the following:

1. **Fibrinogen** has the greatest tendency to cause rouleaux and is the major reason why serum, not plasma, is used in blood bank tests.
2. **γ-Globulin** is a leading cause of rouleaux and is seen in patients with infections, cirrhosis, sarcoidosis, and dysproteinemias.
3. **Dextran** is a high-molecular-weight polysaccharide used as a volume expander and capable of causing rouleaux for 24-36 hr after infusion.

Typically the clumped cells are "stacked like coins" with their flat sides sticking together; microscopic examination should differentiate clumped cells from true immune aggregates. Often, however, rouleaux produce a small irregular clustering of cells that is very difficult to differentiate from agglutination even with the microscope. To differentiate rouleaux from agglutination, the saline replacement technic is recommended.

Saline replacement technic: Saline is added after the antigen-antibody reactions have occurred and there is no danger of diluting out weak or low titered antibodies.

1. When rouleaux are suspected, respin the serum-cell mixture.
2. Remove the serum and replace with an equal volume of saline.
3. Mix. Spin the saline-cell mixture.
4. Resuspend and observe for agglutination. Rouleaux will be dispersed but true agglutination remains.

Wharton's jelly: Cord red cells may clump spontaneously because they have been contaminated by the Wharton's jelly of the umbilical cord. This only occurs if the cord has been stripped instead of using a needle and syringe to obtain cord blood. Typically the clumped red cells appear "stringy" and spontaneously disperse if allowed to stand; they reappear again if agitated. Such cells always appear to belong to group AB on cell testing; this cannot be confirmed with serum tests because of the natural deficiency of isoantibodies at birth. If contamination with Wharton's jelly is suspected, the correct ABO grouping can be obtained by either of the following steps:

1. Repeat ABO tests using well-washed cells to remove the contaminating material; 3 to 5 saline washings are recommended.
2. Add 1 drop of hyaluronidase to the red cell suspension to eliminate the offending hyaluronic acid in the Wharton's jelly.

RHESUS BLOOD GROUP SYSTEM

Outside of the ABO blood group system, the rhesus system is the most important because the D antigen is so immunogenic. Hence, of those recipients who lack the D antigen but receive even 1 unit of donor blood possessing this antigen, 50-80% will become immunized. The Rh blood group system was discovered in 1940 by Landsteiner and Wiener[19] when they injected red cells from the monkey *Macacus rhesus* into rabbits and guinea pigs; the antibody produced reacted with red cells from 85% of the white population. They believed they had discovered human erythrocyte antigens that were identical to some rhesus erythrocyte antigens; the system was named accordingly.

General principles
Genetics and nomenclature

Two theories have been proposed to explain the genetics of the Rh system. The Fisher-Race theory postulates three pairs of genes, closely linked to prevent cross-over.[20] The three pairs are named *Cc, Dd,* and *Ee*. These are codominant genes, and each gene determines the corresponding red cell antigen that can be identified by a specific antiserum. In the years following this proposition, no example of anti-d has been reported and therefore the hypothetical *d* gene probably does not exist; the symbol "d" is still used to denote the absence of the *D* gene or antigen. When the rhesus system expanded beyond the basic five antigens, they were accomodated in the Fisher-Race theory by postulating rare alleles at the three loci; rare phenotypes were explained by cross-over among the genes, but this has actually been proved in exceptional cases.

The Wiener theory postulates eight common allelic genes found at one locus on a chromosome.[21] These common genes are named R^1, R^2, R^0, R^z, r, r', r'', and r^y. Each gene produces an entire complex of blood factors called the **agglutinogen;** the individual factors of the agglutinogen are the red cell antigens and are detected by a specific antiserum. Fig. 14-3 illustrates the basic difference between these two genetic theories.

There are three antigen notations in current use: the CDE nomenclature of Fisher-Race, the Rh-Hr nomenclature of Wiener, and the numeric notation of Rosenfield. Tables 14-8 and 14-9 show comparisons of the two genetic theories and their notations.

One gene or allelic set is inherited from each parent, producing the genotype of the offspring. Although it is difficult to determine the genotype without the aid of

Fig. 14-3. Wiener and Fisher-Race theories to explain most probable genotype of rhesus phenotype CcDEe.

Table 14-8. Red cell antigen notations

Weiner	Fisher-Race	Rosenfield	Wiener	Fisher-Race	Rosenfield
Rho	D	Rh1	Hro	d	—
rh′	C	Rh2	hr′	c	Rh4
rh″	E	Rh3	hr″	e	Rh5

Table 14-9. Common Rh genes and their estimated frequencies

	Wiener		Fisher-Race	Gene frequency (%)	
Gene	Agglutinogen	Blood factors	Allelic set	Whites	Blacks
R'	Rh_1	Rh_o, rh′, hr″	CDe	0.43	0.14
R^2	Rh_2	Rh_o, hr′, rh″	cDE	0.15	0.13
R^0	Rho	Rh_o, hr′, hr″	cDe	0.04	0.46
R^z	Rh_z	Rh_o, rh′, rh″	CDE	< 0.01	0
r	rh	hr′, hr″	cde	0.37	0.25
r'	rh′	rh′, hr″	Cde	0.01	0.02
r''	rh″	hr′, rh″	cdE	< 0.01	0
r^y	rh_y	rh′, rh″	CdE	< 0.01	0

Table 14-10. Common rhesus phenotypes*

RBC reaction with antisera					RBC phenotype		
Anti-Rh_o(D)	Anti-rh′(C)	Anti-rh″(E)	Anti-hr′(c)	Anti-hr″(E)	Fisher-Race	Wiener	Rosenfield
+	+	−	+	+	CcDee	Rh_1 rh	Rh: 1,2,−3,4,5
−	−	−	+	+	ccdee	rh	Rh: −1,−2,−3,4,5
+	+	+	+	+	CcDEe	Rh_1 Rh_2	Rh: 1,2,3,4,5
+	−	+	+	+	ccDEe	Rh_2 rh	Rh: 1,−2,3,4,5
+	−	−	+	+	ccDee	Rh_o	Rh: 1,−2,−3,4,5
+	+	−	−	+	CCDee	Rh_1 Rh_1	Rh: 1,2,−3,−4,5
+	−	+	+	−	ccDEE	Rh_2 Rh_2	Rh: 1,−2,3,4,−5

*+, Agglutination; −, no agglutination.

family studies, all blood is easily characterized by its phenotype: the serologic reactions of the red cells with the five common rhesus antisera: anti-D, anti-C, anti-E, anti-c, and anti-e. In the Fisher-Race nomenclature the phenotype is written by indicating the presence of C, then D, and finally the E antigens. For example, CcDee means agglutination was observed with anti-C, anti-c, anti-D, and anti-e. In the Wiener nomenclature, these observed reactions are written as one of the agglutinogens so defined; in so doing, all the possible genotypes are listed, the most common being selected: Rh₁rh. In the Rosenfield numeric notation,[22] all anti-

gens tested are listed in numeric order, indicating an absence of agglutination with a minus sign: Rh: 1, 2, −3, 4, 5. If certain antigens were not tested, their number is omitted. Table 14-10 lists the most common phenotypes and their designations.

The five common antisera given in Table 14-10 are used only to determine the phenotype of a red cell and are not routinely needed to determine the Rh status of red cells: Cells are Rh positive if the D antigen is present and Rh negative if the D antigen is absent. There is no need to determine the other blood factors in routine procedures.

D^u variant

D^u red cells are cells with a weakened D antigen on their surface so they give only some of the expected reactions with reagent anti-D. The weakest examples will not be agglutinated by anti-D but will absorb it, showing visible clumping only after the addition of antiglobulin serum. The strongest examples may show only a delayed agglutination with reagent antisera.

There are two recognized causes of this phenomenon. In one case the subject has inherited an allelic gene at the Rh locus (D^u or Rh$_0$ gene) that codes for a weakly reactive antigen; this gene is found in 0.02% of the white population and 0.2% of the black population. In the other instance the condition is known as "gene interaction" because a normal D gene on one chromosome has a partially suppressed serologic expression by the gene complex Cde (r') on the opposite chromosome. The latter condition is also often referred to as "high-grade D^u" because it produces a red cell with greater D reactivity than the former genetic condition (called "low-grade D^u"); it is best to avoid these terms entirely.

Because D^u red cells do have the D antigen on their surface, they are capable of immunizing a truly Rh-negative recipient to the D antigen. Although this would be quite uncommon because of the reduced antigenicity of the D^u cells, it is imperative that all Rh-negative donor blood be tested for the D^u phenotype by performing an antiglobulin test (see discussion of Rh typing). Only that blood negative after the addition of antiglobulin serum is considered Rh negative. It is not necessary to test recipient blood for the D^u factor; if a recipient is known to have the D^u phenotype, he may receive Rh-positive or Rh-negative blood.[1]

Minor Rh antigens

A large number of minor antigens exist in this system, most explained as alleles at the rhesus locus or loci. Hence the Rh system is one of the most complex blood group systems. Table 14-11 gives a partial list of these antigens in the three systems of notation. Some of these antigens are **compound antigens:** Ce, CE, cE, ce. These antigens are produced only when the genes governing them are in the **cis** genetic position; i.e., they occur on the same chromosome.

Deleted antigens

Some rare genes may be present that produce a phenotype lacking some or all of the common Rh antigens. Because of the rarity of these genes, persons exhibiting the condition are often the product of a consanguineous mating.

-D-phenotype: Red cells of the -D-phenotype fail to react with anti-C, anti-c, anti-E, or anti-e. Their reaction with anti-D is exceptionally strong because of a great increase in the number of D receptor sites on the red cell surface.[23] In the Wiener notation, it is written $\bar{R}^0$.

Rh null phenotype: Red cells of the Rh null phenotype fail to react with any of the rhesus antisera (written $---$). The condition can result from a rare amorph gene[24] at the rhesus locus or a rare suppressor gene[25] at an unknown locus; the suppressor gene prevents conversion of a basic precursor substance to rhesus precursor substance, and the amorph gene prevents conversion of rhesus precursor substance to the CDE antigens (Fig. 14-4). It is common for persons with the Rh null

Table 14-11. Minor antigens in the rhesus system

Rosenfield	Fisher-Race	Wiener
Rh: 6	f, ce	hr
Rh: 7	Ce	rhi
Rh: 22	CE	—
Rh: 27	cE	—
Rh: 8	C^w	rh^{wl}
Rh: 9	C^x	rh^x
Rh: 11	E^w	rh^{w2}
Rh: 12	G	rh^G
Rh: 10	V ce^s	hr^v
Rh: 20	VS,e^s	—

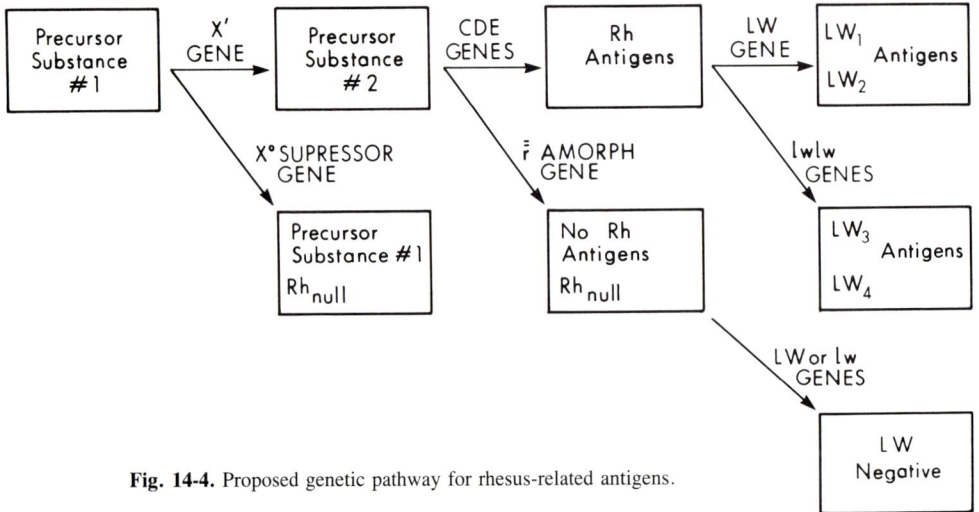

Fig. 14-4. Proposed genetic pathway for rhesus-related antigens.

phenotype to have an associated mild, chronic hemolytic anemia, allowing the speculation that the rhesus antigens are an integral part of the erythrocyte membrane.[26]

LW antigen

It is now realized that Landsteiner and Wiener's antibody to rhesus red cells was not anti-D.[27] As a result of absorption and elution studies, it became evident that both Rh-positive and Rh-negative cells contained the antigen present on rhesus red cells. As a result, the antibody has been renamed anti-LW, in honor of its codiscoverers; the LW antigen is considered a high-incidence antigen present on both Rh-positive and Rh-negative red cells. Generally, Rh-positive cells have more LW antigen than Rh-negative cells[28]; it is for this reason that Landsteiner and Wiener failed to detect their antigen in Rh-negative cells.

The LW antigen is governed by the allelic genes *LW* and *lw* at a genetic locus independent of the Rh locus. These genes act on the CDE antigens to make LW antigen. The LW antigen is considered a group of antigens with quantitative differences analogous to the subgroups in the ABO blood group system. These antigens are named LW_1, LW_2, LW_3, and LW_4 in the order of decreasing antigenicity. Rh-positive cells usually have the LW_1 antigen on their surface; Rh-negative cells have LW_2 antigen on their surface. Those rare red cells that are apparently LW negative belong to one of two categories. One category is red cells with all or some of the normal rhesus antigens; they have the very weak LW antigens LW_3 or LW_4 as proven by their ability to react with some but not all anti-LW antisera.[28,29] The second category is red cells that lack all rhesus antigens (i.e., Rh_{null}); these cells are true serologic negatives for the LW antigens[30] because they lack the CDE substances from which LW antigen is made; they fail to react with all known examples of anti-LW antisera. Hence, except for Rh_{null} cells, all red cells have the LW antigens, even if only in very minute amounts. According to Issitt and Issitt,[31] the LW_1 and LW_2 antigens are the result of the inheritance of the LW gene; the LW_3 and LW_4 antigens are the result of the *lwlw* genotype (Fig. 14-4), the *lw* gene being a less efficient convertor of CDE substance.

Rh antibodies

Most antibodies in the Rh blood group system are IgG immunoglobulins that are unable to agglutinate saline suspended red cells; potentiating media, antiglobulin serum, or enzyme-treated red cells are needed for their routine detection. The antibodies develop as a result of an immune stimulus; the potency of the common rhesus antigens, listed in their order of decreasing immunogenicity, is as follows: D, c, C, E, and e. Occasional examples of naturally occurring Rh antibodies have been reported; in most cases the antibody is anti-E, with fewer examples of anti-C^w and anti-C. Often this naturally occurring antibody is so weak that it is detectable only with the use of enzyme-treated red cells. Rh antibodies do not bind complement, and therefore hemolysis is not expected in serologic assays.

Rh typing technics

For routine purposes blood is typed for the D antigen only. All persons can be classified into three phenotypic types on the basis of the D antigen: Rh positive, Rh negative, and weak Rh positive (D^u variant). All donors must be tested for the D^u phenotype if tests indicate the absence of D antigen; recipients need not be so tested. Antisera for other Rh antigens are used only under special circumstances: if a recipient has a rhesus antibody or if phenotyping is desirable.

Rh typing using incomplete anti-D

Incomplete anti-D is the reagent used most frequently; it is labeled "slide," "modified tube," or "rapid tube test" serum. The reagent contains a high-protein medium and/or other potentiating substances that produce an antiserum capable of rapid, sensitive, and reproducible results. However, these same additions may produce a false positive clumping. To avoid this problem an **Rh control** must be included with each test; the best control consists of all the additives used to enrich the anti-D antiserum but without anti-D itself. The control test must be negative or the cell results cannot be interpreted.

Slide test: The slide test must be performed with high concentrations of protein and red cells. The typing serum should have a protein concentration up to 25-30%. The cells must be suspended in plasma or serum to give a hematocrit value of about 50 vol%. Anemic blood must be concentrated to this hematocrit level by centrifugation of the oxalated specimen and by discarding the appropriate amount of plasma. An Rh viewing box should be used, the electric bulb of which keeps the plate temperature between 45-50° C, allowing the test slide to reach a temperature of 37-39° C during the 2 min required for the test. Since coated red cells may clump in the albumin alone, an albumin control must be included with each test.

Procedure: Label two glass slides for each blood sample to be tested. Prepare a 40-50% suspension of cells in own serum or plasma. On one slide, place 1 drop of anti-D slide or modified test tube serum; on the other slide, place 1 drop of Rh control. Add 2 drops of 40-50% red cell suspension to each slide. With separate applicator sticks, mix each suspension and spread over an area of about 2 × 4 cm. Place both slides on the viewing box and tilt back and forth slowly, observing for macroscopic agglutination over a period of 2 min. Do not read after 2 min. Do not interpret peripheral drying as agglutination.

Modified tube test: The tube test should be run with a 2-5% red cell suspension in serum or saline (follow manufacturer's directions).

Procedure:
1. Prepare a 2-5% suspension of cells.
2. Label two 75 × 10 mm test tubes for each blood sample to be tested.
3. Place 1 drop of anti-D slide or modified test tube serum in one tube and 1 drop of Rh control in the other tube.
4. Add to each tube 1-2 drops of the 2-5% red cell suspension. An applicator stick may be dipped into the clot to approximate a 2-5% concentration.

5. Mix. Centrifuge for 15 sec.
6. Gently resuspend and observe for agglutination with an optical aid.

Interpretation: Agglutination in the test and no agglutination in the control indicates Rh positive. Absence of agglutination in both tubes indicates Rh negative; the D^u test should be performed on donor blood.

Agglutination in the control tube indicates the test must be repeated using saline anti-D. A possible cause for agglutination in the control tube is that the cells are coated in vivo by either antibody or abnormal plasma proteins. If antibody coating is suspected, a direct antiglobulin test is indicated.

Rh typing using saline anti-D

Saline anti-D, or IgM anti-D, will agglutinate cells suspended in saline. It is labeled "for saline," "for saline tube test," or "for tube test." Because high-protein media are not used in the manufacture of this reagent, an Rh control is not needed.

Procedure: Prepare a 2-5% saline suspension of well-washed red cells. Label a 10×75 mm test tube; in it place 1 drop saline agglutinating antiserum. Add 1 drop of 2-5% saline suspended red cells. Mix. Incubate at 37° C for 15-60 min, according to manufacturer's directions. Centrifuge for 15 min. Gently dislodge cells and examine with optical aid for agglutination.

Interpretation: Agglutination indicates Rh-positive cells; absence of agglutination indicates Rh-negative cells.

Errors in Rh typing

False positive tests: False positive tests may be caused by drying (the observation period exceeding 2 min), rouleaux formation, or autoagglutination. Rh antisera are fortified with albumin to obtain the optimal protein concentration required for Rh typing. If the patient's red cells are heavily coated with antibodies, the albumin itself may produce agglutination, leading to a false positive reaction. Suspending the cells in saline and retyping with saline-active antisera will usually lead to correct cell identification. Cold agglutinins usually give spontaneous agglutination.

False negative tests: False negative tests may be caused by old red cells (only fresh cells should be used), wrong concentration of red cells, hemolysis, inadequate mixing of red cells, inactive typing sera, or incorrect temperature. Cells of the Rh_0 variant type (D^u) may also give a false negative test.

False negative tests may also be caused by the presence of blocking antibodies in a high enough concentration to prevent typing of the cells because no binding sites are free on the red cell surface. Incomplete anti-D antisera are usually negative; although saline anti-D can sometimes successfully type these cells, this also may be impossible. To prevent isoagglutinin interference, the antibody can be eluted to liberate binding sites and allow accurate Rh typing. The eluted antibody can then be identified. An example of such a condition is Rh hemolytic disease of the newborn, in which infant red cells are very heavily coated with maternal anti-D.

D^u testing

D^u red cells may give a false negative agglutination pattern with commercial antisera. D^u cells usually are not agglutinated by saline anti-D; they may or may not be agglutinated by incomplete anti-D. However, these cells do absorb the antibody, and this can be easily detected with antiglobulin serum.

Procedure:
1. If Rh testing is initially performed in a test tube, the same tube can be used for D^u testing: begin with step 4 of modified tube test procedure.
2. Label tube and add 1 drop of anti-D slide or modified test tube serum.
3. Add 1-2 drops of 2-5% red cell suspension.
4. Mix and incubate at 37° C for 15-60 min, according to manufacturer's directions.
5. Label a second tube for control and add 1-2 drops of the original cell suspension; or use the Rh control tube from Rh testing.
6. Wash both cell suspensions carefully with at least three changes of large amounts of saline solution.
7. After the final wash, remove all saline solution and blot the rims of tubes dry.
8. Add 1-2 drops of antiglobulin serum to each tube.
9. Mix gently and centrifuge 15 sec.
10. Gently resuspend the cell button and observe for agglutination.
11. Add known sensitized cells as a control for the antiglobulin serum.

Interpretation: Agglutination in the test and absence of agglutination in the control indicates the D^u variant; such blood should be labeled as Rh positive, D^u. Agglutination in the control tube indicates a positive direct antiglobulin test, the cause of which must be determined; the D^u test is invalid under these circumstances.

MNSsU BLOOD GROUP SYSTEM

The MNSsU group was the second blood group system to be discovered. It was the first time in which antibodies were deliberately produced in an animal in an attempt to discover other blood group antigens. This blood group system is used extensively in medicolegal investigations.

Antigens

The MN blood group system was discovered by Landsteiner and Levine by injecting human red cells into rabbits.[32] The two resulting antibodies were called anti-M and anti-N; they divided the population into three distinct groups: those reacting with only one of the antibodies (M or N phenotype) and those reacting with both antibodies (MN phenotype). Later two other antibodies were added to the system: anti-S and anti-s.

The MNSs system is governed by two closely linked sets of allelic genes, *MN* and *Ss*. As a result of close linkage, four gene complexes are possible, which, in the absent of cross-over, are inherited as a pair from each parent: *MS*, *Ms*, *NS*, and *Ns*. From these four gene complexes, 10 common genotypes are possible (Table 14-12).

Table 14-12. Genotype and frequencies in MNSs system

Gene complex	Gene frequency	Phenotype	Phenotype frequency (%)	Possible genotypes	Approximate[33] genotype frequency (%)	Positive (%) with anti-S	Positive (%) with anti-s
MS	0.2311	M	30	MS MS	6	66	80
Ms	0.3090			MS Ms	14		
NS	0.0709			Ms Ms	10		
Ns	0.3890	MN	49	MS NS	4	53	92
				MS Ns ⎱ Ms NS ⎰	22		
				Ms Ns	23		
		N	21	NS NS	0.3	25	99
				NS Ns	5		
				Ns Ns	16		

There is still a third antigen associated with this blood group: U. The U antigen is a high-incidence antigen found in 100% of whites and approximately 98.5% of blacks. This antigen is produced by the gene complexes that produce either S and/or s antigens. In the rare U-negative black, the uncommon phenotype S-s- is usually present. The phenotype S-s- is often written as S^u and is the product of another allele at the Ss genetic locus.

Chemistry of M and N antigens

The M and N antigens are glycoproteins in which approximately 56% is carbohydrate and 44% is protein. Sialic acid constitutes the greatest carbohydrate component, and it appears to confer partial antigenic specificity to the red cells.[34] More recent information suggests the amino acid sequences may be of primary importance in conferring antigenicity.[35,36] At this time there is no universally accepted model of antigenic structure of genetic pathway.

Antibodies

Anti-M and anti-N occur infrequently in human sera; when present they are usually naturally occurring cold agglutinins that react in saline at an optimal temperature of 5-25° C. Anti-M may be formed as an isoimmune antibody after multiple pregnancies and very rarely develops during a pregnancy; in these instances it acts best at 37° C using the antiglobulin technic. Anti-N is much less often encountered than anti-M, perhaps because M red cells possess some N substance, which is believed to be a precursor to M substance.[37] There is a potent anti-N lectin in the seeds of the South American plant *Vicia graminea*.[38] Both anti-M and anti-N exhibit strong **dosage;** i.e., they react most strongly with red cells carrying a double dose of their corresponding antigen; hence, anti-M reacts more strongly with red cells of genotype *MM* than with genotype *MN*.

Anti-S and anti-s are usually immune antibodies reacting optimally at 37° C with antiglobulin serum. They can cause hemolytic disease of the newborn and transfusion reactions.

Anti-U is a rare antibody formed in people who are S-s-. It reacts best by the indirect antiglobulin technic

and can cause hemolytic disease of the newborn and transfusion reactions.

P BLOOD GROUP SYSTEM

The P group was the third blood group system to be discovered. Landsteiner and Levine described it in 1927 as a result of the experiments that led to their discovery of the MN system.

Antigens

There are five phenotypes in the P system and three different antigens that may be present on the red cell surface. Of these phenotypes only two, P_1 and P_2, are common; the other three phenotypes are exceedingly rare (Table 14-13). The five phenotypes are regulated by two independent genetic loci. At one locus are three allelic genes, P_1, P_2, and p, the last one being an amorph gene; individuals homozygous for the p gene lack all antigens of the P system. At the second locus is the gene governing the P^k phenotype; although no universally accepted genetic scheme is available at this time, this gene has been alternately viewed as a rare recessive gene[39] or as a universal public gene.[40] Currently the latter explanation is gaining greater acceptance.

The P_1 antigen is incompletely developed at birth, reaching adult levels at 7 years of age.[41] There is considerable variability of the P_1 antigen strength among P_1-positive adults; this is a quantitative variation that is caused only partially by the genetic constitution of the individual: those having a strong P_1 antigen show a disproportionate increase in homozygosity for the P_1 gene.[42] The P_1 antigen shows rapid deterioration upon storage, so fresh red cells should always be used when searching for P_1-negative donor blood.

P_1 substance is present in hydatid cyst fluid and has allowed chemical analysis of the antigenic substance. In addition, red cell extracts of the P antigens have shown the antigenic specificity to reside in the carbohydrate galactose.[43,44]

Antibodies

Anti-P_1 is the only commonly encountered antibody in the P blood group system. It acts as a cold agglutinin and is found as a naturally occurring antibody in the

Table 14-13. P blood group system

Phenotype	Antigens on red cell	Possible genotype	Genotype frequency (%)	Naturally occurring antibodies
P_1	$P + P_1$	$P_1 P_1$ $P_1 P_2$ $P_1 p$	29 50 0	None
P_2	P	$P_2 P_2$ $P_2 p$	21 0	Anti-P_1
p	None	pp	Rare	Anti-PP_1P^k
P^k_1	$P^k + P_1$	Unknown	Rare	Anti-P
P^k	P^k	Unknown	Rare	Anti-P

serum of two thirds of P_2 individuals. Because the optimal temperature of reactivity is 4° C, the antibody is usually of no clinical significance. Rare examples of anti-P_1 will react at 37° C; if such an antibody is present, it may produce in vivo hemolysis and must therefore be respected in selecting blood for transfusion purposes.

Anti-PP_1P^k is a naturally occurring antibody in the serum of all pp individuals. The antibody is a very potent hemolysin reacting at all temperatures in saline and albumin with antiglobulin serum.

Anti-P is a naturally occurring antibody in the serum of P^k individuals. It can be a potent hemolysin reacting at all temperatures with antiglobulin serum in saline and albumin.

Isolated anti-P^k has never been found in nature but can be produced in the laboratory by absorption of anti-PP_1P^k with P_1 cells.

KELL BLOOD GROUP SYSTEM
Common antigens

There are up to 18 antigens that belong to the Kell system. However, Kell phenotypes are commonly written using only three pairs of allelic genes: Kell *(K)* and Cellano *(k)*, Penny *(Kp^a)* and Rautenberg *(Kp^b)*, and Sutter *(Js^a)* and Matthews *(Js^b)*. The frequencies of these antigens are shown in Table 14-14; the phenotypes and their frequencies are shown in Table 14-15.

Hence, as Table 14-15 shows, the most common Kell phenotype in both white and black populations is written as follows: K−k+ Kp(a−b+) Js(a−b+). Indeed k, Kp^b, and Js^b can be considered high-incidence antigens, i.e., antigens present on the red cells of most persons tested. There are other high-incidence antigens in the Kell system that are present in 99.9% of both whites and blacks; they are KU(K5), KL(K9), Cote (K11), K12, K13, K14, and Kx (K15). Kx is believed to be a precursor in the Kell antigen synthetic pathway; normal red cells have only very small amounts of Kx antigen, most having been converted to the definitive Kell antigens.

K$_0$ and McLeod phenotypes

In 1957 the Kell null phenotype was described and named Peltz (K$_0$).[45] These cells lack all Kell antigens except Kx, which is present in very great amounts. It is believed that the K_0 gene lacks the ability to transform the precursor substance to normal Kell antigens,

Table 14-14. Antigen frequencies in Kell system

Antigen	Numeric designation	Frequency (%)	
		Whites	Blacks
K	K_1	9	3.5
k	K_2	99.8	>99.9
Kp^a	K_3	2	<0.1
Kp^b	K_4	>99.9	>99.9
Js^a	K_6	<0.1	19.5
Js^b	K_7	>99.1	98.9

Table 14-15. Phenotype frequencies in Kell system

Phenotype	Frequency (%)	
	Whites	Blacks
K+k−	0.2	<0.1
K+k+	8.8	3.5
K−k+	91.0	96.5
Kp(a+b−)	<0.1	<0.1
Kp(a+b+)	2.0	<0.1
Kp(a−b+)	98.0	>99.9
Js(a+b−)	<0.1	1.0
Js(a+b+)	<0.1	18.5
Js(a−b+)	>99.9	80.5

leaving most Kx unchanged on the red cell membrane. The red cells of this phenotype appear normal and have a normal survival.

The McLeod phenotype is a rare phenotype written as follows: K−kw Kp(a−bw) Js(a−bw); it was discovered in 1961[46] and has been shown to be the only Kell phenotype completely devoid of Kx antigen and to be morphologically abnormal with reduced survival.[47]

Kx antigen and chronic granulomatous disease

The Kx antigen is the only Kell antigen present on leukocytes and monocytes as well as erythrocytes. The genes controlling the production of this antigen are located on the X chromosome as multiple alleles.[48] Whether the Kx antigen appears on both leukocytes and red cells, on one or the other cell type, or on neither depends on which allele is inherited. In the rare clinical disorder of X-linked chronic granulomatous disease, leukocytes lack the Kx antigen; only some of these cases also lack the Kx antigen on red cells and are therefore of McLeod phenotype. In chronic granulomatous disease the leukocytes are unable to kill the pathogens they have engulfed; it is possible the Kx antigen may serve in a functional capacity in this disease.

Antibodies

The antibodies are generally immune IgG immunoglobulins that react best with antiglobulin serum. Anti-K is a common antibody; 91% of the population lack the Kell antigen and could therefore be sensitized by this very potent antigen. The Kell antigen is second only to the A, B, and D antigens in immunogenicity. Anti-k, anti-Kp^b, and anti-Js^b are rarely encountered because these antigens are present in most of the population. The Kell antibodies can cause transfusion reactions and hemolytic disease of the newborn.

DUFFY BLOOD GROUP SYSTEM
Antigens

The antigen Fy^a is found in about 66% of whites, being present in the homozygous form (*Fy^{a}Fy^a*) in about 17% and in the heterozygous form (*Fy^{a}Fy^b*) in 49% (Table 14-16). Ninety percent of blacks are Fy^a negative, 68% being Fy(a−b−) and 22% being Fy(a−b+). The absence of Fy^a and Fy^b in blacks is explained on the basis of a third gene, *Fy*, which is allelic to *Fy^a* and *Fy^b*. The Fy antigen is easily destroyed by proteolytic enzymes; therefore enzyme treatment of Fy^a or Fy^b test cells is not indicated.

Homozygous (*Fy^{a}Fy^a*) cells are more strongly agglutinated than heterozygous cells and show a marked dosage effect that distinguishes *Fy^{a}Fy^a* from *Fy^{a}Fy^b* cells.

In addition to these common antigens, there are three recently discovered antigens in the Duffy system. In 1971 an antibody was discovered in the serum of a white with the very rare Fy(a−b−) that reacted with all red cells that were Fy(a+) or Fy(b+) but none of the Fy(a−b−) samples.[49] Hence, Fy^3 is a high-incidence antigen in the white population. The Fy^3 antigen is not destroyed by enzyme treatment and, in fact, appears to be enhanced.[49] It has been suggested that Fy^3 may be a precursor substance for both Fy^a and Fy^b antigens.

In 1973 the Fy^4 antigen was discovered and was postulated to be the product of the silent *Fy* gene.[50] Anti-Fy^4 reacts with all Fy(a−b−) cells of blacks and with the majority of Fy(a+b−) and Fy(a−b+) cells of blacks; it fails to react with any Fy(a+b+) cells. Anti-Fy^4 will therefore detect any genotype containing the *Fy* gene. The Fy^4 antigen is enhanced by enzyme treatment.

Fy^5 is an antigen dependent on the simultaneous inheritance of a functioning *rhesus* gene and a *Duffy* gene other than the *Fy* gene. Anti-Fy^5 will react with all Fy(a+) and Fy(b+) cells but fails to react with Rh null cells possessing these Duffy antigens; it fails to react with Fy(a−b−) cells of blacks.[51] The requirement of two functioning genes of different blood group systems is interesting, but all the more so because the *Duffy* and *rhesus* genes are both located on chromosome 1.[52]

Table 14-16. Frequency of Duffy genotypes and phenotypes

Phenotype	Genotype	Frequency (%)	
		Whites	**Blacks**
Fy(a+b−)	*Fy^{a}Fy^a*	17	9
Fy(a+b+)	*Fy^{a}Fy^b*	49	2
Fy(a−b+)	*Fy^{b}Fy^b*	34	22
Fy(a−b−)	*FyFy*	Rare	68

Antibodies

The antibodies of the Duffy blood group system are IgG immunoglobulins that are demonstrated best by the antiglobulin test. Both anti-Fy^a and anti-Fy^b have been implicated in transfusion reaction and in hemolytic disease of the newborn.

Clinical significance

Although 34% of the white population lacks the Fy^a antigen and are therefore at risk of immunization if they receive Fy(a+) donor blood, actual isoimmunization with this antigen is uncommon. This is probably because the Fy^a antigen has low immunogenicity. Fy^b antigen also has very low immunogenicity; anti-Fy^b is even less frequently encountered than anti-Fy^a because a greater proportion of the population possesses the Fy^b antigen. Anti-Fy^a must not be ignored when selecting donor blood, since the antibody can produce a severe transfusion reaction if incompatible blood is administered.

The Fy(a−b−) phenotype offers the red cell protection against invasion by *Plasmodium* organisms.[53]

KIDD BLOOD GROUP SYSTEM
Antigens

The Kidd blood group system was discovered in 1951 during the investigation of a case of hemolytic disease of the newborn.[54] There are two common antigens, Jk^a and Jk^b, which are controlled by codominant allelic genes, *Jk^a* and *Jk^b*. About 75% of whites are Jk^a positive, 25% of phenotype Jk(a+b−) and 50% of phenotype Jk(a+b+); the remainder are Jk^a negative with the phenotype Jk(a−b+) (Table 14-17). The phenotype Jk(a−b−) is very rare in whites and blacks but occurs rather commonly in persons of Mongolian descent. The inheritance of the Kidd null phenotype is attributed to an allele at the Kidd locus, the amorph gene *Jk*.

Antibodies

The antibodies of the Kidd system are IgG immunoglobulins that are complement dependent. They are best demonstrated by an indirect antiglobulin test, provided the antiglobulin serum contains sufficient levels of anticomplement activity. Proteolytic enzymes potentiate the antigens and further aid in identification. If stored serum is tested, complement or fresh compatible serum must be added.

The antibodies are labile, and their titer may rapidly fall to levels too low to be detectable in pretransfusion

Table 14-17. Phenotypes and genotypes of Kidd system

Phenotype	Genotype	Frequency (%)	
		Whites	Blacks
Jk(a+b−)	Jk^aJk^a	25	57
Jk(a+b+)	Jk^aJk^b	50	34
Jk(a−b+)	Jk^bJk^b	25	9
Jk(a−b−)*	JkJk	0	0

*Rare individuals of this type have been found among South American Indians and Chinese.

Table 14-18. Phenotypes and genotypes of Lutheran system

Phenotype	Genotype	Frequency (%)
Lu(a+b−)	Lu^aLu^a	0.15
Lu(a+b+)	Lu^aLu^b	7.5
Lu(a−b+)	Lu^bLu^b	92.3
Lu(a−b−)	See text	Very rare

antibody testing; hence, Kidd antibodies are a frequent cause of delayed transfusion reactions.[55]

LUTHERAN BLOOD GROUP SYSTEM
Antigens

In the Lutheran blood group system there are two codominant allelic genes, Lu^a and Lu^b, which produce the two common antigens, Lu^a and Lu^b. The Lu^b gene is the more common, having an estimated frequency of 0.9646; the gene frequency of Lu^a is estimated to be 0.0354[56] (Table 14-18). Lu(a−b−) is a very rare phenotype and may be caused by a rare amorph gene at the Lutheran locus, Lu,[57] or, more commonly, by a dominant modifier gene at another locus,[58] *In(Lu).*[59] Only the recessive type of Lutheran null is capable of making anti-Lu^{ab}, also called anti-Lu3. The Lutheran genes are linked to the *secretor* genes.

In addition, there are many high-incidence antigens in the Lutheran system, namely, Lu4, Lu5, Lu6, Lu7, Lu8, Lu11, Lu12, Lu13, Lu15, and Lu16; all cells of phenotype Lu(a−b−) lack these antigens, as well as the rare low-incidence Lutheran antigens: Lu9, Lu10, and Lu14. The genes Lu^9 and Lu^6 and allelic at the Lutheran complex locus but are not alleles with Lu^a, Lu^b, and Lu genes.[60] The genetic relationship among the remaining antigens is still unclear.

Antibodies

Anti-Lu^a is an uncommon antibody that reacts as a saline agglutinin at an optimal temperature of 12-20° C. The agglutination pattern observed is that of a mixed-field pattern.[61] Anti-Lu^b is also an uncommon antibody since only 0.15% of the population can form the antibody. Serologically, anti-Lu^b is different from anti-Lu^a; it reacts as an incomplete agglutinin at an optimal temperature of 37° C; it is best detected by the indirect antiglobulin test. Neither antibody causes significant clinical problems.

LEWIS BLOOD GROUP SYSTEM
General principles

The Lewis system is primarily a system of water-soluble antigens found in body fluids and secretions such as saliva. Lewis antigens found on the red cell membrane are not integra parts of the membrane but are acquired from the surrounding plasma. The presence or absence of the Lewis substance in secretion is determined by a pair of allelic genes, *Le* and *le,* respectively.

There are two common antigens is this system: Le^a and Le^b. The inheritance of the *Le* gene, in single or double dose, allows the production of the Le^a antigen. The inheritance of the amorph gene, *le,* in double dose prevents the production of either antigen and results in a null phenotype. The Le^b antigen is explained by the interaction of the dominant *Lewis* gene and the *H* gene, in the presence of the *Se* gene.[62] The biochemistry of the Lewis antigen is well established and supports this theory. Fig. 14-5 shows the biochemistry of the Lewis antigens; Fig. 14-6 illustrates the interactions of the genes at the *H, Se,* and *Le* loci.

The *Le* gene codes for the production of an α-4-L-fucosyltransferase that catalyzes the transfer of fucose to the carbon-4 position of *N*-acetylglucosamine to produce the Le^a active structure. If both the *H* and *Le* gene products are present, the addition of fucose to the carbon-4 position of *N*-acetylglucosamine results in an Le^b active structure, since the *H* gene has transferred fucose to the carbon-2 position of galactose. Hence, Le^b activity is an interaction product of the *H* and *Le* genes in the presence of the *Se* gene, the latter gene allowing the *H* gene to function in secretory cells. This adequately explains why an Le^b gene is not required for the formation of the Le^b antigen.

Of significance in understanding the Lewis system is the realization that there are two types of carbohydrate chain endings in the glycoprotein of the precursor substance. Although the same sugars are present in each type of chain, they have different linkages. In type I chains, the terminal galactose has a β (1-3) linkage with *N*-acetylglucosamine; in type II chains, the sugar has a β (1-4) linkage. Consequently the fucosyltransferase produced by the *Le* gene is unable to act on a type II chain because the number 4 carbon atom is already occupied by the galactosyl structure. Two recently described Lewis antigens, Le^c and Le^d, are postulated to derive from the precursor substance of the type II chain (see below).

Phenotypes

Table 14-19 shows the three common Lewis phenotypes and their frequencies. It can be seen from Table 14-19 that persons of phenotype Le(a+b−) must be nonsecretors unless they are also of the rare Bombay phenotype *(hh);* persons of phenotype Le(a−b+) must be secretors; persons of phenotype Le(a−b−) may be either secretors or nonsecretors, since their null Lewis phenotype derives from the inheritance of the amorph *Lewis* gene. The phenotype Le(a+b+) does not exist except transiently during the first 2 years of life, when the newborn phenotype, which is always Le(a−b−), changes to its adult status.

The concept of an amorph gene in the Lewis system

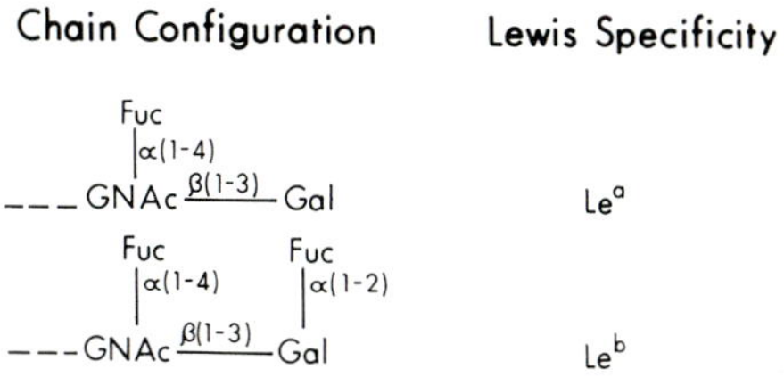

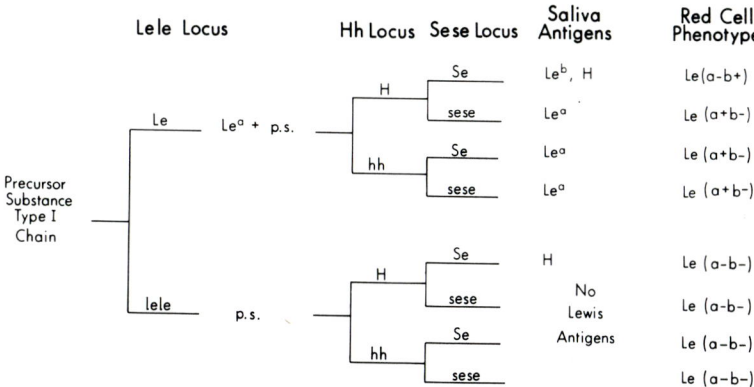

Fig. 14-5. Biochemical structure of Lewis antigen. *GNAc*, N-acetylglucosamine; *Gal*, galactose; *Fuc*, L-fucose.

Fig. 14-6. Genetic pathway of Lewis system.

Table 14-19. Phenotypes and genotypes of Lewis system

Phenotype	Genotype	Frequency (%)	
		Whites	Blacks
Le(a+b−)	*Le, H, sese*	22	23
	Le, hh, Se or sese		
Le(a−b+)	*Le, H, Se*	74	55
Le(a−b−)	*lele, H or hh, Se or sese*	4	22

has recently been challenged. Current data support the theory that the *le* gene may direct the addition of fucose to the number 3 carbon atom of N-acetylglucosamine of a type II precursor chain only; this gives rise to the antigen Le[c].[63] In the presence of *H* and *Se* genes, the *le* gene produces Le[d].[64] Hence, Le[c] and Le[d] antigens have structures similar to those of Le[a] and Le[b], respectively; the only differences are in the sugar linkages. Therefore the null phenotype could be expanded and written Le(a−b−c+d−) or Le(a−b−c−d+) depending on the secretory status. At the present time the implication that the *le* gene controls the production of these additional Lewis antigens is controversial because some Le(a−b−) cells do not react with anti-Le[c] or anti-Le[d].[65,66] Since anti-Le[c] and anti-Le[d] are extremely rare antibodies, there is no practical advantage of classifying cells by these two new Lewis antigens.

Antibodies

Anti-Le[a] and anti-Le[b] are commonly occurring antibodies found in the serum of Le(a−b−) individuals;

they are usually naturally occurring antibodies of IgM immunoglobulin that are capable of fixing complement. The optimal temperature of reactivity is 5-37° C. Most examples are saline agglutinins; the agglutination produced is very fragile, and rough handling will disrupt the small aggregated clumps. Some antibodies react well at 37° C; the indirect antiglobulin test is the best procedure for their detection, provided the antiglobulin serum contains an adequate amount of anticomplement. If old serum is to be tested, complement must be added before attempting the antiglobulin procedure. This method is outlined below. When fresh complement is present in the system, hemolysis may be observed. Both anti-Le[a] and anti-Le[b] are enhanced if the test cells are pretreated with proteolytic enzymes.

There are two types of anti-Le[b]; they are called anti-Le[bH] and anti-Le[bL]. Anti-Le[bH] reacts best with O and A₂ Le(b+) cells; it can be neutralized by the secretion of O Le(a−b−) secretors. Hence, anti-Le[bH] is cross-reacting with the H antigenic substance commonly found in O and A₂ cells. Anti-Le[bL] is the true Le[b] antibody, reacting equally well with all Le(b+) cells of any ABO type and showing neutralization only with saliva of Le(b+) individuals.

Test for Lewis antibody:

Principle: According to Polley and Mollison, the most reliable test for Lewis antibodies is the two-stage antiglobulin test.[67] The test is a method of detecting complement binding with anticomplement globulin serum when the test serum is old, stored, or has anticomplementary properties. There are two stages in the test. In the first stage, Lewis-positive red cells are incubated with EDTA-treated test serum, allowing the cells to take up the Lewis antibody. EDTA treatment of test serum prevents interference by the anticomplementary properties of the stored serum. In the second stage the cells are washed and treated with fresh serum to allow uptake of complement.

Reagents:
1. Anti−γ-globulin that has anticomplement globulin activity
2. EDTA solution

   K_2H_2 EDTA, 4.0 g

   NaOH, 0.3 g

   Mix together in 1 dl distilled water. The final pH must be 7-7.4.
3. Group O red cells of known Lewis phenotype

Procedures: To 1 ml test serum, add 0.1 ml EDTA solution (4 mg/ml serum). Mix well and let stand at room temperature for 10 min.

To a dry button of test red cells, add 4 drops of the EDTA-treated serum. Incubate at 37° C for at least 15 min. Wash the cells three times in saline. Decant thoroughly after the final wash. Add 2 drops of fresh, compatible serum to the washed cells. Incubate at 37° C for 15 min. Wash the cells three times in saline. Decant thoroughly after the final wash. Add 2 drops of antiglobulin serum. Mix well. Centrifuge and observe for agglutination.

Interpretation: Agglutination proves the presence of Lewis antibodies in the serum.

Clinical significance

Lewis incompatibility rarely causes hemolytic transfusion reactions because Lewis antibodies are readily neutralized by Lewis substance in the plasma and because red cells lose their Lewis antigens when transfused into Lewis-negative recipients.[68] However, isolated reports of hemolysis from anti-Le[a] indicate such recipients should ideally receive Le(a−b−) donor blood if at all possible.

Ii BLOOD GROUP SYSTEM
Antigens

The inheritance of the Ii blood group system is still unclear; the antigens produced are I and i. All red cells have both antigens present on their surface, but in variable and reciprocal amounts. In fetal life, i is the main red cell antigen and I antigen is not readily detectable. As the fetus matures more I antigen makes its appearance, and at the time of birth, cord red cells react $0-1+$ with anti-I antiserum but $4+$ with anti-i antiserum. Gradually I antigen replaces i antigen until adult proportions are present at 1-2 years of age; at that time the cells react $4+$ with anti-I antiserum and $\pm$ with anti-i.[69] In contrast, there are very rare adults (0.02%) who retain large amounts of i antigen on their cells throughout life; their phenotype is written i(adult) to distinguish them from the i(cord) phenotype. Depending on the amount of I antigen on their surface, i(adult) cells are subdivided into either i_2 or i_1 cells; i_2 cells are found usually in blacks and have slightly more I antigen than i_1 cells, which have been found only in whites. Fig. 14-7 illustrates the relationship between the I and i antigens. Based on the unproven assumption that at least two allelic genes may be involved in the inheritance of the two antigens, the phenotype I(int) has

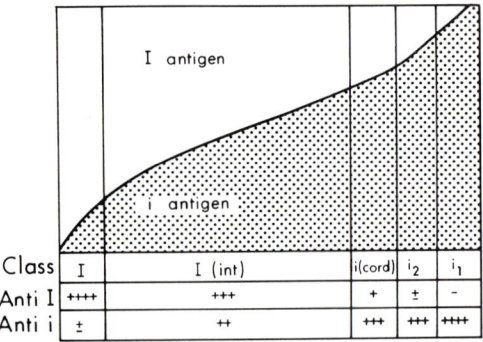

Fig. 14-7. Theoretic amounts of I and i antigen in different classes of I-positive cells. (From Zmijewski, C.M.: Immunohematology, ed. 3, New York, 1978, Appleton-Century-Crofts.)

been used to denote the heterozygous genotype *Ii;* such cells would have less I antigen than those from genotype *II.*

Although 99.98% of adult red cells are I positive, the strength of the antigen varies greatly among the population; this variation is constant throughout the life of the individual. The i antigen is also constant on adult red cells unless increased by hematologic stresses[70]; in such cases there is no concomitant decrease in the amount of I antigen.

Antibodies

Anti-I is a naturally occurring antibody reacting best at cold temperatures (4° C). Agglutinated red cells will spontaneously disperse if exposed to 37° C temperatures and will spontaneously reaggregate when the temperature returns to 4° C. Enzyme treatment of red cells will enhance the reactions of anti-I and therefore allow some positive reactions to be seen at room temperature. All sera contain anti-I in low titers (< 64), and the antibody must therefore be considered an autoantibody because all red cells have I antigen on their surface. At 4° C this antibody will agglutinate the person's own cells. This auto−anti-I has often been called the **harmless cold autoantibody** because it causes no in vivo erythrocyte destruction. Anti-I can be a source of difficulty in routine blood bank procedures if it becomes active at room temperature; this may occur in certain disease states: *Mycoplasma* infections, malignancy, acquired hemolytic anemia, and cold hemagglutinin disease.

Anti-I also occurs regularly in the serum of the rare i(adult); in this instance it is not an autoantibody. This variety is very uncommon because of the rarity of i(adult) phenotype.

Anti-i also a rare antibody that is cold reacting and found in the serum of some persons suffering from reticuloses, infectious mononucleosis, leukemia, and cirrhosis. Under such circumstances the titers are often extremely high (> 200,000).

There is a tendency for the I blood group system antibodies to be of a compound nature, e.g., anti-IH, -IA, -IB, -IP$_1$, -iH, or -iP$_1$. In each instance the compound antibody will react only with red cells having both antigenic specificities on their surface.

Relationship to ABO blood group system

Soluble I blood group substance occurs in some fluids and has allowed biochemical investigations. It is currently believed that the I antigen is closely related to the A, B, H, Le^a, and Le^b antigens, possibly residing at the interior of these antigenic structures.[71] Chemical elucidation of I and i antigens shows a branched and linear glycolipid, respectively, on which the *ABH* genes act.[71a]

SEX-LINKED BLOOD GROUP SYSTEM

The Xg blood group system is inherited as a pair of allelic genes on the X chromosome, *Xg* and *Xg^a;* the former is an amorph gene. These are the only known blood group genes on the X chromosome. Two phenotypes are present in this system: Xg(a+), which is found in 89% of females, and Xg(a−), which occurs in 66% of males. Anti-Xg^a is a weakly reacting antibody detectable best with antiglobulin serum. These antibodies occur frequently in patients who have had multiple transfusions,[72] and one auto–anti-Xg^a has been reported.[73]

LOW-INCIDENCE ANTIGENS

Some blood groups are so rarely encountered that they appear confined to one person or family; they are often referred to as **private antigens.** To qualify for such a designation, the antigens must have an incidence of less than 1/400 population sampled, must not be a part of an established blood group locus, and must be defined by a specific antibody.[74] These antigens are of little clinical importance; persons with antibodies to low-incidence antigens are not difficult to transfuse because random donors usually lack the corresponding antigen. However, a confusing serologic picture may develop in babies suffering from hemolytic disease of the newborn because of a low-incidence antibody (see discussion of hemolytic disease of the newborn).

HIGH-INCIDENCE ANTIGENS

Some antigens are so common in a population that they have been called **public antigens,** since antigen-negative individuals are very rare. The latter individuals, should they become sensitized to a public antigen that they lack, present the blood bank with an almost insurmountable problem, requiring help from reference laboratories with large stocks of rare negative frozen bloods. Brothers and sisters should be typed, since in most cases about one fourth of the siblings will also lack the antigen.

HLA ANTIGENS AND ANTIBODIES[75,76]
General principles

The blood groups described above are mostly confined to red cells. Exception is found in the ABO blood group antigens that are also present on leukocytes, platelets, and tissue cells. The antigens that are most strongly expressed on nucleated cells are those of the HLA system, also called the **major histocompatibility locus antigens.** Because the HLA antigens occur on all nucleated cells of the body and are therefore important in organ transplant survival, they have also been called the **transplantation antigens.** Whenever the HLA antigens of a recipient differ from those of the donor, antibodies to the donor antigens are produced; as a result, HLA antigens are important in many different clinical conditions:

1. In patients who have had multiple transfusions, HLA antigens may be responsible for antileukocytic antibody formation and subsequent febrile, nonhemolytic transfusion reactions.
2. In multiparous women antiplatelet antibodies resulting from fetal-maternal incompatibility may produce neonatal thrombocytopenia.
3. In thrombocytopenic patients receiving large quantities of transfused platelets, there may develop a therapeutic nonresponsiveness because of antiplatelet antibodies.[77]
4. In the organ transplant recipient antitissue antibodies may provoke organ rejection.[78]

In all the above instances, a cellular rejection occurs based on the HLA antigen incompatibility. In addition to these instances, in sophisticated paternity testing the HLA system is a valuable adjunct because of its marked polymorphism.[79]

Antigens

The genes regulating the HLA antigens are located on chromosome 6[80] at the HLA region. This region is composed of four closely linked genetic loci; three of the loci are serologically defined and are called *HLA-A, HLA-B,* and *HLA-C.* At each of these three loci are multiple, codominant, allelic genes. The fourth locus, *HLA-D,* is not serologically defined but is lymphocyte defined; it is commonly called the *LD* locus. Since the antigens at this locus are detected by means of the mixed lymphocyte culture, it has also been called the MLC locus. Fig 14-8 and Table 14-20 show the current status of the HLA system.

Antigen nomenclature is that recommended from the 1975 International Workshop of the World Health Organization.[81] The antigens well established by most participants are given a letter designation for the locus and a number designation that is unique for each antigen. Antigens of provisional status only are written with a "w" preceding the locus number; this letter "w" will be dropped when the antigen becomes officially recognized by the WHO.

Each parent contributes his haplotype of HLA genes as a unit to his offspring. Hence, each individual possesses two genes at each of the four loci, one maternal and one paternal gene. Together these eight genes constitute the individual's complete HLA phenotype. However, the *C* and *D* loci are not included in routine antigen testing; hence, the typical HLA phenotype includes only antigens of the *A* and *B* loci. For example, a phenotype may be written as follows: HLA-A 1,2 B 7,12; the same individual's genotype may be determined and would be written *HLA-A1, B12/A2, B7.* Phenotype determinations can be made by either leukoagglutination or lymphocytotoxicity tests.

Antibodies

HLA antibodies are always the result of alloimmunization. They are IgG immunoglobulins that are either agglutinating or cytotoxic in character. Most of the antibodies are able to fix complement; those antibodies unable to bind complement will not be detected by cy-

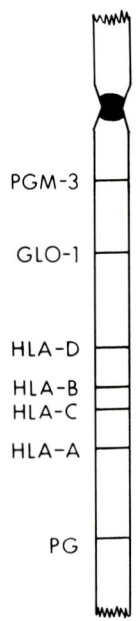

Fig. 14-8. Short arm of chromosome 6. *PGM-3*, Phosphoglu-comutase-3; *GLO-1*, glyoxylase 1; *HLA-A, -B, -C, and -D*, HLA subloci of major histocampatibility complex; *PG*, pepsinogen.

Table 14-20. Presently identified HLA antigens of the HLA system

Alleles at A locus	Alleles at B locus	Alleles at C locus	Alleles at D locus
HLA-A 1	HLA-B 5	HLA-Cw 1	HLA-Dw 1
A 2	B 7	Cw 2	Dw 2
A 3	B 8	Cw 3	Dw 3
A 9	B 12	Cw 4	Dw 4
A 10	B 13	Cw 5	Dw 5
A 11	B 14		Dw 6
A 28	B 18		
A 29	B 27		
HLA-Aw 19	HLA-Bw 15		
Aw 23	Bw 16		
Aw 24	Bw 17		
Aw 25	Bw 21		
Aw 26	Bw 22		
Aw 30	Bw 35		
Aw 31	Bw 37		
Aw 32	Bw 38		
Aw 33	Bw 39		
Aw 34	Bw 40		
Aw 36	Bw 41		
Aw 43	Bw 42		

totoxicity technics. HLA antibodies can be found in the serum of multiparous women and patients who have received multiple transfusions, the latter incidence increasing with the number of units of blood received.

Tests used in defining the HLA locus
Tests to determine the serologically defined antigens

Antisera are used to type the *HLA-A, -B,* and *-C* loci; since antibodies to the *HLA-C* locus are scarce, only the antigens at the *HLA-A* and *-B* loci are usually determined. Antisera can be obtained from a variety of sources including recipients of multiple transfusions, multiparous women, and intentionally immunized volunteers. The most widely used antisera are from multiparous women because these antibodies can be obtained in large amounts from healthy donors and are directed against only a limited number of antigens. Antibodies produced in volunteers may be more monospecific, however.

Leukoagglutination

Leukoagglutination[82] is not used often today but was one of the earlier methods for determination of serologically defined antigens. However, it is still used to detect antibodies to non-HLA leukocyte antigens. A leukocyte suspension is prepared from EDTA-treated blood after adding an erythrocyte-sedimenting agent, e.g., dextran. Known monospecific HLA antisera are incubated with the leukocytes at room temperature for 1 hr; agglutination is observed microscopically. Agglutination indicates the presence of the corresponding antigen on the surface of the white cells. The procedure is not performed today because it has poor reproducibility and is difficult to perform. Furthermore, non-HLA antigen-antibody reactions may interfere with proper interpretation.

Microlymphocytotoxicity

In microlymphocytotoxicity,[83-85] in contrast with leukoagglutination, lymphocytes alone are harvested and tested. The test lymphocytes are incubated with heated antiserum at room temperature for 30 min; complement is added to the cell-serum mixture, and a second incubation at room temperature for 60 min is allowed. If the lymphocytes carry the corresponding antigen, their cell membranes become damaged. The damaged lymphocytes differentially absorb stains (e.g., trypan blue or eosin) and can be easily detected with a phase-contrast microscope. A positive reaction is greater than 30% nonviable cells: 20-29% = ±; 30-49% = weak positive; 50-79% = positive; 80-100% = strongly positive.[85]

Test to determine the lymphocyte-defined antigens
Mixed lymphocyte culture

In a mixed lymphocyte culture[86] no antiserum is used and hence no acutal antigen typing occurs. Instead, this test involves the reactions of lymphocytes from two individuals, one a donor and the other a recipient. Nonidentity at the L_D (HLA-D) locus is indicated by stimulation of the lymphocytes. Usually donor lymphocytes are pretreated with mitomycin C to prevent DNA synthesis; these are the **stimulator cells.** The recipient lymphocytes are untreated and are able to respond by blastogenesis (hence, called **responder cells**) if donor lymphocytes are antigenically different. Mitomycin-treated donor lymphocytes are cultured with recipient lymphocytes in the presence of tritiated thymidine; stimulation of recipient lymphocytes is accompanied by the uptake of radioactivity, which can be subsequently counted.

The procedure requires 3-5 days of lymphocyte culture. Nonidentity at the HLA-SD loci results in no lymphocyte stimulation; only differences at the HLA-LD locus result in mixed lymphocyte culture activation.

Clinical significance
Organ transplantation

It is known that transplanted organs survive longer if the recipient and donor are HLA identical. The best graft prognosis is found with HLA-identical sibling donor-recipient combinations; because of close linkage, such combinations will usually be identical at all four loci of the HLA region. It has been shown that for unrelated donor-recipient pairs, identity at the LD locus is very important for graft survival.[87]

Bone marrow transplantation

Bone marrow transplantation is a specialized type of organ transplantation in which 4-8 dl of aspirated bone marrow are injected intravenously into the recipient. Currently only HLA-identical family members are used as donors. Donor and recipient must be identical for both SD and LD determinants as measured by serologic and mixed lymphocyte culture technics. Successful marrow transplantation has been reported in 33 of 34 patients with aplastic anemia and 63 of 68 patients with acute leukemia.[88]

As a complication unique to the transplantation of immunologically competent cells, graft-versus-host disease can be seen even with SD and LD identical donors. In this condition the infused marrow cells of the donor react against the host. To aid in preventing this phenomenon, a reversed mixed lymphocyte culture test is useful: The donor lymphocytes are the responder cells, and the recipient lymphocytes are the stimulator cells.[89] In addition, it is helpful to pretreat the recipient with various immunosuppressive agents.

Blood component therapy

Thrombocytopenic patients often are treated with pooled platelet concentrates, which allow exposure to hundreds of different donors during periods of hemorrhagic complications. As a result alloimmunization to histocompatibility antigens is a common occurrence. As a consequence the recipient demonstrates a poor therapeutic response to subsequent transfused platelets. The use of HLA-matched platelets results in satisfactory postransfusion platelet increments and in a significant reduction of hemorrhagic phenomena.[90] Further improvement in response has been obtained with leukocyte-poor HLA-matched platelet concentrates.[91]

It is well known that recipients who are sensitized to leukocyte antigens will suffer nonhemolytic, febrile transfusion reactions. This problem can be adequately controlled with the use of leukocyte-poor blood or frozen red cells (see later discussion of blood components). However, alloimmunization to leukocyte antigens can be a significant problem in leukopenic patients requiring granulocyte transfusions. Compatibility at the HLA locus is probably of benefit although clearly defined increments in posttransfusion granulocyte counts are not a reliable indicator of therapeutic effect.

Disease associations

A large number of diseases have been shown to be associated with HLA genes[92]; in the future these associations may help explain pathogenetic processes. A partial list of these diseases is given in Table 14-21.

Paternity testing and the HLA system

Because of the heterogenicity of the HLA system, it is a valuable adjunct to the usual procedures employed

Table 14-21. Disease and HLA association

Disease	HLA-SD antigen	Frequency (%) in patients	Frequency (%) in controls	Average relative risk
Ankylosing spondylitis	B 27	90	7	141.0
Reiter's disease	B 27	76	6	46.6
Acute anterior uveitis	B 27	55	8	16.7
Psoriatic arthritis	B 27			5.0
Psoriasis	Bw 17	29	8	5.0
Graves' disease	B 8	47	21	3.0
Celiac disease	B 8	78	24	10
Addison's disease	B 8			7.0
	D 3			10.5[93]
Dermatitis herpetiformis	B 8	62	27	4.5
Myasthenia gravis	B 8	52	24	4.6
Diabetes mellitus (insulin dependent)	B 8	45		
Multiple sclerosis	A 3	36	25	1.7
	B 7	36	25	1.5
	D 2	60	18	6.7[93]
Chronic active hepatitis	B 8	68	18	9.5

Table 14-22. Exclusion of paternity by ABO groups*

Phenotype of putative mother	Phenotype of putative father			
	O	A	B	AB
O	A, B, AB	B, AB	A, AB	O, AB
A	B, AB	B, AB	None	O
B	A, AB	None	A, AB	O
AB	O, AB	O	O	O

From Wiener, A.S., and Wexler, I.B.: Heredity of the blood groups, New York, 1958, Grune & Stratton, Inc.
*Find the phenotypes of the putative father and mother at the top and side columns of the table and locate the box at which these intersect. In the box are given the groups not possible in children of the mating.

Table 14-23. Exclusion of paternity by M and N types*

Phenotype of putative mother	Phenotype of putative father		
	M	N	MN
M	MN, N	M, N	N
N	M, N	M, MN	M
MN	N	M	None

From Wiener, A.S., and Wexler, I.B.: Heredity of the blood groups, New York, 1958, Grune & Stratton, Inc.
*Find the phenotypes of the putative father and mother at the top and side columns of the table and locate the box at which these intersect. In the box are given the types not possible in children of the mating.

Table 14-24. Exclusion of paternity by Rh-Hr blood types*

Phenotype of putative mother	Phenotype of putative father			
	1 rh Rh_0	2 rh'rh Rh_1rh	3 rh'rh' Rh_1Rh_1	4 rh''rh Rh_2rh
1 rh Rh_0	2, **3, 4, 5,** 6a, 6b, **7, 8**, 9	**3, 4, 5,** 6a, 6b, **7, 8**, 9	**1, 3, 4, 5,** 6a, 6b, **7, 8**, 9	2, **3, 5,** 6a, 6b, **7, 8**, 9
2 rh'rh Rh_1rh	3, **4, 5,** 6a, 6b, 7, **8**, 9	4, **5,** 6a, 6b, 7, **8**, 9	1, 4, **5,** 6a, 6b, 7, **8**, 9	3, **5,** 6b, 7, **8**, 9
3 rh'rh' Rh_1Rh_1	**1, 3, 4, 5,** 6a, **6b, 7, 8**, 9	**1, 4, 5,** 6a, **6b, 7, 8**, 9	**1, 2, 4, 5,** 6a, **6b, 7, 8**, 9	**1, 3, 4, 5, 6b,** 7, **8**, 9
4 rh''rh Rh_2rh	2, **3, 5,** 6a, 6b, **7, 8**, 9	**3,** 5, 6b, **7, 8**, 9	**1, 3, 4, 5, 6b,** **7, 8**, 9	2, **3,** 6a, 6b, **7, 8**, 9
5 rh''rh'' Rh_2Rh_2	**1, 2, 3,** 5, 6a, **6b, 7, 8**, 9	**1, 2, 3,** 5, **6b,** **7, 8**, 9	**1, 2, 3, 4, 5,** **6b, 7, 8**, 9	**1, 2, 3,** 6a, **6b, 7, 8**, 9
6a rh'rh'' Rh_1Rh_2	**1, 3,** 5, 6a, **6b, 7, 8**, 9	**1,** 5, **6b, 7, 8**, 9	**1, 2, 4, 5,** **6b, 7, 8**, 9	**1, 3, 6b, 7, 8**, 9
6b rh_yrh Rh_zrh	2, **3, 4, 5,** 6a, 7, 8, 9	**3, 4, 5,** 6a, 8, 9	**1, 3, 4, 5,** 6a, 6b, 8, 9	2, **3, 5,** 6a, 7, 9
7 rh_yrh' $Rh_z Rh_1$	**1, 3, 4, 5,** 6a, 7, 8, 9	**1, 4, 5,** 6a, 8, 9	**1, 2, 4, 5,** 6a, 6b, 8, 9	**1,** 3, **4, 5,** 7, 9
8 rh_yrh'' $Rh_z Rh_2$	**1, 2, 3,** 5, 6a, 7, 8, 9	**1, 2, 3,** 5, 8, 9	**1, 2, 3, 4, 5,** 6b, 8, 9	**1, 2, 3,** 6a, 7, 9
9 $rh_y rh_y$ $Rh_z Rh_z$	**1, 2, 3, 4, 5,** **6a,** 7, 8, 9	**1, 2, 3, 4, 5,** **6a,** 8, 9	**1, 2, 3, 4, 5,** **6a,** 6b, 8, 9	**1, 2, 3, 4, 5,** **6a,** 7, 9

From Wiener, A.S., and Nieberg, K.C.: J. Forensic Med. **10:**6, 1963.
*Boldface figures represent phenotypes of children for whom **maternity** is excluded. This table is to be applied only to matings in which at least responding to the code numbers are given in the marginal headings, e.g., 1 is the code number for phenotypes rh and Rh_0.

in paternity testing (see later discussion of paternity testing). In fact, using HLA determinations exclusively, there is a 70% chance of excluding paternity.

NON-HLA, LEUKOCYTE-SPECIFIC ANTIGENS

Only a few non-HLA antigens are known that are restricted to leukocytes. The most important is the NAI antigen system; when anti-NAI is present in maternal serum, it is responsible for producing isoimmune neonatal neutropenia.[94]

NON-HLA, PLATELET-SPECIFIC ANTIGENS

Three sets of allelic genes are responsible for platelet-specific antigens: PL^{A1} and PL^{A2}, PL^{E1} and PL^{E2}, and Ko^a and Ko^b. The vast majority of the population (> 95%) possesses the antigens PL^{A1}, PL^{E1}, and Ko^b. Anti-PL^{A1} produces the posttransfusion purpura syndrome.

SERUM ANTIGENS AND ANTIBODIES

Serum factors may act as isoantigens if transfused into an individual who lacks them, leading to the pro-

duction of immune antibodies against the infused plasma factor. This immunization by transfusion usually occurs in patients who have had multiple transfusions (patients with leukemia, thalassemia, etc.) but is of no apparent clinical consequence except perhaps for a febrile transfusion reaction. Pregnancy, because of immunization by the fetus, may also lead to the formation of antibodies against plasma antigens. Some of the inherited serum factors are β-lipoproteins **Ag** and **Lp**; immunoglobulins, including IgG determinant **Gm** and κ-light-chain determinant **Km** (previously **Inv**); α-glycoproteins **Gc**, transferrin **Tf**, and haptoglobin **Hp**; ceruloplasmin **Cp.** Many of these systems serve as genetic markers and are used as tools in the investigation of disputed parentage and in anthropologic studies.

PATERNITY TESTING

Paternity testing is an attempt to prove nonpaternity in an alleged father. It requires blood samples from the baby, the mother, and the alleged father. Generally, there are four possible conclusions that would exclude paternity[95]:

Phenotype of putative father					
5 rh″rh″ Rh_2Rh_2	6a rh′rh″ Rh_1Rh_2	6b rh_yrh Rh_zrh	7 rh_yrh′ $Rh_z Rh_1$	8 rh_yrh″ $Rh_z Rh_2$	9 $rh_y rh_y$ $Rh_z Rh_z$
1, 2, 3, 5, 6a, 6b, **7, 8, 9**	**1, 3, 5, 6a,** 6b, **7, 8, 9**	2, 3, 4, **5, 6a,** **7, 8, 9**	**1, 3, 4, 5,** **6a, 7, 8, 9**	1, 2, **3, 5, 6a,** **7, 8, 9**	1, 2, **3, 4, 5,** **6a, 7, 8, 9**
1, 2, 3, **5**, 6b, 7, **8, 9**	1, **5**, 6b, 7, **8, 9**	3, 4, **5**, 6a, **8,** **9**	1, 4, **5**, 6a, **8, 9**	1, 2, 3, **5, 8,** **9**	1, 2, 3, 4, 5, 6a, **8, 9**
1, 2, 3, 4, 5, **6b, 7, 8, 9**	1, 2, **4, 5,** **6b, 7, 8,** **9**	1, 3, **4, 5**, 6a, **6b, 8, 9**	1, 2, **4, 5,** 6a, **6b, 8,** **9**	1, 2, 3, **4, 5,** **6b, 8, 9**	1, 2, 3, **4, 5,** 6a, **6b, 8, 9**
1, 2, 3, 6a, 6b, **7, 8, 9**	**1, 3**, 6b, 7, 8, **9**	2, 3, 5, 6a, 7, **9**	1, **3, 4, 5, 7,** **9**	1, 2, **3**, 6a, 7, **9**	1, 2, **3, 4, 5,** 6a, **7, 9**
1, 2, 3, 4, 6a, **6b, 7, 8, 9**	**1, 2, 3, 4,** **6b, 7, 8,** **9**	1, 2, 3, **5**, 6a, **6b, 7, 9**	1, 2, 3, **4, 5,** **6b, 7, 9**	1, 2, 3, 4, 6a, **6b, 7, 9**	1, 2, 3, **4, 5,** 6a, **6b, 7, 9**
1, 2, 3, 4, 6b, **7, 8, 9**	1, 2, 4, **6b,** **7, 8, 9**	**1, 3, 5, 6a,** **6b, 9**	1, 2, 4, 5, **6b, 9**	**1, 2, 3, 4,** **6b, 9**	1, 2, 3, 4, 5, 6a, **6b, 9**
1, 2, 3, 5, 6a, 6b, **7, 9**	**1, 3, 5, 6a,** 6b, **9**	2, 3, 4, **5, 6a,** **7, 8**	1, **3, 4, 5,** **6a, 8**	1, 2, **3, 5, 6a,** **7**	1, 2, 3, **4, 5,** **6a, 7, 8**
1, 2, 3, 4, 5, 6b, **7, 9**	1, 2, **4, 5,** 6b, **9**	1, 3, **4, 5**, 6a, **8**	1, 2, 4, 5, 6a, **6b, 8**	1, 2, 3, **4, 5,** **6b**	1, 2, 3, **4, 5,** 6a, **6b, 8**
1, 2, 3, 4, 6a, **6b, 7, 9**	**1, 2, 3, 4,** **6b, 9**	1, 2, 3, **5**, 6a, **7**	1, 2, 3, **4, 5,** **6b**	1, 2, 3, 4, 6a, **6b, 7**	1, 2, 3, **4, 5,** 6a, **6b, 7**
1, 2, 3, 4, 5, **6a**, 6b, **7, 9**	**1, 2, 3, 4, 5,** **6a**, 6b, **9**	**1, 2, 3, 4, 5,** **6a, 7, 8**	**1, 2, 3, 4, 5,** **6a**, 6b, **8**	**1, 2, 3, 4, 5,** **6a**, 6b, **7**	**1, 2, 3, 4, 5,** **6a, 6b, 7, 8**

one of the parents is **Rh₀** positive. Where both parents are **Rh₀** negative, necessarily all **Rh₀**-positive children are excluded. The phenotypes cor-

1. The child possesses a character missing in the phenotype of both the mother and alleged father. This type of exclusion is a first-order, or solid, exclusion.

Example:
Mother   O
Father   A
Child   B

2. The child fails to inherit a character that the alleged father must contribute. This type of exclusion is more tenuous than the first-order exclusion because of the complications introduced by deletions and the modifying, suppressing, or amorph genes.

Example:
Mother   O
Father   AB
Child   O

3. The child possesses a character showing improper linkage with associated genes. Usually other siblings must also be examined to establish the linked antigens.

Example:
Mother MSs   MS/MS
Father MNSs   Ms/NS
Children   MS/NS   MS/NS   Ms/Ms   Ms/Ns

It is clear that the last child has a gene combination, Ns, not present in the alleged father, NS.

4. There is statistical improbability of the mating. The child does not possess an impossible character, nor is missing a required character; however, for the alleged father to have contributed his gene, he would need to be of a very rare genotype.

Example:
Mother   ccddee
Father   CcDEe
Child   ccddee

The most likely genotype of the father is R^1R^2 *(CDe/cDE)*; however, since the child is *rr*, the father would have to be *R²r*, a very rare genotype. To further test the improbability, the alleged father can be tested with anti-f or his family can be studied for rhesus genotype.

In all these instances it is assumed that the mother is actually the biologic mother of the child.

Present-day testing generally includes ABO, Rh, and MNSs blood groups; this allows an exclusion rate of 55%. Examples of exclusions in these blood group systems are found in Tables 14-22 to 14-24.

It is profitable to extend this testing to include the Kell, Duff, Lutheran, and Kidd blood groups; in addition, qualified experts may test erythrocyte enzyme and serum protein polymorphism. Also, HLA testing is very valuable. Together these tests would allow a 98.3% exclusion rate, or a 93.6% exclusion if HLA typing is not used.[96] If paternity has not been excluded by this battery of tests, there is a strong presumption of paternity. It is important to realize that paternity can **never** be absolutely proven, only presumed. In courts of law, therefore, only evidence demonstrating nonpaternity is admissible.

REFERENCES

1. Landsteiner, K.: Wien. Klin. Wochenschr. **14:**1132, 1901.
1a. Miller, W.V., editor: Technical manual of the American Association of Blood Banks, ed. 7, Washington, D.C., 1977, American Association of Blood Banks.
2. Mollison, P.L.: Blood transfusion in clinical medicine, ed. 6, Oxford, England, 1979, Blackwell Scientific Publications, Inc.
3. Prokop, O., and Uhlenbruck, G.: Human blood and serum groups, New York, 1969, John Wiley & Sons, Inc.
4. Erskine, A.G.: The principles and practice of blood grouping, ed. 2, St. Louis, 1978, The C.V. Mosby Co.
5. Barrett, J.T.: Textbook of immunology: an introduction to immunochemistry and immunobiology, ed. 3, St. Louis, 1978, The C.V. Mosby Co.
6. Watkins, W.M., and Morgan, W.T.J.: Vox Sang. **4:**97, 1959.
7. Watkins, W.M.: Science **152:**172, 1966.
8. Marcus, D.M.: N. Engl. J. Med. **280:**994, 1969.
9. Economidou, J., Hughes-Jones, N.C., and Gardner, B.: Vox Sang. **12:**321, 1967.
10. Schacter, H., et al.: Proc. Natl. Acad. Sci. U.S.A. **70:**220, 1973.
11. Issitt, P.D.: In American Association of Blood Banks: A seminar on problems encountered in pretransfusion tests, Washington, D.C., 1972, The Association.
12. Bird, G.W.G., and Wingham, J.: Vox Sang. **26:**163, 1974.
13. Sanger, R., and Race, R.R.: Nouv. Rev. Fr. Hematol. Blood Cells **11:**878, 1971.
14. Cazal, P., et al.: Rev. Fr. Transfus. Immunohematol. **11:**209, 1968.
15. Bird, G.W.G., and Wingham, J.: Vox Sang. **20:**55, 1971.
16. Gerbal, A., Maslet, C., and Salmon, C.: Vox Sang. **28:**398, 1975.
17. Marsh, W.C.: Vox Sang. **5:**387, 1960.
18. Issitt, C.: In American Association of Blood Banks, A seminar on problems encountered in pretransfusion tests, Washington, D.C., 1972, The Association.
19. Landsteiner, K., and Wiener, A.S.: Proc. Soc. Exp. Biol. Med. **43:**223, 1940.
20. Fisher, R.A., and Race, R.R.: Nature **157:**48, 1946.
21. Wiener, A.S.: Proc. Soc. Exp. Bio. Med. **54:**316, 1943.
22. Rosenfield, R.E., et al.: Transfusion **2:**287, 1962.
23. Hughes-Jones, N.C., Gardner, B., and Lincoln, P.J.: Vox Sang. **21:**210, 1971.
24. Ishimori, T., and Hasekura, H.: Transfusion **7:**84, 1967.
25. Levine, P., et al.: Transfusion **5:**492, 1965.
26. Levine, P., et al.: Vox Sang. **24:**417, 1973.
27. Levine, P., et al.: J. Immunol. **87:**747, 1961.
28. White, J.C., et al.: Vox Sang. **15:**368, 1975.
29. Swanson, J.L., et al.: Transfusion **14:**470, 1974.
30. Levine, P., et al.: Nature **194:**304, 1962.
31. Issitt, P.D., and Issitt, C.: Applied blood group serology, ed. 2, Oxnard, Calif., 1975, Spectra Biologicals.
32. Landsteiner, K., and Levine, P.: Proc. Soc. Exp. Biol. Med. **24:**600, 1927.
33. Cleghorn, T.E.: Nature **187:**701, 1960.
34. Springer, G.F., and Ansell, N.J.: Proc. Natl. Acad. Sci. U.S.A. **44:**182, 1958.
35. Lisowska, E., and Duk, M.: Vox Sang. **28:**392, 1975.
36. Walker, M.E., Rubinstein, P., and Allen, F.H., Jr.: Vox Sang. **32:**111, 1977.
37. Springer, G.F., and Huprikar, S.V.: Haematologia (Budap.) **6:**81, 1972.
38. Ottensooser, F., and Silberschmidt, K.: Nature **172:**914, 1953.

39. Race, R.R., and Sanger, R.: Blood groups in man, ed. 6, Oxford, England 1975, Blackwell Scientific Publications, Inc., p. 162.
40. Fellous, M., et al.: Vox Sang. **26:**518, 1975.
41. Heiken, A.: Hereditas **56:**83, 1966.
42. Fisher, R.: Heredity (Lond.) **7:**81, 1953.
43. Naiki, M., and Marcus, D.M.: Biochem. Biophys. Res. Commun. **60:**1105, 1974.
44. Corg, H.T., et al.: Biochem. Biophys. Res. Commun. **61:**1289, 1974.
45. Chown, B., Lewis, M., and Kaita, K.: Nature **180:**711, 1957.
46. Allen, F.H., Jr., Krabbe, S.M.R., and Corcoran, P.A.: Vox Sang. **6:**555, 1961.
47. Taswell, H.F., et al.: Mayo Clin. Proc. **52:**157, 1977.
48. Marsh, W.L., Ragnhild, O., and Nichols, M.E.: Vox Sang. **31:**356, 1976.
49. Albrey, J.A., et al.: Vox Sang. **20:**29, 1971.
50. Behzad, O., et al.: Vox Sang. **24:**337, 1973.
51. Colledge, K.I., Pezzulich, M., and Marsh, W.L.: Vox Sang. **24:**193, 1973.
52. Marsh, W.L.: Mayo Clin. Proc. **52:**145, 1977.
53. Miller, L.H., et al.: N. Engl. J. Med. **295:**302, 1976.
54. Allen, F.H., Jr., Diamond, L.K., and Niedziela, B.A.: Nature **167:**482, 1951.
55. Pineda, A.A., Taswell, H.F., and Brzica, S.M., Jr.: Transfusion **18:**1, 1978.
56. Chown, B., Marion, L., and Hiroko, K.: Vox Sang. **11:**108, 1966.
57. Barnborough, J., et al.: Nature **198:**796, 1963.
58. Crawford, M.N., et al.: Transfusion **1:**228, 1961.
59. Taliano, V., Guevin, R.-M., and Tippett, P.: Vox Sang. **24:**42, 1973.
60. Molthan, L., et al.: Vox Sang. **24:**468, 1973.
61. Callender, S., and Race, R.R.: Ann. Eugen. **13:**102, 1946.
62. Cepellini, R.: Proceedings of the Fifth International Congress on Blood Transfusions, Basel, 1955, S. Karger A.G., p. 207.
63. Iseki, S., Masaki, S., and Shiba, K.: Proc. Imp. Acad. Jpn. **33:**492, 1957.
64. Potapov, M.I.: Probl. Haemathol. **11:**45, 1970.
65. Gandini, E., et al.: Vox Sang. **15:**142, 1968.
66. Savvas, R.S.: Vox Sang. **29:**280, 1975.
67. Polley, M.J., and Mollison, P.L.: Transfusion **1:**9, 1961.
68. Hossaini, A.A.: Am. J. Cin. Pathol. **57:**489, 1972.
69. Marsh, W.L.: Br. J. Haematol. **7:**200, 1961.
70. Hillman, R.S., and Giblett, E.R.: J. Clin. Invest. **44:**1730, 1965.
71. Feizi, T., et al.: J. Exp. Med. **133:**39, 1971.
71a. Hakomori, S.: Semin. Hematol. **18:**39, 1981.
72. Mann. J.D., et al.: Lancet **1:**8, 1962.
73. Vokoyama, M., Edith, D.T., and Bowman, M.: Vox Sang. **12:**138, 1967.
74. Race, R.R., and Sanger, R.: Blood groups in man, ed. 6, Oxford, England, 1975, Blackwell Scientific Publications, Inc., p. 431.
75. Perkins, H.A.: Am. J. Hematol. **6:**285, 1979.
76. Bodmer, W.F.: Br. Med. Bull. **34**(3):213, 1978.
77. Howard, J.E., and Perkins, H.A.: Transfusion **18:**496, 1978.
78. Salvatierra, O., et al.: Transplant. Proc. **9:**495, 1977.
79. Terasaki, P.: J. Fam. Law **16:**543, 1978.
80. Lamm, L.V., et al.: Hum. Hered. **24:**273, 1974.
81. Nomenclature for factors of the HLA system, WHO Bull. **52:**261, 1975.
82. Zmijewski, C.M.: Manual of tissue typing techniques, Department of Health and Human Services publication no. (NIH) 76-545, 1974.
83. Terasaki, P.I., and McClelland, J.D.: Nature **204:**998, 1964.
84. Transplantation and Immunology Branch, NIAID: Manual of tissue typing techniques, Department of Health and Human Services publication no. (NIH) 76-545, 1974.
85. Mittal, K.K.: Vox Sang. **34:**58, 1978.
86. Bach, F.H., and Bach, M.L.: Manual of tissue typing techniques, Department of Health and Human Services publication no. (NIH) 76-545, 1974.
87. Cochrum, K., et al.: Transplant. Proc. **5:**391, 1973.
88. Thomas, E.D., et al.: N. Engl. J. Med. **292:**895, 1975.
89. Miller, W.V.: Prog. Hematol. **10:**173, 1977.
90. Yankee, R.A., Grumet, F.C., and Regentine, G.N.: N. Engl. J. Med. **281:**1208, 1969.
91. Herzig, R.H., et al.: Blood **46:**743, 1975.
92. Bach, F.H., and van Rood, J.J.: N. Engl. J. Med. **295:**927, 1976.
93. Schaller, J.G., and Omenn, G.S.: J. Pediatr. **88:**913, 1976.
94. Boxer, L.A., Yokoyama, M., and Lalezari, P.: J. Pediatr. **80:**783, 1972.
95. Polesky, H.F.: Paternity testing, Chicago, 1975, American Society of Clinical Pathologists.
96. Speiser, P.: Donderdruck aus Osterreichische Richterzeitung, no. 9, 1970.

General methods in blood banking

The entire operation of a blood bank must be under the supervision of a qualified physician; the staff must be adequate in number and competent in the performance of procedures required by the *Standards for Blood Banks and Transfusion Services.*[1] An annually updated, detailed procedure manual is required. For personnel and patient safety, all needles and syringes must be disposable and must be destroyed after a single use.

DONOR SELECTION
Criteria for donor selection

Donors must meet the following criteria to be selected[1]:
A. Age: 17-65 years
   1. Minors considered with written parental consent
   2. After 66 years of age, donors accepted if approved by the blood bank physician

B. Hemoglobin
   1. Male donors: no less than 13.5 g/dl
   2. Female donors: no less than 12.5 g/dl
C. Hematocrit
   1. Male donors: no less than 41%
   2. Female donors: no less than 38%
D. Pulse: between 50-100/min with no irregularities
E. Blood pressure
   1. Systolic: between 90-180 mm Hg
   2. Diastolic: between 50-100 mm Hg
F. Temperature: oral temperature not exceeding 37.5° C
G. Interval between donations: minimum of 8 weeks
H. Weight: Donor weighing 49.5 kg (110 lb) or more may donate a full 450 ± 45 ml unit; donors weighing less than 49.5 kg (110 lb) are bled less and a reduced volume of anticoagulant is used.
I. Absence of any chronic disease: cancer; heart, lung, kidney, or liver disease; bleeding diathesis; convulsions
J. Pregnancy: not within the preceding 6 months
K. Drugs: needs evaluation by blood bank physician

Criteria for donor rejection

Donors are rejected under the following circumstances:
A. Dental surgery: within 72 hr
B. Blood or blood component therapy: within preceeding 6 months (possible source of hepatitis)
C. Immunizations—all acceptable except:
   1. Smallpox vaccination: if scab remains or within 2 weeks
   2. Rubeola, mumps, yellow fever, oral polio, rabies: within 2 weeks
   3. Rubella: within 2 months
D. Infectious diseases
   1. Malaria: applies only to red cell products
      a. Travel to endemic areas: within 6 months if person is asymptomatic and has taken no antimalarial drugs
      b. Symptomatic disease: 3 years after cessation of symptoms or cessation of therapy
      c. Antimalarial prophylaxis: within 3 years
   2. Viral hepatitis
      a. Symptomatic disease: permanent rejection
      b. Known positive hepatitis B surface antigen: permanent rejection
      c. Hepatitis immune globulin recipients: within 9 months of the last therapeutic injection
      d. Recent tattoo: within 6 months
   3. Tuberculosis, clinically active

BLOOD COLLECTION
Anticoagulants

1. ACD solution A (citric acid, 7.3 g; sodium citrate, 22 g; glucose, 24.5 g), 67.5 ml/450 ml blood
2. CPD solution (citric acid, 3.2 g; sodium citrate, 25.8 g; glucose, 25 g; sodium phosphate, 2.18 g), 63 ml/450 ml blood
3. Heparin, 27 ml/450 ml blood
4. CPD-adenine solution (CPD solution except 22.5 g glucose and 0.25 mmole adenine). This soluction was approved for use by the Food and Drug Administration in 1978.[2]

Blood storage
General principles

Blood must be stored in a special blood bank refrigerator that operates between 1-6° C, is well lighted, and is attached to an automatic temperature-recording device equipped with an alarm system. The suggested temperature is 4° C. There is a 21-day limit on storage of ACD and CPD blood bank blood that is meant to assure the survival of at least 70% of the transfused cells 24 hr after transfusion. With the use of CPD-Adenine blood, the shelf life is extended to 35 days. Heparinized blood is also stored at 1-6° C, but its shelf life is only 48 hr because heparin does not support red cell metabolism. Heparin is a useful anticoagulant in blood used for open-heart surgery, because calcium levels will be unaffected. However, to conserve blood it is best to prepare ACD blood for open-heart surgery and to add heparin (27 ml/450 ml) to blood immediately before use, in combination with calcium to replace the ACD-bound calcium (up to 0.6 calcium chloride per unit of blood).

"Storage lesion" of blood bank blood

Red cells stored under artificial conditions, in the liquid state, undergo a progressive loss of intracellular organic phosphates, resulting in decreased function and viability. These changes are referred to as the **storage lesion.**

When compatible stored red cells are infused into a recipient, a small number are expected to be sequestered by the reticuloendothelial system within 24 hr of transfusion; these cells are called *nonviable.* The remaining viable cells have a potential for normal survival with steady sequestration over a period of 110-120 days.[3] The cellular component most important for maintaining this erythrocyte viability is **adenosine triphosphate (ATP),** and stored red cells must be able to regenerate ATP if they are to be viable when transfused. Such regeneration occurs via glucose metabolism. All ACD and CPD anticoagulant solutions contain enough supplemental glucose to allow the red cells continual glycolysis with regeneration of their ATP levels during the 21-day shelf life. ATP is responsible for maintaining the biconcave shape of the red cells, allowing deformability; it is also required for the transport of potassium into and sodium out of the cell, against their concentration gradients. Red cell viability will be maintained if the ATP levels are at least 50% of baseline throughout storage.[4] Calculated ATP levels in ACD and CPD blood, after 21 days of storage, show preser-

vation of greater than 60% of the intitial values. The addition of adenine to the blood preservative mixture prolongs the survival of red cells by accentuating the production of ATP via enzymatic phosphorylation.[5] Calculated ATP levels in CPD-adenine stored blood reveals 60% of the original ATP still present after 42 days of storage.[6] Hence, blood preserved in ACD- or CPD-adenine can be stored for at least 35 days with an expectant 70% 24 hr posttranfusion survival of the red cells.[7]

The other organic compound, **2,3-diphosphoglycerate (2,3-DPG),** is an important regulator of the hemoglobin-oxygen dissociation curve. It is the low levels of 2,3-DPG that account for the increased oxygen affinity of stored blood. During storage, 2,3-DPG levels fall more rapidly than ATP levels, dropping precipitously in the first week of ACD storage. However, CPD solutions preserve 2,3-DPG content better: 100% 2,3-DPG is present after 1 week of storage and 80% after 2 weeks of storage; corresponding values for ACD storage are 60% and 10%, respectively.[8] This beneficial effect from CPD solutions is related to the higher pH values: the alkaline pH favors the mutase responsible for the formation of 2,3-DPG and inhibits the phosphatase responsible for its decomposition.[9] Unfortunately the addition of adenine to either ACD or CPD solutions enhances the decline of 2,3-DPG, so that normal levels of this compound are not maintained beyond the 10 days of storage.[10] On the other hand, the nucleoside inosine has a demonstrably beneficial effect on 2,3-DPG levels, and the addition of inosine to CPD-adenine solutions maintains normal 2,3-DPG levels for 5 weeks of blood storage.[10] 2,3-DPG–depleted red cells will have normal levels restored within hours of transfusion and therefore most recipients do not suffer side effects; however, for patients in shock, those with severe anemia, or those requiring massive transfusions, normal levels of 2,3-DPG are beneficial.

Red cells that are stored in the frozen state show normal ATP and 2,3-DPG levels provided they are processed soon after collection. Hence, such cells are better for oxygen transport than the conventional liquid stored cells.

During storage the most important clinical change in the plasma is the gradual rise in the potassium concentration, which may rise from an initial level of 4-7 mEq/L to 32 mEq/L or more after 21 days. The other plasma changes are of less importance. There is a slight lowering of the pH, associated with some accumulation of lactic acid. There is also about a 1% hemolysis of the red cells, some increase in ammonia, and loss of glucose and sodium, the latter into the red cells. The blood components that are least stable are the white cells, platelets, and coagulation factors II, V, and VIII.

BLOOD AND BLOOD COMPONENTS
Use and administration of blood

Blood and blood components are a form of replacement therapy. The type of blood preparations chosen should be of maximal benefit to the patient, entail the least risk, and treat a specific deficiency. There are dangers inherent in every blood transfusion that burden the physician with the responsibility of carefully weighing the clinical indications vs. the possible untoward reactions.

The patient who is receiving blood should be kept under observation at all times so that the transfusion can be discontinued immediately at the first signs indicative of a transfusion reaction (see later discussion of transfusion reactions). Most patients can tolerate the infusion of a unit of whole blood or packed red cells over a 2 hr period. If there is danger of fluid overload, a slower infusion rate is required. Blood infusion should always be completed by 4 hr to prevent bacterial proliferation. All cellular components and frozen plasma should be administered through a macrofilter to remove debris and fibrin clots; these standard filters have a pore size of 170 μm and easily allow the passage of microaggregates that form during liquid storage.[11] Microaggregate filters with a pore size of 20 μm will prevent their passage thereby prevent the development of the adult respiratory distress syndrome, a condition resulting from the entrapment of microemboli in the lungs.[12] The use of microfilters is still controversial[13] and is used primarily with massive transfusions.[14]

Whole blood preparations
Fresh whole blood[15]

Although blood less than 24 hr old may be used for replacement of deficient coagulation factors, e.g., platelets, factor I (fibrinogen), factor V, and factor VIII (antihemophilic factor), as needed in hemophilia A, thrombocytopenia, and diffuse intravascular coagulation, it is a poor replacement for these factors. Much more efficient specific blood components are available. Futhermore, as pretransfusion tests have become more complex, it is no longer practical to release blood within 24 hr unless the risk of hepatitis is overlooked. In addition, the risk of transmitting syphilis is much greater if such blood is used because the spirochete is unable to survive in citrated blood stored at 4° C for 72 hr.[16] In all the instances mentioned above, fresh whole blood can be adequately replaced by platelet concentrates and fresh frozen plasma. When whole blood is desired for the exchange transfusion of newborns, 4- or 5-day-old blood is still adequate. If it is available, fresh whole blood could be used to advantage in those patients requiring massive whole blood transfusions.

Stored whole blood

There are relatively few indications for the use of whole blood, since its use is restricted to the actual replacement of blood lost in the following situations:
1. Shock caused by blood loss
2. Replacement of surgical blood loss
3. Exchange transfusions
4. Extracorporeal circulation

Component preparations
Red cell preparations

There are four preparations that are primarily intended to supply red cells to the recipient: packed red cells, washed red cells, leukocyte-poor red cells, and frozen red cells.

Packed red cells: Packed red cells is the component remaining after removal of most of the plasma from centrifuged or sedimented whole blood. When red cells are required for their oxygen-carrying capabilities, packed red cells are the preparation of choice. After the plasma has been removed, the packed red cells can be stored at 1-6° C until the shelf life of the original unit has expired; this is true only if the hermetic seal has not been broken, for if the cells have been exposed to the environment, they must be used within 24 hr of preparation. The date and time of expiration must be placed on each bag so prepared. The hematocrit of packed red cells is approximately 70%; the oxygen-carrying capacity of the preparation is identical to the original unit of whole blood since no red cells have been lost. The advantage of this preparation, then, is to supply the same oxygen-carrying capacity in a smaller volume.

The use of packed red cells is indicated in the following circumstances:
1. All conditions in which only the red cell mass is deficient (From each unit of packed red cells, an increase in the hematocrit of 3% is expected in a 70 kg recipient.)
2. Recipients in actual or incipient congestive heart failure
3. The administration of group O blood to nongroup O recipients (The removal of plasma has decreased the amount of anti-A and anti-B present in the donor blood.)

Washed red cells: Washed red cells are useful in those conditions in which very little plasma is tolerated. They may be prepared easily if a continuous-flow cell washer is available. Otherwise, repeated manual washings of lightly packed red cells with normal saline are required. After three or four saline washings, the red cells are ready for use and may be diluted with sterile saline for easier administration.

The indications for this preparation include:
1. Recipients with paroxysmal nocturnal hemoglobinuria
2. Use of group O red cells for non-group O recipients (More isoagglutinins are removed by this method than with packed red blood cells)
3. Recipient hypersensitivity to plasma proteins, especially IgA (Because this condition is attended by such severe reactions when IgA is tranfused, simple saline washing of red cells may not afford adequate protection.)

Leukocyte-poor red cells: Leukocyte-poor red cells are a preparation derived from the deliberate attempt to remove leukocytes from packed red cells. They are useful in recipients suffering repeated, severe febrile transfusion reactions. Such reactions are caused by leukocyte alloantibodies in the serum of the recipient and can be avoided by the transfusion of leukocyte-poor red cells.[17] Many methods are available to prepare this component product.

Inverted centrifugation:

Principle: The blood bag is centrifuged in an inverted position, and the red cells are removed from below the resulting buffy coat; separation occurs by gravity collection of red cells.

Procedure: Place a bag of whole blood in an inverted position in a refrigerated centrifuge and spin at

5000 rpm for 5 min. Remove the bag carefully after centrifugation and hang it inverted on a ring stand. If the transfer packs are no longer present, attach a transfer bag to the centrifuged bag, being careful not to agitate the contents. Allow approximately 80% of the red cells to flow into the transfer bag and discontinue the collection. The transfer bag now contains leukocyte-poor red cells.

Advantages:
1. If the preparation is made without disturbing the original hermetic seal (transfer bags still attached), the shelf life is at least 21 days, depending on the age of the blood when processed and the anticoagulant used.
2. The procedure is simple and economical and can be performed by any blood bank.
3. There is removal of approximately 75% of leukocytes, an amount sufficient to prevent febrile transfusion reactions.

Disadvantages:
1. Initially only 24 hr blood was used. This is probably no longer necessary.[18]
2. There is a loss of at least 20% of the erythrocytes; hence, the expected therapeutic response from each unit of leukocyte-poor red cells is less than the original unit from which it was processed.
3. The hematocrit of the final product is very high and is difficult to infuse; this can be corrected by adding saline prior to its administration.

Filtration:
Principle: Whole blood or packed red cells are filtered through a variety of adsorbents onto which leukocytes are trapped; the blood passing through these filters is leukocyte poor, but the efficiency of their removal varies with the filters used.

Procedures:
Nylon fiber filtration: In the nylon fiber filtration method[19] there is adhesion of granulocytes to the nylon filter but lymphoctes are able to pass through. There is an absolute requirement for very fresh, heparinized blood; it is recommended that filtration be performed within 1 hr of collection and that the filter be prewarmed for maximal efficiency. This method removes 57-73% of granulocytes and sacrifices 6-18% of erythrocytes.[18] The preparation does minimize the occurrence of nonhemolytic transfusion reactions, but the retention of lymphocytes with a long half-life allow likely sensitization of the recipient. Furthermore, it is inconvenient to require heparin as an anticoagulant. The shelf life of this produce is only 24 hr, and no plasma components can be prepared if whole blood is used. A purer red cell preparation is possible if nylon filtration is followed by inverted centrifugation: 95-99% of leukocytes are removed;[18] in addition to the previous disadvantages, the procedure time is now expanded from 20-60 min.[18]

Miscellaneous filters: Danulon fiber filters remove 88% of leukocytes; this can be increased to 95% if the resulting leukocyte-poor blood is washed three times in saline.[20] Various cellulose fiber filters have been used but are either too expensive[21] or contain particulate matter than may be dangerous.[22]

Disposable column filters packed with cotton wool prepared from *Gossypium barbadense* cotton is an effective leukocyte filter, removing 95-100% leukocytes from packed red cells collected in ACD and 92-98% leukocytes from ACD whole blood[23]; there is a 5% loss of erythrocytes. Stored blood can be used with efficiency, and no special anticoagulant is required. Microaggregates that form during blood storage are also removed by the filtration process.

The shelf life of all these products is 24 hr; these miscellaneous filters are difficult to obtain commercially.

Sedimentation:
Principle: The sedimentation of erythrocytes by high-molecular-weight polymers aids in the removal of leukocytes. The two agents that have been used are dextran and hydroxyethyl starch (HES).

Dextran sedimentation[24]: Dextran is a long-chain polymer of glucose units and is available in preparations of variable molecular weights. To be an effective erythrocyte-sedimenting agent, the molecular weight must exceed 120,000. Such preparations are known to be antigenic,[25] and therefore their use has been restricted to experimental and investigational purposes only.

Hydroxyethyl starch sedimentation[26]: HES is derived from a waxy amylopectin starch and is licensed for use as a 6% solution in normal saline. This substance has very low antigenicity,[27] can be safely transfused, and will produce erythrocyte sedimentation equal to that of dextran.

Procedure:
1. The sedimentation can be performed in a 1 L plastic bag with spike lines and an attached satellite bag. One spike is attached to a 5 dl container of 6% HES; another spike line is attached to a 1 L bag of normal saline; the third spike line is attached to the unit of blood to be processed.
2. Allow the blood to enter the 1 L bag; flush the remaining blood from the bag with 30 ml saline and add to the 1 L bag.
3. Clamp and disconnect the spike leading to the emptied blood bag.
4. Add equal volumes of HES and normal saline to the 1 L bag until it is full.
5. Mix the contents of the bag thoroughly by inversion.
6. Place the bag on a plasma extractor and allow sedimentation to occur for 30 min.
7. Express the pink supernatant fluid and the uppermost layer of erythrocytes.
8. Refill the bag with equal volumes of HES and saline and repeat steps 5-7.
9. Mix the remaining blood and allow it to drain into the satellite bag. Transfuse within 24 hr.

Advantages:
1. There is effective leukocyte removal: Ninety-five percent of leukocytes are removed.
2. There is no significant sacrifice of erythrocytes: Less than 10% of erythrocytes are lost.
3. No mechanical equipment is required.
4. No special anticoagulant is required.
5. The procedure is simple and readily adaptable in any blood bank.

Disadvantages:
1. The shelf life is 24 hr after preparation.
2. The residual HES in the processed blood may aggravate bleeding tendencies in thrombocytopenic recipients.[28] To prevent this possibility, HES-sedimented red blood cells can be washed with normal saline prior to infusion in thrombocytopenic recipients.

• • •

Frozen red cells are a very efficient leukocyte-poor preparation; many erythrocytes are sacrificed in its preparation. See the following discussion of frozen red cells.

Frozen red cells: Red cells, in the presence of a cryoprotective agent, can be preserved and stored in the frozen state for extended periods of time and still show normal viability and function when thawed. The most popular cryoprotective agent is glycerol, which is uniformly dispersed in the red cells, reducing ice crystal formation and cell dehydration and thereby protecting the cell membrane from damage.[29] Although glycerol is not metabolically toxic to the red cells, if high levels remain in the erythrocytes, osmotic lysis of the cells will occur when they are infused into the recipient. Therefore after frozen storage and subsequent thawing, all units must be deglycerolized before used. All procedures for freezing erythrocytes therefore involve four steps: glycerolization, storage, thawing, and washing.

There are two basic methods available at this time: a slow freeze, high glycerol content method and a rapid freeze, low glycerol content method. These will be only briefly outlined since most blood banks are not equipped to prepare and handle this blood component. Regardless of which method is to be used, the process begins with a unit of heavily packed red cells having a hematocrit of 85-90%; the plasma so removed is fractionated or frozen. During the process of deglycerolization, the remaining plasma is removed and therefore it is not necessary to issue type-specific blood; group O blood with the appropriate Rh factor is adequate for all recipients.

Slow freeze, high glycerol content: In the slow freeze, high glycerol content method,[30] 4 dl of a 6.2M glycerol solution is added to the heavily packed erythrocytes. The first deciliter is added slowly, mixed, and allowed to equilibrate with the red cells for a period of 5 min; then the remainder of the glycerol is added. The final glycerol concentration is approximately 40%. The bag of glycerolized cells is placed in a protective metal or cardboard canister and stored in a mechanical freezer capable of cooling to −80° C; the rate of cooling is not critical, and freezing to this temperature should occur over a period of 2-10 hr. When thawing is desired, the bag and its canister are immersed in a 37° C water bath for 10-15 min; when completely thawed, the bag is removed from the canister for deglycerolization. Because the content of glycerol is high, mechanical continuous-flow washing is required for deglycerolization. Three wash solutions are used: A 12% sodium chloride solution is followed by a 1.6% sodium chloride solution and then by a 0.8% sodium chloride solution with 0.2 g/dl glucose. The total deglycerolization process requires about 30 min.

Rapid freeze, low glycerol content: In the rapid freeze, low glycerol content method,[31] the glycerol solution is added at one time using a 35% solution equal in amount to the volume of the densely packed red cells to which it will be added. The resulting mixture has a glycerol concentration of approximately 14%. After mixing thoroughly, the bag is placed in a cryoprotective canister and is immersed in liquid nitrogen for rapid freezing: A temperature of −196° C is reached within 2-3 min. The preparation is stored in its canister in a liquid nitrogen freezer. There is no difference in the thaw procedure, but deglycerolization is much faster since the concentration of glycerol is low; batch washings can be performed in a standard refrigerated centrifuge.

• • •

There are disadvantages to each of the above methods. There is greater expenditure involved in the deglycerolization of the high glycerol content red cells, but the less rigid temperature demands provide for more convenient storage and transportation. Recent attempts to simplify the deglycerolization of the high glycerol content red cells involve the removal of much of the glycerol solution prior to freezing and storage; subsequent washings can be performed with a clinical centrifuge in only 45 min.[32]

Advantages:
1. The shelf life is 3 yr.
2. Because of the prolonged shelf life, frozen red cell preparations are the ideal method of storing rare and autologous blood.
3. Previously frozen red cells maintain normal levels of ATP and 2,3-DPG.
4. It is a useful preparation for recipients sensitized to IgA.
5. The risk of transmitting hepatitis is diminished and is directly related to the extensive washing of thawed red cells, thereby greatly diluting any residual plasma.
6. The washing process greatly reduces the number of residual leukocytes and platelets; this is therefore an ideal preparation for potential organ transplant recipients because of the decreased sensitization to HLA antigens.

Disadvantages:
1. The preparation is expensive.
2. A unit of thawed, deglycerolized red cells has a shelf life of 24 hr; if unused in that period of time, the unit must be discarded. Although this is a current requirement of the FDA and must be adhered to, recent evidence has shown that refreezing thawed red cells is not detrimental[33,34] and may, in the future, prevent the loss of blood units of rare types.
3. Because of the time required for deglycerolization, frozen red cells are not available on a "stat" basis.

Leukocyte preparations
Principle

The primary clinical indication for leukocyte transfusions is a patient with severe granulocytopenia (absolute count $< 500/mm^3$) and sepsis that is unresponsive to antibiotic therapy. Most recipients suffer from leukemia, and, prior to the advent of leukocyte transfusions, infection was a major cause of their death.[35] Leukocytes are collected from normal donors through the process of **leukapheresis,** i.e., the mechanical separation of leukocytes from whole donor blood and the immediate return of the leukocyte-poor red cells to the donor. Several mechanical devices are available for this procedure:

Centrifugal leukapheresis can be performed in either an intermittent or a continuous-flow centrifuge. The granulocytes collect in the upper red cell layer near the plasma interface and are skimmed off and collected. The plasma and most of the red cells are returned to the donor. Continuous-flow centrifugation can process 8-10 units of whole donor blood over a period of 4 hr. Centrifugation yields a moderate number of leukocytes. The leukocyte yield can be increased by treating the donor with intravenous dexamethasone[36] 2-3 hr prior to donation and/or by adding hydroxyethyl starch[37] to the input line of the cell separation to allow more efficient red cell separation. With these improvements, an average yield of $1\text{-}3 \times 10^{10}$ granulocytes can be collected in a single procedure.[38]

Filtration leukapheresis[39] utilizes the phenomenon of calcium-dependent adherence of granulocytes to nylon fibers. Trapped granulocytes are subsequently eluted by a plasma or plasma-saline solution.[40] The average yield of granulocytes is $2\text{-}5 \times 10^{10}$ cells over a $2^1/_2$ hr period without the use of additives.[41] Although the yield of leukocytes is very high, some morphologic changes occur, including increased vacuolization and leukocyte membrane disruption; the vacuolization is reversed when the cells are replaced into a physiologic medium.[41] Reports of diminished function in vitro[42] have not been substantiated by all investigators.[43]

Effects on the recipient

Leukocyte transfusions have resulted in the following beneficial and adverse reactions in the recipient.

1. Polymorphonuclear increments: Granulocytes compatible with the recipient in both ABO and HLA antigen systems produce a satisfactory 1 hr posttransfusion increment in the number of circulating cells; a poorer recovery is seen as the number of mismatched HLA antigens increases and no significant increment is present after the infusion of cells having a positive leukoagglutinin test.[44,45]

2. Transfusion reactions: Fever and chills are a more common problem when leukocytes obtained by filtration are used; these reactions are unrelated to compatibility.[44] Compatible leukocytes obtained by centrifugal leukapheresis produce few symptoms. Incompatible leukocytes obtained by either method of collection produce symptoms that increase in number and severity as the degree of incompatibility increases.

3. Leukocyte-directed antibodies: Leukoagglutinins may develop early in the course of treatment and require constant surveillance to provide daily compatible transfusions.

4. Graft vs. host disease: Graft vs. host disease is an uncommon but serious complication resulting from the infusion of viable lymphocytes with their subsequent engraftment and reaction against host tissues. This should theoretically be a greater problem if cells obtained by centrifugal leukapheresis are infused because lymphocytes do not adhere to nylon filters.

Effects on donor

1. Hematologic changes: During leukapheresis, some red cells and platelets are lost and not returned to the donor. A slight fall in hemoglobin and platelet count can therefore be expected.[46] The granulocytes removed are replaced by cells from the marginating leukocyte pool.

2. Discomfort: The donor may experience restlessness, pain at venipuncture site, muscle aches, and chills.

Characteristics of the final product

1. A variable number of erythrocytes are present; hence, ABO group and Rh type must be compatible with the recipient.
2. Serum is present and hence hepatitis testing is required.
3. HLA compatibility is highly desirable.
4. The shelf life is 24 hr from the start of donation.

Platelet preparations
Principle

Platelet transfusions are indicated in hemorrhaging patients with platelet counts less than $50,000/mm^3$ or in surgical candidates with platelet counts less than $100,000/mm^3$. Platelet deficiency can be idiopathic or secondary to chemotherapy, leukemia, aplastic anemia, or increased sequestration (splenomegaly). Idiopathic thrombocytopenia is not treated with platelet transfusions because the immunologic destruction of transfused platelets renders them useless. With the use of platelet transfusion, the rate of fatal hemorrhage is leukemic patients has been reduced by more than 50%. Platelet transfusion is also useful in patients with qualitative platelet disorders.

There are two preparations in use today: platelet concentrates from random donors and plateletpheresis from a single donor.

Platelet concentrates

Principle: When fresh whole blood is *slowly* centrifuged, the resulting plasma is rich in platelets: **platelet-rich plasma.** Although platelet-rich plasma and fresh whole blood are potential sources of platelets, they are not used therapeutically because of the large volume of fluid administered. Rather, platelet-rich plasma is used in the preparation of the definitive therapeutic product, platelet concentrate. When platelet-rich plasma is *heavily* centrifuged, the platelets are sedimented and the resulting **platelet-poor plasma (PPP)** is expressed into a satellite bag for storage as fresh frozen plasma. A small amount of platelet-poor plasma is left behind on the sedimented platelets, and together they constitute the **platelet concentrate.**

Procedure: Collect ACD or CPD blood and maintain at room temperature for no more than 4 hr prior to centrifugation. Centrifuge the fresh whole blood at 2500 rpm for 3 min at 20° C.

Express the platelet-rich plasma into a satellite bag.

Centrifuge the platelet-rich plasma at 3800 rpm for 4 min[47] at 20° C. Express the platelet-poor supernatant into a second satellite bag, allowing 50 ml of platelet-poor plasma to remain with the platelet concentrate. Gently rotate the platelet concentrate on a mechanical rotator for at least 2 hr to allow a uniform resuspension of the platelets. Using continuous gentle agitation.[48] keep at room temperature until ready to transfuse.

One 50 ml bag of platelet concentrate is the extract of 1 unit of whole blood. Platelet concentrates must be used within 72 hr of their preparation; just prior to use, combine up to 6 bags of concentrate into 1 container and transfuse within 4 hr of pooling.

Quality control: Federal regulations require that at least 75% of platelet concentrates must contain at least 5.5×10^{10} platelets per bag.[49]

Use: Platelet concentrates are used to provide platelets to thrombocytopenic patients in the absence of alloimmunization. Whenever possible, ABO-compatible platelets are used; if they are unavailable, ABO-incompatible platelets may be used without reservation. If long-term therapy is anticipated, a single donor preparation is suggested because repeated random donor platelet concentrates result in alloimmunization, generally within 2 months of therapy.[50]

Plateletpheresis

Principle: A large number of platelets can be harvested from a single donor by either repeated, multiple-bag donations or the use of mechanical cell separators. Both methods are pheresis procedures because platelet-poor plasma and erythrocytes are immediately returned to the donor after the collection of platelets.

Procedures:

Multiple-bag donations: Fresh blood is drawn from the donor and collected into a closed system of quadruple double pheresis bags.[51] Each primary bag is weighed during the donation to ensure a 5 dl content (Weight of full bag − Weight of empty bag ÷ 1.06 = Whole blood present [ml]),[97] and the same centrifugation procedures are followed as detailed above for platelet concentrates. The platelet-poor plasma and the sedimented red cells are recombined and returned to the donor before the second primary bag is filled. Each of the platelet concentrates is kept at room temperature with constant agitation and must be used within 72 hr. These single-donor platelet concentrates are pooled prior to use.

Mechanical cell separators[52]: The following description pertains to the Haemonetics Model 30 Blood Processor (Haemonetics Corp., Braintree, Mass.); similar results are obtained with other cell separators. The Model 30 has a conical centrifuge bowl with single input and output ports. Donor blood is allowed to fill the centrifuge bowl at a rate of 60-80 ml/min; the input line is flushed with 3% sodium citrate. While the filling occurs, a clear separation between plasma and red cells is observed with a thin white line of platelets in the center. The plasma is collected first in the plasma bag. When the platelet line approaches the outflow port, the platelet indicator is activated and platelets are diverted into another bag. During platelet collection, blood flow into the centrifuge bowl is reduced to 20 ml/min to re-

duce turbulence. The platelets are collected for approximately $2\frac{1}{2}$ min for a total volume of 50 ml or until the red cells begin to approach the outflow port. The platelet collection is stopped, and the residual red cells and the previously collected plasma are combined and reinfused into the donor. After reinfusion, the procedure is repeated; usually six or seven cycles are attempted, each cycle lasting 15-20 min. For a more distinct separation of platelets from erythrocytes, hydroxyethyl starch is sometimes added to the anticoagulant solution.[53]

Platelet yields: Multiple-bag plateletpheresis yields an average of 0.7×10^{11} platelets per bag collected.[54] Mechanical cell separators yield an average of 4.8-6 $\times$ 10^{11} platelets[52] for the usual six-cycle procedure. The final platelet yield is always directly related to the pretransfusion platelet count of the donor: Greater yields are obtained from donors with high platelet counts.

Donor requirements:
1. The same standards as for whole blood donation apply to random platelet donors.
2. Plateletpheresis donors must have their hemoglobin level and platelet count monitored between phereses; platelet count should not be lower than 150,000/mm[3] immediately prior to any procedure.
3. No aspirin may be ingested for 72 hr before plateletpheresis donation.

Effects on donor: Hematologic changes[55] caused by plateletpheresis include an average drop in hematocrit of 3.5%, most attributable to dilutional effects. The average corrected platelet decrease is 75,000/mm[3]; no significant change in granulocyte counts are observed, although approximately 30% of circulating lymphocytes are removed.

Hypovolemic shock, peroral paresthesia caused by diminished ionized calcium, and anxiety are occasionally encountered.

Effects on recipient: Alloimmunization[56] may occur. The average normal life span of transfused platelets is 8-10 days. The appearance of platelet antibodies in the course of platelet transfusion therapy shortens the life span of the transfused platelets. Once this has occurred, platelet concentrates must be replaced by single donor platelets from HLA-compatible donors; continual transfusion with noncompatible platelets results in a refractoriness to further transfusions and the development of clinical symptoms of transfusion reactions.

Platelet increments are expected; 24 hr posttransfusion increments in platelet counts are the most convenient method of assessing clinical response. These can be calculated from the following equation[57]:

Corrected platelet increment =

$$\frac{\text{Posttransfusion count} - \text{pretransfusion count}}{\text{No. of units of platelets infused}} \times \text{BSA}$$

The above value represents the observed platelet increment adjusted to 1 unit of platelets transfused for each square meter of body surface area (BSA). As a general estimate, 1 unit of platelet concentrates will increase the platelet count by 4,000/mm[3] in an average adult. Smaller increments may indicate alloimmunization, increased splenic sequestration caused by splenomegaly or fever, or acute hemorrhage in the recipient.

Plasma fractions

A number of methods have been developed that allow differential precipitation of plasma proteins and the production of five clinically used plasma fractions:

1. Antihemophilic factor (factor VIII)
2. Fibrinogen (factor I)
3. Prothrombin complex: prothrombin (factor II), proconvertin (factor VII), plasma thromboplastin component (factor IX), and Stuart-Prower factor (factor X)
4. γ-globulins
5. Albumin

The latter two fractions are not associated with hepatitis, but the first three carry the risk of transmitting serum hepatitis. The immunoglobulins are used prophylactically or in the treatment of a variety of infectious diseases; they are also used as anti-Rh_0 immunoglobulins for the prevention of Rh immunization (see discussion of hemolytic disease of the newborn). Albumin is used for volume replacement or for protein replenishment. The remaining fractions are intended as replacement therapy in coagulation factor deficiencies.

Antihemophilic factor

Antihemophilic factor (AHF; factor VIII) is a labile clotting factor present in normal plasma but deficient in the plasma of patients with hemophilia A. Because the clotting factor disappears quickly when plasma or blood is stored at 4° C, all factor VIII preparations utilize *fresh* blood or plasma. It is generally agreed that 1 unit of factor VIII activity is that amount of factor VIII present in 1 ml of citrated fresh normal plasma.[58]

Fresh whole blood and plasma: Between 15-40% of factor VIII activity is lost during the first 12-24 hr of blood storage. It is therefore required that blood or plasma to be used for its factor VIII content be transfused within 6 hr of collection.

Single-donor plasma may be frozen to increase ready availability. Freezing is accomplished with mechanical freezers capable of cooling to −30° C; the plasma must be frozen solid within 6 hr of donor collection. It is then stored at −18° C or lower and has a shelf life of 12 months. When the plasma is to be used, it is thawed at 30-37° C with constant agitation; it must then be infused within 2 hr of thawing. Any fresh frozen plasma that is not used by 12 months can be maintained frozen for an additional 4 years; however, it cannot be administered for its AHF content after the initial 12-month period.

Fresh whole blood, fresh liquid plasma, and fresh frozen plasma each contain approximately 225 ml of plasma. Since each milliliter of fresh plasma contains approximately 1 unit of factor VIII activity, it is expected that 1 container of fresh whole blood or fresh liquid plasma would contain approximately 225 units of factor VIII activity. However, fresh frozen plasma loses a small amount of factor VIII on initial freezing, so 1 ml of fresh frozen plasma contains only 0.8 units of factor VIII activity on thawing; therefore 1 container

of fresh frozen plasma would theoretically contain only 180 units of factor VIII activity (Table 15-1).

The use of any of these preparations for the treatment of hemophilia has limited value because of the large amount of fluid infused. The factor VIII concentrates to be discussed below are the mainstay of treatment today; however, fresh frozen plasma is still used to treat the simultaneous deficiencies of multiple coagulation factors.

Cryoprecipitate: When fresh frozen plasma is thawed, a small precipitate remains adherent to the sides of the bag. This cold insoluble fraction is called the **cryoprecipitate,** and it accounts for approximately 3% of the total plasma protein; it is rich in factor VIII.[59]

Method of preparation: Cryoprecipitate can be easily prepared in any laboratory because no special equipment is necessary. However, extreme care in performing the individual steps is necessary to ensure an adequate yield of factor VIII activity. The following procedure is recommended.[60]

1. Collect blood in a closed, double-bag system as quickly as possible. The American Association of Blood Banks recommends that a collection time of no longer than 8 min be allowed[61] because of the loss of factor VIII with subsequent clotting; if clotting can be avoided, there is no appreciable loss of factor VIII when collection times are slightly delayed.[62] Mix the blood thoroughly at frequent intervals throughout the collection period; if visible clots form, the blood is not acceptable for cryoprecipitate preparation. CPD is the preferred anticoagulant because it produces higher yields of factor VIII.[63]

2. Within 4 hr of collection, separate the red cells from the plasma by centrifugation at 4000 rpm for 5 min in a refrigerated centrifuge.

3. Within 2 hr of separation, freeze the plasma. This may be done with a mechanical freezer (−30° C or lower); if a freezer is not available, the plasma must be wrapped in a protective polyethylene cover and immersed in a bath of 95% ethanol and dry ice chips. If the latter method is used, immersion time should be 45 min.

4. The frozen plasma can be stored at −20° C or lower for 3 months without significant loss of factor VIII activity.

5. When the cryoprecipitate is to be prepared, thaw the frozen plasma overnight in a 1-6° C refrigerator (16-18 hr). Alternatively, the frozen plasma may be placed in a 4° C water bath with constant agitation; it will be thawed in approximately 45 min. In either instance it is important not to redissolve the cryoprecipitate. When the plasma has a mushy consistency, even if a small amount of ice remains, it is ready to be separated.

6. Centrifuge the slushy plasma in a 2° C refrigerated centrifuge at 5000 rpm for 8 min.

7. Immediately after centrifugation, hang the bag in an inverted position and allow the plasma to drain into the satellite bag. The cryoprecipitate will adhere to the wall of the bag.

8. Seal the tubing and separate the cryoprecipitate bag.

9. Store the cryoprecipitate in a $-20°$ C or lower freezer for up to 12 months from the date of blood collection. There is only minimal loss of factor VIII activity during the period of storage, and these losses are further reduced if storage can be maintained at $-30°$ C.

10. When needed, the desired number of cryoprecipitate bags are removed from the freezer and thawed in a $37°$ C water bath; thawing is very rapid. Add 10-20 ml of physiologic saline to each bag and completely resuspend the cryoprecipitate. Pool the contents of the individual bags into a single bag and infuse within 6 hr of reconstitution. The thawed cryoprecipitate must be kept at room temperature prior to use.

Assay of cryoprecipitate: Cryoprecipitate contains about half of the original factor VIII activity in less than 3% of the plasma proteins (Table 15-1). Although it is not practical to assay each bag of cryoprecipitate, all blood banks actively engaged in the preparation of cryoprecipitates must establish a quality control program to monitor their product. Such a program may require a random AHF assay on 1% of the bags produced each week. Properly prepared cryoprecipitates should contain 80 or more units of factor VIII per bag.

Advantages and disadvantages:
1. Cryoprecipitates are a concentrated form of factor VIII and avoid the problem of overhydration; since no significant albumin is present, large amounts can be administered without producing hypervolemia.
2. Cryoprecipitates are inconvenient for home use because of the required storage temperature and the need to pool bags.
3. Factor VIII activity is not standardized, and the content varies from one bag to another, making calculation of dosage more difficult.
4. Uncommonly, reactions may occur to the infusion of this product,[64] including any of the following signs or symptoms: pulmonary edema, fever, urticaria, hypotension, and tachycardia. Hemolysis caused by the administration of blood group antibodies may also occur.

Uses of cryoprecipitate: Cryoprecipitate is an impure preparation and contains many other plasma proteins in addition to antihemophilic factor[65] (Table 15-2). Hence, the preparation can be useful in the treatment of the following conditions:
1. Hemophilia A: as discussed above, a congenital deficiency of AHF and the primary indication for the use of cryoprecipitate.
2. Von Willebrand's disease: a hemorrhagic diathesis characterized by a prolonged bleeding time and diminished AHF activity. The former symptom is caused by a plasma factor producing abnormal platelet retention; this plasma factor is present in cryoprecipitates.[66] Current data indicate the von Willebrand factor may reside on the AHF molecule, distinct from its coagulant and antigenic properties.[67] This concept is strengthened by the long-known fact that hemophiliac plasma contains normal von Willebrand factor.[68]
3. Factor XIII deficiency: a congenital deficiency of fibrin stabilizing factor producing a bleeding disorder

secondary to an instability of clot formation. Although cryoprecipitate only contains an average of 30% of the plasma factor XIII activity, this is sufficient to treat the disorder[69] because only very small quantities are needed for effective hemostasis (0.5%).

4. Decreased fibrinogen levels: see later discussion of fibrinogen.

Commercial antihemophilic factor: There are a number of preparations currently available that offer concentrated, highly potent factor VIII activity. Such preparations include Profilate (Abbott Laboratories, North Chicago, Ill.), Factorate (Armour Pharmaceutical Co., Phoenix), Koate (Cutter Laboratories, Berkeley, Calif.), Humafac (Parke, Davis & Co., Detroit), and Hemofil (Hyland Laboratories, Costa Mesa, Calif.). They are prepared from pooled plasma or cryoprecipitate that is subjected to various extraction procedures to partially remove contaminating proteins, including fibrinogen. See Table 15-1 for average factor VIII content.

Advantages: Commercial preparations of antihemophilic factor have a number of advantages over cryoprecipitates:
1. They are lyophilized and can be stored at $4°$ C.
2. They are reconstituted by adding sterile water; no cumbersome pooling is needed.
3. The therapeutic dose is a smaller volume that can often be administered with a needle and syringe; intravenous tubing is not required.
4. The factor VIII content is always assayed and clearly labeled on the package by its manufacturer.
5. They can be used in the treatment of hemophiliacs with circulating factor VIII inhibitors.

Disadvantages: A major disadvantage of commercial preparations of antihemophilic factor is the greater risk of transmitting serum hepatitis. This is directly related to the increased donor exposure that results from plasma pooling. Other complications of therapy include immune hemolysis secondary to the infusion of blood group antibodies.[70] Rarely, immediate reactions occur after the administration of these concentrates[71]; they consist predominantly of allergic reactions.

Fibrinogen

Fibrinogen is the least soluble of plasma proteins and can be easily isolated when plasma is fractionated. Large plasma pools have been used to prepare fibrinogen commercially. Since fibrinogen cannot withstand the intense heat required to inactivate the hepatitis virus, the use of this preparation has carried a high risk of hepatitis.[72] As a result, the FDA has banned the manufacture of human fibrinogen (June 30, 1978).[73] Cryoprecipitates are now the predominant source of fibrinogen for clinical use, each bag containing approximately 250 mg of fibrinogen.

Fibrinogen replacement has been used with hypofibrinogenemia associated with abruptio placenta, amniotic fluid embolism, intrauterine death, and hereditary afibrinogenemia or dysfibrinogenemia. In many of these conditions, fibrinogen replacement is not the most critical therapeutic measure.

Table 15-1. Comparison of potency and content of human factor VIII preparations

Preparation	Volume (ml)	Units of factor VIII per ml	Units of factor VIII per container
Fresh whole blood	517.5	1	225
Fresh liquid plasma	225	1	225
Fresh frozen plasma	225	0.8	180
Cryoprecipitate	10	10	100
Commercial AHF	20-30	10-33	200-1000

Table 15-2. Clotting factors present in cryoprecipitate

Clotting factor	Original plasma content (%)
Von Willebrand factor	40-75
Antihemophilic factor (VIII)	20-50
Fibrin stabilizing factor (XIII)	30
Fibrinogen (I)	23
Plasma thromboplastin component (IX)	5
Proconvertin (VII)	2
Hageman factor (XII)	2
Prothrombin (II)	1
Proaccelerin (V)	1
Stuart-Prower factor (X)	1
Plasma thromboplastin antecedent (XI)	1

Prothrombin complex

The coagulant factors that make up this complex (II, VII, IX, and X) are characterized by their dependence on vitamin K and their removal from normal plasma by adsorption with various inorganic chemicals, especially $Al(OH)_3$, $Ca_3(PO_4)_2$, $BaSO_4$, and $BaCO_3$. Because of their dependence on vitamin K for synthesis, these factors are decreased in severe liver disease. These factors are relatively stable and could be replaced with bank plasma, but the danger of fluid overload precludes such a practice. Prothrombin complex concentrates are available and are the mode of replacement therapy.

Many commercial preparations are available, all of which rely on adsorption and elution of pooled plasma. Some of these preparations use the chemical adsorption method mentioned above, but removal of the clotting factors is somewhat retarded by the presence of citrate in the plasma. Most preparations therefore employ ionic exchangers (DEAE-cellulose or DEAE-Sephadex [Pharmacia Laboratories, Piscataway, N.J.]) that effectively bind the coagulant factors. The adsorbed factors are then eluted with a buffer and are subsequently purified, concentrated, and lyophilized. The concentrates are stored at 4° C. Factor IX is clinically the most important of the factors in this complex; the yield of factor IX activity is variable with these preparations, ranging from 4-60 units/ml.[74] In the United States, available preparations include Konyne (Cutter Laboratories, Berkeley, Calif.) and Proplex (Hyland Laboratories, Costa Mesa, Calif.).

The prothrombin complex is useful in the treatment of the following clinical conditions:

1. Christmas disease: Christmas disease is a congenital deficiency of factor IX that produces a hemorrhagic diathesis clinically indistinguishable from classic hemophilia.
2. Congenital deficiencies of the other coagulation factors present in the complex: The prothrombin complex can be used in these very rare conditions.
3. Acquired hypoprothrombinemia: Beneficial responses are obtained in cases of vitamin K deficiency and coumarin overdosage; in both these instances, the coagulation deficiencies are limited to the factors present in the concentrate. The hypoprothrombinemia associated with liver disease does not respond as satisfactorily to replacement therapy because the bleeding is partly attributable to deficiencies not corrected by the concentrate, i.e., factor V and platelets.[75]
4. Hemophilia A patients with circulating factor VIII antibodies that cannot be effectively neutralized by high doses of factor VIII concentrates[76]: The prothrombin complex contains activated clotting factors that are active beyond the factor VIII level and therefore can initiate clotting without factor VIII participation. The use of prothrombin in this situation is highly controversial and it is still experimental because of the inherent dangers in the administration of activated clotting factors.[77]

Complications resulting from the use of the prothrombin complex include the following, some of which have proved fatal:

1. Anaphylactic reactions[78]: Anaphylactic reactions can occur in individuals given the prothrombin complex.
2. Development of a hypercoagulable state: Arterial and venous thromboses, as well as disseminated intravascular coagulation,[79,80] may occur. The activation of clotting factors IX and X during the preparation of this concentrate have been shown to account for some of these problems.[81] The complication can be avoided or lessened if antithrombin III and heparin are added to the concentrate during its preparation because these substances effectively neutralize the thrombogenic material.
3. Transmission of serum hepatitis: The occurrence of hepatitis B antigen in pooled plasma that cannot be heat sterilized is high[82]; the risk of hepatitis should decrease with the exclusion of antigen-positive donor.[83]
4. Hemolysis from blood group alloantibodies present in the preparation: Only low titers of antibodies are present,[84] and the risk is minimal.

Plasma and plasma substitutes

Maintenance of a normal blood volume is a significant consideration in tranfusion practices and is especially important in the treatment of **hypovolemic shock**, a shocklike state in which there has been a sudden reduction of intravascular fluid and in which fluid replacement is more critical than red cell replacement. Clinical conditions that may predispose an individual to hypovolemic shock include peritonitis, severe diarrhea, intestinal obstruction, or severe burns. Fluid replacement also plays an important part in the treatment of acute blood loss of mild to moderate degree; the erythrocytes can be replaced with packed red cells and the plasma replaced with volume expanders. Fluid can be replaced by adminitering either crystalloids or colloid solutions.[85]

Crystalloids primarily are saline solutions that have the advantage of little expense and ready availability. Either normal saline (0.85% NaCl) or balanced salt solutions (e.g., lactated Ringer's solution) are available. There is no danger of serologic incompatibility or serum hepatitis when these solutions are used. Approximately 4 volumes of crystalloid must be given to replace 1 volume of lost plasma because of the redistribution of the fluid into the interstitial spaces.

Colloid solutions provide a more accurate volume replacement. Many different preparations are available. The administration of **pooled plasma** as a volume expander is outmoded replacement therapy because of the high risk of transmitting serum hepatitis. In addition, the use of plasma in this way is very wasteful since the essential components are not utilized efficiently.

Albumin preparations allow safe and effective volume expansion. There are three preparations of albumin available:

1. Buffered saline solution, 5%, 12.5 g albumin in 250 ml fluid
2. Salt-poor albumin, 25%, 12.5 g albumin in 50 ml fluid
3. Plasma protein fraction (PPF), 5%, 12.5 g albumin and α- and β-globulin in 250 ml fluid

These preparations are derived from pooled plasma via cold-ethanol fractionation; albumin is isolated as Cohn fraction V, and PPF is isolated from Cohn fraction IV-4 and V. Subsequently, all these preparations are heated for 10 hr at 60° C to inactivate the hepatitis virus[86]; the heating does not destroy the hepatitis virus antigenicity, only its infectivity. Commercial albumin preparations have a shelf life of 3 or 5 years when stored at room temperature or 4° C, respectively.

The following outline* details serum albumin products available for clinical use:

A. Normal serum albumin (NSA) (human)
  1. Protein, 25 ± 1.5%, or 5% ± 0.3%
  2. Purity (At least 96% of the total protein in the final product must be albumin.)
  3. pH: 6.9 ± 0.5
  4. Sodium
    a. 25% NSA: not more than 160 mEq/L
    b. 5% NSA: 130-160 mEq/L

5. Dating
  a. Stored at 2-10° C: 5 years
  b. Stored at room temperature no warmer than 37° C: 3 years
B. PPF (human)
  1. Protein, 5% ± 0.3%
  2. Purity (At least 83% of the total protein in the final product must be albumin; no more than 17% shall be globulins; no more than 1% of globulins shall be γ-globulin.)
  3. pH: 7.0 ± 0.3
  4. Sodium: 100-160 mEq/L
  5. Potassium: no more than 2 mEq/L
  6. Dating
    a. Stored at 2-8° C: 5 years
    b. Stored at no warmer than 30° C: 3 years

The following information is applicable to both NSA and PPF. They should be heated at 60° ± 0.5° C for 10 hr. No preservatives should be used. They should pass standard tests for sterility and for pyrogenic substances. One of the following stabilizers can be used:

1. Sodium acetyl–tryptophanate, 0.16 mmole
2. Sodium acetyl–tryptophanate, 0.08 mmole, and sodium caprylate, 0.08 mmole

Acceptable clinical uses of albumin have been determined[87] and include acute traumatic shock, extensive thermal injuries, the adult respiratory distress syndrome accompanied by pulmonary interstitial edema, and preoperative preparation of cardiopulmonary bypass patients. Albumin may occasionally be beneficial in acute liver failure with or without ascites, acute nephrosis, anemic patients undergoing renal dialysis, as a red cell suspension media, and after radical surgical procedures. It is not beneficial in the treatment of chronic nephrosis or cirrhosis associated with hypoalbuminemia or in the malnutrition states.

Albumin products are free of isoagglutins and therefore require no cross matching prior to use. Albumin is a protein with very low antigenic potential, and NSA, 25% or 5%, has a very low reaction rate in the infused

Table 15-3. Proteins present in PPF and NSA by immunochemical analysis*

Albumin solution (5%)	PPF I	PPF II
Albumin monomer, 9%	Albumin	Albumin
Albumin dimer (trace)	α_1-Antitrypsin	α_1-Antitrypsin
α_1-Antitrypsin	α_1-Antichymotrypsin	IgG
α_1-Antichymotrypsin	α_2-HS globulin	IgM (trace)
IgG (trace)	β_2-Glycoprotein	IgA (trace)
Orosomucoid	IgG	α_1-Lipoprotein
Transferrin (trace)	IgM (trace)	Orosomucoid
	IgA (trace)	Transferrin (trace)
	Transferrin in anodal form (trace)	
	Transferrin, 12 mg/dl	

*From Pennell, R.B.: In Proceedings of the Workshop on Albumin, Department of Health and Human Services publication no. 76-925, Washington, D.C., 1975, U.S. Government Printing Office.
Proteins absent in all preparations: β_1-lipoprotein; complement components C3, C4, C5; fibrinogen; hemopexin; properdin factor B; thyroxine-binding prealbumin.

---

*From Barker, L.F.: In Proceedings of the Workshop on Albumin, Department of Health and Human Services, publication no. 76-925, Washington, D.C., 1975.

patient. PPF contains more proteins than NSA (Table 15-3); known common side effects to this product include urticaria, chills, and fever. In addition, hypotension has been a problem when PPF is administered rapidly in cardiopulmonary bypass patients,[88] and rare cases of systemic anaphylaxis have occurred.[89] These hypotensive reactions are attributed to the presence of bradykinin in heat-treated PPF.[90]

Synthetic colloid preparations can be divided into three groups. The **dextrans** are aqueous solutions of partially hydrolyzed polysaccharides that are synthesized by microorganisms. Native dextrans are glucopyranose units polymerized by α-1,6-glucosidic bonds and have an average molecular weight of several millions. Dextran preparations suitable for clinical use are prepared from native dextran by partial acid hydrolysis, resulting in a variety of average molecular weights: Dextran 70 (Cutter Laboratories, Berkeley, Calif.) and Macrodex (Pharmacia Laboratories) have an average molecular weight of 70,000; Dextran 40 (Cutter Medical) and Rheomacrodex (Pharmacia Laboratories, Piscotaway, N.J.) have an average molecular weight of 40,000. Both of these products are licensed for intravascular use in the United States. The low-molecular-weight products are rapidly excreted in the urine,[91] and therefore the high-molecular-weight preparations are more effective volume expanders.

Hydroxyethyl starch is prepared from the waxy amylopectin found in corn and soybeans after it has been modified by hydroxyethylation to prevent rapid hydrolysis by blood amylase after its infusion.[92] The hydroxyethylated amylopectin is then partially acid hydrolyzed to yield a variety of molecular weight preparations. The hydroxyethyl starches are extremely soluble in solution with no tendency to precipitate. They are eliminated from the body via the kidneys; the intravascular half-life is dependent on the extent of hydroxyethylation and the molecular weight of the preparation. The longer its intravascular half-life, the more effective volume expansion a product will produce; generally, hydroxyethyl starch has a longer intravascular half-life than dextrans of comparable average molecular weight.[93]

Gelatins are produced by animal collagen hydrolysis and have a final viscosity very similar to that of plasma. Those preparations having a molecular size large enough to be well retained in the circulation do not remain fluid at low temperatures. Because of this problem, these solutions were earlier abandoned by the United States. More recent gelatin preparations have been modified to overcome this difficulty[94]; however, gelatin solutions, as presently used in foreign countries, have not received FDA approval for use in the United States. It is recognized that the high-molecular-weight dextrans are more effective volume expanders than the clinical gelatins.

All of these volume expanders will induce bleeding in recipients, the frequency and severity of which are related to the total amount and the molecular size of the material administered.[95] In addition, all three preparations have been associated with allergic reactions, some of which are anaphylactoid in character.[96] Hence, although they are in wide clinical use in Europe, these agents have only limited support in the United States, partly because of the dose-related side effects.[97]

BLOOD PROCESSING FOR COMPATIBILITY
Identification of blood

A numeric system must be established that identifies all blood specimens and blood containers from one particular donation and allows identification of the donor, whose personal information is recorded on a donor's card. It must be possible to trace each unit back to the donor. Proper identification of the intended recipients is also required to ensure that the correct person is transfused. The recipient must be positively identified at the time his blood sample is withdrawn for compatibility testing. This recipient's blood must be stored at 1-6° C for at least 7 days following the transfusion to facilitate retesting if necessary.

Proper selection of blood

Both donor and recipient blood is tested and labeled as to ABO group and Rh type. D^u testing is performed on all Rh-negative donor blood. Generally it is desirable to administer group-specific blood, i.e., the recipient should receive blood of his own ABO group. At times this is not possible, and then compatible, non-group-specific blood may be given according to the following guidelines:

1. A group A recipient may receive group O blood if group A blood is not available; he must not be transfused with group B or AB blood because his serum contains the isoagglutinin anti-B.

2. A group B recipient may receive group O blood if group B blood is not available but must not be transfused with group A or AB blood because of naturally occurring anti-A in his serum.

3. In both of the above instances, if whole blood is to be given, the hemolysin titer of the group O blood must be determined to prevent hemolysis of recipient cells by donor serum (see discussion of transfusion of nonspecific blood).

4. Group AB recipients may receive either group A or group B red cells when AB blood is unavailable. However, only one of these two choices can be used for a recipient because it is dangerous to switch from one group to the other. An AB recipient may also receive group O blood if it is administered as packed red cells. Because AB blood lacks both anti-A and anti-B, all donor red cells are compatible with its serum and such persons have erroneously been regarded as **universal recipients.**

5. Group O recipients must be transfused with group O blood only.

The only other antigen routinely tested is the D antigen; this is a reflection of its extreme immunogenicity. D-positive recipients may receive either D-positive or D-negative blood depending on supply. D-negative recipients should receive D-negative blood to prevent alloimmunization. If D-negative blood is in short supply, the following Rh-negative recipients have priority:

1. Recipients with Rh antibodies in their serum
2. Women of childbearing age
3. Infants with Rh hemolytic disease of the newborn

In emergency situations, any Rh-negative recipient may

receive Rh-positive blood unless he is already immunized.

Cross matching

The cross match consists of a series of tests performed on the blood of the prospective recipient of a blood transfusion and on the blood of the proposed donor (or donors). The purpose is to detect any possible **incompatibility** between the recipient's serum and the donor's red cells; this procedure is termed the **major cross match.** Detecting incompatibility between the donor's serum and the recipient's red cells is termed the **minor cross match.** Only the major cross match is required testing, according to current standards.[1] It is performed on all prospective donor units prior to their transfusion; only compatible units are considered safe for infusion. When a time lapse occurs between subsequent transfusions, fresh recipient serum must be obtained for repeated major cross matches.

The cross match procedures must detect all varieties of antibodies: coating, hemolyzing, and agglutinating antibodies. Therefore the technic must include many phases and temperatures. Many varieties of technic will accomplish this goal, and the actual choice of procedure is the responsibility of the medical director. The ideal procedure will be set up to detect the maximal number of antibodies in the shortest period of time. All procedures include a saline phase at room temperature and a high protein phase at 37° C, which is followed by an indirect antiglobulin phase.

Major cross match

Procedure: Label two 12 × 75 mm test tubes; one is labeled "S" for saline cross match and the other is labeled "P" for protein cross match. Place 2 drops of fresh recipient serum (less than 48 hr old) into each tube. Select donor units of the same ABO and Rh type as that of the recipient. Prepare a 2-5% saline red cell suspension, using the cells in the tail segment. Add 1 drop of donor cells to each tube and mix.

Saline cross match—incubation: Allow tube S to stand at room temperature for 15-30 min. Then centrifuge and observe for hemolysis and agglutination, using an optical aid for the agglutination. Discard this tube.

Saline cross match—immediate spin: Immediately centrifuge tube P and observe microscopically for agglutination.

Protein cross match: Add 2 drops of 22% albumin to tube P; mix and incubate at 37° C for 15-30 min. Centrifuge and observe for hemolysis and agglutination, again using the optical aid for the agglutination.

Antiglobulin cross match: If no agglutination is observed in the protein cross match, wash the cells three or four times with saline, decanting completely after the final wash. Add 1-2 drops antiglobulin serum; mix. Centrifuge immediately and examine for agglutination with an optical aid. Add 1 drop of Coombs' control cells to all negative tubes; spin and read.

Interpretation: If no hemolysis or agglutination is seen in any phase of the cross match, the units are considered **compatible.** An **incompatible cross match** is recognized by agglutination or lysis of the donor's red

cells at any phase of the cross match. The cross match need not be continued to completion if incompatibility is detected unless (1) the behavior of the antibody is to be studied; (2) the agglutination is caused by cold agglutinins; or (3) the "least incompatible" blood is being searched for, as in cases of autoimmune hemolytic anemia.

An incompatible cross match may be caused by any of the following:

1. An error in typing of donor or recipient
2. An error in the identification of the specimen
3. The presence of an irregular antibody in the recipient's serum (see later discussion of detection of irregular antibodies and Table 15-4)
4. Dirty glassware, residual detergents in test tubes and overcentrifugation possibly resulting in false positive reactions

A compatible cross match does not rule out the presence of irregular antibodies, may not prevent immunization of the recipient, and may not detect all errors in ABO grouping and Rh typing.

Agglutination or hemolysis in the **saline cross match** will detect ABO incompatibility, cold agglutinins, and some saline-acting antibodies, e.g., anti-M, anti-N, anti-S, anti-Lu, anti-P, and anti-Le (hemolysis). If difficulties arise in the saline cross match, retype donor and recipient blood for ABO and test for cold agglutinins; suspect anti-Le if hemolysis occurs.

Agglutination or hemolysis in the **protein cross match** at 37° C detects most anti-Rh-Hr antibodies, some anti-M, anti-N, and anti-S antibodies, and some anti-Le antibodies (hemolysis). If difficulties arise in the protein cross match, retype recipient and donor for Rh, test the serum of the recipient on a panel of test cells to screen for an irregular antibody, and if present, identify it (see later discussion of detection of irregular antibodies), and test for autoantibodies; if hemolysis is noted, suspect anti-Le.

Agglutination in the **antiglobulin cross match** detects almost all anti-Rh-Hr antibodies and most immune antibodies; it is the only method to detect anti-Fy, anti-Jk, and most anti-K antibodies. If difficulties arise, test recipient serum with a panel of test cells and identify any irregular antibody encountered.

Abbreviation of major cross match

Routine use: Since the current edition of *Standards for Blood Banks and Transfusion Services*[1] does not specify a procedure for the major cross match, a great variability in technic is common among different blood banks. There are several considerations in routinely shortening the major cross match:

1. Elimination of the antiglobulin phase of the cross match in patients with a negative antibody screen: If it can be assumed that the ABO group and Rh type of both recipient and donor have been correctly performed, then the primary objective of the major cross match is to detect any preformed antibodies in the recipient's serum that are directed against donor cells. However, if in addition the recipient's serum has a negative antibody screen, then the necessity of a cross match rests on the remote possibility that donor red cells possess a low-incidence antigen absent from the

screening test cells. In an evaluation of this problem, it was concluded that only one of 1600 cross matches might fail to detect an incompatibility if the antiglobulin phase was omitted.[98] It is very important that the *antibody screen* include the antiglobulin phase. Two large hospitals have eliminated the antiglobulin cross match under these conditions with no reported problems.[98]

2. Elimination of the incubation step of the saline cross match: Some blood banks have used a one-tube cross match with room-temperature immediate spin in saline followed by the addition of albumin and antiglobulin serum; they believe any antibodies missed by eliminating the saline incubation phase of the cross match are cold IgM antibodies with little clinical significance.[98]

Emergency cross match

At times blood is needed more rapidly than the blood bank can fully process it. In such emergencies, inquire of the doctor how much time you have to select blood; many blood banks require that a legal release be signed whenever the complete compatibility testing cannot be done. Emergencies may be classified on the basis of urgency.

In an extreme emergency, when no time is available for testing, group O, Rh-negative packed red cells may be used along with plasma protein derivations. To issue group O, Rh-negative whole blood without typing or cross matching is dangerous; the danger is lessened somewhat if the blood can be shown to be of a low isoagglutinin titer. If only group O, Rh-positive blood is available, it may be given under these circumstances.

If a 15 min period is available, the patient's ABO group and Rh type should be established and un-cross matched type-specific blood released. While the patient is receiving the blood, the cross match is completed in the usual way.

If a 45 min period is available, the blood is cross matched but the incubation steps can be shortened. It is important that one set of tubes be carried out to completion in the usual manner, even after the blood has been released; any incompatibilities so detected can be indicated to the nursing unit and the transfusion stopped. The use of low−ionic strength solution (LISS) is of particular value in these circumstances.

Minor cross match

Although the minor cross match is no longer a required procedure, many blood banks continue to include it in compatibility testing. This procedure tests the donor serum for incompatibility with recipient cells. It is convenient to perform a one-tube minor cross match along with the two-tube major cross match (Table 15-5).

A third tube is added to the major cross match procedure described above; the tube is appropriately labeled to indicate the minor cross match. To this tube are added 2 drops donor serum and 1 drop 2-5% saline suspended recipient cells. It is then run in unison with the tube P in the major cross match.

Absence of agglutination or hemolysis in this tube indicates compatibility between donor serum and recipient cells. The *Standards for Blood Banks and Transfusion Services*[1] states that the minor cross match is not considered a necessary serologic investigation; careful screening of donor serum for irregular antibodies is prbably more significant.

Detection of irregular antibodies

Recipient and donor blood must be screened for irregular antibodies in advance of the transfusion and as part of compatibility testing. If an antibody is present, it is important to attempt its identification. The actual performance of the antibody screen is most conveniently done simultaneously with the cross match. Donor blood is often screened for antibodies by the collecting agency and then it need not be repeated again. Antibodies in donor blood will not be detected in any other way unless a minor cross match is performed and the recipient happens to have the corresponding antigen. Even if the recipient lacks the antigen corresponding to the donor antibody, donor antibodies may react with the blood of other donors and cause problems; it is advisable to issue such blood only as packed red cells.

In addition, the detection and identification of irregular antibodies are also important in the following instances:

1. In the serum of multiparous women, with or without a history of infants with erythroblastosis fetalis
2. In the serum of blood donors
3. In the serum of recipients of blood transfusions
4. In the red cell eluate to identify antibodies in erythroblastosis fetalis, in acquired hemolytic anemias, and in testing for weak antigens
5. History of transfusion reaction
6. History of infants with erythroblastosis fetalis
7. History of incompatible cross match
8. Failure to confirm red cell grouping by serum grouping
9. Jaundice in the newborn
10. Positive direct antiglobulin test

In all of the above conditions, testing procedures must demonstrate all significant coating, hemolyzing, and agglutinating antibodies active at 37° C.[1] It is also recommended that the routine performance of an autocontrol be run in parallel with the antibody detection tests.

Screening for irregular antibodies

The detection of irregular antibodies is most easily accomplished by using commercially prepared **screening cells.** Screening cells are group O red cells that are pooled to possess those antigens that correspond to the most frequently encountered antibodies. Obviously not all known red cell antigens will be represented, and therefore an important cause of a false negative antibody screen is the failure of the screening cells to have the antigen corresponding to the serum antibody.

It is suggested that the performance of an **autocontrol** be routinely run in parallel with the antibody detection tests. This will detect rouleaux, cold agglutinins, and autoantibodies producing a positive direct antiglobulin test.

Table 15-4. Antibodies encountered in cross matching*

Antibody	Approximate frequency in cross match	Optimal temperature of reaction (°C)	Saline tube	High protein Tube	High protein Slide	Indirect Coombs' test	Approximate percent of blood (white) compatible with antibody	Relation to human disease	Comments
Anti-B	Regular	5-20	Good	Good	Poor	No need	85	HTr-EF†	Natural antibody—immune forms; may be hemolytic
Anti-A	Regular	5-20	Good	Good	Poor	No need	55	HTr-EF	Natural antibody—immune forms; may be hemolytic
Anti-Rh_0 (D)	1 in 400	37	Usually poor	Good	Good	Often no need	16	HTr-EF	Most common immune antibody; enzyme enhanced.
Anti-Rh_6 (D + C)	1 in 600	37	Usually poor	Good	Good	Often no need	15	HTr-EF	rh' (C) alone is rare—combination frequent; enzyme enhanced
Warm autoantibody	1 in 2000	37	Poor	Fair	Fair	Good	0	?	Acquired hemolytic anemia, lupus, occasionally type specific (anti-hr'', anti-hr', etc.); enzyme enhanced
Cold agglutinin	1 in 2000	5	Good	Good	Poor	No need	0	?	Viral pneumonitis; reacts with all cells
Anti-hr' (c)	1 in 5000	37	Fair	Good	Good	Often no need	20	HTr-EF	Most common immunization in Rh-positive persons; enzyme enhanced
Anti-rh'' (E)	1 in 6000	37	Poor	Good	Good	Often no need	80	HTr-EF	Common immunization in Rh-positive persons; enzyme enhanced
Anti-hr' + rh'' (c + E)	1 in 6000	37	Poor	Good	Good	Often no need	19	HTr-EF	Combination can occur in Rh_1Rh_1 (CDe/CDe); enzyme enhanced
Anti-A_1	1 in 10,000	5	Good	Good	Poor	No need	64	HTr ?	Natural antibody occurs in A_2 and A_2B donor and recipient
Anti-K (Kell)	1 in 15,000	37	Poor	Poor	Fair	Good	92	HTr-EF	Potent antibody in erythroblastosis fetalis
Anti-Rh_0'' (D + E)	1 in 15,000	37	Poor	Good	Good	Often no need	15	HTr-EF	Combination found in Rh-negative (rh) persons (cde/cde); enzyme enhanced
Anti-Le_1 (Lewis)	1 in 20,000	20	Good	Good	Fair	Often no need	77	HTr-EF ?	Natural antibody—complex system; may be hemolytic; enzyme may enhance; combination with antiglobulin gives best results
Anti-Fy^a (Duffy)	1 in 20,000	37	Poor	Poor	Fair	Good	35	HTr-EF	Acquired by transfusion and pregnancy; enzyme may destroy
Anti-P	1 in 20,000	5-20	Good	Good	Poor	Often no need	25	HTr ?	Natural—weak—often at refrigerator temperature
Anti-M	1 in 30,000	20-37	Good	Good	Fair	Often no need	22	HTr	Natural—rarely immune; enzyme destroys antigen
Anti-Rh'_0 (C + D + E)	1 in 30,000	37	Poor	Good	Good	Often no need	14	HTr-EF	Acquired antibodies in the Rh-negative person; enzyme enhanced
Anti-Jk^a (Kidd)	1 in 30,000	37	Poor	Poor	Poor	Good	25	HTr-EF	Acquired; enzyme enhanced
Anti-rh' (C)	1 in 50,000	37	Fair	Good	Good	Often no need	33	HTr-EF	Acquired; rare in Rh-negative persons as single antibody
Anti-hr'' (e)	1 in 100,000+	37	Fair	Good	Good	Often no	2	HTr-EF	Acquired by transfusion and pregnancy in

Antibody	Rarity	°C	Saline	Albumin	Enzyme	Coombs	%	Significance	Comments
Anti-rh$_1^w$ (C^w)	1 in 100,000 +	37	Fair	Good	Good	Often no need	98	HTr ?	often with M or MN cells. Acquired; "pure" anti-rh$_1^w$ (anti-C^w) in type Rh$_1$Rh$_1$ or type Rh$_1$rh
Anti-k (Cellano)	1 in 100,000 +	37	Poor	Poor	Fair	Good	0.2	HTr-EF	Acquired; factor allelic to K
Anti-Jk^b (Kidd)		37	Poor	Poor	Poor	Good	25	HTr ?	Acquired; enzyme enhanced; factor allelic to Jk^a
Anti-Fy^b (Duffy)		37	Poor	Poor	Poor	Good	17	HTr	Acquired; enzyme may destroy; factor allelic to Fy^a
Anti-Lu^a (Lutheran)		20-37	Good	Good	Poor	Often no need	92	?	Acquired; enzyme may destroy
Anti-hr (f)		37	Fair	Good	Good	Often no need	35	?	Acquired; positive with cells of individuals having gene r or gene R^0, enzyme enhanced
Anti-N		20-37	Good	Good	Poor	No need	28	HTr ?	Natural; enzyme destroys antigen
Anti-s		37	Poor	Poor	Poor	Good	11	HTr ?-EF	Acquired; related to MN system; factor allelic to S
Anti-Le^H (Le^b)		20	Fair	Fair	Poor	Often no need	22	?	Le^H reactions are reliable with A$_2$ and O cells—difficult to type bloods for this
Anti-U		37	Poor	Fair	Fair	Good	0	HTr-EF	Acquired only by S-negative, s-negative person; compatible donor rare and only black blood
Anti-Tj^a		20-37	Good	Good	Poor	No need	0	? Miscarriages	Natural; related to P system
Anti-Vel		37	Poor	Poor	Poor	Good	0	HTr	Only about 4 in 10,000 fail to react
Anti-H		5	Good	Good	Poor	No need	0	?	Rare as strong antibody—also reacts most strongly with group O and A$_2$ cells; anti-H inhibited by saliva of secretors
Anti-Lu^b (Lutheran)		20-37	Good	Good	Poor	No need	0.2	?	Rare; existence only recently proved
Anti-He (Henshaw)		20	Good	Good	Poor	No need	100	EF	Related to MN system; reacts with a few black bloods
Anti-Di^a (Diego)		37	Poor	Poor	Poor	Good	100	EF	Corresponding factor found in South American Indians and Orientals
Anti-Wr^a (Wright) or anti-Ca		37	Fair	Fair	Fair	Often no need	100	HTr ?-EF	May be natural; antibody may be frequent
Anti-Ven		37	Poor	Poor	Poor	Good	100	EF	Reacts only with family
Anti-Hu (Hunter)		20-37	Good	Good	Fair	No need	100	?	Related to MN system; reacts only with 21% of black bloods

Modified from Dade Diagnostics, Miami.

*Low-frequency factors, e.g., Be^a, Becker, Ca, Gr. Jobbins, Levay, Mi^a, and R$_m$, react with family members and rarely anyone else (private antigens). High-frequency factors, e.g., I, Vel, Yt^a, and Kp^b, react with almost all cells tested (public antigens). Reactions given are those usually found and recorded. Antibodies made by different persons may react differently; e.g., one person's anti-Le may react in saline solution; another Le$_1$ may be detected only by indirect Coombs' test; likewise with anti-S, etc.

Table 15-5. A scheme for compatibility testing*

Test performed	Minor cross match	Major cross match	Antibody screen	Antibody screen	Autocontrol	Conditions of test	Test phase
Test tube set no. 1	Donor serum, 2 drops, + Recipient cells, 1 drop	Recipient serum, 2 drops, + Donor cells, 1 drop	Recipient serum, 2 drops, + Screen cells no. 1, 1 drop	Recipient serum, 2 drops, + Screen cells no. 2, 1 drop	Recipient serum, 2 drops, + Recipient cells, 1 drop	Spin and read. / Add 22% albumin, incubate at 37° C; spin and read. / Add antiglobulin serum; spin and read.	Saline at RT, IS / High protein / Antiglobulin
Test tube set no. 2		Recipient serum, 2 drops, + Donor cells, 1 drop	Recipient serum, 2 drops, + Screen cells no. 1, 1 drop	Recipient serum, 2 drops, + Screen cells no. 2, 1 drop	Recipient serum, 2 drops, + Recipient cells, 1 drop	Incubate at RT. Spin and read.	Saline at RT Incubation

*RT, Room temperature; IS, immediate spin.

The procedure involves mixing 2 drops of fresh serum from the person to be tested with 1 drop of a 5% saline suspension of screening cells; usually two different lots of cells are used separately to encorporate a greater variety of antigens. In the autocontrol, the person's serum is mixed with 1 drop of a 5% saline suspension of his own cells. Both antibody screen and autocontrol are run to parallel the cross match procedure: two tubes with screening cells no. 1, two tubes with screening cells no. 2, and two tubes with autologous cells. One tube of this set is run parallel with tube S and the other tube is run parallel with tube P in the major cross match procedure (Table 15-5). In this manner the following conditions are met:

1. Saline room temperature, immediate spin, and incubation
2. High protein phase, 37° C
3. Indirect antiglobulin test (essentially a direct antiglobulin test in the autocontrol)

Absence of agglutination and hemolysis indicates that no atypical antibodies or autoantibodies are present. After the screening test has established the presence of atypical antibodies, they must be identified by the panel cell technic.

Identification of irregular antibodies

Any unexplained reaction in the antibody screen or compatibility tests must be investigated; this is usually done by testing the serum with a panel of reagent red cells in the same test phases as the antibody screen: saline room temperature, albumin at 37° C, and antiglobulin phase.

Procedure: Label 12 × 75 mm test tubes to accommodate the entire panel of cells; use an additional tube for the autocontrol. Add 1 drop of each panel cell to the corresponding tube; add 1 drop of a 5% saline suspension of autologous cells to the autocontrol. Add 2 drops of the serum to be tested to all tubes. Carry the tubes through the test phases as with the antibody screen.

If a positive result is encountered in any of these phases, record the strength of the reaction; always carry the procedure to completion through the antiglobulin phase.

In some instances, additional test conditions will be useful:

1. A cold temperature phase with saline-suspended cells may be very informative; reduce the incubating temperature to 4° C.
2. An enzyme phase is not used routinely but may be added in special situations requiring very sensitive technics (see discussion of special test procedures: enzyme testing).

Common results:

1. Autocontrol negative, some or all panel cells positive: One or more antibodies are present. If all panel cells are positive, it may indicate an antibody against a high-incidence antigen.
2. Autocontrol negative, all panel cells negative: This may indicate an antibody to a low-frequency antigen; in this instance most cross matches will be compatible and no difficulty is encountered in obtaining compatible blood. It may also indicate

Table 15-6. Antibody identification chart

Patient: Name   Number   Group O   Rh type: Rh neg.   (cde/cde)   Direct Coombs' test: Neg.   Autoagglutinins: Neg.

Test cells	Specificities of panel cells*																	Reactions of unknown serum					

																		Saline			Albumin		
Test cells	Rh_0 (D)	rh' (C)	rh" (E)	hr' (c)	hr" (e)	M	N	S	s	P_1	K	k	Fy^a	Js^a	Jk^b	Le_1 (Le^a)	Le^H (Le^b)	22°	37°	AHG†	37°	AHG†	Bromelin
1	+	+	−	−	+	+	+	+	+	+	−	+	−	+	−	+	−	−	−	±	+	+	+
2	+	−	−	+	+	+	−	−	+	+	−	+	−	−	+	+	−	−	−	±	+	+	++
3	+	−	+	+	−	−	+	+	+	+	+	−	+	+	+	−	−	−	−	+	++	++	++
4	+	−	−	+	+	+	+	+	+	−	+	−	+	−	−	+	−	−	−	−	−	−	−
5	+	+	−	−	+	−	+	−	+	+	+	−	+	+	+	+	−	−	−	−	+	+	+
6	−	−	−	+	+	+	+	+	+	−	+	+	+	−	+	−	+	−	−	−	−	−	−
7	−	+	−	+	+	+	+	+	+	+	−	+	+	+	+	+	−	−	−	−	+	+	−
8	+	+	−	−	−	−	+	+	−	+	−	+	−	−	−	−	−	−	−	−	++	++	+
9	−	−	+	−	−	+	−	−	−	+	−	+	+	+	−	−	−	−	−	−	++	++	−
10					Autologous red cells													−	−	−	−	−	−

Directions for use of antibody identification chart

1. Cross out antigens present on panel cells not agglutinated by unknown serum.
2. Circle remaining antigens.
3. Evaluation:
   a. Antibody(ies) present: anti-Rh_0 (D) and anti-rh" (E)
   b. Antibody(ies) not ruled out: none
4. What panel cells should be used for absorbing?
   a. No. 2 for anti-Rh_0
   b. No. 9 for anti-rh"

*Antigens in panel: D̄,C̄,(E),c̄,ē,M,N̄,S̄,s,P_1,K,k,Fy^a,Js^a,Jk^b,Le^a,Le^b.
†AHG, Anti–human globulin test.

an irregular antibody of the ABO system (e.g., anti-A$_1$) that is not detected because the panel cells are of group O; in this instance many cross matches may be incompatible.

3. Autocontrol positive, some or all panel cells positive: An autoantibody is present, and an alloantibody is also present; or only an autoantibody is present with a broad range of thermal activity.

4. Autocontrol positive, all panel cells positive and both are stronger at 4° C, weaker at 37° C, and weak or absent at the antiglobulin phase: Cold antibodies or rouleaux are present.

Use and interpretation of cell panels: Examine the completed antibody detection work sheet (Table 15-6). Select the first cell that has a negative reaction in all test phases; this is cell no. 4. Cross out the antigenic determinants that are present on that cell: c, e, M, N, S, s, P$_1$, K, and Jk^b.

Repeat the above procedure with the next panel cells that do not react: nos. 6 and 7. The following antigens can be eliminated: Fy^a, Le^a, C, k, Jk^a, and Le^b.

The remaining antigens, i.e., D and E, are both suspect because the antibody specificity may be directed against either one or both of these antigens. Do all the cells containing these antigens react? The answer is "yes." Do all the panel cells reacting contain both factors? The answer is "no": Cell no. 9 reacts but contains only antigen E; the other cells reacting, i.e., nos. 1, 2, 3, 5, and 8 all contain antigen D, and cell no. 3 contains both antigens.

The conclusion is that two alloantibodies are present: anti-D and anti-E.

It can then be determined if the autologous cells lack these antigens; this is done by using specific typing sera.

In some instances all panel cells are reactive and it is very difficult to eliminate antigens from consideration. Then it is very important to examine the reaction patterns that may be present. Generally, if all positive cells react with equal strength, it is suggestive of a single antibody. Variation in strength of reaction may indicate multiple antibodies reacting preferentially in different media; or the variation may indicate an antibody showing **dosage effect**, i.e., an antibody that is stronger with cells carrying a double dose of the corresponding antigen (homozygous). Tables 15-7 and 15-8 characterize many antibodies as a guide to their identification.

In some instances it may be necessary to absorb the suspected antibodies from the serum and identify them by using red cells selected to possess only one of the antigens under consideration.

Table 15-7. Tentative identification of antibody specificity*

| Technic | Temperature (° C) | Frequency (%) of positive reactions with random blood samples | | | | |
		0-10	10-50	50-75	75-90	90-100
Saline and/or albumin	4-22	Lu^a i	Le^a	Le^b N	P$_1$ M	I
Saline and/or albumin	22-37	rh^{wl} (C^w) Lu^a	rh″ (E) Le^a S	rh′ (C) Le^b	Rh$_0$ (D) hr′ (c) s	hr″ (e) Lu^b Ve^a
Saline and/or albumin plus antiglobulin technic	37	rh^{wl} (C^w) K Kp^a Lu^a Di^a Yt^b	rh″ (E) Le^a S Js^a	rh′ (C) Le^b Fy^a Jk^b Xg^a Do^a	Rh$_0$ (D) hr′ (c) Fy^b s Jk^a Au^a	hr″ (e) k U Kp^b Ge^a Lu^b Yt^a Ve^a Js^b Di^b
Enzyme	37	rh^{wl} (C^w)	rh″ (E) Le^a	rh′ (C) Le^b	Rh$_0$ (D) hr′ (c)	hr″ (e)
Enzyme plus antiglobulin technic	37	rh^{wl} (C^w)	rh″ (E) Le^a	rh′ (C) Le^b Jk^b Do^a	Rh$_0$ (D) hr′ (c) Jk^a	hr″ (e)
Hemolysis of saline-suspended cells	37		Le^a	Le^b Jk^b	Jk^a	Ve^a
Hemolysis of enzyme-treated cells	37		Le^a	Le^b Jk^b	Jk^a P$_1$	Ve^a
All technics and temperatures			Le^a			PP$_1$

From Technical methods and procedures of the American Association of Blood Banks, Chicago, 1971, American Association of Blood Banks.
*The special behavior of anti-H should be noted. This antibody usually reacts on saline cell suspensions from 4-22° C. and sometimes by an enzymatic technic at 37° C. It may be found in the sera of A$_1$, A$_1$B, or sometimes B persons. It reacts most strongly with O and A$_2$ cells and weakly or not at all with cells of the same ABO group as the person who made the antibody.

Type and screen only

A common practice in many blood banks is to ABO and Rh type a patient's serum and screen for atypical antibodies without proceeding to a definitive cross match until the actual need for blood replacement is realized. It has been generally accepted that the ratio of the units of blood cross matched to the units of blood transfused (C/T ratio) should be approximately 2.5:1.[99] This means that 2.5 times as many units of blood are cross matched than are actually used. In actual practice, however, the C/T ratio is considerably higher, i.e., in the range of 4:1.[100] This means that many more units are cross matched than used, and this is believed to be a reflection of inefficiency in blood ordering practices. Such inefficiency in blood ordering generally derives from the routine request for cross matching for patient who actually show only a remote possibility for requiring a transfusion. The inefficient ordering practices are a financial deficit and place a severe strain on limited blood supplies.

As a result the type and screen practice has gained popularity in that the patient's blood has been examined and can quickly be cross matched when the need for blood arises. This has been used predominantly for some presurgical cross match orders. At times this necessitates an abbreviated cross match procedure.[101]

Pediatric transfusion

Infants and young children[102] will often require only a portion of a unit of blood; consequently it is necessary to aseptically separate small volumes into transfer packs. The compatibility testing is performed in the usual manner. It is advisable to always include a minor cross match in this age group because donor antibodies are not greatly diluted in the smaller plasma volume of the young recipients. In the pediatric age groups a positive direct antiglobulin test is a common occurrence, and this will result in an incompatibility in the minor cross match procedure.

It may be difficult to obtain enough blood for the compatibility testing by the usual means. One alternative is to perform a skin puncture with a lancet and collect blood into three large nonheparinized capillary tubes (4 mm diameter). One tube is used for ABO and Rh type, another for antibody screen, and the last for cross match procedures. These tubes can be easily centrifuged to yield serum, which can be subsequently aspirated by dry microcapillary tubes.

Table 15-8. Characteristics of certain blood group antibodies

Antibody	Preferred method or medium for detection	Optimal temperature range (° C)
Anti-A Anti-A₁ Anti-B Anti-H	Saline	4-20°
Anti-Rh₀ Anti-hr′	High-protein, antiglobulin, enzyme	37°
Anti-K Anti-k	Antiglobulin	37°
Anti-Fyᵃ Anti-Fyᵇ	Antiglobulin	37°
Anti-Jkᵃ Anti-Jkᵇ	Antiglobulin (anti-non-gamma and complement needed)	37°
Anti-Leᵃ	Saline, enzyme, antiglobulin (anti-non-gamma and complement needed)	20-37°
Anti-Leᵇ	Saline	4-20°
Anti-Luᵃ	Saline	20-37°
Anti-Luᵇ	Saline, antiglobulin	20-37°
Anti-M Anti-N	Saline	4-20°
Anti-S	Saline, antiglobulin	20-37°
Anti-s	Antiglobulin	37°
Anti-U	Saline, antiglobulin	37°
Anti-P₁	Saline	4-15°
Anti-P (Tj)	Saline	20-37°

From Hyland reference manual of immunohematology, Costa Mesa, Calif., 1964, Hyland Laboratories, p. 100.

TRANSFUSION OF NONSPECIFIC BLOOD

Under certain circumstances, group A or B blood is chosen for group AB recipients and group O blood is chosen for group A, B, or AB recipients.

Group A or B blood to AB recipients

If type-specific blood is not available, packed cells of low-titer A or B blood may be given to a group AB patient.

Group O blood for recipients of other blood groups

Group O blood should be given to other than group O recipients only in the following circumstances:
1. A dire emergency (see earlier discussion of emergency transfusions)
2. No other blood is available
3. The recipient's blood group cannot be determined
4. Exchange transfusion in erythroblastosis fetalis
5. The only blood available that lacks the factor to which the patient is sensitized

If time permits, packed red cells only should be administered, since the plasma contains the anti-A and anti-B antibodies. The safety with which group O blood can be administered to individuals of other than group O depends not only on the titer of the saline-acting anti-A and anti-B antibodies but, even more important, on the presence of immune anti-A or anti-B antibodies, which cannot be neutralized by the addition of group-specific substances.

Generally, O blood is considered safe if the titer of both isoagglutinins is less than 1:20. Two tests may be used to determine the **safety of group O blood:** the test for hemolysins and the screening test for isoagglutinin titer.

Test for hemolysins

Procedure: Label two test tubes, A and B. Add 0.5 ml fresh donor serum (complement present) to each tube. Add 0.5 ml 2-4% saline suspension of fresh, washed A cells to tube A and of B cells to tube B. Mix and incubate at 37° C for 15 min. Centrifuge and examine for hemolysis (pink color of supernatant).

Interpretation: Hemolytic activity in the specimen render the donor's blood unsafe for other than group O recipients.

Screening test for isoagglutinin titer of group O blood

Procedure: Dilute donor's serum 1:20 in saline by adding 0.5 ml serum to 9.5 ml saline solution. Label two test tubes, A and B. Add 0.1 ml diluted serum to each test tube. Add 0.1 ml 2% suspension of A cells to tube A and 0.1 ml 2% suspension of B cells to tube B. Mix and allow to incubate at room temperature for 15 min. Centrifuge for 15 sec, dislodge the cell button gently, and observe macroscopically for agglutination or hemolysis.

Interpretation: If agglutination occurs in either tube, the titer is higher than 1:20 and the blood cannot be considered to be of low titer. The saline agglutinin titer does not necessarily reflect the immune antibody titer, which is the more important titer.

Screening test for immune anti-A and anti-B (neutralization test)

Blood group–specific substances A and B (Witebsky substance) are used to neutralize the anti-A and anti-B isohemagglutinins of group O blood. One unit (vial) is sufficient to reduce the anti-A and anti-B in 5 dl of O blood to less than one fourth of its original titer. The A and B specific substances, however, are ineffective against immune anti-A and anti-B. There is evidence that they are antigenic.

A and B blood group–specific substances are found in the saliva and in the gastric juice of most individuals (called **secretors**), as well as in the red cells and tissues. They are found widely distributed in both plants and animals. The commercial products are made chiefly from the gastric mucosa of hogs and horses, the former containing highly potent A but no B and the latter substance containing both A and B and rarely pure B.

Principle: Blood group–specific substances A and B have the capacity to combine specifically with anti-A and anti-B isoagglutinins, thus preventing these antibodies from agglutinating A and B cells.

Procedure: To 0.2 ml serum, add 0.2 ml blood group–specific substances A and B. Add 3.6 ml saline solution to produce a dilution of 1:20. Mix and incubate at room temperature for 5 min.

Test 2 drops of neutralized serum with 2 drops of 2% saline suspension of A cells in a test tube marked A. Repeat the same procedure with B cells in a tube marked B. Mix and incubate at room temperature for 10 min.

Centrifuge for 15 sec and examine macroscopically for agglutination using an optical aid. If agglutination occurs in either tube, repeat the serum neutralization using 0.8 ml group-specific substances A and B to 0.2 ml serum. If no agglutination occurs, test for immune antibodies by incubating the tubes at 37°C for 30 min.

Wash cells three times with saline, decanting well after the final wash. Add 2 drops of antiglobulin serum, spin, and observe for agglutination with an optical aid.

Interpretation: If agglutination occurs after centrifugation, the ABO agglutinins have not been neutralized completely and the test should be repeated as outlined in the next step.

If agglutination does not occur after centrifugation and does not occur in the antiglobulin procedure, nonneutralized antibodies at a titer above 1:20 are present. The blood should not be given to any but a group O recipient.

MASSIVE TRANSFUSIONS

During massive transfusions[103] the following difficulties may develop:

1. Coagulation abnormalities[104]: There is a dilutional thrombocytopenia and a loss of labile coagulation factors V and VIII; diffuse intravascular coagulation and fibrinolysis may be seconday to a major transfusion reaction.

2. Alteration of hemoglobin function: A shift in the oxyhemoglobin dissociation curve is caused by diminished 2,3-DPG levels of stored red cells, resulting in increased oxygen affinity of hemoglobin.

3. Acid-base imbalance: Stored blood has excess acidity because of the citric acid of the anticoagulant and the lactic acid generated by red cell metabolism during storage.

4. Citrate overload and a fall in ionized calcium.[105]

5. Microembolization: Stored blood contains tiny aggregates composed of degenerated platelets and fibrin; these particles pass through common blood filters, presumably lodging in the pulmonary circulation. They have been implicated in the development of acute respiratory insufficiency after massive transfusions. Micropore filters are available to remove much of this accumulated debris.[106]

6. Circulatory overload.

AUTOLOGOUS TRANSFUSIONS

Autologous transfusions refer to the removal and storage of blood or blood components from a donor with subsequent reinfusion.[1] There are two basic types of autologous transfusion: the **predeposit autologous transfusion** and the **intraoperative autologous transfusion.**

Predeposit autologous transfusion

Principle: A patient donates his blood at some time prior to its expected reinfusion. Both the donation and storage of this blood are identical to conventional blood procedures. Usually a large number of units are donated in a short period of time; it is advisable to treat these donors with prophylactic oral iron.[107] Aseptically collected and infused autologous blood is always compatible and free of reactions because the donor and the recipient are one and the same.

Donor criteria[108]:

1. Age: There is no age limitation.

2. Weight: There are no weight requirements. However, it is recommended that no greater than 10-12% of the estimated blood volume be removed at any one time. If the patient-donor weighs less than 45 kg (100 lbs), the amount of anticoagulant must be reduced according to the following formula:

$$\text{Amount of anticoagulant to be used} =$$
$$\text{Normal anticoagulant volume} \times \frac{\text{Donated blood (ml)}}{450 \text{ ml}}$$

3. Hemoglobin: The donor's hemoglobin must be no less than 11 g/dl or the hematocrit no less than 34%.

4. Frequency of donation: Donations must not be any more frequent than every 4 days. A donation should not be allowed within 3 days of the expected reinfusion unless an adequate blood volume can be maintained.

Storage: The duration of storage must not exceed 21 days for ACD- or CPD-anticoagulated blood stored in the liquid phase. It is possible that some autologous blood may become outdated before reinfusion is needed. To prevent wastage, the outdated unit is reinfused immediately after withdrawal of a fresh unit. Because donation is not more frequent than every 4 days, only a limited number of units (5 units maximum) can be collected prior to outdating.[109] Use of CPD-adenine anticoagulant solution with its longer shelf life will increase the number of units available. Freezing autologous red cells allows a great number of units to be stored for very long periods of time.

Pretransfusion testing and labeling: According to the AABB Standards,[1] autologous blood need only be tested for ABO group. The results of this test are then denoted on the label affixed to the unit of autologous blood. An antibody screen and HBsAg test are optional. An ABO test must also be performed on the recipient just prior to infusion, and this result must agree with the label on the unit of donor autologous blood. This latter step is an effort to prevent clerical error with subsequent ABO incompatibility. Autologous blood tested in this manner may only be used for autologous transfusions.

More ideally, therefore, autologous blood should be tested in the same manner as homologous donor blood. Then, if all criteria for blood selection are met, including negative reactions for HBsAg and syphilis serology, this blood may be released for homologous infusion when not used by the autologous donor. Even though more extensive testing has been performed, if the autologous blood shows positivity either for the hepatitis antigen or syphilis serology, this blood is not suitable for homologous use; a label affixed to the unit must clearly indicate that it may be used for **autologous transfusion only**. In this event any unused antologous blood must be discarded.

Routine labeling of autologous blood should include the following information:

1. The ABO group of the donor

2. The donor's name, signature, and identification number

3. The date of donation and date of expiration,

4. The amount of blood collected and the kind and amount of anticoagulant used

5. A special label indicating autologous use, which may be removed when the need for autologous transfusion has passed, providing the blood has met criteria that are required for homologous infusion

Advantages:

1. A source of blood for patients who are difficult to transfuse because of rare blood types or the presence of alloantibodies

2. A source of blood for patients who react adversely to all homologous blood (febrile or allergic transfusion reactions)

3. A source of blood for patients who refuse homologous blood because of religious beliefs

4. The elimination of graft vs. host disease

5. The prevention of alloimmunization to the formed elements in the blood

6. A reduction of demands on an inadequate blood supply

7. The prevention of transmission of blood-borne diseases, especially serum hepatitis

Intraoperative autologous transfusion

Principle: Intraoperative autotransfusion is the reinfusion of blood from the operative field back into the patient. Its greatest application is in surgical procedures involving excessive blood loss; it can also be used in patients suffering trauma with subsequent hemorrhage. In either instance retrieved shed blood can be reinfused without serologic evaluation. The blood is usually reinfused during the operative procedure or immediately afterward; it may not be used if more than 24 hr have elapsed after its collection. Such blood is never available for homologous use.

Procedures: Different commercial devices are available for use,[110] all of which incorporate the following essential steps:

1. Aspiration of blood from the operative field: It is important to prevent red cell hemolysis, which easily occurs from the traumatic aspiration, compression effects of roller pumps, and turbulent flow with foaming in the tubing collection reservoirs. Some of these hazards can be prevented by carefully aspirating only pooled blood.

2. Anticoagulation of the aspirated blood: This can be accomplished by systemic heparinization prior to surgery, or by instilling heparin or CPD into the aspiration line, or both.

3. Filtration of the aspirated, collected blood: It is important to remove as much particulate matter as possible before reinfusion. The procedure usually involves two separate filtration steps, one of which may employ a micropore filter.

4. Reinfusion of the processed blood.

One of the devices available is a continuous-flow centrifugation instrument that removes unwanted debris by high-speed centrifugation, followed by thorough washing of the remaining blood cells. Any excess free hemoglobin or anticoagulant is removed with the wash solutions; the red cells are subsequently resuspended to a desired hematocrit in an electrolyte solution and are reinfused.

Advantages:
1. Serologically compatible blood is always available for hemorrhaging patients regardless of the status of bank blood.
2. A useful product is not wasted, and the demands for homologous blood supplies are reduced.

Complications:[111]
1. Microembolization from fat, denatured protein, and platelet or leukocyte aggregates
2. Air embolism
3. Hemolysis
4. Thrombocytopenia
5. Disseminated intravascular coagulation

Contraindications:
1. Enteric contamination of the shed blood
2. Presence of malignant cells in the operative field
3. A grossly contaminated surgical field
4. Renal or hepatic dysfunction or both

HEPATITIS TESTING

Hepatitis developing after the infusion of blood or blood products is referred to as **serum hepatitis** or **hepatitis B.** The disease characteristically has a long incubation period (6 weeks to 6 months) and can be transmitted by the fecal, oral, and venereal routes, as well as parenterally.[112]

Antigens and antibodies

The hepatitis B virus was isolated in 1965.[113] With the aid of the electron microscope, it has been visualized as a double-shelled particle, 42 nm in diameter.[114] The intact particle is believed to be the infectious agent responsible for the disease; it is referred to as the **Dane particle.** The Dane particle consists of an inner and outer structure, both of which are antigenically distinct. The inner core measures 28 nm; the antigen it contains is called the **core antigen (HBcAg).** The outer protein coat contains another antigen referred to as the **surface antigen (HBsAg).** An excess of surface antigen is produced by the diseased liver and is released into the blood, where it circulates as 20 nm spheric and tubular particles. All the common laboratory tests that are currently used to detect the hepatitis B virus measure the surface antigen. Formerly, the surface antigen was called the **Austria antigen (AuAg)** or the **hepatitis-associated antigen (HAAB).** Antisurface (anti-HBs) and anti-core (anti-HBc) antibodies form in response to these antigens and can be detected in the blood by radioimmunoassay.

Many newer markers have been uncovered. The surface coat of the Dane particle may be subtyped according to the presence of additional protein antigens: **a, d** or **y, w** or **r.**[115] The main subtypes are **adw, ayw, adr,** and **ayr.** Subtypes can be determined by radioimmunoassay and are useful in epidemiologic studies of serum hepatitis. Another antigen, distinct from HBsAg or HBcAg but definitely associated with the hepatitis B virus, is the **e antigen.** The presence of HBeAg has been correlated with active virus replication and infectivity.[116] Both HBeAg and anti-HBe can be measured by radioimmunoassay.[117] Finally, the central core of the Dane particle replicates DNA and a hepatitis B–specific **DNA polymerase** has been isolated that may also be related to infectivity.[118, 119]

Methods of HBsAg testing
Indications

Federal regulations[120] require blood to be tested for hepatitis B virus if it is to be used in any of the following ways:
1. For transfusion
2. For the production of plasma fractions
3. For the manufacture of laboratory reagents
4. For the artificial stimulation of antibody production in donors

In addition, testing is desirable to aid in the diagnosis of clinical hepatitis B disease.

Methods

Many tests have been used to detect the surface antigen of the hepatitis B virus, including the following, listed in the order of increasing sensitivity:
1. Agar precipitation
   a. Agar gel diffusion
   b. Rheophoresis
   c. Counterelectrophoresis
2. Complement fixation
3. Hemagglutination inhibition
4. Reverse passive hemagglutination
5. Enzyme immunoassay
6. Radioimmunoassay, solid phase

These tests have been categorized by the FDA into first, second, and third ''generation'' tests, based on their sensitivity. The first generation test includes only agar gel diffusion, the least sensitive but one of the most specific tests. Second generation tests include rheophoresis, counterelectrophoresis, complement fixation, and hemagglutination inhibition. These tests have similar sensitivity, being approximately 10 times more sensitive than agar gel diffusion. The third generation tests include reverse passive hemagglutination (10 times more sensitive than second generation tests), radioimmunoassay (500 times as sensitive as second generation tests and 1000 times as sensitive as agar gel diffusion), and enzyme immunoassay (sensitivity slightly less than radioimmunoassay).[121]

When the FDA initially required testing for hepatitis B virus, it had to be performed using a method at least equal in sensitivity to counterelectrophoresis. This ruling was supplanted in 1975 when the requirement was changed to demand the use of a third generation test.

Radioimmunoassay:

Principle: A solid phase radioimmunoassay (RIA) utilizing the sandwich technique[122] is the basis of all currently licensed RIA test systems. They all employ antibody bound to a solid matrix surface (tubes or beads manufactured from polystyrene, polyvinyl, or polypropylene). Serum is added to the solid matrix and, if HBsAg is present, it will combine with the bound antibody during a short period of incubation. After the serum is removed and rinsed thoroughly, radioactive anti-HBs is added and allowed to coat the remaining antigen binding sites, thereby completing the sandwich: antibody-antigen-antibody. After a final rinse to remove unbound radioactive antibody, the solid matrix is counted. Both positive and negative controls are run along with the unknown sample; the test is considered positive when the radioactivity of the sample tube is at least 2.1 times greater than that of the average for normal negative controls.

Procedure: Place an antibody-coated tube or bead into each reaction well of a plastic plate, allowing one well for the unknown serum, six or seven wells for negative controls, and three wells for positive controls. Add 0.2 ml serum to the appropriate wells; cover and incubate 2 hr at 45° C. Aspirate serum and wash each tube or bead twice with 5 ml distilled water.

Add 0.2 ml ^{125}I-labeled anti-HBs to the reaction well; cover and incubate 2 hr at 45° C. Aspirate and wash twice with 5 ml distilled water.

Place each tube or bead into a counting tube and count for 1 min in a γ-spectrometer; subtract the background count and calculate the difference between the sample tube and the average of the normal negative controls.

Interpretation: Any serum sample with a count greater than 2.1 times the negative controls is considered to contain HBsAg unless specificity testing proves otherwise (see later discussion of confirmation of positivity).

Advantages:
1. RIA has greater sensitivity than any other third generation test.
2. An objective answer is obtained.
3. It is semiautomated.

Disadvantages:
1. There is a lack of standards for quality control.
2. There may be a lack of reproducibility of borderline results because of the random nature of radioactive emission.
3. There are inherent problems of waste disposal and hazards of radiation.
4. The shelf life of reagents is very short, approximately 45 days.
5. False positive results may occur because of inadequate washings or cross contamination of specimens; it may also depend on the antibody system used. All positive results must be confirmed as positive before the serum can be labeled **positive** for hepatitis B virus.

Confirmation of positivity: All serum specimens that are positive by radioimmunoassay must be confirmed before reporting the result.

1. Repeat the test using RIA. If the test is still positive, perform specificity testing in either of the ways mentioned below.

2. Use another test procedure: counterelectrophoresis or agar-gel diffusion. Agar precipitation is particularly desirable because it may reveal lines of identity to absolutely confirm specificity.

3. Do the neutralization test. If HBsAg is really present in the test sample, it will be neutralized by the addition of high-titer human anti-HBs serum. After incubation of the serums (0.03 ml each) for 2 hr at 37° C, the test serum is again retested with RIA. If the final count is equal to or less than 50% of the original count, specificity is confirmed.

Enzyme immunoassay

Principle: The principle of enzyme immunoassay (EIA)[123,124] is very similar to that for solid phase RIA utilizing the sandwich technic. A solid support is coated with anti-HBs and allowed to react with test serum. If the antigen is present, it will bind to the solid matrix. In this procedure the second antibody is tagged with an enzyme rather than radioactive iodine. A sandwich is again formed. After washing away any unbound enzyme-labeled antibody, an appropriate substrate is added that reacts with the enzyme present. The resulting color is monitored and measured in a spectrophotometer; the intensity of the color is directly proportional to the concentration of the antigen that is present.

Advantages:
1. There is an objective end point.
2. The enzyme-conjugated antibody is more stable than isotopically labeled antibody and has a shelf life of up to 6 months.
3. The sensitivity of the test is very high, similar to RIA.

Disadvantages:
1. Because the test is ultimately based on an enzymatic reaction, temperature of pH variations will affect the sensitivity and specificity of the test.
2. A relatively large volume of serum is required: 0.5 ml.
3. False positive reactions may be related to the antibody system used. In order to confirm positivity, an agar precipitation technic may be used or human anti-HBs may be added for neutralization prior to the final addition of enzyme-labeled anti-HBs.

Reverse passive hemagglutination:

Principle: In reverse passive hemagglutination (RPHA)[125] indicator red cells are coated with purified anti-HBs. When allowed to incubate with serum containing HBsAg, the red cells will agglutinate. An incubation period of 2 hr is required at room temperature, and the reaction plates must be maintained in a vibration-free setting to allow proper settling of the red cells: A solid button indicates a negative test, and an irregular, matted appearance indicates a positive test.

Advantages:
1. The test has high sensitivity, although it is not as sensitive as RIA.
2. It is easy to perform.
3. It is rapid, with results in slightly over 2 hr.
4. The shelf life of the reagents is approximately 6 months.

Disadvantages:
1. The end point is a subjective interpretation, and settling patterns are easily altered, leading to false negative results.
2. False positive results may occur at an incidence of 1-2%. To confirm positivity, an agar precipitation technic can be used. In addition, a neutralization test may be performed in which the test serum is first exposed to human anti-HBs before adding the coated red cells. Positive results are confirmed if the results are four times less than with untreated serum.

Posttransfusion hepatitis

Despite the long-term screening of donor blood for HBsAg by very sensitive methods, transfusion-associated hepatitis still occurs. It is estimated that 5-15% of transfused patients will develop hepatitis, and that 200,000 cases of transfusion-associated hepatitis[126] occur annually, characterized by the following facts:

1. The incidence of the disease is directly related to the number of units of blood or blood products received.

2. Certain blood products have a greatly increased risk of transmitting hepatitis, i.e., fibrinogen, prothrombin complex concentrates,[127] and factor VIII concentrates.[128]

3. Frozen red cells are associated with a reduced incidence of the disease but do not completely eliminate the infectious agent.[129]

4. Pooled plasma products that are heat treated may transmit the disease if improperly prepared,[130] i.e., albumin, plasma protein fraction, and immune serum globulin.

5. Careful donor selection is necessary to reduce the incidence of the disease; volunteer donors have a low prevalence of HBsAg.

6. Posttransfusion hepatitis is not caused by the hepatitis A virus.[131]

7. Most cases of posttransfusion hepatitis are caused by a virus or a group of related viruses, referred to as the **non-A, non-B hepatitis virus** or **hepatitis C virus.**[132] Current tests do not detect these viruses.

REFERENCES

1. Standards for blood banks and transfusion services, ed. 9, Washington, D.C., 1978, American Association of Blood Banks.
2. FDA Drug Bull. **8:**21, 1978.
3. Strumia, M.M., Dugan, A., and Colwell, L.S.: Blood **19:**115, 1962.
4. Dern, R.J., Brewer, G.J., and Wiorkowski, J.J.: J. Lab. Clin. Med. **69:**968, 1967.
5. Lerner, M.H., and Rubinstein, D.: Biochim. Biophys. Acta **224:**301, 1970.
6. Moore, G.L., Ledford, M.E., and Brooks, D.E.: Transfusion **18:**538, 1978.
7. Beutler, E.: Vox Sang. **19:**546, 1970.
8. deVerdier, C.-H., et al.: Communications of the Thirteenth Congress of the International Society for Blood Transfusion, Washington, D.C., 1972.
9. deVerdier, C.-H.: Vox Sang. **16:**361, 1969.
10. Dawson, R.B.: Transfusion **17:**525, 1977.
11. Moseley, R.V., and Doty, D.B.: Ann. Surg. **171:**329, 1970.
12. Fulton, R.L.: Vox Sang. **32:**315, 1977.
13. McDanal, J.T., et al.: Surg. Forum **26:**213, 1975.
14. Reul, G.J., et al.: Arch. Surg. **106:**386, 1973.
15. International Forum: Vox Sang. **31:**368, 1976.
16. Walker, R.H.: In Greenwalt, T.J., and Jamieson, G.A., editors: Transmissible disease and blood transfusion, New York, 1975, Grune & Stratton, Inc.
17. Brittingham, T.E., and Chaplin, H, Jr.: J.A.M.A. **165:**819, 1957.
18. Chapman, R.G., and Dougherty, S.M.: Transfusion **18:**588, 1978.
19. Greenwalt, T.J., Gajewski, M., and McKenna, J.L.: Transfusion **2:**221, 1962.
20. Langfelder, M., Jakschitz, M., and Janossy, A.: Vox Sang. **19:**57, 1970.
21. Nakao, M., Nakayama, T., and Kankura, T.: Nature **246:**94, 1973.
22. Beutler, E., West, C., and Blume, K.-G.: J. Lab. Clin. Med. **88:**328, 1976.
23. Kikugawa, K., and Minoshima, K.: Vox Sang. **34:**281, 1978.
24. Chaplin, H., Brittingham, T.E., and Cassell, M.: Am. J. Clin. Pathol. **31:**373, 1959.
25. Kabat, E.A., and Berg, D.: J. Immunol. **70:**514, 1953.
26. Dorner, I., et al.: Transfusion **15:**439, 1975.
27. Brickman, R.D., et al.: J.A.M.A. **198:**1277, 1966.
28. Lewis, J.H., et al.: Arch. Surg. **93:**941, 1966.
29. Meryman, H.T.: In Spielmann, W., and Seidl, S., editors: Modern problems of blood preservation, Stuttgart, West Germany, 1970, Gustav Fischer Verlag.
30. Meryman, H.T., and Hornblower, M.: Transfusion **12:**145, 1972.
31. Rowe, A.W., Eyster, E., and Kellner, A.: Cryobiology **5:**119, 1968.
32. Meryman, H.T., and Hornblower, M.: Transfusion **17:**438, 1977.
33. Kahn, R.A., Auster, M., and Miller, W.V.: Transfusion **18:**204, 1978.
34. Myhre, B.A., Nakasako, Y.Y., and Schott, R.: Transfusion **18:**199, 1978.
35. Bodey, G.P.: Med. Times **94:**1076, 1966.
36. Higby, D.J., et al.: Vox Sang. **28:**243, 1975.
37. Sussman, L.N., Colli, W., and Pichetshote, C.: Transfusion **15:**461, 1975.
38. Gmür, J.P., Deluigi, J., and Straub, P.W.: Transfusion **15:**565, 1975.
39. Djerassi, I., et al.: Transfusion **12:**75, 1972.
40. Morse, E.E., et al.: Ann. Clin. Lab. Sci. **6:**540, 1976.
41. Roy, A.J., et al.: Transfusion **15:**539, 1975.
42. Herzig, G., Root, R.K., and Graw, R.G.: Blood **39:**554, 1972.
43. Harris, M.B., et al.: Blood **44:**707, 1974.
44. Graw, R.J., Jr., et al.: N. Engl. J. Med. **287:**367, 1972.
45. Appelbaum, F.R., Trapani, R.J., and Graw, R.J., Jr.: Transfusion **17:**460, 1977.
46. Buchholz, D.H., et al.: Transfusion **15:**96, 1975.
47. Kahn, R.A., Cossette, I., and Friedman, L.I.: Transfusion **16:**162, 1976.
48. Murphy, S., and Gardner, F.H.: N. Engl. J. Med. **280:**1094, 1969.
49. Federal Register **40**(20):4300, Jan. 29, 1975.
50. Yankee, R.A.: Puget Sound Blood Center Seminar on Platelet Transfusion, June 16, 1975; reported by Wieckowcz, M.: Transfusion **16:**193, 1976.
51. Schiffer, C.A., Buchholz, D.H., and Wiernik, P.H.: Transfusion **14:**388, 1974.
52. Sussman, L.N.: Ann. Clin. Lab. Sci. **8:**453, 1978.
53. Aisner, J., et al.: Transfusion **16:**437, 1976.
54. Aisner, J.: Med. Clin. North Am. **61:**1133, 1977.
55. Nusbacher, J., Scher, M.L., and MacPherson, J.L.: Vox Sang. **33:**9, 1977.
56. Howard, J.E., and Perkins, H.A.: Transfusion **18:**496, 1978.
57. Yankee, R.A., Grumet, F.C., and Rogentine, G.N.: N. Engl. J. Med. **281:**1208, 1969.
58. Rizza, C.R., and Biggs, R.: Prog. Hematol. **6:**181, 1969.
59. Pool, J.G., and Shannon, A.E.: N. Engl. J. Med. **273:**1443, 1965.
60. Burke, E.R., et al.: Transfusion **15:**307, 1975.
61. Miller, W.V., editor: Technical manual of the American Association of Blood Banks, ed. 7, Washington, D.C., 1977, American Association of Blood Banks, p. 44.
62. Reiss, R.F., and Katz, A.J.: Transfusion **16:**229, 1976.
63. Shanberge, J.N., et al.: Transfusion **12:**257, 1972.

64. Reese, E.P., Jr., McCullough, J.J., and Craddock, P.R.: Transfusion **15**:583, 1975.

65. Blood component therapy, a physician's handbook, ed. 3, Washington, D.C., 1977, American Association of Blood Banks.

66. Weiss, H.J., and Rogers, J.: Am. J. Med. Sci. **53**:734, 1972.

67. Weiss, H.J., Rogers, H., and Brand, H.: Blood **41**:809, 1973.

68. Salzmam, E.W.: J. Lab. Clin. Med. **62**:724, 1963.

69. Ikkala, E.: Ann. N.Y. Acad. Sci. **202**:200, 1972.

70. Orringer, E.P., et al.: Arch. Intern. Med. **136**:1018, 1976.

71. Prager, D., et al.: Blood **53**:1012, 1979.

72. Bove, J.R.: Transfusion **18**:129, 1978.

73. FDA Drug Bull. **8**(2), 1978.

74. Barrowcliffe, T.W., Stableforth, P., and Dormandy, K.M.: Vox Sang. **25**:426, 1973.

75. Sandler, S.G., Rath, C.E., and Ruder, A.: Ann. Intern. Med. **79**:485, 1973.

76. Kurczynski, E.M., and Penner, J.A.: N. Engl. J. Med. **291**:164, 1974.

77. Dreykin, D.: N. Engl. J. Med. **291**:205, 1974.

78. Edell, S.: N. Engl. J. Med. **285**:580, 1971.

79. Blatt, P.M., et al.: Ann. Intern. Med. **81**:766, 1974.

80. Campbell, E.W., Neff, S., and Bowdler, A.J.: Transfusion **18**:94, 1978.

81. White, G.C., et al.: Blood **49**:159, 1977.

82. FDA Drug Bull. **6**:22, 1976.

83. Iwarson, S., Kjellman, H., and Teger-Nilsson, A.C.: Vox Sang. **31**:136, 1976.

84. Seeler, R.A., et al.: J. Pediatr. **89**:87, 1976.

85. Virgilio, R.W., et al.: Surgery **85**:129, 1979.

86. Gellis, S.S., et al.: J. Clin. Invest. **27**:239, 1948.

87. Tullis, J.L.: J.A.M.A. **237**:355, 460, 1977.

88. Bland, J.H.L., Laver, M.B., and Lowenstein, E.: N. Engl. J. Med. **286**:109, 1972.

89. McMillin, R.D., Hood, T.R., and Griffin, W.O.: Am. J. Surg. **135**:706, 1978.

90. Izaka, K., et al.: Transfusion **14**:242, 1974.

91. Arturson, G., et al.: Acta Chir. Scand. **127**:543, 1964.

92. Thompson, W.L., Britton, J.J., and Walton, R.P.: J. Pharmacol. Exp. Ther. **136**:126, 1962.

93. Thompson, E.L.: Prog. Clin. Biol. Res. **19**:283, 1978.

94. Lundsgaard-Hansen, P., and Tschirren, B.: Prog. Clin. Biol. Res. **19**:227, 1978.

95. Alexander, B.: Prog. Clin. Biol. Res. **19**:293, 1978.

96. Ring, J., and Messmer, K.: Lancet **1**(8009):466, 1977.

97. Collins, J.A., et al.: Vox Sang. **36**:39, 1979.

98. Walker, R.: Is a Coombs crossmatch necessary for patients with a negative antibody screen? In Current methods in blood banking and immunohematology, Chicago, 1978, American Society of Clinical Pathologists.

99. Boral, L.I., and Henry, J.B.: Transfusion **17**:163, 1977.

100. Rouault, C., and Gruenhagen, J.: Transfusion **18**:448, 1978.

101. Oberman, H.A., Barnes, B.A., and Friedman, B.A.: Transfusion **18**:137, 1978.

102. Kevy, S.N.: Lab. Med. **10**:459, 1979.

103. Collins, J.A.: Surgery **75**:274, 1974.

104. Miller, R.D., et al.: Ann. Surg. **174**:794, 1971.

105. Perkins, H.A., et al.: Transfusion **11**:204, 1971.

106. Marshall, B.E., Wurzel, H.A., and Ellison, N.: Circ. Shock **2**:249, 1975.

107. Zuck, T.F. and Bergen, J.J.: Adequacy of oral iron to support erythropoiesis during intensive phlebotomy for autologous transfusion. In Thirteenth International Transfusion Congress, Washington, D.C., 1972, p. 53.

108. Autologous transfusions: In Current methods in blood banking and immunohematology, Chicago, 1978, American Society of Clinical Pathologists.

109. Ascari, W.Q., Jolly, P.C., and Thomas, P.A.: Transfusion **8**:111, 1968.

110. Mattox, L.K.: Surgery **84**:700, 1978.

111. Brzica, S.M., Pineda, A.A., and Taswell, H.F.: Mayo Clin. Proc. **51**:723, 1976.

112. Heathcote, J., and Sherlock, S.: Lancet **1**:1468, 1973.

113. Blumber, B.S., Alter, H.J., and Visnich, S.J.: J.A.M.A. **191**:101, 1965.

114. Dane, D.S., Cameron, C.H., and Briggs, M: Lancet **1**:695, 1970.

115. LeBouvier G.: In Symposium on Viral Hepatitis and Blood Transfusion, Hepatitis and blood transfusion, New York, 1972, Grune & Stratton, Inc.

116. Ukkonen, P., Koistinen, V., and Penttinen, K.: Vox Sang. **36**:109, 1979.

117. Frösner, G.G., et al.: J. Med. Virol. **3**:67, 1978.

118. Gerin, J.L., Ford, E.C., and Purcell, R.H.: Am. J. Pathol. **81**:651, 1975.

119. Alter, H.J., et al.: N. Engl. J. Med. **295**:909, 1976.

120. Federal Register **40**:29710, 1975.

121. Hyland, C.A., et al.: Vox Sang. **36**:137, 1979.

122. Ling, C.M., and Overby, L.R.: J. Immunol. **109**:834, 1972.

123. Wolters, G., et al.: J. Clin. Pathol. **29**:873, 1976.

124. Adachi, H., et al.: Vox Sang. **35**:219, 1978.

125. Tuji, T., and Yokochi, T.: Jpn. J. Exp. Med. **39**:615, 1969.

126. Overby, L.R., editor: Hepatitis forum, Chicago, March/April 1979, Abbott Diagnostics Division.

127. Wyke, R.J., et al.: Lancet **1**:520, 1979.

128. Craske, J., Dilling, N., and Stern, D.: Lancet **2**:221, 1975.

129. Alter, H.J., et al.: N. Engl. J. Med. **298**:637, 1978.

130. Patrilli, F.O., Crovari, P., and deFlora, S.: J. Infect. Dis. **135**:252, 1977.

131. Papaevangelou, G., et al.: Br. Med. J. **1**:689, 1978.

132. Feinstone, S.M., et al.: N. Engl. J. Med. **292**:767, 1975.

Special test procedures

In all blood banking procedures, serum should be used rather than plasma for two reasons: the lack of calcium in plasma is anticomplementary and fibrinogen may interfere with clearly visible agglutination. If hemophilic blood fails to clot, add thrombin (50 units/5 ml blood) to induce clotting and serum formation. In afibrinogenemia add 10 mg fibrinogen to 5 ml blood. To remove fibrin from unclotted heparinized blood (e.g., open-heart surgery, dialysis), centrifuge specimen and remove plasma. Add an equal volume of glass or plastic beads and shake well. Centrifuge specimen again and separate serum.[1]

ANTIGLOBULIN (COOMBS') TEST[2-4]

Coombs et al.[2] introduced antihuman globulin serum to detect red cells sensitized by incomplete antibodies (immunoglobulins). Purified human globulin is injected into laboratory animals to produce antibodies against human γ-globulin. If red cells are incubated with an incomplete antibody (a γ-globulin) directed against one of the red cells' antigens, the antibodies attach themselves to the red cells, sensitizing but not agglutinating them. The antigen-antibody reaction taking place on the surface of the red cell remains thus invisible. To confirm the fact that an antibody-antigen reaction has actually taken place on the cell surface, antiglobulin (Coombs') serum is added to the red cells. The antiglobulin serum combines with the antibodies on the red cell surface, causing the red cells to agglutinate. The originally invisible antigen-antibody reaction is thus made visible. Before the addition of the antiglobulin

serum the red cells must be washed with saline solution to remove all traces of free γ-globulin, so that the antiglobulin serum, when added, is not neutralized before it can act on the sensitized red cells.

It is now known that when human globulin is injected into laboratory animals, antibodies are also produced to some non-γ component of the serum globulin, specifically to serum complement. Antiglobulin serum that contains a multitude of antibodies is termed **polyspecific,** a term defined by the Bureau of Biologics as referring to a serum containing at least anti-IgG and anti-C3d but possibly containing other antibody specificities as well.[5] Such polyspecific serum is used to detect red cells sensitized with nonagglutinating antibodies or complement components. Antiglobulin serum, which is produced by injecting animals with purified proteins, e.g., IgG, IgM, IgA, C3, or C4, is termed **monospecific** because only one antibody will be present. After polyvalent antiglobulin serum has detected sensitized red cells, monovalent serum will specifically identify the nature of the sensitizing globulin. It is important to realize that C4 may be ''nonspecifically'' bound to the red cell membrane: complement activation by immune complexes unrelated to erythrocytes or nonspecific binding of C4 by refrigerated clotted blood. Hence, antiglobulin serum containing high levels of anti-C3 activity is more desirable than serum containing anti-C4 because of the possibility of a ''nonspecific'' Coombs' reaction with the latter preparation.

Two types of antiglobulin tests have been described, depending on whether the red cell sensitization takes place (1) in vivo (the direct antiglobulin test) or (2) in vitro (the indirect antiglobulin test).

Direct antiglobulin test

Principle: The direct antiglobulin (Coombs') test will cause the agglutination of human red cells that have been sensitized in vivo by γ-globulin antibodies or complement components. The Coombs' serum, which contains antihuman γ-globulin and anticomplement, will combine with these globulins already present on the surface of the red cell, causing visible agglutination.

Procedure: Washed red cells are directly treated with the antiglobulin serum.

Prepare a 2-5% red cell suspension in saline. With a wooden applicator stick, transfer a small amount of red cells from a clot into a large amount of saline solution; for routine purposes accurate measuring is not necessary provided the technologist is familiar with the density and color of an accurately prepared 2% suspension and compares it occasionally with the estimated "stick suspension."

Place 1 drop of the prepared red cell suspension into a 10 × 75 mm test tube. Wash these red cells thoroughly with saline; at least three or four washings are required. Centrifuge after each wash (3000 rpm) for 15 sec and decant. After the final wash decant as completely as possible by completely inverting the centrifuged tube and blotting the end with absorptive paper. Add 1-2 drops of antiglobulin serum to the cell button and mix well. Centrifuge at 3000 rpm for 15 sec. Gently resuspend cells until all the cells are dislodged; observe for agglutination macroscopically and microscopically. Record results.

To rule out a false negative result, all negative tubes should be retested by adding 1 drop of known IgG-sensitized red cells and recentrifuging. In a valid negative test, the positive control cells should be agglutinated; failure to observe agglutination indicates inactivation of the antiglobulin serum caused by prolonged storage or neutralization because of improper washing of the tested red cells. In either case the test must be repeated.

Interpretation: Agglutination indicates sensitized red cells; a valid negative test indicates lack of in vivo sensitization or insufficient globulin or complement molecules on the red cell surface to allow detection.

Indications:
1. Detection of in vivo red cell sensitization as seen in erythroblastosis fetalis, autoimmune hemolytic anemias, and transfusion reaction because of incompatible blood
2. Diagnosis drug-induced hemolytic anemias

Indirect antiglobulin test

Principle: After allowing a suitable period of time for red cells to become sensitized (incubation time), the indirect antiglobulin (Coombs') test will produce visible agglutination of human red cells. Hence, it measures the in vitro sensitization of red cells. Two procedures are required: first, incubation of the antiserum with red cells of known types to allow the cells to become coated with antibody if present in the serum and, second, testing the cells for sensitization by the application of the direct antiglobulin test.

Procedure: Before using the antiglobulin serum, the red cells are first incubated with test serum and then thoroughly washed.

Prepare a 2-5% red cell suspension in the manner described previously. The red cell antigens must match the suspected serum antibody; e.g., if an anti-Rh_0(D) antibody is suspected in the serum, red cells must be Rh_0(D) positive.

Place 1 drop of the prepared red cell suspension into a 10 × 75 mm test tube. Add 2-4 drops test serum. Incubate for 30 min (15 min in emergency) at 37° C. Some antibodies, e.g., anti-Duffy and anti-Kidd, may require longer incubation.

Centrifuge at 3000 rpm for 15 sec. Wash thoroughly (three or four times) in saline. Decant completely after the last wash by inverting the tube completely and re-

moving all saline at the mouth of the tube with absorptive paper. Add 1-2 drops antiglobulin serum to the cell button and mix well. Centrifuge for 15 sec. Gently resuspend cells as before and observe for macroscopic and/or microscopic agglutination. Record results. As with the direct antiglobulin test, test all negative results with known sensitized cells to be sure the antiglobulin serum was potent and active.

Interpretation: The presence of agglutination indicates the presence of antibodies in the test serum capable of acting with the test cells.

Indications:
1. Cross matching to detect incompatibility
2. Detection and identification of irregular antibodies
3. Detection of antigens, e.g., Rh, Kell, Duffy, and Kidd

Quality control of antiglobulin test

The antiglobulin serum should be checked against known sensitized and nonsensitized red cells. Sensitized red cells may be commercially purchased, or they may be prepared in the laboratory as follows.

Prepare a 2% saline suspension of washed, Rh_0-positive red cells. Dilute 1 part anti-Rh_0 slide typing serum with 9 parts normal saline solution. Mix 0.5 ml 2% cell suspension and 0.5 ml diluted anti-Rh_0 serum; incubate at 37° C for 30 min. Wash the cells at least three times in saline and prepare a 2% suspension. Add 1 drop antiglobulin serum to 1 drop cell suspension, observe for agglutination.

These cells are lightly coated with antibody and serve as a good indicator for subtle loss of anti-IgG activity in the antiglobulin serum; they are preferred over the heavily coated, commercially prepared red cells used as a check in negative Coombs' tests. For nonsensitized red cells, any cells that have not been coated with antibody are adequate.

Sources of error in antiglobulin test
False negative test

1. Very small amounts of human serum protein can neutralize the antiglobulin serum.
   a. Test tube or pipet may be dirty. The use of disposable pipets and test tubes is strongly recommended. They should not be reused.
   b. Red cells may have been inadequately washed. Red cells should be carefully suspended in test tube filled with saline solution which is completely drained after each washing.
   c. Contact with fingers (human protein) must be avoided.
2. Antibody is not absorbed onto red cells because of the following:
   a. Incubation time is too short or too long.
   b. Incubation is at a temperature at which the antibody is not active.
   c. There is a delay in reading the test or in performing the test thus allowing the antibody to be eluted off the red cells.
   d. Test cells are stored improperly, causing them to lose reactivity.
3. The antiglobulin serum is inactive because of im-

proper storage, or it has inadvertently been omitted.

4. Complement-dependent antibodies require complement that may not be available in plasma. Anticoagulants, by removing calcium, are anticomplementary. In the antiglobulin technic, serum should therefore be used rather than plasma.

5. The wrong concentration of cells is used. A 2-5% cell suspension is recommended.

6. The medium must be appropriate for the blood group system investigated: saline albumin etc. Sensitivity of the test cells may have to be increased by enzyme treatment.

7. The manufacturer's instructions regarding the use of his antiglobulin serum must be followed to avoid a **prozone** reaction. A prozone reaction is characterized by the failure of undiluted serum to agglutinate red cells while agglutination occurs when the serum is diluted although progressive dilution, of course, leads to ultimate disappearance of the agglutination.

False positive test

1. Presence of heavy metal ions and of colloidal silica in saline solution used can cause nonspecific agglutination.

2. Bacterial contamination of test cells because of improper storage or septicemia of patient can give rise to agglutination.

3. Test cells giving positive direct antiglobulin test cannot be used for the indirect antiglobulin test.

4. Wharton's jelly may be present in cord blood. Cord red cells should be washed four or five times with saline solution to remove Wharton's jelly.

5. In the past a high reticulocyte count could cause a reaction between the reticulocyte surface transferrin and antitransferrin present in the antiglobulin serum. Such an occurrence is very unlikely now that antiglobulin serum has improved specificity and no longer contains antitransferrin as an impurity.

6. Inadequately absorbed antiglobulin serum can cross react with other antigens.

7. Penicillin antibody may be present.

8. Refrigerated clotted blood causes a nonspecific binding of C4, which will react with the anticomplement components of the antiglobulin serum.

IMMUNOGLOBULIN DIFFERENTIATION

When the technician is working with erythrocyte antibodies it is sometimes important to determine if the antibody is wholly or partly IgG. There are many different procedures that aid in the distinction of γ-globulin classes including fractionation with DEAE-cellulose[6] or Sephadex columns.[6] Other more commonly performed procedures are described in detail below.

Disulfide reduction

Sulfhydryl compounds split IgM antibodies into subunits thereby rendering them incapable of agglutinating red cells.[7] IgG antibodies are unaffected and IgA antibodies are only partially inactivated by such treatment.

Two sulfhydryl compounds are used commonly: 2-mercaptoethanol and dithiothreitol.

Mercaptoethanol treatment of serum[8]

Principle: In a mixture of IgM and IgG antibodies the IgM antibodies are inactivated leaving IgG antibodies to be assayed.

Procedure: Mix 1 ml test serum with 1 ml 0.2M 2-mercaptoethanol in pH 7.4 phosphate buffer and incubate at 37° C for 15 min. For serum control separately mix 1 ml serum with 1 ml pH 7.4 phosphate buffer and incubate at 37° C for 15 min.

Place test and control sera in separate dialysis sacs and dialyze at 4° C against pH 7.4 phosphate buffer for at least 45 min. In some instances overnight incubation may be necessary. This step is considered optional by many.[9] Place dialyzed serum samples into separate tubes, label appropriately, and perform serologic tests.

Dithiothreitol test[10]

Principle: Dithiothreitol is a cyclic structure containing one more reactive group than 2-mercaptoethanol; the cyclic structure eliminates the noxious odor associated with 2-mercaptoethanol. It has the same or greater reducing potency than 2-mercaptoethanol.

Procedure: Prepare 0.01M dithiothreitol by dissolving 154 mg dithiothreitol in 1 dl isotonic saline. This may be stored for 6 months at 4° C in glass containers.

Into a 12 × 75 mm test tube, place 0.1 ml dithiothreitol; add 0.1 ml test serum. As a control, use 0.1 ml saline to 0.1 ml test serum. Mix contents of tubes well. Incubate at 37° C for 15 min. Perform appropriate serologic tests on both the treated and control serum samples.

Interpretation of disulfide reduction

If the serologic activity is identical in the treated and control sera, the antibody is IgG; if treated serum shows diminished activity compared to control serum, the antibody is IgM. If neither treated serum nor control serum is active, the test is invalid.

Indications for disulfide reduction

The test is indicated to study serum antibodies in obstetric patients, since only IgG antibodies can pass the placental barrier and have the potential to cause hemolytic disease of the newborn; also occasionally it is helpful in difficult cases of antibody identification.

Heat inactivation

IgM antibodies are heat labile and can be inactivated by heating serum at 56° C for 3 hr. Such treatment does not inactivate IgG and IgA antibodies.

Neutralization

Principle: Agglutinins (IgM antibodies) are easily neutralized by blood group substances, whereas sensitizing or coating antibodies (IgG antibodies) are resistant to this treatment; IgA antibodies are intermediate in effect. Neutralization of antibodies by group-specific substances is most applicable to the ABO blood group system. IgM anti-A, for example, can be easily neutralized when the serum is mixed with A substances, leaving any IgG or IgA anti-A reactive.

Procedure:

1. Place 1 ml serum to be tested into a 10 × 75 mm test tube. Add 0.2 ml soluble A and B blood group substances. Mix and allow to stand at room temperature for 5 min.

2. Prepare a 1:10 dilution of the neutralized serum with saline.

3. Place 1 drop diluted, neutralized serum into each of two test tubes labeled A and B.

4. Add 1 drop of a 2% saline suspension of A red cells to the A tube and 1 drop of a 2% saline suspension of B red cells to the B tube.

5. Centrifuge and examine for agglutination. If no agglutination is seen, neutralization is complete; proceed with step 6. If agglutination is present, the undiluted previously neutralized serum must be further neutralized by again adding 0.2 ml blood group substance and allowing serum to stand an additional 5 min. The serum must be again diluted 1:10 and retested with 2% saline–suspended cells.

6. Incubate tubes at 37° C for 30 min.

7. Wash red cells three or four times with saline, decanting completely after the last wash. Add 2 drops antiglobulin serum to each tube, mix, and centrifuge. Examine for agglutination. If no agglutination is seen, add sensitized red cells.

Interpretation: If agglutination is seen after the addition of antiglobulin serum, sensitizing anti-A or anti-B is present in addition to the expected IgM antibodies. If no agglutination is seen, no sensitizing antibodies are present at a titer of 10 or higher.

Indications: Immunoglobulin neutralization is used to determine if IgG antibodies of a particular specificity are present when IgM antibodies of the same specificity are known to be present:

1. Hemolytic disease of the newborn
2. Titer IgG anti-A and anti-B in group O serum

ABSORPTION AND ELUTION

Principle: Absorption and elution are two procedures that are frequently used together and serve as a means of extracting and isolating antibodies to allow their identification. An antibody may be extracted from the serum by allowing it to react with red cells having the corresponding antigen; the resulting antigen-antibody complex is then removed from the serum by centrifugation. This process is referred to as **absorption;** the serum remaining after removal of the immunologic complexes is referred to as **absorbed serum.** The temperature at which the serum and red cells are allowed to incubate will vary depending on the type of antibody to be removed: Cold antibodies are absorbed at 4° C and warm antibodies at 37° C. The extracted antibody can then be removed from the red cells through the process termed **elution;** antibodies may also be **eluted** from red cells if absorption has occurred in vivo.

General absorption procedure

Select cells that are homozygous for the antigen that matches the antibody in the serum; wash the cells thoroughly in normal saline solution (six to eight times) to remove any residual serum. If the antibody is a nonspecific cold antibody, the saline solution should be warmed to 37° C. After the final wash, use pipet to remove the saline solution.

Mix 1 volume packed cells with 1 volume serum. If the antibody is weak, the amount of serum may be increased. Dilution of serum with saline solution (1:2 or 1:4) facilitates the absorption of high-titered antibodies.

Place the mixture in a water bath, the temperature of which depends on the type of antibody to be absorbed: for cold antibodies (IgM) the absorption temperature is 4° C; for immune antibodies (IgG) it is usually 37° C. Incubate for 30 min.

Centrifuge at 3400 rpm for 10 min. The centrifuge cups should be prechilled to 4° C or warmed to 37° C, depending on the antibody involved.

Remove serum and test serum for complete absorption of antibody by bringing it in contact with suitable test cells. The direct antiglobulin test on the absorbing cells should be positive.

Indications

1. Removal of an interfering cold or warm autoantibody to allow detection of an alloantibody
2. Removal of anti-A and/or anti-B from the serum to prevent ABO interference
3. Separation of a mixture of alloantibodies
4. Detection of weak erythrocyte antigens by demonstrating their ability to remove the corresponding antibody from the serum
5. Removal of unwanted species-specific antibodies from immune animal sera

Elution procedures

The accuracy of an elution method depends on the complete removal of unabsorbed "contaminating" antibodies. Therefore all elution methods begin with red cells that have been thoroughly washed in saline, i.e., at least four to six times and maybe many more times. Before proceeding with the elution process, the supernatant saline from the last washing should be tested for the presence of unwanted antibody by allowing it to react with appropriate red cells. If the cells reveal the presence of antibody, more saline washings are needed.

Antibody is liberated from the red cell by breaking the antigen-antibody bonds; this can be accomplished in a number of ways: heat, alcohol, ether, or acid. During the process, red cells are often hemolyzed, so the eluate is frequently tinged with hemoglobin. Eluates should be tested immediately, or at least within 24 hr of their preparation. If this is impossible, antibodies should be eluted into group AB serum of 6% albumin rather than saline; it can then be stored at −20° C until testing is performed and no loss of antibody will occur.

Heat elution

The heat elution method of Landsteiner and Miller[11] involves the following procedure.

Procedure: Wash sensitized red cells thoroughly with normal saline. After the last wash, drain the saline solution well. Add an equal volume of saline solution to each volume of packed, washed cells. Mix well.

Place the cell suspension in a 56° C water bath for 10 min, agitating frequently. Centrifuge at high speeds immediately in preheated (56° C water bath) centrifuge cups. Remove the supernatant fluid (eluate).

Alcohol elution

The alcohol elution method of Wiener[12] involves the following procedure.

Procedure: Wash sensitized red cells thoroughly with normal saline. After the last wash, drain the saline solution well. Stopper the tube and freeze the red cells at −6° C to −35° C until the cells are frozen. After freezing, remove the cells from the freezer and thaw at room temperature.

To the thawed cells, add 10 volumes 50% ethanol, precooled to −6° C or lower. Mix well by inversion. Restopper the tube and return to the freezer for an additional 30-60 min. Centrifuge at 3000 rpm for at least 5 min. Remove and discard the supernatant from the sediment.

Add distilled water to fill the tube; break up the sediment with a glass rod if necessary. Shake the tube to mix the sediment thoroughly. Centrifuge at 3000 rpm for 5 min. Discard supernatant.

Add saline equal to the original volume of packed cells to the sediment and thoroughly mix as before. Incubate at 37° C for 30-60 min. Centrifuge at 3000 rpm for 5 min. Transfer the supernatant to a clean tube for testing.

Ether elution

The following procedure is a modification by Hughes-Jones et al.[13] of Rubin's method.[14]

Procedure: Thoroughly wash sensitized red cells with normal saline. After the last wash, drain the saline solution well. Add 1 volume 0.85% saline and 2 volumes diethyl ether to the packed washed cells. Stopper and mix by inversion for 1 min. Remove the stopper slowly to release the volatile ether. Incubate at 37° C for 10 min with the stopper loosely in place. Centrifuge at 3000 rpm for 10 min.

Three layers will be present in the tube: a top layer of clear ether, a middle layer of denatured red cell stroma, and a bottom layer of hemoglobin-stained eluate. Remove the top two layers by aspiration and discard. Centrifuge the eluate at high speed and transfer to another tube.

The eluate can be tested immediately or stored frozen at −20° C. In the latter instance, the eluate should be incubated unstoppered for an additional 15 min in a 37° C water bath to evaporate any residual ether.

Acid elution

Acid elution can be performed on the sensitized red cell stroma or on the intact cell.

Acid stromal elution: The following procedure is that of Jenkins and Moore.[15]

Procedure: To 1.0 ml packed red cells, add 9.0 ml saline and 0.5 ml digitonin suspension (5 mg/ml in saline). Centrifuge for 5 min. Wash stroma with saline until the supernatant is clear (at least three times).

To the packed stroma, add 2.0 ml 0.1M glycine-HC1 buffer, pH 3.0: Dissolve 7.5 g glycine in 8 dl water;

adjust pH to 3.0 with 1.0N HC1; bring the final volume to 1 L; store at 4° C to ensure stability. Mix well with the stroma and allow to stand 1 min. Centrifuge for 5 min; remove supernatant fluid.

To the supernatant, add 0.2 ml 0.8M K_2NaPO_4, pH 8.2: Mix 0.8M K_2HPO_4 with 0.8M NaH_2PO_4 until a pH of 8.2 is achieved. Centrifuge; remove supernatant eluate and test.

Acid elution of intact erythrocytes: The following procedure is that of Rekvig and Hannestad.[16]

Procedure: Mix 1 volume of a washed, prechilled 50% suspension of red cells with 1 volume ice-cold 0.1M glycine-HC1 buffer, pH 3.0. Incubate the suspension in ice-cold water for 2 min with gentle agitation. Centrifuge for 30 sec at 3000 rpm and collect the supernatant. Immediately adjust the pH of the supernatant to 7.0 by adding about 20 μl/ml supernatant of 0.5M tris solution, pH 10.5. Centrifuge the neutralized supernatant to remove any formed precipitate.

The eluate can be tested immediately. If stored, add bovine serum albumin to a final concentration of 10 mg/ml to protect the antibodies.

Indications

1. Demonstration and identification of the antibody on the red cells of infants or cord blood in cases of erythroblastosis fetalis (The eluate of these cells may be used for cross matching for exchange transfusions if the mother's blood is not available.)
2. Identification of the antibody absorbed on the red cells in acquired anemia
3. Investigation of transfusion reactions and demonstration and identification of antibodies absorbed onto the recipient's cells
4. Separation and identification of antibodies in a mixture of antibodies
5. Demonstration of weak variants of group A or B by their ability to absorb homologous antibodies, which are then eluted and identified

SALIVA TESTING FOR SECRETED SUBSTANCES

Principle: Approximately 75% of a random population are genetically capable of secreting water-soluble ABH substances into their body fluids. This is because they are homozygous or heterozygous for the *Se* gene; as a result they all secrete H substance and, in addition, secrete A or B substance, the latter substance depending on their inheritance of an *A* or *B* gene, respectively. To determine if a person is a secretor or not, it is adequate to test for H substance only; on other occasions it may be necessary to test for A, B, and H substances.

In addition, approximately 94% of a random population and 78% of the black population have Lewis substance in their fluids, the result of inheritance of the *Le* gene. All such persons will have Le^a substance in their fluids, although Le(b+) persons have only a small amount. It is possible to test for the presence or absence of the *Le* gene by determining the presence or absence of Le^a substance.

The fluid that is routinely tested is the saliva, and the substances are detected by utilizing the principle of hemagglutination inhibition. Saliva is incubated with appropriate dilutions of antibody; if the soluble antigen is present it will neutralize the antibody, and subsequent addition of indicator red cells containing the corresponding antigen will result in no agglutination. If the saliva does not contain the corresponding soluble antigen, hemagglutination will be observed.

***Collection and preparation of saliva*:** Collect 3-5 ml saliva in a wide-mouthed tube. To stimulate saliva flow, the subject may chew on wax or a rubber band; chewing gum is discouraged because artificially sweetened or flavored gum will affect Le^a activity.

Place the tube in a boiling water bath for 10 min to inactivate salivary enzymes that may destroy the secreted blood group substances. Be careful not to boil for longer than 15 min since then there may be some destruction of the secreted substances as well.

Centrifuge at 3000 rpm for 10 min.

Collect the supernatant fluid and test for blood group substances. Once the fluid is boiled, the blood group substances are relatively stable; refrigerate the supernatant until testing is begun, but if the sample cannot be tested on the day of collection, freeze until ready to use. Frozen samples remain active for several years.

***Procedure*:** Prepare a 1:4 dilution of test and control saliva with saline. Control saliva for ABH secretion is obtained from known *Se* and *sese* persons; control saliva for Lewis testing is obtained from known $Le(a+)$ and $Le(a-b-)$ persons. For reagent control, use saline in place of saliva.

Obtain appropriate antisera: anti-H from *Ulex europaeus* lectin; anti-A and anti-B from normal group B and group A subjects; monospecific anti-Le^a. It is suggested that antisera from normal, nonimmunized group A and B subjects be used rather than commercial antisera because the latter may contain potent IgG antibodies that are difficult to neutralize. Prepare serial dilutions of the antisera and test with the reagent red cells that are to be used later. Use the antisera at the dilution producing a 2+ agglutination of the indicator cells; stronger antisera are not completely neutralized and will reduce the sensitivity of the test.

Set up a maximum of four tubes for each subject to be tested and for each control. Fewer tubes can be used if all four antisera are not needed. Add 1 drop of a different antiserum to each tube.

Add 1 drop saliva to the appropriate tubes and 1 drop saline to the reagent control tube. Incubate 20 min at room temperature.

Add 1 drop of a 5% saline suspension of A_2, B, O, and Le^a cells to the tubes containing anti-A, anti-B, anti-H, and anti-Le^a, respectively. Mix contents well. Incubate at room temperature for 30-60 min. Centrifuge and observe for agglutination macroscopically.

***Interpretation*:** Absence of agglutination in the ABH tubes indicates the subject is a secretor of the appropriate substance. Agglutination in the A or B tubes indicates the subject is not secreting that substance; agglutination in the H tube indicates the subject is a nonsecretor and is genetically *sese*. Absence of agglutination in the Lewis tube indicates the subject is Lewis positive; if that subject is also a secretor, his saliva is assumed to contain Le^b substance also.

LOW–IONIC STRENGTH SALINE SOLUTION

***Principle*:** It is known that many factors can influence the process of hemagglutination, including ionic strength. It has been shown that low ionic strength enhances the rate and extent of erythrocyte antigen-antibody reactions, resulting in an increased sensitivity and reactivity of antibody detection tests.[17] Hence, red cells suspended in low–ionic strength solutions show enhanced specific antibody binding in a shorter period of time than red cells suspended in physiologic saline. Red cells suspended in isotonic saline or bovine albumin require incubation times of 30-60 min for optimal antibody detection; if cells are suspended in a low–ionic strength solution, the incubation time can be reduced to 10 min.[18] To eliminate the possibility of nonspecific uptake of γ-globulin or complement by these red cells, it is recommended that the solution contain an NaCl concentration of at least 30 mM.[19] One of the most popular preparations in use today is a solution of sodium glycinate containing 0.03M NaCl, buffered to pH 6.7 with phosphate.

***Preparation of 0.03M low–ionic strength solution (LISS)*:**
1. Saline, 0.17M, 180 ml
2. Phosphate buffer, 0.15M, pH 6.7, 20 ml
3. Sodium glycinate, 0.3M, pH 6.7, 800 ml

To prepare 0.15M phosphate buffer, mix approximately equal volumes of 0.15M Na_2HPO_4 and 0.15M $Na H_2PO_4$ and adjust the pH to 6.7.

To prepare 0.3M sodium glycinate, dissolve 18 g glycine in approximately 5 dl distilled water; add 1.0M NaOH drop by drop while stirring, until the pH is 6.7.

***Routine use*:** The LISS is used as the final suspending medium for red cells that have been previously washed with physiologic saline. The use of physiologic saline as wash solution helps to eliminate false positive readings.[20] One drop of 3-5% LISS–suspended cells is added to 1 drop serum; the recommended incubation time in the indirect antiglobulin test is 10 min. After preparation of the solution, 1 dl aliquots may be stored frozen and thawed on the day of use; if stored at 4° C, the solution must be discarded after 2-3 days unless previously sterilized. The use of LISS in antibody detection tests has the advantage of uncovering low affinity antibodies.

ENZYME TESTING

***Principle*:** Some enzymes are capable of removing *N*-acetylneuraminic acid (sialic acid) from the red cell surface, thereby enhancing antigen-antibody interactions. Those antibodies that may become easier to detect include anti-Lewis, anti-P_1, anti-I, anti-JK^a, anti-Sd^a, and some anti-Rh. Because cold agglutinins are often enhanced, an autocontrol must be run simultaneously with all test sera. On the other hand, some antibodies may not be detected because their corresponding antigens are destroyed by the use of enzymes; such antibodies are anti-M, anti-N, anti-S, and anti-Fy^a.

The enzymes most commonly used are bromelin, trypsin, papain, and ficin, the latter enzyme being the most potent. Enzymes may be mixed with the red cells and serum directly (one-stage method) or used to pretreat red cells before the serum is added (two-stage method). Although the two-stage method is the more sensitive procedure, it is more difficult to use in routine situations because of the extra time involved.

Enzymes may be commercially obtained, often as lyophilized preparations; after reconstitution, they are stored at refrigerated temperatures but remain stable for only a short time. It is imperative that the manufacturer's instructions be carefully followed. As an alternative, enzyme stock solutions may be prepared by the laboratory and stored frozen until ready to use.

One-stage method using commercial enzyme preparations

Procedure:
1. Place 2 drops patient serum in each of two test tubes.
2. To one tube add 1 drop 2-5% saline–suspended reagent or donor red cells; to the other tube add 1 drop 2-5% saline–suspended patient red cells (autocontrol).
3. Add 1 drop commercial reconstituted enzyme preparation. Always follow manufacturer's instructions if they differ from these procedures.
4. Mix well. Incubate for 15 min at room temperature.
5. Centrifuge for 20 sec. Gently resuspend and observe macroscopically for agglutination.
6. Record results.
7. Resuspend cells and incubate for 15 min at 37° C.
8. Centrifuge for 20 sec. Gently resuspend and observe macroscopically for agglutination.
9. Record results.
10. Wash cells three times with isotonic saline. Decant completely after third wash.
11. Add 1 drop antihuman globulin serum (Coombs' serum).
12. Centrifuge and read as above.

Interpretation: The test results are invalid if agglutination occurs in the autocontrol; further tests are then needed to prove the presence of an antibody in the serum.

Indications:
1. Antibody screening
2. Antibody identification
3. Cross match procedures

Two-stage method using ficin
Preparation of reagents

To prepare the **stock ficin solution**, dissolve 1.0 g ficin in 1 dl phosphate buffered saline, pH 7.3; this will produce a 1% ficin solution. Freeze aliquots of the stock solution until ready to use. Powdered ficin is toxic to sensitive individuals, causing sloughing of mucous membranes[5]; handle with care!

Phosphate buffered saline, pH 7.3, is prepared using the following:
1. Anhydrous Na_2HPO_4, 0.1M, 14.2 g/L
2. Anhydrous KH_2PO_4, 0.1M, 13.6 g/L

To prepare the buffered saline, pH 7.3, mix 7.8 ml Na_2HPO_4 stock solution, 2.2 ml KH_2PO_4 stock solution, and 90 ml saline.

The **working ficin solution** is prepared next. Because ficin is the most powerful enzyme, it is best to use solutions more dilute than 1% ficin. A 0.1% or 0.05% ficin solution is more desirable; if red cells appear to agglutinate spontaneously after treatment with 0.1% ficin solution, the 0.05% solution should be used.

For a 0.1% ficin solution, mix 1 volume 1% ficin stock solution with 9 volumes phosphate buffered saline, pH 7.3.

For a 0.05% ficin solution, mix 1 volume 1% fincin stock solution with 19 volumes phosphate buffered saline, pH 7.3.

Pretreatment of red cells

Wash red cells once with isotonic saline; centrifuge and decant supernatant.

To 1 volume washed, packed red cells, add 1 volume 0.1% ficin solution. Incubate for 15 min at 37° C. Wash red cells two or three times with saline and decant to a dry button.

Use as any other reagent red cells after resuspending to 5% suspension in saline.

Procedure: To 1 drop pretreated saline-suspended red cells, add 2 drops patient serum. Proceed as with one-stage method outlined above, steps 4 through 12.

Indications:
1. Antibody screening
2. Antibody identification

REFERENCES

1. Collymore, M.E.: Am. Assoc. Blood Banks New Briefs, p. 16, May 1973.
2. Coombs, R.R.A., Mourant, A.E., and Race, R.R.: Lancet **2:**15, 1945.
3. Pollack, W., Hager, H.J., and Hollenbeck, L.L., Jr.: Transfusion **2:**17, 1962.
4. Treacy, M.: In Seminar on advanced technics in blood banking, Sixteenth annual meeting of the American Association of Blood Banks, Detroit, 1963.
5. Petz, L.O., and Garratty, G.: Transfusion **18:**257, 1978.
6. Mollison, P.L.: Blood transfusion in clinical medicine, ed. 6, Oxford, England, 1979, Blackwell Scientific Publications, Inc.
7. Deutsch, H.F., and Morton, J.: Science **125:**600, 1957.
8. Freedman, J., et al.: Vox Sang. **30:**231, 1976.
9. Rosner, E.R., Pirofsky, B., and Sheth, K.: Transfusion **14:**47, 1974.
10. Pirofsky, B., and Rosner, E.R.: Vox Sang. **27:**480, 1974.
11. Landsteiner, K., and Miller, C.P., Jr.: J. Exp. Med. **42:**853, 1925.
12. Wiener, W.: Br. J. Haematol. **3:**276, 1957.
13. Hughes-Jones, N.C., Gardner, B., and Telford, R.: Vox Sang. **8:**531, 1963.
14. Rubin, H.: J. Clin. Pathol. **16:**70, 1963.
15. Jenkins, D.E., and Moore, W.H.: Transfusion **17:**110, 1977.
16. Rekvig, O.P., and Hannestad, K.: Vox Sang. **33:**280, 1977.
17. Hughes-Jones, N.C., et al.: Vox Sang. **9:**385, 1964.
18. Rock, G., et. al.: Transfusion **18:**228, 1978.
19. Löw, B., and Messeter, L.: Vox Sang. **26:**53, 1974.
20. Moore, H.C., and Mollison, P.L.: Transfusion **16:**291, 1976.

CHAPTER 17

Antigens and antibodies

Antigens
Antibodies
Immune response
Antigen-antibody reactions
    Complement
    Lectins

ANTIGENS

An antigen is any substance that, when introduced into an animal, causes the production of an antibody that reacts specifically with the antigen. The best antigens are proteins, but high-molecular-weight polysaccharides are also antigenic. Lipids are poor antigens. When the antigen is a glycoprotein or a glycolipid, it is the carbohydrate portion that determines its antigenic specificity, the antigenic specificity of a lipoprotein antigen resides in its protein component. That portion of the antigen that imparts its specificity is the **antigenic determinant site;** this is also the site that combines with the specific antibody.

An antigen has two essential properties: the ability to promote antibody production and the ability to combine, or react, with the formed antibody. Under normal circumstances, an antigen stimulates specific antibody formation only when that antigen is absent from the host; i.e., the antigen must be foreign to the recipient before it is antigenic to that recipient. The term **hapten** was defined by Landsteiner as a compound that by itself cannot evoke antibody formation, but once an antibody is formed, it can combine with it.

Antigens are found on tissue and blood cells and in body fluids. All blood group antigens are located on erythrocyte membranes, some are also present on leukocytes and platelets, and a few are found in soluble form in the body fluids. The erythrocytic antigens serologically characterize groups of individuals as well as single individuals, leading to the recognition of various human blood groups (polymorphism).

ANTIBODIES

Antibodies are serum proteins (γ-globulins) produced by lymphocytes and plasma cells in response to antigenic stimulation. By immunoelectrophoresis, antibodies can be divided into five groups: IgG, IgM, IgA, IgD, and IgE. Table 17-1 summarizes the major characteristics of these immunoglobulins. Antibodies involved in blood group systems are usually IgG and IgM, but occasionally they are IgA; IgD and IgE are never involved. Immunoglobulins are said to be **mon-**

oclonal if a particular class has the same light-chain component; if both light chains are present, the immunoglobulin production is then said to be **polyclonal.**

The immunoglobulins of importance in blood banking exist as monomers or polymers of the basic immunoglobulin structure (Fig. 17-1). IgG is always a simple monomer and therefore possesses two antibody-combining sites. IgM is always a pentamer with 10 potential antibody-combining sites; the five basic units are connected by a joining chain (J chain) to form a ring. IgA exists as two related structural forms: serum IgA and secretory IgA. Serum IgA exists predominantly as a monomer but can form dimers and trimers, the basic units again being linked by J chains. The IgA present in external secretions (e.g., submaxillary and parotid glands and nasal and intestinal secretions) contains a dimer of IgA with an added protein called the secretory piece. The immunoglobulin portion is produced by the plasma cells in these organs, and the secretory piece is produced by the glandular cells. When they come into contact with each other, the secretory piece binds two IgA units to form the characteristic secretory IgA structure. Secretory IgA is then transported across the mucosal membranes. Hence secretory IgA and serum IgA are functionally independent and are not in equilbrium with each other.

IMMUNE RESPONSE

As a result of the introduction of an antigen into a host, active **immunization** occurs. This process can be classified in three ways. **Heteroimmunization** is antibody production against an antigen from another animal species. **Alloimmunization** is antibody production against an antigen within one's own species; this is the process that is primarily studied in the blood bank, the antibodies that have so formed being referred to as **alloantibodies** (previously called **isoantibodies**). **Autoimmunization** is the unusual circumstance in which antibody is produced against self-antigens; it indicates a loss of immunologic tolerance and is usually associated with a disease state. The antibodies involved are referred to as **autoantibodies.**

When a foreign antigen is introduced into the body for the first time, a **primary antibody response** occurs. This is characterized by an initial slow (5-10 days) production of IgM antibody, later changing to IgG antibody. When the same antigen is encountered a second time, the antibody production is much faster (2-7 days), greater in amount, and predominantly IgG in type; this is termed the **secondary antibody response,**

Table 17-1. Characteristics of antibodies

Characteristics	IgM	IgG	IgA	IgD	IgE
Other terminology	Complete "bivalent," natural	Incomplete, "univalent," blocking, immune	Univalent, secretory	—	Reagin
Serum concentration (mg/dl serum)	120 ± 45	1275 ± 280	225 ± 55	3	0.05
Half-life (d)	9-11	25-35	6-8	2-3	2
Synthesis (mg/kg body weight/d)	5-8	28	8-10	0.4	—
Molecular weight	Approximately 900,000	Approximately 150,000	Approximately 150,000 (monomer)	180,000	200,000
Sedimentation coefficient	19S	7S	7-15S	6S	8S
Location by electrophoresis	Between γ and β	γ, slow	Between γ and β	Between γ and β	Between γ and β
Lability to sulfhydryl	High	Low	Moderate	Low	—
Effect of heat (56°C for 3 hr)	Labile	Stable	Stable	Stable	Stable
Optimal medium	Saline	Albumin	Saline	Saline	Saline
Optimal temperature for activity	5-25° C	37° C	5-25° C	—	—
Complement fixation	Yes	Yes	No	No	No
Crosses placenta	No	Yes	No	No	No
Sequence in immunization	First	Last	Intermediate	—	—
Sequence in newborn synthesis	First	Last	Intermediate	—	—

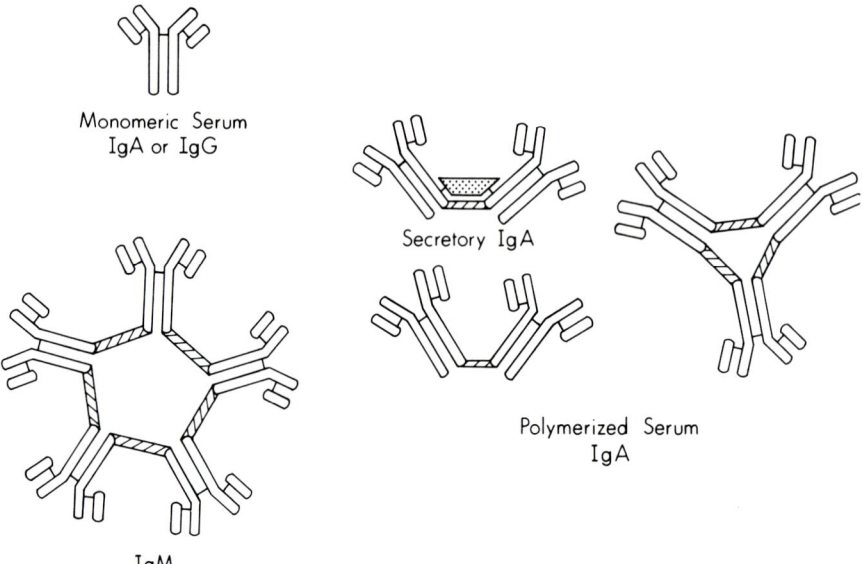

Fig. 17-1. Basic structure of monomeric and polymeric immunoglobulins that are important in blood banks. Basic immunoglobulin unit of two light and two heavy chains can be joined into pairs, triads, or pentamers by means of J chain (*cross-hatched band*). Secretory component of dimeric IgA is diagramatically represented as a speckled rhomboid.

or the **anamnestic response.** Only a small amount of antigen is needed to evoke the secondary antibody response; such a response may be seen for several years after the primary exposure. **Immune tolerance** is an unresponsive state in which the previous exposure to an antigen prevents subsequent antibody formation to that antigen on reexposure. This is believed to be the mechanism by which self-antigens are not recognized by the immune system.

Antibodies that are the result of antigenic stimulation are also termed **immune antibodies.** These antibodies are usually IgG 7S antibodies. Those antibodies that appear in the serum without any apparent antigenic stimulation are termed **natural antibodies.** This is probably a misnomer, because such antibodies probably owe their existence to antigenic stimulation by non-red-cell foreign substances, e.g., bacteria and plants containing blood group–like substances.[1] Blood group systems in which natural antibodies are commonly found include ABO, Lewis, P, MN, and I. These antibodies are usually IgM 19s antibodies. Refer to Table 17-1 for antibody characteristics.

ANTIGEN-ANTIBODY REACTIONS

Antigens and antibodies "react" by forming a physical bond between the antigen determinant group and the antibody-combining site. This reaction is **specific,** i.e., antibody reacts only with the antigen to which it has been directed. Occasionally the antibody will also react with an antigen that did not induce its formation; such **cross-reactivity** is caused by closely similar antigen determinant sites. Although this is a firm union, it is freely dissociable. The combination of antigen with its antibody is an invisible process but can be detected in the laboratory in a number of ways:

1. Complement fixation
2. Neutralization
3. Lysis
4. Precipitation
5. Agglutination
6. Fluorescence
7. Radioimmunoassay
8. Enzyme labeling

The immunoglobulins differ in their ability to participate in these serologic reactions, as shown in Table 17-2. Antibodies that are capable of demonstrating these serologic reactions are named accordingly: **hemolysin, precipitin,** and **agglutinin** are those antibodies demonstrating hemolysis, precipitation, and agglutination, respectively. The antigen participating in the process of agglutination is called the **agglutinogen.**

Both precipitation and agglutination involve the formation of visible complexes by lattice formation. **Precipitation** involves the combination of a soluble antigen with its antibody to form a visible precipitate; **agglutination** involves the combination of a large particulate antigen with its antibody. If the particulate antigen is an erythrocyte, the process is termed **hemagglutination.** In the blood bank, hemagglutination is observed as a clumping of red cells. Most serologic reactions used in the blood bank depend on the process of hemagglutination. Those complexes that aggregate during lattice formation are visible *only* when an optimal concentration of antigen and antibody are present: this is often termed the **equivalence zone.** If antibody is present in excess amounts relative to antigen, then **prozone** exists; if antigen is present in excess amounts relative to the antibody, then **postzone** exists. Both prozone and postzone regions will give a false negative reaction in antibody titration tests.

Although hemagglutination is the mainstay of the blood bank, hemolysis may also be observed and, if present, must also be considered evidence of a serologic union. Most blood banking antibodies are not strong hemolysins, however.

Those antibodies that will agglutinate saline-suspended, antigen-specific red cells are called **saline-agglutinating** or **complete (bivalent)** antibodies. Those antibodies that do not agglutinate red cells suspended in saline solution, even when they are antigen specific, are called **incomplete (univalent)** antibodies; they are able to combine with the antigen but are unable to cause agglutination. Because these antibodies have "coated" the antigen binding sites of the red cells, further addition of an agglutinating antibody will still not produce agglutination; hence these antibodies are also termed **blocking** antibodies. Red cells that are coated with such an antibody are termed **sensitized;** they can be made to agglutinate by the addition of colloids such as bovine albumin or by treatment with proteolytic enzymes. The proteolytic enzymes increase the sensitivity of the erythrocytic antigen to the antibody by removing sialic acid from the red cell membrane and thereby lowering the ζ-potential of the medium and facilitating agglutination. As seen in Table 17-2, IgM antibodies are strong hemagglutinins and can produce agglutina-

Table 17-2. Serologic heterogeneity of the immunoglobulins

Serologic reaction	IgG	IgM	IgA
Precipitation	Strong	Weak	Variable
Agglutination	Weak	Strong	Positive
Hemagglutination	Weak	Strong	Positive
Complement fixation	Strong	Weak	No activity
Hemolysis and bacteriolysis	Weak	Strong	No activity
Virus neutralization	Positive	Positive	Positive
Toxin neutralization	Positive	Negative	Unknown

From Barrett, J.T.: Textbook of immunology: an introduction to immunochemistry and immunobiology, ed.3, St. Louis, 1978, The C.V. Mosby Co.

tion of saline-suspended red cells; IgG antibodies are only weak hemagglutinins and will often require additional treatment of saline-suspended red cells or a different supporting medium before cross-linkage occurs.

An antigen-antibody reaction occurs in two phases: (1) the antibody combines with the antigen, thus sensitizing the antigen (e.g., red cells), and (2) the sensitized antigens come together and agglutinate, or lyse, with the help of complement.

At times special systems have to be used to prove sensitization, e.g., the addition of bovine albumin, antiglobulin serum, or proteolytic enzymes or pretreatment of red cells with such enzymes.

Reporting strength of agglutination reaction

Weak ±	Microscopic aggregates
±	Tiny aggregates, turbid reddish background
1+	Small aggregates, turbid reddish background
2+	Medium-sized aggregates, clear background
3+	Several large aggregates
4+	One solid aggregate

Several factors will influence the in vitro testing of hemagglutination:

1. Antibody.
   a. Concentration. It is possible to determine the concentration of the antibody present through the process of **titration;** i.e., with the antigenic concentration held constant, the concentration of the antibody is changed by a progressive, serial dilution of the serum to be tested. The concentration of the antibody, or **titer,** is the reciprocal of the highest dilution capable of producing a distinct (+) agglutination.
   b. Avidity. The avidity of an antibody is the degree of affinity between it and the corresponding antigen and is determined by the speed and intensity of agglutination.
   c. Type of antibody. Does it require complement, saline medium, bovine albumin, proteolytic enzymes, or antiglobulin serum to demonstrate its existence and activity?
   d. Temperature. Most antibodies have a certain temperature range at which they act best. Cold agglutinins act best at 4° C, and immune antibodies show maximal expression at 37° C. Naturally occurring antibodies act best at 20° C. Testing for antibodies may have to be performed at all three temperature levels: 20° (room temperature), 4°, and 37° C.
   e. Time. After a certain length of time, antigen-antibody complexes may dissociate.
2. Antigen. Not all antigens are equally strong. The strength of an antigen is probably related to the number of sites it occupies on the surface of the red cells. Some antigens are naturally weak, while others may be weakened by age, disease, storage, or presence of other antigens (**competition of antigens**). Homozygosity may strengthen an antigen the so-called **gene dosage effect.**

3. Medium. Antigen-antibody reactions may occur best in saline medium or albumin, in the presence of complement or proteolytic enzymes, or after pretreatment with such enzymes. The addition of albumin standardizes such variables of the medium as pH and ionic strength.
4. Technical factors. The antigen-antibody reaction is influenced by such factors as incubation period, speed and length of centrifugation, and relative amounts of antigen and antibody.

Complement

Complement (C) is a complex system of nine numbered protein components (C1 to C9); they are found in normal serum and account for approximately 10% of the total serum globulins. Many of these proteins exist as proenzymes; when the system is **activated,** the individual components sequentially activate each other. Although there are many substances that can activate this system, the most important is the immunoglobulin molecule. After antigen and antibody have combined, a fragment of the antibody molecule that is capable of binding the first component of complement is exposed. As a result the subsequent cascade of enzymatic events occurs. When red cells are involved and when the cascade is completely activated, hemolysis results; this is because the activated complement components attach to the erythrocyte membrane and cause membrane damage. All nine components must be activated before hemolysis occurs. In some instances the cascade is incomplete, and only some of the components are attached to the red cell membrane; although such cells do not hemolyze, the complement coat may render them liable to early destruction by the reticuloendothelial system. This description refers to the classic pathway for complement activation; there is an alternate pathway for activation in which the early components are bypassed.

IgM antibodies are very efficient complement activators: only one IgM molecule need be present on the membrane to activate the complement system. Most IgG antibodies are also able to activate the system (IgG4 is unable to do this), but it requires two closely placed molecules, 25-40 nm apart. IgA antibodies are unable to activate complement. When complement is bound to the red cell as a result of antigen-antibody reaction, it is termed **fixed.**

Table 17-3. Some commonly used lectins with blood group specificity

Specificity	Lectin
Anti-A$_1$	*Dolichos biflorus*[5]
Anti-A	*Phaseolus limensis*[6]
	Phaseolus lunatus
	Helix pomatia[7]
Anti-H	*Ulex europaeus*[8]
Anti-N	*Vicia graminea*[9]
Anti-T	*Arachia hypogaea*[10]
Anti-Tn	*Salvia sclarea*[11]
Anti-Tn + Anti-Cad	*Salvia horminum*[11]

Complement is thermolabile and can be **inactivated** by heating serum at 56° C for 30 min; this is a reflection of the heat lability of some of the enzymes formed during complement activation. Complement also deteriorates with storage. Normal serum can be stored at 4° C for 2 weeks, −20° C for 2 months, and −55° C for at least 3 months and still maintain 60% or greater complement activity.[2] If kept at room temperature (20-24° C) for 36 hr, serum complement is not reliable; serum kept at 37° C for only a few hours should not be used if complement is required.[2] The addition of 1 drop of fresh serum to an antigen-antibody reaction guarantees adequate complement levels.

Since calcium and magnesium are necessary for the activation of complement, anticoagulants that remove calcium are anticomplementary (EDTA and citrate).

Lectins[3,4]

Within some plants and seeds there are substances that demonstrate specific blood group activity and are able to agglutinate human and animal red cells. Such substances must be properly extracted and carefully diluted to be useful. Table 17-3 lists the more common lectins.

REFERENCES

1. Wiener, A.S.: J. Immunol. **66:**287, 1951.
2. Garraty, G.: Am. J. Clin. Pathol. **54:**531, 1970.
3. Judd, W.J.: Transfusion **19:**768, 1978.
4. Judd, W.J.: CRC Rev. Clin. Lab. Sci. **12:**171, 1980.
5. Bird, G.W.G.: Br. Med. Bull. **15:**165, 1959.
6. Boyd, W.C., and Reguera, R.M.: J. Immunol. **62:**333, 1949.
7. Uhlenbruck, G., and Prokop, O.: Vox Sang. **11:**519, 1966.
8. Cazal, P., and Lalaurie, M.: Acta Haematol. **8:**73, 1952.
9. Ottensooser, F., and Silberschmidt, K.: Nature **172:**914, 1953.
10. Bird, G.W.G.: Vox Sang. **9:**748, 1964.
11. Bird, G.W.G., and Wingham, J.: Vox Sang. **26:**163, 1974.

CHAPTER 18

Immune diseases and the blood bank

HEMOLYTIC DISEASE OF THE NEWBORN

Hemolytic disease of the newborn (HDN) is a condition in which placental transfer of maternal isoantibodies produces hemolysis of fetal red cells. Although the maternal antibody may theoretically be directed against a large number of fetal red cell antigens, in practice, two blood group systems are most often involved: the Rh system (**Rh hemolytic disease of the newborn**) and the ABO system (**ABO hemolytic disease of the newborn**).

Pathophysiology of immunization
Rh incompatibility

Anti-Rh antibodies may be present in maternal serum as a result of previous stimulation by a pregnancy or blood transfusion. The former condition is the more frequent.

During pregnancy, fetal red cells commonly enter the maternal circulation (fetomaternal bleeding); although this can occur at any time, most fetal red cells enter maternal blood during the last trimester, especially during labor and delivery. Under ordinary conditions, only a very small amount of fetal blood (1 ml or less) crosses the placental barrier; however, this amount is often adequate to induce a primary antibody response in the mother. These antibodies, which form after the end of the Rh-positive pregnancy, are harmless because the fetus has been delivered. However, during the second Rh-positive pregnancy, any small amount of Rh-positive fetal red cells that gains entrance into the maternal circulation may easily induce a secondary antibody response; in this instance a large amount of IgG antibody is formed and is capable of crossing the pla-

centa to enter fetal blood. Maternal antibodies attach to the antigenically positive fetal red cells, causing their lysis. The usual sequence of events is as follows: The first Rh-positive pregnancy induces maternal sensitization, and the second Rh-positive pregnancy induces an accelerated antibody response, resulting in HDN.

In a small number of cases (0.4-1.5%), Rh-negative primigravidas with no history of previous transfusion show a detectable level of Rh antibody *during* or at the termination of their first Rh-positive pregnancy.[1] In such cases an unusually early fetomaternal bleeding episode probably occurred, inducing early antibody formation.[2] These cases of early antibody formation are very important because future offspring cannot be protected from disease. Furthermore, if these cases are undetected, they will account for some of the failures observed after the administration of Rh immune globulin (see later discussion of suppression of Rh immunization).

It is important to realize that ABO incompatibility protects against Rh immunization by rapidly clearing incompatible fetal cells from maternal circulation. It is also important to realize that not all Rh-positive pregnancies result in antibody production in an Rh-negative mother (Fig 18-1). In the latter cases the sensitizing

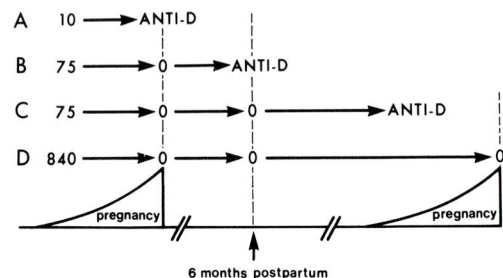

Fig. 18-1. Hypothetical consideration of the pattern of Rh immunization during two pregnancies of 1000 Rh-negative women. The fetuses are all Rh positive and ABO compatible. **A,** Ten women develop antibodies during their first pregnancies. These are usually very weak, demonstrable only with enzyme-treated, Rh-positive erythrocytes. **B,** Seventy-five women develop anti-D antibodies within 6 months postpartum. **C,** Seventy-five women have no antibodies after 6 months; antibodies appear during their second pregnancies as a result of the stimulus of fetal erythrocytes. **D,** The remaining 840 women are not immunized. (From Zipursky, A.: In Nathan, D.G., and Oski, F.A., editors: Hematology of infancy and childhood, Philadelphia, 1974, W.B. Saunders Co.)

dose of fetal red cells may have been too small or the mother may be a **nonresponder,** i.e., a person immunologically incapable of recognizing the Rh antigen as foreign.

Most cases of Rh HDN are caused by maternal isoimmune anti-D; although other antibodies in the Rh system are uncommon, anti-c and anti-E are the most frequently encountered.

ABO incompatibility

ABO incompatibility is initiated by maternal IgG anti-A, anti-B present in a group O mother's plasma; the afflicted infants are almost always group A_1 or B. Since these antibodies are naturally occurring, no antigenic stimulus is needed for induction; hence any pregnancy may be affected, including the first.

Clinical disease
Rh hemolytic disease of the newborn

The severity of Rh HDN is quite variable, producing different clinical sequelae and prognoses. The sequence of events is as follows:

1. Transplacental passage of maternal IgG anti-Rh antibodies
2. Attachment of antibodies to Rh-positive fetal red cells
3. Destruction of antibody-coated fetal red cells in the fetal spleen
4. Metabolism of released heme from lysed red cells with the formation of bilirubin
5. Excess bilirubin removed and metabolized via maternal circulation
6. Anemia
7. Hyperactivity of blood-forming fetal organs, resulting in hepatosplenomegaly

The fetus is not at risk from bilirubin accumulation because the placenta is able to rapidly clear it. However, the fetus is at great risk from anemia, and his prognosis depends directly on the severity of hemolysis. In the most extreme instances the anemia is so great (cord hemoglobin: 3-5 g/dl) that the fetus develops cardiac failure and generalized edema with hypoproteinemia; in this condition, called **hydrops fetalis,** the survival rate is very low (the affected infants are often stillborn).

In the remainder of newborns, survival is good and prognosis now depends on the treatment of anemia and the prevention of hyperbilirubinemia. Unconjugated bilirubin can enter the brain, where it is deposited in large amounts **(kernicterus),** causing neurologic defects and brain damage.

Maternal antibody persists in fetal blood for $2\frac{1}{2}$-3 months, declining with a half-life of 2-3 weeks.[3] Newborns not undergoing an exchange transfusion because their anemia is mild should be frequently tested to rule out the onset of a "delayed anemia" that is partially immunologic in nature.[4]

ABO hemolytic disease of the newborn

ABO HDN is characteristically mild, with slight hemolysis and only rare cases of kernicterus. The sequence of the disease is similar to that listed above; its mild character has been attributed to two factors:

1. There is little hemolysis because the erythrocyte A and B antigens are not fully developed at birth.
2. The effect of maternal antibody is modified by the presence of soluble A or B substance in the plasma of the infant.

Minor antigen incompatibility

In less than 1% of cases, HDN occurs as a result of maternal isoantibodies directed against antigens in blood group systems other than Rh and ABO. Those most often affected are the Kell, Duffy, and Kidd blood group systems. The infrequency of disease in these instances is a result of the low potency of these antigens. When clinical disease is present, it is usually mild, requiring no therapy; however, severe clinical disease has been reported,[5] making proper diagnosis mandatory. Diagnosis of minor antigen incompatibility is identical to that of Rh HDN.

Laboratory testing for diagnosis and management
Rh and minor antigen incompatibility

The diagnosis and investigation of these antigen incompatibilities require prenatal tests with maternal blood and amniotic fluid and neonatal tests with both maternal and cord blood.

Prenatal tests with maternal blood: All pregnant women should have the following tests performed on their blood sample:

1. ABO group.
2. Rh type: If the woman is Rh negative, D^u testing is mandatory and a microscopic end point is required.
3. Screen for irregular serum antibodies: If antibodies are found, they must be identified using panel cells. All IgG antibodies, which are capable of crossing the placenta, should be titered. Antibody titers are run initially and repeated monthly.

All Rh-negative women with initial negative antibody screens should be rescreened at approximately 32 weeks' gestation. If the results are again negative, no further prenatal serologic tests are required.

Antibody titration:

Principle: The tier of a serum antibody is the reciprocal of the highest serum dilution still demonstrating agglutination or hemolysis of test cells positive for the corresponding antigen. An antibody titer is a semiquantitative means of assessing the amount of antibody in the serum: The higher the titer, the more antibody present.

Procedure: Label a row of tubes corresponding to the serum dilution: 1, 2, 4, 8, 16, 32, 64, 128, 256, and 512. Place 0.1 ml saline in the bottom of all tubes except the first (undiluted). Add 0.1 ml test serum to tubes 1 and 2. Mix the contents of tube 2 with a clean pipet and transfer 0.1 ml of the mixture to the tube labeled 4.

Using a clean pipet for each tube, mix and transfer 0.1 ml of each tube mixture into the succeeding tube.

Remove 0.1 ml of the mixture from the last tube and set aside for use if further dilutions are needed.

To each tube, add 0.1 ml of saline-suspended red cells of the appropriate antigen composition. Incubate appropriately according to the antibody being tested.

Centrifuge. Gently dislodge and observe for agglutination with an optical aid. The highest serum dilution revealing agglutination is referred to as the **saline titer.**

Wash all negative and weakly positive tubes in saline three times before adding 1-2 drops of antiglobulin serum. The highest serum dilution revealing agglutination is now referred to as the **antiglobulin titer.**

Comparison of serum sample: During pregnancy, antibody titrations are performed to demonstrate a *change* in the amount of antibody in the mother's serum. To allow this determination, it is imperative that all reported changes in antibody titer be significant, and not the result of artificial variations in laboratory conditions. To achieve this, serum from the previous titration should be saved, frozen, and run in parallel with the repeat specimen. A change in antibody titer that is fourfold or greater is significant.

Clinical significance: Efforts have been made to correlate antibody titer with fetal distress. Although this cannot be done with absolute certainty, some general statements can be made:

1. A constant low or continuous falling titer generally indicates a good prognosis.
2. A constant high titer usually results from earlier sensitization and the prognosis is good but less favorable than above.
3. A constant titer showing a sudden rise at the end of pregnancy may indicate an infant with some degree of hemolysis.
4. A rising titer throughout pregnancy indicates a guarded prognosis; the infant will usually be affected and the titers must be monitored closely to arrange proper management of the fetus.

These statements are only rough guidelines; complete accuracy in predicting infant disease is impossible on an assessment of antibody titers alone, because the antibody level is only *one* of many factors determining clinical severity.[6] Other factors include the maturity of bilirubin excretion, the response of the fetal bone marrow, and the capacity for erythrocyte destruction in the fetal reticuloendothelial system.[6] Fetal phenotype has also been shown to affect clinical severity in rhesus incompatibility.[7]

The best indicator of fetal distress is an evaluation of the amniotic fluid, obtained through the process of **amniocentesis.** Amniocentesis can be a dangerous procedure for both mother and fetus; it is essential therefore that it be performed only when necessary. The primary reason for assessing the strength of maternal antibodies is to determine the need for amniocentesis.

Prenatal tests with amniotic fluid: Amniocentesis is the transabdominal aspiration of amniotic fluid. In suspected cases of HDN, the bilirubin-like content of amniotic fluid serves as an indicator of the extent of fetal hemolysis.[8] It is generally agreed that examination of the amniotic fluid for bilirubinoids is the single best indicator of the magnitude of fetal involvement. Visual inspection of amniotic fluid can give a rough estimate of involvement becuse bilirubinoids impart a bright yellow color to an otherwise colorless fluid. Amniocentesis is performed when maternal antibody titers have risen to dangerous levels (1:32 or higher).

Only small amounts of bilirubin pigment are present in the fluid, even if there is a substantial degree of fetal hemolysis. The usual chemical tests for bilirubin can be performed, but spectrophotometric analysis (optical density [OD] of 450 nm) is often preferred.[9] Because amniotic fluid is not analyzed in the blood bank, details of methodology are given elsewhere (see Chapter 29).

The main objective of this analysis is to avoid intrauterine death of a severely affected baby. This can be done in one of two ways: (1) an early delivery can be planned if the fetus is mature; or (2) an intrauterine transfusion can be attempted if the fetus is incapable of extrauterine survival.

When bilirubin levels are high, amniocentesis must be repeated at weekly or biweekly intervals to allow a sequential bilirubin analysis.

Intrauterine transfusion: Intrauterine transfusion is undertaken to counteract the progressive hemolytic anemia of the fetus that will ultimately lead to hydrops fetalis. It is a dangerous procedure that carries a significant risk of fetal death, and only those fetuses who would otherwise become hydropic before 34 weeks' gestation should be transfused.[10] The immediate fetal hazards from intrauterine transfusion are (1) the infusion of an excess volume of red cells and (2) traumatic injury to fetal blood vessels with hemorrhage.

The transfusion should be made with group O packed red cells that are compatible with the mother's serum. The cells are deposited in the fetal peritoneal sac where they are absorbed intact. To prevent lymphocytes from being introduced into the fetus, which may lead to graft vs. host reaction,[11] and to reduce the risk of hepatitis, the use of frozen washed red cells has been suggested. A protocol for freezing small increments of red cells for pediatric use is available.[12] These infants with Rh HDN may type as Rh negative and have a negative direct antiglobulin test as a result of the intrauterine transfusions.

Neonatal tests with maternal blood: For the patient who has not received a prenatal workup, the following tests are essential to aid in diagnosis:

1. ABO group
2. Rh type including D^u testing
3. Antibody screen with identification of all positive samples

If a minor antigen incompatibility is uncovered, appropriate supportive tests on cord red cells are undertaken. Therapy can be instituted if necessary.

For an Rh-negative mother who has given birth to an Rh-positive infant, the following tests are recommended, most of which are needed to ensure the patient's suitability for Rh immune globulin (RhIG) administration:

1. A repeat serum antibody screen: This will determine if anti-D has been formed in the last phase of pregnancy.
2. An RhIG cross match: FhIG for therapeutic use contains a vial of 1:1000 diluted IgG anti-D to be used in a minor cross match with maternal cells. It serves as a final check to be sure the patient is Rh(D) negative, D^u negative. It may also indicate the presence of fetal red cells.
3. A microscopic D^u test: This has the same purpose

as the RhIG cross match, but the reagent anti-D used is much more sensitive.[13]

4. A demonstration of fetal red cells in maternal circulation: This will confirm the possibility of transplacental bleeding and will enable a quantitation of the amount of fetal blood that has entered the maternal circulation.

Rh immune globulin cross match and D^u testing:

Procedure: RhIG cross match and D^u testing are conveniently run simultaneously.

Label three test tubes for each specimen to be tested: R, D, and C. Place 2 drops of 1:1000 diluted RhIG from the therapeutic kit in the tube labeled R. Place 1 drop slide and rapid tube anti-D serum in the tube labeled D. Place 1 drop 22% albumin in the tube labeled C (control).

Put 1 drop 5% saline–suspended maternal red cells (obtained postpartum) in each of the three tubes. Mix tubes gently and incubate them for 15–30 min. at 37° C. Centrifuge tubes and wash cells three times with saline, decanting completely after the final wash. Add 1-2 drops antiglobulin serum to each tube and mix. Centrifuge tubes and gently resuspend the cell button. Observe tubes for agglutination both macroscopically and microscopically.

Interpretation: Absence of agglutination in all three tubes indicates the mother is Rh(D) negative, D^u negative. Agglutination in either the RhIG cross match or the D^u test can occur in any of the following conditions:

1. The mother is a weak D^u.

2. A fetomaternal hemorrhage has occurred, and the agglutinates represent fetal Rh-positive or fetal D^u-positive red cells reacting with anti-D. This type of reaction usually appears as a weak agglutination that has the characteristics of a mixed-field pattern when viewed under the microscope.

3. The immune sera may contain other weak antibodies that are reacting with the mother's red cells.

Incompatibility in the cross match is not necessarily a contraindication for therapeutic administration of RhIG, provided the mother can be shown to be truly Rh(D) negative and D^u negative and to have no anti-D antibodies in her serum (see later discussion of suppression of Rh immunization).

Kleihauer-Betke acid elution test for fetal red cells:

Principle: When fetomaternal bleeding occurs, fetal red cells enter maternal circulation. The Kleihauer-Betke test[14] is a sensitive indicator of the presence of fetal red cells. The test is based on the fact that hemoglobin F, found in fetal red cells, is resistant to elution by an acid pH; hemoglobin A, found in adult (i.e., maternal) red cells, is readily eluted. If a blood smear is exposed to an acid buffer and subsequently stained, fetal red cells are a pink-red color, whereas maternal red cells are pale ghosts. A simple calculation will allow quantitation of the number of fetal red cells present.

Procedure: Since the procedure is not performed in the blood bank, detailed methodology and reagent preparation are presented elsewhere (see Chapter 4).

Very thin, freshly prepared maternal blood smears (postpartum) are fixed in alcohol. They are then placed in the prewarmed acid buffer for 5 min to allow elution of hemoglobin A. After the slides are washed, they are stained and dried. A total of 2000 adult red cells are counted, and the number of fetal red cells observed during this count is recorded. The percent of fetal red cells is calculated as follows:

No. of fetal red cells ÷ Total red cells counted =
Fetal cells (%) in maternal blood

To estimate the volume of fetomaternal bleeding,[15] calculate as follows:

Fetal red cells (%) × 50 = Whole fetal blood (ml)

Indications: The Kleihauer-Betke stain is useful in the following circumstances.

1. To screen and quantitate fetomaternal hemorrhage

2. To determine the origin of red cells in amniotic fluid

3. To monitor the effectiveness of intrauterine transfusions

Neonatal tests with cord blood: Cord blood must be obtained with a needle and syringe from the umbilical vein of the segment of cord attached to the placenta. The practice of ''stripping'' the cord to extract blood is strictly condemned because of the contamination with Wharton's jelly, a substance containing hyaluronic acid and capable of producing spontaneous clumping of red cells. If HDN is not anticipated at birth, infant blood can be obtained by a lancet puncture of the baby's heel; a micro blood collecting tube is used to collect the blood specimen.

The following tests should be performed on cord or infant blood to establish the diagnosis of HDN:

1. ABO group: Only a direct cell grouping is performed because the infant's maternally occurring antibodies are too low to be detected; in addition, the serum may contain maternal IgG anti-A of anti-B and complicate the results in a reverse serum grouping.

2. Rh type: In Rh HDN, the infant red cells are usually Rh$_0$ positive. Occasional problems in Rh typing are encountered. In one such instance, infant red cells are so coated with maternal antibody that they spontaneously agglutinate in typing sera containing a large amount of albumin—regardless of the antibody content of that antiserum; the reaction is suspected to be falsely positive because a similar agglutination occurs in the albumin control. The problem can be overcome by using IgM reagent anti-D to type the infant red cells. Secondly, in severe Rh HDN, all the D-antigen sites on the red cell may be totally blocked with maternal IgG anti-D. Although a positive albumin control may be observed, the subsequent use of IgM reagent anti-D results in no further agglutination because of the complete binding of all available D-antigen sites. This is a very rare phenomenon; the correct Rh type may be obtained by eluting the antibody from the infant red cells so a routine Rh type may be performed. The antibody so eluted may then be identified.

3. Direct antiglobulin test: Direct agglutination of the infant's red cells by antiglobulin serum indicates sensitization by antibodies. The results are usually strongly positive in both Rh HDN and HDN caused by a minor antigen incompatibility. It must be remembered that a

negative test can occur in Rh HDN after multiple intra-uterine transfusions.

4. Antibody elution and identification: When the direct antiglobulin test is positive, elution of the antibody is mandatory if its identification is desired. Antibody identification is required if the mother's serum is not, available or if it contains multiple antibodies.

In addition to the serologic studies listed above, cord and infant blood should be tested for hemoglobin concentration, a reticulocyte count, and serum bilirubin. The morphology of infant red cells and the presence of normoblasts are important. HDN can be excluded if maternal serum is compatible with fetal red cells in an indirect antiglobulin test.

ABO incompatibility

Prenatal tests: The routine ABO group and Rh type should be performed on all pregnant women during their prenatal visits. Although ABO HDN is found primarily in infants of group O mothers, there is no recognized prenatal workup to indicate which group O mothers will have affected infants. In addition, antibody titration serves no useful purpose in the prenatal management of ABO HDN.

Neonatal tests with cord blood: ABO HDN may be a difficult diagnosis to make because the clinical disease is usually mild and serologic tests, although capable of detecting fetomaternal incompatibility, do not detect clinical hemolysis. ABO HDN should be diagnosed *only* when a fetomaternal ABO incompatibility exists in the presence of clinical and laboratory evidence of hemolysis, e.g., jaundice, anemia, reticulocytosis, or spherocytosis. As a result, some laboratories only test infants of group O mothers if clinical signs of disease are present. It must be remembered that in the presence of clinical hemolysis, irregular antibodies must always be ruled out as the primary cause, because ABO incompatibility is common (15%) and may be only a coincidental finding in association with other serologic incompatibilities.

The following procedures are useful in the diagnosis:

1. ABO group (forward typing only): The most common ABO incompatibility is a group A or B infant born to a group O mother.

2. Rh type.

3. Direct antiglobulin test: In the presence of an ABO incompatibility with clinical signs of hemolysis and in the absence of demonstrable irregular antibodies, this test can be strong supportive evidence of ABO HDN. However, in this disease, the direct antiglobulin test may appear as weakly positive or frankly negative; some estimates indicate that 50% of cases of ABO HDN will give a negative direct antiglobulin test.[16] Hence, a negative test does not eliminate the diagnosis of ABO HDN.

4. Indirect antiglobulin test: The infant's serum is tested against screening cells and adult A_1 and B cells by incubating for 30 min at 37° C and adding antiglobulin serum. In the absence of an irregular antibody (i.e., no agglutination with screening cells), free anti-A or anti-B in the serum of a group A or group B newborn, respectively, is strong confirmatory evidence and allows a tentative diagnosis of ABO HDN.

5. Elution of antibody from infant red cells: Heat elution is the preferred method (see discussion of special test procedures: absorption and elution); the resulting antibody is tested against adult A_1 or B cells and screening cells. The demonstration of homologous antibody on infant red cells (e.g., anti-A on group A red cells) is the ultimate verification of the serologic diagnosis of ABO HDN.

Neonatal tests with maternal blood: Maternal blood is studied primarily to determine the titer of IgG anti-A or anti-B. This is best done by dithiothreitol neutralization of IgM antibodies. Such a procedure is only confirmatory and is not a necessary part of the diagnostic regimen because, irregardless of the strength of immune antibody titers, it does not provide absolute proof of the diagnosis without a positive test on cord blood or cord eluate.

Dithiothreitol determination of IgG anti-A or anti-B:

Procedure: Prepare 0.01M dithiothreitol (DTT) (see discussion of special test procedures: immunoglobulin differentiation). Appropriately mark two 12 × 75 mm test tubes with the patient's name; one tube is then labeled "DTT" and the other "saline." Place 0.1 ml of patient's serum in each tube. Add 0.1 ml DTT and 0.1 ml saline to each appropriate tube. Mix well and incubate at 37° C for 15 min.

Place 2 drops DTT-treated serum in two test tubes, one labeled "DTT-A" and the other "DTT-B." Place 2 drops saline control serum in two test tubes, one labeled "saline-A" and the other "saline-B." Add 1 drop 3-5% suspension of adult A_1 cells to the tubes labeled A and 1 drop 3–5% suspension of adult B cells to the tubes labeled B. Incubate the four tubes at 37° C for 30 min. Wash thoroughly in saline three times, decanting well after the final wash. Add 2 drops antiglobulin serum to each tube. Centrifuge and read macroscopically.

Interpretation: If the neutralized test serum has less activity than the control test serum, the antibody is IgM. If both neutralized and control sera have equal activity, the antibody is IgG. If neither serum shows activity, the test is invalid. If a titer is desired, appropriate serum dilutions are tested, a fall in titer in the neutralized test serum indicates IgM antibody.

Suppression of Rh immunization

Principle: When fetal red cells enter maternal circulation, foreign antigens have the potential of sensitizing the mother. Attempts to prevent such sensitization originated with the principle that passive immunity may suppress active immunization; i.e., in the presence of antibody, the corresponding antigen will not immunize. The validity of this immunologic concept gained support from the clinical observation that ABO incompatibility (group O mother, group A or B fetus) protected the fetus from a simultaneous Rh incompatibility. For example, if the size of a transplacental hemorrhage is unknown, the risk of Rh immunization is approximately 15% if the baby is ABO compatible with the mother, but only 2-3% if the baby is ABO incompatible.[10] This protection is believed to be the result of the rapid removal of ABO-incompatible fetal red cells by maternal anti-A and anti-B; thus the fetal cells are not present long enough to produce Rh immunization. As a direct consequence of these findings, attempts to administer a suitable antibody to the mother were instituted, thus simulating the natural protection afforded by ABO incompatibility.

The concept of suppressing natural immunization has been successfully applied only to Rh incompatibility. IgG anti-D is administered to the Rh-negative mother by intramuscular injection within 3 days of delivery of an Rh-positive infant. A number of different products are available: Gamulin Rh (Parke, Davis & Co., Detroit), MICRhoGAM and RhoGAM (Ortho Diagnostics, Raritan, N.J.), and Rh-D Immune Globulin (Cutter Laboratories, Berkeley, Calif.). Since 1968, RhIG has been available clinically; as a result of its routine use, the incidence of sensitization of Rh-negative mothers has been reduced from 14% to 1%.[17]

Criteria for administration of Rh immune globulin

The following criteria must be met before RhIG is administered:

1. The mother must be $Rh_0(D)$ negative and D^u negative.
2. The mother must not already be immunized to the $Rh_0(D)$ factor, as determined by using reagent red cells designed for the detection and identification of atypical antibodies.
3. The baby must be $Rh_0(D)$ positive or D^u positive.
4. The baby must have a negative direct antiglobulin test because of anti-D.

In addition, all $Rh_0(D)$-negative, D^u-negative women having a spontaneous or induced abortion or undergoing amniocentesis, unless it is known that the father is $Rh_0(D)$ negative, D^u negative also, should be given RhIG.

Determination of appropriate dosage

All the commercial products listed above, with the exception of MICRhoGAM, contain 300 μg of immunoglobulin per vial. It is believed that 20 μg of IgG anti-D will suppress the antigenic effects of 1 ml packed red cells.[18] Hence, one vial of RhIG is sufficient to neutralize up to 15 ml of packed fetal red cells or 30 ml of whole fetal blood. If fetomaternal bleeding has occurred that exceeds this amount, additional RhIG must be given. To calculate the number of vials needed, the Kleihaur-Betke stain must be performed to estimate the quantity of fetomaternal hemorrhage:

$$\text{Fetal RBCs (\%)} \times 50 = \text{Whole fetal blood (ml)}$$

$$\text{No. of vials of RhIG needed} = \text{Volume of whole fetal blood} \div 30 \text{ ml}$$

In some laboratories the Kleihauer-Betke stain is insensitive and, to compensate for this, the calculated number of vials is often doubled. The incidence of fetomaternal hemorrhage requiring multiple vials of RhIG is approximately 0.3%.[19]

After spontaneous or induced abortion or an amniocentesis, a smaller dose is adequate. Namely, 50 μg RhIG is sufficient for amniocentesis or an abortion up to 20 weeks' gestation[20]; an abortion after 20 weeks' gestation is best treated with a full vial of 300 μg RhIG. The commerical product MICRhoGAM is specifically intended for use after abortions, and each vial contains 50 μg antibody.

Failure of immune suppression

With the availability of RhIG, the occurrence of Rh immunization should theoretically be totally eliminated. Yet the formation of anti-D during or after an Rh-positive pregnancy still occurs. Such occurrences are referred to as RhIG failures. The causes of such failures are as follows:

1. Massive fetomaternal hemorrhage: Although the postpartum administration of 300 μg RhIG is far in excess of what is needed for routine deliveries,[21,22] occasional cases of excessive transplacental hemorrhage will require a higher dose. The Kleihauer-Betke stain is essential to avoid this problem.

2. Delayed administration of RhIG[17]: The 72 hr time limit is an arbitrary determination based on the original clinical trials with RhIG. It is probable that effective suppression can still be obtained if administration is delayed for up to 1 or even 2 weeks, although this has not been clinically tested. In some cases, delayed administration may have allowed antibody formation.

3. Failure to treat[23]: Failure to administer RhIG to Rh-negative women after exposure to the Rh_0 antigen, whether from a pregnancy or a blood transfusion, continues to be a problem that is not being adequately surveyed.

4. Immunization during a pregnancy: Approximately 1% of unsensitized Rh-negative women will have anti-D in their serum at the time of delivery of their first Rh-positive baby (Fig. 18-1). Because some women will be immunized *before* the routine postpartum administration of RhIG, this becomes the major reason for the failure to completely eradicate Rh HDN. Clinical trials are currently in progress to evaluate the antenatal administration of RhIG.[24]

5. Failure to protect from obstetric manipulation or early pregnancy termination: Obstetric manipulations such as amniocentesis can produce significant fetomaternal hemorrhage, and therapy must be given to all Rh-negative women undergoing these procedures, even though the Rh type of the fetus is unknown. Abortion, whether spontaneous or induced, and ectopic pregnancies carry a similar risk. Although an abortion at 1 month' gestation carries a negligible risk of immunization, at 2 months' gestational age the risk of abortion is 2% and at 3 months it is 9%.[20] Stated in another way, 3.3% of women who have been Rh immunized in a pregnancy have received their antigenic stimulus from an abortion.[20]

Failure of Rh immunosuppression is determined by the appearance of anti-D in the mother's serum 6 months after delivery. The intramuscular injection of RhIG will produce artificial antiglobulin titers of anti-D from 1:32, if 1 ml of RhIG is injected, to 1:128, if 5 ml of immunoglobulin is injected.[17] Since passive antibody will usually be detectable for at least 3 months in the recipient's circulation,[25] any anti-D present after 6 months of injection represents an RhIG failure.

Table 18-1. Comparison of ABO and Rh hemolytic disease of the newborn

	Rh HDN	ABO HDN
Incidence	Uncommon since advent of RhIG	1-3%
Anemia	Moderate to severe	Absent to moderate
Hemoglobin concentration	Low	Normal to moderately low
Bilirubin	Increased at birth; may be severe	Increased after 24 hr; usually mild
Direct antiglobulin test	Strongly positive	Weakly positive or negative
Eluate of infant cells	Anti-Rh	Anti-A or anti-B
Nucleated red cells	Moderate to marked	Mild to moderate
Reticulocyte count	Moderate to marked increase	Mild to moderate increase
Spherocytes	Inconspicuous	Common
Pregnancy	After the first	First likely
Prenatal testing useful	Yes	No
Therapy required	Often	Rarely
Prevention by antibody	Yes	No

Exchange transfusion

An exchange transfusion consists of the gradual removal of recipient blood and its replacement with compatible donor blood. It is used frequently in newborns who require blood because of a severe anemia or hyperbilirubinemia but who are unable to tolerate the volume of a simple transfusion without sustaining circulatory overload. In the treatment of HDN the principal benefit of an exchange transfusion is the removal of sensitized infant red cells and their replacement by nonreactive red cells that are compatible with maternal antibody and that have a normal oxygen-carrying capacity. The exchange transfusion will simultaneously remove bilirubin and free maternal antibody from the infant's plasma. Exchange transfusion may be required in the treatment of HDN caused by Rh or minor antigen incompatibility but is only rarely needed in ABO HDN.

The choice of blood is governed by three rules:

1. The blood for exchange transfusion must be compatible with the serum of the mother. If the mother is Rh negative, the donor's blood must be Rh negative.
2. If the mother and baby are of the same ABO blood group, that blood group should be used. If they differ, group O cells should be chosen.
3. The blood should be fresh, i.e., 5 days old or less.

If the mother's serum is not available, use an eluate of the baby's cells for the cross match and identification of antibody. If the antibody is anti-Rh_0(D), use Rh_0-negative blood; if it is anti-hr'(c), use type Rh_1Rh_1 blood (DCe/DCe); if it is anti-A or anti-B, use group O blood with low anti-A or anti-B titer, or use group O packed red cells or group O frozen, deglycerolized red cells with compatible group AB plasma; and if it is anti-K, use donor blood compatible with the eluate.

AUTOIMMUNE HEMOLYTIC ANEMIA

An autoantibody is an antibody directed against the host's own tissues. If the antibody is directed against a red cell antigen, hemolysis occurs and an autoimmune hemolytic anemia (AIHA) may result. If the autoantibody is a warm-reacting antibody, the condition is termed **warm antibody autoimmune hemolytic ane-**

mia; if the autoantibody is a cold-reacting antibody, the condition is termed **cold antibody autoimmune hemolytic anemia.** Warm antibody AIHA is much more common than cold antibody AIHA.

Warm antibody autoimmune hemolytic anemia

The causative antibody that is found on the surface of the patient's red cells in warm antibody AIHA[26] is usually an IgG immunoglobulin, but IgM or IgA antibodies may also be involved. Complement components are also often present on the red cell membrane, usually in the form of C3d.[27,28] In approximately 10% of cases, the red cells are coated only with complement; it is assumed the immunoglobulin is present in suboptimal concentrations for detection by monospecific antiglobulin serum.

Immunoglobulin-coated red cells are filtered out in the spleen by the action of macrophages with Fc receptors; complement-coated red cells are filtered out in the liver. As a result such cells are partially or completely phagocytosed, resulting in deformed, fragmented erthrocytes and spherocytes; these cells are more prone to destruction on a second passage through the spleen. Actual intravascular hemolysis of coated red cells is less common but can occur at very high concentrations of the sensitizing antibody.

The specificity of the antibody resides in the rhesus blood group system in most instances.[26,29] It may have very simple specificity, e.g., anti-hr″(e), or be very complex, requiring rare phenotypes for identification.

Proposed theories of pathogenesis of warm antibody AIHA include a breakdown of immunologic tolerance[30] and a possible failure of T cell control over antibody production.[31] The condition may be idiopathic or associated with any of the following diseases: lymphoma, leukemia, collagen diseases, e.g., systemic lupus erythematosus or rheumatoid arthritis, viral infections, and carcinoma.

Diagnosis

The following laboratory tests are useful in diagnosis:

1. Hemoglobin concentration: The anemia may be mild or severe.

2. Plasma and urine hemoglobin: Free hemoglobin in the plasma or urine is a measure of the extent of intravascular hemolysis.

3. Bilirubin: If the bilirubin level is elevated, it is a measure of the extent of hemolysis.

4. Urobilinogen (urine or stool).

5. Direct antiglobulin test: This is the most important test that can be performed. Although the test is usually strongly positive, it is not possible to correlate the strength of red cell sensitization with the severity of hemolysis; this is because there are major differences in hemolytic potential even among antibodies of the same specificity.[32] Occasionally the direct antiglobulin test is negative. One explanation of a negative direct antiglobulin test is the presence of insufficient immunoglobulin molecules, or complement fragments, to react with the antiglobulin serum; approximately 500 IgG or C3 molecules per red cell are required before the antiglobulin test becomes positive.[33] Approximately 2-5% of patients with warm antibody AIHA have a negative direct antiglobulin test. A second explanation for a negative test is the presence of complement fragments only on the red cell surface; if the broad-spectrum antiglobulin serum contains inadequate or inappropriate anticomplement activity, a negative result occurs.

6. Eluate of red cells with antibody identification: If an eluate can be obtained, it may be necessary to use enzyme-treated test red cells for identification, especially if only small amounts of autoantibody are present.

7. Indirect antiglobulin test: The presence of a large amount of free autoantibody is often associated with a poor prognosis; a positive indirect antiglobulin test may be seen in more than 75% of cases with long-standing disease.

Use of blood transfusions

The anemia in some patients with warm antibody AIHA may be sufficiently low to warrant a blood transfusion. However, transfusions should be avoided whenever possible and, in fact, compatible blood may be impossible to find. If donor blood is incompatible with the autoantibody, the donor red cells will be destroyed at a rate similar to the patient's own cells; a frank hemolytic transfusion reaction will not ensue. However, donor blood incompatible with a coexisting alloantibody may provoke extensive hemolysis and a hemolytic transfusion reaction. It is therefore important to detect and identify any alloantibody that may be present and "masked" by the warm autoantibody.

When blood transfusions are absolutely necessary, compatible blood should be used, if possible. In the absence of a complex autoantibody, and in the absence of coexisting alloantibody, compatible blood can usually be found. If the autoantibody is complex, compatible blood will not be possible; the eluate from the patient's red cells should then be titered against random donor units and the least incompatible unit transfused.[34] In the presence of a coexisting alloantibody, units selected for transfusion should be compatible with the alloantibody even if incompatible with the autoantibody.

Detection of alloantibody in the presence of warm autoantibody

Principle: When laboratory personnel are attempting to identify an alloantibody[35] in the serum of a patient, the presence of a warm autoantibody may produce agglutination in all test tubes, thereby masking any alloantibody present. To detect these antibodies, any free autoantibody must be removed first. Usually this is done by absorption, using the patient's red cells that have been eluted to release autoantibody, thereby exposing antigen-binding sites. The eluted cells are enzyme treated to increase the sensitivity of the subsequent absorption. The absorbed serum is then treated in the usual manner to detect and identify alloantibodies.

Procedure:
1. Place 1 ml of the patient's red cells in each of two test tubes.
2. Wash six times with warm (45° C) saline.
3. Heat elute at 56° C for 4 min.
4. Wash eluted cells three times with warm saline.
5. Add 1 volume ficin solution to each volume of washed, eluted, patient's cells.
6. Mix; incubate at 37° C for 30 min, mixing occasionally.
7. Wash four times with saline, decanting completely after the final wash.
8. To one test tube of washed, eluted, enzyme-treated cells, add an equal volume of the patient's serum.
9. Mix; incubate at 37° C for 30-60 min, mixing occasionally.
10. Centrifuge tubes; remove and retain the once-absorbed serum.
11. Add the once-absorbed serum to the second test tube of unused, enzyme-treated, eluted cells.
12. Repeat steps 9 and 10 to complete the second absorption.
13. Use the twice-absorbed serum to detect and identify alloantibodies.

Interpretation: Absence of agglutination in the screening cells indicates an absence of alloantibodies; donor blood may be chosen for compatibility with the autoantibody. Agglutination in the screening cells indicates the presence of alloantibody or incomplete absorption of autoantibody; identification should be attempted and blood selected that lacks the antigenic specificity corresponding to the alloantibody. If identification is not possible, the absorbed serum can be used in a minor cross match to select compatible blood.

Cold antibody autoimmune hemolytic anemia

Cold agglutinins and autoagglutinins are antibodies exhibiting maximal reactivity at low temperature (0-10° C); they can readily activate and fix complement to the surface of the red cell. Cold agglutinins produce two distinct clinical diseases: **cold hemagglutinin disease** and **paroxysmal cold hemoglobinuria,** the former disease being the more common.

Cold hemagglutinin disease

Cold hemagglutinin disease (CHD) may occur as an idiopathic condition unassociated with other clinical diseases, or it may be seen in association with infections, particularly *Mycoplasma* pneumonia[36] and infectious mononucleosis,[37] and with malignancies, especially lymphoma and leukemia[38] but occasionally also solid tumors of parenchymal organs.[39]

CHD is characterized by an acute or chronic hemolytic anemia and/or symptoms relating to peripheral autohemagglutination, e.g., paresthesia or cyanosis of fingers, toes, nose, and earlobes, commonly referred to as **Raynaud's phenomenon.** Either or both of these characteristics must occur in the presence of high titers of IgM cold autoantibody. The *disease* must be distinguished from the occurrence of high titers of cold autoantibodies occurring in postinfectious states that are unassociated with clinical hemolysis or autohemagglutination. In these infections, titers of cold agglutinin in the range of 1000 or more are not uncommon in the acute stages of illness, but they are only rarely associated with clinical hemolysis. It is those occasional instances of simultaneous hemolytic anemia that are categorized as examples of secondary cold hemagglutinin *disease*.

Pathophysiology: Patients with CHD are exposed to the effects of their cold autoantibody when blood circulates in those exposed parts of the body listed above. In these locations the temperature of the circulating blood falls below 37° C. The cold autoantibody then fixes to the erythrocyte and complement activation begins. As the blood continues to circulate into the core (body temperature 37° C), the macroglobulin leaves the surface of the red cell, presumably because of a membrane alteration that occurred in the cold.[40] The complement components remain and continue their activation sequence with the attachment of C3b. Complement-fixed red cells circulate in the body and are readily sequestered in the liver, where some are destroyed but most are released with an antigenically altered C3b receptor, now called C3d; this occurs secondary to the action of C3 inactivator.[41] The C3d-bound cells are capable of normal survival in the circulation and are responsible for the positive direct antiglobulin test. The spleen plays a very small role in the destruction or sequestration of complement-coated red cells. The clinical effects of the autoantibodies depends not only on their titer but also on their thermal amplitude and their ability to fix complement. If enough complement is bound, and if the entire pathway is activated, actual intravascular hemolysis occurs.

Serologic characteristics: The following are the classic serologic findings in patients with CHD:

1. Titer of cold autoantibody: Higher than normal titers are always present, and titers greater than 1000 are common; isolated reports of titers exceeding 100,000 have been reported.

2. Thermal amplitude: Although maximal activity can be demonstrated at cold temperatures (0-10° C), these antibodies do exhibit activity in the range of 32° C and, in the presence of 22-30% albumin, they may often be demonstrated in vitro at temperatures up to 37° C.[42] Hemolytic activity can often be demonstrated at room temperature using untreated cells. The most lytic antibodies are those whose thermal amplitude approaches the thermal activation of complement (optimally 37° C).[43]

3. Antibody specificity: Cold autoantibodies usually have anti-I specificity although those cold agglutinins occurring in infectious mononucleosis and some cases of malignancy are anti-i. Table 18-2 allows characterization of anti-I as it occurs in CHD and in normal serum, where it is known as the "harmless cold autoantibody." To test the specificity of the antibody, cord red cells are a practical source of I-negative cells, although adult i cells are preferable if available. A typical reaction pattern is given in Table 18-3 emphasizing the use of temperature in specificity determination.

4. Clonal proliferation: Primary CHD and many cases of CHD secondary to malignancy show a κ-type monoclonicity; the cold agglutinins seen in postinfectious states are generally polyclonal in character. The postinfective polyclonal antibody formation is always transient and reversible whereas the monoclonal proliferation is permanent.

5. Direct antiglobulin test: The direct antiglobulin test is positive with polyspecific serum. The reaction is caused by complement-coated red cells circulating in the blood; this can be proved by using monospecific antiglobulin serum containing anti-C3d.

6. Eluate of red cells: Red cells properly collected and washed at 37° C will show no antibody activity in the eluate because only complement is present.

Serologic testing:

Collection of blood when cold agglutinins are present: To prevent activation of cold agglutinins, the blood should be collected in a warmed syringe or Vacutainer (Becton-Dickinson and Co., Rutherford, N.J.) tube and placed immediately in a 37° C water bath. If this is not feasible, the blood must be placed in the 37° C water bath immediately *after* collection; any autoabsorption that may have occurred will reverse itself at 37° C.

Blood is collected in EDTA to provide red cells for cell typing, antiglobulin testing, and eluate preparations. A second specimen is allowed to clot to provide serum for antibody identification and, if desired, antibody titrations. EDTA anticoagulant has the advantage of preventing in vitro complement fixation in the event blood is accidently allowed to cool.

The red cells may spontaneously agglutinate when cooled to room temperature, causing much difficulty in those serologic tests run at this temperature. Autoagglutination may be the first clue to the presence of high-titered cold autoagglutinins.

Detection of cold autoagglutinins:

Principle: Cold autoantibodies are optimally reactive at 0-10° C and rarely reactive at 37° C; agglutination observed at cold temperature should be reversed when the autoantibodies are heated to 37° C.

Procedure: Wash the patient's cells (collected and maintained at 37° C) twice in warm saline, draining well after the final wash. Prepare a 2% saline suspension of the patient's cells. Place 2 drops of the patient's serum in a 14 × 75 mm test tube. Add 2 drops of 2% saline–suspended patient's cells to the tube. Incubate tube at 4° C for 60 min.

Table 18-2. Differences between anti-I in health and CHD

	CHD	Normal
Titer at 4° C	>64, often in the thousands	<64
Increased titer after in vitro bovine albumin	Yes	No
Thermal range		
Agglutinin	Up to 32°C	No higher than 22° C
Complement activation	Up to 37° C	No higher than 22° C
Avidity	Fast	Slow
Acts as in vitro hemolysin	Yes	No
Type of antibody	Monoclonal	Polyclonal

Modified from Issitt, P.D.: Prog. Clin. Pathol. 7:137, 1978.

Table 18-3. Identification of auto-anti-I

Patient's serum	Test cells (titer)		
	Cord (i)	Adult (I)	Auto
4° C	256	2048	4096
25° C	0	128	256

Observe tube macroscopically for agglutination. If agglutination is present, place the tube in a 37° C water bath and incubate for 30 min; examine to see if agglutination has lessened or disappeared.

Interpretation: Agglutination of patient's serum and cells at 4° C that is reversed with heating is diagnostic of cold autoagglutination. If agglutination persists at 37° C, poor technic should be considered[44] and the test repeated.

Absorption of cold autoagglutinins:

Principle: Cold autoantibody is removed from the patient's serum by absorbing with autologous red cells at 4° C. Serum free of cold autoantibody can then be used for antibody screening and compatibility testing. The prepared unsensitized red cells can be used for cell testing.

Procedure:

1. Collect the blood specimen from the patient and have at the bedside an ice bath and a 37° C portable water bath. Put half the blood specimen into a clot tube and place the tube immediately into the ice bath. Anticoagulate the other half with EDTA and immediately incubate at 37° C.
2. Allow the iced specimen to continue clotting in a refrigerator for 30 min; then centrifuge it in a refrigerated centrifuge or place it in an ice-filled cup for centrifugation. The serum is immediately removed from the clot; this serum will be referred to as "absorbed serum."
3. Remove the plasma from the anticoagulated, 37° C incubated cells and wash the cells three times in 37° C saline, using warmed centrifuge cups. These cells should be free of autoabsorbed antibody and will be referred to as "patient's cells."
4. Prepare a 2% saline suspension of washed patient's cells. Use these cells for ABO grouping

and Rh typing; they are also used for determining the completeness of serum absorption.

5. Test the absorbed serum against the saline-suspended patient's cells at 4° C. If no agglutination is seen, it is assumed all autoantibodies have been removed and the serum can be used for antibody screening and compatibility testing.
6. If agglutination is observed, further absorption is needed using untreated or enzyme-treated patient cells.
   a. For untreated cells add 1 volume absorbed serum to 1 volume patient's cells (from step 3) and place in an ice bath for 60 min with frequent shaking. Cold centrifuge and retest with the saline-suspended, patient's cells; repeat absorption again if necessary.
   b. For enzyme-treated cells, to 1 volume washed, patient's cells (from step 3) add 1 volume enzyme solution (see discussion of special test procedures: enzyme testing), mix, and incubate at 37° C for 15 min. Wash enzyme-treated cells thoroughly with saline. To 1 volume washed, enzyme-treated, patient's cells add 1 volume absorbed serum, mix, and place in an ice bath for 60 min with frequent shaking. Cold centrifuge and test serum against saline-suspended, patient's cells at 4° C and observe for agglutination. Repeat again with fresh, enzyme-treated patient's cells if necessary.

Identification of cold autoagglutinins:

Principle: This test is used to identify the specificity of cold autoagglutinins by testing against reagent red cell panels or special cell panels.

Procedure: Collect blood from the patient in a clot tube and place immediately in a 37° C water bath for at least 15 min. Allow to clot and centrifuge in tubes surrounded by 37° C water jackets. Remove serum immediately; it contains the cold autoantibody ready for identification. Test 2 drops of serum against 1 drop of 2-5% saline–suspended, patient's cells, cord i cells, adult I cells and, if possible, adult i cells. Incubate at 4° C for 5-6 min and observe for agglutination.

Interpretation: Anti-I agglutinates all adult red cells except adult i cells; weak or negative reactions are seen with cord cells. Anti-i gives the reverse reactions. Proceed with titration, if desired.

Titration of cold autoagglutinins[45]:

Principle: In primary or secondary CHD, it may be desirable to follow the clinical progress by evaluating the amount of antibody present; this is best done by titration of the patient's serum.

Procedure: Collect patient's blood in a clot tube and place immediately in a 37° C water bath; allow to remain at this temperature for at least 15 min while clotting.

Centrifuge in tubes surrounded by 37° C water jackets; remove the serum immediately and place in another tube, appropriately labeled.

Prepare master dilutions of the patient's serum as follows:

1. Label 10 tubes (10 × 75 mm): 1-10.
2. Pipet 1 ml normal saline into each tube.
3. Use a clean pipet for each serum transfer; add 1 ml patient's serum into tube 1 and mix thoroughly.
4. Carefully transfer 1 ml from tube 1 to tube 2; mix and again transfer 1 ml from tube 2 to tube 3. Mix and repeat the process to tube 10.
5. Transfer 1 ml from tube 10 into an extra tube, label, and save to prepare additional dilutions, if needed.

Each tube now contains master dilutions, from which the test dilutions will be taken. The titer correlation is as follows:

Tube no.	Titer
1	2
2	4
3	8
4	16
5	32
6	64
7	128
8	256
9	512
10	1024

Prepare 10 tubes (10 × 75 mm) for titration.

Use the red cell giving the strongest agglutination pattern when identifying the presence of cold atuoagglutinins. Wash the cells once with isotonic saline and decant completely.

Add 2-4 drops of the appropriate master dilution to the respective labeled tubes. Add 1 drop of the washed test red cell; mix, centrifuge, and observe macroscopically for agglutination. The highest dilution demonstrating agglutination is the room temperature titer.

Incubate all tubes at 4° C for at least 60 min. Centrifuge using a refrigerated centrifuge and read macroscopically for agglutination. The highest dilution demonstrating agglutination is the cold incubation titer.

Interpretation: Titers less than 64 are considered nonpathologic.

Blood transfusion in cold hemagglutinin disease: Blood transfusion is rarely needed in patients with CHD; the best way to prevent hemolysis is to avoid exposure to the cold. There are no contraindications to blood transfusion, but it may be difficult to select compatible blood. The primary concern is to unmask significant alloantibodies in the presence of cold antibod-

ies reacting at room temperature. To solve the problem, the cold autoantibody should be completely removed by autoabsorption before compatibility testing is performed. If multiple absorptions are necessary, unabsorbed but prewarmed serum should also be used to identify warm antibodies that may have become excessively dilute during the process of absorption.

If time does not allow a complete autoabsorption (and such instances should be very rare), compatibility testing can be performed using prewarmed serum. It must be remembered that all blood will be incompatible with the auto-anti-I in the patient's serum; however, no transfusion reaction will ensue provided there is no coexisting incompatibility with an alloantibody.

When a patient has a high titer of cold agglutinins with a relatively high thermal amplitude, it is often desirable to transfuse blood through an electric coil.

Paroxysmal cold hemoglobinuria

Paroxysmal cold hemoglobinuria (PCH)[46] is the rarest form of AIHA. The disease is caused by a cold autoantibody that has several peculiar characteristics:

1. Although most cold antibodies are macroglobulins, this cold antibody is a 7S IgG immunoglobulin.

2. The cold autoantibodies of CHD are weakly lytic, and any resulting intravascular hemolysis occurs in the cold, along with complement fixation. The antibody of PCH is biphasic in that complement-dependent, intravascular hemolysis occurs only after warming, even though complement activation may initially occur in the cold.

3. This antibody has anti-P specificity[47] rather than the more common anti-I specificity. It is often called the **Donath-Landsteiner antibody,** named after the men originally describing the disease.

4. The Donath-Landsteiner antibody is extremely lytic, being one of the most potent hemolysins known. As a result, intravascular hemolysis is a characteristic feature of the disease and is present even with low antibody titers (average titer: 2-16; highest titer recorded: 64).

Clinically, these patients experience acute, intermittent but massive, intravascular hemolysis after exposure to the cold; this is frequently accompanied by hemoglobinuria with back and abdominal pain. Although the hemolytic crisis is striking and dramatic, any anemia that develops is usually mild because of the intermittent character of the attacks. The disease was originally associated with congenital syphilis, but this is a very unusual cause in current times. Today most cases are idiopathic or are associated with viral infections; in the latter instance, the disease is transient.

The red cells of a patient with PCH will demonstrate a strongly positive direct antiglobulin test during and for some time after an acute attack; the reactivity is caused by complement components coating the red cell surface. Red cell eluates reveal no antibody specificity, because only complement remains after warming. The Donath-Landsteiner antibodies can be demonstrated in the serum; they will agglutinate normal cells at 4° C to a low titer and will cause in vitro hemolysis if the cells, having been sensitized in the cold, are incubated at 37° C. The Donath-Landsteiner test demonstrates the biphasic nature of hemolysis, which is considered the best indicator for diagnosis.

Donath-Landsteiner test:

Principle: The Donath-Landsteiner test is used to demonstrate the presence of a potent hemolysin, which requires cold incubation for warm hemolysis, in the serum of a patient.

Procedure: Collect 10 ml of patient's blood in a clot tube and place immediately in a 37° C water bath. Allow to clot. Centrifuge the clotted blood in a heated centrifuge and remove the serum immediately.

Place 2 ml of patient's serum in each of two 10 × 75 mm tubes labeled A and B. In 2 additional 10 × 75 mm tubes, place 1 ml of normal compatible serum, as a source of complement. Label the tubes C and D. Add 1 ml of patient's serum to tube C; tube D will remain as a control. Add 1 ml of 50% saline suspension of normal group O, P-positive red cells, or patient's red cells, to each of the four tubes.

Place tubes A, C, and D in an ice bath for 60 min. Place tube B in a 37° water bath. Remove the three tubes from the ice bath, mix, and place in the 37° C water bath for 30 min. Remove all four tubes form the 37° C water bath, mix gently, and centrifuge. Observe for hemolysis.

Interpretation: Visible hemolysis in tubes A and C, with no hemolysis in tubes B and D, constitutes a positive test.

DRUG-INDUCED HEMOLYSIS

Many drugs can stimulate antibody formation by combining with tissue macromolecules (e.g., protein) to render them immunogenic; in some instances a metabolic product of the drug is immunogenic. The anti-

Table 18-4. Drugs involved in immunohemolysis

Type	Drug
Antibiotics and antibacterial and antiprotozoal agents	Stibophen Para-aminosalicylic acid (PAS) Penicillin Sulfonamide Isoniazid (INH) Cephalosporins Streptomycin
Anti-inflammatory and analgesic agents	Phenacetin Mefenamic acid Phenylbutazone Indomethacin
Anti-convulsants and sedatives	Chlorpormazine Phenantoin (Mesantoin) Phenytoin (Dilantin)
Miscellaneous	Quinidine Quinine Methyldopa (Aldomet) Levodopa Sulfonylurea Chlorpropamide Melphalan Insecticides (chlorinated hydrocarbons)

bodies so formed can bind to the red cells and/or bind complement, both resulting in a positive direct antiglobulin test, a hallmark of this condition. In some instances, hemolysis occurs.[49] Table 18-4 lists many of the drugs reported to cause a positive antiglobulin test or hemolysis or both.

Mechanism of drug action

There are four different mechanisms that may cause a positive antiglobulin test or a hemolytic anemia or both.

Immune complex adsorption

Most drugs act by immune complex adsorption. Antidrug antibodies bind firmly to the drug to form an immune complex, which then adsorbs loosely, and in a nonspecific fashion, onto the surface of red cells and, in some cases, white cells and platelets (Fig 18-2). In this process, complement is activated, also becoming bound to the red cell membrane. Because the cell attachment is very loose, the immune complex can readily dissociate from the cell to adsorb to other cells, leaving complement behind. In most instances the positive antiblobulin test is caused by complement alone because any immunoglobulin remaining would be eluted during the wash phase of the antiglobulin test. Long after the offending drug is discontinued, the antiglobulin test remains positive because most complement-coated red cells survive in the circulation without destruction, provided only a small amount of complement is present.

Drug adsorption

Drug adsorption (Fig. 18-3) pertains particularly to the penicillins and, to a lesser extent, the cephalosporins. Penicillin is capable of binding firmly to the surface of red cells, and, in fact, the drug can be detected on the red cell membrane of *all* patients receiving high doses of the drug. In addition, such patients frequently develop antipenicillin antibodies, which circulate in their plasma. Approximately 90% of normal, unselected sera will contain such antibodies if searched for with sensitive technics. Most of these antibodies are IgM immunoglobulins and are considered innocuous. The IgG immunoglobulins that may form can be involved in the process of hemolysis. These latter antibodies may react with the drug-adsorbed red cells, producing a positive antiglobulin test and resulting in destruction in the reticuloendothelial system. Rarely, intravascular hemolysis occurs.[50] Complement is not involved in this type of drug-related hemolysis.

Of all patients treated with high doses of penicillin, only 3% develop a positive antiglobulin test and of these, an even smaller percentage will develop a hemolytic anemia. In the case of cephalosporin therapy, the drug will bind to the red cell membrane and antipenicillin antibodies will cross-react with them or anticephalothin antibodies will form and react with the drug on the red cell.[51]

Nonimmunologic adsorption

Nonimmunologic adsorption (Fig. 18-4) pertains to the cephalosporins only and is the most frequent mech-

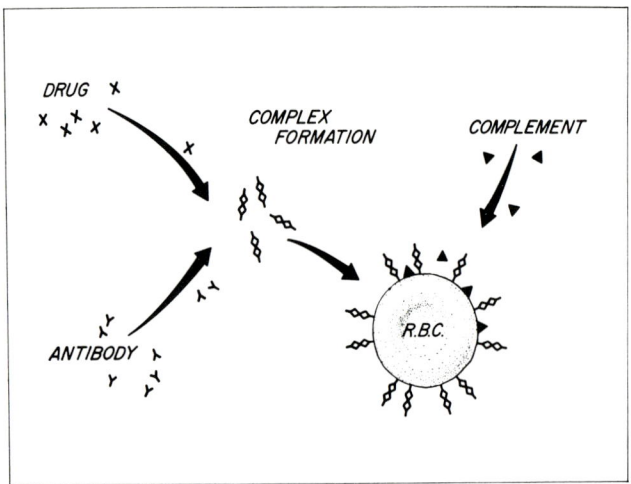

Fig. 18-2. Proposed mechanism of immune complex adsorption. (From Garatty, G.: A seminar on problems encountered in pre-transfusion tests, Washington, D.C., 1972, American Association of Blood Banks.)

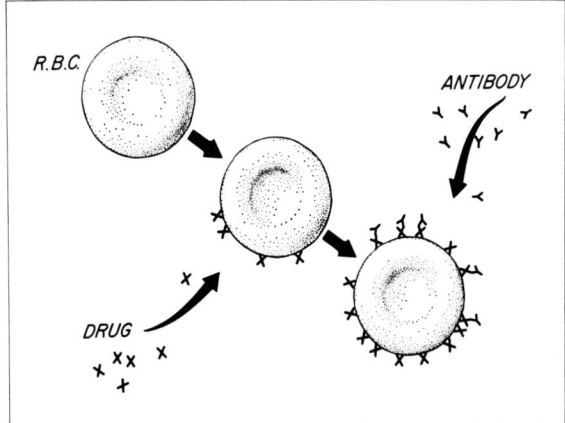

Fig. 18-3. Proposed mechanism of drug adsorption. (From Garatty, G.: A seminar on problems encountered in pre-transfusion tests, Washington, D.C., 1972, American Association of Blood Banks.)

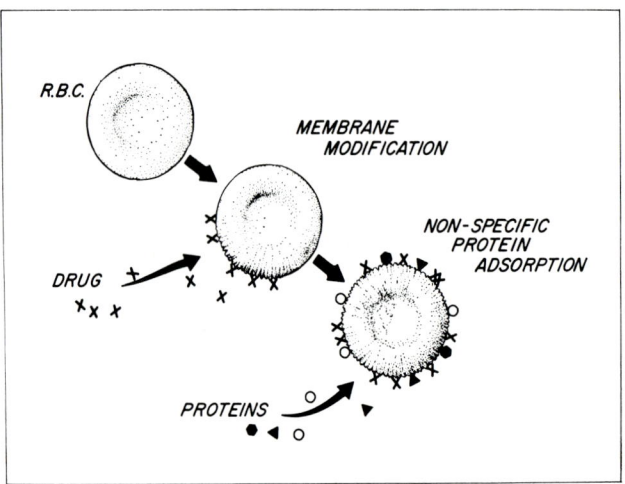

Fig. 18-4. Proposed mechanism of nonimmunologic adsorption. (From Garatty, G.: A seminar on problems encountered in pre-transfusion tests, Washington, D.C., 1972, American Association of Blood Banks.)

anism involved in the development of a positive anti-globulin test after such therapy. The cell membrane is altered by the drug to allow a nonspecific and nonimmunologic uptake by many plasma proteins; albumin, IgG, IgA, IgM, complement, and α-globulins. The condition is suspected if red cells give a positive direct antiglobulin test with a variety of monospecific antiglobulin sera, including anti-IgG, anti-IgA, anti-IgM, and anticomplement. The occurrence of hemolysis by this method is extremely rare.

Development of red cell autoantibodies

Methyldopa (Aldomet) and levodopa can cause the formation of IgG antibodies to normal red cell antigens, usually within the rhesus blood group system. These antibodies will react with normal red cells in the absence of the drug itself and will simulate in all ways the condition of warm antibody AIHA; it can be differentiated from warm antibody AIHA only if the drug history is known. This is the only instance in which a drug can induce an antibody that is primarily directed against an intrinsic red cell antigen; the pathogenesis of this mechanism is unknown. Approximately 15-30% of patients treated with methyldopa develop a positive direct antiglobulin test; less than 1% will develop hemolysis.[52]

Serologic characteristics

1. Antiglobulin testing: The direct antiglobulin test is usually positive using a high-quality, broad-spectrum antiglobulin serum. The use of monospecific antiglobulin serum is helpful in the differentiation of the type of drug reaction present: If only complement is present on the red cells, it is very suggestive of the immune complex group of drugs; if only IgG immunoglobulin

is present, it is suggestive of drug binding of methyldopa therapy; if many classes of immunoglobulin as well as complement are present, it is suggestive of cephalosporin therapy. Positive indirect antiglobulin tests using untreated cells occur only with the methyldopa group because they produce antibodies direct against intrinsic red cell antigens.[53]

2. Antibody screen: The serum should be screened by the usual blood bank procedures, observing agglutination in saline or albumin and using the indirect antiglobulin test. If antibody is detected, specificity tests should be performed to identify any alloantibodies or autoantibodies. If no reaction against normal red cells is observed, the serum should be tested against ABO-compatible cells in the presence of any of the drugs the patient has been receiving. It is best to use a physiologic dose of the drug and to use both untreated and enzyme-treated normal red cells; agglutination, hemolysis, and sensitization to antiglobulin sera are observed.

3. Eluate: An eluate must always be included in the workup of drug-related hemolysis. Only in the case of methyldopa-induced hemolysis will identification of the antibody be possible. In penicillin-related hemolysis, the antibody will react only with penicillin-treated cells, failing to react with those same cells left untreated. In the immune complex group, no antibody may be present, so no reaction will be seen even in the presence of drug.

Preparation of penicillin-coated red cells

Principle: Penicillin is one of the few drugs capable of binding firmly to the red cell membrane; extensive washing will not remove the drug. Penicillin-coated red cells[54] are valuable to detect antipenicillin antibodies.

Table 18-5. Characteristics of drug-induced hemolysis

Mechanism	Drugs*	Direct antiglobulin test (DAT)/coating substance	Indirect antiglobulin test	Clinical importance
Drug-RBC interaction (firm binding between drug and RBC membrane)	Penicillin, possibly carbromal	Positive/IgG	Positive with penicillin-treated normal RBCs	Occasional cause of hemolytic anemia, with extravascular sequestration of cells
Immune complex formation (loose drug-RBC binding)	Quinine, phenacetin, isoniazid	Positive/complement	Positive with quinine-treated normal RBCs	Rare cause of hemolytic anemia, with intravascular hemolysis
Autoantibody production (mainly against Rh antigen)	Methyldopa, mefenamic acid	Positive/IgG	Positive with normal RBCs (i.e., true autoantibodies)	Common cause of positive DAT (20% of methyldopa-treated patients); rare cause of hemolytic anemia, probably with extravascular sequestration
Drug alteration of RBC membrane	Cephalosporins	Positive/IgG, possibly complement	May or may not be positive with cephalosporin-treated normal RBCs	Common cause of positive DAT (4% of cephalothin-treated patients); rare cause of hemolytic anemia

From Horwitz, C.A.: Postgrad. Med. **66:**199, 1979.
*Most common causative agents are listed.

Procedure: Fresh group O red cells are washed three times in isotonic saline. To 1 ml of these washed, packed cells, add 1 × 10⁶ units (approximately 600 mg) K-benzyl penicillin G dissolved in 15 ml barbital buffer, pH 9.6. Incubate at room temperature for 60 min; mix gently. Small clots may form but can be removed with an applicator stick. Wash the cells three times in isotonic saline.

Once prepared, the cells may be stored at 4° C in ACD for up to 7 days.

Preparation of cephalosporin-coated red cells

Principle: The cephalosporins also bind firmly to the red cell membrane and resist removal by repeated washes. Cephalosporin-coated red cells[54] are useful to detect antibodies directed against the drug.

Procedure: Fresh group O red cells are washed three times in isotonic saline. To 1 ml of these washed, packed cells, add 400 mg cephalothin (Keflin) dissolved in 10 ml barbital buffer, pH 9.6. Incubate 2 hr at 37° C; mix gently. Wash the cells in isotonic saline three times.

Detection of antibodies to penicillin and cephalosporin

Procedure: Prepare an eluate from the patient's red cells if the direct antiglobulin test is positive. The eluate and a serial dilution of the patient's serum are tested against normal untreated group O cells and the same group O cells treated with drug. Run a normal control serum.

Incubate 2 volumes eluate or serum dilutions with 1 volume 2-5% saline–suspended, drug-treated, and untreated group O cells. Incubate mixture for 15 min at room temperature. Centrifuge; observe for agglutination. Wash cells four times in isotonic saline. Add antiglobulin serum to the cell button; centrifuge and observe for agglutination.

Interpretation: The drug-coated cells are extremely sensitive, detecting antibody in 97% of random, normal sera; normal sera usually show a low titer (16-32), whereas drug-induced, responsive sera show a titer of 1000 or more.

A positive test is agglutination of drug-treated cells but no agglutination of untreated cells.

Cephalosporin-coated red cells may adsorb other serum proteins, and therefore all normal sera will react in the antiglobulin phase if a sufficiently long incubation was allowed. The highest serum dilutions will usually not have this problem because the serum protein has also been greatly diluted. In addition, the protein content of eluates is usually insufficient to allow such nonspecific adsorption, and agglutination in the eluate indicates anticephalosporin antibodies.

REFERENCES

1. Mollison, P.L.: Am. J. Clin. Pathol. **60**:287, 1973.
2. Scott, J.R., et al.: Obstet. Gynecol. **49**:9, 1977.
3. Mollison, P.L.: Blood transfusion in clinical medicine, ed. 6, Oxford, England, 1979, Blackwell Scientific Publication, Inc., p. 668.
4. Strand, C., and Polesky, H.F.: Minn. Med. **55**:439, 1972.
5. Frigoletto, F.D., and Davies, I.J.: Am. J. Obstet. Gynecol. **127**:887, 1977.
6. Hughes-Jones, N.C., et al.: Vox Sang. **21**:135, 1971.
7. Morley, G.: Vox Sang. **35**:324, 1978.
8. Walker, W., Fairweather, D.V.I., and Jones, P.: Br. Med. J. **2**:140, 1964.
9. Liley, A.W.: Am. J. Obstet. Gynecol. **82**:1359, 1961.
10. Bowman, J.M.: Semin. Hematol. **12**:189, 1975.
11. Parkman, R., et al.: N. Engl. J. Med. **290**:359, 1974.
12. Staples, J.W., and Fritz, G.E.: Transfusion **16**:566, 1976.
13. Polesky, H.F., and Sebring, E.S.: Transfusion **11**:162, 1971.
14. Kleihauer, E., Braun, H., and Betke, K.: Klin. Wochenschr. **35**:637, 1957.
15. Kleihauer, E.: Arch. Kinderheilk. **53**(suppl.):76, 1966.
16. Stratton, F., and Renton, P.H.: Clin. Pediatr. (Phila.) **6**:331, 1967.
17. Freda, V.J., Gorman, J.G., and Pollack, W.: Am. J. Obstet. Gynecol. **128**:456, 1977.
18. Pollack, W., et al.: Transfusion **11**:333, 1971.
19. Sebring, E.S., and Polesky, H.F.: Am. Soc. Clin. Pathol. **72**(suppl. 2):358, 1979.
20. Robertson, J.G.: In Symposium on Rh antibody mediated immunosuppression, Raritan, N.J., May 1975, Ortho Research Institute of Medical Sciences.
21. Hughes-Jones, N.C.: In Symposium on Rh antibody mediated immunosuppression, Raritan, N.J., May 1975, Ortho Research Institute of Medical Sciences.
22. Simonovits, I., and Borocz, I.: Vox Sang. **36**:21, 1979.
23. Berger, G.S., and Keith, L.: In Symposium on Rh antibody mediated immunosuppression, Raritan, N.J., May 1975, Ortho Research Institute of Medical Sciences.
24. Bowman, J.M., and Pollock, J.M.: Can. Med. Assoc. J. **118**:622, 1978.
25. Bowman, J.M.: Obstet. Gynecol. **52**:385, 1978.
26. Dacie, J.V.: Arch. Intern. Med. **135**:1293, 1975.
27. Engelfriet, C.P., et al.: Clin. Exp. Immunol. **6**:721, 1970.
28. Ruddy, S., and Austin, K.F.: J. Immunol. **107**:742, 1971.
29. Vos, G.H., Petz, L.D., and Fudenberg, J.H.: J. Immunol. **106**:1172, 1971.
30. Burnet, M.: Auto-immunity and auto-immune disease, Lancaster, England, 1972, Medical and Technical Publishing Co., Ltd.
31. Allison, A.C.: Boll. Ist. Sieroter Milan **53**(suppl):123, 1974.
32. Constantoulakis, M., et al.: J. Clin. Invest. **42**:1790, 1963.
33. Gilliland, B.C., Baxter, E., and Evans, R.S.: N. Engl. J. Med. **285**:252, 1971.
34. Issitt, P.D., and Issitt, C.H.: Applied blood group serology, ed. 2, Oxnard, Calif. 1975, Spectra Biologicals.
35. Morel, P.A., Bergren, M.O., and Frank, B.: A simple method for the detection of alloantibody in the presence of warm autoantibody, reproduced in current methods in blood banking and immunohematology, Chicago, January 1978, American Society of Clinical Pathologists.
36. Jacobson, L.B., Longstreth, G.F., and Edgington, T.S.: Am. J. Med. **54**:514, 1973.
37. Horwitz, C.A., et al.: Blood **50**:195, 1977.
38. Greally, J.F., et al.: Acta Haematol. **57**:206, 1977.
39. Wortman, J., Rosse, W., and Logue, G.: Am. J. Hematol. **6**:275, 1979.
40. Rosse, W.F., and Lauf, P.K.: Blood **36**:777, 1970.
41. Schreiber, A.D., Atkinson, J.P., and Jaffe, C.J.: Ann. Intern. Med. **87**:210, 1977.
42. Garatty, G., Petz, L.D., and Hoops, J.K.: Transfusion **13**:363, 1973.

43. Schubothe, H.: Semin. Hematol. **3:**27, 1966.
44. Garatty, G.: In Advances in immunohematology, vol. 3, no. 1, Rutherford, N.J., 1973, Becton-Dickson & Co.
45. Branch, D.R.: Lab. Med. **10:**481, 1979.
46. Djaldetti, M.: CRC Crit. Rev. Clin. Lab. Sci. **9:**49, 1978.
47. Levine, T., Celano, M.J., and Falkowski, F.: Transfusion **3:**278, 1963.
48. Donath, J., and Landsteiner, K.: München Med. Wochenschr. **51:**1590, 1904.
49. Petz, L.D., and Garatty, G.: Clin. Haematol. **4:**181, 1975.
50. Ries, C.A., et al.: J.A.M.A. **233:**432, 1975.
51. Spath, P., Garatty, G., and Petz, L.D.: J. Immunol. **107:**860, 1971.
52. Worlledge, S.M.: Br. J. Haematol. **16:**5, 1969.
53. Snyder, E.L., and Spivack, M.: Transfusion **19:**313, 1979.
54. Spath, P., Garatty, G., and Petz, L.D.: J. Immunol. **107:**854, 1971.

Transfusion reactions

The term *transfusion reaction* is usually restricted to untoward reactions occurring during a blood transfusion or shortly afterward and does not include such long-term deleterious effects as the transmission of hepatitis or such immediate effects as acute congestive heart failure or failure to achieve the desired results, e.g., failure to raise the blood count as expected. It cannot be overemphasized that the generally accepted indications for transfusion therapy should be strictly adhered to since every transfusion entails a risk. Whenever a transfusion reaction occurs, the transfusion must be discontinued at once.

Transfusion reactions can be divided into **hemolytic** and **nonhemolytic reactions.** Hemolytic reactions may be either **immediate** or **delayed** in their mode of presentation.

HEMOLYTIC REACTIONS
Immediate hemolytic reactions

Evidence of hemolysis is seen either during or immediately after blood has been infused. It is caused by the destruction of donor red cells by antibodies in the recipient's serum; hence, an in vivo antigen-antibody reaction occurs. The severity of the reaction will depend on the amount of blood transfused and on the type of antibody involved. If the antibody is capable of rapidly activating complement, the hemolysis is **intravascular;** this type of hemolytic reaction is the most severe and most likely to cause the death of the recipient. However, if the antibody does not activate complement or does so very slowly, the red cells will be hemolyzed in the reticuloendothelial system. Such **extravascular** hemolytic reactions are less severe, and fortunately, most hemolytic transfusion reactions are of this type. Antibodies that cause intravascular destruction usually belong to the ABO blood group system[1]; other antibodies include anti-Tj[a], anti-Vel, and some anti-Le[a]. The most common antibodies causing extravascular hemolysis include anti-K, anit-Jk[a], anti-Fy[a], and anti-Rh.[2]

Although most hemolytic transfusion reactions are caused by the destruction of donor red cells by recipient antibody, there are occasions in which recipient red cells may be destroyed by passively transfused donor antibody. Such hemolysis, caused by **minor side incompatibility,** is generally less severe than the hemolysis described above because a small amount of antibody is rapidly diluted by the recipient plasma. Minor side incompatibility can be prevented by accurate antibody screening of donor serum or by a minor cross match. The transfusion of group O blood to a group A, B, or AB recipient is an example of minor side incompatibility; the resulting hemolysis depends on the titer of isoagglutinins in the plasma. Therefore removing much of the plasma from group O blood (i.e., packed red cells) usually renders the unit innocuous; on rare occasions, intravascular hemolysis may still occur even with the use of packed red cells.[3]

Finally, there may be acute hemolysis because of **interdonor incompatibility.**[4-6] In such instances many units of compatible blood are administered to a recipient; an antibody present in one donor unit subsequently reacts with an antigen in another donor unit. All cases of interdonor incompatibility involving atypical antibodies have been associated with the Kell blood group system.[6]

Clinical symptoms of hemolysis include fever, chills, back pain, shock, burning at the infusion site, nausea, and vomiting. Acute renal failure secondary to hemoglobinuria may result from intravascular hemolysis. If the patient happens to be anesthetized at the time of transfusion, most of these symptoms will be masked and the only warnings of hemolysis may be shock, excessive oozing from the operative wound, and/or hematuria.

Causes of an immediate hemolytic transfusion reaction include the following[2]:

1. Failure to recognize antibodies present in the recipient serum prior to transfusion: the most common cause, usually associated with antibodies having weak reactivity or detected only when tested in the antiglobulin phase
2. Failure to recognize donor antibodies before transfusion: no longer a common problem since all donor serum is deliberately screened for atypical antibodies
3. Administration of blood considered compatible on the basis of an incomplete cross match: an emergency cross match may not detect antibodies in time to prevent hemolysis.

4. Erroneous identification of recipient, donor, or both
5. Failure to identify dangerous universal blood donors (group O blood)

Delayed hemolytic reactions

In delayed hemolytic reactions[7] evidence of hemolysis is greatly delayed, following an uneventful transfusion. The insidious character of hemolysis is caused by the presence of a low-titer antibody in the recipient serum, which is undetected despite careful pretransfusion testing. If the transfused cells carry the corresponding antigen, an anamnestic immune response is evoked with a rise in antibody titer several days after the infusion. In all cases the recipient has been primarily immunized either by a previous transfusion or a pregnancy. The delay in hemolysis is variable, ranging from 2-4 days to several weeks. The antibodies most often involved belong to the rhesus and Kidd systems[8]; occasional cases involving anti-K and anti-Fy[a] are recorded. Although only one antibody is usually involved, miltiple antibodies may be found.[9]

The most common clinical symptom associated with delayed hemolytic reactions is fever, which may or may not be associated with chills. Usually the other symptoms of hemolysis are absent; incompatibility is therefore most often suggested by supporting laboratory data, i.e., unexplained anemia after a blood transfusion and mild hyperbilirubinemia (rarely jaundice). In cases with severe hemolysis there may be hemoglobinuria, oliguria, or renal failure.[10]

Delayed hemolytic transfusion reactions are not completely preventable because the antibodies are either not present or are below detectable levels at the time of initial cross match.[11] It is suggested that any recipient who suffers a delayed hemolytic transfusion reaction be issued a card indicating the identity of the antibody involved and/or recording his blood phenotype as completely as possible. Only in this way will subsequent episodes be prevented.

Investigation of hemolytic reactions

Any type of reaction during or after a blood transfusion should be reported to the laboratory, and it is the technologist's duty to investigate each report. As soon as a reaction occurs, the transfusion should be stopped at once, keeping the intravenous line open with a slow saline drip. The entire blood transfusion unit with all unused blood should be returned to the laboratory along with a completed reaction report form. The nursing staff should collect the first urine passed after the reaction and send it to be laboratory for analysis of a possible hemolytic reaction. The technologist should immediately obtain EDTA-anticoagulated and clotted blood samples from the patient (referred to as the **posttransfusion sample**) for analysis.

The American Association of Blood Banks requires that all initial recipient blood samples be stored at 1-6° C for at least 7 days after transfusion[12]; this blood is referred to as the **pretransfusion sample**. After a hemolytic transfusion reaction, the pretransfusion and posttransfusion samples are tested together and compared.

Immediate minimal investigation on all suspected hemolytic reactions

The following minimal steps should clearly indicate if a hemolytic reaction has occurred. If the results of these steps are normal, it is not necessary to proceed further.

1. The following specimens must be collected and used for the investigation: (a) recipient pretransfusion blood sample; (b) recipient posttransfusion blood sample; (c) blood remaining in the bag, or if there is none, the tube segments from the bag; and (d) first posttransfusion urine from the recipient.
2. All the above specimens are examined for visible hemolysis. Compare the color of pretransfusion and posttransfusion sera or plasma; plasma with an approximate hemolglobin content of 20 mg/dl appears faintly pink, whereas plasma containing as much as 100 mg/dl is red in color.[13] If desired, perform a quantitative determination of plasma or serum hemoglobin. Examine the spun urine with reagent chemical strip indicators of hemoglobin.
3. Perform a direct antiglobulin test on the pretransfusion and posttransfusion blood samples; examine microscopically for a mixed-field reaction.
4. Repeat an ABO group and Rh type on all blood samples, including the blood remaining in the bag.
5. Do a complete clerical check to detect identification errors or mislabeling.

Laboratory investigation on all proven hemolytic reactions

If any of the checks described in the preceding section is abnormal, the following steps must be taken:

1. Repeat the major cross match using recipient pretransfusion and posttransfusion blood samples.
2. Repeat the antibody screen on pretransfusion and posttransfusion recipient serum and serum from the bag segments.
3. Identify any antibody detected using panel cells; use enzyme treatment if necessary.
4. Perform appropriate biochemical studies to estimate the patient's status or the severity of hemolysis: serum bilirubin level taken 5-7 hr after the transfusion and BUN and creatinine levels.

Miscellaneous laboratory investigation

The following laboratory investigation is optional.

1. Determine the serum haptoglobin level. Whenever the plasma is discolored by free hemoglobin, the serum haptoglobin measurement will be zero because the haptoglobin-binding capacity has already been exceeded.
2. Determine if methemalbumin is present. Methemalbumin is present 5-24 hr after a hemolytic episode; it discolors the plasma brown.
3. Compare pretransfusion and posttransfusion hemoglobin and hematocrit levels. Within 48-74 hr, each completed transfusion should raise the hemoglobin level by 1.5 g/dl and the red blood cell level by 5,000,000 cells. In the case of a hemolytic transfusion reaction, the expected rise will not take place and there may even be a rapid drop in the red cell count.
4. Examine the patient's plasma for evidence of diffuse intravascular coagulation: low platelet count, pro-

longed activated partial thromboplastin time, thrombin time, prothrombin time test, evidence of fibrin degradation products and of fibrinolysis, and low levels of the so-called clot factors: fibrinogen (I), prothrombin (II), labile factor (V), and antihemophilic factor (VIII).

5. Do a gram stain of donor bag blood if indicated. A culture should be performed if positive.

NONHEMOLYTIC REACTIONS

A variety of nonhemolytic transfusion reactions may occur, most of which are febrile in character and some of which are lethal. These reactions may be caused by recipient or donor leukoagglutinins, recipient antibodies to platelets or plasma protein, or recipient reaction to allergens or bacteria present in donor blood.

Leukoagglutinins

Antibodies to donor white cells may develop after many transfusions and can create difficulties with subsequent transfusions; eventually these recipients will be unable to tolerate further blood transfusions without manifesting recurring, febrile reactions. Leukoagglutinating antibodies are the cause of these reactions,[14] accounting for most cases of **nonhemolytic febrile transfusion reactions** occuring today. The fever may be severe and delayed, becoming evident 1 hr or more after the infusion has begun. Since such a reaction cannot be differentiated from a hemolytic reaction in its early stages, it must be treated as one; however, knowledge of previous, recurrent attacks would aid in differentiation. These patients are best managed by the use of buffy coat–poor red cells or, if needed, frozen red cells.

Leukoagglutinins have also been implicated in another febrile reaction referred to as the **noncardiac pulmonary edema syndrome.** Characteristically the reaction is severe and delayed (1-6 hr after transfusion) with hypotension, dyspnea, cyanosis, moist pulmonary rales, and a nonproductive cough; chest x-ray examination shows bilateral pulmonary infiltrates, and a blood eosinophilia is common. This condition has occurred after the transfusion of whole blood or plasma, and there are isolated reports of it occurring after cryoprecipitate infusion.[15] Although the precise etiology is still unknown, leukoagglutinins in the recipient[16] as well as in the donor[17] have been implicated. The occurrence of leukoagglutinins as well as lymphocytotoxins in women is known to increase with parity[18]; the common association of this syndrome with multiparous donors has led to the routine query of parity in most donor centers or to the selective use of their blood products.

Posttransfusion purpura

A severe, prolonged thrombocytopenia may rarely develop after the administration of blood or platelet-containing components; the thrombocytopenia is usually first detected 7 or more days after the infusion. With the exception of one reported case,[19] all patients lack a very common platelet-specific antigen, PL^{A1}, and their sera contain anti-PL^{A1}. Most patients are women and have a history of many previous pregnancies, suggesting that these patients develop an isoantibody to incompatible platelet antigens. Invariably, the isoantibody causes destruction not only of donor platelets (PL^{A1} positive) but also of autologous platelets (PL^{A1} negative); the cause of the latter phenomenon is unknown.

Diagnosis

The diagnosis of posttransfusion purpura is as follows:

1. Clinical signs: These patients will suddenly present with petechiae, purpuric lesions, "blood blisters," and occult or obvious hemorrhage, all appearing within the appropriate time span of a compatible blood transfusion.

2. Platelet count: A profound thrombocytopenia is present, with values averaging 1000-10,000/mm^3 being common.

3. Demonstration of platelet antibodies: There are a number of laboratory tests that can be performed to assess platelet antibody.

Platelet agglutination[20]

Principle: In the presence of some antiplatelet antibodies, platelets may spontaneously agglutinate; this can be seen as clumping under the light microscope.

Procedure:

1. Mix 1 part normal platelet-rich plasma with 4 parts ACD test plasma.
2. Immediately, and after a 30 min incubation at 37° C, centrifuge slowly.
3. Gently shake the button at the bottom of the tube and observe for clumping under the light microscope.
4. Alternatively, allow the mixture from step 1 to incubate overnight at 4° C before gently resuspending and observing for clumping microscopically.

Interpretation: Normal platelets usually break up when gently rolled; antibody-coated platelets may remain clumped. The test is both nonsensitive and nonspecific. Since false positive reactions do occur, all positive results must be repeated. A negative test does not rule out platelet antibodies because not all platelet antibodies cause agglutination.

Platelet aggregation[21]

Principle: Normal platelets will aggregate when exposed to various stimuli, e.g., adenosine diphosphate (ADP). In the presence of platelet antibodies, spontaneous aggregation occurs, rendering these platelets "ADP nonresponsive." Although platelet aggregation may be assessed by simple visual inspection, spectrophotometers provide a more accurate interpretation. For this purpose, aggregometers are available with a continuous recording strip of the resulting change in optical density. As platelets aggregate, or clump, light transmission through a sample of platelet-rich plasma will increase (optical density will fall); if no aggregation occurs, the plasma remains turbid, with no change in optical density.

Procedure: Prepare normal platelet-rich plasma by centrifuging citrated blood in a silicone glass tube at 2500 rpm for 3 min. Remove platelet-rich plasma from the red cells and place at room temperature for at least 30 min before testing.

Add 1 part heated test serum to 1 part normal platelet-rich plasma in a silicone-coated aggregometer cuvet. Place the cuvet in the light path of an aggregometer, providing a constant temperature and continual stirring of the mixture; record the optical density for a minimum of 3 min. Add 0.5 μM ADP and continue optical density recordings.

If an antibody titer is desired, serial dilutions of the heated test serum can be done, i.e., the reciprocal of the highest serum dilution giving a positive result.

Interpretation: A positive test is an initial fall in optical density with no further fall after the addition of ADP.

Complement fixation

Principle: In the presence of an antigen-antibody complex, complement will be fixed[22,23] and unavailable to lyse sensitized red cells.

Procedure: The test involves the incubation of guinea pig serum (source of complement; commercially obtained), normal platelets (source of antigen), and heated, patient's serum (source of antibody) for 1 hr at 37° C. Then 0.5 ml buffer and 0.1 ml sensitized sheep red cells are added; hemolysis is observed.

Interpretation: Lysis of red cells indicates the presence of complement and the absence of antibody in the test serum. If a platelet antibody is present in the patient's serum, complement will be unavailable to lyse the red cells. False negative results do occur because not all platelet antibodies are complement binding. The test is very cumbersome, requiring difficult serum titrations to achieve proper concentrations of complement; therefore it is not a suitable test for all laboratories.

^{51}Cr release assay[24]

Principle: ^{51}Cr binds to platelet stroma and to low-molecular-weight compounds within the platelet. When an antigen-antibody complex occurs as a result of antiplatelet antibodies, the platelets are damaged and, in the presence of complement, will lyse, releasing the radioactive label.

Procedure: PL^{A1}-positive and PL^{A1}-negative platelets are labeled with the radioactive isotope ^{51}Cr. The isotope-labeled platelets (source of antigen) are mixed with normal EDTA-anticoagulated plasma (source of complement), patient's serum (source of antibody), and MgCl$_2$ (0.1M). The mixture is incubated, 2 ml saline is added, and centrifugation is performed. The supernatant is counted in a γ-counter.

Interpretation: Anti-PL^{A1} antibodies lyse normal PL^{A1} platelets, releasing ^{51}Cr into the supernatant; a count of the supernatant is therefore directly related to the amount of antibody present. This test is very sensitive, exceeding the sensitivity of complement fixation tests[19]; it is easier to perform than the complement fixation test but does require a γ-counter and therefore may not be suitable for all laboratories.

Platelet factor 3 assay

Principle: Platelet factor 3 (PF 3)[25] is a phospholipid that activates the formation of plasma thromboplastin.

In order for PF 3 to be fully expressed, platelets must be "activated" in some way; platelet aggregation, which can be induced by antiplatelet antibodies, is an adequate stimulus for PF 3 release. In the presence of PF 3, the clotting time of plasma will be shortened.

Procedure: Prepare normal platelet-rich plasma by centrifuging citrate blood at 2500 rpm for 3 min. Normal platelet-poor plasma is prepared by centrifuging citrate blood at 4000 rpm for 10 min. Sodium citrate, 40%, 0.1 part, to 10 parts blood is used. The resulting plasma is kept at 22° C.

Prepare test and control sera by allowing the blood to clot completely for 4 hr at 37° C; remove the serum and heat at 56° C for 30 min. Incubate 0.1 ml test and control sera separately with 0.1 ml platelet-rich plasma for 10 min at 37° C.

Place a 0.1 ml aliquot of each reaction mixture into one of two fibrocups; add 0.1 ml platelet-poor plasma to each and allow to incubate 30 sec more at 37° C. Add 0.2 ml CaCl$_2$ (0.025M) to each fibrocup and record the clotting time with a fibrometer.

Interpretation: If the clotting time of the test serum is shorter than that of the control serum, the test is positive, indicating the presence of a large amount of PF 3 that has resulted from platelet injury. The test is highly sensitive yet easy to perform; it represents an adaptation of the original assays utilizing the Stypven clotting time.[26,27] The test can also be used to detect platelet antibodies in idiopathic thrombocytopenic purpura and systemic lupus erythematosus.

Prognosis

The thrombocytopenia in posttransfusion purpura is transient but can be life threatening. Effective therapy includes plasmapheresis,[28,29] exchange transfusion,[30] and corticosteroids.[31]

Antibodies to serum IgA

Of all the selective deficiencies of serum immunoglobulins, IgA deficiency is the most common, occurring approximately 0.1% of random tested blood donors.[32] Although most IgA-deficient persons are healthy, some have associated disorders, including recurrent infections, intestinal disorders, and autoimmune disease. In addition, 10% will develop antibodies to the IgA protein by an obscure mechanism[33] and can suffer acute anaphylactic reactions when infused with blood products containing the protein.[34] The reactions are severe, characterized by flushing, abdominal pain, vomiting, diarrhea, chills and fever, laryngeal edema, shock, and collapse; these symptoms are seen very rapidly after exposure to the IgA protein, often before 10 ml of plasma has been infused. Such patients must be transfused only with IgA-deficient blood, i.e., frozen red cells, autologous blood, or selected IgA-deficient blood obtained through the Rare Donor Files of the American Association of Blood Banks or the National Red Cross.

Laboratory diagnosis

After the appearance of appropriate symptoms following a transfusion, the diagnosis is assumed if an absence of IgA in the recipient's serum can be demonstrated. An absolute diagnosis is possible if the identification of serum anti-IgA is specifically made.

Measurement of serum IgA: Serum IgA is most easily measured with agar gel diffusion using a monospecific anti-IgA serum; absence of a precipitin line is presumptive evidence of an a-IgA globulinemia, which can be confirmed with more sensitive tests, e.g., radioimmunoassay or a hemagglutination inhibition assay utilizing IgA-coated red cells.[35] It is rarely necessary to perform confirmatory tests since the absence of a precipitin band in a patient exhibiting these appropriate symptoms confers a diagnosis of reasonable accuracy.

Those laboratories wishing to maintain their own supply of IgA-deficient donor blood can utilize a recently described latex agglutination slide test as a rapid screening test of the general population. This test utilizes polystyrene beads coated with purified rabbit antihuman IgA antiserum.[36]

Measurement of anti-IgA antibody: Antibodies to IgA can be detected using the **passive hemagglutination assay.**

Principle: Serum containing IgA antibodies will agglutinate indicator red cells coated with purified IgA protein.

Preparation of coated red cells[37,38]: Mix 1 volume washed human group O red cells with 1 volume protein solution at a concentration of 1 mg/ml. A variety of protein solutions are used: IgA myeloma protein, normal human IgG isolated from pooled serum, and IgM protein isolated from patients with Waldenström's macroglobulinemia.

Add 1 volume of 0.05% $CrCl_3$ diluted tris-HCl–buffered saline (pH 7.2). Allow a 5 min incubation at room temperature. Wash the coated red cells four times. Indicator red cells separately coated with IgA, IgG, and IgM protein are now ready for use. They may be stored at 4° C in Alsever's solution for a maximum of 5 days before use.[39]

Procedure[39]: Place 1 drop 0.5% saline–suspended coated red cells on a glass tile. Use 1 drop 0.5% saline–suspended uncoated group O red cells as a cell control. Add 1 drop undiluted test serum, or diluted test serum if performing titration studies. Use 1 drop undiluted normal serum and 1 drop saline as controls.

Incubate slides in a moist chamber at room temperature for 15 min with gentle agitation. Observe for hemagglutination with an optical aid and record the strength of clumping.

Interpretation: Hemagglutination of IgA-coated red cells indicates the presence of IgA antibodies, provided the serum and saline controls are negative and no agglutination is observed with IgG- or IgM-coated cells. The titer of a serum is expressed as the reciprocal of the highest dilution at which at least 1+ agglutination is observed.

Allergic reactions

Allergic reactions are among the most common and, at the same time, the least dangerous reactions. These reactions, which consist of hives and itching, develop during the infusion and can be well controlled with antihistamines; it is usually not necessary to stop the transfusion.

Bacterial reactions

Bacterial reactions are caused by a break in technic and are preventable. The bacteria are usually gram-negative rods (often of the *Pseudomonas* sp.), which are able to multiply at 4° C. *Pseudomonas* bacteremia or endotoxemia or both may result in diffuse intravascular coagulation characterized by profuse bleeding, shock, and death.[40] A Gram stain of the blood taken from the administration set may reveal gram-negative rods.

REFERENCES

1. Buchholz, D., and Bove, J.: Transfusion **15**:577, 1975.
2. Pineda, A.A., Brzica, S.M., and Taswell, H.F.: Mayo Clin. Proc. **53**:378, 1978.
3. Inwood, M.J., and Zuliani, B.: Ann. Intern. Med. **89**:515, 1978.
4. Zettner, A., and Bove, J.R.: Transfusion **3**:48, 1963.
5. Franciosi, R., Awer, E., and Santana, M.: Transfusion **7**:297, 1967.
6. Morse, E.E.: Vox Sang. **35**:215, 1978.
7. Pineda, A.A., Taswell, H.F., and Brzica, S.M.: Transfusion **18**:1, 1978.
8. Howard, P.L.: Ann. Clin. Lab. Sci. **3**:13, 1973.
9. Moncrieff, R.E., and Thompson, W.P.: Am. J. Clin. Pathol. **64**:251, 1975.
10. Meltz, D.J., et al.: Lancet **2**:1348, 1971.
11. Solanki, D., and McCurdy, P.: J.A.M.A. **239**:729, 1978.
12. Standards for blood banks and transfusion services, ed. 9, Washington, D.C., 1978, American Association of Blood Banks.
13. Mollison, P.L.: Blood transfusion in clinical medicine, ed. 6, Oxford, England, 1979, Blackwell Scientific Publication, Inc., p. 587.
14. Hasegawa, T., et al.: Transfusion **15**:226, 1975.
15. Reese, E.P., McCullough, J.J., and Craddock, P.R.: Transfusion **15**:583, 1975.
16. Wolf, C.F.W., and Canale, V.C.: Transfusion **16**:135, 1976.
17. Thompson, J.S., et al.: N. Engl. J. Med. **284**:1120, 1971.
18. Payne, R.: Blood **19**:411, 1962.
19. Ziegler, Z.R., Murphy, S., and Gardner, F.H.: Blood **42**:1023, 1973.
20. VanDerWeerdt, C.M., et al.: Vox Sang. **8**:513, 1963.
21. Deykin, D., and Hellerstein, L.J.: J. Clin. Invest. **51**:3142, 1972.
22. Aster, R.H., Cooper, H.E., and Singer D.L.: J. Lab. Clin. Med. **63**:161, 1964.
23. Shulman, N.R., et al.: Prog. Hematol. **4**:222, 1964.
24. Aster, R.H., and Enright, S.E.: J. Clin. Invest. **48**:1199, 1969.
25. Hirschman, R.J., and Gralnick, H.R.: J. Lab. Clin. Med. **84**:292, 1974.
26. Horowitz, H.I., et al.: Transfusion **5**:336, 1965.
27. Karpatkin, S., and Siskind, G.W.: Blood **33**:795, 1969.
28. Abramson, N., Eisenberg, P.D., and Aster, R.H.: N. Engl. J. Med. **291**:1163, 1974.
29. Laursen, B., et al.: Acta Med. Scand. **203**:539, 1978.
30. Cimo, P.L., and Aster, R.H.: N. Engl. J. Med. **287**:290, 1972.
31. Seidenfeld, A.M., et al.: Can. Med. Assoc. J. **118**:1285, 1978.
32. Koistinen, J.: Vox Sang. **29**:192, 1975.
33. Koistinen, J., and Sarna, S.: Vox Sang. **29**:203, 1975.

34. Pineda, A.A., and Taswell, H.F.: Transfusion **15:**10, 1975.
35. Vyas, G.N., and Fudenberg, H.H.: Clin. Genet. **1:**55, 1971.
36. Newcomb, W., Dibberin, P., and Minard, B.: Lab. Med. **8:**18, 1977.
37. Gold, E.R., and Fudenberg, H.H.: J. Immunol. **99:**859, 1967.
38. Leikola, J., et al.: Blood **42:**111, 1973.
39. Rivat, L., et al.: Clin. Immunol. Immunopathol. **7:**340, 1977.
40. Medal, S.L., et al.: Vox Sang. **6:**170, 1961.

CLINICAL CHEMISTRY

Laboratory principles and instrumentation

Many factors influence the chemical composition of blood and other body fluids in disease. One general factor includes those instances in which blood constituents increase because of alterations of permeable membranes in the excretory organs such as the lungs, kidneys, and liver. The accumulation of nitrogenous waste products in certain forms of nephritis and the hyperbilirubinemia associated with liver disease are examples of retention affected by such processes. In other instances, alterations in blood constituents may be caused by changes in the rate of formation or in the use of these constituents. The accumulation of glucose in the blood of diabetic individuals resulting from a metabolic derangement in the use of this substance is an example. Furthermore, the administration of drugs may alter the concentration of some blood constituents.

Even without more examples it is evident that knowledge of the concentrations of the various blood constituents (and also of other body fluids, e.g., cerebrospinal fluid and urine) is an important aid to the physician not only in diagnosis but also in evaluating the results of therapy. Since the success or failure of the physician's efforts and even the life of the patient may depend on accurate determinations of the blood levels of the important constituents and the transmission of these data to the physician in time for them to be of greatest use to him, the need for accuracy and speed in analysis cannot be overemphasized. However, except for an emergency, accuracy should never be sacrificed for speed. The patient's welfare is as much a trust of the laboratory technicians as of the supervising physician.

During the past 20-30 years there have been tremendous developments in laboratory methods and technics. Constituents for which no satisfactory tests were available a few years ago are now routinely determined in the clinical laboratory. Many new methods have been developed, and improvements are constantly being made. Many methods are available for the commonly determined constituents. Some of these, however, may require special equipment. For each of these constituents, the following sections have endeavored to give the one or two methods that are thought to be most satisfactory for the general clinical laboratory from the point of view of accuracy and simplicity. This does not imply that other equally satisfactory methods may not be available or that those given are the best for every purpose. Every method has its limitations, but those presented are believed to be generally applicable to most laboratories.

In discussing the specific details of the various procedures or tests, mention may be made of an apparatus or component made by a particular manufacturer. This does not mean that products of other manufacturers may not be equally satisfactory. Since it is impractical to mention all possible sources of supply, we have generally mentioned a type that is readily available as a guide to the exact kind of material or apparatus desired. The same is true of reagent chemicals; we may mention that the chemical from a certain manufacturer gives a very low blank. Other brands may also give a low blank, but we have not been able to test all of them and merely mention one that we have found to be satisfactory.

COLLECTION OF BLOOD SPECIMENS

In the analysis of blood constituents the first consideration is collection of the specimen.[1,2] Even if this is not done by the laboratory technician, he should be familiar with the technic and principles involved. The different chemical tests will require different types of specimens, i.e., clotted blood or blood containing a particular anticoagulant or preservative. Usually venous blood is used; sometimes small amounts of capillary blood from the fingertip or earlobe is satisfactory; and occasionally arterial blood is required. For some tests a small amount of hemolysis may not be of great importance, whereas in other tests it must be scrupulously avoided. It is best to develop a technic that will keep hemolysis at a minimum at all times. The technician must be familiar with these factors to advise others as to the type of sample required, even if he does not actually draw the specimen himself.

Venous blood may be obtained by using a hypodermic syringe and a 20- or 21-gauge needle. If many samples are to be drawn, it may be convenient to use the commercially available evacuated blood collecting tubes (e.g., Vacutainers [Becton-Dickinson & Co., Rutherford, N.J.]) obtainable from most laboratory supply houses. This method of securing blood samples eliminates the trouble involved in cleaning the syringes. If glass syringes are used, they must be thoroughly dried before use to prevent hemolysis caused by traces of water. Disposable plastic syringes may also be used. When blood is being transferred from the syringe to a test tube or other container, the needle should be removed first and the blood should not be forced out too vigorously, because this will also cause some hemolysis. To guard against the spread of viral hepatitis disposable needles are used once and then discarded. This also eliminates the necessity of sharpening needles.

Anticoagulants

Whole blood or plasma is required for some tests. This necessitates the use of an anticoagulant to prevent clotting. Not all anticoagulants are equally satisfactory for every test. Some may interfere with the chemical reactions of a given test. Heparin is an excellent anticoagulant but is more expensive than other chemicals used for this purpose. The amount required depends on the potency of the product and should be stated on the vial. Care should be taken to avoid a large excess of anticoagulant, because it may interfere with some chemical tests.

Potassium oxalate is commonly used when oxalate is required, since it is more soluble than sodium or lithium salts; 20 mg of potassium oxalate is sufficient for 10 ml of blood. The use of commercially available evacuated containers that are furnished with a number of different anticoagulants eliminates the trouble of preparing tubes.

Another anticoagulant that is sometimes used is disodium salt of ethylenediamine tetraacetic acid. This is sold under a variety of trade names. It is somewhat less generally applicable than oxalate. About 10 mg is required for 10 ml of blood. When a powdered anticoagulant such as this is used, it must be thoroughly mixed with and dissolved in the blood as soon as possible after the blood is added to the tube.

A special anticoagulant is a 0.1M solution of sodium oxalate, which is made by dissolving 1.34 g of reagent grade sodium oxalate in water to make 1 dl. This is used to secure blood plasma for prothrombin time determinations. In this procedure, 4.5 ml of blood is added to 0.5 ml of the oxalate solution.

Preservation of blood samples

Many constituents of blood may change more or less rapidly in concentration on standing, particularly at room or elevated temperatures. A conspicuous example of this is blood glucose. On standing at room temperature, the glucose in whole blood may be metabolized to the extent of 5% or more per hour. The loss is less at lower temperatures, and blood samples may be kept for several hours without great loss if they are immediately chilled in an ice bath and kept at this temperature. (Merely placing the tubes in the refrigerator may not be satisfactory, since cooling may be very slow, particularly if several tubes are placed together in a small container.) For glucose determinations in which there is to be some delay before analysis it is best to separate the serum by centrifugation after clotting and pour off the serum into another tube. The sample can be left in the original tube after centrifugation if one of the commercially available "barrier" tubes is used. These tubes contain a silicone gel that floats above the clot and below the serum (e.g., SST tubes [Becton-Dickinson & Co., Rutherford, N.J.]). Similar silicone products (e.g., Sur-Sep [General Diagnostics, Morris Plains, N.J.]) are available to be used with tubes with no added silicone.

It is also possible but less desirable to add a preservative that will inhibit glycolysis. Fluoride is generally simple to use and has some anticoagulant properties in itself, but relatively larger amounts are required than for oxalate. Evacuated tubes containing both fluoride and oxalate are available commercially. Fluoride will inhibit enzyme action; therefore it cannot be used when any such reaction is involved (except with amylase or urease if the fluoride is not over 2 mg/ml of blood). However, most enzymatic determinations are made on serum in which no anticoagulant is used.

Other changes may also occur in blood if left standing, e.g., changes in phosphate resulting from hydrolysis of organic phosphate esters, changes in lipids resulting from lipolysis, and changes in chloride resulting from shifts of chloride between cells and serum. Accordingly, it is best to begin analysis as soon as possible after the blood has been drawn. If serum or plasma is to be used for analysis, it should be separated from the cells or clot as soon as possible. (However, at least 30 min should be allowed for complete clotting at room temperature.) After separation, serum or plasma can usually be kept for a somewhat longer time without deterioration. For most tests, including some enzymatic determinations, serum or plasma may be kept for a few days in the refrigerator; for most enzyme tests the frozen serum may be kept for several days. If the serum is frozen, the material must be completely thawed and well mixed again before use. Special precautions for preserving or collecting samples are given in connection with the particular test involved.

BASIC LABORATORY APPARATUS AND PRINCIPLES

A number of basic topics, although directed mainly to the chemistry laboratory, are applicable in other branches of the clinical laboratory as well. Volumetric apparatus, for example, can be used in any part of the laboratory for the accurate preparation and dilution of solutions. The various types of automatic dilutors are also widely applicable. In this and subsequent sections it is impossible to mention all makes of a particular type of instrument or apparatus. If a particular make is mentioned, it is usually to illustrate the type of instrument without implying that the particular instrument is best for all procedures or even for the procedure under discussion. Some information about particular makes of a given instrument type can be found in the catalogs of the larger laboratory supply houses. Another source of information is the *Guide to Scientific Instruments,* which is published annually by the American Association for Advancement of Science as a special issue of the journal *Science.* This contains the names and addresses of the manufacturers of most types of scientific instruments listed by type of instrument. Further information may be obtained by writing directly to the manufacturer.

Quantities and units[3,4]

Many of the results of analyses in the clinical laboratory are expressed in concentration units, e.g., milligrams of glucose per deciliter of serum or milliequivalents of sodium per liter of plasma. The common units used for expressing concentratiions are not always consistent, and different laboratories may use different units. Some of these units are not in accord with the most precise scientific terminology. The older units may have been introduced by different investigators who used different types of units depending on their original training (as physicians, chemists, physicists, etc.). These original units have persisted in common use. The units used in different countries have not always been the same. It is certainly desirable that all laboratories throughout the world report the results for an analysis of a given constituent in the same units. Recognizing these variations, the Commission on Clinical Chemistry of the International Union of Pure and Applied Chemistry (IUPAC) and the International Federation for Clinical Chemistry recommended a set of consistent, scientific units for reporting results in clinical chemistry. These are based on the international system of units (Système International Unité, SIU) in which the basic units are the kilogram, the meter, and the second.

Many of these units have not yet come into common use in the United States and therefore have not been used in this volume. Although many of the commission's recommendations have been adopted by scientific journals, it will take longer for them to attain common usage. A number of the recommendations will be mentioned here, since they do represent a logically and scientifically consistent set of units that undoubtedly will be used increasingly in the future, just as the reporting of serum sodium and potassium as milliequivalents per liter has largely replaced the older expression in terms of milligrams per deciliter.

The term *nanometer* (nm) is used for specification of wavelengths of light in the visible region rather than the older term *millimicron* (mμ). It is also recommended that the term *micron* (μ) be replaced by *micrometer* (μm). Wherever possible the results are to be expressed in multiples of the basic units. A number of prefixes are used for this purpose. For those not familiar with all of these, the following table is given.

Factor	Prefix	Symbol
10^{+9}	giga	G
10^{+6}	mega	M
10^{+3}	kilo	k
10^{-3}	milli	m
10^{-6}	micro	μ
10^{-9}	nano	n
10^{-12}	pico	p
10^{-15}	femto	f

The prefixes giga-, mega-, and femto- are rarely required in the magnitudes usually involved in clinical laboratory work.

Concentration units

The recommendations of the commission also include eliminating expression of concentration as percent. The use of this term can result in confusion and is often not strictly correct. The use of percent should only be taken in its literal meaning, "per hundred," i.e., 5% means 5 units of something per 100 of the same units. Even in expressing the concentrations of simple solutions, an expression such as a 5% (wt/vol) solution of monosodium phosphate can be ambiguous. Does it mean 5 g of NaH_2PO_4/dl of solution or 5 g of $NaH_2PO_4 \cdot 7H_2O$, since both salts are commercially available? One cannot even say that the designation always means the anhydrous salt, since a 5% solution of copper sulfate would almost certainly be understood to mean 5 g of the pentahydrate. In regard to inorganic acids the problem is more complicated. What, for example, is a 5% solution of hydrochloric acid? A 5% (vol/vol) solution is usually taken to mean 5 ml of concentrated acid diluted to 1 dl, and a 5% (wt/vol) solution is one that contains 5 g of pure hydrogen chloride/dl. This latter solution would be made by diluting approximately 12 ml of the concentrated acid to 1 dl. For reagents the best solution is to express the concentrations as molarities when possible. Thus a 0.35M solution of monosodium phosphate will contain the same amount of actual NaH_2PO_4 no matter which salt is used in its preparation. We have tried to follow this procedure in this book in most instances. The IUPAC recommendations include the elimination of expression such as 0.5M, replacing it with 0.5 mole/L, which has generally been done in this book. The IUPAC gave the abbreviation of 1 (lowercase L) for liter, but since this can be confused with the number one, it recommended that the word be spelled out. In the United States the legal abbreviation is L.[5]

The recommendations also include the elimination of the expression *mg%*. This hybrid term is actually meaningless. It should be replaced by *milligrams per 100 milliliters* or, as has been generally used, *milligrams per deciliter* (1 deciliter = 1 dl = 100 ml). The recommendations gave preference to the use of *grams per liter* (or milligrams, micrograms, etc.). This was used earlier in the European countries, but *grams per deciliter* is more commonly used in the United States. Whenever the substance being analyzed or reported consists of a definite molecular species, e.g., glucose, the preferred term is *moles per liter* (or millimoles, micromoles, etc.). This is already required for a number of technical publications in the United States, and these units are given as a secondary expression in parentheses.[6]

The liter has been redefined as exactly 1 cubic decimeter (1000 cubic centimeters). Formerly it was stated to be equal to 1000.028 cubic centimeters; this is of little practical importance because of the small difference. Although the IUPAC discourages the use of the liter, it is still the most convenient means (along with its submultiples) of expressing concentrations.

The units used for expressing enzyme concentrations are discussed in detail in the section on enzymes. As yet it is not possible to express enzymes in mass concentration units (e.g., picograms per milliliter). Furthermore, the basic property of the enzyme in which one is interested is its ability to catalyze a given biologic reaction. Thus the basic unit is the amount of enzyme that will catalyze the decomposition of 1 μmole of substrate per minute under certain specified conditions of temperature, substrate concentration, and pH. If each molecule of the substrate, A, is decomposed into one molecule of product, B, it may be simpler in some instances to measure the amount of B formed rather than the amount of A decomposed, but this does not affect the units. In those instances in which the substrate does not have a definite molecular weight, the unit is usually defined in terms of moles of substrate formed, as in the production of reducing sugars from starch by enzyme analysis. The concentration expression is then given in units (or submultiples) per liter. As will be seen, there are many differently defined units for the different enzymes. When the activity is expressed as above in micromoles per minute per liter, the units are defined as international units.

Volumetric glassware[7]

This category includes graduated cylinders, pipets, volumetric flasks, and burets.

Graduated cylinders

Graduated cylinders are used to measure approximate quantities of reagents or solutions. They should not be used when accurate measurements are required. In the preparation of a reagent solution, for example, the amount of a substance added, e.g., a concentrated acid, may not be critical. It is only required that an excess be added or that the acidity be within a certain range. In such instances graduated cylinders can be used. Even here, for volumes less than 10 ml a measuring pipet is preferable.

Pipets

Pipets may be classified as measuring, serologic, or volumetric. The former are generally cylindric in shape and graduated for measuring different volumes of liquid. These pipets are not very accurate and should not ordinarily be used for measuring standards or samples. Some of these pipets are calibrated to the tip. When measuring the total volume of these pipets, the last drop of solution is blown out after the pipet has drained completely. All "blow-out" pipets have a single sandblasted or frosted ring at the top for identification. When measurement is made of less than the total capacity of the pipet, the delivery is made between appropriate graduations. These pipets may be used for the delivery of reagents to a set of tubes for analysis if care is taken and the same pipet is used for all measurements of a given reagent. Usually the exact volume of reagent added is not as critical as adding the same amount of reagent to all tubes for standards, samples, and blank.

Volumetric pipets have a single graduation to deliver only one specified volume of liquid. Except for the Folin types and the micropipets mentioned later, all volumetric pipets are calibrated for delivery in a definite manner. When the liquid has ceased to flow out, the tip of the pipet is touched to the inner surface of the container into which the liquid has been delivered, and the additional liquid is allowed to flow out by capillary action. The pipet is then removed; any remaining liquid is not blown out. The pipets are marked "TD" for "to deliver" and have no sandblasted rings at the top. Some volumetric pipets of the Ostwald-Folin type are calibrated to blow out the last drop. These are usually used for smaller volumes (0.5-2 ml) of somewhat viscous liquids, e.g., serum. Folin pipets and some others are calibrated "to contain" (marked "TC") and are used for viscous liquids, e.g., whole blood. They are rinsed out with some of the diluting fluid after the blood has flowed out, and the last drop of wash solution is blown out. These are distinguished by two sandblasted or frosted rings at the top. Currently, few analyses are made using whole blood, and these pipets are used much less than formerly.

With all these types, the pipet should be held in a vertical position with the tip touching the side of the solution container. The liquid is then allowed to flow down to the uppermost graduation, reading at the bottom of the meniscus when possible. The tip of the pipet is then carefully wiped off and the solution delivered. All pipets should be throughly cleaned, so that they drain evenly and completely with no drops of liquid remaining on the inner surface. As with all volumetric apparatus, measurements should be made with the liquid at room temperature, since the volume of the liquid and the capacity of the pipet will change with temperature. It is recommended that only those volumetric pipets that, as stated by the suppliers, conform to the class A specifications of the National Bureau of Standards be purchased. Volumetric pipets having a chipped tip should be discarded. Several suppliers have available pipets with class A volume accuracy but with class B flow rates. These pipets do not have the large A on them and under the usual laboratory circumstances of limited time will not give the required class A volume accuracy.

There are a number of different types of micropipets; these may be roughly defined as pipets used for measuring volumes in the range of 10-250 µl. These are usually calibrated "to contain" and are rinsed out with the diluting fluid or other solution to which the contents of the pipet are added. It is not practical to list all the types available. For most work in the clinical laboratory we have found Accupettes (American Scientific Products Div., American Hospital Supply Corp., McGaw Park, Ill.) satisfactory. These are filled in a manner similar to the Sahli diluting pipets, with which most laboratory technicians are familiar. They are available in two types, those having a straight bore and those having a bulb. The latter type is preferred, since it has an accuracy of 0.5% as compared with 1.0% for the straight bore type.

A number of different disposable capillary micropipets are also available. These consist of sections of capillary tubing with a carefully controlled internal diameter. The larger sizes may have a graduation mark; the capillary is filled to this mark. In the smaller sizes the entire capillary is filled. These are filled by capillary action when held in a nearly horizontal position. When the excess of liquid is removed from the outside of the capillary, care must be taken not to remove any liquid from within the capillary. For this procedure the capillary is held nearly horizontal with the end that has been immersed in the liquid at an angle about 15 degrees higher than the other end and the outside carefully wiped off. Facial tissue or similar material is best. The contents of the capillary are then blown out into the diluting fluid and the capillary rinsed several times. The smaller sizes are usually furnished with a holder and a small rubber bulb to assist in this operation. The smaller sizes may also be placed in the tube containing the reagent and the contents eluted by stoppering the tube and shaking. The capillary may be left in the tube during the reactions involved. When the final solution is poured into a cuvet, the capillary will remain behind. These pipets are accurate to only about 1%, and careful use is necessary to attain this accuracy, but they are very convenient.

Volumetric flasks

Volumetric flasks are used for the dilution and preparation of solutions that are made up to a definite volume. It is preferable that only those certified as class A

by the National Bureau of Standards be purchased. In use they should be scrupulously clean, so that no drops will adhere to the neck of the flask above the graduation mark. Preferably, the graduation should not be too high in the neck so as to allow sufficient air space for good mixing. The final dilution to volume must be made with the contents of the flask at room temperature (20-25° C). The flasks are calibrated at 20° C, but if the room temperature is not more than 5° C above this, it usually is not necessary to cool to exactly 20° C before making to volume. Some volumetric flasks may have two graduations: "to contain" (marked "TC") and "to deliver" (marked "TD"). The latter type may be useful if one wishes to dilute a large volume of liquid. For example, to dilute exactly 250 ml of a solution to 1 L, one can fill a 250 ml flask to the "to deliver" mark, pour the contents into the 1 L flask, and allow it to drain completely but without rinsing out the flask. Needless to say, for this the flask must be completely clean. One can obtain the same result by using the "to contain" mark and rinsing out the flask with some of the diluting fluid.

In weighing out salts for the preparation of accurate solutions, it is preferable to weigh the salt on a plastic weighing boat and then transfer most of it to a dry volumetric flask with the aid of a powder funnel (a funnel having a short neck with a relatively large bore). The remaining salt is then rinsed into the flask from the weighing boat and funnel with some of the solvent. The flask is then filled to about 80% of its capacity with the solvent and swirled to dissolve the salt. When the salt has completely dissolved, the flask is allowed to cool (or to warm) to room temperature and is made up to volume. Since rubber stoppers may cause contamination, it is best to use flasks with glass or plastic stoppers. The latter are usually satisfactory, less expensive, and do not break if dropped. Highly alkaline solutions will etch the glass and should not be kept in volumetric flasks longer than necessary. Since volumetric flasks cost more than even the highest quality reagent bottles, it is wasteful to use them to store the solutions.

Burets

Although volumetric methods are not used as much in the clinical laboratory as formerly, burets are needed for some determinations and for the standardization of solutions. Instead of the regular burets with stopcocks, it is preferable to obtain those with Teflon stopcock plugs, because glass plugs tend to freeze if kept in contact with alkaline solutions for any length of time. Also, Teflon stopcocks usually give less trouble with leakage. The burets must be completely clean, so that they will drain evenly with no drops left on the sides. If they are to be used frequently with one solution, they may be kept filled with the solution and capped to prevent evaporation and contamination with dust. Otherwise they may be kept filled with distilled water and capped or they may be rinsed well with water, drained, and kept upside down in the buret holder. For all the uses mentioned in this volume, a 50 ml buret is best suited for the standardization of normal solutions and a 5 ml buret for other purposes. Only those conforming to the National Bureau of Standards class A specifications should be purchased.

Semiautomatic pipets, dispensers, and dilutors

A number of devices are available for rapidly pipetting or dispensing a number of aliquots of the same size.

Semiautomatic micropipets: For micro work there are several different pipets that consist of a spring-activated plunger in a precision bore with a disposable plastic tip. The plunger is depressed to the first stop and the tip inserted in the liquid to be measured. As the plunger is released, a definite volume of liquid is drawn into the plastic tip. After the tip has been wiped off, the plunger is again depressed to transfer the liquid to the desired tube. Some models have a second stop, so that when the plunger is depressed to this stop the liquid remaining in the tip is blown out. For successive sampling only the disposable tip need be changed. Since the liquid to be measured only comes in contact with the tip and is contained entirely within it, contamination and sample carry-over are eliminated. Some models are made to deliver only one specified volume (usually in the range of 20-1000 μl), although the same tips can often be used for pipets measuring different volumes. Other models are constructed so that different volumes can be pipetted by adjusting a stop. These pipets are very simple to use, and with care a precision of 1% can be attained. If the liquid is drawn up too rapidly, small air bubbles may appear in the tip. It is difficult to determine if an actual air bubble has been drawn in or if the correct amount of liquid has been drawn in with some of the air already in the tip and trapped inside the liquid. In the former instance an error would result. Thus it is preferable to release the plunger slowly.

In the use of these pipets it is recommended that the tip first be rinsed out with the solution to be used.[8,9] If sufficient sample is available, an aliquot can be drawn into the tip, discarded, and a second aliquot drawn up for use. If only a small amount of sample is available, an aliquot can be drawn into the tip and expelled back into the original container and the tip refilled. The tip should then be gently wiped off, with care taken not to remove any sample from the interior of the tip. If sufficient samples are available so that first rinse can be discarded, the same tip can be used for successive samplings with negligible carry-over. Prerinsing is imperative if a serum or similar sample is to be compared with an aqueous standard solution delivered with the same pipet. The method of delivery should also be standardized. A satisfactory method is to deliver the solution with the tip against the wall of the test tube, allowing the pipet to drain for a few seconds and then quickly removing it before releasing the plunger.

For small volumes of less than 25 μl the above pipets are not always sufficiently accurate. The SMI pipets (Scientific Manufacturing Industries, Emeryville, Calif.) are more accurate. These have a fine rod as a plunger, which fits into a precision bore glass capillary tube. The capillary tube can be readily changed, although the carry-over between successive samplings with the same capillary is small. These are not as rugged as the previously mentioned type; the wire may be easily bent and the capillaries are not as easily attached as the plastic tips.

Dispensers: To add a definite amount of reagent to a series of tubes, a syringe pipet is helpful. The attachment on the lower part of the syringe contains a two-way valve; the attached tubing with a weight on the end is placed in any vessel containing the reagent to be dispensed. A large-bore needle may be attached to the lower end for ease in delivery. The volume delivered by each stroke can be adjusted as required. It is tedious to adjust it to deliver, e.g., exactly 5 ml, but in many instances the exact volume of reagent may not be as important as delivering the same volume to all tubes. These syringe pipets are not very accurate, particularly when only a fraction of the volume of the syringe is used, but usually they are as satisfactory as regular Mohr pipets. They are inexpensive, and the syringe can be easily replaced. A similar arrangement is available for the SMI pipets mentioned. These are more satisfactory for the repetitive addition of small quantities of reagents.

Pipettors are made of inert material, glass, and Teflon. They are made to fit in the stopper or other closure of a reagent bottle and are generally used for one reagent that is employed daily. The volume delivered can be adjusted by varying the stroke of the piston. Usually the piston must be moved both up and down manually, but the operation is still quite rapid. These are very satisfactory, particularly for delivering strongly acid solutions, which are inconvenient to measure with regular pipets. Models are also made with two syringes. In these the smaller pipet is used to draw up a definite volume of sample, which is then expelled into the test tube, followed by a larger volume of reagent from the larger syringe. These are more fragile and parts are subject to breakage. The glass coil just above the delivery tip offers enough volume so that the sample drawn up never reaches the syringes themselves but remains within the coil where it is completely washed out by the larger volume of reagent or diluting fluid expelled.

Dilutors: A large number of different types of automatic dilutors are available. These usually contain the equivalent of two syringes of different sizes and are operated pneumatically and controlled by a lever. At one position a definite volume of sample is drawn up into the pipet tip; when the lever is moved to the other position, the sample is forced out, followed by a definite volume of diluent or reagent. The volume of sample and the volume of diluent can be regulated over a range of about one tenth of the volume to the total volume of the syringe used, some models having arrangements for replacement of syringes of different sizes. In some models the syringe sizes are fixed, with a range of 0.05-1.0 ml for the sample pickup and from 3-20 ml for the diluent volume. Some models have a fixed delivery pipet, and the tubes must be brought under it. Some models have the delivery tip attached to plastic tubing so that it can be moved from tube to tube. Even more sophisticated models have an arrangement whereby the delivery and pickup volumes can be changed at will merely by pressing the appropriate button. These dilutors are very convenient when a number of samples must be diluted with the same reagent or diluent, as in the determination of sodium and potassium by a manual flame photometer, dilution for hemoglobin determinations, or cell counting in a Coulter counter. In the former determinations the delivery pumps need not be adjusted to give exactly a 1:100 dilution (or whatever dilution is required) provided the samples and standards are diluted in the same dilutor with the same settings. In the hematology dilutions the exact dilution must be known. Usually the settings can be made quite accurately with the better instruments, but they should be checked. One way of doing this is to make several dilutions on a well-mixed blood sample in the usual way on the dilutor and to compare the readings with some manual dilutions made with accurate micropipets. If the usual dilution for hemoglobin is the addition of 0.02 ml of blood to 5 ml of reagent, the accurate manual dilutions can be made by adding 0.10 ml of blood to exactly 25 ml of reagent. The larger dilution can be made more accurately than with the use of only 0.02 of blood. The comparisons should preferably be made on a good spectrophotometer that can be read to 0.001 absorbance. If whole blood is used, one must make certain that it is well mixed before each sampling. It may be better to make a concentrated hemoglobin solution (see directions in the discussion of hemoglobin electrophoresis, but use larger volumes). This solution can be pipetted with less error than whole blood. The dilutor can be adjusted to give the same results as the manual dilution.

Cleaning of glassware

Volumetric glassware requires a much better cleaning method than ordinary glassware. In a few instances, e.g., serum iron and enzyme determinations, all glassware must be scrupulously clean to remove all traces of contaminating iron or heavy metals, but for routine use cleaning with ordinary detergents is satisfactory. Any special cleaning methods are mentioned as precautions for the particular tests involved. A good cleaning solution that has been used for many years is acid dichromate. This may be prepared by dissolving about 50 g of technical grade sodium dichromate in about 50 ml of water and slowly mixing in about 1 L of concentrated sulfuric acid. Since heat is generated in the preparation, it should be done in a heat-resistant flask. The solution may be kept in a tall glass jar with some sort of glass plate as a lid to prevent excessive absorption of moisture by the acid when not in use. Pipets are immersed in the solution for several hours and then removed and rinsed well with water in a regular pipet washer. Before placing pipets in the solution or adding the solution to flasks for cleaning, the glassware should first be rinsed with water to remove as much organic material as possible, because this will prolong the life of the solution. The cleaning solution may be used until the red color has changed to green, indicating that most of the chromic trioxide has been reduced to chromic ions. The solution has the disadvantage that it is extremely corrosive in nature, and great care must be taken in its handling. When the solution is at room temperature, the action is rather slow; it is generally advisable to soak the glassware overnight. Traces of chromic ions may remain on glassware cleaned in this way, even after excessive rinsing with deionized water. A rinse with dilute ammonia can be added before the last several rinses of deionized water to prevent problems with procedures subject to interference by heavy metals (e.g., enzymes).

It is advisable to rinse all glassware with water or a detergent solution immediately after use to remove material that may dry on the glassware and render later cleaning more difficult. Immediately after use, pipets should be placed in a plastic jar containing a mild detergent, e.g., a dilute solution of Acationox (Sherwood Medical Industries, St. Louis). The jar should be tall enough and contain sufficient liquid so that the pipets are immersed above the graduations. Test tubes and small flasks can be placed in a large pan containing a dilute solution of the detergent immediately after use. Glassware that contained strong acids or bases should be rinsed with tap water before being placed in the detergent. Pipets and volumetric flasks that contained organic solvents with dissolved lipid material (e.g., extracts for cholesterol or phospholipid determinations) are best rinsed with some of the solvent before being placed in the detergent solution. In this way, cleaning will be greatly facilitated. Pipets and volumetric flasks that were used with aqueous solutions containing only dissolved inorganic salts may not require cleaning with the chromate–sulfuric acid solution after each use. They can be washed with a detergent such as Alconox (Alconox, Inc., New York) but should be cleaned with acid whenever they begin to show signs of incomplete cleaning (droplets forming on the sides).

Micropipets are easily cleaned by suction by using one of the devices designed for cleaning hematology pipets; these are available from most supply houses. They may usually be cleaned by drawing through them, in order, household bleach, water, Alconox solution, tap water to rinse well, distilled water, acetone or methanol, and air to dry.

In procedures requiring special cleaning, e.g., iron, calcium, or zinc determinations, it is suggested that disposable plastic or glass tubes and pipets be used once and discarded. Usually these are free of contamination, but they should be checked occasionally. The plastic disposable pipets are not highly accurate and care must be taken in their use, because they do not become wet by the solution; the liquid should be allowed to flow out slowly to avoid leaving droplets on the sides. If the same type of pipets are used for samples and standards and care is exercised, fairly good accuracy can be obtained. For micro work, special pipets with disposable plastic tips can be used. These are described later in this chapter.

Distilled and deionized water

Distilled or deionized water should be used in making up all solutions and in all procedures. Sometimes the details of the procedure may merely state that water is used. Distilled or deionized water should always be used unless specifically contraindicated for a heating bath. If the commercial water supply is appreciably hard, it is preferable to use distilled water in heated water baths since this prevents the accumulation of salts as the water evaporates. A good water still will remove all traces of dissolved nonvolatile material but will not necessarily remove traces of volatile substances, e.g., chlorine and ammonia. In the chlorination of water supplies, ammonia is often added to destroy excess chlorine, and traces of ammonia may be found in the distillate. Deionized water is prepared by passing the water through a mixed bed of ion-exchange resins. As the name implies, this removes all ionic compounds but may not always remove all traces of organic compounds.

Cartridges for obtaining good-quality deionized water are commercially available. These are available on a contract basis with the cartridges permanently installed and maintenance and replacement made on a regular basis by the supplier (Culligan USA, Northbrook, Ill.). The larger units have a device that indicates when the capacity of the unit is near exhaustion and the unit should be replaced. With the smaller portable units it is easy to exceed the capacity, and the quality of the water will deteriorate rapidly. The simplest test is to dissolve about 5 g of silver nitrate in about 1 dl of water containing a few drops of nitric acid. If a few drops of this solution are added to about 5 ml of the water to be tested, any visible opalescence resulting from the formation of insoluble silver chloride will indicate a poor quality of water.

In hard-water areas the use of a still involves considerable maintenance and periodic cleaning unless water-softening units are used on the raw-water intake. The laboratory may be located in an institution that already has a large still but that may not produce water of sufficient quality for all chemical tests. The water can usually be used directly for rinsing washed glassware. For use in the preparation of reagents, etc., the water from the still may be passed through a small column of ion-exchange resin such as Amberlite MB-3 (Rohm & Haas Co., Philadelphia). This has an indicator on the resin to distinguish when the column is near exhaustion. Since only small amounts of ions are present in the distillate, a small column may last for several months. Small laboratories may find it simplest to purchase the distilled water from commercial sources but should make certain that it is of good quality. Winstead[10] offers a good discussion of the use of stills and ion-exchange resin beds, together with a number of tests that can be used for checking the purity of water.

COLORIMETERS AND SPECTROPHOTOMETERS[11-13]

In the great majority of tests performed in the clinical chemistry laboratory, quantitation is based on a relationship between the absorption or emission of light and the concentration of the substance being determined. Many of the tests are based on the absorption of light by a solution.

Types of instruments

The instruments used for such measurements are called colorimeters or photometers. Some believe that the term *colorimeter* should be restricted to those instruments in which the comparison of light intensity is made by visual means and the term *photometer* used for those instruments in which the measurements are made by electrical means. Most current instruments isolate a narrow portion of the spectrum using filters,

prisms, or gratings. Those using filters are termed filter photometers, whereas those using prisms or gratings are called spectrophotometers.

The basic equation for the determination of substances by light absorption is known as Beer's law. This is usually given in the form:

$$\frac{I}{I_0} = e^{-k \cdot c \cdot d}$$

where I_0 is the intensity of the light incident on the solution and I is the intensity of the light that has passed through. The light path through the solution is a distance, d in length; c is the concentration of the absorbing substance in solution; and e is the base of the natural logarithms (2.71828 . . .). The value of the constant k depends on the units of c and d. From this we may derive the equation most generally used:

$$A = (2 - \log \%T) = Kcd$$

where:

$$\%T = \frac{I}{I_0} \times 100$$

%T is the percent of the incident light that is transmitted through the solution and K is a different constant from that in the first equation. The expression $(2 - \log \%T)$ is known as the optical density (OD) or absorbance (A). The former term is still in use, but the latter one is now preferred.

The transmitted light is usually measured by means of a photocell or phototube that delivers a small electric current proportional to the intensity of the light falling on it. The current is then measured directly with a sensitive microammeter or after electrical amplification. The meter reading is then taken as a measure of the intensity of the transmitted light and hence of the concentration of the substance being determined.

Conversion table

Most photocells are used in a range such that the electrical output is proportional to the intensity of the light falling on them. Accordingly, the scale of the accompanying meter on older instruments was linear in %T (varies directly with I for a constant I_0) but not linear in absorbance. Therefore it was simpler to interpolate on a linear %T scale and use a table such as Table 20-1 to convert to absorbance for calculations. The equation indicates that the absorbance is directly proportional to the concentration when Beer's law holds. Most of the newer instruments have scales that are linear in absorbance. This is accomplished by extra electric circuits that change the photocell output to a current that is proportional to the logarithm of the light intensity and thus to the absorbance. Such instruments may also have a direct digital readout in absorbance units.

Visible light is only a small part of the totality of electromagnetic radiation, which also includes radio waves, infrared radiation, ultraviolet radiation, and x-rays. These may be characterized in terms of their wavelengths. The wavelength of visible light extends from about 7×10^{-6} cm (red) to about 4×10^{-6} cm

Table 20-1. Conversion table, percent transmittance-absorbance

Transmission (%)	Absorbance (optical density)	Transmission (%)	Absorbance (optical density)	Transmission (%)	Absorbance (optical density)	Transmission (%)	Absorbance (optical density)
1	2.000	26	0.585	51	0.2924	76	0.1192
2	1.699	27	0.569	52	0.2840	77	0.1135
3	1.523	28	0.553	53	0.2757	78	0.1079
4	1.398	29	0.538	54	0.2676	79	0.1024
5	1.301	30	0.523	55	0.2596	80	0.0969
6	1.222	31	0.509	56	0.2518	81	0.0915
7	1.155	32	0.495	57	0.2441	82	0.0862
8	1.097	33	0.482	58	0.2366	83	0.0809
9	1.046	34	0.469	59	0.2291	84	0.0757
10	1.000	35	0.456	60	0.2219	85	0.0706
11	0.959	36	0.444	61	0.2147	86	0.0655
12	0.921	37	0.432	62	0.2076	87	0.0605
13	0.886	38	0.420	63	0.2007	88	0.0555
14	0.854	39	0.409	64	0.1938	89	0.0506
15	0.824	40	0.398	65	0.1871	90	0.0458
16	0.796	41	0.387	66	0.1805	91	0.0410
17	0.770	42	0.377	67	0.1739	92	0.0362
18	0.745	43	0.367	68	0.1675	93	0.0315
19	0.721	44	0.357	69	0.1612	94	0.0269
20	0.699	45	0.347	70	0.1549	95	0.0223
21	0.678	46	0.337	71	0.1487	96	0.0177
22	0.658	47	0.328	72	0.1427	97	0.0132
23	0.638	48	0.319	73	0.1367	98	0.0088
24	0.620	49	0.310	74	0.1308	99	0.0044
25	0.602	50	0.301	75	0.1249	100	0.0000

(violet). Radiation in a range that includes visible light is usually measured in units of 10^{-9} meters, the nanometer (nm). An older term, the millimicron (mμ), is numerically equal to the nanometer, but the latter is now the preferred term. In these units the wavelength of visible light varies between about 700 and 400 nm. The longer wavelengths (infrared) are rarely used in clinical chemistry; measurements are sometimes made at shorter wavelengths (ultraviolet) to about 195 nm.

The fact that ordinary visible white light can be broken down into the familiar red-orange-yellow-green-blue-violet (rainbow) spectrum is well known. A substance that absorbs light usually does not do so equally at all wavelengths. A solution that appears blue-green to the eye does so because it absorbs more strongly in the red end of the spectrum and transmits more of the blue-green. In measuring the absorption of light to determine concentrations, one usually uses light of a wavelength that is more strongly absorbed (red in the above instance) so as to attain the greatest sensitivity (most absorption per unit of concentration). All photometers have some method of isolating the desired portion of the spectrum for use in the analysis.

Use of filters, prisms, and gratings

The light of the desired wavelength is obtained by the use of a glass or other type of optical filter that allows light of only a certain range of wavelengths to pass (filter photometer) or by means of a grating or prism that splits the light into the spectrum and allows only light of the desired wavelength to pass through the absorbing solution (spectrophotometer). The latter method is more convenient. By means of a wavelength scale one can select the desired wavelength within the range of the instrument without the use of an extensive set of filters. Filter photometers are satisfactory for many purposes and are simpler in construction. By measuring the absorbance of the solution to be analyzed at different wavelengths and plotting the results, one obtains an absorption curve. From this one can estimate the wavelength at which the absorption is greatest. This is usually the wavelength selected for the final measurements.

Theoretically, Beer's law holds only for light of a single wavelength. Thus to attain greatest compliance with Beer's law (strict linearity between absorbance and concentration over the widest range) one should use as narrow a wavelength range as possible. Strictly monochromatic light is ideal, approached closely only by the most precise instruments. The usual laboratory photometers give a range or band of wavelengths. Ordinary glass filters may have a bandwidth of 30-50 nm or more. Interference filters are available that have a narrower bandwidth, but they are relatively expensive. Spectrophotometers may have bandwidths from 35 nm down to 5 nm or less, depending on the instrument. The narrower the bandwidth, the smaller the proportion of light from the lamp that will actually reach the photocell. Hence for narrow bandwidths the intensity of the light must be higher or the sensitivity of the photocell greater.

Since the actual absorption of light by the solution will vary with the wavelength used, it is necessary to always use the same wavelength in making measurements on the same type of solution at different times. Photometers using stable glass filters should always give the same wavelength and bandwidth and thus always produce the same absorbance with the same stable solution and cuvet. The interference filters, which are made of several layers of material may deteriorate because of solvents or solvent vapors getting between the different layers of the "sandwich." This can be checked occasionally by visual inspection, if possible, or by periodically measuring the absorbance of a stable solution, e.g., the sulfate solution mentioned later, which is prepared and kept in a tightly sealed cuvet.

Calibration of wavelength scale

In spectrophotometers the wavelength is usually selected by varying the relative positions of the light source, slits, and cuvet by means of cams or levers. The cams or levers are connected to a wavelength scale that indicates the wavelength of light passing through the cuvet. These may slip out of alignment, so that the reading on the scale may not correspond exactly to the actual wavelength being used. In the simpler spectrophotometers merely changing the light source may change the relation between the scale and the wavelength of light reaching the cuvet. These instruments usually include a calibration filter and a method of changing the cam adjustment so that the scale can be set back to the proper wavelength. Other calibration filters are also available. Those made with didymium or holmium oxide glasses have very narrow absorption bands and are most suitable for instruments with a narrow bandwidth.[14] For instruments having a deuterium lamp the emission lines at 486 nm and 656 nm are very suitable for wavelength calibration.[15]

Linearity and accuracy of absorbance scale

In addition to the proper wavelength calibration one should check the linearity of the measurements; that is, will a second solution having exactly twice the concentration of the absorbing substance as found in a first solution give exactly twice the absorbance when measured in the spectrophotometer. A number of solutions have been suggested for this testing, but a very simple and relatively stable one may be used.[16] This is the common green food coloring, which may be purchased in most grocery stores. The colorings manufactured by a number of different companies (R.T. French, Durkee, and McCormick) give the same results. Dilute 0.5 ml of the coloring solution as purchased to 1 L with water. Then carefully prepare dilutions of this as needed. For the highest concentration use the stock solution. For a second concentration carefully dilute (using good quality volumetric pipets) 1 volume of the stock solution with an equal volume of water. This gives a concentration that is one half that of the original. Dilute again a portion of this second solution 1:2 with water, and make a further dilution of this to give final solutions having relative concentrations of the dye of 1.0, 0.5, 0.25, and 0.125. When these are read against water in the spectrophotometer the absorbances should also be in this ratio. The readings are made at 630 nm, 410 nm, and (if available) at 257 nm. If desired, plot the measured absorbances against the relative concentrations to note the deviations from linearity, and make further dilutions to check any divergent samples. The

stock solution is stable for several months when kept in a brown bottle.

Several primary spectrophotometric standards are available from the National Bureau of Standards. These are available as liquids (SRM 931) or neutral density filters (SRM 930) and can be used to check accuracy as well as linearity, since the absolute absorbance is known.

The source of light in most instruments is an incandescent tungsten lamp. The light intensity must be kept as constant as possible. Measurements are usually made by placing a blank solution in the cuvet and adjusting the meter to read I_0 = zero absorbance or 100% T. One then replaces the blank cuvet with one containing the sample and measures A or %T allowing the instrument to calculate I/I_0. Accuracy requires that the actual light intensity from the lamp is the same for both measurements. If it is not, the measured I_0 will not be the same as the actual I_0 at the time the sample is measured and an error will result. Most photometers have a voltage regulator transformer or an internal voltage regulating circuit (or both) to keep the current to the lamp at a constant value. Some instruments compensate for small changes in light intensity by the use of a double-beam arrangement that allows a portion of the light from the lamp to pass through the cuvet to the photocell in the usual way and another portion of the light to traverse another path (which may include a blank cuvet) to a second photocell. The electrical outputs of the two photocells are compared for measurement. Theoretically, since the two photocells are illuminated by light from the same source, slight fluctuations in the light source should not affect the ratio of the two photocell outputs. For example, if the output from the lamp were decreased by 2%, then the output of both photocells would also be decreased by 2% and the ratio would remain the same.

In practically all colorimetric procedures the substances being determined, e.g., glucose, uric acid, or cholesterol, are not themselves colored or are only slightly so, but they form a colored compound through a series of complex chemical reactions. The amount of color formed then depends on the concentrations of the reagents and other conditions, e.g., the time and temperature of heating or incubation. Hence in comparing the concentration of the unknown sample with that of a standard of known concentration, the sample and standard should preferably be run at the same time to ensure that the conditions for color development and measurement are the same. Standards should be run with each set of analyses to avoid errors caused by changes in the conditions mentioned.

The use of precalibrated charts that were often supplied with the instruments lead to serious errors; their use is strongly condemned by all workers in the field of clinical chemistry. MacFate et al.[17] state that in relying on factory calibration of colorimeters one becomes liable for errors from improper calibrations in addition to becoming dependent on methods that may be outmoded or nonspecific. Many workers have found variations between different instruments of the same make in regard to stray light, wavelength calibration, and linearity of response of the photocell, all of which cause deviations from precalibrated charts and serious errors in the final analysis.

Calibration of cuvets

Unless a spectrophotometer has a built-in cuvet (e.g., a flow cell), sample absorbances must be determined in cuvets. The blank absorbance of the cuvet at the wavelength of assay should be checked to ensure that no differences in absorbance are contributed by the cuvets. A series of cuvets to be checked are filled with a solution that has some absorbance at the assay wavelength (e.g., NADH for 340 nm, and biuret solution for 540 nm). The absorbance readings from the cuvets should be ± 0.002. Matched cuvets are commercially available and should be used. Differences in materials used in the manufacture of glass or slight differences in path length are compensated for by using matched cuvets.

Often the reagents themselves give a certain amount of color to the final solution, even when none of the substance being determined is present. This color constitutes the reagent blank. In such circumstances the instrument may be set to zero absorbance (or 100% T) with the blank solution containing all of the reagents but none of the substance being determined. The blank is treated under the same conditions as the samples and standards. Preferably the conditions should be adjusted so that the color resulting from the blank is minimal. If readings are made in terms of absorbance, the samples and blank can be read against water (or other solvents) and the reading of the blank subtracted from that of the sample before calculation. Alternatively one may zero out the blank absorbance by adjusting the spectrophotometer to zero absorbance with the blank in the light path and then read the net absorbance of the samples directly. As mentioned earlier, photometric readings are usually made at the wavelength at which the absorption of the sample solution is greatest. But if the reagents themselves produce colors that are considerably different from those produced by the sample, it may be convenient to read at the wavelength where the difference between the sample and blank is greatest instead of the wavelength where the absorption of the sample solution is greatest.

Calculations with photometric readings

Several methods may be used in the calculations of concentrations from photometric readings. From Beer's law we have $C = KA$ (what follows C refers to concentrations with subscripts to denote sample, standard, etc., and A denotes absorbance with subscripts). From this we find:

$$\frac{C_1}{A_1} = \frac{C_2}{A_2}$$

or

$$C_2 = \frac{C_1}{A_1} \times A_2$$

where subscript 1 refers to the standard and subscript 2 refers to the sample. If one is determining a number of samples with the same standard, it is often convenient to calculate $C_1/A_1 = K$, which is constant for a given standard determination, and $C_2 = K \times A_2$. If several standards of different concentrations are run, the K values calculated from the different standard readings would be the same if Beer's law held exactly. If they are not exactly the same, one could use an average value. If Beer's law does not hold, this is usually indicated by the fact that the K values increase with increasing concentrations. For example, concentrations of 1, 2, and 3 mg/dl might give absorbances of 0.125, 0.236, and 0.333, which would give K values of 8.0, 8.5, and 9.0, respectively. In such a case, the unknown concentration should be determined from a standard curve.

Another way of calculating the results is to run a series of standards and plot the concentration of the standards against the absorbance on linear cross-section paper or against the percent transmission on semilog paper and draw a smooth curve through the points (straight line if Beer's law holds the readings are accurate). One can then read off the concentrations corresponding to other absorbances from the curve. If the standards give slight differences from day to day because of varying conditions, one would need to determine the absorbance of one standard if the assay conformed to Beer's law. If the assay does not conform to Beer's law, as in some AutoAnalyzer methods, then one would need to run an entire standard curve each time the assay was performed. Many instruments have additional circuits that allow the operator to put a K factor directly into the instrument. Results of an assay can then be expressed directly in terms of concentration.

It is important to check each procedure for conformance to Beer's law. Deviations vary from procedure to procedure and with different instruments. Usually conditions are chosen so that conformance is good over the most important range of values. If there are marked deviations, this is usually mentioned in the procedure and one must then run more standards.

In the formulas given, C theoretically refers to the actual concentrations in the spectrophotometer cuvet, which may be quite different from the initial concentrations in the samples. If the standard and sample are treated exactly the same in regard to dilution, addition of reagents, etc., then in the calculations we can use the original concentration of the standard and obtain the concentration in the sample directly. For example, if a sample for glucose determination is diluted 1:10 and 1 ml of the dilution is added to a definite quantity of reagents to develop the color, and if a standard containing 100 mg/dl glucose is similarly diluted and 1 ml is also added to the same quantity of reagents, we could take C_1 in our formula to be 100 mg/dl to calculate the sample concentration directly.

If the standard and sample are diluted differently or are made up to different final volumes for the readings, these facts must be taken into account in the calculations. In such instances it may be more convenient to take C_1 as the actual concentration of standard in the aliquot added or in the final cuvet volume and then multiply by the factors for the dilution of the sample and standard.

In regard to calculations, one other point might be mentioned. Most instrumentation has an uncertainty of about 0.002 A ($\pm$ 0.001) for each reading, and since many assays produce an absorbance of about 0.200 this uncertainty can produce an error of up to 1% in concentration even if all other factors are insignificant.

Since there are many other sources of error in addition to the spectrophotometer reading, it appears that most results could not be accurate to within less than 1% at best. Consequently, it is usually not necessary to report more than three significant figures in the results. It is meaningless to report a result as 136.27 mg/dl when with the routine method one could just distinguish between 136 and 137 mg/dl. Therefore the result should be reported as 136 mg/dl.

FLAME PHOTOMETRY[11,18,19]
Basic principles

When atoms of some chemical elements are introduced into a nonluminous flame, they emit light of definite wavelengths characteristic of the particular element involved. This is illustrated by the yellow light seen when a sodium salt is introduced into the flame of a Bunsen burner. A few of the sodium atoms, after being raised to an excited state (higher energy level) by the thermal energy of the flame, spontaneously revert to the normal (lower or ground state) energy level, producing an emission of light at a characteristic wavelength (for sodium at 589 nm). Within certain limits, the amount of light emitted is proportional to the amount of the element in the flame. Thus if a solution of the element is aspirated into the flame at a constant rate, the amount of light emitted will be proportional to the concentration of the element in the solution. The amount of light emitted will also vary with the flame temperature (amount of thermal energy available). For accurate results all variable factors must be carefully controlled. The flame temperature is kept as constant as possible by carefully regulating the amount of gas and air (or oxygen) fed to the flame with the use of pressure or flow regulators. Since the solution is usually aspirated into the flame by the airflow, this must also be kept constant to keep the rate of aspiration the same. The wavelength of light characteristic of the element being determined is isolated by means of a prism, grating, or filter arrangement similar to those used in spectrophotometers. The intensity of the light is measured with a photocell and meter or other electrical arrangement. Sample determinations are always made in comparison to the light emitted when a standard solution is aspirated in place of the sample.

Since the measurement of the intensity of emitted light is made, the response of the photocell will be directly proportional to the concentration of the emitting atoms. The instrument reads directly in milliequivalents per liter, thus eliminating the need for the mathematical formula used in absorption measurements (Beer's law). The ratio between the concentration of the substance being measured and the light emitted may be linear only over a short range. This must be considered when making the required dilution of the sample. The presence of one element may interfere with the light emission by another element in the flame. For example, the emission of potassium is increased by the presence of relatively large amounts of sodium.

All modern instruments determine simultaneously the amounts of sodium and potassium in a sample in relation to a high concentration of a reference element (usually lithium). The effect of sodium on potassium emission is minimized by the use of a mixed sodium-potassium standard containing concentrations of elements that are similar to those found in serum (140 mEq/L sodium and 5 mEq/L potassium) or urine (50 mEq/L each).

Use in analysis

Details of operation differ somewhat from instrument to instrument. Most use ordinary bottled propane and compressed air, which produce a flame temperature of 1925° C. All instruments use the internal standard principle. An element not ordinarily present in biologic samples (usually lithium or cesium) is added to the standards, samples, and blank dilutions in the same concentration. Three photocells are used as detectors with appropriate filters. One reference photocell will measure the light emitted by the lithium (red), and the other two measuring photocells measure the light emitted by the elements being determined (i.e., the yellow light from sodium and the violet light from potassium). The outputs of the two measuring photocells are compared to the reference photocell for the results. In theory, any fluctuation in flame temperature or aspiration rate should affect the emission of sodium or potassium and lithium equally, thereby maintaining a constant ratio between the readings. In the determination of sodium and potassium the presence of lithium helps to reduce the mutual interference of these two elements.

Most flame photometers have direct reading digital displays for sodium and potassium. Some instruments can also be used to determine the concentration of lithium if potassium is used for an internal standard in place of lithium. Instruments using cesium as an internal standard can determine sodium, potassium, and lithium together.

All biologic fluids (e.g., serum, urine, spinal fluid) are diluted about 1:100 or 1:200 with a nonionic wetting agent and 15 mEq/L lithium ion as an internal reference element to minimize differences in sample-to-sample viscosity. After the diluting solution containing lithium is made up in volumetric glassware, it should be transferred immediately to a polyethylene container for storage. The volumetric glassware has a low content of alkali earth metals (e.g., lithium) and solutions of these ions must be removed from contact with the glassware to prevent the loss of lithium ions from the solution.

Although there are other possibilities, the only elements commonly analyzed by this technic are sodium, potassium, and lithium.

ATOMIC ABSORPTION SPECTROPHOTOMETRY

A newer method for the determination of metallic elements in low concentrations is atomic absorption spectrophotometry.[11,20,21]

Basic principles

The principles on which this method are based are closely related to those of flame emission photometry. The basic difference is that in flame photometry one measures the light emitted by the small fraction of the sample atoms in the flame that are excited to emit their characteristic radiation, whereas in atomic absorption one measures the absorption of light by the unexcited atoms. It has been calculated that for sodium atoms in an ordinary gas flame only a few atoms in every million are actually excited to emit light. If an excited atom emits light of its characteristic wavelength in returning to the lower energy state, atoms in the lower state can be raised to the excited state by the absorption of light of exactly this same wavelength. Thus in the flame at any instant there will be many more atoms theoretically capable of absorbing light than of emitting it.

The light for absorption is obtained from a hollow cathode tube by a glow discharge in helium or argon. The hollow cathode contains some of the element being determined, e.g., calcium. The calcium atoms are vaporized by the glow discharge and caused to emit their characteristic radiation. The sample is aspirated into the flame (usually air-acetylene) in a manner similar to that used for flame photometry. The flame is produced over a long narrow slit, with the incident light passing along the length of the slit to give a long light path through the flame. Some instruments may have an arrangement of mirrors, so that the light is reflected back and passes through the flame several times to give greater absorption.

The burner commonly used for clinical applications is a premix or laminar flow burner, which aspirates and atomizes the sample before burning. In this system large droplets are removed from the stream to the burner, giving a less noisy signal.

The light then passes on to a grating arrangement to isolate the desired wavelength and then to a photocell and measuring device. Since excited atoms in the flame also emit light of the characteristic wavelength, this must be separated from the light of the hollow cathode lamp. This separation is accomplished by interruption of the light from the lamp several hundred times per second before it passes through the flame. Thus the light from the hollow cathode lamp produces a pulsating current in the phototube, whereas the light from the excited atoms in the flame produces a relatively constant current. By electrical means the pulsating current can be separated from the constant current and measured. Thus only the light from the cathode lamp affects the detecting system.

Use in analysis

Atomic absorption may be used for the determination of calcium, magnesium, sodium, potassium, copper, zinc, iron, lead, cadmium, thallium, chromium, mercury, lithium, nickel, bismuth, cobalt, manganese, and some other elements in biologic material. Usually a separate lamp is required for each element being determined, although some multielement lamps, e.g., calcium-magnesium and copper-iron-zinc, are available. Sodium and potassium are still most conveniently determined by flame photometry, but the other elements mentioned are more conveniently determined by atomic absorption. Magnesium, for example, requires a very hot flame for emission photometry but can be easily determined by atomic absorption. Calcium is also more accurately determined by atomic absorption than by flame photometry. As in flame photometry, the presence of other elements may cause some interference with the element being determined. Phosphate, for instance, causes some interference with calcium determinations. This is overcome by adding a constant amount of lanthanum to the samples and standards to combine with the phosphate and eliminate its interference with the calcium determination.

Operating procedures for atomic absorption equipment are similar to those used for flame emission; the details for the various instruments on the market vary somewhat. Since the measurement is that of light absorption, Beer's law will apply and the photocell output will not be proportional to the concentration. In atomic absorption measurements the percent absorption (%A) is often used instead of %T. These are related by the formula %A = 100 − %T. Thus the absorbance, as with other photometers, is proportional to the concentration and may be obtained from tables similar to Table 20-1, in which (100 − %T) is replaced by %A. The calculations are then the same as with other photometry:

$$\frac{\text{Absorbance of sample}}{\text{Absorbance of standard}} \times \frac{\text{Conc. of}}{\text{standard}} = \frac{\text{Conc. of}}{\text{sample}}$$

Some of the more modern instruments may give readings directly in absorbance units.

Simple instruments are available for the determination of such elements as lithium, magnesium, and calcium. For other elements of biologic interest, e.g., lead, iron, and copper, the concentrations normally found are so low that one of the more sophisticated instruments may be required.

Flameless atomic absorption

A recent development is flameless atomic absorption.[20] A hollow carbon tube is positioned horizontally in the space above that normally occupied by the burner, so that the light beam from the cathode lamp passes down the axis of the tube. The ends of the tube are connected to a source of electric current. A small sample is introduced into the center of the tube through a small opening in the top. An electric current is passed through the carbon tube, heating it sufficiently to drive off any solvent present and oxidize any organic matter present without volatilizing the metallic element to be determined. A strong current is then passed through the tube, heating it enough to volatilize the metal. The metallic vapor remains within the tube for a time to give a relatively high concentration of metallic atoms in the light path. The absorption is recorded on a strip-chart recorder attached to the instrument. The peak height produced by the sample is then compared with those produced by a series of standards to calculate the concentration of the element in the sample. In this way, using the appropriate cathode tube, a number of elements, e.g., lead, zinc, or nickel, can be determined on samples of a fraction of a milliliter of serum or other fluid without any preliminary treatment.

FLUOROMETRY

Some chemical compounds have the property of absorbing light energy and then reemitting some of this energy as light of a longer wavelength (less energy) than that originally absorbed. This phenomenon, called fluorescence, can be applied as a mthod of analysis.[11,22,23]

Basic principles

Commonly the exciting light is in the ultraviolet or near-ultraviolet wavelength in the range of 250-400 nm, and the emitted fluorescence is of a longer wavelength, usually in the visible range. Not all wavelengths of light are equally effective in exciting the fluorescence of a given compound, and the fluorescent light emitted is usually concentrated in a certain range of wavelengths. Two filters are generally used in a fluorometer, one to allow only the shorter wavelength exciting light to reach the sample and the second to cut off any scattered exciting light and allow only the emitted fluorescent light to reach the photocell. If prisms or gratings are used instead of filters, the instrument is called a spectrofluorometer. The amount of fluorescent light emitted will be proportional to the concentration of the fluorescent substance in solution and to the intensity of the exciting light. This latter must be kept as constant as possible. Most fluorometers have a voltage-regulating device for the exciting lamp similar to those found in photometers. Even so it is always necessary to compare the fluorescence of the unknown sample with that of a standard run under comparable conditions. The emitted fluorescence of the solution varies much more with temperature than does the actual absorption of light; hence the temperature of the solutions being measured must be controlled more closely than is necessary in photometry. Since the intensity of the fluorescent light and hence of the photocell output will vary directly with the concentration of the substance being determined, the instruments will be read directly without the use of the mathematical transformation (Beer's law) needed in absorption photometry. The meter readings are usually expressed in arbitrary units that are used to compare the reading of the unknown with that of the standard.

The emitted light is measured at right angles to the path of the incident light to avoid interference from transmitted light. This necessitates cuvets that have four equivalent optical sides rather than the cuvets used in absorption spectrophotometry with only two optical windows.

To obtain measurements in the desired range of concentration the amount of exciting light reaching the fluorescent solution is varied by means of variable diaphragms or apertures in front of the exciting lamp and by varying the amount of fluorescent light reaching the photocell by means of apertures or neutral density filters. The intensity of the fluorescent light is usually directly proportional to the concentration of the fluorescent substance over a range of several orders of magnitude. The lower limit of sensitivity is usually limited by the fact that the reagents themselves contain small amounts of fluorescent material, which in lower ranges of concentration of the unknown yield a high blank value. At high concentrations the relation between concentration and fluorescence is nonlinear, because the solution being analyzed absorbs some of the exciting or fluorescent light.

Range of application

The range of application of fluorescent methods is smaller than that of photometric methods in that many more compounds are colored (or can be transformed into colored compounds) than are fluorescent (or can be made into fluorescent compounds). Fluorescent methods can be used to measure concentrations lower than colorimetric methods by a factor of from 10-1000 and thus are desirable for the measurement of very low concentrations. If only a small amount of fluorescent light is emitted, this can be measured with sufficient accuracy by increasing the sensitivity of the photocell and the associated measuring circuitry.

Aside from the occasional high reagent fluorescence mentioned earlier, another interference sometimes encountered in fluorescent measurements is the phenomenon of quenching. Impurities or other foreign substances in the sample will cause a decreased amount of fluorescence of the substance being analyzed. Since this will not be found in the standard, which is usually a simple solution, low results will occur. In extracts of biologic materials the exact nature of the impurity may not be known, so that there is no simple way to correct for it. Here usually an internal standard is used. Two aliquots of the sample are treated similarly to develop the fluorescence. To one of the aliquots is added a known amount of standard. The difference in fluorescence of the two samples with and without added standard would be a measure of the standard, and the difference between the sample without added standard and the blank would be a measure of the sample. It is assumed that the interfering material causes a proportionate decrease in total fluorescence in the two samples.

CHROMATOGRAPHY

Chromatography is a technic used for the separation of relatively small amounts of chemically closely related substances.[11]

Basic principles

A mixture of substances in a suitable solvent is moved past a stationary phase that will adsorb different substances in varying degrees. As the solution moves past the stationary phase, the rates of flow of the more strongly adsorbed substances will be retarded the most and substances that are not adsorbed at all will move directly with the solvent front. Separation is effected because sample components are preferentially retarded by the stationary phase as they are carried past in the mobile phase. If the action of the stationary phase depends solely on the adsorbing power (electrostatic attraction of the sample by ''active'' sites of the adsorbent) of the solid, the process is termed **adsorption chromatography.** If the stationary phase is an inert solid coated with a thin layer of adsorbed liquid so that the separation depends on the partition coefficient of the substances being separated between the solvent and the adsorbed immiscible liquid, the process is termed **partition chromatography. Ion-exchange chromatography** is a refinement of the partition principle in which the stationary phase is a charged resin. If the sample is introduced in a charged state, it will be retarded according to its ability to displace the inorganic ions from the resin. Molecular exclusion, or **molecular sieve chromatography,** refers to the selective exclusion of sample molecules by the porous stationary phase depending on the size and shape of the molecules. This is also called **gel filtration** when the porous material is a gel (the commercial material most widely used is Sephadex, Pharmacia Fine Chemicals, Piscataway, N.J.), which is supplied in a range of particle sizes suitable for many applications. Molecules larger than the pore size pass through the gel, whereas smaller molecules enter the pores and therefore take a longer, more tortuous route. Both ion-exchange and gel-filtration chromatography are most commonly done in columns. All of these processes may occur to some extent in many chromatographic methods, but one usually predominates.

Classification of the type of chromatography can also be based on the nature of the adsorbent (e.g., cellulose, paper, or gel) or on the physical nature of the phases used (e.g., gas-liquid chromatography) or by the process employed (e.g., column chromatography or thin-layer chromatography). These descriptive classifications are more convenient to use, especially when the dominant physical process involved in the separation may not be known.

Column chromatography[24]

The technic first developed was column chromatography. In this method, a stationary phase, e.g., an ion-exchange resin, Sephadex, alumina, or silica gel, in a finely divided form is placed in a column with a fritted disk or other device at the bottom to keep the stationary phase in place but allow the liquid to flow through. Usually the material is added to the column as a slurry in a solvent to obtain an even packing and remove air bubbles.

Simple column chromatography

The substances to be separated are placed on the top of the column in solution. The appropriate solvent is then allowed to flow through the column by gravity or, in some cases, with the aid of applied suction or air pressure.

As the solvent flows through the column, the substances being separated move down the column at different rates, depending on how strongly they are adsorbed by the column material. Eventually they will all be eluted. By successive collection of aliquots of solvent the substances being separated will be in different fractions of the eluate and can be analyzed by the usual chemical methods. Usually, in order to obtain a separation in a reasonable length of time, a number of different solutions are applied to the top of the column in succession to elute different fractions. With aqueous solutions the differences are usually in pH or in buffer or salt concentration. With organic solvents the differences are usually increasing amounts of a polar solvent (e.g., ethyl alcohol) in a nonpolar solvent (e.g., benzene). Since the order in which the substances will be eluted from the column cannot be accurately predicted in advance, the best conditions for separating any particular compounds must be determined experimentally. Column chromatography is often used to separate a particular substance from other impurities that would interfere with its chemical determination. The mixture is applied to a column. The desired substance may be strongly adsorbed and the impurities removed by the passage of a solvent through the column. Then by using a different solvent the desired substance may be eluted in relatively pure form for analysis. Less commonly the impurities may be strongly absorbed and the desired substance eluted first from the column.

Column chromatography may also be used for quantitation. The sample is applied to the column and the eluting solvent pumped through the column. The eluate is analyzed by passage through a spectrophotometer cuvet in which changes in absorbance are measured, or the eluate may be first mixed continuously with a reagent to produce a colored product. The output of the photometer when connected to a recorder will give a series of peaks of absorbance similar in pattern to those shown for protein electrophoresis. Usually a known amount of an internal standard is added. The internal standard is a substance that is known not to be present in the material to be analyzed but which chromatographs similarly to the substances to be separated in the column.

The procedure is calibrated by running a series of analyses with increasing amounts of standards for the substance being analyzed and a constant amount of internal standard. The peak height (or area) ratio of standard to internal standard is plotted against the increasing amounts of the standards used. The analysis of a sample with an unknown concentration is performed by adding the same constant amount of internal standard and determining the peak height ratio. The unknown concentration can then be determined from the graph of peak height ratios previously ascertained.

The use of an internal standard, it if is added to the sample before any separation steps are performed, greatly aids in the analysis. It compensates for incomplete recoveries, and in the case of high-performance liquid chromatography (described below) it compensates for variations in column flow rate or irreversible absorption to the column material.

High-performance liquid chromatography[25,26]

To reduce the amount of sample required for biologic material, smaller colums containing smaller particles of packing are used. The very fine particles of the column packing give greater resolution of materials but require greater pressures to force the eluting liquid through the column. This had led to the development of high-performance liquid chromatography (HPLC), which is sometimes called high-pressure liquid chromacography. In this technic small stainless steel columns (25 cm × 4 mm) and fine packings (5-10 μm) are used, which require pressures of from 1000-3000 lb/in^2 or even more in some applications, to force the mobile phase through the column.

A recent development has been the introduction of small (10 cm × 8 mm) radial compression columns made of high-density polyethylene filled with the usual packing materials. The column is placed in a metal holder that tightly squeezes the polyethylene walls and is said to reduce analysis time and voids or channeling between the packing and the column wall. The columns are somewhat less expensive than the conventional ones made of stainless steel. The quantitation of unknowns is made by light absorption in the ultraviolet or by fluorescent technics using continuously flowing systems, as described for column chromatography.

The adoption of this separation technic has been greatly advanced by the development of improved column packing materials. Ordinary column packing materials (e.g., alumina, silica gel, and ion-exchange resins) are fairly polar materials designed to remove polar analytes from body fluids or extracts of body fluids. The mobile phases that were previously used to reelute these analytes were often mixtures of organic solvents that were somewhat nonpolar and therefore not efficient. The development of reverse phase columns with stable nonpolar materials (e.g., C-18 columns, and octadecyl silane) bonded to inert material allows the use of very polar mobile phases (e.g., water-acetonitrile or buffer-acetonitrile mixtures). The practical result of this reversal of the usual polarity between the stationary column phase and the mobile phase has been to reverse the general order of elution of materials. The most highly polar compounds elute from these columns first, and less polar compounds elute later. Since the compounds of interest are highly polar (e.g., drugs and steroids), a short analysis time is achieved.

In spite of the special high-pressure pumps required, this method has replaced gas chromatography in many applications for the determination of drugs and steroid hormones in body fluids, since it does not require the preparation of a volatile derivative and is usually somewhat simpler and more rapid than gas chromatography (see discussion of gas-liquid chromatography).

Gas-liquid chromatography[11,27-29]

Gas-liquid chromatography (often referred to as gas chromatography) is another type of column chromatography. In this method the substances being analyzed are in the gaseous state. The "solvent" that carries the material through the column is a stream of inert gas, usually helium or nitrogen. The column contains an inert material such as crushed firebrick in which a thin layer of a liquid having a very low vapor pressure is absorbed. The thin layer of liquid acts as the absorbing medium for the substances passing through the column, and this supporting medium does little else. In some types of gas-liquid chromatograms the column is merely a fine capillary tube whose inner walls are coated with the absorbing liquid. The effluent gas containing the eluted material is automatically analyzed by a number of methods, and the results are recorded on a strip chart. Unless the substance being determined is a gas at room temperature (e.g., O_2, CO_2, or CO extracted from blood), all the parts of the apparatus must

be heated to well above room temperature to keep the material being analyzed in the gaseous state. The material to be analyzed is usually injected into the column in a small amount of volatile solvent. Since only very small amounts of material are required, a high enough concentration in the gaseous phase can be obtained for many substances without undue heat, which might decompose them. If the substance to be determined is not sufficiently volatile, it may be converted into a more volatile derivative before analysis. With the use of different column packings a wide variety of biologic materials can be determined. Although the acutal determination in the gas chromatograph may be relatively simple, it often requires considerable time and effort to separate the material from other interfering substances and to prepare a suitable volatile derivative. Since different types of material may require different column packings, the gas chromatograph is most useful when it can be used for the analysis of a relatively large number of similar compounds (e.g., urinary steroids).

Paper chromatography

Paper chromatography[30,31] and thin-layer chromatography are related technics. Paper chromatography is the older technic and, although still in use it has been replaced by thin-layer chromatography for most clinical applications (see discussion of thin-layer chromatography). In paper chromatography the stationary phase is a strip of absorbent paper similar to filter paper. A small amount of solution containing the substances to be separated is applied near one end of the paper strip and the solvent evaporated. If the paper strip is suspended so that the end nearest the point of application of the substances is dipped into a suitable solvent, the solvent will wet the paper and gradually rise through the strip by capillary action. The flow of the solvent will carry the substances along with it at varying rates, depending on the degree to which they are absorbed by the paper. After the solvent has risen to the desired height in the paper, the strip is removed and the solvent is evaporated. The strip can then be sprayed with or dipped into a reagent that will give a color reaction with the substances being determined. If these are separated, a series of distinct spots on the paper will correspond to the individual compounds. The size of the spot or intensity of its color will be roughly proportional to the amount of the particular substance present. These may be compared with the spots obtained with known amounts of standards run similarly.

The process just described is known as **ascending chromatography,** because the solvent rises in the paper strip. In **descending chromatography** the end of the strip containing the applied material is dipped into the solvent, and the strip is then bent over the side of the solvent container and hangs down so that the actual flow of solvent is downward. Both ascending and descending chromatography are carried out in a jar or other closed container, so that the air surrounding the paper is saturated with the solvent vapor. This prevents evaporation from the paper, which would seriously distort the results. A large number of substances have been separated by paper chromatography. The methods must always be standardized with known substances, since the actual rate of migration varies with the conditions. The realtive rates of migration are fairly constant for a given setup and are usually expressed in terms of R_f values. These are the ratios of the rate of migration of the substances in question to that of the solvent front. As the solvent rises in the paper, it carries along the applied substances at slower rates. If, in a given experiment, it were found that the solvent had risen to a height 20 cm from the starting point, and the spot for a particular substance was 10 cm from the starting point, then this substance would have an R_f value of $10/20 = 0.50$ for these particular conditions.

For the separation of a large number of similar substances, e.g., amino acids in plasma or urine, a method known as **two-dimensional chromatography** may be used. A small amount of solution containing the substances to be separated is applied near one corner of a large square of filter paper. This is subjected to ascending chromatography with a particular solvent. The substances will then be distributed along one edge of the paper. If the paper is then dried and the edge dipped into another solvent so that the direction of flow is now at an angle of 90 degrees to the earlier flow, the final result will be a distribution of the spots for the various substances over the entire sheet, because the two solvents are chosen so that most of the compounds have different R_f values. By comparison with the spots obtained from known solutions, the various substances may be identified and the relative amounts estimated.

Thin-layer chromatography

Thin-layer chromatography (TLC) is less cumbersome and faster than paper chromatography. Generally this technic requires a smaller amount of sample. Since it is a simple technic and can be used in any laboratory, general directions applicable to most determinations are discussed, and they are supplemented by specific modifications for particular compounds as needed.

The adsorbents used in TLC are spread in a thin layer on an inert plate of glass, polyester plastic, aluminum, etc., or they can be impregnated in a glass fiber network to make a semirigid sheet. The most commonly used adsorbents are silica gel, silicic acid, alumina, and cellulose powder. A wide variety of TLC media are available commercially. They amy be purchased to meet a variety of needs: with a fluorescent indicator to aid in identification of some compounds; with various thicknesses of adsorbent; and with impregnated substances, e.g., borate, silicate, and phosphate, to modify the character of the adsorbent. Individual requirements must be determined by the character and amount of materials to be studied and by the degree of experience and individual preference. The flexible sheets are easiest to work with and quite adequate for precise quantitative work. Depending on the application, the coatings in TLC plates and sheets may vary from 0.100-0.500 mm in thickness. The plates and sheets are usually made in two sizes, 5 × 20 cm and 20 × 20 cm. Rigid glass plates are sometimes easier to handle, but the various flexible sheets can be readily cut to different sizes with a sharp paper cutter if necessary. The various makes of TLC media differ in the tendency with which the coating will flake or be scratched off, and many must be handled with care for this reason. Some plates are prepared with a binder such as calcium sulfate to help prevent chipping. Care must always be taken to handle the sheets only by the top edge, since contact of the skin with the active surfaces may introduce contamination. TLC plates and sheets should always be stored in a dry place. When indicated, the sheets may be activated in an oven prior to use. Activation is not necessary in partition chromatography but is critical to maintain reporducibility in adsorption systems. The degree of activation is a factor in the ability of the adsorbent to attract other compounds electrostatically. If the adsorbent sites are occupied by water molecules, the electrostatic capacity of the sheet will be reduced. Sheets can generally be activated in a 100-115° C oven for 30-60 min. The time and temperature of activation vary with the *medium and application*. The following list indicates other equipment needed for and TLC method.

Types of equipment

1. Drying oven. A drying oven set at about 100° C is needed. The oven need not be large, but preferably it should have a thermostatic control so that it will not become too hot. Glass plates can be placed directly on the shelves of the oven (coated side up), but less rigid types should be placed on clean glass plates or suspended in the oven with small stainless steel clips to avoid contamination.

2. Source of warm air. Use a small hair dryer (Fisher no. 9-201 [Fisher Scientific Co., Pittsburgh]) or one of the heat guns available from most laboratory supply houses. The latter are more substantially made for continuous laboratory use.

3. Capillary tubes or micropipets for application of samples. We have found that for most purposes the Drummond ''microcaps'' (cat. no. 21805, Sherwood Medical Industries, St. Louis), which hold about 5 µl, are satisfactory. For larger samples, regular plain coagulation capillaries with an inside diameter of 1 mm can be used.

4. Developing chamber. A developing chamber is required for the chromatograms. Glass plates will support themselves in various types of glass jars with tight lids, but more flexible sheets require further support. We have found the Gelman Chromatographic Chamber (cat. no. 51325, Gelman Instrument Co., Ann Arbor, Mich.) to be very satisfactory and convenient for most TLC media.

5. Source of ultraviolet light. Some applications require a source of ultraviolet light. Often both the long wavelength (360 nm) and the short wavelength (254 nm) ultraviolet are required. A multipurpose lamp is best. These are listed in most laboratory supply catalogs. Smaller separate lamps may be purchased at lower cost, but they have a lower intensity.

6. Reagent sprayer. A device for spraying the visualizing reagents on the chromatographic plates or sheets is needed. Small all-glass sprayers that operate on compressed air are available (Fisher Sprayer, cat. no. 5-719-5, Fisher Scientific Co., Pittsburgh). These require a small compressor or other source of compressed air. Sprayers that operate on compressed Freon propellant

(Spra-Tool, cat. no. 15-233, Fisher Scientic Co., Pittsburgh) are more convenient. These sprayers have a 120 ml plastic bottle for holding the reagent. When only a small amount is to be sprayed, it is convenient to keep portions of the stable reagents in 25 × 100 mm tubes with Teflon-lined screw caps. When the cap is removed, the tube fits inside the plastic bottle for spraying. This eliminates the need for transferring the reagent to the holding bottle and washing out the bottle when the spray is changed. The disadvantage of the propellant cans is that one cannot regulate the rate of spraying, and it is easy to add too much spray reagent to thin sheets.

Application of samples

Using a fine lead pencil, make a row of dots 1 cm or more apart along a line 1.5 cm from the lower edge of the sheet. The different samples or standard solutions are applied at these points. The sheet is laid on a clean flat surface and the heater arranged to blow a stream of warm air over the points of application. It is advisable to keep the sheets between clean glass plates during the application of samples, particularly if it has been previously activated. To apply the solution, a capillary tube is tipped into the solution, so that it fills by capillary action. The excess liquid is gently wiped from the outside of the capillary. It is then held in a vertical position and the lower end touched briefly to the application point, so that a small amount of the solution flows onto the sheet. The time of contact should be very short, so that the resulting spot is not more than 2 mm in diameter. Care must be taken not to damage the adsorbent coating. When the solvent has evaporated, the capillary is again touched to the sheet at the same spot to transfer more of the solution. This is continued until the desired amount (usually about 5 μl) has been applied. After all the solutions have been applied to the different spots, the entire sheet may be dried in the oven for a few minutes.

Development of chromatogram

Usually the developing solvent is first added to the developing chamber, which is then closed and allowed to stand for 10-15 min to saturate the air space with the solvent vapors. The sheet is then placed in the chamber with the edge closest to the application points dipping in the solvent. The upper surface of the solvent should be about 0.5 cm below the line of application points. The chamber is then closed and the chromatogram allowed to develop to the required distance. Usually this is about 10 cm above the application points, although this varies with different procedures. The sheet is then removed and the solvent front (the highest point to which the solvent has risen) quickly marked with a pencil line. The sheet is air dried for a few minutes and then may be dried in an oven to remove all the solvent.

For some tests using a coating containing a fluorescent indicator, the sheets are first viewed under short wavelength ultraviolet light. Substances that absorb in the ultraviolet show up as dark spots on the fluorescent background. If fluorescent compounds are present, they show up as bright spots. These spots are carefully outlined with a pencil. Appropriate reagents can then be sprayed on by holding the sheet vertically 15-20 cm from the sprayer, and the reagent applied with a continuous, uniform motion of the sprayer. All the sheet below the solvent front should be evenly moistened with the reagent, but too much must not be applied, because this tends to broaden and distort the spots. With some reagents the color develops almost immediately; with others heating or other treatment is required. The minimal amount of spray that gives a good colored spot should be used.

Calculation of R_f values and identification

The R_f value for a given substance is the ratio of the distance of this substance from the point of application to the distance of the solvent front from the point of application. If, for example, the solvent front were 9.8 cm from the application line and the centers of the spots for two substances were, respectively, 4.9 and 3.5 cm from the application line, then the R_f values for these two substances would be 4.9/9.8 = 0.50 and 3.5/9.8 = 0.36. The R_f value for a given substance varies for different solvent systems. Even with the same solvent system the R_f value of a given compound may change considerably with relative humidity, temperature, and other conditions that may not be easily controlled. Most of the solvent systems used are mixtures of two or more solvents, and slight variations in the composition affect the R_f values. Thus in another run with the two compounds used in the example above it might be found that the solvent front migrated 10.3 cm from the application, and the spots for the two substances were 5.7 and 4.1 cm, respectively. These would have R_f values of 0.55 and 0.40, somewhat higher than in the first example. However, it should be noted that the ratios of the two R_f values in the two experiments, i.e., 0.50/0.36 and 0.55/0.40, are approximately equal. Thus by comparing the measured R_f values with that found for a known compound, the relative R_f values will be essentially constant and can be used for identification more accurately than R_f values alone. R_f values can be made quite reproducible with proper activation and equilibration (saturation of the chamber with solvent vapors), but they may vary considerably among different laboratories. For this reason, R_f values in the literature should be used with caution. They are valuable to indicate the relative order of resolution of compounds but should be determined in each laboratory and preferably checked with each set of determinations. In addition to R_f values, the colors produced with spray reagents are used in the tentative identification of compounds.

RADIOISOTOPES[11,35-37]

Radioactivity measurements are a convenient tool for performing certain types of determinations.

Basic principles

Radioactive atoms are those that spontaneously change into other atomic species with the liberation of energy. In those used in the clinical laboratory the energy is liberated in the form of γ-rays (high-energy electromagnetic radiation similar to high-voltage x-rays) and β-particles (high-velocity electrons). There is another type of decomposition that liberates α-particles (doubly charged helium nuclei), but these particles cannot be measured satisfactorily for ordinary use. Each radioactive atomic species decomposes at a definite fixed rate, which for all practical purposes is not influenced by any external conditions. This rate is usually expressed in terms of the half-life, the time taken for one half of a given number of atoms to decay. The commonly used isotope ^{125}I has a half-life of approximately 60 days. This means that if one starts with a given number of radioactive atoms, in 60 days one half of them will have decomposed into stable atoms and in the next 60 days one half of the remainder will decompose. After 3×60 days only one eighth ($^{1}/_{2}{}^{3}$) of the radioactive atoms will remain. Thus after a certain length of time the amount of radioactivity will have decreased to the point where measurement becomes difficult or inaccurate. For this reason a solution containing a substance such as ^{125}I cannot be kept for an indefinite period of time. It may be calculated that with a half-life of 60 days, approximately eight out of every million radioactive atoms decompose every minute. If this seems like a very small number, it may also be calculated that 1 pg of iodine contains about 5 billion atoms.

Types of application

The use of radioactivity in analysis depends on the fact that the radioactive atoms of a substance such as iodine react chemically just as the nonradioactive iodine atoms, but the former can be readily detected by means of their radioactivity. As will be seen, thyroxine labeled with radioactive iodine is used in some tests of thyroid function. The thyroxine molecule contains four atoms of iodine. Some of these iodine atoms may be replaced by radioactive iodine atoms, giving thyroxine labeled with radioactive iodine. This has no effect on the chemical properties of the thyroxine molecule. Suppose that in our procedure we wish to separate the thyroxine present into two fractions. (This is discussed further in the explanation of competitive protein binding.)

Here we are only concerned with the fact that we wish to make a separation. If the thyroxine contains some radioactive molecules, and after the separation we find that 40% of the radioactivity is in one fraction and 60% in the other, this would mean that 60% of all the thyroxine was in one fraction and 40% in the other. The labeled molecules act just as the unlabeled ones in regard to the separation. Thus we have determined the relative amounts of thyroxine in the two fractions by simple radioactive measurements without having to perform an elaborate chemical analysis. In fact, the solution might contain other substances that would interfere with the chemical determination without affecting the simple fractionation.

Methods of measurement

The determination of the amount of radioactivity present can be relatively simple. For many radioactive elements a crystal scintillation counter is used. This consists of a relatively large crystal of sodium iodide that contains a small amount of an activating substance, e.g., thallium. When a β-particle or γ-ray from the disintegrating atom enters the crystal and is absorbed, a small flash of light is produced. This is detected by a photomultiplier tube attached to the crystal. The resultant electric pulse from the phototube is amplified and counted by electronic means. The total number of pulses detected per unit time is a measure of the radioactivity of the sample. Since the β-particles or γ-rays are emitted randomly in all directions, not all of them will enter the crystal and be counted. If, however, all the samples are counted in exactly the same way, particularly in regard to their position relative to the crystal, the relative activities of the different samples can be accurately determined. Most crystals contain a well into which the vial containing the radioactive material is inserted, so that the radioactive material is more completely surrounded by the crystal and a greater number of particles will be counted.

Even in the absence of any of the radioactive material to be measured, the apparatus will detect a certain amount of radioactivity caused by the natural radioactivity of all materials and extraterrestrial cosmic rays. This "background" count must be subtracted from all measurements. Most instruments have the means to do this automatically. To reduce this background to as low a level as possible, the crystal and phototube are usually surrounded by several inches of lead or iron to absorb these extraneous rays. Different radioisotopes emit particles or rays of different energies, and some counters have provision for measuring only particles of a certain range of energies (depending on the isotope being measured). This further reduces the background count.

Some procedures use radioactive carbon (^{14}C) or hydrogen (^{3}H, tritium). These isotopes emit β-particles whose energy levels are too low to be counted in a crystal counter. For these a liquid scintillation counter is used. The material to be counted is dissolved in an organic solvent containing a scintillator such as naphthalene and certain complex organic compounds as activators. The weak β-particles emitted by the disintegrating atoms cause small flashes of light when absorbed. These flashes are detected by one or more photomultiplier tubes mounted just outside the vial containing the material being counted. The whole assembly is mounted in a heavily shielded, light-tight compartment. With the weak radioactivity it is often necessary to count for extended periods of time to obtain sufficient accuracy. Some of the liquid scintillation counters have an arrangement for automatically counting a series of samples and printing out the results.

The radioactive decay has some of the aspects of an essentially random process. If over a period of time it was found that the average number of disintegrations per minute for a given sample was 600, this would not necessarily mean that there would be 10 disintegrations every second or exactly 1 every $^{1}/_{10}$ sec. The number of disintegrations would fluctuate around this average. If one made a number of 1 min counts, one would obtain values between about 575 and 625, averaging close to 600. In fact the standard deviation (which is a measure of the possible error) of a count is equal to the square root of the number of counts made. The relative standard deviation (RSD) expressed as a percentage is then:

$$\sqrt{N} \times 100/N = 100/\sqrt{N}$$

Thus to make a count to within 1% RSD, a desirable figure, one would have to make 10,000 counts. Another factor must also be considered—the magnitude of the background count. If the background count were, for example, 50 counts/min and the sample count were 10,000 counts in 2 min or 5000 counts/min, then the background correction would only be 1% of the total count. But if it took 20 min to achieve a count of 10,000, this would be at a rate of 500 counts/min and the background correction would now be 10% of this. Just as in colorimetric determinations it is best to keep the blank as low as possible; here the background should be as low as possible relative to the sample count. If possible, the latter should be at least five times the background.

ELECTROPHORESIS[11,30,38-40]

Electrophoresis is a method for the separation of charged particles on the basis of their mobility in an electric field.

Basic principles

In a constant electric field, positively charged particles move toward the negative electrode (cathode), and the negatively charged particles move toward the positive electrode (anode). The rate of migration is inversely proportional to the size (weight) of the particles and directly proportional to their charge. The lightest and most highly charged particles move the most rapidly. Thus particles of different sizes or charges may be separated by migration in an electric field. Theoretically almost any type of charged particles could be separated by this means, but the method is most commonly applied to various types of proteins. Proteins are large molecules consisting of long chains of amino acids, and as such have a number of free amino ($-NH_2$) and carboxyl ($-COOH$) groups attached. These groups acquire a positive or negative charge, depending on the pH of the solution containing the protein. In an acid solution, the carboxyl groups are only slightly ionized, and the amino groups form $-NH_3^+$ ions, giving the molecule a net positive charge. In an alkaline solution the amino groups are only slightly ionized, but the carboxyl groups will form $-COO^-$ to give a net negative charge. Since a protein molecule contains a large number of amino and carboxyl groups with varying degrees of affinity for hydroxyl or hydrogen ions, the net charge on a protein molecule varies with the pH of the solution. Since the protein molecule is positively charged in an acid solution and negatively charged in an alkaline solution, there must be some intermediate point at which the net charge is zero. This is known as the isoelectric point for the protein, and it differs with different proteins. In most protein electrophoresis the pH is kept constant, usually around 8.5 with an appropriate buffer.

Electrophoresis has been used to separate a number of different types of proteins. The principle use is in the separation of the major protein fractions of sera. Other proteins that have been separated by this method include lipoproteins, immunoglobulins, isoenzymes, and different hemoglobins. These are discussed in more detail under specific procedures elsewhere.

Supporting media

Although it is possible by special optical methods to measure the changes in concentration of the protein in different parts of a solution, all the clinical procedures use electrophoresis on some type of supporting medium. An absorbent paper similar to filter paper was first used. The paper strip was moistened with the buffer, the protein mixture applied at one point, and the ends of the strip dipped into containers with buffer and the electrodes connected to the source of electrical potential. After the passage of an electric current for a sufficient time (this required as much as 16 hr with paper electrophoresis), the paper was removed and dried. It was then stained with a dye that would combine with the protein, and thus the various protein fractions would be visible along the strip, the different proteins having different migration rates. By estimating the amount of color at different positions along the strip one can estimate the relative amounts of the different proteins. Paper electrophoresis is rarely used now for proteins, because other methods are more rapid. For serum proteins, most procedures use cellulose acetate. For the other types of protein mentioned, gels of agar, starch, or polyacrylamide are used. For the isoenzymes, after electrophoresis the medium containing the enzyme protein is treated with a substrate that will develop a color with the enzyme being studied. In this way only the enzyme proteins are made visible. Similarly some specificity can be derived by using a lipid stain for lipoproteins and specific antibodies for the immunoglobulins.

Isoelectric focusing[41,42]

Another method that may be used for the separation of protein is isoelectric focusing. The proteins are made to migrate through a solution in which the pH varies along the path of migration, increasing fairly linearly with the distance from one electrode. For example, if the proteins were initially grouped together in a solution of pH 4, all would be positively charged and would tend to migrate toward the cathode. If the pH of the solution increased gradually along the path toward the cathode, the individual proteins would continue to migrate until they reached the point at which the pH was equal to the isoelectric point of the particular protein. At this point the charge on the protein molecule would be zero, and there would be no further migration of that particular protein. It is claimed that proteins differing by as little as 0.01 pH unit can be separated by this method. The pH gradient is obtained by the use of special amphoteric substances (ampholytes) used as buffers. Hydrogen or hydroxide ions also may be made to migrate though the solution causing the change in pH with distance. The method has not been used much in clinical chemistry, but it has been used for the separation of some hemoglobins that are difficult to separate by conventional electrophoresis.[43,44]

ION-SELECTIVE ELECTRODES[45,46]
Basic principles

When dipped into a solution containing a specific ion, ion-selective electrodes develop an electrical potential that is a function of the amount of that ion present.

All ion-selective electrodes require a second indifferent or reference electrode, because two electrodes are required for any measurement. Theoretically the potential developed at the reference electrode does not vary with the changes in concentration of the measured ion. This is generally true, but one should not try to standardize with one reference electrode and make the actual measurement with another. In many instances the two electrodes are combined in a single unit, so the above warning is irrelevant.

Specific applications

One such electrode has been in use for many years—that used to measure the hydrogen ion concentration (pH). It has only been within the past few years that electrodes for the measurement of other ions have been developed to the point that they are useful for routine measurements in the clinical laboratory. Electrodes are now available for the measurement of such commonly determined ions as sodium, potassium, chloride, and calcium, as well as the hydrogen ion. The theoretic relation between the electrical potential developed and the logarithm of the concentration of the ion holds only in very dilute solutions containing no other ions. In practice, an electrode for sodium can be standardized by adding a known amount of sodium ions to a matrix similar to that found in the samples, or both the sample and the standard may be diluted with a diluent such that the total effect on the ion to be determined is the same in both solutions. For sodium, potassium, and chloride, the total concentration of these ions is determined, and the difference between the total concentration and the ionic concentration is adjusted, as mentioned above, to be the same in both sample and standard. For calcium, one is interested in the amount of ionized calcium, and the calcium measured by an ion-selective electrode in solution is the total calcium. The measurement of ionic (or free) calcium can be made by placing the calcium-specific electrode behind a special membrane that physically keeps the electrode from measuring protein-bound or complexed calcium.

The concentration of the above ions in most biologic fluids will usually not vary more than tenfold, and the same is true of the pH of biologic fluids, but a hydrogen ion electrode may be used to measure the pH over a much wider range. A change of pH from 3-9 represents approximately a 1 million−fold change in hydrogen ion concentration. Since most pH meters have a pH range of from 0-14 units, the electrode may be standardized at a pH of 7 and used to measure an acid solution having a pH of around 3. This will not give an accurate result, since the electrodes do not have a linear response over a very wide range. If possible the electrode should be standardized at a value no farther than

2 pH units from the pH of the expected measurement. All the ion-selective electrodes are temperature sensitive; thus the calibration and measurement should be done at the same temperature. Many pH meters have a temperature correction circuit to adjust for temperature differences between the standard and sample, but it is still preferable to use the same temperature for both. In the determination of the pH of blood samples both the standardization and measurement are best done at 37° C. With the electrodes used to measure the sodium, potassium, and chloride ions, the temperature is not so critical, but it should be constant.

One point may be mentioned in regard to the pH electrodes. A substance quite commonly used for a buffer is tris (tris[hydroxymethyl]aminomethane). It has been found that certain reference (calomel) electrodes give a different potential with tris buffers than with phosphate buffers.[47] This would cause an error in the measurement for checking the pH of the buffer. Not all electrodes have this disadvantage, but the manufacturer or supplier of the electrode usually can inform one if the electrodes are suitable for use with tris.

MICROANALYSIS

In many instances, particularly in pediatrics, only very small samples of blood may be available for analysis. In such circumstances, microanalytic methods[48-50] may be helpful. Just what constitutes a micromethod is not always clear. In general, for most blood determinations, those requiring more than 0.5 ml of the sample (whole blood, plasma, or serum) may be considered to be macromethods (ordinary). Those requiring 0.05-0.2 ml of the sample are usually classed as micromethods, and those requiring 0.01-0.025 ml are ultramicromethods. Many of the macromethods can be scaled down by using one fifth to one tenth the amount of the sample and all reagents. A number of precautions must be taken Pipetting small volumes requires extreme care. Pipets can be obtained that have sufficient accuracy (0.5%) but that are somewhat less expensive than the regular micropipets. As with most micropipets these are usually "to contain" types and must be rinsed out. In working with small volumes filtration is usually impracticable, and centrifugation must be used. Because of the much larger ratio of surface to volume in the micromethods, one may encounter more evaporation of solvent, creeping of fluids on wettable surfaces, and absorption onto the glass of diluted ions. Although the micromethods require smaller quantities of blood and reagents, they may be more time-consuming and less precise.

Micromethods are suggested for a number of procedures given in this book. In some instances it is noted that the method can be scaled down by using small volumes. In others separate, different methods are suggested. This may also be helpful in another respect, because occasionally it is advantageous to determine the constituent in a sample by two different methods to find out whether the method or the sample is causing an unexpected result.

Some regular methods given in this volume, e.g., those for glucose and blood urea nitrogen, require at the most 50 μl of serum, and the results can be read in ordinary photometer cuvets. In scaling down other procedures the standards must always be treated in the same way as the samples by using microquantities of standards as well as samples. In making dilutions in small volumes, if, for example, 5 ml volumetric flasks are not available, it is sometimes permissible to add 0.1 ml of sample to exactly 5 ml of water instead of adding the 0.1 ml to a flask and diluting to 5 ml, provided dilutions of the standard are made the same way as for the samples. In this way, if, for example, a 1:200 dilution is used in the flame photometric determination of sodium and potassium, instead of adding 0.1 ml to 20 ml with an automatic diluter, 0.02 ml can be added to 4 ml with a micropipet. The standard must be diluted the same way. If it would require a larger amount of diluted standard to adjust the flame photometer, preliminary adjustments can be made with the regular dilution, but the final comparison must be made between the sample and standard that have both been diluted on a microscale.

LABORATORY INSTRUMENTATION

Complex electronic instruments are coming into use more and more in all branches of the clinical laboratory. It is becoming increasingly necessary that the laboratory technician have some understanding of the electronic and other principles involved in the operation of these instruments. A knowledge of these principles will enable one to make better use of a given instrument; one will also have a better understanding of the advantages and limitations of an instrument for a given type of test. Although the instruments are more reliable, they are still subject to breakdown. The increasing complexity means more components that can fail or malfunction.

Some knowledge of the basic operations of the instrument will enable the technician to perform simple troubleshooting and often return the instrument to operation without calling on the expertise of an electronic serviceman. If the serviceman must be called, the technician may be better able to explain the type of malfunction. A detailed explanation of the electronic and other principles involved in the many instruments is beyond the scope of this book. Some general references with a brief description of the type of material covered in each is given to help one decide which might be the most appropriate for a given situation. Of course, no one book can give all the details of every laboratory instrument available or even of all those in more common use. The instruction manual that accompanies the instrument is the first source of information. It should always be studied carefully. A knowledge of electronic theory and of the principles of operation of the type of instrument are helpful in understanding the manual.

A very simple introduction to electronics is given in the inexpensive programmed text by Jeffers and Lowe.[51] This could serve as an introduction to those who have no knowledge of electrical theory. Lee[52] discusses somewhat more electrical theory and the principles involved in the operation of different classes of common laboratory instruments, including photometers, fluorometers, flame and atomic absorption instruments, electrophoresis equipment, pH meters, radioac-

tive and particle counting instruments, and centrifuges. A brief description is given of a number of the more commonly used instruments in each class together with constructional details on a few of these. White, Erickson, and Stevens[53] discuss the two types of automated analyzers, the continuous flow (Technicon Auto-Analyzer) and the discrete sampler (Robot Chemist), but other models and the more recent developments in this field are not mentioned. Ackermann[11] gives a good introduction to electronic theory. The principles involved in the operation of the various laboratory instruments are discussed, with emphasis on the measurements by electrical means. The various components of the electronic instruments, e.g., voltage supplies, amplifers, and indicating devices (meters and digital readouts) are treated in some detail. There is also an elementary discussion of the theory and operation of computers as applied to the clinical laboratory. Both this book and the one by Lee contain sections on electrical and electronic "troubleshooting" in the various instruments found in the clinical laboratory. Either book should be very helpful in the use of electronic instruments in the laboratory. The book by Ackermann may be somewhat more complete, but it is also written at a somewhat higher level.

Simple but very satisfactory methods for checking the operation of a number of types of instruments, including spectrophotometers, AutoAnalyzers, densitometers, flame photometers, pH meters, and Coulter counters, are given by Winstead.[54] This book is highly recommended as a more detailed and up-to-date treatment of many types of laboratory instrumentation.

AUTOMATED ANALYZERS AND COMPUTERS

Although there is some overlapping, automated analyzers and computers[55-59] may be considered to have different functions. The automated equipment generates the data, e.g., the results of the tests. The computer stores and processes the data, e.g., collects and prints out at one time all the results of the different tests done on a given patient for 1 day or for the entire hospital stay. The computer may have some part in the acquisition of the data; e.g., the raw input to the computer may not be the actual test result in final form but an electrical signal from which the computer calculates the final results. In other instances the automated equipment itself will have what is essentially a small computer that makes these calculations.

Many types of automated and semiautomated equipment are available, for use not only in clinical chemistry but also in hematology, blood typing, serology, and to some extent bacteriology. New instruments are being developed in these latter fields. The obvious advantage of the automated equipment is the ability to handle a much greater work load. Many more tests can be done in the same period of time with the same amount of technical help. In addition, less highly skilled personnel can be trained to handle at least part of the automated procedures, freeing the highly trained technicians for tasks requiring greater expertise.

The semiautomated equipment may require a certain amount of manual operation such as for an initial pipetting of a measured volume of the sample or reagent or some calculations of the final results. In the completely automated systems the sampling, addition of reagents, colorimetric or other measurements, and calculation of final results are all completely automatic. If the automated equipment has a numeric sample identification system, it may be connected directly to a computer. With semiautomated or other equipment it may be necessary to manually arrange the samples in an order given by a computer-generated work list so that the results can be properly correlated with the samples. An intermediate console arrangement may be provided so that the sample identification number can be entered manually. This together with the result is then sent to the computer on the proper signal. A similar arrangement can be used with manual methods. With these the computer must be initially furnished with a list of identification numbers and corresponding patient names.

The automated methods give a greater precision in the analytic methods than do manual ones. The various steps in the determination, pipetting or sampling, addition of reagents, timing of reactions, etc. are done in a much more reproducible manner with automated methods (provided the instrument is operating properly). The increased precision is particularly evident when a large number of samples are analyzed. It has been found that when a technician performs many repetitions of the same test, the precision decreases with the number of tests performed because of fatigue, boredom, and the desire or pressure to obtain the results rapidly. The automated instruments are not subject to these interferences. Changes in conditions or deterioration of reagents causes a drift in results when a large series of tests are done in any method. These factors usually are compensated for by running standards or control sera at regular intervals. In a manual procedure there is greater tendency to omit these controls toward the end of a series because of the aforementioned factors, whereas with automated methods the addition of the extra controls requires only a small additional effort. Also, the correction for the drift may require considerable extra calculation in a manual method. With an automated system this may be done automatically. If the automated procedure gives a direct readout of the results on a chart or as a numeric printout, errors in calculation and transcription of results are also greatly reduced.

With the addition of a computer, the precision and accuracy are further increased. Not only are the calculations made by the computer and the results presented in concentration or other desired units, but corrections for drift are automatically made. Even with some automated methods this latter computation may involve considerable work by the technician. The computer also may be programmed to calculate the means and standard deviations of the different analyses made on the control sera run during the day or on all or selected serum samples. The results of these calculations are available immediately at the end of the run and are often helpful in detecting minor variations in the operation of the analyzer.

The same principles apply in automated procedures for hematology, blood banking, etc. When the results are presented on a chart or printout, clerical errors are greatly reduced. Errors resulting from fatigue, boredom, or improper pipetting or mixing are eliminated, control samples are more readily used, and control results are immediately available for comparison.

The computer is very helpful in handling the large amount of data generated by several automated systems in the same laboratory. With some computer systems the nursing stations can address inquiries concerning the tests directly to the computer and thus save valuable technician time in answering telephone inquiries. Many computer systems automatically mark abnormal results, which is an aid to the physician. Furthermore, with computer printouts all the results of tests done on a given patient during the hospital stay can be printed on one form, which aids the physician in comparing results.

A computer system has another advantage that is not so directly connected with the actual operations within the laboratory—it facilitates the billing for tests done on the patients. With the manual operation that uses charge slips it has been found that often as much as 5% of the tests are not billed because of clerical errors. The computer eliminates this, which results in increased income to the laboratory.

The complete computer installations are relatively expensive but have proved worthwhile for large laboratories. The general opinion is that when the computer system is operating properly the total cost of laboratory operation is not greatly increased because of the savings in clerical technician time and increased billing. Also, larger amounts of test data can be handled with a marked increase in precision and better quality control. The data are more readily and rapidly available to the physician, with consequent benefit to the patient and often decreased hospital stay. The question of direct on-line computer operation versus time-shared operation cannot be discussed here.

One further aspect of highly automated and computerized laboratory operation that can only be mentioned here is reliability. Failure in a highly complex system may result in almost complete shutdown of the laboratory unless adequate backup equipment is available together with a 24 hr technical repair service. A partial solution to some of these difficulties may be a cooperative arrangement between several laboratories to have one laboratory perform the tests for another laboratory in extreme emergencies.

AUTOMATION IN THE CHEMISTRY LABORATORY

With the development of many new tests and the greater use of older ones, many laboratories have had large increases in the work load in recent years. In an attempt to increase the number of tests that can be performed without great increases in personnel and space, consideration must be given to the many automatic and semiautomatic devices[60-64] that have been developed to save both time and effort. Many of these devices are relatively simple and can be adapted to any laboratory, whereas others are more complicated and expensive. The latter may require a certain work load to justify their use. Mention is made of a number of technics and types of apparatus that may be of value in increasing automation in the clinical laboratory.

Although not directly concerned with the performance of the tests themselves, the washing of glassware is an essential part of the laboratory work load. Many of the automatic technics mentioned greatly reduce the amount of glassware used. However, the use of automatic washing machines often proves helpful. Most laboratory personnel are familiar with the pipet washing machines based on the siphon principle that automatically cycle, wash, or rinse water through the pipets. If the work load is large, consideration should be given to the use of an automatic glassware washing machine.

Analytic balances offer a degree of semiautomatic operation. The weights are added or subtracted by turning appropriate knobs, which also indicate the value of the weight on a mechanical scale. The smaller milligram weights are usually read from an optical scale, and the correct weight is easily determined. These balances enable rapid and accurate weighings to be performed by semiskilled persons.

Newer analytic balances are available that are completely automatic (within certain weight limits) displaying the weight of items placed on the weighing pan directly in digital form. Some versions even allow automatic taring; the operator presses a button after an initial weight was obtained (e.g., empty beaker) to display the net weight after a second material was added to the first (e.g., beaker plus solution).

For the colorimetric measurement of samples, recording spectrophotometers and recording attachments for spectrophotometers are available. These devices are also available for some of the smaller instruments, so that readings may be made quite rapidly without the necessity of writing each one down. The results are automatically recorded on a strip chart. This may be conveniently used with another adaptation of the photometer, a cuvet, more or less permanently in place in the photometer, that can be rapidly emptied by suction or gravity flow, so that successive additions and readings on solutions can be made quite rapidly.

In the past decade, revolutionary developments have taken place in the clinical laboratory in terms of automation. This has become a reality as well as a necessity in the laboratory today.

Practically every major instrument company in the country offers a wide choice of automated systems. The laboratory directors are confronted with making the decision of which instrument to choose for their specific needs.

Automated analytic systems are subject to the same problems as those encountered in manual procedures in trying to maintain accuracy and precision. Factors such as sampling, delivery of reagents, removal of interfering materials, heating or incubation of reaction mixtures, and measurement, recording, and quantitation of data must be considered. In this section descriptions of the most commonly used systems and principles of operation are presented. Detailed information that is readily available from the manufacturers is minimal.

Types of automated equipment

The automated chemical analyzers that are available utilize two distinctively different operating principles. The two types are continuous-flow, and discrete sampling.

Continuous-flow systems

Technicon Instruments Corporation is the manufacturer and patent holder of the continuous-flow analyzers. In these systems, in succession, the sample is drawn into the instrument and step by step goes through dialysis if needed, through addition of reagents, into incubation for completion of the reaction, and through the colorimeter flow cell, from which signals are recorded. Samples are separated by air bubbles, and as they flow through the colorimeter flow cell, the reacted sample is read at a "steady state plateau" (the sample is reacted long enough in reference to dimensions of the colorimeter flow cell).

Technicon systems include the AutoAnalyzer II, which is capable of running three different tests and a blank at rates of 60-80 per hour, the SMA II, which can run 18 different tests simultaneously at a rate of 90 per hour, and the SMAC, which can perform simultaneously up to 40 different tests at the rate of 120 per hour. The SMA II and the SMAC are computer controlled with automatic standardization and calibration, and the printout of results with the normal ranges or reference values can be changed as desired by the operator. The SMAC uses ion-selective electrodes for sodium and potassium rather than a flame photometer.

Discrete sampling systems

The other major type of automated analyzers is the discrete system in which each specimen is added separately to a container along with the reagents' and the reaction is carried out followed by colorimetric or other readings. The results are then automatically calculated and printed out. In essence this is similar to what is done in a manual method. The various discrete systems differ in the degree of automation. In the simpler systems a few manipulations may be required, e.g., adding the sample or recording the result; in the more sophisticated systems all the steps are completely automated.

Most discrete automated analyzers follow the same pattern as is generally used in a manual method: the reagents and sample are pipetted into a test tube or other container, mixed, incubated for the required length of time, read in some type of photometer, and the results calculated from the previous similar treatment of standards.

Centrifugal analyzers: The centrifugal analyzers are one special group of automated discrete analyzers. These instruments are provided with special rotors containing compartmentalized cells. The samples and reagents are added to separate compartments, either with a pipetting device or completely automatically. The rotors are then placed in the cenrifugal unit and spun. The centrifugal force moves the sample and reagents into an outer compartment where they are mixed and the reaction takes place. A beam of light passing upward through the transparent portion of the cell measures the absorbance as the rotor is spinning. The results from the separate cells are separated electronically and automatically calculated to give the final result. Although only one constituent can be analyzed at one time for about 20 samples, the reaction time is usually only a few minutes, and while one rotor is spinning another can be filled, so that samples can be processed rather rapidly. These have proved to be quite satisfactory for many laboratories. The amount of sample required per test is generally in the range of 1-50 μl, and the amount of reagent is usually less than 1 ml (often 100-250 μl). The models on the market include the IL Multistat III (Instrumentation Laboratory, Lexington, Mass.), the Cobas Bio (Roche Analytical Instruments Inc., Nutley, N.J.), the Rotochem (American Instrument Co., Silver Spring, Md.), the Centrifi-Chem (Union Carbide Corp., New York), and the EMI Gemsaec (Electro-Nucleonics, Fairfield, N.J.).

Dupont ACA: The Dupont ACA uses a slightly different mode of operation. The reagents for each test are packaged in a special flexible plastic pack with a rigid header. Also, this pack serves as the reaction chamber and test cuvet for the photometric analysis. These packs contain in one or more heat-sealed compartments the reagents necessary for the specific test for which they are designed. Packs for certain tests contain individual disposable chromatographic columns (ion exchange or gel filtration) for removal of interfering substances such as proteins. The rigid header of these packs contains a binary code for the particular tests, which is read by the built-in computer in the system. The programmed computer directs the instrument to draw the specified volume of sample and diluent into each pack and, in succession, mixes the reagents, waits a preset amount of time, forms a precise optical cell within the transparent pack walls, and measures the reaction photometrically. The computer calculates the concentration value for each test and prints out a separate report sheet for each sample, including the patient identification data. The used test packs are discarded automatically into a waste container. In this system only one sample is analyzed at a time, but any of the 42 different tests available can be made consecutively on the same sample.

Abbott Laboratories systems: The systems offered by Abbott Laboratories are the ABA-100, the ABA-200, and the Abbott VP. All these use the principle of measuring the difference in absorbance at two selected wavelengths as a measure of the concentrations. This is said to eliminate much of the interference caused by turbidity and by hemoglobin or bilirubin in serum samples. The ABA-200 is more completely automated than the ABA-100 and can be linked to a data management system for complete automation with complete sample selection, printout, and calculation of averages and standard deviations. The Abbott VP is a newer and more completely automated version of the ABA-100 with a minicomputer.

Coulter analyzers: The Coulter Kem-O-Lab is a small automated instrument that will run profiles of 2-6 analyses at the rate of 540 per hour. The Coulter Chemistry is a larger instrument providing discrete analysis for 22 channels. Tests may be selected individually or in a profile. The instrument will completely analyze 60 specimens per hour. An additional data processing system is also available for billing reports, quality control, and statistical analysis.

Hycel systems: The systems produced by Hycel include the Hycel 17, which is a programmable multichannel analyzer that can perform a 17-test profile or any selection of tests from this on each sample at the rate of 40 per hour. Each test is individually performed in its own tube, eliminating carry-over and increasing accuracy. Only 1.7 ml of sample is required for the total of 17 tests. The Super-17 is an advanced model with larger computer capabilities that can perform the tests at the rate of 60 samples per hour. The newest addition to the Hycel line is the Hycel M, which is a high-speed, 30-channel, completely automated instrument that can process 120 specimens per hour using microtechnics. The computer capabilities include multiple printouts and provision for data collection and quality control procedures. The instrument may be interfaced directly with larger hospital computers.

American Monitor Corporation analyzer: The American Monitor Corporation produces the Monitor KDA, which is a computerized discrete analyzer. As many as 32 different tests can be made on each sample, with a programmed selection of those tests desired for each individual sample. The KDA runs a single procedure at a time as directed by the computer or operator. A larger version, the Parallel, is available, which runs 30 procedures simultaneously, producing a throughput of 240 samples per hour or 7200 tests per hour.

Beckman Company analyzers: The Beckman Company has produced the Astra 4 and 8 (Automated Stat/Routine Analyzer). These analyzers can perform assays for glucose, BUN, sodium, potassium, chloride, carbon dioxide, and creatinine. The Astra 4 assays four or five analytes, usually the electrolytes, and one other, whereas the Astra 8 does all of the listed procedures and three calculated parameters at about 72 samples per hour. Other samples that can be analyzed include amylase, total bilirubin, calcium, and total protein, any two of which can be added to the existing Astra 8.

Instrumentation Laboratory systems: Two new completely automated analyzers were recently introduced by Instrumentation Laboratory systems: the System 504 for the analysis of electrolytes and the System 508 for the analysis of electrolytes plus glucose, BUN, creatinine, and total protein at about 100 samples per hour. These systems are completely automated, including the production of patient reports.

• • •

A number of other instruments, some made by foreign manufacturers, are also discrete automated chemical analyzers. Since the market is continually changing, with new instruments being introduced and older models withdrawn, a complete listing of present models would not be of great value for future use. The preceding discussion should give some idea of the types of instruments available at the time of this writing. A brief description of many of the instruments on the market at any time may be found in the annual publications *Clinical Laboratory Reference* (Medical Economics Co., Oradell, N.J.) or *Guide to Scientific Instruments* (American Association for the Advancement of Science, Washington, D.C.).

REAGENT KITS[65]
Kits for chemical determinations

A considerable number of kits are now on the market containing all the reagents and standards necessary for the determination of a single constituent. Some of these are based on well-established procedures or simple modifications of them. Others may use methods that have not been so well tested. It is not always easy to determine from the explanatory material accompanying the kit or from the advertising brochures how close the actual procedure is to an established method. This material should give literature citations and the actual composition of the reagents. In general it is not advisable to use reagents whose composition is not known. Not all of the kits available are satisfactory. The results of the evaluation of many kits by independent workers have been published. If this has been done and the results were satisfactory, the manufacturer should be able to supply this information. Otherwise it is essential to test the procedures before actual use in the laboratory. A number of samples at different levels of the constituent should be run in parallel by the kit method and with the use of a well-established method such as one of those given in this book. If this is not possible, a number of different control sera should be analyzed with the kit. If only a few samples per day are run, the kits do have the advantage of saving considerable time in the preparation of the reagents. The kit reagents may be more stable than those prepared in the laboratory, often because of special added stabilizers or very pure chemicals. On the other hand, some reagents may have an inherently short life, and if the kit has stood on the supplier's shelf for some time, the reagents may not be satisfactory when received. The kit reagents are usually considerably more expensive than those prepared in the laboratory. If the preparation is simple and requires no accurate weighing of small quantities (e.g., 10 mg of a substance), it may be more economical to prepare the reagent in the laboratory. Some of the kits may contain special reagent chemicals that may be difficult to obtain commercially except in the kit. For some methods, e.g., serum iron, the kits may contain specially purified reagents that give appreciably lower blanks than would ordinary laboratory-prepared reagents.

For kits containing radioactive material such as ^{125}I for the determination of T3 and T4 or ^{51}Fe for the determination of iron-binding capacity the problem is different. It is usually impractical for the laboratory to prepare radioactively labeled thyroxine or the solution containing radioactive iron. Also, the kits may usually be purchased under a general radioactivity license, whereas to obtain the material for preparing the reagents usually would require a special license. For this reason the reagents and supplies must be obtained in kit form. A number of kits are on the market for the thyroid function tests that do not all use exactly the same

methods. All are generally satisfactory provided the directions are followed exactly and the normals given for the particular method are used for comparison. One must be cautious about using the normals given in the literature or for a given kit to compare with the values obtained by a different kit. A general discussion of the evaluation of reagent kits has been given by Logan[66] and Barnett.[67] Evaluation of kits for specific determinations are published from time to time in such journals as *American Journal of Clinical Pathology, Clinical Chemistry,* and *Journal of Clinical Pathology.* Also, *Journal of Laboratory Medicine* publishes frequent short discussions of new reagent kits.

Kits for serologic and immunologic determinations

With these methods, "reagents" such as antigens and antibodies are usually purchased in any event and not prepared by the laboratory. The kits contain not only these reagents but also all other material needed, e.g., diluents or other special substances and usually positive and negative controls. The kit methods may often be modifications of the published methods and thus must be followed exactly.

Reagents

The question of purchasing individual reagents or preparing them in the laboratory must be studied for each reagent and each laboratory. For a very small laboratory it may be more convenient to purchase all but the simplest reagents already prepared. The proportionate amount of time and effort required is much greater when the reagents are prepared in only small quantities. For a moderately sized laboratory, more of the reagents may be made up, depending on the facilities and personnel available. The purchased reagents may be more uniform in quality than those made in the laboratory but this cannot be assumed to be so. Some reagents may not be readily available commercially for the procedure in use in the laboratory. Some reagents containing enzymes or enzyme substrates may be quite unstable in solution and are usually furnished in kits in a lyophilized form for reconstitution just before use. In single test vials these may be rather expensive. To make such reagents in the laboratory usually requires the preparation of a solution that is then placed in aliquots in tightly stoppered tubes and stored frozen until use. For such reagents the trouble involved in their preparation and the possibility of decreased stability may make their purchase in the lyophilized form preferable.

When larger quantities of reagents are used, as in automated multiphasic screening, the problems may be different. The laboratory may well be able to prepare reagents in 1 or 2 L quantities but may not have the facilities for preparation in 20-40 L amounts. If the reagents are relatively stable, it is much more economical in time and labor to prepare them in relatively large quantities. It is sometimes simpler to purchase the reagents at a somewhat higher cost than to obtain additional space and personnel for their preparation on the larger scale. On the other hand, since many of the reagents are actually more than 90% water by weight, if they are not available from a local producer, one may be paying transportation charges on large quantities of water. Some reagents are available in a dry-pack form containing all the chemicals for preparing, e.g., 1 gallon of the final reagent. These may be convenient and save paying the transportation charges on water, but they still require some time for preparation. Many of the automated reagents may be available on a contract basis in which the laboratory agrees to purchase a larger quantity of reagents to be delivered over a period of time such as 1 year. This can result in considerable saving.

The problem of the immediate availability of the reagents in an emergency must also be considered. In some laboratories the purchasing arrangements may be such that it may take a considerable time to obtain the reagents, particularly if ordered from a supplier at some distance. It the reagents are made up in the laboratory, the technicians can theoretically make up reagents during slack periods, so that there are always sufficient quantities on hand. In practice it does not always work out this way. The preparation of a given reagent is often delayed until the last minute. Then the technicians are all busy at other tasks, and it may be found that the supply of a necessary chemical has been exhausted. However, it is usually easier to obtain immediately a necessary quantity of the needed chemical than of the reagent itself.

DRUG INTERFERENCES AND OTHER DIAGNOSTIC CHANGES

The presence of a number of substances in the body may cause the results of a given clinical chemistry determination to be of a value other than that expected or than that which would have been obtained in the absence of the substance. This may interfere with the diagnostic use of the test. Commonly these substances are drugs or their metabolites, but other endogenous substances may also interfere. The common types of interference are mentioned in connection with the discussion of the normal and abnormal values for the separate tests, but a few examples, dealing chiefly with blood glucose, are mentioned here to illustrate the kinds of interference that may be found.

One result of drug administration that is usually not considered an interference is a direct effect of the drug on the concentration of the substance being determined in blood or other body fluid. Usually the physician is aware of this. In fact, a common reason for the chemical determination of the concentration of the compound is to ascertain whether an adequate or satisfactory dose of the drug that affects this concentration has been administered. An example of this is the use of insulin in the treatment of hyperglycemia. The blood glucose is used to determine if an adequate dose of insulin has been administered.

Another result of drug therapy of which the physician may not always be aware is that resulting from the side effects of the drug. The drug may not be given to influence the concentration of the substance being determined, but side effects of the drug may change the concentration. For example, it is known that prolonged administration of some of the oral contraceptives influ-

ences the glucose tolerance curve, giving significantly higher glucose values in the second hour or in later blood specimens. Since these drugs are not administered for any effect on the carbohydrate metabolism, the physician may not be aware of this side effect. This factor must thus be considered in evaluating the results of such tests. Another point must be considered in regard to the drug interferences caused by side effects. A distinction should be made between the relatively mild and possibly transient effects, which disappear when the drug is no longer administered, and more serious changes in blood values resulting from definite pathologic processes brought about by the drug. The mild changes in glucose tolerance that occur as a result of the use of oral contraceptives may be in the former category. These changes may cause some uncertainty in the interpretation of the laboratory results but otherwise probably do not seriously affect the health of the patients. On the other hand, some potent drugs are known to cause, for example, definite liver damage on continued administration. In such cases any increase in alanine aminotransferase or bilirubin must be viewed as a possible indication of early liver damage. These blood changes would not then be considered minor side effects, and the patient should be observed carefully. It may not always be possible to make a clear distinction between the two types, and all changes must be considered in this light when drugs that are known to cause liver or other damage are administered.

A third way in which drugs or their metabolites can affect the results of a determination is by direct interference with the chemical reactions involved. Since this is a purely chemical effect that depends on the actual method used in the determination, the physician usually is not aware of this possibility. Laboratory personnel should keep this in mind when abnormal results are questioned. Often the presence of such interference may be suspected or inferred from an abnormal color or other appearance of the final solution used in the colorimetric readings. For example, the presence of dextran may cause abnormally high values for glucose determined by the o-toluidine method resulting from turbidity caused by the dextran. This may be apparent on visual inspection. With manual methods a little experience should give the technician a good idea of what the appearance of the final solution should be, and one should not uncritically accept readings on solutions that have a highly abnormal appearance, e.g., excess turbidity or a different shade of color. In other instances it is not possible to detect the chemical interference directly. For example, high values of ascorbic acid may cause low glucose values when the sugar is determined by the glucose oxidase method. The ascorbic acid inhibits the production of the chromogen. There is no unusual color; the colorimeter reading is merely less than it should be.

These examples illustrate the various types of drug interference that may be encountered and concerning which the laboratory should be able to advise the physician. Abnormally high values of some endogenous substances may also interfere with the results of other tests. For example, markedly elevated values of uric acid and creatinine (such as may occur in advanced renal disease) cause a spurious elevation of blood sugar when determined by the copper reduction methods. These substances also reduce some of the copper, as does glucose. The influence of high bilirubin levels in increasing the results of cholesterol determinations by the direct methods is also well known. The chemical interference may sometimes be eliminated or reduced by the use of a special blank that might not ordinarily be used or by the use of a different method. These modifications are not always feasible, particularly if the interference is not suspected beforehand.

Literature references to drug interference

Several compilations of drug effects and interferences have been published. The most comprehensive, edited by Young, Pestaner, and Gibberman,[68] was produced as a special issue of *Clinical Chemistry* (April 1975) but may be obtained separately. The listing is very complete, with citations of over 2,000 references, but only partially indicates whether the mentioned interference is common or occurs occasionally. The volumes by Hansten[69] and Garb,[70] while not as comprehensive, list the interferences of the more common tests with some indication as to whether the interference is common or not and its relative importance in diagnostic problems.

Disease-associated changes[71]

Many times the clinician or laboratory personnel are aware of the changes certain diseases produce on the concentration of a given analyte (e.g., high serum glucose is usually associated with diabetes mellitus). The disease, however, may produce a series of changes on other analytes (e.g., decrease of many serum constituents and increase of many urinary constituents secondary to osmotic diuresis), as well as the primary change usually associated with the disease. A comprehensive listing of disease-associated changes has been produced as a special issue of *Clinical Chemistry* (March 1980) and may be obtained separately. The editors have attempted to produce a complete listing with citations to 2002 references and at the same time indicating whether the effect is large or small and if all patients are affected.

WHOLE BLOOD AND SERUM OR PLASMA ANALYSIS

In the early days of clinical chemistry many of the tests were performed on whole blood. These required the preparation of a protein-free filtrate that often still contained interfering materials. For example, the determination of creatinine by the Jaffé reaction is unsatisfactory with a filtrate from whole blood because of the large amount of nonspecific chromogens present. Today there are many methods that use serum (or, in some cases, plasma) directly without the preparation of a filtrate, and such methods are frequently used in automated instruments. When the preparation of a filtrate is required, a more satisfactory solution is obtained from serum. It was found that the amount of total reducing sugars as determined by a copper reduction method on a Somogyi filtrate varied somewhat with the exact method of preparation of the filtrate when whole blood was used. With serum the method of preparation

had no effect. Since most enzyme methods require serum, the use of serum for other determinations enables one to run more determinations on the same sample.

Specific requirements

For most analyses the concentrations of substances of physiologic or clinical interest are those found in the serum (or plasma). The concentrations in the erythrocytes are different and usually of less interest. The serum or plasma concentration could remain constant, yet the concentration in whole blood would appear to vary, depending on the proportion of erythrocytes in the whole blood. One would never try to follow the physiologically active serum concentration of potassium by measuring the totally different concentration in whole blood. This is an extreme example, but the principle applies to many other determinations. For these reasons we feel that the use of serum (or plasma) for analysis is preferable to that of whole blood except in the following special instances:

1. In a few instances the substance of interest is actually present chiefly in the red cells, e.g., glucose-6-phosphate dehydrogenase, galactose-1-phosphate uridyl transferase, and erythrocyte cholinesterase. In such determinations the cells are separated from the plasma, lysed, and the hemolysate used for analysis.

2. For the determination of Pco_2 and pH, heparinized whole blood is preferable. For the determinations of hemoglobin or its derivatives (carboxyhemoglobin and methemoglobin) and oxygen saturation, whole blood is, of course, required.

3. In the determination of lactic and pyruvic acids even the short time required to separate the cells from the serum may result in marked changes in the concentration of these substances. In these determinations a protein-free filtrate may be made from the blood immediately after collection.

4. In some micromethods and ultramicromethods it may be convenient to collect the blood sample in small capillary pipets and introduce this sample directly into the precipitating or other reagents. Thus the use of any anticoagulant is avoided. It has been found that when whole blood is immediately diluted 1:10 with water in this manner, the glucose concentration in the lysed solutions remains quite constant for an hour or more. The precipitating reagents can be added later in the laboratory.

Protein-free filtrates

For the determination of some blood constituents it may be necessary to remove the plasma or serum proteins (and erythrocytes as well if whole blood is used). Although most methods are being introduced that use serum directly, the preparation of a protein-free filtrate is occasionally needed. A number of methods have been used for the preparation of a protein-free filtrate. Some methods are for specific determinations, whereas others are more widely applicable. In these methods a substance is added to combine with and precipitate the proteins, leaving the desired constituents in solution. The most commonly used precipitants are tungstic acid, trichloroacetic acid, and zinc hydroxide. In preparing the filtrates, the blood or serum is diluted in a definite ratio; this factor must be taken into account in the calculations. One milliliter of serum may be added to 9 ml of a solution containing the precipitating reagent. Commonly this is taken to be a 1:10 dilution of the serum, although strictly speaking this is not true. Because of the volume occupied by the precipitate, the constituents from the 1 ml of serum are in a volume of liquid slightly less than 10 ml. The error can be as much as 3-4%, depending on the type of precipitate, but this error has commonly been neglected.

After the protein has been precipitated, the solution is filtered or centrifuged to separate the precipitate. Filtration is often more convenient than centrifugation, but if only a small volume of blood is available, a greater quantity of filtrate can be obtained by centrifugation. Some precipitations made with trichloroacetic acid may filter very slowly and centrifuging is preferred. One difficulty that may be encountered is that a few particles of precipitate may remain floating in the solution. Often these can be removed by filtering through a small filter paper or a small pledget of glass wool.

Folin-Wu filtrate[72]

The Folin-Wu filtrate is used in probably the oldest method of blood deproteinization that is still in use. It was originally designed for the Folin-Wu method for blood sugar and for the determination of nonprotein nitrogen. These particular methods are seldom used now, but modified Folin-Wu filtrates have been used in several other determinations.
Reagents:
1. Sodium tungstate, 0.30 mole/L
   Dissolve 50 g of reagent grade sodium tungstate ($Na_2WO_4 \cdot 2H_2O$) in water to make 5 dl.
2. Sulfuric acid, 0.33 mole/L
   Mix together 2 volumes of 0.5 mole/L sulfuric acid (dilute 1 volume of concentrated acid with 35 volumes of water, adding acid to the water) and 1 volume of water.
Procedure for whole blood: Dilute 1 volume of blood (measured with a "to contain" pipet) with 7 volumes of water. Add 1 volume of sodium tungstate and mix. Then add 1 volume of the sulfuric acid solution and mix well by shaking it in a stoppered tube or flask. Allow it to stand until it turns a chocolate color. Filter or centrifuge.
Procedure for plasma or serum: Plasma and serum contain less protein and require only about half as much of the precipitating reagents. Use 1 volume of serum or plasma, 8 volumes of water, and 0.5 volumes each of sodium tungstate and sulfuric acid. Mix well after the addition of each reagent, allow it to stand for 10 min, and then filter or centrifuge.
Procedure for cerebrospinal fluid: For cerebrospinal fluid or other body fluids such as urine containing only a small amount of protein, use 1 volume of sample, 8.5 volumes of water, and 0.25 volumes each of sodium tungstate and sulfuric acid.

• • •

In some procedures using a Folin-Wu filtrate, different amounts of water may be used to give a dilution other than the 1:10 dilution provided above, or the water and sulfuric acid may be combined as a single reagent.

Somogyi filtrate[73]

The Somogyi filtrate was designed for use with the Somogyi method for glucose in blood. Although this method for glucose is no longer used, a Somogyi filtrate may be suggested for certain other determinations, because it gives a more complete removal of proteins and other interfering substances than do the other precipitation methods.
Reagents:
1. Zinc sulfate solution, 0.175 mole/L
   Dissolve 50 g of reagent grade zinc sulfate ($ZnSO_4 \cdot 7H_2O$) in water and dilute to 1 L. Fresh unefflorescent crystals (nonpowdery) should be used.
2. Barium hydroxide, 0.15 mole/L
   Dissolve 47 g of barium hydroxide ($Ba[OH]_2 \cdot 8H_2O$) in freshly distilled or recently boiled and cooled deionized water and dilute to 1 L. If the solution is cloudy, allow it to stand several days in a tightly stoppered bottle and then decant off the clear supernatant. Protect the solution from contact from air, because it will absorb CO_2 with the precipitation of barium carbonate.

The actual concentrations of the zinc sulfate and barium hydroxide solutions are not as important as the fact that they must exactly neutralize each other. To check this, add exactly 10 ml zinc sulfate solution to a 250 ml flask; add about 50 ml distilled water and 4 drops phenolphthalein indicator (1% in ethyl alcohol). Slowly titrate with barium hydroxide, using continual agitation. Too rapid a titration will give a false end point. The titration is carried out until 1 drop of the barium hydroxide solution turns the solution a faint permanent pink. The results should be that 10 ml zinc sulfate solution requires 10 ± 0.05 ml barium hydroxide.

If one or the other of the solutions is too strong, add distilled water in appropriate quantities and repeat the titration. The bottles containing the barium hydroxide must be protected from air with a soda-lime (sodium hydroxide) tube in the stopper. If the barium hydroxide solution is to be dispensed from a buret, the top of the buret must also be protected with a soda-lime tube, and a buret with a Teflon stopcock plug must be used. The solution should be tested in advance by preparing a trial filtrate with blood. Filtration should proceed rapidly to give a clear solution with little tendency to foam.
Procedure: Add 1 volume of blood (whole blood must always be measured with a "to contain" pipet that is rinsed out) to 5 volume water. Add 2 volumes of barium hydroxide and mix. Add 2 volumes of zinc sulfate solution and mix. Centrifuge or filter. This produces a 1:10 dilution of the blood. The same proportions of serum and reagents are used as for blood.

Trichloroacetic acid filtrate[74]

Trichloroacetic acid filtrate may be used for the determination of inorganic phosphorus and for other procedures requiring an acid filtrate. For a 1:10 dilution one may use 1 ml serum or plasma and 9 ml 0.3 mole/L (5% wt/vol) trichloroacetic acid. After mixing and allowing it to stand for a few minutes, the solution is centrifuged or filtered. Depending on the particular determination, a number of different proportions of acid and serum have been used.

Reagent: Dilute solutions of trichloroacetic acid are not very stable even when kept in the refrigerator. It is preferable to make up a more concentrated solution and dilute as required. The acid may be purchased as a 30% or 40% (wt/vol) solution. Trichloroacetic acid is very corrosive and hygroscopic and thus difficult to weigh out properly. A convenient way to prepare a concentrated solution is to dissolve the entire contents of a previously unopened $^1/_4$ lb. bottle of reagent grade acid in exactly 315 ml water. This will give a 1.8 mole/L solution. As required, 1 volume is diluted with 5 volumes of water to give a 0.3 mole/L solution.

REFERENCES

1. Caraway, W.T.: Am. J. Clin. Pathol. **37:**445, 1962.
2. Winsten, S.: In Meites, S., editor: Standard methods of clinical chemistry, New York, 1965, Academic Press, vol. 5, p. 1.
3. Dybkaer, R., and Jorgensen, K.: Quantities and units in clinical chemistry, Baltimore, 1967, The Williams & Wilkins Co.
4. Dybkaer, R.: In MacDonald, R.D., editor: Standard methods of clinical chemistry, New York, 1970, Academic Press, vol. 6, p. 223.
5. Federal Register Notice: Federal Register, Dec. 10, 1976.
6. Lippert, H., and Lehmann, H.P.: SI units in medicine, Baltimore, 1978, Urban & Schwarzenberg, Inc.
7. National Bureau of Standards Circular C-602: Testing of volumetric apparatus, Washington, D.C., 1959, U.S. Department of Commerce.
8. Wenk, R.E., and Lustgarten, J.A.: Clin. Chem. **20:**320, 1974.
9. Zeman, G.R., and Mathewson, N.S.: Clin. Chem. **20:**497, 1974.
10. Winstead, M.: Reagent grade water, Houston, 1967, American Society of Medical Technologists.
11. Ackermann, P.G.: Electronic instrumentation in the clinical laboratory, Boston, 1972, Little, Brown & Co.
12. Willard, H.H., Merritt, L.L., and Dean, J.A.: Instrumental methods of analysis, ed. 4, New York, 1965, Van Nostrand Reinhold Co.
13. Delory, D.E.: Photoelectric colorimetry in clinical chemistry, London, 1966, Adam Hilger, Ltd.
14. Rand, R.N., Jr.: Clin. Chem. **15:**839, 1969.
15. Frings, C.S.: Clin. Chem. **17:**568, 1971.
16. Frings, C.S., Muscat, V.L., and Waldrop, N.T.: Clin. Chem. **22:**161, 1976.
17. MacFate, R.P., et al.: Am. J. Clin. Pathol. **24:**511, 1954.
18. Dean, J.A.: Flame photometry, New York, 1966, McGraw-Hill Book Co.
19. Dvorak, J., Rubeska, I., and Rezak, Z.: Flame photometry: laboratory practice, Cleveland, 1971, Chemical Rubber Co.
20. Robinson, J.W.: Atomic absorption spectroscopy, New York, 1966, Marcel Dekker, Inc.
21. Slavin, W.: Atomic absorption spectroscopy, New York, 1968, John Wiley & Sons, Inc.
22. Udenfriend, S.: Fluorescent assay in biology and medicine, New York, 1962, 1969, Academic Press, Inc., vols. 1 and 2.
23. Elevitch, F.R.: Fluorometric techniques in clinical chemistry, Boston, 1973, Little, Brown & Co.
24. Snyder, R.L.: Methods Med. Res. **12:**1, 1970.
25. Dixon, P.F., et al., editors: High pressure liquid chromatography in clinical chemistry, New York, 1967, Academic Press, Inc.
26. Hamilton, J.J., and Sewell, P.A.: Introduction to high performance liquid chromatography, New York, 1978, John Wiley & Sons, Inc.
27. Grob, R.L., editor: Modern practice of gas chromatography, New York, 1977, John Wiley & Sons, Inc.
28. Littlewood, A.B.: Gas chromatography: techniques and applications, ed. 2, New York, 1970, Academic Press, Inc.
29. Jones, R.A.: An introduction to gas-liquid chromatography, New York, 1970, Academic Press, Inc.
30. Block, R.J., Durrum, E.L., and Zweig, G.S.: A manual of paper chromatography and paper electrophoresis, ed. 2, New York, 1958, Academic Press, Inc.
31. Zweig, C., and Whitker, R.J.: Paper chromatography and electrophoresis, New York, 1971, Academic Press, Inc.
32. Stahl, E.: Thin-layer chromatography, ed. 2, New York, 1969, Springer-Verlag.
33. Touchstone, J., and Dobbins, M.F.: Practice of thin-layer chromatography, New York, 1977, John Wiley & Sons, Inc.
34. Kirchner, J.C.: Thin layer chromatography, New York, 1976, Interscience.
35. Pasternak, C.A., editor: Radioimmunoassay in clinical biochemistry, London, 1975, Heyden & Son, Ltd.
36. Moss, A.J., Dalrymple, G.V., and Boyd, C.M., editors: Practical radioimmunoassay, St. Louis, 1976, The C.V. Mosby Co.
37. Raires, R.A., and Parks, B.H.: Radioisotope laboratory techniques, New York, 1973, Halsted Press.
38. Chin, H.P.: Cellulose acetate electrophoresis, Ann Arbor, Mich., 1970, Ann Arbor–Humphrey Science Publishers, Inc.
39. Cawley, L.P.: Electrophoresis and immunoelectrophoresis, Boston, 1969, Little, Brown & Co.
40. Gordon, A.H.: Electrophoresis of protein in polyacrylamide and starch gels, Amsterdam, 1975, North-Holland Publishing Co.
41. Catsimpoolos, N.: Ann. N.Y. Acad. Sci. **209:**65, 1973.
42. Radols, N.J., and Graesslin, D., editors: Isoelectric isotactophoresis, proceedings of international symposium, Berlin, 1977, Walter de Gruyter & Co.
43. Monte, M., Breuzard, Y., and Rose, J.: Am. J. Clin. Pathol. **66:**753, 1976.
44. Just, W.W., Leon-V, J.O.: Anal. Biochem. **67:**590, 1975.
45. Durst, R.A., editor: Ion-selective electrodes, N.B.S. spec. pub. no. 814, Washington, D.C., 1973, U.S. Government Printing Office.
46. Bates, R.C.: Determination of pH: theory and practice, ed. 2, New York, 1973, Interscience.
47. Durst, R.A.: Clin. Chem. **23:**238, 1977.
48. Mattenheimer, H.: Micromethods for the clinical and biochemical laboratory, Ann Arbor, Mich., 1970, Ann Arbor–Humphrey Science Publishers, Inc.
49. O'Brien, D., Ibbott, F.A., and Rodgerson, D.O.: Laboratory manual of pediatric micro-biochemical techniques, ed. 4, New York, 1968, Harper & Row, Publishers.
50. Werner, M., editor: Microtechniques for the clinical laboratory, New York, 1976, John Wiley & Sons, Inc.
51. Jeffers, D.M., and Lowe, F.B.: Basic electronics for medical technologists, Houston, 1971, American society of Medical Technologists.
52. Lee, L.W.: Elementary principles of laboratory instrumentation, ed. 4, St. Louis, 1978, The C.V. Mosby Co.
53. White, W.L., Erickson, M.M., and Stevens, S.C.: Practical automation for the clinical laboratory, ed. 2, St. Louis, 1971, The C.V. Mosby Co.

54. Winstead, M.: Instrument check systems, Philadelphia, 1971, Lea & Febiger.

55. Britten, G.M., and Werner, M., editors: Automation and data processing in the clinical laboratory, Springfield, Ill., 1970, Charles C Thomas, Publisher.

56. Krieg, A.F., et al.: Clinical laboratory computerization, Baltimore, 1971, University Park Press.

57. The mechanization, automation and increased effectiveness of the clinical laboratory: status report by the Automation in the Medical Laboratory Sciences—Review Committee of the National Institutes of General Medical Sciences, DHEW pub. no. (NIH) 72-145, Washington, D.C., 1971, U.S. Government Printing office.

58. Kinney, T.D., and Melville, R.S., editors: Conference: evaluation of uses of automation in the clinical laboratory, DHEW pub. no. (NIH) 79-501, Washington, D.C., 1975, U.S. Government Printing office.

59. Enlander, D., editor: Computers in laboratory medicine, New York, 1975, Academic Press, Inc.

60. Alpert, N.L.: Clin. Chem. **15:**1198, 1969.

61. Anderson, N.G.: Clin. Chim. Acta **25:**321, 1969.

62. Winter, S.D., et al.: Am. J. Clin. Pathol. **56:**526, 1972.

63. Findley, P.R., et al.: Adv. Automatic Anal. Tech. Int. Cong. **1:**145, 1969.

64. deHaan, J.B.: In Curtius, C.H., and Roth, M., editors: Clinical biochemistry, Berlin, 1974, Walter de Gruyter & Co., pp. 491-520.

65. Editors: Lab. Manage. **18**(5), 1980 (1981 Gold Book).

66. Logan, J.E.: CRC Crit. Rev. Clin. Lab. Sci. **3:**257, 1972.

67. Barnett, R.N.: Prog. Clin. Pathol. **4:**181, 1972.

68. Young, D.S., Pestaner, L.C., and Gibberman, V.: Clin. Chem. **21**(5):1D-432D, 1975.

69. Hansten, P.D.: Drug interaction, ed. 2, Philadelphia, 1975, Lea & Febiger.

70. Garb, S.: Clinical guide to undesirable drug interactions and interferences, New York, 1970, Springer-Verlag.

71. Friedman, R.B., et al.: Clin. Chem. **26(5):**1D-476D, 1980.

72. Folin, O., and Wu, H.: J. Biol. Chem. **38:**8a, 1919.

73. Somogyi, M.: J. Biol. Chem. **160:**69, 1945.

74. Greenwald, T.: J. Biol. Chem. **34:**97, 1918.

CHAPTER 21

Carbohydrates and nitrogen compounds

GLUCOSE

Historically, glucose was one of the first substances determined in blood, and probably more methods have been suggested for its determination than almost any other blood constituent. In the past, copper or ferricyanide reduction methods have been widely used, but in recent years other methods, including enzymatic ones, have become more popular. Two methods are presented here in detail; one is a condensation method involving o-toluidine, and the other is an enzymatic method using glucose oxidase.

Ortho-toluidine method[1,2]

Principle: When heated with glucose, a solution of the aromatic amine ortho-toluidine(o-toluidine) in strongly acid solution produces a colored product with an absorption maximum at about 630 nm. The aldehyde group of the glucose condenses with the reagent to first form a glucosyl amine, and further rearrangement forms a type of colored product generally termed a Schiff base. The reactions are not specific for glucose. Other aldohexoses, including mannose and galactose, will react, but these are not ordinarily present in the blood in sufficient quantities to cause an appreciable interference. Aldopentoses will also react with the reagent, but they do not produce a product that absorbs at 630 nm. This is advantageous since, as will be mentioned later, the reagent can be used to determine glucose and xylose simultaneously by reading at two different wavelengths. Other aromatic amines have been used for the determination of glucose, o-toluidine has proved generally more satisfactory. Most aromatic amines are potentially carcinogenic, but one study has shown that the toxicity of the reagent is slight when it is used with ordinary precautions.[3]

The original reagent was composed of o-toluidine in glacial acetic acid. This is still widely used, but the strongly acidic and corrosive properties of the reagent are a minor disadvantage. A modification uses an aqueous solution containing an organic acid such as citric acid with borate added to increase the color formation.[4,5] This milder reagent is not always free from turbidity when used in direct determinations. Other modifications use a mixture of approximately 50% glacial acetic acid and 50% of a polyhydric alcohol.[6,7]

The o-toluidine method has been established as the most specific nonenzymatic method for the determination of glucose. The method is simple, rapid, and sensitive because of the intense color that develops.[8]

Reagents: Two formulations for the reagent are given, one with acetic acid alone and one with acetic acid plus a glycol. The latter formulation gives some 40% more color with glucose and may be preferred when this sugar alone is to be determined. The solution is rather viscous, and difficulty may be experienced in completely mixing the small quantity of added sample with the reagent. If it is desired to determine xylose as well by the two wavelength method, the reagent containing acetic acid alone is preferred because it gives more color with xylose. Both reagents contain thiourea as a stabilizing agent.

1. Toluidine reagent A[2]

   Dissolve 1.5 g of thiourea in about 9 dl of glacial acetic acid in a 1 L volumetric flask. Add 60 ml of o-toluidine and dilute to 1 L with the acid. A good grade of o-toluidine is required. The earlier directions specified o-toluidine prepared "from nitrate." The stabilized grade, II-S, obtained from Sigma Chemical Co. (St. Louis) is very satisfactory. The reagent should be allowed to age for at least 24 hr before use and should be stored in a brown bottle at room temperature.

2. Toluidine reagent B[4]

   Dissolve 1.5 g of thiourea in about 4 dl of glacial acetic acid in a 1 L volumetric flask. Add 60 ml of o-toluidine (II-S, Sigma Chemical Co.) and 5 dl of 2,3-butantane diol (Aldrich Chemical Co., Milwaukee). Dilute to the mark with acetic acid and mix well. This reagent should also be allowed to age for a day before use.

3. Benzoic acid solution, 1.4 g/L (12 mmole/L)

   Dissolve 1.4 g of benzoic acid in 8 dl deionized water in a 1 L volumetric flask with warming. Allow to cool and then dilute to volume.

4. Glucose standards

   a. Stock Standard, 1000 mg/dl (55.6 mmole/L)
   Dissolve 1 g of National Bureau of Standards dried D-glucose (SRM-917) in 80 ml of benzoic acid solution in a 1 dl volumetric flask and dilute to volume with benzoic acid solution. This stock standard solution is stable at room temperature, but it may be stored in the refrigerator without crystallization of the benzoic acid. Tightly stoppered, the solution is stable indefinitely.

   b. Working standard, 100 mg/dl (5.56 mmole/L)
   Dilute 5 ml of the stock standard to 50 ml in a volumetric flask with benzoic acid solution to obtain a 100 mg/dl standard. Additional working standards can be made (i.e., to prepare a standard curve) by adding 5 ml of the stock standard to a 50 ml volumetric flask for each 100 mg/dl desired. If a series of standards are prepared using 5, 10, 15, and 20 ml, then standard concentrations of 100, 200, 300, and 400 mg/dl will be obtained.

5. Trichloroacetic acid solution, 3.0% wt/vol (0.18 mole/L)

   Dissolve 3.0 g trichloroacetic acid in 50 ml deionized water in a 1 dl volumetric flask and dilute to volume with water.

Procedure for direct method: Pipet 3 ml of o-toluidine reagent in a series of glass tubes, preferably ones with Teflon-lined screw caps. With accurate micropipets add separately to the tubes 50 μl aliquots of the standard and unknown samples, also reserve one tube of o-toluidine reagent alone as a blank. Mix contents of each tube, cap, and heat tubes in a boiling water bath (or 38° C heating block) for 12 min[9]; remove from heat, cool in ice water, then bring to room temperature, and read standards and samples against blank at 630 nm. Then

$$\frac{\text{Absorbance of sample}}{\text{Absorbance of standard}} \times \begin{matrix}\text{Conc. of}\\\text{standard}\end{matrix} = \begin{matrix}\text{Conc. of}\\\text{sample}\end{matrix}$$

Thus

$$\frac{\text{Absorbance of sample}}{\text{Absorbance of standard}} \times 100 = \text{Glucose (mg)/Sample (dl)}$$

or to express milligram per deciliter results in the SI system

$$\text{mg/dl} \times 0.0556 = \text{mmole/L}$$

Either reagent can be used, and slightly different proportions of reagent and sample may be used to give a better range of readings for the particular cuvets and photometer used. Preferably the absorbance of the 100 mg/dl sample (5.56 mmole/L) should be between 0.2 and 0.25. It is also helpful to occasionally read and record the absorbance reading of the blank against glacial acetic acid. Any significant increase in the blank reading indicates deterioration of the reagent.

Procedure with trichloroacetic acid filtrate: Add 0.5 ml of serum or whole blood to 4.5 ml of the 0.18 mole/L trichloroacetic acid. Mix well, allow to stand for a few minutes, then filter or centrifuge. Add 0.5 ml of the filtrate to 3.5 ml of the reagent. To one tube add 0.5 ml of the trichloroacetic acid solution as a blank. For standards, dilute the standards used in the direct method 1:10 with trichloroacetic acid (0.5 ml of standard + 4.5 ml trichloroacetic acid solution) and add 0.5 ml of the diluted standard to 3.5 ml of reagent. Heat in boiling water bath for 12 min, cool, and read standards and samples against blank as in the direct method. Since the samples and standards are treated similarly, the same calculations are used as in the direct method.

Interferences and limitations: If adjustments are to be made in the relative volumes of reagent and filtrate for use with different size cuvets, too large a volume of filtrate must be avoided. The addition of more than about 15% water will reduce the amount of color formed.

Small amounts of hemolysis or lipemia will not interfere, but for grossly hemolyzed samples (or whole blood, if desired) a trichloroacetic acid filtrate must be made. This problem has been pointed out by several authors[2,8,9] since significant positive errors can occur with hemolyzed, lipemic, or icteric sera. Most laboratories, as judged from Centers for Disease Control (CDC) and College of American Pathologists (CAP) proficiency surveys, report using this method without deproteinization, apparently ignoring this source of interference.

The specificity of the method was examined for normal individuals[9] by treating various samples with yeast to remove glucose and then making trichloroacetic acid filtrates. The apparent glucose found was 5 mg/dl for urine, 4 mg/dl for serum, and 1 mg/dl in spinal fluid. Another study[10] found 13 mg/dl of apparent glucose in yeast-treated pooled serum from uremic patients and 3 mg/dl from normal serum.

The direct method should not be used for glucose determinations for a pediatric population.[11] There are two problems; first, for each 1 mg/dl bilirubin, 1-4 mg/dl of apparent glucose have been observed[8] in various studies with the direct method, and second, the blood galactose in normal neonates can be as high as 15-20 mg/dl.[12,13] Since the reagent reacts with galactose as well as glucose, the error is significant. A comparison of interferences for manual and automated o-toluidine methods has been compiled.[14]

A significant negative interference with the o-toluidine methods is from formaldehyde, which may be present in contrived control specimens containing glucose and uric acid. The formaldehyde is used as a preservative in uric acid solutions and may explain why uric acid has been reported both to interfere and not to interfere with the o-toluidine methods.

Glucose oxidase method[15-17]

Principle: Glucose is oxidized by the enzyme glucose oxidase in the presence of oxygen (air) to glucuronic acid with the formation of hydrogen peroxide. In the presence of the added enzyme peroxidase, the hydrogen peroxide will be decomposed and the liberated oxygen will oxidize a chromogen, which can be measured colorimetrically. The amine o-dianisidine was used in some of the earlier methods, but a better chromogen is a mixture of phenol and aminoantipyrine, which gives a strong red color. The method is very specific for glucose and thus gives results close to true glucose values. High concentrations of reducing substances, particularly ascorbic acid, but also uric acid to some extent, may interfere by competing with the chromogen for the liberated oxygen and thus causing low results. Hemoglobin can interfere by causing a premature decomposition of the hydrogen peroxide, thus giving low results. This interference is apparently not as serious with the phenol-antipyrine chromogen as it was with the older o-dianisidine. For markedly hemolyzed sera and whole blood a Somogyi filtrate must be used.

Reagents:
1. Phosphate buffer, 0.1 mole/L, pH 7.0
   Dissolve 8.5 g of anhydrous disodium phosphate (Na_2HPO_4) and 5.3 g of potassium monophosphate(KH_2PO_4) in about 8 dl of water. Check the pH and adjust to 7.0 ± 0.1 by the addition of a small amount of 1 mole/L NaOH or HCl as required, then dilute to 1 L.

2. Peroxidase reagent
   Dissolve 175 mg (0.75 mmole) of 4-aminoantipyrine (Sigma Chemical Co., St. Louis) (also called 4-aminophenazone) and 2 mg of peroxidase (Sigma type II) in 5 dl of the buffer. This solution will remain stable for approximately 4 weeks in the refrigerator.

3. Glucose oxidase reagent
   Add 2 ml of stock glucose oxidase solution (Sigma type V, 1000 units/ml) to the peroxidase reagent. This solution is stable for 1 week in the refrigerator.

4. Phenol solution
   Dissolve 2.0 g (21.3 mmole) of phenol and 9 g of NaCl in water to make 1 L. This solution is stable at room temperature for several months.

5. Standards
   The same standards are used as in the previous method for the direct procedure.

Procedure and calculations: Add 50 μl of serum or standard to 2 ml of the glucose oxidase reagent in a glass tube and mix. Add 2 ml of the phenol reagent, stopper, and shake (to aerate). Then heat in a bath at 37° C for 15 min, cool, and read samples and standards at 510 nm against a blank of the mixed reagent treated similarly.

Calculations of results are given by the equation:

$$\frac{\text{Absorbance of sample}}{\text{Absorbance of standard}} \times \frac{\text{Conc. of}}{\text{standard}} = \frac{\text{Conc. of}}{\text{sample}}$$

As with the previous method, variations may be made in the amounts of sample and reagents to give the proper absorbance range. For a micromethod using only small amounts of reagent and sample, somewhat greater color development can be obtained by heating at 45° C rather than 37° C.

Limitations: For hyperlipemic sera or those containing somewhat increased levels of bilirubin or slight hemolysis, a serum blank may be prepared by adding the same amount of serum to a reagent composed of the phenol reagent alone diluted with an equal volume of water. This serum blank is read against the reagent alone, and any absorbance measured is subtracted from that for the serum treated with the complete reagent. With sera containing marked hemolysis or high levels of bilirubin it is preferable to make a Somogyi filtrate, preparing a 1:10 dilution and using 10 times the volume of filtrate as of the serum used in the direct method. The standards are similarly diluted 1:10 and added in proportionate amounts so that the calculations remain the same. Acid precipitants, e.g., trichloroacetic acid, are not suitable for use with the glucose oxidase method.[18]

Glucose oxidase is specific for β-D-glucose; however, glucose in solution is distributed into 36% α-form and 64% β-form. The complete oxidation of glucose in solution requires mutarotation of the α-form to the β-form. The rate of this conversion depends on pH and temperature. Some commercial preparations of glucose oxidase contain an enzyme, glucomutarotase, that accelerates this reaction.

The enzymatic procedures for the determination of glucose should not be calibrated with lyophilized serum. The process of lyophilization can cause some of the glucose present to become protein bound. This bound glucose is not available for enzymatic assay under these mild conditions. In contrast, the o-toluidine method with its strongly acid conditions can recover all the glucose of such samples.

The glucose oxidase method is a satisfactory one, but the preparation of the reagents may be troublesome and laboratory personnel may wish to use one of the commercial reagent kits (Biodynamics/Boehringer Mannheim Corp., Indianapolis; Sclavo, Wayne, N.J.; Worthington Biochemical Corp., Freehold, N.J.).

Normal values and interpretation[19-21]

The fasting concentration of glucose in serum or plasma by the methods given here is 70-110 mg/dl (3.9-5.8 mmole/L). The values found by older methods were about 5% higher. The values found in whole blood are somewhat different (see the following discussion). Although the most common methods now in use (enzymatic or o-toluidine) use serum or plasma, one still commonly speaks of fasting blood sugar (FBS); however, unless specifically mentioned, the values given here and in the following sections will actually refer to the concentration in serum.

High fasting glucose values are found in diabetes (up to 500 mg/dl or 28 mmole/L) depending on the severity of the condition. In pancreatitis and pancreatic carcinoma, there may be some increase in the fasting concentration but it is rarely over 150 mg/dl (8.3 mmole/L), except in advanced cases. Moderate increases may be found in infectious diseases and in some intercranial diseases, e.g., meningitis, encephalitis, tumors, and hemorrhage. Anesthesia will also cause an increase in the concentration of glucose. A considerable rise, depending on the duration and degree, may occur, sometimes exceeding 200 mg/dl (11 mmole/L).

Lowered values of glucose (hypoglycemia) occur most often as the result of insulin overdose. The glucose concentration may also be reduced in hypothyroidism, hypopituitarism (Simmonds' disease), and hypoadrenalism (Addison's disease). Values as low as 20 mg/dl (1.1 mmole/L) may be found in the last two conditions. Low concentrations may also be found in glycogen storage disease.

Glucose tolerance tests

In studies of carbohydrate metabolism, particularly in the diagnosis of diabetes mellitus, a glucose tolerance test can be performed. This usually gives more information than can be secured from a fasting blood sugar value alone. The test should be made after the patient has been on a regular mixed diet for several days in order to obtain a true response to the test. Preceding carbohydrate starvation will cause an abnormal increase in blood sugar and a delayed decrease, suggesting a diabetic curve. A preceding very high carbohydrate diet will cause a low blood sugar curve.

Use of serum or whole blood

Many of the earlier studies on glucose tolerance were done using the Folin-Wu or similar methods for the determination of glucose. Later work has shown that some of the methods used determined not only "true" glucose of the blood but also other reducing substances as well.

Although these nonsugar reducing substances might not change markedly during the tolerance test, the use of newer, more precise methods of glucose determination requires the reevaluation of criteria for abnormal glucose tolerance curves. This is particularly true since now the majority of glucose determinations are done on

serum rather than whole blood. Mainly because of the difference in water concentration between the cells and plasma the concentration in serum or plasma is higher than in whole blood. McDonald et al.[22] and Thustison et al.[23] compared the results of determinations on whole blood and plasma. The results may be roughly expressed by the following equation:

$$P = 1.16W + 3$$

where P is the plasma (or serum) concentration and W is that in whole blood (in milligrams per deciliter). Because of differences in analytic methods this expression cannot be expected to hold exactly in all cases, but in general the concentration of glucose in serum is about 15% higher than in whole blood. On the other hand, many of the older studies were made with the Folin-Wu method for glucose in whole blood, which gave values up to 10% higher than the "true glucose" values approached by more modern methods. Thus these older Folin-Wu values for whole blood glucose are not so greatly different than the modern values found in plasma.

Test procedure and factors influencing the test

A committee of the American Diabetic Association has made a number of recommendations for the standardization of the oral glucose tolerance test.[24] The more important points will be mentioned here. It is suggested that they be followed as closely as possible to render the interpretation of the test simpler, particularly in comparison with the results of others, since most laboratories must rely on published criteria.

Diet: A diet containing a minimum of 150 g of carbohydrate per day should be eaten for at least 3 days before the test. The excessive intake of sucrose or glucose (corn syrup, etc.) should be avoided. According to Wilkerson,[25] an individual consuming an average diet should ingest sufficient carbohydrate, but rapid reducing diets would not be satisfactory.

Physical activity: Physical inactivity, e.g., bed rest, over a period of time will influence the glucose tolerance; if possible, the test should be performed on ambulatory patients.

Illness: Infectious diseases and surgical or other trauma will also affect the tolerance test; if possible, several days of recovery should be allowed before the test.

Drugs: A number of drugs will affect the test (see also the later discussion of the effect of drugs on blood glucose concentration). If possible, the drugs should be discontinued for several days before the test. These drugs include particularly oral contraceptives and other hormones as well as large doses of salicylates and the thiazide diuretics. Naturally insulin and the oral antidiabetic drugs will influence glucose tolerance; these should be discontinued for several days before the test if possible or else their effect on the interpretation of the test must be considered.

Pregnancy and endocrine disorders: Pregnancy and endocrine disorders will generally affect the blood sugar concentration. If possible, the endocrine difficulty should be corrected before the test; otherwise, an abnormal glucose tolerance curve could be caused by the endocrine abnormality rather than diabetes mellitus. The effect of any drugs used in treating the endocrine disorder must also be considered. The effect of pregnancy on the glucose tolerance may not be great during the first few months (in the absence of appreciable "morning sickness"), but the test may not be as reliable in the later months.

Prior fasting: The patient should have been fasting for at least 8 and not more than 16 hr before the test. The test is best performed in the morning, beginning between 7 and 9 AM with no food taken after the previous midnight. No alcohol should be taken during the previous evening. Water may be taken freely.

Glucose dosage: The committee recommended a dose of 40 g of glucose per square meter of surface area. If the nomograph for the determination of surface area is not available, a dose of 1 g/kg body weight will be satisfactory. (The report gives a complete table with the recommended dose for various body weights and heights.) Others have used standard doses of 50, 75, or 100 g of glucose for all patients, but a dose varying with the size of the patient seems more logical. The glucose is dissolved in about 3 dl water with lemon juice or other flavoring for increased palatability. There are a number of commercial preparations on the market containing glucose in a flavored solution that may be simple to use. Some preparations do not contain glucose but other carbohydrates labeled in terms of glucose equivalents. The committee recommended that these not be used because of possible differences in absorption,[26] but there seems to be little difference in most individuals.[27]

Procedure: The main points of the technic have been given above. A fasting blood sample is taken, and the patient is given orally the required amount of glucose dissolved in about 3 dl water. The ingestion should be over a period of not more than 5 min. Timing is then started and further blood samples taken at intervals of usually 30, 60, 120, and 180 min, although some prefer to take a 90 min specimen or to continue the test for 4 and 5 hr specimens. Sufficient information can usually be obtained from the fasting and 1, 2, and 3 hr specimens. It is usual to obtain urine specimens with each blood specimen and to test each urine specimen for qualitative sugar.

Collection and analysis

The recommendation is that venous blood be drawn from the antecubital vein and that the analysis be performed by a "true glucose" method on serum or plasma (any of the methods of analysis given in this volume would be satisfactory). Capillary blood is less desirable and may require that the analysis be performed on whole blood, but it may be necessary to use capillary blood in infants and small children. For plasma the preferred anticoagulant is 2 mg sodium fluoride and 1 mg disodium salt of EDTA per tube. Such tubes are available in commercial vacuum tubes. Plasma has the advantage that the cells can be separated more quickly, but there is little change in glucose level if the clot is separated as soon as possible from the serum. After separation from the cells or clot, the glucose content of serum or plasma is quite stable for several hours even at room temperature.

Interpretation of test results

The fasting specimen should be within the limits given earlier. The level may rise to 160-180 mg/dl (9-10 mmole/L), when serum or plasma is analyzed, at the first hour and return nearly to the fasting value by the third hour, as indicated by the following chart of the normal response to the glucose tolerance test.

Serum glucose levels (mg/dl[mmole/L])

Fasting	80 (4.5)
$\frac{1}{2}$ hr	155 (8.6)
1 hr	165 (9.2)
2 hr	140 (7.8)
3 hr	80 (4.5)

Different types of glucose tolerance curves are illustrated in Fig. 21-1. These indicate, as mentioned earlier, that diseases other than diabetes mellitus, particularly hormone conditions, can result in abnormal tolerance curves. Although the curves are not very specific for these other diseases, they may sometimes be helpful in differential diagnosis, if diabetes can be ruled out.

In addition to an inspection of the glucose tolerance curves, more objective criteria have been suggested for the diagnosis of diabetes. These are given below. In the tabulations the times are in hours after the beginning of the test; zero time refers to the fasting specimen. The values given are from the reference cited. They have been calculated from the original data to refer to serum or plasma levels of glucose when determined by "true glucose" methods such as those given in this volume. The values are given in milligrams per deciliter with the results in millimoles per liter following in parentheses. In some instances the data have been adjusted for the glucose loads of 40 g/m[2] used by the original investigators.

Wilkerson point method: In the Wilkerson method,[25] points are assigned to each determination exceeding a certain concentration; a total of over two points is indicative of diabetes.

Time (hr)	Glucose (mg/dl[mmole/L])	Points
0	130 (7.2)	1
1	195 (10.9)	$\frac{1}{2}$
2	140 (7.8)	$\frac{1}{2}$
3	130 (7.2)	1

Fajans and Conn method[28]: In the method of Fajans and Conn,[28] diabetes is considered when any of the glucose levels exceed the values given.

Time (hr)	Glucose (mg/dl [mmole/L])
1	185 (10.3)
$1\frac{1}{2}$	165 (9.2)
2	140 (7.8)

University Group Diabetes Project method: In the University Group Diabetes Project method,[29] the sum of the glucose concentration for 0, 1, 2, and 3 hr is obtained. If this sum exceeds 600 mg/dl (33.3 mmole/L) the diagnosis of diabetes may be considered.

Kobbering and Creutzfeldt[30] have studied these criteria and proposed that diabetes should be suspected when the sum of the concentrations at 1 and 2 hr exceeds 360 mg/dl (20 mmole/L). They found that their criterion gave close to the same percentage of diabetes

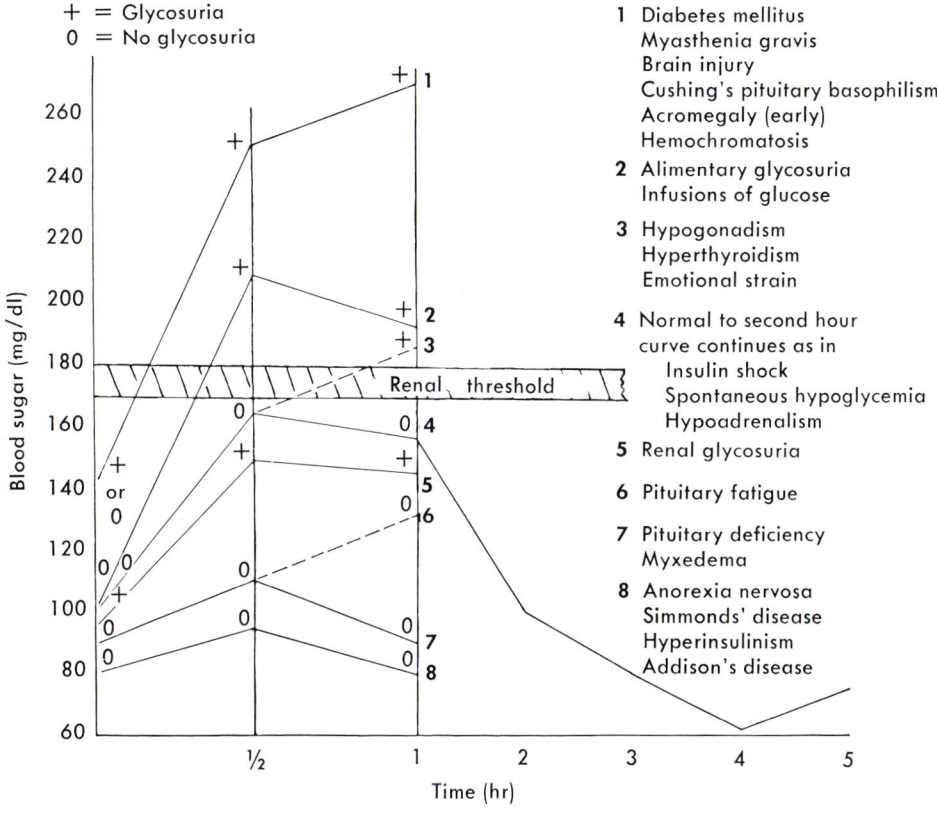

+ = Glycosuria
0 = No glycosuria

1 Diabetes mellitus
  Myasthenia gravis
  Brain injury
  Cushing's pituitary basophilism
  Acromegaly (early)
  Hemochromatosis
2 Alimentary glycosuria
  Infusions of glucose
3 Hypogonadism
  Hyperthyroidism
  Emotional strain
4 Normal to second hour
  curve continues as in
    Insulin shock
    Spontaneous hypoglycemia
    Hypoadrenalism
5 Renal glycosuria
6 Pituitary fatigue
7 Pituitary deficiency
  Myxedema
8 Anorexia nervosa
  Simmonds' disease
  Hyperinsulinism
  Addison's disease

Fig. 21-1. Glucose tolerance curves.

in their group as did the Fajans and Conn method and the University Group Diabetes Project criteria but that the Wilkerson point method gave a somewhat lower percentage.

Another aspect not mentioned previously is that of age. It is known that the glucose levels in a glucose tolerance curve will increase with age in "normal" individuals.[31,32] Most of the work on the criteria mentioned has been done with adults under 50 years of age. For older individuals the values given previously should probably be increased by about 10 mg/dl (0.6 mmole/L) for each decade over 50 years of age. Otherwise, about 50% of older individuals will be diagnosed as having mild diabetes when they are actually normal for their age.

Because of difficulties in standardization of the procedure, the reproducibility of the results, and the many factors influencing the test, there is considerable disagreement between authorities on the usefulness of the test.[33-35] The oral glucose tolerance test should not be used as a "screening test" for diabetes since there is no simple set of criteria to allow total discrimination of normal individuals form abnormal ones.

Classification of glucose intolerance: The National Diabetes Data Group of the National Institutes of Health has proposed a new classification framework for diabetes and other categories of glucose intolerance.[35] The classification has been accepted by the American Diabetes Association and several international groups involved in the study of diabetes, including the World Health Organization. A brief description of the classification framework is given in Table 21-1.

Several important features are recommended. The oral glucose tolerance test (OGTT) load should be standarized to 75 g for nonpregnant adults, 100 g for pregnant women, and 1.75 g/kg for children (not to exceed 75 g). The terminology of juvenile or adult-onset diabetes is considered inappropriate and should be eliminated. Several categories of insulin-dependent and non-insulin-dependent diabetes, impaired glucose tolerance, gestational diabetes, and various risk classes are suggested. Clear diagnostic criteria are given for adults and children for the various categories, and normal concentrations of fasting plasma glucose and OGTT are enumerated.

There is considerable evidence to suggest that there is variability in a subject's response to an OGTT. The individual variation could not be related to age, race, weight, or family history of diabetes. In addition, it is imperative that, before a clinical or laboratory diagnosis of diabetes is made, abnormal fasting plasma glucose or OGTT values be demonstrated on more than one occasion because of the many factors that affect these tests.

Measurements of postprandial or random glucose or nonfasting OGTT are not recommended as definitive procedures although they are useful as "screening" methods. A fasting glucose concentration of <115 mg/

Table 21-1. Classification of glucose intolerance

Class	Former terminology	Diagnostic criteria (adults)
Diabetes mellitus		
Type I: insulin dependent (IDDM)	Juvenile diabetes; ketosis prone; brittle diabetes	Any one of the following*: 1. Classic symptoms and glucose >200 mg/dl 2. Fasting plasma glucose ≥140 mg/dl (7.8 mmole/L) (more than once) 3. OGTT† (75 g) with 2 hr and any other plasma glucose ≥200 mg/dl (11.1 mmole/L)
Type II: NIDDM Nonobese Obese	Adult onset, ketosis resistant; stable diabetes	Same as IDDM
Other types associated with certain conditions Pancreatic disease Hormonal Drug/chemical induced Insulin receptor Genetic syndromes	Secondary diabetes	Same as IDDM
Impaired glucose tolerance		
IGT Nonobese IGT Obese IGT IGT associated with certain conditions	Asymptomatic, chemical, subclinical, borderline, or latent diabetes	All of the following‡: 1. Fasting plasma glucose <140 mg/dl (7.8 mmole/L) 2. ½, 1, 1½ hr OGTT ≥200 mg/dl 3. 2 hr OGTT (75 g) of 140-200 mg/dl
Gestational diabetes (GDM)	Gestational diabetes	OGTT (100 g) and two or more: 1. Fasting glucose >105 mg/dl 2. 1 hr >190 mg/dl 3. 2 hr >165 mg/dl 4. 3 hr >145 mg/dl
Statistical risk classes		
Previous abnormality of glucose tolerance (prev. AGT)	Latent diabetes or prediabetes	Any of the following and prior abnormal FBS or OGTT: 1. FBS§<115 mg/dl 2. OGTT at 2 hr <140 mg/dl 3. OGTT at ½, 1, or 1½ hr <200 mg/dl
Potential abnormality of glucose tolerance (pot. AGT)	Prediabetes; potential diabetes	Same as prev. AGT but no prior abnormalities; generally, first-degree relatives of IDDM or NIDDM

*Children must meet either 1 or 2 and 3.
†Oral glucose tolerance test.
‡Children must meet only 1 and 3.
‡Children must have FBS of <130 mg/dl.

dl is considered normal. The OGTT is not necessary when the fasting glucose concentration is elevated on more than one occasion (≥140 mg/dl [7.8 mmole/L]). The normal glucose tolerance, measured by the OGTT, is considered present when the 2 hr plasma glucose is <140 mg/dl (7.8 mmole/L), with no value between 0 and 2 hr >200 mg/dl (11.1 mmole/L).

It is probable that fasting glucose concentrations between 115-140 mg/dl are abnormal and should not be ignored. However, glucose concentrations above these minimums for either fasting glucose or OGTT but below the criteria for diabetes or IGT are not diagnostic for diabetes or IGT.

Postprandial glucose test

O'Sullivan and Mahan[36] and other investigators have shown that the determination of postprandial glucose concentration is a "screening method" for the detection of diabetes. They have demonstrated that the glucose concentration in serum specimens drawn 2 hr after a meal is rarely elevated in normal individuals, whereas it is significantly increased in diabetic patients. This test has correlated well with other standard tests and is useful as a screening test. It has the advantage of requiring only one blood specimen.

Procedure: For best results the patient should be placed on a high-carbohydrate diet for 2-3 days before the test. The patient should eat a breakfast of orange juice, cereal with sugar, toast, and milk. A blood specimen should be drawn 2 hr after this and the glucose level determined.

Interpretation: A normal response is a serum (or plasma) glucose concentration of less than 145 mg/dl (0.81 mmole/L). An abnormal result is a higher value. As with the glucose tolerance test, this figure applies strictly to individuals under the 50 years of age. The value should be raised to about 160 mg/dl (9 mmole/L) for patients in their sixties and to as much as 180 mg/dl (10 mmole/L) in older individuals. Here also the effects of diet, drugs, hormone disease, etc., as mentioned previously, must be considered in interpreting the results.

Intravenous glucose tolerance test

The intravenous method[37] should be used in sprue, in celiac disese, in hypothyroidism in which absorption is slow, thus giving low flat curves, in thyrotoxicosis in which absorption is accelerated, thus giving hyperglycemic curves, and in patients with gastric resections.

Obtain specimens of blood and urine during the fasting state. Give glucose intravenously, 0.5 g/kg body weight, using a sterile 50% glucose solution and adjusting the rate of flow to require 5 min for its administration. Obtain specimens of blood and urine immediately after administration of the glucose is completed and thereafter at the end of 30, 60, 90, and 150 min. Determine the amount of glucose in each specimen.

Normally the blood sugar concentration will be increased immediately after the glucose infusion is complete, reaching a maximum of about 250 mg/dl (14 mmole/L). The urine may contain glucose. In the 30 min specimen there will be a marked drop in glucose and in the 60 min specimen the amount will return to the fasting value ($\pm$ 10%).

In diabetes mellitus the glucose concentration is still elevated 60 min after the glucose administration has been completed and remains elevated for 3 hr or more. In no specimen of blood does the amount of glucose fall below the fasting value.

In liver insufficiency the return to a normal result may be somewhat delayed—between 1 and 2 hr.

Insulin tolerance test

Insulin administered to a normal person in the postabsorptive state causes a prompt decrease of the blood sugar and then a gradual return to the original value or above. The response to insulin may be used to determine a patient's sensitivity to insulin (ability to store glycogen) and ability to recover after the induced hypoglycemia. The insulin tolerance test[38] is an indirect test of the function of the anterior pituitary and adrenal cortex, both of which produce hormones with antagonistic action to insulin. It is used rarely now that sensitive, direct, and specific assays for various hormones are available.

Take a fasting blood specimen for determination of glucose; then intravenously inject regular insulin 0.1 unit/kg body weight. Take other blood specimens for glucose determinations at 20, 30, 45, 60, and 90 min and 2 hr.

CAUTION: Be prepared to administer glucose promptly if early clinical signs and symptoms of hypoglycemia occur (hunger, sweating, nervousness, tremulousness). Give carbohydrates after a test. If marked symptoms are anticipated, use a smaller dose of insulin.

Normally the blood sugar falls to about 50% of the fasting level in 30 min and returns to the original level or above in 2 hr. The duration of hypoglycemia is more important than the degree. Abnormally there may be only a slight or a delayed fall in blood sugar (insulin resistance) or a delayed rise in blood sugar after the hypoglycemia (hypoglycemic unresponsiveness).

Insulin resistance may occur in hyperfunction of the adrenal cortex or the anterior pituitary and sometimes in diabetes mellitus.

Hypoglycemic unresponsiveness occurs in hyperinsulinism, Addison's disease, hypofunction of the anterior pituitary (Simmonds' disease, pituitary myxedema, pituitary dwarfism), and in some cases of hypothyroidism and glycogen storage disease (von Gierke's disease).

A safer method for determining insulin sensitivity uses the insulin glucose tolerance test. In this procedure glucose is administered orally 30 min after the injection of insulin. In a patient resistant to insulin, the hyperglycemia is not counteracted, and in a normal individual the dose of glucose counteracts the hypoglycemia induced by the insulin.

Epinephrine tolerance test[39]

Epinephrine accelerates glycogenolysis and promptly increases the blood sugar. This increase of blood sugar after the administration of epinephrine is an index of the quantity and availability of liver glycogen for maintaining normal blood sugar.

Take a blood specimen to estimate the fasting blood sugar and then inject intramuscularly 10 minims of 1:1000 solution of epinephrine hydrochloride. Take another blood specimen for glucose at 30 min. Normally the blood sugar will increase over 30 mg/dl in 30 min (over 35 mg/dl in 45-60 min), returning to the fasting level in about 2 hr.

A diminished response occurs when the glycogen store is depleted (hepatocellular damage, including fatty liver and cirrhosis), in glycogen storage disease (von Gierke's disease) in which the glycogen is not readily available, and in hypoglycemia that does not respond normally to the insulin tolerance test (Addison's disease, pituitary cachexia, hyperinsulinism).

Tolbutamide tolerance test[40-44]

The tolbutamide tolerance test is based on the difference in response of normal subjects and diabetic individuals to intravenous administration of a test dose of tolbutamide (Orinase, The Upjohn Co., Kalamazoo, Mich.). Following intravenous injection, the glucose value falls to about 50% of the fasting concentration by 30 min and then returns to normal in a fashion similar to the response of the insulin tolerance test.

The precautions regarding previous dietary intake and severe hypoglycemia symptoms apply here also.

On the morning of the test after an overnight fast, obtain a blood specimen; then inject 20 ml Orinase solution at a constant rate over a 2-3 min period. Obtain blood specimens exactly 20 and 30 min later, timing from the midpoint of the injection. Determine the blood sugar in the three specimens. The test is terminated after the last blood sample, and the patient is fed a high-carbohydrate breakfast.

If the blood glucose value of the 20 min specimen is 90% or more of the fasting value, the patient is definitely diabetic. If the 20 min specimen is in the range of 85-89% of the fasting value, diabetes is probable; the range of 75-84% represents normal. The 30 min specimen is of value in confirming the diagnosis. If it is more than 76% of the fasting value, diabetes is almost certain, but lower values have less significance (Fig. 21-2).

In patients suspected of having functioning adenomas

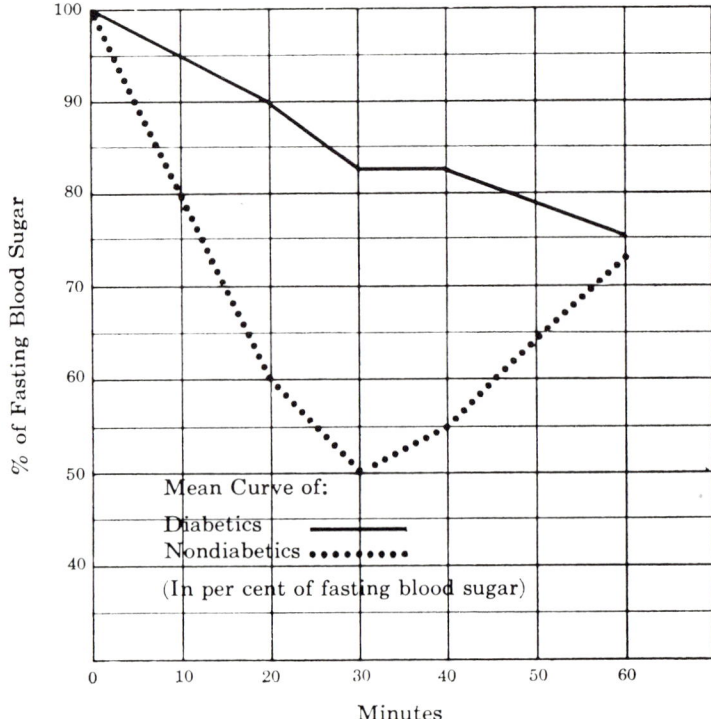

Fig. 21-2. Orinase diagnostic response curves in nondiabetic and diabetic subjects. Blood glucose responses are typical of nondiabetics and of mild diabetics. (Adapted from Unger, R.H., and Madison, L.L.: J. Clin. Invest. **37:**627, 1958.)

of the pancreatic islet cells, the tolbutamide test may be helpful in the differential diagnosis of spontaneous hypoglycemia. For this purpose, after the injection of Orinase, take blood samples at 15 min intervals for the next 2 hr. In normal patients there is a fall in blood sugar for 20-45 min, followed by a rise to normal values during the ensuing 90-180 min. In patients with insulomas the fall in blood sugar is somewhat greater, but more significantly, the hypoglycemia persists for several hours. It is this persistent lowering of blood sugar rather than the magnitude of the fall that is the significant criterion. The blood glucose at 90-180 min is 40-65% of the fasting value as compared with a result of 78-100% in normal individuals.

Effects of drugs on blood glucose levels[35,45-47]

Salicylates: Normal doses of aspirin have little effect on the levels of glucose or on glucose tolerance, but salicylate intoxication may result in hyperglycemia and glucosuria. In infants and young children with carbohydrate depletion from a febrile viral illness or other causes, salicylate overdosage can cause an opposite effect with marked hypoglycemia and coma.

Estrogens and oral contraceptives: Estrogen therapy or administration of oral contraceptives may result in impaired glucose tolerance. The fasting glucose level is usually normal but the levels 2 or $2\frac{1}{2}$ hr after the administration of glucose may be elevated above the normal in up to 40% of patients on oral contraceptives; up to 15% will have mild diabetic types of glucose tolerance curves. The estrogen effect may be the cause of the decreased tolerance found in pregnancy when the endogenous production of estrogen is increased.

Thiazide diuretics: The administration of the various thiazide diuretics may result in hyperglycemia and abnormal glucose tolerance curves, particularly in elderly hypertensive patients with a tendency toward diabetes. The abnormal glucose tolerance curves of such patients are generally of a temporary nature and are usually reversible with continued administration of the drug.

Phenytoin: Overdoses of phenytoin, an anticonvulsive drug, can result in hyperglycemia, glycosuria, and even coma.

• • •

Many other drugs, including corticosteroids, adrenogenic agents, diazoxide, acetazolamide, and reserpine, have been reported to cause hyperglycemia. The effect of drugs must be kept in mind when evaluating abnormal glucose tolerance curves.

Since the methods of glucose determination and the types of drugs in common clinical use keep changing, it is difficult sometimes to state what effect a particular compound will have on a given method or the physiology of the individual. It is best to check for direct effects of drugs in assays by addition of the compound in question to previously analyzed samples at physiologic concentrations and comparision of results after reassay.

Lactose tolerance test

A significant number of healthy adults are found to have a deficiency of small bowel mucosal lactase. These individuals demonstrate an intolerance to ingested lactose manifested by gastrointestinal discomfort and diarrhea following ingestion of milk. The symptoms are usually relieved by removing lactose (milk) from the diet.

Patients can be evaluated using a lactose tolerance test[48-50]; a standard oral 3 hr glucose tolerance test is performed to provide a baseline for comparison. A lactose tolerance test is then performed the following day, substituting the same amount of lactose as was used in the OGTT. Blood samples are taken at 0, 1, 2, and 3 hr and analyzed for glucose.

If the patient has a normal amount of intestinal lactase, the lactose will be split to glucose and galactose and a similar glucose tolerance curve will be observed both days. If the patient has a lactase deficiency, the lactose tolerance curve will be flat with a rise not exceeding 20 mg/dl over the fasting glucose concentration. It is important to conduct the test in an area with a nearby restroom since some patients experience sudden and severe discomfort.

False positive results[51] occur with this procedure since 25-33% of patients who failed to demonstrate a rise in blood glucose of 20 mg/dl within 1 hr had normal lactase activity in biopsy specimens from the small intestine. The common cause of false positive results appears to be slow gastric emptying, which can be verified by instillation of the disaccharide into the duodenum through a tube.

Glycosylated hemoglobin

A test that may be used not for the diagnosis of diabetes but to observe the course of the disease is the determination of the amount of glycosylated hemoglobin (Hb A_{1c})[52] in the red cells. This particular hemoglobin has a glucose derivative combined with the molecule. It is formed slowly and nonenzymatically in the red cells at a rate that is dependent on the concentration of glucose in the cells. When the glucose concentration in the serum is higher than normal, the concentration within the cells will also be higher than normal, and the glycosylated hemoglobin will be formed at an increased rate. Thus individuals (diabetics) with higher than average glucose concentration will also have a higher than average concentration of Hb A_{1c} in the cells. The value of the glycosylated hemoglobin in the cells is thus a measure of the average glucose concentration over a period of several days or more, in contrast to a determination of serum glucose, which gives the status of the patient only at a given time. The differences in concentration depend somewhat on the method of determination, but in general the concentration in normal individuals is between 6.5-7.5% of the total hemoglobin, and in diabetics it is between 11-15%. The methods of determination and further discussion will be found in Chapter 4.

NONGLUCOSE SUGARS

The determination of nonglucose sugars in serum or whole blood is not always simple, since the sample will always contain some glucose. Thus either a very specific, generally enzymatic method must be used or the glucose must first be removed. The problem does not arise to the same extent for urine since the nonglucose sugars are often not utilized by the body and hence are excreted in the urine, whereas glucose, generally speaking, is not excreted. The glucose is most conveniently removed, when required, by treatment with glucose oxidase.

Nonglucose reducing sugars

A general method[53,54] is given for reducing sugars in which the glucose is removed by glucose oxidase and the remaining reducing sugar (i.e., galactose, lactose, fructose) determined by the reduction of an alkaline copper solution.

Reagents:
1. Potassium phosphate, 0.25 mole/L
   Dissolve 3.4 g of monobasic potassium phosphate in water to make 1 dl.
2. Glucose oxidase
   As required, dilute about 500 units of glucose oxidase (Sigma type V [Sigma Chemical Co., St. Louis] supplied as a solution containing about 1000 units/ml; thus use about 0.5 ml) with 2 ml of the phosphate solution.
3. Alkaline copper tartrate
   Dissolve 24 g of anhydrous sodium carbonate and 12 g of sodium potassium tartrate in about 2 dl of water. While stirring, add 40 ml of a solution containing 4 g of $CuSO_4 \cdot 5H_2O$. When this has dissolved completely, add 16 g of sodium bicarbonate and dissolve. Then add 180 g of anhydrous sodium sulfate in 6 dl of water. Heat nearly to boiling, cool, and dilute to 1 L.
4. Acid molybdate
   Dissolve 50 g of ammonium molybdate in 9 dl of water. Add 42 ml of concentrated sulfuric acid and mix. Add 6 g of sodium arsenate ($Na_2HAsO_4 \cdot 7H_2O$) in 50 ml of water. Mix and place in incubator at 37° C for 48 hr. This solution is stable for long periods if kept from contamination by organic matter.
5. Standards
   These are prepared in the same way as the glucose standards given earlier using the appropriate sugar. (For solutions on a millimoles per liter basis use 0.901 g of a hexose or 0.751 g of a pentose for a 50 mmole/L standard.) The stock standards are diluted 1:10 to give standard containing 100 mg/dl (5.56 mmole/L) and are then further diluted as required as given in the procedure directions.
6. Barium hydroxide and zinc sulfate solutions
   These are also required for preparing a Somogyi filtrate.

Procedure: To 0.9 ml of water in a test tube add 0.1 ml of serum and 0.2 ml of the glucose oxidase solution and mix. Incubate at 37° C for 90 min, shaking briefly at intervals to aerate the solution. Set up similarly a reagent blank tube containing 0.1 ml of water (instead of serum), and set up separately a tube containing 0.1 ml of the standard. These are treated the same way as the serum sample. After incubation add 0.4 ml of the barium hydroxide solution and mix well; then add 0.4 ml of the zinc sulfate solution and mix. Centrifuge tubes at high speed for 10 min. Carefully pipet off 1 ml of the supernatant to separate tubes. To each tube add 2 ml of the alkaline tartrate and mix. Heat in a boiling water bath for 20 min and then cool. Add 2 ml of the arsenomolybdate solution and mix. Dilute to 25 ml (or other convenient volume) and read standard and samples against blank at 535 nm.

Calculation: Since the standard is treated similarly to the sample, calculation can be made as follows:

$$\frac{\text{Absorbance of sample}}{\text{Absorbance of standard}} \times 100 \text{ mg/dl} = \frac{\text{Conc. of}}{\text{sample (mg/dl)}}$$

Galactose determination

Galactose may be determined nonspecifically as given above or more specifically by one of the *o*-toluidine reagents given earlier.

o-Toluidine method

If the *o*-toluidine reagent is used, the second formulation for the reagent is preferred since it gives more color with galactose. After the incubation as in the above method, instead of adding the barium hydroxide and zinc sulfate, laboratory personnel should add 0.8 ml of 0.18 mole/L trichloroacetic acid and mix. After centrifugation, 0.5 ml of the filtrate is added to 4 ml of the *o*-toluidine reagent, and the mixture is heated in a boiling water bath for 15 min. Here also, a blank and standard are treated similarly. The samples and standard are then read against the blank at 630 nm. The calculations are the same as in the previous method since the standard and sample are treated similarly.

Galactose oxidase method

The procedure and principles in the galactose oxidase method[55-57] are very similar to the determination of glucose by glucose oxidase given earlier. The galactose is oxidized by air in the presence of the enzyme to galactohexodialdose and hydrogen peroxide. In the presence of the added enzyme peroxidase, the peroxide oxidizes a chromogen to give a colored product. Although the galactose oxidase available may not be free of traces of other oxidases, in a galactose tolerance test this is compensated for by the use of blank specimen taken before the sugar is administered.

Reagents:
1. Phosphate buffer, 0.02M, pH 7.0
   Dissolve 1.06 g KH_2PO_4 and 1.74 g Na_2HPO_4 in about 950 ml water. Check the pH, adjust if necessary to pH 7.0, and then dilute to 1 L.
2. Galactose oxidase
   About 1 mg dry powdered galactose oxidase (equivalent to 30 units of enzyme [Sigma type V, Sigma Chemical Co., St. Louis]) is triturated in a mortar with 50 ml buffered solution and then filtered through Whatman no. 1 paper. This solution is stable for a few days in the refrigerator.
3. Chromogen solution
   Dissolve 10 mg peroxidase (Sigma type II) in 5 dl buffer; then add 50 mg *o*-dianisidine dissolved

in 5 ml methanol. Store in the refrigerator. It should be discarded if it darkens or gives a high blank. If a large number of tests are to be run, these two reagents could probably be made up in glycerin solution similar to the reagents used in the glucose oxidase method.
4. Sulfuric acid, 30%
   Cautiously add 3 dl concentrated sulfuric acid to 7 dl water.
5. Deproteinizing reagents
   Prepare zinc sulfate and barium hydroxide as for making a Somogyi filtrate.
6. Standards
   a. Stock standard
      Dissolve 1 g pure D(+)galactose in water to make 1 dl.
   b. Working standards
      Dilute 1 and 2 ml of the stock solution to 1 dl with water. These standards contain 10 and 20 mg/dl and are equivalent to 100 and 200 mg/dl when treated similarly to a 1:10 blood filtrate.

Procedure: Prepare a Somogyi filtrate. Set up a series of tubes for standards, samples, and blank. To each tube, add 1 ml chromogen solution, 1 ml galactose oxidase solution, and either 1 ml of water (blank), sample filtrate, or working standard. Mix and incubate all tubes for 30 min at 37° C. After incubation, add 2.5 ml 30% sulfuric acid to each tube, mix, and read samples and standards against blank in a spectrophotometer at 530 nm.

Calculation:

$$\frac{\text{Absorbance of sample}}{\text{Absorbance of standard}} \times \frac{\text{Conc. of}}{\text{standard}} = \frac{\text{Conc. of}}{\text{sample}}$$

Although ascorbic acid may interfere slightly to give higher values, this is not important in a galactose tolerance test when a blood sample is taken before any galactose is ingested. The apparent galactose in this sample may be subtracted from all values for the tolerance.

• • •

Measurements of galactose can also be made using a colorimetric galactose procedure that is available in kit form. Galactostat (Worthington Biochemical Corp., Freehold, N.J.) uses this method and galactose oxidase to aid in specificity.

Small amounts of galactose are found in the serum of lactating women and in the urine or newborn infants during the first few weeks of life. Galactosemia and galactosuria also occur in individuals with either of the two inborn errors of galactose metabolism. Screening for the inborn errors of galactose metabolism can be performed using the growth inhibition test of Guthrie and testing urine for galactose several days after birth with commercially available dipsticks. Galactostix (Ames Co., Elkhart, Ind.) can be used with a 1:20 dilution of urine, which will exclude detection of the physiologic excretion of galactose that occurs in newborns. Diagnosis must be made after measuring decreased activity of galactokinase or uridyl transferase in red cell hemolysates. The galactose tolerance test should not be used to confirm or establish the diagnosis.

Oral galactose tolerance test[58,59]

Procedure: With the patient in the fasting state, take a blood sample in the morning for a blank; then give 40 g galactose dissolved in 250 ml water. Take blood samples $1/2$, $1^1/2$, and 2 hr after ingestion of galactose and determine the concentration of galactose in each specimen. The galactose may be determined by one of the methods given above.

Normal values and interpretation: Values for the maximal concentration of galactose in the blood after oral ingestion have been given as 40-80 mg/dl by different investigators. Maclagan[58,59] uses an index that is the sum of the galactose concentrations for the blood samples. In normal individuals this should not exceed 160 mg/dl. Increased values may be found in liver disease. In infectious and toxic hepatitis, values up to 500 mg/dl may be found, decreasing slowly with improvement in the clinical condition. In cirrhosis the values may be 300 or 400 mg/dl or more.

Intravenous galactose tolerance test

An intravenous tolerance test has also been used in which the blood galactose is estimated 5 min and $1/2$, $1^1/2$, and 2 hr after intravenous administration of galactose 0.5 g/kg body weight given as a sterile 50% solution. In this procedure a normal individual should have a curve beginning at about 200 mg/dl and falling steeply, reaching 10 mg/dl or lower at the end of 2 hr. In most cases of obstructive jaundice a normal curve is obtained, whereas with liver damage the curve falls more slowly. Although this test may avoid errors caused by malabsorption, it has no other advantage over the oral test.

Xylose determination in plasma or urine
o-Toluidine method[60-62]

Pentoses may also be determined with the *o*-toluidine reagent. They give a colored compound having a maximal absorbance at about 480 nm in contrast to the hexoses, which give a color having a maximal absorbance at about 630 nm. In the absence of glucose, xylose can be determined with the same *o*-toluidine reagent as given earlier for glucose, reading at 480 nm. In the determination of urinary xylose in the xylose absorption test the urine will ordinarily be free of glucose and the xylose can be determined directly. One could use 0.1 ml diluted urine and 7 ml *o*-toluidine reagent, proceeding as in the glucose method except reading at 480 nm. If the 5 hr urine collection were diluted to 1 L and 0.1 ml of this compared with 0.1 ml of a 100 mg/dl xylose standard, the standard would correspond to an excretion of 1 g of xylose or 20% of a 5 g dose. A blank determination may be made on a specimen of urine collected before the administration of xylose to check on the absence of glucose.

Calculations: Xylose and glucose can be determined in the presence of each other by reading at wavelengths of 630 and 480 nm. For example, add 0.1 ml of standards containing glucose or xylose to 5 ml of *o*-toluidine reagent in separate tubes, heat in a boiling water

bath for 12 min, cool, and read against a blank at both 480 and 630 nm. Then calculate a k value for each reading by dividing the measured absorbance by the concentration of the standard in milligrams per deciliter. Thus:

k_1 = Absorbance of glucose standard at 630 nm/conc. of glucose standard

k_2 = Absorbance of glucose standard at 480 nm/conc. of glucose standard

k_3 = Absorbance of xylose standard at 630 nm/conc. of xylose standard

k_4 = Absorbance of xylose standard at 480 nm/conc. of xylose standard

If more than one glucose standard (or xylose standard) is run, the k values for this substance are averaged. Then, if A_1 is the absorbance of the sample at 630 nm and A_2 is the absorbance of the sample at 480 nm:

$$\text{Glucose in sample (mg/dl)} = \frac{k_4 A_1 - k_3 A_2}{k_1 k_4 - k_2 k_3}$$

and

$$\text{Xylose in sample (mg/dl)} = \frac{k_1 A_2 - k_2 A_1}{k_1 k_4 - k_2 k_3}$$

In these formulas the absorbances of the sample (A_1 and A_2) must be obtained using the same volume of sample as used for the standards (0.1 ml in the procedure suggested above). If a different volume of sample is used, the absorbance inserted in the formula must be that which would have been found if the correct volume were used.

p-Bromoaniline method[63-65]

Xylose has been quantitatively measured in plasma and urine by heating a sample in acetic acid to form furfurol. This is condensed with *p*-bromoaniline to yield a pink-colored compound. The method is fairly specific for pentoses since conditions are too mild to allow glucose, glucuronic acid, or ascorbic acid to form furfurols.

Reagents:
1. *p*-Bromoaniline reagent
   Prepare a saturated solution of thiourea in glacial acetic acid by shaking about 5 g of the material with 120 ml acid. Allow crystals to settle and decant off solution. Dissolve 2 g *p*-bromoaniline in 1 dl of the above acid. Prepare fresh weekly.
2. Xylose standards
   a. Stock standard
      Dissolve 200 mg pure xylose in 1 dl saturated benzoic acid. This stock standard contains 200 mg/dl xylose.
   b. Working standard
      Dilute 1 ml stock solution with 9 ml water on the day required. This working standard contains 20 mg/dl xylose.

Procedure: Have the patient ingest 5 g xylose dissolved in about 250 ml water. Collect all the urine voided during the next 5 hr. Give additional water to drink during this period, if necessary, since a very low urine volume may lead to unreliable results.

Dilute the total urine excreted to 1 L. Then further dilute a portion 1:10. Add to separate tubes 1 ml diluted urine, 1 ml xylose working standard, and 1 ml water as blank. To each tube, add 5 ml bromoaniline reagent and heat in water bath at 70° C for 10 min. Then allow to stand at room temperature in the dark for 90 min. Read standard and sample against blank at 545 nm.

Calculation:

$$\frac{\text{Absorbance of sample}}{\text{Absorbance of standard}} \times 0.2 \times \frac{1000 \times 10}{1000} = \text{Xylose excreted (g)}$$

Since each milliliter of the standard contains 0.2 mg xylose, the urine is diluted to 1 L and then diluted an additional 10 times. The denominator 1000 converts milligrams to grams.

The formula then reduces to:

$$\frac{\text{Absorbance of sample}}{\text{Absorbance of standard}} \times 2 = \text{Xylose excreted (g)}$$

Xylose absorption test

The absorption of D-xylose has been used for the diagnosis of malabsorption states. The pentose, which is not normally present in the blood (except after eating certain fruits [plums]) or urine, is absorbed by diffusion. After a standard dose is given, a low concentration in the blood or urine is considered indicative of a defect in the intestinal absorption process.

Urinary excretion: Some workers have given a 25 g dose of D-xylose, but this amount occasionally causes nausea or diarrhea, and other workers have suggested a 5 g dose, which is sufficient for good results. After giving a 5 g dose to a fasting patient, the amount excreted in the urine during the next 5 hr is measured by collecting the urine and determining the xylose content. Only a small amount is metabolized by the pentose phosphate pathway with most being excreted in the urine.

Within 5 hr the normal individual will excrete 18-24% (0.9-1.2 g) or more of the dose. Children excrete 10-25% depending on age.[12] Liver disease does not affect the test, but impaired renal function results in low excretion and is a source of false positive test results.

After a 25 g dose, normal individuals excrete about 16% (4 g) of the dose; the normal ranges are not identical for different doses. The usefulness of the test has been questioned since abnormal results can be obtained with conditions other than small bowel dysfunction (e.g., bacterial overgrowth) and normal results can be obtained from individuals with celiac disease.

Plasma concentration: After the administration of the standard dose of D-xylose, the plasma concentration can be measured, thus eliminating the difficulties of collecting urine over a 5 hr period. A recent study[66] measured plasma D-xylose concentrations 1 hr after a 5 g dose. The D-xylose was <20 mg/dl in 52 of 53 children with normal bowel biopsy specimens. In addition, 22 children with cystic fibrosis had normal concentrations. The 5 hr urine excretion test had been stated to be abnormal for such groups.[12]

• • •

Interpretation: If both blood xylose concentrations and urinary excretion are considered together, most of the false positive and false negative results can be eliminated.[67] Few patients with small bowel disease demonstrate normal findings for both of these results. At the same time, few individuals without gastrointestinal disorders demonstrate abnormal findings in both cases.

A more complete table of the variation of urinary xylose recovered in children of various ages is given by Meites.[13]

Fructose determination

Fructose is not found in the blood except after ingesting certain fruits or honey. After oral administration of fructose to normal individuals a concentration of 15-30 mg/dl is found. Fructose intolerance occurs in liver disease and in two inborn errors of metabolism, essential fructosuria and hereditary fructose intolerance, as well as in normal newborns presumably because of immaturity of aldolase.

Essential fructosuria is characterized by a lack of fructokinase. Individuals with this condition show a fructosemia and fructosuria without other clinical signs. The condition is apparently harmless.

Hereditary fructose intolerance demonstrates the additional symptoms of a fall in glucose and phosphorus concentration after fructose loading. This condition usually is demonstrated in infancy when sucrose or fructose is added to the diet.

Fructose in serum can be determined by the method for reducing sugars given earlier in this chapter. Fructose in serum cannot be determined by the Selivanoff procedure used for urine since glucose interferes with this procedure. Another method for the determination of fructose involves condensing fructose with indole-3-acetic acid in hydrochloric acid after removal with glucose oxidase.[68]

Fructose tolerance test

In the fructose tolerance test the procedure for the glucose tolerance test is followed, but the patient receives 50 g fructose (levulose) instead of glucose. Blood samples are taken as in the glucose tolerance test, but urine samples are not taken. The total amount of blood reducing sugars is then determined by the method for nonglucose reducing sugars given earlier. This includes both glucose and fructose, but after fructose ingestion there is usually very little increase in the blood glucose, so that the increase, if any, is caused by fructose. In normal individuals the apparent rise in blood sugar is not more than 26-30 mg/dl above the fasting level. In liver disease the rise is greater; the maximal levels may be 60-80 mg/dl above the fasting level, but the differences are never striking.

In either inborn error of fructose metabolism the plasma concentration can rise to >100 mg/dl in response to an oral fructose load.

Intravenous fructose tolerance

An intravenous fructose tolerance test has been used for the diagnosis of hereditary fructose intolerance.[69] Samples are taken every 15 min for 2 hr for glucose, phosphate, and fructose. A prolonged fall occurs in phosphate, then glucose, with a sharp rise in fructose >25 mg/dl in the first 15 min.

In normal subjects or those with essential fructosuria, glucose and phosphorus concentrations do not change.

BLOOD UREA NITROGEN

In the determination of blood urea nitrogen (BUN) urea may be determined colorimetrically by its reaction with diacetyl monoxime in the presence of thiosemicarbazide or by the use of urease. The former method is fairly specific for urea; the latter one is very specific for urea except that any preformed ammonia will be included. Although these methods are both based on the reactions of urea, they are conventionally reported as urea nitrogen (urea $\times$ 0.4665 = urea nitrogen; urea nitrogen $\times$ 2.14 = urea) for historical reasons since this was the largest single contributor to the nonprotein nitrogen discussed later. Although the determinations are most often made on serum, the results are still conventionally reported as BUN. Since the concentrations of urea in whole blood and serum or plasma are quite similar, no clinical significance can be applied to differences between blood and serum determinations.

Oxime method[70,71]

Principle: In the oxime method, diacetyl monoxime in the presence of acid hydrolyzes to produce the unstable compound diacetyl. The diacetyl reacts with urea to produce a yellow diazine derivative. The color of this product is intensified by addition of thiosemicarbazide.

Reagents:
1. Oxime solution
   Dissolve 1 g diacetyl monoxime (also called 2,3-butanedione monoxime), 0.2 g thiosemicarbazide, and 9 g sodium chloride in water and dilute to 1 L.
2. Acid solution
   Cautiously add 60 ml concentrated sulfuric acid and 10 ml 85% phosphoric acid to about 8 dl water. Add 0.1 g ferric chloride and dilute to 1 L.
3. Standards
   a. Benzoic acid, 0.016M
      Dissolve 2 g benzoic acid in 1 L water. Add 0.8 ml concentrated sulfuric acid and mix. Use this solution for preparing and diluting the standard solutions.
   b. Stock standard
      Dissolve 0.644 g urea (SRM 912, National Bureau of Standards) in some of the benzoic acid solution and dilute to 5 dl. This standard contains 129 mg urea/dl or 60 mg urea nitrogen/dl. This standard and a 1:2 dilution to give a 30 mg/dl standard are used for the direct method. (Alternatively, dissolve 0.601 g of urea as above to obtain a standard solution containing 20 mmole urea/L or 9.3 mmole urea nitrogen/L. Some of this standard is also diluted 1:2 to give a standard containing 10 mmole urea/L or 4.7 mmole urea nitrogen/L.)
   c. Diluted standards
      For use with a 1:10 protein-free filtrate the

above standards are also diluted 1:10. When the same aliquots of the diluted standards and protein-free filtrate are used, the calculations are the same as the direct method.

Procedure: The direct determination on serum is more convenient, but a protein-free filtrate can also be used. Place 3 ml of each of the two reagents in test tubes. For the direct procedure, add with a micropipet 0.05 ml of samples and standards (30 and 60 mg urea nitrogen/dl or 10 and 20 mmole urea/L) and reserve one tube of mixed reagent as blank. For use with a filtrate, pipet 0.5 ml of the filtrate or 0.5 ml of the diluted standards to separate tubes containing 3 ml of each of the two reagents. Add 0.5 ml water to one tube as a blank. Heat tubes in boiling water bath for 15 min, cool, and read standards and samples against blank at 520 nm.

Calculation: Since the standards and samples are treated similarly:

$$\frac{\text{Absorbance of sample}}{\text{Absorbance of standard}} \times \frac{\text{Conc. of}}{\text{standard}} = \frac{\text{Conc. of}}{\text{sample}}$$

Ordinarily the two standards given above will be used. Since the reaction may not follow Beer's law at higher concentrations, it is best to always run the two standards as indicated and use the standard having an absorbance nearest that of a given sample for the calculation.

Urease method[72,73]

Principle: Urea is hydrolyzed to ammonium ion and carbonate by urease. The ammonium ion in the presence of base reacts with phenol and sodium hypochlorite to form a blue indophenol. Sodium nitroprusside is added as a catalyst. The intensity of the blue color is proportional to the amount of urea in the sample. Since the final color reaction is very sensitive, ammonia-free water must be used for all reagents and dilutions. It is best to purify the distilled water by passage through a column of ion-exchange resins such as Amberlite MB-3 (Rohm and Haas Co., Philadelphia).

Reagents:
1. Alkaline hypochlorite
   Dissolve 12.5 g sodium hydroxide in about 4 dl water. Cool, add 20 ml sodium hypochlorite solution (any commercial bleach solution containing 5.25% available chlorine), and dilute to 5 dl. Store in a polyethylene bottle in the refrigerator.
2. Phenol reagent
   Dissolve 25 g phenol and 0.13 g sodium nitroprusside in water to make 5 dl. Store in a brown bottle in the refrigerator. This remains stable for several months.
3. Buffer
   Dissolve 5 g disodium salt of EDTA in 2 dl glycerin and 250 ml water. Adjust to pH 6.5 with 4% sodium hydroxide (about 10 ml required) and dilute to 5 dl.
4. Buffered urease
   Dissolve 30 mg urease type III (Sigma Chemical Co., St. Louis) in 1 dl buffer. This remains stable for several weeks when stored in the refrigerator.
5. Standard

Use the stock standard (not diluted) of the oxime method.

Procedure: To 0.5 ml buffered urease, add 0.02 ml serum or standard with a "to contain" micropipet, rinsing well. Incubate all tubes for 15 min at 37° C. Also incubate a blank of 0.5 ml buffered urease alone. After incubation, add to each tube 1 ml phenol reagent and mix well; then add 1 ml alkaline hypochlorite and mix again. Incubate for 15 min at 37° C. Then add 10 ml water and read samples and standard against blank at 620 nm. Conveniently, the 30 mg/dl standard should give a reading of around 0.300 absorbance units. If the color is too intense, dilute the solutions further or use a shorter wavelength, e.g., 580 nm.

Calculation: Since standard and sample are treated similarly:

$$\frac{\text{Absorbance of sample}}{\text{Absorbance of standard}} \times \frac{\text{Conc. of}}{\text{standard}} = \frac{\text{Conc. of}}{\text{sample}}$$

where the same standards are used as in the oxime method.

Modifications of oxime and urease methods for urine

The oxime method can be applied directly to urine. Usually the urine is diluted 1:5 or 1:10 and used in the same way as serum sample. The calculations are the same with a correction for the extra dilution of the urine. If the urine is suspected of having a high or low value it may be advisable to run several different dilutions of the urine at the same time and use for calculations the sample absorbance within the range of the standards.

Since urine contains some preformed ammonia, a slight modification of the **urease method** is required. This method uses an ammonia blank; therefore the urine is diluted 1:5 or 1:10. Determine the preformed ammonia by adding 0.02 ml diluted urine to 0.5 ml water; then add the color reagents and incubate for 15 min along with a water blank. The sample is then read against the water blank. Another aliquot of the dilute urine is treated with urease, as in the procedure for serum, along with a urease blank and standard.

Calculation: For preformed ammonia:

$$\frac{\text{Absorbance of sample}}{\text{Absorbance of standard}} \times D \times 30 = \text{mg/dl ammonia nitrogen}$$

Similarly for the total nitrogen, when the 30 mg/dl standard is used and D is the dilution factor for the urine (D = 5 for a 1:5 dilution, etc.):

$$\frac{\text{Total ammonia}}{\text{nitrogen}} - \frac{\text{Ammonia}}{\text{nitrogen blank}} = \text{Urea nitrogen}$$

Normal values and interpretation

The normal range of BUN is from 10-18 mg urea nitrogen (or 7.14-12.9 mmole urea nitrogen/L).

The most common cause of increased urea concentration in serum is inadequate excretion, usually caused by kidney disease or urinary obstruction. Increased urea nitrogen levels in acute nephritis may vary from 25-160 mg urea nitrogen/dl (or 17.9-114 mmole urea nitrogen/

L). Urea retention also occurs with extensive parenchymatous destruction of kidney tissue, advanced nephrosclerosis, renal tuberculosis, renal cortical necrosis, malignancy, suppuration, and chronic gout. Occasionally very low levels may be found. These are usually indicative of inadequate protein intake.

NONPROTEIN NITROGEN

The nonprotein nitrogen (NPN)[74,75] in the blood was determined as an index of kidney function until the early 1960s. With the introduction of simple methods for BUN determination such as those just presented, the determination of NPN is no longer used in this way. Measurement of BUN and creatinine will usually give more information concerning kidney function than will the NPN. A micromethod is given here since it is also useful in determining the nitrogen (or protein) content of other materials. The sample is digested with sulfuric acid to transform all the nitrogen present into ammonia, which is then determined by the phenol-hypochlorite reaction used for urea. Ordinarily the breakdown of nitrogenous compounds to ammonia requires the use of a catalyst, e.g., copper or mercury. These, however, interfere with the color reaction. By using sufficiently small samples (which is possible because of the great sensitivity of the color reaction), complete conversion can be attained without the use of a catalyst.

Reagents:
1. Phenol and hypochlorite reagents as used in the urease method for BUN.
2. Sulfuric acid and sodium tungstate solutions as used for the preparation of a Folin-Wu protein-free filtrate.
3. Sulfuric acid, 5 moles/L
   Cautiously add 30 ml of concentrated sulfuric acid to about 50 ml of water. Cool and dilute to 1 dl.
4. Stock standard
   Dissolve 0.472 g of reagent grade ammonium sulfate (previously dried at 100° C) in water, add a few drops of concentrated sulfuric acid, and dilute to 1 L. This standard contains 10 mg/dl of ammonia nitrogen. As required, dilute the stock 1:5 to give a working standard containing 2 mg/dl.

Procedure: Prepare a 1:20 Folin-Wu filtrate by adding 0.1 ml of blood, serum, or other fluid to 1.7 ml of water. Add 0.1 ml of the sulfuric acid solution (5 moles/L) and mix; then add 0.1 ml of the sodium tungstate solution (0.3 mole/L), mix, and centrifuge.

Place 0.6 ml water (blank), 0.1 ml sample filtrate plus 0.5 ml water (sample), and 0.1 ml diluted standard solution for standard in three small Pyrex test tubes. Use "to contain" pipets for standard and sample, rinsing well with water. To each tube add 0.1 ml 5 moles/L sulfuric acid and one small glass bead.

Digest carefully over a microburner until the water is driven off and dense white fumes fill the tube. Do not allow the ring of sulfuric acid condensate to rise above half the length of the tube. The digest should be water-clear; if not, digest further.

Cool, add 1 ml phenol reagent to each tube, and mix. Then add 1 ml 1M sodium hydroxide and mix.

Immediately add 1 ml alkaline hypochlorite solution and mix again. Incubate for 15 min at 37° C.

Add 2 ml water to each tube, mix, and read in a spectrophotometer at 600 nm. Read standard and samples against blank. As with the urease method, further dilution or reading at a shorter wavelength may be required to bring the readings of the standard into the desired range (about 0.300 absorbance units).

Calculation: Since 0.1 ml of standard containing 2 mg/dl is treated the same as 0.1 ml of a 1:20 dilution of the blood, the standard is equivalent to $2 \times 20 = 40$ mg/dl; thus

$$\frac{\text{Absorbance of sample}}{\text{Absorbance of standard}} \times 40 = \text{mg/dl nitrogen}$$

Normal values and interpretation[76,77]: The normal range of NPN is from 25-45 mg/dl. A little more than one half of the NPN is derived from urea, uric acid, creatinine, ammonia, and amino acids at normal levels. The remainder is made up of the nitrogen of glutathione, purine, pyrimidine compounds, and unknown constituents. Decreased kidney function is the chief cause of increased NPN. In assessing the course of uremia, most workers have considered it more valuable to determine BUN and creatinine than NPN. Sometimes in the early stages of nephritis the variations in BUN are more readily apparent than changes in the NPN value, since the other constituents change less than urea. In eclampsia, hepatic failure, or some other liver disease, there may be a disproportionate rise in NPN as compared to BUN; but even in such instances the NPN is no longer used because there are more sensitive indicators of liver function. In the assessment of kidney function the urea level is as satisfactory as the NPN and is technically somewhat simpler.

The concentration of NPN (and, similarly, urea) in the blood is chiefly determined by the balance between urinary output of nitrogen and protein catabolism, since the kidneys are the main channel for nitrogen excretion. If, for example, in dehydration the amount of fluid available in the body for urine formation is small, the kidneys may not be able to excrete all the nitrogen metabolites and the NPN will rise. If the concentrating powers of the kidneys become impaired, more than the usual volume of urine will be required to sweep out a given amount of nitrogenous metabolites. Diuresis will tend to increase the excretion of nitrogen and lower the NPN, but only to a limit of about 3 L/day. Further diuresis does not greatly increase nitrogen excretion beyond this. The principal use of urine NPN is in the study of nitrogen balance.

URIC ACID

Many methods for the determination of uric acid are based on the reduction of phosphotungstate by the uric acid with the production of a blue color. Other reducing substances present in the sample may interfere with these methods. Some of these interferences can be eliminated by the use of a protein-free filtrate, but this introduces additional steps in the procedure, which may cause losses of the uric acid. The effects of other reducing substances, e.g., ascorbic acid, may be minimized by allowing the mixture to stand for a short time at a high pH. Two methods for the determination of uric acid are presented. In the first relatively simple method, phosphotungstic acid also serves as a precipitating reagent for the formation of a protein-free filtrate, high alkalinity is obtained by the use of trisodium phosphate and phosphotungstate is reduced by the uric acid. In the second method, uric acid reduces cupric salts at room temperature, and the cuprous ions formed are determined with the sensitive reagent neocuproine. Most interferences are eliminated by measurement using two samples to one of which has been added the enzyme uricase to destroy the uric acid. The difference in color developed between the two samples thus represents the true uric acid content.

Phosphotungstate method[78]

Reagents:
1. Phosphotungstic acid
   Dissolve 50 g of sodium tungstate in 350 ml of water and add 20 ml of 85% phosphoric acid. Reflux the mixture for about 2 hr and then add a drop of bromine. Boil a few minutes in a fume hood to eliminate excess bromine; then cool and dilute to 1 L. This reagent is somewhat troublesome to prepare and preferably should be purchased already prepared.
2. Trisodium phosphate, 0.026 mole/L
   Dissolve 1 g of trisodium phosphate ($Na_3 PO_4 \cdot 12H_2O$) in water to make 1 dl.
3. Alkalizing reagent
   Dissolve 100 g of anhydrous sodium carbonate, 200 g of urea, and 50 g of triethanolamine in water to make 1 L.
4. Uric acid standard
   a. Stock standard, 50 mg/dl
      Dissolve 1.0 g of lithium carbonate in about 5 dl of water in a 1 L volumetric flask. Add 500 mg of pure uric acid (SRM 913, National Bureau of Standards) and swirl until dissolved. Add 5 ml of 40% formaldehyde and 4 dl more of water. Mix and adjust the pH to 5.5 (paper) with the addition, by drops, of diluted acetic acid (1 volume of glacial acetic acid and 3 volumes of water).
   b. Working standard
      Dilute the stock standard 1:10 to give a standard containing 5 mg/dl (0.3 mmole/L). Other concentrations may be prepared if desired to run a calibration curve.

Procedure: To separate tubes (15 ml centrifuge tubes are preferred) add 0.5 ml of serum sample, standard, or water (blank). To each tube add 0.5 ml of the trisodium phosphate solution and mix. Allow to stand for 5 min, then add 1.5 ml of phosphotungstic acid solution, and mix. Allow to stand for a few minutes and then centrifuge (usually the standard and blank need not be centrifuged). Transfer 1 ml aliquots of the supernatants to appropriately labeled tubes, add 3.0 ml of the alkalizing reagent, and mix. After 20 min read samples and standard against blank at 680-700 nm.

Calculation:

$$\frac{\text{Absorbance of sample}}{\text{Absorbance of standard}} \times \frac{\text{Conc. of}}{\text{standard}} = \frac{\text{Conc. of}}{\text{sample}}$$

Modified procedure for urine: If the urine is cloudy or contains a precipitate, warm a well-mixed sample to 60° C for 10 min after adjusting the pH to 10 to dissolve any precipitated urates.[79] Then dilute a portion of the urine 1:10 and proceed as for serum. Since the urine has been diluted 1:10 an additional factor of 10 must be included in the calculations.

Uricase-neocuproine method[80,81]

Reagents:

1. Stock borate buffer, 0.5 mole/L, pH about 9.5
   Dissolve 31 g boric acid, 10 g sodium hydroxide, and 1 g lithium carbonate in water and dilute to 1 L.
2. Working borate buffer
   Dilute the stock solution 1:10 with water as needed.
3. Stock color reagent
   Dissolve 0.3 g copper sulfate ($CuSO_4 \cdot 5H_2O$) and 0.6 g neocuproine (2,9-dimethyl-1,10-phenanthroline) in water in a 1 dl volumetric flask. Add 1 drop of 1 mole/L HCl, then dilute to 1 dl with water, and mix well.
4. Working color reagent
   Dilute the stock reagent 1:10 with water. This should be prepared fresh each day.
5. Enzyme reagent
     Catalase solution in glycerol (Boehringer Mannheim Biochemicals, Indianapolis)
     Uricase solution, 2 mg/ml (Boehringer Mannheim Biochemicals, Indianapolis)
   As needed, mix together 4 volumes of the uricase solution, 1 volume of the catalase solution, and 3 volumes of water. Prepare only the amount needed for the day's work and store mixture in the refrigerator when not used.
6. Standards. The standards are the same as in the previous method.

Procedure: For each sample add 3.0 ml of borate working buffer to each of two tubes; then add 100 μl of sample to each tube. To one of the pair add 20 μl of the enzyme solution and mix. Set up similar pairs using 100 μl of working standard and 100 μl of water (blank). Allow all tubes to stand at room temperature for 10 min. Then add 1 ml of the color reagent to each tube and mix. Allow tubes to stand for 5 min. Read all tubes without enzyme against blank without enzyme and all tubes containing enzyme against the blank with enzyme at 454 nm. Subtract the absorbance of tube containing sample plus enzyme from the absorbance of tube containing sample without enzyme. Do the same for the standard. (The absorbance of the standard tube with enzyme should be essentially zero; if this is true this tube may be omitted in future work.)

Calculation:

$$\frac{A_{(-e)} - A_{(+e)} \text{ of sample}}{A_{(-e)} - A_{(+e)} \text{ of standard}} \times \frac{\text{Conc. of}}{\text{standard}} = \frac{\text{Conc. of}}{\text{sample}}$$

where $A_{(-e)}$ of sample = absorbance of sample without enzyme, $A_{(+e)}$ of sample = absorbance of sample with enzyme, $A_{(-e)}$ of standard = absorbance of standard without enzyme, and $A_{(+e)}$ of standard = absorbance of standard with enzyme.

Urine may be treated similarly except that a preliminary dilution of 1:5 or 1:10 is made and this is taken into account in the calculations. If the urine is cloudy, adjust the pH to 10 and then warm to 60° C to dissolve any precipitated urates before sampling.

Normal values and interpretation for serum

Using the phosphotungstate methods the normal range of uric acid in plasma or serum is from 3.5-8.0 mg/dl (0.21-0.48 mmole/L) for males and from 2.5-7.0 mg/dl (0.15-0.42 mmole/L) for females. Slightly lower results may be obtained using a uricase method. Some of the older values are given for whole blood. Since most of the uric acid is in the plasma, the values for whole blood would vary with the proportion of cells in the blood. Since the cells also contain much more of the interfering substances, it is more satisfactory to determine uric acid in plasma or serum.

Increased levels of uric acid are associated with nitrogen retention and the increase in urea, creatinine, and the other nonprotein nitrogenous constituents of the blood. A uric acid increase must often be interpreted as another indication of decreased kidney function. Uric acid is formed from the breakdown of the cell nucleic acids and is often increased in the blood in conditions in which excessive cell breakdown and catabolism of nucleic acids occur. Increases in the blood level have been reported in the acute stages of infectious diseases, excessive exposure to x-rays, multiple myeloma, and leukemia. Increased levels of uric acid have been found in gout, but the increase may be slight in the early stages of the disease and the amount of the increase is not directly related to the severity of the disease.

Normal values and interpretation for urine

The amount of uric acid excreted in the urine depends in part on the diet. With a diet that is low in purines the amount excreted is usually in the range of 0.3-0.5 g/day (2-3 mmole/day). With an ordinary diet the normal amount excreted may vary more, from 0.4-0.8 g/day (2.5-5.0 mmole/day). Increased excretion is sometimes found in conditions such as leukemia, which also leads to increased blood levels. The excretion of uric acid is usually increased during an attack of gout.

Interference by drugs

When uric acid is determined by a phosphotungstate reduction method, the presence of other reducing agents may give erroneously high results. The usual methods are not greatly affected by normal amounts of ascorbic acid, but excessive amounts may lead to high results. The drugs levodopa and methyldopa are reported to lead to high results because of excessive reduction. Since the uricase method is not affected by these drugs, its use is recommended for these cases. Thiazide diuretics, ethacrynic acid, furosemide, and chlorthalidone all result in increased levels of uric acid when given in the usual doses. Since these drugs act by decreasing uric acid excretion, there will be a lower level in the urine. Mercurial diuretics have little effect. Other drugs that have been reported to increase uric acid levels in serum are quinethazone, acetazolamide, diazoxide, 6-mercaptopurine, and nitrogen mustard.

There are some reports that phenothizines and epinephrine also increase serum uric acid levels. Salicylates in the usual dose are reported to increase the serum level, particularly when given along with phenylbutazone or probenecid. On the other hand, large continued doses of salicylates have been reported to increase uric acid excretion and thus decrease the serum level. A number of drugs have been reported to decrease serum uric acid levels (with an increased urinary excretion of uric acid), but the effect does not appear to be common. Among the drugs mentioned were azathioprine, phenylbutazone, chlorprothixene, acetohexamide, and clofibrate.

CREATININE AND CREATINE

Of the two related compounds creatinine and creatine,[82,83] creatine is the more important biochemically since creatine phosphate plays an important role in muscular contraction. Some of the creatine is converted into the cyclic anhydride creatinine, and the latter substance is excreted by the kidneys as a waste product. The concentration of creatinine in the blood, like that of urea, will increase with decreased kidney function, and the main use of the determination of serum creatinine is in the assessment of kidney function (see the later discussion of renal clearance.

Creatinine method using picric acid

Creatinine is usually determined by the reaction with alkaline picrate to produce a red color (Jaffé reaction). The reaction is not specific, and various methods have been used to increase the specificity. For most clinical purposes, creatinine may be determined directly on a Folin-Wu filtrate or in diluted urine. However, for measurement of creatinine clearance where a slight overestimate of the creatinine concentration in the blood would be of more significance, the creatinine determination in plasma or serum should include the additional purification step of absorption on Lloyd's reagent, which removes some chromogenic impurities. This method is given as an alternative.

Many other technics, depending on the equipment that is available, can be used to increase specificity. One method that has been proposed is to measure the rate of color development of the Jaffé reaction.[84] These kinetic technics are based on the fact that certain pseudocreatinine materials react either much slower (e.g., glucose) or much faster (e.g., protein) than creatinine. By making two absorbance measurements after adding serum or urine to the color reagent, the difference in absorbance can be directly related to the creatinine present. This approach avoids the difficulties of protein-free filtrates and Lloyd's reagent treatment, but the precise timing is difficult to control if done manually.

Since mg creatinine/dl $\times$ 88.4 = μmole creatinine/L, this standard is 13,260 μmole/L (or 13.26 mmole/L). Alternatively, a more convenient stock standard in terms of millimoles per liter is made by using 170 mg creatinine in the same volume as above to give a solution containing 15 mmole/L.

Reagents:

1. Sulfuric acid, 0.33 mole/L, and sodium tungstate,

0.30 mole/L, for the preparation of a Folin-Wu filtrate.

2. Picric acid, 0.04 mole/L

Dissolve 10.5 g of the acid in water to make 1 L.

3. Sodium hydroxide, 0.75 mole/L

Dissolve 30 g of NaOH in water to make 1 L. Store in a tightly closed polyethylene bottle.

4. Creatinine standards

a. Stock standard

Dissolve 150 mg of pure creatinine (SRM 914, National Bureau of Standards) and 0.8 ml of concentrated hydrochloric acid in water to make 1 dl. This solution contains 150 mg/dl (or 1.5 mg/ml) and is stable when kept refrigerated. (Alternately, use 170 mg creatinine in the same volume to give a solution containing 15 mmole/L.)

b. Working standard

Dilute 1 ml of the stock to 1 dl with water. This solution contains 1.5 mg/dl (or 132.6 μmole/L). This solution is not stable and should be prepared as needed.

Procedure for serum creatinine: To 2 ml of serum in a test tube add 3 ml of water and 1 ml of the 0.3 mole/L sodium tungstate solution and mix. Then add 2 ml of the 0.33 mole/L sulfuric acid, stopper, and mix well by inversion. Centrifuge at 2000 rpm for 5 min. Add 3 ml of the supernatant to a test tube. To a second tube add 3 ml of water as blank. Also set up tubes containing 1, 2, and 3 ml of the working standard plus enough water to make 3 ml. To each tube add 1 ml of the picric acid and 1 ml of the sodium hydroxide solution. Mix and allow to stand for 20 min. Read samples and standards against blank at 520 nm.

Calculation:

$$\frac{\text{Absorbance of sample}}{\text{Absorbance of standard}} \times \frac{4}{3} \times S \times V = \frac{\text{Creatinine}}{\text{(mg/dl or }\mu\text{mole/L)}}$$

where the factor 4/3 arises from the fact that 3 ml of a 1:4 dilution of the serum is used, S is the actual concentration of the diluted standard (1.5 mg/dl or 132.6 μmole/L), and V is the actual volume of the standard used (1, 2, or 3 ml). Since Beer's law is not followed closely for this procedure, it is advisable to run all three standards with each group of unknowns and for a given calculation to use the standard giving the reading closest to that of the sample. For normal serum the lowest standard is usually sufficient. If the serum absorbance is much above the absorbance of the highest standard, it is best to repeat the determination using a dilution of the filtrate and making the appropriate correction in the calculations.

Procedure for urine: The urine is diluted 1:100, and 3 ml diluted urine is carried through the same procedure as for the serum supernatant. Since the urine is diluted 1:100 instead of 1:4, the equations given must be multiplied by an additional factor of 25. Because of the greater variation in urine creatinine, it is usually advisable to run all three standards, and one may require another dilution of urine as well. The pH of the urine should be checked; if it is strongly acid or alkaline, add a few drops of acid or base during the dilution so that the diluted sample is approximately neutral.

Creatinine method using Lloyd's reagent

Additional reagents:
1. Lloyd's reagent (a purified fuller's earth)
2. Oxalic acid, saturated solution
   Add about 18 g oxalic acid to 1 dl water and shake until saturated.

Serum creatinine procedure: Prepare a tungstic acid filtrate (as previously described). Set up tubes containing 5 ml water as a blank, 3 ml supernatant plus 2 ml water for sample, and 1, 2, or 3 ml working standard made up to 5 ml with water as a standard. To each tube, add 0.5 ml saturated oxalic acid and approximately 100 mg Lloyd's reagent. Stopper and shake at intervals for 15 min. Centrifuge the tubes strongly, decant off the supernatant, and drain. To each tube, add 3 ml water, 1 ml picric acid solution, and 1 ml 0.75N sodium hydroxide solution. Stopper and shake intermittently for 15 min. Centrifuge strongly, pour off the supernatant into cuvets, and read in a spectrophotometer at 520 nm, reading samples and standards against the blank.

Calculation: The calculation is exactly the same as for the previous method. Because of the greater dilution required for urine, it is rarely necessary to use Lloyd's reagent in the determination.

Direct method for creatinine[85]

In the direct method for creatinine the serum reacts directly with an alkaline picrate solution at two different pH levels. At a pH of 10.0 the protein and other interfering material will react with the picrate but the creatinine does not. At a pH of 11.5 both the creatinine and the protein react. The difference between the absorbance developed at the two pH levels represents that caused by creatinine alone.

Reagents:
1. Picric acid, about 0.05 mole/L
   Add about 15 g of picric acid to 1 L of water. Allow to stand for several hours with shaking at intervals or use a magnetic stirrer; then filter off the excess picric acid.
2. Sodium hydroxide, 1 mole/L
   Dissolve 40 g of NaOH in water to make 1 L.
3. Monosodium phosphate, 1 mole/L
   Dissolve 133 g of $NaH_2PO_4 \cdot H_2O$ in water to make 1 L.
4. Buffer A, pH 10.0
   To a 5 dl volumetric flask add 245 ml of the sodium phosphate solution and dilute to 5 dl with the NaOH solution.
5. Buffer B, pH 11.5
   To a 5 dl volumetric flask add 192 ml of the sodium phosphate solution and dilute to 5 dl with the NaOH solution.
6. Picric acid reagents A and B
   Just before use, mix together 1 volume of the picric acid solution with 4 volumes of the corresponding buffer (A or B).
7. Creatinine standards
   The same stock standard is used as given in the

previous method. Different working standards are used. Dilute 1 and 2 ml of the stock to 50 ml with water, giving standards containing 3 and 6 mg/dl (265 and 530 μmole/L).

Procedure and calculation: To each of a pair of tubes, one containing 3 ml of picric acid solution A and the other containing 3 ml of picric acid solution B, add 0.2 ml of sample. Mix and incubate at 37° C for 45 min. Treat the standards similarly. After incubation read tube B against tube A at 500 nm. The calculations follow the usual form:

$$\frac{\text{Absorbance of sample}}{\text{Absorbance of standard}} \times \frac{\text{Conc. of}}{\text{standard}} = \frac{\text{Conc. of}}{\text{sample}}$$

Normal values and interpretation

The normal values of creatinine in serum are from 0.6-1.2 mg/dl (53-106 μmole/L). In chronic nephritis, when the BUN concentration is above 50 mg/dl, the creatinine rise is roughly proportional and creatinine concentrations over 5 mg/dl (442 μmole/L) are considered of grave diagnostic importance. In obstruction of the urinary tract and in chronic nephritis, the creatinine concentration may be relatively higher than that of urea and high values of 10-15 mg/dl (884-1326 μmole/L) are not so unfavorable. Low levels are found in muscular dystrophy. Bromsulphalein (BSP) and phenolsulfonphthalein (PSP) dyes, if present from previous tests, will interfere with the color reaction. High concentrations of ascorbic acid will also produce interference and give high results as will the presence of ketones.

Determination of creatine in urine

Creatine has been determined in serum or urine. Significant variations in serum creatine have not been found in kidney diseases, so it has little clinical value in these conditions. Elevated concentrations of serum creatine occur in diseases associated with extensive muscle destruction; however, because of analytic difficulties the assay of creatine kinase has replaced measurements of creatine in serum and it is no longer performed.

The analysis of creatine in urine is occasionally used in certain degenerative disorders to measure the rate of muscle catabolism.

Principle: The common method formerly used was to heat the urine with acid to change any creatine present to creatinine. The total creatinine was then determined with the Jaffé reaction. The difference between the creatinine determined with and without the heating was considered to be caused by the creatine originally present. Since the greater part of the potentially chromogenic material present was creatinine, the creatine is determined as the smaller difference between two larger quantities and consequently the accuracy of the procedure is low.

Reagents:
1. Stock sulfuric acid, 0.6N
   Add 17 ml of concentrated sulfuric acid to approximately 9 dl deionized water in a 1 L volumetric flask, mix, and dilute to volume with water.
2. Sulfuric acid reagent, 0.006N

Dilute 1.0 ml of stock sulfuric acid to 1 dl with deionized water.

3. Stock sodium hydroxide, 0.1N
   Dissolve 4 g sodium hydroxide in approximately 9 dl deionized water in a 1 L volumetric flask and dilute to volume with water.

4. Sodium hydroxide reagent, 0.006N
   Dilute 6.0 ml of stock sodium hydroxide to 1 dl with deionized water.

Procedure[86]: Add 1 ml urine to 4 ml of 0.006N sulfuric acid and heat for 90 min at 100° C. Cool and add about 4 ml of sodium hydroxide until pH ~ 7.0. Dilute the solution to a final volume of 20 ml.

Dilute 1 ml urine to 20 ml with water and analyze both solutions for creatinine.

Calculation:

[Creatinine (heated) - Creatinine (unheated)] ×
$20 \times V$ = Creatine (mg) ÷ Time

where 20 is the dilution factor and V is the volume of urine in deciliters for a timed period. The daily ouptut is 0-40 mg for women and 0-80 mg for men.

PLASMA AMMONIA

The production of urea from ammonia occurs in the liver, and the plasma ammonia concentration[87,88] will increase in liver disease. Normally the amount of ammonia in the plasma is very small, and a sensitive and specific method must be used for its determination. Since the amount of ammonia in the blood will increase rapidly after blood is drawn, plasma is preferred to serum since it can be separated more rapidly and then frozen if necessary for preservation. The blood may be collected using oxalate or heparin as an anticoagulant, but obviously the ammonium salt of heparin should not be used. After the blood is drawn it should be cooled in ice and centrifuged as soon as possible, preferably in a refrigerated centrifuge. If the plasma is not analyzed within an hour or so after separation, it should be kept frozen.

Reagents:

1. Ion-exchange resin
   Dowex 50W-X4, 100-200 mesh, resin is used. Add 1 volume of the resin to 2 volumes of 2.5 moles/L NaOH (10 g/dl) and mix. Allow to stand for 15 min with occasional mixing, allow to settle completely, and then decant off the supernatant liquid. Wash the resin several times with 2 volumes of distilled by gentle mixing, allow to settle, and decant the supernatant. Continue the washings until the supernatant is neutral (pH 6.5-7.5 with short range paper). Add 2 volumes of diluted acetic acid (2 ml glacial acetic acid to 1 dl with water) and mix well. Allow to settle and decant the supernatant. Wash the resin again several times with water and finally store the resin under water.

2. Phenol and alkaline hypochlorite reagents
   The same reagents as are used for the urease method for urea can be used.

3. Ammonia standards
   a. Stock standard

Dissolve 69.6 mg of reagent grade ammonium sulfate in water containing a few drops of sulfuric acid and dilute to 1 dl. This contains 15 mg/dl of ammonia nitrogen or 18.2 mg/dl of ammonia. (Alternately, use 65 mg of ammonium sulfate to give a convenient standard in millimoles containing 10 mmole ammonia/L or 17 mg ammonia/dl.)

b. Diluted working standard
   As needed, dilute 0.1 ml of the standard and 0.3 ml of NaCl solution (24 g/dl) to 10 ml with water. This contains 150 μg/dl ammonia nitrogen (or 182 μg/dl of ammonia).

For the preparation of the diluted standard and for dilution of samples and preparation of blank as well as for the washing of the resin as given in the procedure below, ammonia-free water must be used. This is best prepared by adding some of the prepared resin to a bottle of the regular deionized water and shaking. The resin is allowed to settle but remain in the bottle, and the ammonia-free water can be withdrawn as needed.

Procedure: Add 2 ml of plasma to one test tube. Add 2 ml of diluted standard or 2 ml of water (as a blank) to other tubes. To each tube add about 0.5 g of the wet resin. This is most simply done by withdrawing about 1 ml of the wet resin from the bottom of the bottle containing the wet resin (the exact amount is not important) using a wide-tipped pipet (a Mohr pipet with a broken tip can be used). Mix each tube for several minutes by gentle agitation, then add 10 ml of ammonia-free water, and mix. Allow the resin to settle and decant off the supernatant without loss of resin. Wash the resin with two more 10 ml portions of water. After the final washing and decantation, add 1 ml of the phenol reagent to each tube and allow to stand for 3 min with occasional gentle agitation. Add 1 ml of the alkaline hypochlorite and mix well. Incubate at 37° C for 15 min. Add 3 ml more of water, mix, and allow resin to settle. Decant supernatant into spectrophotometer cuvet and read the standard and sample against the blank at 630 nm.

Calculation: The calculations follow the usual form:

$$\frac{\text{Absorbance of sample}}{\text{Absorbance of standard}} \times \frac{\text{Conc. of}}{\text{standard}} = \frac{\text{Conc. of}}{\text{sample}}$$

where the usual concentration for the standard is 150 μg/dl ammonia nitrogen, or expressed as ammonia, 182 mg/dl.

NOTE: If only an occasional determination is to be done, it may be preferable to use one of the commercially available kits, which contain all the reagents, for this purpose.

Normal values and interpretation: The normal range found will depend on the method used; for the resin method the concentrations are in the range of 15-50 μg/dl as ammonia nitrogen (18-60 μg/dl as ammonia).

Some of the toxic symptoms of hepatic coma are believed to be caused by high concentrations of ammonia in the blood, and concentrations of three to five times the upper limits of normal given above are indicative of severe liver damage.

α-AMINO NITROGEN

The α-amino nitrogen[89-91] in plasma or urine is used as a measure of the total amount of amino acids present. These amino acids contribute the second largest source of nonprotein nitrogen in serum. Despite the importance of amino acids in metabolism, determination of α-amino nitrogen is not as useful clinically as might have been expected. It is now understood that it is not the total of all amino acids that is important clinically. The increases or decreases of groups of related amino acids or individual amino acids are diagnostically important and are usually requested. The α-amino nitrogen determination is included for historical reasons and because it may serve as a useful screening procedure.

Principle: The biologically active amino acids contain an α-amino group that reacts differently than other amino groups and thus may be measured separately. Plasma is generally used instead of serum since some amino acids are apparently set free in the process of clotting. A number of different reagents have been used. None of these give exactly the same amount of color with the different amino acids, either on a weight or molar basis, but the differences are not great enough to invalidate the method. The usual standard is an equimolar mixture of glutamic acid and glycine. Ninhydrin, which gives a blue color with the α-amino group, has been used for many years, but it is not very specific. The use of 2,4-dinitrofluorobenzene (DNFB) offers a more specific reagent. Ammonia still interferes but the amount in plasma is too small to cause a measurable error and in urine the ammonia is readily eliminated by making the urine alkaline and gentle boiling. For plasma the proteins are first precipitated by acid tungstate. A special precipitating reagent is used because the usual Folin-Wu precipitants or trichloroacetic acid does not yield consistent results. An aliquot of the filtrate is treated with the reagent in a borate buffer by heating to 70° C, then diluted with acidified dioxane, and read at 420 nm. The actual absorption peak is at a somewhat shorter wavelength, but reading at 420 nm gives better results for a mixture of amino acids.

Reagents:

1. Color reagent
   a. Stock DNFB, 0.1 mole/L
      Dissolve 950 mg (or 0.65 ml if the material is liquid since it has a melting point near 25° C) in 50 ml of acetone. This is stable in the refrigerator for about 2 months.
   b. Borate solution, 0.13 mole/L
      Dissolve 25 g of sodium borate decahydrate in water to make 5 dl. Allow to age overnight before use. This reagent is stable for several months at room temperature.
      Just before use mix together 1 volume of solution a and 9 volumes of solution b.
2. Acid dioxane
   Mix together 10 ml of concentrated hydrochloric acid and 5 dl of dioxane.
3. Plasma protein precipitant
   a. Sodium tungstate, 0.4 mole/L
      Dissolve 33 g of sodium tungstate ($Na_2WO_4 \cdot 2H_2O$) in water to make 250 ml.
   b. Hydrochloric acid, 0.11 mole/L

Dilute 110 ml of 1 mole/L acid (85 ml of concentrated HCl diluted to 1 L) to 1 L with water.
Just before use, mix together 1 volume of solution a with 9 volumes of solution b.

4. Stock amino acid nitrogen standard, 20 mg/dl amino acid nitrogen
   Dissolve 1.050 g of glutamic acid and 0.536 g of glycine in about 8 dl of water. Add 2 g of sodium benzoate and 58 ml of concentrated hydrochloric acid and dilute to 1 L. This solution is stable in the refrigerator.
5. Working standards
   In separate flasks dilute 1, 2, and 4 ml of stock solution to 1 dl with water. These dilutions correspond to 0.2, 0.4, and 0.8 mg/dl of amino acid nitrogen. When compared with a 1:10 dilution of the plasma filtrate, the standards are equivalent to 2, 4, and 8 mg/dl.
6. Sodium chloride, 0.15 mole/L
   Dissolve 9 g of NaCl in water to make 1 L.

Procedure for plasma: To 0.5 ml of plasma in a test tube, add 0.5 ml of NaCl solution and mix. Add 4.0 ml of the precipitating reagent and mix well. Allow to stand for 5 min and then centrifuge strongly. The supernatant is then filtered through a small acid-fast washed paper to remove small amounts of material that does not sediment. To separate tubes add 1 ml of the filtrate, the different standards, and 1 ml of water as blank. To each tube add 1 ml of the color reagent, stopper loosely, and heat in a water bath at 70° C for 15 min. Cool and add 5 ml of acidified dioxane. Mix and read standards and samples against blank at 420 nm.

Calculation:

$$\frac{\text{Absorbance of sample}}{\text{Absorbance of standard}} \times \frac{\text{Conc. of}}{\text{standard}} \times 10 = \frac{\text{mg/dl amino}}{\text{acid nitrogen}}$$

where conc. of standard refers to the actual concentration of the diluted standards used, 0.2, 0.4, and 0.8 mg/dl. With wider-band instruments the absorption may not be linear and the standard having an absorbance nearest that of a sample should be used for the calculation of that sample.

Procedure for urine:

Additional reagents:

1. Sodium hydroxide, 0.2 mole/L
   Dissolve 8 g of NaOH in water to make 1 L.
2. Phenolphthalein solution
   Dissolve 0.1 g of phenolphthalein in 1 dl of 95% ethanol.

Procedure: Place 1 ml of urine and about 15 ml of water in a 50 ml beaker. Add a few drops of phenolphthalein and then add the 0.2 mole/L sodium hydroxide solution by drops until a pink color persists. Add a few glass beads and heat on a hot plate. Boil gently for about 10 min, adding more NaOH if the pink color disappears and more water if the volume is reduced below about 10 ml. Cool and transfer quantitatively to a 25 ml volumetric flask and dilute to the mark with water. Mix well and filter. Treat 1 ml of filtrate the same as the plasma filtrate.

Calculation: The calculations are the same as those in plasma except that the factor of 25 is used instead of 10 since the urine is diluted 1:25. For high results the urine may be diluted further before color development.

mg/ml × Total urine volume (ml/100) = Total amino acid
nitrogen in urine sample (commonly a 24 hr specimen)

Normal values and interpretation: The normal level of amino acid nitrogen is from 3.5-7.0 mg/dl. The values in children are somewhat lower. In those conditions having increased urinary levels as indicated below there may be some increase in plasma levels. Deamination of amino acids occurs in the liver; this is impaired in severe liver damage and the blood level of the amino acids may rise. In acute yellow atrophy, values up to 20 mg/dl have been noted. Slight increases have found in advanced renal failure when the other nonprotein nitrogen constituents are also elevated. In urine the amino acid nitrogen excretion is usually in the range of 2.0-4.5 mg/kg body weight/day, but the amount excreted will depend somewhat on the protein (amino acid) intake. In the congenital aminoacidurias, the α-amino acid nitrogen level is naturally increased. Particularly high values may be found in Wilson's disease, up to five to 10 times normal.

SERUM PROTEINS
Classification

The serum proteins[92,93] may be divided into several different fractions. The number of fractions that may be found depends on the method of analysis used, which in turn may be governed by the particular diagnostic purposes for which the determination is made. For some purposes it may be sufficient to determine only the total serum protein. This may be done with the refractometer or by a simple spectrophotometric method using the biuret reaction. The simplest separation of the proteins is into the albumin and globulin fractions. This was formerly done by salt fractionation methods. A concentrated salt solution (usually sodium sulfate) is added to serum, the salt concentration being adjusted so that almost all of the larger globulin molecules are precipitated but the smaller albumin molecules remain in solution. After separation of the precipitate, the albumin is determined in the solution by the biuret reaction. The globulins are then determined as the difference (globulins = total protein − albumin). Although the separation is never completely clear cut, the method is fairly satisfactory. However, methods have been chosen for the separate determination of albumin and globulins by purely chemical means without prior separation from each other. Usually the total protein and albumin are measured directly and the globulins calculated by subtraction, but for some purposes it may be preferable to determine the globulins directly. Albumin is a relatively simple molecular species, but globulins, on the other hand, are actually composed of a number of distinct proteins. For their separation and determination some type of electrophoresis is commonly used. In the simplest form, using cellulose acetate, the globulins are usually separated into α_1-, α_2-, β-, and γ-globulins. These are the major fractions found in serum. In plasma another protein fraction, fi-

brinogen, is found. The fibrinogen is involved in clot formation and hence is not found in serum. It may be determined separately in plasma if desired. Electrophoresis is usually carried out with serum to avoid the interference that the fibrinogen sometimes causes in the quantitation of the other protein fractions. The principles involved in electrophoresis are mentioned later.

The β- and γ-globulins in particular actually consist of a number of special proteins having separate functions. Most of the immune bodies in serum are found in the γ-globulin fraction. Other special proteins found in the globulin fraction include the hemoglobin-binding protein haptoglobulin and the iron-binding protein transferrin. These special proteins are determined by immunodiffusion or immunoelectrophoresis.

There are a number of other protein-containing molecular species in serum. These include the lipoproteins in which lipids are associated with certain proteins. These are discussed further in the section with the other lipids. There are also a number of glycoproteins or mucoproteins in which the protein chains are linked to a complex carbohydrate moiety.

Total protein
Micro-Kjeldahl method

A main use of the micro-Kjeldahl method[76,94,95] in the clinical laboratory is to check and standardize the nitrogen content of solutions used as protein standards. The method presented here is similar to that used for NPN except that because of the greater difficulty in decomposing proteins as compared with the smaller NPN constituents, a small amount of mercury is added as a catalyst. This is not enough to interfere with the Berthelot reaction when a slightly smaller amount of nitroprusside is used.

Reagents:
1. Alkaline hypochlorite
   This is the same as that used in the urease method for BUN.
2. Phenol solution
   This is similar to the phenol solution used in the urease method except that 0.05 g of sodium nitroprusside is used per 5 dl instead of 0.13 g.
3. Digestion mixture
   Cautiously add 30 ml of concentrated sulfuric acid to about 50 ml of water. Cool, add 30 g of anhydrous sodium sulfate, and dilute to 1 dl. When all the salt has dissolved, add 0.5 g of mercuric chloride and mix.
4. Sodium hydroxide, 2.5 moles/L
   Dissolve 50 g of sodium hydroxide in water and dilute to 5 dl.
5. Nitrogen standard
   The nitrogen standard used for NPN, containing 0.1 mg/ml, is used here. (Since many of the proteins analyzed will not consist of a single molecular species the use of a standard given in millimoles per liter is not appropriate.)

Procedure: As with other methods using the sensitive Berthelot reaction, ammonia-free water must be used throughout. Dilute an aliquot of the serum 1:100 with saline (9 g NaCl per liter). Pipet 1 ml of the dilution into a digestion tube graduated at 50 ml (NPN digestion tube). Add 1 ml of the digestion mixture along with two small glass beads. Digest the mixture over a microburner until the water is removed and fumes of sulfur trioxide begin to fill the tube. Loosely cap the tube with a glass bulb and continue the digestion for 30 min after the mixture has started to boil. Also digest a blank of 1 ml of saline plus 1 ml of the digestion mixture and a standard containing 1 ml of the standard (nitrogen, 0.1 mg/ml) and 1 ml of the digestion mixture. After digestion allow the solutions to cool. While the solutions are still warm add about 10 ml of water to dissolve any crystallized sodium sulfate. Add 4 ml of 2.5 moles/L sodium hydroxide solution; after the solution has cooled to room temperature, dilute to 50 ml and mix well. Alternately, the digestion may be carried out in a somewhat smaller tube, and the contents, after the addition of the sodium hydroxide, carefully transferred to a 50 ml volumetric flask for the final dilution.

Add 1 ml aliquots of the dilutions of the sample, standard, and blank digests to separate tubes. Add 1 ml of phenol reagent to each tube and after mixing add 1 ml of the alkaline hypochloride solution. Mix and incubate the tubes at 37° C for 20 min. Read samples and standards against blank at 625 nm. As mentioned under the urease reaction, a different final dilution can be used if needed to bring the readings into a suitable range for the spectrophotometer and cuvets used.

Calculation: Initially the serum is diluted 1:100, and after this it is treated similarly to a standard containing 0.1 mg/ml or 10 mg/dl. Thus the standard is equivalent to $10 \times 100 = 1000$ mg/dl or 1 g/dl of protein nitrogen in the original serum or other sample. Thus

$$\frac{\text{Absorbance of sample}}{\text{Absorbance of standard}} \times 1 = \text{g/dl protein nitrogen}$$

If the material is a pooled serum, a correction should be made for the small amount of nonprotein nitrogen present. This can be determined by the method given earlier, for for most purposes, a value of 25 mg/dl can be assumed and 0.025 g/dl subtracted from the amount of protein nitrogen calcuated in grams per deciliter. The conventional factor to convert protein nitrogen to protein was 6.25, but for human serum protein pools (i.e., 15.3% by weight) 6.54 is more accurate.[96,97] The factor for crystalline bovine albumin (Armour Pharmaceutical Co., Phoenix) (i.e., 15.6% by weight) is 6.41.

Biuret method[98,99]

Principle: Total protein is commonly determined by some modification of the biuret reaction in which the protein reacts with an alkaline copper tartrate solution to give a violet color. Under carefully controlled conditions the reaction can be used as an absolute method for the determination of protein. Even the purest samples of protein available may contain small amounts of ash, moisture, lipids, and carbohydrate material. To use this protein as an absolute standard one would need to determine the amounts of these various impurities in the sample. It is now possible to use the specific biuret reaction under carefully controlled conditions to calculate the absolute amount of protein in the sample from the measured absorbance. The color developed by the

reaction between a protein and a biuret reagent will depend on the composition and alkalinity of the reagent, the time and temperature of color development, and, to a slight extent, the nature of the protein. By carefully controlling all these factors one can make an absolute determination of the protein. The procedure is given below.[100]

Reagents:
1. Sodium hydroxide, 6 moles/L
   Dissolve 240 g of NaOH from a fresh bottle of the reagent grade material in freshly distilled or recently boiled deionized water and dilute to 1 L. Store in a polyethylene bottle and keep tightly closed.
2. Biuret reagent
   Dissolve 3 g of uneffloresced CuSO4·5H$_2$O in about 5 dl of freshly distilled or recently boiled deionized water. Add 9 g of potassium sodium tartrate and 5 g of potassium iodide and when solution is complete add 1 dl of 6 moles/L sodium hydroxide solution and dilute to 1 L. Store in a tightly closed polyethylene bottle.
3. Biuret blank reagent
   Dissolve 9 g of potassium sodium tartrate and 5 g of potassium iodide in water, add 1 dl of 6 moles/L sodium hydroxide and dilute to 1 L.
4. Sodium chloride solution, 0.15 mole/L
   Dissolve 9 g of NaCl in water to make 1 L.

Procedure for absolute determination of protein: Pipet exactly 5 ml of biuret reagent to two tubes. To one add 100 μl of water as a blank and to the other add 100 μl of the protein test solution. To a third tube add 5 ml of blank solution and 100 μl of protein solution. The protein solution added to the tube should be measured with accurate glass pipets calibrated "to contain" and rinsed out well. Less accuracy is required for the other two additions. Mix the contents of the tubes and incubate for 30 ± 2 min at $25° \pm 1°$ C. Read at 540 nm in cuvets having a 1 cm light path. Measure test and reagent blank against water and measure sample blank against the reagent blank. Then the corrected absorbance, A_c, is

$$A_c = A_t - (A_r + A_s)$$

where A_t is the absorbance of the test protein solution, A_r that of the reagent blank, and A_s that of the sample blank. If cuvets with an exactly 1 cm light path and a spectrophotometer with a narrow bandwidth are used,

$$\text{Protein (mg) in the added sample (100 μl)} = \frac{A_c \times V}{0.295}$$

where V is the volume in milliliters of the final solution and 0.295 is the absorptivity of the pure protein–biuret complex.

The actual light path of the cuvets can be checked by measuring the absorbance of a solution containing 43 g of CoSO$_4$·(NH$_4$)$_2$SO$_4$·6H$_2$0 per liter, which should have an absorbance of 0.556 at 510 nm in 1 cm cuvets, and a solution of exactly 0.05 g of pure potassium dichromate, in 1 L of water containing a few drops of concentrated sulfuric acid, which should have an absorbance of 0.535 at 350 nm. A correction can be made for the difference in light path from 1 cm by multiplying the above equation by the factor f $= A_s/A_m$, where A_s is the standard absorbance of the cobalt or dichromate solution as given above and A_m is the measured absorbance. An average of the two correction factors may be used.

Procedure with use of standard: The reagents used for the routine determination of total protein are the same as given above. The procedure is essentially the same except that the color produced by the samples is compared with that from a standard and thus exactly 1 cm cuvets are not needed. In addition, the timing need not be as accurate as long as the samples and standard are treated similarly. Use 100 μl of standard or sample plus 5 ml of reagent, and 100 μl of water plus reagent as a reagent blank. Standard and sample blanks are made using 100 μl of standard and sample with 5 ml of the blank reagent. The serum blank is essential only for hyperlipemic, hemolyzed, or other highly pigmented sera but accuracy is improved by using it routinely. Inculbate the samples and blanks at 25° C for 30 min and then read at 540 nm. Routinely all the standards and samples may be read against the reagent blank (100 μl water plus 5 ml of complete reagent) and the serum blanks against the blank reagent. Any blank absorbance is subtracted from the biuret absorbance for the same sample. Then

$$\frac{\text{Corrected absorbance of sample}}{\text{Corrected absorbance of standard}} \times \frac{\text{Conc. of}}{\text{standard}} = \frac{\text{Conc. of}}{\text{sample}}$$

As mentioned previously, the concentration of total protein is not expressed in moles per liter but rather in grams per deciliter in the United States and in grams per liter internationally. Bromsulphalein and phenolsulfonphthalein may interfere with the determination of total protein by the biuret reaction because of the color formed in alkaline solution. Dextrans may also interfere by causing a turbidity. Theoretically these interferences should be minimized by the use of an appropriate blank, but a relatively high blank will cause a decrease in accuracy.

Procedure for lipemic serum[101,102]:

Principle: The serum proteins are precipitated with acetone, which keeps the lipids in solution. The precipitate is centrifuged and supernatant removed. The pellet is then dissolved in biuret reagent and protein calculated in the conventional way. The values obtained are in good agreement with the Kjeldahl method and seem superior to several other proposed methods.

Reagents[102]:
1. Biuret reagent
   In a 1 L volumetric flask, dissolve 3.8 g of $CuSO_4 \cdot 5H_2O$ and 6.7 g of Na_2EDTA in 7 dl of deionized water. Prepare a solution of 40 g of sodium hydroxide in 2 dl of deionized water and slowly add this solution to the volumetric flask with constant stirring.
2. Standard
   Any lyophilized control serum without appreciable lipid or bilirubin concentrations can be used.

Procedure: To a glass test tube, add 0.1 ml water and 20 μl serum and then mix. Add 2 ml acetone, shake vigorously for 1 min, and then centrifuge. Pour off the supernatant and invert tube over a paper towel

for 10 min to drain. Add 1.5 ml of biuret reagent and shake to dissolve. Allow to stand 25 min. Mix again and read absorbance at 545 nm within 1 hr.

Calculation:

$$\frac{\text{Absorbance of patient}}{\text{Absorbance of standard}} \times \frac{\text{Conc. of}}{\text{standard}} = \frac{\text{g/dl of}}{\text{patient's sample}}$$

NOTE: The method is linear to 12 g/dl and does not need an alkaline EDTA blank. Samples corrected by this type of blank (or dilution in saline) will be overcorrected by 1-15%.

Refractometer method[103-105]

The American Optical Corporation's TS meter, a hand refractometer, is a convenient method for determining the protein content of serum. It may be obtained with several different scales; one of these is calibrated directly in grams per dl protein. With this instrument one can determine the protein content to within 0.1 g/dl on only a drop of sample. The refractometer measures an entirely different property of the solution than do the chemical methods and is calibrated by reference to a number of standard sera whose protein content has been determined by chemical means; the refractometer may not give correct values when used with reconstituted lyophilized sera that have a somewhat different constitution than normal sera, and these lyophilized sera cannot be used to check the refractometer. Pure albumin solutions cannot be used as a standard for the same reasons.

The normal values and interpretation for total protein will be discussed later along with the protein fractions, albumin, and the globulins.

Albumin by dye binding[106-108]

Principle: When albumin is added to a buffered solution of a dye (indicator), the albumin binds some of the dye, causing a change in color of the solution. Over a certain range the amount of color change is proportional to the amount of albumin present. The other serum proteins react only slightly and much more slowly. A number of different dyes have been used. The method presented here uses bromcresol green, which is less subject to interference by bilirubin than some other dyes that have been used. Earlier methods, such as that given in the last edition of this book, allowed the albumin and dye to react for 5-10 min before measurement. Later work has indicated that values closer to the true albumin content are obtained by reading as rapidly as possible after the mixing of the sample and reagent.[109-111] Albumin reacts very rapidly, whereas the interfering proteins will react to some extent but much more slowly.

Reagents:
1. Color reagent
   Dissolve 8.8 g of succinic acid in about 2 dl of water in a 1 L volumetric flask. Add 85 mg of bromcresol green that has been dissolved in about 5 ml of 0.1 mole/L NaOH and dilute to about 8 dl. Add 1 mole/L NaOH solution (40 g/L) to bring the pH to 4.2 (about 40 ml will be required); then dilute to 1 L with water and mix

well. Store in the refrigerator and warm to room temperature before use.

2. Sodium chloride solution, 0.15 mole/L
   Dissolve 9 g of NaCl in water to make 1 L.

Standards: For occasional use, one of the commercially available lyophilized control sera may be used. The albumin value given for the electrophoretic method should be used. This may be checked by determining the total protein by the reference method given earlier and determining the percentage of albumin by electrophoresis.

Pure albumin standards may be used. These usually will contain 1% or 2% other proteins; the other principal nonprotein material is generally a small amount of moisture. Human serum albumin (Cohn fraction V) is preferable, but bovine albumin may be used.

Determine the moisture content of the standard material by weighing about 0.1 g into a tared weighing bottle, drying for 24 hr at 110° C, and then cooling in a desiccator over phosphorus pentoxide. Reweigh and calculate the precentage of moisture. Preserve the rest of the sample in a tightly stoppered bottle. To prepare the standard, weigh out the equivalent of 10 g of albumin corrected for moisture content and for any labeled amount of globulins present. For example, if the moisture content was found to be 3.5% and the label stated that the material was 98% albumin, 10.00 g/(0.98 × 0.965) = 10.57 g undried material. Dissolve in a solution containing 9 g sodium chloride and 0.5 g sodium azide/L water. The albumin may dissolve very slowly. To best prepare the solution, carefully transfer all of the albumin to a dry 1 dl volumetric flask, adding about 80 ml of the saline solution slowly; then mix by gentle swirling. Allow to stand in the refrigerator with occasional swirling until dissolved. After warming to room temperature, dilute to the mark with the saline solution (avoid excessive foaming) and mix well. This solution is stable for at least 6 months in the refrigerator.

Alternately, the total protein content of the undried material can be determined by the method given earlier; then the proper quantity is weighed out, making a correction for the amount of other proteins present.

Standards of 2, 4, and 6 g/dl albumin can be prepared by diluting 2, 4, and 6 ml of the stock standard to 10 ml with saline solution. This solution could also be used as a protein standard for the biuret reaction. If a correction was made for the amount of other protein (globulins) when weighing out as an albumin standard, this must be taken into account in the use as a protein standard. In the example given above the protein was 98% albumin and 2% globulins (not including the moisture), so when an amount was weighed out sufficient to give exactly 10 g albumin/dl it would contain 10/0.98 = 10.2 g total protein.

If the total protein has been accurately determined by the biuret method then no other correction is needed.

Procedure: Prepare a blank by adding 1 ml of saline to 4 ml of the reagent. Since the absorbance of this does not change with time, it is prepared first and used to set the spectrophotometer to zero absorbance at 632 nm. Add 20 μl of sample to 1 ml of saline in a cuvet and mix. Check the zero absorbance of the spectrophotometer, then rapidly add 4 ml of the reagent to the cuvet containing the sample and mix rapidly but thoroughly. Read the absorbance exactly 30 sec after the addition of the reagent. (If it is convenient, some other short period of time, not exceeding 45 sec, may be used instead, but the time must always be the same for the samples and the standard.) A standard is treated similarly.

Calculation:

$$\frac{\text{Absorbance of sample}}{\text{Absorbance of standard}} \times \frac{\text{Conc. of}}{\text{standard}} = \frac{\text{Conc. of}}{\text{sample}}$$

A bilirubin concentration of up to 20 mg/dl produces negligible interference with this method. Because of the great dilution, small amounts of hemolysis have only a slight effect. Visible hemolysis will have some effect; a concentration of 100 mg/dl of hemoglobin will give a positive error of about 0.1 g/dl in the albumin result. Moderate lipemia has no appreciable effect. An extremely lipemic serum may cause an error of only 0.1 g/dl of albumin. Salicylates were found to have no interference up to about 50 mg/dl.

Direct determination of globulins

Principle: Globulins may be determined directly[112,113] in proteins by means of a color reaction (Hopkins-Cole) in which the tryptophan in the protein reacts with glyoxylic acid in a strongly acid medium to give a color having a maximal absorbance at about 555 nm. The various serum globulins contain about 2.5% tryptophan, whereas albumin contains only about 0.2%. Thus most of the color formed comes from the globulins. Using as a standard a mixture of albumin and globulins approximating normal serum compensates for the contribution to the color of the tryptophan in the albumin. Only in extremely abnormal sera (e.g., one containing 8 g albumin and 2 g globulins) will there be any appreciable error from the tryptophan.

Reagents:

1. Color reagent
   Dissolve 1.0 g copper sulfate pentahydrate in 90 ml water in a 1 L volumetric flask. Add 1 g glyoxylic acid monohydrate. Add at once 60 ml concentrated sulfuric acid slowly with swirling. Cool to room temperature and dilute to the mark with glacial acetic acid. This reagent is stable 1 year in the refrigerator.

2. Globulin standard
   Theoretically any commercially available lyophilized serum having an exactly known globulin content similar to that of normal serum could be used. However, the original developers of the method state that acetyl tryptophan is used as a stabilizing agent in some commercial control sera. If this compound is present, abnormal and misleading results will be obtained from the serum. The protein standard obtainable from Dow Diagnostics, which contains 3.0 g/dl globulins and 4.5 g/dl albumin is recommended and could also be used as a standard for albumin and total protein determinations. An alternative standard can be prepared from 3.0 g dried human γ-globulin (Cohn fraction II, Sigma HG-II Sigma Chemical Co., St. Louis) and 4.5 g human albu-

min (Cohn fraction V, Sigma Chemical Co., St. Louis) with 50 mg NaN_3 diluted to 1 dl with deionized water in a 1 dl volumetric flask. Albumin is added to the standard globulin solution in order to compensate for the color contributed by the albumin in the unknown serum. The globulin would be 7-10% too high without this addition. A synthetic standard can also be prepared. Dissolve 175 mg N-acetyl-DL-tryptophan, CP grade (Schwarz/Mann Div., Becton-Dickinson & Co., Rutherford, N.J.), in 0.8 ml 1N NaOH and dilute to 1 dl with water. This standard was found to be equivalent to 3.0 g/dl globulin. If a different control serum is used, it could be checked against this synthetic standard to determine if it contains any interfering materials.

Procedure: To 4 ml of the reagent in a screwcap test tube, add 0.02 ml (20 µl) of serum and mix well. Prepare a standard similarly. Cap the tubes and heat in a boiling bath for exactly 4 min. After heating, cool in water and read standard and samples against the reagent alone (blank) at 555 nm. The color is stable for at least 1 hr after development.

Calculation:

$$\frac{\text{Absorbance of sample}}{\text{Absorbance of standard}} \times \frac{\text{Conc. of}}{\text{standard}} = \frac{\text{Conc. of}}{\text{sample in g/dl}}$$

Normal values and interpretation for total protein, albumin, and globulins[114]

The normal range for total protein is from 6-8 g/dl; for albumin, 4-5.5 g/dl; and for globulins, 1.5-3 g/dl. The albumin/globulin (A/G) ratio is usually between 1.5:1 and 2.5:1. Since neither the total protein nor the total globulins consist of a single molecular species, their concentrations are not expressible in molar units. Although albumin is generally considered to be a single molecular species with a definite molecular weight, it would seem preferable to express its concentration also in weight units since comparisons are often made between the relative amounts of the different serum proteins.

An increase in total protein is found in hemoconcentration caused by dehydration from loss of fluid (vomiting, diarrhea, etc.). In such cases both the albumin and globulins increase in the same proportion, so that the A/G ratio remains practically unchanged. This is the only instance in which a natural increase in albumin is found. In instances of increased total protein the albumin is unchanged or slightly decreased, whereas the globulin increases; as a result, the A/G ratio falls markedly. Increases in globulins are found in severe liver disease, some infectious diseases, multiple myeloma, and other plasma cell dyscrasias. The changes in liver disease will be discussed further in the section on liver function tests. The increases in infectious diseases may be caused by increases in γ-globulins, which are the protein fractions concerned with antibody formation. The increases in multiple myeloma may be striking, with globulin concentrations of 6 g/dl or more.

Low total protein levels are usually associated with low albumin levels, which are usually accompanied by a smaller change in globulins, so that the A/G ratio

again is low. A low albumin level may be caused by increased loss of albumin in the urine, decreased formation in the liver, or insufficient protein intake. Low serum protein levels may also be found in conditions in which there is severe hemorrhage, since the plasma volume after hemorrhage is restored more rapidly than the protein level.

A low albumin level, if continued for any length of time, is one of the causes of edema, since the oncotic pressure is such that water is able to pass from the serum into the tissue space and edema results. Agammaglobulinemia is a relatively rare condition, often caused by a genetic metabolic defect, in which the γ-globulins are very low or nearly absent. The other blood fractions are relatively normal.

Oral contraceptives containing estrogen-progestin combinations can cause significant decreases in the amount of albumin and, to a smaller extent, in the total protein.

Electrophoresis of serum proteins

Principle: Electrophoresis of serum proteins is a method for the separation of substances by their migration as charged particles in an electric field. It is used not only for serum proteins but also for other substances, e.g., lipoproteins, isoenzymes, and hemoglobin. In routine laboratory methods the electrophoresis is carried out on a supporting medium. Strips of paper or cellulose acetate or thin layers of gels of agar, agarose (a purified agar derivative), starch, or acrylamide may be used. For the simple separation of the major classes of serum proteins, the preferred method is that using cellulose acetate strips. The specific details of the procedure will vary somewhat with the particular apparatus, so only the principles and general details will be given here. The instruction booklet furnished with the apparatus should provide specific instructions. Further details may be found in the manuals by Nerenberg[115] and Cawley.[116]

General procedure: The separation of the proteins is based on the fact that the different proteins have different molecular weights (sizes) and, at a given pH, different net charges. Under the influence of an electric field the different proteins will move at different rates, depending on their charge and size. The protein solution is applied to a strip of cellulose acetate that has been moistened with a buffer. The strip is best moistened by placing it gently on the surface of the buffer in a flat dish and allowing the buffer to soak in from below before immersing the strip completely. The strip is then blotted and the protein solution applied in a thin line with an applicator designed for the particular system used. The strip is then placed in the electrophoresis assembly with the two ends dipping into reservoirs of the buffer. The electrodes in the buffer are connected to a power supply, with the point of application of the serum nearest to the negative electrode. Then a current of 10-30 mA at a potential of 200–300 V is applied (the current and voltage will vary with the particular apparatus used) for about 30-45 min, until the desired migration has been attained.

Different procedures may use slightly different buffers, but a common one is a barbital buffer, pH 8.6,

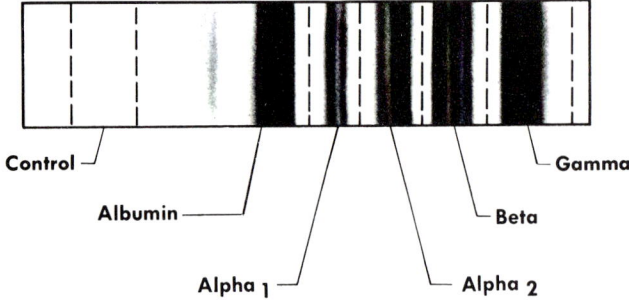

Fig. 21-3. Cellulose acetate electrophoretic pattern of normal human serum. For elution technic, cut fractions at dotted lines.

ionic strength 0.05. This is available commercially as a mixture since the individual components are controlled substances. The barbital may dissolve very slowly; this can be speeded up by gentle heating. A few crystals of thymol may be added as a preservative.

NOTE: Since the electrophoretic pattern is somewhat affected by all the ions present, the buffers are usually specified in terms of ionic strength rather than molarity. The ionic strength is calculated as follows: Multiply the concentration of each ion by the square of the charge, add all ions, and divide by two. For a uni univalent molecule such as sodium chloride the ionic strength would be the same as the molarity, since in a 0.1M solution the ionic strength would be:

$$\frac{0.1 \times 1 + 0.1 \times 1}{2} = 0.1$$

With buffers only the salt form is considered to be ionized. Thus although the above buffer is 0.05M in sodium barbital and 0.01M in the acid, the latter is not ionized, so that the ionic strength is equal to 0.05.

After electrophoresis, the strip is removed and placed in the staining solution for several minutes and then washed several times with 5% acetic acid or a similar solvent. The resulting strip will appear similar to that in Fig. 21-3, showing the stained bands for the different protein fractions. The degree of staining or the amount of color in each band is proportional to the amount of protein present. The staining of cellulose acetate strips is generally done with the dye Ponceau S. The staining solution usually contains a fixative to prevent the protein from washing off. One solution that is used is made by dissolving 1 g Ponceau S, 37.5 g trichloroacetic acid, and 37.5 sulfosalicylic acid in water to make 5 dl. The different manufacturers of cellulose acetate strips may recommend slightly different solutions for their strips.

Estimation of protein fractions: To simply estimate the amount of protein in each fraction from the amount of staining, wash the strip free of excess dye and dry it; then cut it into sections as indicated in Fig. 21-3. Transfer each section to a small tube and completely dissolve both the dye and the cellulose acetate. As a solvent, use either 1 part absolute ethanol and 9 parts chloroform or 1 part formic acid and 9 parts dimethyl-

sulfoxide. Then determine the absorbance of the separate fractions in a spectrophotometer, reading against the blank or control at 520 nm. If the same amount of solvent is added to each tube, the absorbance will be proportional to the amount of protein present in the fraction. The absorbance of a given fraction divided by the sum of all the absorbances yields the fractional amount (in percent) of the given protein. The fractional amount of a given protein multiplied by the total protein content as determined by the refractometer or the biuret reaction gives the total amount of that fraction present.

Usually the proteins are quantitated by scanning the strips in a recording densitometer. Before the strips are scanned, they are cleared by placing them in a clearing solution, so that after drying they will be virtually transparent. Different manufacturers of cellulose acetate may require different clearing solutions for optimal results. The curve obtained by such a scanning is shown in Fig. 21-4. The pips in the lower part of the graph are used to calculate the relative areas under the various portions of the curve, which are divided as shown. As an example of the method of calculation, suppose that the number of pips, relative areas of the separate fractions, were as given in the second column of Table 21-2. The third column gives what percentage each fraction is of the total (95 × 100/176 × 54.0, etc.). The last column gives the absolute amounts of the different protein fractions based on a total protein content of 6.85 g/dl as determined by other means.

Normal values and interpretation[117,118]: Protein electrophoresis has been done with other media, e.g., starch gel and polyacrylamide gel. This latter medium separates the serum proteins into as many as 15 fractions, but the clinical significance of these has not been established. Much of the earlier work on protein electrophoresis was done on paper, but the results with cellulose acetate are similar enough to require no change in interpretation. The average normal values are given in Table 21-3.

Two conditions that give very characteristic electrophoretic patterns are hypogammaglobulinemia and analbuminemia. In hypogammaglobulinemia the γ-globulin fraction is very low, with the rest of the pattern not differing much from normal. The γ-globulins average about 3% of the total protein, or 0.2 g, compared

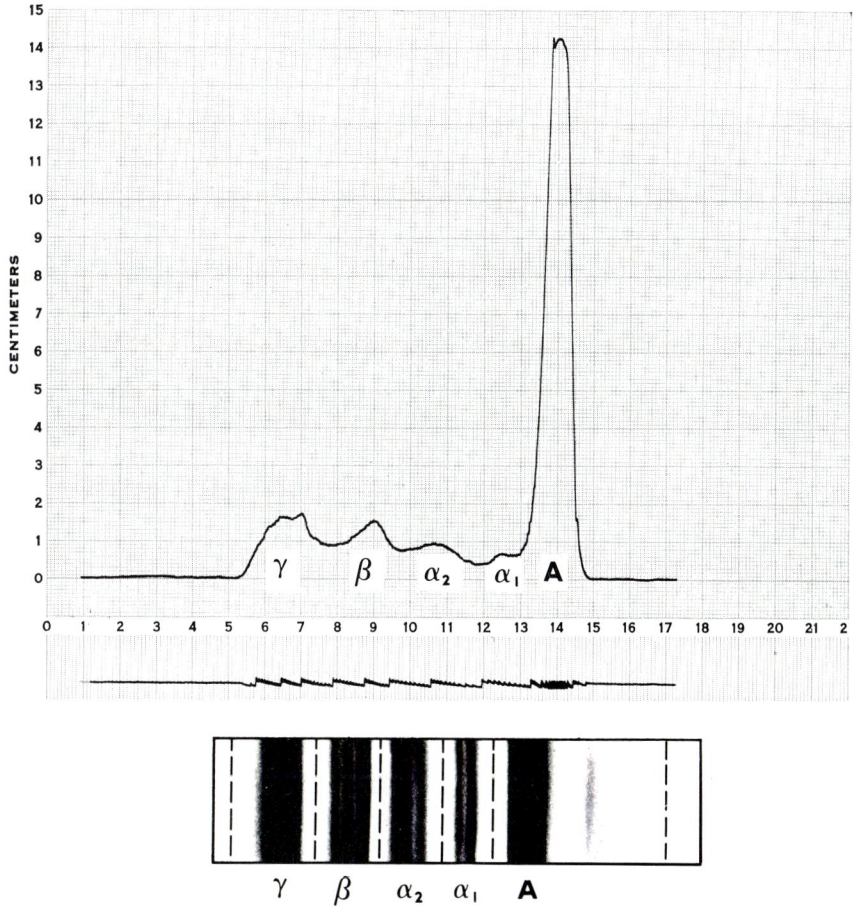

Fig. 21-4. Cellulose acetate electrophoretic pattern of normal human serum. **A,** Albumin; α_1 and α_2, α-globulins; β, β-globulins; and γ, γ-globulins.

Table 21-2. Calculation of protein fractions

Fraction	Relative area	Percent	Protein (g)
Albumin	95	54.0	3.70
Globulin			
α_1	9	3.1	0.34
α_2	16	9.0	0.62
β	25	14.3	0.97
γ	31	17.6	1.21
TOTAL PROTEIN	176	100.0	6.85

Table 21-3. Normal range by cellulose acetate electrophoresis

Fraction	g/dl	Percent of total
Albumin	3.7-5.7	54-74
Globulin		
α_1	0.1-0.3	1.1-4.2
α_2	0.4-1.0	4.6-13.0
β	0.5-1.0	7.3-13.5
γ	0.5-1.5	8.1-19.9
TOTAL PROTEIN	6.5-8.2	100

with a normal value of about 20%, or 1.5 g. In the rare condition of analbuminemia the albumin may amount to not more than 3% of the total protein, which is usually below 5 g.

Various other conditions also give abnormal electrophoretic patterns, although not as striking. Table 21-4 shows the changes in protein fractions with other diseases. Elevated levels of β-globulins are frequently associated with hyperlipemia and hypercholesterolemia and thus may be found in such diseases as the nephrotic syndrome, idiopathic hyperlipemia, uncontrolled diabetes, and obstructive jaundice. The γ-globulins contain most of the immune bodies. Low values of γ-globulins are normally found in infants. At birth the γ-globulin level is characteristically about the same as in the maternal blood (0.9-1.6 g/dl), but it falls sharply during the first few months of life to a low value of 0.3-0.8 g/dl at the age of 3-4 months. It then rises slowly, reaching a level of about 0.5-1.2 g/dl at age 1 year and attaining normal adult levels only after 5-10 years. In multiple myeloma, although the total globulin is markedly increased, the increase is not always chiefly in the γ-globulin fraction. The so-called M globulins of this disease do not always migrate with the γ-globulins, and the increase may sometimes be found in the α- or β-globulins.

Table 21-4. Changes in electrophoretic protein fractions associated with disease*

	Total protein	Albumin	α₁-Globulin	α₂-Globulin	β-Globulin	γ-Globulin
Acute infection		D		I		
Asthma and other allergies with poor response to therapy		D		I		D
Carcinomatosis		D	I	I		
Chronic infection		D				I
Cryoglobulinemia						I
Diabetes mellitus		D	I	I		
Glomerulonephritis	D	D	I			
Hepatic cirrhosis	D	D				I
Hepatitis, viral		D	D	D	I	I
Hodgkin's disease	D	D		I		I
Leukemia, myelogenous		D				I
Lupus erythematosus		D		I		I
Lymphoma and lymphocytic leukemia	D	D				D
Macroglobulinemia	I	D			I	I
Myeloma	I	D				I
Myasthenia		D				I
Myxedema		D		I		I
Nephrosis (highest A₂ elevation)	D	D		I		D
Rheumatic fever		D		I		
Rheumatoid arthritis		D		I		I
Sarcoidosis	I	D		I	I	I
Scleroderma	D	D	D	D	D	D
Ulcerative colitis and other exudative enteropathies	D	D	I	I	D	D

*I, increase; D, decrease.

Macroglobulins

A number of pathologic conditions will cause abnormally high globulin fractions on electrophoresis. One of these conditions is **macroglobulinemia.**

Cryoglobulins

The presence of cryoglobulins[119] will also often give abnormal electrophoretic patterns. When serum or plasma containing cryoglobulin is incubated at 4° C, it will undergo significant changes that are not observed at 37° C.

Fibrinogen

Fibrinogen[120] is the blood protein specially concerned with clotting; its determination is useful in conditions such as myocardial infarction, rheumatic fever, and liver and bleeding disorders. Since fibrinogen is found in the clot, it is not observed in serum electrophoresis.

Immunoglobulins

Most of the antibodies in serum are found in the γ-globulin fraction, and several different immunoglobulins[121-123] have been characterized. These have been designated as IgA, IgG, IgD, IgE, and IgM. The IgA class includes antitoxins, antibacterial agglutinins, cold agglutinins, antinuclear antibodies, and allergic reagins. Included in the IgG class are most of the antibacterial and antiviral antibodies. The IgM class is composed of the ABO blood group isoantibodies, Rh antibodies, the heterophil antibodies of in-

fectious mononucleosis, rheumatoid arthritis factors, and others.

Principles of determination: These γ-globulins may be estimated by radial immuno-diffusion. The procedure is not difficult. Place a thin layer of 2% agar in barbital buffer (pH 8.6) in a Petri dish. The agar also contains antibodies to the particular globulin being determined. Although the plates could be prepared in the laboratory, it is not recommended. The antibody must be purchased and it may require some experimentation to determine the optimal concentration in the agar. Ready-made plates can be obtained from a number of suppliers (Meloy Laboratories, Springfield, Va.; Hyland Laboratories, Costa Mesa, Calif.; and Hoechst-Roussel Pharmaceuticals, Somerville, N.J.), along with the required standards. When making individual plates cut a number of small wells (1 mm diameter) into the agar gel. Place in these wells about 2 μl of the various sera to be determined or various known concentrations of the antigen. Allow the plates to stand at room temperature in a moist chamber for 24-48 hr or until the diffusion is complete. When examined after diffusion, each well will be surrounded by a precipitate ring. Measure the diameters of the various rings with a micrometer microscope or use a calibrated hand magnifying lens. Two different methods of preparing the standard curve have been used. Either plot the square of the ring diameters against the concentrations of the standards or plot the ring diameters against the logarithm of the standard concentration. It may be well to try both methods to find which gives the best result in

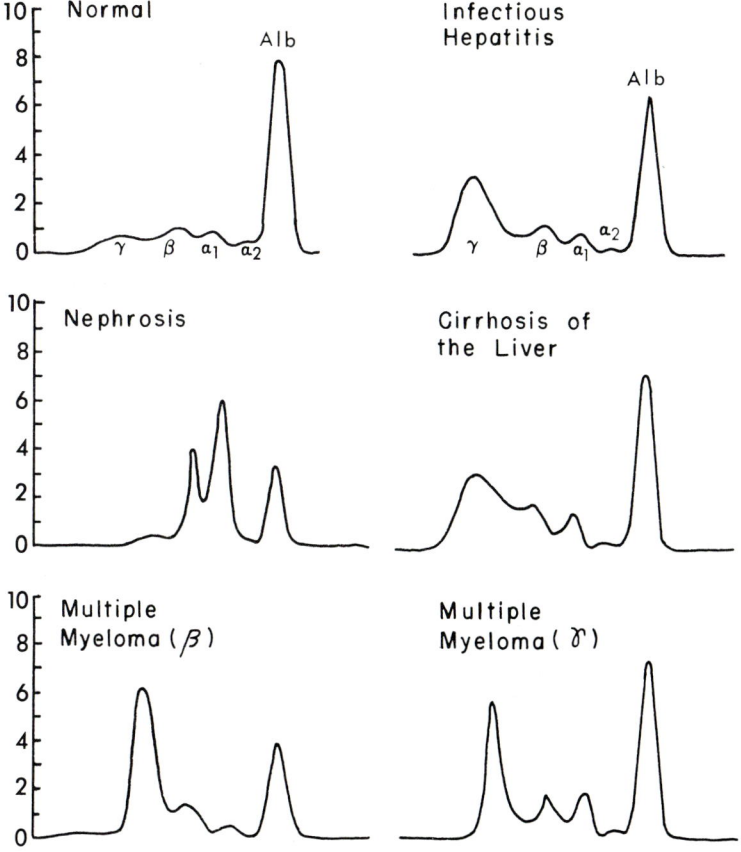

Fig. 21-5. Electrophoretic patterns obtained with cellulose acetate and including normal serum. Infectious hepatitis serum shows slight decrease in albumin and significantly increased γ-globulin; serum from patient with nephrosis shows low level of albumin, significantly elevated α_2-globulin, and elevated β-globulin; serum from patient with cirrhosis shows elevations in β- and γ-globulins with a decrease in albumin; one sample from multiple myeloma shows marked increase of myeloma globulin in β-globulin and the other shows a marked increase in γ-globulin position.

a given determination. The concentrations of the various samples are then determined from the standard curve.

A further treatment of radial immunodiffusion will be found in Chapter 35 on serology.

Normal values and interpretation: The normal values for the immunoglobulins in adults are from 100-220 mg/dl for IgA; 900-1400 mg/dl for IgG; and 70-130 mg/dl for IgM. The levels of IgA and IgM are very low at birth and gradually increase to adult levels at puberty. Immediately after birth the IgG level is equal to that of cord blood but gradually decreases over the next few months to a level of around 400 mg/dl and then increases with age, reaching adult levels at puberty. The levels are generally increased in infectious diseases or other processes that result in antibody formation.

PROTEIN IN CEREBROSPINAL FLUID AND URINE

The biuret color reaction is not sensitive enough for the analysis of protein in cerebrospinal fluid or urine. Here two more sensitive methods are presented. One is a turbidimetric method of Henry and widely used for many years.[124] The other is a more recent dye-binding method.[125]

Turbidimetric method

Principle: The fluid is treated with trichloroacetic acid to precipitate the proteins as a fine suspension. The resulting turbidity is measured spectrophotometrically and compared with a protein standard treated similarly.

Reagents:

1. Trichloroacetic acid, 0.75 mole/L
   Dilute 50 ml of the 1.8 moles/L acid with 70 ml of water. Alternately dissolve 12.5 g of the acid in water to make 1 dl.
2. Sodium chloride, 0.15 mole/L
   Dissolve 0.85 g of sodium chloride in water to make 1 dl.
3. Protein standard
   Any clear normal serum of known protein content or a commercially available control serum may be used. The serum is diluted with the saline solution to a known concentration of around 25 mg/dl. Most serums will have a protein content of 6-7 g/dl. If these are diluted 1:250, the resulting solution will contain around 25 mg/dl; the exact

value calculated from the known concentration of the original serum is used in the calculations.

Procedure for urine: Set up three test tubes labeled standard, sample, and blank. To the standard tube, add 4 ml diluted protein standard; to the sample tube, add 4 ml clear urine (centrifuge if turbid); and to the blank tube, add 4 ml clear urine plus 1 ml water. Add 1 ml trichloroacetic acid to standard and sample tubes and mix immediately. Let stand between 5 and 10 min and read in a photometer at 420 nm. Read the standard tube against water and the sample tube against urine blank. Before the tubes are read, they must be thoroughly mixed and entrapment of air bubbles in the suspension must be avoided.

Calculation: Since 4 ml of urine is treated the same as 4 ml of standard containing 25 mg/dl:

$$\frac{\text{Absorbance of sample} - \text{Absorbance of sample blank}}{\text{Absorbance of standard}} \times 25$$

$$= \text{mg/dl urinary protein}$$

For a 24 hr urine sample:

$$\text{Total urinary protein} = \text{mg/dl} \times \frac{\text{Total volume (ml)}}{100}$$

Some drugs or other products that give a color to the urine may tend to act as indicators, and the addition of the acid will change the color of the urine. In this case the color correction will be very inaccurate. For these samples the phosphotungstate biuret method given below should be used.

Procedure for cerebrospinal fluid: Set up two test tubes labeled standard and sample. Add 4 ml diluted standard to standard tube; add 1 ml clear spinal fluid (centrifuge if cloudy) and 3 ml 0.85% NaCl to sample tube. To each tube, add 1 ml 12.5% trichloroacetic acid and mix immediately. Let stand between 5 and 10 min and read absorbance in a spectrophotometer at 420 nm against a water blank. Tubes must be mixed just before reading, and care must be taken to avoid trapping air bubbles in the suspension.

Calculations: Since 4 ml of standard containing 25 mg/dl is compared with 1 ml of spinal fluid:

$$\text{mg/dl protein} = \frac{\text{Absorbance of sample}}{\text{Absorbance of standard}} \times 4 \times 25$$

Although Beer's law may be obeyed up to an absorbance of about 0.8 or more, the limitations of the photometer should be checked, and for samples giving a higher reading, a determination should be made using a smaller aliquot of sample and making proper adjustment in the calculations.

NOTE: Analysis of xanthochromic spinal fluids may be inaccurate, and it is suggested that a blank similar to that used for urine be run for color correction.

Dye-binding method[126,127]

Principle: The binding of the dye Coomassie Brilliant Blue G-250 to protein causes a shift in the absorption maximum from 465 nm to 595 nm. The change in absorbance at this latter wavelength is used to measure the amount of protein present. The method requires 50 μg or less of protein and thus is quite sensitive.

Reagents:
1. Dye reagent

   Dissolve 150 mg of Coomassie Blue (Sigma Brilliant Blue G, no. B-1131, Sigma Chemical Co., St. Louis) in 50 ml of methanol. Add 1 dl of 85% phosphoric acid and mix. Dilute to 1 L with water and mix well. Allow to stand overnight and then filter through paper. Adjust the filtrate so that the absorbance against water at 595 is about 0.50 with a 1 cm light path. The exact absorbance is not critical, but it is preferable to adjust subsequent batches to the same absorbance to obtain a better duplication of standard curves. The adjustment is made by diluting the dye solution with a mixture of water, methanol, and phosphoric acid in the same proportions as used in preparing the original dye solution. The change in absorbance is not linear with dilution, so care must be taken in the dilution.
2. Sodium chloride, 0.15 mole/L

   Dissolve 8.5 g of NaCl in water to make 1 L.
3. Protein standard

   For the determination of protein in urine and CSF, a dilution of a serum of known protein content is satisfactory. An aliquot of the serum is diluted to a known concentration of approximately 1 mg/ml (100 mg/dl = 1 mg/ml) with 0.15 mole/L NaCl. For example, 1 ml of a serum containing 6.5 g/dl of protein is diluted with exactly 64 ml of saline (50, 10, and 4 ml measured with volumetric pipets) to give a solution containing 1 mg/ml. This may be diluted further to give concentrations of 0.2, 0.4, and 0.6 mg/ml (which equal, respectively, 20, 40, and 60 mg/dl).

Procedure: Add 5 ml of reagent to a number of tubes. Add 100 μl of water to one tube as a blank and then add 100 μl of sample or standard to other tubes. Mix by inversion, capping with Parafilm, allow to stand for 10 min, and then read samples and standards against blank at 595 nm. Depending on the spectrophotometer used the curve may not be linear above an absorbance of about 0.6 units; thus it may be preferable to run several standards with each series of samples and use for the calculations the standard having an absorbance closest to that of the sample.

Preferably one should run a calibration curve when first trying out the procedure. Then, since the actual determination is very simple, whenever the result for a sample is above the linear portion of the curve, one merely repeats the determination using a smaller aliquot of the sample (with a corresponding change in the water added to the blank).

Some error will be caused by very acid urine (as when the urine is collected with acid for other purposes) or very alkaline urine (often found after standing for a long time). In these instances the pH should be adjusted to approximately 7 before determination.

Normal values and interpretation[128,129]

The protein content of normal lumbar spinal fluid ranges between 15-45 mg/dl and contains mostly albumin. Cisternal fluid has on the average a slightly lower

Table 21-5. Dipstick readings

	Neg. or trace	+1	+2	+3	+4
Urine (μl)	20	10	5	2	0.5
Saline (ml)	0	10	15	18	19.5
Dilution factor	1	2	4	10	40

level—about 20 mg/dl. Ventricular fluids have appreciably lower levels—about 10 mg/dl.

The most common abnormality found in spinal fluid is an increase in protein. In many conditions this increase is small, rarely exceeding 100 mg/dl. In different types of meningitis, polyneuritis, and tumors, increases up to 400 mg/dl may be found.

The normal protein content of **urine** is small, ranging from 25-150 mg in a 24 hr specimen. Normal infants may have a significant proteinuria during the first few days of life. Significant increases in urinary protein are found in nephrosis, where the excretion may amount to several grams per day. Variable amounts of protein are found in the urine in various destructive lesions of the kidneys, but these never approach the quantity found in nephrosis. For a discussion of the significance of special proteins such as Bence Jones proteins, see Chapter 27.

Phosphotungstate-biuret method[130]

Principle: Urine proteins are measured by the biuret method after precipitation from urine with ethanolic phosphotungstic acid.

Reagents:
1. Ethanolic phosphotungstic acid
   Transfer 50 ml concentrated HCl (specific gravity of 1.19), 60 ml distilled water, and 770 ml of 95% (vol/vol) ethanol to a 1 L beaker. Add 15 g of phosphotungstic acid and mix until dissolved. Filter and store in the refrigerator at 4° C. The mixture is stable for 1 month.
2. Biuret reagent
   Add 6.4 g potassium sodium tartrate (KNa $C_4H_4O_6\cdot4H_2O$) to 5 dl distilled water in a 1 L volumetric flask. Add 1.6 g $CuSO_4\cdot5H_2O$ and mix until dissolved. Add 240 ml of 2.5N NaOH slowly and then add 0.66 g KI. Dilute to 1 L. Store at 25° C in a plastic bottle. The mixture is stable for 3 years.
3. Alkaline tartrate reagent
   Add 6.4 g potassium sodium tartrate (KNa $C_4H_4O_6\cdot4H_2O$) to 5 dl distilled water in a 1 L volumetric flask. Add 240 ml of 2.4N NaOH slowly and then add 0.66 g KI. Dilute to 1 L with distilled water. Store at 25° C in a plastic bottle. The mixture is stable for 3 years.
4. Protein standard
   A pool of normal serum is collected, mixed well, and centrifuged. The protein concentration in grams per deciliter is determined using the biuret technic. Prepare a 1:250 dilution by adding 1 ml to a 250 ml volumetric flask and dilute to 250 ml with water. The mixture is stable for 1 month at 4° C.

5. Sodium hydroxide, 2.5N
   Dissolve 100 g NaOH in 8 dl distilled water in a 1 L volumetric flask and dilute to the mark with water. Protect from atmospheric CO_2.

Procedure: Measure the volume of a fresh 24 hr urine collection and enter this figure on the data sheet. Transfer an aliquot of 50 ml into a plastic centrifuge tube. Centrifuge at 2000 rpm for 15 min. The supernatant may be saved for later determination in the refrigerator at 4° C. Estimate the protein concentration using a dipstick. Set up the dilutions shown in Table 21-5 in 50 ml centrifuge tubes according to the amount of protein present. Do each in duplicate—one will become a blank for each sample. Enter the dilution factor on the data sheet.

Using 15 ml centrifuge tubes, set up pairs of tubes by adding 5 ml of dilute standard, 5 ml of dilute urine, or 5 ml of saline. Place the tubes in an ice bath for 5 min; then add 5 ml of cold ethanolic phosphotungstate, mix, and allow tubes to stand 15 min in the ice bath. Centrifuge at 2000 rpm for 15 min. Discard supernatants and allow tubes to drain inverted on paper towels for 10 min. Add 1 ml of biuret reagent to one tube of each pair and 1 ml of alkaline tartrate to the other tube of each pair. Allow to stand 5 min; then centifuge and allow to stand 20 min. Read the absorbance at 540 nm against the reagent blank.

Calculation:

Protein concentration (mg/dl) =

$$\frac{\text{Absorbance (unknown} - \text{blank)}}{\text{Absorbance (standard} - \text{blank)}} \times$$
$$\text{Standard conc.} \times \text{Dilution}$$

Protein excreted (mg/24 hr) =

$$\frac{\text{Protein conc.} \times \text{Urine vol. (ml/24 hr)}}{100}$$

NOTE: The method is linear to approximately 30 mg/dl.

REFERENCES

1. Hultman, E.: Nature **183**:108, 1959.
2. Cooper, G.R., and McDaniel, V.: In MacDonald, R.D., editor: Standard methods of clinical chemistry, vol. 6, New York, 1970, Academic Press, p. 159.
3. Thomitzek, V.D., and Bemm, H.: Z. Klin. Chem. Klin. Biochem. **7**:361, 1969.
4. Snegowski, M.C., and Frier, E.F.: Am. J. Med. Technol. **39**:140, 1973.
5. Winkers, P.L.M., and Jacobs, P.: Clin. Chim. Acta **34**:401, 1971.
6. Yamashita, M., and Watanabe, F.: Clin. Chim. Acta **47**:211, 1973.
7. Abraham, C.V.: Clin. Chim. Acta **70**:209, 1976.

8. Cooper, G.R.: CRC Crit. Rev. Clin. Lab. Sci. **4:**101, 1973.
9. Dubowski, K.M.: Clin. Chem. **8:**215, 1962.
10. Powell, J.B., and Djuk, Y.Y.: Am. J. Clin. Pathol. **56:**8, 1971.
11. Pennock, C.A., et al.: Clin. Chim. Acta **48:**193, 1973.
12. O'Brien, D., et al.: Laboratory manual of pediatric micro-biochemical techniques, ed. 4, New York, 1968, Harper & Row, Publishers.
13. Meites, S., editor: Pediatric clinical chemistry, Washington, D.C., 1977, American Association for Clinical Chemistry, Inc.
14. Passey, R.B., et al.: In Cooper, G.R., editor: Selected methods of clinical chemistry, Washington, D.C., 1977, American Association for Clinical Chemistry, vol. 8, p. 9.
15. Trinder, P.: Ann. Clin. Biochem. **6:**24, 1969.
16. Bauminger, B.B.: J. Clin. Pathol. **27:**1015, 1974.
17. Lott, J.A., and Turner, K.: Clin. Chem. **21:**1754, 1975.
18. Hung, V.L.: C.R. Hebd. Sceances Acad. Sci. Ser. D **232:**751, 1976.
19. Forsham, P.H., Steinke, J., and Throne, G.W.: In Harrison, T.R., et al., editors: Principles of internal medicine, ed. 5, New York, 1966, McGraw-Hill Book Co., chap. 86.
20. Seltzer, H.S.: In Ellenberg, M., editor: Diabetes mellitus, theory and practice, New York, 1970, McGraw-Hill Book Co.
21. Henry, R.J., Cannon, F.C., and Winkelman, J.W., editors: Clinical chemistry, principles and techniques, ed. 2, New York, 1974, Harper & Row, Publishers.
22. McDonald, G.W., Fisher, G.F., and Burnham, C.E.: Public Health Rep. **79:**515, 1964.
23. Thustison, W.A., Bowen, A.J., and Crampton, J.H.: Diabetes **15:**775, 1966.
24. Committee on Statistics of American Diabetes Association: Diabetes **18:**299, 1969.
25. Wilkerson, H.L.C.: Diagnosis and glucose tolerance tests in diabetes mellitus diagnosis and treatment, New York, 1964, American Diabetes Association.
26. Searcy, R.L., and Low, E.M.Y.: Diabetes **15:**762, 1965.
27. Leonards, J.R., McCaullagh, E.P., and Christopher, T.C.: Diabetes **14:**96, 1965.
28. Fajans, S.S., and Conn, W.J.: Ann. N.Y. Acad. Sci. **82:**208, 1959.
29. Klint, C.E., et al.: University group diabetes program, a study of relationship of therapy in vascular complications of diabetes, Brook Lodge Symposium, New York, 1967, Excerpta Med. Int. Cong. Ser., no. 149.
30. Kobbering, J., and Creutzfeldt, W.: Diabetes **19:**870, 1970.
31. Andres, R.: Med. Clin. North Am. **55:**835, 1971.
32. Palmer, J.P., and Ensinck, J.W.: J. Clin. Invest. **41:**498, 1975.
33. Siperstein, M.D.: In Stollerman, G.M., editor: Advances in internal medicine, Chicago, 1975, Year Book Medical Publishers.
34. Fajans, S.S., and Siperstein, M.D.: Diabetes Outlook **12:**1, 1977.
35. National Diabetes Data Group: Diabetes **28:**1039, 1979.
36. O'Sullivan, T.B., and Mahan, C.M.: J.A.M.A. **194:**587, 1965.
37. Langer, P.H., and Fies, H.L.: Am. J. Clin. Pathol. **11:**41, 1941.
38. Thorn, G.W., et al.: J. Clin. Invest. **19:**813, 1940.
39. Soskin, S.J.: J. Clin. Endocrinol. Metab. **4:**75, 1944.
40. Unger, H.H., and Madison, L.L.: Diabetes **7:**455, 1958.
41. Unger, H.H., and Madison, L.L.: J. Clin. Invest. **37:**627, 1958.

42. Fajans, S.S., and Conn, J.: J. Lab. Clin. Med. **54:**811, 1959.
43. Swerdlof, H.S., et al.: Diabetes **16:**161, 1967.
44. Kaplan, N.M.: Arch. Intern. Med. **107:**212, 1961.
45. Young, D.S., Pestaner, L.G., and Gibberman, V.: Clin. Chem. **21(5):**1D-432D, 1975.
46. Hansten, P.D.: Drug interactions, ed. 2, Philadelphia, 1975, Lea & Febiger.
47. Garb, S.: Clinical guide to undesirable drug interactions and interferences, New York, 1970, Springer-Verlag New York.
48. Basford, R.L., and Henry, J.B.: Postgrad. Med. **41:**A70, 1967.
49. Friedland, N.: Arch. Intern. Med. **116:**886, 1965.
50. Peternel, W.W.: Gastroenterology **48:**299, 1965.
51. Krasiznikoff, P.A., Gudmand-Høyer, E., and Moltke, H.H.: Acta Paediatr. Scand. **65:**693, 1975.
52. Gabbay, K.H., et al.: J. Clin. Endocrinol. Metab. **44:**59, 1977.
53. Sondergaard, G.: Scand. J. Clin. Lab. Invest. **10:**203, 1958.
54. Waldstein, S.S., et al.: Clin. Chem. **10:**381, 1964.
55. Frings, C.S., and Pardue, H.L.: Anal. Chem. **36:**2477, 1964.
56. Ford, J.D., and Haworth, J.C.: Clin. Chem. **10:**1002, 1964.
57. Hjelm, M.: Clin. Chim. Acta **15:**87, 1967.
58. Maclagan, N.F.: Q. J. Med. **9:**151, 1940.
59. Maclagan, N.F., and Rundel, F.F.: Q. J. Med. **9:**215, 1940.
60. Harris, A.L.: Clin. Chem. **15:**65, 1969.
61. Goodwin, J.F.: Clin. Chem. **16:**85, 1970.
62. Smith, M.B., and Braidword, J.L.: Clin. Biochem. **4:**118, 1971.
63. Roe, J.H., and Rice, E.W.: J. Biol. Chem. **173:**507, 1948.
64. Kerstell, J.: Scand. J. Clin. Lab. Invest. **13:**637, 1961.
65. Santini, R., Jr., et al.: Gastroenterology **40:**772, 1961.
66. Rolles, C.J., et al.: Lancet **2:**1043, 1973.
67. Hindmarsh, J.T.: Clin. Biochem. **9:**141, 1976.
68. Hultman, E.: In Curtiss, H.C., and Roth, M., editors: Clinical biochemistry: principles and methods, vol. 2, Berlin, 1974, Walter de Gruyter & Co.
69. Froesch, E.R., et al.: J. Med. **34:**151, 1963.
70. Coulombe, J.J., and Favreau, L.: Clin. Chem. **9:**102, 1963.
71. Crocker, C.L.: Am. J. Med. Technol. **33:**361, 1967.
72. Fawcett, J.K., and Scott, J.E.: J. Clin. Pathol. **13:**149, 1960.
73. Watson, D.: Clin. Chim. Acta **14:**571, 1966.
74. Searcy, R.L., et al.: Am. J. Med. Technol. **27:**255, 1961.
75. Chaney, A.L., and Marbach, E.P.: Clin. Chem. **8:**130, 1962.
76. Shahinian, A.H., and Reinhold, J.G.: Clin. Chem. **17:**1077, 1971.
77. Mosenthan, H.O., and Bruger, M.: Arch. Intern. Med. **55:**411, 1935.
78. Jung, D.H., and Parekh, A.C.: Clin. Chem. **16:**247, 1970.
79. Landenson, J.E.: In Sonnewirth, A.C., and Jarett, L., editors: Gradwohl's clinical laboratory methods and diagnosis, ed. 8, St. Louis, 1980, The C.V. Mosby Co., p. 181.
80. Bittner, D., Hall, S., and McCleary, M.: Am. J. Clin. Pathol. **40:**423, 1963.
81. Bittner, D.H., and Gambino, S.R.: Uric acid assay, Chicago, 1970, Committee on Continuing Education, American Society of Clinical Pathologists.
82. Taussky, H.H.: J. Biol. Chem. **208:**853, 1954.

83. Hudson, H., and Rappoport, A.: Clin. Chem. **14**:222, 1968.
84. Larsen, K.: Clin. Chim. Acta **41**:209, 1972.
85. Yatzidis, H.: Clin. Chem. **20**:1131, 1974.
86. Van Pilsum, J.F., et al: J. Biol. Chem. **222**:225, 1956.
87. Foreman, D.T.: Clin. Chem. **10**:497, 1964.
88. Kingsley, G.R., and Tager, H.S.: In MacDonald, R.D., editor: Standard methods of clinical chemistry, New York, 1970, Academic Press, vol. 6, p. 115.
89. Dienst, C., and Morris, R.: J. Lab. Clin. Med. **64**:495, 1964.
90. Goodwin, J.F.: Clin. Acta **21**:321, 1968.
91. Goodwin, J.F.: In MacDonald, R.D., editor: Standard methods of clinical chemistry, New York, 1970, Academic Press, vol. 6, p. 89.
92. Oser, B.L., editor: Hawk's physiological chemistry, ed. 14, New York, 1965, McGraw-Hill Book Co., chap. 6.
93. Kachman, J.F., and Grant, G.H.: In Tietz, N., editor: Fundamentals of clinical chemistry, ed. 2, Philadelphia, 1976, W.B. Saunders Co., chap. 7.
94. Dambacher, M., Gubler, A., and Hass, H.G.: Clin. Chem. **14**:615, 1968.
95. Ciaraviglio, E.C., Wolf, A.V., and Prentiss, P.G.: Am. J. Clin. Pathol. **39**:727, 1963.
96. Watson, D.: Clin. Chim. Acta **16**:322, 1967.
97. Sunderman, F.W.: Am. J. Clin. Pathol. **46**:679, 1966.
98. Weichselbaum, T.E.: Am. J. Clin. Pathol. **7**:40, 1946.
99. De la Huerga, J., Smetters, G.W., and Sherrick, J.C.: In Sunderman, F.W., editor: Serum proteins and dysproteinemias, Springfield, Ill., 1964, Charles C Thomas, Publisher.
100. Doumas, B.T.: Clin. Chem. **21**:1159, 1975.
101. Chromy, V., and Fischer, J.: Clin. Chem. **23**:754, 1977.
102. Chromy, V., Fischer, J., and Kulhanek, V.: Clin. Chem. **20**:1362, 1974.
103. Martinek, R.G.: Proc. Assoc. Clin. Biochem. **3**:267, 1965.
104. Lines, J.G., and Raine, D.N.: Ann. Clin. Biochem. **7**:1, 1970.
105. Drickman, A., and McKeon, F.A., Jr.: Am. J. Clin. Pathol. **38**:392, 1962.
106. Doumas, B.T., Watson, W.A., and Biggs, H.G.: Clin. Chim. Acta **31**:87, 1971.
107. Rodkey, F.L.: Clin. Chem. **11**:478, 1965.
108. McPherson, J.G., and Everard, D.W.: Clin. Chim. Acta **37**:117, 1971.
109. Webster, D.: Clin. Chem. **22**:663, 1977.
110. Corcoran, R.M., and Durnan, S.M.: Clin. Chem. **22**:765, 1977.
111. Gustafasson, J.E.C.: Clin. Chem. **22**:616, 1977.
112. Goldenberg, H., and Drewes, P.A.: Clin. Chem. **17**:358, 1971.
113. Saifer, A., and Marven, T.: Clin. Chem. **12**:414, 1966.
114. Korngold, I.: Prog. Clin. Pathol. **1**:398, 1966.
115. Nerenberg, S.T.: Electrophoresis, a practical laboratory manual, Philadelphia, 1966, F.A. Davis Co.
116. Cawley, L.P.: Electrophoresis and immunoelectrophoresis, Boston, 1969, Little, Brown & Co.
117. Sunderman, F.W., Jr.: Am. J. Clin. Pathol. **42**:21, 1964.
118. Sheperd, H.G., and Mason, C.C.: Am. J. Clin. Pathol. **43**:464, 1965.
119. Stephanini, M., and Dameshek, W.: The hemorrhagic disorders, New York, 1955, Grune & Stratton, Inc.
120. Reiner, M., and Chung, H.I.: Clin. Chem. **5**:414, 1959.
121. Fahey, J.L., and McKelvey, E.M.: J. Immunol. **94**:84, 1965.
122. McKelvey, E.M., and Fahey, J.L.: J. Clin. Invest. **44**:1778, 1965.
123. Stiehm, E.R., and Fudenberg, H.H.: Pediatrics **37**:715, 1966.
124. Henry, R.J., Sobel, C., and Segalove, M.: Proc. Soc. Exp. Biol. Med. **92**:748, 1956.
125. Tinncy, D.J.: Can. J. Med. Technol. **39**:97, 1977.
126. Bradford, M.M.: Anal. Biochem. **72**:248, 1976.
127. McIntosh, J.C.: Clin. Chem. **23**:1939, 1977.
128. Ellis, A.W.: Lancet **1**:1, 1942.
129. Poortmans, J.R.: Protides Biol. Fluids Proc. Colloq. **16**:603, 1968.
130. Savory, J., Pu, P.H., and Sunderman, F.W., Jr.: Clin. Chem. **14**:1160, 1968.

CHAPTER 22

Inorganic elements and blood gases

CALCIUM
Colorimetric determination of serum calcium[1-3]

Cresolphthalein complexone forms a colored product with calcium, which may be determined in a spectrophotometer at 575 nm. Hydroxyquinoline is added to reduce the interference by magnesium. The method requires only a small amount of serum and has been used in some automated methods. Because of the great sensitivity of the reagent, one disadvantage of the manual method is the contamination caused by minute amounts of calcium adsorbed on glassware that is not scrupulously clean. It is preferable to use disposable plastic tubes and store the reagents in polyethylene bottles. If it is necessary to use glass tubes or cuvets, these should be washed well with hydrochloric acid, and preferably a few tubes should be reserved for calcium determinations alone.

Reagents:
1. Cresolphthalein complexone (CPC) reagent, 0.063 mmole/L
   Add 40 mg cresolphthalein to a small beaker, followed by 1 ml concentrated hydrochloric acid. Swirl it until it dissolves, and then rinse it into a 1 L volumetric flask with 1 dl dimethyl sulfoxide. Add 2.5 g 8-hydroxyquinoline and 1 dl water. When all the material has dissolved, dilute to 1 L with water and mix well.
2. Diethylamine solution, 0.4 mole/L
   Dissolve 40 ml reagent grade diethylamine and 0.5 g potassium cyanide in water to make 1 L.
3. EGTA solution, 0.13 mole/L
   Dissolve 0.5 g ethyleneglycol-bis-(β-aminoethyl ether)-N, N^1-tetraacetic acid (EGTA) in water to make 1 dl.

4. Stock calcium standard, 100 mg/dl = 25 mmole/L

   Dissolve exactly 2.500 g pure calcium carbonate (National Bureau of Standards, SRM-915) in 1 dl water and 8 ml concentrated hydrochloric acid by warming. When all the carbonate has dissolved, rinse into a 1 L volumetric flask and dilute to the mark with water.

5. Working standard, 10 mg/dl, 2.5 mmole/L

   Dilute the stock solution 1:10 with water.

Procedure: Add 20 μl serum or standard to 1.0 ml CPC reagent contained in a plastic tube. Mix and then add 1.0 ml diethylamine solution. Mix and allow to stand for a few minutes. Read at 575 nm against a blank of a mixture of equal volumes of the two reagents.

With turbid, hyperlipemic, or hemolyzed samples, a correction may be made. Add 20 μl EGTA solution to both blank and sample and read again. Subtract any absorbance obtained from that of the initial readings. The absorbance of the sample is corrected as below if required. The method is linear to 20 mg/dl.

Calculation:

$$\frac{\text{Absorbance of sample}}{\text{Absorbance of standard}} \times \frac{\text{Conc.}}{\text{of standard}} = \frac{\text{Conc.}}{\text{of sample}}$$

Colorimetric determination of urine calcium

The colorimetric method for serum calcium can also be used with urine. Because of the wider range of the concentration of calcium in urine it may be necessary to make a dilution of the urine to bring the concentration of calcium in the sample to not more than about 15-20 mg/dl, which is 3.8-5.0 mmole/L. Because of the simplicity of the procedure it is easy to make a preliminary reading on the undiluted urine and then to make a dilution if needed.

Procedure: Since some calcium may be precipitated in alkaline urine, this must first be dissolved. Measure the total volume of the well-mixed urine and withdraw an aliquot to about 10 ml. Acidify with a few drops of concentrated hydrochloric acid to a pH of about 1 (wide-range paper). Warm the acidified mixture for about 15 min at 60° C, mixing occasionally. Then determine the urine calcium as for serum calcium using 20 μl sample. If the absorbance of the sample is more than twice that of the standard, dilute the urine and run again.

Calculation: The calculation is the same as for serum, multiplying by any dilution factor.

$$\frac{\text{Absorbance of sample}}{\text{Absorbance of standard}} \times \frac{\text{Conc.}}{\text{of standard}} = \frac{\text{Conc.}}{\text{of sample}}$$

Then

mg/dl calcium × 10 × volume of urine (L) = mg excreted

or

mmole/L × volume (L) = mmole excreted

Special procedure for patients on EDTA or other chelators: A problem may be encountered in the determination of calcium with patients who have been treated with EDTA, which interferes with the colorimetric (but not the atomic absorption) method for calcium. In this case the calcium may first be separated by precipitation as the oxalate.

Additional reagents:

1. Ammonium oxalate, 0.7 mole/L

   Dissolve 10 g ammonium oxalate in water to make 1 dl.

2. Hydrochloric acid, 1 mole/L

   Dissolve 8.3 ml concentrated hydrochloric acid in water to make 1 dl.

3. Acetic acid, 1.6 mole/L

   Dissolve 10 ml glacial acetic acid in water to make 1 dl.

4. Sodium citrate, 0.05 mole/L

   Dissolve 1.5 g sodium citrate dihydrate in water to make 1 dl.

5. Ammonium hydroxide, concentrated

6. Bromcresol green indicator

   Dissolve 0.1 g in 1 dl 95% ethanol.

Procedure: Place 1 ml serum or urine in a 15 ml conical centrifuge tube. Add 0.2 ml ammonium oxalate solution. Add 2 drops of the indicator, then ammonium hydroxide by drops to a green color. Then add acetic acid by drops with mixing until the color just changes to yellow. Heat the tube in a boiling water bath for 15 min; then cool and centrifuge. Decant off the supernatant and invert the tube on filter paper to drain completely. Dissolve the precipitate in 0.5 ml of 1 mole/L hydrochloric acid. Then add 0.5 ml citrate solution and mix. Treat 20 μl of this like the original sample. Since 1 ml of the original sample is made up to 1 ml, there is no change in the calculations.

Determination by atomic absorption

Calcium may also be determined by flame photometry[4,5] or by atomic absorption spectrophotometry.[6-8] The flame emission photometric methods suffer from interference by sodium and require the addition of normal amounts of sodium (140 mEq/L) to standards and blanks. These methods generally have been superseded by advances in atomic absorption instrumentation.

Principle: When a dilute solution of calcium is introduced into a hot flame the element dissociates from its chemical bonds as free atoms of calcium. If a light beam from a hollow calcium cathode lamp is passed through the flame, some of the light at 422.7 nm will be absorbed by the calcium atoms as they are excited to higher energy levels. The decrease in light intensity is proportional to the calcium concentration. The air-acetylene fuel generally used is not hot enough to dissociate some fractory compounds of calcium such as the phosphates or sulfates. Lanthanum or strontium solutions are added to the dilution medium, since these ions bind phosphates and sulfates more strongly than calcium. Lanthanum is preferred, since it forms a tighter complex than strontium with phosphate. Acid is also added to the dilution medium to release calcium from the protein and eliminate protein precipitation. Hydrochloric acid appears to be superior to nitric, phosphoric, or trichloracetic acids for this purpose.

Since serum contains large amounts of protein, which binds calcium, alternative methods have been proposed that precipitate the protein and free the bound calcium; however, the losses on precipitation and volume displacement errors are avoided by direct measurement on large dilutions (e.g., 1:50 or 1:100) with lanthanum solution. The details of the procedure vary somewhat with the instrument used, but some general directions can be given.

Reagents:
1. Stock lanthanum, 50 g/L La (0.36 mole/L) in 3 moles/L HCl
   Place 58.7 g high purity La_2O_3 and 5 dl water in a 1 L volumetric flask. Add 250 ml concentrated HCl and mix until clear. Cool and dilute to the mark with water.
2. Working lanthanum diluent, 1.0 g/L La (7.2 mmole/L) in 60 mmole/L HCl
   Dilute 20 ml stock lanthanum solution to 1 L with water.
3. Blank reagent
   Place 8.2 g NaCl, 0.373 g KCl, and 0.072 g Na_2HPO_4 in a 1 L volumetric flask. Add water to the mark and dissolve. The solution contains 140 mmole/L Na, 5.0 mmole/L K, and 1.4 mg/dl P.
4. Stock calcium standard, 100 mg/dl Ca (25 mmole/L) in 60 mmole/L HCl
   Add 2.5 g dry $CaCO_3$ (National Bureau of Standards, SRM-915) to a 1 L volumetric flask containing 3 dl water and 5 ml concentrated HCl. Mix until clear; then cool and dilute to the mark with water.
5. Working calcium standard, 10 mg/dl Ca (2.5 mmole/L)
   Dilute 10.0 ml stock calcium standard to 1 dl using volumetric glassware and the blank reagent.

General procedure: Turn on the atomic absorption instrument and follow the manufacturer's directions for lighting and adjusting the burner and flow rates. Set the wavelength for 422.7 nm.

Prepare a blank by diluting 0.1 ml blank reagent with 9.9 ml working lanthanum diluent, and zero the instrument while aspirating this solution. Dilute samples, controls, and standards by using 0.1 and 9.9 ml working lanthanum diluent. No calculation is necessary, because most instruments have direct readouts in concentration terms. The procedure is linear to approximately 20 mg/dl Ca on several instruments, but it is best to determine the linearity limits by running several samples over a wide range of concentrations.

Procedure for urine calcium: These same methods may also be used for urine, although a further dilution may be required. There may be some interference from the large amount of phosphate present in spite of the added lanthanum. This is not a serious problem, because it is not necessary to know the urine calcium to the same degree of precision as in the serum calcium procedure.

Ionized calcium[9-12]

About half of the calcium present in the serum is bound to proteins in a nondiffusible form. A small amount of the remainder is complexed with citrate or phosphate, and the rest is present as ionized calcium (Ca^{++}). Only the ionized calcium is physiologically ac-

tive. Thus it would seem more logical to measure the ionized calcium rather than the total, unless the two were always present in the same ratio (which they are not). However, the measurement of ionized calcium is not as simple as that of total calcium.

Calculation from protein and calcium content

The amount of ionized calcium has been estimated from the following equation of McLean and Hastings[13]:

$$\text{Ionized calcium (mg/dl)} = \frac{(6 \times C) - P/3}{P + 6}$$

where C is the total calcium concentration in milligrams per deciliter and P is the total protein content in grams per deciliter. This equation does not hold too well for abnormal sera, which are of most interest.

Determination with calcium ion electrode

The amount of ionized calcium is readily determined by the use of the calcium electrode, although the sample must be treated anaerobically and processed and measured without delay. The measurement is sensitive to both temperature and pH. These instruments are now readily available and quite reliable. However, they are relatively expensive, and since measurement of ionized calcium is of value in only a small proportion of the patients in a general hospital, the instrument would have a place in only the larger institutions.

Determination by membrane filtration

Recently a disposable membrane filtration system has become available (Worthington Biochemical Corp., Freehold, N.J.). A sample of serum is filtered through a special membrane, and the calcium is determined on the filtrate by any conventional total calcium method. Since the filtration process is fairly rapid, the equilibrium between protein and calcium is not greatly disturbed, and calcium determined on the filtrate is similar to results determined by ion-specific electrodes. The device should allow any hospital doing calcium determinations to do ionized calcium determinations.

Normal values and interpretation
Serum calcium

The normal range of total calcium in serum is 8.9-10.3 mg/dl (2.2-2.6 mmole/L).[14] Increases in serum calcium are relatively uncommon. The highest values are found in hyperparathyroidism, in which values of 20 mg/dl (5 mmole/L) may be reached, although individuals with this condition may have values under 12 mg/dl (3 mmole/L). Excesssive administration of vitamin D or ingestion of large amounts of milk and alkali as treatment for peptic ulcers may also raise the serum calcium value to 15 mg/dl (3.8 mmole/L) at times. Similar values may also be reached in some cases of multiple myeloma and in carcinoma metastatic to bones. A number of tumors exhibit parathyroid-like activity leading to hypercalcemia.

Low values are found in hypoparathyroidism, in which the concentration may be as low as 6 mg/dl (1.5 mmole/L). Values do not fall this low in diseases involving impaired calcium absorption. In rickets the phosphorus concentration is depressed, but the calcium value may be normal or only slightly lowered to around 8 mg/dl (2 mmole/L). A low serum calcium value is found in adults with rickets and osteomalacia. In steatorrhea the serum calcium value is normal or only slightly lowered. In advanced renal failure the high inorganic phosphate concentration is accompanied by a lowered calcium concentration that may be as low as 6 mg/dl (1.5 mmole/L). In conditions in which the serum protein valve is increased or decreased from normal values there is often an accompanying increase or decrease in calcium concentration. Since about one half of the calcium in the serum is bound to protein, one might expect that decreased protein values, for example, would result in decreased amounts of calcium in the serum. There has been considerable discussion in the medical literature as to whether one should "correct" the measured calcium value for the lowered protein to give a better indication of the "true" calcium status. Thus it has been found that there is a good correlation between the calcium result and that of albumin (the calcium is bound chiefly by the albumin). A correction of 0.09 mg/dl of calcium may be added to the determined calcium for every 0.1 g/dl the albumin level is below 4.6 g/dl and the same proportion subtracted when the albumin is above this value,[15,16] but not all investigators are convinced of the value of the correction.[17] It would seem preferable to measure the ionized calcium by using the membrane filtration technic and thus determine the actual calcium status directly rather than make an approximate correction.

Ionized calcium

Normal values for ionized calcium measured by the calcium ion–specific electrode are 4.7-5.5 mg/dl (1.175-1.375 mmole/L)[9] or about 48-56% of total calcium. A better correlation of ionized calcium concentration (than total calcium concentration) and disease state was found by Ladenson and Bowers[10] in a series of patients with various types of hyperparathyroid disease.

Urine calcium

The normal range for urine calcium is 50-250 mg (1.3-6.3 mmole) per day. The amount varies with the calcium in the diet, and unless this is at least approximately known, the measurement of the output is not of great value.

INORGANIC PHOSPHORUS

Although most of the phosphorus in blood exists as inorganic **phosphate** or organic **phosphate esters** because of the diversity of compounds, it is usually reported as phosphorus (P) but often spoken of as phosphates. The phosphorus in blood exists in a number of different types of compounds, which include (1) **inorganic phosphate,** the phosphates of alkalies, and alkaline earths; (2) **lipid phosphate** and phosphorus in such lipid substances as lecithin, cephalin, and sphingomyelin; and (3) organic or **ester phosphate,** including glycerophosphate, hexose phosphate, nucleotide phosphate, etc. Ester phosphates are chiefly in the cells, whereas the other two groups of compounds are present in somewhat similar concentrations in the cells

and plasma. Usually determinations are made only of inorganic phosphorus and lipid phosphorus; proteins are precipitated with trichloroacetic acid, and phosphate is determined in the filtrate. In an acid solution, phosphate together with molybdate (or tungstate) produces a blue color in the presence of a reducing agent. Many of the phosphate methods differ mainly in the use of different molybdate and acid concentrations and different compounds as the reducing agent.

Organic phosphates, which are susceptible to hydrolysis, are found chiefly in erythrocytes, and the inorganic phosphate content of whole blood can increase markedly on standing at room temperature. Hence the serum should be separated from the cells as soon as possible. After separation the inorganic phosphate content of serum or plasma is stable for several days in the refrigerator. Acidified urine is quite stable for phosphate when kept in the refrigerator. To determine phosphate in urine the specimen must be acidified before sampling to dissolve any precipitated calcium or magnesium phosphates.

Two methods for the determination of inorganic phosphate are given.

Determination of inorganic phosphate with acid filtrate

Principle: Serum proteins are precipitated by means of trichloroacetic acid, and the phosphate is converted to a phosphomolybdate complex. The addition of *p*-phenylenediamine and sodium bisulfite reduces the phosphomolybdate complex to a blue-colored complex. The absorbance of the blue complex at 690 nm is proportional to the serum phosphate concentration. In this method the trichloroacetic acid used to precipitate the proteins is combined with the molybdate solution, so that only two reagents are needed.[18]

Reagents:
1. Acid molybdate.
   Cautiously add 30 ml concentrated sulfuric acid to about 60 ml water. Cool and dissolve in this 5 g ammonium molybdate (82% MoO_3) and dilute to 1 dl.
2. Trichloroacetic acid, 30%.
   See discussion of precipitating reagents.
3. Combined reagent.
   Mix 3 volumes of acid molybdate, 2 volumes of 30% trichloroacetic acid, and 4 volumes of water.
4. Reducing agent.
   Dissolve 0.5 g *p*-phenylenediamine hydrochloride and 5 g sodium bisulfite ($Na_2S_2O_5$) in water and dilute to 1 dl.
5. Phosphorus standard:
   a. Stock standard, 50 mg/dl P(16.1 mmole/L).
      Dissolve 0.439 g anhydrous potassium dihydrogen phosphate (KH_2PO_4) in water to make 2 dl. (For a standard containing 15 mmole/L use 0.408 g of the salt.)
   b. Working standard. Dilute the stock 1:10 to give a standard containing 5 mg/dl (1.61 mmole/L).

Procedure: In centrifuge tubes add 0.2 ml sample, standard, or water (blank). To each tube, add 1.8 ml combined reagent, mix well, allow to stand for 5 min, and then centrifuge strongly. Add 1 ml aliquots of the supernatants to separate tubes; then add 4 ml reducing agent to each tube, mix well, allow to stand for 20 min, and read samples and standard against the blank at 690 nm.

Urine samples, diluted if necessary, may be treated similarly.

Calculation:

$$\frac{\text{Absorbance of sample}}{\text{Absorbance of standard}} \times 5 = \text{mg/dl P}$$

For lipid phosphorus see discussion of phospholipid determination.

Direct determination of inorganic phosphate[19]

Principle: A direct method is presented for phosphate that does not require precipitation of the proteins. The phosphomolybdate complex is formed by the addition of the reagent to the serum diluted by the reducing solution. The addition of ethanolamine dissolves the precipitated protein and allows the development of the color. High levels of bilirubin and marked hemolysis cause some interference, but the method is quite suitable for ordinary serum samples.

Reagents:

1. Reducing solution
   Dissolve 5 g *p*-methylaminophenol sulfate and 15 g sodium bisulfite in water to make 1 L. This solution is stable for several months at room temperature.
2. Acid molybdate
   Dissolve 64 g ammonium molybdate (82% MoO_3) and 90 ml concentrated sulfuric acid in water to make 1 L. This solution is stable for several months. It should be discarded if a blue color develops.
3. Monoethanolamine
   A good grade of this reagent should be used. It may darken slightly with age, but this does not interfere with the determination.
4. Phosphorus standard
   The same stock standard as used in the previous method is again diluted 1:10 for a working standard.

Procedure for serum: To a series of tubes that each contain 3 ml reducing solution, add 100 µl standard, serum sample, or water as blank. To each tube add 1 ml molybdate solution and mix well. (The precipitate formed in the tubes containing serum will dissolve on the addition of the ethanolamine.) To each tube now add 0.5 ml ethanolamine and mix well. Pour into spectrophotometer cuvets and allow to stand undisturbed for 10 min. Then read samples and standard against blank at 630 nm.

Agitation after the alkalizing agent is added may cause some loss in blue color. Thus, after mixing well, pour the solutions into the cuvets and allow to stand undisturbed for full color development. Agitation should also be avoided during the readings.

Calculation: The calculation is as usual:

$$\frac{\text{Absorbance of sample}}{\text{Absorbance of standard}} \times \frac{\text{Conc.}}{\text{of standard}} = \frac{\text{Conc.}}{\text{of sample}}$$

Procedure for urine: The method for serum can also be applied to urine. The 24 hr or other collection is well mixed and the volume measured. If is is alkaline, the pH is adjusted to 1-2 (on paper) to dissolve any precipitated phosphates. Depending on the volume a 1:10 or 1:20 dilution of the urine is made with water, and the dilution is treated the same as for serum.

Calculation: The calculation is the same as for serum, with the additional multiplication by the dilution factor. The excretion is given by the following calculation:

mg/dl P × 10 × Urine volume (L) = Total mg P excreted

or

mmole/L P × Urine volume (L) = Total mmole P excreted

Normal values and interpretation

The normal range of inorganic phosphorus in adults is 2.5-4.8 mg/dl (0.8-1.5 mmole/L). The level is from 25-50% higher in growing children. In severe nephritis the inorganic phosphate value may rise as high as 15 mg/dl (5 mmole/L). In rickets the level may be as low as 2 mg/dl (0.65 mmole/L) or less. In hyperparathyroidism the level is also decreased to about this same concentration. A moderate increase in the value occurs in hypoparathyroidism. The product of the concentrations of calcium and inorganic phosphate appears to be more constant than the concentration of either, so that a fall in the concentration of one usually means an increase in the concentration of the other. Some decrease to below 3 mg/dl (1 mmole/L) occurs in active carbohydrate metabolism because of the utilization of phosphates in the glucose metabolic cycle and the absorption of glucose into the cells as during a glucose tolerance test.

The use of purgatives or enemas containing large amounts of sodium phosphate causes an increase in the amount of inorganic phosphate in the serum. The value may increase as much as 5 mg/dl (1.5 mmole/L) 1-2 hr after the dose, but the increase is usually temporary, rarely lasting more than 4-6 hr. This factor should be kept in mind when abnormal results that cannot be explained otherwise are obtained.

The amount of inorganic phosphate in the urine largely depends on the dietary intake, but the daily excretion is usually about 1 g/day (as P) (300 mmole/d).

Phosphate clearance

Phosphate clearance is increased in hyperparathyroidism and is decreased in hypoparathyroidism. Some tests have been suggested on this basis for the diagnosis of these disease, but they have proved to be of limited value. They are based on the ratio of creatinine clearance to phosphate clearance.

$$R = \frac{\text{Phosphate clearance}}{\text{Creatinine clearance}} = \frac{P_c U_p}{P_p U_c}$$

P and U refer to plasma and urine concentrations, and the subscripts c and p refer to creatinine and phosphate. One index that has been used is the **tubular reabsorbed phosphate** (TRP).

$$\text{TRP} = (1 - R) \times 100$$

The normal values are given as 84-95%. Reduced values occur in hyperparathyroidism.

Another index is the **phosphate excretion index** (PEI).

$$PEI = R - (0.055 \times Serum\ P - 0.07)$$

Normal values range from -0.09 to $+0.09$. Higher values occur in hyperparathyroidism.

MAGNESIUM
Colorimetric determination of magnesium

The following colorimetric method for magnesium is not too accurate, but it may be used if the preferred atomic absorption method is not available.[20-22]

Principle: In alkaline solutions magnesium forms a colored compound (lake) with the dye **titan yellow.** The amount of color formed is proportional to the amount of magnesium present. Since the colored product is actually colloidal in nature and is not a true solution, polyvinyl alcohol is added to stabilize the color. The final solution is rather highly colored even in the absence of any magnesium. If too much dye is present, the blank will be high enough to increase the error in the readings. If too little dye is present, the magnesium color will not develop properly. It may be necessary to experiement with different lots of dye to find the best concentration. In the method presented proteins are first removed by precipitation with trichloroacetic acid.

Reagents:
1. Sodium hydroxide, 2.5 moles/L
   Dissolve about 55 g sodium hydroxide in 5 dl water. Check the concentration by titration with a standard acid and dilute to 2.50 ± 0.05 moles/L.
2. Polyvinyl alcohol, 0.1 g/dl
   Suspend 1 g polyvinyl alcohol (Elvanol 70-05, E.I. DuPont de Nemours & Co., Wilmington, Del.) in about 40 ml ethyl alcohol and pour into about 5 dl water while swirling. Then warm to dissolve and dilute to 1 L.
3. Titan yellow solutions
   a. Stock solution. Dissolve 75 mg titan yellow (Titan yellow, Eastman no. P4454 is the same as Clayton yellow, Eastman no. 1770.) in 1 dl 0.1 g/dl polyvinyl alcohol. Store in a brown bottle. It will remain stable for 2 months at room temperature.
   b. Working solution. Dilute stock solution 1:10 with the polyvinyl alcohol solution as needed. It will remain stable for 1 week when stored in a brown bottle.
4. Trichloroacetic acid, 0.3 mole/L
   Dissolve 25 g trichloroacetic acid in water to make 5 dl.
5. Magnesium standards
   a. Stock standard. Dissolve 2.465 g unefflo-resced crystals of magnesium sulfate ($MgSO_4 \cdot 7H_2O$) in water to make 1 L. This solution contains 20 mEq/L Mg (10 mmole/L). Alternatively, dissolve 2.205 g magnesium gluconate (National Bureau of Standards, SRM-929) in water to make 1 L of 20 mEq/L stock magnesium standard.

   b. Working standard. Dilute the stock solution 1:10 as required to give a solution containing 2 mEq/L (1 mmole/L).

Procedure: To 5 ml (0.3 mole/L) trichloroacetic acid in a test tube, add 1 ml serum and mix. Allow to stand for 10 min and centrifuge for 5 min at 2000 rpm. Pipet 3 ml supernatant for the tests. Also set up a blank with 0.5 ml water and 2.5 ml (0.3 mole/L) trichloroacetic acid and a standard with 0.5 ml diluted standard plus 2.5 ml (0.3 mole/L) trichloroacetic acid. To each tube add 2 ml titan yellow working solution, mix, and add 1 ml (2.5 moles/L) sodium hydroxide. Read standard and samples against the blank at 540 nm. It is preferable to read within 10-15 min after the addition of alkali.

Calculation: Since 1 ml serum is diluted with 5 ml trichloroacetic acid to 6 ml, then 3 ml supernatant is equivalent to 0.5 ml serum. This is treated the same as 0.5 ml working standard containing 2 mEq/L (1 mmole/L). Hence

$$\frac{Absorbance\ of\ sample}{Absorbance\ of\ standard} \times \frac{Conc.}{of\ standard} = \frac{Conc.}{of\ sample}$$

The magnesium content of red cells is about three times that of serum; therefore hemolyzed samples should be avoided. As previously mentioned the optimal amount of dye to use may be determined by experiment. One should also check the linearity of the procedure up to about 5 mEq/L (2.5 mmole/L).

Determination by atomic absorption[23]

General procedure: Preferably magnesium should be determined by atomic absorption. For this a simple dilution of the serum samples with water is satisfactory. It may be convenient to use the same dilution as for calcium (which contains lanthanum), but the addition of lanthanum is not necessary for the determination of magnesium alone. Depending on the sensitivity of the instrument a 1:50 or 1:100 dilution of serum is satisfactory. One merely aspirates dilutions of the serum and standard along with a water blank into the flame and determines the concentration by using the 285.2 nm line of magnesium.

A convenient standard can be made by dissolving 284.8 mg magnesium acetate (Ultrex, no. 4833, J.T. Baker Chemical Co., Phillipsburg, N.J.) in a 1 L volumetric flask with 2 dl water. Add 1 ml glacial acetic acid and dilute to the mark. The standard contains 4.0 mEq/L and can be diluted to give other standards of 1.0, 2.0, and 3.0 mEq/L.

Normal values and interpretation

The normal level of serum magnesium in adults is 1.5-2.2 mEq/L (0.75-1.10 mmole/L). In the older literature results may be expressed as 1.8-2.6 mg/dl. About 30% of the serum magnesium is bound to albumin, and the remaining 70% is free or ionized magnesium. At birth, magnesium values are approximately 0.2 mEq/L lower than adult values, but adult values are reached after 7 days.[24] Decreased magnesium concentrations have been found in the malabsorption syndrome, acute pancreatitis, and chronic alcoholism. Increased concentrations have been found in dehydration, severe diabetic acidosis, and Addison's disease. Decreased kidney function leading to decreased magnesium excretion may lead to high serum values.

Thiazide diuretics and ethacrynic acid cause an increase in urine magnesium excretion and may lead to low serum values. Large doses of magnesium-containing products (antacids, milk of magnesia) can lead to markedly elevated serum values in patients with renal insufficiency. Gluconic acid (given as calcium gluconate) may interfere with the color reaction in the colorimetric method for magnesium, leading to erroneously low results.

Urine magnesium

Little is known concerning the significance of urine magnesium. Its determination may be helpful in assessing magnesium deficiency states, since the plasma value does not ordinarily fall below 1 mEq/L until at least 25% of the cellular magnesium has been lost. The titan yellow method could probably be adapted to urinary determinations, and the analysis could certainly be done by atomic absorption. The 24 hr urine excretion of magnesium is between 6 and 9 mEq when the patient is on a normal diet.

IRON AND IRON-BINDING CAPACITY
General principles

Iron is transported in the serum from the point of absorption in the intestines to the point of use in the erythropoietic system in combination with a fraction of the β-globulins known as **transferrin.** This is the iron available for the formation of hemoglobin and that measured in serum iron determinations. Usually the transferrin is not saturated with iron; i.e., it could absorb and transport much more iron than is actually in the serum. The amount of iron that the protein could absorb to be fully saturated is the latent or **unsaturated iron-binding capacity** (UIBC). Thus serum iron added to unsaturated iron-binding capacity gives the **total iron-binding capacity** (TIBC) (serum iron + UIBC = TIBC).

The serum iron may be determined by adding acid to split the iron from the protein and trichloroacetic acid to precipitate the proteins. The iron is determined in the supernatant by a colorimetric procedure. Since the usual reagents give the color only with ferrous iron, a reducing agent is added. Also, the pH of the strongly acid supernatant must be adjusted to around 3.0-5.0 (depending on the particular color reagent used). The buffer commonly used for this is sodium acetate. In another procedure the iron is split from the protein at a controlled pH such that the proteins will not be precipitated and the color developed in the solution will still contain the proteins. This requires a serum blank to compensate for the absorption by the serum. In lipemic serum or reconstituted control sera the turbidity may be very high with a consequently high blank, a disadvantage of this method.

Determination of serum iron[25]

There are two general methods for the determination of serum iron. In one the iron is split off from the serum-binding proteins by hydrochloric acid and the proteins precipitated with trichloroacetic acid. After centrifugation the iron is determined colorimetrically with any of several chromogens in the supernatant. This is the more accurate procedure and has been recommended as the reference method by the International Committee for Standardization in Hematology.[26] The disadvantages are that it is a rather lengthy procedure and unless very pure reagents are used a high blank is obtained. In the second method the iron is determined directly on the serum without precipitation of the proteins. A correction is made for the absorbance caused by the serum. In slightly hemolyzed, hyperlipemic, or other turbid serum samples, including most lyophilized serum samples, which are often used as controls, the correction for serum absorbance can be relatively high, and a decrease in the accuracy is found. The sensitive color reagents for iron react only with ferrous iron, and a reducing agent must be included. In the methods that are presented here ascorbic acid is used as the reductant.

A very good grade of deionized or distilled water must be used for all reagents. Iron free solutions of some reagents can be obtained from some suppliers (G. Frederick Smith Co., Columbus, Ohio), but good grades of analytic grade reagents are generally satisfactory. Sometimes it may be necessary to try several lots of a reagent produced by several different manufacturers to obtain one with a satisfactory low blank. Glassware and plasticware should be rinsed with dilute nitric acid (1:4) and then copiously rinsed with distilled water. Disposable plastic tubes can be used without treatment and are generally preferred for use whenever possible.

Serum iron with protein precipitation

First a method is presented for determination of serum iron using a trichloroacetic acid precipitation.[27]

Reagents:
1. Trichloroacetic acid–hydrochloric acid reagent
   Dissolve 50 g trichloroacetic acid in about 3 dl water in a 5 dl volumetric flask. After the acid has dissolved, add 60 ml concentrated hydrochloric acid and dilute to 5 dl with water.
2. Sodium acetate solution, 2 moles/L
   Dissolve 136 g sodium acetate trihydrate in water and dilute to 5 dl.
3. Sodium acetate–ascorbic acid reagent
   Just before use dissolve 250 mg ascorbic acid in 50 ml sodium acetate solution.
4. Stock iron standard, 50 mg/dl (8.96 mmole/L Fe)
   Dissolve exactly 250 mg pure iron (National Bureau of Standards, SRM-937) in about 3 ml concentrated hydrochloric acid in a 5 dl volumetric flask. When all the iron has dissolved, dilute to 5 dl with water, or dissolve 1.755 g pure reagent grade $Fe(NH_4)_2(SO_4)_2 \cdot 6H_2O$ in water with a few drops of concentrated hydrochloric acid and dilute to 5 dl.
5. Iron intermediate standard, 5 mg/dl (0.9 mmole/L)
   Dilute 10 ml stock to 1 dl with water.
6. Iron working standards
   Dilute 1, 2, 3, and 4 ml of the intermediate standard to 1 dl with water. These will give solutions containing 50, 100, 150, and 200 µg/dl Fe. These

solutions may be used to check the calibration curve and linearity. Routinely one would use only the 100 μg/dl (~20 μmole/L) standard.

7. Ferrozine reagent

Dissolve 250 mg ferrozine (Hack Chemical Co., Ames, Iowa) (3-[2-pyridyl]-5, 6-bis[4-phenylsulfonic acid]-1,2,4-triazine) in water in a 50 ml volumetric flask. Then dilute to the mark and mix well. The solution is stable for a few months when stored in a brown bottle.

Procedure: Into plastic tubes labeled "blank," "test," and "standard" pipet respectively 1 ml water, 1 ml serum, and 1 ml standard (100 μg/dl Fe or 20 μmole/L Fe, as desired). To each tube add 1 ml trichloroacetic acid–hydrochloric acid reagent and mix on a Vortex mixer. Allow the tubes to stand for 20 min at room temperature. Then centrifuge tubes containing serum (blank and standard need not be centrifuged) at 2000 rpm for 10 min. The supernatant in the serum tube should be perfectly clear. If it is hazy, heat the tube to 56° C for 15 min and then recentrifuge. Transfer 1 ml supernatant from each tube to other suitably labeled tubes. To each tube add 1 ml sodium acetate–ascorbic acid followed by 0.3 ml ferrozine reagent. Mix the contents of the tubes and allow them to stand for 10 min at room temperature. Read the sample and standard tubes against the blank at 562 nm. The amounts of all the solutions may be proportionately increased if larger volumes are required for the cuvets used.

Calculation:

$$\frac{\text{Absorbance of sample}}{\text{Absorbance of standard}} \times \frac{\text{Conc.}}{\text{of standard}} = \frac{\text{Conc.}}{\text{of sample}}$$

The concentration of standard usually used is 100 μg/dl Fe (or 20 μmole/L Fe).

Serum iron without precipitation[28]

Principle: This method is simple and rapid and requires less serum than the previous one, but it is not as accurate. It may give somewhat high results on slightly hemolyzed, hyperlipemic, or turbid serum samples. The serum is treated with a pH 4.5 acetate buffer, which splits off the iron without precipitating the proteins. A blank absorbance measurement is made to correct for the absorbance of the serum, then the color reagent is added, and after color development a second reading is taken.

Reagents:

1. Acetate buffer, 0.8 mole/L, pH 4.5
   Dissolve 42.9 g sodium acetate trihydrate and 28.3 ml glacial acetic acid in about 8 dl water. Check the pH and, if necessary, adjust the pH to 4.5 by the addition of small amounts of sodium acetate or acetic acid as required. Then transfer to a 1 L volumetric flask, dilute to the mark with water, and mix well.

2. Acetate-ascorbate solution
   Just before use dissolve 250 mg ascorbic acid in 50 ml acetate buffer.

3. Iron standards
   Same as in the previous method.

4. Ferrozine solution
   Same as in the previous method.

Procedure: The reaction is carried out directly in the spectrophotometer cuvets. To each of a number of cuvets add 1.5 ml acetate-ascorbate solution. Then to properly labeled tubes add 0.3 ml water (blank), 0.3 ml iron working standard, and 0.3 ml serum. Read the absorbance of the cuvet containing the serum against the blank at 562 nm. Record this reading as A(serum blank). Now add 0.2 ml ferrozine reagent to each cuvet and mix. Place the cuvets in a water bath at 42° C for 20 min (40 min at 37° C may be used, but this may yield less consistent results). Then carefully wipe the cuvets dry and allow them to stand at room temperature for 10 min. Read the serum and standard cuvets against the blank at 562 nm, giving readings recorded as A(serum) and A(standard).

Calculation:

$$\frac{\text{A(serum)} - 0.9 \text{ A(serum blank)}}{\text{A(standard)}} \times \frac{\text{Conc.}}{\text{of standard}} = \frac{\text{Conc.}}{\text{of sample}}$$

The serum blank is multiplied by a factor of 0.9, since the solution is diluted between readings. If the cuvets require a larger volume of solution, one may use 2.5 ml acetate-ascorbate, 0.5 ml serum and standard, and 0.3 ml ferrozine reagent.

Determination of serum iron–binding capacity
Serum iron–binding capacity[28]

The first method is a direct method in which the serum is mixed with a buffer at a pH of 7.8. A known excess of iron is then added to saturate the transferrin in serum. At this pH the excess iron not bound to the serum will react with the color reagent, but the iron bound to the serum will not react. The difference between the known amount of added iron and that determined after binding represents the iron bound by the serum, the latent (LIBC) or unsaturated (UIBC) iron-binding capacity.

Reagents:

1. Tris buffer, 0.2 mole/L, pH 7.8
   Dissolve 24.2 g tris(hydroxymethyl)aminomethane in about 7 dl water. Add diluted hydrochloric acid (165 ml concentrated acid diluted to 1 L) to bring the pH to 7.8 (about 60 ml is required in all); then dilute to 1 L.

2. Tris-ascorbate buffer
   Just before use dissolve 250 mg ascorbic acid in 50 ml tris buffer.

3. Ferrozine reagent
   Same as in the previous methods.

4. Iron standards
   Same intermediate standards as described earlier. From this a working standard containing 400 μg/dl Fe (or 80 μmole/L Fe) is prepared by diluting the intermediate standard 4 ml to 50 ml with water.

Procedure: To each of a number of cuvets add 1.5 ml tris-ascorbate buffer. Then to appropriately labeled cuvets add 0.3 ml water (reagent blank), 0.1 ml water and 0.2 ml working standard (standard), and 0.1 ml serum and 0.2 ml working standard (sample). After thorough mixing incubate the tubes at 42° C for 10 min. Then read the absorbance of the sample cuvet against water at 562 nm and record as A(sample blank). Add 0.2 ml ferrozine reagent to each tube, mix the contents, and incubate the tubes at 42° C for 20 min more. Allow the cuvets to stand at room temperature for 10 min. Then read the standard and samples against the reagent blank at 562 nm, recording the results as A(sample) and A(standard).

Calculation:

$$\text{Serum UIBC} = B - \frac{A(\text{sample}) - 0.9\,A(\text{sample blank})}{A(\text{standard})} \times B$$

where the result will be in micrograms per deciliter when B is taken as 800 (twice the 400 µg/dl Fe standard) or in micromoles per liter when B is taken as 160 (twice the 80 µmole/L Fe standard). The value of B is taken as twice that of the standard, since 0.2 ml standard is compared with 0.1 ml serum. The total iron-binding capacity is calculated as follows:

$$\text{TIBC} = \text{UIBC} + \text{Serum iron}$$

Serum iron–binding capacity, resin method[29]

The following method for serum iron–binding capacity, which can also be used for serum iron, uses an ion-exchange resin to separate the serum saturated with iron from the excess iron before colorimetric determination. Serum iron can also be determined by omitting the addition of the saturating iron solution. Although this method has no precipitating step, it gives good results with most turbid or lipemic serum samples.

Reagents:
1. Sodium chloride–bicarbonate solution
   Dissolve 8.2 g NaCl and 1.68 g $NaHCO_3$ in water to make 1 L.
2. Saturating iron solution
   a. Stock iron. Dissolve 810 mg $FeCl_3 \cdot 6H_2O$ and 1.2 ml concentrated hydrochloric acid in water to make 2 dl.
   b. Stock tartrate solution. Dissolve 18.5 g ammonium tartrate in water to make 1 dl. These two stock solutions are stable.
   c. Saturating solution (about 0.75 mmole/L). On the day of use mix together 0.1 ml iron solution (a), 0.4 ml water, and 0.1 ml tartrate solution (b).
3. Disodium catechol-3,5-disulfonate (CDS)
   Dissolve 630 mg of the salt (sold as a reagent for iron under the name of Tiron [Fisher Scientific Co., Pittsburgh]) in water to make 1 dl. This solution is stable for about 1 week in the refrigerator. Just before use mix together 1 volume of the CDS solution with 9 volumes of the sodium chloride–bicarbonate solution.
4. Ferrozine solution
   Prepare an acetate buffer by dissolving 10.9 g sodium acetate trihydrate and 13.8 ml glacial acetic acid in water to make 1 dl. Just before use dissolve 23 mg ferrozine and 88 mg ascorbic acid in 5 ml acetate buffer.
5. Iron standard
   Same standards as used in the previous methods.

Routinely only the 100 µg/dl Fe (or 20 µmole/L Fe) standard is used.
6. DEAE cellulose
   Mix thoroughly 4 g DEAE cellulose A-50 with about 2 dl sodium chloride–bicarbonate solution in a 250 ml cylinder. Allow the cellulose to settle, and decant off or aspirate the supernatant. Repeat the washing six times to thoroughly equilibriate the cellulose with the solution. The cellulose is finally made up into a slurry with the sodium chloride–bicarbonate solution such that the total volume is about 1.8 times the volume of the settled cellulose. This may be stored in the refrigerator for several months. It should be brought to room temperature before use.

Preparation of columns: The columns are prepared from the barrels of disposable 1 ml plastic syringes. For convenience in adding solutions to these small columns Eppendorf-type pipets are used, with capacities of 0.2, 0.5, and 1.0 ml. A piece of polyvinyl tubing with an internal diameter of about 1.5 mm and which will just fit inside the barrels is attached to the regular tips supplied with the pipets. A length of about 2.5 cm is attached to the 0.2 and 0.5 ml pipets, and a length of about 8 cm is attached to the tip of the 1 ml pipet.

A small disk of acid-washed filter paper is placed in the syringe barrel next to the tip and the barrel clamped in a vertical position with the tip down. One milliliter of the well-mixed suspension of the DEAE cellulose is taken up in the tubing attached to the tip of the 1 ml pipet. The end of the tubing is pushed down to the bottom of the barrel, and the suspension is delivered slowly while raising the tubing, so that no air bubbles are trapped in the suspension. After excess liquid has drained from the column, 0.25 ml CDS solution is added to the column. Then sufficient additional cellulose is added to the column in the same manner, so that a column of 0.8-0.9 ml is formed (about 0.6-0.7 ml additional suspension will be needed). The column is then washed with 0.5 ml sodium chloride–bicarbonate solution. In the preparation of the columns and the subsequent additions the solutions must be added slowly, 10-15 sec for the addition of 0.5 ml, with minimal disturbance of the column. The columns should be used within 90 min after preparation. They are conveniently prepared while the serum is incubating with the saturating solution (see below).

Procedure: To 0.5 ml serum add 0.1 ml saturating solution and allow to stand for 30 min. Then add 0.5 ml of the mixture to a column and collect all the eluate in a tube, or preferably in the spectrophotometer cuvet. When the last traces of liquid have disappeared from the top of the column, add five successive 0.5 ml portions of the sodium chloride–bicarbonate solution to the column, allowing each portion to enter the column completely before adding the next. Collect all the eluate in the same tube as used for the first eluate. As noted above, add each portion slowly over a 10-15 sec interval. If it is desired to run the serum iron by this method, add 0.5 ml serum without prior treatment to a column, and follow the same elution procedure.

A standard tube is set up containing 1 ml standard (usually 100 µg/dl Fe or 20 µmole/L Fe) and 2 ml water and a blank tube containing 3 ml water. If any of the eluate tubes appears colored, the absorbance of this solution can be measured as a serum blank by reading against water at 562 nm. If the solutions appear colorless a serum blank need not be run. Add 0.1 ml ferrozine solution to each tube and mix. Allow the tubes to stand at room temperature for 20 min. The standard and the eluates are read against the blank at 562 nm.

Calculation:

$$\frac{A_x}{A_s} \times 2 \times C = \text{Serum iron concentration}$$

and

$$\frac{A_x}{A_s} \times C \times 2 \times \frac{6}{5} = \text{Total iron-binding capacity}$$

where A_x is the absorbance of the sample (corrected by subtracting any serum blank) and A_s is the absorbance of the standard. C is the concentration of the standard, usually 100 μg/ml Fe or 20 μmole/L Fe. The factor of 2 arises from the fact that 1 ml of standard is compared with 0.5 ml of serum, and the additional factor of 6/5 for the iron binding arises from the fact that 0.5 ml of serum is mixed with 0.1 ml of the saturating solution and only 0.5 ml of this is added to the column. Note that here the total iron saturation is measured and again: UIBC = TIBC − Serum iron.

Normal values

The normal range of serum iron generally is 70-150 μg/dl Fe (12.5-27.0 μmole/L) in men and about 10-15% lower in women, but recent studies[30] indicate that normal individuals may actually have a somewhat wider range than this. Lower values are found in patients with hyperchromic anemias and often in individuals suffering from various infectious diseases. High values have been found in patients with those anemias characterized by decreased hemoglobin production not caused by iron deficiency, such as pernicious anemia.

At birth the serum iron value is somewhat higher, 150-200 μg/dl (27-36 μmole/L), but it falls rapidly to below the adult value and does not regain this concentration for several years. A diurnal variation occurs in serum iron concentration, which can be as much as 50% or more. It is highest in the morning, 8:00 AM to noon, and falls during the day, reaching the lowest value between 8:00 PM and midnight. There appear to be other random fluctuations in the serum iron concentration as well. A single specimen taken at an unspecified time of the day is not satisfactory. If comparisons are to be made on the serum iron in a patient over a period of time, e.g., in following the course of a disease or the results of therapy, all the samples should be drawn at the same time of day. A convenient time is in the morning when other fasting samples are drawn.

The TIBC averages about 300 μg/dl Fe (54 μmole/L Fe) in normal subjects with about 40% saturation in men and about 35% in women. Rather wide ranges of TIBC have been given by different investigators, so that values of 200-400 μg/dl Fe (36-72 μmole/L Fe) are not considered abnormal. The TIBC is a measure of the iron-binding protein, transferrin, and indirectly storage iron (ferritin). The TIBC is apparently not subject to the large variations found in serum iron values; however, the UIBC will vary with serum iron value.

In iron deficiency anemia the TIBC is normal or even elevated, but if the serum iron value is low, the UIBC is increased and is usually over 300 μg/dl (54 μmole/L) in iron deficiency anemia and under 150 μg/dl (27 μmole/L) in pernicious anemia. In hemochromatosis

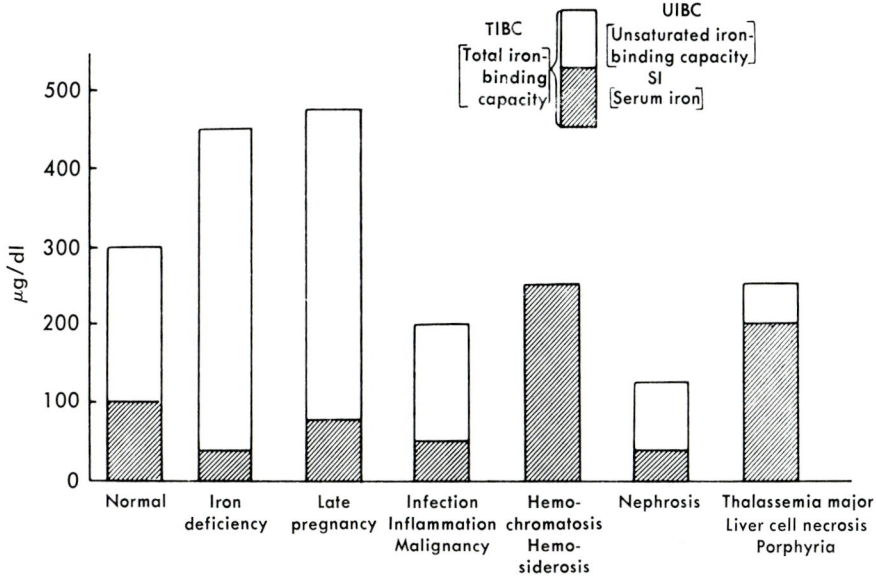

Fig. 22-1. Relationships of serum iron, unsaturated iron-binding capacity, and total iron-binding capacity in various clinical conditions. (From Brown, E.B.: Clinical aspects of iron metabolism, Semin. Hematol. **3:**314, 1966. By permission.)

the serum iron value is markedly elevated (200 μg/dl or 36 μmole/L) and the UIBC is low.

The administration of steroids is said to cause a decrease in the serum iron value, and the use of estrogens and oral contraceptives is claimed to increase iron levels. The administration of EDTA derivatives (as occasionally used in heavy metal poisoning) interferes with the color reactions for iron and iron-binding capacity tests. The parenteral administration of iron compounds causes erroneously high results for possibly several days after the dose.

Transferrin saturation

The percent saturation of serum transferrin can be calculated from the serum iron and TIBC concentrations as follows:

$$\text{Saturation (\%)} = \frac{\text{Iron (μg/dl Fe)}}{\text{TIBC (μg/dl Fe)}} \times 100\%$$

The normal values found are 20-45%, with values in men slightly higher than those in women. Some representative clinical conditions are shown in Fig. 22-1.

Determination of serum iron by atomic absorption

Serum iron has also been determined by atomic absorption spectrophotometry.[31] Because of the low concentration of iron present in serum the use of the direct flame methods presents difficulties, but the "flameless" methods using the carbon graphite furnace show more promise.[32,33]

COPPER

Although the exact role of copper in the body has not been completely explained, it probably acts as an essential part of or as an activator for a number of enzymes. Most of the serum copper is combined with a transport protein known as ceruloplasmin, which is probably related to or identical to the enzyme ferroxidase I. This enzyme is probably one of those involved in the production of hemoglobin, as it has been known for many years that copper is necessary for hematopoiesis. However, serum copper is not generally determined in the study of the anemias. A small amount (about 6%) is bound to albumin and forms the direct reacting pool of copper in serum.

A problem in the determination of copper, as well as iron, zinc, and other trace metals, is the elimination of contamination from the measuring reagents and glassware. Deionized water is used in the preparation of reagents, and it may be helpful to try several different brands of analytic reagents if unduly high blanks are obtained. Glassware is a frequent source of contamination. Preferably, disposable plastic tubes and pipets should be used, as well as plastic syringes for blood collection. For copper and zinc, stainless steel needles should be used if available. Any glassware used should be rinsed well with diluted nitric acid (1:10) and then rinsed well with deionized water.

Determination of serum or urine copper[34]

Hydrochloric acid is added to split the copper from the serum proteins. The latter are then precipitated with trichloroacetic acid, and the copper is determined in the filtrate by reaction with the color reagent.

Reagents:
1. Hydrochloric acid, 2 moles/L
   Dilute 165 ml concentrated hydrochloric acid with water to make 1 L.
2. Trichloroacetic acid, 1.38 moles/L
   This is best prepared by dissolving the contents of a ¼ lb bottle of reagent grade trichloroacetic acid in water to make 5 dl.
3. Color reagent
   Dissolve 8 mg dicyclopentamethylenethiuram disulfide (cat. no. 85,778-5, Aldrich Chemical Co., Milwaukee) in 1 dl glacial acetic acid.
4. Copper standard
   Dissolve 1.965 g clear uneffloresced crystals of copper sulfate ($CuSO_4 \cdot 5H_2O$) in water to make 5 dl. This solution contains 100 mg/dl. A fresh working standard (100 μg/dl) is prepared weekly by diluting 1 ml stock to 1 L. If preferred one may use 1.873 g to obtain a stock solution containing 15 mmole/L, which is diluted 1:1000 to obtain a working standard containing 15 μmole/L. Alternatively, one may purchase a standard made up for atomic absorption work that contains 1 mg/ml (or 100 mg/dl).

Procedure: Using a 1 ml disposable plastic pipet, transfer 1 ml serum to a plastic test tube. Similarly set up a standard tube containing 1 ml working standard and a blank tube containing 1 ml water. To each tube add 1 ml acid reagent and mix. Allow to stand at room temperature for 10 min. To each tube add 1 ml precipitating reagent and mix. Cap to prevent evaporation and centrifuge sample tubes. (The blank and standard tubes need not be centrifuged.) Transfer 2 ml supernatant to a second tube and add 1 ml reagent. Mix and read sample and standard against blank at 420 nm 10 min after the addition of the reagent.

Calculation:

$$\frac{\text{Absorbance of sample}}{\text{Absorbance of standard}} \times \frac{\text{Conc.}}{\text{of standard}} = \frac{\text{Conc.}}{\text{of sample}}$$

• • •

The above method may be used for urine, without modification. Occasionally there may be interfering substances that are not removed by the trichloroacetic acid. In that event the following extraction method should be used.

Determination of urine copper by extraction[35]

In this method the copper is complexed with the color reagent and extracted into carbon tetrachloride for separation and color quantitation.

Reagents:
1. Zinc dibenzyldithiocarbamate (DBDC) (K & K Laboratories, Plainview, N.Y.)
   Dissolve 75 mg of this reagent in 5 dl reagent grade carbon tetrachloride.
2. Standard
   Same diluted standard as in the previous method.

Procedure: Pipet 10 ml aliquots of the urine into separate tubes. (If a 24 hr urine specimen is used, it is collected in a plastic container rather than glass.) Add 1 ml concentrated hydrochloric acid to each tube, and heat in a water bath to just below boiling (95° C) for 15 min; then cool and transfer to separate funnels. To one funnel add 5 ml DBDC reagent (urine sample), and to the other add 5 ml carbon tetrachloride (urine blank). Also add to separate funnels 5 ml DBDC reagent plus 1 ml hydrochloric acid and 10 ml water (reagent blank), and in another funnel add 5 ml reagent plus 2 ml dilute copper standard, 8 ml water, and 1 ml hydrochloric acid. Shake funnels vigorously for 1 min. Allow layers to separate; draw off lower layer into separate tubes. Centrifuge tubes briefly to clarify; read in spectrophotometer at 436 nm. Read urine sample against urine blank and standard against reagent blank.

Calculation: Since 2 ml standard is compared with 10 ml urine,

$$\frac{\text{Absorbance of sample}}{\text{Absorbance of standard}} \times \frac{\text{Conc. of standard}}{5} = \frac{\text{Conc.}}{\text{of sample}}$$

Determination of serum copper without precipitation[36]

Principle: In this method copper and iron can be determined simultaneously in 0.4 ml serum without protein precipitation. The sensitive ferrous ion–TPTZ reaction occurs over a narrow pH range, and the iron measurement is made at pH 4.8. The pH is then adjusted to above 8, and copper is allowed to react with the second chromogen in the presence of iron with no extraction or masking steps. The copper and iron are released from protein binding by guanidine hydrochloride, which disrupts the tertiary structure of protein without causing precipitation.

Reagents:
1. Stock TPTZ (G. Frederick Smith Co., Columbus, Ohio), 10 g/L
   Dissolve 100 mg 2,4,6-tripyridyl-s-triazine in 1.0 ml of 1.0 mole/L hydrochloric acid (8.5 ml concentrated hydrochloric acid to 1 dl), and dilute to 10.0 ml with distilled water.
2. Stock tris, 2.0 moles/L
   Dissolve 121.1 g tris(hydroxymethyl)aminomethane in water to make 5 dl.
3. Stock acetate buffer, 2.0 moles/L, pH 4.8
   Dissolve 96.8 g sodium acetate (or 160.5 g sodium acetate trihydrate) and 47.2 ml glacial acetic acid in about 8 dl water. Check the pH and, if necessary, adjust the pH to 4.8 by the addition of small amounts of sodium acetate or acetic acid as required. Transfer to a 1 L volumetric flask, dilute to the mark with water, and mix well.
4. Copper reagent, 1 g/L
   Dissolve 100 mg disodium 2,9-dimethyl-4,7-diphenyl-1,10-phenanthroline disulfonate in stock tris and dilute to 1 dl.
5. Stock guanidine solution, 6.0 moles/L in 0.1 mole/L acetate, pH 4.8
   Dissolve 286 g guanidine hydrochloride and 25 ml stock acetate buffer, pH 4.8, in 4 dl water in a 5 dl volumetric flask. Add 5 ml stock TPTZ solution, dilute to the mark, and mix well.
6. Iron reagent

Dissolve 250 mg ascorbic acid in 50 ml stock guanidine solution just before use, using volumetric glassware.
7. Stock blank solution
   Dissolve 286 g guanidine hydrochloride and 25 ml stock acetate buffer, pH 4.8, in 4 dl water in a 5 dl volumetric flask. Dilute to the mark and mix well.
8. Reagent blank solution
   Dissolve 250 mg ascorbic acid in 50 ml stock blank solution just before use, using volumetric glassware.
9. Standard 100 μg/dl copper and iron
   Prepare this mixed standard by using 2 ml intermediate iron standard and 100 μl stock copper standard, and dilute to 1 dl with volumetric glassware.

Procedure: Prepare a series of plastic tubes as follows:

Solution	Reagent blank (ml)	Standard Fe/Cu (ml)	Sample blank (ml)	Sample (ml)
Serum	—	—	0.2	0.2
Standard	—	0.2	—	—
Water	0.2	—	—	—
Blank reagent	—	—	1.0	—
Iron reagent	1.0	1.0	—	1.0

Allow tubes to stand for 5 min; then pour into labeled cuvets, zero spectrophotometer at 593 nm with the reagent blank, and record the absorbance of the other solutions. Then add to the cuvets:

Solution	Reagent blank (ml)	Standard Fe/Cu (ml)	Sample blank (ml)	Sample (ml)
Tris stock	—	—	0.2	—
Copper reagent	0.2	0.2	—	0.2

Allow to stand for 5 min; then zero spectrophotometer at 485 nm with the reagent blank and record the absorbance of the other solutions.

Calculation:

$$\text{Fe or Cu (μg/dl)} = \frac{A(\text{sample}) - A(\text{sample blank})}{A(\text{standard})} \times 100$$

where A is the absorbance. To calculate Fe results use the absorbance values at 593 nm, and to calculate Cu results use the absorbance values at 485 nm.

Determination of copper by atomic absorption[37,38]

Principle: The direct determination of serum copper by atomic absorption spectrophotometry at 324.7 nm is a simpler, faster, and more precise technic. The addition of glycerol compensates for the low viscosity of the standards in comparison to diluted serum.

Reagents:
1. Glycerol, AR, 10% v/v
   Dilute 1 dl glycerol in a 1 L volumetric flask to the mark with water.
2. Copper, stock standard, 500 μg/ml
   In a 1 L volumetric flask dissolve 0.500 g copper metal in a small volume of 6N hydrochloric acid.

Dilute to the mark with 0.12N hydrochloric acid (1 ml concentrated hydrochloric acid/dl). A similar standard containing 1 mg/ml (1000 μg/ml) is commercially available (Fisher Scientific Co., Pittsburgh).

3. Copper, intermediate standard, 500 μg/dl
   Dilute 10.0 ml stock copper standard to 1 L with 10% glycerol in volumetric glassware.

4. Copper, working standards
   Dilute 5, 10, 15, and 20 ml intermediate copper standard to 50 ml with 10% glycerol in volumetric glassware to give 50, 100, 150, and 200 μg/dl standards. These correspond to apparent concentrations of 100, 200, 300, and 400 μg/dl copper in serum because of the 1:1 dilution.

Procedure: Dilute serum samples with an equal volume of distilled or deionized water. Aspirate the working copper standards and set instrument at 324.7 nm to read apparent concentration directly. Alternatively plot values from strip chart recorder against apparent concentration, and determine sample results from the standard curve.

Normal values and interpretation

Published reports on normal serum copper values vary somewhat, but an average range is 95-130 μg/dl (14.9-20.4 μmole/L) for men and 95-140 μg/dl (14.9-22 μmole/L) for women.[39] The range is somewhat lower in children; having been reported as 15-65 μg/dl (2.5-10 μmole/L) in newborns and 30-150 μg/dl (5-25 μmole/L) in children. Increased values are found in pregnancy or in any condition in which there is an increased concentration of estrogen in the blood. Women on oral contraceptives[39] have a range of 150-245 μg/dl (23.6-38.5 μmole/L). Hypercupremia has also been reported in myocardial infarction, cirrhosis, rheumatoid arthritis, and many acute and chronic infections. Hypocupremia is associated with certain nutritional disorders, nephrosis, and Wilson's disease. Wilson's disease is the one in which there is most interest in connection with serum copper concentrations. Values in the range of 40-60 μg/dl (6-9 μmole/L) are common.

The urinary excretion of copper shows considerable variation, but the normal range is 15-50 μg/day (0.25-0.8 μmole/day). The excretion tends to be higher when there is proteinuria or aminoaciduria, because these substances tend to carry copper bound to them into the urine. In Wilson's disease, in which there is a marked aminoaciduria, the excretion of copper is greatly increased, as much as 500-1000 μg/day (7.5-15 μmole/day).

ZINC

Zinc is another trace element that is a constituent of many enzymes and is essential to growth. A number of symptoms, e.g., growth retardation, hypogonadism, rough, dry skin, poor appetite, and mental lethargy, have been observed in men on zinc-deficient diets.[40,41]

Supplemental zinc administered orally has been shown to reverse many of these symptoms.[42]

The relation of zinc concentrations in the blood and several other tissues to human disease states has been clearly established. A recent review of the nutritional importance of both copper and zinc in neonates and growing children covers much about the metabolic roles of these elements and the clinical manifestations of trace element deficiencies.[43] Zinc deficiency has been shown in children on limited meat diets[44] and in individuals with alcoholic cirrhosis, malabsorption syndrome,[45] acrodermatitis enteropathica, and sickle cell disease.

Determination of zinc in plasma[46]

Principle: Fasting specimens are preferable. Plasma should be rapidly separated from red cells, because zinc concentrations in the erythrocytes are 10-15 times greater than those found in plasma. Plasma is preferred to serum, since zinc is released from platelets during clotting, producing higher results. Zinc may be determined colorimetrically using the reagent 4-(2-pyridylazo)resorcinol (PAR). This reagent forms colored complexes with a number of metals. The addition of cyanide inhibits the formation of the colored complexes, but the addition of chloral hydrate activates the formation of the color with zinc but not with other metals; thus a specific colorimetric determination can be made. The addition of guanidine allows the determination to be made without precipitation of the plasma proteins.

The same precautions in regard to contamination as mentioned under the determination of copper should also be observed here—the use of metal-free water and plastic pipets and test tubes whenever possible.

Reagents:

1. Stock guanidine solution, 6.0 moles/L
   Dissolve 286 g guanidine hydrochloride and 12.1 g tris(hydroxymethyl)aminomethane in water to make 5 dl.

2. Working guanidine solution
   Dissolve 75 mg sodium cyanide and 0.25 g ascorbic acid in 50 ml stock solution.

3. Color reagent, 5 mmole/L
   Dissolve 0.5 g 4-(2-pyridylazo)resorcinol (PAR) in water to make 5 dl. Store in a brown bottle in the refrigerator.

4. Chloral hydrate, 3.6 moles/L
   Dissolve 300 g chloral hydrate in water to make 5 dl.

5. Stock standard, 1 mg/ml
   Dissolve 1.245 g pure zinc oxide in 10 ml water and 1 ml concentrated nitric acid; then dilute to 1 L with water. For a 15 mmole/L solution use 1.221 g zinc oxide, or purchase a standard made up for atomic absorption containing 1 mg/dl (Fisher Scientific Co., Pittsburgh).

6. Working standard
   Dilute an aliquot of the stock 1:500 to give a standard containing 200 μg/dl (or 30 μmole/L).

Procedure: In a series of plastic tubes set up the amounts as indicated in the chart at the top of p. 519.

Mix and allow to stand for 5 min; then read in a spectrophotometer at 497 nm after zeroing the spectrophotometer with the reagent blank.

Tube	Serum (ml)	Standard (ml)	Water (ml)	Guanidine (ml)	PAR (ml)	Chloralhydrate (ml)
Sample	0.2	—	—	1.0	0.1	0.05
Sample blank	0.2	—	0.1	1.0	—	0.05
Standard	—	0.2	—	1.0	0.1	0.05
Reagent blank	—	—	0.2	1.0	0.1	0.05

Calculation:

$$\frac{A(sample) - A(sample\ blank)}{A(standard)} \times \frac{Conc.}{of\ standard} = \frac{Conc.}{of\ sample}$$

where A is the absorbance.

Determination of zinc by atomic absorption[47]

Principle: The direct determination of plasma zinc using air-acetylene atomic absorption spectrophotometry at 213.8 nm is a simple, precise, and rapid technic. The addition of glycerol to aqueous standards compensates for the difference in viscosity between the standards and diluted plasma.

Reagents:
1. Glycerol solution, 5% v/v
   Dilute 50 ml glycerol to 1 L with deionized water.
2. Stock standard zinc, 1000 mg/L
   Dilute 10 ml concentrated nitric acid to 50 ml with deionized water, and dissolve 1.000 g Zinc powder (Alfa Inorganics, Beverly, Mass.) in this solution and further dilute to 1 L.
3. Working standards, 10, 20, 30, and 40 μg/dl
   Dilute 1.0 ml stock zinc standard in a 1 dl volumetric flask with 5% glycerol to the mark and mix well. Further dilute this intermediate standard (1, 2, 3, and 4 ml) into four 1 dl volumetric flasks with 5% glycerol. The standards obtained are 10, 20, 30, and 40 μg/dl, which correspond to apparent standards of 50, 100, 150, and 200 μg Zn/dl plasma because of the 1:5 dilution.

Procedure: Dilute plasma samples with four parts deionized water. Aspirate a blank solution of 5% glycerol to zero the instrument and between samples to reduce protein buildup. Aspirate the zinc standards; set the concentration readout to read the apparent concentration of the standards, or plot the instrument response against the apparent concentration and determine sample results from the curve. The method is linear to 200 μg/dl.

Normal values

The normal range of zinc in plasma is 74-130 μg/dl (11.3-20 μmole/L)[47] in men and 76-110 μg/dl (11.6-16.8 μmole/L) in women. The value is somewhat lower during pregnancy. Since red cells contain roughly 10 times as much zinc as plasma, any appreciable hemolysis in the sample produces unacceptably high results.

SODIUM AND POTASSIUM[48]
Determination by flame photometry

Sodium and potassium are usually determined by flame photometry. A general discussion of this method has been given, but a few comments on these particular determinations may be helpful.

A solution of plasma or serum is diluted 1:100 or 1:200 and aspirated into a hot flame, generally of air and propane (1925° C). The elements of the alkaline earth group Na^+, K^+, Li^+, and Cs^+ are temporarily activated by the heat of the flame, and as they return to the ground state they emit light of characteristic wavelengths. The emitted light can be isolated by a series of filters, one for each element and a series of phototubes. Many instruments incorporate dilute lithium solutions (e.g., $LiNO_3$ or LiCl) as an internal standard and measure the amounts of sodium and potassium in relation to the amount of lithium to compensate for minor variations in aspiration rate or flame temperature.

Some instruments use diluted cesium solutions as an internal standard, and this can measure sodium, potassium, and, if needed, lithium simultaneously. With instruments that measure only sodium and potassium in relation to lithium, some manufacturers allow the operator to reverse the lithium and potassium circuits. This result in the ability to measure sodium and lithium in relation to an internal standard of potassium, as well as the usual sodium and potassium in relation to lithium. The only difficulty with this process is that the operator must rinse the system thoroughly between groups of sodium and potassium determinations and sodium and lithium determinations, since the internal standards will interfere with subsequent assays.

Solutions of standards or internal standards should be stored in plastic bottles. The lithium solution in particular should be quickly transferred to a polyethylene bottle after being made in volumetric glassware to prevent the loss of lithium ions into the borosilicate glass.

Even with an internal standard, marked variations in the aspiration rate will have some effect on the determination; the manufacturer's directions should be followed quite closely in regard to fuel and air pressure, aspiration rate, cleaning the burner and atomizer, and the use of a nonionic detergent if needed. All modern instruments have a direct readout, and the calibrating solutions usually contain 140 or 150 mmole/L sodium and 5 mmole/L potassium. The SI unit of measure is millimoles per liter, and since this is numerically the same as milliequivalents per liter for sodium, potassium, and chloride, only the former unit will be used. Usually the standards are available with the instrument, but if desired they can be made up by dissolving 8.182 g NaCl and 0.373 g KCl (National Bureau of standards, SRM-919 sodium chloride, SRM-918 potassium chloride; both salts that have been previously dried for several hours at 110° C) in water to make 1 L.

The determination of sodium and potassium in urine may also be requested. The concentrations of these ions are quite different in urine than in serum, and a different standard is required. One containing 100 mmole/L of both sodium and potassium is suggested (5.84 g NaCl and 7.45 g KCl to 1 L). If the instrument used will not simultaneously measure the two elements in this range, different dilutions may be required for the sodium and potassium. Because of the wide variation in the amounts found in urine, great accuracy is not necessary.

Sodium and potassium may be determined by atomic absorption spectrophotometry, but this is rarely done since the flame photometry methods are simpler.

Determination by ion-selective electrodes

Sodium and potassium ions in serum and urine can also be determined by ion-selective electrodes. These electrodes develop an electrical potential that is proportional to the activity of sodium or potassium ions, the way a glass electrode responds to the activity of hydrogen ions.[49-51] Potassium electrodes also have been developed that contain a membrane impregnated with the antibiotic valinomycin, which complexes with potassium to produce a voltage potential poroportional to the potassium activity in solution.[52] The electrode has a selectivity of 5000:1 for potassium over sodium.

These various types of electrodes are used in continuous flow systems (NOVA Biomedical, Newton, Mass.; Technicon Instruments Corp., Tarrytown, N.Y.) in which a diluted solution flows past the electrodes[53,54] and also in discrete analyzers (Beckman Instruments, Fullerton, Calif.; Instrumentation Laboratory, Lexington, Mass.; Photovolt Corp., New York) in which a single sample is diluted and measured.[55-59] Many varieties of automated systems using these electrodes are now available with from two to eight or more analytes being assayed from a single sample.

Perhaps one of the most novel approaches to the assay of sodium and potassium with ion-selective electrodes is the use of a disposable pair of electrochemical half cells (Eastman Kodak Co., Rochester, N.Y.) contained in a small slide mount.[60] Each slide contains two many-layered, thin-film, ion-selective electrodes connected by a small paper bridge. The sample is added, and it interacts with the various layers to create an electrical potential that is related to the electrolyte concentration of the sample. After measurement the slide is discarded.

Normal values and interpretation[61]
Effect of drugs

A large number of drugs will influence the serum concentration of sodium and potassium. These include particularly the corticosteroid hormones and diuretics or other drugs that cause a marked increase or decrease in urine flow, leading to an excessive loss or retention of salts. The intravenous use of potassium penicillin may cause hyperkalemia, whereas the use of the use of the sodium salt may cause an increased excretion of potassium. The physician may not always be aware that these or other drugs are given as sodium or potassium salts and that significant amounts of these ions can be thus administered. In patients with heart disease there may be a decrease in serum potassium of as much as 0.4 mEq/L during a glucose tolerance test or the ingestion of large amounts of glucose.

Sodium

The normal level of sodium in serum is from 136-145 mmole/L, with values up to 2 mmole/L lower in patients older than 60-65 years. Sodium is the principal ion of the plasma, and its function appears to be chiefly physiochemical in connection with the maintenance of osmotic pressure and acid-base balance. The body has a strong tendency to maintain a constant total base content and only slight changes are found even under most pathologic conditions. Significant decreases in sodium content of serum have been noted in pregnancy, pyloric obstruction, severe nephritis, and Addison's disease. Since the loss of sodium is usually accompanied by the loss of chloride, reference may be made to the discussion of the chloride concentration, particularly in regard to Addison's disease.

It is not generally realized that the method of dilution[62,63] can have a slight effect on the values obtained for sodium by flame photometry. The normal values were generally established using manual dilution or one of the syringe type of dilutors mentioned earlier. Many of the automated flame photometers use roller tubes for dilution. If the viscosity of the standard (simple aqueous solution) is different than that of the sample (serum), a positive error of up to 3 mmole/L in the value for sodium may result, since the dilutions of the standard and sample are not exactly the same. This may not seem large, but in view of the narrow range of normal values for sodium, it may be significant in some cases. Even greater errors can occur with hyperproteinemic serum samples such as those found in multiple myeloma and Waldenström's macroglobulinemia. Generally this error will not occur if one uses a serum-based standard or increases the viscosity of the standard solution. Most manufacturers of commercial standards have adjusted the viscosity of their standards to be similar to that of normal serum. Presumably the same effect will occur with the potassium measurements, but because of the much wider normal range the error is of less consequence.

In extreme hyperlipemia the measured values of sodium, potassium, and chloride in serum may be artifactually lowered.[64] The actual amounts of ions per milliliter of water in the serum may be normal, but because of marked hyperlipemia the measured volume of sample will contain much less than the usual amount of water and hence of the ions. A simple method of correcting for this has been suggested, using the level of triglycerides as an index of the hyperlipemia. The factor, F, by which the measured electrolyte concentrations must be multiplied to obtain the true concentration is given by

$$F = 1 + (0.021 \times TG) - 0.006$$

where TG is the triglyceride concentration in grams per deciliter. Ordinary concentrations of triglycerides of a few hundred milligrams per deciliter will have no effect, but for a triglyceride level of 2500 mg/dl or 2.5 g/dl the factor would be

$$1 + (0.021 \times 2.5) - 0.006 =$$
$$1 + 0.053 - 0.006 = 1.047$$

The measured concentrations of the ions will be about 5% too low.

Potassium

The normal range of serum potassium is 3.8-5.4 mmole/L. An increase in serum potassium is often found in severe cases of Addison's disease (adrenal cortical insufficiency), particularly in the crisis of that disease. Values of up to 8 mmole/L have often been found, and concentrations of over 10 mmole/L have been reported. Some increases in serum potassium have been reported in uremic coma and acute intestinal obstruction.

A decrease in serum potassium may be produced by severe diarrhea and vomiting and has been reported in Cushing's syndrome. In patients with familial periodic paralysis, a rare disease with intermittent attacks of paralysis of the somatic muscles, the serum potassium level is lowered during the attacks, usually to about 2.5 mmole/L, but it is normal in the intervals between attacks.

Since the potassium content of erythrocytes is about 20 times that of plasma, any **hemolysis** during collection of the sample will give erroneously high results. It has been calculated that a just barely visible hemolysis will increase the potassium concentration of serum by about 0.2 mmole/L. Hence samples containing a readily noticeable hemolysis should not be used. Even without visible hemolysis there may be a shift of potassium from the cells to the serum when the latter stands in contact with the clot for a long time. Therefore the serum should be separated from the cells as soon as possible. After separation the serum is stable for a week or more, even at room temperature.

In an emergency a potassium determination may be made on a slightly hemolyzed serum sample, but the fact should be noted on the report form. In some instances the result so obtained may be of value to the physician. If, for example, a serum sample with slight hemolysis was found to have a potassium value of 5.2 mmole/L, the physician would know that the actual concentration could not be markedly elevated.

It has been reported that opening and closing[65] the fist 10 times with a tourniquet in place results in an increase in the potassium level of the sample by 10-20%, that this increase is caused by forearm exercise, and that restricted blood flow persists for about 2 min. Hence the blood sample should be taken without a tourniquet, or the tourniquet should be released after the needle has entered the vein and 2 min allowed to elapse before the sample is taken.

Although potassium is usually analyzed in serum, plasma is the preferred sample. Hartmann[66] has reviewed the problem of pseudokalemia in serum; it is most commonly caused by potassium release from

platelets during clotting, although white cells can also be a source of potassium release. The difference between plasma and serum averages 0.4 mmole/L, but it is not constant for all patients and cannot be predicted from platelet and white cell counts.[67] It is recommended that heparinized plasma be used for the most accurate potassium determinations. The time of sampling affects the potassium values (0.2-0.4 mmole/L), with the highest concentrations obtained in the afternoon and early evening.[68,69]

CHLORIDE
Determination by mercuric nitrate titration[70,71]

Chloride ions may be determined by titration with **mercuric nitrate.** The mercuric chloride formed is so slightly ionized that it does not react with the indicator **diphenylcarbazone.** When an excess of mercuric ions has been added, they react to give a violet-blue color with the indicator.

Reagents:
1. Mercuric nitrate solution
   Dissolve 1.7 g reagent grade mercuric nitrate and 2.6 ml concentrated nitric acid in 2 dl water; then dilute to 1 L. This solution is quite stable.
2. Indicator solution
   Dissolve 100 mg s-diphenylcarbazone in 1 dl 95% ethyl alcohol. Store in a brown bottle in the refrigerator. This solution slowly deteriorates, especially on exposure to light, and should be prepared fresh monthly.
3. Sodium tungstate and sulfuric acid
   These are the same as used for the preparation of Folin-Wu filtrate.
4. Chloride standard (National Bureau of Standards, SRM-919)
   Dry sodium chloride at 110° C for several hours. Weigh out exactly 584.5 mg of the salt and dissolve in water to make 1 L. This solution contains 10 mmole/L chloride.

Procedure: Pipet 2 ml 1:10 Folin-Wu filtrate (= 0.2 ml serum) into a 25 ml Erlenmeyer flask and add 2-3 drops indicator. Titrate with mercuric nitrate solution from a buret calibrated in 0.01 ml intervals. (Some burets have small hypodermic needles as tips; these have proved unsatisfactory, because mercuric nitrate solution tends to react with the metal, thereby causing errors.) The buret should have a fine glass tip that delivers about 100 drops/ml. The clear solution becomes an intense violet on the addition of the first drop of excess mercuric nitrate (end point). To standardize the mercuric nitrate solution, similarly titrate 2 ml standard chloride solution. Although the mercuric nitrate solution is stable, standardizations should be run frequently as a check.

Calculation: Since 2 ml of a 1:10 dilution and 2 ml of a 10 mmole/L standard are titrated, this is equivalent to titrating 2 ml serum and 2 ml of a 100 mmole/L standard. Hence:

$$\frac{\text{ml titration of filtrate}}{\text{ml titration of standard}} \times 100 = \text{mmole/L chloride}$$

The serum may also be titrated directly. Add 0.2 ml serum to 1.8 ml water in a flask, add indicator, and titrate. When the first drops of mercuric nitrate are added, the solution will turn blue. As the titration is continued the blue color will disappear to a pale pink, and with blue color appearing again at the end point. The end point may not be quite so sharp as with the titration of the filtrate. For this quantity of serum the calculation is the same as previously given. Cerebrospinal fluid may be titrated without deproteinization, similar to serum.

Urinary chloride: Titrate 2 ml diluted urine (1:10 is usually satisfactory) as described for the filtrate of serum. If the chloride concentration is very low, the titration may be repeated using a different dilution of urine. The urine sample must not be alkaline at the start of the titration (test with paper). If the diluted urine is alkaline, add a few drops of diluted nitric acid (1:20) to a 2 ml aliquot to bring the pH to approximately 4.0. If the acidity is too high, the indicator loses sensitivity. It may be convenient to add the acid by drops to an aliquot of the diluted urine and count the drops required to bring the pH to 4.0. Then add the same number of drops to the aliquot to be titrated.

This method sometimes gives slightly high results in urine specimens that have been standing for several days, even if refrigerated. Hence only fresh specimens should be used.

Calculation: When 2 ml standard and 2 ml of a 1:10 dilution of urine are titrated, the calculation is the same as for serum. If another dilution of urine is used and 2 ml standard is titrated, then

$$\frac{\text{Titration of sample}}{\text{Titration of standard}} \times 10 \times \frac{B}{A} = \text{mmole/L chloride}$$

where "A" ml urine is diluted up to a volume of "B" ml. Usually the total excretion per day is required.

$$\text{mmole/L} \times 24 \text{ hr urine vol (L)} = \text{Total mmole excreted}$$

The excretion of chloride can be expressed in terms of grams of sodium chloride:

$$\text{mmole} \times 0.0585 = \text{g sodium chloride}$$

Determination with chloridometer[72,73]

Principle: The chloridometer is a very convenient instrument for the determination of chloride. The chloride in solution is titrated with silver ions, which are formed at a constant rate by the passage of an electric current. The silver ion concentration in the solution is monitored by a silver electrode. As long as any chloride ions are present, the concentration of silver ions remains low. When sufficient silver ions have been generated to combine with all the chloride present, the concentration of silver ions begins to rise. This is detected by the silver electrode, and an associated circuit automatically stops the titration. A timing device is connected in the circuit so that one actually measures the time required for the constant current to generate sufficient silver ions to combine with all the cloride in the solution. By comparing the time required to titrate the sample and a known standard, the concentration of the sample can be readily calculated. Most instruments now in use have a direct readout in which the concentration of chloride is displayed directly in millimoles per liter. Some instru-

ments may have several ranges for use with different sizes of samples or concentrations of chloride. The titration is usually carried out in a solution containing 1.7 moles/L acetic acid and 0.1 mole/L' nitric acid with a small amount of gelatin added to allow smoother operation.

The different instruments (American Instrument Co., Silver Spring, Md.; Buchler Instruments, Fort Lee, N.J.; Corning Medical, Medfield, Mass.; The London Co., Cleveland; Beckman Instruments, Fullerton, Calif.; etc.) may require slightly different reagents or procedures, but here the details on usage are presented using the Buchler Chloridometer, which are similar to those originally proposed by Cotlove.[72]

Reagents:
1. Diluting fluid.
   Add 1 dl glacial acetic acid and 6.4 ml concentrated nitric acid to about 8 dl water in a 1 L volumetric flask, mix, dilute to the mark with water, and mix well. This reagent is quite stable when stored in a glass bottle with a glass or plastic stopper.
2. Gelatin solution
   Dissolve 6 g gelatin (Knox, unflavored no. 1), 0.1 g water-soluble thymol blue, and 0.1 g thymol in 1 L hot water. Cool and transfer approximately 10 ml aliquots to test tubes that are tightly stoppered and kept in the refrigerator. The gelatin solution is not stable at room temperature, and solutions that have been standing at room temperature for more than 1 day should not be used. Vials containing 6.2 g of the mixed reagents are obtainable from the instrument manufacturers.
3. Chloride standard (National Bureau of Standards, SRM-919)
   Sodium chloride (100 mmole/L) is dried for several hours at 110° C and then cooled in a desiccator. Exactly 5.845 g is weighed out and dissolved in water to make 1 L. A 100 mmole/L standard is more convenient, particularly for the direct readout instruments.

Procedure for serum, plasma, and cerebrospinal fluid: Pipet 4 ml diluting fluid to a titration vial and add 4 drops gelatin solution. At the beginning of each day titrate several standards to condition the electrodes. Set the blank correction index to zero and titrate several blanks. Set the blank correction index to the average value of the blanks. Then add 0.1 ml standard of 4 ml diluting fluid plus gelatin and titrate standards. If necessary adjust so that the standard reading is 100 mmole/L. Then titrate samples similarly, noting the result for each. Some other instruments may use different amounts of diluent and sample.

Procedure for urine: Since the concentration of chloride in urine may vary much more than in serum, a different size of sample may be required to obtain a titration in the optimal range (at least one third and no more than twice the titration of the standard). If the chloride concentration is too high, the urine may be diluted 1:2 or 1:5 with water and 0.1 ml titrated, or one may use 0.05 or 0.02 ml sample. The results obtained are then multiplied by 2 or 5. If the concentration is too low, 0.2 or even 0.5 ml sample may be titrated and the result divided by 2 or 5, respectively.

Determination with chloride electrode

Chloride may also be determined by the chloride electrode.[54,74,75] This electrode is used principally in a number of automated instruments in conjunction with the sodium and potassium ion-selective electrodes mentioned earlier. The chloride electrode is also used for the determination of chloride in sweat in the diagnosis of cystic fibrosis.

Interference of other elements

Bromides interfere chemically with the determination of chloride, since the two elements react similarly with most reagents. The interference is apparently greater when the chloride is determined by the mercuric thiocyanate method (as in some automated procedures), because the bromide apparently gives more color than an equivalent amount of chloride. In the titration methods the two ions act similarly, and the net result is the determination of chloride plus bromide. Since the bromide does not replace the chloride physiologically, an erroneous result for chloride would be obtained. Theoretically, iodides could interfere in the same way, but these are rarely present in a sufficiently high concentration to give a noticeable interference. In the electrical titration traces of sulfides will interfere to give erratic results. Ordinarily sulfides are not a serious contamination in blood, but they may occur in the reagents, one source being rubber stoppers.

Normal values and interpretation

The normal values for serum chloride are 98-109 mmole/L and for spinal fluid 122-132 mmole/L.[76] The urinary excretion of chloride depends on the dietary intake and other factors and may be subject to wide variation. A normal range for individuals on an average diet may be taken as 170-250 mmole/24 hr. Drugs influencing diuresis and electrolyte excretion affect the serum and urine levels similar to the effect on sodium discussed earlier.

Because of the relatively high concentration of chloride in the gastric secretion, prolonged vomiting from whatever cause may lead to considerable chloride loss and lowered serum value. In pyloric obstruction the value may fall to as low as 50 mmole/L. When there is vomiting in gastric disease in which there is achlorhydria, the loss is less. Severe diarrhea may also cause loss of chloride, but to a lesser extent. In ulcerative colitis the serum value may fall as low as 70 mmole/L.

The urinary excretion of chloride falls to a very low value whenever the serum value is much below 100 mmole/L.

Although the reason is not clear, low plasma chloride levels have been observed in a number of acute infections. The plasma chloride is rather variable in renal disease. It is sometimes increased in acute glomerulonephritis; in nephrosis it may be almost normal. When renal failure is present, it may be reduced. This is a common finding in the later stages of chronic glomerulonephritis. Plasma chloride can be maintained for years near normal limits even when a considerable de-

gree of renal failure is present. Hence chloride determinations are of limited value in renal disease.

The chloride value in cerebrospinal fluid is said to be decreased in meningitis, but its determination in this condition is of doubtful diagnostic significance.

In some conditions the urinary excretion of chloride is appreciable even when the serum value is as low as 85 mmole/L or less. The chief condition of interest in this regard is Addison's disease, in which there is a deficiency of the adrenal hormone that controls the excretion of both sodium and chloride. The Robinson-Power-Kepler test had been used, but it is both obsolete and dangerous. The ACTH stimulation tests are preferable with the direct measurement of the steroid hormones.

CARBON DIOXIDE CONTENT AND CARBON DIOXIDE–COMBINING POWER[77-79]
General principles

Carbon dioxide (CO_2) may be determined by acidifying the plasma or serum with lactic acid and extracting the gas, which is measured in the Natelson Microgasometer or other device.

The plasma CO_2 content is used as an indicator of the acid-base balance in the blood. It is not too sensitive an indicator (see the later discussion in the section on blood pH), but the manometric method is quite simple. For accurate results the plasma should be collected anaerobically. The simplest method to do this is to use heparinized Vacutainers. The blood is collected with a minimum of stasis and the tube filled as completely as possible. After thorough mixing, the blood is centrifuged while still warm and with the stopper in place. The stopper is not removed until one is ready for sampling for the determination. A less satisfactory method is to collect the blood in a heparinized syringe and, after mixing, to transfer the blood to a small test tube with a minimum of agitation but as rapidly as possible. The tube should be filled completely and a stopper inserted so that the tube may be centrifuged at once with the stopper in place.

The determination of CO_2-combining power has been used in the past instead of the CO_2 content. This is defined as the CO_2 content of the plasma after it has been equilibrated with gas containing CO_2 at a partial pressure of 40 mm Hg. It has the advantage that no special precautions are needed in the collection or separation of the plasma. As usually run, the determination lacks accuracy. The gas containing the CO_2 at a pressure of 40 mm Hg is customarily taken as the alveolar air from the technician's lungs. The actual alveolar air in healthy individuals may vary as much as 20% from the assumed value, and often the technician does not exhale completely enough to bring true alveolar air in contact with the sample. This method is not often used and is not recommended because of the inaccuracies of the technic.

A theoretically correct method, equilibrating the plasma with tank gas containing CO_2 at exactly 40 mm Hg and at 37° C, would not be as simple as even the determination of the CO_2 content. It has been found that the CO_2 content of plasma in samples collected without special precautions is usually only about 1-1.5

mmole/L lower than the CO_2-combining power and is sufficiently accurate for a rough estimate of the acid-base balance.

Determination using Natelson Microgasometer[78]

Reagents:
1. Lactic acid, 1 mole/L
   Add 90 ml 85% lactic acid to water and dilute to 1 L.
2. Sodium hydroxide, 3 moles/L
   Dissolve 60 g sodium hydroxide in water and dilute to 5 dl.
3. Caprylic alcohol

The reagents are conveniently kept in small screw-capped vials. The lower third of one vial is filled with mercury and above this is added about an equal volume of lactic acid with a layer of caprylic alcohol on top. A second vial will contain water and mercury, and a third vial will contain mercury and sodium hydroxide solution. Other vials may be used for lactic acid and water for washing the chamber. One should also have some sort of broad vessel below the measuring tip to collect any drops of mercury that may fall out.

Procedure: The procedure for transferring a reagent from a vial to the chamber of the apparatus is as follows: Dip the sampling tip below the surface of the liquid in the vial, and with the upper stopcock open, advance the plunger slightly so that a small droplet of mercury is forced from the tip. Then draw the appropriate amount of liquid into the tip, measuring by the graduations on it. Then lower the tip below the surface of the mercury in the bottom of the vial and draw about 0.03 ml mercury into the tip if another reagent is to be added next. If the material in the capillary is to be transferred to the chamber, keep the tip in the mercury and the plunger retracted so that the liquids are carried completely into the extraction chamber by the flow of mercury. Do not hold the sampling tip forcibly against the bottom of the vial so as to impede the flow of mercury. Also, the bore of the stopcock should be precisely aligned with the other capillaries: otherwise there is a tendency for the mercury to break up into drops on entering the chamber. The same procedure can be used for adding the serum sample if the serum overlays some mercury in a small tube. Add the mercury to the tube first and then the serum. If the serum is already in the tube, the mercury will be broken up into drops and it will be difficult to add the mercury to the chamber. Another method for the addition of serum is to add serum to somewhat above the 0.03 ml mark, then place the tip in mercury, expel the excess serum exactly to the mark, and draw up some mercury.

The procedure for CO_2 analysis is as follows: Add successively, measuring with the tip and sealing with mercury after each addition, 0.03 ml sample, 0.03 ml lactic acid, 0.01 ml caprylic alcohol, and then 0.1 ml water. After adding the water, draw the mercury in to carry all the solutions into the extraction chamber. The mercury should be brought down to the top of the extraction chamber. Close the stopcock and lower the mercury to near the bottom of the extraction chamber. Shake for 2 min. If a small bubble of liquid remains in

Table 22-1. Factors for determination of CO_2 in Natelson Microgasometer*

Temp. (°C)	Factor	Temp. (°C)	Factor
17	0.242	25	0.232
18	0.240	26	0.231
19	0.238	27	0.230
20	0.237	28	0.229
21	0.236	29	0.228
22	0.235	30	0.227
23	0.234	31	0.225
24	0.233	32	0.224

*Results calculated as millimoles per liter.

the tube above the extraction chamber, warm above the bubble by holding the glass stem with the fingers. This will cause the gas to expand and expel the bubble. Raise the level in the chamber to the 0.12 ml mark and read the pressure (P_1). Advance the mercury to release the pressure and add 0.03 ml 3N sodium hydroxide (be sure that the sampling tip is in the sodium hydroxide solution before opening the stopcock), followed by mercury to bring the sodium hydroxide solution into the chamber. Lower the liquid briefly to the bottom of the chamber and then bring it up to the 0.12 mark. Read the pressure (P_2).

Calculation: The amount of CO_2 is then calculated with the use of the appropriate factor (Table 22-1).

$$mmole/L = (P_1 - P_2) \times F$$

Formerly the results were sometimes expressed in volume percent, the milliliters of CO_2 (at standard conditions) liberated from 1 dl blood, but this expression is now obsolete. The CO_2 content was also expressed in milliequivalents per liter calculated as bicarbonate. Since all the CO_2 in the blood is not present in this form, the expression millimoles per liter is preferred. Numerically this is the same as the older milliequivalents per liter.

Gambino and Schreiber[80] have suggested a method for the preservation of plasma samples for CO_2 content analysis. This method was primarily intended for the AutoAnalyzer, but there is no reason why it could not be used for other methods. It was found that 1 drop 1N ammonium hydroxide added to 1 ml plasma would keep the CO_2 content constant for at least 4 hr. In the automated method the same amount of ammonia was added to the standards, so that no dilution effect need be considered, but if the technic were applied to gasometric analysis, this would have to be taken into account. It was found that 1 drop ammonia from a disposable pipet added to 1 ml plasma caused a volume change of no more than 1-2%, so that a correction of 1.5% would reduce the error to a negligible amount.

The procedure can be standardized by using 25 mmole/L sodium carbonate solution. This is made by dissolving in water (to make 1 dl) 0.265 g reagent grade anhydrous sodium carbonate that has been dried for several hours at 110° C. Unless kept in a well-filled, tightly stoppered bottle, this solution will change in concentration with time. When the sodium carbonate solution is run in the apparatus as a check, the addition of the caprylic alcohol should be omitted.

Determination using Harleco CO₂ apparatus[81,82]

Principle: The CO_2 dissolved in a serum or plasma sample may be liberated by addition of lactic acid. The volume of gas produced is measured at 1 atm by displacing a calibrated syringe barrel. For the small laboratory or as a backup method for few samples, the device is excellent.

Procedure: The Harleco CO_2 apparatus (Item no. 64837, Harleco, Philadelphia) consists of a small reaction vessel and a syringe, which may be clamped to the reaction chamber. The 1.0 ml serum sample is added to the chamber, and the syringe containing lactic acid is clamped on. The lactic acid is added to the serum and the apparatus agitated. The amount that the plunger rises is taken as a measure of the liberated CO_2, and a comparison is made with a standard bicarbonate solution treated similarly. The apparatus is quite simple, and the results compare favorably with analysis on the Natelson Microgasometer. A disadvantage of the device is that it requires 1 ml serum. Using diluted serum leads to inaccurate results, except that for levels over 40 mmole/L in which a 1:2 dilution with saline can be used.

Determination using CO₂ electrode[83]

The measurement of total CO_2 in serum or plasma is carried out when a sample is added to a sulfuric acid reagent. The CO_2 is determined as the rate of change of pH of a buffer inside a P_{CO_2} electrode when compared with a reference P_{CO_2} electrode. The device (Cl/CO_2 Analyzer, Beckman Instruments, Fullerton, Calif.) requires a 10 μl sample and measures the CO_2 concentration and Cl concentration by a modified coulometric titration technic within 30 sec. Both manual and automated versions of the instrument are available. Manual instruments using electrode technology have rapidly taken over in the small- and medium-sized laboratories that were previously using the microgasometer, and automated versions have greatly encroached on the dominance of the AutoAnalyzer in large laboratories.

Normal values

The CO_2 content of arterial plasma is 21-28 mmole/L and of venous plasma 23-30 mmole/L. The CO_2-combining power for plasma is 24-32 mmole/L. For a further discussion of the significance of the CO_2 determinations see the following discussion on acid-base balance.

BLOOD GAS ANALYSIS

As a means of evaluating the acid-base balance of the patient and the functioning of alveoli of the lung in gas exchange (e.g., loss of CO_2 and gain of O_2), blood gases are determined by using pH, P_{CO_2}, and P_{O_2} electrodes. These determinations are generally carried out by semiautomated or completely automated blood gas analyzers.*

*Technicon Instruments Corp., Tarrytown, N.Y.; Instrumentation Laboratory, Lexington, Mass.; The London Co., Cleveland; Corning Medical, Medfield, Mass.

Principle

Measurements are usually made on arterial blood drawn anaerobically into a syringe that is capped. Capillary blood that has been "arterialized" by intensive warming of the collection area for 10 min prior to sampling is an acceptable alternative. The measurements of pH, P_{CO_2}, and P_{O_2} are made on whole heparinized blood on an instrument within a few minutes of collection or within 20-30 min if the sample is placed in ice to reduce the rate of cellular metabolism.

The technic of blood gas analysis is simply a modern extension of gasometric analysis, and, although not currently in widespread use, some comments on the technic are included for historic reasons. The manual methods for measurement of P_{CO_2} using the microgasometer are included as an alternative to modern blood gas instrumentation, although they are considerably more time consuming and require a very careful technic to give acceptable results.

Gasometric analysis[77]

Chemical analyses can be made by measuring the amount of gas liberated in a reaction. In theory any chemical reaction that will produce a stoichiometric amount of gas could be used. A number of methods were developed by Van Slyke using this technic, but in recent years the gasometric methods have been limited chiefly to the determination of the gases combined in blood: oxygen, carbon dioxide, and carbon monoxide. The gas liberated from the blood by an appropriate reagent is extracted by shaking under a partial vacuum. The amount of gas liberated is then measured by compressing it to a definite known volume and measuring the absolute pressure exerted by the gas. In accordance with the gas laws:

$$PV = nRT$$

where P is the pressure of the gas; V its volume; n the number of moles of gas present; R a constant that depends on the units of measurement used; and T the absolute temperature (°C + 273). When P is expressed in millimeters of mercury, as is customary, and V is expressed in milliliters, then

$$\text{Gas (mmole)} = PV/(62.21T)$$

The volume, V, is a constant specified by the apparatus used, so that at a given temperature there is a direct relationship between the amount of gas present and the pressure.

The measured pressure results not only from the gas being determined but also from the water vapor present. The vapor pressure of water varies not only with the temperature but also with the amount of dissolved salts in the aqueous solution. Even when the determination is made using the difference in pressure before and after the absorption of the gas being measured, the water vapor pressure may vary slightly between the two measurements because of the added reagent. A correction must also be made for the solubility of the gases in the aqueous solution of the reagents. When the extracted gas is compressed for measurement, a small amount of gas may redissolve (this is particularly true for CO_2). Finally, the gases may not follow the gas laws exactly. The corrections for these deviations are all included in the factors given for the calculation of the amount of gas from the measured pressure. The factors also include the volume of sample taken and are applicable only when the directions as to volumes of sample and reagents are followed exactly. If in the Natelson apparatus, for example, 0.02 ml sample is used instead of the recommended 0.03 ml, it may suffice to multiply the final figure obtained by $^3/_2$, but if markedly different volumes of the reagents are added, the corrections for solubility will not be the same and an error will result. Since the factors vary with the temperature, the one corresponding to the ambient temperature must always be used.

The Natelson Microgasometer is an instrument that is much more rapid and requires a smaller sample than the older Van Slyke apparatus. All the samples and reagents are introduced through the tip, which is calibrated at 0.01, 0.02, 0.03, and 0.10 ml. The mercury is moved by means of a plunger attached to a handwheel, thus doing away with all leveling bulb manipulations. The extraction chamber has a volume of 3 ml, and the gas is measured at a volume of 0.12 ml. The shaking of the sample for extraction of the gas may be done by hand, or a mechanical shaker attachment is available. This is quite convenient if a number of samples are to be run. Newer models have a motorized handwheel for raising and lowering the mercury level and a small magnetic stirrer for gas extraction, but the basic principles remain the same.

Determination using Natelson Microgasometer[78]

The details of collecting and preserving blood samples are given in Chapter 4, along with the details for the preparation of the fully oxygenated blood. Since the gasometric methods in effect measure the oxygen (O_2) associated with the red cells, it is essential that the two samples for O_2 content and O_2 capacity have the same proportion of red cells (hematocrit). The difficulty is that when the blood is rotated in the glass vessel to saturate it with O_2, more of the plasma than of the cells is adsorbed by the glass walls, so that the sample as finally taken may have a slightly different hematocrit than initially.

Reagents:
1. Saponin-ferricyanide
   Prepare a solution of 1.2 g potassium ferricyanide in 1 dl water. This is stable when stored in the refrigerator. Also dissolve 1 g reagent grade saponin in 1 dl normal saline solution; this solution must be prepared weekly. On the day of use, mix together 1.5 ml ferricyanide solution with 10 ml saponin solution. Place in a small bottle, cover the solution with a layer of caprylic alcohol, and deaerate as described below.
2. Sodium hydroxide 3 moles/L
   Dissolve 12 g sodium hydroxide in water, cool, and make up to 1 dl. Store in a polyethylene bottle. Transfer a portion to a 20 ml vial, cover with mineral oil, and add mercury to a height of 2 cm, delivered to the bottom of the vial. This solution must also be deaerated.

3. Potassium hydroxide, 1 mole/L
   Dissolve 6 g potassium hydroxide in water and make up to 1 dl. Store in a polyethylene bottle.
4. Sodium hydrosulfite solution
   Place 1 g sodium hydrosulfite in a 20 ml vial and cover with mineral oil. Add 5 ml 1 mole/L potassium hydroxide and 2 ml mercury. The hydrosulfite will dissolve as the solution is being deaerated.

Since the solutions cannot be deaerated in the apparatus, this must be done beforehand. One method is to place the vials, with the liquid covered with light mineral oil or caprylic alcohol, in a vacuum desiccator and evacuate to a pressure of 25-35 mm. The pressure should not be so low that the liquids will tend to boil over. If a desiccator is not available, the individual vials may be connected to a vacuum source through small, one-hole rubber stoppers and a glass manifold. Deaeration should be continued for between 25 and 30 min.

Procedure: Rinse the chamber with water and expel. Draw up 0.1 ml 1 mole/L actic acid into the bottom of the lower bulb. Shake for a few seconds and expel. Close the stopcock, move the poston back until the mercury is in the lower bulb, and then expel any trapped gases. Draw up 0.01 ml caprylic alcohol, then 0.1 ml saponin-ferricyanide mixture, and 0.01 ml caprylic alcohol as a seal. Now draw up 0.03 ml well-mixed blood, then 0.01 ml caprylic alcohol, followed by 0.1 ml saponin-ferricyanide and 0.01 ml caprylic alcohol. This is followed by mercury to reach the 0.12 ml mark. The stopcock is closed and the liquid brought down about halfway in the reaction chamber. Run piston back and forth several times to ensure complete mixing. Shake the gasometer for 3 min to release the oxygen. Raise the caprylic alcohol meniscus to the 0.12 ml mark and take the pressure reading (P_1). Lower the liquid and repeat the shaking; then take another reading to ensure complete extraction of the oxygen.

The pressure is released by advancing the piston. Add 0.03 ml 3 moles/L sodium hydroxide, followed by mercury to reach the 0.11 ml mark. Lower the mercury to the 3 ml mark and shake the gasometer for 3 min. Raise the caprylic alcohol meniscus to the 0.12 ml mark and take a reading (P_2).

Next, the O_2 is absorbed by introducing 0.03 ml hydrosulfite solution, followed by mercury. Lower the mercury in the extraction chamber and shake the gasometer for 3 min. Raise the caprylic alcohol meniscus again to the 0.12 ml mark and take a reading (P_3). A blank is run using all the reagents and steps but no blood. The $P_2 - P_3$ value for the blank is the correction C. Then the corrected pressure is

$$P_2 - P_3 - C = P$$

and

$$P \times F = Vol\% \ O_2$$

The factor for O_2 at various temperatures is given in Table 22-2.

A correction must be made for the O_2 physically dissolved in the blood (not combined with hemoglobin). This amounts to 0.1 vol% for venous blood, 0.3 vol%

Table 22-2. Factors for calculating O_2 concentration in vol% using Natelson Microgasometer

Temp. (°C)	Factor (vol% O_2)
18	0.494
19	0.492
20	0.490
21	0.488
22	0.486
23	0.485
24	0.483
25	0.481
26	0.480
27	0.478
28	0.476
29	0.475
30	0.473
31	0.472
32	0.470
33	0.468
34	0.467
35	0.465

for arterial blood, and 0.6 vol% for blood saturated by equilibration with pure O_2.

Since the O_2 capacity varies with the hemoglobin content, the determination of O_2 capacity gives little information that is not given by the hemoglobin content.

The usual blood gases, O_2 and CO_2, as well as others such as carbon monoxide and nitrous oxide have been determined by gas-liquid chromatography using special columns. These methods are only used for research purposes rather than in the regular clinical laboratory, although there are some special small gas chromatographs that are made for this latter use.

Normal values and interpretation: The O_2 capacity of blood is 1.34 ml/g hemoglobin. In the absence of significant amounts of carboxyhemoglobin or methemoglobin the O_2 capacity can be estimated quite well from an accurate hemoglobin determination, and, conversely, O_2 capacity measurements have been used to calibrate hemoglobin methods. The O_2 capacity is normally about 20.7 vol% (15.4 g Hb) for men and 19 vol% (14.2 g Hb) for women. It is increased in polycythemia and anhydremia and is decreased in anemia. As determined by gasometric methods, the O_2 saturation of arterial blood in normal individuals has been considered as 95%. Somewhat higher values, approaching 98%, are obtained by spectrophotometric methods. This is partially because of the hematocrit error in the saturation of the blood, as previously mentioned. The O_2 saturation of venous blood is 60-85%.

PO_2 ELECTRODE[84,85]

The PO_2 electrode, used for the measurement of the partial pressure of oxygen in the blood and hence of oxygen saturation, is generally found in most types of blood gas apparatus along with the electrodes for the measurement of pH and PCO_2 and is discussed briefly here. In this electrode the reaction chamber is separated from the sample by a plastic membrane that will allow the diffusion of oxygen gas through the membrane but not the diffusion of ions. The electrode itself consists of two platinum electrodes in a potassium chloride solution, which is 0.01 mmole/L in potassium hydroxide. The passage of a small current at a potential of about 0.7 V causes some electrolysis of the water with the formation of hydrogen at the cathode. This tends to insulate (polarize) the electrode, thus reducing the amount of current flow. Oxygen from the sample diffusing through the membrane will react with the hydrogen, thus depolarizing the electrode and increasing the current. Within certain limits the changes in current will be proportional to the amount of oxygen diffusing in and thus to the amount of oxygen in the sample. Since the reaction at the electrode uses oxygen, the electrodes and electrode current is made small, so that the rate of diffusion of the oxygen will not be a limiting factor. The amplified electrode current is then indicated on a meter that is graduated directly in PO_2. The electrode is usually calibrated by the use of gases of known PO_2 (PO_2 = Mol fraction × Total pressure; in accordance with the gas laws, mol fraction is the same as percent by volume for gases). From the measured PO_2 and simultaneously measured pH, the oxygen saturation can be calculated by means of a table or nomogram. These are usually furnished with the instrument, or it may calculate the oxygen saturation and report it directly.

Oxygen content, oxygen capacity, and saturation

The oxygen content of blood is the amount of O_2 actually present, chiefly combined as oxyhemoglobin but with a small amount of physically dissolved oxygen. The O_2 capacity is the amount of O_2 that would be found if the blood were completely saturated with the gas. The ratio of the content to the capacity (multiplied by 100%) represents the percent of saturation of the blood. When determined volumetrically, the content and capacity are conventionally reported as volume percent, the volume of O_2 (in milliliters at standard conditions) that is combined with 1 dl blood. Other units such as millimoles per liter could also be used, but the main interest is in the calculation of the percent of saturation, which is independent of the units.

The spectrophotometric methods for the determination of O_2 have been given in Chapter 4. These methods are quite simple if one has the required instrument. Another method for the determination of oxygen saturation is by the use of the O_2 electrode, which measures the PO_2 (the partial pressure of O_2), from which the oxygen saturation can be calculated when the pH of the blood is also known.

PCO_2 ELECTRODE

Another method for determining the CO_2 content of blood or serum is by measuring the partial pressure of CO_2 with the PCO_2 electrode.[86-89] This is a small pH electrode system immersed in a carbonate-bicarbonate buffer. This is separated from the sample by a plastic membrane that is permeable to gaseous CO_2 but not to the ions in solution. The CO_2 from the sample diffuses through the membrane and changes the pH of the buffer solution (see following discussion of pH and buffers). The change in pH is read directly as Pco$_2$. A solution having a Pco$_2$ of 30 mm Hg is defined as one that would be in equilibrium with a gaseous phase that also has a Pco$_2$ of 30 mm Hg. (For the gaseous phase the Pco$_2$ equals the mol fraction of CO_2 in the gas multiplied by the total pressure). Since the greater the partial pressure of the CO_2 in the gaseous phase the greater the amount of CO_2 that will be dissolved in the liquid phase, the Pco$_2$ is thus a measure of the amount of CO_2 in the sample. In fact, the Pco$_2$ electrodes are generally calibrated by equilibrating with a gaseous mixture containing a known percentage of CO_2. The Pco$_2$ is generally reported in millimeters of mercury (torr). The new SI unit is the kilopascal (kPa), but almost all instruments are still scaled in millimeters of mercury (1 mm Hg = 1 torr = 0.133 kPa). These electrodes can be used by themselves, but they are generally found in blood gas apparatus along with the pH and Po$_2$ electrodes.

HYDROGEN ION CONCENTRATION (pH) IN BLOOD
Determination with glass electrode

The determination of the pH is usually made by means of the glass electrode and an electronic measuring device. The simpler pH meters suitable for checking the pH of chemical solutions are not accurate enough for blood measurements in which the range of values is not large. For blood measurements, microelectrodes are commonly used; these are kept at 37° C, since the blood should be measured at this temperature, and the electrodes prevent the exposure of the blood to the air, since loss or gain of CO_2 will change the pH.

A number of accurate pH meters are on the market, together with thermostated microelectrodes, that are suitable for blood pH determinations. With these electrodes, the solution to be measured (blood or plasma) is drawn up into a fine capillary made of the electrode glass, and the known solution is in a small jacket around the capillary. This enables one to use small samples of blood and also protects the blood from exposure to air during measurement. These electrodes are also jacketed with a circulating water bath or heating device to keep them at a constant temperature. The operating details vary somewhat from instrument to instrument. The blood may be drawn up into the capillary by gentle suction through a thin capillary tip. The tip is then dipped into a potassium chloride solution connected to the reference electrode for measurement, or the blood may be drawn into a small chamber where the pH, Po$_2$, and Pco$_2$ are measured simultaneously (with different electrodes). With care, reproducible measurements can be made to within 0.005 pH unit or better. Since the electrodes may not be quite linear, they are usually standardized with buffers of two different pH values. The pH should be measured at 37° C.

The normal values for the pH of arterial blood are 7.35-7.45; for venous blood the values are about 0.03 unit lower. The significance of blood pH changes will be discussed in relation to acid-base balance.

ACID-BASE BALANCE

An evaluation of the acid-base balance[90-92] in blood requires a knowledge of the factors involved in the blood carbonic acid–bicarbonate buffer (a mixture of a weak acid and its salt) system.

Definitions of terms

According to the Henderson-Hasselbalch equation, the general mathematic formulation for any buffer may be expressed as follows:

$$pH = pK' + \log \frac{[Salt]}{[Acid]}$$

where the brackets denote concentrations.

The pK′ for carbonic acid is 6.1; then for the bicarbonate buffer this is

$$pH = 6.1 + \log \frac{[HCO_3^-]}{[H_2CO_3]}$$

Normally the bicarbonate [HCO$_3^-$] concentration is about 24 mmole/L and the carbonic acid [H$_2$CO$_3$] concentration is about 1.2. Then

$$pH = 6.1 + \log \frac{24}{1.2} = 6.1 + \log 20 = 6.1 + 1.3 = 7.4$$

The equation indicates that there are three variables that must be considered in the assessment of acid-base balance: pH, concentration of bicarbonate, and concentration of carbonic acid. When two of these variables have been measured, the third may be calculated. The actual measurements are usually of the total CO_2 content (as may be determined on the Natelson Microgasometer), pH, and Pco$_2$. The Pco$_2$ is a measure of the carbonic acid concentration; when Pco$_2$ is expressed in millimeters of mercury (as is customary), then [H$_2$CO$_3$] = 0.03 Pco$_2$. Since the total CO_2 concentration, T, is the sum of [HCO$_3^-$] and [H$_2$CO$_3$], the equation may be written as follows:

$$pH = 6.1 + \log \frac{T - 0.03 \, Pco_2}{0.03 \, Pco_2}$$

Siggaard-Andersen nomogram

When two of the values have been measured, the third may be calculated by means of a nomogram. There are several variations of the nomongram originally devised by Siggaard-Anderson.[93] One such nomogram is given in Fig. 22-2. Thus from a measurement of pH and Pco$_2$, the changes in [HCO$_3^-$]/[H$_2$CO$_3$] as shown in Table 22-3 can be calculated.

The nomogram also contains a variable denoted as base excess. This is defined as the number of millimoles of acid (or base if the base excess is negative) required to be added to 1 L of blood to bring the sample back to the standard conditions of a pH of 7.40 and a total CO_2 content of 25 mmole/L. Since the system, reduced hemoglobin–oxidized hemoglobin, exerts some buffer action, the amount of hemoglobin in the sample is included in the nomogram. The base excess is used as a measure of the imbalance of the acid-base equilibrium. Many other acid-base nomograms have been devised. Weisberg[93a] cites more than 100 such

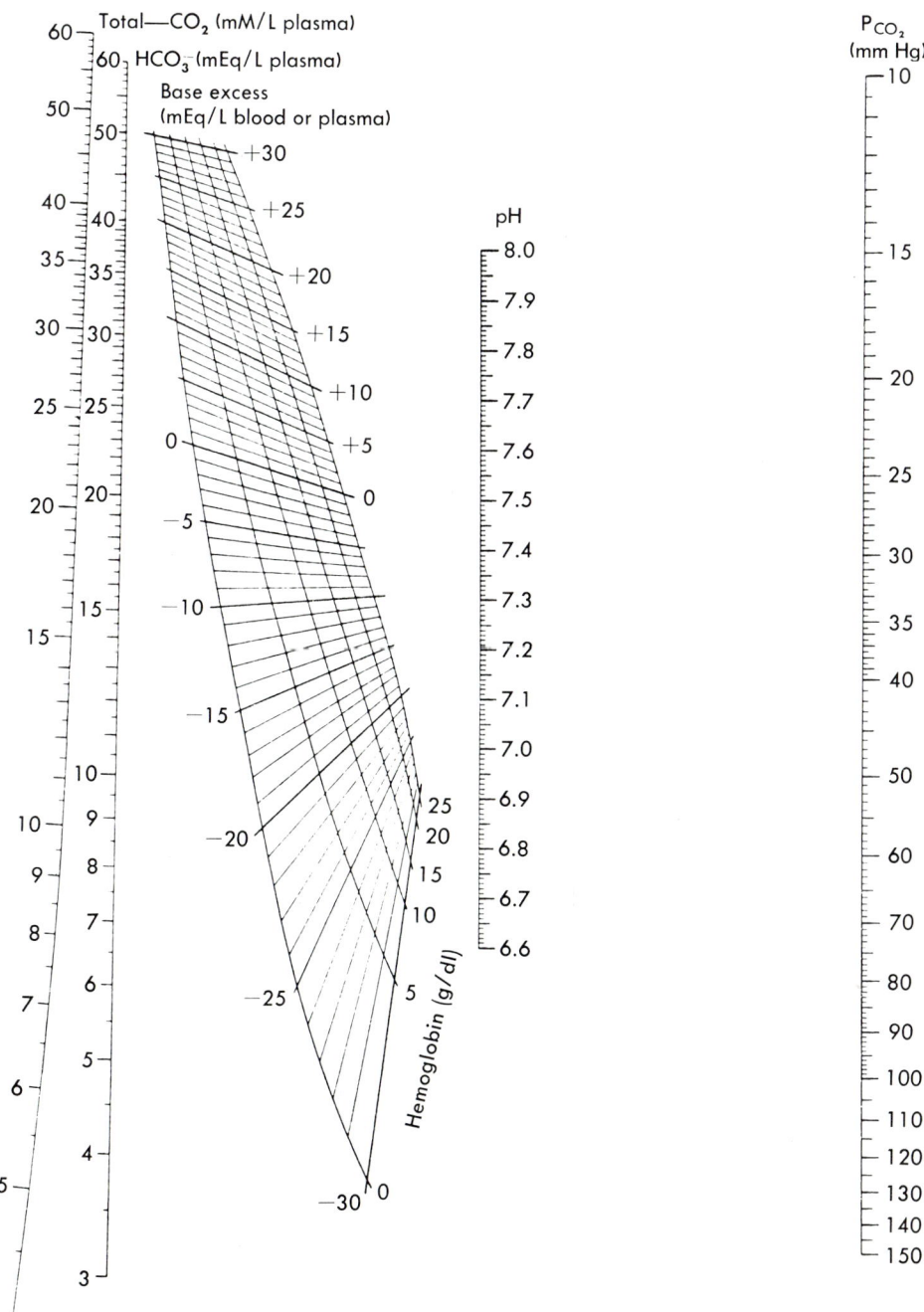

Fig. 22-2. Siggaard-Andersen nomograph. (Copyright by Radiometer A/S.)

Table 22-3. Acidosis and alkalosis: changes in blood pH and CO_2 content caused by changes in bicarbonate buffer $\left(\dfrac{HCO_3^-}{H_2CO_3}\right)$

Clinical condition	Change in denominator H_2CO_3	Change in numerator HCO_3^-	Common causes
Respiratory acidosis (CO_2 content and P_{CO_2} high, pH low)	Increases as result of pulmonary retnetion of CO_2*	May be increased late in compensation†	Impaired pulmonary function (asthma, emphysema, etc.)
Metabolic acidosis (CO_2 content and P_{CO_2} low, pH low)	May be decreased late in compensation‡	Decreases as result of loss of $NaHCO_3$* or displacement by other ions	Loss of base through diarrhea or impaired renal function and in diabetes and starvation
Respiratory alkalosis (CO_2 content low, pH high)	Decreases as result of hyperventilation*	May be decreased late in compensation†	Hyperventilation
Metabolic alkalosis (CO_2 content high, pH high)	May be increased in compensation‡	Increased as result of loss of Cl or ingestion of $NaHCO_3$*	Loss of HCl (vomiting), ingestion of alkali (peptic ulcer treatment)

*Primary changes that occur as result of abnormal conditions.
†Changes made by homeostatic mechanisms of body to restore a normal pH and compensate for abnormality. Changes in bicarbonate are chiefly mediated by an increase or decrease in renal excretion of bicarbonate.
‡Changes in H_2CO_3 brought about by changes in respiratory function to accelerate or decrease elimination of CO_2.

nomograms or slide rules of varying degrees of difference.

Astrup method

Another procedure for the measurement of the acid-base parameters is that devised by Astrup and associates.[94,95] In this method, only pH measurements are made. The pH of the original blood sample is determined, and then the pH is determined on other aliquots of the sample after they have been equilibrated at 37° C with two different gas mixtures of different known CO_2 content; usually these are about 4% and 8% CO_2. From these three pH measurements and a special nomogram, the other acid-base parameters can be determined. This method also calculates some other parameters, e.g., standard bicarbonate and base excess, which are claimed to be helpful in diagnosing acid-base imbalance. This method does not require the P_{CO_2} electrode but does necessitate the use of standard gases and a good tonometer for eqilibration.

Interpretation of changes in acid-base balance

Table 22-3 illustrates the changes in blood pH and CO_2 content in various pathologic conditions. Note that in both respiratory acidosis and metabolic alkalosis the CO_2 content is high, so that a measurement of this would not assist in diagnosis as would the measurement of pH. In metabolic acidosis and respiratory acidosis the pH is low, so that this measurement would not distinguish between them, although a measurement of CO_2 content would. In compensated respiratory acidosis there would be a gradual retention of HCO_3^- to bring the pH to near normality. At this time a measurement of pH would not indicate the true condition of the patient, but a determination of CO_2 content would indi-

cate a level even above that of the uncompensated condition. Other examples indicating that the single measurement of CO_2 content or pH alone is not sufficient to accurately assess the acid-base balance could also be given.

Gambino[96] has pointed out that many patients with severe intra-abdominal or intracerebral diseases (peritonitis, liver coma, hypertensive encephalopathy) may have a normal CO_2 content of the serum (26-31 mmole/L) but have a high pH (over 7.5). An abnormal level of the CO_2 content alone does not indicate any serious disease process in such cases.

Complete discussions of acid-base balance are found in two of the references already cited.[90,92]

Temperature correction tables

In modern blood gas measuring instruments the measurements are usually made at 37° C. If the body temperature of the patient is different than 37° C, the measured values of pH, P_{CO_2}, and P_{O_2} will not be the same as those actually existing in the patient, since these values are all temperature dependent. To obtain the true values a correction must be applied to the measured values. Tables 22-4 and 22-5 give values for the corrections. Table 22-4 for pH and P_{CO_2} is simple. Note that the corrections are applied differently depending on whether the patient's temperature is above or below 37° C. If desired, interpolation may be made in the tabulated values, but for most purposes this is not necessary.

Since the value for P_{O_2} depends on the oxygen saturation as well as the temperature, Table 22-5 gives both the temperature and the percent saturation to obtain the required correction factor. The factor changes only slightly with oxygen saturations below 70%, and the

Table 22-4. Temperature corrections for pH and P_{CO_2}

Temp. (° C)		pH F*	P_{CO_2} F*	Temp. (° C)		pH F*	P_{CO_2} F*
37.0		0	1				
36.5	37.5	0.007	1.023	30.0	44.0	0.103	1.359
36.0	38.0	0.015	1.045	29.5	44.5	0.110	1.388
35.5	38.5	0.023	1.068				
35.0	39.0	0.029	1.091	29.0	45.0	0.118	1.419
34.5	39.5	0.037	1.116	28.5	45.5	0.125	1.451
				28.0	46.0	0.132	1.483
34.0	40.0	0.044	1.140	27.5	46.5	0.140	1.515
33.5	40.5	0.051	1.165	27.0	47.0	0.147	1.549
33.0	41.0	0.059	1.191				
32.5	41.5	0.066	1.218	26.0		0.162	1.618
32.0	42.0	0.074	1.245	25.0		0.176	1.690
				24.0		0.191	1.766
31.5	42.5	0.081	1.272	23.0		0.206	1.845
31.0	43.0	0.088	1.300	22.0		0.221	1.928
30.5	43.5	0.096	1.329				

Correction for pH
1. When temperature is greater than 37° C, subtract pH F from measured pH.
2. When temperature is less than 37° C, add pH F to measured pH.

Correction for P_{CO_2}
1. When temperature is greater than 37° C, multiply measured P_{CO_2} by P_{CO_2} F.
2. When temperature is less than 37° C, divide measured P_{CO_2} by P_{CO_2} F.

*F = factor.

Table 22-5. Temperature corrections for P_{O_2}

Temp. (° C)		Oxygen saturation (%)								
		100	99	98	96	94	92	90	85	70
36.5	37.5	1.006	1.014	1.020	1.028	1.032	1.035	1.036	1.037	1.038
36.0	38.0	1.012	1.028	1.041	1.057	1.066	1.070	1.073	1.075	1.076
35.5	38.5	1.018	1.043	1.062	1.086	1.100	1.108	1.112	1.116	1.117
35.0	39.0	1.024	1.058	1.083	1.116	1.135	1.146	1.152	1.157	1.158
34.5	39.5	1.030	1.072	1.105	1.148	1.172	1.186	1.193	1.200	1.202
34.0	40.0	1.037	1.088	1.127	1.180	1.210	1.227	1.236	1.245	1.247
33.5	40.5	1.043	1.103	1.150	1.213	1.249	1.269	1.280	1.291	1.294
33.0	41.0	1.049	1.118	1.173	1.247	1.289	1.313	1.326	1.339	1.343
32.5	41.5	1.056	1.134	1.196	1.281	1.319	1.358	1.374	1.389	1.393
32.0	42.0	1.062	1.150	1.220	1.317	1.347	1.406	1.423	1.444	1.446
31.5	42.5	1.068	1.166	1.245	1.345	1.418	1.454	1.475	1.490	1.500
31.0	43.0	1.074	1.183	1.270	1.392	1.464	1.505	1.528	1.550	1.555
30.5	43.5	1.081	1.199	1.295	1.431	1.511	1.557	1.582	1.107	1.614
30.0	44.0	1.087	1.216	1.321	1.471	1.560	1.611	1.639	1.667	1.675
29.5	44.5	1.094	1.233	1.348	1.512	1.610	1.666	1.698	1.729	1.738
29.0	45.0	1.101	1.251	1.375	1.554	1.662	1.724	1.759	1.793	1.802
28.5	45.5	1.107	1.268	1.403	1.597	1.715	1.784	1.822	1.865	1.871
28.0	46.0	1.114	1.286	1.431	1.642	1.771	1.846	1.888	1.929	1.941
27.5	46.5	1.120	1.304	1.460	1.688	1.828	1.909	1.956	2.001	2.014
27.0	47.0	1.127	1.323	1.489	1.735	1.887	1.976	2.025	2.075	2.089
26.0		1.141	1.360	1.550	1.833	2.010	2.115	2.174	2.238	2.249
25.0		1.155	1.399	1.613	1.937	2.143	2.264	2.333	2.401	2.417
24.0		1.168	1.438	1.678	2.047	2.283	2.423	2.504	2.583	2.605
23.0		1.182	1.479	1.746	2.163	2.432	2.594	2.687	2.779	2.802
22.0		1.197	1.531	1.817	2.285	2.591	2.777	2.884	2.989	3.020

1. When temperature is greater than 37° C, multiply measured P_{O_2} by F.*
2. When temperature is less than 37° C, divide measured P_{O_2} by F.*

*Obtain the proper factor, F, from table by interpolation if necessary from measured or calculated oxygen saturation and temperature. For saturations below 70% use the values in column labeled 70.

values given in this column may be used for all lower saturations. The figures in these tables are calculated from the equations given by Burnett.[97]

OSMOLALITY[98-101]

To illustrate the concept of osmotic pressure and related phenomena, suppose that one has an aqueous solution of a solute separated from pure water by a membrane that will allow the free passage of water molecules but that is impermeable to the solute molecules. The water will then tend to diffuse through the membrane into the solution (thus increasing its volume and decreasing the concentration of the solute in the solution). If a positive pressure could be applied to the solution, this would tend to decrease the flow of water into it, because the increase in volume would be opposed by the applied pressure. If the membrane were capable of withstanding the pressure used and the latter were gradually increased, an equilibrium point would be reached at which there would be no net flow of water into the solution. This equilibrium pressure could be defined as the osmotic pressure of the solution. The same phenomena would occur if the membrane separated two solutions of different concentrations; the water would tend to diffuse from the dilute into the concentrated solution. The driving force would be the difference in osmotic pressure between the two solutions. The phenomenon of osmosis is of biologic importance, since the osmotic pressure is one of the factors regulating the flow of water through cell membranes.

Although the measurement of osmotic pressure by the use of a semipermeable membrane is of theoretic importance, it is impractical for biologic systems. Membranes that withstand the pressures needed and that are close to ideal in allowing only the passage of water and being equally impermeable to all solutes in a biologic system are very difficult to obtain. Also the attainment of equilibrium is usually very slow. It is known that the osmotic pressure is closely related to the other colligative properties of a solution: vapor pressure, freezing point, and boiling point, which vary with changes in solute concentration. These changes in colligative properties vary somewhat differently with the solvent concentration than do such other properties as specific gravity, conductivity, or refractive index. The changes in osmotic pressure or freezing point with concentration depend only on the number of particles in solution and not on their size, weight, or charge. Thus a solution of 60 mg urea (mol wt 60) in a given volume of water has the same osmotic pressure or depression in freezing point as a solution containing 180 mg glucose (mol wt 180) in the same volume of water, since each yields the same number of particles (molecules). With substances that form ions when dissolved in water (e.g., sodium chloride), it is found that each ion acts like a separate particle in its effect on the colligative properties. Thus a solution containing 0.1 mole of NaCl would yield 0.2 mole of particles (if it were completely ionized, which is not strictly true) and thus would exert the same osmotic pressure as a solution of 0.2 moles of urea, which yields one particle per molecule. Because of this effect the concentrations are usually expressed in osmols. A solution containing 1

osmol of any substance would have the same number of particles (in terms of the effect on the colligative properties) as a solution containing 1 mole of a substance that forms exactly one particle per molecule when dissolved (e.g., does not ionize or otherwise dissociate or associate in solution). The concentrations are conventionally expressed as osmolalities (osmols per kilogram of solvent [water in biologic systems]) and not as molarities (moles per 1000 ml solution). Usually the values for serum and urine are expressed in milliosmols per kilogram.

The osmolalities may be measured by determining the changes in boiling point, freezing point, or vapor pressure of the solution as compared with these constants for pure water. Although the measurement of changes in boiling point is simple, it is not practical for most biologic systems, since at the boiling point of water many of the substances would be decomposed or otherwise changed. The osmotic pressure may be measured by changes in the vapor pressure or freezing point. The latter is the more common method, although one instrument on the market uses the change in vapor pressure (Wescor, Logan, Utah). A number of instruments (Advanced Instruments, Needham Heights, Mass.; Fiske Associates, Uxbridge, Mass.; Precision Systems, Sudbury, Mass.) are on the market using the freezing point lowering, and since this is still the more common method a few remarks follow.

The technic may vary slightly with the instrument used, but in general the sample is placed in a cooling bath at about $-5°$ C and slowly cooled to slightly below its freezing point. It is then stirred or otherwise agitated so that freezing takes place, and the temperature of freezing is measured. Most instruments are calibrated with solutions of known osmolality and are designed to read in milliosmols directly rather than temperature. (A 100 mOsm solution should have a freezing point $0.186°$ C below that of pure water.)

The normal range of serum osmolality is 280-300 mOsm/kg for males and about 5 mOsm/kg lower than this in females. In cases of dehydration from whatever cause, the osmolality will be increased, and in excessive water intake the osmolality will be decreased. The ratio between the serum sodium level in millimoles per liter and the osmolality in milliosmoles per kilogram is normally between 0.33 and 0.50. Values lower than 0.33 generally have an unfavorable prognostic significance. Actually, in some instances this unfavorable ratio could result from a high value of urea in the serum (as in severe kidney disease) or a very high value of glucose in the serum (as in uncontrolled diabetes). Another method of comparison is to calculate the osmolality by multiplying the sodium value in millimoles per liter by 1.86, add to this the figures obtained by dividing the urea nitrogen value in milligrams per deciliter by 2.8 and the glucose value in milligrams per deciliter by 18. The measured osmolality is generally only 5-10 mOsm/kg higher than that calculated by the above method. A larger difference is said to indicate an abnormal condition. In comparing a number of formulas for calculating the osmolality, Dorwart and Chalmers[102] concluded that the formula given above is as satisfactory as any, but that the predictive value of the calculated osmolality compared with the actual measured value was small. Another cause of increased osmolality is alcohol intoxication. Alcohol is a relatively small molecule, so that a concentration of 0.1 g/dl would theoretically cause a rise in osmolality of about 22 mOsm/kg, a significant change compared with the normal value of around 290 mOsm/kg. In fact, the measurement of osmolality has been suggested as a simple screening test for this condition.[103] The serum osmolality is also useful in following the course of patients on intravenous therapy. An increase in osmolality above normal might indicate that the patient is receiving too great a quantity of electrolytes relative to the amount of water, and a decrease in osmolality might indicate that the patient is receiving relatively too much water. Another use of osmolality is in interpreting the electrolyte levels found in extremely hyperlipemic sera. The electrolytes are dissolved only in the serum water and not in the lipids. Thus the amount of sodium per milliliter of serum water might be within normal limits, but because of the large amounts of lipids present the amount of sodium present per milliliter of total serum volume would be low. A normal serum osmolality (which would be only slightly affected by the presence of the lipids) indicates that the apparently low sodium level resulted from the hyperlipemia and not from any disturbance in the electrolyte metabolism.

The normal range of urine osmolality is 390-1090 mOsm/kg for males (average 840) and 300-1090 mOsm/kg for females (average 750). Hospital patients usually have somewhat lower values, in the range of 280-900 mOsm/kg. The corresponding values for 24 hr urinary output are 770-1630 mOsm/24 hr for males and 430-1150 mOsm/24 hr for females, with somewhat lower values for convalescent bed patients. As with the excretion of sodium and chloride, the urinary osmolality varies with the dietary intake.

REFERENCES

1. Zak, B., Epstein, E., and Baginski, E.S.: Ann. Clin. Lab. Sci. **5:**195, 1975.
2. Morin, L.C.: Am. J. Clin. Pathol. **61:**114, 1974.
3. Baginski, E.S., et al.: Clin. Chim. Acta **46:**46, 1974.
4. Brandstein, M., Castellano, A., and Mezzacappa, C.: Am. J. Clin. Pathol. **40:**583, 1963.
5. Sardou, R.: Ann. Biol. Clin. **21:**593, 1963.
6. Trudeau, D.L., and Freier, E.F.: Clin. Chem. **13:**101, 1967.
7. Lott, J.A.: CRC Crit. Rev. Anal. Chem. **3:**41, 1972.
8. Bowers, G.H., Jr., and Pybus, J.: In Cooper, G.R., editor: Standard methods of clinical chemistry, New York, 1972, Academic Press, Inc., vol. 7, p. 143.
9. Ladenson, J.H., and Bowers, G.W., Jr.: Clin. Chem. **19:**565, 1973.
10. Ladenson, J.H., and Bowers, G.H., Jr.: Clin. Chem. **19:**575, 1973.
11. Robertson, W.C.: Ann. Clin. Biochem. **13:**540, 1976.
12. Husdan, H., et al.: Clin. Chem. **23:**1775, 1977.
13. McLean, E.C., and Hastings, A.B.: J. Biol. Chem. **108:**285, 1958.
14. Ladenson, J.H.: In Sonnenwirth, A.C., and Jarett, L., editors: Gradwohl's clinical laboratory methods and diagnosis, ed. 8, St. Louis, 1980, The C.V. Mosby Co., chap. 16.
15. Willis, H.B., and Lewin, M.B.: J. Clin. Pathol. **24:**856, 1971.
16. Payne, R.B., et al.: Med. J. **4:**643, 1973.
17. Phillips, P.J., et al.: Clin. Chem. **23:**1938, 1977.
18. Parekh, A.C., and Jung, D.H.: Clin. Chim. Acta **27:**373, 1970.
19. Drewes, P.A.: Clin. Chim. Acta **39:**81, 1972.
20. Orange, M., and Rhein, H.C.: J. Biol. Chem. **189:**379, 1951.
21. Andreasen, K.: Scand. J. Clin. Lab. Invest. **9:**170, 1957.
22. Basinski, D.H.: In Meites, S., editor: Standard methods of clinical chemistry, New York, 1965, Academic Press, Inc., vol. 5, p. 137.
23. Hansen, J.L., and Freier, E.F.: Am. J. Med. Technol. **33:**158, 1967.
24. David, L., and Anast, C.S.: J. Clin. Invest. **54:**287, 1974.
25. Bauer, J.D.: In Sonnenwirth, A.C., and Jarett, L., editors: Gradwohl's clinical laboratory methods and diagnosis, ed. 8, St. Louis, 1980, The C.V. Mosby Co., chap. 37.
26. International Committee for Standardization in Hematology: J. Clin. Pathol. **24:**334, 1971, and Br. J. Haematol. **38:**291, 1978.
27. Horak, E., Hohnadel, D.C., and Sunderman, F.W., Jr.: Ann. Clin. Lab. Sci. **5:**303, 1975.
28. Horak, E., and Sunderman, F.W., Jr.: Ann. Clin. Lab. Sci. **4:**87, 1974.
29. Ramsey, W.N.M.: J. Clin. Pathol. **28:**156, 1975.
30. Fiet, J., et al.: Ann. Biol. Clin. **35:**305, 1977.
31. Dreux, C., Bouchet, R., and Girard, M.L.: Ann. Biol. Clin. (Paris) **29:**251, 1971.
32. Glenn, M.T., et al.: Anal. Chem. **45:**203, 1973.
33. Yeh, Y-Y., and Zee, P.: Clin. Chem. **20:**360, 1974.
34. Carter, P.: Clin. Chim. Acta **39:**497, 1972.
35. Giorgio, A.G., Cartwright, G.E., and Wintrobe, M.M.: Am. J. Clin. Pathol. **41:**22, 1964.
36. Williams, H.L., Johnson, D.J., and Hant, M.J.: Clin. Chem. **23:**237, 1977.
37. Dawson, J.B., Ellis, D.J., and Newton-John, H.: Clin. Chim. Acta **21:**33, 1968.
38. Analytical methods for atomic absorption spectrophotometry, Norwalk, Conn., 1976, Perkin-Elmer Corp.
39. Hohnadel, D.C., et al.: Clin. Chem. **19:**1288, 1973.
40. Prasad, A.S., et al.: J. Lab. Clin. Med. **61:**531, 1963.
41. Prasad, A.S., et al.: Arch. Intern. Med. **111:**407, 1963.
42. Halsted, J.A., et al.: Am. J. Med. **53:**277, 1972.
43. Walravens, P.A.: Clin. Chem. **26:**185, 1980.
44. Hambridge, K.M., et al.: Pediatr. Res. **6:**868, 1972.
45. McMahon, R.A., et al.: Med. J. Aust. **2:**210, 1968.
46. Johnson, D.J., et al.: Clin. Chem. **23:**1321, 1977.
47. Smith, J.C., Jr., Butrimovitz, G.P., and Purdy, W.C.: Clin. Chem. **25:**1487, 1979.
48. Teloh, H.A.: In Sunderman, F.W., and Sunderman, F.W., Jr., editors: Clinical pathology of the serum electrolytes, Springfield, Ill., 1966, Charles C Thomas, Publisher.
49. Durst R.A., editor: Ion-selective electrodes, N.B.S. spec. pub. no. 314, Washington, D.C., 1969, U.S. Government Printing Office.
50. Neff, C.: Clin. Chem. **16:**781, 1970.
51. Eisenman, G., Rudin, D.O., and Casby, J.W.: Science **126:**831, 1957.
52. Pioda, L.A., et al.: Clin. Chim. Acta **29:**289, 1970.
53. Westgard, J.O., et al.: Clin. Chem. **22:**489, 1976.
54. Durst, R.A.: Clin. Chim. Acta **80:**225, 1977.
55. Fievet, P., et al.: Clin. Chem. **26:**138, 1980.
56. Finley, P.R., et al.: Clin. Chem. **24:**2125, 1978.
57. Lustgarten, J.A., et al.: Clin. Chem. **20:**1217, 1974.
58. Truchaud, A., et al.: Clin. Chem. **26:**139, 1980.

59. Hartmann, A.E., and Fillbach, J.R.: Am. J. Clin. Pathol. **74:**275, 1980.

60. Galen, R.S.: Diagn. Med. **4:**79, 1981.

61. Leaf, A.: N. Engl. J. Med. **267:**24, 1962.

62. Haven, G.T., and Haven, M.C.: Clin. Chem. **19:**791, 1973.

63. Vink, C.L.J.: Clin. Chim. Acta **65:**379, 1975.

64. Steffes, M.W., and Freier, E.F.: J. Lab. Clin. Med. **88:**683, 1976.

65. Romano, A.T., and Young, G.W., Jr.: Clin. Chem. **23:**303, 1977.

66. Hartmann, R.C.: In Brinkhous, K.M., Shermer, R.W., and Mosotifi, F.K., editors: The platelet, Baltimore, 1971, The Williams & Wilkins Co.

67. Ladenson, J.H., et al.: Am. J. Clin. Pathol. **62:**545, 1974.

68. Wesson, L.G., Jr.: Medicine **43:**547, 1964.

69. Böing, D., Schweigart, U., and Kunze, M.: Eur. J. Appl. Physiol. **32:**239, 1974.

70. Schales, O., and Schales, S.S.: J. Biol. Chem. **140:**879, 1941.

71. Schales, O.: In Reiner, M., editor: Standard methods of clinical chemistry, New York, 1953, Academic Press, Inc., vol. 1, p. 37.

72. Cotlove, E.: In Seligson, D., editor: Standard methods of clinical chemistry, New York, 1961, Academic Press, Inc., vol. 3, p. 81.

73. Cotlove, E.: In Glick, D., editor: Methods of biochemical analysis, New York, 1964, Interscience, vol. 12.

74. Bray, P.T., et al.: Clin. Chim. Acta **77:**69, 1977.

75. Szabo, L., Kenney, M.A., and Lee, W.: Clin. Chem. **19:**727, 1973.

76. Smetters, G.W., Sherrick, J.C., and de la Huerga, J.: In Sunderman, F.W., and Sunderman, F.W., Jr., editors: Clinical pathology of the serum electrolytes, Srpingfield, Ill., 1966, Charles C Thomas Publisher, p. 253.

77. Peters, J.P., and Van Slyke, D.D.: Quantitative clinical chemistry. Vol. 2. Methods, Baltimore, 1932, The Williams & Wilkins Co.

78. Natelson, S.: Techniques of clinical chemistry, ed. 3, Springfield, Ill., 1971, Charles C Thomas, Publisher.

79. Holaday, D.A., and Verosky, M.: J. Lab. Clin. Med. **47:**634, 1956.

80. Gambino, S.R., and Schreiber, H.: Am. J. Clin. Pathol. **45:**406, 1966.

81. Buttery, J.E., Loh, G.W., and Mok, S.L.: Clin. Biochem. **10:**102, 1977.

82. Grens, R.J., and Koch, B.H.: Am. J. Med. Technol. **40:**50, 1977.

83. Beckman Instruments, Inc.: Carbon dioxide chemistry module operating and service instructions, Brea, Calif., 1979, Beckman Instruments, Inc.

84. Hamilton, L.H.: Prog. Clin. Pathol. **2:**284, 1969.

85. Torres, C.R.: J. Appl. Physiol. **18:**1008, 1963.

86. Gelder, R.I., and Neville, J.R., Jr.: Am. J. Clin. Pathol. **55:**325, 1971.

87. Severinghaus, J.W.: Scand. J. Clin. Lab. Invest. **17:**614, 1965.

88. Hahn, E.E.W., and Smith, A.C.: Br. J. Anaesth. **67:**559, 1975.

89. Gill, P.E., and Brown, S.S.: CRC Crit. Rev. Clin. Lab. Sci. **7:**99, 1976.

90. Natelson, S., and Natelson, E.A.: Principles of applied clinical chemistry. Vol. 1. Maintenance of fluid and electrolyte balance, New York, 1975, Plenum Press, pp. 13-39.

91. Durst, R.A., editor: Blood pH, gases and electrolytes, N.B.S. spec. pub. no. 450, Washington, D.C., 1977, U.S. Government Printing Office.

92. Filley, G.F.: Acid-base and blood gas regulation, Philadelphia, 1971, Lea & Febiger.

93. Siggard-Andersen, O.: Scand. J. Clin. Lab. Invest. **15:**211, 1963.

93a. Weisberg, H.F.: In Durst, R.A., editor: Blood pH, gases and electrolytes, N.B.S. spec. pub. no. 450, Washington, D.C., 1977, U.S. Government Printing Office, p. 103.

94. Astrup, P., et al.: Ann. N.Y. Acad. Sci. **133:**59, 1966.

95. Astrup, P., and Siggard-Andersen, O.: Adv. Clin. Chem. **6:**3, 1963.

96. Gambino, S.R.: J.A.M.A. **198:**250, 1966.

97. Burnett, R.W.: Clin. Chem. **24:**1850, 1978.

98. Johnston, R.B., Jr.: In Meites, S., editor: Standard methods of clinical chemistry, New York, 1965, Academic Press, Inc., vol. 5, p. 159.

99. Ehrmantraut, H.C.: In Sunderman, F.W., and Sunderman, F.W., Jr., editors: Clinical pathology of the serum electrolytes, Springfield, Ill., 1966, Charles C Thomas, Publisher.

100. Hendry, R.B.: Clin. Chem. **6:**246, 1968.

101. Albrink, M.J., et al.: J. Clin. Invest. **34:**1483, 1955.

102. Dorwart, W.V., and Chalmers, L.: Clin. Chem. **21:**191, 1975.

103. Robinson, A.C., and Loeb, J.N.: N. Engl. J. Med. **284:**1253, 1971.

CHAPTER 23

Liver function, lipids, and other miscellaneous tests

LIVER FUNCTION TESTS

The liver is the largest organ in the human body and possesses a large and varied array of biochemical activities that are essential to proper function of the body. The liver plays a central role in the metabolism of carbohydrates and in the formation of proteins and other aspects of protein metabolism. It is concerned with detoxification of drugs and other harmful substances and with the metabolism of steroid hormones. It plays an important role in the production of some of the substances necessary for the coagulation of blood and in the metabolism of iron and the formation and breakdown of hemoglobin. It is also concerned with the production of bile, which aids in the digestion of fats and the absorption of fat-soluble vitamins. The liver has a great reserve capacity; nearly four fifths of the liver can be removed without seriously affecting its function. On the other hand only a mild diffuse lesion (affecting the whole organ) may alter the results of liver function tests. In severe liver damage all of the functions will be decreased to some extent. This depends on the type of disease; some functions may be affected more than others.

Liver function tests can be classified on the basis of the principal metabolic process or type of function with which they are concerned, on the basis of their sensitivity in detecting liver damage, or on the basis of the clinical conditions in which they are most useful. All three methods would have some validity for the purposes of this volume, but a classification has been adopted based mainly on the first—the specific function or metabolic process involved.

TESTS BASED ON BILIRUBIN
Bilirubin metabolism

Bilirubin is formed by the breakdown of hemoglobin by the cells of the reticuloendothelial system (spleen, bone marrow, Kupffer's cells of the liver), and it circulates in the blood in low concentrations. A small amount is excreted by the kidneys into the urine. Bilirubin is excreted by the liver cells into the bile and passes with the bile into the intestines, where it is reduced by bacterial action to **urobilinogen.** The major portion of the urobilinogen is excreted in the feces. Some is reabsorbed into the blood and reexcreted by the liver as urobilinogen. A portion of the absorbed urobilinogen is also excreted by the kidneys into the urine.

An increased bilirubin concentration in the bloodstream results in the clinical condition of jaundice (Table 23-1). This increase may result from a number of causes. Because of increased hemoglobin destruction, the liver may not be able to properly excrete the greater load of pigment present and the bilirubin level in the blood will rise. This is a prehepatic condition known as **hemolytic jaundice;** the liver function may be relatively normal but is unable to cope with the pigments

from the marked increase in erythrocyte destruction. The second type of jaundice, **hepatogenous jaundice,** is caused by intrahepatic damage to the liver parenchyma, which may be of a toxic, infectious, or mechanical nature. Excretion of bile is greatly decreased, and the concentration of bilirubin in the blood rises. In the third type of jaundice the liver cells may have a normal or nearly normal ability to excrete bilirubin, but because of obstruction in the biliary tract, the proper flow of bile is inhibited and the bile capillaries are dilated and even disrupted by the back pressure. The bile flows into the perilobar lymphatics and hence into the bloodstream. This extrahepatic condition has been designated as **obstructive jaundice.**

Bilirubin tests

Principle: Bilirubin reacts with diazotized sulfanilic acid to give a color that is red-violet in acid solution and blue in alkaline solution. It has been known for many years that not all of the bilirubin present in serum reacts at once with the diazo reagent in an aqueous solution. To obtain a complete reaction, the addition of a fairly high concentration of alcohol (ethyl or methyl) or some other solubilizing agent is necessary. Bilirubin

Table 23-1. Early laboratory findings in jaundice

	Hemolytic (prehepatic)	Hepatogenous (intrahepatic)	Obstructive (extrahepatic)
Bile pigments			
Urine			
Urobilinogen and urobilin	Markedly increased	Slight to moderate increase	Not increased
Bilirubin	Negative	Positive	Positive
Serum			
Direct bilirubin	Normal	Increased	Increased
Total bilirubin	Moderate increase	Moderate to marked increase	Marked increase
Feces			
Urobilinogen compounds	Marked increase	Normal or variable	Low or negative (acholic)
Serum enzymes			
Alkaline phosphatase	Normal or slight increase	Normal or slight increase	Marked increase
Glutamic oxalacetic transaminase (GOT), aldolase, isocitric dehydrogenase (ICDH)	Normal or slight increase	Marked increase	Slight increase
Leucine aminopeptidase (LAP), γ-glutamyl transpeptidase	Normal	Slight increase	Marked increase
Glutamic pyruvic transaminase (GPT), ornithine carbamyl transferase (OCT), guanase	Normal or slight increase	Marked increase	Slight increase
Pseudocholinesterase	Normal	Decreased	Decreased
Serum proteins			
Albumin	Normal	Slight decrease	Normal or slight decrease
Globulins	Normal	Increased	Normal or slight increase
Albumin/globulin (A/G) ratio	Normal	May be reversed	Normal
Other tests			
Serum cholesterol	Normal	Decreased	Marked increased
Bromsulphalein retention	Usually negative	Usually positive	Positive
Prothrombin time	Normal	Increased	Normal, later increased
Response to vitamin K	Normal	Decreased or none	Normal

exists in the serum in two forms—a "free" form (absorbed on albumin) and a conjugated form (chiefly as glucuronides). The so-called **direct-reacting bilirubin** is the **conjugated form** that is more soluble in water and reacts relatively rapidly in aqueous solution. The free bilirubin is much less soluble in water and does not react (or reacts very slowly) in simple aqueous solution. The addition of methyl alcohol to a concentration of 40-50% will dissolve the bilirubin sufficiently to react with diazo reagent. This is the basis for the commonly used Malloy-Evelyn method. A solution containing a relatively high concentration of caffeine and sodium benzoate will also dissolve the free bilirubin for reaction. This is used in the method of Jendrassik and Grof.

Although the method of Malloy and Evelyn is widely used, it has several disadvantages that are not always kept in mind. The diazo color is slightly different in hue and intensity when the test is run on diluted serum than when it is run on a chloroform standard containing no serum or protein, as is often done with this method. Although a chloroform standard is convenient, it may introduce a slight error. Furthermore, unreacted bilirubin has some absorption at the wavelength used, so that in the standardization the blank should contain the same amount of bilirubin as the diazotized standard. The diazotized bilirubin is actually an indicator in which the color changes with the pH. As ordinarily run, the final solution is only slightly buffered, so that changes in pH can occur, particularly if the serum sample used is one in which the pH has changed on standing. The high concentration of alcohol in the reaction for total bilirubin often causes some turbidity that is not always the same in the diazotized sample as in the serum blank. The presence of more than traces of hemoglobin will also interfere with the color reaction.

The method of Jendrassik and Grof suffers less from these disadvantages. The final color is read in a highly buffered alkaline medium in which changes in pH are negligible. This reduces the effects of varying protein content; the effects of hemolysis are also markedly reduced. Since the method of Malloy and Evelyn is still widely used, both methods will be presented.

It should also be mentioned that bilirubin is markedly **sensitive to light.** This applies to all methods; samples for bilirubin determination should not be exposed to strong light at any time. When serum samples that are not to be analyzed immediately are stored in the refrigerator, the effect of light is no problem; however, exposure to ordinary light in the laboratory for several hours could reduce the bilirubin content by 10% or more.

Jendrassik-Grof method[1-3]

Reagents:

1. Caffeine solution
   Dissolve 50 g caffeine, 75 g sodium benzoate, and 125 g crystalline sodium acetate (trihydrate) in warm water. Cool and dilute to 1 L. This solution is stable for at least 6 months. Other accelerator solutions have been suggested,[4] but they possess no marked advantages over the solution used here.

2. Diazo I
   Dissolve 5.0 g sulfanilic acid and 15 ml concentrated HCl in water to make 1 L.

3. Diazo II
   Dissolve 0.1 g sodium nitrite in 20 ml of water. This solution is stable for several weeks when kept in the refrigerator. It may be convenient to weigh 0.1 g portions of the salt into small stoppered vials, which can be added to 20 ml of water as needed.

4. Diazo mixture
   Mix 10 ml of diazo I and 0.25 ml of diazo II. This solution has been found to be stable for 24 hr at room temperature and up to 72 hr when kept at 4° C.[5,6] It is convenient to make up daily. A more stable diazo reagent has been suggested,[7] but this is somewhat more trouble to prepare.

5. Hydrochloric acid, 0.05 mole/L
   Dilute 4.5 ml concentrated hydrochloric acid to 1 L.

6. Ascorbic acid, 4 g/dl
   Dissolve 200 mg ascorbic acid in 5 ml water. This should be freshly prepared on the day of use. A convenient method for obtaining the ascorbic acid solution is to use sterile ampules of ascorbic acid for parenteral injection. One ampule is opened and diluted with water as required for use, but this is more expensive than preparing the reagent directly.

7. Alkaline tartrate
   Dissolve 100 g sodium hydroxide and 350 g potassium sodium tartrate in water and dilute to 1 L. Store in a polyethylene bottle.

Procedure for total bilirubin (macromethod): In the macromethod for each serum sample set up two tubes, sample and serum blank. Also set up one reagent blank, using water instead of diluted serum. Dilute 1 ml serum with 4 ml saline solution; this will give sufficient diluted serum for both direct and total bilirubin. For total bilirubin place 1 ml diluted serum and 2.1 ml caffeine mixture in test tubes and mix. To serum sample and reagent blank, add 0.5 ml diazo mixture; to serum blank, add 0.5 ml diazo I. Allow mixture to stand for exactly 10 min. To each tube, add 1.5 ml alkaline tartrate. Read the serum and serum blank against the reagent blank at 600 nm 5-10 min after the addition of the tartrate. Note that although the diazotized bilirubin is blue in alkali, the solutions appear green because of the yellow color from the reaction of the diazo reagent and the caffeine mixture. This yellow color has negligible absorbance at 600 nm. Subtract the absorbance of the serum blank from that of the serum for calculation. Experience will show that, except for noticeably hemolyzed serum samples, the blank reading is fairly constant and that a constant blank may be used without great error with unhemolyzed serum samples.

For hemolyzed samples the effect of hemoglobin may be reduced by using 2 ml caffeine solution and then adding 0.1 ml ascorbic acid just before the alkaline tartrate solution, as in the direct bilirubin method.

Procedure for direct bilirubin: The setup for direct bilirubin is similar to that for total bilirubin, using 1 ml diluted serum, 2 ml 0.05 N hydrochloric acid, and 0.5

ml diazo mixture. After exactly 10 min, add 0.1 ml ascorbic acid solution, mix, and then add at once 1.5 ml alkaline tartrate. Also set up a serum blank and reagent blank as before, adding diazo I instead of the diazo mixture to the serum blank. Read as for total bilirubin.

Procedure for micromethod: For the micromethod to 0.25 ml water and 1 ml caffeine mixture, add 0.05 ml serum from a micropipet. Add 0.25 ml diazo mixture and let stand exactly 10 min; then add 0.75 ml alkaline tartrate and read against blank as for macromethod. A serum blank and reagent blank should also be set up as in the macromethod. The solution is sufficient for reading in standard 10 mm cuvets.

Direct bilirubin can also be run by the micromethod, using 1 ml 0.05N hydrochloric acid, 0.2 ml water, 0.05 ml serum, 0.25 ml diazo mixture, 0.5 ml ascorbic acid, and finally, 0.75 ml alkaline tartrate.

Calculation: Bilirubin values are often read from a calibration chart. The preparation of a chart will be discussed in the section on standardization. If a standard of a serum of known bilirubin content is used, then

$$\frac{\text{Absorbance of sample}}{\text{Absorbance of standard}} \times \frac{\text{Conc.}}{\text{of standard}} = \frac{\text{Conc.}}{\text{of sample}}$$

where the absorbances of standard and sample have been corrected for any blank readings. In the United States the concentration of bilirubin in the lyophilized serum samples is usually given in milligrams per deciliter. To convert to micromoles per liter multiply by 17.1.

All standards are calibrated in terms of total bilirubin only and are used to calibrate both the direct bilirubin and total bilirubin in the sample.

$$\text{Total bilirubin} - \text{Direct bilirubin} = \text{Indirect bilirubin}$$

Malloy-Evelyn method[8-10]

Reagents:
1. Diazo mixture
   Prepare the same as for the previous method.
2. Hydrochloric acid, 1.5%
   Dilute 15 ml concentrated hydrochloric acid to 1 L.
3. Methyl alcohol

Procedure: Add 2 ml serum to 18 ml normal saline solution and mix. For **direct bilirubin** pipet 4 ml diluted serum to each of two tubes, A and B. To tube A, add 1 ml diazo mixture and mix immediately. To tube B, add 1 ml 1.5% hydrochloric acid and mix. Read tube A against tube B in a spectrophotometer at 540 nm after 1 min.

For **total bilirubin** proceed as for direct bilirubin, but after the addition of diazo reagent, add 5 ml methyl alcohol, mix, and allow to stand for 30 min before reading. Read tube A against tube B as for direct bilirubin.

Calculation: Note that in this procedure the final volume for total bilirubin is twice the final volume for direct bilirubin. Hence, if a known serum is used as a standard for total bilirubin, then for direct bilirubin:

$$\frac{\text{Absorbance of sample}}{\text{Absorbance of standard}} \times \frac{\text{Conc. of standard}}{2} = \frac{\text{Conc.}}{\text{of sample}}$$

For total bilirubin:

$$\frac{\text{Absorbance of sample}}{\text{Absorbance of standard}} \times \frac{\text{Conc.}}{\text{of standard}} = \frac{\text{Conc.}}{\text{of sample}}$$

$$\text{Total bilirubin} - \text{Direct bilirubin} = \text{Indirect bilirubin}$$

As mentioned earlier, the methyl alcohol may cause some turbidity and this can result in an apparent negative value for low bilirubin levels.

Bilirubin standardization

Many commercial bilirubin preparations are by no means pure, and all bilirubin solutions are subject to deterioration on storage. Consequently, the standardization[8] of a bilirubin assay is not simple. Chloroform solutions of bilirubin are relatively stable and have been used as standards, but they are not applicable to all methods. It has also been shown that absorption of diazo-bilirubin is different in the presence of protein (as in a serum sample) and in the absence of protein (as in a chloroform standard). It has been stated that this difference depends somewhat on the type of instrument used (spectrophotometer or filter instrument). The best method seems to be the preparation of a standard curve using dilutions of a commercial lyophilized control serum (American Monitor Corp., Indianapolis). The serum should be used for bilirubin determination within 2 hr after reconstitution and should not be exposed to bright light at any time. If the method used is sensitive to protein concentration (as is the Malloy-Evelyn method), it is preferable to use not only dilutions of a high bilirubin serum with saline solution but mixtures of a low bilirubin serum and a high bilirubin serum to keep the protein content approximately constant. For example, if the one control serum contained 0.6 mg/dl bilirubin (serum A) and the other serum contained 6 mg/dl bilirubin (serum B) and the method required that 1 ml serum be diluted with 9 ml saline solution, then setting up the tubes as given in Table 23-2 would give a series of standards.

It is desirable to have an independent check on the bilirubin curve, and the Harleco Dripak bilirubin standard (Harleco, Philadelphia) is satisfactory for this purpose. The material is quite stable in the dry form. Standardization using this material is rather tedious and hence is most suitable as an occasional check on the calibration curve.

The Harleco bilirubin is supplied in plastic containers that hold exactly 40 mg pure bilirubin each. The entire packet is dropped into exactly 40 ml 0.1M sodium carbonate (10.6 g anhydrous salt/L) and swirled until dissolved. The bilirubin should form a clear solution within a few minutes. The entire standardization procedure should be carried through as rapidly as possible and in as dim a light as practicable.

Table 23-2. Preparation of bilirubin standards

Tube no.	1	2	3	4	5	6
Serum A (ml)	1.0	0.8	0.6	0.4	0.2	0.0
Serum B (ml)	0.0	0.2	0.4	0.6	0.2	1.0
Equivalent	0.60	1.68	2.76	3.84	4.92	6.00

In each of two test tubes place a dilution of a clear serum of low bilirubin content. Use the same volume of solution and the same dilution of serum as in the regular bilirubin procedure. To one tube, add 0.05 ml bilirubin solution, using an accurate "to contain" micropipet that has been rinsed well. To the other tube, add 0.05 ml sodium carbonate. The regular procedure for total bilirubin is then carried out for both tubes. The difference in absorbance for the readings of the two tubes is the diazo color caused by 0.05 mg bilirubin (the bilirubin solution contains 1 mg/ml). If the method under calibration regularly uses 0.4 ml serum, then the color would be equivalent to that from a serum containing $(0.05 \times 100)/0.4$, or 12.5 ml/dl. One could carry out a calibration curve by this method with different pipets and dilutions of the strong bilirubin solution, but ordinarily this is used to check one or two points on the curve.

Bilirubin obtained from other suppliers (Pfanstiel Laboratories, Waukegan, Ill.; J.T. Baker Chemical Co., Phillipsburg, N.J.) and the National Bureau of Standards (SRM-916, National Bureau of Standards, Washington, D.C.) may also be used. These are not supplied in preweighed amounts. The material furnished by the NBS is the primary standard and is recommended although it is more expensive. The solution made up in sodium carbonate is stable for only a short time. If one desires a standard that can be used on several occasions, the following procedure may be used.[6,11]

Procedure: Accurately weigh about 20 mg of the bilirubin and transfer to a 1 dl volumetric flask. Dissolve the bilirubin in 4 ml of 0.1 mole/L sodium carbonate solution. Some samples of bilirubin are not readily soluble in the sodium carbonate solution. These are first suspended in 1 ml of dimethylsulfoxide in the flask and then 2 ml of the sodium carbonate solution added. When the bilirubin has dissolved, about 80 ml of a protein solution, 4 g/dl of bovine serum albumin, human serum albumin, or clear pooled serum of known low bilirubin content, is added. Next, 2-4 ml of 0.1 mole/L hydrochloric acid is added to neutralize the alkali. The exact amount of acid to exactly neutralize is determined beforehand by titrating 4 ml of the sodium carbonate solution with the hydrochloric acid solution to the phenolphthalein end point. The solution is then made up to 1 dl with the protein solution. After mixing is finished, aliquots of the solution are transferred to small, plastic, capped tubes, which are then stored frozen. The frozen material is stable for about 3 months when stored at $-20°$ C and for about 9 months when stored at $-70°$ C. This solution will contain about 20 mg/dl, depending on the exact amount of bilirubin weighed, together with any bilirubin in the pooled serum if used. This latter should not be more than about 1 mg/dl. An aliquot may then be thawed, mixed well, and dilutions made to check a calibration curve.

Direct spectrophotometric method[12]

Principle: The total bilirubin in the serum of newborns is proportional to the absorbance of bilirubin at 455 nm. The absorbance of hemoglobin at 455 nm is corrected by subtracting the absorbance at 575 nm. The determination cannot be used in adults or newborns older than a few weeks because of the presence of other lipochromes, e.g., carotene, that increase the nonbilirubin absorbance at 455 nm.

Reagents:
1. Phosphate buffer, 0.067 mole/L, pH 7.4
   Dissolve 9.541 g $Na_2HPO_4 \cdot 2H_2O$ and 1.777 g KH_2PO_4 in water and make up to 9 dl in a 1 L volumetric flask. Check pH with meter and adjust if necessary; then dilute to volume.
2. Bilirubin standard
   Prepare a series of bilirubin standards from 2-20 mg/dl as described previously.
3. Hemoglobin standard
   Prepare a series of dilute hemoglobin standards from 10-200 mg/dl from washed red cells that have been lysed with water.

Procedure: Pipet 1.0 ml phosphate buffer into separate tubes for each sample or control to be analyzed. Add 50 µl serum or control serum, mix, and measure the absorbance against a water blank at 455 nm and 575 nm.

Calculation:

$$\text{Total bilirubin (mg/dl)} = (K_1 A_{455} - K_2 A_{575}) \times \text{Dilution}$$

where K_1 and K_2 are absorption constants for bilirubin and hemoglobin, A_{455} is absorbance at 455 nm, and A_{575} is absorbance at 575 nm. The constants are determined by using several standards of bilirubin and, separately, several standards of hemoglobin and reading the absorption of each solution after dilution in the procedure at both 455 and 575 nm. In each case the absorption is divided by the standard concentration in milligrams per deciliter to give an absorbance per milligrams per deciliter. The absorbance results per milligrams per deciliter for several bilirubin concentrations are then averaged for each wavelength. The same process is carried out for hemoglobin. After this has been done one will have two constants for bilirubin, K_{b455} and K_{b575}, and two constants for hemoglobin, K_{h455} and K_{h575}. These are combined in the final equation as follows:

$$\text{Total bilirubin (mg/dl)} =$$
$$\frac{(K_{h575} \times A_{455}) - (K_{h455} \times A_{575})}{(K_{b455} \times K_{h575}) - (K_{b575} \times K_{h455})} \times \text{Dilution}$$

For the example given in Tietz[13] this is as follows:

$$\text{Total bilirubin (mg/dl)} =$$
$$(1.30 A_{455} - 1.37 A_{575}) \times \text{Dilution}$$

The constants will be slightly different for each spectrophotometer and must be determined on each instrument.

There are several commercially available instruments (Advanced Instruments, Needham Heights, Mass.; American Optical Corp., Buffalo, N.Y.) that use the above principles to give direct readings of total bilirubin on diluted serum.

Normal values and interpretation

The normal values for the bilirubin fractions are as follows:

Direct bilirubin, 0.1-0.4 mg/dl (1.7-6.8 μmole/L)
Indirect bilirubin, 0.2-0.8 mg/dl (3.4-13.7 μmole/L)
Total bilirubin, 0.1-1.3 mg/dl (1.7-22.2 μmole/L)

In hemolytic jaundice the increase in indirect bilirubin is greatest, whereas in obstructive jaundice the increase in direct bilirubin is more pronounced. This may be explained by the fact that bilirubin is produced in the reticuloendothelial cells by the breakdown of hemoglobin and is transported in the blood in the form of unconjugated or indirect-reacting bilirubin to the liver, where it is conjugated to form the water-soluble direct-reacting bilirubin. Thus in jaundice caused by increased destruction of red cells there will be more indirect bilirubin in the serum, whereas if the jaundice is caused by the fact that the bilirubin already conjugated by the liver cannot be properly excreted, the amount of direct-reacting bilirubin will rise. In jaundice caused by liver parenchymal damage, both fractions may be greatly elevated. The ratio of direct to indirect bilirubin is still only of limited value in the differential diagnosis of jaundice. In infectious hepatitis the serum bilirubin level rises to a peak and then steadily returns to normal when recovery ensues.

NOTE: Hemolysis will interfere with the chemical determination of bilirubin, particularly with the Malloy-Evelyn method, giving high or variable results. The use of ascorbic acid in the Jendrassik and Grof method will eliminate interference by moderate amounts of hemolysis. Interference has been noted from the contamination of the reagents by free chlorine (hypochlorite cleaners). The previous administration of dextran may produce a turbidity that cannot be entirely corrected for by a blank. Radiopaque contrast media remaining in the serum can interfere with the color reaction. Bilirubin is sensitive to light and the exposure of the serum to high light intensities may result in a decrease in the apparent bilirubin level.

A large number of drugs have been reported to be hepatotoxic, resulting in high bilirubin levels after more or less prolonged administration. Among the drugs that have been stated to produce liver damage in some individuals are erythromycin, nitrofurantoin, phenothiazine, chlordiazepoxide, ethionamide, phenylbutazone, imipramine, ethacrynic acid, methotrexate, and oxyphenisatin. This list is not complete and many other drugs may have similar effects. The possibility must be considered that an increased bilirubin level resulted from liver damage by an administered drug and not from some preexisting liver disease.

Other tests based on bile pigments are the determination of urinary **bilirubin** and urinary and fecal **urobilinogen.** Bilirubin is found in urine in obstructive jaundice but is usually not present in hemolytic jaundice, since the kidneys excrete the water-soluble direct-reacting bilirubin more readily. Urinary bilirubin is usually tested for only qualitatively, but a semiquantitative test for urinary and fecal urobilinogen is included here.

Urobilinogen in urine and feces[14-16]

Principle: Urobilinogens found in urine and feces will give a red color with **Ehrlich reagent.** For a quantitative determination any urobilin present is reduced to urobilinogen by the use of alkaline ferrous sulfate. Ascorbic acid is added as a reducing agent to maintain urobilinogen in a reduced state and prevent the formation of urobilin. The use of sodium acetate inhibits the color formation from indole and skatole and intensifies the urobilinogen color. Although there was no urobilinogen standard available and the material designated as urobilinogen may be more than one definite chemical compound, it has been found that the color produced with Ehrlich reagent approximates that produced by phenolsulfonphthalein (PSP) in alkaline solution; therefore this reagent has been used as an artificial standard. In alkaline solution, 0.20 mg/dl PSP will give the same color as 0.35 mg/dl urobilinogen when treated with Ehrlich reagent under the prescribed conditions.

Studies by Henry et al.[16] indicated that the quantitative method using petroleum ether extraction of urine gives erratic recoveries from 40-68% of urobilinogen or urobilin added to urine. Similar recovery problems and poor reproducibility occur in low and normal urine samples, suggesting that only the semiquantitative method[15] should be used.

Reagents:
1. Modified Ehrlich reagent (Watson)
   Dissolve 0.7 g *p*-dimethylaminobenzaldehyde in 150 ml concentrated hydrochloric acid. Add 1 dl water.
2. Ferrous sulfate, 20 g/dl
   Add 5 g ferrous sulfate to 23 ml water to dissolve. This solution must be made up fresh as needed.
3. Sodium hydroxide, 10 g/dl
   Dissolve 50 g sodium hydroxide in water and dilute to 5 dl.
4. Sodium acetate (saturated solution)
   Add about 60 ml water to 100 g crystalline sodium acetate trihydrate, warm to dissolve, and then allow to cool. Some excess sodium acetate should crystallize out.
5. Sodium hydroxide, 50 mg/dl
   Dilute 1 ml of reagent 3 (above) to 2 dl with deionized water.
6. Ascorbic acid, powder
7. Artificial standard
   Dissolve 20 mg PSP (phenolsulfonphthalein [phenol red], acid form) in 1 dl of 50 mg/dl sodium hydroxide. For the working standard required, pipet 1 ml of this solution to a 1 dl volumetric flask and dilute with 50 mg/dl NaOH. As mentioned, this solution containing 0.20 mg/dl PSP gives the same color in alkaline solution as 0.35 mg urobilinogen treated with Ehrlich reagent and made up to the same volume. PSP salts or solutions for intravenous injection should not be used to prepare the standard.

Procedure for urine: The test can be applied to any urine sample but is usually performed on one collected from 2 PM to 4 PM since higher and more consistent values seem to be obtained. The analysis must be performed without delay and the urine protected from bright light before and during the analysis.

Measure the volume of the 2 hr urine sample and record. Test the urine for bilirubin; if positive, mix 2.0

ml of 10 g/dl $BaCl_2$ with 8.0 ml urine and filter. Dissolve 100 mg ascorbic acid in 10 ml clear urine (centrifuge if needed) and place 1.5 ml in each of two test tubes. Label one blank tube and one sample tube.

To the blank tube add 4.5 ml of a freshly prepared mixture of 5 ml of reagent 1 and 10 ml of reagent 2 and mix.

To the sample tube add 1.5 ml of reagent 1 and mix; then immediately add 3.0 ml of reagent 2.

Adjust the spectrophotometer to zero with water at 562 nm and within 5 min measure the absorbance of the blank and sample solutions. Measure the absorbance of the working PSP standard against water as well.

Calculation:

$$\text{mg urobilinogen/dl} = \frac{A(\text{sample}) - A(\text{blank})}{A(\text{standard})} \times$$
$$0.35 \times (6/1.5)$$
$$= \frac{A(\text{sample}) - A(\text{blank})}{A(\text{standard})} \times 1.38$$

$$\text{mg urobilinogen/2 hr} = \frac{A(\text{sample}) - A(\text{blank})}{A(\text{standard})} \times$$
$$1.38 \times \frac{\text{Volume (ml)}}{100}$$

where A = absorbance. These calculations should be multiplied by 1.25 if bilirubin was removed with $BaCl_2$.

Normal values and interpretation. The normal values found by this method for women are 0-1.1 mg/2 hr and 0.3-2.1 mg/2 hr for men. There is considerable day-to-day and hour-to-hour fluctuation apparently related to diet. The output is much lower at night and higher in the afternoon. The normal daily excretion is 0-4 mg. Results are sometimes expressed as Ehrlich units (EU) where 1 EU = 1 mg urobilinogen.

Urinary urobilinogen is increased in hemolytic jaundice, and values up to 10 mg/day have been found. In obstructive jaundice the level is normal or low depending on the degree of obstruction, often less than 0.3 mg/day. In infectious hepatitis the amount excreted may be normal or somewhat increased.

Procedure for feces: Use either a portion of a single stool specimen or, for a more accurate interpretation, an aliquot of a homogenized 24 or 48 hr specimen.

Weigh out 1 g ($\pm$ 0.01 g) of stool. Grind into a paste in a small flask using a glass rod with 19 ml water. Add 10 ml of 20 g/dl ferrous sulfate solution and mix. Add 10 ml of 10 g/dl sodium hydroxide and mix. Stopper and allow to stand at room temperature in the dark for 1-3 hr. Mix contents of flask well and filter part of contents; then dilute 5.0 ml to 50 ml with water. Dissolve 100 mg ascorbic acid in 10 ml clear filtrate and place 1.5 ml in each of two test tubes. Label one tube as blank and the other as sample.

To the blank tube add 4.5 ml of a freshly prepared mixture of 5 ml of reagent 1 and 10 ml of reagent 2 and mix. To the sample tube add 1.5 ml of reagent 1 and mix; then immediately add 3.0 ml of reagent 2 and mix. Adjust the spectrophotometer to zero at 562 nm with water and within 5 min measure the absorbance of the blank and sample solutions. Measure the absorb-

ance of the working PSP standard against water as well.

Calculation:

mg urobilinogen/100 g stool
$$= \frac{A(\text{sample}) - A(\text{blank})}{A(\text{standard})} \times 0.35 \times$$
$$(6/1.5) \times [(40 \times 10)/1 \text{ g}]$$
$$= \frac{A(\text{sample}) - A(\text{blank})}{A(\text{standard})} \times 560$$

where A = absorbance.

Normal values and interpretation: The normal range is given as 75-350 mg/100 g stool. Fecal urobilinogen is increased in those conditions in which there is an increased breakdown of hemoglobin, e.g., hemolytic jaundice. Values of 400-1400 mg/d have been found in such conditions. Fecal urobilinogen is reduced when there is any obstruction to the flow of bile into the intestines. In obstructive jaundice, values as low as 5 mg/d have been found. In conditions such as infectious hepatitis the fecal levels may be low but not as low as in obstructive jaundice. In cirrhosis of the liver the levels are low but are usually in the normal range. Urobilinogen is rarely found in the feces of newborns before the age of 3 weeks, and some infants fail to excrete urobilinogen for up to 6 months.

TESTS BASED ON CHANGES IN PLASMA PROTEINS

The liver plays an important role in the production of plasma proteins. The procedures for the determination of total protein, albumin, and globulin are given elsewhere. Their determination often gives useful information in cases of chronic liver disease. In advanced stages of the disease, albumin is decreased and the globulins are increased, so that the A/G ratio may be reversed. Albumin may fall to 2-3 g/dl, total globulins may increase to 4-5 g/dl, and an examination of protein electrophoresis patterns may be of some help. In the early stages of acute hepatitis, examination reveals the protein levels to be normal.

Fibrinogen

The procedure for the determination of fibrinogen has also been given. This protein is produced exclusively by the liver. Except in very severe forms of liver disease, e.g., acute yellow atrophy, poisoning from phosphorus or carbon tetrachloride, and advanced stages of liver cirrhosis, the fibrinogen content of the blood is not altered greatly from normal values, so this is not a sensitive liver function test.

Amino acids

Along with changes in plasma proteins, changes in the plasma amino acids have been reported in liver disease. A marked increase is found only in severe liver damage. The increased plasma levels also lead to increased urinary excretion. In severe liver disease the increase in amino acid excretion in the urine may be sufficient to cause the formation of leucine and tyrosine crystals in urinary sediment. There is a marked increase in urinary amino acid excretion in Wilson's disease (hepatolenticular degeneration).

Flocculation and turbidity tests

In the past a number of flocculation and turbidity tests have been used in the study of liver disease. These were based on the formation of a turbidity or flocculation when an aliquot of the patient's serum was added to the reagent. In general, the tests were only semi-quantitative in nature and not very specific. They were merely an indication of an abnormal ratio of globulin to albumin in the serum, which is often found in liver disease. A much more satisfactory examination of the changes in types and amounts of proteins is by protein electrophoresis. One study[17] states that if paper electrophoresis is available it is preferred to the turbidity tests. With the widespread use of the simpler and more rapid cellulose acetate electrophoresis, there is even less need for these tests. The electrophoretic tests have also been suggested in screening for liver disorders, but some enzyme tests are just as simple and much more specific.

TESTS BASED ON CARBOHYDRATE METABOLISM

The liver plays an important role in carbohydrate metabolism, especially in the formation of **glycogen** from glucose. When the liver function is impaired in this respect, more of the ingested sugar absorbed from the intestines into the portal circulation passes into the peripheral circulation. The administration of glucose cannot be used as a test for this function because it is difficult to separate the part played by the liver from other factors (insulin, etc.) in glucose metabolism. Historically, other sugars have been used instead, principally galactose and fructose. **Galactose** is rapidly converted by the liver into glucose, and much of the latter is changed to glycogen. In a normal individual very little galactose appears in the blood after a test dose. **Fructose (levulose)** is also converted into glucose, chiefly in the liver.

Tolerance tests have been used to evaluate the metabolic function of the liver, and they are abnormal in a high percentage of cases of cirrhosis and acute hepatitis but are normal in biliary obstruction. These tests are not very sensitive, however, since extensive impairment of liver cells or necrosis is required before a disturbance in metabolic function is observed. Further information on tolerance tests of this type is covered in Chapter 21.

TESTS BASED ON DETOXIFYING FUNCTIONS

One of the important functions of the liver is its role in the **detoxification** of injurious substances. One of the mechanisms by which it performs this function is by chemical reactions to form substances that are less toxic or more readily excreted by the kidneys through conjugation with glucuronic acid, glycine, or other compounds.

Hippuric acid test[18-22]

Principle: Detoxification is the basis of the hippuric acid test in which a dose of sodium benzoate is given and the amount of hippuric acid formed by the reaction of benzoic acid and glycine is determined. Since the test is based on the amount of hippuric acid formed as measured by the amount excreted in the urine, inaccurate results will be obtained if renal function is greatly impaired.

Benzoate may be given either orally or intravenously. For the oral test the patient ingests 6 g sodium benzoate dissolved in about 250 ml water. All the urine passed during the next 4 hr is saved, together with the urine obtained by emptying the bladder at the end of the period.

Because impaired absorption and nausea may occur when sodium benzoate is given orally, an intravenous test may be used. Sodium benzoate is available in sterile ampules containing 1.77 g sodium benzoate (equivalent to 1.5 g benzoic acid) in 20 ml water. Have the patient empty the bladder and drink a glass of water. Inject the sodium benzoate, taking at least 5 min for the injection. The bladder is emptied after 1 hr, and this urine is taken for analysis.

In the analysis for hippuric acid the urine is saturated with sodium chloride, acidified with sulfuric acid, and cooled to precipitate out the hippuric acid that is only slightly soluble. The precipitated hippuric acid is centrifuged, washed, and titrated with alkali. A correction is made for the slight solubility of the acid.

Reagents:
1. Sodium chloride, 5.1 moles/L
   Dissolve 30 g sodium chloride in water to make 1 dl. Since this solution should be cold when used, it is convenient to store it in the refrigerator. A slight crystallization is of no importance.
2. Sodium hydroxide, 0.1 mole/L
   Accurately standardize by titration with standard acid.
3. Concentrated sulfuric acid
4. Sodium chloride crystals

Procedure: Measure the total volume of the urine obtained and take an aliquot amounting to $^1/_{10}$ of the total volume for the oral test or $^1/_5$ the volume for the intravenous test. It may be simpler to take a definite volume, e.g., 10 or 20 ml, that is approximately the desired aliquot ratio. Transfer the aliquot to a suitably sized centrifuge tube. Add 3 g sodium chloride for each 10 ml aliquot. Dissolve completely and warm slightly if necessary. Add 0.1 ml concentrated sulfuric acid for each 10 ml aliquot, mix well, and place in the refrigerator for at least $^1/_2$ hr. If precipitation of hippuric acid has not occurred at the end of this time, scratch the inside of the tube below the surface of the liquid with a glass stirring rod and return to the refrigerator for another 30 min or longer. If convenient, it may be left overnight in the refrigerator. Centrifuge at high speed and carefully pour off and discard the supernatant. Wash the precipitate by adding 10 ml cold sodium chloride solution (5.1 moles/L) and rinse down the sides of the tube. Mix the contents of the tube and recentrifuge. Pour off supernatant and repeat the washing. Dissolve the final precipitate in about 10 ml boiling water, transfer to a small flask, and titrate with 0.1 mole/L sodium hydroxide, using phenolphthalein as an indicator. Some of the hippuric acid may precipitate out and redissolve slowly; therefore one must be certain that the final end point of the titration has been reached.

Calculation: Since 1 ml of 0.1 mole/L alkali is equal to 0.0179 g hippuric acid:

$$\text{Hippuric acid (g)} = 0.0179 \times \text{Alkali (ml)}$$

Add 0.12 g to the calculated amount for each 1 dl of total volume of urine sample to correct for the solubility of hippuric acid.

Normal values and interpretation: For the intravenous test, 0.7-1.6 g should be excreted in the 1 hr period. For the oral test at least 3-3.5 g hippuric acid should be excreted in the 4 hr period. Amounts excreted above the limits have no significance. Excretion is normal in hemolytic jaundice and in uncomplicated gallbladder disease and obstructive jaundice. It is decreased in hepatitis, tumors, cirrhosis, and obstructive jaundice with liver impairment.

Liver function test using dye (Cardio-Green) excretion

For many years the excretion of the dye Bromsulfphalein (BSP) has been used as a test of liver function. The dye sometimes causes adverse reactions, and the manufacturer is replacing it by the dye indocyanine green (Cardio-Green).[23] As the name indicates, this dye has been used previously in studies on cardiac output. No adverse reactions have been reported from the use of this dye.[24] Since BSP may not be available for parenteral administration in the future, the procedure using Cardio-Green is presented.

The dye is not stable in aqueous solution and must be made up just before use. It is supplied in sterile lyophilized ampules along with sterile buffer for preparation of the solution. Because the preparation and administration of the dye are not within the duties of the laboratory technician, the details of this procedure as outlined in the package insert are not given here. Although the aqueous solution is not stable, at the lower concentration found in the serum after injection the solution is more stable and the serum samples obtained after the injection of the dye may be kept in the refrigerator for a day or two before analysis without deterioration.

The dye is usually made up to a concentration of 5 mg/ml and given at a dose of 0.5 mg/kg body weight or 1 ml of the solution per 10 kg. A small amount of the dye solution as injected should be obtained by the laboratory for use as a standard. If the analysis cannot be made within a few hours, the dye should be mixed with serum as outlined in the procedure for analysis; in this form it is relatively stable.

Procedure: The procedure requires no reagents nor any standard other than the injected dye itself. The procedure given by the manufacturer is as follows. Before the injection of the dye obtain a blood sample of 6 ml of whole blood, allow it to clot, centrifuge at 2000 × *g* for 10 min, and remove 2.5 ml of the clear serum for use. The dye is injected in the amount given in the package insert. Exactly 20 min later, obtain a blood sample from the opposite arm, allow it to clot, centrifuge, and separate the serum.

Set up a series of 1.0 ml microcuvets with a 1 cm light path as follows:

	Blank	50% Standard	Sample
Preinjection serum	1.0 ml	1.0 ml	—
Injected dye	—	1 μl	—
Postinjection serum	—	—	1.0 ml

The standard is equivalent to 50% retention. Blank the spectrophotometer at 805 nm with the blank cuvet and read the absorbance of the standard and sample cuvets.

Calculation: Since the standard corresponds to 50% retention:

$$\frac{\text{Absorbance of sample}}{\text{Absorbance of standard}} \times 50\% = \text{Retention (\%)}$$

Normal values and interpretation: In normal individuals not more than 4% should be retained after 20 min.

In contrast to the simple procedure formerly used for BSP, smaller laboratories may experience difficulties with some aspects of procedure for Cardio-Green given above. The spectral range of the spectrophotometer may not reach 805 nm, microcuvets with a volume of 1 ml and with a light path of 1 cm may not be available, the instrument may not give accurate or linear readings at an absorbance of about 1.3, which is that obtained with the 50% retention standard,[25] and finally the measurement of 1 μl of dye solution cannot always be done accurately. Suggestions for overcoming some of these difficulties are given below.

Alternate procedure: The modified procedure requires the use of about 8 ml of a clear pooled serum as well as 4 ml of preinjection serum and 2 ml of postinjection serum. Excess serum from other determinations may be used provided it is not hemolyzed, lipemic, or icteric. Just before use centrifuge the pooled serum to remove clots or other debris. Take 5.0 ml of pooled serum, add 10 μl of the injected dye, and mix well. Set up 3.0 ml cuvets with a 1 cm light path as follows:

	Blank	50% Standard	Sample
Pooled serum	1.0 ml	—	1.0 ml
Preinjection serum	2.0 ml	2.0 ml	—
Dyed pooled serum	—	1.0 ml	—
Postinjection serum	—	—	2.0 ml

With this dilution of the serum the standard will have an absorbance of about 0.85 with a 1 cm light path, which may allow more accurate measurement. If the instrument does not have a scale up to 805 nm, read at the longest possible wavelength. At longer wavelengths there will be less interference from hemolysis.

If one wishes to measure only the amount retained after 20 min, a 25% retention standard may be preferred, which is made by adding 10 μl of dye solution to 10 ml of pooled serum and proceeding as above.

Disappearance rate: The measurement of the disappearance rate using several samples is more accurate than the single measurement at 20 min but requires four blood samples after the injection rather than just one. Obtain blood samples exactly 5, 10, 15, and 20 min after injection of the dye. Measure the absorbance of the serum samples and calculate the percent retention for each as above. Plot the percent retention against the time on log-linear paper, or the logarithm of the percent retention against the time on linear paper. By visual inspection draw the best straight line through the points, including 100% retention at zero time. From the curve read off the time corresponding to exactly 10% retention. Then the disappearance rate as percent per minute is calculated as R = 230/T where T is the time in minutes required to obtain exactly 10% retention. For example, if the curve reaches the 10% line at $11^1/_2$ min, then the disappearance rate is $230/11^1/_2$ = 20%/min. In normal individuals the rate will be between 18-24%. With decreased liver function, the rate will be lower (i.e., the dye is eliminated at a slower rate). The figure given above of 4% retention in 20 min corresponds to a disappearance rate of about 16%/min.

Normal values and interpretation: In healthy adults[26] not more than 4% of the dye should remain in the serum after 20 min (disappearance rate of 18-26%/min). Removal of the dye proceeds more slowly when liver function is impaired; and in advanced cirrhosis, the amount remaining may be over 10%, corresponding to a disappearance rate of 11.5%/min. Since the dye is removed in the bile, the test is accurate only when there is no obstruction to bile flow. It is most useful in liver cell damage without jaundice, in cirrhosis, and in acute hepatitis. In these chronic liver diseases it may be one of the most sensitive liver function tests available.

MISCELLANEOUS LIVER FUNCTION TESTS

A number of tests given elsewhere in this volume are also of value in the study of liver disease. Brief mention will be made of these tests, together with their application to liver function testing.

Cholesterol

The liver is concerned with the metabolism of lipids, especially cholesterol. Hypercholesterolemia is found in obstructive jaundice. The increase in cholesterol often parallels the increase in bilirubin during the course of the disease. In parenchymatous liver disease the findings are variable; the value is normal in many instances. Very high cholesterol values are found in xanthomatous biliary cirrhosis. Changes in the ratio of free to esterified cholesterol are often found in liver disease. In infectious hepatitis and other conditions involving liver damage the amount of esters tends to fall relatively more than the total cholesterol, which may remain relatively constant. In severe acute liver necrosis the total serum cholesterol value is usually low and may fall below 100 mg/dl, with a marked reduction in the percentage of the esters.

Prothrombin time

Prothrombin time is used chiefly for the control of anticoagulant therapy; it has also been used as a test of liver function. Prothrombin is formed by the liver cells, which require vitamin K for the process. In liver disease the prothrombin formation may be reduced in two

ways. In obstructive jaundice the absence of bile salts severely reduces the absorption of vitamin K from the intestines. In severe liver damage the liver is less able to form prothrombin, even in the presence of adequate amounts of the vitamin. These two conditions may be distinguished by the vitamin K tolerance test.

Vitamin K tolerance test

Determine the prothrombin time on several different days to find the range or level for the patient. Then give intramuscularly 76 mg Synkayvite (Roche Diagnostics, Nutley, N.J.) (2-methyl-1,4-naphthohydroquinone diphosphate) for 4 consecutive days. Determine the prothrombin time daily just before the injection and on the day following the last injection.

In normal individuals there is a normal prothrombin time and no change occurs after administration of vitamin K. If an increased initial prothrombin time returns to normal (vitamin K deficiency), the liver function is not seriously impaired.

Liver impairment may result in failure of an increased prothrombin time to return to normal.

Enzymes in diagnosis of liver disease

A number of different enzymes have been used in the diagnosis of liver disease. Not all of them are equally valuable. A good review of the subject is given by Zimmerman and Seeff.[27] These authors divide the enzymes into a number of groups that are useful in differentiating the various types of liver disorders. Thus alkaline phosphatase, leucine aminopeptidase, and γ-glutamyl transpeptidase are all only slightly elevated in hepatitis or alcoholic cirrhosis, markedly elevated in some forms of metastatic carcinoma of the liver, and very markedly elevated in intrahepatic cholestasis and extrahepatic obstructive jaundice. On the other hand, the enzymes glutamic oxalacetic transaminase, aldolase, isocitric dehydrogenase, and malic acid dehydrogenase are markedly increased in hepatitis, somewhat increased in infectious mononucleosis and metastatic carcinoma, and only slightly increased in cholestasis or obstructive jaundice. The enzymes glutamic pyruvic transaminase, sorbitol dehydrogenase, and ornithine carbamyl transferase are usually markedly increased only in hepatitis. Serum pseudocholinesterase is the enzyme that is sometimes decreased in liver disease. Further discussion of the use of the various enzymes in the diagnosis of liver disease is given under the separate enzymes, since these are the most sensitive indicators of liver disease yet discovered.

The determination of the isoenzymes is also sometimes helpful in the diagnosis of liver disease.[28] The isoenzymes of lactate dehydrogenase and alkaline phosphatase are most often determined in trying to elucidate the nature of liver disease. For a further treatment of this see the discussion of the separate enzymes in the following chapter.

OTHER SPECIAL TESTS
Humoral antibodies

The study of humoral antibodies[29] may sometimes be helpful in the diagnosis of liver disease, although the role of autoimmune processes in liver disease is not clear. These antibodies may be detected in serum by the usual fluorescent antibody technics. Antimitochrondrial and anti-smooth-muscle antibodies have been studied.

α-Fetoglobulin (AFP)

A distinct protein, α_1-fetoglobulin,[30-32] sometimes termed α-fetoprotein (AFP), has been noted in the serum of about two thirds of patients with primary hepatocellular carcinoma. This protein is present in fetal serum during the development of the fetus but falls to a low level by birth and usually disappears completely by the first week after birth. The protein has been most often quantitated by immunodiffusion and electroimmunodiffusion. More recently, much more sensitive technics have been employed, including radioimmunoassay, enzyme-linked immunoassay,[33] latex fixation[34] and hemagglutination inhibition,[35] some of which produce sensitivities in the nanogram per milliliter range.

The test is quite specific for primary liver cell carcinoma and gives few false positive results but will not be positive in all patients with the disease. Fetoglobulin is also present in the serum of some patients with testicular tumors, particularly teratoblastomas, but these can usually be distinguished from liver carcinomas by other means.

The primary use of AFP concentration measurements is not in diagnosis but in clinical management where serial measurements can be related to surgical or chemotherapeutic success as well as recurrence of the disease.

With the more sensitive RIA test method, AFP concentrations are found to be elevated in cirrhosis and infectious hepatitis[36] but at a concentration below the sensitivity of immunodiffusion tests. This increase is usually transient and may indicate liver regeneration.

SERUM LIPIDS

The lipids are fats and fatty acid derivatives together with some other substances of similar solubility properties that are concerned with fat metabolism. Reference is sometimes made to blood lipids, but usually the substances determined are contained in serum (or plasma). There are some lipids in the erythrocytes (chiefly in the cell membrane), but these are not concerned with fat metabolism.

Classification of lipids

The main constituents of total serum lipids are **cholesterol** and **cholesterol esters, phospholipids,** and **triglycerides.** There are also small amounts of free (unesterified) fatty acids, monoglycerides and diglycerides, bile acids, and other sterols together with the fat-soluble vitamins. The lipids are relatively insoluble in aqueous solution and are present in serum either in combination with certain proteins (lipoproteins) or in an emulsified form (chylomicrons).

In the study of serum lipids there are two general methods employed. One is the determination of the separate constituents, e.g., cholesterol, cholesterol esters, phospholipids, and triglycerides as well as the total lipids; the other method is the determination of the relative amounts of the different lipoproteins by electrophoresis or other means. The substances present in the largest amounts are cholesterol (and cholesterol esters) with normal serum concentrations of total cholesterol of 150-300 mg/dl (4-8 mmole/L), phospholipids with serum concentrations of lecithin of 125-300 mg/dl or of phosphorus of 5-12 mg/dl (1.6-3.9 mmole/L), and the triglycerides with normal concentrations of 30-150 mg/dl (triolein concentration of 0.55-1.65 mmole/L). There are also some other lipids present in much smaller amounts.

Approximately 70% of the serum cholesterol is esterified with long-chain fatty acids; the remainder is unesterified (free). Esterification is carried out chiefly in the liver, and the relative amounts of esterified and unesterified cholesterol have been used as a test for liver function. There are many other more satisfactory tests for this purpose. Cholesterol values tend to be elevated in hypothyroidism, and its determination has been used as a test for this disease, but it is not a very reliable one. Elevations in cholesterol concentrations along with abnormalities in the amounts of the other lipid fractions have been implicated in the pathogenesis of atherosclerosis and heart disease, and this is probably the best reason for its determination.

The triglycerides are glycerol esters of long-chain fatty acids. They are what might be called the "true" fats, substances such as olive oil and lard being largely triglycerides. The dietary fats are at least partially hydrolyzed in the intestines before absorption but are mainly reconverted into triglycerides before entering the bloodstream as emulsified particles (chylomicrons). There are very small amounts of monoglycerides and diglycerides in the serum along with some glycerin and unesterified fatty acids.

The phospholipids are glycerol derivatives in which two of the hydroxyl groups are esterified with long-chain fatty acids. The third hydroxyl is combined with a phosphate radical to which is attached another grouping, which in the common serum phospholipids is either choline or ethanolamine. There are a number of other special phospholipids that are found in nervous tissue. These may occur in the serum in such conditions as Tay-Sachs disease and Gaucher's diease, but they are not commonly determined in the usual clinical laboratory.

CHOLESTEROL

In the past the main methods for the determination of cholesterol required the use of strongly acid and potentially corrosive reagents, either in the Liebermann-Burchardt reaction using a mixture of acetic anhydride, acetic acid, and sulfuric acid, or modifications of a method using a ferric salt in the presence of acetic and sulfuric acids. More recently developed methods use the enzyme cholesterol oxidase. The reactions involved here are quite similar to those for the determination of glucose using glucose oxidase. The oxidase methods are relatively simple, use no corrosive reagents, and are somewhat more specific than the older method. A minor disadvantage of the oxidase method is that, being more specific, the normal range of cholesterol in serum would be slightly lower than the ranges formerly used when the acid reagents were used. In kit form, the oxidase method is not easily adapted to the determination of cholesterol esters instead of total cholesterol. However, this latter determination is not now requested since there are far more sensitive methods of assessing liver function. Here three methods are presented: a method using ferric ions and acetic acid, which is adapted to the determination of the cholesterol esters as well as total cholesterol, an enzymatic oxidase method, and the current reference method (Abell).

Free and total cholesterol (method of Parekh and Jung)[37,38]

Principle: The serum is added to an acetic acid solution containing small amounts of ferric acetate and uranyl acetate. The proteins are precipitated and the cholesterol extracted by the acetic acid. The uranyl acetate aids in the complete precipitation of the proteins. After centrifugation an aliquot of the supernatant is transferred to another tube and concentrated sulfuric acid containing a small amount of ferrous sulfate is added. The addition of the concentrated acid develops the color, which is then read at 560 nm. The method is less subject to interference by bilirubin than other direct ferric chloride methods and, as with other methods using ferric salts, gives close to the same amount of color with cholesterol and cholesterol esters.

Reagents:

1. Ferric acetate–uranyl acetate solution
   Dissolve 0.5 g $FeCl_3 \cdot 6H_2O$ in about 10 ml water in a centrifuge tube. Add about 3 ml concentrated ammonium hydroxide to precipitate the iron as ferric hydroxide. Centrifuge, decant the supernatant, wash the precipitate several times with water, and then dissolve in acetic acid. Transfer the solution to a 1 L volumetric flask and dilute to volume with acetic acid. To this, then add 0.1 g powdered uranyl acetate ($UO_2[C_2H_3O_2]_2 \cdot 2H_2O$) and mix the contents well. Allow the solution to stand overnight; then mix well again. This solution is stable for at least 6 months when stored in a brown bottle.

2. Sulfuric acid–ferrous sulfate solution
   In a 1 L volumetric flask, dissolve 0.1 g anhydrous ferrous sulfate in 1 dl glacial acetic acid. Then add 1 dl concentrated sulfuric acid while swirling. After cooling to room temperature, dilute the solution to volume with concentrated sulfuric acid. Mix the mixture well and store in a tightly closed reagent bottle.

3. Cholesterol standards
   a. For total cholesterol dissolve 250 mg pure cholesterol in 1 dl chloroform to make a standard containing 250 mg/dl (6.47 mmole/L).
   b. For free cholesterol dissolve 75 mg pure cholesterol in isopropanol to make 1 dl. This gives a standard containing 75 mg/dl (1.94 mmole/L).

4. Digitonin solution for free cholesterol
   Dissolve 1 g digitonin in 1 dl 50% ethanol warmed to about 56° C with gentle agitation. The

solution is stable for about 6 weeks at room temperature.

Procedure for total cholesterol: To separate tubes (screw-capped tubes with Teflon-lined caps), add 50 µl serum or standard. Add 10 ml ferric acetate–uranyl acetate solution to each tube. Cap, mix by inversion a few times, and then mix well with a vortex mixer. Allow to stand for about 5 min, then centrifuge at 2000 × *g* for 5 min. Transfer 3 ml aliquots of the supernatant to another set of tubes, including one tube with 3 ml ferric acetate–uranyl acetate solution as a blank. To each tube, add 2 ml sulfuric acid–ferrous sulfate solution, preferably from a dispenser, cap, and mix well. Allow tubes to stand for 20 min, then read samples and standard against blank at 560 nm.

Calculation: Since equal amounts of standard and samples are treated similarly:

$$\frac{\text{Absorbance of sample}}{\text{Absorbance of standard}} \times \text{Conc. of standard} =$$
$$\text{Conc. of sample (mg/dl) (total cholesterol)}$$

Procedure for free cholesterol: Add 0.2 ml serum or standard to separate screw-capped centrifuge tubes. Add 2.0 ml isopropanol to each. Mix by inversion a few times; then mix well on a vortex mixer. Allow to stand for about 5 min and centrifuge for 10 min.

Transfer 1 ml aliquots of the supernatants to a second set of tubes. To each tube, add 0.5 ml of the digitonin solution, mix, and place in a refrigerator for 30 min. Centrifuge at 2000 × *g* for 10 min; then carefully decant and discard the supernatant. Wash the precipitate twice with 10 ml portions of acetone. After decanting the second wash, add 5 ml of ferric acetate–uranyl acetate solution to the precipitate. Mix thoroughly to dissolve. Pipet 3 ml of this solution to a reaction tube, and add 2 ml of sulfuric acid–ferrous sulfate solution by running it down the side of the tube. Cap the tube and mix by holding the capped end and swinging the tube at a 180-degree angle 10 times. Allow the tubes to stand for 20 min and then read standards and samples against a blank of 3 ml ferric acetate–uranyl acetate solution and 2 ml sulfuric acid–ferrous sulfate solution at 560 nm.

Calculation: Since samples and standard are treated similarly:

$$\frac{\text{Absorbance of sample}}{\text{Absorbance of standard}} \times \text{Conc. of standard} =$$
$$\text{Conc. of sample (mg/dl) (free cholesterol)}$$

Esterified cholesterol = Total cholesterol − Free cholesterol

Total cholesterol (enzymatic method)[39-41]

Principle: The determination of cholesterol by the use of cholesterol oxidase is a relatively simple, accurate, and specific method. Cholesterol is oxidized by atmospheric oxygen in the presence of the enzyme cholesterol oxidase with the formation of hydrogen peroxide. In the presence of the enzyme peroxidase the peroxide liberates oxygen, which oxidizes phenol and aminoantipyrine to form a red color, which is read in a spectrophotometer. Cholesterol esters must be hydrolyzed before oxidation. This is done by adding the enzyme cholesterol esterase to the reaction mixture, if cholesterol esterase is omitted, the method will measure free cholesterol.[42] Although the method itself is very simple, the preparation of the reagents, which are not too stable, is not as easy. Although directions for the preparation of the reagents are presented, it is recommended that the reagents be purchased, either in a completely lyophilized form or as stablized solutions that are mixed just before use (Calbiochem-Behring Corp., San Diego; Sclavo, Wayne, N.J.; SKI, Sunnyvale, Calif.; Worthington Biochemical Corp., Freehold, N.J.). The commerical reagents are more stable than those prepared in the laboratory since they contain extra stabilizing agents. The cholesterol oxidase and cholesterol esterase enzymes are relatively expensive, and in the laboratory preparation there may be some waste. If one wishes to make the reagent, the following procedure may be used.

Reagents:
1. Dissolve 0.70 g sodium cholate, 0.90 g 4-aminoantipyrine, 3.75 g Na_2HPO_4, 3.65 g NaH_2PO_4 · H_2O, and 0.5 g polyethylene glycol 6000 in water to make 5 dl. Store in refrigerator.
2. Dissolve 0.7 g phenol in 10 ml of 50% ethanol.
3. Add 18 units of cholesterol ester hydrolase (E.C. 3.1.1.13) and 35,000 units of peroxidase (E.C. 1.11.1.7) in water to make 10 ml. This will form a suspension of the enzymes, not a true solution, and should be mixed thoroughly before withdrawing a portion. Store at 4° C.
4. Suspend 65 units of cholesterol oxidase (E.C. 1.1.3.6) in water to make 5 ml. Store at 4° C.
5. To prepare the complete reagent, mix together 50 ml of reagent 1, 1 ml of reagent 2, 1 ml of reagent 3, and 0.5 ml of reagent 4. This may be stable for several days if kept in the refrigerator.
6. Cholesterol standard may be used with all cholesterol oxidase methods. Dissolve 250 mg of pure cholesterol in isopropanol to make 1 dl (6.47 mmole/L cholesterol).

Procedure: Generally this procedure may be used with any of the cholesterol oxidase reagents. Slightly different proportions of the reagent to sample may be used to give the proper absorbance with the cuvets and spectrophotometer used. Add 3 ml of reagent to a number of tubes. To separate tubes add 50 μl of standard or sample, reserving one tube as a blank. Incubate all tubes at 37° C for 10 min. Then read standard and samples against blank at 500 nm.

Calculation:

$$\frac{\text{Absorbance of sample}}{\text{Absorbance of standard}} \times \frac{\text{Conc.}}{\text{of standard}} = \frac{\text{Conc.}}{\text{of sample (mg/dl)}}$$

The cholesterol oxidase is specific for sterols having a 3 β-hydroxyl group and a double bond between C4 and C5 or C5 and C6.[43] There are other naturally occurring steroids with these structures, but this is not an important source of error since their concentrations are low and do not seem to vary.

Total cholesterol (method of Abell)

The definitive reference method for cholesterol has been that of Abell.[44,45] Eventually it may be replaced by an enzymatic method, but this has not yet been done. This reference method is presented, although it is ordinarily not used for routine determinations but rather to check reference and control sera.

Principle: The cholesterol esters are first saponified by heating with alkali. The cholesterol is then extracted from the serum with petroleum ether. Next an aliquot of the ether extract is evaporated to dryness. This is then treated with Liebermann-Buchardt reagent consisting of acetic acid, acetic anhydride, and sulfuric acid. The color development is carried out in a water bath at 25° C in the ark, since both light and temperature variations will affect the results.

Reagents:
1. Stock potassium hydroxide, 33% (w/w)
   Dissolve 20 g potassium hydroxide in 40 ml water.
2. Working solution
   Just before use, dilute 6 ml of the stock solution with 94 ml ethyl alcohol.
3. Color reagent
   Prepare just before use. Transfer 1 dl acetic anhydride to a glass-stoppered bottle. Cool in an ice bath and add while swirling 5 ml concentrated sulfuric acid. Cool for several minutes more and then add 50 ml glacial acetic acid. Allow to come to room temperature before use.
4. Cholesterol standard, 250 mg/dl
   Dissolve 250 mg pure cholesterol in ethyl alcohol to make 1 dl.

Procedure: To a series of 25 ml glass-stoppered centrifuge tubes, add 5 ml of the working KOH solution. Add to the separate tubes, 0.5 ml of serum samples or standard. Stopper tubes and mix well. Place in a water bath at 37° C for 1 hr. During the incubation mix the tubes by inversion on several occasions. Then cool the tubes to room temperature and add exactly 10 ml petroleum ether and 5 ml water to each tube. Stopper the tubes and shake vigorously for at least 1 min; then allow to stand until the layers separate. Draw most of the lower aqueous layer off with a Pasteur pipet and centrifuge the tubes. Pipet and transfer exactly 4 ml of the supernatant ether layer to labeled tubes. Evaporate the petroleum ether by placing tubes in a water bath with a stream of clean air to hasten evaporation. (CAUTION! No flames.) While the petroleum ether is evaporating, the color reagent may be prepared. Place the tubes containing the evaporated extract, an empty tube for a blank, and the color reagent in a water bath at 25° C in a dark place. Add 6 ml of the color reagent to the separate tubes at timed intervals. (One-half minute intervals are commonly used.) The incubation is continued for exactly 30 min; then the tubes are removed in the same order and read against the blank at 630 nm.

Calculation: Since the sample and standard are treated similarly:

$$\frac{\text{Absorbance of sample}}{\text{Absorbance of standard}} \times 250 = \text{mg/dl} \begin{array}{l}\text{cholesterol}\\\text{in sample}\end{array}$$

Normal values and interpretation

Most of the normal values for cholesterol tabulated in the literature are based on the chemical determinations. The enzymatic methods give values about 10 mg/dl (0.25 mmole/L) lower in normal individuals. Since the enzymatic methods are less subject to interferences by bilirubin and hyperlipemia, the differences may be greater in abnormal serum samples. The range of values for normal healthy young adults has been given as 150-270 mg/dl (3.9-7.0 mmole/L). It may be lower in children. The concentration increases somewhat with age until about age 60 years. The concentration in women is generally somewhat lower than in men up to the time of menopause when the values increase and may exceed that in men of the same age. Healthy individuals over 70 years of age may have lower values, approaching those of young adults. The proportion of total cholesterol present as esters is usually between 68-74%.

Cholesterol, along with other lipids, is markedly increased in uncontrolled diabetes, but the concentration does not appear to be related to the severity of the disease. Cholesterol as well as other lipids may reach extremely high values in the nephrotic syndrome, but the mechanism of this increase is not well understood. Little if any disturbance of the cholesterol value occurs in other renal diseases, but elevated results are observed in patients undergoing long-term dialysis. Total cholesterol values in diseases of the liver may be increased or decreased, depending on the nature and duration of the condition. Marked deviations from the normal ratio of free to esterified cholesterol occur in diseases of the liver and biliary tract, infectious diseases, and extreme hypercholesterolemia.

The cholesterol value tends to vary inversely with the basal metabolic rate, and its estimation has been used in the study of thyroid function. The cholesterol concentration may be increased in hypothyroidism and decreased in hyperthyroidism, but because of the wide range of normal values, serum cholesterol can only be considered a secondary aid in the diagnosis of thyroid dysfunction especially with the widespread availability of direct measurement of thyroid hormones.

Marked increases in cholesterol are found in most cases of lipoidosis and xanthomatosis as well as in instances of familial or idiopathic hypercholesterolemia.

Cholesterol values are not greatly affected by ordinary dietary changes, but they may be low in wasting diseases such as tuberculosis and terminal cancer.

In recent years much attention has been focused on the possible role of hypercholesterolemia in the pathogenesis of atherosclerosis. There is some evidence that populations consuming a smaller amount of their total calories as fats and ingesting vegetable rather than animal fats have a lower cholesterol value and a lower incidence of atherosclerosis and coronary artery disease than do populations with a higher fat intake. The exact role of hypercholesterolemia in the development of atherosclerosis is still the subject of some controversy. It would appear that it is not necessarily the total amount of cholesterol per se, as the amounts of certain lipoprotein fractions, all of which contain cholesterol, which are more indicative of the tendency toward atherosclerosis.

PHOSPHOLIPIDS

The simplest phospholipids consist of a glycerol molecule with two of the hydroxyl groups esterified with long-chain fatty acids as in the true fats and the third hydroxyl group esterified with phosphoric acid to which is attached an amine such as choline. There are other phospholipids of somewhat different structure, but they all contain fatty acids, phosphate, and amine groups. They apparently play an important role in the metabolism of the true fats (i.e., triglycerides).

General procedure: The phospholipids may be extracted from the serum by an organic solvent. After separation of the precipitated proteins, an aliquot of the extract is evaporated to dryness and digested with sulfuric or nitric acid to oxidize all organic material; the phosphorus is determined in the digest by the usual method. Alternately the phospholipids can be precipitated along with the proteins by trichloroacetic acid. The precipitate is then digested to oxidize organic matter, and the inorganic phosphorus is determined. The conventional factor for conversion of lipid phosphorus (in milligrams per deciliter) to phospholipid (in milligrams per deciliter) is 25. This can be only an average value but is commonly used. No conversion is needed when the concentration is expressed in moles per liter since the phospholipids in general contain one atom of phosphorus per molecule.

Phosphorus method of Baginski et al.[46,47]

Principle: The phospholipids are extracted from the serum with alcohol ether. After separation of the precipitated protein, an aliquot of the extract is evaporated to dryness and then treated with nitric acid containing a small amount of calcium. The calcium prevents the possible loss of phosphorus during digestion and the formation of pyrophosphates. The organic material in the residue is destroyed by evaporating the nitric acid completely. The residue is dissolved in a trichloroacetic acid–ascorbic acid mixture, and the molybdate and arsenite are added to form the blue-colored product with the phosphate. The excess molybdate is combined with citrate to prevent turbidity.

Reagents:

1. Phosphate stock standard
   Dry reagent grade potassium dihydrogen phosphate (KH_2PO_4) at 100° C for several hours. Dissolve 438.1 mg in water to make 1 dl to give a stock standard containing 100 mg P/dl (28 mmole P/L). For a working standard dilute 5 ml of the stock to 1 dl with water, giving a standard containing 5 mg P/dl (1.4 mmole P/L).
2. Ascorbic acid–trichloroacetic acid solution Dissolve 2 g ascorbic acid and 10 g trichloroacetic acid in water and make up to 1 dl.
3. Ammonium molybdate
   Dissolve 1 g ammonium molybdate ($[NH_4]_6Mo_7O_{24} \cdot 4H_2O$) in water to make 1 dl.
4. Arsenite-citrate solution
   Dissolve 20 g trisodium citrate dihydrate and 20 g anhydrous sodium arsenite in water, add 20 ml glacial acetic acid, and dilute the solution to 1 L.
5. Extraction mixture
   Mix together 3 volumes absolute alcohol and 1 volume ether.

6. Nitric acid–calcium solution
   Dissolve 30 mg calcium carbonate in 1 L concentrated nitric acid.
7. Antibumping BOH granules
   Prewash these granules (Gallard-Schlesinger Chemical Mfg. Corp., Carle Place, N.Y.) by boiling with nitric acid for several minutes; then rinse thoroughly with water and dry.

Procedure: Place 2 ml of the extraction mixture in a small test tube and add 50 μl serum with continuous mixing. A fine precipitate should be obtained, or extraction will be incomplete. Then thoroughly mix the suspension on a vortex mixer, allow to stand for a few minutes, and centrifuge at 2500 rpm for 5 min.

Pipet a 1 ml aliquot of the clear supernatant to a 25 × 150 mm Pyrex test tube and evaporate the extract to dryness. Set up two other tubes, one containing 50 μl of the working standard and the other a blank. To each tube add 2 ml of the nitric acid–calcium solution and a few antibumping granules. Heat the tubes over a microburner until the yellow-brown fumes of nitrous oxide are completely gone. The acid should be completely evaporated. A slight additional heating will do no harm, but prolonged extra heating should be avoided.

Then cool the tubes and add 1 ml of the ascorbic acid–trichloroacetic acid solution to each tube and agitate to dissolve any precipitate. Add 0.5 ml of the ammonium molybdate solution and mix well. Then add 1 ml of the arsenite citrate solution and mix well. Allow the solutions to stand for about 20 min and then read the standard and samples against the blank at 700 nm.

Calculation: In the extraction 0.05 ml of serum is added to 2.0 ml of extraction fluid giving a dilution of 2.05:0.05 or 41:1. Then 1 ml of the dilution is compared with 1/20 (= 0.05) ml of standard; thus

$$\frac{\text{Absorbance of sample}}{\text{Absorbance of standard}} \times \frac{41}{20} \times \frac{\text{Conc.}}{\text{of standard}} = \frac{\text{Conc.}}{\text{of sample}}$$

where the concentration of standard is that of the working standard: 5 mg/dl (1.4 mmole/L); or

$$\frac{\text{Absorbance of sample}}{\text{Absorbance of standard}} \times 10.25 = \text{mg P/dl in sample}$$

By convention the term *mg P/dl* may be converted to phospholipid by multiplying by 25.

Many detergents used for cleaning glassware contain phosphates; accordingly, all glassware must be thoroughly rinsed with distilled water before using. It may be advisable to avoid the use of detergents entirely and to clean the tubes with sulfuric acid–chromic acid cleaning solution alone.

Normal values and interpretation

The normal value of serum lipid phosphorus is from 5-12 mg P/dl (1.6-3.9 mmole P/L). This corresponds to a lecithin range of 125-300 mg/dl.[48] The phospholipid concentration in serum parallels the serum cholesterol value in most instances. For low lipid concentrations the ratio of cholesterol to phospholipid is approximately 0.8 when concentrations are in milligrams per deciliter and about 1.6 when the concentrations are in millimoles per liter. At higher lipid concentrations the ratio approaches 1 for results in milligrams per deciliter and

2.0 for results expressed in millimoles per liter. An increase in the ratio has been held by some investigators to be a more reliable index of a tendency toward atherosclerosis than the cholesterol concentrations alone.

FATTY ACID ESTERS

Since all but 2-5% of the fatty acids in serum are esterified (as cholesterol esters, phospholipids, or triglycerides), the simple colorimetric procedure given here to determine the esterified fatty acids[49,50] is often satisfactory as a measure of the total fatty acids of the serum. The method is presented for historical reasons, since the measurement of total fatty acid esters does not offer any additional clinical information over that which is obtained from direct measurement of the individual components.

Principle: The test is based on the formation of hydroxamates from the reaction of the esters with hydroxylamine in alkaline solution and the formation of a colored complex on the addition of ferric chloride.

Reagents:
1. Alcohol-ether, 3:1
   Mix together 3 volumes 95% ethanol and 1 volume diethyl ether.
2. Sodium hydroxide, 3.5 moles/L
   Dilute 115 ml of 50% (w/w) sodium hydroxide to about 5 dl with water. Titrate with standard acid and dilute to exactly 3.5 moles/L. The commercial 50% (w/w) solution is preferable to the pellets for making the solution since the former contains less carbonate. Store the sodium hydroxide solution in a tightly stoppered polyethylene bottle.
3. Hydrochloric acid, 4.2 moles/L
   Dilute 2 dl concentrated hydrochloric acid to 5 dl with water. Titrate with standard base and dilute to 4.2 moles/L.
4. Ferric chloride, 0.37 mole/L
   Dissolve 10 g ferric chloride ($FeCl_3 \cdot 6H_2O$) and 1 ml concentrated hydrochloric acid in water to make 1 dl.
5. Hydroxylamine hydrochloride, 2 moles/L
   Dissolve 14 g hydroxylamine hydrochloride in water to make 1 dl. Store in the refrigerator.
6. Standards
   a. Stock standard. Dissolve 110 mg triacetin or 321 mg cholesteryl acetate in alcohol-ether mixture (3:1) to make 1 dl. This contains 15 mmole/L.
   b. Working standard. As required dilute a ml of the stock standard to 50 ml with the alcohol-ether mixture.

Procedure: Prepare an alcohol-ether extract using 1 ml serum and 50 ml alcohol-ether mixture. Add, with constant swirling, 1 ml serum to about 35 ml warm alcohol-ether in a 50 ml volumetric flask. Carefully heat just to boiling on a steam bath. Cool to room temperature and dilute to 50 ml with alcohol-ether. Mix well and then filter through paper into a small flask, covering the top of the funnel with a watch glass to prevent evaporation. Pipet 3 ml of the filtrate to a test tube. Add 3 ml alcohol-ether mixture to another tube as a blank. To a third tube add 3 ml of the working standard.

Add 0.5 ml hydroxylamine solution to each tube and mix; then add 0.5 ml sodium hydroxide solution, mix, stopper tightly, and allow to stand at room temperature for 30 min. Add 0.5 ml hydrochloric acid solution, mix, and then add 0.5 ml ferric chloride solution. Mix and read in a photometer at 520 nm, setting to zero with the blank.

Calculation: Since the serum sample is diluted 1:50 in making the extract, the stock standard is diluted in the same proportion to make the working standard, and equal amounts of the extract and working standard are used:

$$\frac{\text{Absorbance of sample}}{\text{Absorbance of standard}} \times 15 = \text{mmole/L}$$

where 15 is the concentration of stock standard. If high values are obtained, e.g., in extremely hyperlipemic serum, repeat the test using 1 ml of the extract and 2 ml of alcohol-ether and multiply the result obtained by 3.

Normal values and interpretation: The normal range of fatty acids is 7-14 mmole/L. Since a considerable portion of the fatty acids are esterified with cholesterol and phospholipids, the total fatty acids will be high when the levels for these substances are elevated. The remainder of the fatty acids are chiefly triglycerides.

NONESTERIFIED FATTY ACIDS

The nomenclature of this lipid fraction is confused and controversial. The terms *nonesterified fatty acids* (NEFA),[51-54] *unesterified fatty acids* (UFA), and *free fatty acids* are in widespread use. This group of fatty acids, which are not covalently bound to protein or other lipids in serum but which are tightly bound, should not be termed *free fatty acids* as they have been historically called, since current convention uses the term *free* to mean "not protein bound."

Principle: Nonesterified fatty acids are present in relatively small amounts and are determined after extraction from plasma by titration. The extract must be washed with dilute acid to remove lactic acid and other interfering material.

Reagents:

1. Isopropyl alcohol, spectrograde
2. Heptane, spectrograde
3. Sulfuric acid, 0.5 mole/L
   Dilute 28 ml concentrated sulfuric acid to 1 L with distilled water.
4. Extraction mixture
   Mix together 40 volumes isopropyl alcohol, 10 volumes heptane, and 1 volume 0.5 mole/L sulfuric acid.
5. Thymolphthalein indicator, 0.01% in 90% ethanol
   Mix 1 volume of 0.1 g/dl aqueous thymol blue and 9 volumes of 100% ethanol.
6. Dilute sulfuric acid, 0.009 mole/L
   Dilute 0.5 ml concentrated sulfuric acid to 1 L with distilled water.
7. Sodium hydroxide solution, 0.018 mole/L
   Prepare fresh daily by diluting 1 ml of 50% sodium hydroxide to 1 L with boiled, cooled distilled water. It is not necessary to standardize this

solution since standards are used in the procedure.

8. Stock standard
   Palmitic acid (Sigma Chemical Co., St. Louis) (99% purity) is used. The standard is made by dissolving 64 mg of the free acid in 25 ml heptane to give a concentration of 10 mmole/L.
9. Working standard
   Dilute stock standard 1:10 with heptane to give a concentration of 1.0 mmole/L.

Procedure: As soon as possible after the separation of plasma, add 5 ml extraction mixture to 1 ml plasma in a glass-stoppered tube and shake vigorously for a moment.

Allow to stand 10 min or longer; then divide the system into two phases by mixing into it an additional 2 ml heptane and 3 ml water. The phases should separate rapidly without centrifugation and form a sharp interface.

Transfer a 5 ml aliquot of the upper phase to glass-stoppered centrifuge tubes and shake vigorously with an equal volume of dilute sulfuric acid solution. Centrifuge at 200 rpm for 5 min.

Transfer a 3 ml aliquot of the upper phase to a 15 ml conical centrifuge tube containing 1 ml titration mixture. Nitrogen gas, delivered to the bottom of the tube with a fine glass capillary, expels the carbon dioxide from the sample and keeps the two phases mixed during titration. Titrate with the sodium hydroxide solution. As the yellow-green end point is approached, interrupt the gas stream from time to time to examine the indicator color in the alcoholic phase.

Run a blank using 1 ml water instead of 1 ml plasma and carry through the same procedure. Run a standard by adding to a glass-stoppered tube 1 ml working standard, 4 ml isopropyl alcohol, 0.1 ml 0.5 mole/L sulfuric acid, and 1 ml water. Shake the mixture and allow to stand for 10 min. Separate the phases by adding 2 ml heptane and 3 ml water as in the sample procedure. Titrate a 3 ml aliquot of the heptane layer.

Calculation: Since the working standard contains 1.0 mmole/L of palmitic acid and since 1 ml each of standard and plasma is used, then:

$$\text{mmole/L nonesterified fatty acids} = \frac{A - B}{C - B}$$

where A is the milliliters of sodium hydroxide required for titration of the sample; C, that required for the standard; and B, that required for the blank.

NOTE: The extraction must be carried out as soon as possible after drawing the blood to prevent any lipolysis on standing that might increase the NEFA concentration. Since heparinized plasma can be separated much more rapidly than serum from clotted blood, its use is preferable. If serum must be used or the extraction cannot be carried out immediately, the tubes containing the blood should be stored in an ice bath.

Normal values and interpretation: The normal range of NEFA in plasma is 0.45-0.90 mmole/L. The value is decreased somewhat after an ordinary meal but shows some increase after a fat meal or the injection of epinephrine.

Unusually high values are found in diabetes mellitus.

These values return to normal with treatment, and it has been shown that the response of the NEFA to treatment occurs more rapidly than do the responses of blood sugar, plasma carbon dioxide, or excretion of urinary ketones.[55,56]

SERUM TRIGLYCERIDES

The triglycerides are the true fats, glycerol esters of long-chain carboxylic acids. Their determination is important in the study of conditions involving fat metabolism including diabetes and atherosclerosis. There are two general methods for their determination. In one the triglycerides are extracted from the serum by a solvent that does not remove the other glycerol esters, e.g., the phospholipids. The triglycerides are hydrolyzed by transesterification with heat and alkali, and the glycerol formed is determined colorimetrically. In the other method the triglycerides are hydrolyzed enzymatically and the glycerol determined by means of enzymatic reactions. When the reagents are available, the latter method is much simpler and rapid but suffers from the disadvantage that since the determination is made directly on the serum, the small amount of free glycerol in the serum is also determined. Either a correction can be made for this or the free glycerol can be determined separately.

Modified colorimetric method of Soloni[57]

Principle: The triglycerides are extracted from the serum by a solvent that does not extract the phospholipids or other interfering materials. The extracted triglycerides are hydrolyzed by heating with alkali, and the resulting glycerol is oxidized to formaldehyde with periodate. The formaldehyde is determined by the Hantzsch condensation with ammonia and acetylacetone. The resulting yellow diacetyldihydrolutidine is determined spectrophotometrically at 410 nm.

Reagents:
1. *n*-Nonane, reagent grade
2. Isopropanol, reagent grade
3. Sulfuric acid, 0.04 mole/L
   Dilute 80 ml of 0.5 mole/L acid to 1 L.
4. Sodium methylate
   Dissolve 50 mg sodium methylate in 1 dl isopropanol. Prepare fresh as needed.
5. Sodium metaperiodate, 0.025 mole/L
   Dissolve 0.535 g sodium metaperiodate ($NaIO_4$) in 1 mole/L acetic acid and dilute to 1 dl. The acid is prepared by diluting 58 ml glacial acetic acid to 1 L with water.
6. Acetylacetone
   Dissolve 0.75 ml of 2,4-pentanedione and 2.5 ml isopropanol in 2 moles/L ammonium acetate (154 g/L in water) to make 1 dl. The solution is stable for about 1 month when stored in a brown bottle in the refrigerator.
7. Triolein standard 300 mg/dl
   Dissolve 300 mg pure triolein in isopropanol to make 1 dl. This solution is quite stable in the refrigerator.

Although the triglycerides are actually a mixture, they are conventionally calculated as triolein. Since triolein is a liquid at room temperature, it is difficult and unnecessary to try to weigh exactly 300 mg. One should accurately weigh as close to this amount as possible and then use the actual weight in the calculations, e.g., 317 mg/dl. In the procedure as given it is assumed that the standards are made up to the exact amount, but any corrections in the calculations can easily be made.

Procedure: To 16 × 150 test tubes with Teflon-lined screw caps, add 0.5 ml serum, 2.0 ml *n*-nonane, 3.5 ml isopropanol, and 1.0 ml sulfuric acid. Set up standard using 0.5 ml standard, 0.5 ml water, 2.0 ml *n*-nonane, 3.0 ml isopropanol, and 1.0 ml sulfuric acid. Also set up a blank similar to the sample, substituting water for the serum. Mix the tubes well on a vortex mixer for 30 sec. Allow the layers to separate completely, and use aliquots of the upper layer for analysis.

Into separate tubes, add 0.2 ml aliquots of the *n*-nonane layers from sample, standard, and blank. To each tube, add 3 ml sodium methylate solution and incubate at 60° C for 15 min. Add 0.2 ml metaperiodate solution, mix, and then add 1.0 ml acetylacetone reagent. Mix and incubate at 60° C for 15 min. Cool to room temperature and centrifuge. Using the upper phase, read standard and samples against blank at 410 nm.

The linearity of the spectrophotometer and the procedure should be checked periodically (i.e., monthly) by running a calibration curve. Prepare a series of standards by adding 1, 2, 3, and 4 ml of the standard to separate tubes and adding isopropanol to each to make 5 ml, using accurate volumetric pipets. These dilutions together with the original standard correspond to 60, 120, 180, 240, and 300 mg/dl (or 0.68, 1.34, 2.03, 2.71, and 3.4 mmole/L). Run standards and blank as given in the procedure. Plot the absorbance against the concentration. If the calibration curve is not linear, it may be preferable to run several standards with each group of samples using for the calculations for each sample the standard having an absorbance closest to that of the sample. If the reading for the sample is more than about 1.2 times that of the highest standard, it is best to repeat the determination using a 1:3 dilution of the supernatant (with isopropanol) and multiplying the result obtained by 3. For very high levels it is better to dilute a portion of the original serum 1:5 or 1:10 with saline before extraction.

Calculation:

$$\frac{\text{Absorbance of sample}}{\text{Absorbance of standard}} \times 300 = \frac{\text{Conc.}}{\text{of sample (mg/dl)}}$$

since equal volumes of the sample and serum are treated similarly.

To convert milligrams per deciliter triolein to millimoles per liter, use the following:

$$\text{mmole/L} = \text{mg/dl} \times 0.0113$$

where 0.0113 = (10 dl/L) × 1/(885 mg/mmole).

Enzymatic method

Principle: In the enzymatic method[58-60] the glycerides are first hydrolyzed by the action of glycerol lipase. Then the glycerol is determined by a series of reactions such as:

$$\text{Glycerol} + \text{ATP} \xrightarrow[\text{kinase}]{\text{Glycerol}} \text{Glycerol-3-phosphate} + \text{ADP}$$

$$\text{Phosphoenolpyruvate} + \text{ADP} \xrightarrow[\text{kinase}]{\text{Pyruvate}} \text{Pyruvate} + \text{ATP}$$

$$\text{Pyruvate} + \text{NADH} + \text{H}^+ \xrightarrow[\text{dehydrogenase}]{\text{Lactate}} \text{Lactate} + \text{NAD}^+$$

The extent of the reaction is then measured by the change in absorbance at 340 nm where NADH has a high absorbance but NAD^+ does not.

The enzymes for the preparation of the reagents are not all readily available, and the same disadvantages apply as discussed under the glucose oxidase method. It is advisable to purchase the complete reagents in kit form (see suppliers listed under the glucose oxidase method). As mentioned, these methods also determine the free glycerol in the sample. Some of the kits may have a provision for separately determining the free glycerol, but this is inconvenient and requires a relatively large sample. Often a correction is made of the supposedly average value of free glycerol. One study[61] found an average of 1.33 mg/dl of glycerol in serum. This corresponds to 13 mg/dl of triglycerides (as triolein), or 0.14 mmole/L. Although there was a fairly wide range of values, the concentration did not appear to be related to the total triglycerides present. If, in the enzymatic methods, the free glycerol is not actually determined but only an empiric correction is used, it is important to know whether the concentration of free glycerol increases on storage of serum. The increase has been both stated[62] and denied.[63] It is suggested that if serum is to be stored for some time, it first be heated to 56° C for 20 min to inactivate enzymes that may presumably cause a slow hydrolysis of triglycerides.[61] Freezing is sufficient for storage up to a week.

Normal values and interpretation

The normal range of values for serum triglycerides by the chemical methods is from 40-145 mg/dl (0.45-1.64 mmole/L). The values by the enzymatic methods if corrected for free glycerol are slightly lower, but without the correction they approximate the values for the chemical methods. Values below the normal range are of little clinical significance. Elevated concentrations are often found in disturbances of lipid metabolism and in atherosclerosis and coronary artery disease.

TOTAL LIPIDS

The determination of total lipids in serum has been used for many years in the study of lipid metabolism. The commonly used gravimetric method is rather lengthy and requires careful technic. The determination of total lipids is not a very specific test because of the number of different compounds that are included. It is generally agreed that the most information concerning derangements of lipid metabolism is obtained by determinations of cholesterol, triglycerides, and lipoprotein phenotyping. A simple and rapid method for the determination of total lipids would be of some value. The colorimetric method presented below, although somewhat lacking in specificity, is simple and rapid and probably gives just as much information as the gravimetric method.

Principle: When the blood lipids, particularly those containing monounsaturated fatty acids, are heated with concentrated sulfuric acid, they are oxidized to ketones that subsequently give a color with a phosphovanillin reagent. The different lipid components will give different amounts of color, so that the method is not very specific, but it has been found to give good correlation with the gravimetric method. The reaction can be carried out either on a serum extract or directly on serum. The use of the extract may give slightly better precision and sensitivity, but in view of the empiric nature of the reactions involved and the wide range of normal values, the direct method is satisfactory for almost all purposes.[64-67]

Reagents:
1. Concentrated sulfuric acid
2. Phosphovanillin reagent
   Dissolve 0.52 g vanillin in about 2 dl water in a 5 dl volumetric flask. Add with stirring 150 ml of 85% phosphoric acid. Cool and dilute to 5 dl with water. The reagent is stable for about 2 months stored in a brown bottle at room temperature.
3. Standards
   Dissolve 1 g pure olive oil in absolute ethanol to make 1 dl. This solution contains 1000 mg/dl of lipids. Lower concentrations are prepared by diluting 10, 15, and 20 ml to 25 ml with ethanol. These solutions contain 400, 600, and 800 mg/dl. These standards together with the 1000 mg/dl standard may be used to prepare a calibration curve. If it is found to be linear over this range only the 600 mg/dl standard need be run routinely. Since the total lipids represent a collection of totally unrelated chemical substances, the use of moles per liter is inappropriate. If desired, the results may be expressed in grams per liter by dividing by 100.

Procedure: Add 20 μl of water (blank), standard, or sample to labeled test tubes. To each tube add 0.2 ml concentrated sulfuric acid, mix well, and place in a boiling water bath for 10 min. Cool in water for about 10 min. then add 10 ml of the phosphovanillin reagent. Mix well and then incubate at 37° C for 15 min. Cool for about 5 min and then read standard and samples against the blank at 540 nm within 30 min.

Calculation: Since standard and sample are treated similarly:

$$\frac{\text{Absorbance of sample}}{\text{Absorbance of standard}} \times \frac{\text{Conc.}}{\text{of standard}} = \frac{\text{Conc.}}{\text{of sample in}}$$
$$\text{mg/dl total lipids}$$

or the results may be obtained from a calibration curve.

Normal values and interpretation: The normal value of total lipids may be taken as 400-1000 mg/dl. Published estimates of ranges vary rather widely. At birth the concentrations are usually in the range of 100-250 mg/dl and increase to about twice this value within a few days, reaching the adult value after about 1 year. The total lipid value will be increased after a fat meal.

It may be decreased in steatorrhea or other malabsorption syndromes, but a determination of some of the separate constituents (fatty acids, cholesterol, etc.) will give more valuable information.

LIPOPROTEINS AND LIPOPROTEIN PHENOTYPING
Use of cellulose acetate electrophoresis

The lipids in the serum are combined with the protein fractions as lipoproteins. The presence of abnormal amounts of some of the lipoproteins has been implicated in the pathogenesis of atherosclerosis. The lipoproteins have been separated into a number of classes by means of ultracentrifugation. This method requires special equipment that is found only in a few research laboratories. For the ordinary clinical laboratory the most practical method of separation is by some type of electrophoresis. In theory this is similar to protein electrophoresis, except that a stain is used that combines with the lipid rather than with the proteins. Lipoprotein electrophoresis has been carried out with the use of paper, cellulose acetate, agar or agarose gel, starch gel, or polyacrylamide gel. Each method is said to have ad-

vantages. It is most convenient to use the same general method in the laboratory for both regular protein and lipoprotein electrophoresis. A method is presented using cellulose acetate,[68] since this is now probably the most commonly used method for regular protein electrophoresis. However, not all types of cellulose acetate membranes that are suitable for protein electrophoresis may be suitable for lipoprotein electrophoresis.[69] The differences appear to be the result of the method of manufacture. Since these methods are continually being improved, the results of this study may not necessarily be valid today. One must use a membrane designated specifically for lipoprotein electrophoresis.

Apparatus: Any of the systems available for the separation of serum proteins using cellulose acetate membranes can also be used for lipoprotein electrophoresis.

Reagents: Most manufacturers of the membranes will furnish the powder for preparing the buffer, the staining solution, and, if used, the decolorizing solution. These may vary with the manufacture and are generally adapted to a specific type of membrane. In general, these solutions are similar to those listed on p. 554.

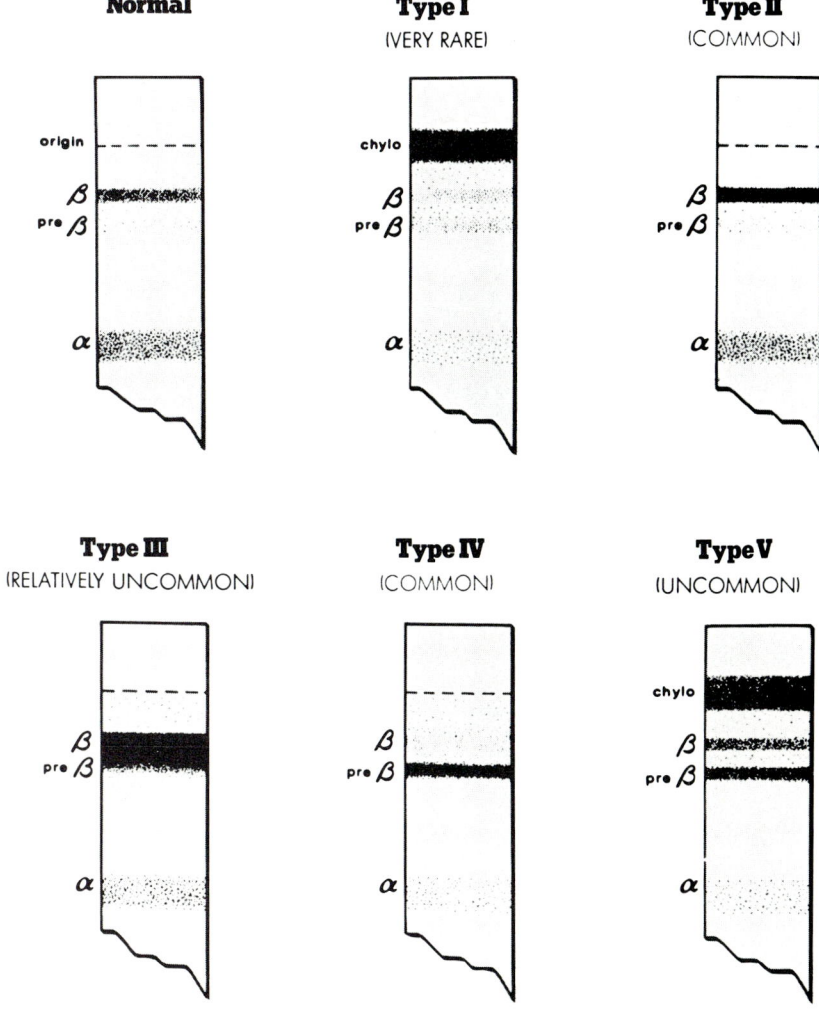

Fig. 23-1. Lipoprotein patterns.

1. Buffer

    The buffer is usually a barbital buffer of 0.075 μm ionic strength and a pH of 8.6. To make this, dissolve 15.4 g sodium diethylbarbiturate and 2.76 g diethylbarbituric acid in about 9 dl water with the aid of heat; cool and dilute to 1 L.

2. Staining dye

    Dissolve 0.4 g oil red O (C.I. 26125) in a mixture of 7 dl methanol and 3 dl water by boiling for a few minutes. Cool and store at 37° C. Use without filtering.

3. Decolorizing solution

    Mix 5 ml commercial sodium hypochlorite (liquid bleach, 5.25% available chlorine) with 1 dl of 5% acetic acid (5 ml glacial acetic acid to 1 dl with water).

Procedure: Carry out the electrophoresis in accordance with the directions furnished with the particular instrument. It may be necessary to use more sample (two or more applications) than for protein electrophoresis. This must be determined by experiment if not specified in the directions with the instrument.

After electrophoresis, stain at 37° C overnight. Then immerse in decolorizing solution for 60-90 sec. Scan as directed with the instrument without clearing. Note that for regular protein electrophoresis on cellulose acetate the protein is also stained with a (different) red dye so that the same filter can be used for lipoprotein scanning.

The electrophoretic pattern will show four bands, as illustrated in Fig. 23-1. There will be a band at the origin caused by the chylomicrons; this band may not be as distinct with cellulose acetate electrophoresis as when some of the other supporting media are used. There will be three other bands labeled, in order, β, pre-β, and α. There may also be a faint band at the albumin position caused by staining of the free fatty acids and a small amount of other lipids bound to the albumin. This band is not considered in the interpretation.

Lipoprotein patterns

The different lipoprotein patterns are illustrated in Fig. 23-1. In most instances one need not scan the bands in a densitometer as one does for serum proteins; rather, one can merely classify the pattern as one of the types shown in the illustration by visual inspection.

On the basis of the lipoprotein pattern, together with a consideration of the cholesterol, triglyceride, and chylomicron content of the serum, the lipid abnormalities may be classified into several types. The usual classification is based on that of Fredrickson and associates,[70-72] as indicated in Table 23-3. A number of the abnormal types have a significant genetic basis, and the classification is often spoken of as lipoprotein phenotyping.[73-74] It is probable that certain of the abnormal types indicate an increased tendency toward atherosclerosis and heart disease.[75] Lipoprotein electrophoresis is often done on a routine basis as a screening procedure, but not all workers are convinced of the need for this.

High-density lipoprotein cholesterol (HDLC)

When the lipoprotein fractions are separated by the ultracentrifuge,[76] the various fractions are known as the chylomicrons, the low-density lipoprotein (LDL), very low–density lipoproteins (VLDL), and high-density lipoproteins (HDL) on the basis of their relative motions under the influence of centrifugal force. One particular high-density fraction (HDL) seems to be inversely related to the tendency toward heart disease.

Principle: It has been found that by a simple chemical procedure, polyanionic precipitation, the low- and very low–density lipoproteins may be precipitated and removed by centrifugation. The high-density lipoprotein remains in the supernatant. Since a certain amount of cholesterol is associated with each of the lipoprotein fractions, the determination of the cholesterol remaining in the supernatant is a measure of the amount of the high-density lipoprotein present. A number of different precipitating agents have been used[76-80]; the procedure given here uses magnesium chloride and sodium phosphotungstate.[80] The cholesterol in the supernatant is determined by the cholesterol oxidase method.

Reagents:

1. Magnesium chloride solution, 2 moles/L

    Dissolve 40.6 g $MgCl_2 \cdot 6H_2O$ in water to make 1 dl.

2. Sodium phosphotungstate

    Add 4 g phosphotungstic acid and 8 ml of 1 mole/L NaOH to about 80 ml of water. Adjust pH to 6.15 by the addition of more of the NaOH solution and dilute to 1 dl.

3. Reagent for cholesterol determination

    The reagent for cholesterol determination is the same as the previous reagent. The determination by the cholesterol oxidase method is preferred. It

Table 23-3. Frederickson's classification of lipid abnormalities

Type	Cholesterol	Triglycerides	Chylomicrons	β (LDL)	Pre-β (VLDL)	α (HDL)
Normal	N	N	±	+	±	+
I	+	+ +	+ +	+	±	+
IIa	+	N	±	+ +	±	+
IIb	+	N	±	+ +	+ +	+
III	+	+	±	+ + + +		+
IV	N or +	+	±	+ +	+ +	+
V	N or +	+ +	+ +	+ +	+ +	+

N, normal level (under 250 mg/dl for cholesterol and under 150 mg/dl for triglycerides); +, elevated level. For electrophoretic bands, ±, faint band; +, visible band of about the same intensity as found in normal individual; + +, much darker band. In type III there is a strong band covering both β and pre-β positions, termed *floating* or *broad* β-*band*.

is not necessary to add EDTA when magnesium-phosphotungstate is used as a precipitating agent. This would be absolutely necessary if manganese-heparin were used as a precipitating agent,[77-80] since the manganese inhibits the enzymatic reactions used to determine cholesterol.

4. Cholesterol standard

This is the same as in the cholesterol methods. Since the cholesterol value in the supernatant is low, it is best to dilute the standard to about 50 mg/dl (1.3 mmole/L).

Procedure: Recentrifuge the serum if necessary to remove all traces of red cells. To 1 ml of serum (preferably in a plastic tube with stopper) add 100 µl of the sodium phosphotungstate solution and mix briefly on a Vortex mixer. Add 25 µl of the magnesium chloride solution and mix. Allow the tubes to stand for 30 min and then centrifuge at 3000 rpm for 30 min. Immediately after centrifugation remove about 0.5 ml of the supernatant and reserve for analysis. If the analysis cannot be done immediately, store the supernatant in the refrigerator. Also prepare a sample blank by mixing together 1 ml saline, 100 µl phosphotungstate, and 25 µl magnesium chloride solution. Set up tubes containing the cholesterol reagent and saline (reagent blank), sample blank, standard and sample, using twice the volume of sample, and diluted standard and blank solutions as called for in the method for total cholesterol.

Calculation: After color development read standard against reagent blank and sample against sample blank. Then

$$\frac{\text{Absorbance of sample}}{\text{Absorbance of standard}} \times \frac{\text{Conc.}}{\text{of standard}} \times 1.125 = \frac{\text{Conc.}}{\text{of sample}}$$

where the factor of 1.125 corrects for the fact that the original serum sample was diluted by the added precipitating reagents.

Normal values and interpretation: Studies[81,82] have indicated that when the high-density lipoprotein cholesterol (HDLC) value is *lower* than 45 mg/dl (1.2 mmole/L) in men and lower than 55 mg/dl (1.4 mmole/L) in women there is an increased risk for heart disease and the relative risk increases with lower HDLC concentrations. Higher HDLC concentrations may be associated with decreased coronary risk and increased longevity.

• • •

Calculated very low–density lipoprotein cholesterol and low-density lipoprotein cholesterol

When chylomicrons are absent and triglycerides are less than 400 mg/dl, the LDL-cholesterol and VLDL-cholesterol values[82,83] can be estimated from the following relationships:

$$\text{VLDL}_{\text{chol}} = \frac{\text{Plasma triglycerides}}{5}$$

$$\text{LDL}_{\text{chol}} = \text{Total cholesterol} - \text{HDLC} - \frac{\text{Triglyceride}}{5}$$

All concentrations are expressed in milligrams per deciliter.

MISCELLANEOUS TESTS AND INFORMATION

VITAMIN A AND CAROTENE[84-86]

Principle: Carotene is the precursor of vitamin A and is usually determined along with the vitamin. The proteins in the serum are precipitated with ethanol, and the carotene and vitamin A are extracted with hexane. Carotene is determined directly by its absorbance at 450 nm. Vitamin A is determined by reaction with trifluoroacetic acid to give a transient blue color. Since carotene also produces some color with the reagent, a correction must be made. The preparation of all standards and all analytic processes must be performed in areas with low light levels.

Reagents: Spectrograde solvents are preferred for this determination.

1. Trifluoroacetic acid (TFA) reagent

Mix together 1 volume of trifluoroacetic acid and 2 volumes of chloroform. Prepare fresh as needed and just before use add 1 drop of acetic anhydride for each 10 ml of the mixture.

2. Absolute ethanol

3. *n*-Hexane

4. Chloroform

5. β-Carotene standards

a. Stock standard. Dissolve 20 mg β-carotene (Eastman Organic Chemicals, Rochester, N.Y.) in 4 ml chloroform and dilute to 1 dl with hexane. This solution contains 200 µg/ml.

b. Working standards. Prepare a solution of 20 µg/ml by diluting the stock standard 1:10 with hexane. Into 1 dl volumetric flasks pipet 0.5, 1.0, 1.5, 2.5, 5.0, and 10.0 ml of 20 µg/ml standard and dilute to volume with hexane to give working standards of 10, 20, 30, 50, 100, and 200 µg/dl. These standards are stable 5 days if kept at 5-8° C in the dark in containers with little air space.

6. Vitamin A (retinol) standards

a. Stock standard, 20 mg/dl (200 µg/ml). Dissolve 22.9 mg vitamin A acetate (trans-retinyl acetate, equivalent to 20 mg vitamin A) in chloroform to make 1 dl. The acetate is preferred as a standard since it is more stable and gives the same amount of color on a molar basis as does the alcohol.

b. Working standards. Prepare a solution of 20 µg/ml by diluting the stock 1:10 with chloroform. Into 1 dl volumetric flasks pipet 0.5, 1.0, 2.5, and 5.0 ml of 20 µg/ml standard and dilute to volume with chloroform to give working standards of 10, 20, 30, 50, and 100 µg/dl. These standards are stable for 5 days if kept at 5-8° C in the dark in containers with little air space.

All the carotene and vitamin A standards should be kept in tightly stoppered brown bottles in the refrigerator.

Extraction procedure: Place 1 ml of fasting plasma or serum sample in a screw-capped test tube with a

Teflon-lined cap and add 2 ml absolute ethanol by drops with agitation. Add 3 ml hexane, stopper, and shake vigorously for 3 min. Centrifuge at 2000 rpm for 10 min to separate the phases completely. Pipet as much as possible of the upper hexane layer to a second tube, taking care not to include any of the aqueous layer. Cap tube containing hexane layer to prevent evaporation.

Carotene determination: Transfer 2.0 ml of the hexane extract to a cuvet and read against a blank of hexane at 450 nm. Retain the sample cuvet is for later determination of vitamin A. To a series of cuvets add the 10, 20, 30, 50, 100, and 200 μg/dl carotene working standards and read them against the blank. Since the 3 ml hexane contains the carotene from 1 ml of serum (a 1:3 dilution) the standards are equivalent to 30, 60, 90, 150, 300, and 600 μg/dl of apparent carotene in the serum.

Calculation:

$$\frac{\text{Absorbance of sample}}{\text{Absorbance of standard}} \times \frac{\text{Apparent}}{\text{conc.}} = \frac{\text{Conc.}}{\text{in sample (μg/dl)}}$$
$$\text{of standard}$$

One can choose the standard with the absorbance nearest the sample for the calculations or plot a calibration curve and read the sample concentration from the curve.

Vitamin A determination: Carefully evaporate to dryness the solution in the cuvet used for the determination of carotene. Place cuvet in a water bath at 60° C and evaporate with the aid of a small stream of nitrogen or carbon dioxide. Dissolve the residue in exactly 0.1 ml chloroform. Adjust the spectrophotometer to zero absorbance with a chloroform blank at 620 nm. Add 1 ml of the TFA reagent quickly to the sample and read at once in the spectrophotometer. The color develops rapidly, reaching a maximum in 5-10 sec, and then fades. Record the maximal reading. Make similar readings with a series of vitamin A working standards by adding to a series of cuvets 0.1 ml of each diluted vitamin A standard. These standards are treated in the same manner as the extract equivalent to $^2/_3$ ml of serum. Thus they are equivalent to 15, 30, 45, 75, and 150 μg/dl vitamin A in the serum (Original standard concentration $\times$ $^3/_2$; i.e., 10 μg/dl $\times$ $^3/_2$ = 15 μg/dl).

Calculation: Thus:

$$\frac{\text{Absorbance of sample}}{\text{Absorbance of standard}} \times \frac{\text{Conc.}}{\text{of standard}} = \text{μg/dl vitamin A}$$

or one may plot a calibration curve and obtain the unknown values from the curve.

A correction must be made for the amount of carotene present, which gives a slight amount of color with the reagent. For this, transfer 1 ml diluted carotene standard (200 μg/dl) to a cuvet, evaporate the solvent, dissolve in 0.1 ml chloroform, and treat with the reagent as with the vitamin A samples and standards. To correct for the amount of color contributed by the carotene, calculate as follows:

$$F = \frac{A_{620} \text{ of carotene in vitamin A procedure}}{A_{450} \text{ of carotene in carotene procedure}}$$

$$F \times \text{μg/dl carotene in sample} = \text{μg vitamin A}$$

where A_{620} = absorbance at 620 nm and A_{450} = absorbance at 450 nm. The vitamin A calculated from the above formula is subtracted from the total vitamin A. Thus, if F were 0.05 and the carotene concentration were 150 μg/dl, then 150 × 0.05 = 7.5 μg/dl. This figure would be subtracted from the measured value of vitamin A.

• • •

The above procedure is sufficient for most clinical purposes. If greater specificity and accuracy are desired, the following modification may be used.[87] Prepare an approximately 10 moles/L solution of potassium hydroxide in water to make 1 dl. As needed mix 1 volume of this with 9 volumes of absolute ethanol. Add 2 ml of this solution by drops to 1 ml of serum, mix by shaking, and then incubate at 60° C for 30 min. Cool, add 3 ml hexane, and proceed as given above.

Normal values and interpretation:

Carotene: The normal range for carotene may be taken as from 50-250 μg/dl. The concentration in the blood is influenced by the amount of carotene in the diet and may be high in a diet rich in vegetables such as carrots. Increased values have been reported in patients with diabetes mellitus, myxedema, and chronic nephritis. Low values have been found in patients with steatorrhea or malabsorption syndrome.

Vitamin A: The range of normal values reported in the literature varies considerably but may be taken as from 25-75 μg/dl in adults and 15-60 μg/dl in infants. If the concentration is above 20 μg/dl, it may be assumed that there is no vitamin A deficiency.

The absorption of vitamin A is decreased when there is a decreased fat absorption as in steatorrhea; a tolerance test with vitamin A has been used to determine decreased fat absorption. The technics used vary somewhat, but in general, a dose of about 7500 IU vitamin A/kg body weight is given orally and the blood levels are determined at several timed intervals after the ingestion. Usually if the blood level rises over 500 IU (150 μg/dl) 4 or 5 hr after ingestion, steatorrhea may be excluded. Failure of the serum value to increase this much is not conclusive evidence of the disease.

Vitamin A dosage forms are usually given in terms of international units. One international unit is equivalent to 0.3 μg of pure vitamin A alcohol, to 0.344 μg vitamin A acetate, or to 0.60 μg pure β-carotene.

ASCORBIC ACID[88,89]

Principle: The dye 2,6-dichlorophenol-indophenol is reduced from a blue to a colorless form by ascorbic acid. When excess dye is added to a solution containing ascorbic acid the decrease in color, determined in a spectrophotometer, is a measure of the amount of ascorbic acid present. Because ascorbic acid is not stable in blood, plasma (oxalate is satisfactory as anticoagulant) is preferable to serum, since the former can be separated from the cells more rapidly. Ascorbic acid is stable in plasma for only about 30 min at room temperature, so the analysis should be performed as soon as possible after the sample is obtained. Sulfhydryl compounds will interfere with the determination. The interference is only slight for plasma and may be neglected.

For the determination in urine the interference is minimized by the addition of hydroxymercuribenzoate. The dehydroascorbic acid found in urine will not be measured by this method.

Proteins are precipitated by metaphosphoric acid, which aids in the stabilization of the ascorbic acid. The protein-free filtrates are stable for several hours.

Reagents:

1. Stock indophenol solution, 3.4 moles/L
   Dissolve 100 mg of the sodium salt of 2,6-dichlorophenol-indophenol (Eastman Organic Chemicals, Rochester, N.Y.) in water to make 1 dl. This solution is stable for several months when stored in the refrigerator.

2. Working indophenol dye solution
   Just before use dilute 5 ml of the stock solution to 50 ml with water. This solution is not stable and should be prepared fresh each day it is to be used. If necessary, the concentration of the dye can be adjusted so that the reagent blank (see below) gives an initial absorbance of about 0.65 in the cuvets used.

3. Sodium citrate solution, 0.15 mole/L
   Dissolve 4.4 g sodium citrate dihydrate in water to make 1 dl.

4. Mercuribenzoate solution, 5.5 mmole/L
   Dissolve 200 mg of the sodium salt of *p*-hydroxymercuribenzoate in water to make 1 dl.

5. Metaphosphoric acid, 0.38 mole/L
   Dissolve 3 g reagent grade metaphosphoric acid (containing 35% HPO_3) in water to make 1 dl. This solution is stable for about 1 week in the refrigerator.

6. Ascorbic acid standards
   a. Stock standard, 40 mg/dl. Dissolve 40 mg of ascorbic acid in 40 ml deionized water and dilute to 1 dl with the metaphosphoric acid solution. This is stable for about 1 month in the refrigerator (2.3 mmole/L).
   b. Working solution. Just before use dilute 1 ml of the stock solution to 50 ml with a mixture of 3 volumes metaphosphoric acid solution and 2 volumes deionized water. This solution contains 0.8 mg/dl (45.4 μmole/L). A good grade of deionized water must be used, since small traces of metals will interfere.

Procedure for plasma: Add 3 ml of 0.38 mole/L metaphosphoric acid to 2 ml plasma, mix well, and centrifuge to obtain a clear supernatant. In separate cuvets set up the following:

1. Reagent blank: 1.2 ml metaphosphoric acid solution, 0.8 ml water, and 0.5 ml sodium citrate solution. Mix well.

2. Standard: 2.0 ml working standard and 0.5 ml sodium citrate solution. Mix well.

3. Sample: 2.0 ml protein-free supernatant, 0.2 ml sodium citrate solution, and 0.3 ml water. Mix well.

To each tube, add 1.0 ml of the working dye solution, mix, and read after 30 sec against a water blank at 520 nm. To each tube then add a few crystals of ascorbic acid to completely decolorize, and read again. For each tube, subtract the absorbance obtained after the addition of the excess ascorbic acid from that obtained initially. (This serves to correct for any turbidity, which sometimes occurs.) These differences are then recorded as the corrected absorbances for the reagent blank, standard, and sample.

Calculation:

$$\frac{\text{Corr. abs. of reagent blank} - \text{Corr. abs. of sample}}{\text{Corr. abs. of reagent blank} - \text{Corr. abs. of standard}} \times$$

$$2.5 \times \text{Conc. of standard} = \text{Conc. of sample}$$

The factor of 2.5 arises from the fact that 2 ml of standard is compared with 2 ml of a 1:2.5 dilution of the serum sample (2-5 ml). The concentration of the standard is 0.8 mg/dl, or 45.4 μmole/L, depending on which units are used.

If the initial absorbance of the sample tube is very low (indicating a high concentration of ascorbic acid, which reduces nearly all of the added dye) repeat the determination using 1 ml of supernatant, 0.6 ml of the phosphoric acid solution, and 0.4 ml of water instead of 2 ml of supernatant and multiply the answer by an additional factor of 2.

Normal values and interpretation: The normal range in plasma is from 0.5-2.0 mg/dl (28.4-114 μmole/L).[90] The concentration is slightly higher in women than in men and in children as compared with adults. The value is also said to be lower in smokers than in nonsmokers. Symptoms of scurvy may be seen in individuals with values below 0.2 mg/dl (11.4 μmole/L), and individuals with values below 0.4 mg/dl (23 μmole/L) may be considered at risk in regard to scurvy. High values are indicative only of massive vitamin intake.

Procedure for urine: Mix 3 ml metaphosphoric acid solution with 2 ml urine and centrifuge. To 3 ml of the supernatant, add 1 ml of the mercuribenzoate solution, mix, and allow to stand for about 10 min. Centrifuge and use 2 ml of this supernatant plus 0.5 ml sodium citrate solution; then proceed as for plasma, using the same standard and reagent blank solutions. The calculated result is multiplied by four thirds to correct for the extra dilution of the urine.

Normal values and interpretation: The daily urinary output of ascorbic acid varies with the intake; it is approximately half the intake. The average daily intake ranges from 30-80 mg, with an output of 20-30 mg/day. In vitamin C deficiency, the urinary ascorbic acid level is significantly reduced and may disappear completely. Since ascorbic acid is not very stable in urine, the analysis of a 24 hr urine specimen is of little value.

In addition, this method does not measure the dehydroascorbic acid form, which is biologically active and found in appreciable amounts in urine.

Ascorbic acid saturation tests

Ascorbic acid saturation tests are based on the assumption that previous intake of ascorbic acid has been insufficient; when large doses of the vitamin are administered, the tissues will take up most of the vitamin so that little or none is excreted in the urine. If the intake has been adequate, the individual will excrete appreciable amounts of the administered vitamin.

Ascorbic acid may be given orally or intravenously,

and different times may be used for urine specimen collection. Normally, when 500 mg ascorbic acid (in 5 ml sterile distilled water) is given intravenously, at least 200 mg should be excreted 4 hr after injection.

Procedure: A dosage of 11 mg ascorbic acid/kg body weight is given orally. Only one urine specimen is needed for the period of 4-6 hr after ingestion of the vitamin, which is the time when excretion is at its maximum.

The test is carried out as follows: At a designated time, 11 mg ascorbic acid/kg body weight dissolved in 120-180 water is given orally. For an average individual weighing 70 kg this will correspond to 770 mg. Have the patient empty the bladder completely 4 hr later and discard the urine; 2 hr later have patient empty the bladder completely and determine ascorbic acid content with the method previously described.

Repeat test daily until a normal response is obtained.

Normal values and interpretation: Normal individuals excrete approximately 0.8 mg/kg or about 50 mg. In vitamin C deficiency the excretion may be below 10 mg.

ANALYSIS OF BILIARY CALCULI[91]

Procedure: Grind up calculi in mortar. Extract one portion with ether (about 10 ml) and filter. Test filtrate for cholesterol as follows:

1. Add equal parts of ether extract and alcohol, let evaporate, and examine microscopically for cholesterol crystals.

2. When dry, dissolve in about 2-3 ml chloroform and add 1 ml acetic anhydride and 2-3 drops concentrated sulfuric acid. Cholesterol gives a greenish blue color.

Test small portions of residue on microslides as follows:

1. For calcium dissolve in 3 moles/L hydrochloric acid and adjust to pH of 5 with ammonium hydroxide. Then add 4-5 drops of a saturated solution of ammonium oxalate and examine microscopically for calcium oxalate crystals.

2. For phosphates dissolve in 1 drop concentrated nitric acid. Add a few drops of saturated ammonium molybdate solution and heat. A yellow precipitate indicates phosphates. An alternate method is to dissolve in acetic acid and add ammonia. Phosphates give a white precipitate that is crystalline if triple phosphates are present and amorphous if earthy phosphates are present.

3. For iron dissolve in 3 moles/L hydrochloric acid by heating to dryness. Add potassium ferrocyanide; ferric iron gives a blue color (precipitate). Add potassium ferricyanide; ferrous iron gives a blue color (precipitate). An alternate method is to heat with 1 drop of nitric acid, evaporate to dryness, and add 1 drop potassium thiocyanate. A salmon-red color indicates iron.

4. For bile pigment test another portion of the powder as follows: Extract a portion with chloroform. Place a few drops on filter paper and add 1 drop Fouchet reagent. A green color indicates bile. Evaporate a portion and take up with water. Test with yellow nitric acid. A green color indicates bilirubin.

Extract again with hot alcohol and test with yellow nitric acid. A green color indicates biliverdin.

BUFFERS AND INDICATORS

General principles: The hydrogen ion concentration is an important factor in many biologic systems and reactions. It is usually expressed in terms of pH. This may be defined by the following equation:

$$pH = -\log [H^+] = \log 1/[H^+]$$

where the brackets represent molar concentrations. Pure water will ionize to a slight extent to give equal amounts of hydrogen and hydroxyl ions:

$$H_2O \rightleftharpoons H^+ + OH^-$$

At room temperature the concentration of each ion is about 1×10^{-7} M. Thus pure water would have a pH of 7.0. This is taken as the neutral point; solutions having a greater number of hydrogen ions (lower pH) are acidic, and those having a smaller number of hydrogen ions are basic. Since the product of the concentrations of H and OH ions is always equal to 1×10^{-14} (at room temperature), a basic solution having an OH concentration of 10^{-4} would have an H^+ concentration of $10^{-14}/10^{-4} = 10^{-10}$, and thus a pH of 10.

Mechanism of buffer action: Since the pH is so important in many reactions, one needs methods for keeping the pH relatively constant. Solutions that are used for this purpose are called buffers. These are usually composed of a weak acid (or weak base) and its salt. Suppose one has a solution containing both sodium acetate and acetic acid. The sodium acetate will be almost completely ionized into sodium ions and acetate ions, and the acetic acid will be only very slightly ionized, particularly in the presence of the acetate ions from the salt. Thus the concentration of acetate ions will be equal to the amount of sodium acetate added, and the concentration of the undissociated acetic acid will be equal to that added to the solution. Under these conditions one can derive the following expression:

$$pH = pK' + \log \frac{[Salt]}{[Acid]}$$

where the brackets again indicate molar concentrations and pK' is a constant that is different for different acids. This expression, known as the Henderson-Hasselbalch equation, is fundamental in the discussion of buffers. To illustrate the action of buffers, consider a solution that is 0.1M in both acetic acid and sodium acetate. Since the pK' for acetic acid is 4.64, the pH of the solution will be as follows:

$$pH = 4.64 + \log \frac{[0.1]}{[0.1]} = 4.64$$

Suppose that to the buffer solution is added the equivalent of 0.01M hydrogen ions; then some of the salt will be changed into acid and the pH will now be as follows:

$$pH = 4.64 + \log \frac{[0.1 - 0.01]}{[0.1 + 0.01]} = 4.55$$

If the solution has been originally brought to a pH of 4.64 by the addition of acid alone (pH 4.64 = H^+ concentration of 2.3×10^{-5}), then the addition of 0.01M hydrogen ions would bring the pH down to 2.0, a much greater change. Thus a buffer tends to keep the hydrogen ion concentration relatively constant. Buffers act best when the concentrations of acid and salt are approximately equal. Theoretically, the greater the concentration of acid and salt, the greater the buffering capacity (more hydrogen ions required for a given pH change), but in use, e.g., in enzyme reactions, a very high concentration of salts may have an inhibiting effect on the enzymes, so that a more dilute buffer must be used.

The pK′ is not an invariable constant but will change somewhat with the total concentration of dissolved salt and with the temperature. Thus a solution that is 0.1M in acid and salt will not have exactly the same pH as one that is 1M in both. Ordinarily a tenfold dilution of a buffer will change the pH by about 0.1 unit. Similarly, for most buffers, the pH at 37° C will not be the same as at 25° C. Again the change is often about 0.1 pH unit, usually less at the higher temperature. This is sometimes of importance in enzyme determinations when the buffer may be made up and checked at 25° C and used at 37° C.

A number of buffer solutions have been used, some of them for specialized purposes. The following directions are for a few of the more common buffers, which cover a wide range of pH. In the buffers given, the pH is that measured at room temperature (about 25° C). The phthalate buffer will show no appreciable change with temperature, the acetate and phosphate buffers will have a pH 0.03-0.05 less at body temperature, and the tris and barbital buffers will have a pH about 0.1 less at 37° C. The directions are given for preparing buffers with a definite concentration of salt and acid. The pH value will change somewhat on dilution of the buffer. A twofold dilution may change the pH value by 0.05 unit or more, depending on the buffer. For many purposes these changes are unimportant, but they should be kept in mind when making up buffers of different concentrations. Unless great care is taken in weighing and using pure chemicals, the pH of the final solution may vary somewhat from the desired value. Hence it is best to check the buffers with a pH meter against known commercial pH standards unless only an approximate pH is desired. In Tables 23-4 to 23-8 the pH values are given in increments of 0.2 unit; interpolation may be readily made to obtain the amounts of solutions required for intermediate values. Simple explanations of the calculation of the pH of acid, bases, and buffers as well as other laboratory calculations will be found in the books by Remsen and Ackermann[92] and Blankenship and Campbell.[93] For a more detailed explanation of the changes in pH of buffers with dilution see Segal.[94]

Preparation of phthalate buffer, 0.05M, pH 2.2-3.8: Weigh out 40.83 g reagent grade potassium acid phthalate that has been previously dried at 110° C for several hours, dissolve in water, and dilute to 1 L. This solution is 0.2M in potassium acid phthalate. Also prepare a 0.2N solution of hydrochloric acid as directed in the section on the preparation of standard acid. To prepare the buffer solutions, add 50 ml phthalate solution to a 2 dl volumetric flask. Add the amount of 0.2N hydrochloric acid given in Table 23-4 and dilute to the mark.

Preparation of acetate buffer, 0.2M, pH 3.6-5.8: Prepare a 0.2M solution of sodium acetate by dissolving 27.22 g crystalline sodium acetate trihydrate in water to make 1 L. Prepare a solution of 0.2N acetic acid by diluting 11.5 ml glacial acetic acid to 1 L. Standardize against sodium hydroxide as outlined in the section on preparation of standard acids, using phenolphthalein as indicator, and dilute to exactly 0.2N. To prepare the buffer solutions mix together the required amounts of the two solutions as given in Table 23-5.

Preparation of phosphate buffer, 0.067M, pH 5.4-8.2: Prepare a solution of 0.067M disodium phosphate by dissolving 9.47 g reagent grade anhydrous Na_2HPO_4 in water to make 1 L. Prepare a 0.067M solution of monopotassium phosphate by dissolving 9.08 g reagent grade KH_2PO_4 in water and diluting to 1 L. To prepare

Table 23-4. Phthalate buffer

pH	0.2N HCl (ml)	pH	0.2N HCl (ml)
2.2	46.7	3.2	14.8
2.4	39.6	3.2	9.95
2.6	33.0	3.6	6.0
2.8	26.5	3.8	2.65
3.0	20.4		

Table 23-5. Acetate buffer

pH	0.2M sodium acetate (ml)	0.2N acetic acid (ml)
3.6	7.5	92.5
3.8	12.0	88.0
4.0	18.0	82.0
4.2	26.5	73.5
4.4	37.0	63.0
4.6	48.0	52.0
4.8	59	41
5.0	70	30
5.2	79	21
5.4	86	14
5.6	91	9
5.8	94	6

Table 23-6. Phosphate buffer

pH	0.067M Na_2HPO_4 (ml)	0.067M KH_2PO_4 (ml)
5.6	5.0	95.0
5.8	7.8	92.2
6.0	12.0	88.0
6.2	18.5	81.5
6.4	26.6	73.4
6.6	37.5	62.5
6.8	49.8	50.2
7.0	61.1	38.9
7.2	71.5	28.5
7.4	80.6	19.4
7.6	87.0	13.0
7.8	91.5	9.5
8.0	94.6	5.4
8.2	97.0	3.0

Table 23-7. Tris buffer

pH	0.1N HCl (ml)	pH	0.1N HCl (ml)
7.2	45.0	8.2	23.3
7.4	42.0	8.4	17.5
7.6	38.9	8.6	12.8
7.8	34.0	8.8	9.0
8.0	29.0	9.0	6.3

Table 23-8. Barbital buffer

pH	0.1M Na barbital (ml)	0.1N HCl (ml)
6.8	52.2	47.8
7.0	53.6	46.4
7.2	55.4	44.6
7.4	58.1	41.9
7.6	61.5	38.5
7.8	66.2	33.8
8.0	71.6	28.4
8.2	76.9	23.1
8.4	82.3	17.7
8.6	87.1	12.9
8.8	90.8	9.2
9.0	93.6	6.4
9.2	95.2	4.8
9.4	97.4	2.6

Table 23-9. Nontraditional buffers

Trivial name	pK' (25° C)	Useful range
ACES	6.8	6.1-7.5
ADA	6.6	6.0-7.2
BES	7.1	6.4-7.8
Bicine	8.3	7.6-9.0
Bis-tris propane	6.8, 9.0	6.3-9.5
CAPS	10.4	9.7-11.1
EPPS	8.0	7.3-8.7
HEPES	7.5	6.8-8.2
MES	6.1	5.5-6.7
MOPS	7.2	6.5-7.9
PIPES	6.8	6.1-7.5
TAPS	8.4	7.7-9.1
TES	7.5	6.8-8.2
Tricine	8.1	7.4-8.8

the buffer solutions, mix together the amounts of the two solutions as given in Table 23-6.

Preparation of tris buffer, 0.05M, pH 7.2-9.0: Prepare a 0.1M solution of tris(hydroxymethyl)-aminomethane by dissolving 12.11 g tris in water and diluting to 1 L. Also prepare a 0.1N solution of hydrochloric acid. To prepare the buffers, add 50 ml tris solution to a 1 dl volumetric flask, add the required amount of hydrochloric acid as given in Table 23-7, and dilute to 1 dl.

Preparation of barbital buffer, 0.1M, pH 6.8-9.4: Prepare a 0.1M solution of sodium diethylbarbiturate (sodium barbital) by dissolving 20.6 g salt in water and diluting to 1 L. Also prepare a 0.1N solution of hydrochloric acid. To prepare the buffers, mix togeter the amounts of solutions given in Table 23-8.

Nontraditional buffers: In an attempt to provide buffers in the physiologic pH range, Good and co-workers[95] in 1966 developed a series of compounds with pK' values between 6.1 and 10.4. These compounds are available commercially (Sigma Chemical Co., St. Louis) and provide an alternative to the traditional compounds with pK' values near neutrality. Table 23-9 lists the trivial name, pK', and usable pH range for each compound.

Indicators: An indicator is the salt of a weak acid (or base) that exhibits one color in the free un-ionized form and another color in the ionized salt form. The Henderson-Hasselbalch equation will hold in this instance also. Here the pH is regulated by the other buffers in the solution and is not affected by the small amount of indicator present. By this equation, the pH

determines the relative proportion of the salt and acid forms of the indicator. The indicator bromcresol green has a pK' of approximately 4.8 and at this pH will exist in solution in approximately equal proportions of the salt and acid forms. Since the acid form is colored yellow and the salt form blue, the solution will appear green. At pH 3.8, there will be 10 times as much of the acid as of the salt form and the solution would appear yellow; at pH 5.8, there would be 10 times as much of the blue salt form as of the acid form. Thus in this range one could estimate the approximate pH by the color of the solution. By using different indicators, different ranges may be covered, and with the use of a mixture of several indicators, a series of color changes over a considerable range of pH may be found.[96] The pK' and hence the color of an indicator solution at a given pH can be affected by high concentrations of salts, the indicator having slightly different colors in solutions of the same pH but different total salt concentrations.

Indicator colors may also be affected by the presence of proteins through absorption or other means. This is in fact the basis of one method for the determination of albumin. The indicator bromcresol green in a buffered solution of the proper pH will change color in the presence of albumin, and the amount of color change is, over a certain range, proportional to the amount of albumin present. With this and some other indicators, the effect is not produced by other proteins such as globulins, so the method is fairly specific for albumin. The dipsticks used for the determination of urinary protein are based on this principle and may ordinarily detect albumin (which is the chief urinary protein in most instances) but will not detect other proteins (e.g., Bence Jones proteins).

Determination of pH

Accurate determinations of pH[97] are usually made with the aid of the glass electrode. Such an electrode consists essentially of a small bulb made of a special glass and containing a solution of known pH. When this bulb is dipped into another solution, a potential will be developed across the glass membrane that is related to the difference in hydrogen ion concentration of the inner and outer solutions. This potential is amplified and measured electronically. In order to measure an electric potential, two electrodes are needed. One of these is a wire of an inert metal dipping into the solution within the bulb. The other electrode that dips into the solution being measured is usually a calomel electrode. This consists of mercury in contact with a saturated solution of mercurous chloride (calomel) and is connected to the solution being measured by means of a tube filled with saturated potassium chloride. The measured potential (EMF) may be expressed by the following formula:

$$EMF = E_o + kT \log \frac{[H_o^+]}{[H_i^+]}$$

where H_o^+ and H_i^+ are hydrogen ion concentrations on the two sides (outer and inner) of the glass membrane, k is a constant, T is the absolute temperature (°C + 273), and E_O represents the potential developed by the reference electrode and the various liquid interfaces in the system. In theory, in the equation one should use not the actual hydrogen ion concentration but the "effective" hydrogen ion concentration (activity or thermodynamic potential), which takes into account the effect of other ions and the number of actual hydrogen ions on the action of the electrode. Then instead of the concentration of hydrogen ions one could use the term $a \cdot x[H^+]$ where a, the activity coefficient, is unity for very dilute solutions and less than 1 for more concentrated solution. In actual practice at the pH levels in biologic systems and most reagents used in the laboratory (with pH between 3 and 10) the activity coefficient is close to unity. The only instance in the clinical laboratory where the activity coefficient might be used is in the determination of the actual hydrogen ion concentration from pH measurement in gastric juice, which may have a pH as low as 1.

Theoretically all the terms of the equation should be constant in a given case except for $[H_o^+]$, and thus the measured potential would be directly proportional to the pH, the logarithm of the hydrogen ion concentration. Because of the fact that E_o will vary with the experimental conditions and cannot be accurately determined by itself, the pH electrode is always standardized by the use of bufferes of known pH. Note that this equation contains the factor T, which means that the measured potential will vary with the temperature. The commercially available standardizing buffers usually give the pH of the buffer at different temperatures, and preferably the standardization and measurement of the unknown should be made at the same temperature. Most instruments have a temperature-compensating control so that one can standardize at one temperature and make the measurements at a different one.

In the following chapter on enzymes it will be found that solutions for the determination of enzymes contain a buffer to maintain a definite pH value, usually the optimal one for the particular enzyme. Although the determination of the enzyme activity may be made at 37° C, the pH of the reagent solution is usually checked at room temperature (25° C). This is allowable because in the original specification of the optimal conditions for the particular buffer the pH of the solution was measured at 25° C even though the measurements of

activity were to be made at a different temperature.

In making pH measurements the electrode system should be standardized at a pH fairly close to that expected in the measurements. The change in potential with the change in pH is not always equal to the theoretic value (kT = 0.0591 V at 25° C), so that an error may be made if the measured pH is different from the standardization value by more than about 2 pH units.

The compound known as tris (tris [hydroxymethyl] aminomethane) is often used in the preparation of buffers. These buffers are quite satisfactory, but it has been found that some pH electrode systems do not give the same values for the tris buffer as with the phosphate buffers that are commonly used as standards. The difference is usually not more than 0.1 pH unit which may be allowable in some instances, but for accurate work the possibility of a difference should be kept in mind. The problem apparently arises from the liquid junction used in the reference electrode. Not all electrodes have this error, and information on this can be obtained from the manufacturer or distributor. At least one supplier (Sigma Chemical Co. St. Louis) of tris furnishes a list of some electrodes that are satisfactory. For almost all purposes in the laboratory the combination electrodes in which the glass electrode and the reference electrode are combined are more convenient to use and will measure smaller volumes of liquid.

STANDARD SOLUTIONS OF ACIDS AND BASES

Standard acids and bases of known concentration are of great importance in analytic procedures. If only small amounts are used, they may be purchased already standardized. If larger amounts are used, it is often more convenient, besides being less expensive, to use standardized solutions made up in the laboratory. Since sulfuric acid solutions are probably the most stable and accurate solutions, this acid is the best for a secondary standard against which the other acids and bases can be standardized.

A normal solution contains 1 g replaceable hydrogen or its equivalent per liter; i.e., it contains 1 g equivalent weight (the molecular weight divided by the number of hydrogen atoms or hydroxyl radicals) per liter.

To make approximately 1N solutions of the common acids and bases, the following amounts are required (for many purposes, such as reagents, exact normality is not required.

Acids

Dilute the following amounts of concentrated acids to 1 L with distilled water:
1. Sulfuric acid, 28 ml
2. Hydrochloric acid, 86 ml
3. Nitric acid, 67 ml
4. Glacial acetic acid, 58 ml

Bases

1. Ammonium hydroxide. Dilute 68 ml concentrated solution to 1 L.
2. Sodium hydroxide. Dissolve 40 g in water to 1 L.
3. Potassium hydroxide, 60 g. Dissolve in water to 1 L.

Preparation of standard acids and bases

Sulfuric acid, 1N: For most purposes requiring accurately known normality, acids stronger than 1N will not be required. Hence if a 1N solution is accurately prepared, lower normalities can be prepared by dilution, using volumetric pipets and flasks. Add 60 ml concentrated sulfuric acid to 2 L distilled water (this solution will be slightly stronger than 1N). For standardization use tris(hydroxymethyl)aminomethane. This compound is now available in a very pure form for use as a primary standard (Trizma Base, Sigma Chemical Co., St. Louis; Tham, Fisher Scientific Co., Pittsburgh; SRM-922,923, National Bureau of Standards, Washington, D.C.). Accurately weigh approximately 3 g tris; any weight between 3 and 3.5 g is satisfactory, but the exact weight must be accurately known. Transfer quantitatively to a beaker with about 50 ml distilled water and titrate with the sulfuric acid, using a few drops of ethyl orange as indicator (0.2 g in 1 dl 22% methyl alcohol). Calculate the exact normality of the sulfuric acid solution from the following formula:

$$\text{Normality} = \frac{\text{wt of tris}}{(\text{ml titration}) \times 0.12114}$$

Calculate the amount of distilled water necessary to dilute to exactly 1N by means of the following formula:

$$\frac{\text{Actual normality} - \text{Desired normality}}{\text{Desired normality}}$$
$$\times \text{ Vol of solution to be diluted}$$

If, for example, the actual normality was 1.065 and it was desired to dilute 2 L of this normality to exactly 1N, the required amount of water to be added would be as follows:

$$\frac{1.065 - 1.000}{1.000} \times 2000 = 130 \text{ ml water to be added}$$

Add slightly less than the calculated amount of distilled water to the sulfuric acid solution, mix well, repeat the standardization with another weighed sample of tris, and calculate the new normality. If the normality is now between 1.005 and 1.000, repeat the standardization with two additional samples of tris and calculate the normality from average of the three values. Add the calculated amount of additional water to bring to exactly 1N; mix well. Solution is stable indefinitely if kept well stoppered in a glass-stoppered bottle.

Sodium hydroxide standard solution: Sodium hydroxide standard solution is best prepared from 50% (w/w) solution that is available commercially and is practically carbonate free. For a 1N solution, dissolve 80 g solution in recently boiled and cooled distilled water to make 1 L. The concentrated solution should be weighed rapidly, avoiding excess contact with air, but need not be accurately weighed. Accurately pipet 25 ml cooled sodium hydroxide solution to a beaker, add 50 ml water, and titrate with the 1N sulfuric acid to the methyl red end point. Calculate the normality from the relationship:

$$\text{Normality of base} = \frac{\text{Acid (ml)} \times \text{Normality of acid}}{\text{Base (ml)}}$$

Adjust to approximately 1N by the same method as used for the sulfuric acid, make several titrations, calculate the average normality, and adjust to exactly 1N. The sodium hydroxide solution should be kept in a well-stoppered polyethylene bottle. In preparing more dilute solutions of sodium hydroxide it is well to use distilled water that has been recently boiled and cooled.

Hydrochloric acid standard solution, 1N: Dilute 86 ml concentrated hydrochloric acid to 1 L with water. Standardize either as for sulfuric acid or against the sodium hydroxide solution. Adjust to exact normality.

ATOMIC WEIGHTS

Table 23-10 gives the atomic weights for a number of elements that may be used in the clinical laboratory. The weights, based on IUPAC 1973 values, have been rounded off to four significant figures since greater accuracy than this is not needed.

FORMULAS FOR CALCULATIONS

$$\text{g/dl} = \text{sp gr} \times \text{\% by wt}$$

Approximate normality =
$$\frac{10 \text{ (g/dl) } \sqrt{}}{\text{mol wt}} = \frac{10 \text{ (sp gr } \times \text{ \% by wt) } \sqrt{}}{\text{mol wt}}$$

where $\sqrt{}$ is the valence.

The number of milliliters required to make 1 L approximately normal solution is given as follows:

$$\frac{\text{mol wt} \times 100}{\sqrt{} \text{ (g/dl)}} = \frac{\text{mol wt} \times 100}{\sqrt{} \text{ (sp gr } \times \text{ \% by wt)}}$$

where $\sqrt{}$ is the valence.

The results of the calculations in Table 23-11 are approximately as shown in Table 23-12.

Milliequivalents and millimoles

The results for the determination of the univalent ions such as Na^+, K^+, Cl^-, and HCO_3^- are often expressed in equivalents (or submultiples) per liter. The preferred SI unit is moles per liter. The univalent ions in the two expressions are numerically the same: milliequivalents per liter equal millimoles per liter. The divalent ions, e.g., Ca^{++}, Mg^{++}, $SO_4^=$, and $HPO_4^=$, were usually expressed in terms of milligrams per deciliter (or in the case of phosphate, milligrams P per deciliter) Some preferred to use milliequivalents per liter for calcium and magnesium; then

$$\text{mEq/L} = \frac{\text{(mg/dl)} \times 10}{\text{Atomic weight/}\sqrt{}}$$

where $\sqrt{}$ is the valence (e.g., 2). The preferred unit for these is now also millimoles per liter and thus for these two ions

$$\text{mmole/L} = \text{(mg/dl)} \times 10/\text{Atomic weight}$$

Thus, since calcium has an atomic weight of 40, a concentration of 10 mg/dl = 100/20, or 5, mEq/L = 100/40, or 2.5, mmole/L.

Table 23-10. International atomic weights* (1973)

Element	Symbol	Atomic weight	Element	Symbol	Atomic weight
Aluminum	Al	26.98	Magnesium	Mg	24.31
Antimony	Sb	121.8	Manganese	Mn	54.94
Arsenic	As	74.92	Mercury	Hg	200.6
Barium	Ba	137.3	Molybdenum	Mo	95.94
Bismuth	Bi	209.0	Nickel	Ni	58.70
Boron	B	10.81	Nitrogen	N	14.01
Bromine	Br	79.90	Oxygen	O	16.00
Calcium	Ca	40.08	Phosphorus	P	30.97
Carbon	C	12.01	Platinum	Pt	195.1
Cerium	Ce	140.1	Potassium	K	39.10
Chlorine	Cl	35.45	Selenium	Se	78.96
Chromium	Cr	52.00	Silicon	Si	28.09
Cobalt	Co	58.93	Silver	Ag	107.9
Copper	Cu	63.55	Sodium	Na	22.99
Fluorine	F	19.00	Strontium	Sr	87.62
Gold	Au	197.0	Sulfur	S	32.06
Hydrogen	H	1.008	Tin	Sn	118.7
Iodine	I	126.9	Tungsten	W	183.9
Iron	Fe	55.85	Uranium	U	238.0
Lead	Pb	207.2	Vanadium	V	50.94
Lithium	Li	6.941	Zinc	Zn	65.37

*Rounded to four significant figures.

Table 23-11. Strengths of concentrated acids and bases

Grade CP		Molecular weight	Specific gravity	Percent by weight
Hydrochloric acid	HCl	36.5	1.19	37.0
Sulfuric acid	H_2SO_4	98.1	1.84	96.0
Nitric acid	HNO_3	63.0	1.42	70.0
Phosphoric acid (syrupy)	H_3PO_4	98.0	1.69	85.0
Acetic acid	CH_3COOH	60.0	1.06	99.5
Ammonium hydroxide	NH_4OH	35.0	0.90	28.0(NH_3) 57.6(NH_4OH)

Table 23-12. Dilution of concentrated acids and bases

	Normality (approximate)	ml/L to make 1.0N solution (approximate)
HCl	12.1	83.0
H_2SO_4	36.0	28.0
HNO_3	15.7	64.0
H_3PO_4	44.0	23.0
CH_3COOH	17.4	57.5
NH_4OH	14.8	67.5

EQUIVALENTS

Table 23-13. Table of equivalent measures

1 gr (grain)	0.065	g	65	mg	
1 oz (avoirdupois)	28.350	g	437.5	gr	
1 oz (troy, apothecaries')	31.103	g	480.0	gr	
1 lb (avoirdupois)	453.59	g			
1 lb (troy, apothecaries')	373.2	g			
1 mg	1/65	gr	1000	µg	
1 g	15.43	gr	1000	mg	
1 kg	2.2	lb (avoirdupois)	1000	g	
1 fl oz	29.573	ml			
1 pt	473.176	ml			
1 qt	0.946	L			
1 gal	3.785	L	231.0	in^3	
1 ml	16	minims			
1 L	1.0567	qt	0.2642	gal	
1 in^3	16.387	ml			
1 ft^3	28.3	L	7.48	gal	
1 in	25.4	mm			
1 ft	0.3048	m			
1 yd	0.9144	m			
1 m	39.37	in	3.2808	ft	
1 mm	1000	micrometers (µm)			
1 Ångstrom (Å or A)	0.1	nm	0.0001	µm	

	Autoclave			
Pressure (lb)*	**°C**	**°F**	**Temperatures**	
5	107.7	226	Degrees F = (Degrees C $\times$ 1.8) + 32	
10	115.5	240	Degrees C = (Degrees F $-$ 32) $\div$ 1.8	
15	121.6	251		
20	126.6	260		

*Gauge pressure at sea level. To reach the indicated temperature, the guage pressure must be increased 0.5 lb for each 1000 ft altitude above sea level.

REFERENCES

1. Gambino, S.R., and Di Re, J.: Bilirubin assay, Chicago, 1968, Commission on Continuing Education, American Society of Clinical Pathologists.
2. Gambino, S.R.: In Meites, S., editor: Standard methods of clinical chemistry, New York, 1965, Academic Press, Inc., vol. 5, p. 55.
3. Jendrassik, L., and Grof, P.: Biochem. Zeit. **297**:81, 1938.
4. Lolekha, P.H., and Limpavithayskul, K.: Clin. Chem. **23**:778, 1977.
5. Gambino, S.R., and Freda, V.J.: Am. J. Clin. Pathol. **46**:198, 1966.
6. Doumas, B.T., et al.: Clin. Chem. **19**:984, 1973.
7. Biggs, H.G., Ledyard, P., and Kasper, S.: Clin. Chem. **21**:451, 1975.
8. Malloy, H.T., and Evelyn, K.A.: J. Biol. Chem. **119**:481, 1937.
9. Malloy, H.T., and Evelyn, K.A.: J. Biol. Chem. **122**:597, 1938.
10. Kingsley, G.R., Getchell, G., and Schaffert, R.R.: In Reiner, M., editor: Standard methods of clinical chemistry, New York, 1953, Academic Press, Inc., vol. 1, p. 11.
11. Henry, R.J., Jacobs, S.L., and Chaimori, N.: Clin. Chem. **6**:529, 1960.
12. Meites, S., and Hogg, C.K.: Clin. Chem. **6**:421, 1960.
13. Routh, J.I.: In Tietz, N., editor: Fundamentals of clinical chemistry, ed. 2, Philadelphia, 1976, W.B. Saunders Co., p. 1042.
14. Watson, C.J., and Hawkinson, V.: Am. J. Clin. Pathol. **17**:108, 1947.
15. Watson, C.J., et al.: Am. J. Clin. Pathol. **14**:605, 1944.
16. Henry, R.J., Fernandez, A.A., and Berkman, S.: Clin. Chem. **10**:440, 1964.
17. Troeger, E., and Koeltsch, V.: Deutsch. Gesungheitsw, **27**:586, 1972.
18. Quick, A.J.: Am. J. Med. Sci. **135**:630, 1933.
19. Gaebler, O.H.: Am. J. Clin. Pathol. **15**:452, 1945.
20. Lavers, G.D., et al.: J. Lab. Clin. Med. **34**:965, 1949.
21. Weichselbaum, T.E., and Probstein, J.G.: J.Lab. Clin. Med. **24**:636, 1939.
22. Mateer, J.G., et al.: Am. J. Dig. Dis. **9**:13, 1942.
23. Paumgartner, G.: Schweiz. Med. Wochenschr **105**:1, 1975.
24. Leevy, C.M., et al.: J.A.M.A. **200**:236, 1967.
25. Romach, M., Giles, H.G., and Sellers, E.M.: Clin. Chem. **23**:780, 1977.
26. Martin, J.G., et al.: Proc. Soc. Exp. Biol. Med. **150**:612, 1975.
27. Zimmerman, H.J., and Seeff, L.B.: In Coodley, E.L., editor: Diagnostic enzymology, Philadelphia, 1970, Lea & Febiger, p. 1.
28. Wilkinson, J.H.: Isoenzymes, ed. 2, Philadelphia, 1970, J.B. Lippincott Co.
29. Doniach, D., et al.: Clin. Exp. Immunol. **1**:237, 1966.
30. Smith, J.B., and Todd, D.: Lancet **2**:833, 1968.
31. Abelev, G.I.: Adv. Cancer Res. **14**:295, 1971.
32. Masseyeff, R.: Pathol. Biol. (Paris) **20**:703, 1972.
33. Belanger, L., et al.: Clin. Chem. **22**:198, 1976.
34. Cahill, J., et al.: Am. J. Obstet. Gynecol. **119**:1095, 1974.
35. Lehmann, F.G., and Lehmann, D.: J. Clin. Chem. Clin. Biochem. **11**:339, 1973.

36. Waldmann, T.A., and McIntire, K.R.: Cancer **34:**1510, 1974.
37. Parekh, A.C., and Jung, D.H.: Anal. Chem. **42:**1423, 1970.
38. Parekh, A.C., et al.: Ann. Clin. Lab. Sci. **8:**423, 1976.
39. Richmond, V.: Clin. Chem. **19:**1350, 1973.
40. Slikers, K.A.: CRC Crit. Rev. Clin. Lab. Sci. **8:**198, 1977.
41. Allain, C.C., et al.: Clin. Chem. **20:**470, 1974.
42. Lie, R.F., et al.: Clin. Chem. **22:**1627, 1976.
43. Richmond, W.: Clin. Chem. **22:**1579, 1976.
44. Abell, L.L., et al.: In Seligson, D., editor: Standard methods of clinical chemistry, New York, 1958, Academic Press, Inc., vol. 2, p. 26.
45. De la Huerga, J., and Sherrick, J.C.: Ann. Clin. Lab. Sci. **2:**360, 1972.
46. Baginski, E.S., Foa, P.P., and Zak, B.: Clin. Chem. **13:**326, 1967.
47. Baginski, E.S., Epstein, E., and Zak, B.: Ann. Clin. Lab. Sci. **2:**255, 1972.
48. Wybenga, D.R., and Inkpen, J.A.: In Henry, R.J., Cannon, D.C., and Winkleman, J.W., editors: Clinical chemistry, principles and techniques, ed. 2, New York, 1974, Harper & Row, Publishers, p. 1470.
49. Stern, I., and Shapiro, B.: J. Clin. Pathol. **6:**158, 1953.
50. Galletti, F.: Clin. Chim. Acta **6:**749, 1961.
51. Dole, V.P.: J. Clin. Invest. **35:**150, 1956.
52. Trout, D.L., Estes, E.H., Jr., and Friedberg, S.J.: J. Lipid Res. **1:**199, 1960.
53. Goss, J.E., and Lein, A.: Clin. Chem. **13:**36, 1967.
54. Parijs, J., Barbier, F., and Elewaut, A.: Clin. Chem. **12:**767, 1966.
55. Laurell, S.: J. Clin. Invest. **8:**81, 1956.
56. Bierman, E.L., Dole V.P., and Roberts, T.N.: Diabetes **6:**475, 1957.
57. Soloni, F.G.: Clin. Chem. **17:**529, 1971.
58. Bucolo, G., and David, H.: Clin. Chem. **19:**476, 1973.
59. Ziegenhorn, J.: Clin. Chem. **21:**1627, 1975.
60. Mueller, P.H., et al.: J. Clin. Chem. Clin. Biochem. **15:**457, 1977.
61. Spandrio, L., and Pradini, B.D.: Quad. Sclavo Diagn. **9:**77, 1973.
62. Rehkaemper, H.: Clin. Chem. **20:**87, 1974.
63. Frings, C.S., Neri, B.P., and Fendley, T.W.: Clin. Chem. **20:**87, 1974.
64. Frings, C.S., and Dunn, R.T.: Am. J. Clin. Pathol. **53:**89, 1970.
65. Frings, C.S., et al.: Clin. Chem. **18:**683, 1972.
66. Johnson, E.R., Ellis, G., and Toothill, C.: Clin. Chem. **23:**1669, 1977.
67. Epstein, E., Baginski, E.S., and Zak, B.: Ann. Clin. Lab. Sci. **2:**244, 1972.
68. Fletcher, M.J., and Styliou, M.H.: Clin. Chem. **16:**362, 1970.
69. Beckering, R.E., Jr., and Crowson, M.: Am. J. Clin. Pathol. **56:**765, 1971.
70. Fredrickson, D.S., and Lees, R.S.: Circulation **31:**321, 1965.

71. Fredrickson, D.S., Levy, R.L., and Lees, R.S.: N. Engl. J. Med. **276:**34, 94, 148, 215, 273, 1967.
72. Fredrickson, D.S., Goldstein, J.L., and Brown, M.S.: In Stanbury, J.B., Wyngaarden, J.B., and Fredrickson, D.S., editors: The metabolic basis of inherited disease, ed. 4, New York, 1978, McGraw-Hill Book Co.
73. Beaumont, J.L., et al.: Bull. WHO **43:**891, 1970.
74. Lipo, J.F., and Preston, J.A.: CRC Crit. Rev. Clin. Lab. Sci. **2:**461, 1971.
75. Harlan, W.R., and Shaw, W.A.: CRC Crit. Rev. Clin. Lab. Sci. **3:**451, 1972.
76. Manual of laboratory operations, Lipid Research Clinics Program, vol. 1, lipid and lipoprotein analysis, DHEW pub. no. NIH 76-628, Bethesda, Md., 1974, National Heart and Lung Institute, National Institutes of Health, pp. 51-59.
77. Iammarino, R.M.: Clin. Chem. **21:**300, 1975.
78. Bachorik, P.S., et al.: Clin. Chem. **22:**1828, 1976.
79. Lopes-Virella, M.F., et al.: Clin. Chem. **23:**882, 1977.
80. Grove, T.H.: Clin. Chem. **25:**560, 1979.
81. Glueck, C.J., et al.: Metabolism **24:**1243, 1975.
82. Friedewald, W.T., Levy, R.I., and Fredrickson, D.S.: Clin. Chem. **18:**499, 1972.
83. Burstein, M., and Samaille, J.: Clin. Chim. Acta **5:**609, 1960.
84. Neeld, J.B., Jr., and Pearson, W.N.: J. Nutr. **79:**454, 1963.
85. Bieri, J.G.: In Sunderman, F.W., editor: Applied seminar on the clinical pathology of the lipids, Philadelphia, 1971, Association of Clinical Scientists.
86. Rogers, W.E., Jr.: In Association of Vitamin Chemists: Methods of vitamin assay, ed. 3, New York, 1966, Interscience Publishers, Inc.
87. Roels, O.A., and Trout, A.: In Cooper, G.R., editor: Standard methods of clinical chemistry, New York, 1972, Academic Press, Inc., vol. 7, p. 215.
88. Roe, J.H.: Ann. N.Y. Acad. Sci. **92:**277, 1961.
89. Pellietier, O.: J. Lab. Clin. Med. **72:**674, 1968.
90. Sauberlich, H.E.: Ann. N.Y. Acad. Sci. **258:**438, 1975.
91. Reiner, M., Cheung, H.L., and Thomas, J.L.: In MacDonald, R.P., editor: Standard methods of clinical chemistry, New York, 1970, Academic Press, Inc., vol. 6, p. 193.
92. Remsen, S.T., and Ackermann, P.G.: Calculations for the medical laboratory, Boston, 1977, Little, Brown & Co.
93. Blankenship, J., and Campbell, J.B.: Laboratory mathematics: medical and biological applications, St. Louis, 1976, The C.V. Mosby Co.
94. Segal, I.H.: Biochemical calculations, ed. 2, New York, 1977, John Wiley & Sons, Inc.
95. Good, N.E., et al.: Biochemistry **5:**467, 1966.
96. Weast, R.C., editor: Handbook of chemistry and physics, ed. 56, Cleveland, 1975, CRC Press, p. D-136.
97. Bates, R.G. Determination of pH: theory and practice, ed. 2, New York, 1973, John Wiley & Sons, Inc.

Enzymology

NATURE OF ENZYMES

Enzymes are complex naturally occurring proteins that catalyze many biologic reactions; i.e., they speed reactions that might otherwise proceed very slowly. There are hundreds of different enzymes in each cell, attached to the cell walls and membranes, in the cytoplasm, in the nucleus, and in the many other specialized subcellular organelles (i.e., microsomes, mitochondria, lysosomes). A few of the enzymes that are found in the plasma or other extracellular fluids seem to have a function in these fluids, but most enzymes function inside cells.

Changes in enzyme concentrations in tissue cells should reflect changes in states of health and disease of the tissue. However, it is not technically feasible to assay cellular enzyme concentrations in intact tissues on a routine basis. At best, changes in enzyme concentrations in the plasma (or serum) can be followed with the assumption that these changes reflect parallel changes that have taken place in specific organs or tissues. In a few special cases enzyme concentrations are measured in lysates of tissues (red or white cell enzymes) since these tissues are relatively easily sampled and the contents can be assayed without too much difficulty.

SPECIFICITY OF REACTION

Some enzymes will react with many related types of compounds and are said to have a broad specificity (i.e., alkaline phosphatase). In contrast, most enzymes are quite specific in their action in that they will only catalyze a definite type of chemical reaction or act on a particular compound or substrate. Many enzymes were first named for the type of substrate on which they act: urease hydrolyzes urea, lipase hydrolyzes lipids, and phosphatases act on organic phosphates.

ENZYME KINETICS

The concentration of an enzyme in plasma or serum cannot be determined directly in micrograms per liter because the concentrations are very low and there is no direct way to measure a particular enzyme the way one measures glucose or sodium concentrations. Quantitation is provided by measuring the specific catalytic activity that is related to the concentration of a particular enzyme.

The general reaction involving an enzyme may be written as follows:

$$E + S \rightleftharpoons ES \rightarrow E + P$$

where E represents the enzyme; S, the substrate on which the enzyme acts; ES, the postulated enzyme-substrate complex; and P, the reacted substrate or product that may represent a changed molecular species of S or the splitting of S into two or more different molecules. The enzyme thus represents a true catalyst in that it is not changed in the reaction. The speed with which this reaction takes place depends, as in all chemical reactions, on the concentration of the reacting substances, E and S. If the concentration of the substrate, S, is sufficiently high in comparison with that of the enzyme, so that it remains relatively constant, then the rate will be proportional to the concentration of the enzyme and the amount of product, P, formed in a given period of time will be proportional to the amount of active enzyme present; or, looking at it in another way, if the concentration of the substrate, S, is sufficiently high so that practically all of the enzyme is in the form of the enzyme-substrate complex, ES, the reaction rate will be proportional to the amount of ES present and therefore to the amount of enzyme.

The reaction rate or velocity of reaction has been studied for many enzyme reactions. The description of the velocity or the kinetics of the reaction has been related to the concentration of substrate by the Michaelis-Menten equation:

$$v = \frac{V_{max} [S]}{K_m + [S]}$$

where [S] is the concentration of substrate, v is the velocity or rate (i.e., enzyme activity), V_{max} is the maximal rate of reaction when the enzyme is saturated with substrate (i.e., a constant), and K_m, the Michaelis-Menten constant, is that substrate concentration that produces one half the maximal velocity.

At a fixed high substrate concentration, the velocity, v, approaches V_{max} and is proportional to the amount of enzyme present since all other factors are constant. The common convention used for assaying activity is at high substrate concentration (i.e., about S = 10 × K_m). The rate at this substrate concentration is given by the following equation:

$$v = \frac{V_{max} (10 \times K_m)}{K_m + (10 \times K_m)} = V_{max} \frac{10 \times K_m}{11 \times K_m} = 0.91 \, V_{max}$$

Thus at S = 10 × K_m the rate produced is greater than 90% of V_{max}. If all other factors are present in similar excess the rate is said to follow zero order kinetics; i.e., it is independent of all other factors and depends only on the amount of enzyme present.

The other principal factors that influence enzyme rates are temperature, pH, activators, cofactors, coupling enzymes, and buffer concentration. Like all chemical reactions, the rate of enzyme reactions increase with increasing temperature. However, enzymes are complex protein molecules and are inactivated by too high a temperature (usually over 40° C). Enzymes have been measured at 25°, 30°, 32°, and 37° C. The recommended standard temperature is now 30° C, although many determinations are still made at 37° C, because greater sensitivity is achieved.

The results of an enzyme determination are expressed in terms of the amount of product formed per unit of time, under specified conditions, for a given amount of sample (usually serum) and are conventionally given in units. Thus one unit of enzyme activity might be that amount which would, under certain specified conditions, cause the formation of 1 mg of the product, P, per minute when 1 ml of sample was used. In the older procedures quite arbitrary units were employed.

The enzyme activity was reported in the units of measure utilized by the authors who developed the assay; i.e., for alkaline phosphatase using β-glycerol phosphate as a substrate, 1 Bodansky unit = 1 mg P formed/dl serum/hr; and using phenolphosphate as a substrate, 1 King-Armstrong unit = 1 mg phenol formed/dl serum/30 min. The units were expressed as so many King-Armstrong units or Bodansky units after the authors who developed the assay. Each time an assay was modified a new unit would be created taking on the name or names of the authors who proposed the modified assay. The use of such units is discouraged, and new assays will not use private units since the preferred unit for all enzymes is the international unit (IU), defined as that amount of activity that will transform 1 μmole of substrate per minute. In those instances where one molecule of substrate is transformed into a number of molecules of product, the definition is per mole of product formed. The Système International (SI) originally defined a unit of enzyme activity as the katal (K) as 1 mole/sec of substrate changed, but this unit has met with little acceptance as yet.

To convert international units to katals:

$$1 \, IU = \frac{\mu mole}{min} \times \frac{10^{-6} \, mole}{\mu mole} \times \frac{1 \, min}{60 \, sec} = 1.67 \times 10^{-8} \, K$$

Thus 10 IU = 167 nK (nanokatals).

Although these international units have been adopted by most workers in the field of clinical enzymology and journals such as *Clinical Chemistry* require the use of international units in papers presented for publication, the use of the new units in the clinical laboratory has been slower in gaining acceptance since physicians are more familiar with the older units. When the determination of new enzymes is introduced, these will presumably be expressed in international units from the beginning. In some instances, at least, the use of the international unit would make for better comparison between methods.

ENZYME NOMENCLATURE

With an ever-increasing number of enzymes being discovered and studied, a completely systematic nomenclature of the enzymes was needed. The Enzyme Commission (EC) of the International Union of Biochemistry (IUB) developed and proposed a systematic convention for the naming of enzymes.[1] Many of the clinically important enzymes are still known by trivial names that arose from historic circumstances and will continue to pervade the literature because of their simplicity.

IUB names and code

The IUB systemic name describes the reaction catalyzed. The IUB also recognized that tirvial names were important and assigned practical names to many enzymes. For each individual enzyme the system provides a numeric code designation consisting of four numbers separated by periods. The first number assigns the enzyme to one of six categories of reaction. The next two numbers are subclasses of reaction, and the last is a serial number unique to the enzyme. A more complete description is given below.

Nonstandard abbreviations

A variety of simple abbreviations containing four or fewer capital letters are also used to describe the enzymes in common usage. These abbreviations are not part of the IUB system but have been suggested by Baron et al.[2,3]

EC classification

Since the EC classification of the enzymes will be used increasingly in the future, a brief description of its basis will be given. All enzymes are placed in one of six classes depending on the type of reaction they catalyze. The first class includes the oxidoreductases, those enzymes that catalyze oxidation-reduction (electron transfer) reactions. If the reaction involves the transfer of hydrogen, as in the change from lactate to pyruvate, the enzymes are known as dehydrogenases. If the reaction involves a direct participation of oxygen, the enzymes are termed oxidases. The second group of enzymes contains the transferases, those enzymes that

catalyze the transfer of a group, e.g., a methoxy or an amino group, from one molecule to another. Aspartate aminotransferase (EC 2.6.1.1), to be discussed later, is an example of this group; this enzyme catalyzes the transfer of an amino group from aspartate to ketoglutarate. A third group are the hydrolases, which catalyze the cleavage of C—O and other bonds with the addition of water. An example of this group is alkaline phosphatase, which catalyzes the hydrolysis of a number of organic phosphate esters. A fourth group contains the lyases, which cleave C—C, C—O, and C—N bonds with the formation of a double bond or the reverse reaction, the addition of a group to a double bond. It will be seen that this and the subsequent groups contain relatively few enzymes that are used in clinical diagnosis. An example of this group, which is mentioned later, is aldolase (EC 4.1.2.13). The fifth group are the isomerases, which catalyze structural or geometric changes in a molecule. An example of this group is the enzyme triosephosphate isomerase (EC 5.3.1.1), which catalyzes the change of glycerol-3-phosphate into dihydroxyacetone phosphate; it can be seen that the two compounds mentioned have exactly the same number of different atoms except that they are arranged in a slightly different structure. A sixth and last group are the ligases (synthetases), none of which are currently used in clinical diagnosis.

In the systemic number the second number denotes the type of group, e.g., amino group or hydroxyl

Table 24-1. Enzyme nomenclature

EC code	Practical name	Abbreviation	Systemic name	Trivial name
Oxidoreductases				
1.1.1.27	Lactate dehydrogenase	LD	L-Lactate: NAD oxidoreductase	—
1.1.1.37	Malate dehydrogenase	MD	L-Malate: NAD oxidoreductase	—
1.1.1.42	Isocitrate dehydrogenase	ICD	L-Isocitrate: NADP oxidoreductase	—
1.1.1.49	Glucose-6-phosphate dehydrogenase	G-6-PD	D-Glucose-6-phosphate: NADP oxidoreductase	—
1.4.1.2	Glutamate dehydrogenase	GMD	L-Glutamate: NAD oxidoreductase	—
Transferases				
2.1.3.3	Ornithine carbamoyltransferase	OCT	Carbamoylphosphate: ornithine carbamoyltransferase	Ornithine carbamyltransferase
2.3.2.2.	γ-Glutamyl transpeptidase	GGT	γ-Glutamyl transferase	—
2.6.1.1	Aspartate aminotransferase	AST	L-Aspartate: 2-oxoglutarate aminotransferase	Glutamic oxaloacetic transaminase
2.6.1.2	Alanine aminotransferase	ALT	L-Alanine: 2-oxoglutarate aminotransferase	Glutamic pyruvic transaminase
2.7.1.40	Pyruvate kinase	PK	ATP: pyruvate phosphotransferase	—
2.7.3.1	Creatine kinase	CK	ATP: creatine phosphotransferase	—
Hydrolases				
3.1.1.3	Lipase	LPS	Glycerol ester hydrolase	—
3.1.1.8	Cholinesterase	CHS	Acylcholine: acyl hydrolase	—
3.1.3.1	Alkaline phosphatase	ALP	Orthophosphoric monoester phosphohydrolase	—
3.1.3.2	Acid phosphatase	ACP	Orthophosphoric monoester phosphohydrolase	—
3.1.3.5	5'-Nucleotidase	NTP	5'-Ribonucleotide phosphohydrolase	—
3.2.1.1	α-Amylase	AMS	α-1,4-Glucan-4-glucanohydrolase	Diastase
3.4.1.1	Leucine aminopeptidase	LAS	L-Leucylpeptide hydrolase	Arylaminidase
Lyase				
4.1.2.13	Aldolase	ALS	Fructose-1,6-diphosphate: D-glyceraldehyde-3-phosphate-lyase	—

group, that takes part in the reaction. The third number of the systemic number indicates the different subclass of reaction, and the last number is merely the serial number of the particular enzyme in the subgroup. Thus for the enzyme creatine kinase (EC 2.7.3.2) the first number, 2, indicates that the enzyme is a transferase; the second number, 7, indicates that the group transferred is a phosphate group; the third number, 3, indicates that the acceptor is an amino group; and the fourth number, 2, is merely the serial number of the enzyme in the 2.7.3._ group. The actual reaction is as follows:

$$\text{Adenosine triphosphate (ATP)} + \text{Creatine} \overset{CK}{\rightleftharpoons} \text{Adenosine}$$
$$\text{diphosphate (ADP)} + \text{Creatine phosphate}$$

A few clinically important enzymes are listed in Table 24-1 along with the IUB code and systemic names.

ENZYME ASSAY CONDITIONS

The rate of reactions involving enzymes is markedly influenced by temperature, pH, concentration of substrate, and a number of other factors. Accordingly, all the details of a given procedure must be followed exactly in order to give accurate results. The time as well as the temperature of incubation must be closely controlled.

With most enzymatic procedures the reaction rate is not constant with time, if they are examined carefully. There is an initial "lag" phase with little change per unit time when the reactants are mixed and reach thermal equilibrium, then a linear phase of constant change per unit time, and finally a phase of substrate exhaustion with little change per unit time. If in the assay the lag phase is very short and the linear phase is relatively long and the assay is stopped before the phase of substrate exhaustion, then halving or doubling the time of assay will halve or double the amount of product produced. However, one cannot always compensate for increased activity by halving the incubation time and then multiplying the number of units found by 2. This may be true for some enzyme reactions, but not all. It cannot be assumed to be true unless specifically stated in the procedure.

There are a number of enzyme systems that involve the conversion of **nicotinamide adenine dinucleotide** (NAD) to its reduced form (NADH), or vice versa. The reduced form, NADH, has a much greater absorption at 340 nm than does the oxidized form, and consequently the reactions may be followed by measuring the change in absorption at this wavelength. In addition, many other enzyme reactions that do not involve the NAD-NADH change directly can be coupled with another reaction involving NAD, so that the change in NAD becomes a measure of the enzyme reaction. A good example of this is the reaction catalyzed by the enzyme lactate dehydrogenase:

$$\text{Lactate} + \text{NAD}^+ \overset{LD}{\rightleftharpoons} \text{Pyruvate} + \text{NADH} + \text{H}^+$$

Since the NAD is essential to the reaction, it is sometimes termed a coenzyme. In some instances the NAD may be replaced by NADP (nicotinamide adenine di-

nucleotide phosphate), which has similar properties. Thus a number of enzyme reactions can be followed by measuring the absorbance change at 340 nm. Some older photometers may not operate in the ultraviolet range, but with the increasing use of this method for enzyme analysis there are a number of good simple instruments on the market with this capacity. Usually with this method one assumes that at 340 nm, NADH has an molecular absorption coefficient of

$$A/(d \times C) = 6.22 \times 10^3$$

where A is the actual absorbance of a solution, d is the light path (in centimeters) through the solution, and C is the concentration (in moles per liter) of the absorbing substance. Thus for a 1 cm light path, $C = A \times 10^{-3}/6.22$, and when the concentration is expressed in millimoles per liter (micromoles per milliliter), $C = A/6.22$. Thus from the absorbance change and the volume of the solution measured, one can readily calculate the number of micromoles of NADH formed or used up during the enzyme measurement period. There is some evidence[4,5] that the absorption coefficient differs from 6.22 by a small amount (less than 2%), but the figure of 6.22 is still used in all calculations. In using a particular instrument, one must be certain that the wavelength scale and bandwidth are such that the absorbance of NADH as measured gives the correct value and that the light path is accurately known.

Fixed time and kinetic assays

Enzymes have been measured by several different approaches. The two most commonly employed methods are fixed time and kinetic assays. Most older methods employed a fixed time approach, often for 30 or 60 min and in some cases for several hours. It is now known that many of these time periods were too long and that some enzyme degradation occurred. Fixed time assays are still used in some cases, but generally shorter time periods are employed. In these assays a reaction is started and allowed to incubate at a constant temperature for a fixed time period (i.e., 30 min). The reaction is then stopped, and the amount of product is measured. The assumption of the assay is that a constant amount of product is produced throughout the entire time period.

If the rate of reaction is followed as a function of time, the assay is termed a kinetic assay. Usually the reaction time is short (i.e., some seconds to a few minutes), and there is little danger of enzyme degradation. Current instrumentation often permits multiple readings to be made automatically for the determination of the enzyme rate; with some instruments, hundreds of readings can be taken and averaged to determine the rate. The use of multiple readings allows the analyst to determine when the lag phase is over and also if the enzyme activity in the sample is so high that substrate exhaustion occurs within the usual measurement time period. Such refinements are not possible with fixed time assays.

Optimal assays

Assays of enzyme activity should be performed under zero order kinetics (i.e., with the rate dependent only on the amount of enzyme). If experiments are not carried out to determine the substrate concentration that gives maximal activity, it may be that an assay will give different results if the substrate concentration is increased. It has been shown that one of the substrates used in the original assay conditions for alanine aminotransferase (ALT [SGPT]) was suboptimal for maximal activity. If the determination of ALT activity is run at the optimal substrate concentration, a considerably higher value is obtained.

To optimize an assay, e.g., the lactate dehydrogenase reaction given earlier, a series of assays would be set up with increasing concentrations of lactate but at high fixed NAD^+ concentration and the rates measured. Then a series of assays would be set up with increasing concentrations of NAD^+ but at a fixed high lactate concentration determined from the first series of assays and the rates measured again. This same type of experiment would be carried out for each item of the assay mixture (i.e., metal ions, pH) until all the variables have been evaluated for maximal enzyme activity. The final assay conditions determined from this series of experiments would be the optimal assay. Such experiments have been done for the current clinically important enzymes, and diagnostic kits are available with all the materials at optimal concentrations.

At times optimal conditions cannot be used, i.e., the substrate might have a limited solubility or might inhibit a secondary enzyme used in a coupled assay, and then compromises must be made.

pH: Changes in pH will markedly affect the enzyme reaction rate. For most enzymes there is a definite pH at which the enzyme is most active, and this is the pH usually specified for the measurement of that particular enzyme. The optimal pH is different for different enzymes. Reduced activity is observed at pH levels greater and less than the optimal.

Buffer: Buffers may not only serve to regulate the pH of an assay, they may take part in the reaction as well. Alkaline phosphatase, assayed using p-nitrophenol phosphate as a substrate, uses the buffer 2-amino-2-methyl-1-propanol to regulate pH to 10.2 in the Bowers and McComb procedure.[81] The enzyme cleaves the substrate into p-nitrophenol and phosphate in a multistep process, part of which involves a temporary phosphorylation of the enzyme. The final and rate-limiting step involves hydrolysis of the enzyme—p bond to regenerate free enzyme. At similar pH levels buffers that are phosphate acceptors in a transphosphorylation process with the enzyme will produce higher rates of alkaline phosphatase activity than buffers that do not act as phosphate acceptors. Thus AMP buffer produces higher rates of alkaline phosphatase activity at pH 10.2 than glycylglycine buffer at pH 10.2 because glycine is not a phosphate acceptor.

Cofactors: Many enzymes require a nonprotein, often dialyzable, material for maximal activity. In the lactate dehydrogenase reaction, NAD+ is such a cofactor, and although it reacts in a simlar fashion on a mole basis with lactate it is not a substrate. This is because it is regenerated from its reduced form, NADH, in order to participate in the reaction again

rather than be passed on in a series of metabolic reactions. If the cofactor is an organic compound, it is called a coenzyme; if it is an inorganic ion, it is called an activator.

Activators: Many enzymes require divalent metal ions for maximal activity. All phosphate transferring enzymes (i.e., hexokinase) require Mg^{++} ions. Other common metal ion activators are Mn^{++}, Ca^{++}, Zn^{++}, Fe^{++}, and K^+. Amylase requires Cl^- for maximal activity, and there are enzymes that require several ions for maximal activity (i.e., pyruvate kinase requires K^+ and Mg^{++}). In each case the concentration of activator must be determined by experimentation just as the optimal substrate concentration is determined.

Coupling enzymes: Some enzyme reactions of interest (i.e., the transaminases alanine aminotransferase [ALT] and aspartate aminotransferase [AST]) do not involve NAD^+ or $NADP^+$ and thus cannot be followed directly. One may couple the initial enzyme reaction to a second indicating enzyme reaction that does contain the $NAD^+/NADH$ conversion to make a convenient assay. Thus the AST rate can be coupled to malic dehydrogenase (MD):

$$\text{L-Aspartate} + \alpha\text{-Ketoglutarate} \overset{\text{AST}}{\rightleftharpoons}$$

$$\text{L-Glutamate} + \text{Oxaloacetate}$$

$$H^+ + \text{Oxaloacetate} + NADH \overset{\text{MD}}{\longrightarrow} \text{L-Malate} + NAD^+$$

This gives the following net reaction:

$$\text{L-Aspartate} + \alpha\text{-Ketoglutarate} + NADH + H^+$$

$$\rightarrow \text{L-Glutamate} + \text{L-Malate} + NAD^+$$

In this case the MD enzyme must be present in excess as well as the substrate and other activators in order to have an optimized assay.

ISOENZYMES

Many enzymes are found in two or more slightly different forms known as isoenzymes, a term recommended by the IUB. These different forms of a given enzyme all catalyze the same reaction and hence are all classified as the same enzyme. The protein moiety of the different isoenzymes may vary somewhat giving the different isoenzymes slightly different chemical or physical properties.

The isoenzymes of creatine kinase and lactate dehydrogenase have been the most extensively studied and characterized. The isoenzymes can be separated by electrophoresis, by differences in absorptive properties, or by reaction with specific antibodies. CK is a protein that is made up of two distinctly different subunits. The subunits are of two types, M and B; thus three combinations of the two subunits are possible: CK_3 = MM (skeletal muscle type), CK_2 = MB (heart muscle type), and CK_1 = BB (brain type). LD is a protein that is made up of four subunits, and there are two types of subunit: M and H. There are five combinations of these four subunits from H_4 for LD_1 to M_4 for LD_5, and five isoenzymes are commonly found in sera. It is not clear at present if all enzymes that have isoenzyme forms will fit this pattern of different combinations of subunits or whether it will be demonstrated that several proteins exist with changes in amino acid sequence or conformational changes for a portion of the enzyme that does not affect the catalytic activity.

The clinical significance of the isoenzymes is that for a given enzyme different proportions of the different isoenzymes may be found in different organs or types of tissue. By determining which isoenzyme is most increased in the serum or other body fluid, one may obtain information as to which organ or type of tissue is responsible for the increased enzymatic activity. The enzyme alkaline phosphatase, for example, consists of several different isoenzymes, one of which is most active in bone metabolism and another originating chiefly in the liver. Thus if one can distinguish between the isoenzymes, one can decide whether the increase in total alkaline phosphatase as measured by the usual methods is caused by bone or liver disease. In some instances the determination of the relative amounts of the different isoenzymes may offer no clear-cut distinction between the different possibilities but will give valuable information to aid in the diagnosis.

Isoenzymes have been separated in a number of different ways. Since the differences between the isoenzymes are in the protein part of the molecule or in the relative amount of various subunits, the isoenzymes may often be separated by electrophoresis or column chromatography. In some instances the protein portions of the isoenzymes are sufficiently different that they can be distinguished immunologically by means of specific antisera to the different isoenzymes. The different isoenzymes must first be separated and purified in some other way to be able to form the specific antibodies.

In some instances the isoenzymes may be separated or identified by heat inactivation, one particular isoenzyme being much more or less sensitive to inactivation by heat than another. The placental form of alkaline phosphatase is much more resistant to heat inactivation than the other alkaline phosphatase isoenzymes. In other instances one isoenzyme may be more resistant to inhibition by an added chemical agent. Thus the acid phosphatase from the prostate is much more strongly inhibited by added tartrate than are the other isoenzymes of acid phosphatase. Or one may use a slightly different substrate to distinguish between the isoenzymes. Thus some of the isoenzymes of lactate dehydrogenase under suboptimal conditions will also catalyze the reduction of α-ketobutyric acid, which is chemically quite similar to lactic acid. Some specific examples of the determination of isoenzymes will be given in connection with certain of the enzymes.

ENZYME STORAGE

Most enzymes in biologic fluids are stable at refrigerator temperature for 2-3 days to a week and at room temperature for a shorter time (Table 24-2). When storage for longer periods is required, serum or plasma should usually be frozen. Exact pipetting, incubation time, and temperature must always be observed, and extreme cleanliness of the glassware must be ensured.

Because no primary standards are available, it is of extreme importance that all conditions for enzyme assays be maintained exactly the same each time they are run and that a quality control serum of a known value be included.

Only enzymes recognized as having clinical significance will be described in this chapter. Others will be mentioned briefly.

Table 24-2. Stability of some serum enzymes under storage (no more than 10% change during specified time)

	Room temp. (25° C)	Refrigerator (0-4° C)	Frozen (−25° C)
Aldolase	2 days	2 days	Unstable*
α-Hydroxybutyrate dehydrogenase	Unstable	3 days	Unstable*
Amylase	1 mo	6 mo	2 mo
Ferroxidase I	1 day†	2 wk	2 wk
Creatine kinase (activated, creatine phosphokinase)	2 days	1 wk	1 mo
Isocitrate dehydrogenase	5 hr	3 days	3 wk
Lactate dehydrogenase	1 wk	2 days‡	2 days‡
Leucine aminopeptidase (LAP, not leukocyte alkaline phosphatase)	1 wk	1 wk	1 wk
Lipase	1 wk	3 wk	3 wk
Phosphatase, acid	4 hr	3 days§	3 days§
Phosphatase, Alkaline	2 days‖	2 days‖	1 mo
Aspartate aminotransferase (serum glutamic oxaloacetic transaminase)	3 days	1 wk	1 mo
Alanine aminotransferase (serum glutamic pyruvic transaminase)	3 days	1 wk	Unstable*

*Change caused by thawing.
†Variable.
‡Isoenzyme pattern will change, particularly on freezing and thawing.
§With added acetic acid.
‖Change may be caused by change in pH on standing.

CLINICAL USE OF ENZYMES

The enzymes normally found in plasma can be divided into two classes.[6] The **plasma-specific** enzymes include those enzymes that have a very definite and specific function in plasma. Plasma is their normal site of action, and they are present in higher levels than most tissues. Among these are the enzymes involved in blood coagulation, the immune response, as well as **ferroxidase I** and **pseudocholinesterase.** These enzymes are synthesized in the liver and are constantly liberated into the plasma to maintain a steady state concentration. They are of clinical interest when present in plasma at values that are below normal as a result of impaired liver function or absent as a result of an inborn metabolic error. Hepatolenticular degeneration (Wilson's disease), for example, is associated with a deficiency of ferroxidase, a copper-containing oxidase, and very low values of serum copper and ferroxidase are generally found.

The second group, the **non-plasma-specific** enzymes, has no known physiologic function in plasma. They are present in plasma at concentrations much lower than their concentrations in certain tissues. In many cases plasma is deficient in activators or coenzymes necessary for the optimal activity of these enzymes. This group contains the **enzymes of secretion** and the **enzymes associated with cellular metabolism.** Among the enzymes of secretion are such enzymes as **amylase, lipase,** and the **phosphatases.** Although secreted at high rates, they are rapidly disposed of through the usual excretory channels, e.g., the urine, the bile, and the intestinal tract, and normal plasma concentrations are relatively low and constant. If, however, any of the usual pathways of excretion are blocked, or the rate of liberation into the extracellular fluid is suddenly accelerated, or the rate of production is increased, a significant increase in plasma concentrations of these enzymes will occur.

The enzymes of cellular metabolism are located within the tissue cells and are present there at very high concentrations. Some exist free in the cellular fluid, and others are contained in cellular structures such as the mitochondria and lysosomes. As long as the cell membrane is intact, such enzymes are contained within the cell walls, and the value of these enzymes in the extracellular fluid and the plasma is extremely low or absent. The cell membranes are impermeable as long as the cells are metabolizing normally. It was formerly thought that the increase in serum transaminases that occurs in acute hepatitis is mediated by cellular necrosis with the release of the contents of the necrotic cells into the circulation. It is now clear that cellular necrosis is **not** necessary for the release of cellular enzymes and that inflammatory lesions accompanied by reversible changes in membrane permeability can also lead to release of cellular enzymes. If cell activity is impaired or destroyed as a result of deficiencies in oxygen or glucose or if the cell is damaged in some way (bacterial or viral infection), the membrane becomes permeable or ruptures. The cell contents, including their enzyme complement, are released into the extracellular fluid and eventually reach the plasma. If a large volume of

cells is so affected, the plasma value of the enzymes may increase very suddenly to activities many times greater than normal.

Of the thousands of known enzymes only a few hundred have been studied in humans and of these only 15-18 have been routinely established as valuable diagnostic tools. Modern clinical enzymology is only about 25 years old and is still in an active state of development. The concept of a specific enzyme as a "marker" for a particular disease has not been generally realized. The greater utility of clinical enzymology has developed in the form of tissue-specific markers. Since most cells contain most enzymes, it is difficult to be specific in an absolute sense. However, the concentrations of enzymes are not the same in different organs, and a comparison of several different enzymes may serve to pinpoint the affect tissue. If the enzymes are derived from a given cell type (i.e., liver or heart), their ratio in serum will approximate that in the tissue of origin. Different tissues with the same total enzyme activity may have different distributions of isoenzyme activity, and thus the isoenzyme pattern in serum has been used to help reflect tissue of origin.

The isoenzyme patterns obtained from heart muscle and liver are quite different even though both organs have large amounts of total lactate dehydrogenase activity. Most of the serum enzymes have been found to be composed of isoenzymes.

The material on the diagnostic use of enzymes has been subdivided into several broad categories. The principle diagnostic enzymes are then considered under each heading as appropriate, and methods of assay are included the first time an enzyme is presented.

DIAGNOSIS OF MYOCARDIAL INFARCTION

When a small portion of cardiac muscle dies because of an obstructed arteriole, a myocardial infarct occurs and the affected cells leak their contents into the surrounding tissue fluids. This material ends up in the plasma adding to existing materials present from other sources.

An examination of several enzyme activities that can be used as tissue markers can be helpful in establishing the diagnosis. The major diagnostic enzymes for this use are creatine kinase (CK), creatine kinase isoenzymes, lactate dehydrogenase (LD), lactate dehydrogenase isoenzymes, and aspartate aminotransferase (AST). Samples taken at one point in time are of little use since many tissues contain these enzymes and even some of the isoenzymes. What is important is the serial sampling of plasma or serum over a period of a few days to watch the changes in several enzymes and isoenzymes. Several enzymes appear early in the course of myocardial damage whereas others appear later, and the dynamic changes that are observed with several enzymes can increase the specificity of the diagnosis. The specific time course will be covered with each specific enzyme determination.

Creatine kinase (CK) (EC 2.7.3.2; ATP: creatine phosphotransferase)

Principle: The enzyme creatine kinase catalyzes the following reaction:

Creatine + Adenosine triphosphate (ATP) $\overset{CK}{\rightleftharpoons}$

Phosphocreatine + Adenosine diphosphate (ADP)

Like most kinases the enzyme requires magnesium ions for activation. The enzyme activity has been measured in a number of ways. In an older method the reaction was run in the direction indicated above. After a timed interval, acid was added to stop the reaction and the phophocreatinine formed was allowed to spontaneously decompose into creatine and inorganic phosphate. The latter substance was then determined colorimetrically. This method was rather insensitive and required a correction for the inorganic phosphate originally present in the serum. In another method the ADP formed was determined by means of a series of coupled reactions. The reaction may be run in the reverse direction, and the creatine formed determined colorimetrically be reaction with diacetyl and α-naphthol. In the most common method now used, the reaction is run in the reverse direction and the ATP formed is measured by means of a series of coupled reactions:

ATP + Glucose $\overset{Hexokinase}{\rightleftharpoons}$ Glucose-6-phosphate + ADP

Glucose-6-phosphate + NADP$^+$ $\overset{G\text{-}6\text{-}PD}{\rightleftharpoons}$

6-Phosphogluconate + NADPH + H$^+$

The second reaction above is catalyzed by the enzyme glucose-6-phosphate dehydrogenase.

As usual the reaction is followed by the change in absorbance at 340 nm. The procedure given here is based on that of Swanson and Wilkerson[7] with some modifications as suggested by Szasz et al.[8] for optimization.

Reagents:

1. Imidazole buffer, 115 mmoles/L, pH 6.7
   Dissolve 7.49 g imidazole in about 9 dl water. Adjust the pH to 6.7 by the addition of 6 moles/L hydrochloric acid (concentrated hydrochloric acid diluted with an equal volume of water) (about 12 ml of the acid will be required); then dilute to 1 L and mix well. This buffer is preferably kept in the refrigerator.

2. Buffered reagent mixture
   Dissolve the following in 1 dl of the buffer: magnesium acetate tetrahydrate, 246 mg; glucose, 415 mg; creatine phosphate disodium salt, hydrate, 1.13 g; adenosine monophosphate (AMP), sodium salt, 224 mg; and adenosine diphosphate sodium salt, 103 mg. After these chemicals have dissolved, the pH should be checked and adjusted if necessary. The solution is not too stable and is best preserved by pipetting 2.6 ml aliquots into small tubes, tightly stoppering these, and freezing. The tubes are then thawed as needed.

3. NADP solution, 4.6 mg/ml in buffer
   This is prepared as needed, which is best done by adding 1.1 ml of buffer to a preweighed vial containing 5 mg NADP.

4. Thiol solution
   Dissolve 980 mg N-acetylcysteine in 10 ml of buffer. This solution may be stored in the refrigerator for a few days.

5. Enzyme solution
   Dilute a suspension of hexokinase to a concentration of 50 units/ml (50,000 units/L) and a suspension of glucose-6-phosphate dehydrogenase to a concentration of 30 units/ml (30,000 units/L); then mix equal volumes of the two solutions. The resulting mixture is stable for about a week when kept in the refrigerator.

Procedure: To a series of cuvets having a 1 cm light path add 2.6 ml of the buffer reagent mixture and 0.1 ml each of the NADP solution, thiol solution, and enzyme solution, mix and warm in a water bath to 30° C for about 5 min; then add 0.1 ml of serum sample, mix, and incubate at 30° C. After 5 min, read absorbance at timed intervals of 30 sec or 1 min for 5-10 min and calculate the average absorbance change per minute. If needed for icteric serum samples readings may be made against a blank solution, replacing serum by buffer, or against a dichromate solution. The activity is then calculated in the usual way as follows:

$$\text{Units/L} = \frac{\Delta A}{\min} \times \frac{1000 \times 3.0}{6.22 \times 0.1} = \frac{\Delta A}{\min} \times 4823$$

For highly active samples the best procedure is to repeat the analysis using a smaller aliquot of serum, since dilution with water, saline, or heated serum gives an apparent increase in activity.[9] If when using smaller aliquots, additional buffer is added to the cuvet to make the total volume exactly 3.0 ml then the factor 4823 as given above for 100 μl of serum is replaced by 9646, 19,293, and 48,232 for aliquots of 50, 25, and 10 μl respectively. If, as is more convenient, the extra buffer is not added and less serum is used, the factors are 9486, 19,132, and 48,071, respectively. Various lyophilized reagents are available commercially: Worthington Biochemical Corp., Freehold, N.J.; Abbott Laboratories Diagnostics Div., South Pasadena, Calif.; and many others) and are very convenient to use, but it must be remembered that these may not contain exactly the same proportions of the reagents as given above so that they may not give exactly the same normal ranges, although the differences will usually be slight.

Normal values and interpretation: The normal range for adults by this method at 30°C 20-70 units/L for men and 10-50 units/L for women. Children over 1 year of age usually have the same range as adults; two to five times higher values have been found in neonates and during the first months of life.[10] Values below the lower limit have no clinical significance.

Garcia[11] has suggested that normal CK activities for apparently healthy men may be related to muscle mass, and muscular individuals may have upper limits of normal of about 100-120 units/L. Meltzer[12] has observed that CK activity appears high in black men than white men, 110 units/L vs. 70 units/L. This may reflect a difference that is genetic, or it may be a consequence of a difference in physical labor of the two groups.

Elevated CK values have been reported after the onset of myocardial infarction; elevations occur about 6 hr after the onset of symptoms and reach peak values in about 18-36 hr. There is usually a rapid return to normal values by the fourth day. Extremely elevated values have been reported in Duchenne's muscular dystrophy; somewhat lower values have been reported in muscular dystrophy affecting the limbs and girdle. Following strenuous exercise, elevations of up to three times the normal CK values have been observed. These elevations disappear within 24-48 hr.

Comment: The preferred samples for CK assay are serum or heparinized plasma. CK is inhibited by EDTA, citrate, and fluoride and is not stable for long periods at room temperature or refrigerator temperature. Much of the older literature using nonactivated methods of assay comments on the need for rapid analysis. However, most or all of the CK activity is regained by adding sulfhydryl agents (i.e., N-acetylcysteine) to the assay mixture to give an activated assay, making rapid assays less necessary.

Some hemolysis can be tolerated because red cells have no CK activity, but since adenylate kinase and other materials that contribute to the lag phase or undesired side reactions are liberated, it is best to avoid hemolyzed samples if possible.

Creatinine kinase isoenzymes

The conditions causing elevated CK values may often be distinguished by determining the relative amounts of the CK isoenzymes. Three main isoenzymes have been found; these are generally labeled as MM (CK_3), MB (CK_2), and BB (CK_1). The CK_1 (BB) isoenzyme is the most negatively charged and migrates furthest to the anode ($+$) during electrophoresis (Fig. 24-1) or is the isoenzyme most tightly bound and requiring the highest salt concentration to elute it during column chromatography. The CK_3 (MM) isoenzyme is found largely in skeletal muscle and is generally responsible for most of the total activity in serum. The amount and proportion are increased in Duchenne muscular dystrophy. The CK_1 (BB) isoenzyme is found in brain tissue and generally constitutes only a small fraction of the total activity in serum. It may be elevated in some types of brain injury if the blood-brain barrier is damaged or in cases of infarcted bowel or carcinoma. The MB isoenzyme is specific for myocardial tissue, and increased amounts are usually found in the serum after myocardial infarction and other cardiac damage.

The isoenzymes have been separated in a number of different ways: by electrophoresis on cellulose acetate[13] or agarose gel,[14] by differential inhibition,[15,16] by column chromatography[13,17] or batch absorption,[18] and by radioimmunoassay.[19,20] The electrophoretic methods require some special equipment and are rather time consuming but are technically simple and demonstrate all the isoenzyme bands at once (Fig. 23-1). There remains some controversy as to the accuracy of the inhibition methods. The column chromatography or batch absorption methods remain the most promising as rapid methods for small numbers of samples but these suffer from the disadvantages that the original activity is diluted considerably in the procedure and either the eluate must be concentrated or relatively large volumes used in the analysis. In addition, bleeding over of CK_3 (MM) into CK_2 (MB) fractions can occur with unsatisfactory columns or samples of high CK_3 (MM) activity. Because of the increasing number of reports of unusually migrating isoenzymes that are potentially seen as CK_2 (MB) it seems prudent to examine the serum samples of positive column chromatographic MB patients by electrophoresis to eliminate this source of false positive results.

The radioimmunoassays give good results but again require special equipment unless the laboratory already is performing other radioactive immunoassays, and these assays are as time consuming as the electrophoresis assays.

Electrophoresis (Corning Medical, Medfield, Mass.; Helena Laboratories, Beaumont, Tex.) with fluorometric detection and column chromatographic (Roche Diagnostics, Nutley, N.J.; Worthington Biochemical Corp., Freehold, N.J.) methods are the most widely used methods. The preparation of agarose films or DEAE-Sephadex columns is troublesome, and commercially available materials are recommended since they are convenient and reproducible.

Normal values and interpretation: The normal range of CK_2 (MB) isoenzyme may vary somewhat with the method of determination, but usually the amount of the CK_2 (MB) isoenzyme in normal individuals determined by electrophoresis or column chromatography is between very low and trace. Values of 0-5 units/L are found,* which represent less than 5% of the total CK activity. Slightly higher values are found by immunoinhibition.[16]

After a myocardial infarction, especially with a point

---

*See references 13, 14, 17, 21, and 22.

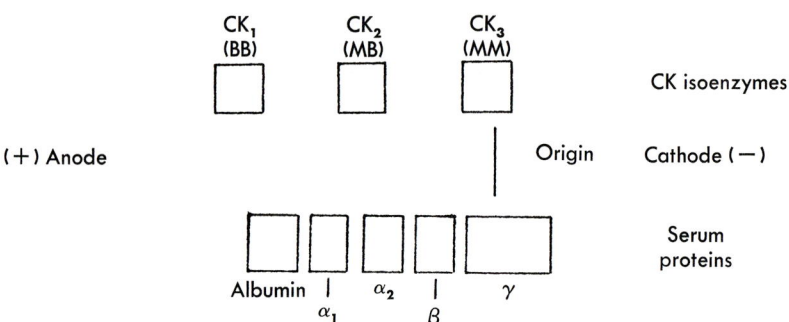

Fig. 24-1. Comparison of electrophoretic mobilities on agarose.

of acute onset of symptoms, a series of increases in enzyme activity is seen.[23-27] The total CK and CK_2 (MB) concentrations become abnormal within the first 48 hr.[15] Usually within 24-36 hr after an acute myocardial infarction, sometimes within 6 hr, the percentage of CK_2 (MB) isoenzyme may rise to >5% of the total, along with a marked increase of total CK. The average peak times after infarction in 47 patients were 6 hr for CK_2 (MB), 18 hr for CK, 24 hr for AST, and 48 hr for LD.[26] The actual times are not as important as the sequence, since it may be difficult to pinpoint the time of infarction.

Blood samples should be obtained on admission and 12 and 24 hr after the onset of symptoms,[27] so that the increased CK_2 (MB) concentration will not be missed. Subsequent samples may be taken at 24 hr intervals to evaluate changes in LD isoenzymes.

Myocardial infarct extension or reinfarctions may change the time course of enzyme abnormalities. Suggestions by Shell et al.[28] and Roe[29] that the size of the infarction may be related to the amount of CK_2 (MB) remain to be fully evaluated.

Although the most widely used isoenzyme for diagnosis is CK_2 (MB), there are a number of reports of elevations of CK_1 (BB). This isoenzyme, which is not often observed in normal serum samples evaluated by agarose electrophoresis, has been found to be associated with gastrointestinal[30] or prostatic carcinoma,[31-33] muscle neoplasms,[34] oat cell carcinoma,[35] hemorrhagic strokes,[36] infarction of the bowel,[37] renal dialysis,[38] malignant pyrexia,[39] hypothermia,[40,41] Reye's syndrome,[42] and various hematologic disorders.[43] Elevations have also been seen during coronary bypass surgery[44] and in women during labor.[45] The most common condition associated with an elevated level of CK_1 (BB) is infarcted bowel.

Unusual creatine kinase isoenzymes: A number of atypically migrating CK isoenzyme bands have occasionally been described in serum. Yuu et al.[46] and Liu et al.[47] reported the presence of a "macro-CK" band cathodal to CK_3 (MM) on agarose for breast carcinoma. The band does not appear to be a complex of CK and IgM, IgG, IgA, or β-lipoprotein. Preliminary data suggest it is a tetramer of four dimeric CK isoenzymes and may be produced in patients exposed to radiation.

Another unusual band (or bands) appears on agarose electrophoresis between CK_1 (MM) and CK_2 (MB). Sax et al.[48] reported several patients with these atypical bands, which gave false positive MB results by DEAE-Sephadex column chromatography. Later studies[49,50] have shown that at least some of these abnormal bands can be characterized as CK_1 (BB) complexed with IgG. The bands do not seem to have an underlying common disease process or condition, and recent studies[49] dispute the suggestion of Lim[51] that the bands are present in cases of severe angina pectoris.

Comment: The same precautions that apply to CK also apply to the assay of isoenzymes. Exercise has been shown to increase CK_3 (MM) values when CK increases. Intramusculature injections produce temporary increases in CK values, which is CK_3 (MM); the CK_2 (MB) value remains normal. Myocarditis produces a pattern of enzyme changes that mimic acute myocar-

dial infarction, probably because of increased membrane permeability during inflammation. Minor heart rhythm disturbances usually do not lead to the release of enzymes in the blood. Electrical countershock to correct rhythm disturbances, cardiac catheterization, and coronary arteriography may produce elevations in CK values in about half of these patients studied. The elevations seen are in CK_3 (MM) with only occasional CK_2 (MB) elevations, which are usually smaller in magnitude than those changes observed in individuals with acute myocardial infarctions.

Lactate dehydrogenase (LD) (EC 1.1.1.27; L-lactate: NAD oxidoreductase)

Principle: The enzyme lactate dehydrogenase catalyzes reversibly the following reaction:

$$\text{Lactate} + \text{NAD}^+ \overset{LD}{\rightleftharpoons} \text{Pyruvate} + \text{NADH} + \text{H}^+$$

In the simple spectrophotometric method the reaction is followed by measuring the change in absorbance at 340 nm as a result of the conversion of NAD to NADH or vice versa. The reaction may be run in either direction. In the procedures mentioned here the reaction is run in the so-called reverse direction. The two methods may be designated as LD-L and LD-P, the final L or P designating whether lactate or pyruvate is used as substrate. The Enzyme Commission has recommended 30° C as the preferred temperature for enzyme assay, but other temperatures are often used, e.g., 25°, 32°, and 37° C. As mentioned, the rate of reaction increases with the temperature, so that for a given amount of actual enzyme, the absorbance change will be greater at a higher temperature. Since the result in terms of enzyme units is usually proportional to the absorbance difference, a given amount of enzyme will yield a higher measured activity at a higher temperature. In comparing the results for LD assays when run at different temperatures, Table 24-3 has been used. It gives the relative activities at different temperatures compared with that at 30° C. The formula for calculating the activity at different temperatures is as follows:

$$\text{Activity at } T_1 \text{ (units)} = \text{Measured activity at } T_2 \times F_2/F_1$$

where F_1 is the factor in Table 24-3 associated with T_1 and similarly for T_2.

It must be emphasized that the above figures are only approximate since the factor will vary with the details of the methods used, but they can serve as a rough guide in comparing results at different temperatures.

Table 24-3. Factors for temperature correction of LD activity*

°C	F	°C	F	°C	F
25	1.44	30	1.00	35	0.70
26	1.34	31	0.92	36	0.65
27	1.24	32	0.86	37	0.60
28	1.15	33	0.80	38	0.56
29	1.17	34	0.75	39	0.52

*Based on data from Henry et al.: Am. J. Clin. Pathol. **34**:381, 1966.

Determination in serum

The spectrophotometric method is quite simple and rapid and differentiates with certainty between normal and elevated serum LD activities. It requires one of the simple photometers, reading at 340 nm, with a thermostated cuvet chamber and a recorder attachment to have excellent sensitivity and accuracy. There is no ideal buffer for use with LD since it has been shown that the different isoenzymes of the enzyme react somewhat differently with different buffers, even at the same pH.[52] A method is presented here using tris buffer at a pH of 7.4.[53]

Since the erythrocytes contain about 150 times as much of the enzyme as is found in serum, hemolyzed samples should not be used. It has also been reported that the presence of an appreciable number of platelets or traces of many types of detergents used in washing glassware interfere with the assay.[54]

Reagents:

1. Tris buffer, 0.5 mole/L, pH 7.40 at 30° C
   Dissolve 60.6 g tris(hydroxymethyl)aminomethane in about 7 dl water. Add 1 mole/L hydrochloric acid (83 ml of concentrated acid diluted to 1 L with water) to the tris solution to bring the pH to 7.4 at 30° C (about 1 dl will be required); then dilute to 1 L.

2. Working buffer, tris, 57.5 mmole/L, pH 7.4
   Dilute 57.5 ml of the 0.5 mole/L buffer to 5 dl with water. Check pH after warming to 30° C and adjust if necessary with 1 mole/L hydrochloric acid or sodium hydroxide.

3. NADH solution, 5.58 mmole/L in tris buffer, pH 7.4
   Dissolve 21.8 mg of β-NADH (disodium salt, trihydrate) in 5.0 ml of 57.5 mmole/L tris buffer. Solution is stable for 72 hr in the refrigerator, but it is recommended that only a sufficient amount for 1 day be prepared at any time. As a convenient method of preparation, preweighed vials containing 10 mg (and other sizes as well) may be purchased (Sigma Chemical Co., St. Louis) and 2.25 ml of the working buffer added to a 10 ml vial.

4. Pyruvate solution, 14 mmole/L
   Dissolve 155 mg sodium pyruvate in 1 dl working buffer. This is stable for several weeks if kept refrigerated.

For enzymatic reactions involving the NAD-NADH couple or with other unstable reagents, a number of manufacturers (Calbiochem-Behring Corp., San Diego; Worthington Biochemical Corp., Freehold, N.J.; Smith Kline Instruments, Sunnyvale, Calif.) provide the complete reagent system in tablet or lyophilized form that may be dissolved in water as needed. These are very convenient and can usually be obtained in different sizes for different numbers of tests. They are simplest to use for the small laboratory. One must check if the normal range as given by the manufacturer is the same as given here or use the former values.

Procedure: To a cuvet with a 1 cm light path add 2.6 ml of the working buffer, 100 μl of the NADH solution, and 100 μl of serum sample. Mix and incubate at 30° C for about 10 min. Then add 200 μl of the pyruvate solution, mix by gentle inversion, and take readings in the spectrophotometer at 1 min intervals for several minutes. Calculate the average change in absorbance per minute during the period in which the absorbance change is relatively constant. (NOTE: With some older instruments the initial absorbance of the solution when read against water may be too high for accurate readings. In this case read against a blank of a dichromate solution. Dissolve 150 mg potassium dichromate and a few drops of concentrated sulfuric acid in water to make 5 dl. Dilute this further, usually between 1:5 and 1:10, so that the initial reading of the solution is around 0.7 absorbance units. This can be checked during the preincubation period, and once the proper dilution is found, a larger amount can be diluted since the dichromate solution is quite stable when protected from contact with organic matter.)

Calculation: Then the activity in units per liter is as follows:

$$\text{units/L at 30° C} = \frac{\Delta A}{\text{min}} \times \frac{3.00 \times 1000}{6.22 \times 0.1} = \frac{\Delta A}{\text{min}} \times 4823$$

since the total volume is 3.00 ml and 0.1 ml of serum is used. For samples of high activity a smaller aliquot of serum can be used with the appropriate change in the factor; e.g., for 0.05 ml of serum the factor would be 9486.

Normal values and interpretation: The normal range of the enzyme in serum by this method is 95-200 units/L. Many different results for the normal values of LD may be found in the literature. Not only may the reaction be run at different temperatures, which leads to different numeric values, but the forward reaction may be used with lactate as the substrate and a pH of about 9. Values by this method are generally in the range of 35-90 units/L at 30° C.

LD increases in value later than the changes reported for CK after myocardial infarction. This increase often becomes abnormal in 24-48 hr, peaks in 3-6 days, and returns to normal in 8-14 days. The increase somewhat parallels the extent of cardiac damage.

Elevations have been reported in leukemia, hemolytic anemias, pernicious anemia, pulmonary infarction, sickle cell anemia, malignant lymphoma, trauma to striated muscle, and liver disease, as well as renal disease.

Because LD activity is **not** much elevated in pulmonary infarction and the AST value remains almost normal, these tests may be used for the differential diagnosis of pulmonary embolism and myocardial infarction.

Cerebrospinal fluid may also be assayed for enzyme activity. Since the activity is generally lower than in serum, one may use 0.2 ml of fluid (total volume of 3.1 ml) with the factor of 2492. The expected value of enzyme activity in the fluid is in the range of from 10-30 units/L. Elevations are seen in subarachnoid hemorrhage and with cerebrovascular thrombosis and hemorrhage.

Comment: Serum or heparinized plasma may be used, but oxalate and EDTA plasma should not be used. The various isoenzymes of LD show differing temperature stabilities but the least loss occurs at 25°

C,[55] and samples can be stored for 48 hr at 25° C with only a 6% loss and minimal change in isoenzyme patterns.

The colorimetric assays of LD activity are less precise and less accurate than the continuous kinetic methods since they are often standardized with control serum samples. Their use as assays of LD is discouraged in view of the large number of kinetic assays that are available for directly observing the reaction.

Determination in urine

For the determination of the enzyme in urine, the urine must first be dialyzed to remove interfering substances. The dialysis is carried out against water using the readily available cellophane dialysis tubing (6 mm diameter). Wash tubing for several hours in three changes of distilled water heated to about 90° C. Rinse with distilled water and store in distilled water in the refrigerator. Obtain an accurately timed 8 hr overnight urine specimen (no preservatives are needed). Measure and record the volume in milliliters. Then centrifuge about 10 ml for about 10 min at 2000 rpm.

Transfer 6 ml of the centrifuged urine sample to a dialysis sack as follows: Squeeze excess water from the dialysis sack and tie a knot at one end. Add 6 ml urine to the sack by using a pipet or small graduated cylinder. With a squeezing action of the fingers, expel the air from the sack above the urine and tie a secure knot in the sack about 3 in above the level of urine. Weigh on balance to nearest 0.1 g and place the sack into a 250 ml Erlenmeyer flask. Fasten length of soft rubber tubing to a cold water tap; adjust flow to at least 50 ml/min. Insert the rubber tube into flask so that the end is at the bottom. Set the flask so that the overflow runs down the drain and allow to dialyze for 2 hr. Remove the sack from the flask, wipe off the outside, and reweigh. Transfer the liquid to a test tube and centrifuge if there is any precipitate. The assay is carried out in a similar way to that for serum, except than one uses a somewhat more concentrated buffer made by diluting 18 ml of the stock to 1 dl with water. To the cuvet one then adds 1.7 ml of the concentrated buffer, 1 ml of the dialyzed urine, and 100 μl of the NADH solution. After incubation for about 15 min, the 200 μl of pyruvate solution is added and absorbance readings determined as for serum. The factor for conversion to units per liter is now $\Delta A/min \times 482$. Then total units of LD activity per 8 hr is as follows:

$$\text{units/L} \times 8 \text{ hr urine volume} \times \frac{\text{Wt after dialysis}}{\text{Wt before dialysis}}$$

Normal values and interpretation: The normal urinary LD activity is 480-1900 units in 8 hr specimens. Considerably elevated values have been reported by Wacker and Dorfman[56] and Dorfman et al.[57] in cases of carcinoma of the kidney or bladder. Significant elevations have also been reported in several other diseases involving the urinary system, including malignant hypertension, glomerulonephritis, lupus nephritis, acute tubular necrosis, and possibly pyelonephritis. However, these diseases are readily differentiated from malignant lesions. Urinary LD increases as much as 5000% in carcinoma of the kidneys or bladder.

Spurious elevations may result from urologic instrumentation, hemolysis, and menstrual contamination. Low activities may result from incomplete urine collection or the use of unclean glassware, as well as inhibitors found in urine.

Lactate dehydrogenase isoenzymes

Because of the wide distribution of LD throughout the various tissues of the body, an elevated serum LD level is of limited value in establishing the specific site of tissue damage. Studies have shown that serum LD is composed of five fractions (isoenzymes) that can be separated by electrophoretic or other methods. All of the five isoenzymes catalyze the same reaction and thus are considered to be the same enzyme in the EC classification. The enzymes are generally referred to as LD_1, LD_2, LD_3, LD_4, and LD_5, in the order of decreasing mobility during electrophoresis at a pH of 8.6. The enzyme LD is a tetramer composed of four subunits. The subunits are of two types: the heart, H subunit, and the muscle, M subunit. Combinations of four of these subunits give rise to the five isoenzymes found in serum: LD_1 (H_4), LD_2 (H_3M), LD_3 (H_2M_2), LD_4 (HM_3), and LD_5 (M_4).

It has been found that different types of tissue may contain different proportions of the various isoenzymes, and the proportions are often characteristic of the different types of tissue. For example, liver contains a relatively large proportion of LD_5 and only small amounts of the other isoenzymes. Cardiac muscle, on the other hand, has a relatively high content of LD_1 and LD_2 with only very small amounts of the other isoenzymes. Other tissues may contain other different proportions of the isoenzymes. Pancreatic tissue, for example, contains a fairly high proportion of LD_3. When a particular type of tissue is damaged by a disease process, the proportion of the isoenzymes characteristic of that tissue will increase in the serum; i.e., when the liver is damaged by a disease process, a relatively large increase in the LD_5 content of the serum will be observed and after myocardial infarction, the serum LD_1 and LD_2 values are increased. This may serve as a means for differential diagnosis of these two conditions. These two types of tissue show the greatest differences in LD isoenzyme proportions, and the method has not been applied to other types of tissue to any great extent.

Methods of determination: There are a number of ways these LD isoenzymes can be differentiated. Wilkinson et al.[58-60] introduced the measurement of α-hydroxybutyrate dehydrogenase (HBDH) activity as a test that measured the cardiac isoenzymes LD_1 and LD_2 and the HBDH/LD ratio as a more sensitive and specific test for myocardial infarction. It is now known[61] that the LD isoenzymes have varying affinities for 2-ketobutyrate, the substrate of HBDH, which depends on temperature. Any departure from the original suboptimal LD assay and HBDH assay at 25° C results in the loss of any clinically useful ratio. With the availability of the routine electrophoretic separation of the 5 LD isoenzymes, HBDH assays should be abandoned.

Other methods of differentiating isoenzymes include heat,[62] ion-exchange chromatography,[63] and electrophoresis.[64] For routine use, electrophoresis on agarose, polyacrylamide, or cellulose acetate is preferred since all isoenzymes are seen at one time.

Lactate dehydrogenase isoenzymes by electrophoresis: The LD isoenzymes can be accurately differentiated by electrophoresis. Electrophoresis has been carried out on agar gel, polyacrylamide gel, and cellulose acetate strips. The serum is applied to the gel or strip and the electrophoresis allowed to proceed for the required time. The strip may then be stained. The stain may be essentially the same as the substrate used for a colorimetric method for LD activity using tetrazolium blue and phenozine methosulfate. The staining occurs on the strips only in positions where the enzyme is present, and the amount of staining produced will be proportional to the amount of enzyme present at a given point. After fixing, the bands may be evaluated in a densitometer as in protein electrophoresis. Alternately the bands may be treated with a reagent similar to that used in the ultraviolet method for LD. NADH will then be formed on the strip at positions where the enzyme is present. If the strip is then scanned by ultraviolet light the NADH will fluoresce and the amount of fluorescence will be measured as an indication of the amount of enzyme present. The method to be used will depend on the equipment available. Cawley[65] gives details on the use of agarose gel electrophoresis, De Giorgio[66] and Myers and Van Remortel[67] discuss the use of two different systems for the use of cellulose acetate as supporting medium and Dietz et al.[68] give details for the polyacrylamide gels.

Normal values and interpretation: Current fluorometric detection technics after agarose electrophoresis (Corning Medical, Medfield, Mass.) easily demonstrate all five isoenzyme bands. The approximate percentages are as follows: LD_1, 16-28%; LD_2, 29-37%; LD_3, 17-23%; LD_4, 9-15%; and LD_5, 8-20%. After myocardial infarction the LD_1/LD_2 ratio is greater than one, or "flipped," about 12-24 hr after infarction and remains greater than one for as long as 7 days. Samples of serum after a suspected myocardial infarction should be drawn every 24 hr for LD isoenzyme analysis. Only about two or three samples are needed since the "flip" will occur within 48 hr of a myocardial infarction.

Liver disease produces an elevated LD_4 and LD_5 pattern with LD_5 generally the most elevated. In pulmonary infarcts the LD_3 is elevated to approximately the same value as LD_2.

Generalized elevations of many isoenzymes have been called isomorphic patterns. These patterns have been reviewed[69] and seem consistent with multisystem disease as seen in shock, anoxia, trauma, and neoplasm.

About 50% of patients with malignancy show increased LD activity in serum. The increases are generally in the slower isoenzymes (LD_4 and LD_5), but they are not specific and not always used in clinical practice. The increases reflect the rapidity of tumor growth, the cellularity of the tumor, and its metastatic activity.[70-72] The values may be normal in early or localized malignancy. A favorable response to therapy may be accompanied by a fall in the serum enzyme value, and recurrence of the tumor may be signaled by a rise in the total LD and its isoenzymes. The differences in patterns between tissues are not always great, and the normal variations between individuals are such that exact differentiation is at times difficult.

Renal LD is not helpful in the diagnosis of urinary tract malignancy,[73] since several nonneoplastic conditions give rise to increased urine LD values. Similar considerations limit the value of cerebrospinal fluid LD in detecting tumors of the central nervous system[74] and the value of LD in effusions in determining malignancies of the lung and abdominal organs.[75]

The transaminases: aspartate aminotransferase and alanine aminotransferase[76-78]

Principle: The older names and abbreviations "SGOT" and "SGPT" aspartate aminotransferase and alanine aminotransferase are still frequently used, but the newer EC names and abbreviations "AST" and "ALT" are preferred. Note that the reactions catalyzed by the enzymes and the assays are generally used in the direction written for the determinations as follows:

$$\text{Aspartate} + \alpha\text{-Ketoglutarate} \overset{\text{AST}}{\rightleftharpoons} \text{Glutamate} + \text{Oxalacetate}$$

and

$$\text{Alanine} + \alpha\text{-Ketoglutarate} \overset{\text{ALT}}{\rightleftharpoons} \text{Glutamate} + \text{Pyruvate}$$

Thus the EC names are more descriptive.

The enzymes may be assayed by measuring the change in absorbance at 340 nm by adding coupling enzymes. For AST the enzyme MD and the coenzyme NADH are added so that the following reaction occurs:

$$\text{Oxalacetate} + \text{NADH} + \text{H}^+ \overset{\text{MD}}{\rightleftharpoons} \text{Malate} + \text{NAD}^+$$

For ALT, LD and NADH are added, and the reaction is

$$\text{Pyruvate} + \text{NADH} + \text{H}^+ \overset{\text{LD}}{\rightleftharpoons} \text{Lactate} + \text{NAD}^+$$

In both instances the coupling enzyme must be added in large amounts so that the limiting reaction is the first (transaminase) reaction. In the reagents for the determination of AST, some LD is added to accelerate the competing endogenous reactions and thus shorten the preincubation time. Both enzyme reactions are influenced by the presence of pyridoxal-5-phosphate, and thus the measured activity will vary somewhat with the amount of this substance in the serum sample. To eliminate this source of variability an excess of the compound is added to the reaction mixtures for both enzymes.

Determination of aspartate aminotransferase (AST)   (EC 2.6.1.1; L-aspartate: 2-oxoglutarate aminotransferase)

Reagents:
1. Stock tris solution, 1 mole/L
   Dissolve 60.5 g tris(hydroxymethyl)aminomethane in water to make 5 dl. This stock solution is also used in the preparation of the ALT reagents.
2. Working tris buffer for AST, 92 mmole/L, pH 7.8
   In a 250 ml volumetric flask add 23 ml stock buffer and about 150 ml water. Add 1 mole/L hydrochloric acid to bring the buffer to a pH of

7.8 at 30° C. (Alternately one may adjust to a pH of 7.9 at 25° C with little error.) Dilute to the mark and mix well. Store at 4° C.

3. Aspartate solution

To a 250 ml volumetric flask place 10.87 g L-aspartic acid, 23 ml stock tris solution, 33 ml 2.5 moles/L sodium hydroxide solution (100 g/L) and about 1 dl of water. Dissolve the aspartate by heating, cool, and adjust the pH to 7.8 at 30° C (or 7.9 at 25° C) with the addition of small amounts of 1 mole/L hydrochloric acid or sodium hydroxide as required; then dilute to 250 ml and mix well. Store at 4° C.

4. α-Ketoglutarate solution

In a 1 dl volumetric flask add 10 ml of the stock tris solution, 2.63 g oxoglutaric acid and about 50 ml of water. Adjust the pH to 7.8 at 30° C (or 7.9 at 25° C) by the addition of 2.5 moles/L hydroxide sodium and then dilute to 1 dl. Store in the refrigerator. This solution is stable for about 2 weeks.

5. NADH solution

Dissolve 5 mg NADH in 1.3 ml working buffer. It is convenient to use the preweighed vials containing 5 mg NADH. This solution should be prepared just before use. If kept cold at all times, it may be used for 2 or 3 days.

6. Pyridoxal-5-phosphate solution (P-5-P)

Dissolve 7.5 mg pyridoxal-5-phosphate in 10 ml working buffer. This is stable for 1 week in the refrigerator.

7. LD suspension, 500 units/ml

Dilute a suspension of LD (e.g., Sigma type XV [Sigma Chemical Co., St. Louis], 5 mg protein at 500 units/mg). This enzyme and MD are supplied as suspensions in ammonium sulfate solution. These are diluted with a mixture of equal volumes of glycerol and water to avoid adding appreciable amounts of ammonium sulfate to the reaction mixture. If the vial supplied contains 2500 units it is diluted to 5 ml with the diluent. Alternatively one can use sigma type XVII in 50% glycerol and dilute as above. Both enzymes are stable for several months if stored in the refrigerator and kept on ice when out of the refrigerator. The suspensions should be well mixed before being pipetted.

8. MD suspension, 250 units/ml

Dilute a suspension of MD (e.g., Sigma vial containing 5000 units) to the above concentration with the water-glycerol diluent.

Procedure: To a cuvet with 3 ml capacity and a 1 cm light path add the following: 2.2 ml aspartate solution (no. 3 above), 0.1 ml NADH solution (no. 5 above), 0.1 ml P-5-P solution (no. 6 above), 0.1 ml LD suspension (no. 7 above), 0.1 ml MD suspension (no. 8 above), and 0.2 ml serum sample. Mix and warm to 30° C. Incubate for 10 min and then add 0.2 ml of the α-ketoglutarate solution (no. 4 above) previously warmed to 30° C, mix rapidly, and measure change in absorbance per minute for about 10 min. If desired the enzyme solution may be read against a dichromate blank as given earlier with the LD assay. The average absorbance change per minute is then obtained.

Calculation: The activity is calculated in the usual manner as follows:

$$\text{units/L at 30° C} = \frac{\Delta A}{\min} \times \frac{1000}{6.22} \times \frac{3.0}{0.2} = \frac{\Delta A}{\min} \times 2412$$

where the volume of solution in the cuvet is 3.0 ml and the sample aliquot is 0.2 ml. With new batches of reagents, particular the enzymes, it is advisable to run a blank using 0.2 ml of water instead of the serum and subtract any blank value obtained from the actual ΔA measurements.

When a large number of samples are to be run, it may be convenient to mix the reagents together in larger quantities. One may mix together 22 ml of the aspartate solution and 1 ml each of the NADH solution, P-5-P solution, LD suspension, and MD suspension. Then 2.6 ml of the mixture is added to a number of cuvets, and 0.2 ml of serum is added after preliminary incubation of 0.2 ml of the oxoglutarate solution.

Determination of alanine aminotransferase (ALT)
(EC 2.6.1.2; L-alanine: 2-oxoglutarate aminotransferase)

Similar solutions as have been used for AST are used for determination of alanine aminotransferase with the changes as indicated below.

Reagents:

1. Alanine reagent

To a 250 ml volumetric flask add 15.19 g L-alanine, 29 ml stock tris buffer, about 1 dl water, and 65 ml of 2.5 moles/L sodium hydroxide solution. Dissolve the L-alanine with the aid of gentle heat if necessary; then cool and adjust the pH to 7.5 at 30° C (or 7.6 at 25° C); then dilute to the mark and mix well. Store at 4° C.

2. α-Ketoglutarate solution

In a 1 dl volumetric flask add 10 ml of the stock tris solution, 3.29 g of α-ketoglutaric acid, and about 50 ml of water. Adjust the pH to 7.5 at 30° C (or 7.6 at 25° C) by the addition of 2.5 moles/L sodium hydroxide solution; then dilute to 1 dl and mix. Store in the refrigerator.

3. NADH solution

This solution is the same as that used for the determination of AST.

4. P-5-P solution

This solution is the same as that used for the determination of AST.

5. LD suspension

This suspension is the same as that used for the determination of AST.

Procedure: To cuvets add 2.2 ml of the L-alanine solution, 0.1 ml each of the NADH and P-5-P solutions, and 0.2 ml of the LD suspension. Mix and incubate at 30° C for about 10 min. Then initiate the reaction by the addition of 0.2 ml of the L-alanine solution and measure the change in absorbance per minute.

Calculation: The activity is calculated as follows:

$$\text{units/L at 30° C} = \frac{\Delta A}{\min} \times \frac{1000}{6.22} \times \frac{3.0}{0.2} = \frac{\Delta A}{\min} \times 2412$$

The lyophilized reagents mentioned under LD are also available commercially for the determination of

AST and ALT. These reagents may not be in the optimized concentrations and may not contain added P-5-P. Without the latter, the normal range is about 25% lower than that given below. When using the method given here, care must be taken in the interpretation of the results obtained with some control sera. It has been found[79] that with some control sera (but not all) the values obtained with added P-5-P were over twice as great as without the added pyridoxal. Since the "optimized" method is used more often, the manufacturers may give results using this method. If there is any question concerning a given control serum, one can analyze the serum with and without added P-5-P (replacing the P-5-P solution by buffer alone in the formulation) and the difference in results noted.

Normal values and interpretation

The normal levels of AST by this method at 30° C are 12-30 units/L, and for ALT they are 7-30 units/L. The upper limits are slightly lower in women than in men. Elevations in transaminase activity occur in myocardial infarction, infectious mononucleosis, and infectious hepatitis. Other conditions that often show some elevation are cirrhosis and biliary obstruction with active hepatic necrosis, acute interstitial pancreatitis, metastatic carcinoma of the liver, extensive traumatic injuries, prolonged shock, and muscle injury. Although the AST value is always increased in acute myocardial infarctions, the ALT value does not always increase proportionately. In acute liver necrosis the ALT value often exceeds that of AST.

The serum AST starts to rise 6-12 hr after a myocardial infarction. The peak value is usually seen in 24-48 hr and returns to normal by the fourth to sixth day.

Comment: AST may also be determined by a colorimetric method in which the oxalacetate formed reacts with a diazonium salt to give a colored product.[80] This method is subject to interference in that ketones in the blood (e.g., in diabetic ketosis) will also react with the color reagent, giving falsely high results. This error can be minimized by running a separate serum blank with every unknown. However, since the procedure must be standardized as well either against a known control serum or with standard solutions of oxalacetate, and there are excellent more direct methods available, such colorimetric methods are discouraged and should not be used.

DIAGNOSIS OF LIVER DISEASE

The evaluation of serum enzyme activity is helpful in the diagnosis and management of a variety of liver diseases. Numerous enzyme tests have been proposed for this evaluation. The most commonly employed are alkaline phosphatase (ALP), aspartate aminotransferase, (AST), and alanine aminotransferase (ALT). Used less often are 5'-nucleotidase (NTP), γ-glutamyl transferase (GGT), alkaline phosphatase isoenzymes, and lactate dehydrogenase isoenzymes. Generally several samples are taken at several points in time to observe the course of treatment, but unlike the creatine kinase (CK) isoenzymes used for myocardial infarctions, timing is less important. Samples can be taken at 24-48 hr intervals to examine changes that have occurred.

Some information is provided on a group of enzymes used less often; this group includes ceruloplasmin, ornithine carbamyl transferase (OCT), malate dehydrogenase (MD), isocitrate dehydrogenase (ICD), sorbitol dehydrogenase (SD), glutamate dehydrogenase (GMD), arginase, guanosine deaminase (GDS), and adenosine deaminase (ADS).

Alkaline phosphatase (ALP) (EC 3.1.3.1; orthophosphoric monoester phosphohydrolase)

Alkaline phosphatase[81-83] has an optimal activity at a pH of approximately 10. It is found in a number of tissues but is used in clinical diagnosis chiefly in connection with bone and liver diseases.

Phosphatases are usually determined by measuring the amount of phosphatase ester split by the enzyme under specified conditions. A number of different substrates have been employed, since the natural substrate is unknown. Glycerophosphate was used in earlier methods (Bodansky). Disodium phenylphosphate has been widely employed (King-Armstrong). The more modern substrates produce chromogens as products and thus the enzyme rate can be followed kinetically. Of the two methods presented, the first is preferred. A comprehensive monograph on this enzyme gives many analytic and clinical details.[83]

Nitrophenyl phosphate method[82]

Principle: The method given here uses a substrate (p-nitrophenyl phosphate) that has a colored reaction product (nitrophenol) so that it can be determined directly in the solution.

$$p\text{-Nitrophenyl phosphate} + H_2O \xrightarrow{\text{Alkaline phosphatase}}$$
(colorless in acid and alkali)

$$p\text{-Nitrophenol} + H_3PO_4$$
(yellow in alkali)

Reagents:
1. Alkaline buffer solution, 2-amino-2-methyl-1-propanol, 0.89 mole/L, pH 10.33 at 30° C
   Warm the 2-amino-2-methyl-1-propanol to about 35° C until it is liquefied; then weight out exactly 78.5 g of the liquid and transfer it to a 1 L volumetric flask with about 5 dl water. Next add exactly 160 ml of exactly 1.00 mole/L hydrochloric acid (or the proportionate amount of a different known concentration of acid). Dilute nearly to 1 L and mix well. Bring the solution to 25° C, dilute to the mark, and mix well. This solution should have a pH of 10.33 at 30° C. (NOTE: When checking the pH with a glass electrode assembly, the latter should be one that is stated by the supplier to be suitable for use with tris buffers. Sigma Chemical Co. [St. Louis], Beckman Instruments [Fullerton, Calif.], and other distributors supply such electrodes. An accurate standard with a pH near 10 should be used for calibration, and the electrode should be well rinsed with water after immersion in the alkaline buffer solution before again being placed in the standard solution.) The solution should be kept well stoppered to prevent absorption of carbon dioxide from the air. The solution is stable for about 1 month without rechecking the pH.

2. Magnesium chloride solution, 1.5 mmole/L

   Dissolve 30 mg $MgCl_2 \cdot 6H_2O$ in water to make 1 dl. This solution is stable indefinitely.

3. Substrate solution, p-nitrophenyl phosphate, 225 mmole/L

   Dissolve disodium p-nitrophenyl phosphate hexahydrate (Sigma Chemical Co., St. Louis) in an aliquot of the magnesium chloride solution in the following proportion: 83.5 mg p-nitrophenyl phosphate per milliliter of magnesium solution. This solution should be made up fresh each day and is stable for about 8 hr at room temperature. The pH should be between 8 and 9.

4. Stock standard, p-nitrophenol, 1 mmole/L

   Dissolve 139.1 mg pure p-nitrophenol in water at 25° C to make 1 L. (The stock standard obtained from Sigma Chemical Co. [St. Louis] is satisfactory.) If the material appears to be markedly discolored, it may be purified by recrystallization from hot water and drying the crystals overnight in a vacuum dessicator over silica gel. The solution is stable for several months if it is stored in the dark.

Procedure: Prepare a blank by mixing together 2.8 ml of buffer and 0.2 ml of the substrate solution. For each sample determination, mix together 2.7 ml of buffer and 0.1 ml of serum. Warm to 30° C; then add 0.2 ml of the substrate solution (also previously warmed to 30° C), mix, and read sample against blank in 1 cm cuvet at 402.5 nm at 1 min intervals for 5-8 min.

Calculation: Calculate the absorbance change per minute. The activity is then calculated by the usual formula:

$$\mu\text{mole/min/L} = \frac{\Delta A}{\min} \times \frac{3.0 \times 1000}{18.8 \times 0.1} =$$
$$\frac{\Delta A}{\min} \times 1596 = \text{units/L}$$

where ΔA is the absorbance change per minute and 18.8 the absorptivity of p-nitrophenol. If convenient the sample may be read against water and a correction made, if necessary, for any slight change in the absorbance of the blank during the time of the test. If the instrument does not have a constant temperature cuvet or cuvet chamber it should not be used for short time kinetic assays. The temperature variation will produce imprecise and unacceptable results.

For cuvets with a light path other than 1 cm (and as a check on the 1 cm cuvets used and the reagent) the absorbance factor may be calculated as follows.

Dilute 2, 3, and 4 ml of the stock p-nitrophenol standard to 1 dl with buffer at 25° C. Read these solutions against a blank of the buffer at 402.5 nm and 30° C; then calculate the absorptivity factor for use with the cuvets as follows:

$$A' = A \times \frac{100}{a}$$

where A' is the absorptivity and A is the actual absorbance when *a* milliliters of the stock standard is diluted to 1 dl. The average absorptivity may be used in the calculations. With exactly 1 cm cuvets and a narrow

bandwidth instrument the determined absorptivity should be close to the theoretic value of 18.8.

Normal values and interpretation: The normal value of ALP by this method may be taken as 20-100 units/L in adults with slightly lower values below 50 years of age in women than in men. The activity in children varies greatly. In general the values rise markedly after birth to three to four times the adult values. The values fall somewhat at about 2-3 years of age to about two to three times the adult values where they remain until about 13 years of age. In females the values remain fairly constant until about 12-14 years of age when they gradually decrease, reaching the adult values at about 18 years of age. In males the values at 12-14 years of age are somewhat higher than in females and remain elevated longer. They do not reach the adult values until about 20-22 years of age.

ALP is elevated in liver disease with cholestasis (see discussion of liver function tests). In bone disease the alkaline phosphatase value is increased in those conditions in which bone regeneration is taking place. It is not found when there is bone destruction unless there is simultaneous formation of new bone or osteoid tissue. In rickets the increase is very marked, with the increases roughly paralleling the severity of the disease. Values from 800-2400 units/L may be found. In osteomalacia (adult rickets) there is some increase, but it is not as marked as in children. In Paget's disease, values over 1200 units/L are not unusual. In hyperparathyroidism the increase may be less marked (600 units/L). In bone tumors the findings are variable. The serum ALP value is usually normal in multiple myeloma.

Thus increased ALP activity is seen in all cases where increased osteoblastic activity occurs. This category includes children's normal rapid skeletal growth periods and the bone disorders described above as well as hyperparathyroidism where Ca^{++} is mobilized from bone. Under these conditions 5'-nucleotidase (NTP) activity is normal and can be used to distinguish the ALP elevations caused by bone disorders from those that occur as a result of hepatobiliary causes. During the third trimester of pregnancy, ALP elevations occur normally because of the placental isoenzyme.

Comment: Serum or heparinized plasma is the preferred sample since ALP is inhibited by oxalate, citrate, and EDTA, presumably by chelation of the Mg^{++} ion required for optimal activity. Hemolysis has little effect on most assays since red cells have low activity of ALP.

Phenolphthalein monophosphate method[84]

Principle: In the phenolphthalein monophosphate method the substrate is hydrolyzed to yield phenolphthalein, which gives a strong red color in alkaline solution. If has the advantages that the color is somewhat more intense than that from nitrophenol and the absorption maximum is much further from that of bilirubin, so that the interference from a high initial absorbance by this compound and from hemoglobin would be less if it is present in serum samples.

Phenolphthalein monophosphate + $H_2O \rightleftharpoons$

Phenolphthalein + Phosphoric acid

Reagents:

1. Stock substrate

   Dissolve 73.2 g 2-amino-2-methyl-l-propanol and 21.9 ml concentrated hydrochloric acid in water to make 250 ml. Dissolve in this 0.39 g of dicyclohexylamine salt of phenolphthalein monophosphate (Warner-Chilcott Laboratories, Morris Plains, N.J.). The concentration of the active substrate is then 26 mmole/L. This stock solution is stable for several months in the refrigerator. It should be warmed to room temperature before diluting.

2. Color stabilizer, phosphate buffer, 0.1 mole/L, pH 11.2

   Dissolve 9.3 g $Na_3PO_4 \cdot 12H_2O$ and 12.8 g $Na_2HPO_4 \cdot 2H_2O$ in water to make 1 L.

3. Stock standard

   Dissolve 79.5 phenolphthalein in ethanol and dilute to 1 dl in a volumetric flask. Store in refrigerator in brown tightly stoppered bottle. This contains 2.50 mmole/L phenolphthalein.

4. Working standard

   As required dilute a portion of the stock standard 1:50 with water. This contains 50 μmole/L.

Procedure: Dilute a portion of the stock substrate 1:10 with water and transfer 1 ml aliquots to a number of test tubes. Place in water bath to warm to 37° C. To one tube add 0.1 ml serum, mix, and replace in water bath. Incubate for exactly 20 min; then add 5 ml of the color stabilizer and mix. When a number of samples are run the sera can be added to the successive tubes at 1 min intervals and the color stabilizer added exactly 20 min later for each tube.

The tubes are then read in a spectrophotometer at 550 nm against a blank; 0.1 ml of water is added to 1 ml of the substrate followed by 5 ml of the color stabilizer.

The results are then read from a standard curve obtained as follows. To separate tubes add, respectively, 1, 2, 3, and 4 ml of the working standard. To these tubes add, respectively, 5.1, 4.1, 3.1, and 2.1 ml of the color stabilizer. This will give a total volume of 6.1 ml in each tube, the same as in the sample tubes, which contain 0.1 ml serum, 1 ml substrate, and 5 ml color stabilizer. Read the absorbance of these tubes at 550 nm against the same blank as used for the serum samples.

Calculation: The lowest standard contains 1 ml of a solution containing 50 μmole/L. The definition of the international unit (IU) is that amount of enzyme that will decompose 1 μmole of the substrate per minute per liter of serum. Since the samples contain 0.1 ml of serum and are incubated for 20 min, the lowest standard is equivalent to 50/(0.1 × 20), or 24 units/L, and the other standards are equivalent to 50, 75, and 100 units/L, respectively. The absorbances are plotted against the units and the activity of the samples read off from the curve. If the activity of one sample is above the upper limit of the curve, the solution may be diluted 1:2, the absorbance measured, and the result from the curve multiplied by two. For even higher values the determination should be repeated using a 1:5 dilution of the serum.

Initially the standards should be run with every batch of serum samples. If there is good agreement between the successive sample runs, they may be omitted for routine work but the sample curve should be checked occasionally.

Normal values: The normal range by this method is 9-35 units/L.

Alkaline phosphatase isoenzymes

Serum ALP may be derived from the liver, bone, intestinal mucosa, placenta, and certain tumors.[85] The placental ALP will be found only during pregnancy and is heat stable. It is not inactivated by heating for 30 min at 56° C. The serum ALP activity is elevated in a number of diseases of bone and liver.

In order to differentiate the tissue of origin, many technics have been used. Elevations of total activity are more meaningful if the source of isoenzyme contributing to the elevation can be identified. Isoenzymes have been evaluated by inhibition studies,[85-87] electrophoresis,[88] and sensitivity to heat.[89,90]

The most commonly used methods are electrophoresis and sensitivity to heat, but electrophoresis has poor resolution. The sensitivity to heat method is simple to perform but can be difficult to interpret because of the overlap between bone and liver isoenzymes.

Heat inactivation[90]: One method for distinguishing between the ALP isoenzymes from **bone** and those from **liver** is by heat inactivation. Using tissue extracts, the bone isoenzyme was found to be about 90% inhibited by heating at 55° C for exactly 16 min, while the isoenzyme from liver is only about 50% inhibited. Thus if in a serum with an elevated ALP value, more than 70% activity is lost on heating as described, the rise is probably caused by bone disease. If the percent inhibition is less than 65%, the increased ALP value is probably caused by liver disease. Unfortunately, although the bone isoenzyme seems to be fairly constant in degree of inhibition, the liver and the intestinal isoenzymes are more variable, thus detracting from the value of the method.

Moss and Whitby[90] have studied procedure and suggest using two time points to eliminate some of the variability of the one point method. They suggest removing an aliquot at 15 min and at 25 min. ALP activity is determined by the *p*-nitrophenyl phosphate method and the results plotted on semilog paper. The 15 min and 25 min activities are extrapolated to zero time to determine the percent "liver" ALP. The "liver" ALP so determined will be composed of liver as well as intestinal and placental forms.

At most the heat inactivation or other methods could serve as a guide but not as a positive diagnostic test.

One other ALP isoenzyme might be mentioned. The **placenta** is the source of an isoenzyme that is very heat stable. Even heating at 55° C for 30 min will cause no appreciable inhibition. The value of placental ALP has been suggested as a measure of placental function. Some of the albumin solutions used for intravenous administration are prepared from cord blood, which contains a large amount of placental ALP. After the administration of such a solution the patient may have an elevated ALP value. If this is suspected, it can be checked by heating a portion of the serum to 55° C for 30 min. If an appreciable amount of enzyme activity remains, the serum contains some placental ALP.

Tumors involving bone increase the bone ALP fraction, provided they lead to osteoblastic proliferation[91]; purely osteolytic lesions are not accompanied by ALP elevations.

The presence of elevated liver isoenzyme values does not distinguish between primary or metastatic liver carcinoma or other liver diseases resulting in extrahepatic or intrahepatic biliary obstruction.

A heat-stable placental type of ALP isoenzyme has also been identified in the serum in a variety of cancers and is called the **carcinoplacental antigen.**[92,93]

Increased urinary ALP levels have been reported in 90% of patients with renal cell carcinomas,[94] although similar levels are found in a low percentage of nonneoplastic urinary tract diseases.[95]

γ-Glutamyl transferase (GGT) (EC 2.3.2.2; [γ-glutamyl] peptide: amino acid γ-glutamyl transferase)

Principle: The enzyme γ-glutamyl transferase[96,97] catalyzes the transfer of a γ-glutamyl group from a γ-glutamyl peptide to an amino acid or other peptide. The usual method for determining the reaction is as follows:

γ-Glutamyl nitroanilide + Glycylglycine $\overset{GGT}{\rightleftharpoons}$

4-Nitroaniline + Glutamyl glycylglycine

The reaction is followed by measuring the absorbance of the liberated nitroaniline at 405 nm. Usually a blank is run to compensate for the small amount of spontaneous hydrolysis of the substrate.

Reagents:

1. Buffer, 110 mmole/L, pH 8.6 25° C
   Dissolve 5.78 g 2-amino-2-methyl-1,3-propanediol in about 4 dl water. Adjust to a pH of 8.6 by the addition of 1 mole/L hydrochloric acid (8 ml of concentrated acid diluted to 1 dl). This will require about 35 ml of acid. Then dilute to 5 dl and mix well. This buffer is stable for several months in the refrigerator.

2. Combined reagent
   Dissolve 126 mg γ-glutamyl nitroanilide (4.4 mmole/L) and 727 mg glycylglycine (55 mmole/L) in 1 dl of the buffer by warming to about 50° C with constant stirring. The material dissolves very slowly but should not be warmed above 60° C, since this will tend to decompose the nitroanilide. The material tends to crystallize out on standing and should be stored at room temperature. The solution is stable for only 3-5 days and should not be used if any material has crystallized out or if the absorbance read vs. buffer is more than 0.7 units. (NOTE: A different substrate, γ-glutamyl-3-carboxy-4-nitroanilide is available commercially [Biodynamics/bmc, Boehringer Mannheim Corp. Indianapolis]. It is more soluble than the reagent used above and thus avoids some of the problems encountered with the usual substrate, but it has no other great advantage.)

Procedure: Place 1.0 ml of the combined reagent in a cuvet having a 1 cm light path and warm to 30° C. Add 100 μl serum and mix. Read the absorbance against water at 405 nm at 2 min intervals for 10-15 min. Calculate the change in absorbance per minute. Run a blank by adding 100 μl water to 1.0 ml of the reagent, warm to 30° C, and measure the change in absorbance at 0 and 15 min. Calculate the change in absorbance per minute for the blank and subtract this from the sample absorbance change per minute.

Calculation: If the cuvet has an exactly 1 cm light path then

$$\text{units/L} = \frac{\Delta A}{\text{min}} \times 1110$$

where ΔA is the corrected absorbance change per minute. The factor "1110" is obtained in a similar manner to those given earlier, with 0.1 ml serum, 1.1 ml total volume, and 9.9 for the absorbance factor.

To determine the factor experimentally, dissolve 68.1 mg pure p-nitroaniline in about 90 ml of water using a minimum (5-10 drops) of 1 mole/L hydrochloric acid to aid solution, and dilute to 1 dl. This contains 500 μmole/L. To three cuvets add 1 ml of the complete reagent. To one add 100 μl water. To the other two add 100 μl of the above standard. Mix and read the two standards against the blank. Average the absorbance of the standard tubes. Since an absorbance change per minute of the amount measured would be equivalent to 500 units/L, the factor to use in place of the 1110 given earlier would then be F = 500/A where A is the average of the two absorbance measurements with the standard.

Normal values and interpretation: Using the above method the normal range is 4-25 units/L at 30° C for women and 7-40 units at 30° C for men. Increased values of the enzyme in human serum have been found almost entirely in hepatobiliary diseases, except that values up to 140 units/L at 30° C may be found in neonates (with values to 250 units/L at 30° C in premature infants). The results decrease to the adult values within the first 2 years of life. Very high values (up to 2000 units/L) of enzyme indicate cholestasis. In the absence of obstructions to biliary flow, high values indicate toxic liver damage. The value is not increased in bone disease or pregnancy, and this helps to differentiate the cause of high values of ALP. Other conditions that cause decreased hepatic blood flow, e.g., myocardial infarction, may cause some increase in the value of the enzyme.

5'-Nucleotidase (NTP) (EC 3.1.3.5; 5'-ribonucleotide phosphohydrolase)

Principle: The enzyme 5'-nucleotidase[98] hydrolyzes a large number of nucleotides by the following reaction:

5'-Nucleotide + H_2O $\overset{NTP}{\rightleftharpoons}$ Nucleoside + Orthophosphate

The above reaction with adenosine 5'-monophosphate as a substrate is used in the present determination. The liberated phosphate is determined by a simple method that does not require the precipitation of the proteins.

Other nonspecific phosphatases will also hydrolyze some of the nucleotide. The determination is made more specific by performing the reaction twice, once in the presence of manganous ions, which activate the nucleotidase, and a second time in the presence of nickel ions, which strongly inhibit only the nucleotidase. Thus the difference in the phosphate released in the two tests is a measure of the nucleotidase present.

Reagents:
1. Barbiturate buffer, 50 mmole/L, pH 7.5
   Dissolve 10.31 g sodium diethylbarbiturate in about 8 dl water in a 1 L volumetric flask. Adjust to a pH of 7.50 by the addition of 0.1 mole/L hydrochloric acid (about 30 ml will be required); then dilute to volume with water and mix well. Store in the refrigerator.
2. Buffer, 50 mmole/L, with nickel, 7.6 mmole/L
   Dissolve 951 mg nickel chloride hexahydrate in buffer to make 5 dl.
3. Buffer, 50 mmole/L, with manganese, 2 mmole/L
   Dissolve 168 mg manganous sulfate monohydrate in buffer to make 5 dl.
4. Adenosine monophosphate (AMP), 13.3 mmole/L
   Dissolve 52 mg AMP sodium salt (Sigma type II, Sigma Chemical Co., St. Louis) in 10 ml buffer. This may be kept in the refrigerator for a few days, but it is preferably made up fresh as needed.
5. Stock phosphate standard, 20 mmole/L
   Dissolve 1.361 g dried reagent grade KH_2PO_4 in water to make 5 dl.
6. Working phosphate standard, 0.2 mmole/L
   Dilute the stock standard 1:100 with water. Make up fresh as required.
7. Ascorbic acid, 0.23 mmole/L
   Prepare a solution of approximately 0.35 mmole/L sulfuric acid by diluting 10 ml of concentrated acid to 5 dl with water. As needed dissolve 1 g ascorbic acid in 25 ml sulfuric acid solution. This solution is stable for only a few days in the refrigerator.
8. Teepol 610*
   Dilute an aliquot of this solution with an equal volume of water.
9. Molybdate solution
   Dissolve 5 g ammonium molybdate in water to make 5 dl.
10. ACD solution
    Dissolve 20.0 g anhydrous sodium arsenite and 20.0 g sodium citrate dihydrate in about 3 dl water, add 20 ml glacial acetic acid, and mix. Then add 4 dl dimethyl sulfoxide and dilute to 1 L with water.

Procedure: For each determination set up two tubes. To the sample (s) tube add 500 μl of the buffer with manganese; to the sample blank (SB) tube add 500 μl of the buffer with nickel. Place tubes in 37° C water bath for about 5 min. Then add 25 μl of serum sample

*A sulfonated fatty acid detergent made by Shell Oil Co.

to each tube, mix, and incubate for exactly 30 min at 37° C.

While the samples are incubating prepare a standard tube (STD) by adding 500 μl of the working standard to one tube, and a reagent blank (RB) by adding 500 μl of water to another tube. These tubes are not incubated but are treated exactly like the tubes containing serum after incubation.

After incubation add, in order, to each tube, with brief vortex mixing between additions, 0.5 ml ascorbic acid solution, 0.25 ml Teepol, 0.5 ml molybdate solution, and 1.0 ml ACD reagent.

Allow tubes to stand for 10 min and then read in a spectrophotometer at 700 nm.

Calculation: Read sample (S) against sample blank (SB) and standard (STD) against reagent blank (RG); then if A_x is the absorbance reading of the sample and A_s is the absorbance reading of the standard:

$$units/L = \frac{A_x}{A_s} \times \frac{0.2}{0.025} \times \frac{0.500}{30} = \frac{A_x}{A_s} \times 133$$

since 0.500 ml of standard containing 0.2 mmole/L (0.2 μmole/ml) is compared with 0.25 ml of sample and the incubation period is 30 min. The above procedure gives a final total volume of 2.78 ml. If this is not sufficient for the spectrophotometer used, all the quantities in the procedure may be doubled.

Normal values and interpretation[99-102]: The normal range by this method has been reported as 0-12 units/L at 37° C. The enzyme is markedly increased in liver disease, especially when the hepatobiliary tree is involved. The enzyme is at the most only slightly elevated in bone disease and thus is of value in distinguishing between liver and bone disease. The enzyme is much more sensitive to metastatic liver carcinoma than ALP since it is not markedly elevated in other conditions, e.g., pregnancy, or in childhood, both of which cause increases in ALP. Some increase in the enzyme activity may be noted after surgery.

Ferroxidase I (EC 1.16.3.1; iron [II]: oxygen oxidoreductase)

Principle: The enzyme ferroxidase I was commonly known as ceruloplasmin. It is a protein containing a relatively large amount of copper, and when isolated it has a blue color—hence its name. It is now classified as an iron oxidase catalyzing the following basic reaction:

$$4\text{-Iron (II)} + 4H^+ + O_2 \rightleftharpoons 4\text{-Iron (III)} + 2H_2O$$

It catalyzes the oxidation of a number of aromatic amines to colored products, and this is the usual basis for its determination.[103,104] *p*-Phenylenediamine has been used, but *o*-dianisidine is preferred since the latter is less subject to nonenzymatic oxidation in the analysis.

Reagents:
1. Acetate buffer, pH 5.0, ionic strength 0.1
   Add about 9 dl water to a 1 L volumetric flask. Dissolve 13.61 g sodium acetate trihydrate and 2.6 ml glacial acetic acid in the flask. Check the pH and adjust to 5.0 by the addition of small

amounts of 0.1 mole/L sodium hydroxide or acetic acid, then dilute to 1 L, and mix well. Store in the refrigerator.

2. Sulfuric acid, 9 moles/L
   Cautiously add, with mixing, 2 dl concentrated sulfuric acid to an equal volume of water.

3. o-Dianisidine dihydrochloride, 8 mmole/L
   Dissolve 253 mg o-dianisidine hydrochloride in water and dilute to 1 dl. Store in refrigerator in amber bottle.

Procedure: To two tubes labeled blank and sample add 0.75 ml of the buffer and 50 µl of serum. Place tubes in water bath at 30° C for about 5 min to allow temperature equilibrium; then add at timed intervals 0.2 ml of the dianisidine solution to each tube. Exactly 5 min after the addition of the dianisidine to the blank tube remove it from the water bath and add 2 ml of the sulfuric acid solution and mix well. Exactly 15 min after the addition of the dianisidine to the sample tube remove it from the water bath and add 0.2 ml of the sulfuric acid solution. After tubes have cooled to room temperature, read sample against blank at 540 nm in cuvets with a 1 cm light path.

Calculation:

$$\text{units/L at 30° C} = \frac{\Delta A}{\min} \times 625$$

The factor "625" is derived as given earlier using a 10 min incubation time, 0.05 ml sample, 3 ml total volume, and 9.6 as the absorption coefficient for the colored substance formed.

Normal values and interpretation: By this method the range of normal values is 60-140 units/L. Concentrations below the lower limit have been reported in patients with Wilson's disease, in the neonatal period, in the nephrotic syndrome, and occasionally in unaffected relatives of patients with Wilson's disease. There may be a deficiency of ferroxidase I in patients with kwashiorkor and tropical sprue and in certain infants with a syndrome of anemia and hypoproteinemia.

Increased concentrations of ferroxidase I have been noted in pregnancy, subacute or chronic infection, myocardial infarction, hepatic cirrhosis, hyperthyroidism, aplastic or refractory anemia, Hodgkin's disease, acute leukemia, and cirrhosis and in patients receiving estrogen therapy, including oral contraceptives. The ferroxidase I activity generally parallels the copper content of the serum.

In Hodgkin's disease a fall in ferroxidase I activity may be the first sign of successful therapy.[105]

The physiologic function of the enzyme has been unclear. The principle function now seems to be that of a catalyst which oxidizes Fe^{++} to Fe^{+++}, helping to transport iron across the intestinal wall. The enzyme thus enables the iron to bind to apotransferrin, forming transferrin, and helps to mobilize iron from storage.[106] A noneeruloplasmin ferroxidase (ferroxidase II), which has no amine oxidase activity has been isolated from serum samples.[107] This material has been said to account for 15% of the total ferroxidase activity in humans and nearly 100% of the activity in patients with Wilson's disease.

• • •

The following enzyme assays for hepatic evaluations are used much less frequently than the preceding assays. In many uncomplicated cases no additional information is gained by using these assays.

Ornithine carbamyltransferase (OCT)

(EC 2.1.3.2; carbamoyl phosphate: L-ornithine carbamoyl transferase)

Principle: The enzyme ornithine carbamyltransferase catalyzes the following reaction:

Ornithine + Carbamoyl phosphate ⇌
Citrulline + Orthophosphate

This reaction is involved in the synthesis of urea. The usual method for the determination of the citrulline formed is to add urease to remove any urea present and then react the citrulline with diacetyl monoxime and antipyrine in a method similar to that used for serum urea. A method[108,109] is given using a timed reaction, which is stopped by the addition of trichloroacetic acid. The proteins are precipitated, and the citrulline is determined in an aliquot of the supernatant after centrifugation.

Reagents:

1. Triethanolamine buffer, 0.4 mole/L, pH 7.7
   Dissolve 74.2 g triethanolamine hydrochloride in about 9 dl water. Adjust to a pH of 7.7 with 1 mole/L sodium hydroxide (4 g sodium hydroxide to 1 dl water) and then dilute to 1 L.

2. Buffered urease
   Dissolve 200 mg urease (Sigma type IX [Sigma Chemical Co., St. Louis], 5000 units/g) in 2 dl triethanolamine buffer.

3. Carbamyl phosphate, 50 mmole/L
   Just before use dissolve 150 mg carbamyl phosphate, dilithium salt, in 20 ml of buffer.

4. Diacetyl monoxime, 100 mmole/L
   Dissolve 10.1 g diacetyl monoxime in water to make 1 L.

5. Antipyrine reagent
   Dissolve 12.2 g (65 mmole) antipyrine and 3.4 g $FeCl_3 \cdot 6H_2O$ (12.5 mmole) in a mixture of 625 ml phosphoric acid (85%) and 375 ml water.

6. Citrulline standard, 15 mmole/L
   Dissolve 263 mg citrulline in water to make 1 dl.

7. Trichloroacetic acid, 0.67 mole/L
   Dissolve 22 g trichloroacetic acid in water to make 1 dl.

Procedure: For the determinations set up a series of tubes as given in Table 24-4. A sample blank must be run for each sample, but one reagent blank can be used for a whole series. Warm the tubes to 30° C; then at timed intervals add 0.4 ml carbamyl phosphate solution to tubes 1 and 3 and 0.4 ml urease solution to tube 2. Mix well and incubate for 30 min; then stop reaction by addition of 1.0 ml of the trichloroacetic acid to each tube. Mix and centrifuge at 5000 rpm for 10 min. Transfer 1 ml of the supernatant to marked tubes and add 4 ml antipyrine reagent and 1 ml diacetyl monoxime reagent. Heat in a boiling water bath for 20 min. Then place tubes in cold water in the dark for 10 min. Bring to room temperature and read against a water blank at 460 nm.

Table 24-4. Tube setup for determination of ornithine carbamyl transferase

	1 (sample)	2 (sample blank)	3 (reagent blank)
Buffer (ml)	—	0.4	0.1
Ornithine solution (ml)	0.4	—	0.4
Serum or plasma	0.1	0.1	—

Calculation: For calculations subtract the absorbances of tubes 2 and 3 from that of tube 1. Then calculate the activity by means of a factor determined as outlined below.

Standardization: Dilute the stock solution of citrulline 1:50 and 1:100 giving solutions containing 150 and 300 μmole/L. Treat 0.1 ml aliquots of these the same as for serum except that the 30 min incubation is not required and centrifugation is not necessary after the addition of the trichloroacetic acid. Since 1 unit is defined as the activity that produces 1 μmole of citrulline per minute per liter or 30 μmole/30 min/L, the above standards correspond to 150/30 = 5 and 300/30 = 10 units/L. A factor, K, may be calculated as K = absorbance of standard/units of standard and an average value of K used in the calculations as units in sample = K × net absorbance of sample. When the procedure is first set up a number of standards should be run (including, if desired, a higher standard such as a 1:25 dilution of the stock standard, which would be equivalent to 20 units). Later an occasional standard may be run to check the factor.

Normal values and interpretation: Normally the activity of the enzyme in serum is very low, often below 2 units/L. The normal range is 0-5 units/L.

Serum levels are markedly elevated in patients with acute viral hepatitis and those with other forms of hepatic necrosis. Only small elevations occur in obstructive jaundice, cirrhosis, or metastatic carcinoma. Slight elevations may sometimes occur after myocardial infarction if there is congestive liver involvement. Serum levels are usually normal in muscular dystrophy and bone diseases.

Isocitrate dehydrogenase (ICD) (EC 1.1.1.41; threo-D-isocitrate: NADP oxidoreductase [decarboxylating])

Principle: The enzyme isocitrate dehydrogenase catalyzes the conversion of isocitrate into oxalosuccinate, which is immediately decarboxylated to α-ketoglutarate (hence the qualification, decarboxylating, in the EC name).

$$\text{Isocitrate} + \text{NADP}^+ \underset{\text{ICD}}{\rightleftharpoons} \text{NADPH} + \\ \text{H}^+ + \alpha\text{-Ketoglutarate} + \text{CO}_2$$

This enzyme is activated by manganese ions, which are added to the reaction mixture. The reaction is usually followed by noting the change in absorbance at 340 nm.[110,111]

Reagents:
1. Tris buffer, 100 mmole/L, pH 7.4
   Dissolve 12.1 g tris (hydroxymethyl)aminomethane in about 750 ml of water. Adjust pH to 7.4 by the addition of 1 mole/L hydrocloric acid (83 ml concentrated acid diluted to 1 L); about 80-90 ml will be required.
2. Manganous chloride, 50 mmole/L
   Dissolve 1.0 g $MnCl_2 \cdot 4H_2O$ in water to make 1 dl. Store in the refrigerator.
3. NADP, 13 mmole/L
   Dissolve 20 mg NADP sodium salt in 2 ml water. This must be made up fresh as required. It is convenient to use preweighed vials containing 10 mg of the salt (Sigma Chemical Co., St. Louis). Add 1 ml water to a vial as needed.
4. Substrate solution: D,L-isocitrate, 68 mmole/L
   Dissolve 100 mg D,L-isocitrate, trisodium salt, in 5 ml of the buffer.

Procedure: Because of the low values found in normal serum samples and the large amount of sample used, it is preferable to run a blank with every determination. For each patient set up a pair of cuvets with a 1 cm light path and add 1.2 ml of buffer, 0.1 ml of manganese solution, 0.1 ml of the NADP solution, and 1.0 ml of serum. Incubate at 30° C for 10 min; then add 0.6 ml of the substrate solution to the sample cuvet and 0.6 ml of the buffer to the blank. Allow mixture to incubate for 5 min and then read at 340 nm at 1 min intervals to obtain the average absorbance change per minute. Either the sample can be read against the blank, or the sample and blank may be read separately against water and the difference in absorbance change determined.

Calculation: The results are calculated using the following equation:

$$\text{Units/L} = \frac{\Delta A}{\min} \times 480$$

Normal values and interpretation: By the method given the normal range is 1.5-7.0 units/L. It is higher in newborns but decreases to the adult value within a few weeks. Significantly elevated values have been reported in viral hepatitis and in about half of patients with metastatic carcinoma of the liver. However, the determination of this enzyme does not appear to offer any marked advantage over the more commonly determined AST and ALT in liver disease.

Malate dehydrogenase (MD) (EC 1.1.1.37; L-malate: NAD oxidoreductase)

The enzyme malate dehydrogenase[112,113] catalyzes the following reaction:

$$\text{Malate} + \text{NAD}^+ \underset{\text{MD}}{\rightleftharpoons} \text{Oxalacetate} + \text{NADH} + \text{H}^+$$

The reaction may be run in the direction indicated and the course followed by the change in absorbance at 340 nm, or the oxalacetate formed may be determined by reaction with a diazotized dye intermediate. In some methods the reaction is run in the reverse direction. Since oxalacetate is not very stable it is formed as required by the addition of α-ketoglutarate, aspartate, and the enzyme aspartate aminotransferase (AST); the following reaction occurs:

$$\alpha\text{-Ketoglutarate} + \text{Aspartate} \overset{\text{AST}}{\rightleftharpoons} \text{Glutamate} + \text{Oxalacetate}$$

In general the changes in MD levels with disease are similar to those with the more commonly determined AST and LD, and the determination is not widely used.

Sorbitol dehydrogenase (SD; iditol dehydrogenase) (EC 1.1.1.14; iditol: NAD$^+$ 5-oxidoreductase)

The enzyme sorbitol dehydrogenase[114,115] also catalyzes the oxidation of some other isomeric polyalcohols. The reaction generally used for the determination is as follows:

$$\text{Fructose} + \text{NADH} + \text{H}^+ \overset{\text{SD}}{\rightleftharpoons} \text{Sorbitol} + \text{NAD}^+$$

The reaction is carried out in a tris buffer (0.09 mole/L; pH 6.6) with a substrate concentration of 0.5 mole/L and an NADH$^+$ concentration of 250 μmole/L at 37° C. Under these conditions the normal range is 0-2.6 units/L.

The enzyme is markedly elevated in hepatitis, moderately elevated in obstructive jaundice, and only slightly increased in other liver diseases. It is said to be a good index of acute hepatic anoxia. The enzyme activity is generally normal in nonhepatic diseases.

Glutamate dehydrogenase (GMD) (EC 1.4.1.3; L-glutamate: NAD[P] oxidoreductase [deaminating])

The reaction catalyzed by the enzyme glutamate dehydrogenase[116,117] is as follows:

$$\text{Glutamate} + \text{NAD}^+ + \text{H}_2\text{O} \overset{\text{GMD}}{\rightleftharpoons} \alpha\text{-Ketoglutarate} +$$
$$\text{NADH} + \text{NH}_4^+$$

The NAD(P) in the EC name means that either NAD or NADP can be used in the reaction. An amino group is removed from the glutamate, hance the qualification of "deaminating" in the EC name. The most common method for the determination of glutamic dehydrogenase is by measuring the change in absorbance at 340 nm in accordance with the above equation.

GMD is another of the enzymes present chiefly in the liver, and the activity in serum is usually normal in nonhepatic diseases. In liver disease the relative increase in the serum value is usually less than that of AST. The ratio of GMD to AST is usually higher in hepatitis and other diseases involving extensive diffuse parenchymal damage and lower in conditions involving localized but more severe damage. The determination of the enzyme is still used to some extent in Europe but is seldom used in the United States.

Arginase (EC 3.5.3.1; L-arginine amidinohydrolase)

The enzyme arginine[118-120] catalyzes one of the steps in the formation of urea in the liver:

$$\text{Arginine} + \text{H}_2\text{O} \rightleftharpoons \text{Ornithine} + \text{Urea}$$

The enzyme is usually determined by measuring the amount of urea formed when the enzyme is incubated with a substrate of arginine and manganous ions as an activator. The urea formed may be determined by the use of diacetyl monoxime or urease and phenol-hypochlorite as given earlier in the methods for the determination of blood urea nitrogen. A blank determination is carried out to correct for the amount of preformed urea in the added serum. Since this enzyme, like ornithine carbamoyl transferase, is concerned with the formation of urea in the liver, changes in the blood level of the two enzymes may be expected to be similar in liver disease. The determination of this enzyme has no practical advantage over other more commonly determined enzymes in liver disease, and it is rarely determined. The enzyme may be decreased in serum in a rare congenital condition involving the enzymes of arginine metabolism in which there is an excessive amount of arginine in the blood and urine.

Guanine deaminase (GDS) (EC 3.5.4.3; guanine aminohydrolase) and adenosine deaminase (ADS) (EC 3.5.4.4; adenosine aminohydrolase)

The enzymes guanine deaminase[121-123] and adenosine deaminase[124-126] are both concerned with purine metabolism and are found chiefly in the liver. They catalyze similar reactions:

$$\text{Guanine} + \text{H}_2\text{O} \longrightarrow \text{Xanthine} + \text{Ammonia}$$

and

$$\text{Adenosine} + \text{H}_2\text{O} \longrightarrow \text{Inosine} + \text{Ammonia}$$

The enzyme activities are usually determined by measuring the amount of ammonia formed on incubation of the enzyme with the appropriate substrate. The ammonia is usually determined by means of the Berthelot reaction (see the determination of serum BUN [ammonia] given earlier). A blank determination may be made to correct for the small amount of ammonia originally present in the sample or formed by other reactions. It has been claimed that 8-azaguanine is a better substrate than guanine for the determination of guanase, but neither enzyme is commonly determined. The values of both enzymes are said to be elevated in liver disease, particularly in the acute forms with marked hyperbilirubinemia, with marked elevations occurring particularly with guanase. A number of isoenzymes of guanase have been found by agar gel electrophoresis, but the clinical value of these isoenzymes has not been established.

DIAGNOSIS OF MUSCLE DISORDERS

Elevated values of serum enzyme activity occur in neurogenic muscle atrophies, and results are temporarily elevated after muscle trauma, surgery, and intramuscular injections. The three enzymes used diagnostically are creatine kinase (CK), aspartate aminotransferase (AST), and aldolase (ALS), all of which are elevated in all types of muscular dystrophy. The largest changes are seen with Duchenne muscular dystrophy with CK activity sometimes becoming 50 times the upper limit of normal and AST and ALS becoming, respectively, 10 and six times the upper limit of normal. These activity levels fall with progression of the disease as muscle mass is decreased.

Aldolase (ALS; fructose diphosphate aldolase)
(EC 4.1.2.13; fructose-1,6-diphosphate: glyceraldehyde-3-phosphate lyase)

Principle: There are a number of aldehyde lyases that may properly be considered to be different aldolases, but the one given here is the one most commonly called merely aldolase. This enzyme takes part in the breakdown of glucose at the level of fructose-1,6-diphosphate. The reaction is as follows:

Fructose-1,6-diphosphate $\rightleftharpoons$ Dihydroxyacetone phosphate +

Glyceraldehyde-3-phosphate

In the procedure given below,[127] the enzyme triosephosphate isomerase is added; it converts the dihydroxyacetone phosphate into glyceraldehyde-3-phosphate. With the addition of glycerophosphate dehydrogenase and NADH the following reaction takes place:

Glyceraldehyde-3-phosphate + NADH + H$^+$ $\rightleftharpoons$

Glycerol phosphate + NAD$^+$

The reaction if followed by measuring the change in absorbance at 340 nm.

Reagents:
1. Tris buffer, 0.1 mole/L, pH 7.4
   Dissolve 12.1 g tris(hydroxymethyl)aminomethane in about 8 dl water. Add 1.0 mole/L hydrochloric acid (8.3 ml concentrated acid diluted to 1 dl with water); about 80 ml of acid will be required to bring the pH to 7.4. When pH has been adjusted to 7.4, dilute to 1 L and mix well.
2. NADH, 0.9 mmole/L
   Since this solution is very unstable and interfering substances may develop even when the solution is kept frozen, it is preferable to use the preweighed vials (Sigma Chemical Co., St. Louis) containing 5 or 10 mg NADH. Add 0.8 ml water to a vial containing 5 mg (or 1.6 ml to a 10 mg vial if a larger number of tests are to be run at one time).
3. Fructose-1,6-diphosphate (FDP), 22 mmole/L
   Dissolve 1.1 g FDP trisodium salt (Sigma Chemical Co., St. Louis) in 1 dl tris buffer. Dispense into 2 ml aliquots in vials, stopper tightly, and store at -20° C. Thaw only a sufficient amount for 1 day's use and store thawed material at 4° C.
4. Glycerophosphate dehydrogenase: triosephosphate isomerase (GD:TI), 10 mg/ml as an ammonium sulfate suspension
   That reagent obtained from Calbiochem-Behring Corp., San Diego, is satisfactory.

Procedure: In suitable cuvets having a 1 cm light

path, place 2.5 ml of buffer, 0.1 ml NADH solution, and 0.05 ml GD:TI enzyme mixture. Mix and then add 0.2 ml of serum. Warm to 30° C and allow to stand for 5 min. Then add 0.2 ml FDP solution previously warmed to 30° C, mix, and measure the absorbance change at 340 nm for 5 min or more.

Calculation: For calculations the usual formula is used:

$$\text{units/L} = \frac{3.05 \times 1000}{0.2 \times 6.22} \times \frac{\Delta A}{\min} = \frac{\Delta A}{\min} \times 2450$$

where ΔA is the absorbance change per minute.

Normal values and interpretation[128-130]: The normal values by this method are 7-14 units/L for females and 8.5-20 units/L for males. Significant elevations are found in acute infectious hepatitis, usually up to 20 times the average normal. Normal results are usually obtained in portal cirrhosis and obstructive jaundice.

A significant increase is also found in progressive muscular dystrophy (primary myopathy) and severe traumatic injury. No elevation is found in muscular dystrophy secondary to alterations of the nerves or nerve centers.

Increases in ALS activity have been reported after myocardial infarction, advanced prostatic carcinoma, hepatoma, large pulmonary infarcts, hemorrhagic pericarditis, erythroblastosis fetalis, acute pancreatitis, hemolytic anemia, chronic myelogenous leukemia, and polycythemia vera.

DIAGNOSIS OF PANCREATIC DISEASE

In inflammatory diseases of the pancreas, particularly acute pancreatitis, several enzymes have been used as diagnostic probes. Serum amylase (AMS), urine amylase, and serum lipase (LPS) have been the most widely used enzymes to help elucidate the diagnosis of pancreatitis. Many factors, including infections, obstruction, toxins, and trauma, may lead to a partial proteolytic pancreatic tissue destruction and subsequent release of these enzymes into the serum.

Amylase (AMS) (EC 3.2.1.1; α-1,4-glucan 4-glucanohydrolase)

Amylase is a low-molecular-weight (about 45,000) digestive enzyme that hydrolyzes starch into smaller molecular units. Starch is a long-chain, highly crosslinked polymer of glucose molecules. α-Amylase attacks the chain at random α-1,4-positions, breaking it down into smaller units and eventually into maltose, some glucose, and limit dextran. These former compounds will react with alkaline copper reagents, and the amount of reducing sugars formed is one method of determining AMS activity (saccharogenic method). Although this method is not used as much as formerly, it is still the reference method against which other methods are compared. Starch gives an intensely blue color with dilute iodine solutions. This is used in the determination of AMS activity by measuring the decrease in blue color formed after the action of the enzyme. Newer methods use a dye combined with a starch product in a relatively insoluble form. As the combined dye-starch is acted on by the enzyme, some of the dye is liberated into solution. At the end of the reaction period the excess dye-starch is removed and the amount of liberated dye in the solution is measured spectrophotometrically. These methods are usually calibrated against the saccharogenic method.

Saccharogenic method

Principle: A saccharogenic method[131,132] of Somogyi modified by Henry and Chiamori is given based on the determination of the amount of reducing sugars formed as AMS acts on a buffered starch solution.

Reagents:

1. Phosphate buffer, 0.1 mole/L, pH 7.0
   Dissolve 4.55 g KH_2PO_4 and 9.35 g Na_2HPO_4 in water to make 1 L. Check pH and adjust if needed.
2. Starch solution
   Add 1.5 g soluble starch (Lintner) to 1 dl of the phosphate buffer and heat to boiling for about 3 min. Cool and then add further buffer to a total volume of 140 ml. Add 1.2 g sodium benzoate as a preservative and dissolve. This solution should be stable at room temperature for several months if kept sterile.
3. Sodium chloride solution, 0.15 mole/L
   Dissolve 9 g sodium chloride in water to make 1 L.
4. Sodium tungstate, 0.3 mole/L, and sulfuric acid, 0.33 mole/L
   Dissolve 10 g sodium tungstate in 1 dl water. Separately add 5.5 ml concentrated sulfuric acid to 3 dl water.
5. Glucose standard, 200 mg/dl
6. Copper reagent
   Dissolve 40 g anhydrous sodium carbonate in about 4 dl water in a 1 L volumetric flask. Add 7.5 g tartaric acid and dissolve. Then add 4.5 g copper sulfate pentahydrate, dissolve, and dilute to volume.
7. Phosphomolybdic acid reagent
   Dissolve 40 g sodium hydroxide in about 8 dl water. Add 70 g molybdic acid and boil for about 30 min. Cool, add 250 ml of 85% orthophosphoric acid, mix, cool further if necessary, and dilute to 1 L.

Procedure: Generally the test may be run on undiluted serum or plasma; a 1:2 dilution of urine or a 1:25 dilution of duodenal contents is common, although with high activity, further dilutions may be required; in all cases saline is the diluent. To two tubes labeled sample and sample blank add 3.5 ml buffered starch solution. Warm to 37° C; then add 0.5 ml of the patient's serum to sample tube, mix, and incubate for exactly 30 min. At the end of the period add 0.75 ml sulfuric acid and 0.25 ml sodium tungstate to each tube and mix. Then add 0.5 ml of the patient's serum to sample blank tube and mix. While the above tubes are incubating, prepare standard and reagent blank tubes by adding 3.5 ml of the buffered substrate to each tube, 0.5 ml water to reagent blank tube, and 0.5 ml of the 200 mg/dl glucose standard to the standard tube. Add 0.75 ml sulfuric acid and 0.25 ml sodium tungstate to each tube and mix well. Centrifuge all tubes and if supernatant is not perfectly clear, filter through paper.

Pipet 1 ml of the separate filtrates to appropriately labeled 15 × 125 mm tubes. To each tube add 1 ml

alkaline copper reagent, mix, and heat in boiling water bath or heating block at 100° C for 6 min. Cool to room temperature and add 1 ml phosphotungstic acid and place in a boiling water bath for 5 min. Cool tubes and then add 10 ml water to each tube. Read sample tube, sample blank tube, and standard tube against reagent blank at 420 nm. If some readings are too low, readings may be made at a longer wavelength, but all tubes must be read at the same wavelength.

Calculation:

Somogyi units/dl =

$$\frac{\dfrac{\text{Absorbance}}{\text{of sample}} - \dfrac{\text{Absorbance}}{\text{of sample blank}}}{\text{Absorbance of standard}} \times 200$$

Normal values: The normal range is 60-180 units/dl.

Iodometric method

Principle: In the iodometric method[133,134] the amount of starch and the incubation time are adjusted so that only a portion of the starch is hydrolyzed when the reaction is stopped by the addition of iodine. The difference between the amount of blue color formed in the incubated sample and a blank prepared by the addition of the serum after incubation will be a measure of the amount of starch hydrolyzed and hence of the AMS activity of the sample.

Reagents:

1. Buffered starch substrate, pH 7.0
   Dissolve 4.30 g benzoic acid and 13.30 disodium phosphate (Na_2HPO_4) in about 250 ml water and heat to boiling. Mix 0.2 g soluble starch with 5 ml cold water in a small beaker. Add the starch suspension to the boiling solution while stirring. Rinse out the beaker with additional water to transfer all of the starch to the boiling solution. Boil for an additional minute. Allow the solution to cool and dilute to 5 dl. Store in the refrigerator. This solution is fairly stable, but there will be a tendency for molds to form. It may be preferable to use sterile water and sterile containers in the preparation, and the solution should be transferred aseptically to small sterile bottles. Usually containers that have been well washed and dried by heating in an oven will be sufficiently sterile. Not all brands of soluble starch will be equally satisfactory. Harleco's starch powder (Smith and Roe) and Harleco's starch reagent labeled "prepared according to Caraway" have been found satisfactory as well as Merck's soluble starch (Lintner). The starch labeled "prepared according to Somogyi" and some other starches may not be satisfactory for this method since they may cause turbidity in the final solution, which should be perfectly clear.
2. Stock iodine solution
   Dissolve exactly 3.567 g reagent grade potassium iodate and 45 g potassium iodide in about 8 dl water. Slowly add 9 ml concentrated hydrochloric acid while stirring. Cool and dilute to 1 L. Store in a brown bottle in the refrigerator. This solution is quite stable.

3. Working iodine solution
Dilute the stock 1:10 with water. Store in a brown bottle in the refrigerator. This solution should be prepared fresh each month.

Procedure: Add 5 ml buffered starch substrate to each of two 50 ml volumetric flasks, labeling one test and the other blank. If available, it may be convenient to use large test tubes graduated at 50 ml, e.g., nonprotein nitrogen digestion tubes. Place the two flasks in a water bath at 37° C for 5 min. Add 0.1 ml serum to test flask and mix well. Replace in bath and incubate for exactly 7.5 min. Remove from bath and add about 35 ml water and 5 ml working iodine solution. Remove blank tube from bath, add 0.1 ml serum, and then add at once 35 ml water and 5 ml iodine solution. Dilute contents of flasks to 50 ml and mix well. Read solutions in a spectrophotometer at 660 nm against water. Then

$$\frac{\text{Absorbance of blank} - \text{Absorbance of test}}{\text{Absorbance of blank}} \times 800 =$$

$$\text{Amylase units/dl}$$

If the reading is equivalent to over 400 units, an aliquot of the serum should be diluted with 0.9% sodium chloride and the test repeated, multiplying the result obtained by the appropriate dilution factor. Several samples can be run in one series by making the additions at timed intervals. A serum blank is required for each sample, since the serum proteins decrease the amount of color produced by the starch-iodine complex and this will be different for each serum. Urine or other body fluids can be run in a similar manner. At least once each day it is advisable to run a reagent blank, carrying out the above procedure on one flask without the addition of any serum. The resulting absorbance should be constant from day to day. A decrease in absorbance would indicate deterioration of the starch solution.

The upper limit of normal by this method is 60-180 units/dl thus the results are quite comparable with those by the saccharogenic method.

Dye methods*

A method was introduced for the determination of AMS that involves the use of a starch-dye complex. As the starch is hydrolyzed by the action of the AMS, some of the dye is liberated in free form. After incubation, the excess starch-dye complex is separated from the solution by precipitation with acid or alcohol or in some cases merely by centrifugation. The amount of dye remaining in the clear supernatant, as determined spectrophotometrically, is a measure of the amount of starch that has been hydrolyzed and thus of the enzyme activity. A number of different red and blue dyes have been used by several manufacturers.[135-139] At present this starch-dye complex is available commercially only as a component of a kit for AMS determination. Some kits require calibration against commercially available control sera or against sera that have been analyzed by

the saccharogenic method. Other kits may include a chart giving the activity in dye units that may not necessarily be the same as the customary Somogyi units.

Normal values and interpretation

The normal range of AMS by methods calibrated in Somogyi units is 60-180 units. Serum AMS is greatly increased in acute nonhemorrhagic pancreatitis early in the course of the disease, usually within 2-3 hr, and returns to normal usually within 3-6 days.[140,141] Values can rise as high as 500-600 units and in some cases 2000-3000 units. Increased activity may also be found in patients with perforated gastric or duodenal ulcers. Since AMS is normally cleared by glomerular filtration, renal disease may produce elevated serum values. Urine AMS also rises early in the course of pancreatitis but remains elevated longer.

Low serum values are seen in chronic pancreatitis and pancreatic carcinoma. The injection of morphine causes a temporary rise in serum AMS levels (up to 24 hr). Other narcotic analgesics may have a similar effect. Some increase in serum AMS activity has been reported following the ingestion of relatively large amounts of alcohol. Thiazide diuretics have also been reported to cause increases in serum AMS of up to 200%.

Since AMS is also produced by salivary glands, mumps leads to increased AMS levels.

Persistently elevated AMS values have been associated with pancreatic pseudocyst[142,143] and carcinoma.

Urine amylase

The same methods just described may be used merely by substituting urine for serum. A clean-voided, accurately timed specimen ranging from 2-24 hr is required. Thus

$$\text{units/hr} = \text{units/dl} \times \frac{\text{Total urine volume (ml)}}{100 \times \text{collection time (hr)}}$$

Normal values range from 35-260 units/hr.

Assays of urine AMS are useful[140] since the enzyme is found in urine for about 10 days after an attack of acute pancreatitis. Thus, when serum AMS activity is normal and pancreatitis is still suspected, the measurement of urine AMS with or without the creatinine ratio may be useful. Urine AMS may be used to distinguish rare cases of macroamylasemia[144,145] in which AMS is bound to IgG or IgA and is too large to be filtered normally. An increased serum AMS value in the presence of normal renal function suggests this condition. Hydroxyethyl starch, which has been used as a plasma expander, has been reported to induce macroamylasemia.[146,147]

There are a number of conditions in addition to macroamylasemia where an increased AMS value occurs in the absence of pancreatitis[143,148]; these include biliary tract disease, gastrointestinal disease, and some ectopic pregnancies.

Amylase creatinine clearance ratio

The ratio of the clearance of AMS to the clearance of creatinine[149] is about 1-4% in normal individuals.

---

*Dyamyl, General Diagnostics, Morris Plains, N.J.; Phadebas Amylase, Pharmacia Laboratories, Piscataway, N.J.; Amylochrome, Roche Diagnostics, Nutley, N.J.

$$\frac{\text{Urine AMS (units/dl)}}{\text{Serum AMS (units/dl)}} \times \frac{\text{Serum creatinine (mg/dl)}}{\text{Urine creatinine (mg/dl)}} \times$$

$$100\% = \text{Ratio}$$

In cases of pancreatitis, this ratio often rises to about 6% regardless of the method used to measure serum and urine AMS, and it was originally thought to be diagnostically very specific.[150]

This change is not specific for pancreatitis since other acute states, including diabetic ketoacidosis,[151] burns[152] severe renal insufficiency,[153] and duodenal perforation,[154] show increased ratios as well. About one third of individuals with pancreatitis do not show an increase in this ratio,[155] and the original authors have questioned the validity of using this ratio diagnostically.[156]

Amylase isoenzymes

By the use of cellulose acetate electrophoresis, serum AMS can be shown to be composed of six isoenzymes. There are three salivary isoenzymes (S_1-S_3) and three pancreatic isoenzymes (P_1-P_3),[157] but unlike CK and LD, the changes in isoenzyme patterns with disease do not necessarily reflect the tissue of origin.[158] The predominant isoenzyme pattern in normal individuals is S_1 and P_2[157,159] with 65% of the activity being salivary and the remainder pancreatic.[160,161]

Studies by Legaz and Kenny[159] found no AMS isoenzyme P_3 in 25 blood donors, but 40 patients with acute pancreatitis had substantial amounts of the P_3 band. None of 85 patients with nonpancreatic disease had the P_3 isoenzyme band except 37% of patients with severe renal disease. Assays of AMS isoenzymes remain to be more fully evaluated.

Comment

An important consideration in all methods for the determination of AMS is to take extra precautions to avoid any contamination of the reaction mixtures by saliva during pipetting, since saliva contains large amounts of the enzyme. Heparinized plasa or serum yields similar results, but citrate and EDTA anticoagulants are to be avoided because of the binding of Ca^{++}, which is essential for activity. The recovery of added AMS to lipemic serum samples depends on the method of assay. Iodometric procedures have low recoveries (i.e., 5%) of AMS activity, whereas saccharogenic or dye-binding methods give appropriate or high recoveries.[162]

Newer methods of AMS assay involve the use of defined substrates; i.e., maltopentose, as in the DuPont ACA method and assays (E.I. DuPont de Nemours & Co., Wilmington, Del.), coupled to glucose oxidase or hexokinase. Several of these methods have been evaluated in an attempt to produce a kinetic AMS assay.[163]

Lipase (LPS) (EC 3.1.1.3; triacylglycerol acyl-hydrolase)

Lipase is an enzyme that hydrolyzes fats into fatty acid and glycerol. Usually an aliquot of serum is incubated with a buffered emulsion of olive oil as substrate. The liberated fatty acids are then determined as a measure of the amount of hydrolysis. Methods have been tried using glycerol esters of short-chain fatty acids, e.g., glycerol butyrate, but it has been found that other enzymes in the serum will also hydrolyze these esters, and for a measure of true pancreatic lipase a true fat must be used as substrate.

Titrimetric method

Principle: In the titrimetric method the fatty acids liberated in the reaction are titrated with 50 mmole/L sodium hydroxide. Preferably the titration is carried out potentiometrically using a pH meter to determine the end point, or thymolphthalein can be used as the indicator. The amount of sodium hydroxide solution required to neutralize the liberated fatty acids is equivalent to the lipase units per milliliter of serum.[164-166]

Reagents and equipment:
1. Olive oil emulsion
   To 1 dl distilled water, add 200 mg sodium benzoate and 7 g gum arabic (acacia). Mix in a blender at low speed until dissolved. With the blender at low speed, slowly add 1 dl pure olive oil. Mix for an additional 10 min at high speed. This reagent should be kept at refrigerator temperature. Freezing or exposure to excessive heat will destroy the emulsion. A creamy layer on top of the emulsion may form during storage; shake the reagent thoroughly before using. Discard the reagent if excessive separation occurs after mixing. Olive oil should be purified as follows: To 3 dl pure olive oil, add 60 g aluminum oxide while stirring. Stir at 10 min intervals for 1 hr. Let the aluminum oxide settle and filter through Whatman no. 1 filter paper. The olive oil may be checked by mixing 5 ml purified oil with 5 ml ether and 5 ml 95% ethanol and titrating with thymolphthalein as indicator. If the titration requires more than 0.5 ml 0.05N sodium hydroxide, repeat the purification.
2. Stock tris buffer solution, 0.8 mole/L
   In a 5 dl volumetric flask dissolve 48.55 g tris(hydroxymethyl)aminomethane and dilute to volume.
3. Working buffer solution, 200 mmole/L
   Dilute 50 ml of the stock buffer and 21 ml of 1 mole/L hydrochloric acid to nearly 2 dl. Adjust the pH with additional hydrochloric acid as required to a value of 8.0 and dilute to 2 dl.
4. Sodium hydroxide, 50 mmole/L
   Dilute 5 ml of standardized 1 mole/L sodium hydroxide to 1 dl with water in a volumetric flask.
5. Thymolphthalein indicator
   Dissolve 1 g thymolphthalein in 1 dl of 95% ethanol.
6. Ethanol, 95%

As mentioned, the end point is best determined using a good pH meter and electrodes accurate to 0.01 pH. Also convenient is a magnetic stirrer with a small stirring bar.

Procedure: Into each of two test tubes labeled blank and test, pipet 2.5 ml water, 10 ml olive oil emulsion, and 1 ml working buffer. Mix; to the tube marked test add 1 ml serum and mix. Place both tubes in a water bath at 37° C for 3 hr. Next immediately pipet 1 ml of the serum into a 50 ml Erlenmeyer flask and store it in the refrigerator.

At the end of the incubation period, pour the contents of the blank tube into the cold blank flask containing test serum and pour the contents of the "test" tube into a clean Erlenmeyer flask labeled test. Rinse both tubes with 3 ml ethanol. Add washings to the respective flasks. Mix the contents of the flasks by rotation and add 4 drops thymolphthalein. With the use of an accurate buret, titrate both flasks with 0.05N sodium hydroxide to a light but distinct blue color (the test and blank must be titrated to the same color intensity). Icteric sera and some lighting conditions may cause the end-point color of titration to be grayish green rather than blue.

For potentiometric titration the procedure is similar although it may be more convenient to use large (25 mm diameter) test tubes for the titration vessels, clamping them above a magnetic stirrer with a small stirrer in the bottom of the tube. The indicator is also added, so that the pH need not be measured until the end point is approached. The titration is continued to a measured pH of 10.5. Preferably the electrodes should be standardized at a pH near 10 and the electrodes checked to determine that the magnetic stirring does not interfere with the electrode readings; i.e., the same pH reading is obtained with the stirrer on and off. If any interference is noted the stirrer should be turned off when pH readings are taken.

Calculation: The titration (in milliliters) of the blank is subtracted from that of the sample. The difference is then the number of milliliters of 50 mmole/L sodium hydroxide required to neutralize the fatty acids liberated from the lipid during the 3 hr incubation period. This figure is taken to be the numeric value of the enzyme activity in "conventional" units.

$$\text{Conventional units} = \text{ml in sample} - \text{ml in blank}$$

The factor for converting conventional units to international units is derived as follows; since 1 ml of serum was used, and since 1 ml of 50 mmole/L sodium hydroxide contains 50 μmole NaOH and thus is equivalent to 50 μmole fatty acid titrated, and since this fatty acid is liberated during a 3 hr period:

$$\frac{50 \times 1000}{3 \times 60} = 278$$

Thus international units per liter = conventional units × 280.

Normal values: The normal range by the method presented is 0-0.85 conventional units, which corresponds to 0-240 IU.

Spectrophotometric method[167-169]

The following alternative method for LPS requires an incubation time of only 30 min and eliminates the subjective errors in determining the titration end point. It requires more manipulations and careful technic to obtain good results.

Principle: The fatty acids liberated by the hydrolysis of the substrate are extracted with petroleum ether and an aliquot of the ether extract is evaporated to dryness. A buffered indicator solution is added to the residue of

the extracted fatty acids. The change in color of the indicator solution as a result of the acids is measured photometrically.

Reagents:
1. Olive oil

   Free a good-quality olive oil (reagent grade) from traces of fatty acids by mixing 25 ml oil with an equal volume of chromatography grade alumina for several minutes. Then filter the alumina out with a pledget of glass wool. Check the blank value by adding 0.05 ml oil to 3 ml methyl red reagent, shaking well, and then centrifuging to remove the excess oil (similar to the corresponding steps in the procedure below). The absorbance of the solution in 10 mm light path cuvets should not be more than 0.08 greater than the reagent alone. If it is greater, the oil should be further purified.

2. Buffer

   Add, in order, to about 8 dl water in a 1 L volumetric flask 2.42 g tris(hydroxymethyl)aminomethane, 3.5 g deoxycholic acid, and 0.2 g sorbic acid. When dissolved, dilute to 1 L and mix well.

3. Substrate

   Homogenize 5.0 ml purified olive oil with 1 dl buffer in a high-speed household blender. The blending should be done in short intervals of 30-60 sec, with periods of cooling between to avoid overheating the solution and consequent hydrolysis of some of the oil. The blending is continued until no film of oil is seen after the foam settles. The pH is now adjusted to 8.5 by the addition of 1 mole/L sodium hydroxide or hydrochloric acid. This solution is stable for at least 2 months in the refrigerator.

4. Absolute ethanol, reagent grade

5. Ethanol, 95%, reagent grade

6. Sulfuric acid, 0.14 mole/L

   Dilute 4 ml concentrated sulfuric acid to 5 dl with water.

7. Petroleum ether, reagent grade

8. Acid-alcohol mixture

   Mix together 3 volumes absolute ethanol and 2 volumes 0.14 mole/L sulfuric acid. This solution should be prepared fresh as needed.

9. Methyl red, 0.2%

   Dissolve 200 mg methyl red (reagent grade, free acid, not the sodium salt) in 1 dl 95% alcohol. The indicator dissolves rather slowly, requiring a day or more. This can be speeded up by using a magnetic stirrer.

10. Methyl red reagent (buffered indicator solution)

    Add 10 ml 1 mole/L to 1 L 95% alcohol. After mixing, add sufficient 0.2% methyl red solution (usually 10-13 ml is required) to bring the absorbance to 0.095-0.100 in 10 mm cuvets when read against alcohol at 500 nm. Then add 1 ml 1 mole/L sodium acetate (13.6 g trihydrate diluted to dl with water) while mixing with a magnetic stirrer. With continued mixing, add 1 mole/L hydrochloric acid, by drops, until a faint orange-red tinge remains. Measure the absorbance of the solution and carefully add further acid until the absorbance is 0.200 ± 0.005 in 10 mm cuvets. If too much acid has been added, carefully add 1 mole/L sodium hydroxide to bring the solution to the proper absorbance. The color of the solution may fade slightly at first, but it should then remain stable for at least 1 month when kept in a brown bottle at room temperature.

11. Standard solution

Dissolve 14.3 mg reagent grade stearic acid in 1 dl petroleum ether or hexane. The latter is preferred because of its somewhat higher boiling point. This solution contains 0.5 μmole/L.

Procedure: Use screw-capped culture tubes (16 × 100 mm) with Teflon-lined caps throughout.

Warm aliquots of the serum and substrate to 37° C in a water bath. To one tube (sample), add 1.0 ml substrate and 0.050 ml serum, cap, and incubate at 37° C for exactly 30 min. To a second tube (blank), add 1.0 ml substrate and incubate for 30 min. This will serve as a serum blank, and a separate tube must be set up for each sample. Also incubate separately at 37° C for 30 min a portion of the serum. After incubation, add 3.3 ml acid-alcohol to sample and blank tubes and then add 0.050 ml incubated serum to blank tube. Add 4 ml petroleum ether to all the tubes. Then cap and shake vigorously for 2 min and centrifuge at 2000 rpm for 5 min. Carefully pipet a 2.0 ml aliquot of the upper petroleum ether layer off and transfer to another tube. Take care not to pick up the slightest trace of the aqueous layer. Evaporate the ether at 50° C with the aid of a gentle stream of air. Set up three standards by carefully pipetting 0.25, 0.50, and 0.75 ml of the standard solution to tubes and evaporating off the solvent. Several sets of standards can be prepared at one time, since the evaporated residue is stable for several weeks in the refrigerator when kept in tightly stoppered tubes.

Add 3 ml methyl red reagent to each tube of standards, samples, and blanks. Then tightly cap the tubes and shake vigorously for 1 min. Centrifuge the samples and blanks for a short time at 2000 rpm to remove suspended oil. If the room temperature is too high, difficulty may be experienced in completely centrifuging down the oil. This can be remedied by cooling the tubes in the refrigerator for several minutes before centrifuging. The standards are not centrifuged, but care must be taken that all the material is dissolved.

Read standards, samples, and blanks at 502 nm against alcohol.

Calculation: Plot the absorbances of the three standards against the concentrations on linear graph paper. Since an aliquot of half of the original petroleum ether extract was used, the standards are equivalent to 0.25, 0.50, and 0.75 μmole in the sample. Read the concentration of each sample and its respective blank from the calibration curve.

Then

$$\left(\begin{array}{c} \text{μmole} \\ \text{in sample} \end{array} - \begin{array}{c} \text{μmole} \\ \text{in blank} \end{array} \right) \times 1 \times \frac{60}{30} = \text{Units of lipase}$$

since in this method the unit was defined as micromoles of fatty acid liberated per hour per milliliter of serum. To convert to international units, multiply the above

result by 1000/60 (= 16.67) to give micromoles per minute per liter.

If the sample reading is higher than that of the highest standard, dilute the sample tube and its corresponding blank with an equal volume of the reagent and read against alcohol. Calculate the units of activity as above and multiply the result by 2 to take into account the dilution. If necessary, a second dilution can be made with the appropriate change in the calculation.

Normal values and interpretation: The normal range by this method is 2.0-7.5 units as defined above, or 30-125 IU.

Elevated serum LPS values of 10 times the upper limit of normal and higher are found in acute pancreatitis. This enzyme rises as fast as AMS and remains elevated for about 7-10 days,[140,168] generally paralleling the increase and time course found for serum AMS. Either LPS or AMS or both enzymes rise in all cases of pancreatitis during the course of the disease.[170] In chronic pancreatitis the LPS level may be normal. Moderate increases are found in some cases of pancreatic carcinoma. Occasionally elevated values are found in kidney diseases, high intestinal obstruction, and duodenal ulcers penetrating into the pancreas.

LPS determination is an underutilized procedure that can help in the differential diagnosis when elevated serum AMS values are obtained. LPS values are normal in salivary diseases and macroamylasemia.

Comment: The results obtained on dilution are not always linear since the enzyme is acting at an oil-water interface. The pathologic changes observed in pancreatitis are large enough to make this a relatively unimportant problem.

Hemolysis at significant concentrations (i.e., 0.5 g/dl) produces a 50% inhibition of activity,[171] and therefore normal results from hemolyzed samples are probably incorrect.

Leucine arylamidase (LAP; amino acid arylamidase) (EC 3.4.1.1; aminoacyl-peptidase [cytosol])

Although the enzyme leucine arylamidase[172-174] has been known as leucine aminopeptidase (LAP) for many years, it is now classified under a more general term as an arylamidase. It is a proteolytic enzyme whose exact function in the body is unknown, and it apparently catalyzes a number of reactions of the following type:

$$\text{Aminoacyl-peptide} + H_2O \longrightarrow \text{Amino acid} + \text{Peptide}$$

Principle: The reaction used in the determination of leucine arylamidase is as follows:

$$\text{Leucyl-}p\text{-nitroanilide} + H_2O \longrightarrow \text{Leucine} + p\text{-Nitroaniline}$$

The amount of *p*-nitroaniline produced is measured at 405 nm.

Reagents:

1. Phosphate buffer, 0.1 mole/L, pH 7.2

Dissolve 2.04 g Na_2HPO_4 and 0.77 g KH_2PO_4 in water and dilute to 1 L. Check the pH and adjust to 7.2 by the addition of small amounts of 1 mole/L hydrochloric acid or sodium hydroxide as needed. This solution is stable for 1 year if kept refrigerated.

2. Leucine-*p*-nitroanilide reagent, 25 mmole/L
Dissolve 63 mg leucine-*p*-nitroanilide in 10 ml reagent grade methanol. This solution is stable for 6 months when stored in an amber bottle in the refrigerator.

Procedure: To several cuvets add 3 ml of buffer and 0.1 ml of the leucine-*p*-nitroanilide solution. Warm to 30° C; then add 0.1 ml of each unknown serum to separate cuvets and mix. Read absorbance at 405 nm for 2 min intervals for at least 10 min or until a linear rate is obtained.

Calculation: Calculate the absorbance change per minute. Then

$$\text{units/L} = \frac{\Delta A}{\min} \times \frac{1000 \times 3.2}{9.9 \times 0.1} = \frac{\Delta A}{\min} \times 3232$$

Procedure for urine: An overnight specimen is collected and the volume measured. An aliquot of 10 ml of the centrifuged urine is dialyzed against running deionized water in a cellulose casing for about 90 min. The dialysis is carried out similar to that for urinary LD. After dialysis use 0.1 ml urine in place of the serum and proceed exactly as given for serum, making a correction for any change in volume during dialysis as follows:

$$\text{units/L} \times \frac{\text{wt after dialysis}}{\text{wt before dialysis}}$$

Normal values and interpretation: The normal range for serum is 11-30 units/L with possibly slightly higher levels in men than in women. For an overnight (8 hr) urine specimen the normal range is 0.8-6.2 units/L for men and 0.2-4.7 units/L for women.

It was originally believed that elevations of leucine arylamidase were consistently found in carcinoma of the pancreas. However, this enzyme may be elevated in carcinoma of the pancreas, stomach, lungs, and particularly the liver. The enzyme is also elevated in other liver conditions, e.g., viral hepatitis, biliary obstruction, and infectious mononucleosis. Elevations are also found after estrogen-progesterone therapy or the use of oral contraceptives and in acute pancreatitis. Increases in serum activity give rise to increases in urinary values.

Trypsin (EC 3.4.4.4; no systemic name)

Trypsin is a proteolytic enzyme secreted by the pancreas. It acts preferentially in hydrolyzing peptide bonds containing arginine or lysine. The enzyme is secreted as the inactive trypsinogen. The intestinal mucosa secretes a small amount of the enzyme enterokinase, which activates the trypsinogen to trypsin by hydrolytic removal of a single peptide. The removal of a second peptide will form trypsin. The presence of a small amount of active trypsin will also catalyze the formation of trypsin from trypsinogen. In the in vitro determination as given below, a small amount of active trypsin is added to activate the trypsinogen present.

In cases of suspected pancreatic insufficiency, trypsin may be determined in a duodenal aspirate or in the feces. The value of the latter has been questioned, since not only may the intestinal bacteria degrade the trypsin in the passage through the lower intestinal tract, but the bacteria themselves may also secrete proteolytic enzymes. It has been shown, for example, that germ-free rats have much larger amounts of trypsin in their feces than conventional rats.

Principle: A quantitative method for the determination of trypsin in duodenal contents is given here.[175] This uses the substrate benzoyl-arginine-*p*-nitroanilide. The reaction product, *p*-nitroaniline, can be readily determined by its absorbance at 405 nm. The trypsinogen in the duodenal contents is first activated by incubation with a very small amount of trypsin.

Reagents:

1. Tris-HCl buffer, 0.1 mole/L, pH 7.6 with 20 mmole/L calcium chloride
   a. Tris, stock solution, 0.5 mol/L. Dissolve 30.3 g tris(hydroxymethyl)aminomethane in water to make 5 dl.
   b. Hydrochloric acid, 0.5 mole/L. Dilute 21 ml concentrated hydrochloric acid to 5 dl with water.
   c. Calcium chloride, 0.1 mole/L. Dissolve 7.35 g $CaCl_2 \cdot 2H_2O$ in water to make 5 dl.
   To prepare buffer, add 1 dl stock tris and 1 dl calcium chloride solution to a 5 dl volumetric flask. Add about 2 dl water, then bring to a pH of 7.6 by the addition of 0.5 mole/L hydrochloric acid (about 78 ml will be required), and dilute to 5 dl.

2. Tris buffer, 0.05 mole/L, pH 8.2 with 20 mmole/L calcium chloride
   To a 5 dl volumetric flask add 50 ml stock tris, 1 dl calcium chloride solution, and about 250 ml water. Bring to a pH of 8.2 with the addition of the 0.5 mole/L hydrochloric acid (about 23 ml will be required) and dilute to 5 dl.

3. Activating solution
   Just before use dissolve 10 mg crystalline trypsin in 1 dl of the pH 7.6 buffer. Dilute 100 μl of this with 10 ml of the buffer to give a solution containing 1 μg/dl trypsin.

4. Substrate solution
   Dissolve 43.5 mg benzoyl-arginine-*p*-nitroanilide (BAPNA, Aldrich Chemical Co., Milwaukee) in 1 ml dimethylsulfoxide (Aldrich Chemical Co., Milwaukee) and dilute to 1 dl with the pH 8.2 buffer.

5. Trypsin standards
   Just before use dissolve 20 mg crystalline trypsin in 20 ml of 1 mmole/L hydrochloric acid (dilute 1 ml of 0.5 mole/L to 5 dl with water). Prepare working standards by diluting 0.5, 1.0, 2.0, and 3.0 ml to 10 ml with the pH 7.6 buffer. These solutions contain 50-300 μg/ml but since the sample is diluted 1:2 in the procedure these standards correspond to 100, 200, 400, and 600 μg/ml.

Procedure: Mix 1 ml of the sample with 1 ml of the pH 7.6 buffer and incubate for 20 min at 37° C. For the assay add 100 μl of the incubated sample to 3 ml of the substrate previously warmed to 37° C, mix, and read against a blank of 3 ml of the substrate and 100 μl of pH 7.6 buffer. Read at 405 nm at 1 min after addition of sample and again at 5 and 10 min later, incubating at 37° C between readings.

Calculation: Prepare a standard curve by treating similarly 100 μl samples of the working standards and plot absorbance at 405 nm against micrograms per milliliter. Read samples from the curve.

Alternatively, results can be expressed in international units per liter as follows:

$$IU/L = \frac{\Delta A}{min} \times \frac{3.05}{0.05} \times \frac{1000}{9.9} = \frac{\Delta A}{min} \times 6160$$

where 3.05 is the total volume, 9.9 the absorbance factor for *p*-nitroaniline, and 0.05 the amount of serum added, since the 100 μl contains 50% serum and 50% buffer.

Normal values and interpretation: The normal values of the enzyme in duodenal contents are 150-600 μg/ml. Fat malabsorption has been observed with enzyme values below 50 μg/ml. No normal values have yet been established if international units per liter are used.

DIAGNOSIS OF PROSTATIC DISEASE

The prostate gland is an excellent source of acid phosphatase (ACP), and normally serum has a very low activity of this enzyme. During metastasis of carcinomas of the prostate, outside the capsule, a large elevation of serum ACP is observed. Other tissues also contain large amounts of this enzyme, notably red cells and platelets. The enzyme activity of these other tissues must be distinguished to pinpoint the source of the elevated enzyme activity. Assays using specific substrates or specific enzyme inhibitors are used to confirm the tissue enzyme source.

Acid phosphatase (ACP) (EC 3.1.3.2; orthophosphoric monoester phosphohydrolase)

Since the determination of acid phosphatase is of interest chiefly in the diagnosis of prostate malignancies, a test as specific as possible for the prostatic ACP is desirable.

p-Nitrophenyl phosphate and tartrate inhibition method[176-177]

Principle: The enzyme acid phosphatase hydrolyzes orthophosphate esters at an acidic pH. The substrate used in this assay is *p*-nitrophenyl phosphate, and citrate buffer maintains an acid pH.

p-Nitrophenyl phosphate (colorless) + $H_2O \rightleftharpoons$

p-Nitrophenol (yellow in alkali) + Phosphoric acid

In the method presented here the determination is run in the presence and the absence of tartaric acid, which strongly inhibits the prostatic ACP but has little effect on the other isoenzymes. If only the total ACP is desired, the inhibition step may be omitted.

Reagents:

1. Citrate buffer, 0.09 mole/L, pH 4.85 at 37° C
   Dissolve 18.91 g citric acid in about 5 dl water in a 1 L volumetric flask. Add 180 ml of 1 mole/L sodium hydroxide solution and mix to dissolve.

Then add 1 dl of 10 mmole/L hydrochloric acid and dilute to nearly 1 L. Check the pH at 37° C and adjust if necessary with acid or base to bring to 4.85. Dilute to 1 L and mix well. A few drops of chloroform may be added as a preservative. Store in the refrigerator.

2. Citrate-tartrate buffer, 0.09 citrate and 0.04 mole/L tartrate, pH 4.85
   Dissolve 1.5 g L(+) tartaric acid in 250 ml of the buffer and adjust pH again if necessary.

3. Stock substrate, *p*-nitrophenyl phosphate, 15 mmole/L
   Dissolve 40.0 mg disodium salt of *p*-nitrophenyl phosphate in water containing 1 or 2 drops of 0.1 mole/L hydrochloric acid and dilute to 10.0 ml. This solution is not stable and should be prepared only in the amount needed.

4. Acid substrates
   a. For citrate only, mix together equal volumes of citrate buffer (no. 1) and the stock substrate. This solution is not stable and is best kept by pipetting 1 ml aliquots to small test tubes, which are then stoppered well and kept frozen until needed.
   b. For citrate-tartrate, mix together equal volumes of the citrate-tartrate buffer (no. 2) and the stock substrate. Dispense 1 ml aliquots into tubes, stopper well, and keep frozen. Be sure to label the tubes well to distinguish between the two types of substrates.

5. Sodium hydroxide solution, 100 mmole/L
   Dissolve 4.0 g sodium hydroxide in water to make 1 L.

6. Stock standard of *p*-nitrophenol
   Dissolve 167 mg pure *p*-nitrophenol in water to make 1 dl. Sigma (Sigma Chemical Co., St. Louis) spectrophometric grade is satisfactory. The solution contains 12 mmole/L. It is stable for several months if kept refrigerated in a brown bottle.

Procedure: Set up a series of tubes in accordance with Table 24-5. Read tubes 2, 3, and 4 (Table 24-5) against tube 1 (reagent blank) at 410 nm. For total activity subtract absorbance of tube 4 (serum blank) from that of tube 2 and read result from calibration information given in the following section. For activity after inhibition (nonprostatic) subtract absorbance of tube 4 from that of tube 3 and read result from chart. For prostatic ACP subtract (nonprostatic) activity from total activity.

Calibration: Although the procedure was developed to give readings in terms of B-L-B units it is preferable to standardize the assay in terms of international units (1 B-L-B unit = 16.7 IU or 1 IU = 0.067 B-L-B units). Dilute 1, 2, 4, 6, 8, and 10 ml of the stock standard to 1 dl with water. Transfer 200 μl of these dilutions to separate tubes each containing exactly 5 ml of the sodium hydroxide solution. Mix and read against a blank of the alkali alone at 410 nm. The stock standard contains 12 mmole/L (= 12,000 μmole/L) nitrophenol; thus the dilutions contain 120-1200 μmole/L. Since these are used in the same proportions as the serum, the equivalent in micromoles per minute per liter of color for the standards would be 120/30 to 1200/

Table 24-5. Tube setup for determination of acid phosphatase

	Tube no.			
	1* (reagent blank)	2 (total ACP)	3† (nonprostatic)	4 (serum blank)
Citrate buffer (substrate; ml)	1.0	1.0	0	1.0
Citrate-tartrate buffer (substrate; ml)	0	0	1.0	0
H_2O (ml)	0.2	0	0	0
Mix and warm all tubes to 37° C. Then add at timed intervals:				
Serum sample (μl)	0	200	200	0

Incubate for exactly 30 min and then add 4 ml sodium hydroxide solution (100 mmole/L) to each tube and mix; then add 200 μl serum to serum blank tube.

*Only one tube of this blank need be made for each series of tests.
†This tube is omitted if only the total activity is to be determined.

30 or 4, 8, 16, 24, 32, and 40 μmole/min/L = 1 IU. Plot absorbance at 410 nm vs. international units on linear graph paper.

Normal values and interpretation: The normal range for total acid phosphase is 2.5-11 IU for men and 0.3-9 IU for women. For prostatic ACP (tartrate inhibited) the ranges are 0.2-3.5 IU for men and 0-0.8 IU for women. ACP (and particularly the tartrate-inhibited fraction) is markedly elevated in prostatic carcinoma. Small increases in the total ACP are found in conditions such as acute myelogenous leukemia, liver damage, metastizing carcinoma, thrombocythemia, and Paget's disease in which there are very high levels of ALP.[178] There is a fairly good correlation between the changes in ACP levels in serum and the results of therapy. A decrease in phosphatase activity usually indicates satisfactory therapy.

Comment: Prostatic ACP is very unstable. Blood should be refrigerated immediately after drawing. Centrifuge after standing 30 min and separate serum. Do not use if hemolyzed. Keep serum at 0-5° C at all times or add 20 μl 20% acetic acid to each 2 ml of serum to stabilize the enzyme.

Thymolphthalein monophosphate method

Principle: Thymolphthalein monophosphate[179] has been found to be much more specific for prostatic acid phosphate than *p*-nitrophenyl phosphate. The procedure is similar to the previous method in that the decomposition of the substrate yields a substance that is highly colored, in this instance blue, in alkaline solution.

Reagents:
1. Citrate buffer, 0.1 mole/L, pH 5.95
   A. Dissolve 29.41 g trisodium citrate dihydrate in about 9 dl water. Add 17 ml of a 30% (w/v) solution of Brij-35 (Fisher Scientific Co., Pittsburgh) and dilute to 1 L.
   B. Dissolve 4.2 g citric acid monohydrate in about 180 ml water, add 3.4 ml Brij-35 solution, and dilute to 2 dl.
   To 9 dl solution A add a sufficient amount of solution B to bring the pH to 5.95. This solution is stable in the refrigerator for about 6 months.
2. Buffered substrate
   Dissolve 0.185 g sodium thymolphthalein mono-

phosphate in 1 dl of the buffer. This is stable in the refrigerator for about 2 months.
3. Color developer
   Dissolve 2 g (0.05 mole) sodium hydroxide and 5.3 g (0.05 mole) anhydrous sodium carbonate in water to make 1 L.
4. Stock standard, 22.5 mmole/L thymolphthalein
   Dissolve 969 mg of thymolphthalein in ethanol to make 1 dl.
5. Acetate buffer, 5 moles/L, pH 5.0
   To a 1 dl volumetric flask add 43.5 g sodium acetate trihydrate, 50 ml water, and 13 ml glacial acetic acid. Add water to about 95 ml and swirl to dissolve the salt. Adjust the pH to 5.0 at 37° C by the dropwise addition of glacial acetic acid and then dilute to 1 dl.

Procedure: Since ACP is not stable at the pH of serum in vitro, if the analysis is not be done immediately, the above acetate buffer should be added as a preservative in the ratio of 20 μl for each milliliter of serum.[180] With this addition the enzyme is stable for several days in the refrigerator.

Add 1 ml aliquots of the buffered substrate to a number of tubes and warm for 5 min in a water bath at 37° C. To one tube add 200 μl of sample, mix, and incubate for exactly 30 min. When a number of samples are run they may be added to the respective tubes at 30 sec or 1 min intervals.

After exactly 30 min incubation add 5 ml of the color developer to each tube and mix by inversion. Read each tube at 590 nm against the corresponding serum blank prepared by mixing 1 ml substrate, 5 ml color developer and 200 μl serum, added in that order. The activity is then read from a standard curve or calculated by use of the appropriate factor.

Calibration: Dilute 1 ml of the stock standard to 50 ml with ethanol. This will contain 0.45 mmole/L. Prepare a series of standards by diluting 1, 2, 4, 6, 8, and 10 ml of the above diluted standard with sufficient alcohol to make 10 ml. To 200 μl of each of these add 1 ml of the buffered substrate and 5 ml of the color developer and mix. Read at 590 nm against a blank obtained by using 0.2 ml alcohol instead of the diluted standard. The highest standard contains 0.45 mmole/L, which is thus equivalent to the formation of 0.45/30

= 0.015 mmole/L/min or 15 μmole/L/min, which by definition is 15 IU. Thus the series of standards are equal to 1.5, 3, 6, 9, 12, and 15 IU. If the curve obtained is linear in this range, only one or two standards need be run with every batch of samples.

If the reading for the sample is above the reading of the highest standard but less than twice this value, the sample and its blank may be diluted with an equal volume of water and read again, multiplying the result obtained from the curve by 2. For high values it is best to repeat the determination using a 1:10 dilution of the serum with saline.

Normal values: The range of normal values is 0.1-0.6 IU/L, which correlates well with the prostatic fraction of ACP measured by the *p*-nitrophenol method.

DIAGNOSIS OF GENETIC ABNORMALITIES

A number of enzymes are found in the red cells. Their measurements may be used to study certain inborn metabolic errors.[181,182] These enzymes are all controlled by **autosomal recessive genes.** Usually an individual who is homozygous for the defective gene will have very low levels of the particular enzyme involved. A heterozygous individual will have values intermediate between those of homozygous and normal individuals. Usually a heterozygous individual shows no clinical signs of the enzyme deficiency. The determinations may be of value in the diagnosis of the particular enzyme deficiency involved and in the detection of heterozygous carriers for genetic counseling.

Glucose-6-phosphate dehydrogenase (G-6-PD)
(EC 1.1.1.49; D-glucose-6-phosphate: NADP$^+$ 1-oxidoreductase) **and phosphogluconate dehydrogenase (PGD)** (EC 1.1.1.1.44; 6-phosphogluconate: NADP$^+$ 2-oxidoreductase [decarboxylating])

The enzymes glucose-6-phosphate dehydrogenase and phosphogluconate dehydrogenase take part in the following reactions involving glucose metabolism:

D-Glucose-6-phosphate +

$$\text{NADP}^+ \xrightleftharpoons{\text{GPD}} \text{D-Gluconolactone-6-phosphate} +$$

$$\text{NADPH} + \text{H}^+$$

$$\text{D-Gluconolactone-6-phosphate} \xrightleftharpoons{\text{Gluconolactonase}}$$

$$\text{6-Phosphogluconate}$$

and

6-Phosphogluconate +

$$\text{NADP}^+ \xrightleftharpoons{\text{PGD}} \text{Ribulose-6-phosphate} + \text{NADPH} +$$

$$\text{H}^+ + \text{CO}_2$$

They are determined in red cell hemolysates, since a deficiency of these enzymes is one of the most common causes of impaired red cell glucose metabolism and thus shorter cell life.

Principle: In the overall reactions, two (or nearly two) molecules of NADP are consumed for each molecule of glucose-6-phosphate transformed. The total reaction is used in the simple WHO method for detecting G-6-PD deficiency (old name, G-6-PDH), but the two

enzymes may be estimated separately, first by measuring the total activity by the WHO method and then by measuring the PGD activity alone by the use of 6-phosphogluconate as substrate.

In the following procedure,[183,184] provision is made for the determination not only of the total enzymatic activity, but also of the separate activity of the two enzymes. For most purposes the simple WHO determination is all that is needed since a deficiency of G-6-PD is probably the most common erythrocyte enzyme deficiency, whereas that for 6-phosphogluconic acid dehydrogenase is relatively rare.

Reagents:

1. Tris buffer, 107 mmole/L, with magnesium chloride, 10.7 mmole/L
   Dissolve 3.22 g tris(hydroxymethyl aminomethane and 545 mg MgCl$_2$·6H$_2$O in about 2 dl water in a 250 ml volumetric flask; add 1 mole/L hydrochloric acid to a pH of 7.5 at 30° C (or 7.62 at 25° C) (this will require some 20-25 ml of the acid). The solution is stable at room temperature for several months.

2. NADP solution, 3 mmole/L
   Dissolve 4.6 mg of the sodium salt of NADP in 2 ml of the buffer or alternately use a preweighed vial containing 5 mg of the salt and add 2.2 ml of buffer solution. This solution is not stable, but it may be stored frozen and thawed once.

3. Glucose-6-phosphate, 9 mmole/L
   Dissolve 5 mg of the monosodium salt in 2 ml of buffer. This should be prepared fresh as required.

4. 6-Phosphogluconate, 12 mmole/L
   Dissolve 9 mg of the trisodium salt in 2 ml of buffer. Prepare fresh as required.

5. Saponin solution, 0.01%
   Dissolve 100 mg of a good grade of saponin in water to make 1 L.

Preparation of hemolysate: Any common anticoagulant can be used for the collection of the blood sample, but if the analysis is not to be done immediately it is preferable to use ACD solution. Centrifuge the blood and remove supernatant plasma. Wash packed cells several times with 5 volumes of acid citrate dextrose (ACD) or 0.15 mole/L sodium chloride solution. After the final wash, suspend the cells in an equal volume of 0.15 mole/L sodium chloride solution. Obtain the red cell count or hemoglobin concentration of the well-mixed cell suspension (depending on whether the result is to be reported in terms of grams of hemoglobin or in terms of 10^{12} red cells [the latter is preferred]). Add 200 μl well-mixed cell suspension to 3.8 ml saponin solution. Mix and place in a 30° C water bath for about 5 min for lysis and then centrifuge. Use the supernatant for the test. The test should be carried out as soon as possible after the preparation of the hemolysate.

Procedure: For each blood sample place in cuvets labeled 1, 2, 3, and 4 the amounts given in Table 24-6.

Depending on the type of equipment available, the readings can be done in two ways. One can add the final reagent to tube 2 only and read the absorbance against the blank at 1 or 2 min intervals for 5 or 6 min

Table 24-6. Tube setup for determination of G-6-PD and PGD

	Tube no.			
	1	2	3	4
Tris buffer (ml)	2.6	2.4	2.4	2.2
NADP solution (ml)	0.2	0.2	0.2	0.2
Red cell hemolysate (ml)	0.2	0.2	0.2	0.2

Place in bath at 30° C for 5 min and then add the following, prewarmed to 30° C:

Glucose-6-phosphate solution (ml)	—	0.2	—	0.2
6-Phosphogluconic acid (ml)	—	—	0.2	0.2

Then read tubes 2, 3, and 4 against tube 1 (blank) at timed intervals at 340 nm.

(or longer if the activity is low), then add the final reagent to tube 3, and repeat the process, and finally add reagent to tube 4 and make readings on this tube; or one can add the final reagents to tubes 2, 3, and 4 at timed (e.g., 30 sec) intervals and take absorbance readings on the tubes at the corresponding timed intervals. In any event one finally calculates the absorbance change per minute for each tube.

The activity in the diluted hemolysate is then calculated as usual:

$$units/L = \frac{\Delta A}{min} \times \frac{1000 \times 3}{6.22 \times 0.2} = \frac{\Delta A}{min} \times 2410$$

As mentioned earlier, the reactions in tube 2 consume more than 1 mole of NADP per mole of glucose-6-phosphate, but in accordance with the convention, the factor of 1 is used for the WHO method. Tube 3 measures the activity of the PGD and tube 4 the activity of G-6-PD + PGD, and thus the difference in activity between the two tubes represents the "true" activity of the G-6-PD. For most purposes the WHO activity is all that is necessary and for this only tubes 1 and 2 are needed.

If the activity of the hemolysate prepared by a 1:20 dilution of the erythrocyte suspension is that containing "H" grams of hemoglobin per liter (H/10 per deciliter), then the activity expressed per gram of hemoglobin is as follows:

$$units/L \text{ (in hemolysate)} \times \frac{20}{H} = units/g \text{ Hb}$$

If the erythrocyte suspension contained $C \times 10^6$ cells/μl, then the activity per 10^{12} cells would be as follows:

$$units/L \text{ (in hemolysate)} \times \frac{20}{C} = units/10^{12} \text{ cells}$$

since 10^6 cells/mm^3 = 10^6 cells /μl = 10^{12} cells/L.

Interpretation: The normal ranges in terms of units per gram hemoglobin are 5.9-12.0 units G-6-PD by the WHO method, 3.9-7.8 units for "true" G-6-PD and 4.3-6.9 units for 6-phosphogluconate dehydrogenase. In terms of units per 10^{12} red cells the corresponding values are 200-420 units, 135-270 units, and 150-240 units, respectively.

G-6-PD deficiency is the most common enzymatic deficiency in the red cell. There are a large number of genetically controlled enzyme variants, some of which result in a marked deficiency in enzyme activity, causing sensitivity to drug-induced hemolytic anemia, neonatal icterus, and favism.

Pyruvate kinase (PK) (EC 2.7.1.40; ATP: pyruvate phosphotransferase)

Principle: Pyruvate kinase[185,186] is an important enzyme in the glycolytic pathway. It catalyzes the phosphorylation of adenosine diphosphate (ADP) to adenosine triphosphate (ATP) by phospho(enol)pyruvate (PEP).

$$PEP + ADP \rightleftharpoons ATP + Pyruvate$$

The rate of formation of the pyruvate is usually measured by means of the following coupled reaction:

$$Pyruvate + NADH + H^+ \rightleftharpoons Lactate + NAD^+$$

which is catalyzed by adding LD. As in other methods involving the NAD-NADH change, the change in absorbance at 340 nm is used to quantitate the reaction.

Leukocytes contain relatively large amounts of PK, and it is essential, particularly in cases of suspected enzyme deficiency in the red cells, that the leukocytes be separated as completely as possible from the red cells. In removing the plasma and washing the cells, the buffy coat should be removed as completely as possible each time. Thus it is helpful to have a sufficient blood sample so that after each centrifugation a small amount of the packed red cells can be removed from the top to aid in complete separation of the red cells.

Reagents:
1. Tris buffer, 1.0 mole/L, pH 8.0 with 5 mmole/L EDTA
   Dissolve 60.6 g tris(hydroxymethyl)aminomethane in about 1 dl water and 300 ml of 1 mole/L hydrochloric acid (83 ml concentrated acid diluted to 1 L), add 0.84 g disodium ethylenediaminetetraacetate, and dissolve. Bring the pH to 8.0 by the addition of more 1 mole/L hydrochloric acid (about 40 ml additional will be required) and then dilute to 5 dl. The buffer is stable at room temperature.
2. Magnesium chloride, 100 mmole/L
   Dissolve 2.03 g $MgCl_2 \cdot 6H_2O$ in water to make 1 dl.
3. Potassium chloride, 1 mole/L
   Dissolve 7.46 g potassium chloride in water to make 1 dl.
4. ADP, 15 mmole/L
   Dissolve adenosine diphosphate, sodium salt, in water in the proportion of 7 mg/ml. Since this solution is not stable even when frozen, only an amount sufficient for the day's analyses should be prepared at one time.
5. NADH, 2 mmole/L
   Dissolve NADH in water in the proportion of 1.5 mg/ml. Since the solution is not stable, it is best prepared by purchasing the preweighed vials (Sigma Chemical Co., St. Louis) and adding the required amount of water.

6. LD, 60 units/ml)
The enzyme is purchased as a suspension in about 2 moles/L ammonium sulfate. A preparation free of PK should be obtained. A small amount is diluted to the required concentration as needed.

7. Phospho(enol)pyruvate, 60 mmole/L
Dissolve 1.24 g of the monopotassium salt to make 1 dl.

Preparation of hemolysate: The blood may be collected with heparin, EDTA, or ACD solution as an anticoagulant. As mentioned above, all leukocytes must be removed. A more satisfactory procedure than simple washing is to pass the blood through a cellulose column. Equal amounts of cellulose and microcrystalline cellulose (Sigmacell-50 [Sigma Chemical Co., St. Louis]) are made into a slurry with 0.15 mole/L sodium chloride. A 5 ml disposable plastic syringe is used as the column. It is placed in an upright position and the slurry poured in to give a column to the 2 ml mark. The column is washed with about 15 ml of the sodium chloride solution and the eluate discarded. About 1 ml of whole blood is allowed to pass through the column, and the effluent is collected in a tube. The remaining cells are washed through with about 2 ml of saline. The tube is centrifuged and the cells washed with two additional portions of ice-cold sodium chloride solution. The packed cells are then diluted to a hematocrit of about 50%. The hemoglobin content of the cell suspension is then determined in the usual manner. If it is desired to express the results in terms of enzyme units per milliliter of packed cells or per 10^{12} red cells, the hematocrit and cell count must be determined on the cell suspension.

Hemolysis is produced by mixing 1 volume of the well-mixed cell suspension with 9 volumes of a solution containing 9 mg disodium EDTA and 5 µl mercaptoethanol per 1 dl. The hemolysate is then rapidly frozen by placing the tube in acetone or methanol previously cooled to $-20°$ C. After thawing in a water bath at 25° C, the hemolysate is ready for use. It is not centrifuged to remove stroma since some of the enzyme will be bound to the stroma.

Procedure: Just before use, mix together 1 ml of each of the first six reagents listed and 3 ml of water. (When a number of samples are to be run, a larger quantity may be made up, but the mixture should be used within a few hours.) Add 2.7 ml of the mixture to each of several cuvets and place in a 37° C water bath. To one cuvet add 50 µl water as a reagent blank and to the other tubes add 50 µl hemolysate from sample or control. Mix and warm in a water bath for about 10 min. Then at timed intervals add 250 µl of the PEP solution to cuvets and read about 15 sec after mixing and exactly 5 and 10 min later. When the spectrophotometer is zeroed against water, the initial readings should be between 0.7 and 0.9 absorbance units. If they are higher than this the readings may be made against a dichromate solution as described under the LD procedure to bring the readings in the proper range. For each unknown determine the change in absorbance per minute and subtract from this the corresponding reading for the blank. This gives the ΔA used in the calculations.

Calculation:

$$\text{IU/L of hemolysate} = \frac{\Delta A}{\min} \times \frac{3 \times 1000}{6.22 \times 0.05} = \frac{\Delta A}{\min} \times 9650$$

where 3 is the total volume in the cuvet and 0.05 is the volume of hemolysate added.

To calculate the activity in terms of international units, milliliters per gram of hemoglobin, milliliters of packed cells, or 10^{12} red cells, respectively, multiply by 1000/Hb, 1000/Hct, or 10,000/RBC, respectively, where Hb is the hemoglobin in grams per deciliter, Hct is the hematocrit in percent, and RBC is the red cell count in 10^{12}/L in the suspension of washed cells used to prepare the hemolysate; the extra factor of 10 arises from the fact that the cell suspension is diluted 1:10 in the preparation of the hemolysate.

Galactose-1-phosphate uridyl transferase
(EC 2.7.7.12; UDP-glucose-galactose-1-phosphate uridyl transferase; hexose-1-phosphate uridyl transferase)

The enzyme galactose-1-phosphate uridyl transferase[187] catalyzes the following reaction:

Uridine diphosphate glucose + Galactose-1-phosphate ⇌
Uridine diphosphate galactose + Glucose-1-phosphate

This is an important step in the metabolism of galatose by which it is converted into glucose. A deficiency of this enzyme is the basis for an inborn error of metabolism with the inability to utilize galactose. The test for this enzyme has been used in the study of this genetic trait, particularly in the detection of heterozygous carriers in which the level of the enzyme is about one half that of normal adults.

Principle: Although galactose-1-phosphate uridyl transferase is concerned with the metabolism in other body tissues, particularly the liver, it is usually determined in the red cells as a convenient source of the enzyme. The enzyme may be determined by incubating a hemolysate of the red cells with galactose-1-phosphate and uridine diphosphate glucose so that the above reaction takes place. After this reaction has taken place the unchanged uridyl diphosphate glucose (UDPG) is measured by means of the following reaction:

$$\text{UDPG} + \text{NAD}^+ \xrightleftharpoons{\text{UDPG dehydrogenase}} \text{NADH} + \text{H}^+ +$$

Uridine diphosphate gluconate

Although this enzyme is important in the study of galactose intolerance, its determination is technically rather difficult. Details of a method are given by Beutler.[184]

Glutathione reductase (EC 1.6.4.2; reduced NAD[P]: oxidized glutathione oxidoreductase)

Glutathione reductase[184,188] is also implicated in some types of congenital **nonspherocytic hemolytic anemia.** It is not concerned directly with the glucolytic process as are the previously mentioned erythrocyte enzymes, but it is necessary for the functional integrity of the cell membrane. The enzyme maintains glutathione in the reduced state in the presence of NADPH. It may be determined by incubating a dialyzed hemolysate under aerobic conditions with the oxidized form of glutathione and NADPH. The reduced glutathione formed may be determined colorimetrically by reaction with sodium nitroprusside or by the change from NADPH to NADP, which is observed by measuring the changes in absorption at 340 nm. The enzyme requires activation by preincubation with flavine adenine dinucleotide (FAD) before analysis.

Glucose phosphate isomerase (GPI)
(EC 5.3.1.9)

Glucose phosphate isomerase, one of the enzymes in the glycolytic (Embden-Meyerhof) pathway, catalyzes the interconversion of glucose-6-phosphate and fructose-6-phosphate. It is said to be more consistently elevated in various types of neoplasia than any of the commonly determined enzymes involved in glycolysis, and it often decreases with effective therapy.[189,190] In addition, it is second in frequency to PK deficiencies and is associated with hemolytic anemia when it is deficient in an individual.

α₁-Antitrypsin

Principle: A method for the determination of α_1-antitrypsin,[191] an enzyme inhibitor, is presented. It is an inhibitor of trypsin activity that is present in the serum in abnormally large amounts in certain pathologic conditions. The method is based on the inhibition of a standard trypsin sample by the α_1-antitrypsin present in the added serum sample. The method uses the same synthetic substrate as in the BAPNA method for trypsin. The blood sample should be collected with EDTA as anticoagulant and should be free from hemolysis. The separated serum is stable for a few days at 4° C, but for longer storage it should be kept at $-20°$ C.

Reagents:
1. Tris buffer, pH 8.2
   This is the same as the buffer no. 1 of the BAPNA method for trypsin, except that the pH is adjusted to 8.2 (only about 45 ml of the 0.5 mole/L hydrochloric acid will be required).
2. Stock substrate
   Dissolve 100 mg BAPNA (benzoyl-arginine-*p*-nitroanilide) in 2.3 ml dimethyl sulfoxide. This is stable for about 1 week at 4° C.
3. Working substrate
   Just before use dilute 1 ml of the stock substrate with buffer to 1 dl.
4. Trypsin
   Crystalline trypsin from any of a number of suppliers can be used, but it should be substantially free of chymotrypsin. To prepare a stock solution, dissolve 50 mg of trypsin in 50 ml of 1 mmole/L hydrochloric acid (1 ml of 0.5 mole/L hydrochloric acid diluted to 5 dl). This solution is stable for about 2 weeks at 4° C. Prepare a working solution by diluting about 1 ml of the stock to 25 ml with the buffer. The dilution may be adjusted so that when the procedure is carried through to the end the absorbance of the control tube is about 0.5.

5. Albumin solution, 4 g/dl
   Prepare a stock solution by dissolving 2 g bovine serum albumin in 50 ml of the buffer. For the control assay dilute 1 ml of the stock solution to 1 dl with the buffer.
6. Acetic acid, 5.2 moles/L
   Dilute 30 ml glacial acetic acid to 1 dl with water.

Procedure: Dilute the serum sample 1:100 with the tris buffer. For each serum to be assayed label one of a pair of tubes test and the other blank. Also label one pair of tubes control and blank. (If desired the test and control may be run in duplicate.) To each tube add 5 ml working substrate and place in a water bath at 37° C. For each serum to be assayed, mix together 2 ml of the 1:100 dilution of the serum and 2 ml of the working trypsin solution and allow to stand at room temperature for 10 min.

For the control similarly mix 2 ml of the diluted albumin solution and 2 ml of the working trypsin solution and allow to stand at room temperature for 10 min. (These times need not be exact.)

To the tube containing 5 ml of the warmed substrate and labeled "serum test" add 1 ml of the incubated mixture of diluted serum and incubate for exactly 10 min at 37° C. Similarly to the tube marked "control" add 1 ml of the incubated mixture of diluted albumin solution and substrate and incubate for exactly 10 min. Add nothing to the blank tubes at this time.

After the 10 min incubation add 1 ml of the 5.2 moles/L acetic acid to each tube including the blanks. Then add to the serum blank 1 ml of the incubated serum substrate mixture, and to the control blank add 1 ml of the incubated diluted albumin plus substrate. Mix and read each serum or control tube against the corresponding blank at 400 nm. Preferably the readings should be made in cuvets with a 1 cm light path.

Calculation: Then, taking the molar absorbance of the liberated nitroaniline as 10,500:

$$\mu\text{mole/min/ml} = \frac{\Delta A \times 7 \times 1000}{10.5 \times v \times t}$$

where ΔA is the difference in absorbance between the control and serum readings, 7 is the total volume in milliliters, v is the volume of the serum sample, and t is the time of incubation. As outlined above, t = 10 min, v = 5 μl (serum was diluted 1:100 and 1 ml of an additional 1:2 dilution was used), and the equation reduces to

$$\mu\text{mole/min/ml} = \Delta A \times 13.3$$

The control reading represents the activity of the trypsin standard, and the serum reading represents the activity of the trypsin after inhibition by the antitrypsin present. The difference represents the amount of inhibition and thus the amount of antitrypsin present. When the absorbance of the serum tube is very low, representing a large amount of inhibition, the assay should be repeated using a greater dilution of the serum. Routinely, when the absorbance of the serum tube is less than 0.07, the test should be repeated using an original

1:250 dilution of the serum instead of 1:100. For this the above factor will be 33.3 instead of 13.3.

Normal values and interpretation: By this method the normal levels for men are 2.1-3.5 μmole/min/ml and for women from 2.4-3.8 μmole/min/ml. About 20% of the antitrypsin activity of serum as measured by the above method is caused by α_2-antitrypsin, and the remainder results from the more common α_1-antitrypsin. Acute or chronic inflammatory diseases will cause marked increases in the α_1-antitrypsin activity and thus in the activity as measured by the above procedure.

The chief interest lies in the congenital deficiency of α_1-antitrypsin.[192] In the infant this may result in the development of emphysema at an early age and an increased incidence of neonatal hepatitis, often progressing to cirrhosis. The normal gene is usually designated as M and the abnormal as Z. The homozygotes, MM, have the normal values given above, whereas the heterozygotes, MZ, will usually have values by the above method of between 1.0 and 2.1 μmole/min/ml. These individuals may or may not have respiratory symptoms as infants, but they are more likely than the healthy individuals to develop emphysema as adults. The homozygotes, ZZ, will have enzyme values in the range of 0.5-0.7 μmole/ml/min and will very frequently develop the respiratory and hepatic difficulties mentioned above.

Cholinesterase (CHS)

True cholinesterase (EC 3.1.1.7; acetylcholine hydrolase; acetylcholinesterase) **and pseudocholinesterase** (EC 3.1.1.8; acylocholine acylhydrolase; cholinesterase)

There are two different enzymes called cholinesterases—"true" cholinesterase (EC 3.1.1.7) is found in red cells and nervous tissue and is fairly specific for acetylcholine; pseudocholinesterase (EC 3.1.1.8) is found in serum and hydrolyzes a number of choline esters. The determination of "true" cholinesterase in red cells is of importance only in assessing the exposure to certain potent insecticides related to the "nerve gases." The determination of pseudocholinesterase is more frequently performed, and two methods will be given here.

Principle: In the first simple method,[193] acetylcholine is hydrolyzed by the enzyme to choline and acetic acid. The reaction is followed by noting the change in an indicator color caused by the liberated acetic acid.

Reagents:
1. Buffered m-nitrophenol
   Dissolve 6.65 g anhydrous disodium phosphate (Na_2HPO_4) and 0.43 g potassium dihydrogen phosphate (KH_2PO_4) in about 2 dl distilled water. Dissolve 0.30 g metanitrophenol in about 2 dl distilled water (with the aid of slight heating if necessary). Mix the two solutions and adjust to pH 7.8 with 0.1 mole/L sodium hydroxide solution; then dilute to 1 L.
2. Acetylcholine solution, 1.9 moles/L
   Dissolve 15 g acetylcholine in water to make 1 dl. Store in the refrigerator.

3. Sodium chloride solution, 0.15 mole/L.
   Dissolve 9 g sodium chloride in water and make up to 1 L.

Procedure: To each of two tubes, add 0.1 ml of 0.15 mole/L sodium chloride solution and 0.1 ml serum. Heat one tube to 60° C in a water bath for 3 min. This is the blank tube; the heating inactivates the enzyme. The other tube is the sample tube. To each tube, add 2.5 ml buffered nitrophenol and 0.1 ml acetylcholine solution. Mix and incubate at 25° C for 30 min. Then read both tubes in a spectrophotometer at 420 nm, setting to zero with water. Read sample exactly 30 min after addition of acetylcholine. Subtract the absorbance of the sample tube from the absorbance for the blank.

Calibration curve: Dilute 58 ml glacial acetic acid to 1 L with distilled water. Titrate against standard alkali solution with phenolphthalein indicator and adjust to exactly 1 mole/L. Dilute 1, 2, 3, 4, and 5 ml of the 1 mole/L acid to 50 ml in volumetric flasks. These solutions will correspond to 20, 40, 60, 80, and 100 units, respectively. Pipet 2.5 ml buffered nitrophenol and 0.1 ml pooled inactivated serum (heated to 60° C for 3 min) to each of six tubes. Do not use hemolyzed, icteric, or turbid serum. To one tube add 0.1 ml distilled water; this is the blank. To the other tubes add 0.1 ml diluted acetic acid solutions made up to correspond to 20, 40, 60, 80, and 100 units. Mix and read in a spectrophotometer at 420 nm, setting to zero absorbance with water. Subtract the reading of each standard tube from that for the blank. Plot the values obtained against the units of standard. The unknown samples are read from this curve. A new standard curve must be made up for every new batch of reagents. For values higher than 120 units, dilute the serum with an equal volume of sodium chloride solution and repeat the test, taking 0.1 ml diluted serum and multiplying the result obtained by 2.

Normal values and interpretation: The normal values by this method are 40-80 units. Low values have been found in anemia, tuberculosis, hypoproteinemia, uremia, and shock. Low serum pseudocholinesterase levels are also found in most liver diseases, although the decrease may only be slight in infectious mononucleosis, cirrhosis, and metastatic carcinoma. The organic phosphorus insecticides are potent cholinesterase inhibitors, and exposure to these may result in low levels of the enzymes in both the serum and the red cells. The level of the enzyme may thus be used as an index of exposure to the insecticides. Another important use of the determination of pseudocholinesterase is in measuring the susceptibility to succinylcholine. In major surgery the compound succinylcholine is often given as a muscle relaxant. This compound is slowly hydrolyzed by the pseudocholinesterase in the serum. If the value of the enzyme is low, the inactivation of the succinylcholine is slow and the patient may experience a period of dyspnea in the recovery room. It is often helpful for the anesthetist to know whether the value of the enzyme is low. The value may be low because of an acquired disease or because the patient is one of the small percentage of individuals who have a genetically determined low pseudocholinesterase activity.

Increased values have been found in hyperthyroidism and diabetes but are of little diagnostic value in these conditions.

Cholinesterase enzyme variants

Decreased values of pseudocholinesterase activity in the serum may also be caused by genetic variant enzymes, which will lead to low enzyme activity in the absence of any disease or other abnormal state. The preceding simple method, while adequate for the simple detection of low values, is not satisfactory for the distinction between the various enzyme variants. For this purpose the following somewhat more complicated method is preferred.

Principle: In this assay the substrate used is propionylthiocholine.[194] The free thiol groups formed by the hydrolysis are determined by reaction with the reagent 5,5'-dithiobis-(2-nitrobenzoic acid) to yield a colored product, which is measured at 410 nm. After incubation, quinidine is added to stop the enzymatic reaction. For detection of the enzyme variants, benzocaine or sodium fluoride is added to the reaction mixture. These two substances inhibit the different enzyme variants by different amounts, allowing a distinction to be made between the variants.

Reagents:

1. Phosphate buffer, pH 7.6, ionic strength 0.1 μm
   Prepare a 0.1 mole/L solution of KH_2PO_4 by dissolving 3.40 g of the anhydrous salt in water to make 250 ml. Prepare a 0.033 mole/L solution of Na_2HPO_4 in water to make 1 L. To 5 dl of the Na_2HPO_4 solution add a sufficient amount of the KH_2PO_4 solution to bring the pH to about 7.7 at room temperature (about 20-25 ml will be required). Warm the solution to 37° C and check the pH; adjust if necessary to bring the pH to 7.6 at this temperature.
2. Substrate solution: propionylthiocholine iodide (PTCI; Sigma Chemical Co., St. Louis), 20 mmole/L
   Dissolve 606 mg of the salt in 1 dl water. This solution may be stored frozen, but it is preferable to make up the amount required fresh each day.
3. Color reagent: 5,5'-dithiobis-(2-nitrobenzoic acid) (DTNB; Sigma Chemical Co., St. Louis) 0.42 mmole/L
   Dissolve 83 mg DTNB in sufficient buffer solution to make 5 dl. This solution should be stored in a brown glass bottle in the refrigerator.
4. Dibucaine, 0.3 mmole/L
   Dissolve 57 mg of dibucaine hydrochloride (Nupercaine hydrochloride, Ciba Pharm. Co., Summit, N.J.) in water to make 5 dl. This solution is stable at room temperature.
5. Sodium fluoride, 40 mmole/L
   Dissolve 84 mg sodium fluoride in water to make 50 ml. This solution should be prepared fresh as needed.
6. Quinidine sulfate, 12 mmole/L
   Dissolve 0.5 g quinidine sulfate in water to make 1 dl.

Procedure: For the simple test without inhibitor, dilute an aliquot of the stock substrate solution with an equal volume of water. Dilute an aliquot of the serum to be used 1:100 with water. If low values of activity are expected, a 1:50 or 1:25 dilution may be used. To each of two tubes labeled test and blank add 3 ml of the DTNB solution and warm to 37° C. Then add to each tube 1 ml of the substrate solution previously warmed to 37° C and mix. To the tube marked test add 1 ml of the diluted serum (also previously warmed to 37° C), mix rapidly, and start timing. Exactly 3 min later add 1 ml of quinidine solution to both tubes and mix at once. Then add 1 ml of the diluted serum to the blank tube and mix. Remove from the bath and read the "test" tube against the blank one within 30 min at 410 nm. It is preferable to standardize the procedure by making all readings at a definite time, e.g., 15 min after the addition of the quinidine.

Calculation: The activity is then calculated in the usual way:

$$\text{units/ml} = \mu\text{mole/min/ml} = \frac{V \times D \times \Delta A}{13.6 \times t}$$

where V is the final volume in milliliters, D is the dilution factor, 13.6 is the millimolar absorptivity of the colored compound formed, and t is the time of incubation in minutes.

For cuvets with a 1 cm light path and for spectrophotometers having a narrow bandwidth, and using the volumes and time given above, the expression reduces to the following:

$$\text{IU/L} = \frac{\Delta A \times 6 \times 100}{13.6 \times 3} = \Delta A \times 14.7$$

where ΔA is the difference in absorbance between the blank and test solutions. If desired the tubes for the "test" may be prepared and run in duplicate.

Inhibition test: For the inhibition test the procedure is similar except that the stock solution of substrate is diluted with an equal volume of the inhibitor solution (dibucaine or fluoride) instead of water. The percent inhibition is then calculated as follows:

$$\text{Inhibition (\%)} = 100(1 - [A'/A''])$$

where A' is the activity with inhibitor and A'' is the activity without inhibitor. A number of other inhibitors have also been used, but dibucaine is the most commonly used and some values for this inhibitor are given below. There are a number of genetic variants of the enzyme; the homozygous pheno-types are designated as U (usual), A (atypical), S (silent), F (fluoride resistant).[181,195,196]

Normal values and interpretation: By this method the normal values for the common U phenotype are 5-12 units, with 81-86% inhibition by dibucaine and 77-82% by fluoride. In general, individuals having an activity less than 4 units/ml will have prolonged apnea after the use of succinylcholine. This includes individuals with the genotypes A and AS and some individuals with the genotypes AF and UA. There are a number of acquired conditions that may also result in increased suceptibility to succinylcholine. These include parenchymal liver disease, the later stages of pregnancy, estrogen therapy in women, and sometimes chronic renal disorders and a variety of wasting and cachectic states.

Exposure to organophosphorus insecticides, either in the manufacture or use, will also result in lowered activity of the enzyme. These acquired conditions can be distinguished from the genetic disorders by measuring the dibucaine inhibition. Patients with the acquired conditions will generally have the same dibucaine inhibition as normal individuals, whereas those with the genetic variants will have lower amounts of inhibition. Usually if the activity in serum is greater than 4 units/ml, it is not necessary to perform the inhibition test. If it is desired to establish the exact genotype of an individual with a lowered level of activity, inhibition studies must be made.[181,195,196]

MISCELLANEOUS ENZYMES
Porphobilinogen synthase (EC 4.2.1.24; aminolevulinate dehydratase)

The enzyme porphobilinogen synthase catalyzes the synthase following reaction:

$$5\text{-Aminolevulinate} \rightleftharpoons \text{Porphobilinogen} + 2\ H_2O$$

The above reaction is one of the steps in the synthesis of the porphyrins in the body. The enzyme is inhibited by the presence of heavy metals, particularly lead, and its determination is used in the study of lead poisoning.

Principle: In the procedure used here,[197,198] the activity of the enzyme is measured with and without the addition of dithiothreitol, which neutralizes the inhibition by lead, and thus the difference between the two determinations is a true measure of the inhibition by lead. In the collection of the specimen and preparation of the reagents, contamination by trace amounts of lead must be avoided. The blood is collected with a plastic syringe with heparin as anticoagulant and placed in a new plastic tube or an acid-washed glass one. Some of the lead-free Vacutainers contain EDTA as the anticoagulant, which is unsatisfactory for this test. As soon as the specimen is collected, it is placed in an ice bath. Two samples of well-mixed blood are then withdrawn for hematocrit determination. The blood may be kept for several days if it is stored frozen in a well-capped tube. The sample for immediate use is hemolyzed by freezing and thawing several times, preferably with the aid of dry ice and acetone.

Reagents:
1. Phosphate buffer, 0.1 mole/L, pH 5.8
   Dissolve 1.78 g disodium phosphate dihydrate ($Na_2HPO_4 \cdot 2H_2O$) in water to make 1 dl. Dissolve 7.80 g of $NaH_2PO_4 \cdot 2H_2O$ in water to make 5 dl. The sodium salts are preferred since potassium salts will form a precipitate with the perchloric acid of the Ehrlich's reagent. Warm the above solutions to 37° C and add about 40 ml of the solution of the disodium salt to the 5 dl of the solution of the monosodium salt. Check the pH and adjust to 5.8 by the careful addition of more of the disodium salt. This buffer is stable for several weeks at 4° C.
2. Buffered substrate with aminolevulinic acid (ALA), 4 mmole/L
   To 1 dl of the buffer add 67 mg δ-aminolevulinic acid hydrochloride. (Sigma Chemical Co., St. Louis). Warm to 37° C and check pH and adjust

if necessary. This solution is stable for 1 month in the refrigerator.
3. Buffered substrate with dithiothreitol, 20 mmole/L
   Add 31 mg dithiothreitol (Sigma Chemical Co., St. Louis) to 10 ml of the buffered substrate. This solution should be prepared fresh just before use.
4. Protein precipitant
   Dissolve 0.635 g N-ethylmaleimide in about 40 ml warm water, add 4 g trichloroacetic acid, and dilute to 1 dl. This solution is stable.
5. Modified Ehrlich's reagent
   In a 250 ml volumetric flask add about 180 ml glacial acetic acid and 45 ml of 70% perchloric acid. Dissolve 4.56 g p-dimethylaminobenzaldehyde in this solution and then dilute to 250 ml with glacial acetic acid. The reagent is stable for about 1 week in the refrigerator.

Preferably, new plastic test tubes should be used. If glass tubes are used, they should be washed with 1:1 nitric acid and rinsed well with water. (NOTE: Since lead interferes only with the enzymatic reactions, these precautions are not necessary for the steps after the protein has been precipitated and the reaction stopped.)

Procedure: For each test set up four tubes, labeled 1, 2, 3, and 4. To tubes 1 and 2 add 100 μl of buffered substrate (reagent no. 2); to tubes 3 and 4 add 100 μl of substrate with dithiothreitol (reagent no. 3). Place tubes in an ice bath and add 100 μl hemolyzed blood sample to each. Mix each tube briefly with vortex mixer. Place tubes in water bath at 37° C and start timer. Exactly 5 min later add 4 ml of the protein precipitant to tubes 1 and 3, mix on a vortex mixer and centrifuge. Incubate tubes 2 and 4 for 60 min more and then add the protein precipitant. Mix the tubes on a vortex mixer and then centrifuge. Add 2 ml aliquots from each of the four tubes to separate cuvets. To each cuvet then add 2 ml of the modified Ehrlich's reagent and mix the contents.

Tube 2 is read against tube 1 and tube 4 against tube 3 at 553 nm. The color is not stable, and the tubes must be read between 15 and 20 min after the reagent is added. The absorbance reading for tube 4 will be higher than that for tube 2 since the lead inhibition has been eliminated.

Calculation: If the light path in the cuvets is 1 cm, the enzyme activity for the two tubes may be calculated as follows:

$$\frac{\Delta A \times 138,000}{H} = \text{Activity in nmole/ml RBC/hr at 37° C}$$

where A is the absorbance reading for tube 2 or 4 and H is the hematocrit of the sample (as percent). The ratio of the activities in tube 4 to that in tube 2 is known as the activation ratio and may be a better index of lead exposure than the actual value of the inhibited enzyme (tube 2).

Normal values and interpretation: In children having lead concentrations of less than 40 μg/dl, the activation ratio varied from 1.5-4.9. The ratio increased to a range of 3.3-8.8 at a level of 60 μg/dl of lead, and there was a linear relation between the ratio and the lead concentration. Thus a ratio over 6 would be a definite indication of lead poisoning. The range of the lead-inhibited activity was much wider. In "healthy" individuals the activity ranged from 240-1180 units, expressed as given above; and in individuals with a lead concentration of about 60 μg/dl, the range of enzyme activity was 65-350 units.

Lysozyme (EC 3.2.1.17; mucopeptide N-acetylmuramyl hydrolase)

The activity of the enzyme lysozyme[199,200] is increased in inflammatory states and infections and in some types of leukemia. Urinary levels may be increased in a number of renal diseases.

Principle: The enzyme is usually determined by its action of hydrolyzing the cell walls of the microorganism *Micrococcus lysodeikticus* thereby decreasing the turbidity of a suspension of the organism. The enzyme is present in relatively large quantities in egg white, and the pure enzyme has been isolated from egg white for use as a standard.

Reagents:

1. Phosphate buffer, 0.067 mole/L, pH 6.2
   Dissolve 1.75 g Na_2HPO_4 and 0.740 g KH_2PO_4 in water to make 1 L. Check the pH and adjust to 6.2 with the addition of a small amount of 1 mole/L sodium hydroxide or hydrochloric acid as required.

2. Sodium chloride, 0.15 mole/L
   Dissolve 9 g sodium chloride in water to make 1 L.

3. Substrate
   Add 15 mg dried cells of *Micrococcus lysodeikticus* to 10 ml sodium chloride solution and mix. Dilute to 1 dl with the buffer. Mix on a vortex mixer to ensure that the cells are completely disbursed without any clumps. The substrate is stable for about 30 hr and should be prepared 12 hr in advance of the assay.

4. Enzyme standard
   The enzyme used should be crystallized at least three times and then dialyzed free of salt and lyophilized. Sigma grade I (Sigma Chemical Co., St. Louis) may be used (25,000-50,000 units/mg protein).
   a. Stock standard. Dissolve 10 mg of the enzyme in 25 ml of the sodium chloride solution. This is stable for 1 week at 4° C.
   b. Intermediate standard. Dilute a portion of the stock 1:10 with saline (20 μg protein/ml). This solution is not stable and should be prepared fresh as needed.
   c. Working standards. Dilute 1, 2, 3, and 4 ml of the intermediate standard to 10 ml with saline. These contain 2, 4, 6, and 8 μg/ml protein. Prepare dilutions just before use.

Procedure: In one cuvet place 5 ml of saline as blank. To similar cuvets for standards and samples add 5 ml of the substrate. Place all cuvets in a water bath at 37° C and allow to equilibrate at this temperature. Set spectrophotometer at 540 nm and zero with a blank. Treat one cuvet at a time. To a cuvet with 5 ml of substrate warmed to 37° C add 0.5 ml of sample or standard also previously warmed to 37° C and mix by inversion. Start stopwatch and take reading exactly 30 sec after addition of sample. Return to 37° C water bath for about 100 sec and then take second reading exactly 150 sec after the first. Use the same procedure for each standard or sample.

Calculation: For the standards plot the ΔA (difference between two readings) against the concentration of standards (in micrograms per milliliter). Note that the concentrations are expressed in micrograms of enzyme and not in enzyme units. The samples are read from the calibration curve. Serum or plasma may be used, but heparin should not be used as an anticoagulant because it interferes with the reaction. Urine samples should be centrifuged before the assay is performed. If the instrument has a thermostated cuvet well, the procedure can be simplified by leaving the cuvet in the well between readings. If the sample is too high it should be diluted with saline and the assay repeated.

Normal values and interpretation: The normal range for serum by this method is 3-8 μg/ml and less than 3 μg/ml for urine. In view of the variations in the standards available, it is advisable to check the determinations with a number of normal serum samples.

Serum lysozyme is elevated in acute and chronic microcytic leukemia[201] and in renal disease. High urinary levels are found in a number of renal diseases.

REFERENCES

1. Enzyme Nomenclature: Recommendations on enzyme nomenclature of the Commission on Nomenclature and Classification of the Enzymes of the International Union of Biochemistry, Amsterdam, 1973, Elsevier Publishing Co.
2. Baron, D.N., et al.: J. Clin. Pathol. **24:**656, 1971.
3. Baron, D.N., et al.: J. Clin. Pathol. **28:**592, 1975.
4. Bowers, G.N., Jr., et al.: In Amido, G., et al.: editors: Quality control in clinical chemistry, Berlin, 1973, Walter de Gruyter and Co.
5. Bergmeyer, H.U.: Med. Lab. **30:**57, 1977.
6. Hess, B.: Enzymes in blood plasma (translated by K.S. Henley), New York, 1963, Academic Press, Inc.
7. Swanson, J.R., and Wilkerson, J.H.: In Cooper, G.R. editor: Standard methods of clinical chemistry, New York, 1972, Academic Press, Inc., vol. 7, p. 33.
8. Szasz, G., Gruber, W., and Bernt, E.: Clin. Chem. **22:**650, 1976.
9. Dobosz, I.: Clin. Chim. Acta **50:**301, 1974.
10. Meites, S., editor: Pediatric clinical chemistry, Washington, D.C., 1977, American Association for Clinical Chemistry, p. 84.
11. Garcia, W.: J.A.M.A. **228:**1395, 1974.
12. Meltzer, H.Y.: J.A.M.A. **229:**1169, 1974.
13. Yasmineh, W.G., and Hanson, N.Q.: Clin. Chem. **21:**381, 1975.
14. Roberts, R., and Sobel, B.E.: Am. Heart J. **95:**521, 1978.
15. Obzansky, D., and Lott, J.A.: Clin. Chem. **26:**150, 1980.
16. Gerhardt, W., and Waldenström, J.: Clin. Chem. **25:**1274, 1979.
17. Nealon, D.A., and Henderson, A.R.: Clin. Chem. **21:**392, 1975.
18. Henry, P.D., Roberts, R., and Sobel, B.E.: Clin. Chem. **21:**844, 1975.
19. Willerson, J.T., et al.: Proc. Natl. Acad. Sci. U.S.A. **74:**1711, 1977.

20. Roberts, R., Sobel, B.E., and Parker, C.W.: Clin. Chim. Acta **83**:141, 1978.
21. Klein, B., et al.: Clin. Chem. **23**:504, 1977.
22. Roberts, R., et al.: Am. J. Cardiol. **33**:650, 1974.
23. Ahumada, G., Roberts, R., and Sobel, B.E.: Prog. Cardiovasc. Dis. **18**:405, 1976.
24. Navin, T.R., and Hager, D.W.: Curr. Probl. Cardiol. **3**:1, 1979.
25. Roe, C.R.: Ann. Clin. Lab. Sci. **7**:201, 1977.
26. Blomberg, D.J., Kimber, D.W., and Burke, M.D.: Am. J. Med. **59**:464, 1975.
27. Irvin, R.G., Cobb, F.R., and Roe, C.R.: Arch. Intern. Med. **140**:329, 1980.
28. Shell, W.E., et al.: J. Clin. Invest. **52**:2579, 1973.
29. Roe, C.R.: Clin. Chem. **23**:1807, 1977.
30. Lederer, W.H., and Gertsbrein, H.L.: Clin. Chem. **22**:1748, 1976.
31. Silverman, L.D., et al.: Clin. Chem. **25**:1432, 1979.
32. Forman, D.T.: Ann. Clin. Lab. Sci. **9**:333, 1979.
33. Feld, R.D., and Witte, D.L.: Clin. Chem. **23**:1930, 1977.
34. Hoag, G.N., et al.: Clin. Biochem. **13**:1949, 1980.
35. Coolen, R.B., and Pragay, D.: Clin. Chem. **22**:1174, 1976.
36. Koste, M., et al.: Arch. Neurol. **34**:142, 1977.
37. Doran, G.R.: Clin. Chim. Acta **92**:415, 1979.
38. Gerson, B., and Petersen, K.: Clin. Chem. **24**:1518, 1979.
39. Zsigmond, E.K., et al.: Anesth. Analg. (Cleve.) **51**:220, 1972.
40. Weyman, A.E., et al.: Am. J. Med. **56**:13, 1974.
41. McDaniel, R.C., and Devine, J.E.: Ann. Clin. Lab. Sci. **10**:155, 1980.
42. Rock, R.C., et al.: Clin. Chim. Acta **62**:159, 1975.
43. Cornbleet, P.J., and Evans, M.D.: Clin. Chem. **26**:1635, 1980.
44. Vladutiu, A.O., et al.: Clin. Chim. Acta **75**:467, 1977.
45. Laboda, H.M., and Britton, V.J.: Clin. Chem. **23**:1329, 1977.
46. Yuu, H., et al.: Clin. Chem. **24**:2054, 1978.
47. Liu, T.Z., et al.: Clin. Chem. **25**:1765, 1980.
48. Sax, S.M., et al.: Clin. Chem. **22**:87, 1976.
49. Ljungdahl, L., and Gerhardt, W.: Clin. Chem. **24**:832, 1978.
50. McClellan, S.L., Lee, N., and Madiedo, G.: Am. J. Clin. Pathol. **73**:799, 1980.
51. Lim, F.: Clin. Chem. **21**:975, 1975.
52. Buhl, S.N., et al.: Clin. Chem. **23**:200, 1977.
53. Kieding, R.: Scand. J. Clin. Lab. Invest. **33**:291, 1974.
54. Bais, R., Prior, M.P., and Edwards, J.B.: Clin. Chem. **23**:1056, 1977.
55. Lott, J.A., and Turner, K.: In Cooper, G.R., editor: Selected methods for the small clinical laboratory, vol. 9, Washington, D.C., 1981, American Association for Clinical Chemistry.
56. Wacker, W.E.C., and Dorfman, L.E.: J.A.M.A. **181**:972, 1962.
57. Dorfman, L.E., Amador, E., and Wacker, W.E.C.: J.A.M.A. **184**:1, 1963.
58. Elliott, B.A., and Wilkinson, J.H.: Lancet **1**:698, 1961.
59. Rosalki, S.B., and Wilkinson, J.H.: Nature **188**:1110, 1960.
60. Elliot, B.A., and Wilkinson, J.H.: Clin. Sci. Mol. Med. **24**:343, 1963.
61. Smith, F.A.: Clin. Chim. Acta **35**:498, 1971.
62. Plagemann, P.G.W., et al.: Biochem. Z. **2**:334, 1961.
63. Schlabach, T.D., Alpert, A.J., and Regneis, F.E.: Clin. Chem. **24**:1351, 1978.
64. Gregory, K.F., and Wroblewski, F.: Ann. N.Y. Acad. Sci. **94**:912, 1961.
65. Cawley, L.P.: Electrophoresis and immunoelectrophoresis, Boston, 1969, Little, Brown & Co.
66. De Giorgio, J.: Clin. Chem. **17**:326, 1971.
67. Myers, R.C., and Van Remortel, H.: Clin. Chem. **14**:1131, 1968.
68. Dietz, A.A., et al.: In Cooper, G.R., editor: Standard methods of clinical chemistry, New York, 1972, Academic Press, Inc., vol. 7, p. 49.
69. Jacobs, D.S., et al.: Ann. Clin. Lab. Sci. **7**:411, 1977.
70. Zondag, H.A., and Klein, F.: Ann. N.Y. Acad. Sci **151**:578, 1968.
71. Wroblewski, F.: Am. J. Med. Sci. **234**:391, 1957.
72. Goldman, R.D., Kaplan, N.O., and Hall, T.C.: Cancer Res. **24**:389, 1964.
73. Mirabile, C.S., Bowers, G.N., Jr., and Berlin, B.B.: J. Urol. **95**:79, 1966.
74. Glennon, J.A., and Healy, M.K.: Conn. Med. **30**:183, 1966.
75. Raabo, E., Rasmussen, K.N., and Terkildsen, T.C.: Scand, J. Respir. Dis. **47**:150, 1966.
76. Bergmeyer, H.U., Scheibe, P., and Wahlefeld, A.W.: Clin. Chem. **24**:58, 1978.
77. London, J.W., et al.: Clin. Chem. **21**:1939, 1975.
78. Moss, D.W.: J. Clin. Chem. Clin. Biochem. **15**:719, 1977.
79. Burger, F.J., and Potgeiter, G.F.: Clin. Chem. **24**:841, 1978.
80. Morin, L.G., and Prox, J.: Clin. Chem. **19**:776, 1973.
81. Bowers, G.N., Jr., and McComb, R.B.: Clin. Chem. **12**:70, 1966.
82. Bowers, G.N., Jr., McComb, R.B., and Kelley, M.L.: In Cooper, G.R., editor: Selected methods of clinical chemistry, Washington, D.C., 1977, American Association for Clinical Chemistry, vol. 8.
83. McComb, R.B., Bowers, G.N., Jr., and Posen, S.: Alkaline phosphatase, New York, 1979, Plenum Publishing Corp.
84. Babson, A.L., et al.: Clin. Chem. **12**:482, 1966.
85. Fishman, W.H., et al.: Cancer Res. **28**:150, 1968.
86. Fernlez, H.N., and Walker, P.G.: Biochem J. **116**:543, 1970.
87. Kellen, J.A., and Lustig, V.: Oncology **25**:239, 1971.
88. Epstein, E., Baginski, E.S., and Zak, B.: Ann. Clin. Lab. Sci. **8**:34, 1978.
89. Whitby, L.G., and Moss, D.W.: Clin. Chim. Acta **59**:361, 1975.
90. Moss, D.W., and Whitby, L.G.: Clin. Chim. Acta **61**:63, 1975.
91. Taswell, H., and Jeffers, D.: Am. J. Clin. Pathol. **40**:347, 1963.
92. Nathanson, L., and Fishman, W.: Cancer **27**:1388, 1971.
93. Fishman, W., Inglis, N., and Green, S.: Cancer Res. **31**:1054, 1971.
94. Fishman, W., Zimmermann, T.S., and Wacker, W.E.C.: J.A.M.A. **185**:769, 1973.
95. Gault, M.H., et al.: Br. J. Urol. **39**:296, 1967.
96. Szasz, G.: Clin. Chem. **22**:2011, 1976.
97. Szasz, G.: In Cooper, G.R., editor: Selected methods of clinical chemistry, Washington, 1977, American Association for Clinical Chemistry, vol. 8.
98. Baginski, E.S., et al.: Ann. Clin. Lab. Sci. **7**:469, 1977.
99. Young, I.I.: Ann. N.Y. Acad. Sci. **75**:357, 1958.
100. Schwartz, M.K., and Bodansky, O.: Am. J. Clin. Pathol. **42**:886, 1965.
101. Bodansky, O., and Schwartz, M.K.: In Bodansky, O., and Stewart, C.P., editors: Advances in clinical chemistry, New York, 1968, Academic Press, Inc., vol. 2, p. 278.

102. Kim, N.K., et al.: Clin. Chem. **23**:2034, 1977.
103. Schosinsky, K.H., Lehman, P.E., and Beeler, M.F.: Clin. Chem. **20**:1556, 1974.
104. Lehman, P.L., Schosinsky, K.H., and Beeler, M.F.: Clin. Chem. **20**:1654, 1974.
105. Hrgovic, M., et al.: Cancer **21**:743, 1968.
106. Lee, G.R., et al.: J. Clin. Invest. **47**:2058, 1968.
107. Topham, R.W., and Frieden, E.: J. Biol. Chem. **245**:6698, 1970.
108. Bagrel, A., Museur, C., and Siest G.: Clin. Chem. **21**:1716, 1975.
109. Vassef, A.A.: Clin. Chem. **24**:101, 1978.
110. Bowers, G.N., Jr.: Clin. Chem. **5**:509, 1959.
111. Ellis, C., and Goldberg, D.M.: Clin. Biochem. **2**:175, 1971.
112. Wacker, W.E.C., Ulmer, D.D., and Vallee, B.L.: N. Engl. J. Med. **255**:449, 1955.
113. Bergmeyer, H.U., and Bernt, E.: In Bergmeyer, H.U., editor: Methods of enzymatic analysis, New York, 1965, Academic Press, Inc., p. 757.
114. Wiesner, I.S., et al.: Am. J. Dig. Dis. **10**:147, 1965.
115. Rose, C.L., and Henderson, A.R.: Clin. Chem. **21**:1619, 1975.
116. Jung, K., Sokolowski, A., and Egger, E.: Enzyme **14**:44, 1973.
117. Jung, K.: Clin. Chim. Acta **36**:231, 1972.
118. Mellerup, B.: Clin. Chem. **13**:900, 1967.
119. Loeb, W.F., and Stuhlman, R.A.: Clin. Chem. **15**:162, 1969.
120. Jorgovic, L., et al.: Clin. Chim. Acta **30**:765, 1970.
121. Ellis, G., and Goldberg, D.M.: Clin. Chim. Acta **37**:47, 1972.
122. Mandel, E.E., et al.: Am. J. Gastroenterol. **54**:253, 1970.
123. Coodley, E.L.: Am. J. Gastroenterol. **50**:55, 1968.
124. Goldberg, D.M.: Br. Med. J. **1**:353, 1965.
125. Karker, H.: Scand. J. Clin. Lab. Invest. **16**:570, 1964.
126. Nishihara, H., et al.: Clin. Chim. Acta **30**:251, 1970.
127. Sibley, J.A.: Ann. N.Y. Acad. Sci. **75**:399, 1959.
128. Drefus, J.C., Schapira, G., and Schapira, F.: J. Clin. Invest. **33**:794, 1954.
129. Volk, B.W., et al.: Am. J. Med. Sci. **232**:38, 1956.
130. Beck, W.S.: J. Biol. Chem. **212**:38, 1955.
131. Somogyi, M.: Clin. Chem. **6**:23, 1960.
132. Henry, R.J., and Chiamori, N.: Clin. Chem. **6**:434, 1960.
133. Caraway, W.T.: Am. J. Clin. Pathol. **32**:97, 1959.
134. McNair, R.D.: In MacDonald, R.P., editor: Standard methods of clinical chemistry, New York, 1970, Academic Press, Inc., vol. 6, p. 183.
135. Sax, S.M., Bridgewater, A.B., and Moore, J.J.: Clin. Chem. **17**:311, 1971.
136. Babson, A.L., Tenney, S.A., and Megraw, R.E.: Clin. Chem. **16**:39, 1970.
137. Klein, B., Foreman, J.A., and Search, R.L.: Clin. Chem. **16**:32, 1970.
138. Hathaway, J.A., Hunter, D.T., and Barrett, C.R.: Clin. Biochem. **3**:217, 1970.
139. Hall, F.F., et al.: Am. J. Clin. Pathol. **53**:627, 1970.
140. Saxon, E.I., et al.: Arch. Intern. Med. **99**:607, 1957.
141. Song, H., Teitz, N.W., and Tan, C.: Clin. Chem. **16**:264, 1970.
142. Gambill, E.E.: Pancreatitis, St. Louis, 1973, The C.V. Mosby Co., p. 50.
143. Banks, P.A.: Pancreatitis, New York, 1979, Medical Book Co., p. 65.
144. Berk, J.E., et al.: Am. J. Gastroenterol. **53**:211, 1970.
145. Barrows, D., Berk, J.E., and Fridhandler, L .: N. Engl. J. Med. **286**:1352, 1972.
146. Kohler, H., et al.: Eur. J. Clin. Invest. **7**:205, 1977.
147. Duerr, H.K., et al.: Eur. J. Clin. Invest. **8**:189, 1978.
148. Stefanini, P., et al.: Am. J. Surg. **110**:866, 1965.
149. Levitt, M.D., et al.: Ann. Intern. Med. **71**:919, 1969.
150. Warshaw, M.D., and Fuller, A.F.: N. Engl. J. Med. **292**:325, 1975.
151. Murry, W.R., and MacKay, C.: Br. J. Surg. **64**:189, 1977.
152. Levine, R.I., et al.: N. Engl. J. Med. **292**:329, 1975.
153. Morton, W.J., et al.: Gastroenterology **68**:961, 1975.
154. Berger, G.M.B., et al.: S. Afr. Med. J. **50**:1559, 1976.
155. Duerr, H.K., et al.: N. Engl. J. Med. **296**:635, 1977.
156. Levitt, M.D., and Johnson, S.G.: Gastroenterology **75**:118, 1978.
157. Benjamin, D.R., and Kenny, M.A.: Am. J. Clin. Pathol. **62**:753, 1974.
158. Lehrner, L.M., et al.: Am. J. Clin. Pathol. **66**:576, 1976.
159. Legaz, M.E., and Kenny, M.A.: Clin. Chem. **22**:57, 1976.
160. Levitt, M.D.: Mayo Clin. Proc. **54**:428, 1979.
161. Gillard, B.K.: Clin. Chem. **25**:1919, 1979.
162. Ladenson, J.H., et al.: Clin. Chem. **24**:815, 1978.
163. Kaufman, R.A., and Tietz, N.W.: In Goldberg, D.M., and Werner, M., editors: Progress in clinical enzymology, New York, 1980, Masson Publishing U.S.A., Inc., p. 219.
164. Arst, H.E., Manning, R.T., and Depl, M.H.: Am. J. Med. Sci. **238**:598, 1959.
165. Tietz, N.W., Broden, T., and Stapleton, J.D.: Am. J. Clin. Pathol. **31**:148, 1959.
166. Tietz, N.W., and Fiereck, E.A.: In Cooper, G.R., editor: Standard methods of clinical chemistry, New York, 1972, Academic Press, Inc., vol. 7, p. 19.
167. Massion, C.G.: Lab. Med. **2**:26, 1961.
168. Massion, C.G., and Seligson, D.: Am. J. Clin. Pathol. **48**:307, 1967.
169. Massion, C.G., and McNeely, M.D.D.: Ann. Clin. Lab. Sci. **2**:444, 1972.
170. Lifton, L.J., et al.: J.A.M.A. **229**:47, 1974.
171. Yang, J.S., and Biggs, H.G.: Clin. Chem. **17**:512, 1971.
172. Szasz, G.: Am. J. Clin. Pathol. **47**:607, 1967.
173. Willig, F., et al.: Klin. Wochenschr. **45**:474, 1967.
174. Joesch, W., and Dubach, U.C.: J. Clin. Chem. Clin. Biochem. **5**:59, 1967.
175. Erlanger, B.F., Kokowsky, N., and Cohen, W.: Arch. Biochem. Biophys. **95**:271, 1961.
176. Fishman, W.H., and Lerner, F: J. Biol. Chem. **200**:89, 1953.
177. Sudhof, H., Meumann, G., and Oloffs, J.: Dtsch. Med. Wochenschr. **89**:217, 1964.
178. Lepow, H., et al.: J. Urol. **87**:991, 1962.
179. Roy, A.V., Brower, M.E., and Hayden, J.E.: Clin. Chem. **17**:1093, 1971.
180. Doe, R.D., Mellinger, G.T., and Seal, U.S.: Clin. Chem. **11**:943, 1965.
181. Hsia, D.Y.Y.: Inborn errors of metabolism, ed. 2, Chicago, 1966, Year Book Medical Publishers, Inc.
182. Stanbury, J.B., Wyngaarden, J.B., and Fredrickson, D.S., editors: The metabolic basis of inherited disease, ed. 4, New York, 1978, McGraw-Hill Book Co.
183. Bishop, C.: J. Lab. Clin. Med. **68**:149, 1968.
184. Beutler, E.: Red cell metabolism, New York, 1971, Grune & Stratton, Inc.
185. Blume, K.G., Loehr, G.W., and Beutler, E.: Clin. Chim. Acta **43**:443, 1973.
186. Morse, E.E.: In Sunderman, F.W., editor: Seminar on clinical enzymology, Philadelphia, 1976, Institute for Clinical Science, p. 233.

187. Carson, P., Brewer, G.J., and Ickes, C.: J. Lab. Clin. Med. **58:**804, 1961.
188. Hormbeck, C.L., and Bradley, D.W.: Clin. Chem. **20:**512, 1974.
189. Ratliff, C.R., Culp, T.W., and Hall, F.F.: Am. J. Gastroenterol. **56:**199, 1971.
190. Schwartz, M.K.: Clin. Chem. **19:**10, 1973.
191. Dietz, A.A., Rubinstein, H.M., and Hodges, L.V.: In Cooper, G.R., editor: Selected methods of clinical chemistry, Washington, D.C., 1977, American Association for Clinical Chemistry, vol. 8, p. 149.
192. Heidelberger, K.P.: Ann. Clin. Lab. Sci. **6:**110, 1976.
193. Rappaport, F., Fischl, J., and Pinto, N.: Clin. Chim. Acta **4:**227, 1959.
194. Dietz, A.A., Rubenstein, H.M., and Lubrano, T.: In Cooper, G.R., editor: Selected methods of clinical chemistry, Washington, D.C., 1977, American Association for Clinical Chemistry, vol. 8, p. 41.
195. Rubenstein, H.M., et al.: J. Clin. Invest. **48:**479, 1971.
196. Bearn, A.G., and Litwin, D.S.: In Stanbury, J.B., Wyngaarden, J.B., and Frederickson, D.S., editors: Metabolic basis of inherited disease, ed. 4, New York, 1978, McGraw-Hill Publishing Co., p. 1712.
197. Lubran, M.M.: In Sunderman, F.W., editor: Seminar on clinical enzymology, Philadelphia, 1976, Institute for Clinical Science, p. 237.
198. Mitchell, H.A., et al.: Clin. Chem. **23:**105, 1976.
199. Reimer, S.M.: In Sunderman, F.W., editor: Seminar on clinical enzymology, Philadelphia, 1976, Institute for Clinical Science, p. 245.
200. Zuker, S., and Webb, A.W.: In Cooper, G.R., editor: Standard methods of clinical chemistry, New York, 1972, Academic Press, Inc., vol. 7, p. 9.
201. Perillie, P.E., et al.: J.A.M.A. **203:**317, 1968.

CHAPTER 25

Hormone analysis

NATURE OF HORMONES[1-3]

A hormone may be broadly defined as any substance normally produced by specialized cells in some part of the body and carried by the bloodstream to other parts of the body where it may affect other specialized cells or exert a more general effect other specialized cells or exert a more general effect on the body processes. Because hormones play an essential role in body metabolism, a deficiency or excess may lead to serious derangement of body function. Since the majority of the hormones are carried in the bloodstream to their sites of action, measuring the blood concentration of a particular hormone would seem to be the simplest and most direct method of determining abnormal levels. Unfortunately most of the hormones are present in blood in such small amounts that their measurement is very difficult. Before the introduction of the competitive protein-binding and radioimmunoassay methods, only very few hormones were routinely determined in blood (usually in serum or plasma).

Some of the hormones or their metabolites are excreted in the urine and in many instances their concentration in urine is much greater than in blood. Since it is much easier to obtain a few hundred milliliters of urine, than, say, 20 ml of blood, some hormone analysis may be done with urine. Since the hormone excretion rate may vary during the day, the use of a 24 hr urine specimen gives more accurate results. Not all hormones are excreted in the urine in appreciable amounts; those of lower molecular weight, e.g., the steroids, are more likely to be found in the urine in

measurable amounts than are larger molecules such as the pituitary hormones. In some instances the hormone itself may not be excreted in the urine in large quantities, but various metabolites of the hormone may be found. The measurement of these metabolites sometimes gives a satisfactory estimate of the amount of original hormone present in the blood.

A number of different methods have been used for hormone analysis. The older methods are generally colorimetric or fluorometric. The hormone is extracted from the blood or urine by the use of an immiscible organic solvent or by the use of a chromatographic column. In urine, hormones may be present primarily as conjugated glucuronides or sulfates, and these must be hydrolyzed before extraction. After some further purification the extracted hormone or its metabolites are treated with a reagent to produce a color or fluorescence for measurement. The problem here is that it is often difficult to remove all interfering substances that would also react with the reagent, and the reagents are usually not very specific for a single hormone or metabolite. The urinary steroid hormones and metabolites can be better separated by gas chromatography[4] (see p. 456 for some details on the principle of this method, which is not yet adapted to routine clinical laboratory determinations). Recent methods that have been adapted for the determination of a number of different hormones are those using competitive protein binding and radioimmunoassay. Since the principles involved are somewhat different from the familiar colorimetric procedures, a brief survey of the general method is given.

Competitive binding methods

Several methods based on the principle of competitive binding are used for the determination of hormones and a number of other substances, including some drugs, in body fluids. For convenience, in the following discussion the substance being determined is referred to as a hormone, although there are applications for the determination of other substances as well. The method is based on the principle of using some substance or compound that will selectively absorb or combine with the hormone being determined. In addition, there is some method for labeling or otherwise distinguishing between the hormone present in the original sample and the added amount of labeled hormone, and there is some method of separating the hormone that is bound to the binding substance from that which

Table 25-1. Examples of competitive protein binding

Mixture		Bound	Free
1.	90 B + 100 A*	90 A*B	10 A*
2.	90 B + 100 A*	60 A*B	40 A*
	+ 50 A	30 AB	20 A
3.	90 B + 100 A*	45 A*B	55 A*
	+ 100 A	45 AB	55 A
4. 90 A*B +	90 A	45 A*B	45 A*
		45 AB	45 A
5.	90 B + 70 A*	70 A*B	
6.	90 B + 70 A*	70 A*B	
	+ 20 A	20 AB	
7.	90 B + 50 A* ⎱	45 A*B	5 A*
	50 A ⎰	45 AB	5 A
8.	90 B + 50 A* ⎱	30 A*B	20 A*
	50 A ⎰	60 AB	40 A
	50 A		

remains free. Table 25-1 and the following explanation will help to make this more clear. In the following brief discussion, A will designate the molecules of the substance being determined, with A* the added A molecules that are labeled or identified in some way in which they may be measured, and B the binding substance. The exact nature of the labeling and of the binding substances will be different for the different methods, and these will be treated later. In addition, there is a requirement that the binding substance B combine equally well with the A molecules and with the A* molecules. Also, some method is needed to separate the bound AB and A*B molecules from the unbound A and A* molecules. The methods of separation may differ from assay to assay. For simplicity, small numbers are used for the explanation, although actually 1 ng of a hormone may contain around 10^{12} molecules. In some instances the binding substance B may be a large molecule that actually binds several A molecules; however, this makes no difference in the illustration if B is considered to be the number of binding sites rather than the number of binding molecules.

Suppose that 90 molecules of B are mixed with 100 molecules of A* (line 1 of Table 25-1). Then 90 molecules of the complex A*B will be formed and 10 molecules of A* will remain uncombined. If the AB complex is now separated from the uncombined A molecules by some means, 90% of the A* molecules would be in the bound fraction and 10% in the free fraction. (A number of different methods of separation have been used and are discussed later, but generally the AB molecules are much larger than either component, and the separation is often based on this.) If to the same amounts of B and A* molecules we add, as a standard, 50 molecules of unlabeled A (line 2 of Table 25-1), then since one of the requirements of the test is that the B molecules combine equally well with the A and with the A* molecules, we see that now 40% of the labeled molecles are in the free fraction and 60% in the bound fraction. (line 2). Similarly, when 100 molecules of A are added (line 3), 45% of the labeled molecules will be in the bound fraction and 55% in the free fraction. As the amount of A is increased, the distribution of the labeled A* molecules between the two fractions

changes. By plotting the amount of A* in one fraction against the amount of added standard, a calibration curve may be constructed that can be used to obtain the amounts of A in added samples. In practice, somewhat more sophisticated methods of plotting are used, but the principle remains the same.

The molecules of A* and B may be added to the solution as the complex A*B. When the unlabeled molecules of A are then added and equilibrium is established, the final results are the same as seen by comparing lines 3 and 4 of Table 25-1. In the procedure a sufficient amount of the labeled material designated by A* must be added to combine with all the binding agent present. This is illustrated in lines 5 and 6. If only 70 molecules of A* are added to 90 molecules of B, all the A* will be found in the bound fraction, as indicated in line 5. Even when 20 molecules of A are added (line 6), all the labeled molecules still remain in the bound fraction; the addition of the extra A molecules produces no change.

In practice the labeled material designated by A* in Table 25-1 may not consist entirely of labeled molecules but of a mixture of labeled and unlabeled molecules. This makes no difference as long as the proportion of labeled and unlabeled molecules remains the same. This is illustrated by comparing lines 1 and 2 with lines 7 and 8. In lines 7 and 8 the 100 A* of the first two lines has been replaced by 50 A + 50 A*; the ratio of A* in the free and bound fractions is the same in lines 1 and 7 and in lines 2 and 8, although the actual amounts are different.

Labeled molecules

The most common method of labeling compounds (A* Table 25-1) is with a radioactive atom, usually ^{125}I, ^{14}C, or ^3H (tritium), although for special purposes other atoms may be used. The ^{125}I is the easiest to measure and is often used. It can be measured in a simple γ-counter. The carbon and hydrogen isotopes require a more complicated scintillation counter, so that the use of ^{125}I is preferred when it is available. An increased use of nonisotopic competitive binding assays is seen in more recent developments. These include enzyme and fluorescent markers used in both homogeneous and heterogeneous assay systems. These nonisotopic methods are relatively simple to perform, do not require sophisticated or expensive equipment, and can often achieve a sensitivity equal to that of radioimmunoassay (RIA) methods. These procedures are discussed in more detail later.

Competitive protein-binding methods

A number of hormones and hormonelike substances are bound by specific proteins in the serum.[5,6] The binding protein may serve a definite physiologic purpose as the thyroxine-binding globulin, which serves to transport the thyroxine from the thyroid gland to its sites of action in the cells, or it may serve a less obvious purpose, e.g., as a protein in the serum of pregnant women that has been found to strongly bind the hormone testosterone. If available, such binding proteins can be used as the binding agent in the assay of a hormone. The labeling of the hormone is usually done by means of a radioactive isotope, often ^{14}C or ^{3}H. The practical difficulty with the method is obtaining the binding protein in a sufficiently pure form. In some instances serum can be used directly or with only a simple purification step. The separation of the free and bound portions may be made by gel filtration with Sephadex by an ion-exchange resin, by precipitation of the bound fraction, or by absorption on solid particles such as dextran-coated charcoal. Many procedures formerly done by this method have now been replaced by radioimmunoassay methods.

Radioimmunoassay

In radioimmunoassay (RIA) methods[7,8] the binding agent B is an antibody to the A molecules and the combined AB complexes can usually be easily separated from the unbound A molecules. In cases in which the A molecules are too small to form a satisfactory antibody they may be coupled to a larger molecule to form a satisfactory antigen. In the competitive protein-binding methods the binding protein was often simply obtained from a suitable serum specimen by easy manipulations. In the radioimmunoassay methods the binding antibodies usually must be obtained commmercially, because it is difficult to prepare them in the laboratory. The antibody-antigen complex is separated from the uncombined antigen by methods similar to those used in competitive protein-binding methods, e.g., gel filtration, precipitation, and absorption. A refinement sometimes used is to add a second antibody to combine with the AB and A*B complexes to form a larger complex that is more readily separated by centrifugation or filtration (double antibody technic).

Another variation of RIA is solid-phase immunoassay. This makes use of the fact that some proteins, including many antibodies, are strongly absorbed by certain plastics such as plystyrene and polypropylene. Plastic tubes may be obtained that are already coated on the lower inside portion with the required antibody, or the serum with the antibody may be added to the tubes and the absorption of the antibody will take place during the incubation period. In any event, after the desired reactions have taken place, the antibody and the combined antigens (represented by AB and A*B of Table 25-1) will remain firmly absorbed on the walls of the tubes, and the unbound material may be separated by merely pouring off the solution in the tubes and rinsing the tubes briefly with a wash solution. The radioactivity in the tubes may be measured to give the bound fraction in the tubes. Thus the separation is easily made without any centrifugation or other treatment.

A recent publication, "Chemists' guide to radioassay products," ed. 2, which is found in *Clinical chemistry,* vol. 24, no. 7, 1978, pp. 1222-80, contains a list of products for radioimmunoassay listed by analyte, with the manufacturers' addresses and phone numbers, a bibliography of the literature, and an essay on troubleshooting."

A number of instruments are now available for the automation of RIA procedures.[9] Useful for laboratories with relatively large sample volumes, these instruments

can be adapted for a number of RIAs, greatly increasing the precision over that in manual assays.

Enzyme immunoassay

One type of enzyme immunoassay (EIA) is similar to RIAs except that the A* molecules of Table 25-1 are labeled not with a radioactive atom but with an enzyme. The enzyme is coupled with the A molecule in such a way that this does not interfere with its action as an antigen (coupling with the B molecules) nor with the activity of the enzyme. Then after separation, as in the previous methods, the amound of A* in either fraction is estimated by determining the enzymatic activity in the fraction in the usual manner. Enzymes that are simple to measure, e.g., peroxidase or lysozyme, may be used. When such methods are applicable, the EIA has several advantages over the RIA: (1) there is no radioactive material and hence no precautions need be taken in this regard; (2) the reagents may have a longer shelf life with proper care; and (3) the enzymes used are easily determined in the usual clinical laboratory, are readily adapted to automated methods already available in the laboratory, and do not require expensive equipment such as γ-counters.

These methods have not yet been adapted to as wide a variety of hormones as have competitive protein binding methods or RIAs, but further developments may be expected.

A variation of the heterogeneous method described above is the homogeneous EIA. This procedure is often referred to as an enzyme multiplied immunoassay technic or EMIT (registered trade name of Syva Corp., Palo Alto, Calif.). In this method the enzyme is coupled to the antigen in such a way that the complex (equivalent to A* of Table 25-1 and here labeled A-E) inhibits the action of the enzyme; i.e., the enzyme in the form A-E is not active as an enzymatic agent because of the nature of the binding between A and E. However, when the A-E complex combines with the binding substance (B of Table 25-1) to form B-A-E (A*B of Table 25-1), the enzyme becomes active; the combination of B-A somehow removes the inhibition of the enzyme because of the binding with A. This is equivalent to stating that only the A*B molecules are enzymatically active and are measured by the enzymatic analysis, whereas the A* molecules are not. Referring again to Table 25-1, we see that it is not necessary for the determination to separate the "bound" and "free" fractions, since the total amount of A*B in both fractions together is different in lines 1, 2, and 3, which correspond to zero and two different standards. Thus the measurements can be made without any separation of the fractions. This simplifies the procedure and thus offers many advantages when applicable.

Advances in both EIA systems, EMIT and enzyme-linked immunosorbent assay (ELISA) (in which the enzyme is often linked to antibody), have occurred, resulting in a wide spectrum of the type of antigen that can be measured. These include small, nonprotein hormones as well as the protein hormones. Many of these EIA procedures achieve a level of precision and sensitivity equal to that of RIA.

Fluorescent immunoassays

The use of enzymes as labels for substrates in immunoassays has more recently been paralleled by the use of fluorescent compounds as labels. The fluorescent immunoassays (FIA) are also available in both homogenous[10,11] and heterogeneous[12,13] systems. A major consideration of all FIAs is background fluorescence. The removal of serum in the heterogeneous FIAs may be advantageous for the measurement of compounds present in physiologic concentrations, e.g., hormones.

Homogeneous FIAs for serum proteins have also been developed that utilize the technic of fluorescent protection.[11] In this type of competitive immunoassay the fluorescence of a labeled analyte is inhibited when immune complexes are formed with antibodies to the fluorescer. The simplest model of this assay requires the fluorescent-tagged antigen and the antibodies to both the antigen and the fluorescer. In the absence of a competing, unlabeled antigen, immune complexes between a labeled antigen and antibodies to that antigen are allowed to form, protecting the fluorescer from reacting with its antibodies, resulting in a maximal fluorescent signal. As the concentration of competing, unlabeled antigens increases, more labeled antigens remain free to react with the antibody to the fluorescent tag, resulting in a decreased signal. The increased antigen concentrations in the sample are related to a decreasing fluorescent signal. Future modifications may allow this type of assay to be available for smaller molecules.[14]

The ability of FIAs to achieve a sensitivity comparable to RIAs may also result from the increased sophistication of the instrumentation. Newer fluorometers have the ability to count individual photons with reduced background signals, giving a theoretic counting rate approaching that of RIAs.[15]

High-performance liquid chromatography

The use of high-performance liquid chromatography (HPLC) to measure analytes present in pharmacologic doses has achieved widespread acceptance. However, the use of HPLC for the measurement of hormones present in physiologic concentrations (nanograms to micrograms per milliliter range) has lagged. This is primarily because of the lack of sensitivity of the HPLC detection systems. However the development of sensitive spectrofluoromter detectors and the increasing use of electrochemical detectors (ECD) may result in a more widespread use of this versatile technic. Several assays for the measurement of hormones in urine are already available, and assays for the measurement of serum constituents may be available soon (see below).

THYROID HORMONES

The hormones of the thyroid gland, **thyroxine** (tetraiodothyronine) and **triiodothyronine,** are unusual in that the molecules contain a relatively large percentage of iodine (65.4% for thyroxine). Most of the methods of assaying these hormones are based on the direct chemical determination of the iodine or on the use of radioactive iodine as a tracer. The synthesis and utilization of the thyroid hormones in the body involves a number of steps. These may be conveniently listed as follows:

1. Iodides in the blood derived from the dietary intake are absorbed by the thyroid gland.
2. The iodide in the gland is oxidized and combined with tyrosine derivatives to form triiodothyronine (T3) and tetraiodothyronine (T4, thyroxine).
3. The T3 and T4 are combined with protein and stored in the gland as thyroglobulin.
4. Under the influence of the pituitary hormones, T3 and T4 are released in the free form and secreted into the bloodstream.
5. In the plasma the hormones combine with certain protein (thyro-binding globulins) and are carried to the various organs and tissues of the body where they are released from the binding proteins and exert their metabolic effect.

The rate at which several of these different steps occur may be used to measure the activity of the thyroid gland.

Radioactive iodine uptake

The radioactive iodine (RAI) uptake measures step 1 above, the absorption of iodide by the thyroid gland. When a solution containing RAI is administered orally, it is rapidly absorbed into the bloodstream. Here the RAI acts similarly to the nonradioactive material, and both are absorbed by the thyroid gland. The rate of absorption of the RAI (increase in radioactivity of the gland) is then a measure of the ability of the thyroid gland to concentrate iodide from the plasma. The increase in radioactivity may be measured after 2, 6, or 24 hr, the last being the period most generally used. A comparison is usually made of the percentage of the administered dose that is absorbed by the thyroid in normal individuals and in the patients. In normal individuals, 1-13% will be absorbed after 2 hr, 2-25% after 6 hr, and 15-45% after 24 hr. This procedure measures only the first step in the production of the hormone. The absorption of iodine could be normal, and yet the actual production of the hormone could be low because of a deficiency in one of the subsequent steps. The RAI uptake is lower than normal in hypothyroidism and high in hyperthyroidism.

A number of substances inhibit the uptake of iodine. These include the previous administration of inorganic or organic iodine compounds, including many contrast media, thiocyanate, thiouracil and similar drugs, cortisone, ACTH, and estrogens. Also a number of foods contain inhibiting substances; cabbage and other members of the *Brassica* genus are particularly active. The urinary excretion of RAI has also been used as a measure of thyroid activity, since almost all of the RAI that is not absorbed by the thyroid gland is eventually excreted in the urine, but the test is not too reliable.

Since the in vivo use of radioactive materials requires a special Atomic Energy Commission license and the supervision of a qualified physician, this test is usally not run in the clinical laboratory but in a separate isotope laboratory or by a radiologist.

Since the advent of the immunoassays for the thyroid

hormones, the older chemical methods are now rarely used. However, for those who may require the estimation of the total thyroid hormone without the use of radioactive material, the following method is presented.

Thyroxine-binding index (TBI) and T3 uptake[16-18]

The thyroid hormones in plasma are bound to a specific plasma protein, the thyroxine-binding globulin (TBG). Under usual conditions TBG is not saturated with the thyroid hormones, and additional binding sites are available to combine with further hormone if it were present. Except in cases of severe dysproteinemia, the amount of TBG is relatively constant. Thus the number of unsaturated binding sites depends on the amount of endogenous hormone already present and bound to the plasma. The greater the amount of endogenous hormone present in the plasma, the smaller will be the number of sites available for binding by added exogenous hormone. Thus the determination of the number of binding sites present in a plasma sample is an inverse measure of the amount of endogenous hormone present.

The binding sites may be measured by adding an excess of ^{131}I-labeled T3 to a plasma sample to completely saturate the binding sites. The conditions are adjusted so that the added T3 will not displace any of the endogenous thyroid hormone present but merely add on to all the unsaturated sites. After equilibration, the excess unbound labeled T3 is removed, and the radioactivity of the saturated plasma is measured. The excess T3 may be removed by use of an ion-exchange resin by filtration through a Sephadex column, which will separate the smaller T3 molecules from the larger entities of the TBG-T3 complex. The radioactivity of the saturated plasma is compared with that of the original labeled T3 added and the proportion of the added radioactivity that is absorbed by the serum is calculated.

A number of different kits are available for the determination of the TBI. These may use different sequences in the addition of the reagents and sample, but, as pointed out in earlier discussions of Table 25-1, after equilibrium is established the result is the same irrespective of the order of addition. Also, there are two different methods for expressing the results of the TBI determination, again depending on the kit used.

In one procedure the radioactivity of the saturated TBG from the sample is compared with that obtained with a standard control serum that has been treated similarly. This gives an index, the TBI, which is the ratio of the amount of labeled T3 bound by the sample to that bound by the standard control serum. Since a smaller absorption of radioactive T3 means a greater amount of T4 originally present in the sample, the calculation of the TBI gives an inverse proportion; an index greater than 1 means a decreased amount of endogenous thyroid hormone present, and vice versa.

In the other method of presentation the result is calculated as the percentage of a standard amount of added radioactive T3 taken up by the resin, i.e., not taken up

by the sample. Originally the method used erythrocytes to absorb the excess T3, but an ion-exchange resin was found to be superior. Expressed in this way, the smaller the amount of radioactive T3 taken up by the resin, the greater is the amount absorbed by the sample and thus the greater the number of binding sites and accordingly the smaller the amount of endogenous thyroid hormone present.

Although the different kits are all satisfactory for distinguishing between hypothyroid, euthyroid, and hyperthyroid patients, the numeric values themselves are not always directly comparable between different kits. If the normal range for the TBI is taken as 0.9-1.1 and the normal range for the T3 uptake as 25-36%, then theoretically

$$\text{Percent uptake} = 100 - 50(\text{TBI})$$

and

$$\text{TBI} = 1.60 - (\text{Percent uptake}/50)$$

but actually this can serve only as a rough guide for comparison.

An EIA procedure has been developed that also can estimate the degree of saturation of TBG. In this competitive binding assay (Thyrozyme, Abbott Diagnostics, North Chicago, Ill.) the amount of enzyme activity expressed is directly related to the degree of TBG unsaturation.[19] Preliminary results indicate that this procedure compares very well with radiolabeled assays.

Normal values and interpretation: Since the values for the TBI are generally standardized with a normal control serum and reported as the ratio of the observed value to that of the control serum, the normal level is thus 0.9-1.1. In hyperthyroidism, values are less than 0.9, and, in hypothyroidism, values are greater than 1.1. Note that a decreased value of the TBI indicates a smaller than normal number of binding sites available, which results from an increased level of endogenous T4 in the blood. Normal values for the T3 uptake are generally taken as 25-35%; hyperthyroid patients have values greater than 35% and hypothyroid patients less than 25%. However, not all the kits given the same ranges, depending on the exact procedure used, and the package insert should be consulted for the normal range for the procedure used.

In pregnancy, even in euthyroid individuals, there is a marked increase in the TBI and an increase in T3 uptake (decreased index of thyroid activity) resulting from an increase in TBGs caused by increased estrogen secretion. This change in the TBI usually occurs around the fifth or sixth week of pregnancy and remains until delivery. Oral contraceptives and estrogens produce similar changes.

Various clinical conditions also show changes in TBI findings. Apparent increases in thyroid activity (decreased TBI values and increased T3 uptake values) are found in nephrosis, severe liver disease, anticoagulant therapy (bishydroxycoumarin, heparin), metastatic malignancies, pulmonary insufficiency, and hyperandrogenic states.

The TBI test follows the clinical state of the patient very closely. As the hyperthyroid patient improves clinically under iodine or propylthiouracil therapy, the TBI increases to more normal levels. A decrease in the TBI value occurs during the administration of thyroid hormones. The administration of various iodine compounds, whether organic or inorganic, usually does not affect the TBI or T3 uptake values significantly. This is a very important advantage, since these compounds are known to cause spuriously high values in many T4 determinations. Trypan blue, sometimes used for diagnostic studies, is known to interfere with the TBI by combining with the TBGs and causing false low TBI results.

Determination of thyroxine by competitive protein-binding[20-23]

Thyroxine (T4) may be determined by the general method of competitive protein-binding described earlier. The binding protein used is the thyroxine-binding globulin (TBG). This method was formerly one of the most commonly used methods for the determination, but it is now largely replaced by radioimmunoassay. The T4 was usually separated from the serum by precipitation with alcohol in which the T4 was soluble. After centrifugation an aliquot of the supernatant is evaporated and the binding protein and an excess of radioactively labeled T4 are added. After equilibration, the bound and free fractions are separated, and the radioactivity of the fractions is measured. The separation may be made by means of a Sephadex column or dextran-coated charcoal. If standards of pure thyroxine are used, a correction may be made for incomplete extraction. The extraction is generally about 80% and can be checked by measuring the T4 content of a known control serum. If standards of serum of known T4 content are used, any correction for incomplete extraction is automatically made. Some methods have been used in which the aliquot of the alcoholic extract is added directly to the reaction mixture without evaporation of the alcohol, provided that the standards are similarly treated. Kits for the determination of T4 by this method are available from some manufacturers, although the radioimmunoassay kits are much more common. The normal values and interpretation of results of this procedure are the same as for T4 by radioimmunoassay, which are given later.

Determination of thyroxine and triiodothyronine by radioimmunoassay[24]

A number of kits are available for the determination of thyroxine (T4) and triiodothyronine (T3) by radioimmunoassay (RIA). As with the competitive protein-binding methods, the kits differ in the method used to separate the free and bound radioactive material. In the RIA methods, hormone present in the sample may combine with the thyroid-binding globulin (TBG) also present in the sample; this will inhibit the binding of the hormone with the added antibody. A substance may be added to the reaction mixture to inhibit the binding of the T4 by the TBG. The sodium salt of 8-anilino-1-naphthalenesulfonic acid (ANSA is commonly used for this purpose,[25] although human serum albumin has also been used. Among the methods used for the separation of the free and bound fractions are polyethylene glycol precipitation,[26] Sephadex gel filtration,[27] and polyacrylamide gel filtration.[28] A newer method uses a solid-phase absorbent in which the antibody is strongly absorbed on the walls of a polyethylene test tube.[28] The other reagents and samples are added to the tubes, and equilibration is carried out. The solution is then poured out and the tube rinsed with a small amount of buffer. The proportion of the radioactive T4 or T3 that is then combined with the immobilized antibody is measured. This method is relatively simple and requires few manipulations. Some have questioned whether by this method one always has the same amount of antibody attached to the tube wall to the same extent as one would obtain by adding the antibody with a pipet. As mentioned in the earlier discussion of the general principles of this method, the order in which the reactants are added makes no difference as long as a true equilibrium is finally obtained.

A large number of different kits are on the market, and no study has compared more than a few of these.[29] One can merely try a few kits and adopt one that appears most suitable to the needs and facilities of the laboratory and appears to give good precision and agreement with the generally accepted normal values.

Another recent development is the determination of T4 in small samples of blood dried on filter paper for the screening of neonates for hypothyroidism.[30] Not all kits are sensitive enough for this purpose, and a number of precautions must be taken in the collection and preservation of the dried blood samples. Suggestions for the correct use of the blood spots have been given.[31,32]

T4 may also be determined by the homogeneous enzyme immunoassay (EMIT) method,[33,34] the principles of which have been discussed earlier. Although it has not as yet been widely used, it appears to give results that compare well with RIA methods. An advantage of the enzyme method is that the kits have a much longer shelf life because there is no radioactive decay factor. In addition, the standard curves appear to be more constant from batch to batch with the same lot of reagents.[35]

Normal values and interpretation: The manufacturers of the different kits may give slightly different normal values for T4; a satisfactory range is 4.5-13.5 µg/dl (60-175 nmole/L). In the earlier literature when the determination was made of protein-bound iodine, the results were usually expressed in terms of iodine, and the above range would correspond to 3.0-9.0 µg/dl of thyroxine iodine. Now it is preferable to express the results in terms of thyroxine in micrograms per deciliter or in SI units (nanomoles per liter). Increased levels of T4 are found in hyperthyroidism, ranging from 15-35 µg/dl (190-380 nmole/L). Moderate increases are found in pregnancy and following the administration of estrogens or oral contraceptives. These latter increases are generally caused mainly by increases in the TBG content of the serum proteins. Decreased serum levels are found in hypothyroidism (0-4 µg/dl). Lowered levels may be found in nephrosis and other conditions characterized by low levels of serum protein (and consequently of TBG).

In infants the T4 level ranges from 11-23 μg/dl (140-300 nmole/L) during the first few days of life and from 9-18 μg/dl (115-230 nmole/L) after 1 month, gradually falling to the adult level in a few years. The TBI is only slightly decreased in infants as compared to that in adults (65-105% as compared to a normal of 85-115%). The level of T3 is also somewhat elevated in newborns. The level in the first days of life is 180-240 ng/dl, gradually falling to a normal adult level of 70-200 ng/dl.

Determination of free thyroxine

The free (unbound) thyroxine (FT4)[36-38] may be the moiety that actually determines the thyrometabolic state of the patient. FT4 activity is independent of TBG concentration. However, FT4 is present in a rather low concentration (about 0.05% of the total T4, or 4 ng/dl in normal individuals). The methods for the actual determination of TF4 in serum are rather complicated for routine use. These determine the percentage of FT4, which must be multiplied by the total T4 to determine the actual amount of FT4.

Other indices have been used that may be more indicative than T3 or T4 of true thyroid function.[39] One of these is known as T7, which is obtained by multiplying the T3 uptake (expressed as a decimal) by the T4 (as micrograms per deciliter). This gives a normal range of 1.3-4.4. Another suggestion is to divide the T4 value by the TBI. When T4 is expressed as micrograms per deciliter, this gives a normal range of 4.6-13.5. These various calculated indices are claimed to be better measures of true thyroid function, since they are apparently less influenced by pregnancy or the administration of drugs, including estrogens and oral contraceptives.

Antithyroid antibodies

Several different antithyroid antibodies[40,41] may be found in the serum of patients with Hashimoto's disease (autoimmune thyroiditis). Apparently, damage to the thyroid gland releases "foreign" antigens into the serum, and the body forms antibodies to these. Several different antibodies may be present, and the test results may depend on the test procedure used and the type of antigen used. The antibodies usually determined are the thyroglobulin antibody and a throidal microsomal antibody. The most commonly used procedures are a hemagglutination test with tanned red cells (Ames Co., Elkhart, Ind.) and an immunofluorescent method (BioDx, Morristown, N.J., Clinical Sciences, Whippany, N.J.). The general principles of such tests are discussed in Chapter 35. High titers are found in more than 80% of patients with Hashimoto's disease, but titers above the normal range are also found in about 15% of patients without clinical evidence of the disease.

STEROID HORMONES

A large number of hormonal substances, found chiefly in the gonads and adrenal cortex, have a similar basic chemical structure and are known as the steroid hormones.[42,43] The basic steroid nucleus is as follows:

In the female hormones **estrogens,** the methyl group at position 19 is missing (hence these are sometimes known as the C-18 steroids), and the ring A has a benzenoid structure, giving these compounds more acidic properties; therefore they may be separated from the other steroids by extraction with dilute alkali. For the most part the androgenic hormones have the basic structure just shown and are thus referred to as the C-19 steroids. The **adrenocortical hormones** and the progesterone derivatives (corpus luteum hormone) have an additional 2-carbon chain attached to carbon 17 and are referred to as the C-21 steroids. Within each group there are usually several different hormones secreted by a given endocrine gland (testes, ovary, adrenal cortex), and often several more chemically similar metabolites are found in the urine. The procedure to determine a single individual compound was formerly often quite complicated, and it was usually deemed sufficient for most clinical purposes to determine a number of similar compounds together, e.g., ketosteroids, corticosteroids, and total estrogens. With the newer radioimmunoassay and enzyme immunoassay methods it is now sometimes easier to determine individual compounds, but for some purposes the group tests are still used. It might be mentioned that the cholesterol molecule also contains the same steroid nucleus with a longer carbon chain at position 17. Cholesterol is believed to be a precursor in the synthesis in vivo of many of the steroid hormones.

Steroid hormones influence the entire body. They control salt and water metabolism; affect carbohydrate, protein, and fat metabolism; control the development of the primary and secondary sex characteristics; and affect the distribution of hair and the development of the muscular and skeletal systems. The physiologic differences of the various hormones result from variations in the nature and position of side chains.

Estrogens

Estrogens[44,45] and estrogen metabolites have been isolated from the ovaries, placenta, testes, and adrenal cortex. In males and postmenopausal women the total amount of estrogen excreted in the urine is usually less than 15 μg/day, and the determination of such small amounts is technically difficult. In males, estrogen excretion may be increased by estrogen-producing tumors of the adrenal cortex or testes, in cirrhosis when the liver fails to inactivate the estrogens normally produced, and in certain cases of male infertility. In females the estrogen excretion is increased in ovarian tumors. There is a cyclic variation during the menstrual cycle and an enormous increase in pregnancy.

In the normal cycle the excretion may vary from a low of 10-20 μg/day at the beginning of the cycle to a high of 40-100 μg/day at ovulation. In pregnancy the excretion may rise to near 30 mg/day at term. The determination of the larger quantity of estrogens in urine is not difficult and has been used for monitoring high-risk pregnancy patients. The fetal adrenal gland synthesizes dehydroepiandrosterone, which is hydroxylated by the fetal liver and converted into **estriol** by the placenta. Thus estriol excretion increases progressively during the third trimester of pregnancy. This increase probably reflects the competency of the developing fetoplacental unit. Any sharp decrease in the amount of estriol excreted or a failure of the amount of hormone excreted to rise progressively is evidence of a complicated pregnancy. Since estriol accounts for 80-90% of the total estrogens excreted during late pregnancy, the determination of total estrogens is usually made rather than attempting to separate the three estrogens (estrone, estradiol, estriol), which is much more difficult and would yield little additional clinical information (see also p. 747).

Determination of urinary estrogens

The urinary estrogens[46,47] may be determined separately by means of gas-liquid chromatography (see reference 2, pp. 435 and 480), but this requires special equipment and is best used when a considerable number of samples are to be run daily. The plasma estrogens may be determined by competitive protein-binding or by radioimmunoassay. However, this is usually done using tritium-labeled (^{3}H-labeled) antigens (see reference 2, pp. 402 and 409), which requires a scintillation counter not available in most laboratories.

The estrogens are excreted chiefly as glucuronides. These must be hydrolyzed before extraction. The hydrolysis may be carried out enzymatically or by heating with acid. The enzymatic method is somewhat lengthy; the acid treatment is quite commonly used for the determination of estrogens in pregnant women. Although the acid hydrolysis may cause the loss of 15-20% of the total estrogens, this is not serious, particularly if the normal ranges have been established by a method using acid hydrolysis. After hydrolysis the estrogens are extracted with ether. The ether layer is washed to remove some impurities and evaporated to dryness. The residue is treated with sulfuric acid and hydroquinone to give a colored product, which is determined in a spectrophotometer. Normally the colorimetric readings are made at three wavelengths to correct for some impurities (Allen's test). Estriol is used as a standard, since this compound accounts for most of the estrogens.

Reagents and equipment:

1. Hydrochloric acid, concentrated, about 12 moles/L
2. Diethyl ether, reagent grade, preferably freshly distilled in an all-glass apparatus
3. Sodium sulfate crystals, anhydrous
4. Ethanol, reagent grade
5. Sodium bicarbonate–carbonate buffer, pH 10.6, 1.5 moles/L
   Dissolve 69.5 g $NaHCO_3$ in about 850 ml water. Add 130 ml of 5 moles/L sodium hydroxide solution (200 g/L) and dilute to 1 L.
6. Sulfuric acid solution, 12 moles/L
   Cautiously add 250 ml concentrated sulfuric acid to 135 ml water; cool before use.
7. Hydroquinone solutions, 0.18 mole/L
   a. Dissolve 0.5 g hydroquinone in 25 ml diethyl ether. Preferably this is made up fresh as needed.
   b. Dissolve 0.5 g hydroquinone in 25 ml of the 12 moles/L sulfuric acid.
8. Estriol standards
   a. Estriol, 100 μg/ml. Dissolve 10 mg estriol in 1 dl ethanol. This is the "internal standard" used in the procedure.
   b. Estriol μg/ml. Dilute 5 ml solution A to 1 dl with ethanol. This is the "external standard" used in the procedure.
   If it is desired to express the final results in micromoles rather than in milligrams, the above standards can be used by multiplying the final results by the conversion factor (see calculation).
9. Small glass beads or other "boiling chips" for the evaporation of the ether solutions
10. Test tubes with ground glass stopper, having a capacity of around 20 ml (Screw-capped tubes with caps having Teflon linings can also be used.)

Procedure: Collect a 24 hr urine specimen; measure and record the total volume. Dilute the total urine volume to 2 L with water and mix well. Add 2 ml of the diluted urine to each of three glass-stoppered tubes; then add 0.3 ml concentrated hydrochloric acid to each tube. Stopper the tubes and heat them in a boiling water bath for 1 hr. (NOTE: If the total urine volume collected is more than 2 L make up to the next nearest liter with water, and mix and use 1/1000 of the volume for hydrolysis, increasing the amount of added hydrochloric acid proportionately.)

After hydrolysis cool the tubes to about 10°C. Add 10 ml ether to each tube. Label two of the tubes S_1 and S_2 (samples); to the third tube add 0.2 ml of the internal standard (A above) and label "Standard." Stopper the tubes tightly and shake vigorously for 30 sec, or mix well on a vortex mixer. Allow the layers to separate completely and remove the lower aqueous layer by suction. Then add 0.5 ml of the sodium bicarbonate–carbonate buffer to each tube, stopper, and shake (or mix on a vortex mixer). Then add 2 g anhydrous sodium sulfate and shake again.

To two additional clean, glass-stoppered tubes labeled "Sample 1" and "Sample 2" add 3 ml of the ether extract from the corresponding extraction tubes. To two additional tubes add 3 ml each of the ether extract from the standard tube. To an additional tube labeled "Control" add 2 ml ether and 1 ml external standard (B above) (5 μg/ml). To each of these tubes add 0.2 ml of the 2% hydroquinone in ether. Also add the same amount of hydroquinone to a sixth tube to serve as a blank.

Evaporate the ether completely in a fume hood by using a water bath or heating bent glass tubing connected to a suction manifold.

After complete evaporation of the ether, cool the tubes to room temperature and add 2 ml of the hydroquinone solution in sulfuric acid to each tube. Then stopper the tubes and place them in a boiling water bath or a heating block at 100° C for 40 min, with occasional agitation.

Then cool the tubes to room temperature and add 1.7 ml water to each tube. Mix the contents of each tube; then allow them to stand at room temperature for 15 min.

Each of the other tubes is then read against the blank at 472, 514, and 556 nm.

Calculation: The corrected absorbance for each tube is then calculated:

$$A(corr.) = A_{514} - \left(\frac{A_{472} + A_{556}}{2} \right)$$

where A is the absorbance. The mean of the two tubes from the urine sample is obtained, and the mean of the two tubes from the standard is obtained. Then

$$\text{Total estrogen (as estriol) (mg/24 hr)} = \frac{20 \times A_u}{A_s - A_u}$$

where A_u is the average corrected absorbance for the urine sample, and A_s is that for the urine plus added standard. Note that 1/1000 of the total 24 hr sample is taken for analysis and that the added standard is 20 μg corresponding to a sample of 1/1000 of the total; thus 20 μg in 1/1000 of the total equals 20 mg in the total sample. If it is desired to convert milligrams to micromoles, miltiply by the factor 3.47.

As a check on the procedure, read the control tube against the blank and calculate the corrected absorbance. Then the percent of recovery of the added standard may be calculated as

$$\frac{5 \, (A_s - A_u) \times 100}{6A_c}$$

where A_c is the corrected absorbance of the control tube. (The figures arise from the fact that 20 μg estriol is found in the 10 ml ether extract of the standard tube and 3 ml of this [6 μg] is taken for analysis and compared with 5 μg added in the control tube.) If the recovery is less than 75% or more than 110%, this indicates some error in the procedure as performed and the test should be repeated. Often the estrogen/creatinine ratio in the urine is used instead of the estrogen excretion alone, because the former ratio may show less variation from day to day. The ratio may be expressed as

$$E/C = \frac{\text{Estrogen (μg/ml)}}{\text{Creatinine (mg/ml)}}$$

or, if both are expressed as 24 hr excretion, the ratio is

$$E/C = \frac{\text{Estrogen (mg/24 hr)}}{\text{Creatinine (g/24 hr)}}$$

Normal values and interpretation: Both the E/C ratio and the 24 hr estrogen excretion increase from very low values at the beginning of pregnancy to much higher values at term. The increase is only slight until about the twentieth week of gestation.

Table 25-2. Variation in estrogen excretion with gestational age

Gestation (wk)	Normal range	
	E/C ratio	24 hr estrogen excretion (mg)
20	2-8	3-7
24	4-12	4-10
28	6-18	5-15
32	10-22	8-20
36	14-30	10-30
40	18-40	15-42

Table 25-2[48] gives the variation in estrogen excretion with gestational age. Values even below these ranges have been found in apparently normal women, so a single low value is not so important from a diagnostic point as the failure to show a gradual rising trend. A sudden drop from a normal level is a grave prognostic sign and indicates fetal distress. A continued drop to below the normal range may indicate the need for induced delivery. A decline to very low values in the later weeks of gestation usually indicates fetal death.

Serum estrogens

Since the urinary concentration of estriol is dependent on both maternal and fetal placental function, the measurement of unconjugated serum estriol has been proposed as a more satisfactory test.[49] The serum concentration of unconjugated estriol is only dependent on fetal-placental function and thus can more accurately reflect changes over a short period of time. Radioimmunoassay procedures are available for this assay and a high-performance liquid chromatography method using electrochemical detection has been suggested.[50] The advantage of the latter method is that its relative simplicity and speed can allow measurement of unconjugated serum estriol during parts of the day when most laboratories cannot perform the radioimmunoassay procedure.

Luteal hormones

The corpus luteum of the ovary also produces some hormones. The principal steroid is progesterone, which is also a 21-carbon steroid similar to the adrenal steroids. The chief metabolite of this hormone found in the urine is **pregnanediol.** It is present in quantities of 2-10 mg/day during the latter half of the menstrual cycle. Smaller amounts are found in the earlier part of the cycle, in the urine of men, and in postmenopausal women. The chemical methods for the determination of pregnanediol are rather complicated involving enzymatic hydrolysis, extraction with toluene, purification by chromatography on an alumina column, preparation of an acetyl derivative, further purification, and final formation of the chromogen with sulfuric acid. The usual method of determination is by gas-liquid chromatography. The results of the assays have not proved to be of striking diagnostic value. There is a rise during pregnancy to a peak excretion of 30-100 mg/day, but there are much simpler and more reliable tests for pregnancy. Lower excretion values during pregnancy have been associated with threatened abortion or toxemia of pregnancy, and increased levels of progesterone-like compounds have been found in adrenal hyperplasia.

Androgens

The androgenic hormones have methyl groups at positions 18 and 19 and an OH or =O group at position 17. Those with the C=O structure at position 17 are the 17-ketosteroids. The most important testicular hormone, **testosterone,** is actually not a ketosteroid, but a number of its metabolites such as androsterone, dehydroepiandrosterone, and etiocholanolone are ketosteroids found in urine. Thus the 17-ketosteroid concentration will in part represent androgenic activity.

Testosterone itself has been determined by competitive protein binding or radioimmunoassay. The older methods use tritium-labeled (^{3}H-labeled) compounds, which are difficult to measure, but kits are now available using ^{125}I labels. These can be used in most clinical laboratories, but the determination of testosterone is not yet a routine procedure. Procedures for the separation and quantification of testosterone by gas chromatography technology have also been reported.[51]

Adrenocortical hormones: corticosteroids

As previously mentioned, corticosteroids have an additional 2-carbon side chain attached to position 17 of the steroid nucleus. They are excreted partially as C-21 steroids and partially as C-17 ketosteroids. A number of methods have been used for the determination of various groups of the corticosteroids. One of the methods presented here involves the change of the corticosteroids into 17-ketosteroids by oxidation; hence the group of compounds determined is known as the **ketogenic steroids.** These include most of the important corticosteroids and the method is quite satisfactory for most clinical purposes because the level of ketogenic steroids reflects the adrenal cortex activity quite well.

There is a decrease in ketogenic steroid (and ketosteroid) excretion in Addison's disease, hypopituitarism, Simmonds' disease, and cretinism. An increased level of ketogenic steroid excretion is found in Cushing's syndrome, precocious puberty caused by adrenal hyperplasia, and physiologic stress (surgery, burns, infectious diseases).

Determination of ketosteroids and hydroxysteroids (ketogenic steroids)[52-54]

Ketosteroids are excreted in the urine chiefly as conjugated sulfates and glucuronates. These are usually hydrolyzed by heating with acid, a method not entirely satisfactory, since the acid causes some alteration of the steroids. It is still generally used when only the total ketosteroids are being determined.

After hydrolysis the ketosteroids are extracted from the urine with an organic solvent. Ether is used in the method given here. This solvent has some disadvantages because of its volatility and flammability, but it usually extracts less interfering chromogens and gives less trouble with emulsions during extraction than other solvents. The ether extract is washed with sodium hydroxide solution, which removes some interfering color

as well as the estrogens extracted from the urine. The ether is then dehydrated by means of solid sodium hydroxide, filtered, and an aliquot evaporated to dryness for the colorimetric determination.

Steroids having a ketone (> C=O) grouping at position 17 in the molecule (17-ketosteroids) will react with metadinitrobenzene in alkaline solution to form a purple-red color. Numerous modifications of the reagents have been used. The ones given here are relatively stable and yield a low blank value. After development of the color (usually 1 hr or more at room temperature in the dark), the solution is somewhat diluted and read in the colorimeter.

Usually some interfering brown color is present. This can be corrected by various methods. The absorbance can be measured at two or more different wavelengths and an empirically determined correction formula can be used, or the colored solution can be diluted with alcohol, water, and chloroform (or ethylene dichloride) in such proportions that two immiscible layers are formed. The desired ketosteroid color is found in the lower solvent layer; the interfering color in the upper aqueous layer is discarded. If a good spectrophotometer is available, the two-wavelength method is simpler, but if only a filter photometer is available, the extraction method is necessary.

Many of the important adrenocrotical steroids and their metabolites have a hydroxyl group and a short carbon chain at position 17 (17-hydroxysteroids) in the following molecule:

$$> C\genfrac{}{}{0pt}{}{-OH}{-CH_3}$$

These hydroxysteroids can be oxidized to ketosteroids by the use of sodium bismuthate or sodium periodate. If the urine is first reated with the reducing agent sodium borohydride, the ketosteroids originally present are reduced to compounds that no longer give the color with the reagent even after subsequent treatment with an oxidizing agent. Thus, by successive treatment with borohydride and periodate, the original ketosteroids are eliminated as chromogens and the hydroxysteroids are oxidized to ketosteroids and determined as such (**ketogenic steroids).** Appreciable amounts of glucose in the urine will interfere, but this can usually be overcome by using larger quantities of the two reagents.

Reagents:
1. Methyl alcohol, AR, acetone free
2. Potassium hydroxide, 4 moles/L in methanol
   Add 34 g potassium hydroxide pellets to 120 ml purified methanol and dissolve, preferably with the aid of a magnetic stirrer. Filter through hardened paper or centrifuge if necessary and transfer the clear liquid to a polyethylene bottle. Add exactly 2 ml solution to about 20 ml water and titrate with standard acid with phenolphthalein indicator. Calculate the normality and dilute to 4.00 ± 0.15 moles/L. This reagent is quite stable. A small amount of potassium carbonate may settle out, but this is not harmful.
3. Ethylene glycol monomethyl ether (Methyl Cellosolve)
   The reagent grade of the solvent may be used.

4. Dinitrobenzene, 60 mmole/L
   Dissolve 1 g dinitrobenzene (recrystallized from alcohol or special Sigma grade [Sigma Chemical Co., St. Louis]) in 1 dl Methyl Cellosolve. Store in refrigerator.

5. Sodium hydroxide, 5 moles/L
   Dissolve 100 g sodium hydroxide in water to make 5 dl. This solution need not be standardized.

6. Sodium hydroxide, 1 mole/L and 0.1 mole/L
   Prepare from the 5 moles/L solution by appropriate dilution (1:5 and 1:50).

7. Sulfuric acid, 0.05 mole/L
   Add 14 ml concentrated acid to about 4 dl water; cool and dilute to 5 dl.

8. Acetic acid, 4.4 moles/L
   Mix 1 dl glacial acetic acid with 3 dl water.

9. Acetic acid, 1 mole/L
   Dilute 30 ml glacial acetic acid to 5 dl with water.

10. Sodium borohydride, 10 g/dl
    Just before use dissolve 1 g sodium borohydride in 10 ml of 0.1 mole/L sodium hydroxide solution.

11. Sodium metaperiodate, 0.47 mole/L
    Just before use dissolve 2 g sodium metaperiodate in 20 ml water. This solution is near saturation, and the salt may dissolve slowly.

12. Steroid stock standard, 2.5 mg/ml steroid
    Dehydroepiandrosterone is commonly used as a standard for ketosteroids. Dissolve 250 mg of this steroid in methyl alcohol and dilute to 1 dl. Store in refrigerator in a tightly stoppered bottle. (NOTE: Since the ketosteroids extracted and determined do not represent a single definite compound but rather a mixture, there may be some question as to the applicability of the use of the SI units. However, in the use of the conventional units the report really means, though not explicitly stated, milligrams of ketosteroids [calculated as dehydroepiandrosterone], and likewise the report in SI units would mean "micromoles of ketosteroids calculated as dehydroepiandrosterone." To convert milligrams of ketosteroids to micromoles multiply by the factor 3.47.)

13. Working standard
    Dilute 2 ml stock standard to 1 dl with methyl alcohol. This standard contains 25 μg in 0.5 ml. Store in the refrigerator and make up fresh monthly.

14. Ether, AR

15. Sulfuric acid, 9 moles/L
    Cautiously add 1 dl concentrated sulfuric acid to 1 dl water. Mix and cool.

General procedure: Measure the total volume of a well-mixed 24 hr urine specimen. Record the volume and reserve a few hundred milliliters for analysis. Run determinations in duplicate. Perform extractions in 25 × 150 mm screw-capped tubes with rubber-lined caps. During extraction procedure with ether, keep tubes cooled in ice water or cold, running tap water except during actual manipulations. During warm weather it is helpful to cool the solutions used for washing the ether extract. This is conveniently done by storing bottles of these solutions in the refrigerator. Care must be taken in the evaporation of ether extracts; even a hot plate can ignite high concentrations of ether vapors. The lower aqueous layer is removed from the ether extract in the tubes by means of a 1 ml serologic pipet attached with rubber tubing to a source of suction and trap. Suction is controlled by pressure on the rubber tubing at the top of the pipet.

Ketosteroids: To the extraction tube, add 7.5 ml urine and 1 ml of 9 moles/L sulfuric acid. Heat in a boiling water bath for 15 min; then cool well. Add exactly 25 ml ether, cap tightly, and shake for 3 min. Allow the layers to separate while cooling; then remove the lower aqueous layer. Add 5 ml of cold 1 mole/L sodium hydroxide solution, cap, and shake for 15 sec. Allow the layers to separate and remove the lower aqueous layer. Add 20-30 pellets solid sodium hydroxide, cap, and shake at intervals during the next 10 min. Cool well and centrifuge briefly. Filter ether extract through rapid paper, covering top of funnel with watch glass to prevent evaporation. Transfer a 10 ml aliquot of the filtrate (corresponding to 3 ml urine) to a 25 × 150 mm tube. (A large aliquot may be used if the original total urine volume was over 1500 ml, although in this case it may be advisable to evaporate the ether in portions, adding a second portion to the tube after most of the first has evaporated.) Evaporate the ether on a water bath under a fume hood. CAUTION! No flame! Dissolve the residue in 0.5 ml methyl alcohol and again evaporate to dryness on a water bath. Similarly, evaporate a standard of 25 μg steroid in 0.5 ml alcohol and a blank of 0.5 ml methyl alcohol. Allow the tubes to cool to room temperature before proceeding with color development. Prepare a sufficient quantity of color reagent just before use by mixing 3 volumes of 4 moles/L alcoholic potassium hydroxide and 4 volumes of 60 mmoles/L metadinitrobenzene. Add 0.7 ml of the mixture to each tube of sample, standard, or blank. After agitating ently to dissolve the residue, allow to stand for 1 hr at room temperature in the dark. Then add to each tube 5 ml Methyl Cellosolve and mix. Read standards and samples against blank at 520 and 430 nm. Calculate the corrected readings for each tube:

$$\text{Corr. A} = \frac{A_{520} - (0.6 \times A_{430})}{0.73}$$

NOTE: The corrected absorbance (A) for the standard should be close (5%) to the uncorrected A_{520}. A lower corrected reading usually indicates faulty reagents. Then

$$\frac{\text{Corr. A sample}}{\text{Corr. A standard}} \times \frac{\mu g \text{ standard}}{\text{ml urine excreted}} \times \frac{\text{Vol ether added}}{\text{Vol ether evaporated}} = \mu g \text{ steroid/ml urine}$$

Since μg/ml = mg/L, then

$$\mu g/ml \times \text{Vol (L)} = \text{Total mg ketosteroids excreted}$$

For the aliquots used as given

$$\frac{\text{Corr. A sample}}{\text{Corr. A standard}} \times \frac{25 \times 25 \times \text{urine}}{7.5 \times 10} \times \text{Vol (L)} =$$

Total mg excreted

As an alternative to reading at two wavelengths, proceed as follows: When the color has been developed after standing 1 hr, add to each tube 2.5 ml Methyl Cellosolve and mix. Add 2 ml water and mix. Then add 2.5 ml ethylene dichloride and mix. The reagents must be added in the order given, mixing after each addition. Then agitate strongly and transfer to a smaller test tube and centrifuge at high speed. Remove the top aqueous layer completely. If the lower layer is not perfectly clear, add a few drops of methyl alcohol. Transfer the lower layer to a cuvet and read at 520 nm only. The calculations are the same except that the absorbance at 520 nm is used without any correction.

Hydroxysteroids (ketogenic steroids): Test urine for sugar with Clinistix or similar test strip. If no more than a trace of sugar is present, proceed as outlined. If more sugar is present, see notes at end of section for necessary modifications Pipet 7.5 ml urine to 25 × 150 mm tube. Check the pH and adjust to 6.5-7.5 with short-range paper, using 1 mole/L sodium hydroxide or 6% acetic acid as needed. Add a few milliliters of ether to aid in reducing foaming; then add 0.9 ml freshly prepared sodium borohydride solution. Allow the tubes to stand at room temperature for 1 hr. Cautiously add 0.5 ml 4.4 moles/L acetic acid, adding a few more milliliters of ether if necessary to prevent foaming. Allow to stand for a few minutes, check the pH, and add a few more drops of acid if necessary to bring the pH to near 7.0. Allow to stand for 15 min with occasional swirling. Add 3 ml of 0.47 moles/L sodium metaperiodate solution and 0.5 ml 1 mole/L sodium hydroxide. Incubate at 37° C for 1 hr. Add 0.5 ml of 5 moles/L sodium hydroxide and incubate for 15 min more. Cool tubes well, add exactly 25 ml ether, cap tubes, and shake for 3 min. Remove the lower aqueous layer. It may be necessary to centrifuge briefly at this point to break any emulsion formed on shaking. Gently stir up any white precipitate in the bottom of the tube and remove as much of it as possible along with the aqueous layer. Add 3 ml of 1 mole/L sulfuric acid, cap, and shake vigorously. Allow the layers to separate while cooling; then remove the aqueous layer. Wash the ether layer with 5 ml of cold 1 mole/L sodium hydroxide solution, shake again for about 15 sec, allow the layers to separate, and remove the lower layer by suction. Add 20-30 pellets of solid sodium hydroxide to the ether. From this point proceed exactly as with the ketosteroids. All final details and calculations are the same.

NOTE: If more than a trace of sugar is present in the urine, proceed as follows: After the addition of the borohydride, allow to stand for 45 min and add 0.3 ml of 4.4 moles/L acetic acid and about 60-70 mg more solid borohydride. Allow to stand for an additional 45 min. Then add 0.5 ml 4.4 moles/L acetic acid as in the regular procedure and allow to stand for 10 min. More acetic acid may be necessary to bring the pH to 7.0.

After the addition of the periodate, incubate for at least 1½ hr, add an additional 200 mg periodate after 45 min, and then agitate to dissolve the salt after addition.

NOTE: The same comments in regard to the use of SI units apply to the ketogenic steroids as to the ketosteroids, and the same conversion factor may be used.

Normal values and interpretation: Increases in the ketosteroids are found in testicular or other virilizing tumors (Cushing's syndrome, adrenal hyperplasia, etc.) and in precocious puberty. Decreased levels are found in gonadal agenesis or dysgenesis and in hypothyroidism. A fraction of the ketosteroids measured in the urine also are metabolites of the various hormones secreted by the adrenal cortex; hence changes in the secretion of these hormones will also cause changes in the urinary excretion of ketosteroids. The normal levels of the ketosteroid excretion per day are as follows: birth to 3 yr, less than 1 mg; 3-8 yr, 0.5-2.5 mg; 12-16 yr, 4-9 mg; adult men, 10-18 mg; and adult women, 6-15 mg. After the age of about 50 yr, excretion of the ketosteroids begins to decrease and may be only in the range of 4-8 mg/day in either sex after the age of 65. The changes in ketosteroids as reflections of the changes in adrenocortical hromones are included in the discussion of those hormones.

Determination of urinary 17-hydroxysteroids: modified Porter-Silber method[55,56]

As with the two previous methods, this one also determines a group of related steroids and metabolites with possibly a somewhat greater proportion derived from the adrenocortical hormones. Since cortisol is used as a standard, the same comments apply as to the use of SI units. The corticosteroids are excreted mainly as glucuronide conjugates. These are hydrolyzed by glucuronidase at a pH of 6.8. The steroids are then extracted with chloroform and reacted with a reagent of phenylhydrazine in alcholic sulfuric acid to form a yellow chromogen. A control is run with each urine specimen to compensate for the nonsteroid chromogenic substances present in the urine.

Reagents:
1. Chloroform, reagent grade
   If redistilled before use, add 0.1% ethanol to prevent formation of phosgene.
2. Sodium hydroxide, 0.1 mole/L
3. Absolute ethyl alcohol
4. Sulfuric acid, 11.5 moles/L
   Add 640 ml concentrated sulfuric acid of 11.5 moles/L to 360 ml distilled water.
5. Alcoholic sulfuric acid reagent
   Mix 1 dl sulfuric acid with 50 ml absolute ethanol.
6. Recrystallized phenylhydrazine hydrochloride
   (If Baker's phenylhydrazine is used, there is no need for recrystallization. Phenylhydrazine hydrochloride may be twice recrystallized from absolute ethanol and dried in a desiccator over calcium chloride.)
7. Phenylhydrazine–alcoholic sulfuric acid reagent
   Dissolve 50 ml recrystallized phenylhydrazine hydrochloride in 50 ml alcoholic sulfuric acid reagent. This reagent must be freshly prepared before use.

8. Glucuronidase (bacterial), 1000 units/ml in distilled water
   Prepare fresh before use or keep frozen.
9. Phosphate buffer, pH 6.8, 0.5 mole/L
   Dissolve 68 g K_2HPO_4 in about 6 dl water. Adjust the pH to 6.8 by the addition of 1 mole/L sodium hdroxide solution (40 g/L) and dilute to 1 L.
10. Stock standard, 100 μg/ml
    Dissolve 25 mg cortisol (hydrocortisone alcohol) in absolute ethanol and dilute to 250 ml.
11. Working standard, 5 μg/ml
    Dilute 5 ml stock to 1 dl with distilled water.

Procedure: A 24 hr urine specimen is collected in a bottle containing 10 ml toluol as a preservative. The total volume is measured and approximately 1 dl is retained for analysis. To a 1 dl glass-stoppered cylinder, transfer 10 ml urine, 1 ml β-glucuronidase enzyme (1000 units/ml), 2 ml of 0.5 mole/L phosphate buffer, and 1 ml chloroform.

The reagent blank and standard samples are prepared in like manner by using 10 ml water and 10 ml working standard instead of urine. Samples are mixed well and incubated at 37° C for 18-24 hr. Add to each cylinder 50 ml chloroform. The contents of the cylinders are mixed by repeated inversion for 30 sec and then allowed to stand until the organic and aqueous phases have separated. Remove the aqueous supernatant by aspiration. Add 10 ml of 0.1 mole/L sodium hydroxide to each cylinder and shake for 30 sec. The two phases are allowed to separate, and the alkali layer is removed by aspiration. In the same manner the chloroform extracts are washed twice with 10 ml water. Two 20 ml aliquots of the chloroform extracts from the blank and the urine are transferred to 50 ml glass-stoppered cylinders. One 20 ml aliquot of the standard is transferred to a 50 ml cylinder. One aliquot of the blank and the unknown control. The other aliquots serve as the reagent blank, standard, and unknown.

Add 5 ml alcoholic sulfuric acid reagent to the cylinders containing the control blank and the urine controls. Add 5 ml phenylhydrazine–alcoholic sulfuric acid to the cylinders containing the reagent blank, standard, and unknowns. Stopper the cylinders tightly, shake vigorously for 30 sec, and allow to stand for 15-20 sec.

Transfer the supernatants from each cylinder to a small cuvet and incubate in a 60° C water bath for 45 min.

Read the unknown controls against the control blank; read the standard and the unknowns against the reagent blank at a wavelength of 410 nm.

Calculation:

$$\text{17-OH corticosteroids (mg/24 hr)} = \frac{U - C}{S} \times 0.005 \times V$$

where U = absorbance of unknown, C = absorbance of control, S = absorbance of standard, 0.005 = concentration of standard in milligrams per milliliter, and V = volume of urine in milliliters.

Normal values:
Adults: 10-15 mg/24 hr
Children: 0-1 yr, 0.5 mg/24 hr
    1-5 yr, 1-2 mg/24 hr

Note that the three tests just presented, ketosteroids, ketogenic steroids, and the Porter-Silber hydroxysteroids, give not greatly differing values for the normal 24 hr excretion. Thus the determination of one or more of these can be and has been used in the adrenal function tests given below.

Adrenal function tests[57,58]

The adrenal cortex secretes its hormone on stimulation by the pituitary hormone (ACTH). If the output of the adrenal cortex is low, this may be caused by failure of the pituitary gland to secrete the necessary ACTH or failure of the adrenal cortex to respond to the ACTH produced by the pituitary gland. The administration of exogenous ACTH will aid in differentiating between these two conditions. If the administered ACTH causes a marked rise in the excretion of ketosteroids and ketogenic steroids (in normal individuals the urinary output of ketosteroids may be increased two to three times and that of ketogenic steroids three to four times), then

Table 25-3. Summary of adrenal function tests

	Hormonal changes in urine		Tests	
Disease	**17-Ketosteroids**	**Ketogenic steroids**	**ACTH stimulation**	**Cortisone suppression**
Cushing's disease (hyperplasia)	± to N	+ +	+ + +	50%
Adenoma (unilateral) functioning	+ + variable	+ + variable	KGS + KS variable	None
Carcinoma (unilateral) functioning	+ +	+ +	None	None
Adrenogenital syndrome	+ + + Dehydroepian-drosterone in urine	Depends on whether it results from hyperplasia, adenoma, or carcinoma (see above)		
Congenital adrenal hyperplasia	+ Pregnanetriol in urine	+	None	Yes
Addison's disease	Not indicated	Low	None	Not indicated

+ = Increased; − = decreased; ± = variable; N = normal; KGS = ketogenic steroids; KS = ketosteroids.

the original low level is a result of the failure of the pituitary gland to secrete ACTH. If the exogenous ACTH causes little rise in the steroid excretion, the adrenal gland is at fault.

Stimulation test: Collect a 24 hr urine specimen before the test and assay for 17-ketosteroids and 17-hydroxysteroids. On the day of the test start collection of 24 hr urine specimen at 8:00 A.M. and begin intravenous drip of saline solution containing 20 units ACTH. This should be allowed to run for a period of 8 hr. Intramuscular injection of 80 units ACTH on 2 successive days can also be utilized. The response to the stimulation test is related to the mass of the cortical tissue, the number of units of ACTH, and the sensitivity of the patient to ACTH. A 24 hr urine specimen is again collected and assayed for 17-ketosteroids and 17-hydroxysteroids.

Suppression test: The theoretic basis for this test is the so-called **feedback mechanism.** Cortisone derivatives decrease the output of adrenal cortical hormone by depressing the anterior pituitary gland.

A 24 hr urine specimen is obtained before the test. It is assayed for 17-ketosteroids and 17-hydroxysteroids. The test is performed by administering 1 mg 1-α-fluorohydrocortisone, 0.5 mg dexamethasone (Decadron), or 2.5 mg prednisolone daily for each 3 mg of 17-hydroxycorticoids in the urine. The dose is divided and given every 6 hr after meals for 3 days. Then a 24 hr urine specimen is collected again and assayed for 17-ketosteroids and 17-hydroxysteroids. Table 25-3 summarizes the results obtained in the various adrenal function tests.

Metyrapone test: The metyrapone test[59] may also be employed to assess the pituitary function in regard to ACTH production. This drug inhibits the action of an enzyme that converts 11-deoxycortisol into cortisol. Thus the production of cortisol but not other corticosteroids is decreased. Since the feedback mechanism controlling the production of ACTH is influenced chiefly by cortisol, the decrease in cortisol level will tend to stimulate the pituitary gland to secrete more ACTH, with the consequent production of more ketosteroids and ketogenic steroids if both the pituitary and adrenal glands are active.

Usually 750 mg metyrapone is administered orally every 4 hr for 48 hr. If the pituitary and adrenal glands are both active, the result will be similar to the administration of ACTH—a marked increase over the basal level in urinary steroid excretion. In patients with pituitary insufficiency no such increase is noted.

Cortisol is the principal substance involved in the feedback mechanism that regulates the production of ACTH; thus it seems best to measure the actual amount of cortisol in the plasma or urine in the study of adrenal function. Kits are available for the determination of cortisol by radioimmunoassay or competitive protein binding (see reference 8 and the publication mentioned on p. 610). A simple fluorometric determination follows.

Fluorometric determination of cortisol in plasma and urine[60-63]: Cortisol (hydrocortisone) is one of the steroids secreted by the adrenal cortex and is the most physiologically active of the glucocorticoids. In plasma it is largely bound by plasma proteins. A small amount exists in the free state and is excreted in the urine. The free cortisol may be extracted from the plasma or urine by dichloromethane and determined fluorometrically. Thus the amount of free cortisol found in the plasma or urine serves as a measure of the total amount of the hormone secreted and thus of the adrenocortical activity. The fluorometric determination is not absolutely specific for cortisol, and the substance (or substances) determined might more properly be called 11-hydroxycorticosteroids, but the term *cortisol* is used here. The plasma or serum is made alkaline with sodium hydroxide and the cortisol extracted with methylene chloride. After separation a fluorescent reagent, consisting of a mixture of ethanol and concentrated sulfuric acid, is added to a portion of the extract. Since the fluorescence developed varies slowly with time, the standards and samples are all read in the fluorometer at definite time intervals after the addition of the reagent. The extraction solvent and other reagents must be of the highest purity to reduce the blank fluorescence as much as possible. The glassware used must be cleaned with chromic acid or a nonfluorescent detergent.

Procedure for cortisol in urine:
Reagents:
1. Sodium hydroxide, 0.1 mole/L
   Dissolve 1 g sodium hydroxide in 250 ml water.
2. Extraction solvent, methylene chloride (dichloromethane), spectrograde
3. Fluorescent reagent
   Place 35 ml absolute ethanol in a flask, cool in an ice bath, and slowly add, with swirling, 65 ml concentrated sulfuric acid. The acid should be added slowly, so that the temperature does not rise above 24° C. It is stable for several months if stored in the refrigerator.
4. Cortisol standard
   a. Stock standard. Dissolve 20 mg hydrocortisone in absolute ethanol to make 1 dl. This contains 200 μg/ml. If a standard containing 600 μmole/L is desired, use 21.7 mg. The solution is stable for 1 year if stored in the refrigerator.
   b. Intermediate standard, 1 μg/ml. Dilute 1 ml stock standard to 2 dl with water. If the other standard is used, the intermediate standard will contain 0.30 μmole/L.) Prepare fresh monthly and store in the refrigerator.
   c. Working standard, 0.25 μg/ml (0.75 μmole/L). Dilute 25 ml intermediate standard to make 1 dl with water. Prepare this fresh daily as needed. When used as given in the directions, this standard is equivalent to 250 μg/L free cortisol (or, with the other standard, 750 nmole/L).

Specimens: Twenty-four hour urine specimens are collected, with boric acid as the preservative. If the specimen is not analyzed shortly after collection, it may be stored frozen for some time.

Procedure: Prepare unknown, standard, and blank tubes by adding 2.0 ml urine, working standard, or water to labeled 50 ml glass-stoppered centrifuge tubes, respectively. Add 15.0 ml dichloromethane to each tube and shake thoroughly. Finish the extraction by mixing on a vortex mixer for 1 min. Allow the layers to separate; then remove and discard the upper aqueous layer. Add 2 ml of the 0.1 mole/L sodium hydroxide to each tube and mix on a vortex mixer for 1 min. Allow the layers to separate, and remove and discard the upper alkaline layer. Wash the extract with 2.5 ml water by mixing on a vortex mixer for 30 sec; then remove and discard the upper layer.

The following steps must be done at accurately timed intervals, so that the fluorescent readings are taken exactly 15 min after the reagent is added to the extract. Usually the additions can be made at 1 min intervals. Warm the fluorescent reagent to room temperature and add 5 ml to a number of labeled tubes. Add 10.0 ml of an extract to one tube, start the timer, stopper the tube, and mix for 30 sec on a vortex mixer. Immediately remove the upper dichloromethane layer and discard. Transfer the lower portion to fluorescent cuvets. With a spectrofluorometer read the fluorescence with an exciting wavelength of 475 nm and a emission wavelength of 530 nm. With the Turner Model 111* use nos. 3 and 48 as primary filters and no. 16 as the secondary filter. Set the instrument to zero with pure water.

Calculation:

$$\frac{F_u - F_b}{F_s - F_b} \times 250 \times \text{Urine vol (L)} = \text{Cortisol } (\mu g/24 \text{ hr})$$

Or, if the other standard is used, replace 250 by 750 to give the result in nmole/24 hr. F_u, F_s, and F_b are the fluorescent readings for the unknown, standard, and blank, respectively.

Normal range: The following values have been obtained for the normal limits of cortisol excretion:
Men: 90 265 $\mu g/24$ hr or 250-730 nmole/24 hr
Women: 70-180 $\mu g/24$ hr or 195-500 nmole/24 hr
Procedure for cortisol in plasma:
Reagents:
1. Sodium hydroxide, 0.25 mole/L
   Dissolve 2.5 g sodium hydroxide in 250 ml water.
2. Extraction solvent
   Same as for urine.
3. Fluorescent reagent
   Same as for urine.
4. Cortisol standards
   Stock, intermediate, and working standards are the same as for urine.
Procedure: Set up sample, standard, and blank as in the method for urine, using 1 ml heparinized plasma or serum, 1 ml standard, and 1 ml water as blank. To each tube add 0.1 ml sodium hydroxide solution, mix briefly on a vortex mixer, and allow to stand for 5 min. Then add 10 ml extraction solvent and mix on a vortex mixer for 30 sec.

Filter the contents of each tube through Whatman phase-separating paper (no. 1 PS, 9 cm). Transfer 6 ml aliquots of the filtrates to clean test tubes. At timed intervals, add 4 ml fluorescent reagent and mix on a vortex mixer for 10 sec. Allow the tubes to stand for a

*G.K. Turner Associates, Palo Alto, Calif.

few minutes to allow the phases to separate; then remove and discard the upper layer. Transfer the lower layer to fluorescent cuvets and read exactly 30 min after addition of the reagent. The readings are done the same as for urine, and the calculations are similar.

Calculation:

$$\frac{F_u - F_b}{F_s - F_b} \times 25 = \text{Cortisol } (\mu g/dl)$$

since the working standard contains 0.25 $\mu g/ml$ or 25 $\mu g/dl$.

Normal range: The normal range for healthy adults for specimens collected between 8:00 AM and 10:00 AM is 11-26 $\mu g/dl$ (300-720 nmole/L). Although these procedures are not completely specific for cortisol, they are satisfactory for most clinical purposes in comparing normal and abnormal adrenal function.

Since plasma cortisol levels show a marked circadian pattern (the 8:00 AM sample having the highest level of the day, and the 8:00 PM sample level being approximately two thirds that of the morning specimen), serum samples should be obtained at both times on several successive days. Loss of circadian differences in the presence of elevated cortisol levels is usually seen in Cushing's syndrome. Procedures for measuring serum cortisol by more specific radioimmunoassay and high-performance liquid chromatography methods have also been reported.[64]

Spironolactone treatment may result in an increase in nonspecific fluorescence in the extract, leading to erroneously high results. Urinary steroids determined by colorimetric methods are not affected by the drug. The administration of oral amphetamine or parenteral methamphetamine has been stated to cause increases in plasma cortisol levels, particularly in morning specimens. This should be kept in mind in interpreting the results. It has also been claimed that large doses of alcohol or heavy smoking cause increases in plasma cortisol levels.

Aldosterone

Aldosterone is an adrenocortical hormone that appears in the urine in amounts up to 15 $\mu g/24$ hr. The amount of aldosterone varies with the state of electrolyte balance of the individual. Sodium depletion raises the level, whereas administration of sodium lowers it. These changes are controlled by the extracellular fluid volume rather than by the serum or total body sodium. Administration of potassium also increases the aldosterone level, whereas potassium deficiency lowers it. An increase in aldosterone is referred to as aldosteronism and occurs as primary aldosteronism and secondary aldosteronism.

Primary aldosteronism: In this condition the high aldosterone excretion results from adrenal tumors, e.g., adenoma and carcinoma. Laboratory findings include normal 17-ketosteroids and 17-OH excretion, low serum potassium, alkalosis, low specific gravity of urine, increased 24 hr volume of urine, and elevation of serum sodium. The clinical findings are hypertension, weakness, polyuria, and tetany.

Secondary aldosteronism: In this condition the characteristic elevated aldosterone excretion results from salt depletion, cardiac failure, cirrhosis, pregnancy, and lower nephron nephrosis.

Assay of aldosterone: Because of its importance in the regulation of electrolyte balance, many attempts have been made to find an adequate assay method for aldosterone. The compound is present in the urine in minute amounts representing less than 1% of the total corticosteroid metabolites in the urine. Thus for chemical methods extremely elaborate separation and purification schemes are required. The older methods used at least one separation by column chromatography followed by additional separations using paper or thin-layer chromatography before the final colorimetric or fluorometric determination. More recent methods use double isotope dilution methods. Since these use tritium-labeled (^{3}H-labeled) compounds, these are also beyond the scope of the usual clinical laboratory. (See, for example, reference 2, p. 258.)

CATECHOLAMINES[65-68]

The adrenal gland consists of the cortex and the medulla. The cortical hormones have been described previously in the discussion of steroids. The adrenal medulla consists of cells that have affinity for chrome salts and are therefore called chromaffin cells and belong to the chromaffin system. This system embraces not only the adrenal medulla but also the extramedullary chromaffin tissue in the paraganglia. The adrenal medulla produces two pressor amines called **epinephrine** and **norepinephrine** that belong to the group of catecholamines. Tumors arising in the adrenal medulla and in the extra-adrenal chromaffin tissue are called **pheochromocytomas.** These tumors, a small percentage of which are malignant, give rise to hypertension, either paroxysmal or sustained, resulting from their production of the pressor amines.

These pressor substances are found within the red cells and serum. In the serum, epinephrine is partially bound to albumin. In the urine, catecholamines appear either free or conjugated to glucuronides. Of the free catecholamines in the urine, 80% are norepinephrine and the remainder are epinephrine. In patients with pheochromocytoma there is an increased excretion of urinary catecholamines.

Determination of epinephrine and norepinephrine or total catecholamines

A method is presented for the determination of either epinephrine and norepinephrine separately or together as total catecholamines. The latter determination is quite simple and can be used in any laboratory possessing a simple fluorometer. The former determination is somewhat more complicated and may require a more sophisticated fluorometer. Since usually some 80% of the catecholamines are norepinephrine, the determination of the total is sufficient for most clinical purposes. The catecholamines are isolated from the urine by batch absorption on alumina at a pH of 8.6, the alumina is then washed, and the catecholamines are eluted with acid. For the total amines the eluate is oxidized at an alkaline pH with ferricyanide to produce a fluorescent compound. This is compared with a similarly oxidized norepinephrine standard.

For the separate catecholamines the epinephrine is determined by carrying out the oxidation at a pH of 2, and the fluorescence is read. The fluorescence of each oxidation is compared with the respective standard. An empirically determined equation is then used to calculate the amounts of norepinephrine and epinephrine, since oxidation at the two pH values does not completely separate the two amines. The procedure described should properly be labled ''free'' catecholamines, since the urine also contains some conjugated amines that are not determined, but the free amines are most commonly determined and the designation of ''free'' is often omitted.

Reagents:

1. Perchloric acid, 70% (16.5 moles/L)
2. Perchloric acid, 0.4 mole/L
   Dilute 12 ml of the concentrated acid to 5 dl with water.
3. Perchloric acid, 0.1 mole/L
   Dilute the 0.4 mole/L acid 1:4 as needed.
4. Aluminum oxide (chromatographic grade; activity, grade I)
   This is purified and activated as follows: Suspend 100 g aluminum oxide in 5 dl of 2 moles/L hydrochloric acid (165 ml concentrated acid to 1 L) and heat to about 95° C for 45 min, stirring frequently. Discontinue the heating and stirring and allow the alumina to settle for about $1^1/_2$ min; then pour off the supernatant along with the fines. Wash the alumina twice with 250 ml hydrochloric acid at 70° C for 10 min, then twice at 50° C for 10 min, each time stirring during the heating and allowing the alumina to settle for $1^1/_2$ min after stirring and decanting the supernatant and fines. Then wash the alumina, repeated with 2 dl portions of distilled water until the pH of the supernatant reaches 3.5; dry the alumina at 120° C for 1 hr and at 200° C for 2 hr. Store tightly stoppered at 37° C.
5. EDTA (disodium salt of ethylenediaminetetraacetic acid)
6. Sodium metabisulfite crystals ($Na_2S_2O_5$)
7. Sodium hydroxide, 5 moles/L
   Dissolve 20 g sodium hydroxide in water to make 1 dl.
8. Buffered perchloric acid, 0.1 mole/L
   To 1 dl of 0.1 mole/L perchloric acid, add a sufficient amount of 5 moles/L sodium hydroxide to bring the pH to 2.1.
9. Phosphate buffer, pH 7.0, 0.5 mole/L
   Dissolve 13.6 g KH_2PO_4 in about 1 dl water. Adjust to a pH of 7.0 by the addition of 1 mole/L sodium hydroxide (5 moles/L diluted 1:5).
10. Buffer, pH 2.0
    Dissolve 0.37 g potassium chloride in about 50 ml water. Cautiously add 0.2 mole/L hydrochloric acid (1.6 ml concentrated acid plus 1 dl water) to bring the pH to 2.0, and dilute to 1 dl.
11. Ascorbic acid, 0.11 mole/L
    Dissolve 1 g ascorbic acid in water to make 50 ml. This solution should be prepared within a few hours of use and kept on ice.
12. Alkaline ascorbic acid

Just before use mix together 9 ml of 5 moles/L sodium hydroxide, 0.2 ml ethylenediamine, and 1 ml of fresh 0.11 mole/L ascorbic acid solution.

13. Potassium ferricyanide solution, 7.5 mmole/L
Dissolve 0.25 g potassium ferricyanide in water to make 1 dl. This solution should be prepared fresh on the day of use.

14. Sodium hydroxide–ethylenediamine mixture
Mix 9 ml of 5 moles/L sodium hydroxide solution with 0.2 ml ethylenediamine.

15. Norephinephrine stock standard, 200 μg/ml
Dissolve 39.8 mg norepinephrine bitartrate in 1 dl of 0.1 mole/L perchloric acid. Store in refrigerator and prepare fresh monthly.

16. Norepinephrine working standard
Dilute 100 μl of the stock with the buffered 0.1 mole/L perchloric acid. Prepare fresh as needed. When used in the assay, 500 μl of the standard contains 100 ng norepinephrine.

17. Epinephrine stock standard, 200 μg/ml
Dissolve 36.4 mg epinephrine bitartrate in 1 dl of 0.1 mole/L perchloric acid. Store in the refrigerator and prepare fresh monthly.

18. Epinephrine working standard
Dilute 100 μl of the stock to 1 dl with the buffered 0.1 mole/L perchloric acid. When used in the assay, 500 μl of the standard contains 100 ng epinephrine. Prepare fresh as needed.

Procedure: The 24 hr urine specimen is collected in a glass or plastic bottle containing about 15 ml concentrated hydrochloric acid. Refrigeration is not necessary, but the pH of the urine should be kept below 3. The 24 hr specimen is mixed well and the total volume measured.

To a 25 ml aliquot of the urine add 0.6 ml of 16.5 moles/L perchloric acid and agitate for 5 min. Then centrifuge strongly to remove all suspended material. Decant the urine into a 150 ml beaker, and add 40 ml of 0.4 mole/L perchloric acid. Add 700 mg alumina, 400 mg EDTA, and 20 mg sodium metabisulfite; then mix.

With continuous stirring add 5 moles/L sodium hydroxide to bring the pH to 8.6 (use a pH meter). Keep at a pH of 8.6 with gentle stirring for 5 min. It is pref-

erable not to use a magnetic stirrer because of its abrasive action. If the pH goes above 8.6, it can be brought back with a few drops of hydrochloric acid. After 5 min discontinue the stirring and allow the alumina to settle. Remove as much as possible of the supernatant by aspiration or decantation.

Add about 75 ml water to the beaker, mix well, and allow the alumina to settle. Decant the supernatant and transfer the almina to a large centrifuge tube with the aid of about 25 ml water. Stopper the tube and shake well; then centrifuge strongly and decant or aspirate the supernatant. Repeat the washing once more.

After the final washing remove as much water as possible; then add 5 ml of 0.1 mole/L perchloric acid, stopper the tube, and shake well. Centrifuge strongly, decant off the supernatant, and save for analysis.

For analysis and standardization set up the tubes as shown in Table 25-4. If only the total of catecholamines is required, only the tubes designated by the asterisk (*) need to be run. In the protocol as given below, the standard or sample eluate is added to small tubes and mixed. The ferricyanide solution is added at timed 30 sec intervals, and exactly 3 min after the addition of the ferricyanide the alkaline solution is added. Mix after each addition. After 10 min read in fluorometer with an excitation wavelength of 395 nm and an emission wavelength of 505 nm.

For epinephrine standards, repeat exactly as in Table 25-3, labeling the tubes E_1 to E_4 and using the diluted epinephrine standard (reagent no. 18 above). For samples, repeat exactly as in Table 25-4, using 500 μl of the eluate in each tube and numbering the tubes S_1 to S_4. (For the total of catecholamines only, run only tubes S_1 and S_2.)

Calculation: After all the tubes have been run, calculate the following by subtracting the corresponding blanks:

$$X = S_1 - S_2$$

and

$$Y = S_3 - S_4$$

where S_1 is the fluorometer reading for the tube labeled S_1, etc., and $a = N_1 - N_2$, $b = N_3 - N_4$, $c = E_1 - E_2$, and $d = E_3 - E_4$.

Table 25-4. Analysis and standardization of norepinephrine

	Tube no.			
	N_1*	N_2*	N_3	N_4
Diluted norepinephrine standard (16)	500 μl	500 μl	500 μl	500 μl
Buffer, pH 7.0 (9)	250	250	—	—
Buffer, pH 2.0 (10)	—	—	250	250
Ferricyanide solution (13)	25	25	25	25
Alkline ascorbic acid (12)	500	—	500	—
Sodium hydroxide–ethylene diamine mixture (14)	—	500	—	500
Ascorbic acid solution (11) (add after 15 min)	—	25	—	25

*N = Treatment of norepinephrine standard.
Subscripts: 1 = oxidation at pH of 7.0, and 2 = corresponding blank; 3 = oxidation at pH of 2.0, and 4 = corresponding blank.
The numbers after the reagents represent the numbers of the particular reagents given earlier.

The standards added to each tube contain 100 ng norepinephrine or epinephrine. The amount of eluate added (500 µl) represents one tenth of the total eluate, which contains the catecholamines from 25 ml urine. Thus an eluate that gave the same reading as a standard would represent 100 ng amine in 2.5 ml urine or 40 ng/ml. Thus for total catecholamines only

$$\text{Urine (ng/ml)} = 40 \times \frac{X}{A}$$

For the separate amines more complicated formulas are needed, because corrections are made for the interference of norepinephrine on the estimation of epinephrine and vice versa. The formulas are

$$\text{Norepinephrine (ng/ml)} = \frac{(40 \times X \times d) - (Y \times c)}{(a \times d) - (b \times c)}$$

and

$$\text{Epinephrine (ng/ml)} = \frac{40 \times Y}{d} - \frac{N - b}{40 \times d}$$

where N represents the actual amount of norepinephrine calculated in the first equation.

$$\text{Total excreted} = \text{ng/ml} \times \text{Vol (L)} = \mu g/24 \text{ hr}$$

To convert micrograms to nanomoles multiply by 5.46 for epinephrine and 5.91 for norepinephrine, or use an average value of 5.8 for both without serious error.

Normal values and interpretation: The range of total catecholamines in normal individuals is 30-70 µg/24 hr, of which about 80% is norepinephrine. In screening for pheochromocytoma a 24 hr excretion of up to 100 µg total free catecholamines is considered normal, 100-200 µg is borderline, and above 200 µg may be considered suggestive of disease. Ordinarily about 20% of the total is epinephrine and the remainder norepinephrine.

A number of drugs may interfere with the determination of the catecholamines, usually giving erroneously high results. A number of these, e.g., quinine, quinidine, and the B complex vitamins, may produce interfering fluorescence. Drugs such as methenamine compounds that liberate formaldehyde in the urine also interfere. The excessive use of epinephrine inhalation or the use of isoproterenol or levodopa can also produce high results.

The foregoing drugs produce interfering chemical effects. Other drugs may produce elevated catecholamine levels by their physiologic action. These include caffeine, aminophylline, and ethanol. It is advisable to limit the intake of these drugs for several days before the collection of the urine specimen.

In children an elevation of epinephrine output often indicates an adrenal source, whereas an increase in urinary norepinephrine is seen in children with extraadrenal tumors.

Urinary free norepinephrine, epinephrine, and dopamine by high-performance liquid chromatographic analysis

High-pressure liquid chromatography (HPLC) allows for the specific separation and quantification of all three

compounds by using electrochemical detection. The HPLC assay described by Moyers et al.[69] is very satisfactory. This procedure requires the use of both alumina and cation-exchange columns to sufficiently purify the biogenic amines before analysis. Although labor is intensive and requires rigorously controlled technic, this method can easily process 4-5 specimens per day. The advantage of this technic is an increased specificity. With this assay the patient does not have to be on a specially controlled diet before urine collection.

This method, with minor modifications, can also be used to assay for total urinary normetanephrine and metanephrine (metabolites of norepinephrine and epinephrine, respectively).[70] The measurement of urinary metanephrines plus VMA (see below) have been suggested as the best screening procedure for the detection of pheochromocytomas.

The use of a plasma catecholamine assay has also been advocated. The radioenzymatic assay currently available may be too tedious and time consuming for many laboratories. However, an HPLC technic for plasma catecholamines has been developed,[71] although the actual efficiency of such measurements will have to be determined in the future.

Determination of vanillylmandelic acid (3-methoxy-4-hydroxymandelic acid)

Vanillylmandelic acid (VMA)[72-74] is a metabolite of epinephrine and norepinephrine found in the urine in amounts 10-100 times the amount of pressor amines. Its determination is used as a measure of endogenous secretion of catecholamines. Urinary excretion of VMA is highly elevated in the urine of patients with pheochromocytoma and related tumors. Because the concentration of VMA in urine is much greater and methods for its determination are simpler and more adaptable to the average laboratory, it is preferred over the more intricate catecholamine determination.

There are three general methods for the determination of VMA. In one method the VMA is extracted from acidified urine, reextracted with sodium carbonate solution, and then treated with diazotized p-netroaniline to give a colored product. The color is extracted with butanol and the absorbance measured. Since the reaction is not very specific, the difference in the absorption at 450 nm and 540 nm is often used. The method is not too specific but may be satisfactory as a screening test.

In the second method, the VMA, after extraction, is oxidized to vanillin and the absorbance read at 360 nm. Although this method is more specific, it requires a spectrophotometer that can measure absorbance at 360 nm in the ultraviolet.

The third method, an HPLC method, is becoming increasingly popular.[75] The analysis requires a liquid-liquid extraction with ethyl acetate. The combined extracts are reduced to dryness and, when reconstituted, are analyzed on reverse-phase HPLC with ultraviolet detection. The procedure is more specific than the colorimetric assays and shows good precision and ease of analysis.

The procedure presented here combines some features of the two colorimetric methods.[76] The urine is extracted as in the other methods, and one aliquot is oxidized to vanillin. The oxidized and unoxidized aliquots are then both treated with diazotized *p*-nitroaniline. The difference in absorption between the two aliquots is then proportional to the amount of VMA present.

Reagents:

1. Ethyl acetate, AR
2. *n*-Butanol, AR
3. Sodium chloride, crystals
4. Hydrochloric acid, 2 moles/L
   Dilute 17 ml concentrated hydrochloric acid to 1 dl with water.
5. Citrate buffer, pH 4.0, 0.2 mole/L
   Dissolve 21.04 g citric acid monohydrate in about 4 dl water. Add 1 mole/L sodium hydroxide (40 g/L) to a pH of 4.0 (about 50 ml is required); then dilute to 5 dl.
6. Carbonate buffer, pH 10.4, 2 moles/L
   Dissolve 106 g anhydrous sodium carbonate in water to make 5 dl. Dissolve 21 g $NaHCO_3$ in water to make 250 ml. Add about 20 ml of the bicarbonate solution to 1 dl of the carbonate solution. Check the pH and add more bicarbonate as required to bring the pH to 10.4.
7. Stock VMA standard, 1 mg/ml
   Dissolve 50 mg of 3-methoxy-4-hydroxymandelic acid in 50 ml water. This solution is stable if kept refrigerated. Dilute the stock standard 1:50 to give a solution containing 0.2 mg/dl as needed. This working standard contains 1.01 mmole/L and can also be used as a standard for SI units.
8. Metaperiodate solution, 0.2 mole/L
   Dissolve 4.3 g sodium metaperiodate ($NaIO_4$) in water to make 1 dl. This solution is stable for several months.
9. Diazotized *p*-nitroaniline, 7 mmole/L
   Prepare a solution of 300 mg *p*-nitroaniline and 2 ml concentrated hydrochloric acid in water to make 1 dl. This solution is stable for several months in the refrigerator. Just before use dissolve 0.3 g sodium nitrite in 10 ml water. For the reagent, mix together 3 ml *p*-nitroaniline solution, 3 ml water, and 1 ml sodium nitrite solution. This final solution should be used within 30 min of preparation.

Procedure: To one 15 ml glass-stoppered centrifuge tube add 2 ml of the 24 hr urine specimen and 0.2 ml hydrochloric acid solution; label it "U" (unknown). To a second tube add 2 ml urine, 0.2 ml hydrochloric acid, and 0.1 ml VMA working standard; label it "S" (standard). To each tube add 1.5 g sodium chloride crystals and 5 ml ethyl acetate. Stopper and shake for 5 min.

Centrifuge the tubes and pipet 4 ml of the upper ethyl acetate layer into separate, labeled tubes. To each tube add 5 ml citrate buffer; stopper and shake for 5 min. Centrifuge to separate the layers; then remove and discard the upper ethyl acetate layer.

Pipet 2 ml of the solution from the unknown tube to each of two tubes labelled "U" and "B1" (blank no. 1). Similarly, pipet 2 ml aliquots of the contents of tube S to each of two tubes labled "S" and "B2" (blank no. 2). Add 3 ml carbonate buffer to all four tubes, mix.

Treat tubes U and S as follows: To each tube add 0.5 ml metaperiodate solution and mix briefly; then add at once 0.2 ml of the diazotized *p*-nitroaniline, mix, and after 15 sec add 3 ml *n*-butanol and shake well. Allow the layers to separate; then transfer 2 ml of the upper *n*-butanol layer plus 1 ml additional *n*-butanol (not used in the extraction) to labeled cuvets for reading.

Treat tubes B1 and B2 as follows: To each tube add 0.5 ml metaperiodate solution and mix. Incubate B1 for 6 min and B2 for 12 min at 30° C. Then add 0.2 ml diazotized *p*-nitroaniline to each tube, followed in 15 sec by 3 ml *n*-butanol, and shake. Transfer 2 ml supernatant plus 1 ml additional *n*-butanol to labeled tubes for reading.

Calculation: Read tubes U and S against B1 at 575 nm. Also read B1 against B2. Then if u and s are the readings for tubes U and S and b is the value obtained by reading B1 against B2,

$$\frac{u - b}{s - u} \times A \times V = \text{VMA excreted per day}$$

where V is the 24 hr urine volume in liters, A is 10 for the result in milligrams per day, and A is 50 for the result in micromoles per day.

Normal values and interpretation: By this method the urinary excretion of VMA in the normal adult is 2-8 mg/24 hr (10-40 μmole). A marked increase is found in functioning pheochromocytoma, with concentrations reaching as high as 150 mg/day. Increased levels are also seen in neuroblastomas, retinoblastomas, carcinoid tumors, ganglioneuromas, carotid body tumors, and stress. Drugs such as epinephrine, norepinephrine, and levodopa could be excreted as VMA or related compounds, but usually the dosage of these drugs is not high enough to cause a marked increase in the VMA excretion. Monoamine oxidase inhibitors may inhibit the conversion of catecholamines to VMA and thus cause a decrease in excretion. A similar effect is said to occur after the administration of imipramine. The pesence of phenolsulfonphthalein or bromsulphalein in the urine may give an interfering color. Some foods such as bananas, chocolate, coffee, tea, and those containing vanilla extract also give increased color not caused by VMA and thus a false positie reaction. On the other hand, meprobamate, dextroamphetamine, ephedrine, and isoproterenol apparently do not affect the VMA determination.

Determination of serotonin and 5-hydroxyindoleacetic acid[77-79]

Serotonin (5-hydroxytryptamine) is derived from the amino acid tryptophan by hydroxylation and deamination. This occurs mainly in the enterochromaffin cells of the intestines, although small amounts are found in some other organs. In patients with carcinoid syndrome the production of serotonin is markedly increased. The serotonin is further deaminated and excreted primarily as 5-hydroxyindoleacetic acid (5-HIAA). The increased excretion of the 5-HIAA has been used in the diagnosis of the carcinoid syndrome. The 5-HIAA is generally determined by the reaction with nitrous acid and 1-nitroso-2-naphthol to produce a purple color.

Presented first is a simple screening test in which the reaction is carried out directly in the urine sample. A negative result with this test indicates that the 5-HIAA excretion is very probably normal. A positive screening test should be followed by the quantitative procedure in which the urine sample is first treated with dinitrophenylhydrazine and extracted to remove some interfering material, and the test should be compared with standards to give a quantitative determination. Some drugs may interfere, as is indicated later in the discussion of the interpretation of the test.

Collection of specimen: Although a random specimen can be used for the screening test if analyzed within a few hours, preferably a 24 hr specimen should be collected, because it can be used later for the quantitative test if needed. Since the 5-HIAA is not stable in alkaline solution, the specimen should be collected with the addition of 25 ml glacial acetic acid.

Screening test:
Reagents:
1. 1-Nitroso-2-naphthol, 5.8 mmole/L
   Dissolve 0.1 g 1-nitroso-2-naphthol in 95% ethanol to make 1 dl.
2. Sodium nitrite, 0.36 mole/L
   Dissolve 2.5 g sodium nitrite in water and dilute to 1 dl. Store in the refrigerator and prepare fresh at biweekly intervals.
3. Sulfuric acid, 1 mole/L
   Carefully add 14 ml concentrated sulfuric acid to about 2 dl water; cool and dilute to 250 ml.
4. Nitrous acid solution
   Just before use mix 0.2 ml sodium nitrite solution and 5 ml sulfuric acid solution.
5. Ethylene dichloride, reagent grade

Procedure: Prepare in duplicate a test tube containing 0.8 ml water and 0.2 ml urine sample. To one of these tubes add 0.2 ml of 5-HIAA standard (see below) to serve as a positive control. Add an additional 0.2 ml water to the remainder of the tubes. Add 0.5 ml freshly prepared nitrous acid to each tube and mix. Allow the tubes to stand for 10 min; then add 5 ml ethylene dichloride to each tube and shake well. Allow the tubes to stand so that the layers will separate. If an emulsion forms, centrifuge briefly. A positive test is indicated by a purple color in the top layer. The negative control should be only slightly yellow.

The positive control is run, since several compounds can be present in urine that can act to inhibit color formation. The following compounds are reported to interfere with this procedure:
Inhibition: methenamine, phenothiazine, prochlorperazine, and promethazine
False positive results: acetanilid, acetophenetidin, glyceryl guaiacolate, mephenesin, and methocarbamol (diagnostic reagents kit information, Hycel, Houston)

Quantitative test: For the quantitative test the urine is treated with dinitrophenylhydrazine to remove any keto acids that might interfere. The solution is then extracted with chloroform to remove 5-HIAA. The solution is then saturated with sodium chloride and the 5-HIAA extracted with ether. The 5-HIAA is then reextracted back into the buffer for the color reaction, as in the qualitative test. The color is read in a photometer at 540 nm and the absorbance compared with that of a standard.

Additional reagents (in addition to those already used for the qualitative test):
1. Sodium chloride crystals
2. Chloroform, reagent grade
3. Ethyl acetate, reagent grade
4. Diethyl ether, peroxide free
5. Dinitrophenylhydrazine, 25 mmole/L in hydrochloric acid (2 moles/L.)
   Dissolve 0.5 g dinitrophenylhydrazine in 1 dl of 2 moles/L hydrochloric acid (17 ml concentrated acid to make 1 dl with water), with gentle warming if needed.
6. Phosphate buffer, pH 7.0, 0.5 mole/L
   Dissolve 8.67 g Na_2HPO_4 and 5.30 g KH_2PO_4 in about 190 ml water. Check the pH and adjust if necessary with a small amount of 1 mole/L sodium hydroxide or 1 mole/L hydrochloric acid as required; then dilute to 2 dl and mix well.
7. Standards
   a. Stock standard. Dissolve 10 mg pure 5-HIAA or 20 mg monodicyclohexyl ammonium salt in 10 ml of the phosphate buffer. Store in the refrigerator.
   b. Working standard, 20 μg/ml (105 μmole/L). Dilute 1 ml stock standard to 50 ml with water. Prepare fresh as needed.

Procedure: Transfer 6 ml urine to a 50 ml glass-stoppered centrifuge tube. Also set up a blank of 6 ml water and a standard of 3 ml working standard and 3 ml water. Carry sample, blank and standard all through the same procedure. To each tube add 6 ml dinitrophenylhydrazine reagent and mix. Allow to stand for 30 min; then add 25 ml chloroform, stopper, and shake well for a few minutes.

Centrifuge to separate the layers; then remove and discard the chloroform layer. Repeat the extraction with a second 25 ml portion of chloroform and also discard this extract.

Transfer 10 ml aqueous solution to another tube containing 4 g solid sodium chloride. Add 30 ml ether, shake well, and centrifuge. Transfer 20 ml ether extract to a third stoppered centrifuge tube, add 3 ml phosphate buffer, and shake for 5 min. Centrifuge; then remove the ether layer by aspiration. Transfer 2 ml of the aqueous phase to a 15 ml glass-stoppered centrifuge tube, add 1 ml 1-nitroso-2-naphthol reagent, and mix. Add 1 ml of the nitrous acid solution and mix.

Incubate for 5 min at 37° C; then cool, add 5 ml ethyl acetate, and shake well. Allow the layers to separate (centrifuge if necessary) and remove the ethyl acetate layer by aspiration and extract with a second 5 ml portion of ethyl acetate. After separation of the phases remove the ethyl acetate layer and discard.

Transfer aqueous solution to a cuvet and read at 540 nm against the blank. Also, read the standard against the blank.

Calculation: The standard contains 10 μg/ml of 5-HIAA (3 × 20 μg in 6 ml), and 6 ml standard is treated exactly the same as 6 ml urine. Then, since micrograms per milliliter equals milligrams per liter,

$$\frac{A(\text{sample})}{A(\text{standard})} \times 10 \times \text{Urine vol (L)}$$

$$= \text{Total 24 hr urine specimen (mg)}$$

where A is the absorbance. If the initial qualitative test gives a very strong reaction (deep purple to almost black), it is advisable to run a 1:10 and a 1:50 dilution of the urine along with the undiluted urine to avoid having to repeat the test.

Normal values and interpretation: Normally, small amounts of the serotonin metabolite 5-HIAA can be found in the urine. The normal range of excretion is 2-9 mg/24 hr. In the presence of a carcinoid or islet cell type of tumor the level rises to 25-1000 mg/24 hr. A number of drugs are said to cause lowered levels of 5-HIAA excretion; these include monoamine oxidase inhibitors, methyldopa, imipramine, and *p*-chlorophenylalanine. It is not clear whether the decrease is sufficient to interfere with the diagnosis of a carcinoid tumor. Methenamine and phenothiazines when excreted in the urine may result in some chemical interference with the test, leading to low values. The metabolites of some drugs such as acetanilid, phenacetin, mephenesin, and methocarbamol when excreted in the urine may cause a chemical interference that gives erroneously high values. It is also stated that ingestion of certain foods high in serotonin may lead to elevated levels of 5-HIAA in urine. Foods said to contain large amounts of serotonin include eggplant, avocados, bananas, pineapple, and plums.

REFERENCES

1. Loraine, J.A., and Bell, E.T.: Hormone assays and their clinical applications, ed. 4, Baltimore, 1976, The Williams & Wilkins Co.
2. Breuer, H., Hamel, D., and Krueskemper, H.L., editors: Methods of hormone analysis, New York, 1976, John Wiley & Sons, Inc.
3. Dorfman, R.I., editor: Methods in hormone research, ed. 2, New York, 1968, Academic Press, Inc., vol. 1.
4. Porter, R., editor: Gas chromatography in biology and medicine, London, 1969, J. & A. Churchill.
5. Odell, W.D., and Daughaday, W.J., editors: Steroid assay by competitive protein binding, Philadelphia, 1971, J.B. Lippincott Co.
6. Ransom, J.P.: Practical competitive binding assay methods, St. Louis, 1976, The C.V. Mosby Co.
7. Kirkham, E.E., and Hunter, W.M., editors: Radioimmunoassay methods, Edinburgh, 1971, Churchill Livingstone.
8. Moss, A.J., Jr., Dalrymple, G.V., and Boyd, C.M., editors: Practical radioimmunoassay, St. Louis, 1976, The C.V. Mosby Co.
9. Chen, I.W.: Radioligand Review 2:46-50, 1980; 2(3):46-48, 1980.
10. Boguslaski, R.C., et al.: In Nakamura, R.M., editor: Laboratory and research methods in biology and medicine: immunoassays for clinical laboratory techniques for the 1980's, New York, 1980, Alan R. Liss, Inc., vol. 4.
11. Zuk, R.F., Rowley, G.L., and Ullman, E.F.: Clin. Chem. 25:1554-1560, 1979.
12. Curry, R.E., et al.: Clin. Chem. 25:1591-1595, 1979.
13. Harte, R.A.: In Kaplan, L.A., and Pesce, A.J., editors: Non-isotopic methods and techniques in clinical chemistry, New York, 1981, Marcel Dekker, Inc.
14. Tuttle, C., Hsa, C.J., and Winfrey, L.: Clin. Chem. 26:1070A, 1980.
15. Franklin, M.L., Horlick, G., and Malmstadt, H.V.: Ann. Chem. 41:2-10, 1969.
16. Boerner, W., et al.: Nucl. Med. 9(suppl):799, 1971.
17. Braverman, V.A., and Williams, C.M.: J. Nucl. Med. 12:55, 1971.
18. Clark, F.: J. Clin. Pathol. 20:344, 1967.
19. Stein, E.A., et al.: Clin. Chem. 27(abstract): 1070, 1981.
20. Murphy, B.P., and Pattee, C.J.: J. Clin. Endocrinol. Metab. 24:187, 1964.
21. Murphy, B.P., Pattee, C.J., and Gold, A.: J. Clin. Endocrinol. Metab. 26:247, 1966.
22. Guaron, A.: J. Nucl. Med. 10:532, 1969.
23. Murphy, P.B.: Semin. Nucl. Med. 1:301, 1971.
24. Chopra, I.J.: J. Clin. Endocrinol. Metab. 34:938, 1972.
25. Hoertner, M., and Hesch, R.D.: Clin. Chim. Acta 44:106, 1973.
26. Farid, N.R., and Kennedy, C.: Clin. Chem. 23:1333, 1974.
27. Goedemans, W.T., et al.: Clin. Chem. 23:2324, 1977.
28. Rugg, N.E., et al.: Clin. Chem. 23:851, 1977.
29. Backala, H.R., Leavelle, D.E., and Hamberger, H.A.: Clin. Chem. 23:2177, 1977.
30. Bell, A.B., and Coleman, L.H.: Clin. Chem. 24:1755, 1978.
31. Davis, G.: Clin. Chem. 23:2356, 1977.
32. Davis, G., and Poholek, R.: Clin. Chem. 25:24, 1979.
33. Schall, R.F., Jr., et al.: Clin. Chem. 24:1801, 1978.
34. Finley, P.H., and Williams, R.J.: Clin. Chem. 24:165, 1978.
35. Van Lente, F., and Fink, D.J.: Clin. Chem. 24:387, 1978.
36. Ingbar, S.H., et al.: J. Clin. Invest. 44:1679, 1965.
37. Sterling, K., and Brenner, M.A.: J. Clin. Invest. 45:155, 1966.
38. Lee, N.D., Henry, R.J., and Golub, O.J.: J. Clin. Endocrinol. Metab. 24:486, 1966.
39. Clark, I.F., and Horn, D.B.: J. Clin. Endocrinol. Metab. 25:39, 1965.
40. Rose, N.R., and Witebsky, E.: J. Immunol. 76:417, 1956.
41. Doniach, D., and Rott, I.M.: Clinical aspects of immunology, ed. 2, Philadelphia, 1968, F.A. Davis Co.
42. Heftman, E.: Steroid biochemistry, New York, 1970, Academic Press, Inc.
43. Dorfman, R.I., and Ungar, F.: Metabolism of steroid hormones, New York, 1965, Academic Press, Inc.
44. Breuer, H., and Nocke-Finck, L.: In Curtius, H.C., and Roth, M., editors: Clinical biochemistry, Berlin, 1974, Walter de Gruyter & Co., p. 790.
45. Dickey, R.P., et al.: Am. J. Obstet. Gynecol. 94:591, 1966.
46. Oakey, R.E., et al.: Clin. Chim. Acta 15:35, 1967.
47. Oakey, R.E.: In Breuer, H., Hamel, D., and Krueskemper, H.L., editors: Methods of hormone analysis, New York, 1976, John Wiley & Sons, Inc., p. 469.
48. Scommegna, A., and Chattoraj, S.C.: Am. J. Obstet. Gynecol. 99:1087, 1967.
49. Kirkish, L.S., et al.: Clin. Chem. 24:1830-1832, 1978.
50. Kaplan, L.A., and Miller, J.: In Kaplan, L.A., and Pesce, A.J., editors: Non-isotopic methods and techniques in clinical chemistry, New York, 1981, Marcel Dekker, Inc.
51. Chattoraj, S.C.: In Tietz, N., editor: Fundamentals of clinical chemistry, Philadelphia, 1974, W.B. Saunders Co., pp. 749-756.
52. Callow, N.H., Callow, R.K., and Emmons, C.W.: Biochem. J. 32:1213, 1938.
53. Few, J.D.: J. Endocrinol. 72:31, 1961.
54. Larsen, K.: Acta Endocrinol. 57:228, 1968.
55. Silber, R.H., and Busch, R.D.: J. Endocrinol. 16:1333, 1956.

56. Silber, R.H., and Porter, C.C.: Methods Biochem. Anal. **4:**139, 1957.

57. Williams, R.H., editor: Textbook of endocrinology, Philadelphia, 1968, W.B. Saunders Co.

58. Lauler, D.P., and Thorn, G.W.: In Harrison, T.R., et al., editors: Principles of internal medicine, ed. 5, New York, 1966, McGraw-Hill Book Co.

59. Cope, L.C.: Proc. Roy. Soc. Med. **58:**551, 1965.

60. Mattingly, D.: J. Clin. Pathol. **15:**374, 1962.

61. Verjee, Z.H.M.: Clin. Chim. Acta **33:**268, 1971.

62. Pirke, K.M., and Stamm, D.: J. Clin. Chem. Clin. Biochem. **10:**243, 1972.

63. Ratliff, C.R., and Hall, F.F.: Sel. Meth. Clin. Chem. **8:**115, 1977.

64. Frey, F., Frey, B.M., and Benet, L.Z.: Clin. Chem. **25:**1944-1947, 1979.

65. Weil-Malherbe, H.: Methods Biochem. Anal. **16:**203, 1968.

66. Sandhu, R.S., et al.: Stand. Meth. Clin. Chem. **7:**231, 1972.

67. Anton, A.H., and Sayre, D.F.: J. Pharmacol. Exp. Ther. **145:**326, 1964.

68. Bohuon, C.: In Curtius, H.C., and Roth, M., editors: Clinical biochemistry, Berlin, 1974, Walter de Gruyter & Co., p. 855.

69. Moyers, T.P., et al.: Clin. Chem. **25:**256-263, 1979.

70. Shoup, R.E., and Kissinger, P.T.: Clin. Chem. **23:**1268-1274, 1977.

71. Goldstein, D.S., and Feverstein, G.: Clin. Chem. **27:**508, 1981.

72. Mahler, D.J., and Humoller, F.L.: Clin. Chem. **8:**47, 1962.

73. Pisano, J.J., Crout, J.R., and Abraham, D.: Clin. Chim. Acata **7:**285, 1962.

74. Jacobs, S.L., Sobel, C., and Henry, R.J.: J. Clin. Endocrinol. Metab. **21:**315, 1961.

75. Soldin, S.J., and Hill, J.G.: Clin. Chem. **26:**291-294, 1980.

76. Gumboldt, G.: Clin. Chem. **23:**1949, 1977.

77. Peart, W.S., Andrews, T.M., and Robertson, J.I.S.: Lancet **1:**577, 1961.

78. Udenfriend, A., Titus, E., and Weisbach, H.: J. Biol. Chem. **216:**499, 1955.

79. Pernow, B., and Waldenstriem, J.: Lancet **2:**951, 1954.

Toxicology and therapeutic drug monitoring

Simply stated, toxicology is the study of poisons. More specifically, toxicology is concerned with the chemical and physical properties of toxic substances, their physiologic effects on living organisms, qualitative and quantitative methods of analysis of toxicants in biologic and nonbiologic materials, and methods for the treatment of poisonings including the development of specific antidotes. The best definition of a poison is that given by the sixteenth century physician Paracelsus: "All substances are poisons; there is none which is not a poison. The right dose differentiates a poison from a remedy."

This definition indicates that toxicology is essentially a quantitative science which is seeking to determine what amount of substance under what conditions will result in toxicity in a given individual. The major ap-

plication of toxicology in the clinical laboratory is the determination of drugs and poisons in blood, gastric contents, or urine collected from living persons. Emergency toxicologic analysis identifies toxicants that may be responsible for illness or coma in emergency room patients. Therapeutic drug monitoring serves as an adjunct to effective drug therapy. This chapter presents procedures that enable a clinical laboratory to meet both of these roles with a minimum of sophisticated analytic instrumentation. To perform all the presented analyses, a laboratory needs only microdiffusion dishes, thin-layer chromatographic equipment, a visible ultraviolet recording spectrophotometer, and a fluorometer. This excludes determinations of lead and mercury, which require an atomic absorption spectrophotometer. The chapter is divided into two sections: toxicology and therapeutic drug monitoring.

TOXICOLOGY

Toxicologic analyses assist the clinician to (1) resolve a diagnostic dilemma, (2) indicate the prognosis of the poisoned patient, and (3) provide information that may influence therapeutic measures. The detection and quantitative determination of a toxicant in blood or urine may indicate if a patient's symptoms or coma is the result of drugs, trauma, or illness. In the intoxicated patient, quantitative toxicology results may indicate the severity and course of the poisoning. In patients suffering multiple trauma, e.g., as in automobile accidents, the presence of alcohol or drugs may be an important consideration to the neurologist, surgeon, and internist providing emergency therapy.

The drugs and poisons most commonly encountered in cases of drug overdose or intoxications, excluding ethanol and carbon monoxide, and the analytic methods employed in this chapter are presented in Table 26-1. These toxicants represent approximately 90% of emergency or fatal drug intoxications.[1-6] Utilizing the procedures presented, personnel in the clinical laboratory may provide dependable, qualitative drug analyses for the toxicants listed. Quantitative procedures capable of measuring toxic concentrations in blood, plasma, or serum are presented for the majority of these agents. It should be noted that therapeutic concentrations will not be detected by many of the procedures. To perform the necessary test, a minimum of 10 ml of blood, plasma, or serum and 40 ml of urine should be submitted to the

Table 26-1. Analytic procedures*

Drug	Urine color test	TLC drug screen (confirmation)	Specific TLC	UV blood drug screen	Specific UV	Specific blood colorimeter
Acetaminophen	+					+
Amitriptyline		+(UV)		+	+	
Amphetamines		+(Fl)				
Barbiturates		+(UV)		+	+	
Benzodiazepines			+			
Chlordiazepoxide				+		
Diazepam				+		
Flurazepam				+		
Chloral hydrate	+					+
Cocaine		+(UV)	+			
Codeine		+(UV)				
Desipramine	+	+(UV)		+		
Ethchlorvynol	+	+				+
Glutethimide		+(UV)				
Hydromorphone		+(UV)				
Imipramine	+	+(UV)		+		
Meperidine		+(Fl)				
Meprobamate						+
Methadone		+(UV)				
Methamphetamine		+(Fl)				
Methapyrilene		+(UV)		+		
Methaqualone		+(UV)	+	+	+	
Methyprylon						+
Morphine		+(Fl)	+			
Nicotine		+(UV)				
Nortriptyline		+(UV)	+	+		
Oxycodone		+(UV)				
Pentazocine		+(UV)				
Phencyclidine		+(UV)				
Phenothiazines	+			+		
Chlorpromazine	+	+(Fl)				
Thioridazine	+	+(Fl)				
Phenylpropanolamine		+(UV)				
Propoxyphene		+(UV)		+		
Quinine/quinidine		+(UV)				
Salicylate	+				+	

*Fl, Fluorescent spectrophotometry; TLC, thin-layer chromatography; UV, ultraviolet spectrophotometry.

laboratory. Blood alcohol analysis and the qualitative screening of urine should initially be performed. Once the toxicants have been identified in urine, their quantitative determinations in blood, plasma, or serum should be undertaken.

COLOR TESTS FOR URINE DRUG SCREENING

A color test is a chemical procedure in which the substance tested for is acted on by a reagent that produces an observable color or color change in the reagent. Color tests may be used to determine the presence of specific compounds or a general class of compounds. The methods are usually rapid, inexpensive, and easy to perform. A positive reaction indicates the presumptive finding of a drug or group of drugs. A negative finding eliminates the probability of the presence of a particular drug or drug group. The major disadvantages of color tests are lack of specificity, false positive or false negative reactions, and the difficulty of interpreting the results.

Acetaminophen

Acetaminophen,[7] phenacetin, and their urinary metabolites are hydrolyzed in acid solution to *p*-aminophenol, which is coupled with *o*-cresol to produce a distinctive indophenol blue color.

Reagents: All chemicals should be analytic reagent grade.
1. Saturated *o*-cresol reagent
   Shake 10 ml *o*-cresol with 1 L distilled water. Allow to stand for 24 hr before use.
2. Ammonium hydroxide, 4N
   Dilute 284 ml concentrated ammonia to 1 L with distilled water.
3. Concentrated hydrochloric acid
4. Reference urine
   Use an aliquot of a urine sample obtained from a patient who took 1 g acetaminophen in the previous 24 hr period. The reference urine may be divided into 2 ml aliquots and stored frozen.

Procedure: Pipet 1 ml of sample (test urine), reference urine, and water (as a reagent blank) into separate test tubes. Add 1 ml of concentrated hydrochloric acid and heat in a boiling water bath for 10 min. Dilute 0.1 ml of this solution to 10 ml with *o*-cresol reagent and add 2 ml of 4N ammonium hydroxide. Observe color; a blue color is an indication that acetaminophen may be present.

Interfering substances: Acetaminophen and *p*-aminophenol are metabolites of phenacetin; hence this reaction can give positive results after ingestion of phenacetin.

Interpretation: The formation of the indophenol blue is extremely sensitive. A strong positive result can be obtained with urine samples from volunteers who have taken 1 g of acetaminophen previously. Therefore if a positive test result is obtained, acetaminophen serum concentrations should be determined (see discussion of blood analysis).

Chloral hydrate and halogenated hydrocarbons[8,9]

Halogenated hydrocarbons heated with sodium hydroxide and pyridine produce an intense red color.
Reagents:
1. Sodium hydroxide, 20%
2. Pyridine
   Store in a dark tightly closed bottle in a room free of halogenated hydrocarbons. If pyridine is wet (cloudy), do not use.
3. Standard
   Dissolve 500 mg chloral hydrate in 1 dl ethanol. Store in a dark bottle in a refrigerator.

Procedure: To 1.0 ml of sample (test urine) standard and water as a reagent blank add 1.0 ml of 20% sodium hydroxide and 1.0 ml of pyridine. Heat in a boiling water bath for 1 min. (Do not carry out procedure in a laboratory room where chloroform or other halogenated hydrocarbons are used for extractions.)

A pink to red color in the pyridine layer indicates the presence of chloral hydrate or other halogenated hydrocarbon.

Interpretation: Chloral hydrate is the commonly used prescription drug that will produce a positive reaction. However, numerous halogenated hydrocarbons will be detected if present, including chloroform, carbon tetrachloride, ethylene dichloride, trichlorethylene, perchlorethylene, and methylene dichloride.

Ethchlorvynol

Ethchlorvynol[10] reacts with diphenylamine to form a pink color.
Reagents:
1. Diphenylamine sulfate
2. Concentrated sulfuric acid
3. Standard
   Dissolve 10 mg ethchlorvynol in 50 ml ethanol and dilute to 1 dl with water. Dilute 1 ml of this stock standard with 25 ml water for test standard. An alternate reference urine may be prepared from the early morning urine of a volunteer who has ingested 500 mg ethchlorvynol the previous evening.

Procedure: Place 2.0 ml of urine (standard and water as a reagent blank) in a test tube and sprinkle a spatula full of diphenylamine sulfate crystals onto the surface. Incline the tube and carefully trickle in 1.0 ml sulfuric acid.

A red color on the surface of the crystals indicates the presence of ethchlorvynol.

Interfering substances: Phenothiazines and imipramine will react with the sulfuric acid. The presence of these drugs may be ruled out by the following color test for these compounds.

Occasionally an orange or blue color may develop because of urinary constituents or other drugs. A pink or red color indicates ethchlorvynol or phenothiazines. Neutral drugs of similar chemical structure do not produce false positive results, e.g., methyprylon or ethinamate.

Interpretation: A positive result indicates ingestion of ethchlorvynol. No meaningful interpretation can be ascribed to the patient's behavior or severity of intoxication.

Imipramine

In the presence of strong oxidizing acids, imipramine[11,12] and its metabolites are converted to green oxidation products.

Reagents: CAUTION: When preparing acid solutions, always add acid in small portions to water and stir constantly.
1. Potassium dichromate, 0.2%
   Dissolve 200 mg potassium dichromate in 1 dl water.
2. Sulfuric acid, 30%
   Dilute 30.0 ml concentrated sulfuric acid to 1 dl of water.
3. Perchloric acid, 20%
   Dilute 20.0 ml concentrated perchloric acid to 1 dl water.
4. Nitric acid, 50%
   Dilute 50.0 ml concentrated nitric acid to 1 dl with water.
5. Imipramine reagent
   Mix equal volumes of the above four reagents. Store the mixture in an amber glass bottle.
6. Standard
   Dissolve 25 mg imipramine hydrochloride in 1 dl water.

Procedure: Add 1.0 ml imipramine reagent to 1.0 ml sample (urine, standard, and water as a reagent blank). Gently shake the mixture. Immediately observe if a green or blue color is produced.

Interfering substances: A positive reaction will occur with imipramine and chemically related drugs: desipramine and trimipramine. Development of a purple color may indicate phenothiazine drugs.

Interpretation: A positive reaction is only seen in urine from patients receiving high therapeutic doses or who have overdosed with imipramine.

Phenothiazines

In the presence of strong oxidizing acids, the phenothiazines[12-15] and their metabolites are converted to colored oxidation products.
Reagents:
1. Ferric chloride, 5%

Dissolve 0.25 g ferric chloride in 5.0 ml water.
2. Perchloric acid, 20%
Dilute 9.0 ml perchloric acid to 45 ml with water.
3. Nitric acid, 50%
Dilute 25.0 ml nitric acid to 50 ml with water.
4. FPN reagent
Mix the solutions prepared above (1:9:10, by volume). Store in a dark bottle. The reagent is stable without refrigeration for 1 year.
5. Standard
Dissolve 25 mg chlorpromazine hydrochloride in 1 dl water.

Procedure: Add 1.0 ml FPN reagent to 1.0 ml sample (urine, standard, and water as a reagent blank) and mix. **Note color immediately after adding FPN reagent.** Disregard all colors appearing after a delay of 10 sec or more. The reaction of various phenothiazines is given in Table 26-2.

Interfering substances: Occasionally false positive results arise in drug-free urines. The color is usually orange and may be confused with trifluoperazine (Stelalazine) or promazine (Sparine) positive urine samples. False positive results may also occur in urine samples from patients with impaired liver function or phenylketonuria. False positive results may arise in urine from patients receiving *p*-aminosalicylic acid or estrogen therapy.

Interpretation: The FPN test will detect phenothiazine overdoses (1.0 g) and high and medium therapeutic doses (50-800 mg/day) from urine samples collected within 24 hr of ingestion. However, low therapeutic doses (20 mg/day) may yield inadequate color reactions.

Fluphenazine (Prolixin), promethazine (Phenergan), trifluoperazine (Stelazine), and triflupromazine (Vesprin) are only detected after overdose. Urine from patients receiving both chlorpromazine and trifluoperazine gives a purple color.

Additional phenothiazine test

Chlorpromazine and thioridazine are the most widely used phenothiazines. An additional test may be run for these drugs.

Chlorpromazine reagent[16,17]: Mix 20 parts 5% ferric chloride and 80 parts 10% sulfuric acid. Add 1.0 ml of this reagent to 1 ml of sample (as described above) and note color within 20 sec. A violet to deep purple color indicates the presence of chlorpromazine. Promazine and mepazine will also react.

Thioridazine reagent[18]: Mix 1 part 5% ferric chloride with 49 parts 30% sulfuric acid. Add reagent to 1 ml of sample and note color that appears within 15 sex of mixing. A pink to blue color indicates thioridazine. Other phenothiazines may also react.

Salicylates

This method is applicable to the quantitative determination of salicylates[19] in numerous biologic samples: blood, plasma, serum, tissue homogenates, and urine. The procedure is based on the formation of a violet-colored complex between ferric ions and phenols. The test is not specific for salicylates, but false negative results do not occur. The color developing solution contains acid and mercuric ions to precipitate protein.

Reagents:
1. Color reagent (Trinder's reagent)
Dissolve 40 g mercuric chloride, AR, in 850 ml of water by heating. Cool the solution and add 120 ml of 1N hydrochloric acid and 40 g ferric nitrate. When all the ferric nitrate has dissolved, dilute the solution to 1 L with water. It is stable indefinitely.
2. Salicylate standard stock
Dissolve 580.0 mg sodium salicylate (500 mg salicylate acid) in water and dilute to 250 ml. Add a few drops of chloroform as a preservative. This solution contains 2.0 mg salicylic acid/ml. Store the solution in the refrigerator; it is stable for 6 months.
3. Working standard, 200 μg/ml
Dilute 10.0 ml stock salicylate solution to 1 dl with water. Add a few drops of chloroform as a preservative. Store the solution in the refrigerator; it is stable for about 6 months.

Procedure: Pipet 1.0 ml specimen into a 15 ml centrifuge tube and add 50 ml Trinder's reagent while shaking the tube. Continue shaking until precipitate is finely dispersed.

Prepare a blank consisting of 1.0 ml water and 5.0 ml Trinder's reagent. Also prepare a standard consist-

Table 26-2. Reaction of phenothiazines with FPN reagent

Phenothiazine*	Color	Sensitivity (μg/ml)
Chlorpromazine (Thorazine)	Pink	5
Fluphenazine (Prolixin)	Pink	20
Methdilazine (Tacaryl)	Pink	5
Perphenazine (Trilafon)	Pink	4
Prochlorperazine (Compazine)	Pink	5
Promazine (Sparine)	Orange	5
Promethazine (Phenergan)	Pink	10
Thiopropazate (Dartalan)	Pink	5
Thioridazine (Mellaril)	Blue	5
Trifluoperazine (Stelazine)	Orange	10
Triflupromazine (Vesprin)	Pink	20

*Trade name given in parentheses.

ing of 1.0 ml of 200.0 μg/ml working standard and 5.0 ml Trinder's reagent. Beer's law is followed over a range of 100-500 μg/ml using the procedure as described. Dilute specimens with water if necessary.

Centrifuge the tubes at 2000 rpm (moderate speed) or filter through Whatman no. 42 filter paper. Urine solutions may not require centrifuging or filtering.

Transfer the clear supernatant to a cuvet and read absorbance against the reagent blank at *540* nm with a spectrophotometer. The resultant absorbance is stable for 1 hr.

For urine only, after reading the absorbance of the unknown, obtain a sample blank by setting the instrument with water and reading the absorbance of a solution prepared by mixing 1.0 ml urine, 5.0 ml Trinder's reagent, and 0.1 ml phosphoric acid (specific gravity 1.75), using the same cuvets as before.

Calculation:

$$\mu g/ml = \frac{\text{Absorbance of unknown } (\mu g/ml)}{\text{Absorbance of standard}}$$

For urine subtract the sample blank absorbance from the unknown abosrbance before making the calculations.

Interfering substances: Phenothiazines in high concentration may react with the reagent. Chlorpromazine (20 μg/ml) and thioridazine (20 μg/ml) will produce pink and blue colors, respectively. Acetoacetic acid in urine from diabetics may produce a faint false positive reaction; 500 μg/ml of acetoacetic acid gives an absorbance of 10 μg/ml salicylate. Boiling urine prior to analysis removes acetoacetic acid.

Interpretation: Salicylamide, salicylic acid, and methyl salicylate all give a positive reaction. A positive reaction in urine indicates only ingestion of aspirin or salicylates. Ingestion of two 5-grain aspirins will produce a grossly positive urine. In adults a common therapeutic dose of 600 mg aspirin will result in a serum concentration of 50 μg/ml salicylate.[20] Maximal concentrations occur within 2 hr of ingestion.[21] Arthritic patient receiving aspirin or sodium salicylate may have therapeutic serum concentrations up to 250 μg/ml. At concentrations greater than 300 μg/ml, tinnitus and other overt signs of toxicity may occur. Respiratory alkalosis and metabolic acidosis occur at concentrations greater than 500 μg/ml. At toxic concentrations, plasma elimination mechanisms become saturated, resulting in protracted elevated serum concentrations. The plasma half-life may increase from the norm for several hours to as long as 25 hr.[22]

THIN-LAYER CHROMATOGRAPHY FOR URINE DRUG SCREENING[23-28]

In thin-layer chromatography (TLC) the stationary phase is a thin layer of an absorbent, usually silica gel, which is spread on a solid support, e.g., a glass plate. Concentrated sample extracts and drug standards are applied as a series of spots along the bottom of the plate and allowed to dry. The plate is then placed in a closed tank in which the absorbent layer makes contact with a developing solvent (mobile phase) below the applied spots. The solvent moves up the plate by capillary action, dissolving and separating the components of the

extracts. When the solvent has reached the top of the plate or ascended a predesigned distance, the plate is removed from the tank and the solvent evaporated from the plate. Each individual drug in the standard mixture and in the extracts will separate during migration, producing a series of spots or narrow bands extending from the bottom to the top or solvent front on the plate. The migration of compounds is expressed by the retardation factor (R_f), which is defined as the ratio of the distance moved by the compound to the distance the mobile phase ascends the plate from the point of application of the compound. The presence of a drug is visualized by spraying the plate with various reagents that produce colored reactions with particular components. Several sprays may be used in sequence to aid in identification of compounds. Some drugs will react with certain sprays but not with others. If a compound from the extract migrates the same distance and reacts to the applied sprays in the same manner as one of the drug standards, a tentative identification is obtained for the compound. However, this identification must be confirmed by other chemical tests.

Preparation of urine extract

Numerous procedures have been proposed for the isolation of drugs from urine. By manipulation of pH and extracting solvent, drugs may be isolated in several extract fractions: strong acids, weak acids, amphoterics, and bases. However, only two procedures will be presented. These methods were selected based on their speed of analysis, simplicity of sample manipulation, and, with the exception of morphine, their ability to isolate the major drugs of interest in cases of drug overdose. Each procedure yields a single extract for TLC analysis. Morphine is excreted in urine as sulfate and glucuronide conjugates, which require a hydrolysis step to free the morphine for extraction. A three-fraction procedure for the analysis of morphine and the other drugs of interest is presented below under morphine. An alternate two-fraction procedure is presented under cocaine.

Materials:
1. Developing tank: standard glass tank for 20 × 20 cm TLC plates
2. Drying oven
3. Fume hood
4. TLC plates: silica gel 0.25 mm thick on 20 × 20 cm glass plates
5. Ultraviolet view box or hand-held ultraviolet lamp
6. Visualizing spray applicator: glass atomizer or aerosol spray cans
7. Warm air blower: hair dryer

Reagents:
1. Developing systems
   a. Ethyl acetate–chloroform–methanol–ammonia (50:30:12:1.5). Prepare fresh.
   b. Ethyl acetate–methanol–ammonia (85:10:5). Prepare fresh.
   c. Methanol-ammonia (100:1.5). Prepare fresh.
   d. Chloroform-acetone (90:10). Prepare fresh.
2. Developing tank sealant
   Mix 27 g soluble starch and 99 g glycerin in a

porcelain dish and heat to exactly 130° C. Remove the mixture from the heat and cool with stirring. (NOTE: This sealant is water soluble and can be easily removed from the tank. Never seal tank with silicon grease. If tanks are soaked with other glassware during washing, silicon grease will coat all glassware and may interfere with more sensitive analyses, e.g., gas chromatography.)

3. Visualizing spray reagents
   a. Ninhydrin spray. Dissolve 1 g ninhydrin in 1 L isopropyl-methanol (700:300). Store in a tightly capped, dark bottle.
   b. Diphenylcarbazone spray. Dissolve 10 mg diphenylcarbazone in 1 dl acetone-water (1:1) before use. This solution is stable for 1 week when refrigerated.
   c. Mercuric sulfate spray. Dissolve 2.5 g mercuric oxide in 1 L of 10% sulfuric acid.
   d. Iodoplatinate spray. Dissolve 1 g chloroplatinic acid in 1 dl water to make solution A. Dissolve 20 g potassium iodide in 1 dl water to make solution B. Mix equal parts of A and B before use. The mixed spray is stable for 2 weeks if refrigerated.

Thin-layer chromatography standards:
1. Standard 1. Dissolve 100 mg morphine hydrochloride, codeine phosphate, meperidine hydrochloride, hydrochloride, and methadone hydrochloride in 50 ml methanol. Label as "Narcotic ladder" and store in refrigerator.
2. Standard 2. Dissolve 100 mg amphetamine sulfate, cocaine hydrochloride, propoxyphene hydrochloride, chlordiazapoxide hydrochloride, and chlorpromazine hydrochloride in 50 ml methanol. Label as "Basic ladder" and store in refrigerator.
3. Standard 3. Dissolve 100 mg meprobamate, glutethimide, phenobarbital, and pentobarbital in 50 ml methanol. Label as "Acid ladder 1" and store in refrigerator.
4. Standard 4. Dissolve 100 mg amobarbital, phenytoin, and secobarbital in 50 ml methanol. Label as "Acid ladder 2" and store in refrigerator.
5. Internal standard. Dissolve 200 mg scopolamine hydrobormide in 1 dl methanol-water (1:1).
6. Control urine. Prepare individual drug solutions each having a concentration of 1 mg/ml MeOH/water (1:1); then prepare a mixture of these solutions in the following proportions:
   Scopolamine hydrobromide (internal standard), 4 ml
   Morphine, 2 ml
   Quinine, 1 ml
   Pentobarbital, 8 ml
   Amphetamine, 5 ml
   Glutethimide (Doriden), 5 ml
   Phenobarbital, 8 ml
   Phenothiazine, 3 ml
   Methadone, 10 ml
   Dilute the mixture with MeOH-water (1:1) to 1 dl. A working drug control is prepared by adding 1 ml of the diluted mixture to 20 ml of drug-free urine.

Direct extraction
Reagents:
1. Extracting solvent: chloroform-methanol (9:1)
2. Saturated sodium bicarbonate
   Dissolve 2.5 g sodium bicarbonate in 50 ml water. Prepare fresh.
3. Solid anhydrous sodium sulfate

Procedure:
1. Place 20 ml urine in a 125 ml separatory funnel, add 20 μl internal standard, and add small portions of solid sddium bicarbonate until effervescence ceases. Swirl the funnel after each addition. Add a small amount in excess of the amounts given above. The pH should not exceed 9.5.
2. Add 60 ml of the extracting solvent to the funnel, cap, and gently shake for 5 min. Occasionally tilt the funnel upside down and open the stopcock to relieve pressure in the funnel.
3. Place the funnel in a stand and allow sufficient time for the aqueous and organic phases to separate.
4. Prepare a second 125 ml separatory funnel by placing on top a filter funnel containing Whatman no. 1 filter paper.
5. Drain the organic phase into the second funnel and add 15 ml of the saturated sodium bicarbonate solution. Extract as in step 2.
6. Allow the phases to separate, drain off the bottom organic layer into a 1 dl beaker, and discard the aqueous layer. Pour the organic solution back into the funnel and repeat step 5.
7. Repeat step 6, but add 15 ml water to the funnel. Shake and allow phases to separate.
8. Prepare a filter funnel with Whatman no. 1 paper and add solid anhydrous sodium sulfate to the funnel. Drain the organic layer through the sulfate into a clean, dry 1 dl beaker.
9. Evaporate the organic solution just to dryness on a water bath.
10. Dissolve the residue in 2.0 ml ethanol. Add 1 drop of 10N hydrochloric acid.
11. Transfer ethanol solution into micro test tubes (or evaporation cups) and evaporate on warm water bath, passing a stream of air over the surface.
12. The resultant residue is dissolved in 3 drops of methanol and applied to TLC plates using a microcapillary tube (5-20 μl).

Amberlite XAD-2 column extraction

Buffered urine is passed through a column of XAD-2 resin, which adsorbs the drugs present. The drugs are then desorbed from the column by an eluting solvent. The solvent is then evaporated to prepare the extract residue for the TLC analysis. Numerous methods employing various absorbent materials have been applied to drug separations.[29-31] The procedure below closely follows that recommended by Eppendorf-Brinkman, Inc., Westbury, N.Y.[29]

Automatic instrumentation based on this procedure is also available (PREP I Automated Sample Processor, DuPont Clinical Systems Div. Wilmington, Del.).

Reagents:
1. Acetone
2. Amberlite XAD-2
   Prepare Amberlite XAD-2 resin (20-50 mesh) by washing with stirring four times with four bed volumes of acetone and three times with three bed volumes of distilled water. Store the resin in distilled water until transferred to the columns.
3. Buffer solution, pH 9.0
   Dissolve 81 g sodium bicarbonate in 1 L water and adjust to pH 9.0 by adding portions of solid sodium carbonate.
4. Control urine
   See reagent no. 5 under direct extraction procedure above.
5. Eluting solvent
   Mix 120 ml isopropanol with 7 dl dichloromethane.
6. Methanol
7. Preparation of column
   Prepacked XAD-2 resin columns are commercially available.[29] Alternately, fill empty polypropylene and glass columns (13.5-15.0 × 0.1 cm) with sample reservoir chambers (3 × 5 cm) with the resin prepared as described above in no. 2. Plug the columns with fine glass wool and pour an aqueous slurry of resin into the column to provide a resin bed filling approximately 40% of the lower portion of the column. Apply a small glass plug to the top of the resin, and store the column in distilled water until use.

Procedure: Wash the column with several milliliters of pH 9.0 buffer. Add 20 ml urine, quickly followed by 3 ml of pH 9.0 buffer, to the sample reservoir. Allow the urine to slowly flow through the column. Apply pressure or suction to remove excess urine.

Transfer the columns* to a 50 ml centrifuge tube containing 1 ml of aqueous saturated sodium bicarbonate solution (5% w/v). Elute the resin with 20 ml of the eluting solvent in two portions of 10 ml followed by a final 10 ml.

After elution, remove the column and shake the organic-aqueous phases in a centrifuge tube on a vortex mixer for 2 min. Allow the phases to separate and then remove the aqueous phase by aspiration. Prepare a residue for TLC analysis by treating the organic phase as described above under the direct extraction procedure starting with step no. 9.

Identification

The TLC plates may be developed as in system A or B (Table 26-3). TLC standard mixtures 1-4 and the control urine extract should be applied to the same plate as the sample urine extracts. After the solvent has migrated 12 cm from the points of extract application, remove the plate from the tank and dry it with hot air from the hair dryer. The ammonia from the developing

---

*Commercial XAD-2 systems have a cartridge affixed to the bottom of the column. The organic-aqueous phases are trapped following elution from the column. Special phase separating paper then permits only the eluting solution to pass through the cartridge into an evaporating cup.

system is removed by heating the plate at 75° C for 10 min in a drying oven.

Identification of the extracted drugs is by R_f (Table 26-3) and color reaction with spray reagents (Table 26-4). Gently outline all positive spots with a lead pencil. Note which spray reagents visualized the spots.

Remove the plate from the oven and while still hot, spray it lightly with ninhydrin reagent. Place the plate in the ultraviolet view box for 2-3 min. Primary amines (e.g., amphetamine, phenylpropanolamine) will appear as pink or red spots. Metabolites of methadone and amitriptyline may also react.

Then spray the plate with diphenylcarbazone, allow the reagent to air dry, and spray with mercuric sulfate reagent. Barbiturates and glutethimide will appear as purple spots. Secobarbital is a whitish-blue spot that fades quickly.

Dry the plate with a hair dryer and spray again with diphenylcarbazone reagent. Low concentrations of barbiturates will now be visible. Place the plate in the drying oven for 2-3 min. The barbiturate spots will disappear. Sulfuric acid in the mercuric sulfate reagent will react with phenothiazine drugs to produce a series of brightly colored spots. The phenothiazines are extensively biotransformed and are present in the urine as numerous metabolites. Chlorpromazine and metabolites are red and pink. Thioridazine and metabolites are blue and greenish blue.

Observe the plate in the ultraviolet view box. Quinine and its metabolites produce a bright blue fluorescence. Benzodiazepine drugs have a yellow-green fluorescence.

Remove the plate and spray with iodoplatinate reagent. Nitrogeneous bases will appear as yellow-brown, purple, or bluish spots.

Compare the R_f and color reactions of the drugs from the urine extracts with those of the TLC standards.

Interpretation

All apparent drug identifications should be confirmed by other chemical methods. Several additional analyses for specific compounds are presented below. The analyst should bear in mind that the presence of a drug or its metabolites in urine indicates only that at some time before the collection of the specimen, the drug had been administered. The concentration of a drug in urine does not correlate with the pharmacologic activity of the drug. Once excreted into the urine and stored in the bladder, drugs are not reabsorbed into the general circulation and hence do not exert a physiologic effect on the body. Pharmacologic activity is generally, although not always, related to drug blood or plasma concentration. If a single urine specimen is collected, the urine drug concentration cannot be related to the plasma concentration. Urinary excretion of drugs is subject to numerous variables. In certain instances urine drug concentrations may be related to plasma drug concentrations but only under controlled conditions involving multiple sampling, e.g., pharmacokinetic studies. However, the single urine specimen provided to the laboratory by emergency rooms, medical examiners, or methadone clinics does not meet necessary criteria for

Table 26-3. $R_f \times 100$ of drugs in TLC developing systems*

Drug	System†			
	A	**B**	**C**	**D**
Amitriptyline	48	98	49	
Amphetamine	38	48	48	
Barbiturates				
Amobarbital	75	75		48
Butabarbital		73		42
Butalbital		71		50
Pentobarbital	75	75		47
Phenobarbital	53	46		33
Secobarbital	75	75		55
Benzodiazepines				
Chlordiazepoxide	61	56	67	
Diazepam	88	75	75	
Flurazepam		72	62	
Oxazepam	43	56	63	
Chlorpromazine	78	73	49	
Cocaine	92	76	60	
Benzoylecgonine	3	3	21	
Codeine	30	32	35	
Desipramine		40	24	
Ethchlorvynol	92			95
Glutethimide	90	99		80
Hydromorphone	16		24	
Imipramine		64	43	
Meperidine	60	75		
Methadone	84	78	37	
Methapyriline		70	48	
Methaqualone		77	70	
Morphine	15	15	34	
Nicotine	68	61	57	
Nortriptyline		51	28	
Oxycodone			53	
Pentazocine		72	60	
Phencyclidine		80	59	
Phenylpropanolamine	27	27	52	
Phenytoin	66	45		30
Propoxyphene	91	91	66	
Norpropoxyphene	50		3	
Quinine	38	45	52	
Scopolamine	55		54	
Thioridazine	77	72	47	

*For system for separation of nitrogenous bases, see basic fractions from cocaine and morphine TLC procedures. For system for separation of acid and neutral drugs, see acid fraction of morphine TLC procedure.
†For description of developing systems, see p. 634.

Table 26-4. Visualizing procedure for TLC

Drugs	Ninhydrin	Diphenylcarbazone in mercuric sulfate	Heat at 75° C for 2 min	UV light	Iodoplatinate
Amitriptyline					Brown
Amphetamine	Pink	Disappears			
Barbiturates					
Amobarbital		Purple	Disappears		
Butabarbital		Purple	Disappears		
Butalbital		Purple	Disappears		
Pentobarbital		Purple	Disappears		
Phenobarbital		Purple	Disappears		
Secobarbital		Whitish blue	Disappears		
Benzodiazepines					
Chlordiazepoxide				Yellow-green	Brown
Diazepam				Yellow-green	Brown
Flurazepam				Yellow-green	Brown
Oxazepam				Yellow-green	Brown
Chlorpromazine			Red		Violet
Cocain					Red-brown
Benzoylecgonine					Red-brown
Codeine					Brown
Desipramine					Brown
Ethchlorvynol		Aqua	Disappears		
Glutethimide		Purple	Disappears		
Hydromorphone					Brown
Imipramine					Light brown
Meperidine					Brown
Methadone					Red/brown
Methamphetamine					Blue
Methapyrilene					Yellow-brown
Methaqualone					Blue
Morphine					Blue
Nicotine					Blue
Nortriptyline					Brown
Oxycodone					Brown
Pentazocine					Brown
Phencyclidine					Brown
Phenylpropanolamine	Red				Brown
Phenytoin		Purple	Disappears		
Propoxyphene					Red-brown
Norpropoxyphene					Red-brown*
Quinine				Blue	Brown
Scopolamine					Brown
Thioridazine			Blue		Brown

*May have a green halo around the spot.

physiologic interpretation. One can state with certainty only the presence or absence of the drug.

Confirmation analysis of thin-layer chromatography positive drugs
Ultraviolet spectrophotometry

Spots on the TLC chromatogram may be scraped from the plates and subjected to ultraviolet analysis.[32] The analyst should bear in mind that many drugs have identical ultraviolet spectra and also that the absorbance of mixtures is additive. If a spot contains more than one drug or a coextracted urinary constituent, a distorted spectrum may be observed. The entire spectrum, from 320-220 nm, of the sample should match that of drug standards. The absorbance maximum and minimum, as well as absorbance shifts in acid and basic solution, should be noted (Table 26-5 and Figs. 26-1 to 26-16).

Elution of mercuric sulfate–positive spots (barbiturates, acidic drugs): Scrape spots into small screw-top tubes. Add 1 ml of 0.1N sulfuric acid. Break up spots with applicator sticks. Add 8-9 ml of chloroform-isopropanol (9:1) mixture and shake for 10 min. Centrifuge the mixture for 5 min. Remove the top (aqueous) layer with a Pasteur pipet and discard. Filter the bottom (chloroform) layer through Whatman no. 2

filter paper into larger tubes. Add 1 ml of 0.5N sodium hydroxide. Shake for 5 min and centrifuge. Remove the aqueous (pH 13) upper layer with a Pasteur pipet and place in an ultraviolet microcuvet. Discard the bottom layer.

In a recording spectrophotometer, scan the upper layer against the plate blank from 340-220 nm. Add 0.1 ml of saturated ammonium chloride, mix, and check the pH. The pH should be between 10.3 and 10.5. Rescan from 340-220 nm. Compare the resultant ultraviolet spectrum with that of similarly treated known drug standards. The absorbance maximum and $E_{1\%}$ of acidic or neutral drugs of toxicologic interest are presented in Table 26-5.

Elution of iodoplatinate-positive spots (basic drugs): Scrape spots into small screw-top tubes. Scrape a control spot from a portion of the plate below the solvent line that shows no reaction. Add 1 ml water and a pinch of sodium bisulfite to each tube. Break up the spot with an applicator stick. Add sodium hydroxide, 8N, until pH 11 is obtained (approximately 6-8 drops). For the elution of morphine and dihydromorphone, add sodium bicarbonate until saturated, until a pH of 8-8.5 is obtained. Add 8-9 ml of chloroform-isopropanol (9:1) and shake for 10 min. Centrifuge to separate the phases. Discard the aqueous (top) layer.

Text continued on p. 644.

Table 26-5. Ultraviolet absorbance maximums of drugs of toxicologic interest

Drug	Sulfuric acid 0.1N		Sodium hydroxide, 0.45N	
	$E_{1\%}$*	Maximum	$E_{1\%}$	Maximum
Amitriptyline	500	240	185	242
Amphetamine	26	257 (254, 263)†	30	258
Benzodiazepines				
Chlordiazepoxide	1100	245	1100	262
Diazepam	1100	240		231
Flurazepam	600	239	452	231
Oxazepam	950	237	824	235
Chlorpromazine	1200	255	500	278
Cocaine	520	233	335	225
Benzoylecgonine	392	234		
Desipramine	307	251	299	254
Hydromorphone	50	281		292
Imipramine	240	251		251
Meperidine	12	257 (254, 263)	12	257
Methadone	19	259	65	290
Methapyrilene	640	238	640	240
Methaqualone	1185	233		228
Morphine	255	280	192	298
Nicotine	343	259	260	261
Nortriptyline		240		
Oxycodone	31	280		
Pentazocine	112	278	67	298
Phencyclidine	12	263		
Phenylpropanolamine	10	257 (254, 263)		258
Propoxyphene	13	257 (254, 263)		
Norpropoxyphene	13	257 (254, 263)		
Quinine	853	250	980	230
Theophylline	530	270	575	274
Thiopental	930	305	760	288
Thioridazine	1240	263	900	276

*$E_{1\%}$ = Absorbance of a 1 g/dl solution.
†Numbers in parentheses indicate secondary peaks.

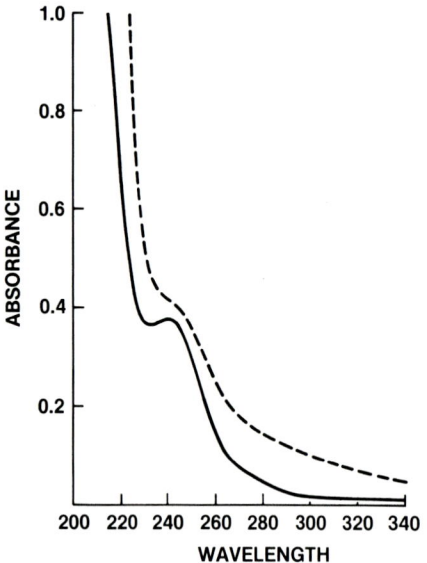

Fig. 26-1. Amitriptyline: solid line, 7.5 μg/ml in 0.5N sulfuric acid; dotted line, 2 drops of 40% sodium hydroxide added to acid solution. Similar spectrum produced by nortriptyline.

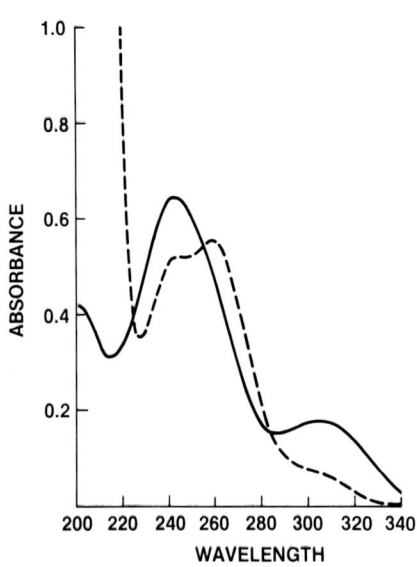

Fig. 26-2. Chlordiazepoxide: solid line, 6 μg/ml in 0.5N sulfuric acid; dotted line, 6 μg/ml in 0.5N sodium hydroxide.

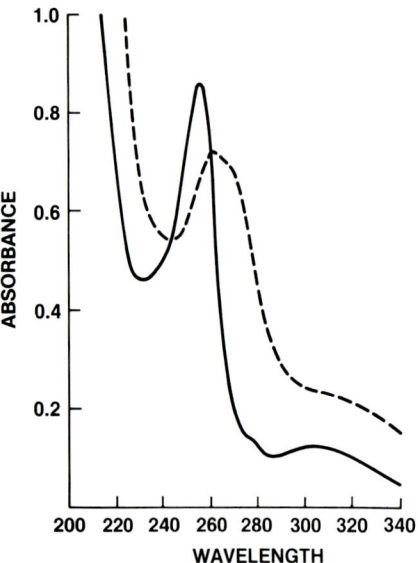

Fig. 26-3. Chlorpromazine: solid line, 7 μg/ml in 0.5N sulfuric acid; dotted line, 2 drops of 40% sodium hydroxide added to acid solution. Similar spectra produced by other phenothiazines.

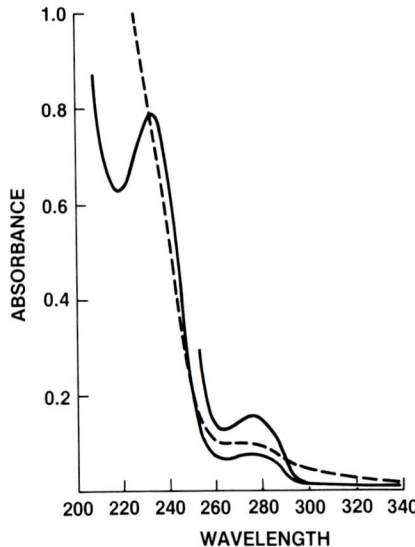

Fig. 26-4. Cocaine: solid line, 15 μg/ml in 0.5N sulfuric acid; dotted line, 2 drops of 40% sodium hydroxide added to acid solution. Similar spectrum produced by benzoylecgonine.

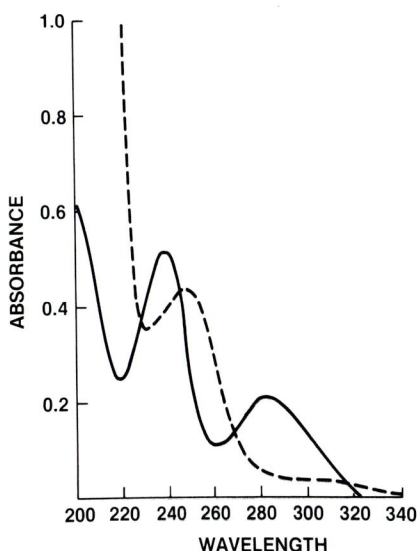

Fig. 26-5. Diazepam: solid line, 5 µg/ml in 0.5N sulfuric acid; dotted line, 5 µg/ml in 0.5N sodium hydroxide. Similar spectra produced by flurazepam, oxazepam, and other benzodiazepine drugs and metabolites.

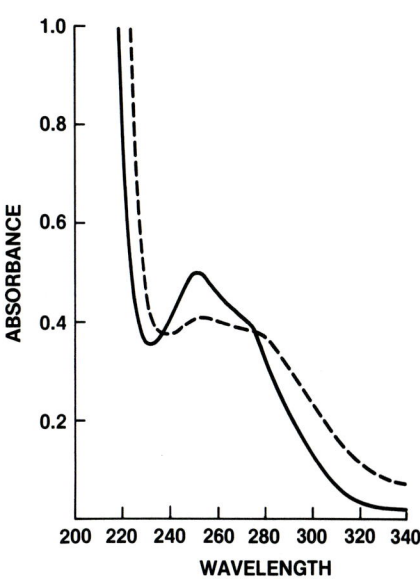

Fig. 26-6. Imipramine: solid line, 20 µg/ml in 0.5N sulfuric acid; dotted line, 2 drops of 40% sodium hydroxide added to acid solution. Similar spectrum produced by desipramine.

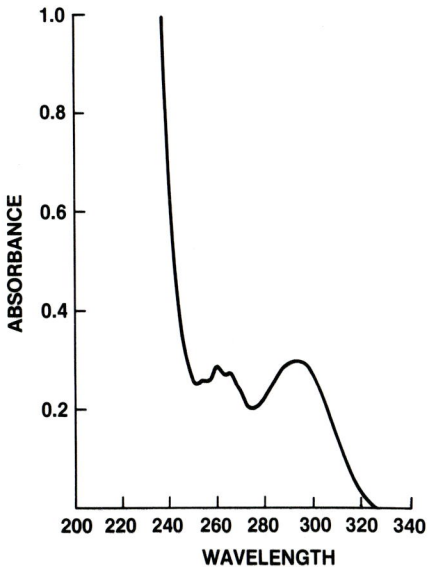

Fig. 26-7. Methadone: 175 µg/ml in 0.5N sulfuric acid.

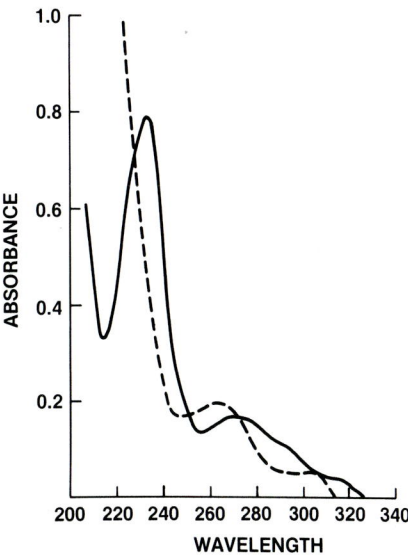

Fig. 26-8. Methaqualone: solid line, 7.5 µg/ml in 0.5N sulfuric acid; dotted line, 2 drops of 40% sodium hydroxide added to acid solution.

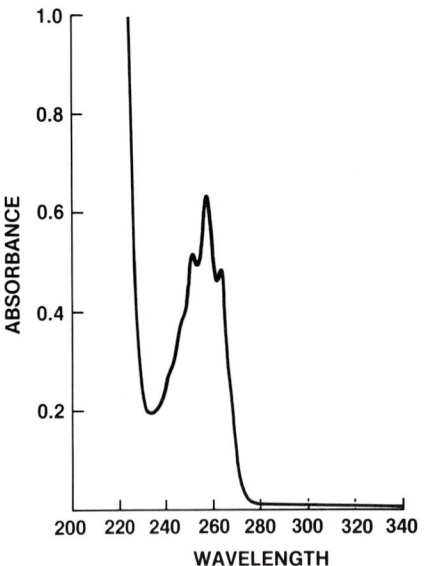

Fig. 26-9. Propoxyphene: 500 μg/ml in 0.5N sulfuric acid; Similar spectra produced by amphetamine, methamphetamine, meperidine, and phencyclidine.

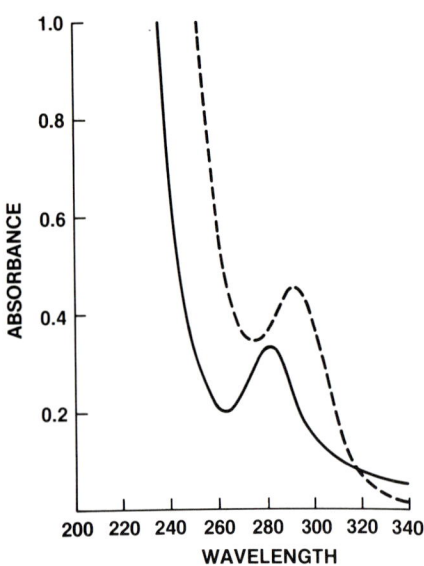

Fig. 26-10. Morphine: solid line, 12 μg/ml in 0.5N sulfuric acid; dotted line, 2 drops of 40% sodium hydroxide added to acid solution. Similar spectra produced by morphine analogs such as hydromorphone and oxymorphone.

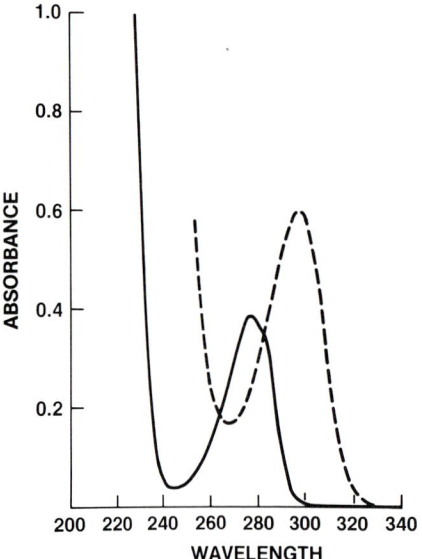

Fig. 26-11. Pentazocine: solid line, 55 μg/ml in 0.5N sulfuric acid; dotted line, 2 drops of 40% sodium hydroxide added to acid solution. Similar spectrum produced by hydroxyamphetamine.

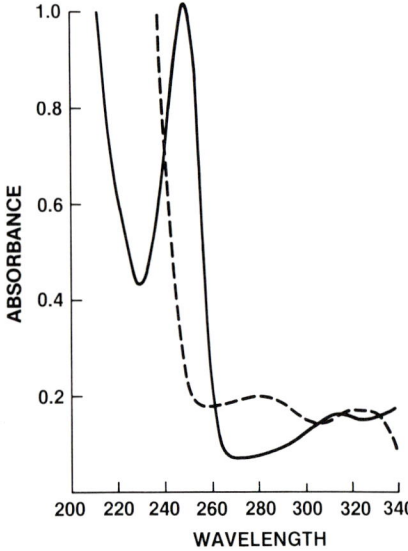

Fig. 26-12. Quinine: solid line, complete spectrum, 12 μg/ml in 0.5N sulfuric acid; dotted line, 2 drops of 40% sodium hydroxide added to acid solution. Similar spectrum produced by quinidine.

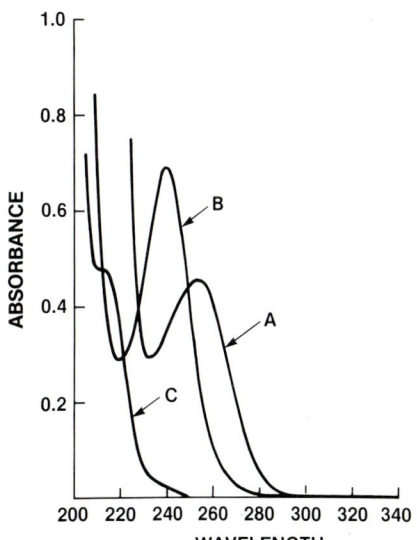

Fig. 26-13. Secobarbital: 30 μg/ml. *(A),* Buffered solution, pH 13; *(B),* 0.45N sodium hydroxide, pH 10; *(C),* acid solution, pH 2. Similar spectra produced by barbiturates in Table 26-14.

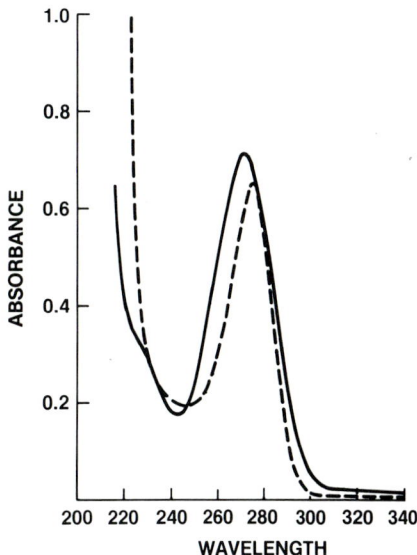

Fig. 26-14. Theophylline: solid line, 15 μg/ml in 0.1N sulfuric acid; dotted line, 2 drops of 40% sodium hydroxide added to acid solution. Similar spectra produced by other xanthine derivatives, e.g., caffeine and theobromine.

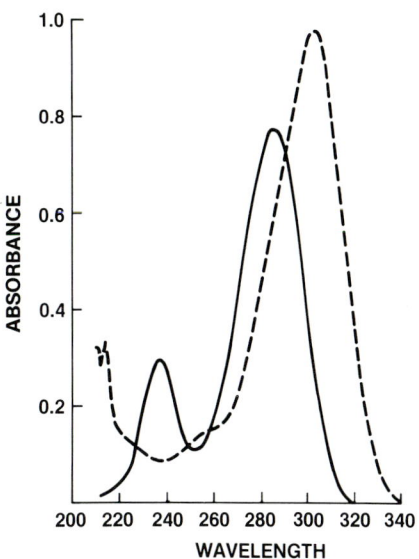

Fig. 26-15. Thiopental: solid line, 10 μg/ml in 0.5N sulfuric acid; dotted line, 2 drops of 40% sodium hydroxide added to acid solution.

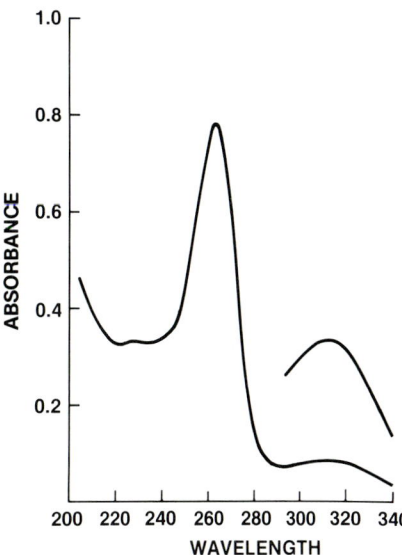

Fig. 26-16. Thioridazine (complete spectrum): 7 μg/ml in 0.5N sulfuric acid. Maximum at 313 nm is 21 μg/ml.

Filter the chloroform (bottom) layer through Whatman no. 2 filter paper into larger tubes. Add 1.5 ml of 0.1N sulfuric acid. Shake for 5 min and centrifuge. Remove the acid (top) layer with a Pasteur pipet and place in an ultraviolet microcuvet. Discard the bottom layer.

In a recording spectrophotometer, scan the acid solution against the acid plate blank from 340-220 nm. Pour the acid extract and acid blank into separate small clean test tubes. Make the solutions basic by the addition of 1 drop of 40% sodium hydroxide. The pH should exceed 10. Transfer back to the cuvets and rescan. Compare the resultant ultraviolet spectrum with that of similarly treated known drug standards. The absorbance maximum and $E_{1\%}$ of basic drugs of toxicologic interest are presented in Table 26-5.

Fluorometry

Amphetamine and methamphetamine confirmation[33-35]:

Reagents:
1. Chloroform
2. Copper sulfate solution
   Dissolve 7 g copper sulfate in 1 dl water.
3. NBD solution
   Dissolve 1 mg/ml NBD (7-chloro-4-nitrobenzene-2-oxa-1,3-diazole) in chloroform.
4. Sodium bicarbonate solution
   Dissolve sodium bicarbonate in water until saturated, approximately 5%.

Procedure: To 2 ml of the urine specimen and a urine blank, add 2 ml copper sulfate solution. Mix and let stand for 10 min. Centrifuge the mixture at 2000 rpm for 5 min and transfer 3 ml of the supernatant liquid to a screw-cap test tube. Add 2 ml of saturated sodium bicarbonate solution and 5 ml of chloroform, shake for 15 min, and centrifuge for 5 min. Remove the upper aqueous layer. Then transfer 4 ml of the chloroform layer to a clean dry test tube. Add 1 ml of NBD solution, mix, and then evaporate the extract to dryness in an oven at 110° C. Let cool to room temperature and dissolve the residue in 4 ml chloroform.

In a spectrofluorometer, record the spectrum of the chloroform extract from 480-540 nm, using an excitation of 468 nm. If a fluorescence peak with a greater intensity than that in the urine blank appears at 520 nm, an excitation spectrum must be obtained.

If the observed excitation maximum is at 468 nm and the emission maximum is at 520 nm the chloroform is evaporated to dryness in a small cup and the residue spotted on a silica gel TLC plate. NBD reacts with many primary and secondary amines. Positive identification is made by comparing known amphetamine-NBD and methamphetamine-NBD derivatives to the sample spots after TLC development in isopropyl ether. The spots are yellow under ultraviolet light. In room light, amphetamine (R_f of 0.42) is yellow and methamphetamine (R_f of 0.24) is orange.

Meperidine confirmation[36]:

Reagent: Use Marquis reagent. Add 10 drops of 40% formaldehyde solution to 10 ml of concentrated sulfuric acid.

Procedure: A urine extract residue or the spot suspected to be meperidine scraped from the TLC plate is placed in a 5 ml beaker. Add 5 drops of Marquis reagent to the scraping and heat the mixture in an oven at 110° C for 10 min. Add 1 ml distilled water and observe under a long-wave ultraviolet light. A blue fluorescence indicates that meperidine may be present. Add 2 ml water, shake, and centrifuge the mixture. Place 2 ml of the clear solution in a spectrofluorometer and record the emission spectrum from 380-480 nm using an excitation at 270 nm. Meperidine is indicated by a doublet with maximums at 420 and 440 nm.

Morphine confirmation[37,38]:

Reagents:
1. Ammonium hydroxide
2. Sulfuric acid

Procedure: To a urine extract residue in a 30 ml beaker add 0.2 ml concentrated sulfuric acid. Mix throughly and allow to stand for 15 min. Add 2 ml of water, mix, and then immediately add, with continuous stirring, 2 ml concentrated ammonium hydroxide. Place the mixture in a pressure cooker and autoclave for 15 min at 120° C under 15-18 pounds of pressure. Remove the beaker and allow the mixture to cool. The mixture is transferred to cuvets and placed in a spectrofluorometer. The emission spectrum is recorded between 400 and 510 nm using an excitation of 392 nm. An emission spectrum of morphine has a maximum at 425 nm. If TLC appears positive for morphine but fluorometry is negative, hydromorphone may be considered.

Phenothiazine confirmation[39-41]:

Reagents:
1. Acetic acid, 50%
2. Hydrogen peroxide, 30%

Procedure: To a urine extract residue in a 10 ml beaker, add 2 ml of 50% acetic acid and 1 ml of 30% hydrogen peroxide. Heat the mixture in a boiling water bath for 10 min. Allow mixture to cool and transfer to a cuvet for spectrofluorometric analysis. The emission and excitation maximums for various phenothiazines is indicated in Table 26-6. Chlorpromazine and thioridazine are two derivatives most often encountered in cases of drug overdose. This procedure can be utilized in conjunction with the color test discussed earlier and TLC.

Benzodiazepine confirmation[42-45]:
Benzodiazepines and their metabolites are acid hydrolyzed to aminochlorobenzophenones. *N*-1-alkyl substituted benzophenones are converted to various secondary aminochlorobenzophenones, while those lacking such *N*-1-alkyl groups are converted to a primary 2-amino-5-chlorobenzophenone. Following extraction from hydrolyzed urine and chromatographic separation, the alkyl substituted benzophenones appear as visible yellow spots, and the primary amines are visualized as purple spots with Bratton-Marshall reagent. The benzodiazepines most often encountered in emergency screening, their primary urinary metabolites, corresponding benzophenones, and chromatographic data are presented in Table 26-7.

Reagents:
1. Hydrochloric acid
2. Ammonium hydroxide
3. Diethyl ether
4. Benzene

Table 26-6. Emission and excitation maximums for various phenothiazines

| | Wavelength maximum (nm) | |
Phenothiazine	Excitation	Emission
Promazine	344	372
Trifluopromazine	348	396
Chlorpromazine	344	390
Prochlorperazine	338	398
Trifluoperazine	356	412
Thioridazine	362	435

Table 26-7. TLC identification of benzophenone derivatives of benzodiazepines

Parent benzodiazepine metabolite	Benzophenone*	Benzophenone R_f	Visualization
Chlorazepate	ACB	0.54	Violet
Nordiazepam	ACB	0.54	Violet
Oxazepam	ACB	0.54	Violet
Chlordiazepoxide	ACB	0.54	Violet
Demoxepam	ACB	0.54	Violet
Norchlordiazepoxide	ACB	0.54	Violet
Diazepam	MACB	0.66	Yellow (visible)
3-Hydroxynordiazepam	ACB	0.54	Violet
Nordiazepam	ACB	0.54	Violet
Oxazepam	ACB	0.54	Violet
Flurazepam	DECFB	0.08	Yellow (visible)
Desalkylflurazepam	ACFB	0.49	Violet
Hydroxydesalkylflurazepam	ACFB	0.49	Violet
Hydroxyethylflurazepam	HEFB	0.34	Yellow (visible)

*ACB, 2-amino-5-chlorobenzophenone; MACB, 2-methylamino-5-chlorobenzophenone; DECFB, 2-diethylamino-ethylamino-5-chlor-2′ fluorbenzophenone; ACFB, 2-amino-5-chlor-2′ fluorbenzophenone; HEFB, 2-hydroxyethylamino-5-chlor-2′ fluorbenzophenone.

5. Acetic acid
6. Bratton-Marshall spray
   a. Sulfuric acid, 50%
   b. Sodium nitrate, 1% w/v, freshly prepared
   c. Ammonium sulfamate, 5% w/v
   d. N-1-naphthylethylenediamine hydrochloride. Dissolve 1 g in 80 ml acetone and 20 ml water.
7. Standards: diazepam, chlordiazepoxide, N-1-hydroxyethylflurazepam
   Dissolve separately 10 mg of the hydrochloride salt of each benzodiazepine in 1 dl water.
8. Benzodiazine control urine
   Prepare three different control urine specimens by adding 0.5 ml of each standard solution to 4.5 ml of drug-free urine.

Procedure:
1. Place 5.0 ml patient's urine and the benzodiazone control urine specimens in a series of hydrolysis bottles with Teflon cap inserts.
2. Add 3.0 ml of concentrated hydrochloric acid to all hyrolysis bottles, cap tightly, and boil under pressure in pressure cooker for 15 min. Alternately, place the samples in a round bottom flask with a condenser affixed and reflux for 40 min.
3. Cool bottles to room temperature and then carefully add 5 ml of concentrated ammonium hydroxide.

4. Cool bottles again to room temperature and then transfer the contents to a screw-top 25 ml centrifuge tube.
5. Add 10 ml diethyl ether to each tube, cap tightly, and shake slowly for 10 min.
6. Centrifuge tubes at 2000 rpm for 5 min and then aspirate lower (aqueous) phase from tubes.
7. Carefully pour ether into a small beaker or evaporation tube. If any of the aqueous phase is carried over, remove it with a capillary pipet.
8. Evaporate ether to dryness.
9. Dissolve residue in a few drops of methanol and apply the entire residue to a silica gel TLC plate. Develop the chromatogram in benzene–acetic acid (97:3).
10. Remove the developed plate, allow to dry, and outline the yellow spots on the chromatogram.
11. The primary aminochlorobenzophenones are seen as violet spots by spraying the chromatogram with Bratton-Marshall reagent. Spray the plate successively with reagents 6(a), 6(b), 6(c), and 6(d), drying the plates between sprays with warm air.

Interpretation: A violet spot from the patient's urine that has the same R_f as the violet chlordiazepoxide spot indicates the presence of benzodiazepine drugs. The method is quite sensitive; after ingestion of a single therapeutic dose of the benzodiazepines in Table 26-7 a positive result may be obtained in urine collected 18-

24 hr later. At therapeutic doses, diazepam will not be present in urine in detectable amounts; diazepam metabolites produce the same violet spots as chlordiazepoxide and oxazepam. However, in cases of overdose, diazepam (Valium) and flurazepam may be distinguished from chlordiazepoxide and oxazepam by the presence of N-1-alkyl substituted benzophenones (yellow spots). Compare the R_f of these yellow spots with those of the diazepam and N-hydroxyethylflurazepam control urine specimens.

Cocaine confirmation[46]: Cocaine is extensively biotransformed, and following therapeutic use of doses associated with recreation-abuse of the drug, only trace amounts of cocaine are available for detection in urine. The major urinary metabolite is benzoylecgonine and, to a lesser extent, ecgonine.[47,48] These metabolites are water soluble and are not easily isolated by resin or organic solvent extractions.

Numerous methods for the isolation of cocaine metabolites have been proposed. These procedures involve "salting out" metabolites and extraction with polar solvents. If chloroform-ethanol (7:3) is used as the extracting solvent in the TLC urine drug screening procedure above, benzoylecgonine may be extracted. However, recovery of the cocaine metabolites is often poor and coextracted urinary constituents may interfere with detection of the other drugs in the TLC analysis. The procedure presented below results in good recoveries of the cocaine metabolites and separation by TLC. The method is based on the butylation of the metabolites and identification of these derivatives. It may be used as a secondary confirmatory urine analysis for benzoylecgonine detected in the urine drug screening procedure. The method results in two fractions: one containing cocaine and other basic drugs of toxicologic interest and one containing the cocaine metabolites.

Reagents:
1. Butanol
2. Control urine
   Add 0.025 ml of each standard to 10 ml drug-free urine.
3. Cyclohexane
4. Developing systems
   a. Ethyl acetate–methanol–water (7:2:1)
   b. Methanol–ammonia (100:1.5)
   c. Benzene–ethyl acetate–methanol–ammonia (80:20:1.2:0.1)
   d. Chloroform-acetone-ammonia (5:94:1)
5. Extracting solvent: chloroform-ethanol (3:2)
6. Hydrochloric acid, 6N
7. Standard solutions
   Dissolve 20 mg cocaine in 10 ml methanol to make a 0.2% stock standard. Dissolve 20 mg benzoylecgonine in 10 ml methanol to make a 0.2% stock standard.
8. Solid anhydrous potassium carbonate
9. Solid sodium bicarbonate
10. Sulfuric acid, concentrated
11. TLC plate: silica gel, 0.25 mm
12. Visualizing spray: iodoplatinate reagent (see reagents under discussion of TLC urine drug screen)

Procedure:
1. Place 10 ml of sample and control urine specimens in separate test tubes and add 250 mg of solid sodium bicarbonate to adjust the pH between 8 and 9.
2. Add 5 ml of extracting solvent, shake on a vortex mixer for 20 sec, and then centrifuge at 1100 g for 10 min.
3. With a Pasteur pipet, transfer the upper (aqueous) layer to a clean test tube. The remaining (organic) layer contains unmetabolized cocaine and other basic drugs. Treat this extract as described in the above TLC drug screen: direct extraction; start at step no. 9.
4. To the ethanolic aqueous layer containing cocaine metabolites, add solid anhydrous potassium carbonate until saturated. Shake on a vortex mixer and let stand for 5 min. A dark brown suspension will float on the surface of the tube.
5. Centrifuge the mixture at 1100 g for 10 min to separate the ethanol phase. With a Pasteur pipet, transfer the ethanol layer to a 40 ml centrifuge tube. Add 6N hydrochloric acid 1 drop at a time until the pH is below 7.
6. Butylate the cocaine metabolites by adding 2 ml of 1-butanol and 0.1 ml of concentrated sulfuric acid and heating the mixture to 120-130° C for 30 min. Allow the solution to cool to room temperature.
7. Add 5 ml of toluene and transfer the entire mixture to a clean test tube. Wash the centrifuge tube with water and add the wash to the toluene-butanol mixture.
8. Shake the mixture for 10 sec, centrifuge at 275 g for 5 min, and aspirate the upper organic layer.
9. Saturate the remaining aqueous layer with solid sodium bicarbonate and extract for 3 min with 10 ml cyclohexane.
10. Centrifuge the mixture at 275 g for 5 min, transfer the organic layer to a clean test tube, and evaporate to dryness on a water bath.
11. Dissolve the residue in 15 μl chloroform and apply to a TLC plate. Develop the plates in solvent system A or B (Table 26-8).
12. Following development, air dry the plate for 30 min and then heat in an oven at 90° C for 5 min.

Table 26-8. TLC detection of butylated cocaine metabolites

R_f	System	
	A*	B†
Morphine	.34	.00
Butylated metabolites		
Ecgonine	.52	.14
Benzoylecgonine	.64	.32
Benzoylnorecgonine	.58	.07

*Methanol-ammonia (100:1.5).
†Benzene–ethyl acetate–methanol–ammonia (80:20:1.2:0.1).

Visualize the matabolites by spraying with io-doplatinate reagent. Spray once and then respray it 5 min later.

Interpretation: Detection of cocaine metabolites is by R_f (Table 26-8) and color reaction. Butylated ecgonine is a bluish purple spot while butylized benzoylecgonine and benzoylnorecgonine provide a purple-brown spot. The glucuronide conjugate of morphine is extracted in the ethanol extract. Morphine is freed during butylation of cocaine metabolites. Cocaine may be detected in overdose cases by treating the chloroform extract in step no. 3 as indicated in the TLC urine drug screen procedure above.

Methaqualone confirmation[49,50]: Methaqualone is extensively biotransformed into a series of hydroxylated metabolites. These metabolites are excreted into urine as highly polar, water-soluble conjugates. Following acid hydrolysis to destroy the conjugates, the hydroxylated metabolites are extracted from urine and chromatographed. The presence of methaqualone is indicated by a characteristic pattern of metabolites separated by TLC.

Reagents:
1. Hydrochloric acid
2. Ammonium hydroxide
3. Diethyl ether
4. Sulfuric acid, 5%
5. Iodoplatinate reagent (see discussion of TLC drug screening)
6. DSA reagent
   Dissolve 0.4 g diazotized sulfanilic acid (DSA) in 1 dl of 2 moles/L sodium hydroxide. Prepare fresh as needed.
7. Standard
   a. Methaqualone. Dissolve 10 mg methaqualone hydrochloride in 1 dl water.
   b. Methaqualone metabolites. Pure metabolites may be available through the manufacturer of methaqualone; prepare these as the methaqualone standard. However, it is more convenient to use the control urine indicated below.
8. Control urine
   a. Methaqualone. Add 0.5 ml methaqualone standard to 9.5 ml drug-free urine.
   b. Methaqualone metabolites. Collect several morning voidings of urine from a patient (or

volunteer) who was given a 250 mg tablet of methaqualone the previous night. Divide into aliquots of 10 ml each and store frozen.

Procedure: Place 10 ml of patient's urine, methaqualone, and methaqualone metabolite control urine specimens in separate hydrolysis bottles and carry through steps 2-8 as outlined above for benzodiazepines.

Dissolve the residue in a few drops of methanol and apply the entire residue to a silica gel TLC plate. Develop the chromatogram in diethyl ether (system 1 in Table 26-9) or chloroform–diethyl ether–ammonium hydroxide, 50:50:2 (system 2 in Table 26-9).

Allow the plate to dry in a safety hood. Then visualize the chromatogram by spraying the plate in the following sequence: 5% sulfuric acid; iodoplatinate reagent; or DSA reagent. Dry the plate between applications with warm air.

Interpretation: The R_f and color development of methaqualone and its metabolites are presented in Table 26-9. After ingestion of therapeutic dosages, only the metabolites may be present; however, in overdose cases, the parent drug is detected.[51] System 1 will permit identification of parent methaqualone if present; however, metabolites 3 and 4 (Table 26-9) are not resolved. System 2 will resolve the four metabolites, but methaqualone migrates too close to the solvent front to permit clear identification.

Morphine confirmation[52,53]: About 90% of morphine excreted in urine is present as a glucuronic acid conjugate.[54,55] The conjugate is highly polar and is not readily extracted from urine into organic solvents. This necessitates hydrolysis of the conjugates in order to free the morphine before extraction of the specimens. This may be accomplished by enzymatic hydrolysis using commercially available β-glucuronidase or by acid hydrolysis. Generally, acid hydrolysis will result in a greater yield of free morphine than enzymatic methods.[56] However, acid strength, temperature, and the time period of hydrolysis will influence the resultant yield of morphine. The hydrolysis procedure must be adjusted to sufficient temperature, time, and acidity to break the conjugate but not result in further breakdown of the freed morphine. The hydrolysis procedure will destroy many drugs (e.g., cocaine, propoxyphene) and diminish the sensitivity of detection of others (amphetamines,

Table 26-9. TLC identification of methaqualone and methaqualone metabolites

| Compound | R_f | | Visualization | |
	System 1	System 2	Iodoplatinate	DSA*
Methaqualone	.64	.90	Violet-brown	—
Metabolite 1†	.35	.65	Violet-brown	—
Metabolite 2‡	.57	.56	Violet-brown	Yellow
Metabolite 3§	.49	.46	Violet-brown	Orange-red
Metabolite 4‖	.50	.34	Violet-brown	Red

*Diazotized sulfanelic acid.
†2-Methyl-3-(2'-hydroxymethylphenyl)-4(3H)-quinazolinone.
‡2-Methyl-3-(2'-methyl-3'-hydroxyphenyl)-4(3H)-quinazolinone.
§2-Methyl-3-(2'-methyl-4'-hydroxyphenyl)-4(3H)-quinazolinone.
‖2-Methyl-3-0-tolyl-6-hydroxy-4-(3H)-quinazolinone.

barbiturates). It should be kept in mind that morphine is an amphoteric drug soluble in both acidic and basic solutions; therefore before extraction the pH of the specimen should be adjusted close to the pK_a of morphine.

Reagents:
1. Extracting solvent: chloroform-ethanol (9:1)
2. Control urine
   See TLC drug screen.
3. Sodium hydroxide pellets, reagent grade
4. Solid sodium bicarbonate, reagent grade
5. Sulfuric acid, 8.3%.
   Add slowly 8.3 ml concentrated sulfuric acid to sufficient water to make 1 dl.

Hydrolysis procedure: Measure 20 ml urine into a graduated cylinder and transfer into a 50 ml screw-top tube (or 3-4 oz pharmacuetical jar with screw top). If the sample is less than 20 ml, add water to obtain the necessary volume. Wash the cylinder with 10 ml of 8.3% sulfuric acid and transfer to the sample tube. Cap and mix the solution, which is now approximately 5% sulfuric acid.

Place the tube in a pressure cooker containing 6 mm of water and set the control for 250° C. Place the lid on the cooker and once the cooker begins to pressurize, close the control valve on top. Allow the solution to hydrolyze for 20 min.

Alternately, reflux the acidic urine solution in a round-bottom flask with a reflux condenser attached. Adjust the sulfuric acid concentration to approximately 10%. Carry out refluxing for 40 min.

After hydrolysis, filter the sample while it is still warm through Whatman no. 12 filter paper into a 1 dl beaker. The samples may be a dark red-brown and contain some granular material. Wash the filter paper two times with warm acidic water and allow the hydrolysate to cool.

Extraction procedure: Treatment of the resultant hydrolysate now depends on the particular extract method employed (see TLC drug screen above). If XAD-2 resin is used, the hydrolysate is neutralized by the addition of 20% sodium hydroxide, 7.5-8.0 ml. The end point is reached when turbidity disappears. The hydrolysate is then treated as a urine sample in the Amberlite XAD-2 Resin Column Extractor described above.

If solvent extraction is to be used for the isolation of morphine, transfer the hydrolysate to a 125 ml separatory funnel and extract three times with an equal folume of ether. If only morphine is sought, discard the ether and proceed to the following paragraph. If additional drugs are to be considered, combine the ether extracts in a 125 ml separatory funnel and extract three times with 10 ml of freshly prepared 5% sodium bicarbonate solution. Discard the bicarbonate solutions. Wash the ether with 10 ml of water and allow the phases to separate. Discard the water. Filter the ether into a 125 ml beaker or evaporating cup through Whatman no. 1 filter paper containing solid anhydrous sodium sulfate. Label the beaker "Acids" and evaporate to dryness on a steam bath. This extract will contain weakly acidic and neutral drugs.

To the ether-washed hydrolysate, add sodium hydroxide pellets until the pH of the solution exceeds 10.

Extract the hydrolysate three times with an equal volume of chloroform. If only morphine is sought, discard the chloroform and proceed to the following paragraph. If other drugs are to be considered (particularly other narcotics), filter the chloroform through Whatman no. 1 filter paper containing solid sodium sulfate into an evaporating cup. Label the cup "Bases." Add 1 drop of 10N hydrochloric acid and evaporate the chloroform to dryness on a water bath. This extract will contain basic drugs.

To the basic hydrolysate, add, by drops, sufficient concentrated sulfuric acid until the solution is just acid, pH 5-6. Then add small portions of solid sodium bicarbonate with swirling after each addition. Continue adding bicarbonate until effervescence ceases and then add a small excess amount. The pH of the mixture should not exceed 9.5.

Extract the hydrolysate three times with an equal volume of chloroform-ethanol (9:1). Combine extracts and filter through anhydrous sodium sulfate into a 125 ml beaker. Label the beaker "Morphine" and evaporate just to dryness on a steam bath.

Prepare the extracts for TLC as described under the direct extraction procedure, step 10, for TLC urine drug screening.

The morphine and "Bases" extract may be chromatographed in TLC systems A, B, and C (Table 26-3). The "Acids" extract should be developed in system D (Table 26-3). Visualize morphine with iodoplatinate reagent; the spot is blue.

Interpretation: Identification of morphine is based on Rf and color development. The presence of morphine indicates administration of morphine or heroin. Heroin is rapidly biotransformed to morphine and is not present in urine. After administration of codeine, trace amounts of morphine may be detected.

ANALYSIS OF TOXICANTS IN BLOOD

Specific procedures for the quantitative determination of various commonly encountered toxicants are presented. Also presented are two general procedures: one for the determination of alcohols (ethanol, isopropanol, and methanol) and one for the determination of psychoactive drugs. Essentially two analytic technics are utilized in these procedures: microdiffusion analysis and visible or ultraviolet spectrophotometry.

Microdiffusion analysis[57-61] is used for the rapid isolation and detection of volatile poisons. A simple microdiffusion apparatus consists of a small porcelain dish with two separate compartments, an inner well, which is formed between the periphery of the wall of the inner compartment and the higher outer well of the dish. The outer well is the sample cell, to which a small quantity, 1-5 ml, of blood or urine is added. To the inner well an "absorbent" is added. The absorbent is a reagent or solvent in which particular volatile substances will readily dissolve. After the sample and absorbent are added to the proper cell, the dish is sealed with a viscous sealant material and a ground glass cover plate. If allowed to sit at room temperature or gently heated, the volatile poison will diffuse from the sample into the atmosphere of the dish and be entrapped by the absorbent solution. As the compound is liberated from the sample, color change in the absorbent in the inner well may be observed. Numerous volatile poisons and gases may be detected by this technic. Specific microdiffusion procedures for carbon monoxide, cyanide, and ethanol are presented below. The microdiffusion dishes are readily available (Fisher Scientific Co., Pittsburgh; Arthur H. Thomas Co., Philadelphia).

Spectrophotometry is based on the absorption of radiant energy.[62-64] The absorption of radiation is a characteristic of all molecules; however, the wavelength of the absorbed radiation may vary from x rays through ultraviolet, visible, and infrared wavelengths to microwave and radio frequencies. Therefore the interaction between radiation and a chemical compound depends on its molecular structure and the wavelength of the radiation. When the absorption of radiation by a compound is determined relative to the wavelength of the radiation, an absorption spectrum is observed that is a characteristic of that compound. There is a direct relationship between the magnitude of the absorption of radiant energy and the quantity of absorbing material present. By experimentally choosing the wavelength of maximal absorption, the concentration of a compound present in a sample can be determined.

The spectrophotometer used to measure the absorption of radiant energy consists of a radiation source, a sample cell through which the radiation passes, and a detector for measuring the absorption of the radiation. The wavelengths most applicable to toxicologic analysis are the ultraviolet and visible. The commercial instruments used for measuring the absorption of these forms of light may vary from simple colorimeters, used to measure absorption in the visible range, to highly sophisticated spectrophotometers employing monochromatic light and sensitive electronics to detect, amplify, and record low levels of radiation.

Absorption of ultraviolet light may result in electronic transitions in organic molecules causing the promotion of electrons in low energy to high energy orbitals. The actual wavelength of maximal absorption will depend on the chemical groups present in the molecule, the solvent in which the compound is dissolved, and the pH and temperature of the solution. Aqueous solutions and extracts are the most common solvents used by toxicologists. Plotting or electronically graphing the absorbance of a compound vs. wavelength (210-350 nm) results in an ultraviolet absorption spectrum. The majority of drugs of toxicologic interest absorb light in the ultraviolet region or may form color complexes that absorb in the visible region. The ultraviolet spectrum is characteristic of a compound under controlled experimental conditions and may be used as tentative identification for the presence of a given drug. However, identification is not conclusive since numerous compounds display the same ultraviolet spectrum. For example, amphetamine, ephedrine, methamphetamine, phenylethylamine, propoxyphene, and many other drugs possess ultraviolet absorption maximums in acidic solution at 263, 257, and 252 nm. Also, if other ultraviolet-absorbing compounds are present in a sample, a mixed spectrum, i.e., the composite spectrum of all compounds, will be observed. The concentration of the drug may be determined by comparing the magnitude of absorption (absorbance) at the maximal wavelength of absorption to that of a series of concentrations of pure drug standards analyzed under the same experimental conditions.

Toxicologists generally express the magnitude of absorbance in terms of the $E_{1\%}$ of a drug. The $E_{1\%}$ is defined as the absorbance of 1 g of compound per liter of solution. The $E_{1\%}$ is constant for each drug. It depends on the pH and the solvent in which the compound is dissolved. The $E_{1\%}$ divided by 100 will give the absorbance of 10 μg/ml of compound.

If both urine and blood specimens are submitted to the laboratory, a qualitative analysis should first be performed on the urine specimen. Once the toxicant has been identified, then a quantitative determination of the agent in blood should be performed. The absorbance maximum and approximate $E_{1\%}$ of commonly encountered toxicants are presented in Table 26-5. Specific ultraviolet spectra of various drugs are presented in Figs. 26-1 to 26-16.

General screening for alcohols and acetone by gas chromatography[64,65]

Apparatus:
1. Gas chromatograph equipped with a flame ionization detector
2. Column: 6 ft × ⅛ in internal diameter; stainless steel packed with Porapak-S (80-100 mesh; Waters Associates, Milford, Mass.)

Operating conditions:
1. Detection temperature: 240° C
2. Injector temperature: 220° C
3. Column temperature: 160° C
4. Electrometer settings
   a. Range of 10
   b. Air tank set at 155 psi, 330 ml/min
   c. Hydrogen tank set at 30 psi, 45 ml/min
   d. Nitrogen (carrier gas), 55 psi, 45 ml/min
5. Recorder
   a. Input: 1 mV
   b. Chart speed: 1 cm/min

Specimens:
1. Blood
   Add sodium fluoride if analysis is not immediately performed.
2. Urine

Reagents:
1. Triton X-100, 12% v/v
   With a magnetic stirrer, mix 12 ml Triton X-100 with 80 ml water.
2. Internal standard (IS)
   Add 1.2 ml Triton X-100, 12%, and 0.2 ml acetonitrile to water. Mix thoroughly and dilute to 1 dl. Store tightly capped at room temperature. This solution is stable for 60 days.
3. Ethanol standard
   a. Commercial standard (Sigma Chemical Co., St. Louis), 80 mg/ml
   b. Commercial standard (College of American Pathologists, Skokie, Ill.), 150 mg/ml
4. Acetone standard
   a. Acetone standard, 50 mg/dl. Dilute 0.65 ml acetone to 1 L with water.

b. Acetone standard, 100 mg/dl. Dilute 1.3 ml acetone to 1 L with water.

5. Methanol standard
   a. Methanol standard, 100 mg/dl. Dilute 0.125 ml methanol to 1 dl with water.
   b. Methanol standard, 200 mg/dl. Dilute 0.250 ml methanol to 1 dl with water.

6. 2-Propanol standard
   a. 2-Propanol standard, 100 mg/dl. Dilute 0.125 ml 2-propanol to 1 dl with water.
   b. 2-Propanol standard, 200 mg/dl. Dilute 0.250 ml 2-propanol to 1 dl with water.

Keep all standards tightly capped and refrigerated.

Procedure: To separate disposable test tubes add 0.05 ml of IS, followed by 0.05 ml of each standard and test specimen. Cap immediately. Mix on a vortex mixer and centrifuge. Inject approximately 2-4 μl into the gas chromatograph and record each chromatogram for 5 min. Compare the retention times of the specimen components to that of the standards to determine the presence of acetone or alcohols.

Retention times:
1. Methanol: 1.0 min
2. Ethanol: 2 min
3. Acetone: 3 min
4. 2-Propanol: 3 min 40 sec

Calculation:

$$\frac{\dfrac{\text{Peak height of unknown}}{\text{Peak height of IS}}}{\dfrac{\text{Peak height of standard}}{\text{Peak height of IS}}} \times \frac{\text{Conc.}}{\text{of standard}} = \frac{\text{Conc.}}{\text{of unknown}}$$

$$\text{Conc. of unknown} =$$
$$\frac{\text{Peak height of unknown}}{\text{Peak height of IS}} \times \frac{\text{Peak height of IS}}{\text{Peak height of standard}} \times$$
$$\text{Conc. of standard}$$

For each standard a proportion factor, K, may be calculated:

$$K = \frac{\text{Peak height of IS}}{\text{Peak height of standard}} \times \text{Conc. of standard}$$

$$\text{Conc. of unknown (mg/dl)} = K \times \frac{\text{Peak height of unknown}}{\text{Peak height of IS}}$$

General screening for alcohols and acetone by microdiffusion[66,67]

Principle: Alcohols, aldehydes, and other volatile reducing substances are oxidized by potassium dichromate. The dichromate is reduced, producing a color change from orange to green or blue.

Apparatus: Microdiffusion dishes.

Specimens: Blood or urine.

Reagents: All chemicals should be analytic reagent grade.

1. Potassium dichromate reagent
   Dissolve 1.0 g potassium dichromate in 5 dl water and add 0.1 g silver nitrate to the solution. Carefully add 5 dl concentrated sulfuric acid. Store in a tightly capped dark bottle. This solution is stable for 1 year.

2. Control solution
   Add 1.8 ml ethanol to 1 L water (approximately 150 mg/dl).

Procedure: Add 0.5 ml potassium dichromate reagent to the center well of each microdiffusion dish. In the bottom of the middle ring of a dish, place 1-2 ml of specimen, and in the second dish place 1-2 ml of control solution. Add with gentle mixing 1 ml of saturated aqueous potassium carbonate solution. Place the covers on the dishes and heat at 50° C in an oven or at 60-70° C on a hot plate. A green color developing in 30 min indicates the presence of alcohols or other reducing substances.

Confirmation of positive reactions: A positive reaction is not specific for ethanol; other reducing substances, including methanol, isopropanol, paraldehyde, and acetone, may react. Methanol can be ruled out by the methanol formaldehyde procedure. If isopropanol has been ingested, acetone will be present in the patient's urine. One can test for acetone by adding 1 drop of urine to an Acetest tablet (Ames Co., Div. of Miles Laboratories, Elkhardt, Ind.). Confirmation by the gas chromatographic procedure for alcohols and acetone is strongly recommended.

Ethanol alcohol dehydrogenase procedure[68,69]

Principle: Blood ethanol concentrations may be determined by commercially available enzymatic kits (Sigma Chemical Co., St. Louis; Calbiochem-Behring Corp., San Diego). The procedure is based on the method of Bonnichsen and Theorell,[68] which uses alcohol dehydrogenase (ADH) and nicotinamide-adenine dinucleotide (NAD). At pH 9, alcohol is converted to acetaldehyde, and NAD is reduced to NADH. The reaction is forced to completion by reacting the acetaldehyde with semicarbizide to form a Schiff base (acetaldehyde semicarbazone). The concentration of alcohol present is directly proportional to the absorbance of the NADH formed.

Apparatus: Spectrophotometer.

Specimens:
1. Blood
2. Serum
3. Urine

Reagents:
1. NAD-ADH single assay vial (stock no. 330-1, Sigma Chemical Co., St. Louis)
2. Ethanol standard solution (contains 0.08% ethanol) (stock no. 330-20, Sigma Chemical Co., St. Louis)
3. Pyrophosphate buffer solution (stock no. 330–30, Sigma Chemical Co., St. Louis)
4. Trichloroacetic acid solution, 6.25% (stock no. 331-7, Sigma Chemical Co., St. Louis)

Procedure: The following procedure uses whole blood, serum, and urine (with deproteinization).

Prepare protein-free supernatant as follows:
1. Pipet into centrifuge tube 2.0 ml of 6.25% trichloroacetic acid solution.
2. While swirling tube, slowly add 0.5 ml of sample.
3. Stopper and mix well by inverting.
4. Centrifuge for 5 min at 3000 rpm.

All solutions must be at room temperature.

To labeled single assay vials (i.e., Blank; Std. 80; Std. 150; Tests) pipet 3.0 ml pyrophosphate buffer. Add 100 μl clear supernatant fluid. Cap vials and mix gently by inversion. Allow vials to stand capped for 45 min at room temperature. Transfer the contents of vials to cuvets. Record absorbance at 340 nm of each test vs. blank as reference. Read at room temperature or 25° C if temperature-controlled cells are available.

Calculation:

Ethanol (%) (w/v) in original sample = Absorbance at 340 nm × 0.115.

Explanation of calculation:

Ethanol (%) (w/v) in original sample =

$$\frac{\text{Absorbance at 340 nm} \times 3.1 \times 0.000046}{6.22 \times 0.02} \times 100 =$$

Absorbance at 340 nm × 0.115

where 3.1 represents the volume of liquid in the cuvet; 0.000046 is the weight in grams of 1 μmole of ethanol; 100 converts grams per milliliter to percent (w/v); 6.22 is the absorbance at 340 nm of a solution containing 1 μmole of NADH per milliliter; and 0.02 is the volume of specimen per test.

Possible interferences: The ADH method will give false positive results if certain straight-chain alcohols are present.[70,71] The rate of oxidation of these alcohols decreases in the following order: ethanol = allyl alcohol > n-propanol > n-butanol > n-amyl alcohol > isopropanol. Acetone, methanol, sec-butyl, and isobutyl alcohols are not oxidized. The possibility of a false positive result using the ADH method can be eliminated if the specimen to be analyzed is first subjected to gas chromatographic screening under conditions that will indicate the presence of interfering alcohols, most commonly, isopropanol.[72]

Blood ethanol concentrations determined simultaneously by enzymatic methods and gas chromatography display good correlation.[72,73]

Interpretation: Ethanol is rapidly absorbed directly from the stomach. Absorption is complete 60-90 min after ingestion. Approximately 90% of absorbed ethanol is eliminated from the body by oxidation in the liver by the enzyme alcohol dehydrogenase.[74] Urinary excretion of unchanged ethanol proceeds at approximately 0.48% to total body alcohol per hour.[75] Additionally, small quantities are also eliminated in breath and sweat. The average rate of elimination of ethanol from blood is 16.4 mg/dl/hr[76]; however, individual rates may vary from 13-37 mg/dl/hr.[76] At equilibrium the concentration of ethanol in any body tissue or fluid is related to the water content of that specimen.[77] The

Table 26-10. States of acute alcoholic influence/intoxication[74]

Ethyl alcohol concentration (mg/dl blood)	Stage of alcoholic influence	Clinical signs/symptoms
10-50	Sobriety	No apparent influence Behavior nearly normal by ordinary observation Slight changes detectable by special tests
30-120	Euphoria	Mild euphoria, sociability, talkativeness Diminution of attention, judgment, and control Increased self-confidence, decreased inhibitions Loss of efficiency in finer performance tests
90-250	Excitement	Emotional instability; decreased inhibitions Loss of critical judgment Impairment of memory and comprehension Decreased sensory response; increased reaction time Some muscular incoordination
180-300	Confusion	Disorientation, mental confusion, dizziness Exaggerated emotional states (fear, anger, grief, etc.) Disturbance of sensation (diplopia, etc.) and of perception of color, form, motion, and dimensions Decreased pain sense Impaired balance; muscular incoordination
270-400	Stupor	Apathy; general inertia, approaching paralysis Markedly decreased response to stimuli Marked muscular incoordination; inability to stand or walk Vomiting; incontinence of urine and feces Impaired consciousness; sleep or stupor
350-500	Coma	Complete unconsciousness; coma; anesthesia Depressed or abolished reflexes Subnormal temperature Incontinence of urine and feces Embarrassment of circulation and respiration Possible death

Prepared by Kurt M. Dubowski, Ph.D., F.A.I.C., Director, Department of Clinical Chemistry and Toxicology, University of Oklahoma School of Medicine.

plasma/whole blood ratio varies from 1.10-1.35 with a mean ratio of 1.18.[78] During the elimination phase (point in time where the rate of alcohol absorption is less than the rate of elimination and alcohol is now in equilibrium with all body tissues), the urine/blood ratio is approximately 1.30.[79]

The physiologic effects of ethanol are related to the concentration in blood (Table 26-10). In a few states a blood ethanol concentration (BEC) of 80 mg/dl is the legal limit; however, in most states, a BEC of 100 mg/dl is prima facie evidence of legal impairment to operate a motor vehicle.[80]

Methanol (methyl alcohol) and formaldehyde[81]

Apparatus: Spectrophotometer.
Specimens:
1. Blood (plasma or serum), 2 ml
   Do not use EDTA or heparin for anticoagulants. These will give false positive results.
2. Urine, 2 ml
Reagents:
1. Trichloroacetic acid, 20%
2. Potassium permanganate reagent
   Dissolve 3 g potassium permanganate in 15 ml concentrated phosphoric acid. Add to 85 ml distilled water.
3. Sodium bisulfite
4. Chromotropic acid (powder)
5. Sulfuric acid (concentrated)
6. Standards same as GC alcohol procedure: 80 mg/dl and 150 mg/dl
7. Reagent blank

Procedure: In separate labeled tubes place 2 ml water (reagent blank), 2 ml of each standard, and 2 ml of each specimen. To all tubes add 4 ml trichloroacetic acid with mixing to precipitate proteins. Centrifuge and filter through Whatman filter paper no. 2.

Label two tubes for blank, each standard, and each specimen. Into each tube pipet 0.1 ml of filtrate. To one tube of each set add 2 drops of permanganate solution and mix. Let stand exactly 2 min and decolorize excess permanganate with a pinch of sodium bisulfite. To all tubes add a pinch of chromotropic acid and mix.

Carefully underlay solution in all tubes with 3 ml sulfuric acid. A purple ring at the interface of solutions in tubes oxidized with permanganate solution is positive for methanol. A purple ring in tubes not oxidized is a positive test for formaldehyde. High concentrations of ethanol may produce a brown color.

Mix and diffuse the purple color. Let stand for 20 min for the color to develop. Spin for 5 min and then read against a reagent blank at 570 nm.

Calculation:

$$K = \frac{\text{Conc. of standards}}{\text{Absorbance of standards}}$$

Conc. of unknown = K × Absorbance of unknown

Interpretation: Ingestion of 1-2 dl of methanol is fatal to most adults and as little as 10 ml may cause permanent blindness.[82] Normal blood methanol concentrations, derived from endogeneous production and dietary sources, are 0.15 mg/dl or less.[83] Methanol is biotransformed by alcohol dehydrogenase and aldehyde dehydrogenase to formic acid. The severe metabolic acidosis and ocular toxicity of methanol are attributed to this metabolite.[84] Ethanol, by competitive inhibition, slows the biotransformation of methanol and is the recommended antidote for methanol poisoning.[85] Toxicity may be evident at blood methanol concentrations as low as 20 mg/dl, but concentrations may be as high as 450 mg/dl. It should be noted that blood methanol concentrations are not a good prognostic index.

Analysis of other drugs and intoxicants
Bromide[86,87]

Apparatus: Spectrophotometer.
Specimen: Serum or plasma.
Reagents: All chemicals should be analytic reagent grade.
1. Trichloroacetic acid, 10 g/dl
   Dissolve 10 g trichloroacetic acid and 120 mg sodium chloride in 1 dl water.
2. Gold chloride, 500 mg/dl
   Dissolve 1 g gold chloride in distilled water and then dilute to 2 dl. Store the solution in a glass-stoppered brown bottle.
3. Bromide stock solution, 300 mg/dl
   Dissolve 0.386 g sodium bromide (0.447 g potassium bromide) in water and then dilute to 1 dl.
4. Bromide reference solutions
   Transfer 5.0, 15.0, and 25.0 ml of the bromide stock solution to 50 ml volumetric flasks; then add distilled water to the calibration marks. The resulting solutions have bromide concentrations of 30.0, 90.0, and 150.0 mg/dl, respectively.

Procedure: Place 1.0 ml serum in a test tube. Slowly add 4.0 ml trichloroacetic acid solution and mix well. Process 1.0 ml of each bromide reference solution and 1.0 ml of water for a reagent blank in the same manner. After about 15 min, centrifuge the tubes. Filter the clear supernatant, protein-free solutions through Whatman no. 1 filter paper or its equivalent. Place 2.0 ml of each filtrate into a cuvet and add 0.5 ml of the gold chloride solution. Determine the absorbance of each mixture at 440 nm in a suitable spectrophotometer using the reagent blank as the reference solution.

Calculation: Calculate K as follows:

$$K = \frac{\text{Conc. of standards}}{\text{Absorbance of standards}}$$

Conc. of unknown = Absorbance of unknown × K

Interpretation: Serum bromide concentrations higher than 50 mg/dl are compatible with mental confusion. With bromide concentrations between 150 mg and 250 mg per deciliter of serum, incoordination and emotional instability may occur. Concentrations above 300 mg/dl may be fatal.

Accuracy and precision: Recovery of bromide added to serum is 92-95%. Results are reproducible to within ±5% over the range from 50-200 mg/dl.

Carbon monoxide (microdiffusion method)[88,89]

Principle: Carbon monoxide is released from carboxyhemoglobin by acid. The free carbon monoxide reduces palladium chloride to metallic palladium, which appears as a black film. If the black film is visible, a carboxyhemoglobin saturation greater than 30% is present.

Apparatus:
1. Microdiffusion dish
2. Ultraviolet spectrophotometer

Specimen: Whole blood. Refrigerate immediately.

Reagents: All chemicals should be analytic reagent grade.
1. Hydrochloric acid, 0.1N
   Dilute 8.3 ml concentrated hydrochloric acid to 1 L with water.
2. Palladium chloride, 0.005N
   Dissolve 0.44 g palladium chloride in 5 dl of 0.1N hydrochloric acid in a 1 L flask. Mix the solution, allow it to stand overnight, and then dilute it to 1 L with 0.1N hydrochloric acid. One milliliter of 0.005N palladium chloride is equivalent to 0.056 ml of carbon monoxide.
3. Sulfuric acid, 3.6N
   Dilute 10.0 ml concentrated sulfuric acid to 1 dl with water.
4. Lead acetate–acetic acid solution
   Dilute 10.0 ml glacial acetic acid to 1 dl with water. Saturate this solution with lead acetate.

Procedure: On the lid of the microdiffusion dish spread a thin layer of sealant in a circle comparable to the outer rim of the dish.

Pipet 3.0 ml palladium chloride into the center well of the dish. Pipet 1.0 ml of 3.6N sulfuric acid into the outer well and place the cover over the dish, leaving an opening to permit the addition of the blood specimen. Add 0.5 ml blood and then slide the cover over the opening to seal the dish. Mix the contents of the outer well by gentle rotation; then allow the dish to stand at room temperature for 2 hr. (At this time a semiquantitative estimate of carboxyhemoglobin can be made by observing the extent of the reduction that has occurred. The black film of metallic palladium that forms is a function of the amount of carbon monoxide released from the specimen.)

Transfer the contents of the center well to a 50 ml volumetric flask, rinsing three times with 3.0 ml of 0.1N hydrochloric acid. Dilute the flask contents to 50.0 ml with 0.1N hydrochloric acid and mix well Determine the absorbance of this solution in a 1 cm silica cuvet at 278 nm; use 0.1N hydrochloric acid as the reference solution. Then determine the absorbance of 3.0 ml of the 0.005N palladium chloride solution diluted to 50.0 ml with 0.1N hydrochloric acid.

Standardization and calculation: Dilute 0.5, 1.0, 1.5, 2.0, 2.5, and 3.0 ml of the 0.005N palladium chloride to 50.0 ml with 0.1N hydrochloric acid and mix well. Determine the absorbance of the palladium chloride solutions against 0.1N hydrochloric acid at 278 nm. Plot the absorbances obtained as the ordinate against the volumes of carbon monoxide per deciliter on the abscissa. The respective carbon monoxide values are as follows:

Volumes of palladium chloride (ml/50 ml)	Volumes of carbon monoxide (ml/dl)
3.0	0.0
2.5	5.6
2.0	11.2
1.5	16.8
1.0	22.4
0.5	28.0

Determine the carbon monoxide volumes from the reference curve. If the absorbance of the palladium chloride solution differs (at zero volume) from that shown on the curve, draw a new reference curve parallel to the old one, passing through the new zero point.

Perform a hemoglobin determination on an aliquot of the original specimen; then complete the calculation as follows:

$$\frac{\text{Volume of carbon monoxide} \times 100}{\text{Hemoglobin (g/dl)} \times 1.35} =$$

Hemoglobin (%) carbon monoxide saturated

Interpretation: See discussion of carboxyhemoglobin (spectrophotometric procedure) below.

Carboxyhemoglobin (spectrophotometric procedure)[90,91]

Principle: A blood hemolysate is prepared by diluting a blood sample with 0.4% ammonium hydroxide. Addition of sodium dithionite deoxygenates hemoglobin. Comparison of the 541 nm/555 nm absorbance ratio for the hemolysate with the ratio obtained for solutions of known concentrations of carboxyhemoglobin serves as a means to determine the percent of carboxyhemoglobin present in the sample.

Apparatus: Spectrophotometer.

Specimen: Whole blood. Refrigerate immediately.

Reagents:
1. Ammonium hydroxide, 0.4%
   Dilute approximately 8.0 ml concentrated ammonium hydroxide to 500 ml with deionized water. Prepare this solution fresh daily.
2. Sodium hydrosulfite (sodium dithionite)
   Preweigh 10 mg portions of sodium dithionite, place into individual small test tubes, and stopper or cover with Parafilm.
3. Carbon monoxide, CP (Union Carbide Corp.)
4. Oxygen, CP (Union Carbide Corp.)

Procedure:

Preparation of hemolysate and spectophotometric measurement: Add 100 μl whole heparinized blood to 25 ml of 0.4% ammonium hydroxide. Mix the solution and allow to stand for 2 min. As a control, treat a normal blood specimen (no significant carbon monoxide concentration) as the sample.

Transfer 3 ml ammonium hydroxide and 3 ml hemolysate, respectively, into 1 cm cuvets. Record the absorption spectrum from 600-450 nm. The classic oxyhemoglobin (Oxy-Hb) spectrum should be observed. There should be a sharp peak at approximately 577 nm and 541 nm.

Add to each cuvet 10 mg sodium dithionite. Cover

the cuvets with Parafilm and gently invert 10 times. Exactly 5 min after the addition of the dithionate, record the absorption spectrum from 600-450 nm. In the absence of carboxyhemoglogin, the classic hemoglobin spectrum is observed with an absorption maximum at 555 nm. (If a number of samples are analyzed, the addition of the reducing agent is spaced so that each spectrum may be recorded after exactly 5 min.)

Calculate the 541 nm/555 nm absorbance ratio for the dithionate-treated sample and determine the percent of carboxyhemoglobin from the calibration curve.

Preparation of the standard curve: CAUTION: Use a fume hood when working with carbon monoxide gas.

Collect 20 ml heparinized blood from a healthy nonsmoker. Transfer 4 ml portions of the fresh, heparinized blood sample into each of two 125 ml separatory funnels. Treat one sample with pure oxygen and the other with pure carbon monoxide for 15 min while gently rotating the funnels. After the addition of the gas, close the separatory funnels and rotate gently for an additional 15 min. Then immediately analyze the fully saturated samples in triplicate according to the procedure above. Calculate the ratios of the absorbance at 541 nm/555 nm for the 0% and 100% carboxyhemoglobin samples.

Prepare intermediate standards by first filling the funnel containing the 100% carboxyhemoglobin with nitrogen gas and rotating for 5 min. Treatment with nitrogen removes the physically dissolved carbon monoxide from the sample, but only a small amount of carbon monoxide will dissociate from hemoglobin. Prepare intermediate standards by mixing appropriate proportions of the nitrogen-treated sample with the oxygen-treated sample.

Analyze each of the diluted blood samples in triplicate. Then plot the calculated concentrations against the observed absorbance ratios. The curve is linear over the range of 10-100% saturation.

Interpretation: The symptoms of acute carbon monoxide poisoning depend on the concentration of carbon monoxide in the inspired air, the duration of exposure, and the age and state of activity of the person exposed. The relationship between percent carboxyhemoglobin and symptoms of carbon monoxide poisoning is presented in Table 26-11. In healthy adults, inhalation of

Table 26-11. Carboxyhemoglobin (%) vs. symptoms

Carboxyhemoglobin (%)	Symptoms*
0-2%	None (normal nonsmoker)
3-5%	None (normal smoker)
10%	None (heavy smoker)
20%	Shortness of breath, nausea, vomiting
30%	Headache, dizziness, tinnitus, fatigue, collapse
40-60%	Death possible
60% and higher	Level at which most persons die

*Toxicity may develop at a much lower percent of saturation in elderly or diseased persons.

60 ppm carbon monoxide for 1 hr will cause headaches; 100 ppm for 2 hr may be fatal; and 3000 ppm (automobile exhaust) may cause death within minutes.

Comments: The major source of error in this and other similar methods is that sulfhemoglobin interferes. Sulfhemoglobin is not affected by reducing agents and although two of its absorption peaks are near those of carboxyhemoglobin, sulfhemoglobin has an additional peak at 620 nm that may be used for its quantitation. In cases of carbon monoxide poisoning, it is generally assumed that sulfhemoglobin is not present and that only the two pigments, carboxyhemoglobin and oxyhemoglobin, are present. In reality, other interfering pigments may be present and could reduce the accuracy of this method.

Cyanide

Principle: Cyanide[92,93] may be liberated from biologic fluids by acidification. The evolved hydrogen cyanide is absorbed in alkali, and the sodium cyanide thus formed is qualitatively and/or quantitatively determined by measuring the absorbance of chromophores formed by interaction of the cyanide ion with suitable reagents.

Apparatus:
1. Microdiffusion dishes
2. Spectrophotometer or colorimeter

Specimens:
1. Whole blood
2. Urine

Reagents: All reagents should be analytic reagent grade.
1. Sodium hydroxide, 0.1N
   Dissolve 4 g sodium hydroxide in water and dilute to 1 L with water.
2. Cyanide stock standard, 100 mg/dl
   Dissolve 0.250 g potassium cyanide in approximately 50 ml water. Add 2.0 ml of 0.5N sodium hydroxide (20 g/L) and dilute to 1 dl. Store in polyethylene container. **Discard after 3 months.**
3. Cyanide working standards (freshly prepared)
   a. Cyanide, 10 μg/ml. Dilute 0.1 ml to 10 ml with water.
   b. Cyanide, 2 μg/ml. Dilute 0.1 ml to 50 ml with water.
4. Sulfuric acid, 3.6N
   Dilute 10 ml concentrated sulfuric acid to 1 dl with water.
5. Monobasic sodium phosphate, 1M
   Dissolve 13.8 g monobasic sodium phosphate in water and dilute to 1 dl.
6. Chloramine-T, 0.25%
   Dissolve 0.25 g of chloramine-T in water and dilute to 1 dl. Store in refrigerator.
7. Color reagent
   Prepare fresh. To a 25 ml volumetric flask add 0.3 g barbituric acid, 15 ml pyridine, and 3.0 ml concentrated hydrochloric acid. Mix to dissolve and dilute to volume with water. Filter before using. This is a saturated solution.

Procedure: Place water in outer rim of diffusion dish to facilitate sealing. To inner compartment of each dish add 0.5 ml of 0.1N sodium hydroxide. To outer compartment of each dish add 0.5 ml of 3.6N sulfuric acid.

To outer chamber of each labeled dish add 0.5 ml water (for blank), each standard, and each specimen without mixing with the acid. Quickly cover each dish after addition of standard or specimen and rotate to mix acid and specimen.

Allow sample to diffuse a minimum of 2 hr at room temperature. To labeled test tubes add 0.1 ml of the contents of the inner chamber. To each tube add 1 ml of 1M sodium phosphate and 0.5 ml chloramine-T solution. Mix and let stand for 2-3 min. To each tube add 1.5 ml of color reagent. Mix and let stand for 10 min. A red color indicates cyanide ions are present. Determine the absorbance of each solution against the reagent blank at 580 nm.

Calculation:

$$\frac{\text{Absorbance of unknown}}{\text{Absorbance of standard}} \times \frac{\text{Conc.}}{\text{of standard}} = \frac{\text{Conc.}}{\text{of unknown}}$$

Interpretation: Blood concentrations of cyanide in healthy adults are usually less than 0.1 μg/ml in non-smokers and up to 0.20 μg/ml in heavy cigarette smokers.[94] Acute toxicity may occur as blood cyanide concentrations approach 0.5 μg/ml. Fatalities are usually associated with concentrations exceeding 1.0 μg/ml. Any oral dose of 250 mg potassium cyanide is usually lethal; however, as little as 60 mg has resulted in death.[95] Inhalation of 120 ppm cyanide will cause death within 1 hr; inhalation of twice this concentration will be immediately fatal.

Serum drug screen by ultraviolet spectrophotometry[96,97]

Apparatus: Ultraviolet spectrophotometer.
Specimen: Serum, 5 ml.
Reagents:
1. Buffer, pH 8.5
   Dissolve 53.5 g ammonium chloride in 950 ml water. Add 18 ml concentrated ammonium hydroxide. Mix. Adjust pH to 8.5 with hydrochloric acid or ammonium hydroxide.
2. Sodium hydroxide, 0.5N
   Dissolve 20 g sodium hydroxide in water in a sufficient quantity to make 1 L.
3. Ammonium chloride, saturated
   Dissolve 20 g ammonium chloride in 1 dl water.
4. Sulfuric acid, 2N
   Add 56 ml concentrated sulfuric acid to water, let cool, and add water to make 1 L.
5. Chloroform
6. Hexane
7. Alcoholic sulfuric acid, 0.5%
   Add 0.5 ml concentrated sulfuric acid to 1 dl reagent alcohol (ethanol).
8. Activated charcoal
9. Stock standards
   All stocks standards are 1 mg/ml prepared in reagent alcohol.
10. Working standards, 10 μg/ml
    a. To 5 ml water add 0.05 ml each of phenobarbital, chlordiazepoxide, and diazepam.
    b. To 5 ml water add 0.05 ml methaqualone.

Procedure: To separately labeled 40 ml screw-top tubes, add 5 ml water for blank. To separate tubes add 5 ml of each standard and 5 ml of each test specimen. To all tubes add 5 ml of buffer and 30 ml of chloroform.

Shake for 10 min and centrifuge. Remove and discard upper aqueous layer and add a small pinch of charcoal. Mix. Filter into 25 ml graduated cylinders through Whatman no. 2 filter paper. Add 25 ml aliquots of chloroform to separately labeled 40 ml tubes. To blank add 8.0 ml of 0.5N sodium hydroxide; to all other tubes add 4.0 ml. Shake tubes for 5 min and centrifuge. Remove alkaline layer and save chloroform in tubes.

To determine barbiturate content perform the following:
1. Scan 3 ml of the alkaline extract from standard 10(a) above and all test serum specimens against blank from 310-220 nm. A positive barbiturate level will exhibit a peak at approximately 255 nm. Read the absorbance of 260 nm and record.
2. To a 3.0 ml alkaline extract of blank, standards, and all specimens add 0.5 ml saturated ammonium chloride. This changes the pH from 14 to 10.3. Rescan the standard and test serum specimens from 310-220 nm. The absorption peak will shift to approximately 240 nm. Read and record the absorbance at 260 nm (Fig. 26-13).
3. The calculation is as follows:

$$\text{Absorbance at pH 14} - \text{Absorbance at pH 10.3} \times \frac{3.5}{3} = \Delta$$

$$\frac{\Delta \text{ unknown}}{\Delta \text{ standard}} \times 10 \text{ μg/ml} = \text{Conc. of unknown}$$

To the chloroform remaining in the tubes add 3.0 ml of 2N sulfuric acid. Shake for 10 min and centrifuge. Remove acid layer and save the chloroform layer. The acid will have extracted the chlordiazepoxide from the standard. Chlordiazepoxide, amitriptyline, or nortriptyline and other basic drugs can be detected in this fraction. Scan each acid extract from 340-220 nm. Chlordiazepoxide will exhibit an absorption peak at 245 nm and a minor peak at 306 nm (Fig. 26-2). Amitriptyline and/or nortriptyline will have a single peak at 240 nm (Fig. 26-1). If amitriptyline, nortriptyline, and other basic drugs are detected, a 10 μg/ml standard of drug should be carried through the procedure. Check absorbance maximums observed with those presented in Table 26-4.

The calculation is as follows:

$$\frac{\text{Absorbance of unknown}}{\text{Absorbance of standard}} \times \frac{\text{Conc.}}{\text{of standard}} = \frac{\text{Conc.}}{\text{of unknown}}$$

Filter remaining chloroform layers into labeled beakers or evaporation cups and add 2 drops of alcoholic acid. Evaporate to dryness under the hood at low temperature or at room temperature. After evaporation add 2 ml hexane to each cup and with a transfer pipet wash down the sides of the cup and transfer the hexane to a labeled 10 ml screw-top tube. Repeat with another 2 ml of hexane. To each tube add 2.5 ml of 2N sulfuric acid. Shake by hand for 90 sec and centrifuge.

Diazepam and methaqualone will be extracted in this fraction. Scan each acid extract (lower phase) from

Table 26-12. Blood serum concentration (μg/ml)

Drug	Therapeutic concentration	Toxic concentration	Lethal concentration
Amitriptyline	0.05-0.20	0.40	1-20
Chlordiazepoxide*	1-3	5	—
Chlorpromazine	0.5-1.0	2-4	+5
Desipramine	0.15-0.25	0.40	3-10
Diazepam*	0.5-2.0	5-20	—
Flurazepam*	0.05	1.0	—
Imipramine	0.15-0.25	0.40	1-10
Methapyrilene	2-4	30-50	+50
Methaqualone	5	10-30	+30
Nortriptyline	0.15-0.15	0.50	5-10

*As single agents, these drugs seldom cause life-threatening central nervous system depression. Severe toxicity is usually related to coingestion of alcohol or other psychoactive or depressant drugs.

340-200 nm. Diazepam exhibits an absorption peak at 241 nm with a minor peak at 284 nm and a minimum at 265 nm (Fig. 26-5). Methaqualone has a major peak at 234 nm (Fig. 26-8).

The calculations are as follows. For diazepam:

$$\frac{\text{Absorbance at 241 nm} - \text{Absorbance at 265 nm of unknown}}{\text{Absorbance at 241 nm} - \text{Absorbance at 265 nm of standard}}$$
$$\times \text{ Conc. of standard} = \text{Conc. of unknown}$$

For methaqualone:

$$\frac{\text{Absorbance at 234 nm of unknown}}{\text{Absorbance at 234 nm of standard}} \times \text{Conc. of standard} =$$
$$\text{Conc. of unknown}$$

Interpretation: Blood concentrations of drugs that may be detected by this procedure are correlated with physiologic activity in Table 26-12. Those with limited experience in toxicology should be aware that this table is not an absolute or ultimate guide for interpretation. Numerous factors will influence both the blood concentration of a drug and the resultant response in any individual. Blood drug concentrations per se do not preclude the careful observation and management of any poisoned patient. Therapeutic blood concentrations are those obtained after administration of a therapeutically effective dosage in humans. Toxic blood concentrations are those associated with serious toxic symptoms in humans. Lethal blood concentrations are those usually detected in cases of fatal intoxication.

Acetaminophen[98]

Apparatus:
1. Boiling water bath
2. Spectrophotometer (visible) or colorimeter

Specimens:
1. Serum, 1 ml
2. Urine, 1 ml (not suitable for intensely colored urine)

Reagents:
1. Trichloroacetic acid, 20%
   Dissolve trichloroacetic acid in 50 ml water and dilute to 1 dl.
2. Hydrochloric acid, concentrated
3. Ammonium hydroxide, 4N

Dilute 142 ml concentrated ammonium hydroxide to 5 dl with water.
4. Phenol, 2%
   Mix 23 ml liquefied phenol with water and dilute to 1 L. Store in the refrigerator. This solution is stable for 2 months.
5. Color reagent
   Prepare fresh. Mix 7 parts of 2% phenol with 3 parts of 4N ammonium hydroxide. Five milliliters is needed for each test, standard, and blank.
6. Stock standard, 1000 μg/ml
   Dissolve 100 mg in water and dilute to 1 dl. Refrigerate. This solution is stable for 6 months.
7. Working standard, 1 mg/dl and 5 mg/dl
   a. For 1 mg/dl (10 μg/ml) working standard, dilute 0.05 ml stock solution to 5 ml with water.
   b. For 5 mg/dl (50 μg/ml) working standard, dilute 0.5 ml stock solution to 10 ml with water.

Procedure: Label 10 ml test tubes for blank, standards, and unknown serum specimens; add 1 ml water for blank, 1 ml of each standard, and test serum specimens to proper tubes. To all tubes add 2.0 ml of 20% trichloroacetic acid. Mix well and centrifuge.

To labeled 10 ml test tubes transfer 1 ml of supernatant from blank and standards. For each unknown, transfer a 1 ml aliquot and a 0.1 ml aliquot; bring to volume with 0.9 ml of water. To all tubes add 0.2 ml concentrated hydrochloric acid. Place in a boiling water bath for 10 min. Cool to room temperature and add 5 ml color reagent. Allow color to develop for 20 min and then read the absorbance at 620 nm against a blank.

Calculation:

$$\frac{\text{Absorbance of unknown}}{\text{Absorbance of standard}} \times \frac{\text{Conc.}}{\text{of standard}} = \frac{\text{Conc.}}{\text{of unknown}}$$

Alternatively, one can calculate a K factor. Then

$$\text{K} \times \text{Absorbance of unknown} = \text{Conc. of unknown}$$

If a 0.1 ml aliquot is used for calculation, the final answer will be times ten.

Interpretation: The manifestations of acetaminophen poisoning are characterized by three stages. The first stage, occurring within 24 hr of ingestion, consists of nausea, vomiting, and diaphoresis. No acute distress is exhibited at this time. In the second phase, occurring from 24-72 hr after ingestion, the patients seems to improve but serum hepatic enzymes (SGOT) increase dramatically. The right upper quadrant abdominal area is tender to palpation. In the third stage, 3-7 days after ingestion, signs of hepatic necrosis (jaundice, increased prothrombin time, and hypoglycemia), hepatic encephalopathy, and renal failure can occur.

Acetaminophen poisoning is one of the few occurrences in which serum concentrations may have a direct effect on the continuance of antidotal therapy. Hepatotoxicity resulting from ingestion of an overdose of acetaminophen may be avoided by oral administration of N-acetylcysteine (Mucomyst), 10-20% solution; an initial dose of 140 mg/kg is followed every 4 hr by 70 mg/kg for 17 doses.[99]

The probability of hepatotoxicity is related to serum concentration vs. time after ingestion. Hepatotoxicity is probable at serum acetaminophen concentrations (1) greater than 200 μg/ml up to 4 hr after ingestion, (2) between 100-200 μg/ml from 4-8 hr after ingestion, and (3) between 50-100 μg/ml from 8-12 hr after ingestion. The antidote should be administered for all 17 doses if these situations occur. The patient's prognosis may be determined by analysis of two or more samples drawn first on admission and then at 3 hr intervals. The plasma half-life (time necessary for a 50% decrease in drug concentration) may be determined by plotting the log of plasma acetaminophen concentration against time. A plasma half-life of 2-4 hr is normal; 5-8 hr indicates hepatotoxicity; and greater than 12 hr indicates that hepatic coma may develop.

Amitriptyline and nortriptyline[100]

Apparatus: Ultraviolet spectrophotometer.
Specimen: Serum or plasma, 5 ml.
Reagents:
1. Ethyl ether
2. Buffer, pH 11
   Dissolve 21 g sodium carbonate and 420 mg sodium bicarbonate in water. Dilute to 1 L. Check the pH and adjust with solid sodium carbonate or sodium bicarbonate as necessary.
3. Sulfuric acid, 0.5N
   Add 14 ml concentrated sulfuric acid to water. When solution is cool, dilute to 1 L.
4. Stock standards
   Dissolve 114.5 mg amitriptyline hydrochloride in ethyl alcohol and dilute to 1 dl.
5. Working standards
   a. For the 5 μg/ml working standard, dilute 0.05 ml to 10 ml with water.
   b. For the 10 μg/ml working standard, dilute 0.10 ml to 10 ml with water.

Procedure: To separate 40 ml screw-top tubes add 5 ml water for blank, 5 ml of each standard, and 5 ml of each unknown. To all tubes add 5 ml carbonate-bicarbonate buffer. To all tubes add 30 ml ether. Shake for 5 min and centrifuge. Aspirate and discard aqueous (lower) layer. Filter the ether through Whatman no. 2 filter paper into labeled graduated cylinders. Collect 25 ml.

Transfer solvent to clean, labeled 40 ml screw-top tubes. To each tube add 3.0 ml of 0.5N sulfuric acid, shake for 5 min, and centrifuge. Remove acid (lower) phase to labeled test tubes and place in 80° C water bath **(not on a hot plate)** to expel ether. Scan standards and unknowns against blank from 300-220 nm. Record absorbance at 240 nm.
Calculation:

Conc. of unknown = Absorbance of unknown × K

$$K = \frac{\text{Conc. of standards}}{\text{Absorbance of standards}}$$

• • •

To confirm and differentiate amitriptyline and nortriptyline make acid extracts basic with 50% sodium hydroxide (check pH). Extract with 20 ml ether and centrifuge and discard aqueous (lower) phase. Wash ether with 10 ml water two times. (Discard water after each washing.) Filter ether through Whatman no. 2 filter paper into evaporation cups and add 2 drops of alcoholic 0.5% sulfuric acid. Evaporate and spot on TLC plates with amitriptyline and nortriptyline standards. Use the same solvent system and visualization sprays as for a routine drug screen.

Interpretation: Any overdose of amitriptyline is a potentially life-threatening situation. No direct correlation has been established between serum concentrations and severity of toxicity. Patients with greater than therapeutic serum concentrations (Table 26-12) should be kept under close observation.

Barbiturates

Principle: All the 5,5-substituted barbiturates[101,102] display a shift in their ultraviolet absorbance maximum between pH 10 and pH 13. Therefore identification of a specific barbiturate is not possible by ultraviolet spectrophotometry. However, of immediate clinical importance in overdose cases is the pharmacologic classification of the barbiturates, whether long, intermediate, or short acting. The quantitative procedure presented here allows the rapid identification of barbiturates by pharmacologic class. Following ultraviolet analysis, the specific barbiturates may be identified by TLC (also see ultraviolet drug screen and Fig. 26-13).

Reagents:
1. Borate buffer, 0.6M
   Dissolve 37.1 g boric acid and 44.7 g potassium chloride in distilled water and dilute to 1 L.
2. Chloroform, spectroanalyzed grade
3. Norit-A (animal charcoal)
4. Phosphate buffer, pH 7.4
   a. For solution A dissolve 17.0 g dibasic potassium phosphate in distilled water and dilute to 250 ml making a 0.5M solution.
   b. For solution B dissolve 179.1 g monobasic sodium phosphate (hydrate salt 12 water) in distilled water and dilute to 1 L making a 0.5M solution. Various hydrated forms of monobasic sodium phosphate are available. Use an equivalent weight of other hydrated forms.
   c. Prepare pH 7.4 buffer by mixing 19.2 ml of

solution A with 80.8 ml of solution B. Check with a pH meter.

5. Sodium hydroxide, 0.45N
   Dissolve 18.0 g sodium hydroxide in distilled water and dilute to 1 L. Store in a polyethylene bottle.

6. Barbiturate control
   a. For stock standard (1 mg/ml) dissolve 100 mg phenobarbital in reagent ehtanol and dilute to 1 dl with ethanol.
   b. For control (10 μg/ml) dilute 0.10 μl stock standard to 10 ml with drug-free blood, plasma, or serum if available; alternately, dilute with water.

Procedure:

1. To separate 125 ml separatory funnels, add 10 ml water for blank, 10 ml of control, and 10 ml of sample.

2. Extract each three times with 30 ml chloroform each time. (If an emulsion occurs, add a few milliliters of chloroform in excess and invert separatory funnel gently several times. The layers should separate readily. Filter the combined chloroform extracts through a piece of Whatman no. 1 paper into a second 125 ml separatory funnel. Save the filter funnel.)

3. Wash the chloroform with 5.0 ml of phosphate buffer solution. Draw off the chloroform into a 150 ml beaker. Decant the phosphate solution into a test tube for salicylate analysis; otherwise, discard this solution.

4. Transfer the chloroform back into the same separatory funnel and wash with another 5.0 ml portion of phosphate buffer solution. Repeat step 3.

5. Return the chloroform to the separatory funnel and add approximately 50 mg Norit-A. Shake vigorously.

6. Filter the chloroform through Whatman no. 1 filter paper into a third separatory funnel.

7. Add 10.0 ml of 0.45N sodium hydroxide and extract for 5 min. If neutral drugs (e.g., glutethimide, ethchlorvynol, or meprobamate) are suspected, the chloroform may be transferred to a 150 ml beaker, evaporated to dryness, and subjected to TLC analysis; otherwise, draw off the chloroform and discard. Draw off the 0.45N sodium hydroxide into a clean 15 ml test tube and centrifuge for 5 min.

8. Prepare two test tubes for each sample, control, and blank. Lable test tubes as follows:
   a. NaOH sample (1, 2, etc.)
   b. Borate sample (1, 2, etc.)
   c. NaOH blank
   d. Borate blank
   e. NaOH control
   f. Borate control

9. Pipet 2.0 ml of 0.45N sodium hydroxide into each tube labeled NaOH and 2.0 ml of borate buffer solution into each tube labeled borate.

10. Pipet 2.0 ml of 0.45N sodium hydroxide sample extract into each tube labeled sample or control and 2.0 ml of 0.45N sodium hydroxide blank extract into each tube labeled blank. Mix thoroughly.

11. Record the ultraviolet spectra of the extracts from 300-220 nm as follows:
    a. Borate samples and control against the borate blank as reference
    b. Sodium hydroxide samples and control against the sodium hydroxide blank as reference
    NOTE: Save the blank solutions.

12. The criteria for barbiturate identification are as follows (Fig. 26-13):
    a. Borate buffer: absorbance maximum of 238-240 nm
    b. Sodium hydroxide: absorbance maximum of 252-255 nm and minimum of 234-237 nm
    c. Isobestic points: 227-230 nm and 247-250 nm

13. If a typical barbiturate spectrum is obtained and the identity of the barbiturate is known, proceed to the second calculation below.

14. If the identity of the barbiturate is not known, place a centrifuge tube containing 5.0 ml of 0.45N sodium hydroxide sample and control extracts in a boiling water bath for 15 min (time exactly).

15. Remove the tubes and cool in an ice-water bath. Prepare two test tubes for each sample and control and label as follows:
    a. NaOH-hydrolyzed sample
    b. Borate-hydrolyzed sample
    c. NaOH-hydrolyzed control
    d. Borate-hydrolyzed control

16. Pipet 2.0 ml of 0.45N sodium hydroxide fresh solution into the sodium hydroxide tube and 2.0 ml of borate buffer into the borate tube.

17. When the sodium hydroxide–hydrolyzed extract has cooled to room temperature, adjust the volume to 5.0 ml with distilled water. Mix well. Pipet 2.0 ml of this solution into each of the above two tubes. Run ultraviolet absorption spectra as before, using the appropriate blank solutions as references.

Calculation: In the following calculations A1 = absorbance of 0.45N sodium hydroxide solution at 260 nm, A2 = absorbance of borate solution at 260 nm, A3 = absorbance of 0.45N sodium hydroxide–hydrolyzed solution at 260 nm, and A4 = absorbance of borate-hydrolyzed solution at 260 nm.

Table 26-13. F and R values of classes of barbiturates

Barbiturate pharmacologic class	F	R
Long acting	43.7	20-40
Intermediate	41.7	40-65
Short and intermediate	44.4	65-75
Short or intermediate and short	44.4	75-85
Short acting	47.8	85-100

$$R = \frac{A3 - A4}{A1 - A2} \times 100$$

From Table 26-13 find the barbiturate and its F value corresponding to R. If the F value cannot be determined, use F = 44.1 (mean). (For an explanation of F see reference 101).

$$C = F \times (A1 - A2) \times 2.0 = \text{Barbiturate } (\mu g/ml)$$

If 5.0 ml of sample is used and the hydrolysis step is to be omitted, (i.e., type of barbiturate is known) use 5.0 ml of 0.45N sodium hydroxide for extraction of chloroform and calculate using the equation just given.

If 5.0 ml of sample is used and the hydrolysis step is to be included, use the following equation:

$$C = F \times (A1 - A2) \times 4.0 = \text{Barbiturate } (\mu g/ml)$$

If amounts of sample (or 0.45N sodium hydroxide extract) used are other than those given above use the following equation:

$$C = F \times (A1 - A2) \times 2.0 \times \frac{0.45N \text{ NaOH (ml)}}{\text{Sample (ml)}} =$$

$$\text{Barbiturate } (\mu g/ml)$$

If the sample consists of urine or stomach contents, use 10-25 ml of sample, acidify with sulfuric acid, and proceed with the chloroform extraction as before. Calculate using the equation just given.

Differentiation of barbiturates:
1. Acidify unknown extracts with 50% sulfuric acid. Check pH.
2. Extract all unknowns with 25 ml chloroform. Centrifuge and discard aqueous (upper) phase.
3. Wash chloroform twice with 10 ml water. (Discard water after each washing.)
4. Filter chloroform through Whatman no. 2 filter paper into evaporation cups.
5. Evaporate and spot on TLC plate with barbiturate standards. Use solvent system D in TLC urine drug screen given earlier. Visualize spots with diphenylcarbazone and mercuric sulfate reagent.

Interpretation: The relationship between blood concentrations and physiologic effect for various barbiturates is presented in Table 26-14. The definition of the terms *therapeutic, toxic,* and *lethal* is explained in the discussion of the serum drug screen: interpretation. Individual patients may vary greatly in their response to a given blood barbiturate concentration. Those on long-term barbiturate therapy or those who are addicted to barbiturates will be tolerant to concentrations that may produce severe central nervous system depression in nontolerant persons.

Chloral hydrate and metabolites; trichloroacetic acid and trichloroethanol[103]

Apparatus: Spectrophotometer.
Specimen: Plasma or serum.
Reagents:
1. Chloral hydrate
2. Trichloroacetic acid (TCA)
3. Pyridine
4. Potassium hydroxide, 10M
   Dissolve 56 g potassium hydroxide in 1 dl water.
5. Hydrochloric acid
6. Potassium hydroxide, 16M
   Dissolve 89.9 g potassium hydroxide in 1 dl water.
7. Standards
   a. Stock chloral hydrate standard, 1 mg/ml. Dissolve 100 mg chloral hydrate in water and dilute to 1 dl.
   b. Working chloral hydrate standard. For 10 μg/ml dilute 0.05 ml stock standard to 5 ml with water. For 20 μg/ml dilute 0.10 ml stock standard to 5 ml with water.
   c. Stock trichloroacetic acid standard, 1 mg/ml. Dilute 4 ml Sigma 6.25% trichloroacetic acid (Sigma Chemical Co., St. Louis) to 250 ml with water.
   d. Working trichloroacetic acid standards. For 10 μg/ml dilute 0.05 ml stock standard to 5 ml with water. For 20 μg/ml dilute 0.10 ml stock standard to 5 ml with water.
   e. Stock trichloroethanol (TCE) standard, 1 mg/

Table 26-14. Interpretation of blood serum barbiturate concentrations

Barbiturates by pharmacologic class	Blood concentration (μg/ml)		
	Therapeutic	**Toxic**	**Lethal***
Short acting (less than 3 hr)			
Heptabarbital	1	5-10	+10
Pentobarbital	1†	5-10	+10
Secobarbital	1	5-10	+10
Intermediate acting (3-6 hr)			
Allybarbituric acid	1-5	10-30	+30
Amobarbital	1-5	10-30	+30
Butibarbital	1-5	10-30	+30
Long acting (6 or more hr)			
Phenobarbital			
Anticonvulsant therapy	10-30	80	150
Nighttime sedation	8-19	40-60	80-150

*Even at a concentration often encountered in fatal poisoning, some individuals may only exhibit drowsiness or stupor.
†In neurologic therapy for head trauma or Reye's syndrome, therapeutic concentrations may range from 10-20+ μg/ml (see discussion of thiopental).

ml. Dilute 0.4 ml trichloroethanol to 250 ml with water.

f. Working trichloroethanol standards. For 10 µg/ml dilute 0.05 ml stock standard to 5 ml with water. For 20 µg/ml dilute 0.10 ml stock standard to 5 ml with water.

Procedure: Label screw-top test tubes and add amounts as follows:

1. Blank: Add 1 ml water.
2. Chloral hydrate, 10 µg/ml: Add 1 ml of 10 µg/ml standard.
3. Chloral hydrate, 20 µg/ml: Add 1 ml of 20 µg/ml standard.
4. TCA, 10 µg/ml: Add 1 ml trichloroacetic acid 10 µg/ml standard.
5. TCA, 20 µg/ml: Add 1 ml trichloroaceitc acid 20 µg/ml standard.
6. TCE, 10 µg/ml: Add 1 ml of trichloroethanol 10 µg/ml standard.
7. TCE, 20 µg/ml: Add 1 ml trichloroethanol 20 µg/ml standard.
8. Test 1-A: Add 1 ml serum.
9. Test 1-B: Add 1 ml serum.

(Set up tubes A and B for each unknown.)

To the blank, chloral hydrate standards, trichloroethanol standards, and test A tubes, add 5 ml of pyridine and mix on a vortex mixer. Place these tubes in an ice bath; after 3 min add 2 ml of 10M potassium hydroxide, mix with a vortex mixer, and transfer to a boiling water bath for 5 min. After 5 min, return tubes to an ice bath for 5 min. Transfer a 3 ml aliquot of the pyridine to clean labeled test tubes and keep these in the ice bath.

To trichloroacetic acid standards and test B tubes add 2 ml of 10M potassium hydroxide, mix with a vortex mixer, and place in a boiling water bath for exactly 2 min. Transfer these tubes to an ice bath and after 5 min add 5 ml pyridine. Mix on a vortex mixer and place in a boiling water bath for 5 min. Transfer a 3 ml aliquot of the pyridine to clean labeled test tubes and keep in an ice bath. Immediately before transferring pyridine aliquots to cuvets, add 0.5 ml water and mix. Scan each standard and test or tests from 600-350 nm. Record the absorbance at 440 nm and 540 nm.

Calculation:

Chloral hydrate: Calculate K for chloral hydrate standards at 540 nm; where

$$K = \frac{\text{Conc. of standard}}{\text{Absorbance of standard}}$$

then

K × Absorbance of test A tube at 540 nm =

Conc. of chloral hydrate and TCA

Trichloroacetic acid: Calculate K for trichloroacetic acid standards at 540 nm as follows:

K × Absorbance of test B tube at 540 nm = Conc. of TCA

For tests only subtract concentration of trichloroacetic acid from concentration of trichloroacetic acid plus chloral hydrate to obtain concentration of chloral hydrate.

Trichloroethanol: Calculate K for trichloroethanol standards at 440 nm as follows:

K × Absorbance of test A tube at 440 nm = Conc. of TCE

Interpretation: Chloral hydrate is rapidly reduced in the body to trichloroethanol so that virtually no parent drug is observed in the blood or plasma after therapeutic doses.[104] Serum trichloroethanol concentrations following a dose of 1 g range between 3-12 µg/ml and are consistent with sedation.[105] Severe central nervous system depression may occur at concentrations of 50-100 µg/ml. Death may occur at concentrations exceeding 100 µg/ml, but values of 200-400 µg/ml are more commonly detected in fatal intoxications.

Ethchlorvynol[106]

Apparatus: Spectrophotometer or colorimeter.

Specimens:
1. Serum or plasma, 2 ml
2. Gastric contents, 2 ml
3. Urine, 2 ml

Reagents:
1. Trichloroacetic acid, 10%
   Dissolve 10 g trichloroacetic acid in water and dilute to 1 dl.
2. Color reagent
   Dissolve 1.0 g diphenylamine in 50 ml concentrated sulfuric acid. Slowly add this solution, while stirring, to a mixture of 50 ml water and 50 ml glacial acetic acid.
3. Control reagent
   Slowly add 50 ml concentrated sulfuric acid, while stirring, to a mixture of 50 ml water and 50 ml glacial acetic acid.
4. Stock standard, 1 mg/ml
   Dissolve 100 mg ethchlorvynol in reagent alcohol (ethanol). Dilute to 1 dl with alcohol.
5. Working standards
   a. For 5 µg/ml dilute 0.05 ml to 10 ml with water.
   b. For 10 µg/ml dilute 0.10 ml to 10 ml with water.

Procedure: To 2 ml serum or plasma add 4 ml trichloroacetic acid, mix on a vortex mixer, and centrifuge. Transfer supernatants to clean labeled tubes. Set up the following labeled tubes:

1. Reagent blank: 2 ml water
2. Standard of 5 µg/ml: 2 ml of 5 µg/ml working standard
3. Standard of 10 µg/ml: 2 ml of 10 µg/ml working standard
4. Serum blank: 2 ml supernatant
5. Serum test: 2 ml supernatant
6. Urine blank: 2 ml centrifuged urine
7. Urine test: 2 ml centrifuged urine
8. Gastric blank: 2 ml centrifuged gastric contents
9. Gastric test: 2 ml centrifuged gastric contents

Add 3 ml control reagent to each blank. Add 3 ml color reagent to each test. Mix on a vortex mixer and let stand at room temperature.

After 2 hr (for color development) measure the absorption of each standard and test against its corresponding blank at 510 nm. The test is linear from 2-10 μg/ml. If the concentration exceeds this amount, repeat using smaller volume of trichloroacetic acid filtrate, urine, or gastric contents and bring to 2 ml volume with water.

Formaldehyde, acetaldehyde, acetone, or paraldehyde in concentrations of 100 mg/dl will inhibit color development. If any of these substrates is present, extract the color complex with chloroform.

Calculation:

$$K = \frac{\text{Conc. of standard}}{\text{Absorbance of standard}}$$

Serum:

Absorbance at 510 nm × K × 3* = Ethchlorvynol (μg/ml)

Urine or gastric contents:

Absorbance at 510 nm × K = Ethchlorvynol (mg/ml)

Interpretation: After a single therapeutic oral dose of 200 mg ethchlorvynol, peak plasma concentrations range from 0.6-1.8 μg/ml at 1 hr after ingestion.[107] At higher therapeutic doses (750 mg) peak plasma concentrations may reach 8 μg/ml.[108] Severe central nervous system depression after ingestion of several grams may develop at concentrations of 20-30 μg/ml. Fatalities are associated with concentrations exceeding 50 μg/ml. From time to time drug addicts have injected ethchlorvynol intravenously. The drug is much more toxic by this route of administration and life-threatening pulmonary edema may rapidly develop. Plasma concentrations are not well correlated with the severe toxicity caused by intravenous use.

Methyprylon[109]

Apparatus: Spectrophotometer.
Specimens:
1. Serum or plasma, 2 ml
2. Urine, 2 ml
Reagents:
1. Folin-Ciocalteu reagent (obtain commercially)
   Dilute 1 ml with 2.5 ml water just before use.
2. Diethyl ether
3. Chloroform
4. Sodium hydroxide, 5N (20%)
   Dissolve 200 g sodium hydroxide in water and dilute to 1 L.
5. Sodium hydroxide, 0.5N
   Dissolve 20 g sodium hydroxide in water and dilute to 1 L.
6. Sodium hydroxide, 0.8N
   Dilute 80 ml of 1N sodium hydroxide to 1 dl or dissolve 3.2 g sodium hydroxide in water and dilute to 1 dl.
7. Stock standard, 1 mg/ml
   Dissolve 100 mg methyprylon in reagent alcohol and dilute to 1 dl.
8. Working standard
   a. For 5 μg/ml dilute 0.05 ml stock standard to 10 ml with water.

b. For 10 μg/ml dilute 0.10 ml stock standard to 10 ml with water.

Procedure:
1. To separate screw-top tubes add 2 ml water for blank, 2 ml of each standard, and 2 ml of each test specimen.
2. To all tubes add 0.6 ml of 5N sodium hydroxide and 20 ml ether. Put in shaker for 20 min and centrifuge.
3. With a Pasteur pipet remove and discard aqueous layer.
4. Add 1 ml of 0.5N sodium hydroxide and shake by hand for 1 min. Centrifuge. Remove and discard alkaline layer.
5. Repeat step 4.
6. Filter ether through Whatman no. 1 filter paper into a graduated cylinder. Collect 15 ml.
7. Transfer the ether to separate tubes and place in a 60° C water bath to evaporate. **Do not place on a hot plate.**
8. After evaporation dissolve the residue in 1.5 ml water by shaking on a vortex mixer for 30 sec. Add 0.5 ml of dilute Folin-Ciocalteu reagent and 0.5 ml sodium hydroxide, 0.8N. Mix and let stand at room temperature for 10 min for color development.
9. To each tube add 2 ml chloroform and shake vigorously for 30 sec. Centrifuge.
10. Transfer the aqueous (top) layer to a cuvet and read the absorbance against a blank at 600 nm.

Calculation:

$$K = \frac{\text{Conc. of standard}}{\text{Absorbance of standard}}$$

K × Absorbance of test = Methyprylon (μg/ml)

Interpretation: After a single therapeutic dose of 650 mg, peak plasma methyprylon concentrations average 10 μg/ml and are consistent with sedation.[110] Concentrations greater than 30 μg/ml may produce coma.[111] Fatalities may occur at 50 μg/ml.

Meprobamate[112]

Apparatus: Spectrophotometer.
Specimens:
1. Serum, plasma, or whole blood, 1 ml
2. Urine, 1 ml
3. Filtered gastric contents, 1 ml
Reagents:
1. Sodium hydroxide, 0.5N
   Dissolve 20 g sodium hydroxide in water and dilute to 1 L.
2. Chloroform
3. AAA reagent
   Add 10 ml glacial acetic acid to 30 ml acetone. This solution is stable indefinitely if stored in a brown bottle.
4. DMB reagent
   Dissolve 500 mg *p*-dimethylaminobenzaldehyde in benzene. Dilute to 50 ml with benzene. This solution is stable for 1 month if stored in a brown bottle.
5. ATA reagent

---

*Two milliliters of specimen + 4 ml trichloroacetic acid = ×3 dilution.

Combine 2 g antimony trichloride with 8 ml chloroform and 2 ml acetic anhydride. Prepare fresh as needed.
6. Benzene
7. Stock standard, 1 mg/ml
   Dissolve 100 mg meprobamate in reagent alcohol and dilute to 1 dl with alcohol.
8. Working standards
   a. For 10 μg/ml dilute 0.05 ml stock standard to 5 ml with water.
   b. For 20 μg/ml dilute 0.10 ml stock standard to 5 ml with water.

Procedure: To separate screw-top tubes pipet 1 ml of water for blank, 1 ml of each standard, and 1 ml of each test specimen. To all tubes add 0.1 ml sodium hydroxide, 0.5N, and 10 ml chloroform. Place all tubes on the mechanical shaker for 5 min and centrifuge. Remove and discard aqueous (upper) layer from each tube.

Transfer a 5 ml aliquot of the chloroform layer from the blank and the standards to evaporate cups. For each test sample, set up two cups: to one add a 5 ml aliquot and to the second add a 0.5 ml aliquot. Place cups in the evaporator with the temperature set at 50° C. Evaporate to dryness.

After evaporation add the following to each cup:
1. 0.2 ml of AAA reagent
2. 0.2 ml of DMB reagent
3. 1.0 ml of ATA reagent

Replace cups in the evaporator at 50° C for 10 min. Do not turn on the vacuum pump. Remove cups from the evaporator or heating block and add 2 ml benzene to each cup. Using a Pasteur pipet mix and wash down the sides of the cup. Transfer the contents of the cup to a cuvet and read against the blank at 550 nm.*

Calculation:

$$K = \frac{\text{Conc. of standards}}{\text{Absorbance of standards}}$$

$$K \times \text{Absorbance of unknown} \times \frac{5}{\text{Aliquot of chloroform of test used}} =$$

$$\text{Meprobamate (μg/ml)}$$

Interpretation: After oral therapeutic doses up to 800 mg, peak plasma meprobamate levels range from 10-20 μg/ml.[113] Plasma concentrations of 60-120 μg/ml may induce light coma, while 100-240 μg/ml produce deep coma.[114] Fatalities are associated with concentrations greater than 200 μg/ml.

Methaqualone[115]

Apparatus: Ultraviolet recording spectrophotometer.
Specimen: Serum or plasma, 1.0 ml.
Reagents:
1. Hexane
2. Sodium hydroxide, 1.0N
   Dissolve 40 g sodium hydroxide in water and dilute to 1 L.
3. Sodium hydroxide, 0.5N

Dissolve 20 g sodium hydroxide in water and dilute to 1 L.
4. Hysdrochloric acid, 1.0N
   Add 83.0 ml concentrated hydrochloric acid to water. Cool and dilute to 1 L.
5. Stock standard, 1 mg/ml
   Dissolve 115 mg methaqualone hydrochloride (equivalent to 100 mg methaqualone base) in methanol in a 1 dl volmetric flask. Dilute to volume with methanol. Store in a brown glass bottle in the refrigerator.
6. Working standards
   a. For 5 μg/ml dilute 0.05 ml stock to 5 ml with water.
   b. For 10 μg/ml dilute 0.10 ml stock to 5 ml with water.

Procedure: To separately labeled 15 ml centrifuge tubes, transfer 1 ml water for blank, 1 ml of each standard, and 1 ml of each test serum. To each tube add 0.2 ml of 1N sodium hydroxide and 5.0 ml hexane. Shake for 3 min and centrifuge.

With a Pasteur pipet transfer upper hexane layer to a clean labeled tube. Reextract each specimen with 5 ml hexane. Shake for 3 min. Centrifuge. Remove hexane from each tube and combine with first extraction. To all pooled hexane extracts add 3 ml of 0.5N sodium hydroxide. Shake for 3 min and centrifuge. Transfer 8 ml hexane (upper) layer to clean labeled 20 ml screw-top tubes. Add 3.0 ml of 1N hydrochloric acid. Shake for 3 min and centrifuge. Scan each hydrochloric acid extract against blank from 340-200 nm. Record the absorbance at 235 nm (Fig. 26-8).

Calculation:

$$K = \frac{\text{Conc. of standard}}{\text{Absorbance of standard}}$$

$$K \times \text{Absorbance of unknown} = \text{Methaqualone (μg/ml)}$$

Interpretation: See interpretation under discussion of serum drug screen.

Propoxyphene (Darvon)[116]

Principle: The toxic concentration of propoxyphene in blood is usually only several micrograms per milliliter. The $E_{1\%}$ of propoxyphene is only about 13; therefore the observed absorbance of 10 ml of blood containing 2 μg/ml of propoxyphene extracted and concentrated into 2 ml of acid solution would be 0.013 or essentially undetectable. In the following procedure the extracted propoxyphene is converted by ultraviolet radiation to a derivative with strong absorbance in the ultraviolet region.

Apparatus:
1. Ultraviolet recording spectrophotometer
2. Ultraviolet light source, 257 nm
Specimen: Serum or plasma, 10 ml.
Reagents:
1. Hydrochloric acid, concentrated
2. Sodium hydroxide, 50%
   Dissolve 50 g sodium hydroxide in water and dilute to 1 dl.
3. Diethyl ether
4. Hydrochloric acid, 0.25N
   Add 2 ml concentrated hydrochloric acid to water and dilute to 1 dl.

5. Stock standard, 1 mg/ml
   Dissolve 100 mg propoxyphene hydrochloride in reagent alcohol and dilute to 1 dl.
6. Working standard, 10 μg/ml
   To a 30 ml Pyrex tube, add 0.5 ml stock standard and 4.5 ml water. Add 2.5 ml concentrated hydrochloric acid and place in a boiling water bath for 20 min. Cool in an ice bath for 5 min and add 50% sodium hydroxide (2.0-2.5 ml) until solution is alkaline. Then acidify with hydrochloric acid. Dilute to 50 ml with water.

Procedure:
1. Place 10 ml serum or plasma in a 40 ml screw-top Pyrex tube. To the serum or plasma add 15 ml concentrated hydrochloric acid.
2. Heat in a boiling water bath for 20 min. Stir occasionally with a glass stirring rod.
3. Cool the tubes in an ice bath for 5 min. Then while tubes are still in the ice bath **slowly** add 15 ml of 50% sodium hydroxide.
4. When the solution has cooled to room temperature, transfer to a 250 ml separatory funnel and add 150 ml diethyl ether.
5. Shake funnel for 5 min. Allow layers to separate. Drain off the lower aqueous layer.
6. Add 10 ml water to the funnel and shake for 2 min. Allow to separate and drain off lower layer. Repeat wash with additional 10 ml of water
7. Filter ether through Whatman no. 1 filter paper into a graduated cylinder. Record volume of ether recovered.
8. Transfer the ether extract to a clean 250 ml separatory funnel and add 5 ml of 0.25N hydrochloric acid.
9. Shake funnel for 5 min. Allow the layers to separate. Filter acid (lower) layer through small filter paper.
10. Scan the standard and unknwon from 310-200 nm using 0.25N hydrochloric acid as a blank. Record absorbance at 254 nm. If absorbance exceeds 0.4, dilute with 0.25N hydrochloric acid and rescan and record the absorbance at 254 nm.
11. Place the cuvets containing the blank, standard, and unknown within a few centimeters of a 257 nm ultraviolet light source for 5 min.
12. Scan the irradiated solutions as in step 10 and record the absorbance at 254 nm. The irradiated product has a sharp peak at 254 nm with a shoulder at 247 nm and minor peaks at 277, 287, and 298 nm.

Calculation: Determine the Δ absorbance (ΔA) at 254 nm for the standard and unknown.

$$\Delta A = A \text{ of irradiated product} - A \text{ of nonirradiated product}$$

$$\frac{\Delta A \text{ of unknown}}{\Delta A \text{ of standard}} \times 10 \text{ μg/ml} \times \frac{1}{2} \times$$

$$\frac{150}{\text{Volume of ether recovered}} =$$

Propoxyphene (μg/ml)

$$\frac{\text{Final volume of hydrochloric acid (5.0 ml)}}{\text{Original volume of serum (10 ml)}} = \frac{1}{2}$$

Interpretation: After a single 130 mg oral dose of propoxyphene hydrochloride, peak blood concentrations of propoxyphene range from 0.24-0.75 μg/ml at 2 hr.[117] Peak norpropoxyphene blood concentrations are two to three times that of the parent drug at 4 hr. Serious toxicity may develop at blood propoxyphene levels of 1 μg/ml. Fatalities have been associated with concentrations as low as 2 μg/ml[118] but generally range from 5-20 μg/ml. The concentration obtained by this procedure is the total of propoxyphene and norpropoxyphene present.

Screening for toxic metals (arsenic, lead, and mercury)

The accurate and precise determination of toxic metals in biologic materials requires a consistent effort to minimize contamination of glassware and samples. Few laboratories that analyze metals only on rare occasions are able to produce accurate results. Generally, toxic metal determinations are best left to laboratories dedicated to their routine analysis. In the past the dithizone colorimetric method was routinely used for metal determinations; however, this procedure is only reliable in the hands of an experienced analyst.[119]

Where applicable, atomic absorption spectrophotometry (AAS) is the method of choice for metal determinations.[120] The basic principle of AAS is absorbance of discrete emission radiation by a vapor of unexcited, unionized atoms of the metal analyzed. The radiation source is a hollow cathode lamp constructed of the metal of interest. The lamp emits the radiation spectrum of the desired metal. An acetylene flame converts the radiation to atomic vapor, which absorbs the resultant radiation. A monochromator or filter set at the analytic wavelength (a spectral line characteristic of the metal) directs the radiation passing through the vapor into a photodetector. The photodetector sees the minimized intensity of the lamp signal radiation. The reduction in intensity is proportional to the concentration of metal atoms vaporized.

Reinsch test: general screening method[121,122]

Principle: Certain metals, e.g., arsenic, antimony, bismuth, and mercury, in an acid medium and with heat can be deposited on a copper wire. Arsenic can be differentiated from antimony and bismuth.

Specimens:
1. Urine, 20 ml
2. Filtered gastric contents, 20 ml
3. Tissue homogenate (Tissue specimens [liver or kidney] are finely macerated with water, or they may be homogenized in a kitchen blender by using 10 ml tissue to 10 ml water.)

Reagents:
1. Copper wire, 20 gauge
   Make a 7 mm coil of the wire by wrapping it around a glass stirring rod.
2. Nitric acid, 2.5N
   Dilute 15.0 ml concentrated nitric acid to 1 dl with water.
3. Ethanol, 95%
4. Hydrochloric acid, concentrated
5. Ether
6. Potassium cyanide, 10%

Dissolve 10 g in water and dilute to 1 dl.

Procedure: Into a 50 ml Erlenmeyer flask place 20 ml specimen and 4 ml concentrated hydrochloric acid. Wash the copper wire successively with 2.5 N nitric acid, ethanol, and ether; then add to flask. Heat the flask and contents in a boiling water bath (100° C) for 1 hr. After cooling remove the copper coil and examine for a dark deposit, which may be caused by arsenic, antimony, or bismuth. If mercury is present, the color of the deposit ranges from grayish to shiny silver. To confirm the presence of arsenic place the copper wire into a test tube containing 2.0 ml of 10% potassium cyanide. Arsenic will dissolve in the cyanide solution, but bismuth or antimony will remain on the coil.

Interpretation: If a positive test is observed for arsenic or mercury, the specimen should be reanalyzed by the appropriate quantitative procedure given below.

Arsenic[123,124]

Principle: The organic compounds in the specimen matrix are completely destroyed by digestion with strong acid solutions. Arsenic in the digest is converted to the trivalent form and then liberated as arsine gas by treatment with zinc and hydrochloric acid. The arsine is chelated by diethyldithiocarbamate, forming a colored complex whose absorbance is measured in a spectrophotometer at 540 nm.

Apparatus:
1. Glass boiling beads
2. Hot plate
3. Generator flask (Fisher Scientific Co., Pittsburgh)
4. Ice bath
5. Spectrophotometer

Specimens:
1. Serum or whole blood, 10 ml
2. Urine, 24 hr specimen, 50 ml

Reagents:
1. Sulfuric acid, concentrated
2. Nitric acid, concentrated
3. Caprylic (octyl) alcohol
4. Perchloric acid
5. Arsenic standard, 2 μg/ml
   Dilute 0.5 ml stock solution (1 mg/ml) to 25 ml with water.
6. Hydrochloric acid, concentrated
7. Potassium iodide, 15%
   Dissolve 15 g potassium iodide in 1 dl water.
8. Stannous chloride, 40%
   Dissolve 40 g stannous chloride in 1 dl water.
9. Lead acetate, 10%
   Dissolve 10 g lead acetate in 1 dl water.
10. Color reagent
    Dissolve 250 mg silver diethyldithiocarbamate in 50 ml pyridine.
11. Zinc granules

Procedure:
1. In a 125 ml Erlenmeyer flask, place 50 ml urine or 10 ml serum (add an equal amount of water to the serum or whole blood).
2. Add 5 ml concentrated sulfuric acid and mix.
3. Add 20 ml concentrated nitric acid and mix.
4. Add 6-8 glass boiling beads and begin heating **gently** (a setting of 2 on a hot plate).

5. When the contents of the flasks have been gently boiling for a few minutes with no evidence of foaming, increase the heat gradually and boil until charring occurs. If excessive foaming occurs, add caprylic alcohol by drops until the foaming ceases.
6. When charring occurs, remove the flasks from the hot plate and allow to **cool** completely. Then add 10 ml nitric acid and 2 ml perchloric acid and return the flasks to the hot plate.
7. Boil until charring again occurs or, if no charring occurs, until the flask is filled with dense white fumes and the contents of the flask are clear or pale yellow-green.
8. If charring occurs, repeat steps 6 and 7.
9. When the flask has cooled, quantitatively transfer the contents to a generator flask and dilute to approximately 35 ml.
10. To another generator flask, add 1 ml arsenic standard (2 μg/ml) and 34 ml water.
11. To both flasks, add 5 ml concentrated hydrochloric acid and 2 ml of 15% potassium iodide.
12. Wait 1 min and then add 10 drops of 40% stannous chloride and mix. Place flasks in an ice bath for 15 min.
13. Assemble remaining portion of generator, placing glass wool in scrubber. Saturate glass wool with 10% lead acetate.
14. Place on generator flasks and support to avoid tipping.
15. After 15 min in the ice bath, add 3 ml color reagent to the reservoir of each generator.
16. Add zinc granules to the flask and allow gas to bubble through color reagent for 30 min.
17. Record the absorbance of the colored complex at 525 nm against the color reagent as a blank.

Calculation:
Urine:

$$\frac{\text{Absorbance of unknown}}{\text{Absorbance of standard}} \times 2 = \text{μg/50 ml urine}$$

$$\frac{\text{μg/50 ml urine}}{50} = \text{μg/ml urine}$$

Blood:

$$\frac{\text{Absorbance of unknown}}{\text{Absorbance of standard}} \times \frac{2}{10} = \text{Conc. of unknown (μg/ml)}$$

Interpretation: Arsenic is present in trace amounts in body tissues and fluids. Blood concentrations in healthy adults vary as a result of dietary (seafood contains relatively high concentrations of arsenic) and environmental influences and range from 0.002-0.062 μg/ml.[125] The largest source of arsenic exposure is occupational exposure from arsenic pesticides and herbicides. Workers using dimethylarsinic acid herbicide may display no symptoms of arsenic poisoning at blood concentrations as high as 0.27 μg/ml.[126] Arsenic toxicity is usually associated with blood concentrations of 0.5-1.0 μg/ml. Fatalities have occurred at concentrations ranging from 0.6-9.3 μg/ml.[127]

The kidney is the major route of excretion of arsenic. Urinary excretion of a single administered dose is complete within 6 days and accounts for 90% of the dose.[128] Urine arsenic concentrations in unexposed adults range from 0.01-0.30 µg/ml.[129] Concentrations in persons eating a diet high in seafood may be as high as 1-1.5 µg/ml.[129] Urine concentrations greater than 2 µg/ml may indicate arsenic exposure in persons who have no occupational association with arsenic. This concentration may be obtained with no symptoms of poisoning in industrial or agricultural workers.[130,131]

Lead in blood[132,133]

Principle: Lead is chelated in hemolyzed blood by ammonium pyrrolidinedithiocarbamate (APDC). The lead APDC is extracted into methylisobutylketone (MIBK), which is aspirated into an acetylene flame. An atomic vapor of lead is produced in the flame. The absorbance of the lead is determined in an atomic absorption spectrophotometer.

Apparatus:
1. Atomic absorption spectrophotometer with air-acetylene flame (analytic wavelength, 283.3 nm)
2. Lead-free, acid-washed glassware (test tubes and stoppers)
3. Lead hollow cathode lamp or electrolyte discharge lamp

Specimen: Whole blood, 5 ml, collected in lead-free, heparinized collection tube.

Reagents:
1. Triton X-100, 5%
   Prepare a 5% v/v solution with deionized water.
2. Ammonium pyrrolidinedithiocarbamate (APDC), 2%
   Prepare a solution of 2% w/v in 5% Triton X-100 and refrigerate. It will remain stable for 1 month.
3. Methylisobutylketone (MIBK), water saturated
4. Lead stock standard, 1000 µg/ml (purchase prepared)
   a. Intermediate working standard. Dilute stock standard to 50 µg/ml by adding 5 ml to a 1 dl volumetric flask and dilute to 1 dl.
   b. Working standards. Prepare in duplicate 25, 50, 75, and 100 µg/dl standards by adding 25, 50, 75, and 100 µl, respectively, of dilute stock standard (intermediate) to 1 ml deionized water. Two sets of duplicate blanks are also prepared with deionized water. To each of these tubes add 5 ml pooled whole blood.

Sample preparation: To a tube containing 1 ml deionized water, add 5 ml of the unknown whole blood specimen. Add 1 ml APDC solution to the unknown, blanks, and standard tubes and mix. Add 3 ml MIBK; stopper and shake vigorously about 60 times to ensure complete extraction. Centrifuge for 10 min at 2000 rpm.

Analytic procedure:

Instrument setup: Install the lead lamp in the lamp compartment. Turn the power switch on and adjust the cathode lamp source to the required current (10 mA). Set the analytic wavelength to 283.3 nm and maximize the lead line to obtain the maximal deflection of the energy needle. Then turn the gain so that the energy needle is at midscale. Install the standard air-acetylene burner head, and substitute an organic solvent cork gasket in the nebulizer port for the aqueous neoprene gasket. Turn on the compressed air and adjust the burner

regulator to 30 psi and the flowmeter to 50 psi. Open the valve on the acetylene tank and adjust the outflow pressure to 8 psi. Adjust the fuel flowmeter to 30 psi. Make sure that the loop in the burner drain tube is filled with water and that the end of the tube is at least 4 in. below the surface of the water in the waste receptacle to prevent flashback. Turn the air and acetylene switches on at the control unit. Activate the "gases on" switch and press "ignite" to light the flame. With the nebulizer aspirating distilled water, allow the flame to stabilize for 5 min. Then quickly switch from aspirating deionized water to aspirating saturated MIBK. The flame will become intensely yellow. Immediately, carefully turn the fuel mixture flow valve on the control unit clockwise to obtain a lean blue flame. Depress the sensor override switch on the gas control unit. If, when adjusting the flame, the burner goes out, immediately turn the gases off and wait 1 min before attempting to relight the flame. When the MIBK flame has stabilized, depress "auto zero" to zero the atomic absorption spectrophotometer in the absorbance mode.

Sample analysis: Aspirate each standard (blank and unknown). Allow the scale to maximize with "10 average" key depressed. When maximized, depress "100 average" key. Record absorbance. Depress the "10 average" key, replace capillary in water-saturated MIBK, and analyze the next sample when the display has returned to zero.

Calculation: Average four blank absorbance values to obtain the mean blank value. Subtract the average blank value from the absorbance of each standard to correct for any lead present in the pooled blood. Prepare a standard calibration curve by plotting the corrected absorbance against the concentration of the lead standards. Determine the concentrations of the unknown from the observed absorbance compared to the corresponding lead concentration on the calibration curve.

Interpretation: In healthy adults, normal blood lead concentrations range from 0.10-0.30 µg/ml, with 0.40 µg/ml considered the upper limit of normal. Concentrations exceeding 0.40 µg/ml may indicate abnormal exposure to lead. Toxicity is generally associated with concentrations of 0.60 µg/ml or greater. In children, normal blood lead concentrations range up to 0.20 µg/ml. If values of between 0.20-0.40 µg/ml are obtained, a second blood specimen should be drawn and analyzed. Concentrations of 0.30 µg/ml may indicate abnormal exposure, and concentrations of greater than 0.40 µg/ml may indicate toxicity for children. Such children should receive clinical attention.

Lead in urine[132]

Principle: See discussion of lead in blood.

Apparatus:
1. Atomic absorption spectrophotometer with air-acetylene flame (analytic wavelength, 283.3 nm)
2. Centrifuge
3. Lead-free, acid-washed glassware
4. pH meter with combination electrode

Specimens: Twenty-four hour urine specimen collected in lead-free collection vessel, 30 ml.

Reagents:
1. Hydrochloric acid, 6N

Add 498 ml concentrated hydrochloric acid to a 10 dl volumetric flask containing 3 dl water. Allow to cool and dilute to 1 L. Mix thoroughly.
2. Ammonium pyrrolidinedithiocarbamate (APDC), 2%
   See reagents list under discussion of lead in blood.
3. Triton X-100, 5%
   See reagents list under discussion of lead in blood.
4. Methylisobutylketone (MIBK), saturated
5. Stock standard, 1000 μg/ml (purchase prepared)
   a. Intermediate standard, 50 μg/ml. Add 5 ml stock standard to a 1 dl volumetric flask and dilute to 1 dl with water.
   b. Working standards. To each of five separately labeled 40 ml screw-topped, acid-washed tubes, add 30 ml deionized water that has been adjusted to a pH of 2.2-2.8 with 6N hydrochloric acid. Add 0, 25, 50, 100, and 300 μl of intermediate lead standard to the five tubes. These standards are equivalent to 0 (blank), 0.04, 0.08, 0.16, and 0.48 μg lead/ml, respectively.

Sample preparation: Transfer 30 ml urine to a 40 ml acid-washed, screw-topped tube and adjust the pH to 2.2-2.8 with hydrochloric acid. Determine the pH with a pH meter. Add 1 ml APDC to the blank, standards, and unknowns. Mix well. Add 3 ml MIBK, cap, and mix by inversion for 2 min. Centrifuge at 2000 rpm for 10 min. Transfer the organic phase (and emulsion layer, if present) to 10 × 100 mm tubes, using acid-washed transfer pipets. Stopper and centrifuge for 5 min.

Analytic procedure:

Instrument setup: Refer to setup under analytic procedure in discussion of lead in blood.

Sample analysis: Refer to sample analysis under analytic procedure in discussion of lead in blood.

Calculation: Average blank values to obtain a mean blank value. Subtract average blank value from each standard value to correct for any lead contamination in the water source or reagents. Prepare a standard curve by plotting the corrected absorbance against the concentration of the lead standards. Determine the concentration of the unknowns from the observed absorbance compared to the corresponding lead concentration on the calibration curve.

Interpretation: Urine lead concentrations vary greatly in healthy adults with a total of 0.08 mg in a 24 hr urine specimen as the upper limit of normal. In most adults a total of 0.15 mg in a 24 hr specimen is consistent with lead poisoning. A total of 0.1 mg indicates abnormal exposure.

Mercury in blood and urine[134]

Principle: Inorganic and organic mercury in blood or urine is reduced to elemental mercury by reaction with sodium borohydride in a sealed vessel. The released mercury vapor is flushed through the absorption cell of an atomic absorption spectrophotometer.

Apparatus:
1. Atomic absorption spectrophotometer with flow-through quartz absorption cell (analytic wavelength, 253.7 nm)
2. Mercury hollow cathode lamp
3. Reaction vessel. A reaction vessel and washing vessel are connected in series to the spectrophotometer absorption cell by polyvinyl chloride tubing. The vessels are made of 15 × 2.5 cm test tubes, and each inlet tube comes to within 0.5 cm of the bottom of the vessel and ends in a fine tip. The first vessel is initially empty, and the second contains 10 ml water and 3 drop of antifoam and is immersed in ice water. An air source capable of delivering a constant 3 L/min flow is connected to the inlet of the reaction vessel.

Reagents:
1. Antifoam (tri-*n*-butyl phosphate)
2. Borohydride reagent
   Dissolve 50 g sodium borohydride in 1 L of 4% sodium hydroxide.
3. Stock standard, 1 mg/ml (commercial source)
4. Working standard
   Prepare dilute stock standard by diluting 1.0 ml stock to 1 dl with water. Working standards of 0.1, 0.5, 1.0, and 2.0 ml of dilute stock standard are prepared by adding 0.10, 0.50, 1.0, and 2.0 ml of dilute stock standard to acid-washed 10 ml volumetric flasks and diluting to volume with distilled water.

Procedure: Samples should be analyzed in sequence: a blank, a standard, a blank, test specimen, etc. A reagent blank should be analyzed between each specimen or standard to monitor contamination from reagents, glassware, and residual mercury in the analytic apparatus. With the air flow off, transfer 2 ml of specimens to the reaction vessel. Add 3 ml water and 1 drop of antifoam and close the vessel with the stopper containing the inlet and outlet tubes. Inject 1 ml borohydride reagent through the rubber stopper of the reaction vessel by using a hypodermic syringe. Mix on a vortex mixer for 2 min. Turn on the air supply and read the absorbance peak of the mercury vapor as it passes through the absorption cell of the spectrophotometer. Clean the reaction vessel and flush the system with air before analyzing the next sample.

Calculation: Average the blank absorbance readings to obtain a mean blank value. Subtract the mean blank value from the absorbance of each standard. Prepare a standard curve by plotting the corrected absorbance against the concentration of the standard. Determine the concentration of the unknowns from the observed absorbance compared to the corresponding mercury concentration on the standard curve.

Interpretation: In healthy adults blood mercury concentrations range up to 0.020 μg/ml in persons with low fish consumption, up to 0.50 μg/ml in persons eating moderate amounts of fish, and up to 0.20 μg/ml in those whose diet is primarily predatory marine fish.[135] Toxicity may develop at concentrations exceeding 0.4 μg/ml. Lethal concentrations are generally greater than 1.0 μg/ml. Urine concentrations of 0.09-0.25 μg/ml are consistent with acute toxicity.[136] Normal urine concentrations in industrial workers range from 0.05-0.10 μg/ml.[137,138]

THERAPEUTIC DRUG MONITORING

Therapeutic drug monitoring (TDM) is the determination of plasma drug concentrations for those drugs that display a high degree of correlation between their plasma concentrations and their pharmacologic activity. Today TDM is a well-established adjunct to rational drug therapy. The biologic effects of drugs result from the interaction of the drug and an endogeneous tissue receptor that controls a particular response. The intensity of the response (pharmacologic activity) is proportional to the concentration of the drug at the receptor. This concentration is in equilibrium with drug concentrations in the extracellular fluid, which in turn is in equilibrium with the plasma drug concentration. Therefore the plasma concentration is an indirect measure of the concentration of drug interacting with the receptor and thus is related to the intensity of pharmacologic activity. Numerous factors influence the plasma drug concentration obtained following a given drug dosage. These factors include the rates of drug absorption, the distribution throughout body tissues and fluids, excretion, and biotransformation. The route of administration, the pharmaceutic formulation of the drug, the co-administration of other drugs, and the patient's age and health are important additional factors affecting plasma drug concentrations. Discussion of the pharmacokinetic basis of TDM is beyond the scope of this chapter; however, the interested reader may wish to consult references for additional information.[139-144] Laboratory personnel should be familiar with the following terms: plasma half-life, peak plasma concentration, and "steady state" concentration. The plasma half-life is the time required for a 50% decrease in plasma drug concentration. Peak plasma concentration is the maximal drug concentration obtained following a given dose of a drug. It is observed when the rate of drug absorption equals the rate of drug elimination. Steady state concentrations occur following long-term drug administration. When oral, long-term drug therapy is initiated, a drug will continue to accumulate in the body until the rate of elimination is equal to the rate of administration. The resultant plasma concentration is the steady state concentration for the drug. It generally requires four to seven drug half-lifes for this concentration to be obtained. The usual dosage, plasma half-lifes, and therapeutic steady state plasma concentrations of commonly monitored drugs are presented in Table 26-15.

Specimens for analysis should be collected just before the next scheduled administration of the drug. At this time the drug will be at its lowest plasma concentration. Monitoring will determine if this concentration is still therapeutically effective. If a toxic response occurs during the initial therapy, wait at least 4-8 hr before collecting a specimen. This is to allow adequate time for the complete drug absorption and distribution to the body tissues. If a specimen is collected before this time, a deceptively high concentration may be obtained, because the drug is not yet in equilibrium in the body tissues and fluids. At the initiation of drug therapy, wait the equivalent of at least five drug half-lifes to allow time for the steady state concentration to be obtained.

Plasma drug concentrations should be determined in the following situations: (1) after therapy is initiated and time has passed for the drug to achieve steady state concentrations, (2) when the patient responds inadequately or excessively to a standard recommended dosage, (3) following any change in drug source, dose, or dosage, (4) immediately after the appearance of symptoms of toxicity (excluding the initial drug dose), and (5) every 4-6 months, even in therapeutically responsive patients.

Analytic methods recommended for TDM include immunoassay technics, gas-liquid chromatography, and high-pressure liquid chromatography. Most clinical laboratories lack the necessary instrumentation and analytic expertise to apply the chromatographic methods. The immunoassay procedures are commercially available, self-contained kits (EMIT, Homogenous Enzyme Assays, Syva Corp., Palo Alto, Calif.; Radioimmunoassay, American Diagnostics Corp., Newport Beach, Calif.; Clinical Assays, Travenol Laboratories, Cambridge, Mass.; Wien Laboratories, Succasunna, N.J.). Presented below are several procedures that may be applied to the majority of TDM specimens. The required equipment is an ultraviolet spectrophotometer and a fluorometer.

PHENOBARBITAL

See discussion of barbiturates above for ultraviolet spectrophotometric procedure.

PHENYTOIN (DIPHENYLHYDANTOIN)[145-148]

Principle: Phenytoin is extracted from serum and oxidized to a benzophone derivative with sufficient ultraviolet absorbance ($E_{1\%} \sim 500$) to permit accurate determinations of the drug at therapeutic concentrations.

Apparatus:
1. Aeration manifold of glass tubing and rubber stoppers to fit the flasks (Attach the inlet to a source that will release a continuous flow of clean air.)
2. Centrifuge
3. Erlenmeyer flasks with 24/40 joints, 125 ml
4. Magnetic stirrer with hot plate
5. Reflux condenser with 24/40 joint
6. Tubes, screw-topped, 25 × 150 mm, or separatory funnels, 125 ml
7. Ultraviolet spectrophotometer
8. Water bath

Specimen: Plasma or serum, 5 ml.

Reagents:
1. Chloroform, ultraviolet spectrograde
2. Phenytoin stock standard, 80 μg/ml
   Dissolve 87.3 mg sodium phenytoin in water and dilute to 1 L.
3. Phenytoin working standard, 8 μg/ml
   Dilute 10.0 ml phenytoin stock standard to 1 dl with water.
4. *n*-Heptane
5. Phosphate buffer, pH 6.8
   Dissolve 13.6 g anhydrous potassium phosphate, monobasic, and 14.2 g anyhdrous sodium phosphate, diabasic, in water and dilute to 1 L.
6. Potassium permanganate, 5 g/dl

Table 26-15. Blood concentrations and pharmacologic parameters of some drugs associated with therapeutic monitoring

Pharmacologic indication (drug)	Drug or metabolite determined	Recommended dosage (mg/kg/day)	Plasma half-life (hr)	Therapeutic concentration (μg/ml)
Antidepressants				
Amitriptyline	Same	0.7-1.4	17-40	0.12-0.25
	Nortriptyline	0.7-1.4	18-93	0.05-0.150
Desipramine	Same	1-2	12-54	0.15-0.25
Doxepin	Same		12	0.200
	Desmethyl-doxepin		12	0.100
Imipramine	Same	0.7-1.4	9-24	0.15-0.25
	Desipramine	1-2	12-54	0.15-0.25
Nortriptyline	Same	0.7-1.4	18-93	0.05-0.150
Antiepileptics				
Carbamazepine	Same			
Adults		10-20	10-30	8-12
Children		15-30	8-19	8-12
	10,11-Epoxide carbamazepine			
Adults		—	5-16	0.2-20
Ethosuximide	Same			
Adults		10-30	40-60	40-100
Children		30-60	30-50	40-100
Phenobarbital	Same			
Adults		2-4	58-120	10-40
Children		4-8	40-70	10-30
Phenytoin	Same			
Adults		5-6	18-30	10-30
Children		5-10	12-22	10-30
Primidone	Same			
Adults		10-20	3-12	5-15
Children		15-30	4-6	5-12
	Phenobarbital			
Adults		—	50-120	12-40
Children		—	40-70	10-30
Valproic acid	Same			
Adults		30-60	8-15	50-100
Children		30-60	6-15	50-100
Antiarrhythmics				
Digoxin	Same	0.003-0.005	36-51	0.008-0.012
Disopyramide	Same	8.6	5-6	2-5
Lidocaine	Same	1.5 (IV load)	1-2	1.5-5
	Monoethylglycine-xylidide	—	Not established	
Procainamide	Same	32 mg	2-4	4-8
	N-Acetylprocainamide		3-6	2-6
Propranolol	Same	1-1.7	3-6	0.04-0.25
	4-Hydroxylpropanol		4-8	0.008-0.07
Quinidine	Same	10-20	2-5	3-6
Bronchodilator				
Theophylline	Same			
Adults		16-30	3-8	10-20
Children		25-40	1-8	10-20

Dissolve 25 g potassium permanganate in water and dilute to 5 dl.

7. Sodium hydroxide, 1N
   Dissolve 40 g sodium hydroxide in water and dilute to 1 L.
8. Sodium hydroxide, 9N
   Dissolve 360 g sodium hydroxide in water and dilute to 1 L.

Procedure: To a 25 × 150 mm screw-topped tube or to a 125 ml separatory funnel add 5 ml specimen. To a second tube or separatory funnel add 5 ml phenytoin reference standard. Add 5 ml phosphate buffer to each tube. Add 30 ml chloroform; then mix for 2 min.

Discard the upper layers. Filter the chloroform layers into clean tubes or separatory funnels. Add 6 ml of 1N sodium hydroxide and shake each mixture for 2 min. Aspirate and discard the lower layers. Centrifuge the aqueous layers.

Place 4 ml of each centrifugate into a 125 ml Erlenmeyer flask with 24/40 joint. Aerate the contents of each flask for 15 min at 60° C. Add 16 ml of 9N sodium hydroxide, 6 ml postassium permanganate, and 5 ml *n*-heptane. Reflux each mixture for 30 min, stirring continually. Prepare a heptane blank, refluxing *n*-heptane with potassium permanganate and sodium hydroxide in another flask. Cool the contents of each flask to room temperature before removing the condenser. Aspirate most of the lower layer from each flask; then transfer the *n*-heptane (upper) layers to stoppered 1 cm silica cells. Determine the absorbance of standards and unknown heptane solutions from 340-220 nm against the heptane blank. The oxidation product of phenytoin has an absorption maximum at 247 nm.

Calculation:

$$\frac{\text{Absorbance of standard}}{\text{Absorbance of unknown}} \times 8 =$$

Phenytoin concentration (μg/ml)

Interpretation: See Table 26-15.

PROCAINAMIDE AND N-ACETYLPROCAINAMIDE[149,150]

Principle: Procainamide and its metabolite are extracted from alkalinized plasma into toluene. After back extraction into aqueous acid the two substances are measured individually in the fluorometer at different pH values.

Apparatus: Fluorescence spectrophotometer.

| | **Analytic conditions** | |
	Excite	**Analyze**
N-acetylprocainamide	282 nm	340 nm
Procainamide	298 nm	358 nm

Specimen: Plasma or serum, 2 ml.
Reagents:
1. Extraction solvent (toluene–isoamyl alcohol [98.7:1.3])
2. Hydrochloric acid, 0.1N
   Dilute 8.25 ml concentrated hydrochloric acid to 1 L with water.
3. Sodium chloride, solid
4. Sodium hydroxide, 20%

Dissolve 20 g sodium hydroxide in 1 dl water.
5. Stock standards
   a. Procainamide, 1 mg/ml. Dissolve 100 mg procainamide in 1 dl methanol.
   b. *N*-Acetylprocainamide (NAPA), 1 mg/ml. Dissolve 100 mg NAPA in 1 dl methanol.
6. Working plasma standards
   Prepare a working stock standard of 0.1 mg/ml by dissolving 10 ml of each stock standard in 1 dl methanol. Prepare working standards of 2, 5, and 10 μg/ml of procainamide and NAPA by adding 20, 50, and 100 μl of the working stock standard to a 5 ml volumetric flask and diluting with drug-fee plasma or serum (obtained data specimens for blood bank).

Procedure: Transfer 2 ml serum to a 15 ml screw-topped tube. Add about 250 mg sodium chloride and 0.25 ml of 20% sodium hydroxide and mix on a vortex mixer. Add 10 ml extraction solvent and shake for 30 sec. Centrifuge and transfer 8 ml of the solvent layer to a clean tube. Add 3 ml of 0.1N hydrochloric acid and shake to extract. Centrifuge and transfer 2.5 ml of the aqueous layer to a quartz cuvet. Determine *N*-acetylprocainamide by reading the fluorometer against a plasma blank under the specified conditions above. Add 0.1 ml of 20% sodium hydroxide to each cuvet and mix. Determine procainamide by reading the fluorometer against a plasma blank under the conditions above.

Calculation: Prepare a standard curve for procainamide and *N*-acetylprocainamide by plotting the fluorometer readings for each against the concentrations of their respective standards. Determine the concentrations of the unknowns for the observed fluorometer reading compared to the corresponding procainamide and NAPA concentrations on the calibration curve.

SERUM QUINIDINE[151]

Principle: An organic base, quinine, or its analog, quinidine, can be extracted from an alkaline solution of the biologic matrix. Reextraction of this extract into dilute acid produces a solution whose emission fluorescence spectrum can be used to identify and quantitate either drug.

Apparatus: Spectrophotofluorometer.
Specimen: Serum, 1 ml.
Reagents:
1. Buffer solution, pH 8.5
   Dissolve 53.3 g ammonium chloride in 950 ml water. Add 10 ml concentrated ammonium hydroxide and adjust the pH to 8.5 with ammonium hydroxide or hydrochloric acid.
2. Chloroform–isopropyl alcohol mixture (3:1)
   Mix 3 volumes of chloroform with 1 volume of isopropyl alcohol.
3. Sulfuric acid, 0.1N
   Dilute 2.8 ml concentrated sulfuric acid to 1 L with water.
4. Quinine sulfate stock solution
   Dissolve 1 g quinine sulfate in 1 L water.
5. Quinine standards (1.0 and 0.5 mg/dl quinine sulfate)
   a. Quinine sulfate, 1.0 mg/dl or 10 μg/ml. Dilute 100 μl stock solution to 10 ml with water.

b. Quinine sulfate, 0.5 mg/dl or 5 μg/ml. Dilute 50 μl stock solution to 10 ml with water.

Procedure: In appropriately labeled screw-topped tubes add 100 μl water for blank, 100 μl of 1.0 mg/dl standard, 100 μl of 0.5 mg/dl standard, 100 μl control sera for quality control, and 100 μl test sera. To all tubes add 1 ml buffer and 10 ml solvent mixture. Place on a mechanical shaker for 10 min. Centrifuge for 5 min. With a volumetric pipet, transfer 4 ml of the solvent layer from each tube to a clean, labeled, screw-topped tube. To each tube add 3 ml of 0.1N sulfuric acid; shake by hand for 90 sec and centrifuge. With the spectrofluorometer set at 365 nm excitation and 440 nm emission, adjust the blank to zero, 1.0 mg/dl standard to 100, and 0.5 mg/dl to 50. Read control and tests. Then determine the relative fluorescence of the unknown by recording the fluorometric reading.

Calculation:

$$\frac{\text{Relative fluorescence of unknown}}{10} =$$

$$\text{Concentration of quinidine (μg/ml)}$$

THEOPHYLLINE[152]

Apparatus: Ultraviolet recording spectrophotometer.
Specimen: Serum or plasma, 3 ml.
Reagents:
1. Chloroform-isopropanol (95:5)
   Add 50 ml isopropanol to 950 ml chloroform and mix.
2. Phosphate buffer, 0.5M, pH 7.4.
   Dissolve 69 g sodium phosphate in water and dilute to 1 L.
3. Sodium hydroxide, 0.1N
   Dissolve 4 g sodium hydroxide in water and dilute to 1 L.
4. Ammonium chloride, 2M
   Dissolve 11.7 g ammonium chloride in water and dilute to 1 dl.
5. Theophylline stock standard, 1 mg/ml
   Dissolve 100 mg theophylline in 1 dl reagent alcohol.
6. Theophylline working standard
   a. Theophylline, 10 μg/ml. Dilute 0.1 ml stock to 10 ml with water.
   b. Theophylline, 20 μg/ml. Dilute 0.1 ml stock to 5 ml with water.

Procedure: To separate screw-topped tubes add 3 ml water for blank, 3 ml of each standard, and 3 ml test serum. To each tube add 2 ml phosphate buffer and 30 ml chloroform-isopropanol mixture. Shake for 5 min and centrifuge. Aspirate off and discard aqueous (upper) layer. Filter the solvent through Whatman no. 2 filter paper into a graduated cylinder. To separate, clean test tubes transfer 25 ml of each solvent extract. Add 3 ml of 0.1N sodium hydroxide. Shake for 5 min and centrifuge. Transfer 2 ml of the aqueous (upper) layers to separate test tubes and add 0.1 ml of 2M ammonium chloride. Mix. Scan the standards and serum extracts from 320-220 nm against a blank. Record the absorbance at 300 nm and 275 nm.

Calculation: Subtract the absorbance at 300 nm from

the absorbance at 275 nm to get the corrected absorbance.

$$K = \frac{\text{Conc. of standard}}{\text{Corrected absorbance at 275 nm}}$$

K × Corrected absorbance of test = Theophylline (μg/ml)

Interferences: Phenylbutazone and the sulfonamides are weakly acidic ultraviolet-absorbing drugs and may produce an overlapping spectrum. However, it is not likely that they would be co-administered with theophylline. Phenobarbital and caffeine do not interfere with this method.

THIOPENTAL[153]

Apparatus: Ultraviolet spectrophotometer.
Specimens:
1. Serum or plasma, 5 ml.
2. Urine, 5 ml.
Reagents:
1. Chloroform
2. Sodium hydroxide, 0.5N
   Dissolve 20 g sodium hydroxide in 1 L water.
3. Buffer (1.5M sodium dihydrogen phosphate)
   Dissolve 20.8 g sodium dihydrogen phosphate in water and dilute to 1 dl.
4. Sulfuric acid, 50%
5. Stock standard
   Dilute 100 mg/dl in ethanol.
6. Working standards
   a. For 1 μg/ml dilute 10 μl stock to 10 ml in water.
   b. For 5 μg/ml dilute 50 μl stock to 10 ml in water.
   c. For 10 μg/ml dilute 100 μl stock to 10 ml in water.

Procedure: In appropriately labeled 40 ml screw-topped tubes add 5 ml water for blank, 5 ml of each standard, and 5 ml of each unknown. To all tubes add 30 ml chloroform. Shake for 10 min and centrifuge. Remove aqueous (upper) layer from each tube and discard. To each tube add 15 ml phosphate buffer. Shake for 3 min and centrifuge. Remove aqueous (upper) layer from each tube and discard. Filter the chloroform into separately labeled 25 ml graduated cylinders. Collect 25 ml and transfer to clean, labeled 40 ml screw-topped tubes. To blank add 8 ml of 0.5N sodium hydroxide and to each of the other tubes add 4 ml of 0.5N sodium hydroxide. Shake for 5 min and centrifuge. Remove the aqueous phase and scan against a 3 ml aliquot of the blank from 320-220 nm. Record the absorbance at 305 nm. To a 3 ml aliquot of blank add 4 drops of 50% sulfuric acid. Add 4 drops of 50% sulfuric acid to test or standard solutions. Rescan and record the absorbance of the acid solution at 305 nm. Repeat for all standards and unknowns.

Calculation: To calculate the change in absorbance (ΔA), subtract the absorbance of the acid solution from the absorbance of the basic solution at 305 nm.

$$\frac{\text{Concentration of standard}}{\Delta A \text{ of standard}} = K$$

Concentration of unknown = K × ΔA of unknown

Interpretation: Within the last few years, high-dosage barbiturate therapy has become a useful adjunct in the control of intracranial hypertension that is refractory to other methods of therapy.[154] Patients suffering from head injury, subarachnoid hemorrhage, intracranial hemorrhage, Reye's syndrome, and viral, metabolic, or posthypoxic encephalopathies may be candidates for high-dosage barbiturate therapy. Pentobarbital (see discussion of barbiturates) and thiopental are two barbiturates commonly employed in this treatment. Plasma pentobarbital concentrations range greatly, from 15-30 μg/ml. Plasma thiopental concentrations vary greatly, from 20-50 μg/ml. It should be noted that these concentrations are generally considered lethal; however, all patients receiving this therapy are on respirators and are closely monitored.

REFERENCES

1. O'Brien, J.P.: Arch. Gen. Psychiatry **34**:1165, 1977.
2. Walberg, C.B., Pantilik, V.A., and Lundberg, G.D.: Clin. Chem. **24**:507, 1978.
3. Bailey, D.N., and Guba, J.J.: J. Anal. Toxicol. **3**:133, 1979.
4. Poklis, A., and Gantner, G.E.: Mo. Med. **76**:588, 1979.
5. Bailey, D.N., and Manoguerra, A.S.: J. Anal. Toxicol. **4**:199, 1980.
6. Bailey, D.N.: J. Anal. Toxicol. **4**:204, 1980.
7. Berry, D.J., and Grove, J.: In Sunshine, I., editor: Methodology for analytical toxicology, Cleveland, 1975, CRC Press, p. 13.
8. Fujiwara, K.: Abhandl. Naturforsch. Ges. Rostock. **6**:33, 1914.
9. Kaye, S., and Goldbaum, L.: In Gradwohl, R.B.H., editor: Legal medicine, St. Louis, 1954, The C.V. Mosby Co., p. 620.
10. Fiorese, F.F., and Carella, T.: Riv. Clin. Tossicol. **1**:51, 1971.
11. Forrest, F.M., Forrest, I.S., and Mason, A.S.: Am. J. Psychiatry **118**:300, 1961.
12. Forrest, F.M., Forrest, I.S., and Mason, A.S.: Am. J. Psychiatry **116**:1021, 1960.
13. Forrest, I.S., and Forrest, F.M.: Clin. Chem. **6**:362, 1960.
14. Forrest I.S., Forrest F.M., and Kanter, S.L.: Clin. Chem. **12**:379, 1966.
15. Frings, C.S.: CRC Crit. Rev. Clin. Lab. Sci. **4**:357, 1973.
16. Forrest, F.M., and Forrest, I.S.: Am. J. Psychiatry **113**:931, 1957.
17. Forrest, F.M., and Forrest, I.S.: Am. J. Psychiatry **114**:931, 1958.
18. Forrest, I.S., Forrest, F.M., and Mason, A.S.: Am. J. Psychiatry **116**: 928, 1960.
19. Trinder, P.: Biochem. J. **57**:301, 1954.
20. Leonards, J.R.: Clin. Pharmacol. Ther. **5**:476, 1963.
21. Done, A.K.: Pediatrics **26**:800, 1960.
22. Levy, G., Tsuchiya, T., and Amsel, L.P.: Clin. Pharmacol. Ther. **13**:258, 1972.
23. Davidow, B., Petri, N.L., and Quame, B.: Am. J. Clin. Pathol. **38**:714, 1966.
24. Fujimoto, J.M., and Wang, J.H.: Toxicol. Appl. Pharmacol. **16**:186, 1970.
25. Clarke, E.C.G.: Isolation and identification of drugs, London, 1969, Pharmaceutical Press, p. 43.
26. Treiber, L.R.: In Sunshine, I., editor: Handbook series in clinical laboratory science, section B: toxicology, Cleveland, 1978, CRC Press, p. 157.
27. Cochin, J.: Psychopharmacol. Bull. **3**:53, 1966.
28. Berry, D.J., and Grove, J.: J. Chromatogr. **80**:205, 1973.
29. Drug Screen II Procedure Manual, Westbury, N.Y., 1978, Eppendorf-Brinkman, Inc.
30. Mule, S.J., et al.: J. Chromatogr. **63**:289, 1971.
31. Meola, A., and Vanko, J.: Clin. Chem. **20**:184, 1974.
32. Freimuth, H.C.: In Sunderman, F.W., and Sunderman, F.W., Jr., editors: Laboratory diagnosis of diseases caused by toxic agents, St. Louis, 1970, Warren H. Green, Inc., p. 90.
33. Monforte, J., Bath, R.J., and Sunshine, I.: Clin. Chem. **18**:1329, 1972.
34. Van Hoof, F., and Heyndrickx, A.: Anal. Chem. **46**:286, 1974.
35. Hudson, J.C., and Rice, W.P.: J. Chromatogr. **117**:449, 1976.
36. Dal Cortivo, L.A., De Mayo, M.M., and Weinberg, S.B.: Anal. Chem. **42**:941, 1970.
37. Matuisak, W., and Dal Cortivo, L.A.: One hundred fifty-sixth National Meeting of the American Chemical Society, Atlantic City, N.J., September 1968.
38. Monforte, J., and Turk, R.F.: In Sunshine, I., editor: Methodology for analytical toxicology, Cleveland, 1975, CRC Press, p. 267.
39. Ragland, J.B., and Kinross-Wright, V.J.: Anal. Chem. **36**:1356, 1964.
40. Tompsett, S.L.: Acta Pharmacol. **26**:303, 1968.
41. Pacha, W.L.: Experientia **25**:103, 1969.
42. de Silva, J.A.F., et al.: Anal. Chem. **36**:2099, 1964.
43. Schuetz, H.: J. Anal. Toxicol. **2**:147, 1978.
44. Poklis, A.: J. Anal. Toxicol. **5**:174, 1981.
45. Palermo, S.F., and Poklis, A.: Can. Soc. Forensic Sci. J. **10**:77, 1977
46. Bastos, M.L., Jukofsky, D., and Mule, S.J.: J. Chromatogr. **89**:335, 1974.
47. Woods, L.A., McMahon, F.G., and Seevers, M.H.: J. Pharmacol. Exp. Ther. **101**:200, 1951.
48. Fish, F., and Wilson, W.D.C.: J. Pharm. Pharmacol. **21**:135S, 1969.
49. Heyndrickx, A., and deLeenheer, A.: J. Eur. Toxicol. **1**:56, 1969.
50. Sleeman, H.K., et al.: Clin. Chem. **21**:76, 1975.
51. Bonnichsen, R., et al.: Clin. Chim. Acta **60**:67, 1975.
52. Curry, A.: Poison detection in human organs, Ed. 3, Springfield, Ill., 1975, Charles C Thomas, Publisher, p. 74.
53. Mule, S.J.: J. Chromatogr. **12**:245, 1974.
54. Boerner, U., Abbott, S., and Roe, R.L.: Drug Metab. Rev. **4**:39, 1975.
55. Yeh, S.Y.: J. Pharmacol. Exp. Ther. **192**:201, 1975.
56. Fish, F., and Hayes, T.D.: J. Forensic Sci. **19**:676, 1974.
57. Conway, E.J.: Microdiffusion analysis and volumetric error, London, 1950, Crosley, Lockwood and Sons.
58. Feldstein, M., and Klendshoj, N.C.: J. Forensic Sci. **2**:39, 1957.
59. Sunshine, I.: Handbook of analytical toxicology, Cleveland, 1969, CRC Press, p. 1015.
60. Feldstein, M.: In Stewart, C.P., and Stolman, A., editors: Toxicology mechanisms and analytical methods, New York, 1960, Academic Press, vol. 1, p. 639.
61. Feldstein, M.: In Stewart, C.P., and Stolman, A., editors: Toxicology mechanisms and analytical methods, New York, 1960, Academic Press, vol. 1, p. 463.
62. Siek, T.J.: J. Forensic Sci. **19**:193, 1974.
63. Siek, T.J., and Osiewiez, R.J.: J. Forensic Sci. **20**:18, 1975.
64. Dubowski, K.M.: In Sunshine, I., editor: Methodology for analytical toxicology, Cleveland, 1975, CRC Press, p. 149.

65. Jain, N.C., and Cravey, R.H.: J. Chromatogr. Sci. **10**:262, 1972.
66. Kozelka, F.L., and Hine, C.H.: Ind. Eng. Anal. Ed. **13**:905, 1941.
67. McConnell, W.B.: Am. J. Clin. Pathol. **22**:1223, 1952.
68. Bonnichsen, R., and Theorell, H.: Scand, J. Clin. Lab. Invest. **3**:58, 1951.
69. Bucher, T., and Redetzki, H.: Klin. Wochenschr. **29**:615, 1951.
70. Vasiliades, J., Pollack, J., and Robinson, C.A.: Clin. Chem. **24**:383, 1978.
71. Barron, E.S.G., and Levine, S.: Arch. Biochem. **41**:175, 1952.
72. Poklis, A., and Mackell, M.A.: J. Anal. Toxicol. **3**:183, 1979.
73. Poklis, A., and Mackell, M.A.: Clin. Chem. **27**:1106, 1981.
74. Harger, R.N., Hulpieu, H.R., and Lamb, E.B.: J. Biol. Chem. 120:689, 1937.
75. Harger, R.N.: In Stewart, C.P., and Stolman, A., editors: Toxicology mechanism and analytical methods, New York, 1961, Academic Press, Inc., vol. 2, p. 85.
76. Harger, R.N., and Forney, R.B.: In Stolman, A., editor: Progress in chemical toxicology, New York, 1961, Academic Press, Inc., vol. 1, p. 54.
77. Widmark, E.M.P.: Die theoretischen Grundlagen und die partische Verwendbarkeit der gerichtlich-medizinschen Alkolbestimmung, Berlin, 1932, Verlag Urban & Schwarzenberg.
78. Gruner, O.: Deutsch. Z. Ges. Gerichtl. Med. **46**:10, 1957.
79. Lundquist, F.: Acta Pharmacol. Toxicol. (Copenh.) **18**:231, 1961.
80. Alcohol and the impaired driver, Chicago, 1968, American Medical Association.
81. Hindberg, S.J., and Weith, J.O.: J. Lab. Clin. Med. **61**:355, 1963.
82. Baselt, R.C.: Disposition of toxic drugs and chemicals in man, Davis, Calif., 1978, Biomedical Publications, vol. 2, p. 154.
83. Eriksen, S.P., and Kulkarni, A.B.: Science **141**:639, 1963.
84. Makar, A.B., and Tephly, T.R.: J. Toxicol. Environ. Health **2**:1201, 1977.
85. Roe, O.: Acta Med. Scand. **9**:182S, 1946.
86. Weith, O.J.: J.A.M.A. **88**:2013, 1927.
87. Sunshine, I., editor: Manual of analytical toxicology, Cleveland, 1971, CRC Press, p. 56.
88. Kaye, S.: Handbook of emergency toxicology, ed. 3, Springfield, Ill., 1970, Charles C Thomas, publisher, p. 38.
89. Berka, I.: Acta Med. Scand. **157**:129, 1957.
90. Tietz, N.W., and Fiereck, E.A.: Ann. Clin. Lab. Sci. **3**:36, 1973.
91. Maehly, A.: In Lundquist, F., editor: Methods of forensic science, New York, 1962, John Wiley & Sons, Inc., vol. 1, p. 539.
92. Wawschinek, O., Paletta, H., and Beyer, W.: Arch. Toxicol. **23**:52, 1968.
93. Rieders, F.: In Sunshine, I., editor: Methodology for analytical toxicology, Cleveland, 1975, CRC Press, p. 114.
94. Ballantyne, B.: Forensic toxicology, Bristol, England, 1974, John Wright & Sons Ltd., p. 99.
95. Polson, C.J., and Tattersall, R.N.: Clinical toxicology, Philadelphia, 1969, J.B. Lippincott Co., p. 143.
96. Goldbau, L.R.: Clin. Toxicol. **17**:319, 1980.
97. Wallace, J.E., Blum, K., and Singh, J.M.: In Singh, J.M., and Lal, H., editors: Drug Addiction, Miami, Beach, Fla., 1974, Symposia Specialists, vol. 4, p. 175.

98. Welch, R.M., and Conney, A.H.: Clin. Chem. **11**:1064, 1965.
99. Peterson, R.G., and Rumack, B.H.: J.A.M.A. **237**:2406, 1977.
100. Wallace, J.E., and Dahl, E.V.: J. Forensic Sci. **12**:484, 1967.
101. Broughton, P.M.G.: Biochem. J. **63**:207, 1956.
102. Goldbaum, L.R.: Anal. Chem. **24**:1604, 1952.
103. Cabana, B.E.: Anal. Chem. **39**:1449, 1967.
104. Baselt, R.C.: Drug disposition of toxic drugs and chemicals in man, Canton, Conn., 1978, Biomedical Publications, vol. 1, p. 277.
105. Kaplan, H.L., et al.: J. Forensic Sci. **12**:295, 1967.
106. Andryauskas, S., Matusiak, W., and Dal Cortivo, L.A.: Int. Microfilm J. Legal Med., vol. 2, card 4, 1967.
107. Maes, R., et al.: J. Forensic Sci. **14**:235, 1969.
108. Cummins, L.M., Martin, Y.C., and Scherfling, E.E.: J. Pharm. Sci. **60**:261, 1971.
109. Roche Laboratories Products Reference Manual, Nutley, N.J., 1970, Roche Laboratories.
110. Randall, L.O.: Arch. Int. Pharmacol. Ther. **106**:388, 1956.
111. Bailey, D.N., and Jatlow, P.I.: Clin. Toxicol. **6**:563, 1973.
112. Hoffman, A.J., and Ludwig, B.J.: J. Am. Pharm. Assoc. **48**:740, 1959.
113. Hollister, L.E., and Levy, G.: Chemotherapy **9**:20, 1964.
114. Maddock, R.K., and Bloomer, H.A.: J.A.M.A. **210**:999, 1967.
115. Bailey, D.N., and Jatlow, P.I.: Clin. Chem. **19**:615, 1973.
116. McBay, A.J., et al.: J. Forensic Sci. **19**:18, 1974.
117. Verebely, K., and Inturrisi, C.E.: Clin. Pharmacol. Ther. **15**:302, 1974.
118. McBay, A.J.: Clin. Chem. **22**:1319, 1976.
119. Keenan, R.G., et al.: Indust. Hyg. J. **12**:481, 1963.
120. Kahn, H.L.: In Advances in chemistry series, no. 73, Washington, D.C., 1968, American Chemical Society, p. 183.
121. Kaye, S.A.: Am. J. Clin. Pathol. **14**:83, 1944.
122. Gettler, A.O., and Kaye, S.A.: J. Lab. Clin. Med. **35**:146, 1950.
123. Hoffman, L., and Gordon, A.D.: J. Assoc. Off. Agric. Chem. **46**:245, 1963.
124. George, G.M., Frahm, L.J., and McDonnell, J.P.: J. Assoc. Off. Anal. Chem. **56**:793, 1973.
125. Heydorn, K.: Clin. Chim. Acta **28**:349, 1970.
126. Wagner, S.L., and Weswig, P.: Arch. Environ. Health **28**:77, 1974.
127. Rehlig, C.J.: In Stolman, A., editor: Progress in chemical toxicology, New York, 1967, Academic Press, Inc., vol. 3, p. 363.
128. Hunter, F.T., Skip, A.F., and Irvine, J.W., Jr.: J. Pharm. Exp. Ther. **76**:207, 1977.
129. Schrenk, J.J., and Shreibers, L., Jr.: Am. Indust. Hyg. Assoc. J. **19**:225, 1958.
130. Pinto, S.S., and Nelson, K.W.: Ann. Rev. Pharm. **16**:95, 1976.
131. Tarrant, R.F., and Allard, J.: Arch. Environ. Health **24**:227, 1972.
132. Pierce, J.O., and Cholak, J.: Arch. Environ. Health **13**:208, 1966.
133. Hessel, D.W.: At. Absorption Newsletter **7**:55, 1968.
134. Baselt, R.C.: Biological monitoring methods for industrial chemicals, Davis, Calif., 1980, Biomedical Publications, p. 181.
135. Clarkson, T.W.: In Brown, S.S., editor: Clinical chemistry and chemical toxicology of metals, New York, 1977, Elsevier Scientific Publishing Co., Inc., p. 189.

136. Gerstner, H.G., and Huff, J.E.: Clin. Toxicol. **11**:131, 1977.
137. Dreisbach, R.H.: Handbook of poisoning: diagnosis and treatment, ed. 6, Los Altos, Calif., 1969, Lange Medical Publications, p. 183.
138. Nakayama, E., Momotaru, H., and Ishizu, S.: In Brown, S.S., editor: Clinical chemistry and chemical toxicology of metals, New York, 1977, Elsevier Scientific Publishing Co., Inc., p. 209.
139. Lab. Med. **11**(12)(special issue), December 1980.
140. Kalman, S.M., and Clark, D.R.: Drug assay: the strategy of therapeutic drug monitoring, New York, 1979, Masson.
141. Pippenger, C.E., Penry, J.K., and Kutt, H.: Antiepileptic drugs: quantitative analysis and interpretation, New York, 1978, Raven Press.
142. Werner, M., Sutherland, E.W., and Abramson, F.P.: Clin. Chem. **21**:1368, 1975.
143. Avery, G.S.: Drug treatment principles and practice of clinical pharmacology and therapeutics, Sydney, Australia, 1976, Adis Press.
144. Melmon, K.L., and Morelli, H.J.: Clinical pharmacology: basic principles in therapeutics, ed. 2, New York, 1978, MacMillan Publishing Co.
145. Wallace, J.E., Biggs, J.D., and Dahl, E.V.: Anal. Chem. **37**:410, 1965.
146. Wallace, J.E.: J. Forensic Sci. **11**:552, 1966.
147. Wallace, J.E.: Clin. Chem. **15**:323, 1969.
148. Wallace, J.E.: J. Pharm. Sci. **63**:1795, 1974.
149. Matusik, E., and Gibson, T.P.: Clin. Chem. **21**:1899, 1975.
150. Baselt, R.C.: Analytical procedures for therapeutic drug monitoring and emergency toxicology, Davis, Calif., 1980, Biomedical Publications.
151. Mule, S.S., and Hushin, P.L.: Anal. Chem. **43**:708, 1971.
152. Jatlow, P.: Clin. Chem. **21**:1518, 1975.
153. Sunshine, I., editor: Methodology for analytical toxicology, Cleveland, 1975, CRC Press, p. 373.
154. Dalessio, D.J.: J.A.M.A. **243**:2195, 1980.

CHAPTER 27

Urinalysis

STRUCTURE OF KIDNEY AND FORMATION OF URINE

Urine, the liquid excreted by the kidneys, contains water and various metabolic end products: urea from deaminated amino acids, uric acid from the breakdown of purines, creatinine from muscle breakdown, and porphyrins and their precursors from heme synthesis. Other end products are derived from the catabolism of hormones, drugs, and foreign chemicals. The kidney is also an endocrine organ producing renin and the erythropoietic factor.

The composition of the urine not only reflects the state of the kidneys (physiologic or pathologic) but also changes in the acid-base and electrolyte balance and in the metabolism of hormones, carbohydrates, proteins, salts, and many other physiologic and nonphysiologic substances and drugs.

Bisecting the kidney along its long axis reveals its essential gross anatomic features (Fig. 27-1). The outer layer of the parenchyma is the cortex, which houses the glomeruli, the short loops of Henle, and the supporting vascular network. The inner layer forms the medulla and the pyramids, which house the long loops of Henle, and the collecting ducts, which drain into the renal pelvis. The ureter guides the urine into the bladder, where it is temporarily stored and then eliminated via the urethra.

The functional unit of the kidney is the **nephron,** of which there are about 1 million in each human kidney. The nephron, which is best studied by light and electron microscopy, is composed of a vascular tuft (the glomerulus) and a fluid-collecting and -modifying apparatus (Bowman's capsule and the tubules) (Fig. 27-2). The glomerulus consists of a network of capillaries that invaginates the blind end of the nephron to create Bowman's capsule, the double-walled slitlike space of which marks the beginning of the proximal convoluted tubule. The afferent arteriole carries blood from the renal artery to the glomerular capillary network, which is drained by the efferent arterioles, the diameter of which is smaller than that of the afferent vessels. The efferent arterioles break up into the peritubular capillaries, which cuff the tubules and rejoin to drain into the renal vein. The pressure differential between the afferent and efferent arterioles is responsible for the filtra-

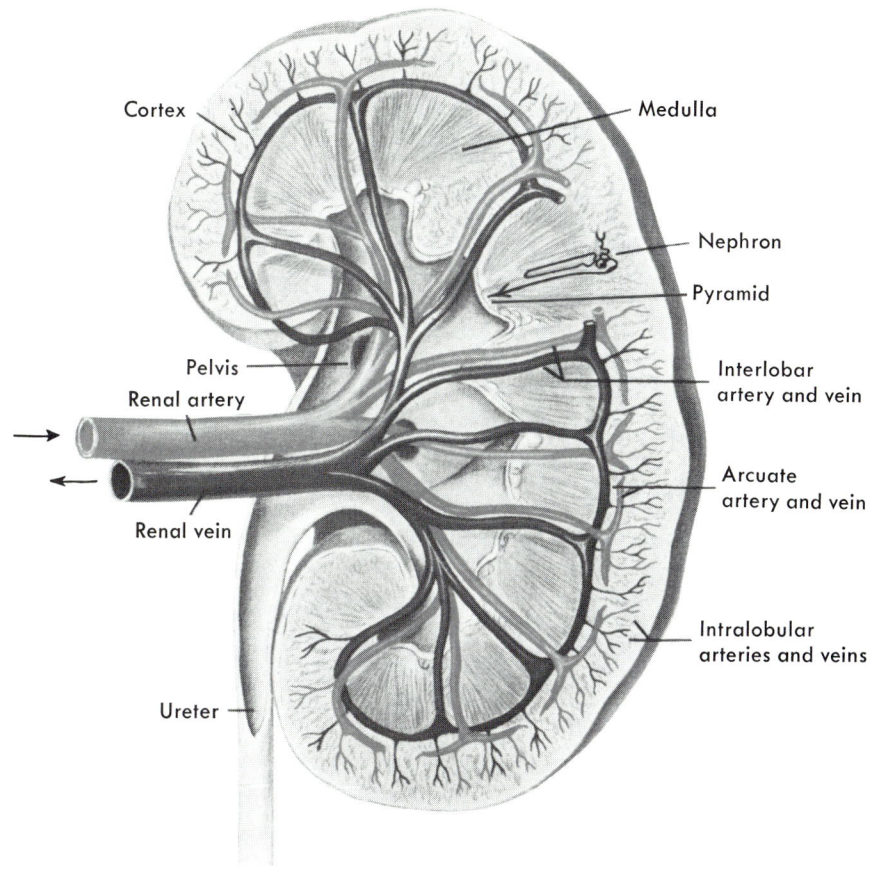

Fig. 27-1. Anatomy of the kidney. (From Medical Department, G.D. Searle & Co.: Research **40**:3, 1955.)

tion and escape of fluid from the plasma within the glomerular capillaries into Bowman's space, thus producing the glomerular filtrate. The proximal convoluted tubule guides the glomerular filtrate into the straight, thin descending limb of **Henle's loop,** which after dipping into the medulla curves upward and returns toward the cortex as the thin ascending limb of the loop of Henle. Before it connects with the distal convoluted tubules, it dilates to form the thick ascending limb of the loop of Henle. The distal convoluted tubules of neighboring glomeruli join to form collecting ducts that traverse the medulla and discharge their contents into the renal pelvis at the tip of the pyramids.

The **formation of urine** begins with the filtration of the blood plasma through the glomerular capillaries. As the filtrate flows down the tubules it is concentrated, and its composition is altered by resorption (transfer) of substances from the tubules into the peritubular capillaries and stroma and by active secretion of substances into the tubular lumina. The **glomerular filtrate** is the result of the interaction of the permeability of the glomerular capillary and of the opposing hydrostatic and osmotic pressures within the capillary and Bowman's capsule. The hydrostatic pressure in the capillary is about 75 mm Hg, which is opposed by 25 mm Hg osmotic pressure in the capillary and by 20 mm Hg hydrostatic pressure and 0 mm Hg osmotic pressure in

Bowman's capsule and the adjoining tubule.[1] Thus the net filtration pressure in the afferent capillary is about 25 mm Hg.

One liter of blood is filtered each minute, giving a glomerular filtration rate of 120 ml/min. The glomerular filtration rate is controlled by a number of factors, e.g., plasma flow, blood pressure, anatomic changes within the arterioles, number of glomeruli functioning at any given time, and resistance to tubular flow.[2] The glomerular filtrate has the same composition as the blood plasma, except that it is essentially protein free except for less than 1% albumin. It contains about 100 mg/dl glucose, 150 mEq/L sodium, 15 mg/dl urea, and 1 mg/dl creatinine. As the glomerular filtrate passes down the tubules, various substances are absorbed by the tubular lining cells, whereas others are added to the filtrate by tubular secretion, so that the concentration of solvents in the urinary end product is quite different from the concentration of solvents in the glomerular filtrate. The secretion or absorption of solvents is accomplished by passive diffusion along gradients or by active transport against such gradients.[1] Up to 80% of the glomerular filtrate is absorbed by the proximal tubules. Sodium, chloride, and water diffuse passively into the tubular lining cells, but sodium is actively transported into the intercellular space.[2] Water and chlorides follow passively. The absorbed salt and water reach the peri-

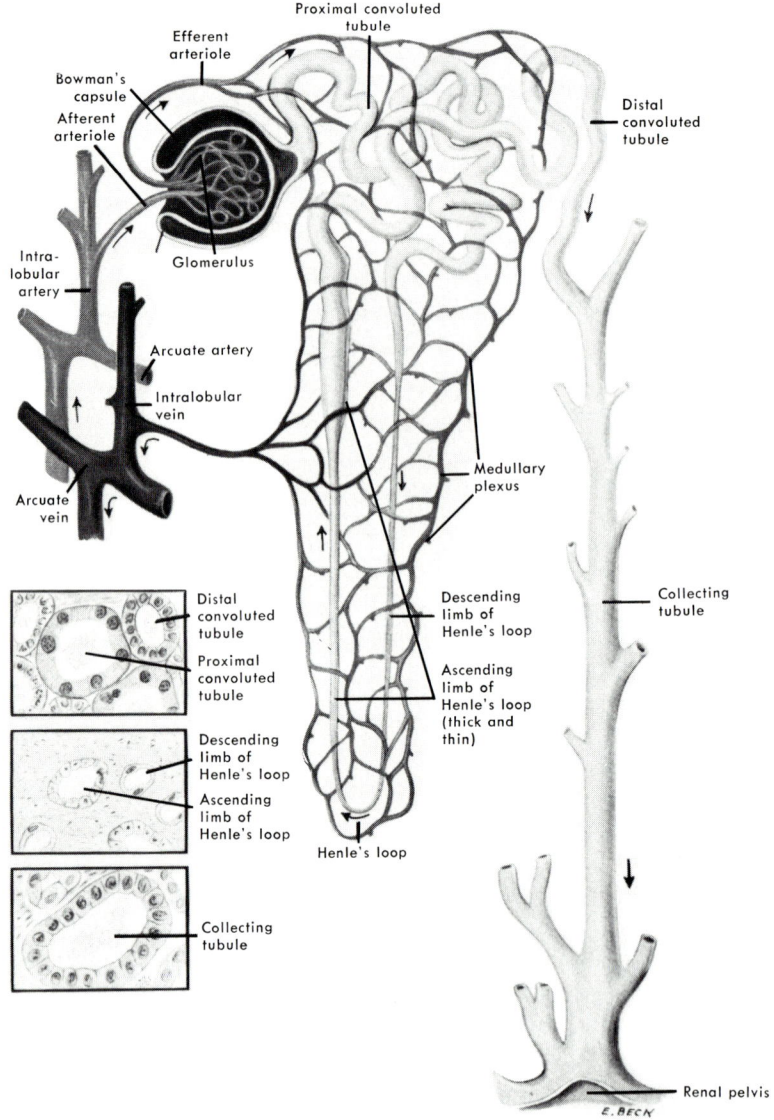

Fig. 27-2. The nephron. (From Medical Department, G.D. Searle & Co.: Research **40:**3, 1955.)

tubular space and the peritubular capillaries. The proximal tubule absorbs and thus removes from the filtrate all glucose, potassium, and amino acids, as well as 80% of sodium, chloride, water, urea, and uric acid. It shares with the distal convoluted tubule the absorption of calcium, phosphorus, and magnesium. The proximal tubule also absorbs bicarbonates and secretes uric acid, ammonia, and protein-bound drugs. Water, chlorides, urea, and uric acid are absorbed passively in the direction of the osmotic gradient, whereas sodium, potassium, and glucose are absorbed actively against a pressure gradient. Substances that are completely absorbed by the tubules when their plasma concentration is normal and not completely absorbed if their plasma concentration exceeds normal levels are called **threshold substances.** If a substance is not absorbed or only slightly absorbed, it is a low-threshold substance (e.g., creatinine, urea, and uric acid). A high-threshold sub-

stance, on the other hand, is completely absorbed (e.g., glucose and amino acids). The maximal rate at which a high-threshold substance can be absorbed is designated Tm; TmG = tubular maximum for glucose, which amounts to 350 mg/min.

In the descending loop of Henle the filtrate becomes increasingly hypertonic, a phenomenon explained by the **countercurrent theory** of urine concentration.[3-5] The maximal concentration of the fluid is reached as it passes through the most distal curve of the loop of Henle. On its return toward the cortex it is rendered hypotonic. The interstitial fluid of the medulla surrounds a number of structures, e.g., both limbs and the curved tip of the loop of Henle, the collecting ducts, and the accompanying vessels. The osmolality of the interstitial fluid of the medulla increases progressively from the level of the corticomedullary junction toward the apex of the pyramid (Fig. 27-3), because its con-

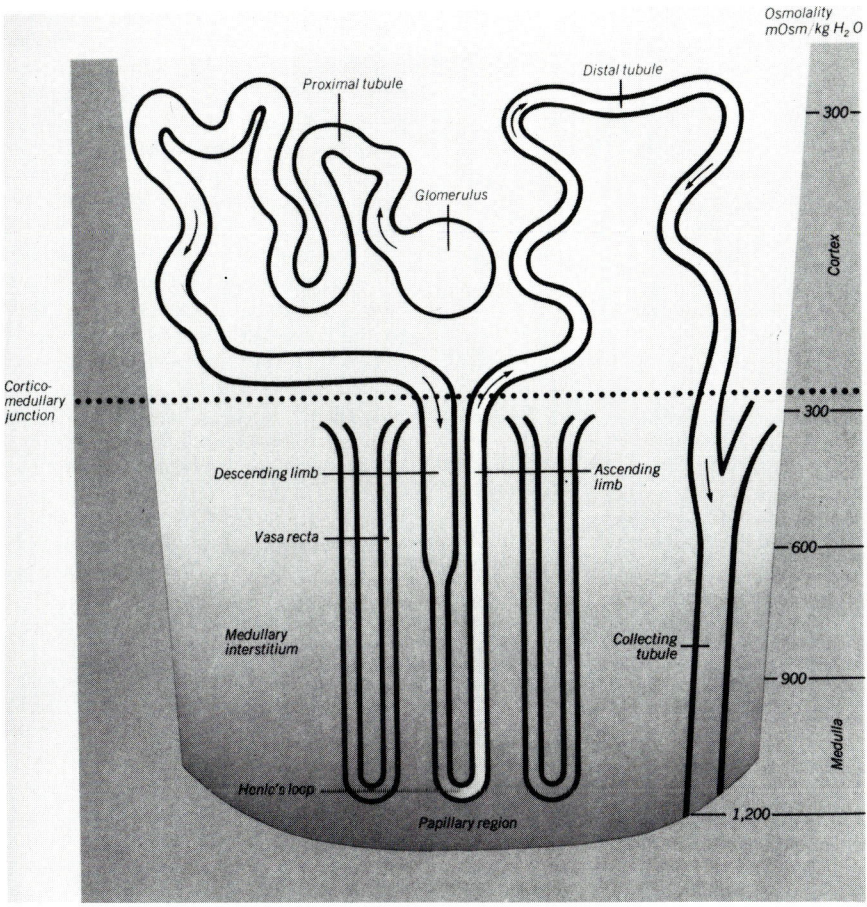

Fig. 27-3. Sketch of interstitial fluid of medulla and of tubular fluid, the basis of the countercurrent theory. (From Oken, D.E.: Urinalysis in the 70s—a new Medcom total learning system, Elkhart, Ind., 1973, Ames Division, Miles Laboratories, Inc.)

centration of sodium, chloride, and urea increases. Because of the high medullary osmotic pressure, water passively leaves the hypertonic tubular fluid for the medullary interstitium, allowing the tubular fluid to become increasingly concentrated. The ascending and descending limbs of Henle's loop differ in the way that they handle sodium, chloride, and water. The ascending limb actively pumps sodium into the medullary interstitial fluid but retains water, since it is impermeable to water. The descending limb, on the other hand, is permeable to water but lacks the sodium and chloride pump. As the medullary osmolality rises in response to sodium forced into it, water leaves the descending loop to dilute the medullary interstitial fluid, leaving behind a progressively more concentrated tubular fluid. When the fluid enters the ascending limb it becomes progressively hypotonic in response to the sodium loss. The peritubular plexus, which is permeable to water and solutes, equilibrates with the interstitial fluid and thus maintains the medullary osmolality gradient. By the time the fluid reaches the distal tubule the flow is slowed down, and 90% of the water and sodium have been absorbed.[6] In the distal tubule the sodium transport is under the influence of the adrenal steroids (aldosterone).[7] Potassium, hydrogen, and ammonia are secreted into the tubular fluid of the distal segment. The hydrogen ions lower the pH of the tubular fluid from the proximal tubular level of 6.8 to 4.4. Ammonia is produced by the distal tubular lining cells as the major buffer for hydrogen ions. The collecting tubules are also under the influence of the antidiuretic hormone of the pituitary gland, which responds to the state of hydration of the individual and renders the collecting tubules permeable to water and urea. In the absence of antidiuretic hormone in response to hyperhydration the collecting tubule is rendered poorly permeable to water, so that water is not absorbed (despite the osmotic gradient) and dilute urine is excreted.

URINE COLLECTION

Urine specimens should be collected in labeled, chemically clean, sterile, disposable, clear, graduated plastic containers with wide mouths protected by tightly fitting lids. The lips of the container should allow easy spill-free pouring. If the collection receptacles fulfill the above criteria, no special containers are needed for the culture of the urine. The label should contain not only the necessary identification information but should also mention whether the specimen was obtained by spontaneous voiding or by catheterization. The voided specimen, if at all possible, should be a midstream specimen so as to avoid contamination by bacteria and cells of the foreskin or vagina.[8,9]

Instructions for midstream collection of urine specimens

Men:

1. Retract foreskin (if not circumcised).
2. Using one of the towelettes provided (e.g., Clinipad-iodophor prep, Clinipad Corp., Guilford, Conn.), cleanse the urethral opening with a single stroke directed from the ring of the glans toward the tip, discard towelette.
3. Repeat cleansing procedure with two more towelettes.
4. Void into toilet and continue to void but interrupt the stream to collect urine into the supplied container.
5. Close container, complete information on label, and attach it to the specimen container.

Women:

1. While seated on the toilet spread the outer folds (labia majora).
2. Using one of the towelettes provided (see step 2 above), wipe the inner side of one inner fold (labium minor) by using a single stroke from front to back; discard towelette.
3. Using a second towelette, repeat step 2 on the opposite side.
4. Using a third towelette, cleanse urethral (urinary) opening with a single front-to-back stroke.
5. Void into the toilet and continue to void, but interrupt stream to collect urine into the supplied container.
6. Close the container, complete information on the label, and attach it to the specimen container.

Some urologists modify the above procedures and collect urine in two or three separate containers. Clouding of the urine in only the first container may be indicative of urethral disease, whereas clouding in only the second or third specimen suggests localization of the pathologic process in the bladder or kidneys.

For bacteriologic and cytologic investigations specimens obtained by catheterization may be preferable, although there is always the danger that this procedure may introduce bacteria into the bladder.

Collection of urine in children

The collection of urine of young children, newborns, and infants is aided by commercially available plastic bags with adhesive strips. Suprapubic aspiration of the bladder is suggested for obtaining critical urine specimens for culture from neonates, because the quality of specimens obtained by catheterization in this age group does not exceed that of clean voided specimens.[10]

Types of specimens

Most of the urine samples obtained in hospitals (''admission urines'') and in physicians' offices are midstream random specimens and generally are quite satisfactory for analysis. The main disadvantage is the variability in dilution and concentration of solutes. In a very dilute specimen, solutes of low concentration, but nevertheless of pathologic significance, may be missed. On the other hand, the random specimen, which is usually an early afternoon or midafternoon postprandial sample, offers the advantage of allowing the detection of pathologic postprandial concentrations of solutes, e.g., glucose and protein.

In general, the first morning specimen is the preferred sample, because the night urine specimen is less variable in dilution, more concentrated, of higher osmolality, and more acidic than the day specimen. The low pH aids in the preservation of casts and other formed elements, and the high osmolality reflects the concentrating power of the kidneys. The overnight growth of bacteria in the bladder urine may aid in the diagnosis of urinary tract infection but may be responsible for the lowering of the glucose contents and for changes in the pH. The first morning specimen is usually a fasting specimen and is therefore of value in the diagnosis of diabetes.

Since urobilinogen reaches its highest concentration in the urine between 2:00 PM and 4:00 PM, it should be assayed in a specimen voided shortly after 4:00 PM.

Twenty-four hour urine specimen

If it is necessary to measure the total amount of solutes excreted in 24 hr, a strictly timed 24 hr specimen is required, because many solutes exhibit diurnal variations. The lowest concentrations of catecholamines, 17-hydroxysteroids, and electrolytes are found in the early morning, whereas maximal levels can be demonstrated at noon or shortly thereafter.[11]

Instructions for collection of 24 hr urine specimens:

1. Empty the bladder at 8:00 AM (beginning of collection) and discard the specimen.
2. Save all urine voided during the next 24 hr.
3. At 8:00 AM the next day empty the bladder and add this specimen to the total volume.
4. Keep the urine under refrigeration in a wide-mouth, capped, clean, transparent, graduated, plastic collection bottle that is large enough to hold about 30 dl. Such bottles are commercially available from Midwest Medical Supply Co., St. Louis.
5. If a special preservative is required, add it to the collection bottle before the beginning of the urine collection.
6. The label on the collection bottle must state, in addition to the patient's identification, etc., the preservative used and the test requested. If spillage of the preservative could harm the patient, add a suitable warning to the label.

Other specimens

A variety of other types of timed specimens are occasionally examined for special purposes. These include, but are not restricted to, 2 hr, 4 hr, and 12 hr (day or night) samples.

Sources of error

Some of the following points also apply to single urine specimens (see also discussion of quality control in urinalysis in Chapter 1):

1. Bacterially or chemically contaminated containers
2. Wrong or inadequate preservative
3. Partial loss of specimen or too much specimen because of the inclusion of two morning specimens in a 24 hr collection
4. Inadequate mixing of specimen before examination
5. Careless measuring of the 24 hr volume

Errors in the collection and handling of 24 hr urine specimens are so common that it is suggested to employ serum tests whenever possible or to utilize random urine specimens instead of 24 hr specimens. The adequacy of a 24 hr urine specimen cannot be evaluated on the basis of its creatinine concentration as was once thought. Chemical analysis of 24 hr urine specimens has a 20% risk of error.

For many years the completeness of 24 hr urine collection or the excretion of a constituent (e.g., urine estriol) has been related to the 24 hr creatinine excretion. The amount of creatinine produced is fairly constant at 1.0-1.6 g/24 hr in an individual. Although widely used, this method of checking for completeness of collection has been questioned,[12-14] and an alternative method being examined has been to use the ratio of the test substance to creatinine in first morning specimens rather than 24 hr specimens.[15-17] It remains to be seen whether or not this will prove to be a more useful parameter.

Preservation of urine specimens

Preservation prevents the following:
1. Bacterial growth
2. Instability of solutes
3. Degeneration of sediments such as pus, blood, and casts

Single urine specimens should be examined within 1 hr of voiding so that no method of preservation is required, but if immediate examination is not possible, one of the methods described below must be utilized.

Methods of preservation

Refrigeration at about 5° C prevents growth of bacteria, thus maintaining the original pH for up to 8 hr,[18] and helps to preserve casts and red, white, and epithelial cells. Some urine specimens turn cloudy when refrigerated but clear when brought to room temperature, at which temperature they should be analyzed.

Chemical preservation is necessary when the urine specimen needs to be mailed or transported over long distances and cannot be refrigerated. Such specimens are unsuitable for cytologic and bacteriologic investigations, and their pH value may be erroneous. The preservative must be chosen carefully, because it may influence the test result, and not all preservatives are satisfactory for all tests. Formalin (40%) is a good preservative; 1 drop is added to each 10 ml urine specimen, or 10 ml is added to each 24 hr urine specimen. It interferes with the Obermayer test for indican and reduces alkaline copper solutions used in some tests for glucose (Clinitest, Ames Co., Elkhart, Ind.). Tablets that produce formaldehyde are commercially available and easier to handle than formalin. One tablet is used per 60 ml urine, and in this concentration it does not interfere with the Clinistix (Ames Co., Elkhart, Ind.) or Clinitest for glucose.

One or two drops of toluene form a thin surface layer, which by excluding air prevents oxidative changes.

Concentrated hydrochloric acid (10 ml/24 hr specimen) is an excellent preservative for hormones such as adrenalin, noradrenalin, catecholamines, vanillylmandelic acid, and steroids. It lowers the urinary pH, destroys any formed elements, and may precipitate uric acid.

Thymol, one 5 mm crystal/dl urine, inhibits bacterial and fungal growth. An excess may give a false positive result for the precipitation test for albumin when heat or acetic acid is employed, but it does not interfere with the colorimetric test based on protein error of indicators (Albustix, Ames Co., Elkhart, Ind.).

Other preservatives: Sodium carbonate (5-10 g) has been used as a preservative for porphyrin determination, and samples must be protected from light by wrapping them in foil. Glucose in 24 hr urine specimens has been preserved for periods of 6 weeks at room temperature by the addition of 5 ml Hibitane (chlorhexidine gluconate, 200 g/L).

Urine identification

Specimen identification is sometimes a problem for the analyst. Table 27-1 contains concentrations of several constituents that can be used to distinguish the specimen type. Although no single test is diagnostic, except perhaps urea nitrogen, the results of measuring several constituents can unequivocally designate the type of specimen. The most useful procedures for identifying urine involve measuring the following constituents: total protein, uric acid, creatinine, urea nitrogen, potassium, and osmolality.

Tests to identify a liquid as urine

In certain clinical situations a liquid must be identified as urine and differentiated from a serous exudate, spinal fluid, or amniotic fluid. The presence of considerable amounts of urea nitrogen (600 mg/dl) and creatinine (50 mg/dl) is highly suggestive of urine, because most other body fluids contain only small amounts of these substances.[19] The characteristics of serous exudate and of spinal and amniotic fluids are discussed in Chapter 29.

Quality control in urinalysis

The urinalysis area of the laboratory needs to have the reported results evaluated for accuracy and precision in the same way as do other laboratory sections. The presumption of the laboratory that similar samples will always have similar results reported is not consistent with studies of quality control in this area of the laboratory.[20] Because many of the determinations are qualitative in nature and since "screening" methods are usually employed, a variety of results are sometimes possible on a single sample. In addition, the examination of urine sediment is difficult to control because of the many factors involved and the instability of the formed elements. The sediment examination has been shown to be more imprecise than previously believed.

Table 27-1. Distinguishing characteristics of several body fluids

Constituent	Serum	Urine*	Amniotic fluid	Cerebrospinal fluid†
Total protein (g/dl)	5.6-8.3‡	0.01-0.02§	0.2-1.7‡	35.0
Uric acid (mg/dl)	2.1-5.6‡	17-50§	1.9-9.0‡	0.25
Creatinine (mg/dl)	0.5-0.9‡	66-130§	0.5-1.7‡	1.2
Urea nitrogen (mg/dl)	4-18‡	800-1300§	5-14‡	13.1
Glucose (mg/dl)	60-165‡	<30§	20-65‡	60.0
Sodium (mEq/L)	133-141‡	25-150§	130-150‡	138.0
Potassium (mEq/L)	3.1-4.9‡	16-80§	3.3-4.3	2.8
Urobilinogen (mg/dl)	Negative	<1	Negative	Negative
pH	7.35-7.45	4.8-7.8§	7.0-7.25‡	7.33
Specific gravity	—	1.005-1.030‡	1.025-1.050‡	—
Total bilirubin (mg/dl)	0.2-1.0§	Negative§	0.025-0.075§	Negative
Osmolality (mOsm/L)	289-308§	>600§	240-280	295

*Apparent concentrations are 24 hr excretion divided by a 1.5 L approximate volume.
†Data from Fishman, R.A.: Cerebrospinal fluid in diseases of the nervous system, Philadelphia, 1980, W.B. Saunders Co.
‡Data from Natelson, S.L., Socommegna, A., and Epstine, M.B., editors: Amniotic fluid, New York, 1974, John Wiley & Sons, Inc.
§Data from Tietz, N.W., editor: Fundamentals of clinical chemistry, ed. 2, Philadelphia, 1976, W.B. Saunders Co.

More accurate and reproducible results are found for chemical and sediment analysis[21] with experienced individuals who are performing the tests regularly. Studies of routine urinalysis performed by ward and clinic staffs[22] rather than by laboratory personnel reflect a 26% error rate of false positive or false negative results. Such statistics support centralized laboratory testing, where quality control programs can help to produce more reproducible and accurate test results.

The design of a quality control program must include several aspects: (1) using control materials at least once each day that a procedure is performed, (2) noting the results of all determinations, (3) keeping track of the lot number and expiration date of all control materials, and (4) noting internal inconsistencies between screening and confirmatory tests when differences in sensitivities are excluded. The most complete quality control system would employ several samples of urine or simulated urine, with various concentrations of each major constituent, including sediment.[23] Included in such a system would be one or several samples with trace positive results. When results of such samples become consistently negative, examination of the procedure (chemicals or dipsticks) is in order, since sensitivity has been lost. This is a particular problem of dipsticks[24] exposed to moisture and is hard to eliminate, because sinks and dipsticks are both necessary in the urinalysis laboratory (see also Chapter 1).

Control materials

A variety of control preparations are commercially available in lyophilized, tablet, or liquid form with varying concentrations of constituents. These include QC-U (General Diagnostics, Morris Plains, N.J.), Tek-Chek (Ames Co., Elkhart, Ind.), UR-Sure (Hyland Laboratories, Costa Mesa, Calif.), Urintrol (Harleco, Philadelphia), Kovatrol (ICL Scientific, Fountain Valley, Calif.), and Chemstrip control (Biodynamics/bmc, Boehringer Mannheim Corp., Indianapolis).

The laboratory may make its own controls by using a normal urine supplemented with various materials at considerable savings over the commercially available products. One urine control formula[25] is as follows: to 5 dl of 0.9% (w/v) sodium chloride add 5 ml of 50% (w/v) glucose, 2 ml acetone, 25 ml serum, and 0.1 ml whole blood lysed in 0.1 ml water. Adjust the pH to 6 by using 0.1N sodium hydroxide or 0.1N hydrochloric acid. The solution should give a pH of 6; protein, +3; glucose, medium; ketones, moderate; blood, moderate; and specific gravity, 1.010. The solution is stable for about 2 weeks if refrigerated and capped tightly; it is stable longer if frozen. Several other mixtures are available[23,26] with similar results expected and containing sediment. The use of a small amount of chloroform as a preservative allows solutions to remain at room temperature. This preservative should not be added to those solutions containing fixed sediment or to those solutions whose refractive index is determined by the falling drop method (Clinilab, Ames Co., Elkhart, Ind.).

Volume of urine

Procedure: Measure the exact amount of urine in a calibrated cylinder.
Normal values of 24 hr urine specimens:
Newborns:

Birth to 3 days	20-50 ml/24 hr
5-10 days	100-350 ml/24 hr

Children:

1 year	300-600 ml/24 hr
10 years	750-1500 ml/24 hr

Adults: 750-2000 ml/24 hr

The ratio of night excretion to day excretion in adults is usually 1:2 or 1:3. In children the ratio is not reliable.

Interpretation: The urinary volume depends on the following:

1. The amount of fluid intake
2. The load of solutes to be excreted, primarily sodium and urea
3. The loss of fluid in perspiration and exhaled air
4. The cardiac and renal status of the individual

Increased volume (polyuria): Increased amounts of urine are excreted under the following conditions:

1. In response to excessive fluid intake (orally or intravenously), the administration of diuretics, or the consumption of diuretic drinks, e.g., alcohol, tea, and coffee
2. During absorption of edema, transudates, and exudates
3. In anxiety states
4. In chronic kidney disease in which the kidneys are unable to concentrate (specific gravity of 1.010), in diabetes mellitus (high specific gravity), in diabetes insipidus (low specific gravity), and in tumors with inappropriate antidiuretic hormone secretion

Frequent emptying of the bladder, as seen in cystitis, must not be mistaken for polyuria.

Decreased volume: Decreased amounts of urine are excreted under certain conditions.

Anuria (absence of excretion of urine): Anuria occurs under the following conditions:

1. Total suppression of urine formation as the kidneys fail to function and the urinary bladder remains empty. The most common etiology is renal agenesis, bilateral cortical necrosis, or acute glomerulonephritis.
2. Obstructive uropathy. The kidneys produce urine (at least for a limited time), but it cannot escape because of total obstruction of the outflow tract. The most common etiology is stones in both ureters, bladder neck obstruction (prostate in older men and valve in children), or prostatic hypertrophy.

Oliguria: In oliguria there is a scanty urinary volume, an output of about 50-300 ml/24 hr. The most common etiology is acute renal failure, acute glomerulonephritis, acute tubular necrosis resulting from hemoglobinuria, myoglobinuria, shock and trauma (hypoxia), cortical and tubular necrosis (nephrotoxins), or renal vein or artery thrombosis.

ANALYSIS OF SPECIMEN

Urinalysis consists of noting the physical characteristics of the urine, e.g., color, transparency, hydrogen ion concentration (pH), and the concentration of solutes (specific gravity and osmolality), and the presence of abnormal amounts (and types) of protein and of reducing substances, ketone bodies, hemoglobin, urobilinogen, bile, and formed elements.

Physical characteristics[27]

Variations in odor, color, and turbidity may be caused by the handling of the specimen (standing, refrigeration) and may not reflect pathologic changes. If the physical appearance is important, a fresh specimen should be requested and examined immediately after voiding.

Odor

The normal odor of urine may be modified by the presence of acetone (as in diabetes mellitus, starvation, and dehydration), which imparts a fruity odor, or by bacterial decomposition, which produces an ammoniacal odor. Maple syrup urine disease is characterized by a maple syrup–like odor of urine. An offensive odor may be the result of bacterial action in the presence of pus. Some foods (garlic and asparagus) and some medications (menthol) also affect the odor. In phenylketonuria the odor has been described as "mousy," but, in general, the odor is not of diagnostic significance.

Color

Normally, urine is some shade of yellow because of a mixture of pigments such as uroerythrin, urochrome, and porphyrins. The color varies with the specific gravity; if the urine is diluted, it is straw colored, and, if concentrated, almost deep orange. It is influenced by a variety of metabolic products, foods, drugs, and pigments.[28] On standing, urine darkens because of oxidation of the colorless urobilinogen to colored urobilin. The color of urine varies according to the following conditions:

Very pale yellow or greenish yellow, almost colorless:
  Chronic kidney disease
  Diabetes insipidus
  Diabetes mellitus
  High dilution
  Severe iron deficiency
Yellow:
  Atabrine (Winthrop Laboratories, New York)
  Azulfidine (Pharmacia Laboratories, Piscataway, N.J.)
  Cascara
  Food color
  Normal urine
  Phenacetin
Orange:
  Azo Gantrisin (Roche Laboratories, Nutley, N.J.)
  Carotene
  Concentrated urine (fever, inadequate water intake, excessive water loss)
  Food color
  Furoxone (Norwich-Eaton Pharmaceuticals, Norwich, N.Y.)
  Rhubarb
  Riboflavin
Green or blue-green (often caused by blue mixed with yellow of urine:
  Bile pigment
  Blue diaper syndrome
  Elavil (Merck Sharp & Dohme, West Point, Pa.)
  Indican (increased amounts)
  Methylene blue (kidney pills)

Robaxin (A.H. Robins Co., Richmond, Va.)
Vitamin B complex
Pink, red, or reddish orange:
  Azo Gantrisin
  Beets
  Blood (smoky if red cells are intact)
  Chromogenic bacteria (e.g., *Serratia marcescens*)
  Dilantin (Parke-Davis, Morris Plains, N.J.)
  Food color
  Hemoglobin (see discussion of hemoglobinuria)
  Myoglobin (see discussion of myoglobinuria)
  Phenolsulfonphthalein
  Porphyrin
  Povan (Parke-Davis, Morris Plains, N.J.)
  Pyridium (in acid urine) (Parke-Davis, Morris Plains, N.J.)
  Rhubarb (in alkaline urine)
Black, gray, or brown:
  Alkapton bodies (ochronosis, homogentisic acid, alkaptonuria)
  Aralen (Winthrop Laboratories, New York)
  Bilirubin
  Iron compounds (injectable)
  Melanin
  Methemoglobin
  Phenol poisoning
  Porphyrin

Transparency and turbidity

Freshly voided urine is clear.
Causes of turbidity:
1. Temperature and pH. Diffuse clouding may occur or a sediment may form on standing because of changes in the pH and in the temperature, which may be responsible for the precipitation of solutes from a supersaturated solution. For this reason about 50% of normal urine specimens received in the laboratory are cloudy.
2. Amorphous phosphates and carbonates. They are soluble in acid urine but may precipitate in alkaline urine. They dissolve on addition of 5-10% acetic acid, amorphous phosphates without and carbonates with gas formation.
3. Urates. They are soluble in neutral or alkaline urine but may precipitate in acid urine. They are often pink and dissolve on heating. If protein is present, the cloudiness may increase on heating.

4. Oxalates. Clearing is produced by 12% hydrochloric acid.
5. Pus (pyuria), blood, and epithelial cells. In alkaline urine, pus is usually mucoid; it is crumbly in acid urine. About 200 white cells/mm^3 or about 500 red cells/mm^3 produce turbidity.
6. Bacteria. They are not removed by filtration through filter paper unless some inert substance such as kaolin is added first; even then the results are not always satisfactory.
7. Fat (lipuria). Fat globules impart a milky appearance to the specimen but may be removed and cleared by extraction with ether.
8. Chyle. Chyluria may be parasitic (filarial) or nonparasitic (as in thoracic duct obstruction, trauma, and tumor) in origin and imparts a cream color to the urine. Obstructed lymph vessels may force chylous fluid and cholesterol into the excretory urinary apparatus and into the urine. Shaking the specimen with ether will clear the urine sample.

Reagent strips

The introduction of reagent strips has streamlined urinalysis. The strips are specific, rapid, sensitive, easy to use, accurate, and time and cost saving, but, despite their simplicity, certain precautions must be observed. Mix the urine well, strictly observe correct timing, remove the strip immediately after insertion into the specimen, and remove the excess urine by touching the rim of the container with the strip. Compare the test results with the correct color chart. The manufacturer's instructions with regard to storage of the strips, for example, in brown, tightly capped containers in a cool, moisture-free atmosphere, must be strictly observed.

There are a substantial number of reagent strips that are commercially available, ranging from one to nine test pads. A few of the combination reagent strips are listed in Table 27-2.

Hydrogen ion concentration (pH)

The concentration of free hydrogen ions in solutions is most conveniently expressed in terms of pH. The pH is defined as the negative or the logarithm of the hydrogen ion concentration.

The standard method of accurately measuring hydro-

Table 27-2. Comparison of reagent test pads for selected dipsticks

Test item	Bililabstix*	Multilabstix*	N-multilabstix*	Chemstrip 8†	Chemstrip 9†
pH	X	X	X	X	X
Protein	X	X	X	X	X
Glucose	X	X	X	X	X
Ketones	X	X	X	X	X
Bilirubin	X	X	X	X	X
Blood	X	X	X	X	X
Urobilinogen		X	X	X	X
Nitrite			X	X	X
Leukocytes					X

*Ames Co., Elkhart, Ind.
†Boehringer Mannheim Corp., Indianapolis.

gen ion concentration or pH is with the glass electrode. This is an unnecessary refinement in urinalysis, since small changes in pH are of little clinical significance, and the pH may be estimated much more rapidly with sufficient accuracy by the use of strips impregnated with an indicator or a mixture of indicators. These are dyes that change color with changes in pH. By the use of the proper mixture of indicators a noticeable change in color is seen over a range of several pH units. The indicator strips should be checked at intervals by the use of a urine of known pH as determined with the glass electrode or by the use of a commercial buffer solution, which is available in several pH ranges. Urinary pH measurements are only accurate if the specimen is freshly voided, since the pH becomes alkaline on standing because of loss of carbon dioxide and the conversion of urea into ammonia by bacteria. The pH measurement of the "routine" urine specimen is of little clinical significance, but if extreme acid or alkaline values are encountered, they are usually indicative of careless and irresponsible handling and collection of a clinical specimen.

Measurement of urinary pH

A number of pH papers are available, e.g., nitrazine paper (E.R. Squibb, Princeton, N.J.) and pHydrion paper (Micro-Essential Laboratories, Brooklyn, N.Y.), but the most widely used method employs the pH indicator block of multitest reagent strips, which utilizes two indicators. They are methyl red and bromthymol blue, providing a pH range from 5.0-9.0 that is expressed in a color change from orange to green to blue.

Normal value: Random specimen, pH 5.0-8.0 (average 5.5-6.5).

Discussion: Acid urine results from starvation, a high-protein diet, metabolism of fat, drugs used in the prevention of calcium carbonate or calcium phosphate stone formation, acid-producing bacteria, metabolic and respiratory acidosis, and sleep.

Alkaline urine results from a vegetable diet, respiratory and metabolic alkalosis, drugs used in the prevention of uric acid and oxalate stone formation, and ammonia-producing, urea-splitting bacteria.

Urinary pH is used to monitor the adequacy of treatment in a number of conditions. The pH should be kept alkaline during sulfonamide and streptomycin therapy to prevent precipitation of the drugs in the kidneys and the formation of uric acid, cystine, and oxalate stones. The alkaline pH is also maintained during the treatment of transfusion reactions and salicylate intoxication. The pH is kept acid to combat bacteriuria and to prevent the formation of "alkaline stones," e.g., calcium carbonate or calcium phosphate stones.

Kidney in acid-base metabolism[29]

The pH of urine depends largely on the acid-base composition of the blood. Normal metabolism produces an excess of acids (H ions) consisting mainly of mineral acids such as sulfuric and phosphoric acids, which are excreted by the kidneys (**fixed acidity**). Carbonic acid produced by metabolism of carbohydrates is eliminated by the lungs (**volatile acidity**). In pathologic conditions, nonmetabolized organic acids such as β-hy-

droxybutyric acid (diabetes) or lactic, citric, and pyruvic acids significantly add to the acidity of the urine. Because of the very adequate buffering systems of human urine (NaH_2PO_4, creatinine, β-hydroxybutyric acid, etc.), the kidney can excrete up to 480 mEq acid/day. Most titratable acidity is present as acid phosphate (NaH_2PO_4), which forms part of a reversible reaction:

$$H^+ + Na_2HPO_4 = NaH_2PO_4 + Na^+$$

In **acidosis** most phosphate is excreted as NaH_2PO_4 and in **alkalosis** as Na_2HPO_4. Normally the largest number of H ions is excreted as NH_4 (**ammonium**), which is synthesized in the kidney and excreted in amounts depending on the systemic acid-base balance. Microelectrodes have recently been used to measure Po_2 and Pco_2 in the urine of the renal pelvis and of the urinary bladder. The Pco_2 varies greatly in acidosis and alkalosis. In **respiratory acidosis** (CO_2 retention) and in **metabolic acidosis** (diabetic ketosis, starvation, and uremia) the urine is usually acid, whereas in **respiratory alkalosis** (hyperventilation) and **metabolic alkalosis** (vomiting and administration of alkalies) the urine is usually alkaline. In metabolic acidosis there is an increased titratable acidity (total excretion of acid) of the freshly voided urine, whereas in metabolic alkalosis the titratable acidity is decreased. There are exceptions to this rule, e.g., renal failure (inability to form ammonia) and renal tubular diseases (e.g., Fanconi and Milkman's syndromes), in which weakly alkaline urine may be excreted in the presence of systemic acidosis because of the increased urinary loss of bicarbonates.

Potassium deficiency and hyperaldosteronism produce alkaline urine.

Specific gravity

Specific gravity is defined as the ratio of the weight of a fixed volume of solution to that of the same volume of water at a specified temperature, usually 20° C. For most chemical substances an increase in the amount dissolved in a fixed volume of water causes an almost linear increase in the specific gravity of the solution. The specific gravity of urine has been used for years as a measure of the total amount of material dissolved in it (total solids) and thus of the concentrating and excretory power of the kidneys.

Measurement of specific gravity

The specific gravity may be determined by means of a special hydrometer, often called a urinometer, or a refractometer.

Urinometer: Mix urine well and allow it to come to room temperature. Float the instrument in the specimen, giving it a slight twist to see that it is completely free. Read the bottom meniscus and correct the figures for temperature, protein, sugar, and any dilution. If the amount of urine is too small to measure with the urinometer, use the refractometer.

Sources of error:

Temperature differences: Most urinometers are calibrated at 20° C. A difference of 3° C between urine temperature and calibration temperature requires a correction of 0.001, to be added if above and subtracted if below the proper temperature.

Proteinuria: For each 1% of protein in the urine the specific gravity is increased 0.003 and should be corrected for this increase, because it does not reflect the concentrating ability of the kidney.

Glycosuria: For each 1% of glucose in the urine the specific gravity is increased 0.004 and should be corrected, because the increase does not reflect the concentrating power of the kidney.

X-ray contrast media: The specific gravity may exceed 1.050 if the urine contains contrast media.

Urinary preservatives: Preservatives increase the urinary specific gravity.

Disadvantages of urinometer procedure:

1. The mass-produced urinometers are often inaccurate and should always be checked against solutions of known specific gravity (see urinometer controls below), and the appropriate corrections should be applied to all measurements.
2. At least 15 ml urine is required to float the instrument, an amount not always available.
3. Turbid urine may make reading of the scale difficult.

The use of the urinometer should be discontinued and it should be replaced by the refractometer (see below).

Urinometer controls: The following solutions, which are quite stable if kept in well-stoppered bottles, may be used to check urinometers. The salts should be weighed to the nearest 10 mg and the solution made up in a volumetric flask. All measurements are made at 20° C.

Solution	Specific gravity
Pure water	1.000
Sodium chloride solution (2.50 g/dl)	1.018
Sodium chloride solution (5.00 g/dl)	1.035
Sodium chloride solution (7.5 g/dl)	1.051

It is important to check the accuracy of the urinometer. A couple of matched instruments to cover the entire range from 1.000-1.040 is preferable to a single urinometer.

An error of ±0.003 renders a urinometer reading unsatisfactory.

Refractometer: The refractive index of a solution, defined as the ratio of the velocity of light in the solution to that in a vacuum, is a property of a solution that increases at a fairly linear rate with increases in the amount of dissolved solute. Thus the measurement of the refractive index of urine serves the same purpose as a measurement of the specific gravity, an index of the amount of solids excreted by the kidneys. As with specific gravity the increase with concentration is not the same for all substances, but an average value serves as it does for specific gravity. Generally, physicians are not familiar with the refractive index, and a statement about the refractive index of a urine specimen being 1.3385 would be meaningless to them. Thus the refractometers are calibrated in terms of specific gravity (when used for urine) by measuring the specific gravity (with a hydrometer) and the refractive index of a large number of urine samples and calculating an average

empiric relation between the two. This is then used to construct a specific gravity scale for the refractometer.

The commercial hand refractometers for urinalysis (Total Solids Meter, TS meter, American Optical Corp., Scientific Instrument Division, Buffalo, N.Y.) are convenient, accurate, and rapid. They require only a few drops of urine, and the measurement takes only a few seconds. The instrument also has a built-in temperature compensator, so that one does not need to make any correction for temperature in the usual range from 20-30° C. However, as with the hydrometer, one should make a correction for glucose and protein in the urine. For glucose the same correction may be used as with the hydrometer, but for protein a slightly higher correction of 0.004 is probably more accurate.

Quality control with refractometer: The instrument is relatively sturdy and should not get out of alignment. It has an adjustment screw for checking the zero point with pure water. If it is desired to check other points on the scale, the sodium chloride (NaCl) solutions mentioned earlier for use with the urinometer can be used here. The important point is that these solutions will not read 1.018, 1.035, and 1.051 on the refractometer scale but should read 1.011, 1.022, and 1.033 on it. The reason for this is that the specific gravity scale on the refractometer is an empirically derived scale relating the refractive index to the specific gravity of a typical urine specimen. A solution of NaCl having a specific gravity of 1.018 will have quite a different composition than a typical urine specimen of the same specific gravity, and the two cannot be expected to have the same refractive index, because the refractive index and the specific gravity are entirely different properties of the solutions and vary in different ways with the type of solute. If the refractive index were actually reported as such, to check a point, say, 1.3340, on the scale, one would use a solution known to have that refractive index. To check the specific gravity scale on the refractometer at, say, 1.020, one would use a solution that is known to have the same refractive index (since this is the property of the solution being measured) as a typical urine specimen having a specific gravity of 1.020. Thus the NaCl solutions containing 2.5, 5.0, and 7.5 g/dl have specific gravities of 1.018, 1.035, and 1.051, as mentioned, and would be used as such to check a urinometer, but their respective refractive indices are the same as typical urine specimens of specific gravities of 1.011, 1.022, and 1.033, and these figures would be used to check the refractometer.

Normal values of specific gravity

Newborns: Random specimen, 1.002-1.004

Adults:

   Random specimen, 1.005-1.030 (highest in the morning)

   24 hr specimen, 1.015-1.018

Middle age and over: Progressive decrease of specific gravity

Interpretation of specific gravity measurements

Normal specific gravity is primarily influenced by the electrolytes and nitrogenous waste products, e.g., urea and creatinine dissolved in the urine. The first morning specimen should have a specific gravity between 1.015 and 1.025.

Increase of specific gravity: Values over 1.020 are seen in decreased fluid intake, fever, sweating, vomiting, and diarrhea. The increased values are also encountered in diabetes mellitus (glycosuria), congestive heart failure, adrenal insufficiency, and proteinuria and when preservatives or x-ray contrast media are added to the urine specimen. Tumors that secrete abnormal quantities of antidiuretic hormone increase the concentration of solutes and thus the specific gravity. See sources of error (earlier) for correction for proteinuria and glycosuria.

Decrease of specific gravity: Low specific gravity (less than 1.009) is seen in exaggerated oral or intravenous fluid intake, following the administration of diuretics, and in hypothermia. The renal concentrating power is impaired or lost in glomerulonephritis, in pyelonephritis, and in the absence of antidiuretic hormone (diabetes insipidus).

Fixed specific gravity: In severe renal damage the specific gravity is fixed at 1.010, the value of the glomerular filtrate.

• • •

Concentration and dilution tests are discussed under renal function tests (p. 724).

Osmolality

Another technic for the measurement of the amount of dissolved material is the determination of the osmolality.[30] Osmolality is a measure of the so-called colligative properties of a solution. These properties depend on the number of particles in the solution and not on their size or weight. A solution containing 0.1 gram-molecule urea in 1 kg water will give a solution of 0.1 osmolality. Conventionally, the concentrations are expressed as moles per kilogram of solvent rather than as moles per liter of solution; hence they are designated as molal solutions rather than molar. A solution containing 0.1 gram-molecule of dissolved material as the above-mentioned urea solution (5.85 g NaCl as compared with 6.00 g urea) would have quite a different osmolality. If the NaCl were completely ionized in solution, it would yield 0.2 mole of particles (0.1 mole of sodium ions and 0.1 mole of chloride ions). Each of these particles (ions) would have the same effect on the colligative properties as a molecule of urea. Hence the NaCl solution should have twice the osmolality of the urea solution; its osmolality should be 0.2. Actually the "effective" ionization of the NaCl would be somewhat less than 100%, so that the solution would actually be about 0.16 osmolality. The concentrations in body fluids are usually expressed in milliosmoles per kilogram (of water), and the above examples would be given as 100, 200, and 160 mOsm/kg, respectively.

Measurement of osmolality

Osmometer: The use of the freezing point osmometer is based on the fact that, as a solute is dissolved in a solvent, the freezing point is lowered.[31] One molecular weight (mole) of any nonionizing solute dissolved in 1 kg water (the solvent in urine) lowers the freezing point of the water 1.86° C. In clinical practice, osmolality is expressed in milliosmoles. One milliosmole depresses the freezing point by 0.00186° C. The freezing osmometer consists of a refrigerated bath to freeze the body fluids, an electric thermistor probe, which changes its resistance with temperature, and a Wheatstone bridge and a galvanometer to translate temperature changes into milliosmoles per kilogram of water.

The vapor pressure osmometer (product literature, Wescan Instruments, Santa Clara, Calif.) uses a thermocouple hygrometer to measure osmolality as a function of vapor pressure depression over a sample in a closed chamber. The urine is absorbed by a filter paper disk, which is then inserted into the sample chamber. This step initiates a programmed sequence: (1) equilibration of the sample and electronic nulling of the ambient reference temperature, (2) cooling the thermocouple sensor to a temperature below the dew point, (3) convergence of the thermocouple temperature to the dew point, and (4) the measured temperature differential establishing the final reading expressed in milliosmoles per kilogram.

Normal values[32]

Infants: 213 mOsm/kg
Adults: 300-1200 mOsm/kg

Interpretation

The urine osmolality varies greatly with the diet and should always be considered in relation to the serum osmolality. The urine osmolality/serum osmolality ratio should exceed 1.0 and after an overnight fast should be 3.0 or greater. About 500-600 mOsm solute is caused by urea. Sodium phosphate, potassium, sulfate, and other ions are responsible for the remaining milliosmoles.

The kidneys' ability to dilute concentrated urine depends on a complex set of renal functions and on the antidiuretic hormone titer. The concentrating capacity of the kidneys is impaired in most renal diseases, so that the osmolality of even a maximally concentrated fasting urine specimen is reduced, e.g., to 400 mOsm/kg vs. 800 mOsm/kg of a normal control specimen. Osmometry also lends itself to the investigation of inappropriate antidiuretic hormone secretion as seen in some tumors or in central nervous system diseases, which raises the osmolality of the small amount of urine secreted significantly higher than the serum osmolality, irrespective of the patient's water intake.

CHEMICAL EXAMINATION OF URINE
Measurement of urinary proteins
Qualitative methods

Two methods (dipsticks and sulfosalicylic acid) are presented, which are not interchangeable, and both should be utilized on the same specimen.

Dipstick method (protein area of multiple strips): This protein test is based on the phenomenon of "protein error of indicators," the principle of which is that at a fixed pH certain indicators will have one color in the presence of protein and another color in the absence of protein. At pH 3.0 the indicator (tetrabromphenol blue) is yellow, but in the presence of protein the color changes from yellow to green to greenish blue, depending on the amount of protein.

Procedure: Dip the strip into well-mixed urine and immediately compare with color chart. Results may vary from negative to trace to 1-4 +. Trace readings indicate 5-20 mg protein (albumin)/dl urine. Plus readings correspond to 30, 100, 300, and 1000 mg protein (albumin)/dl urine.

Normal value: Negative for protein.

Discussion: The dipstick method responds semiquantitatively to increasing concentrations[33] of urinary albumin only and fails to react with γ-globulins, Bence Jones protein, and other serum proteins.[33] The test is therefore falsely negative in Bence Jones proteinuria and in globulinuria. This lack of sensitivity of the strips to proteins other than albumin has to do with the binding characteristics of the indicator dye used.[34] The dipstick readings are also affected by the salt concentration and the pH of the specimen. Salt concentrations that are sufficient to increase the specific gravity reduce the reading of the protein concentration.[33] If the urine is highly alkaline (over pH 10) and highly buffered, the test will be falsely positive. To give accurate results the pH should be reduced to 7 by the addition of acid before testing.[33] The dipstick method may record false positive trace and 1 + values in specimens in which no protein can be detected by the sulfosalicylic acid method. These two values must always be confirmed by the turbidity method.

Sulfosalicylic acid semiquantitative turbidity method (Kingsbury-Clark)[35]:

Principle: Protein, denatured by acid, precipitates and renders the urine specimen progressively more turbid as its concentration increases.

Reagents and equipment:
1. Sulfosalicylic acid, 3% aqueous (3 g acid/dl deionized water)
2. Kingsbury-Clark standards
3. Test tubes, 13 × 100 mm

Procedure: To 1 ml centrifuged urine add 3 ml reagent. Mix and allow to stand for 5 min. Observe the degree of turbidity and compare the test sample with the original urine specimen in 13 × 100 mm tube and with Kingsbury-Clark standards.

Normal value: No turbidity.

Method of reporting: See Table 27-3.

Discussion: The sulfosalicylic acid method is sensitive to 20 mg protein/dl urine and has a broad specificity reacting with all types of proteins but also with iodine containing x-ray contrast media, plasma volume expanders, intravenous albumin, and sulfisoxazole (Gantrisin).

Combined use of dipstick and sulfosalicylic acid test: If both methods are positive, proteinuria is present; if both tests are negative, proteinuria is absent. If the dipstick is 1 + and the sulfosalicylic acid test is negative, there is probably no pathologic concentration of protein in the urine. If the reverse is found (i.e., the dipstick is negative and the sulfosalicylic acid test is positive), then the protein may be Bence Jones protein or one of the heavy-chain proteins and should be confirmed by immunologic (electrophoretic) methods (see below).

Table 27-3. Method of reporting of sulfosalicylic acid semiquantitative turbidity method for urinary proteins

Turbidity	Protein range (mg/dl)
None	7.5
Trace (when sample placed in beam of light)	20
1 + (print can be easily seen and read when viewed through test tube)	30-100
2 + (print can be seen but not easily read when viewed through test tube)	100-250
3 + (print cannot be seen when viewed through test tube)	250-450
4 + (precipitate formed)	>450

Quantitative methods

Trichloroacetic acid method: See p. 501.

Immunologic methods: Immunologic methods measure urinary protein concentration according to the molecular size of the protein. Low concentrations of albumin may be measured by using radial immunodiffusion Endoplates (Kallestad Laboratories, Chaske, Minn.), which are devised for quantitation of low concentration of albumin in cerebrospinal fluid.[36] The disadvantage of this method is that the plates are specific for albumin. Electrophoresis of concentrated urine specimens[37] on a number of media, e.g., agarose gel, cellulose acetate, polyacrylamide gel containing sodium dodecyl sulfate, can be utilized to distinguish glomerular from tubular proteinuria.[38-40] Prior to electrophoresis, the 24 hr urine specimen is concentrated fiftyfold in the Minicon B-15 concentrator (Amicon Corp., Lexington, Mass.). If cellulose acetate plates[41] are used, the electrophoresis is performed on Titan III (Zip Zone Plates, Helena Laboratories, Beaumont, Tex.) for 15 min at 180 V in barbital buffer (125 mmole/L, pH 8.8). The plates are then stained with Ponceau S and cleared. For acrylamide gel electrophoresis the Beckman model R-113 is used (Beckman Instruments, Fullerton, Calif.).[42] See "Selectivity of protein excretion" below.

Proteinuria

Proteinuria implies the presence of proteins in the urine in a high enough concentration to be detected by clinical laboratory methods. A trace amount of protein (up to 150 mg/24 hr) may be present in the urine of healthy individuals, but it remains undetected by clinical laboratory methods. Twenty-three percent of this protein is albumin,[43] and the remainder is **Tamm-Horsfall protein**[44] and other nonplasma proteins. The Tamm-Horsfall protein is excreted by distal tubules and collecting ducts and forms the matrix of renal casts.[45] Since most of the abnormal protein found in the urine is albumin, the protein excretion is often called albuminuria.

Selectivity of protein excretion

Selectivity[46] is not related to the amount of proteinuria but to the type of protein lost in the urine. In the face of equal degrees of proteinuria, selectivity is related to the type of glomerular damage and to its response to steroid therapy. Selectivity is high in lipoid nephrosis **(minimal change disease),** which responds to steroid therapy, and is low in nephrosis complicating various forms of glomerulonephritis, which is nonselective.

The differentiation of urinary proteins on the basis of their molecular size also allows the distinction of renal disease of glomerular etiology from that of tubular origin.[42] Glomerular damage allows the escape of serum proteins of intermediate molecular size (50,000-200,000), e.g., albumin, α-macroglobulins, transferrin, and IgG,[47] whereas tubular proteins excreted into the urine are made up of such components as lysozyme, L chains, β_2-microglobulins, and α_2-microglobulins, all proteins of a molecular weight of less than 44,000.[47] In glomerular proteinuria, the ratio of albumin to low-molecular-weight proteins is 20:1, whereas in tubular proteinuria the ratio is about 1:1.[42]

Proteinuria may be classified on the basis of pore size:

1. Prerenal proteinuria. Low-molecular-weight proteins, e.g., hemoglobin (mol. wt., 65,450), myoglobin, or Bence Jones protein, accumulate in the plasma and are filtered out by the kidney in such concentrations as to block their tubular absorption.

2. Glomerular proteinuria. It is caused by increased permeability of the glomerular capillary membrane to normal plasma proteins, resulting from glomerular injury inflicted by immune complexes, antibodies, toxins, and bacteria. Increasing glomerular permeability (increasing pore size) allows proteins of varying sizes to escape into the filtrate. The proteins of low molecular weight pass through the injured glomerulus first, e.g., hemoglobin (mol. wt., 68,000) and albumin (mol. wt., 70,000), followed by middle-molecular-weight proteins (mol. wt., 100,000), e.g., globulins (mol. wt., 90,000), which as the glomerular damage increases are followed by high-molecular-weight proteins (mol. wt. over 100,000), e.g., fibrinogen (mol. wt., 400,000) and globulin (mol. wt., 156,000). In nonselective (global) proteinuria all serum proteins from low to high molecular weight are found in the urine, indicating severe glomerular damage. In selective proteinuria only serum components of low molecular weight (less than 100,000), e.g., transferrin and albumin, are found in the urine, indicating minimal change disease.[48]

Glomerular proteinuria is encountered in orthostatic or postural proteinuria, membranous and acute proliferative glomerulonephritis, chronic pyelonephritis, polycystic disease, diabetic glomerulosclerosis, amyloidosis, systemic lupus erythematosus, Goodpasture's syndrome, nephrosclerosis, renal vein thrombosis, and lipoid nephrosis.

3. Tubular proteinuria. Tubular proteinuria is encountered in heavy metal poisoning, Fanconi's syndrome,[49] Wilson's disease, renal tubular acidosis, and galactosemia. The proteins are of low molecular weight, and the diagnosis requires immunologic methods.

4. Nonpathologic proteinuria. Nonpathologic forms are seen in postural (orthostatic) proteinuria, transient proteinuria, and proteinuria after muscular exertion.

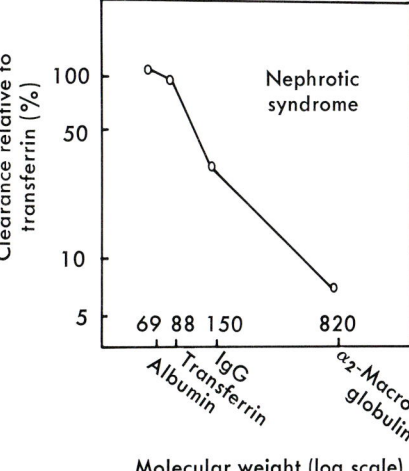

Fig. 27-4. Relative clearances of four plasma proteins plotted against molecular weight ($\times 10^{-3}$). (From Rennie, D.I.: Med. Clin. North Am. **55**:213, 1971.)

These proteins are not derived from plasma proteins but originate in the prostate, vagina, semen, seminal vesicles, pus, or periurethral glands.

Technics of pore sizing and selectivity measuring

The clearance of IgG as compared to that of albumin or transferrin is used as an index of selectivity (Fig. 27-4). The molecular weight of IgG is about twice that of albumin and transferrin; the percent of related clearance is determined from the following equation:

$$\frac{C_1}{C_a} \times 100 = \%$$

where C_1 = clearance of IgG, and C_a = clearance of albumin. The clearance is determined on the basis of the clearance formula, C = UV/P (see p. 726). As in the calculation of the ratio the volume of urine cancels out, the clearance formula is reduced to C = U/P, where C = clearance, U = urinary concentration of test substance, and P = the concentration in plasma (or serum). The concentration of the proteins is determined by the immunologic method described above or by the recently introduced nephelometry.[50,51]

Aminoaciduria

The renal threshold for plasma amino acids is high, so that only small amounts of amino acids are normally found in urine. Amino acids are excreted by the glomeruli but are readily reabsorbed by the tubules. The amino acids that normally occur in larger quantities (25-200 mg/24 hr) in urine are glycine, taurine, histidine, and glutamine. The other amino acids (e.g., tryptophan, tyrosine, serine, leucine, cystine, arginine, and phenylalanine) occur in much smaller amounts (0-25 mg/24 hr).

Dent's classification of aminoaciduria[52]

Renal aminoaciduria: Renal aminoaciduria results from defective tubular reabsorption of certain amino acids and leads to increased renal excretion. The classification is as follows:

1. Generalized
   Fanconi's syndrome
   Cystinosis
   Wilson's disease
   Galactosemia
2. Specific
   Cystinuria
   Glycinuria

Overflow aminoaciduria: Overflow aminoaciduria results from increased plasma amino acid concentration, which accounts for hypersecretion of urinary amino acids. The classification is as follows:

1. Generalized
   Liver disease
   Premature and newborn infants
   Megaloblastic anemias
   Lead poisoning
   Muscular dystrophies
   Wilson's disease
   Leukemia
2. Specific
   Maple syrup urine disease
   Hartnup disease
   Phenylketonuria (phenylalaninemia)

Abnormal excretion of products derived from amino acids: The classification is as follows:

1. Alkaptonuria
2. Oxalosis
3. Tyrosinosis
4. Pyridoxine deficiency
5. Folic acid deficiency

Tests for amino acids[53]

The total excretion of amino acids can be evaluated by measuring the total free α-amino acid nitrogen in urine and determining its ratio to total nitrogen or creatinine. Specific amino acids can be determined by paper, column, and thin-layer chromatography as well as by thin-layer electrophoresis (low and high voltage).

Test for amino acid nitrogen:

Procedure: See chemistry section, p. 492.

Normal values: The average adult excretes about 50-200 mg amino acid nitrogen in the urine in 24 hr, the full-term infant about 8 mg/kg/day, and the premature infant about four times as much. Throughout childhood a value of about 3 mg/kg/day is maintained. The total value of amino acid nitrogen is not as important clinically as the amounts of the individual amino acids. Total amino acids are increased in "overflow aminoaciduria" (see Dent's classification above). It must be differentiated from renal aminoaciduria in which only certain amino acids fail to be reabsorbed.

Thin-layer chromatography of urinary amino acids[53-58]:

Principle: The method is based on the different speeds with which compounds travel in two phases: a solid phase and a liquid phase. The liquid or mobile phase is usually an organic solvent saturated with water, whereas the solid or stationary phase is water saturated with organic liquid held stationary within a silica base.

For a complete separation of urinary amino acids, two-dimensional chromatography is best. However, if a particular amino acid or group of amino acids is suspected of being present in abnormal concentrations, this can often be detected by one-dimensional chromatography. Comparison is made by chromatographing on the same sheet the unknown sample, a normal urine specimen, and a normal urine specimen to which the suspected amino acids are added. If chromatograms are run with two or three different solvents, the identification can usually be made in a few hours. This method requires some idea as to the nature of the amino acid abnormality, e.g., cystinuria (cystine), phenylketonuria (phenylalanine), maple syrup disease (leucine, isoleucine, and valine), or Hartnup disease (glutamine, histidine, and alanine). Since the offending amino acids are usually excreted in amounts that are many times normal, they can usually be readily recognized. The amino acid standards are made up in concentrations of 0.5 mg/ml in a solvent of 8 ml concentrated hydrochloric acid and 1 dl isopropanol made up to 1 L with water. These solutions are quite stable in the refrigerator.

Concentration of urine for chromatography or electrophoresis: The sample is concentrated in a disposable, multiple ultra filter intended for concentrating the macromolecular constituents of dilute specimens (Minicon, SC 15, Amicon Corp., Lexington, Mass.).

One-dimensional chromatogram:

Procedure: Apply standards and urine to a Brinkmann SIL-N-HR sheet (Brinkmann Instruments, Westbury, N.Y.) as outlined in the general procedure (p. 457). Apply 2 μl standard and not more than 5 μl urine (less if the urine is concentrated). If microcapillaries are used, fill nearly full; then touch the end to a piece of filter paper until the desired amount remains in the capillary (assuming the total capacity is 5 μl).

When the specimen sample is first applied to the sheet, the spot will appear dark. As the liquid evaporates, the spot will appear brighter (whiter) than the background. With further evaporation of the solvent the difference in appearance between the spot and the background will decrease until the spot is barely visible. It is then dry enough for a second application if necessary. Keep the size of the spots as small as possible by making small applications. Care must be taken in handling the sheets. Touching the surface with the fingers will leave material (amino acids from the skin) that will produce spots with the ninhydrin spray reagent. The unknown urine specimen, control urine specimens, and standard can be applied to a 5 × 20 cm sheet. Develop with chloroform-methanol–concentrated ammonium hydroxide (4:4:1) or butanol-ethanol-water (7:2:2) for about 10 min. Remove from the chamber, air dry for a short time, and then heat in an oven to dry completely. Spray with ninhydrin reagent (0.3 g ninhydrin in 1 dl butanol and 3 ml glacial acetic acid). Take care not to spray on too much liquid, because this may cause the spots to run. Air dry the sheet again for a few minutes and then place it in an oven at 105-110° C. After heating for a few minutes remove it from the oven and inspect it for faint spots, carefully marking them with a pencil. After several more minutes repeat the heating process. In this way, spots that may become confluent on prolonged heating can be identified separately. Finally, heat for 15-20 min to develop the less sensitive spots. Compare the pattern developed by the unknown sample with those of the control urine and the control plus added amino acid.

The intensity of the spots will be roughly proportional to the amount of amino acid present. With the ninhydrin, most of the amino acid spots will be shades of purple. Proline will give a yellow spot and should be marked with a pencil, because it may fade. The chromatogram may be preserved for a while by spraying with a protective lacquer. (Krylon, clear spray, Krylon, Morristown, Pa.) Here also, avoid too much spray, which will cause the spots to run. It is best to apply several thin coats, allowing the chromatogram to dry between each application.

Two-dimensional chromatogram: Although two-dimensional chromatograms give a better separation of the many different amino acids, the disadvantage is that only one specimen can be run on a sheet; hence, if standards or controls are desired, they must each be chromatographed separately.

Procedure: Apply the sample at a point near the lower right-hand corner of a 20 × 20 cm sheet at a distance of 1.5 cm from each edge. After drying, place the sheet in the chamber, with the point of application at the lower right-hand corner just above the solvent. Chromatograph with the chloroform-methanol-ammonia solvent for a distance of 12-13 cm. Remove from the chamber and dry completely in the oven. Then replace the sheet in the developing chamber, turning it 90 degrees clockwise from its original position, so that the point of application is now at the lower left-hand

corner, just above the solvent. Develop with the butanol-ethanol-water solvent for a distance of about 12-13 cm. Remove from the chamber, dry, and spray with the ninhydrin reagent. Heat as described for the one-dimensional chromatogram.

Since the R_f values for the different amino acids will vary somewhat under the exact conditions, it is best to run known amino acids or controls. However, Fig. 27-5 will serve as a guide. If a few normal urine controls are run, one will have a guide as to what the normal pattern should be and thus be able to recognize an abnormal one.

There are now well over 100 known conditions attributable to "errors of metabolism"[56] in which there is a defect at the molecular or enzymatic level. Since treatment, which should be initiated as early as possible, is available for some of these conditions, early screening of newborns for the "treatable" conditions (phenylketonuria, branched-chain ketoaciduria, etc.) is essential (Table 27-4).

High-voltage electrophoresis[59,60]: High-voltage electrophoresis (exceeding 400 V) using paper or thin-layer material has advantages and disadvantages as compared with conventional thin-layer chromatography. The advantages are (1) better separation of smaller molecular substances, which is not possible by conventional chromatography, and (2) increasing voltage increases the migration speed so that the analysis time is shortened.

The disadvantages involve (1) expensive equipment with an elaborate cooling system and (2) danger of high voltage.

Renal aminoaciduria
Fanconi's syndrome[61]

Fanconi's syndrome, transmitted by an autosomal recessive gene, is divided into an infantile and an adult type according to the time of its clinical appearance. The infantile type is frequently associated with cystinosis.

Laboratory diagnosis: Although the clinical manifestations differ in the two types, the laboratory findings are essentially similar. Aminoaciduria of 10 or more amino acids occurs as part of the multiple renal transport mechanism defect, which also leads to glycosuria, polyuria with fixed specific gravity, and increased excretion of potassium, phosphorus, and uric acid with corresponding lowering of their serum levels. In the infantile type, cystine deposits can be found in the reticulum cells of bone marrow aspirates and of kidney or liver biopsy specimens.

Cystinosis

Cystinosis is an inherited metabolic disorder characterized by deposition of cystine crystals in tissue (Fig. 27-6); it is part of Fanconi's syndrome and must not be confused with cystinuria.

Cystinuria

Cystinuria[62] represents a congenital defect involving reabsorption of four amino acids—cystine, lysine, ornithine, and arginine—by the kidney tubules. The demonstration of cystine and the other three amino ac-

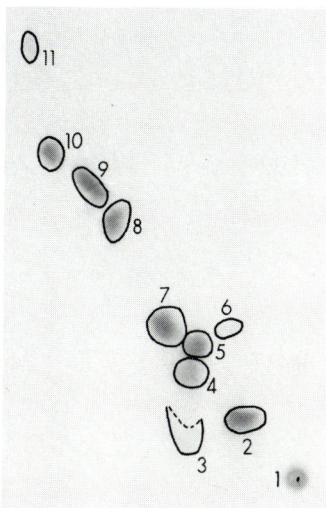

Fig. 27-5. Urinary two-dimensional thin-layer amino acid chromatogram.

1 Starting point	**7** Glutamine
2 Lysine	**8** Valine
3 Glutamic acid	**9** Leucine isoleucine
4 Glycine	**10** Marker
5 Alanine	**11** Peptide
6 Histidine	

(Courtesy C. Utz.)

Table 27-4. Characteristics of some genetically determined aminoacidurias

Condition	Amino acids excreted in urine	Other substances excreted in urine	Pathogenesis	Main clinical features	Heredity	Heterozygote expression
Cystinuria	Cystine, lysine, arginine, ornithine	—	Specific renal tubular defect	Urinary calculi	Recessive	*
Phenylketonuria	Phenylalanine	Phenylpyruvic acid and metabolites, indolyllactic and indolylacetic acids	Absence of phenylalanine hydroxylase	Mental defect	Recessive	†
Maple syrup urine disease (branched-chain ketoaciduria)	Leucine, valine, isoleucine	α-Keto acids, α-hydroxy acids, indolyllactic and indolylacetic acids	Missing enzyme(s)	Cerebral degeneration	Probably recessive	‡
Hypophosphatasia	Phosphorylethanolamine	—	Lack of phosphatase	Bony changes	Recessive	*
Galactosemia	As in plasma§	Galactose, protein	Absence of transferase	Liver damage, cataracts, mental defect	Recessive	†
Wilson's disease	? As in plasma§	Copper, sometimes glucose	Defect in copper metabolism	Cirrhosis, lenticular degeneration	Recessive	†
Cystinosis	As in plasma§	Glucose, phosphate, K^+, HCO^-, protein	?	Dwarfing, rickets, acidosis, early death	Recessive	‡
β-Aminoisobutyric aciduria	β-Aminoisobutyric acid	—	Probably missing enzyme	Benign in character	Recessive	‡
Cystathioninuria	Cystathionine	—	Probably missing enzyme	? Mental defect	?	‡
Argininosuccinic aciduria	Argininosuccinic acid	—	?	Mental defect	?	‡
Hartnup syndrome	Tryptophan and many others	Indican, indolylacetic acid and its conjugates	Defects in amino acid transport	Pellagra (variable)	Recessive	‡
Benign familial aminoaciduria	As in plasma§	Glucose, protein, sometimes phosphate	Renal tubular defect	Benign in character	Dominant	*
Glycinuria	Glycine	? Oxalate	Specific renal tubular defect	Urinary calculi	Dominant	*
Lowe-Terrey-MacLachlan syndrome	Lysine, arginine, histidine, tyrosine, and many others	Organic acids, protein, glucose	Multiple congenital abnormalities	Cerebroocular malformations	?	‡
Infantile hepatic and renal dysfunction	As in plasma, but all in very high concentration, tyrosine prominent§	Glucose, phenolic acids, protein, phosphate, HCO_3^-	?	Jaundice, early death, rickets, acidosis, cirrhosis	?	‡
De Toni-Debré-Fanconi syndrome	As in plasma§	Glucose, phosphate, HCO^-	Variable	Rickets, acidosis	Recessive	‡
Osteomalacia with aminoaciduria	As in plasma§	Glucose, phosphate	Renal tubular defects	Osteomalacia	Recessive	‡

From Woolf, L.J.: Br. Med. Bull. **17:**225, 1961.
*Some or all heterozygotes spontaneously show aminoaciduria.
†Heterozygotes show abnormality on a loading test.
‡No heterozygote expression detected.
§All the amino acids present in plasma appear in the urine in approximately the same concentrations, relative one to another, as in plasma.

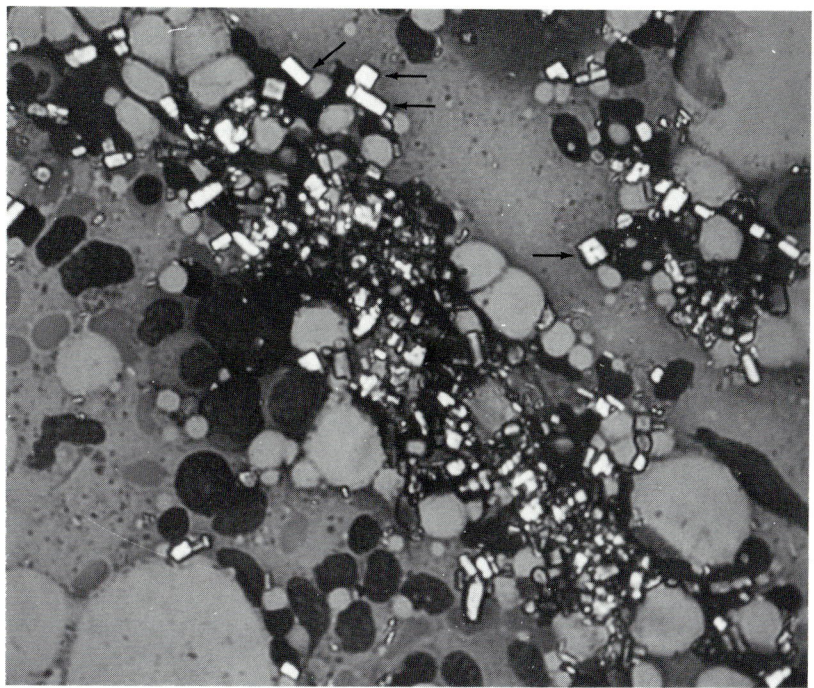

Fig. 27-6. Cystine crystals in bone marrow aspirates of child with cystinosis. Under polarized light, crystals (arrows) light up.

ids in urine helps to distinguish this disease from cystinosis (see above), a generalized disease involving 10 or more amino acids and leading to cystine deposits in the organs of the reticuloendothelial system (liver, bone marrow, etc.) and in the kidneys. The main clinical feature of cystinuria is recurrent cystine calculus formation, which does not occur in cystinosis. The blood levels of the four amino acids involved are normal or low.

Laboratory diagnosis:

Thin-layer amino acid chromatography: Thin-layer chromatography reveals a characteristic four-amino-acids pattern with increased amounts of cystine, lysine, ornithine, and arginine.

Crystals in urinary sediment: In acid urine, colorless, hexagonal, transparent crystal plates are seen (Fig. 27-7); these are insoluble in water, alcohol, and acetic acid. The presence of cystine crystals can be confirmed by the cyanide nitroprusside test.

Cyanide nitroprusside test (Lewis)[63]:

Principle: Cystine is reduced to cysteine by alkaline cyanide, which gives a purple-red compound when nitroprusside is added.

Reagents:
1. Sodium cyanide aqueous, 5% (5 g/dl)
2. Sodium nitroprusside, 5% (5 g/dl)

Procedure: To 5 ml urine add 2 ml of 5% sodium cyanide solution. Mix and allow to stand for 10 min. Add 5% sodium nitroprusside drop by drop and shake.

Result: The presence of cystine leads to a red color.

Modification of cyanide nitroprusside test: Fischl[64] and Humbel and Kutter[65] modified the cyanide nitroprusside test by using a finely **powdered reagent.**

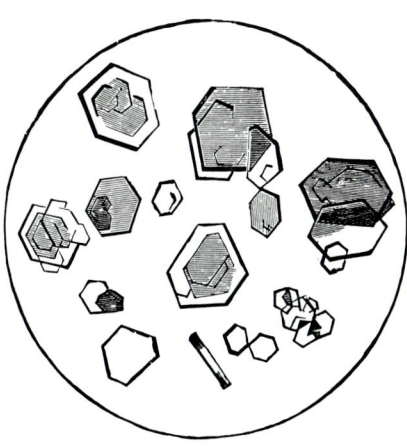

Fig. 27-7. Cystine crystals from patient with cystinuria. (From Gershenfeld, L.: Urine and urinalysis, Philadelphia, 1948, Lea & Febiger.)

Reagent: The reagent consists of the following:
1. Sodium nitroprusside, powdered, 1 g
2. Sodium carbonate, anhydrous, powdered, 200 g
3. Sodium ammonium sulfate, powdered, 200 g
Mix in mortar. To 50 g mixture, add:
1. Sodium cyanide, powdered, 5 g
2. Aluminum hydroxide, 200 g

Procedure: Build a small mound of powder with a central depression and add 3 drops of urine.

Result: The presence of cystine leads to a red ring around the urine spot.

Interpretation: See discussion of Acetest (below).
Acetest tablet procedure:
Principle: The Acetest (Ames Co., Elkhart, Ind.) tablet procedure[66] represents a modification of the Lewis test in which sodium cyanide in 1N sodium hydroxide and Acetest tablets are used as the source of nitroprusside and buffer.
Reagents:
1. Acetest tablet
2. Sodium hydroxide, 1N
3. Sodium cyanide, 10%, in 1N sodium hydroxide (10 g/dl)
Procedure: Place an Acetest tablet on a spot plate. Add 1 large drop of sodium cyanide reagent to the tablet, immediately followed by 1 drop of urine.
Result: A cherry-red color at 1 min in solution around the tablet indicates presence of cystine.
Interpretation: According to Free and Free,[57] a positive test indicates 25 mg or more of cystine per 1 dl urine. The normal excretion of cystine is 40-80 mg/day. In patients with cystinuria the amount increases to 700-1500 mg/day. The intensity of the color is proportional to the amount of cystine. Homocystine, which may occur as the result of an inborn error of metabolism, also gives a red color with the Acetest tablet technic. Ketone bodies that give a positive "powder test" do not give a false positive reaction with the Acetest tablet.

Wilson's disease (hepatolenticular degeneration)[67]

Wilson's disease is a genetically determined metabolic disorder of low incidence associated with the following laboratory findings: low serum copper levels (hypocupremia), high urinary copper excretion, aminoaciduria, glycosuria, phosphatemia and phosphaturia, hypouricemia, uricosuria, and often proteinuria. The plasma ceruloplasmin level is usually decreased. Clinically, there is evidence of mental retardation, slowing of movement, and a gray-green ring at the periphery of the cornea (Kayser-Fleischer ring).
Laboratory diagnosis: The procedures related to copper metabolism are sensitive enough to discover asymptomatic cases (homozygous and heterozygous) as well as to confirm any clinically proved cases. The most useful screening tests are the determination of (1) 24 hr urinary copper levels before and during oral penicillamine administration, (2) plasma ceruloplasmin levels, and (3) SGOT and SGPT levels (nonspecific). For all these procedures, see the chemistry section.
Results: In Wilson's disease the urinary copper levels are consistently elevated, the plasma copper levels are low, the ceruloplasmin level is usually low, and the transaminases may show nonspecific elevations.

Galactosemia

Galactosemia is an inherited disease transmitted by an autosomal recessive gene that is characterized by the inability to metabolize galactose to glucose. If untreated, the disease leads to liver and brain damage. The urine not only contains increased levels of galactose but also excessive amounts of amino acids.
Diagnosis: See urinary sugars, p. 696.

Overflow aminoaciduria
Maple syrup urine disease (branched-chain ketoaciduria)

Maple syrup urine disease is an inherited disorder characterized by the inability to metabolize branched-chain amino acids (leucine, isoleucine, and valine) so that they and their respective α-keto acids accumulate in the plasma and urine.
Diagnosis: Thin-layer chromatography of plasma and urine reveals increased levels of branched-chain keto acids (Table 27-4).

Hartnup disease

Hartnup disease, named after a patient, is a congenital disorder characterized by skin rash and cerebellar ataxia. The defect lies in the failure of the kidney tubules to reabsorb tryptophan.
Diagnosis: Aminoaciduria, diagnosed by thin-layer chromatography involving 10 or more amino acids and associated with the clinical manifestations mentioned, provides the basis of the diagnosis.
Screening test: Dinitrophenylhydrazine test.
Reagents:
1. 2,4-Dinitrophenylhydrazine, 0.1%, in 2N hydrochloric acid
2. Hydrochloric acid, 2N (168 ml concentrated hydrochloric acid per 10 dl)
Procedure: Centrifuge fresh urine, add 1 ml reagent, and allow to stand for 10 min before reporting results.
Results: A heavy white precipitate indicates excess α-keto acids, which is indicative of Hartnup disease.

Phenylalaninemia[68]

The degradation of phenylalanine, one of the essential alimentary amino acids, occurs in a number of steps, each of which is catalyzed by an enzyme system.[69]
1. Phenylalanine is converted to tyrosine by phenylalanine hydroxylase. The deficiency of this enzyme leads to increased levels of phenylalanine in the blood and to **phenylketonuria**.
2. Tyrosine is metabolized to homogentisic acid with the help of p-hydroxyphenylpyruvic oxidase. The deficiency of this enzyme leads to **tyrosinosis**.
3. Homogentisic acid is converted to maleylacetoacetic acid with the help of homogentisic oxidase. The deficiency of this enzyme leads to **alkaptonuria**.
4. Tyrosine is converted by tyrosinase to 3,4-dihydroxyphenylalanine (dopa) and to melanin. Absence of this enzyme leads to **albinism**.

Types of phenylalaninemia: A number of conditions and combinations contribute to the heterogeneous pattern of phenylalaninemia. Menkes,[70] Carpenter, Auerbach, and DiGeorge,[71] and Hsia[72] proposed various classifications of phenylalaninemic types according to the laboratory findings.

Phenylketonuria

Phenylketonuria (PKU)[68,73] is a hereditary form of mental retardation associated with the appearance of

phenylpyruvic acid in the urine and of increased levels of **phenylalanine** in the blood and spinal fluid. It is caused by a congenital hereditary deficiency of hepatic phenylalanine hydroxylase (heat-labile fraction),[74] which normally oxidizes alimentary phenylalanine to tyrosine, so that under normal conditions only minute amounts of phenylalanine are transaminated to phenylpyruvic acid. In phenylalanine hydroxylase deficiency, tyrosine is not produced.

The diagnosis is based on the following measures: (1) screening test for phenylpyruvic acid in urine, (2) screening test for increased levels of phenylalanine in blood, and (3) quantitative measurement of phenylalanine in blood.

Urine tests for phenylpyruvic acid:

Ferric chloride test[75]:

Reagent: Ferric chloride, 10% (10 g/dl). Store in refrigerator.

Procedure: Add 3-5 drops of reagent to 5 ml fresh acid urine.

Results: A positive test is indicated by a grayish green or blue-green color appearing in 1-90 sec and fading again in the same period of time.

Discussion: The test depends on the following conditions[76]:

1. The concentration of phenylpyruvic acid in the urine. It is therefore necessary to avoid low specific gravity (diluted urine).

2. Temperature. Phenylpyruvic acid is unstable when standing at room temperature. Tests should therefore be performed on fresh urine or on urine that has been refrigerated immediately after voiding. At refrigerator temperature, phenylpyruvic acid is stable, but the urine must be allowed to come to room temperature before it is tested for the presence of phenylpyruvic acid.

3. pH. The method suggested gives a final pH of about 2.3.[77]

Interpretation: The test is sensitive enough to detect over 40-50 μg phenylpyruvic acid/ml urine. In children with PKU the output may vary from 100-300 μg/ml urine with no diurnal variation.[1]

The test has many disadvantages, including the following: (1) for various reasons it may not detect up to 50% of children with PKU; (2) urine is difficult to collect in newborns; (3) there are interfering substances, e.g., high levels of phosphates and many other substances, that give color reactions with ferric chloride (Table 27-5)[78,79]; (4) the test is negative even in affected children in the first week of life when the diagnosis is important; and (5) PKU reflects the phenylalanine level in the plasma, and this level depends on the diet and on the presence or absence of infection, during which it usually increases.

Phenistix: Phenistix (Ames Co., Elkhart, Ind.) is a reagent strip impregnated at one end with ferric ammonium sulfate, a buffer, and a magnesium salt.

NOTE: Neither the ferric chloride test nor the Phenistix should be used to screen newborns for PKU.

Blood phenylalanine screening test: bacterial inhibition test (Guthrie)[80]:

Principle: Germination of spores of *Bacillus subtilis* is markedly enhanced by the presence of phenylalanine

Table 27-5. Reactions of ferric chloride with various substances in urine

Substance	Reaction
Phenazopyridine (Azo Gantrisin)	Red-brown
Diacetic acid	Purple
Homogentisic acid (alkaptonuria)	Transient green
Melanin (melanogen)	Gray-black precipitate
p-Aminosalicylic acid	Red-brown
Phenacetin	Reddish
Phenylpyruvic acid	Transient green
Salicylates	Purple
Thiocyanates	Red-brown
Thorazine	Purple to red-brown

Based on data from Lancaster, R.G., and Marsh, H.H.: Urinalysis workshop, New Orleans, 1968; and Gibbs, N.K., and Woolf, L.I.: Br. Med. J. 2:532, 1959.

in a medium containing an inhibitor to spore germination. One drop of blood taken from the infant's heel is collected on a special filter paper disk, which is then placed on the streaked medium. The area of bacterial growth around the specimen disk is compared with areas of growth around control disks containing known amounts of phenylalanine. Elevated phenylalanine plasma levels may be found before urine levels are increased.

Interpretation: The test is fairly specific, inexpensive, and relatively accurate in concentrations below 20 mg phenylalanine/dl blood. The blood specimen should be obtained 24 hr after the first milk feeding of the infant.

Quantitative fluorometric phenylalanine determination in blood[81]: Quantitative fluorometric phenylalanine determination in blood is the method of choice, because both the Guthrie test and the Phenistix method may produce false positive results.

Principle: The test is based on the fact that the fluorescence of the phenylalanine-ninhydrin-copper complex is greatly enhanced when formed in the presence of a peptide such as leucylalanine. Since the test is often performed on infants, the directions are given for use of only a small amount of serum. With microtechnics, even smaller amounts can be used.[82]

Reagents:

1. Succinate buffer, 0.6M, pH 5.88
   Dissolve 16.21 g sodium succinate ($Na_2C_4H_4O_4 \cdot 6H_2O$) in water containing 8 ml 1N hydrochloric acid and dilute almost to 1 dl. Mix well and check the pH. Adjust if necessary and dilute to 1 dl. Store in refrigerator.

2. Ninhydrin, 0.03M
   Dissolve 0.534 g ninhydrin in water to make 1 dl. Store in refrigerator.

3. Leucylalanine, 0.005M
   Dissolve 0.1 g of the peptide in 1 dl water. This solution is not stable. Divide into small aliquots and keep frozen until needed. If the test is run only occasionally, it may be more convenient to use either sterile ampules containing 1 mg/ml

peptide (Schwarz-Mann Laboratories, New York) or preweighed vials containing 2 mg of the peptide (Sigma Chemical Co., St. Louis) to be dissolved just before use.

4. Fluorescence reagent
On the day of use mix 5 volumes of solution 1 (succinate buffer), 2 volumes of solution 2 (ninhydrin), and 1 volume of solution 3 (peptide).

5. Copper diluent
Prepare daily by mixing 3 volumes of solution containing 2.66 g anhydrous sodium carbonate and 113 mg Rochelle salt in 1 L, and 2 volumes of solution containing 200 mg crystalline copper sulfate/L.

6. Trichloroacetic acid, 0.6M
Dissolve 9.8 g trichloroacetic acid in water and dilute to 1 dl.

7. Phenylalanine standards
Dissolve 5, 10, and 20 mg phenylalanine in 1 dl solution containing 7.5% bovine albumin. Also prepare a blank solution containing only the bovine albumin. Divide the standards and blank in small aliquots in test tubes, stopper securely, keep frozen, and thaw as needed. The standards are made up in bovine albumin, so that when the standards are treated like the serum samples, the final pH will be the same in all.

Procedure: Add 0.1 ml serum or heparinized plasma to 0.1 ml trichloroacetic acid in a small test tube. Mix well and allow to stand for 10 min. Treat 0.1 ml aliquots of the blank and standards similarly. After they stand for a while, centrifuge strongly. To 0.05 ml supernatant add 0.80 ml mixed reagent and incubate at 60° C for 2 hr. Cool by immersion in tap water; then add 5 ml copper diluent. Mix and determine the fluorescence within 1 hr. Use filters with an activating wavelength of 365 nm and a secondary filter at 515 nm. Either read standards and samples against blank or read all tubes against water and subtract blank reading from that of standards and samples.

Calculation:

$$\frac{\text{Sample reading}}{\text{Standard reading}} \times \frac{\text{Conc. of}}{\text{standard}} = \frac{\text{Conc. of}}{\text{sample}}$$

The readings are corrected for the blank and the standard reading closest to the sample reading is used. The three standards used are equivalent to 5, 10, and 20 mg/dl phenylalanine.

Normal values and interpretation: By this method the normal range for adults is 0.9-2.2 mg/dl; for newborn infants, it is 1.6-2.6 mg/dl. Newborn infants with low birth weights have a slightly higher range, 3.7-4.7 mg/dl. In contrast, children with PKU have levels of 16-46 mg/dl. Heterozygous parents of children with PKU have slightly higher values than the normal adult population, with a range of 1.4-2.5 mg/dl.

Elevated serum tyrosine may contribute to the fluorescence, but in infants with PKU, tyrosine levels are usually low.[83] Therefore in doubtful cases the **quantitative tyrosine level** (low) may add to the diagnostic armamentarium.

Phenylalanine tolerance test[84]: This test is useful for the diagnosis of heterozygotes. A dose of 200 mg/kg L-phenylalanine is divided into two portions; one-half is given initially and the other half is given 30 min later and the blood tyrosine response or the phenylalanine/tyrosine ratio is measured on the amino acid analyzer. The best method for the detection of the individual heterozygous for PKU is the determination of the phenylalanine/tyrosine ratio before lunch after breakfast.[84a]

PHENYLKETONURIA: ITS DIAGNOSIS AND VARIANTS

The hepatic phenylalanine hydroxylase system consists of two enzymes and two nonprotein cofactors.[85] In classical PKU the affected component is phenylalanine hydroxylase. Despite 10 yr of experience with screening programs for hyperphenylalaninemia in newborn infants, there is still some problem in identifying the infant who must be treated to prevent mental retardation and convulsions.[86] Not all infants who have a positive screening test have classical PKU, because 85% of those infants have normal phenylalanine concentration (up to 20 mg/dl) on regular diets and do not develop mental retardation.[87] Between 5% and 10% of infants who ultimately develop PKU are not detected by screening methods. There are a number of reasons for these false negative results:

1. In the first 4 days of life the blood phenylalanine concentration in infants with PKU is only minimally elevated[88] and may remain undetected by poorly controlled screening tests.

2. Many infants do not eat well the first 4 days, and most infants are screened on the third day.

3. A PKU variant may be present.

Recently, several variants of PKU have been identified that result from defects of the other two components of the hydroxylase system: dihydropteridine reductase and tetrahydrobiopterin or a related pterin. In some of these infants retardation is severe and is unresponsive to dietary restrictions of phenylalanine.[89] Screening tests are negative or inconclusive, because the blood concentration of phenylalanine in the face of a regular diet rises only minimally.[90]

Abnormal excretion of products derived from amino acids
Alkaptonuria

Alkaptonuria is a rare congenital (single recessive gene) metabolic disease in which the enzyme homogentisic acid oxidase is absent. The error in the metabolism leads to the accumulation and excretion of homogentisic acid (a normal intermediary metabolite of phenylalanine and tyrosine), which cannot be metabolized. The patient is clinically well until the later years of life when black pigments are deposited in the bones and joints (**ochronosis**).

Diagnosis: The diagnosis is based on the demonstration of homogentisic acid, which is not normally present in urine.

Urine may appear normal on voiding but turns reddish brown or black on standing or on becoming alkaline. The reaction begins on the surface.

Ferric chloride test:

Reagent: Ferric chloride, 10% (10 g/dl).

Procedure: Add reagent drop by drop; if homogentisic acid is present, a bluish black color develops, which rapidly fades.

Tyrosinosis (tyrosinuria)

Tyrosinosis is a rare congenital defect in which *p*-hydroxyphenylpyruvic acid appears in the urine and gives a positive Millon reaction. Clinically, there is cirrhosis of the liver with abdominal distention and splenomegaly.

Millon test:

Reagent: Dissolve 1 ml mercury and 9 ml concentrated nitric acid with the aid of heat. Dilute with equal parts of water and allow to stand for several hours; filter.

Procedure: Mix equal parts of urine and reagent; heat the mixture to the boiling point.

Results: A red precipitate appears if tyrosine or *p*-hydroxyphenylpyruvic acid is present. Since Millon reagent also precipitates proteins, the test cannot be used on urine containing protein.

Homocystinuria

Homocystinuria[91] results from a congenital (recessive gene) defect in the metabolism of methionine, leading to excessive amounts of homocystine in the urine. Clinically, the disease is characterized by mental retardation associated with ocular, vascular, and skeletal changes. Cystinuria and homocystinuria can be distinguished by high-voltage paper electrophoresis.

MUCOPOLYSACCHARIDOSES[92]

Gene-determined disorders not only involve the enzymes controlling amino acid metabolism but may also involve the enzymes associated with the metabolism of mucopolysaccharides.

Mucopolysaccharides are large molecular substances found in various connective tissues, e.g., cartilage, the umbilical cord, the aorta, and heart valves, and are responsible for the physical characteristics of these tissues. According to their chemical composition, mucopolysaccharides are grouped into dermatan sulfate, heparan sulfate, keratan sulfate, chondroitin-6-sulfate, and cholesterol sulfate, which are excreted in abnormally large amounts in mucopolysaccharidoses (MPS). MPSs are divided into several groups such as Hurler's, Hunter's, Sanfilippo's, and Morquio's syndromes or into MPS I, II, III, IV, VI, and VII.[93] The outstanding abnormality in the metabolism of individuals with MPS is the excretion of about 100 mg mucopolysaccharides/day as compared to less than 15 mg mucopolysaccharides/day in normal individuals. The excretion pattern varies in the different types of MPS (Table 27-6).

Screening test:

Principle: Paper is impregnated with azure A dye, which forms purple metachromatic complexes with MPS.[94] The test is commercially available as MPS test papers (Ames Co., Elkhart, Ind.).

Reagents:
1. Test paper
2. Wash solution
    Dissolve 20 ml methanol and 0.1 ml glacial acetic acid in distilled water to make 2 dl.

Procedure: Use a fresh random or 24 hr refrigerated (without preservative) urine specimen. Cloudy urine must first be filtered or centrifuged. Place 1 drop of urine in the middle of the test paper. After 3 min transfer it to a Petri dish filled with wash solution. Rinse for 20 min, remove, and blot dry.

Results: A positive result is indicated by a distinct purple color where urine has been applied. A negative result is indicated by a pale blue background color only. A positive screening test should be confirmed by measuring the cetylpyridinium chloride–precipitable MPS[95] or by column chromatography.[96]

Table 27-6. The mucopolysaccharidoses*

Class	Eponym	Enzyme defect	Urinary mucopolysaccharides	Mental retardation	Corneal clouding	Skeletal dysplasia	Life expectancy (yr)
I-H	Hurler's disease	α-L-Iduronidase	DS, HS	+ +	−	+ + +	<10
I-S	Scheie's disease	α-L-Iduronidase	DS, HS	−	−	+	Normal
I-H/S	H/S compound	α-L-Iduronidase	DS, HS	+	−	+ +	20s
II-Severe	Hunter's disease	Iduronate sulfatase	DS, HS	+ +	−	+ +	<15
II-Mild	Hunter's disease	Iduronate sulfatase	DS, HS	+	−	+	Adulthood
III-A	Sanfilippo's disease	Heparan *N*-sulfatase	HS	+ + +	−	+	<20
III-B	Sanfilippo's disease	*N*-Acetyl-α-D-glucosaminidase	HS	+ + +	−	+	<20
III-C	Sanfilippo's disease	Heparin *N*-acetyl transferase	HS	+ +	−	+	Adulthood
IV	Morquio's syndrome	Hexosamine-6-sulfatase	KS, CS	−	−	+ + +	20-40
VI	Maroteaux-Lamy syndrome	Galactosamine-4-sulfatase	DS	−	+	+ +	20s
VII	Sly's disease	β-Glucuronidase	DS	+	+ −	+	?
Mucosulfatidosis		Multiple sulfatases	DS, HS Cholesterol S, sulfatide	+ +	−	+	3-12

From Kolodny, E.H.: Storage diseases of the reticuloendothelial system. In Nathan, D.G., and Oski, F.A., editors: Hematology of infancy and childhood, ed. 2, Philadelphia, 1981, W.B. Saunders Co., vol. 2.

*DS = Dermatan sulfate; HS = heparan sulfate; KS = keratan sulfate; CS = chondroitin-6-sulfate; cholesterol S = cholesterol sulfate.

Table 27-7. Screening for inborn errors of metabolism

Disease	Ferric chloride test	Benedict test	MPS test papers	Dinitrophenyl-hydrazine test	Amino acid test	Metachromatic stain
Phenylketonuria	+	±	−	+	+	−
Tyrosinuria	+	±	−	−	+	−
Histidinemia	+	−	−	−	+	−
Maple syrup urine disease	−	−	−	+	+	−
Lowe's syndrome	−	−	−	+	+	−
Hartnup disease	−	−	−	− (?)	+	−
Wilson's disease	−	−	−	−	+	−
Arginosuccinic aciduria	−	−	−	− (?)	+	−
Hyperglycinemia	−	−	−	+	+	−
Joseph's disease	−	−	−	−	+	−
Citrullinuria	−	−	−	−	+	−
Homocystinuria	−	−	−	−	+	−
Hyperlysinemia	−	−	−	+	+	−
Cystathioninuria	−	−	−	−	+	−
Lead poisoning	−	+	−	−	+	−
Galactosemia	−	+	−	−	+	−
Fructosuria	−	+	−	± (?)	−	−
Metachromatic leukodystrophy	−	−	−	−	−	+
Amaurotic familial idiocy	−	−	−	−	−	±*
Hurler's syndrome	−	−	+	−	−	−
Morquio-Ullrich syndrome	−	−	+	−	−	−
Marfan's syndrome	−	−	±	−	−	−
Murdoch's syndrome	−	−	+	−	−	−
"Forme-fruste gargoylism"	−	−	+	−	−	−

Modified from Renaurt, A.W.: N. Engl. J. Med. **274:**385, 1966.
*Rare.

From the laboratory point of view, the following two aspects of MPS should be mentioned: (1) giant granules occur in neutrophils (**Alder-Reilly anomaly**) (see section on hematology, p. 158) and (2) by **tissue culture** methods these disorders can be diagnosed in utero (see section on amniotic fluid, p. 771). When cultured fibroblasts of affected individuals are stained with toluidine blue, pink metachromatic granules develop within the cells. Normal cells are devoid of these granules.[97]

Summary of screening for inborn errors of metabolism: Numerous disease entities resulting from enzymatic defects have been described,[98] many of which can be investigated by the methods already outlined (Table 27-7).

TESTS FOR URINARY REDUCING SUBSTANCES (SUGAR AND NONSUGAR)

The following is a suggested scheme for identification of reducing substances (Fig. 27-8):

1. A nonspecific copper reduction method such as Clinitest (Ames Co., Elkhart, Ind.) is used to establish the presence of a reducing substance.
2. An enzymatic reagent strip such as Clinistix (Ames Co., Elkhart, Ind.) is used to identify glucose.

If 1 and 2 are positive, glucose is present. If 1 is positive and 2 is negative, reducing substances other than glucose are present.

3. Thin-layer chromatography is used to identify other reducing sugars such as lactose, fructose, galactose, and pentose.

If 3 is negative, the reducing substance is not a sugar but most likely a drug or drug metabolite.

The most important urinary reducing agents are as follows:

1. Glucose
2. Other reducing sugars: lactose, fructose, galactose, and pentose
3. Organic compounds: homogentisic acid and possibly very high levels of glucuronic acid, creatinine, and uric acid
4. Drugs and drug metabolites[99]: salicylates, chloral hydrate, ascorbic acid, NegGram, Skelaxin, and Keflin
5. Preservatives: formaldehyde

Tests to demonstrate presence or absence of reducing substances
Clinitest tablets

Principle: Soluble blue cupric ions of copper sulfate ($CuSO_4$) in heated, strongly alkaline solution are reduced by urinary reducing agents to yellowish red insoluble cuprous ions of cuprous oxide (Cu_2O) as follows:

$$\text{Cupric ions} \quad\quad \overset{\text{Heat}}{\longrightarrow} \quad \text{Cuprous ions}$$

Cupric ions   Heat   Cuprous ions
$CuSO_4$ + Glucose $\longrightarrow$ Cu_2O + Oxidized
Blue   Alkali Orange-red   glucose

In addition to copper sulfate, the tablet also contains sodium carbonate, citric acid, and sodium hydroxide. When the tablet is added to a water and urine mixture it dissolves with the evolution of carbon dioxide and

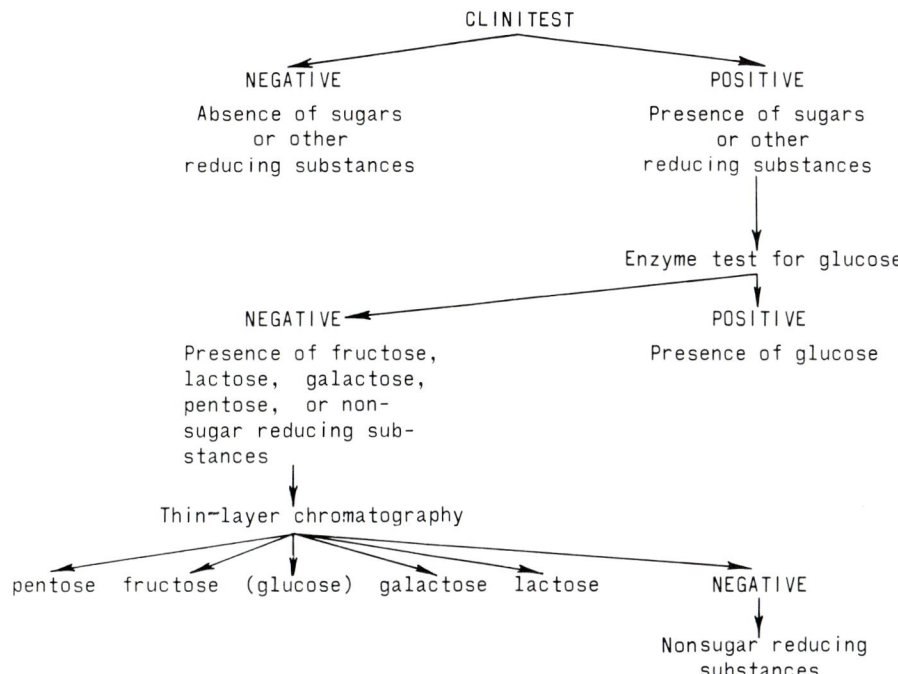

Fig. 27-8. Scheme for identification of reducing substances in urine.

heat. The latter results from the interaction of sodium hydroxide with citric acid, and the carbon dioxide liberated from the sodium carbonate acts as a mixer for the reagents. After 15 sec the bubbling stops and the orange produced by a reducing substance is compared with a reference color chart. The test is based on the time-honored Benedict test.[100]

Procedure: The original procedure requires 5 drops of water and 5 drops of urine, both delivered into a test tube from a standardized dropper, followed by the addition of the tablet. Most internists prefer the Clinitest 2-drop method reagent tablet, which uses only 2 drops of water and is more sensitive than the 5-drop method. The reaction mixture must be handled so as not to interfere with the heat production.

Normal value: No reducing substance is present (see discussion of glucosuria).

Interpretation: The lower limit of glucose detection by the Clinitest is 200 mg glucose/dl urine. The test is thus 50% less sensitive than the enzymatic test (lower limit of sensitivity is 50-100 mg glucose/dl urine). The Clinitest is nonspecific for glucose, because other reducing substances, e.g., ascorbic acid, other reducing sugars, drug metabolites, Keflin, and NegGram, also reduce the test tablets and may be responsible for a positive reduction test in the face of a negative enzymatic test. On the other hand, a negative reduction test and a positive enzymatic test indicate a glucose concentration between 100 and 200 mg/dl urine. The day-to-day control of diabetic patients depends almost completely on the home monitoring of urinary glucose. In selected diabetics (e.g., in pregnancy) home monitoring of blood glucose is essential[101] (Dextrostix [Ames Co.,

Elkhart, Ind.] used with the Eyetone Reflectance Colorimeter [Ames Co., Elkhkart, Inc.]). In the nonpregnant patient with diabetes the control depends on the accuracy with which urinary glucose measurements reflect blood glucose concentrations.[102] Readings of 0% glucose in urine indicate blood glucose concentrations below the renal threshold since the last urine specimen was analyzed; 2% indicates about 180 mg glucose/dl, and 5% indicates more than 210 mg glucose/dl in the blood.[102]

Enzymatic test for glucose

The enzymatic test for glucose can be performed with Clinistix and the glucose area on Bili-Labstix, N-Multistix, Uristix, Diastix (Ames Co., Elkhart, Ind.), or Chemstrip-8 and 9 (Boehringer-Mannheim Corp., Indianapolis).

Principle: The test is highly specific and is based on the following reaction:

Glucose + O_2 + Glucose oxidase $\longrightarrow$
    Gluconic acid + Hydrogen peroxide

Hydrogen peroxide + *o*-Tolidine + Peroxidase $\longrightarrow$
    Oxidized *o*-tolidine (blue) + H_2O

Glucose oxidase reacts with glucose in the urine to remove two hydrogen ions, forming gluconolactone, which is then hydrated to gluconic acid. The removed hydrogen ions combine with atmospheric oxygen to form hydrogen peroxide. The hydrogen peroxide in the presence of peroxidase oxidizes *o*-tolidine, an oxygen-accepting chromogen (indicator) to yield the blue color of the oxidized dye. The chromogen in N-Multistix and

Diastix is iodide, and in Chemstrip-8 and Clinistix it is *o*-tolidine.

Interpretation: The N-Multistix is sensitive to 100 mg glucose/dl urine, whereas Chemistrip-8 is sensitive to 50 mg glucose/dl urine. The first has an exceedingly wide range extending to 4 + readings at a concentration of 2000 mg glucose/dl urine.[103] Recent investigations[104] prove Chemstrip-8's superior sensitivity and lower rate of false negative results, whereas N-Multistix displays superior specificity and a lower rate of false positive results. False negative results of enzyme tests may be expected in the presence of large concentrations of ascorbic acid, ketones, and homogentisic acid. It should be noted that tetracycline contains vitamine C (ascorbic acid). False positive results may be caused by residual hypochlorite or peroxide in the urine container.[105] The dipstick glucose assay should be accepted as a specific qualitative test only and should not be interpreted quantitatively.[104,106]

Thin-layer chromatographic detection of urinary sugars

For thin-layer chromatography of urinary sugars,[107] good results have been obtained using the Gelman-type SA impregnated glass fiber sheets (Gelman Instrument Co., Ann Arbor, Mich.). These are first sprayed with 0.1M potassium phosphate (13.6 g KH_2PO_4/L water). After spraying until well moistened, the sheets are dried at 110° C for 1 hr.

Known standard: A standard containing 1 mg/ml each of a number of sugars is made up in 0.1% benzoic acid. Convenient standards are glucose, galactose, and lactose, and, if pentosuria is suspected, rhamnose or xylose.

Developing solution: Mix 30 volumes of chloroform, 35 glacial acetic acid, and 5 volumes of water.

Color reagent: Dissolve 1 g diphenylamine and 1 ml aniline in 1 dl acetone. Just before use, add 15 ml of 85% phosphoric acid. The precipitate that first forms should dissolve on mixing.

Procedure: The general directions given on p. 457 should be followed. Apply 5 μl mixed standard and 5-15 μl urine, depending on the concentration. The urine should be added in small increments to keep the spot as small as possible. The sheets are developed in the solvent for a distance of about 10 cm and then removed from the chamber, air dried to remove most of the solvent, and dried in an oven to completely remove the solvent.

The sheets are either sprayed with or dipped in the color reagent. Dipping has proved satisfactory. The sheets are air dried to remove most of the acetone and then heated in the oven to develop the colors. It may be helpful to place a beaker of hot water in the oven to increase the humidity during color development. The sugars are then identified by their R_f values and to some extent by the different colors developed (Fig. 27-9 and Table 27-8).

Impurities in the urine may cause some diffuse background color, but this should not be mistaken for a definite spot. The R_f values cited are somewhat larger than those cited by Haer,[108] but the relative R_f values are approximately the same and the order is the same.

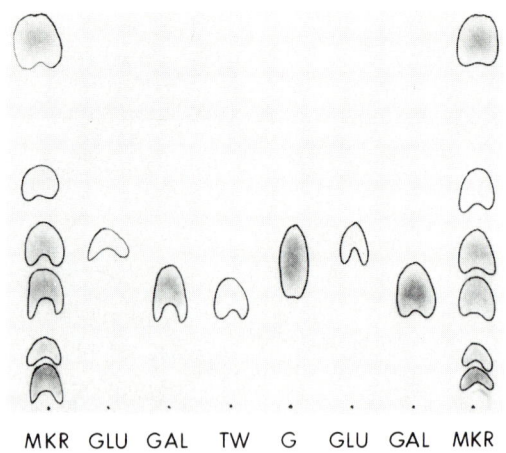

Fig. 27-9. One-dimensional chromatogram of sugar in urine. *MKR*, Marker; *GLU*, glucose; *GAL*, galactose; *TW*, unknown; *G*, unknown. (Courtesy C. Utz.)

Table 27-8. Identification of sugars

Sugar	R_f	Color of spot
Rhamnose (pentose)	0.68	Gray-green
Fructose	0.56	Reddish brown
Glucose	0.50	Gray-blue
Galactose	0.47	Gray-blue
Sucrose	0.36	Gray-blue
Lactose	0.26	Gray-blue

Other pentoses will have an R_f value and color similar to rhamnose. Glucose and galactose have similar R_f values and may be difficult to distinguish by chromatography. Glucose will give a positive result with the reagent test strip (Clinistix), but galactose will not. If galactose is suspected in the presence of glucose, it may be detected by one of the chemical tests (Tollens), or the spot test for galactosemia may be applied (see discussion of galactose).

Glucosuria

Glucose is not normally excreted and detected in the urine, because the amount filtered is almost completely absorbed by the tubules, leaving less than 20 mg glucose/dl urine, which is not detected by clinical methods. The absorption of glucose is effected by phosphorylation in the tubular cells, a process that is enzymatically catalyzed and limited by the enzyme concentration. In the face of an elevated blood glucose level, the filtrate may contain more glucose than can be absorbed, so that the excess passes into the urine to produce glucosuria (glycosuria). The **renal threshold level** for glucose is reached when the venous blood glucose concentration reaches 180 mg/dl.

Glucosuria occurs under the following conditions:
1. When the blood glucose level is elevated as a result of insulin deficiency (diabetes mellitus)
2. When excessive glycogenolysis follows severe physical and emotional stress

3. When the glucose transport mechanism of the renal tubules is defective because of a congenital or acquired tubular disease (nephrosis) that allows glucose to spill into the urine at normal blood glucose levels (renal glucosuria)

To evaluate glucosuria urine and blood sugar specimens should be collected at the same time, e.g., 2 hr postprandial, and be assayed for glucose.

IDENTIFICATION OF SUGARS OTHER THAN GLUCOSE

Meliturias involving sugars other than glucose are uncommon but include fructosuria, pentosuria, galactosuria, and lactosuria. These sugars reduce copper in hot alkaline solution and must therefore be differentiated from glucose, so that an erroneous diagnosis of diabetes is not made. The recommended method of differential diagnosis of nonglucose meliturias is thin-layer chromatography[109] (see p. 457), but selected confirmatory tests are mentioned with each reducing substance.

Fructose

Levulose (fructose) may appear in the urine after eating large amounts of fruit or honey (alimentary levulosuria), especially if the liver function is impaired. Essential fructosuria is caused by a harmless enzyme deficiency (ketohexokinase), whereas hereditary fructose intolerance resulting from fructose-L-aldolase deficiency produces severe liver and kidney diseases.[110] Levulose gives a positive Selivanoff test.

Selivanoff test:

Principle: Boiling with concentrated hydrochloric acid converts fructose to oxymethyl furfurol, which gives a red color when condensed with resorcinol.

Reagents: Dissolve 50 mg resorcinol in 3 ml concentrated hydrochloric acid.

Procedure: To 3 ml reagent add 6 ml urine and heat in a boiling water bath.

Result: Intense orange-red color and a dark precipitate develop immediately if fructose is present. The precipitate is soluble in ethanol.

Normal value: Negative for fructose.

Control: Fructose, 50 mg/dl water.

Pentose

Pentose occurs in the urine after the ingestion of fruits, e.g., cherries (alimentary pentosuria or L-xylulosuria), and as a congenital anomaly of metabolism (idiopathic pentosuria) characterized by the inability to metabolize L-xylose, which results from a deficiency in L-xylulose reductase.[111]

Bial orcinol test:

Principle: Heating pentose with mineral acids leads to the formation of furfurol, which combines with orcinol to produce a colored compound.

Reagent: Mix 0.2 g orcinol, 1 dl concentrated hydrochloric acid, and 5 drops of 10% ferric chloride.

Procedure: Bring 5 ml reagent to a boil and add 1 ml urine drop by drop.

Result: Pentose turns olive green and is soluble in amyl alcohol.

Normal value: Negative for pentose.

Control: Xylose, 500 mg/dl water.

Interpretation: Fructose gives a red color with the Bial orcinol test, and glucose interferes with the color reaction.

Galactose

Galactose is formed by the hydrolysis of lactose. It is converted to glucose in the liver and is metabolized as glucose with the aid of insulin. The ability of the liver to convert galactose into glucose forms the basis of the galactose tolerance test, a hepatic function test.

Galactosuria occurs as an acquired condition in liver disease and as a congenital disease in infants. In congenital galactosemia there is an impaired ability to convert galactose to glucose, so that the blood galactose level is elevated and galactose appears in the urine. The basic defect lies in the inability to convert galactose-1-phosphate to glucose-1-phosphate because of a hereditary congenital absence of the enzyme galactose-1-phosphate uridyl transferase. This enzyme is normally present in the red cells, which may therefore be used as indicators of galactosemia. In the congenital form the disease expresses itself in the first week of life when the infant starts vomiting and develops diarrhea, hepatomegaly, and jaundice. If the disease is allowed to progress, it leads to cirrhosis of the liver, mental retardation, and blindness. Early diagnosis is imperative.

Screening spot test for galactosemia[112]:

Principle: Whole blood (or, for the micromethod, a strip of filter paper with dried capillary blood) is added to a reaction mixture containing α-galactose-1-phosphate (Gal-1-P), uridine diphosphoglucose (UDPG), triphosphopyridine nucleotide (TPN), buffer, and saponin. If Gal-1-P uridyl transferase is present, β-glucose-6-phosphate is formed by way of several intermediate steps. Glucose-6-phosphate dehydrogenase in the hemolysate oxidizes it to 6-phosphogluconate, which in turn is oxidized to ribulose-5-phosphate. These reactions lead to the reduction of TPN. Reduced TPN fluoresces when activated with long-wavelength ultraviolet light. The reaction mixture is spotted on Whatman no. 1 filter paper and allowed to dry.

Reaction mixture (6 ml):
1. UDPG sodium salt (6 mg/ml), 0.2 ml
2. Gal-1-P dipotassium salt (10 mg/ml), 0.4 ml
3. TPN, 5 mg/ml, 0.6 ml
4. Trisacetate buffer, pH 8.0, 2.0 ml
   Mix 81 g tris, 7 dl distilled water, and glacial acetic acid to pH 8.0; dilute with water to make 10 dl.
5. Saponin, 1%, 0.8 ml
6. Disodium EDTA (1 mg/dl), 0.03 ml
7. Distilled water, 1.97 ml

Reagents and positive and negative controls for the ultraviolet determination of Gal-1-P uridyl transferase are available from Sigma Chemical Co., St. Louis, Sigma Technical Bulletin no. 195.

Procedure: Add 0.02 ml heparinized blood to 0.2 ml reaction mixture with a pipet that is left in the reaction mixture while it is incubated at 37° C for 2 hr. Then spot the solution on Whatman no. 1 filter paper, covering an area of 3-15 mm, allow it to dry, and examine it under long-wavelength ultraviolet light. Repeat with positive and negative controls.

Interpretation: Bright fluorescence indicates a normal specimen or samples from individuals heterozygous for galactosemia or homozygous for the Duarte variant.[113] Blood from homozygous galactosemia patients fails to fluoresce. Heterozygotes for galactosemia and homozygotes for the Duarte variant can be discovered by spotting the filter paper after 1 hr incubation, of the blood sample at which time they show less fluorescence than normal.

Lactose

Lactose may appear in the urine in the last months of pregnancy and in the postpartum period. Lactose intolerance may be congenital and may be the cause of the failure of an infant to thrive, or it may be an acquired abnormality of the older population. In both cases, lactose appears in the urine following oral administration of sugar.

Test for lactose (Woehlk):
Principle: If the pH is highly alkaline, lactose reduces potassium hydroxide.
Reagents:
1. Ammonium hydroxide, concentrated
2. Potassium hydroxide, 15% (15 g/dl)
Procedure: To 5 ml urine add 2.5 ml ammonia and 5 drops of potassium hydroxide. Warm in a water bath (do not boil).
Result: Lactose turns red.

Disacchariduria

Lactose and sucrose are the disaccharides that may be found in the urine in a number of congenital and acquired gastrointestinal disorders. They can be demonstrated by thin-layer chromatography. Lactose is a reducing agent, but sucrose is not and is therefore not detected by routine clinical laboratory methods for sugars.

KETONE BODIES

Ketone bodies consist of acetoacetic acid (diacetic acid), β-hydroxybutyric acid, and acetone. In small amounts (25 mg/24 hr) these substances appear together normally as intermediary compounds of fat metabolism. The normal liver produces free acetoacetic acid from condensed acetyl-CoA units. This β-keto acid is converted to β-hydroxybutyric acid and acetone. Normally ketones are rapidly metabolized by entering into the citric acid cycle. If the latter is depressed by "intracellular carbohydrate starvation,"[114] the ketone bodies cannot be metabolized and accumulate in the bloodstream, showing approximately the following distribution: 78% β-hydroxybutyric acid, 20% acetoacetic acid, and 2% acetone. If the specimen is allowed to stand, the ketones may evaporate. In ketosis the ketones may increase to 5 g/dl, as compared to the normal level of about 1 mg/dl. Any urine that contains glucose must be tested for ketone bodies.

Tests for ketone bodies

Dipstick tests (Ames Co., Elkhart, Ind.):
Principle: Alkaline nitroprusside turns purple with acetoacetic acid. The test is based on the original Rothera test, which has been modified many times and is difficult to standardize.

Sensitivity: The test detects 10 mg acetoacetic acid/dl urine and is primarily sensitive to the presence of acetoacetic acid, as indicated by the purple color, but it also reacts with acetone. It is not sensitive to β-hydroxybutyric acid. The test should be performed on fresh urine before the acetoacetic acid decomposes to acetone.

Acetest, a reagent tablet, is more sensitive than Ketostix (Ames Co., Elkhart, Ind.), detecting as little as 5 mg acetoacetic acid/dl urine. For performance of the test, follow the manufacturer's instructions. The tablet may be used with serum and whole blood.

Interfering substances: False positive results may occur with phthaleins, as after sodium sulfobromophthalein (Bromsulphalein) and phenolsulfonphthalein tests, because of interfering color. Aspirin may be responsible for a false negative result.[115]

Interpretation: Ketosis occurs in starvation, fat feeding, and uncontrolled diabetes.

BILIRUBIN

Bilirubin is the pigmentary constituent of bile, which consists of bile acids, phospholipids, bile salts, cholesterol, calcium, inorganic electrolytes, and the previously mentioned bilirubin pigment.

Metabolism[116,117] (Fig. 27-10)

Eighty-five percent of bilirubin is formed by the reticuloendothelial system (liver, spleen, and bone marrow) from the heme (porphyrin) moiety of the hemoglobin molecule of senescent red cells. As the red cells are destroyed, the globin portion of the hemoglobin is split off and heme is converted to biliverdin first followed by its conversion to bilirubin. A smaller amount (15%) of bilirubin, called "early labeled" bilirubin,[118] because it is detected by the administration of radioactive heme precursors, is the result of bilirubin formed from cytochromes, myoglobins, and ineffective erythropoiesis in the bone marrow. The heme portion originating from the nonhemoglobin sources (cytochromes, myoglobins, etc.), bound to a glycoprotein in the plasma called **hemopexin,**[119] is also transported to organs of the reticuloendothelial system to be converted to bilirubin. "Shunt" pathways have been described where bilirubin is formed directly from pyrrole rings without heme as the precursor. Bilirubin is carried in the plasma as "free," unconjugated, but albumin-bound bilirubin to the liver cells, where it is conjugated with glucuronic acid to form **bilirubin monoglucuronides** and **diglucuronides,** which are excreted into the bile ducts and into the duodenum as one of the constituents of bile. The "free," unconjugated bilirubin in the plasma gives the **"indirect" van den Bergh** reaction, since it is methyl alcohol soluble but insoluble in water. The bilirubin–glucuronic acid conjugation in the liver cell is catalyzed by the enzyme bilirubin glucuronyl transferase. **Conjugated bilirubin** is water soluble and gives the **"direct" van den Bergh** reaction. In the intestinal tract the bacteria normally present hydrolyze the bilirubin conjugate and reduce bilirubin to colorless

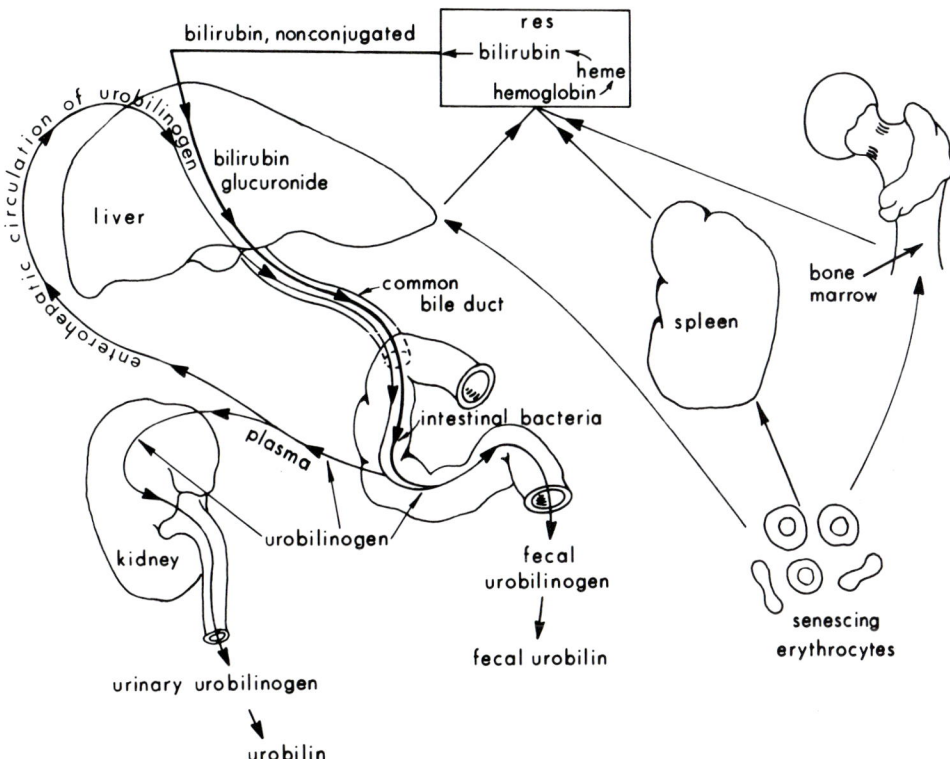

Fig. 27-10. Bilirubin metabolism. *res,* Reticuloendothelial system.

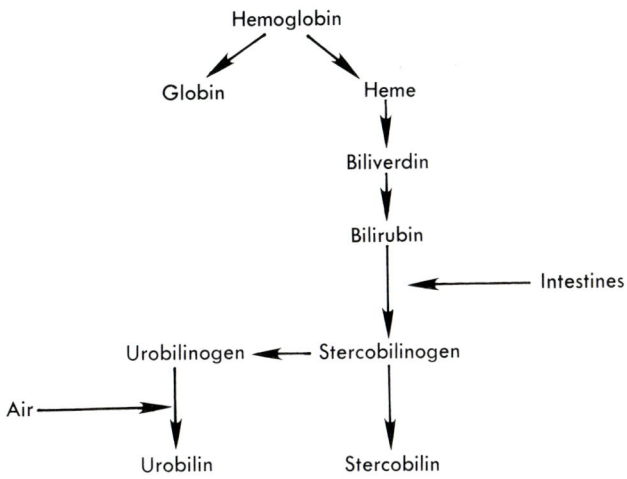

Fig. 27-11. Formation of urobilin.

urobilinogen (stercobilinogen) and to colored urobilin (stercobilin). The latter is excreted in the feces and is responsible for their color. The major portion of the urobilinogen is absorbed into the portal circulation and excreted unchanged into bile (enterohepatic circulation) and urine. The urinary urobilinogen after autooxidation gives rise to urobilin (Fig. 27-11). The kidney does not excrete unconjugated bilirubin since it is insoluble in water, but it is able to excrete urobilinogen and conjugated bilirubin because both are water soluble.

Normal urine contains a small amount of urobilinogen (urobilin after standing) but no bilirubin. Examination of the urine for bile (bilirubin) and urobilinogen is useful in the investigation of jaundice (Table 27-9).

Tests for urine bilirubin

Three types of tests are available: (1) oxidation tests (oxidizing bilirubin to green biliverdin and other pigments), (2) diazotization tests (diazotizing bilirubin to a highly colored compound), and (3) the shake test.

Oxidation tests

Principle: The principle employed in the oxidation test is the oxidation of bilirubin to biliverdin and other pigments.

Gmelin test:

Reagent: Concentrated yellow nitric acid (place several wooden applicator sticks into concentrated nitric acid).

Procedure: Pour about 2 ml unfiltered urine into a test tube and run 1 or 2 ml yellow nitric acid under the urine.

Result: Bile gives a play of colors, with green on the periphery, then blue (bilicyanin), and red and yellow (choletelin) nearest the acid.

• • •

This test may be adapted to filter paper, through which larger quantities of urine can be filtered. When the filter paper is nearly dry, drop yellow nitric acid on it.

Table 27-9. Differential diagnosis of jaundice based on urine bilirubin and urobilinogen tests

Liver pathology and type of jaundice	Urine bilirubin	Urine urobilinogen
Normal	0	Trace
Hepatitis (viral, toxic, drug); hepatocellular jaundice	↑	↑
Biliary obstruction (extrahepatic and intrahepatic); obstructive jaundice	↑	0
Hemolytic jaundice	0	↑
Liver cell dysfunction (cirrhosis, infections, metastases, heart failure, hyperthyroidism)	0	↑

0 = Absent; ↑ = increased.

Interfering substances: Formalin, indican, thymol, and potassium iodine.

Fouchet test (Harrison's modification of Gmelin test):

Principle: Barium chloride precipitates phosphates that entrain and concentrate bile pigments, which are tested for by the oxidation reaction.

Reagent: To make Fouchet reagent mix 25 g trichloroacetic acid, 1 dl, distilled water, and 10 ml 10% aqueous ferric chloride.

Procedure: To about 10 ml urine, add about 1 g barium chloride, mix, and filter. Spread the filter paper out and, when partly dry, drop a little Fouchet reagent or yellow nitric acid on the precipitate.

Result: A green color of biliverdin is positive and indicates the presence of bile (bilirubin) in the urine.

Interfering substances: Salicylates and phenazopyridine give an interfering purple color.

A test for bilirubin should be included in every routine urinalysis and has been suggested for all blood donors. A positive test for bile may be the first finding in hepatitis without jaundice.

Diazotization tests

Diazotization tests that employ diazo salts to form colored complexes are more specific than oxidation tests. Ictotest (Ames Co., Elkhart, Ind.), a tablet test using sulfosalicylic acid plus a diazo salt, is more sensitive than the easier to use and more convenient reagent strips and should be used to confirm the dipstick tests.

Reagent strip test:

Principle: In the case of the Ames strips (Ames Co., Elkhart, Ind.), the test area of the strip is impregnated with stabilized diazotized 2,4-dichloroaniline, which is colored brown by bilirubin. The BMC product (Table 27-2) (Boehringer Mannheim Corp., Indianapolis) utilizes a diazotized salt that allows coupling with bilirubin.

Sensitivity: A positive reaction is produced by 0.5 mg bilirubin/dl urine.

Discussion: The test should be performed on fresh urine only, since urinary bilirubin glucuronide is unstable at room temperature and may hydrolyze or oxidize when exposed to light. The resulting bilirubin is less reactive or not reactive at all to diazotization tests.

Interfering substances: Large quantities of chlorpromazine and phenazopyridine (red color).

Shake test

If the urine contains bile, shaking of the test tube produces yellow foam. The test is neither sensitive nor specific.

Interpretation of urinary bilirubin tests

Normal urine does not contain bilirubin. Bilirubin appears in the urine as the result of intrahepatic and extrahepatic obstruction, as seen in chronic and acute hepatitis, infectious mononucleosis, hyperthyroidism, drug-induced hepatitis, alcoholic hepatitis, cirrhosis, obstructing tumors, and septicemia.

UROBILINOGEN

Significance: See discussion of urine bilirubin and urobilinogen tests in the differential diagnosis of jaundice, below, and metabolism of bilirubin, p. 700.

Qualitative methods

Dipstick method: The dipstick methods of the Ames Co. (Table 27-2) (Elkhart, Ind.) utilizes *p*-dimethylaminobenzaldehyde, which produces a pink color with urobilinogen. False negative results may be caused by pyridium and azo dyes in the urine, whereas false positive reactions are produced by porphobilinogen and *p*-aminosalicylic acid. The lower limit of sensitivity of the dipstick method is 1.5 mg urobilinogen/dl urine. The BMC dipsticks (Table 27-2) (Boehringer Mannheim Biochemicals, Indianapolis) develops a red azo dye color when urobilinogen acts on *p*-methoxybenzene-diazonium-fluoroborate. Bilirubin may interfere with the recognition of the red color but otherwise there are fewer interfering substances than there are with the Ames dipsticks.

Ehrlich benzaldehyde test:

Principle: The colorless urobilinogen is changed into a colored compound with Ehrlich reagent.

Type of specimen: Use only fresh urine, since urobilinogen changes to urobilin on exposure to light. The specimen should be a 2 hr sample collected between 2:00 and 4:00 PM. If a 24 hr specimen is used or if a fresh specimen is not available, the oxidation of urobilinogen to urobilin can be prevented by collecting the urine in a brown bottle containing 5 g anhydrous sodium carbonate.

Reagent: To make, Ehrlich dimethylaminobenzaldehyde mix 1 dl concentrated hydrochloric acid, 1 dl distilled water, and 4 g *p*-dimethylaminobenzaldehyde.

Procedure: To 10 ml urine, add 1 ml Ehrlich benzaldehyde reagent; mix and let stand for about 10 min. Observe color by looking down into the tube held over a white surface.

Normal values: The trace of urobilinogen normally present gives only a very slight pink color or no color at all.

When the qualitative test shows an apparent increase in urobilinogen, repeat the test with urine dilutions of 1:10, 1:20, etc., and report the highest dilution giving a positive test.

False reactions: Ehrlich reagent reacts with substances other than urobilinogen, e.g., phenazopyridium (bright red), porphobilinogen (bright red), formaldehyde (yellow), bilirubin (greenish yellow), and indole (red).

Interpretation: A cherry-red color indicates increased amounts of urobilinogen; absence of color indicates a decreased or normal amount of urobilinogen.

Decreased urobilinogen: Urobilinogen is absent in newborn infants (absence of reducing intestinal bacteria) and in complete obstruction of the common bile duct. It may be absent after administration of antibiotics that suppress the intestinal flora. It is diminished in incomplete obstruction of the common bile duct, in hepatitis with cholestasis, and because of reduced bile formation in starvation.

Increased urobilinogen: Urobilinogen is increased in augmented bilirubin formation caused by accelerated blood destruction in hemolytic anemias and in infarction and liver cell dysfunction.

Quantitative method

See p. 540.

Urine bilirubin and urobilinogen tests in differential diagnosis of jaundice

Three types of jaundice are usually described—obstructive, hepatocellular, and hemolytic. Obstructive jaundice caused by cholestasis or complete obstruction of the common bile duct leads to bilirubin in the urine not accompanied by urobilinogen; in partial obstruction and in hepatocellular disease, both urobilin and urobilinogen are present. In hemolytic jaundice (increased blood destruction), urobilinogen without bilirubin is found in urine (Table 27-9). The normal serum bilirubin level is 1.1 mg/dl. Jaundice (icterus) is the result of hyperbilirubinemia so that bilirubin accumulates in the skin, sclerae, and all other organs of the body, which take up a yellowish hue. Clinically, jaundice is noticeable if the plasma bilirubin level exceeds 2 mg/dl. Obstruction to the flow of bile in the common bile duct renders the stool acholic (clay colored) and prevents the formation of urobilinogen, so that the urine urobilinogen is absent. The water-soluble, direct-acting esterified bilirubin is pushed back into the bloodstream since it cannot escape via the bile duct and is responsible for conjugated hyperbilirubinemia and bilirubinuria. Unconjugated hyperbilirubinemia is seen in hemolytic processes in which excessive amounts of free bilirubin are formed from rapidly catabolized hemoglobin. Free bilirubin is not excreted by the kidneys but is responsible for increased amounts of urobilinogen in urine and feces, because the liver esterifies some of the additional supplies of the free bilirubin. In hepatocellular jaundice there are varying degrees of obstruction so that conjugated bilirubin is partially retained and partially released into the intestines.

UROBILIN

See discussion of metabolism of bilirubin, p. 700. Urobilin is derived from urobilinogen on exposure to air and light or on addition of Lugol solution and has the same significance as urobilinogen. If the urobilinogen test is negative, the urine should be examined for urobilin, since all urobilinogen may have been oxidized to urobilin.

Schlesinger test:

Principle: Urobilinogen is oxidized to urobilin by the addition of Lugol solution. The addition of zinc acetate leads to the production of a green color.

Reagents:
1. Saturated alcoholic zinc acetate solution
   a. Zinc acetate, 10 g
   b. Ethyl alcohol, 90%, 1 dl
      Mix well before use.
2. Lugol solution
   a. Iodine, 5 g
   b. Potassium iodide, 10 g
   c. Water, 1 dl

Procedure: To 5 ml urine, add 2 or 3 drops Lugol solution and let stand for 10 min to convert all urobilinogen to urobilin. Add 5 ml saturated absolute alcoholic zinc acetate solution and filter.

Results: If urobilin is present, a greenish fluorescence is noted. The reaction is more marked after 1-2 hr. Normally there is no urobilin present in fresh urine. If bilirubin is present, precipitate bile pigments by adding 5 g calcium chloride powder, mix, and filter. Test the filtrate as above.

INDICAN

Indican, indoxyl sulfate, is the result of intestinal decomposition of tryptophan. It is absorbed into the blood stream and excreted into the urine.

Obermayer test:

Principle: Indoxyl sulfate is hydrolyzed by strong mineral acids and the resulting indoxyl is oxidized to indigo blue.

Reagents:

1. Obermayer reagent
   a. Concentrated hydrochloric acid, 1 dl
   b. Ferric chloride, 0.8 g
2. Chloroform

Procedure: To 6 ml urine, add 6 ml Obermayer reagent, mix, and allow to stand for 5 min. Add 4 ml chloroform and mix well by inverting several times until all color is taken up by the chloroform.

Result: Indican turns indigo blue.

Normal values: Normally the color is light sky blue, indicating not more than a trace of indican in the urine.

Interpretation: Pathologically, the indican level is increased whenever there is increased intestinal putrefaction, e.g., in enteritis, pancreatic insufficiency, common bile duct obstruction, or intrahepatic biliary obstruction. Indican is also increased whenever there is accelerated protein decomposition anywhere in the body, e.g., septicemia with abscess formation. Intestinal obstruction with necrosis and ulceration of the intestinal mucosa leads to increased indican absorption into the bloodstream.

BLOOD IN URINE: HEMATURIA AND HEMOGLOBINURIA

Terminology: The term *hematuria* implies the presence of more or less intact red cells in the urine; the term *hemoglobinuria* denotes the presence of dissolved hemoglobin. Hematuria is usually accompanied by some degree of hemoglobinuria because of the disintegration of red cells in the urine on standing.

Hematuria

Gross hematuria may color the urine red or brown or produce a "smoky" appearance. Urine that contains red cells, as seen by microscopic examination of the sediment, also contains hemoglobin in solution. Hemolysis of red cells is more rapid in alkaline than in acid urine.

Measurement of urine hemoglobin

Dipstick test: Both the Ames (Table 27-2) (Ames Co., Elkhart, Ind.) and BMC (Table 27-2) (Boehringer Mannheim Corp., Indianapolis) methods utilize the peroxidase-like activity of hemoglobin. The hemoglo-

bin pad contains *o*-tolidine, peroxide, and buffers. Hemoglobin that is freed from the confines of the red cells by the lytic action of the reagents releases oxygen from the hydrogen peroxide so that it becomes available to oxidize *o*-tolidine into its blue form.

$$H_2O_2 + \begin{array}{c} \text{Chromogen} \\ (o\text{-tolidine}) \end{array} + \begin{array}{c} \text{Hemoglobin} \\ \text{(peroxidase} \\ \text{activity)} \end{array} \rightarrow \begin{array}{c} \text{Oxidized} \\ \text{chromogen} \\ \text{(blue)} \end{array} + H_2O$$

Sensitivity of the Ames dipstick is about 190,000 RBC/ml for intact cells and 35,000 RBC/ml for hemoglobin. Sensitivity of the BMC product is about 4000 erythrocytes/ml for intact cells and 10,500 cells/ml for hemoglobin.[120] The BMC product distinguishes between hemoglobinuria and hematuria by lysing the intact erythrocytes first and then producing a color reaction that is homogeneous in hemoglobinuria and spotty in hematuria.

Interpretation: A positive test may be caused by the presence of red cells, hemoglobin, or myoglobin. **False positive** tests may be caused by pus (peroxidase of white cells), iodides, bromides, or sodium hypochlorite used to disinfect containers. Ascorbic acid, which is added to some antibiotics in large quantities, inhibits the color reaction (**false negative** reaction). The screening tests also detect **myoglobin,** which occurs in urine less often than hemoglobin.

Microscopic method: In hematuria, red cells or their "envelopes" can be seen in the sediment. In pure hemoglobinuria and in myoglobinuria no red cells are seen in the sediment.

Causes of hematuria

1. Kidney diseases: glomerulonephritis, pyelonephritis, tumors, polycystic kidney, infarcts, tuberculosis, trauma, and necrotizing papillitis
2. Blood diseases: thrombocytopenia, leukemia, hemophilia, and sickle cell trait
3. Drugs: bishydroxycoumarin, heparin, and salicylates
4. Bladder diseases: cystitis, tumors, and prostatic hypertrophy
5. Iatrogenic: catheterization

Hemoglobinuria

Hemoglobinuria (free hemoglobin in urine) is related to hemoglobinemia (free hemoglobin in serum), the level of which is determined by the plasma **haptoglobin** level (see below).

Dipstick methods for detecting free hemoglobin in the urine are the same as for blood except for the microscopic examination of the urinary sediment, which is negative unless the hemoglobinuria is caused by lysis of red cells in alkaline urine, in which case the sediment will show red cell envelopes.

Hemoglobinuria and haptoglobins[121]

Haptoglobin, a serum mucoprotein, unites stoichiometrically with free hemoglobin in the serum, so that hemoglobin is excreted into the urine only after all haptoglobin is saturated. Plasma hemoglobin normally does not exceed about 5 mg/dl plasma, at which level the hemoglobin concentration is not adequate to color the plasma pink. The kidney threshold for haptoglobin is about 100-140 mg/dl. Since the haptoglobin-hemoglobin complex is not excreted by the kidneys, hemoglobinuria does not occur until all plasma haptoglobin is saturated and the hemoglobin concentration exceeds 140 mg/dl. Since the hemoglobin-haptoglobin molecule is destroyed by the reticuloendothelial system and haptoglobin is not rapidly replaced, the plasma haptoglobin level falls during continued hemolysis, and free hemoglobin appears in the urine at plasma hemoglobin levels much lower than 140 mg/dl. (See discussion of haptoglobin on p. 104.)

Causes of hemoglobinuria

1. Incompatible blood transfusions
2. Hemolytic anemias associated with intravascular hemolysis, e.g., drugs, chemicals, parasites (malaria), and antibodies
3. Severe burns
4. Poisoning (snake venom, spider bites, etc.)
5. Paroxysmal nocturnal hemoglobinuria
6. Paroxysmal cold hemoglobinuria
7. Severe physical exercise, e.g., march hemoglobinuria

Hemosiderin

Hemosiderin is a yellow to brown granular pigment, an iron containing hemoglobin derivative, which is deposited in the tubular cells of the kidneys in the course of chronic hemoglobinuria. Hemosiderin-laden macrophages and epithelial cells may be found in the urinary sediment. (See discussion of Prussian blue reaction on hemosiderin in urinary sediment, p. 724.)

MYOGLOBIN

Myoglobin[122] is a ferrous porphyrin similar to hemoglobin, except that it has a molecular weight one fourth that of hemoglobin (17,000 vs. 68,000) and only one iron molecule as compared to the four iron molecules of hemoglobin. Free myoglobin in plasma is not bound to haptoglobin; its plasma level is kept low (renal threshold of 20 mg/dl plasma) because of its rapid excretion by the kidneys, which prevents myoglobin from reaching plasma concentrations visible on gross examination.

Measurement of myoglobin

Myoglobin (like hemoglobin) gives a peroxidase-like reaction with the chromogens used for the detection of blood in urine. When the urine is pink from hemoglobinuria, the plasma is also pink but in the case of myoglobinuria the plasma is colorless, since all myoglobin has been cleared. The best test for qualitative and quantitative evaluation of myoglobinuria is the radial immunodiffusion with specific antiserum that can also be utilized in the radioimmunoassay procedure. Adams[123] developed an agglutination procedure using latex particles tagged with either myoglobin or hemoglobin.

Causes of myoglobinuria

1. Traumatic myoglobinuria: occurs after crush injuries and muscle trauma (postoperative)

2. March hemoglobinuria: appears after severe muscular exercise and is a mixture of myoglobinuria and hemoglobinuria; not complicated by anemia
3. Alcoholic myoglobinuria: probably results from a direct toxic action of alcohol on muscle
4. Electric shock
5. Ischemic myoglobinuria: caused by arterial occlusion and diminishing blood supply (myocardial infarct)
6. Progressive muscle diseases
7. Idiopathic paroxysmal myoglobinuria

PORPHYRINS

Porphyrins consist of four pyrrole rings linked by methane bridges to which various side chains are attached. This chemical configuration is responsible for their ability to fluoresce under ultraviolet light, a physical characteristic that is used in most of the assay methods. Porphyrins form complexes with metal ions to produce various compounds, e.g., hemoglobin, an iron protoporphyrin attached to globin; myoglobin, an iron protoporphyrin occurring in muscle; and cytochrome, an iron-containing transfer agent.

Porphyrin synthesis[124-126] (Fig. 27-12)

Porphyrins are synthesized in the living cell from glycine from the general amino acid pool and from active succinate (succinyl coenzyme A) from the Krebs cycle (α-ketoglutaric acid of the citric acid cycle). The first precursor is δ-aminolevulinic acid (ALA), which is the result of the combination of glycine and coenzyme A by the enzyme δ-aminolevulinic acid synthetase. Two molecules of ALA are combined by the enzyme ALA dehydrase to form mainly uroporphyrinogen III, which is destined to become heme. A minimal amount of uroporphyrinogen I is also produced but is not available for heme production. Uroporphyrinogen III is transformed to coproporphyrinogen III by enzymatic decarboxylation and is further modified to protoporphyrinogen III by oxidation and decarboxylation. Protoporphyrinogen III is then oxidized to protoporphyrin IX. The incorporation of one iron atom into the protoporphyrin molecule produces the metalloporphyrin heme. The combination of protein and heme leads to the formation of **hemoglobin.** ALA, porphobilinogen, and the porphyrinogens are colorless, nonfluorescing compounds. After autooxidation the porphyrinogens (uroporphyrinogen and coproporphyrinogen) form red fluorescing porphyrins when viewed under ultraviolet light.

Laboratory diagnosis of porphyria

Two screening tests are available: the Watson-Schwartz test for porphobilinogen in the urine and the screening tests for porphyrins (coproporphyrins and uroporphyrins). They may be followed by quantitative determinations.

Test for porphobilinogen (Watson-Schwartz test)[127]:

Principle: Porphobilinogen (PBG) turns red with Ehrlich *p*-dimethylaminobenzaldehyde reagent, which is similar to the color produced by urobilinogen and indole but differs in solubility.

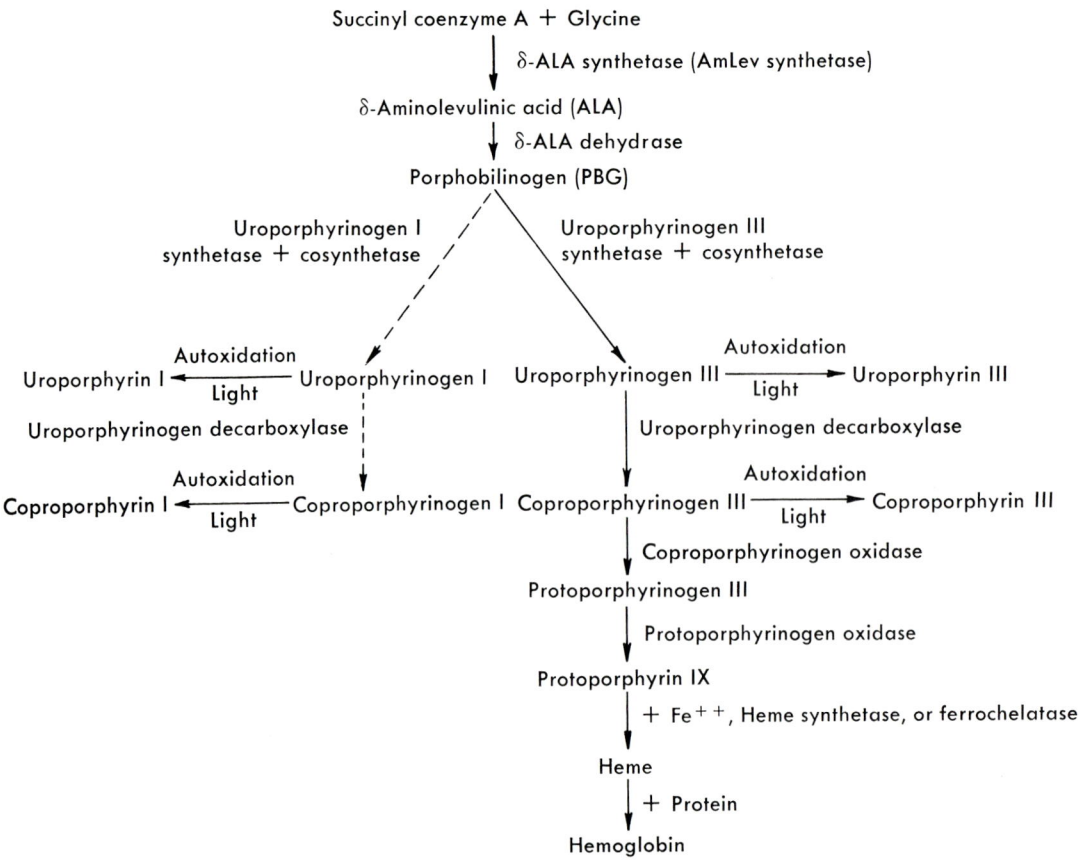

Fig. 27-12. Synthesis of porphyrins, heme, and hemoglobin from glycine and succinate.

Specimen: A random specimen is adequate. If coproporphyrin and uroporphyrin levels are also requested, a 24 hr specimen should be collected in a brown bottle (to protect it from light) containing 5 g sodium carbonate; it should be stored in the refrigerator to prevent the loss of PBG. The pH should be 6.5-9.5. It is best to perform the assay as soon as possible.

Reagents:
1. Fisher's modification of Ehrlich reagent
   a. *p*-Dimethylaminobenzaldehyde, 0.7
   b. Concentrated hydrochloric acid, 150 ml
   c. Distilled water, 1 dl
      Keep in dark bottle.
2. Sodium acetate, saturated, aqueous
3. Chloroform
4. *n*-Butanol

Procedure: Combine 2.5 ml fresh urine with 2.5 ml Fisher's modification of Ehrlich reagent; shake for 30 sec. Add 5 ml saturated solution of sodium acetate and mix well. Test resulting solution with pH paper and adjust to pH 5.5 by adding more sodium acetate if necessary. With PBG the major color development occurs immediately after addition of Ehrlich reagent; with urobilinogen, it occurs after addition of sodium acetate. If no pink color develops, PBG is not present and the test does not need to be carried any further. If a pink color develops, continue with the extraction procedure.

Extraction. Combine the test solution with 5 ml chloroform and shake. Allow to stand for a few moments. Two layers will separate—the chloroform forms the lower layer and the water the upper layer. PBG remains in the aqueous phase, whereas urobilinogen and indole are extracted into the lower chloroform layer.

Results: The test is positive for PBG if the upper (aqueous) layer is red or deep pink and the lower layer (chloroform) is colorless or pale yellow-brown. If the upper (aqueous) layer is pink or red, decant and shake with $\frac{1}{2}$ volume of *n*-butanol. Allow solution to separate into an upper butanol layer and a lower aqueous layer. Red or pink remaining in the aqueous layer is caused only by PBG.

Interpretation: Normally no PBG or only traces are found. PBG is increased in congenital hepatic prophyrias (acute intermittent porphyria, acute variegate porphyria, and hereditary coproporphyria) and is normal in acquired and erythropoietic porphyrias (Table 27-10). A number of substances produce interfering colors, e.g., aminosalicylic acid, phenothiazine, and phenazopyridine.[99]

Quantitative determination of porphobilinogen: See discussion of quantitative ALA determination, p. 88.

Procedure: Elute the porphobilinogen from the Dowex-2 column with 2.5 ml of 1M acetic acid (6 ml

Table 27-10. The porphyrias: chemical findings and clinical aspects*

Disorder	Inheritance	Age of clinical onset	Primary organ involvement	Chemical findings	Urine	Feces	Red Cells	Primary symptoms
Congenital erythropoietic porphyria	Autosomal recessive	Birth to 5 yr	Erythropoietic	ALA	N	—	—	Severe photosensitivity
				PBG	N	—	—	
				Uroporphyrin	↑↑	↑	↑↑	
				Coproporphyrin	↑	↑↑	↑	
				Protoporphyrin	N	N	N	
Acute intermittent porphyria	Autosomal dominant	Adult	Hepatic	Acute phase				Mild to severe neurologic-visceral symptoms
				ALA	↑↑	—	—	
				PBG	↑↑	—	—	
				Uroporphyrin	↑-↑↑	↑-↑↑	N-↑	
				Coproporphyrin	↑	↑	N-↑	
				Protoporphyrin	N-↑	N-↑	N	
				Remission				
				ALA	N-↑	—	—	
				PBG	N-↑	—	—	
				Uroporphyrin	N-↑	N	N	
				Coproporphyrin	↑-↑↑	↑↑	N	
				Protoporphyrin	—	↑↑	N	
Hereditary coproporphyria	Autosomal dominant	Adult	Hepatic	Acute phase				Similar to variegate porphyria
				ALA	↑↑	—	—	
				PBG	↑↑	—	—	
				Uroporphyrin	↑↑	↑	N	
				Coproporphyrin	↑↑	↑↑	N	
				Protoporphyrin	↑↑	N	N	
Variegate porphyria	Autosomal dominant	Adult	Hepatic	Acute phase				Mild to severe photosensitivity and neurologicvisceral symptoms
				ALA	↑↑	—	—	
				PBG	↑↑	—	—	
				Uroporphyrin	↑↑	↑↑	N	
				Coproporphyrin	↑-↑↑	↑↑	N	
				Protoporphyrin	↑↑	↑↑	N	
				Remission				
				ALA	N	—	—	
				PBG	N	—	—	
				Uroporphyrin	N-↑	—	N	
				Coproporphyrin	N-↑↑	↑↑	N	
				Protoporphyrin	↑↑	↑↑	N	
Porphyria cutanea tarda	Unknown	Adult	Hepatic	ALA	N	—	N	Similar to variegate porphyria
				PBG	N	—	N	
				Uroporphyrin	↑↑	↑↑	N	
				Coproporphyrin	↑↑	↑↑	N	
				Protoporphyrin	—	N	N	
Protoporphyria	Autosomal dominant	Usually childhood	Erythropoietic	ALA	N	—	—	Mild photosensitivity
				PBG	N	—	—	
				Uroporphyrin	↑↑	↑↑	N	
				Coproporphyrin	↑↑	↑-↑↑	N	
				Protoporphyrin	N	N-↑	N	
Acquired porphyria	Acquired	Adult	Hepatic	ALA	N	—	—	Mild photosensitivity
				PBG	N	—	—	
				Uroporphyrin	↑-↑↑	N-↑	N	
				Coproporphyrin	↑-↑↑	N-↑	N	
				Protoporphyrin	—	—	↑	

↑, Increase; ↑↑, marked increase; N, normal; ALA, δ = aminolevulinic acid; PBG, porphobilinogen.
*Modified from Levere, R.D., and Kappas, A.: Hosp. Pract. **5**:61, 1970.

glacial acetic acid diluted to 1 dl with water), followed by 2.5 ml of 0.2M acetic acid (1M diluted 1:5). Collect the eluate in a 10 ml volumetric flask, make up to volume with water, and mix well. To 2 ml of diluted eluate, add 2 ml Ehrlich reagent as used for the ALA determination. Mix the solution well and read at 553 nm after 15 min against a blank of equal parts water and Ehrlich reagent. If the measurements are made in cuvets having an exact 1 cm light path,

$$\text{Absorbance} \times 0.33 = \text{µmole PBG/ml urine}$$

and

$$\text{Absorbance} \times 75 = \text{µg PBG/ml urine}$$

If other cuvets are used, ALA standards may be run, as in the determination of this substance with the following factors:

$$\text{µmole ALA} \times 0.94 = \text{µmole PBG}$$
$$\text{µg ALA} \times 1.60 = \text{µg PBG}$$

Screening procedures for total porphyrins (coproporphyrins and uroporphyrins):
Principle: Coproporphyrins are extracted from urine by ethyl ether and uroporphyrins are extracted with ethyl acetate.
Reagents:
1. Ethyl ether
2. Ethyl acetate
Procedure: Acidify 1 dl urine with 10 ml glacial acetic acid, mix, and allow to stand overnight.
Coproporphyrins: Extract the acetic acid–urine mixture three times with two to three times the volume of ethyl ether, using a separatory funnel. Combine the ether extracts and wash once with 50 ml distilled water, which is returned to the original urine sample. Extract the ether three times with 2 ml 25% aqueous hydrochloric acid. Combine the acid extracts and examine for red fluorescence under long-wavelength ultraviolet light. If red appears, coproporphyrins are present.
Uroporphyrins: Adjust the acidity of the acetic acid–urine mixture to pH 3.0 by adding 1% aqueous hydrochloric acid. Extract the urine three times with one to two times the volume of ethyl acetate. Combine these extracts and wash with 50 ml distilled water. Then extract the ethyl acetate extracts three times with 2 ml of 25% hydrochloric acid. Combine the acid extracts and examine for red fluorescence under long-wavelength ultraviolet light. If red appears, uroporphyrins are present.
Screening test for fecal porphyrins (Dean)[128]: Routine testing for increased porphyrin excretion in stool is more reliable than routine testing for urinary porphyrins, since the latter may not be detected in a dilute urine.
Principle: Porphyrins are extracted by a special solvent, which is then examined for fluorescence.
Reagent (solvent): Mix 1 part amyl alcohol, 1 part glacial acetic acid, and 1 part ether.
Procedure: Collect a small fragment of stool on a finger stall, glass rod, or wooden stick. Insert stool into a tube containing 2 ml solvent. Stir the solvent until it becomes light brown. Then decant the liquid into a clean test tube. Examine the solution under ultraviolet light in a darkened room or box.
Result: The porphyric stool under ultraviolet light will show a brilliant pink fluorescence, persisting even if the solvent is diluted several times. If the patient is not porphyric, the solution will be green, gray, or perhaps slightly orange when examined by long-wavelength ultraviolet light.
Interpretation: A false positive test caused by chlorophyll can be distinguished from a positive test for coproporphyrin and protoporphyrin as follows: add 2 ml 1.5N hydrochloric acid to the solvent, shake the mixture, and allow the acid to settle to the bottom of the tube. Coproporphyrin and protoporphyrin will be in the bottom of the test tube in the hydrochloric acid, while the chlorophyll will remain in the top of the tube in the ether solution. Fecal porphyrins are increased in erythropoietic porphyria, protoporphyria, variegate porphyria, hereditary coproporphyria, and porphyria cutanea tarda. They are usually within normal limits in acute intermittent porphyria.
Urine screening test for coproporphyrins: Increased excretion of porphyrin in urine is seen in porphyria, lead poisoning, and liver disease. The test described is used chiefly as a screening test for lead intoxication.
Reagent (solvent): Mix 1 part amyl alcohol, 1 part glacial acetic acid, and 1 part ether.
Procedure: To 10 ml fresh urine in a test tube add 1 ml solvent. Invert the tube several times to ensure adequate mixture and extraction. Allow the tube to stand for a few minutes so that the solvent floats to the top. Examine in a dark room under long-wavelength ultraviolet light.
Interpretation: If excess porphyrin is present, the ether solution at the top of the test tube will show red fluorescence. In lead poisoning, porphyrin is found in the urine earlier than stippling is seen in the peripheral blood. Excessive porphyrin may be found in the urine even after exposure to lead has been discontinued.
Quantitative determination of urinary coproporphyrins and uroporphyrins[129-131]: Two methods are presented for the determination of urinary porphyrins. The first is a spectrophotometric method in which the coproporphyrins and uroporphyrins are separated by selective solvent extraction before spectrophotometric determination. The second method is a fluorometric one in which the porphyrins are separated by the use of a column of ion-exchange resin. This requires fewer manipulations and a smaller amount of urine.

If a 24 hr urine specimen is collected it should be stored in a brown bottle containing 25 ml of 2 moles/L sodium carbonate (210 g anhydrous sodium carbonate/L) and kept refrigerated.
Method 1 (solvent extraction):
Reagents:
1. Saturated sodium acetate solution
   Dissolve 300 g sodium acetate trihydrate in 2 dl hot water. Allow to cool to room temperature. Some sodium acetate should crystallize out.
2. Sodium acetate buffer, pH 4.8
   As required, mix together 5 volumes glacial

acetic acid, 15 volumes water, and 20 volumes saturated sodium acetate solution.

3. Sodium acetate, 0.13 mole/L
   Dissolve 1.7 g sodium acetate trihydrate in 1 dl water.

4. Acetic acid, 0.09 mole/L
   Dilute 5 ml glacial acetic acid to 1 L with water.

5. Hydrochloric acid, 1.5 moles/L
   Dilute 125 ml concentrated hydrochloric acid to 1 L with water. (NOTE: Add acid to water.)

6. Iodine solution
   a. Stock solution 40 mmole/L. Dissolve 1 g iodine crystals in 1 dl 95% ethanol. Store in the refrigerator.
   b. Working solution, 200 μmole/L. Just before use dilute 0.5 ml of the stock to 1 dl with water.

7. Ethyl acetate

8. *n*-Butanol

9. Pertroleum ether

10. Coproporphyrin standard, 1 μg/ml (1.53 μmole/L)
    This is most conveniently prepared from pre-weighed vials containing 5 μg coproporphyrin I. Add exactly 5 ml of 1.5 moles/L hydrochloric acid to a vial, stopper tightly, heat in hot water for a few minutes with gentle agitation, and then cool. The standard is fairly stable in the refrigerator, but because of the relatively low cost and ease of preparation, it may be made up fresh monthly.

Procedure: Measure the total volume of urine collected and mix well. If the urine has been collected with sodium carbonate, adjust the pH of an aliquot of 1 dl to 5.5 (paper) by adding drops of glacial acetic acid. Check the fluorescence of the urine with long-range (360 nm) ultraviolet light. If a red fluorescence is plainly visible, dilute the urine 1:5 (or greater if a very strong fluorescence is noted).

Coproporphyrins: Add 50 ml urine (or diluted urine) and 25 ml acetate buffer to a 250 ml separatory funnel. Add 75 ml ethyl acetate, stopper, and shake gently. Some urine specimens tend to form emulsions very readily. These should be shaken only gently for 5 min. If only a small amount of emulsion is formed, the urine may be shaken more vigorously for a shorter time.

Allow the layers to separate completely. If a troublesome emulsion is formed that separates very slowly, add a few drops of amyl alcohol to aid in breaking the emulsion. Withdraw the lower aqueous layer and save for the determination of uroporphyrin. Wash the ethyl acetate phase by shaking gently with several 2.5 ml portions of the 0.13 mole/L sodium acetate solution until the washings show no fluorescence with ultraviolet light. Add the washings to the aqueous layer previously saved for the determination of uroporphyrin.

Shake the ethyl acetate phase gently with 5 ml freshly prepared working iodine solution. The iodine solution should not remain in contact with the ethyl acetate for more than 5 min. Withdraw and discard the iodine solution. NOTE: This step is not necessary for urine specimens that have been standing for 24 hr or more in alkaline solution (sodium carbonate preserva-

tive) but is required for freshly voided samples.

Extract the ethyl acetate layer with successive 2.5 ml portions of 1.5 moles/L hydrochloric acid until the extract shows no fluorescence under ultraviolet light. Usually three or four extractions are sufficient. Combine the acid extracts in a graduated cylinder or centrifuge tube and record the total volume of the extract, or, if desired, make up to a definite volume, e.g., 10 or 15 ml, with additional hydrochloric acid. Mix the extracts well and centrifuge if not optically clear.

Measure the absorbance of the extract in a spectrophotometer having a narrow bandwidth (less than 5 nm) against a blank of 1.5 moles/L hydrochloric acid. Take readings at 380 and 430 nm and at 1 nm intervals in the range of 400-408 nm. Then calculate:

$$A^* = (2 A_m - [A_{420} + A_{380}])$$

where A_m is the maximal absorbance in the range from 400-408 nm, A_{420} is the absorbance at 420 nm, A_{380} is the absorbance at 380 nm, and A^* is the corrected absorbance. If the instrument has a very narrow band path and exactly 1 cm cuvets are used, the amount of coproporphyrin may be calculated directly as follows:

$$\mu g/ml \text{ in extract} = A^* \times 0.81$$

or

$$\mu mole/L = A^* \times 1.24$$

For other instruments it is better to repeat the measurements with the standard and calculate A^* for the standard. Then as usual

$$\frac{A^*(\text{sample})}{A^*(\text{standard})} \times \frac{\text{Conc. of}}{\text{standard}} = \frac{\text{Conc. of}}{\text{sample}}$$

If the standard is made up as above, it contains 1.0 μg/ml, or 1.53 μmole/L. Then

$$\frac{\mu g/ml \text{ in extract} \times \text{Vol. of extract} \times \text{Total vol. of urine}}{\text{Vol. of urine used}} =$$

$$\mu g \text{ in total vol. of urine}$$

All volumes are expressed in milliliters. For micromoles per liter a similar expression is used except that the total volume of urine is now expressed in liters.

If the maximal absorbance near 404 nm is too high for accurate reading, the extract may be diluted 1:3 with 1.5 moles/L hydrochloric acid and the appropriate correction made in the calculation. If the reading on the diluted solution is still too high it is better to repeat the determination with a smaller amount of urine, e.g., 50 ml of a 1:10 dilution, with the appropriate changes in the calculations.

Uroporphyrins: To the combined aqueous layers saved for the uroporphyrin determination, add concentrated hydrochloric acid to a pH of 2.8-3.2 (measured with a pH meter or narrow-range indicator paper). Transfer the acidified extracts to a separatory funnel and add 10 ml butanol. Shake for 1 min. Use the same procedure as with the ethyl acetate extraction if an emulsion tends to form. Allow the layers to separate and transfer the butanol layer to a second separatory funnel.

Extract the aqueous layer with three additional 5 ml

portions of butanol. Combine the butanol extracts in a separatory funnel and wash with two 5 ml portions of 0.13 mole/L acetic acid. Discard the washings.

Add 15 ml petroleum ether and 0.5 ml concentrated hydrochloric acid to the combined butanol layers and shake. Withdraw the lower aqueous layer into a graduated centrifuge tube. Extract the solvent layer with an additional 1 ml of 1.5 moles/L hydrochloric acid and add to previous extract. Mix combined extracts, measure volume, and centrifuge if not optically clear.

Extract the solvent layer with an additional 3 ml of 1.5 moles/L hydrochloric acid, place in a separate tube, and centrifuge if not clear. Use this as a blank in reading the uroporphyrin extract. Make readings at 380 and 430 nm and at 1 nm intervals between 403 and 410 nm, using the maximal reading in this range in the calculations. Use the standard reading obtained in the coproporphyrin determination. The calculations are exactly the same except that the final results are multiplied by an additional factor of 1.1 to correct for the difference in absorbance between uroporphyrin and the coproporphyrin standard.

Normal values: The normal excretion of coproporphyrin in adults is 20-200 µg/day (30-300 nmole/day); for uroporphyrin it is 5-50 µg/day (7.5-75 nmole/day).

Method 2 (column chromatography):

Principle: In the column chromatography method the coproporphyrin and uroporphyrin are separated by the use of a small column of ion-exchange resin. The separation is not complete, but a small correction is made for this. The separated extracted porphyrins are then determined fluorometrically. A simple fluorometer such as the Turner model III (Turner Associates, Palo Alto, Calif.) is satisfactory, but a more sensitive instrument will give greater accuracy, particularly in the lower ranges. Any column having an internal diameter of about 5 mm, space for a column about 4 cm in height, and an upper reservoir may be used. A convenient type is the plastic column often used for drug screening, e.g., the Evergreen no. 3077-78 (Evergreen Scientific Co., Los Angeles).

Reagents:
1. Anion exchange resin, Dowex 1-X2, 200-400 mesh, chloride form. This can be used as received, but it is preferable to remove any fines present, which will tend to slow up the flow of liquid through the column. Suspend a portion of the resin in about 10 volumes of water in a graduated cylinder. Allow most of the resin to settle and decant the supernatant with any fines. Repeat the operation several times. The resin is kept in the refrigerator as a 50% slurry in water. When the column is prepared, a small plug of cotton or glass wool is placed in the bottom of the column and the slurry added to form a column of resin about 4 cm high.
2. Wash solution
   In a 1 L volumetric flask add about 5 dl water, 8.3 ml concentrated hydrochloric acid, 150 ml absolute ethanol, and 57 ml glacial acetic acid and mix. Dilute to the mark with water and mix well.
3. Coproporphyrin eluting solution
   In a 1 L volumetric flask place 5 dl water, add 8.3 ml concentrated hydrochloric acid, 250 ml isopropanol, and 1 dl absolute ethanol. Dilute to the mark with water and mix well.
4. Uroporphyrin eluting solution
   In a 1 L volumetric flask add about 5 dl water and 8.3 ml concentrated hydrochloric acid. Mix, add 250 ml isopropanol, and mix again. Dilute to the mark with water and mix well.
5. Coproporphyrin stock standard
   This is the same as that used in the previous method and contains 1 µg/ml, or 1.53 µmole/L. The working standards are made up by dilution with the appropriate elution solvent as noted in the procedure.

The 24 hr urine specimen is collected with sodium carbonate as noted in the previous method. Since the treatment with iodine is not available for this method, it is essential that the urine is allowed to stand for 24 hr before analysis. Adjust a portion of the urine to a pH of 7.0-7.5 (by paper measurement) before use. As in the previous method the urine should be first viewed under ultraviolet light, and if a noticeable fluorescence is seen the urine is diluted 1:5 before analysis.

Procedure: For extraction allow a prepared column to drain completely and then add 1 ml urine to the top of the column (2 ml may be used if low values are expected or the 24 hr volume was very large; 1 ml of a diluted urine may be used if high values are expected). To a similar column add 1 ml water as a blank. Allow the urine or blank to enter the column, then add 15 ml wash solution, and allow to drain completely. Next add 5 ml water to each column and allow to drain completely. Discard these washings.

Place a test tube of about 20 ml capacity under each column and add 15 ml coproporphyrin eluting solution to each column. Collect the entire eluate. Label the tubes as coproporphyrin eluates and coproporphyrin blank; stopper and mix well. Place fresh tubes under the column and add 15 ml uroporphyrin eluting solution to the top of each column. Collect the entire eluate, label tubes, stopper, and mix well.

Prepare standards by adding 0.1 ml stock standard to a 4.9 ml aliquot of coproporphyrin and uroporphyrin blanks; mix each well.

For fluorometric measurements set the exciting wavelength to 405 nm or use a filter peaking at this wavelength (Turner no. 405 [Turner Associates, Palo Alto, Calif.]). Set the secondary wavelength at 600 nm or use a filter passing wavelength longer than 595 nm (Turner no. 25 [Turner Associates, Palo Alto, Calif.]). Set to zero with the coporporphyrin blank and adjust sensitivity to read approximately half scale with the coproporphyrin standard; then read the coproporphyrin sample. Repeat using the uroporphyrin blank, standard, and sample. If an eluate reading is off scale, dilute the eluate 1:3 with a portion of the blank solution. If the reading is still off scale, it is best to repeat the extraction using a greater dilution of the urine.

Calculation:

Coproporphyrin (µg/ml [µmole/L]) =
$$\frac{R_x}{R_s} \times 15 \times 1.09 \times D \times C_s$$

R_x is the reading of the sample eluate, R_s is the reading of the standard, 15 is the volume of the eluate in milliliters, the factor 1.09 corrects for the coproporphyrin not eluted, D is the total dilution factor (for dilution of original urine or eluate or both), and C_s is the concentration of the standard. If the standard is diluted as given, $C_s = 0.02$ μg/ml, or 0.0314 μmole/L. If this standard is used along with 1 ml urine and no dilutions are made, the above expression reduces to the following:

$$\text{Coproporphyrin (μg/ml)} = \frac{R_x}{R_s} \times 0.327$$

For micromoles per liter replace the factor 0.327 by 0.500. Uroporphyrin in the sample (not corrected for the small amount of coproporphyrin included) is given by a similar equation where the uroporphyrin is read against the corresponding blank and standard and the factor 1.09 is replaced by the factor 1.14, which corrects for the fact that 1 μg coproporphyrin gives the same amount of fluorescence as 1.14 μg uroporphyrin. Again, using the standard as given above and 1 ml urine with no dilutions, the expression reduces to the following:

Uroporphyrin (μg/ml) (corrected) =
$$\text{Uroporphyrin (μg/ml) (uncorrected)} - \frac{\text{Coproporphyrin (μg/ml)}}{10}$$

Exactly the same equation is used when the concentrations are in micromoles per liter. For both

$$\text{Porphyrins (μg/ml)} \times \text{Urine vol. (ml)} = \text{μg/day}$$

or

$$\text{μmole/L} \times \text{Urine vol. (L)} = \text{μmole/day}$$

Normal values: The normal values are the same as for the previous method.

Estimation of δ-aminolevulinic acid: δ-Aminolevulinic acid (ALA) is a precursor in the synthesis of porphobilinogen (PBG) and hence of porphyrins (Fig. 27-12). The enzyme responsible for the conversion of ALA into PBG, ALA dehydratase, is inhibited by heavy metals such as lead and mercury. Thus the conversion of ALA to PBG is decreased in lead poisoning. Since the synthesis of ALA itself is not affected, ALA will tend to accumulate in the body fluids and more will be excreted in the urine. The increased urinary excretion of ALA is thus considered a good index of lead poisoning.

Principle: In the method described, ALA is separated from interfering material by means of ion-exchange resin columns. The urine sample is first passed through a column that absorbs the interfering PBG and allows the ALA to pass through. The ALA is then absorbed on a second column, whereas impurities and interfering materials are washed through. The ALA is eluted with a sodium acetate solution and heated with acetylacetone to form a pyrrole, giving a red color with modified Ehrlich reagent. The method is essentially that of Mauzerall and Granick[132] as modified by Wilkinson[133] and Davis and Andelman.[134]

Reagents:

1. Dowex 2-X8 resin (200-400 mesh). Suspend the resin in water and wash until the supernatant is clear. Then suspend in several volumes of 3M sodium acetate, stirring occasionally, for about 30 min. Pour off the supernatant after the resin has settled and repeat the treatment. Then wash the resin several times with about 5 volumes of distilled water and store as a slurry in water.
2. Dowex 50-X4 resin (200-400 mesh). Suspend the resin in water and wash until the supernatant is clear. Then allow it to stand overnight in about 3 volumes of 2N sodium hydroxide. Decant the supernatant and wash the resin several times until the supernatant is nearly neutral. Then wash twice with about 4 volumes of 2N hydrochloric acid and finally wash several times with distilled water.
3. Sodium acetate, 3M
   Dissolve 408 g sodium acetate trihydrate in distilled water and make the volume up to 1 L.
4. Sodium hydroxide, 2N
   Dissolve 80 g sodium hydroxide in water and dilute to 1 L.
5. Hydrochloric acid, 4N
   Dilute 336 ml concentrated hydrochloric acid with water to make 1 L.
6. Acetate buffer, pH 4.6
   Dissolve 136 g sodium acetate trihydrate and 57 ml glacial acetic acid in water and dilute to 1 L.
7. Modified Ehrlich reagent
   Dissolve 6 g p-dimethylaminobenzaldehyde in 26 ml concentrated hydrochloric acid and dilute to 1 dl with glacial acetic acid.
8. Acetylacetone
9. ALA standards
   a. Stock standard, 0.001M. Dissolve 13.1 mg of the amino acid in acetate buffer and make up to 1 dl. This solution is stable for 1 month when stored in the refrigerator.
   b. Working standard. Dilute 1 ml stock standard to 10 ml with the acetate buffer.

Preparation of chromatographic columns: Inexpensive columns may be made from disposable 10 ml plastic syringes. Remove the plunger and discard. Place a disk of rapid filter paper at the bottom of the syringe. Pour a slurry of the ion-exchange resin in water to give a column height of 2 cm. Place another disk of filter paper on top of the column. The preparation of the columns is somewhat time consuming, and care must be taken beforehand to wash the resin well. The disposable columns (along with all the reagents) can be purchased as a kit (Bio-Rad Laboratories, Richmond, Calif.), which may be more convenient.

Collection of sample: It has been found[135] that the urine for ALA determination is best collected with tartaric acid (1 g/dl). This may be obtained by adding 10 g tartaric acid to the original collection bottle if the usual volume is expected. The specimen should be kept refrigerated until used, and a portion of the urine should be adjusted to a pH of 6.0-7.0 just before use.

Procedure: It is convenient to arrange the two columns so that the eluate from the Dowex-2 column passes directly into the top of the Dowex-50 column. Alternately, eluate from first column is transferred in small portions to second column as collected.

Wash the columns first with several 5 cm portions of water and discard the washings. Add 1 ml urine to the Dowex-2 column. Add three 4 ml portions of water to the column and allow the eluate to drip directly into the Dowex-50 column or transfer to the top of this column as collected. Discard the Dowex-2 column now or save it for quantitative determination of PBG.

Wash the Dowex-50 column with two additional 4 ml portions of water. Discard all the washings. Elute the ALA from the column by adding 8 ml of 1M sodium acetate (made by diluting the 3M solution) and collect the eluate in a 10 ml volumetric flask or a test tube graduated at 10 ml. In a separate flask, add 7 mm of 1M sodium acetate and 1 ml working standard.

To each tube, add 0.2 ml acetyl-acetone and dilute to the mark with the acetate buffer. Stopper the flasks or tubes and heat in a boiling water bath for 10 min. Transfer 2 ml aliquots of the treated sample and standard to test tubes, add 2 ml modified Ehrlich reagent, and mix well. Allow to stand for 15 min and then read standard and sample against a blank composed of equal parts acetate buffer and Ehrlich reagent.

Calculation:

$$\frac{\text{Absorbance of sample}}{\text{Absorbance of standard}} \times 1 = \mu\text{mole/ml ALA}$$

$$\mu\text{mole/ml} \times 131 = \mu\text{g/ml}$$

$$\mu\text{mole (or } \mu\text{g)/ml} \times 24 \text{ hr vol. (ml)} = \mu\text{mole or } \mu\text{g/24 hr}$$

Normal values:

Children: About 0.3-0.6 mg (2.2-4.5 μmole)/24 hr at 5 years of age, generally increasing to adult levels at about 15 years of age

Adults: From 1.5-4.0 mg (11-23 μmole)/24 hr, or 0.2 mg/dl

Discussion: The urinary excretion of ALA is markedly increased in **lead intoxication** (up to five times the normal level). There may be an increase in ALA excretion without increased coproporphyrin excretion. Increased excretion of ALA may also be found in the congenital hepatic porphyrias.

In children ALA determination in urine is the method of choice for the detection of **lead poisoning** and is superior to the determination of blood lead levels. In periods of bone growth, blood is rapidly cleared of lead, which is either deposited together with calcium in the growing ends of the long bones or is excreted in the urine. The blood lead level may therefore be within

normal limits in a child who has osseous lead deposits, which produce lead intoxication when mobilized in periods of acidosis. ALA reflects the effect of immobilized lead on heme production rather than the level of circulating lead.

Determination of level of δ-aminolevulinic acid in erythrocytes: The activity of the enzyme ALA dehydratase in the erythrocytes is measured as a test for lead intoxication.[136,137] As mentioned, this enzyme is necessary for the conversion of ALA to PBG and is inhibited by lead and other heavy metals.

Principle: The method is relatively simple; hemolyze 50 μl blood in water and add buffered substrate containing ALA. After incubation, precipitate the proteins with trichloroacetic acid; any PBG formed is measured by adding a modified Ehrlich reagent. Then calculate the activity in units per deciliter of red cells based on the hematocrit determination. Up to blood lead levels of about 60-70 μg/dl, there is a fairly good correlation between the lead level and the decrease in ALA dehydratase activity, but higher levels of lead seem to cause little additional decrease in activity. This test has not been extensively studied, but it seems to be somewhat simpler than the ALA determination and in theory is more specific.

Porphyrias

Porphyrias[138] are a group of hereditary and acquired diseases that have in common the excessive excretion of one or more porphyrins, porphyrinogens, or porphyrin precursors, e.g., δ-aminolevulinic acid (δ-ALA) and porphobilinogen (PBG) in the urine or feces or both. Each type of hereditary porphyria is caused by an abnormally low activity of one of several enzymes involved in the porphyrin metabolism (Table 27-11). The congenital porphyrias are divided into two groups: those with erythropoietic abnormalities and those with hepatic abnormalities.

Congenital erythropoietic porphyria: Congenital erythropoietic porphyria is a rare hereditary disease that is transmitted as an autosomal recessive trait and is found in infancy and early childhood. It is characterized clinically by extreme sensitivity to light resulting in blistering and scarring of the skin. Porphyrins become deposited in the tissues, especially in the bones and teeth, staining them deep brown. The defect lies in a reduction of the enzyme uroporphyrinogen III cosynthetase, which leads to an imbalance between the con-

Table 27-11. Enzyme defects of porphyrias

Porphyrias	Enzyme defects
Erythropoietic porphyria	
Congenital erythropoietic porphyria	Uroporphyrinogen III cosynthetase
Hepatic porphyrias	
Acute intermittent porphyria	Uroporphyrinogen I synthetase
Hereditary coproporphyria	Coproporphyrinogen oxidase
Variegate porphyria	Protoporphyrinogen oxidase
Porphyria cutanea tarda	Uroporphyrinogen decarboxylase
Protoporphyria	Ferrochelatase
Toxic porphyria	Variable

centration of uroporphyrinogen III cosynthetase and uroporphyrinogen I synthetase, with the latter exceeding the former. Although the genetic defect is present in all cells, it is expressed mainly in the erythropoietic tissue. Since uroporphyrinogen I is readily converted into the corresponding porphyrin, large quantities of uroporphyrin I and coproporphyrin I are found in the urine, which varies in color from reddish to black, reflecting variations of the porphyrin excretion (Table 27-10).

Acute intermittent porphyria: Acute intermittent porphyria is the most common type of porphyria; it occurs in adult life and is more common in women than in men. Clinically, it is characterized by abdominal and nervous symptoms that may mimic acute abdominal emergencies and mental disorders. It is an autosomal dominantly inherited disease resulting from a deficiency of uroporphyrinogen I synthetase, so that large amounts of porphyrin precursor substances are excreted in urine rather than porphyrins. The increased urinary uroporphyrin sometimes seen can be explained on the basis of polymerization of porphobilinogen.

Urine examination reveals increased amounts of ALA and PBG. A marked increase in PBG detected by the Watson-Schwartz method is pathognomonic of the disease.

Patients with acute intermittent porphyria can be divided into two groups: those in the acute phase and those in remission (Table 27-10).

Hereditary coproporphyria: A defect of the coproporphyrinogen oxidase is inherited as an autosomal dominant trait that produces a variegate porphyria–like clinical picture and results in an increased excretion of porphyrin precursors. Fecal coproporphyrin III and porphobilinogen are fairly constantly increased.

Variegate porphyria: Variegate porphyria is an autosomal dominant disorder that blocks the conversion of protoporphyrinogen III to heme, a defect that is responsible for increased concentrations of porphyrins and their precursors in urine and increased uroporphyrins and coproporphyrins in feces.

Porphyria cutanea tarda: Porphyria cutanea tarda is the most common form of porphyria since it is associated with liver disease, a rather frequent malady. The metabolic defect probably consists of a deficiency in the uroporphyrinogen decarboxylase, the predictable effect of which is an increase in urinary and fecal uroporphyrins and coproporphyrins.

Protoporphyria: Despite the fact that protoporphyria is more common than erythropoietic porphyria, it was not clearly defined until 1961, presumably because it lacked abnormal urinary findings. The disease is caused by a dominant inherent deficiency of ferrochelatase activity in all tissues[139] leading to an accumulation of protoporphyrin in tissues. Since protoporphyrin is not excreted by the kidneys there are no urinary findings in protoporphyria. The diagnosis is based on increased protoporphyrin levels in feces and in red cells, which fluoresce when viewed under the fluorescent microscope, but neither the fluorescence nor the fecal protoporphyrin increase is pathognomonic of protoporphyria.

Acquired porphyria: The acquired form of porphyria results from the effect of drugs, alcohol or toxic heavy metals such as gold, lead, and arsenic. They inhibit some of the enzyme systems of heme synthetic pathways, e.g., δ-ALA synthetase, uroporphyrinogen synthetase, or ferrochelatase. The list of drugs that are able to produce a hepatic porphyria-like clinical picture of varying intensity includes barbiturates, penicillin G, procaine, sedatives, hypnotics, sulfonamides, and stilbestrol. The durgs exert their influence against a background of previously damaged liver parenchyma. Urine examination reveals an increase in porphyrins.

MELANIN

Twenty percent of patients with disseminated malignant melanoma excrete black melanin or its colorless precursor, melanogen, in the urine. The urine darkens and becomes black on standing (oxidation), and the colorless melanogen changes into the black pigment melanin.[140]

Ferric chloride test:

Principle: Tyrosine, the precursor of melanin, is oxidized to melanogen and to melanin by ferric chloride (Table 27-5).

Reagents:
1. Ferric chloride, 10% (10 g/dl)
2. Hydrochloric acid, 10% (10 ml/dl)

Procedure: To 10 ml urine add sufficient 10% ferric chloride solution 1 drop at a time to precipitate all phosphates. Add drop by drop enough 10% hydrochloric acid to dissolve the precipitated phosphates. Centrifuge at 2000 rpm for 5 min.

Result: A gray or black precipitate indicates melanin.

Thormahlen test:

Principle: Sodium nitroprusside is reduced to ferrocyanide (Prussian blue) by melanogen.

Reagents:
1. Nitroprusside, 5% (5 g/dl)
2. Sodium hydroxide, 25% (25 g/dl)
3. Glacial acetic acid

Procedure: Add 2 ml 5% aqueous sodium nitroprusside solution to 5 ml urine. Add 2 ml 25% sodium hydroxide. Add 2 ml glacial acetic acid.

Result: If melanogen is present, the red color changes to blue-green.

Discussion: As already stated, melanin occurs in the urine because of the presence of melanotic tumors, especially if they have metastasized to the liver. The differential diagnosis includes **alkaptonuria,** a defect in amino acid metabolism that leads to the excretion of homogentisic acid and to dark discoloration of urine on exposure to air (p. 682). In patients with melanoma the urinary excretion of phenylalanine and other catechols is increased.[141]

URINARY SEDIMENT
Microscopic examination

Principle: The formed elements suspended in the urine are precipitated by centrifugation and analyzed under the microscope. Crystalline structures are of relatively little importance, but the shed cellular elements and casts often give valuable information as to the pathology of urinary tract disease.

Specimen: The first morning specimen is the specimen of choice and should be examined within a few hours. Preservative tablets are suggested as a means of preserving formed elements in the urine if the specimen is to be mailed. Acid urine stored in the refrigerator will preserve almost all cellular elements, crystals, and casts fairly well for a few hours.

Procedure: Mix specimen thoroughly. Fill 15 ml centrifuge tube to fingerbreadth of top and centrifuge for 3 min at 1800 rpm. Pour off supernatant fluid by inverting tube without wiping lip of tube. Mix sediment with the small amount of urine that remains in the tube (by holding the top of the tube with one hand and striking the bottom of the tube with a finger of the other hand). With a capillary pipet, transfer 1 small drop onto a slide, apply coverslip (24 × 32 mm), and under subdued light examine the entire coverslip area.

Casts are reported as the average number per 10 low-power fields (lpf). The high-power objective is used to identify the type and composition of the casts. Structures smaller than casts, red cells, white cells, and epithelial cells are reported as the average number per 10 high-power fields (hpf). Other structures that may be seen in the sediment, e.g., yeast, bacteria, mucous threads, spermatozoa, and fat droplets, are reported as many, moderate, or few.

Since amorphous deposits may cover up important structures such as casts, they should be removed. If urine contains many amorphous urates, warm specimen gently before centrifuging to dissolve the urates. If urine contains many amorphous phosphates and carbonates, add just enough 10% acetic acid to dissolve the amorphous sediment before centrifuging. Urinary microscopy is difficult to standardize, to assay, and to establish quality control for. In a given institution it is essential that the microscopy is performed under as standardized conditions as possible by technicians well trained in the recognition of the various structures that make up urinary sediment.[142] The Kova system (ICL Scientific, Fountain Valley, Calif.) offers one approach to the standardization of urinary microscopy.

Urinary microscopy is usually performed on unstained wet preparations that are examined by means of conventional light microscopy. Better details are obtained by the use of phase-contrast microscopy of unstained wet preparations.[143,144] To improve the reproducibility and accuracy of the method some investigators have suggested special stains such as the Sternheimer-Malbin or the Kova stain, the use of interference-contrast microscopy, the use of Millipore filters,[145,146] or the combination of the cytocentrifuge and Papanicolaou technic.[147]

Appearance of sediment stained with Sternheimer-Malbin stain[148]:

Cellular elements: Squamous cells stain pale purple with dark purple nuclei; renal cells have an orange-purple cytoplasm and dark nuclei; leukocytes are pale pink with purple nuclei; glitter cells stain pale blue; erythrocytes may not stain at all or they may stain pale pink; and yeast cells may stain dark purple, or they may not take the stain at all.

Casts: Hyaline and waxy casts may not stain at all or are pale pink; granular casts have a pink matrix and purple granules; and red cell casts are red-purple.

Crystals: Crystals do not stain.

Bacteria: Bacteria vary in color.

Spermatozoa: Spermatozoa stain blue.

Trichomonas: Trichomonas take a pale blue dye; the nucleus is purple.

Cytocentrifuge-Papanicolaou technic[147]:

Reagents and equipment:

1. Papanicolaou stains
2. Parlodion
   Ethyl alcohol, 95%, 2 dl
   Ether, anhydrous, 2 dl
   Parlodion, 1 g
3. Fixative
   Glacial acetic acid, 1 part
   Ethanol, 95% 9 parts
4. Cytocentrifuge (Shandon Southern Instruments, Sewickley, Penn.)

The combination of cytocentrifuge and Papanicolaou staining allows rapid identification of (1) hematopoietic elements, e.g., granulocytes and lymphocytes, (2) urinary casts,[149] e.g., hyaline, erythrocytic, and hemoglobin casts, (3) epithelial cells, e.g., squamous, metaplastic, and transitional cells, and (4) viral inclusions, as seen in infections with herpes simplex virus and cytomegalovirus.

Procedure: Obtain an early morning, well-mixed, clean-catch specimen and prepare wet preparation as described above, but retain about 1 ml supernatant in which the sediment is resuspended. With a cytocentrifuge prepare at least two slides, using 4 drops of resuspended urinary sediment per chamber. Centrifuge at 900 rpm for 3 min. Apply 1-2 drops of parlodion to cellular area on slide after discarding the filter paper. Fix the slide in acetic acid alcohol. Stain by the Papanicolaou technic. Count the formed elements in 10 high-power fields (hpf) (×430).

Addis count

The Addis count technic, an attempt to quantitatively measure the excretion rate of formed urinary elements in a given period, is theoretically sound, but the execution of the test in the laboratory is time-consuming, tedious, lacking in precision and control, and probably inaccurate, because some of the elements of the sediment disintegrate during the collection period. The Addis count has no diagnostic significance anymore since it has been replaced by the kidney biopsy, but it can be used to follow the clinical course of patients. A detailed description of the test procedure is omitted, because a carefully performed urinalysis of the first morning midstream specimen provides the same information as the tedious, nonspecific Addis count.

Leukocytes

In the centrifuged specimen there is usually an occasional leukocyte, not more than 1/hpf in specimens from men and 1-5/hpf in specimens from women and children. Larger numbers, if found consistently, indicate inflammation (pyuria).

Most of the white cells are granulocytes, which may show ameboid movements in a fresh specimen or adopt a spheric, often distended outline in toxic surroundings. The other white cells are lymphocytes and macrophages. Clumping of granulocytes should be noted. The Sternheimer-Malbin stain differentiates large, pale blue, so-called renal leukocytes (glitter cells) from the smaller pink leukocytes of the lower urinary tract.

Glitter cells: Glitter cells are phagocytic polymorphonuclear cells, the granules of which show brownian movement. They can be found in a variety of kidney diseases but are most closely related to pyelonephritis. The Sternheimer-Malbin gentian violet–safranin stain will stain glitter cells a faint blue.

Leukocytes are found in the urine in acute infections of the urinary tract, acute prostatitis, tuberculosis of the urinary tract, acute and subacute glomerulonephritis, lupus nephritis, interstitial nephritis,[150] and acute allograft rejection. Fifty percent of leukocytes lyse in hypotonic alkaline urine within 2-3 hr.[150]

A **Gram stain** of the urinary sediment provides valuable microbiologic information. Wilson[150] reports that occasional bacteria per oil-immersion field of an unspun specimen indicate about 10,000 bacteria/ml. If there are bacteria in most fields, there are 100,000 bacteria/ml in the urine.

Blood (erythrocytes)

Red cells are highly refractile, round, yellowish structures that can be distinguished from fat droplets by

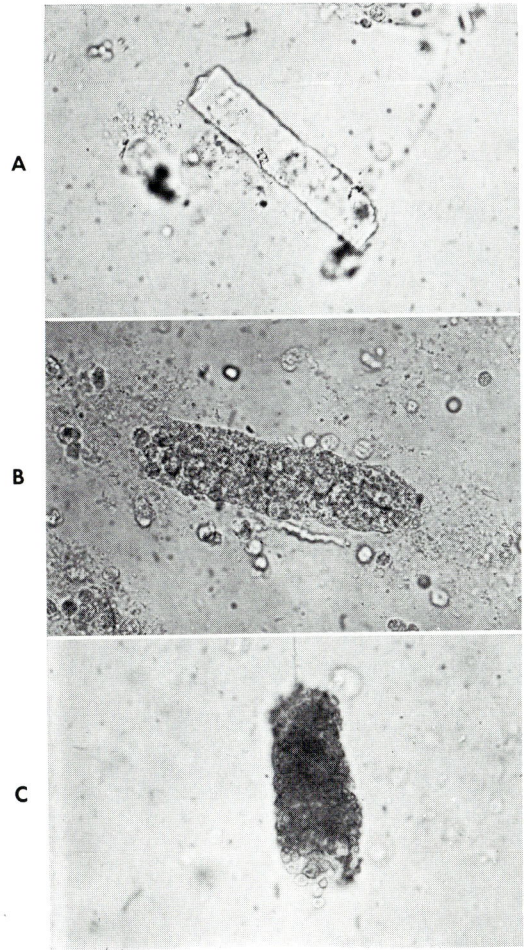

their color and by the fact that they do not stain with Sudan III; they can be distinguished from yeast by the addition of dilute acetic acid, which dissolves them (Fig. 27-13). For a reliable evaluation of erythrocytes in the sediment the urine must be not too dilute and not very alkaline.[150] An erythrocyte count of 60,000 cells/ml is needed for recognition of an increase of red cells in the sediment.[150]

Causes of hematuria: The causes of hematuria may be grouped as follows: (1) prerenal, indicating purpura, infections, and drugs; (2) renal, resulting from inflammation, tumors, tuberculosis, calculi, and trauma to kidney; and (3) postrenal, resulting from inflammation, tumors, and parasites of the urinary bladder.

Red cells may be evidence of vaginal contamination or may follow catheterization, but with these two exceptions they always represent an important finding. It is of no clinical importance whether they are crenated (as in hypertonic urine) or pale and distended (as in hypotonic urine).

Urinary casts

Casts in the urine (cylindruria) are almost always pathologic and are a tool in the evaluation and diagnosis of kidney disease[151] and renal allograft rejection.[152] Casts are the result of the gelling of a specific renal mucoprotein common to all casts, immunologically identified as Tamm-Horsfall protein,[153] although IgG and IgM have also been identified.[153] Their formation is poorly understood but is probably related to such factors as urinary stasis, volume, pH, and osmolality. The widths of casts are determined by the dimensions of the tubules in which they form. Typically, casts are cylindric structures with parallel sides and blunt, rounded ends, but they may be straight or convoluted. Castlike structures with long, thin, tapering tails or without the protein base have no significance.[149] Casts are classified on the basis of appearance, physical properties, and the nature of the embodied material (Table 27-12).

Hyaline casts: Hyaline casts are the most frequent casts and are clear cylinders, often difficult to visualize by bright-field microscopy, because their refractive index is nearly that of the surrounding medium.[154] The protein matrix is hyaline and composed mainly of Tamm-Horsfall protein, which is probably secreted by

Table 27-12. Classification of casts

Cast	Significance
Hyaline	Changes in pH and osmolality, normal exercise, mild renal disease
Cellular	
Red cell	Acute glomerulonephritis
Hemoglobin	Intravascular hemolysis
White cell	Pyelonephritis
Epithelial cell	Tubular damage
Granular	Chronic renal disease
Fatty	Chronic renal disease
Waxy	Chronic renal disease
Mixed	Chronic renal disease

Fig. 27-13. Urinary casts. **A,** Hyaline cast. **B,** White cell cast. **C,** Red cell cast. (Courtesy Ames Co., Elkhart, Ind.)

Data from Haber, M.H., and Lindner, L.E.: Am. J. Clin. Pathol. **68:**547, 1977.

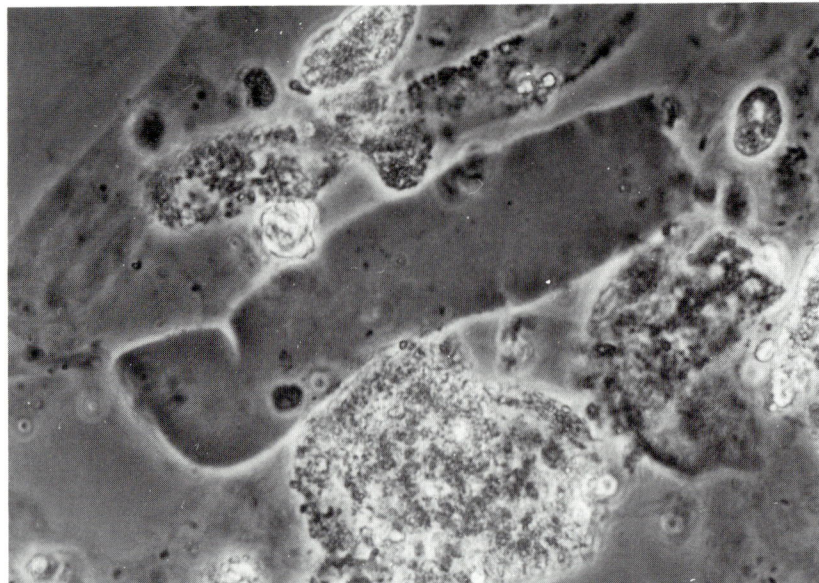

Fig. 27-14. Multiple casts, phase microscopy. In center of photograph is a broad waxy cast with one red cell on it. Around this cast there is a broad granular cast at 6-o'clock position, a hyaline cast at 11-o'clock position, and a granular cast at 2-o'clock position. Renal epithelial cells and amorphous urates are seen in background. (Courtesy L.H. Brody.)

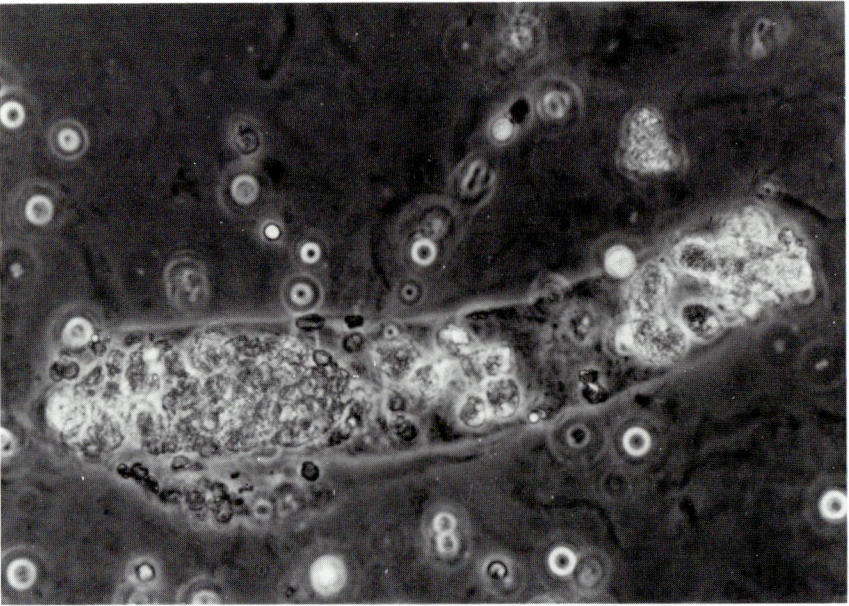

Fig. 27-15. Mixed cellular cast, phase microscopy. Left end of cast is packed with red cells, whereas in center of cast there are six white cells, and in right end of cast there are many renal epithelial cells. Around the cast there are many red cells. (Courtesy L.H. Brody.)

the lining cells of the distal convoluted tubules.[155] They therefore may be straight or serpentine, broad or slim, and varying in length (Figs. 27-13, *A*, and 27-14). A variety of inclusions may be detected within the protein gel, representing material such as cells or unidentifiable structures trapped when the gelling of the protein occurred.

Significance: An occasional hyaline cast (less than 1/hpf) may be detected in the sediment of healthy individuals, but their number increases in progressive renal disease and may reach values of 20-30 per low-power field (1pf).[156]

Cellular casts: The protein matrix of cellular casts contains a variety of cellular inclusions that may undergo successive changes from coarsely granular to finely granular and finally to waxy, each stage signifying one step in the progressive degeneration of the inclusions.[157]

Red cell casts: Red cell casts are granular, dark red to red-orange cylinders composed of a matrix containing red cells in various stages of degeneration and visibility (Figs. 27-13, *C*, and 27-15).

Significance: Red cell casts are always pathologic, since they are characteristic of glomerular disease, indicating severe injury to the glomerular basement membrane, which allows red cells and protein to escape into the urine. They are seen in acute glomerulonephritis, lupus nephritis, Goodpasture's syndrome, subacute bacterial endocarditis, Wegner's granulomatosis, periarteritis and polyarteritis, and sickle cell disease.

Hemoglobin casts: Hemoglobin casts are orange to yellow-red casts and must be distinguished from bile or drug-stained casts. On the dry slide they can be stained for hemoglobin.[158]

Significance: Hemoglobin casts are indicative of intravascular hemolysis, e.g., following a mismatched transfusion or *Clostridium* bacteremia.

White cell casts: Polymorphonuclear leukocytes are enmeshed in the cast matrix (Figs. 27-13, *B*, and 27-15) and usually allow recognition of their multilobed nuclei. As these cells degenerate, the cytoplasm becomes granular, the cell boundaries disappear, and a granular cast is born, which in different segments may reflect the stages of its development.

Significance: White cell casts are associated with acute pyelonephritis, interstitial nephritis, and acute glomerulonephritis.

Epithelial casts: Cells shed by the tubular lining cells are caught within or on the surface of the hyaline matrix to form the cast, the epithelial component of which may undergo sequential degenerative changes to form granular and waxy casts. The epithelial casts must be differentiated from all other cellular casts, a task made easier by the large, rounded or oval nuclei of the incorporated cells, which are often arranged in parallel rows rather than haphazardly, although the latter pattern is also seen and may indicate desquamation from different and separate portions of the tubules.[156] The nuclei may contain nucleoli surrounded by thin shells of cytoplasm, giving these cells a polyhedral outline. As the cells degenerate they lose their nuclear and cytoplasmic membranes and become granular. The matrix also fills with granular material, resulting in a coarse granular cast.

Significance: Epithelial casts, which are relatively infrequent, owe their existence to damaged or necrotic renal tubular epithelium as seen in nephrosis or in the nephrotic phase of acute and chronic glomerulonephritis. Epithelial necrosis is also produced by nephrotoxic agents, e.g., ethyl glycol, bichloride of mercury, lead, and bismuth, or by viruses such as cytomegalovirus and hepatitis virus.[156]

Granular casts: Granular casts owe their existence to the progressive degeneration of the inclusions of various cellular casts. As the cells within the cast deteriorate, the nucleus becomes pyknotic and fragmented and loses its membrane. The cytoplasm is also stripped of its membrane and assumes a granular appearance. The granulation is coarse at first, at which time intact remnants of the original inclusion may still be found. As the degenerative process progresses, a finely granular pattern appears, the source of which may not be ascertainable. Since the different cellular casts have different clinical connotations, it is important to correctly identify them before they have degenerated beyond recognition. As the degeneration proceeds, cholesterol esters and fat may be incorporated into the shed cells, giving a characteristic picture under polarized light (Fig. 27-15). The appearance of waxy casts marks the final phase of degeneration of the finely granular casts in which the inclusions become homogeneous and unidentifiable.

Significance: The significance of granular casts depends on their etiology before their degeneration (e.g., the clinical implications of epithelial casts are different from those of white cell casts). Granular casts are frequently seen in chronic kidney disease and in the recovery phase from acute renal failure. The differentiation of coarsely granular from finely granular casts is of no clinical significance.

Fat: Fat[159] may be present in urine (lipiduria) (1) as free fatty globules, (2) as fat globules within the cytoplasm of shed tubular lining cells, and (3) in fatty casts.

Under low-power magnification free fat globules appear as floating, spheric or ovoid, dark, glistening structures. Under polarized light these droplets are doubly refractile and show a Maltese cross pattern (Fig. 27-16). The Maltese cross pattern is not pathognomonic of fat, because some crystals may give an identical picture. Interference contrast microscopy assists in the recognition of fat in urine by revealing highly refractile yellowish to brown spheric structures devoid of any inclusions. If there is any doubt as to the lipid nature of the material, special stains for fat should be employed, e.g., oil red O fat stain.[160]

Significance: Free fat in urine is an expression of hyperlipidemia or fat embolism. Hyperlipidemia, although it may be primary in about 15% of patients, is secondary to underlying disorders such as the nephrotic syndrome, hypothyroidism, uncontrolled diabetes, alcoholism, acute pancreatitis, primary biliary cirrhosis, and alcoholism.

Oval fat bodies: Oval fat bodies[159] are degenerated epithelial cells that contain fat droplets within their cytoplasm. The fatty nature of these inclusions is demonstrated by the methods used for documentation of free fat in urine.

Significance: Fatty degeneration of renal epithelial

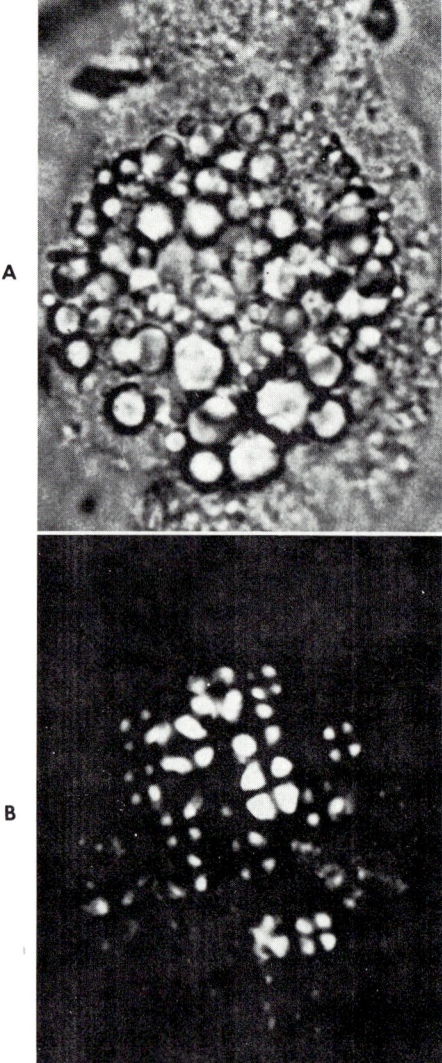

Fig. 27-16. Oval fat body viewed under ordinary light, **A,** and under polarized light, **B,** showing Maltese cross patterns. (From Daysog, A., and Dobson, H.L.: Am. J. Clin. Pathol. **39:**419, 1963.)

cells may be an expression of hyperlipidemia, the etiology of which is mentioned above, but most frequently is associated with anoxia (heart failure), advanced kidney disease, and toxic conditions, e.g., toxemia of pregnancy.

Fatty casts: Fatty casts[159] contain a variable number of fat droplets of various sizes within the hyaline matrix and are demonstrated by the methods described.

Significance: Fatty casts are indicative of intrinsic renal disease, e.g., diabetic nephropathy and chronic renal disorders.

Waxy casts: Waxy casts have a characteristic appearance (Fig. 27-14). They are prominent, often wide, opaque, and yellowish to tan, with slightly undulating edges and squared ends, which may appear to be "broken off". No inclusions are present. Waxy casts are

the final stage in the degeneration of granular casts, and their formation is discussed under granular casts.

Significance: Waxy casts are found in chronic kidney disease, diabetic nephropathy, and renal amyloidosis.

Mixed casts: The term *mixed casts* refers to casts having more than one distinct component (Fig. 27-15), e.g., as seen in the evolution of waxy casts from cellular casts in which mixed pictures of epithelial and granular inclusions frequently and readily arise.

Significance: Depending on the mixture of the inclusions present, a mixed cast may indicate damage to several anatomic areas of the kidney, e.g., the glomerulus (red cells), the tubules (epithelial cells), and the interstitium (white cells).

The term *telescoped urinary sediment* is used to describe a sediment that contains a variety of casts and other pathologic components and is frequently encountered in acute glomerulonephritis.

Epithelial cells

Squamous cells in the urinary sediment are derived from the vagina or the anterior urethra and prepuce and are of no clinical significance. Since they should not be present in a well-collected midstream specimen, their presence indicates a poor collection technic.

The recognition of renal tubular cells is of clinical importance, because their presence is one of the indicators of acute renal allograft rejection.[160] Schumann, Palmieri, and Jones[160] divide the exfoliated renal cells into five types: type I, a large cell with abundant, granular, eosinophilic cytoplasm arises from the proximal convoluted tubules; type II, a smaller cuboidal cell with granular, eosinophilic cytoplasm, represents the distal convoluted tubules; type III, an even smaller cuboidal cell with a light eosinophilic cytoplasm, originates in the collecting tubules; type IV cells, which also arise in the collecting tubules, occur in castlike tissue fragments; and type V cells represent the urothelium. In siderosis or hemochromatosis the tubular cells contain hemosiderin, which is brown and may be confirmed by histologic stains for iron.

Exfoliative cytology

The Papanicolaou technic is used to demonstrate the above-mentioned type of epithelial cells and malignant cells in urine.

Procedure: A fresh urine specimen is concentrated by the cytocentrifuge technic immediately after voiding (within 1 hr) and is then subjected to the various steps of the Papanicolaou staining technic.

Mucous strands or threads

Mucous strands or fibers are present in small numbers normally. Increased numbers are found in chronic inflammation of the urethra and bladder.

Bacteria

Bacteria are of no significance except in fresh or catheterized specimens. They should be studied by Gram stain and culture. Normally fewer than 1000 bacteria/ml urine are present in the uncentrifuged specimen. In wet preparations of the centrifuged specimen they are only detectable if their number exceeds 10,000/ml urine. The observer should pay special attention to the presence or absence of associated pus cells.

Yeast

On microscopic examination, double-walled, oval to pear-shaped budding organisms, which are smaller than red cells, are seen (Fig. 27-17, *D*). Urinary yeast infections are common in patients with diabetes, on birth control pills, or undergoing intensive antibiotic or immunosuppressive therapy.

Viruses and other inclusions

Desquamated cells may contain the large inclusions of salivary gland virus disease or the small, acid-fast inclusions of heavy metal (lead and bismuth) intoxication[161] or of herpes simplex virus.

Semen

Well-preserved spermatozoa are not infrequently found (Fig. 27-18).

Parasites

Animal parasites are rare. Flagellates (*Trichomonas hominis* [Fig. 27-19] and *Chilomastix mesnili*), *Schistosoma haematobium*, and filaria may be found (Fig. 27-19). Ova of intestinal parasites may be present as a contamination, e.g., ova of *Enterobius vermicularis* (Fig. 27-20).

Amorphous sediment

Amorphous phosphates, sometimes neutral or amphoteric, are found in alkaline urine specimens and appear as colorless, granular masses. They are soluble in 10% acetic acid, without formation of gas. Granular masses of calcium carbonate are rare and dissolve in 10% acetic acid with effervescence. In acid urine specimens, **amorphous urates** appear as very fine granules, usually colored by urinary pigments. The granules appear yellowish microscopically and pink grossly. They disappear on warming or on the addition of acetic or hydrochloric acid.

Crystals

Crystals are not usually present when urine is voided but form after it cools, either because the urine is supersaturated at the cooler temperature or because changes in the reaction alter the solubilities of the substances. The presence of albumin and other substances often interferes with crystallization.

Crystals are of little clinical significance except for cystine, uric acid, leucine, and tyrosine crystals. The type of crystal depends largely on the pH of the freshly voided urine, and time should not be wasted on the identification of crystals.

Crystals in acid urine (Plate 12, p. 720): **Calcium oxalate crystals** are colorless, octahedral, so-called envelope crystals with a highly refractile cross connecting the corners; more rarely they appear as oval spheres or biconcave disks with a dumbbell shape when viewed from the edge. They are soluble in hydrochloric acid and not in acetic acid (Fig. 27-21).

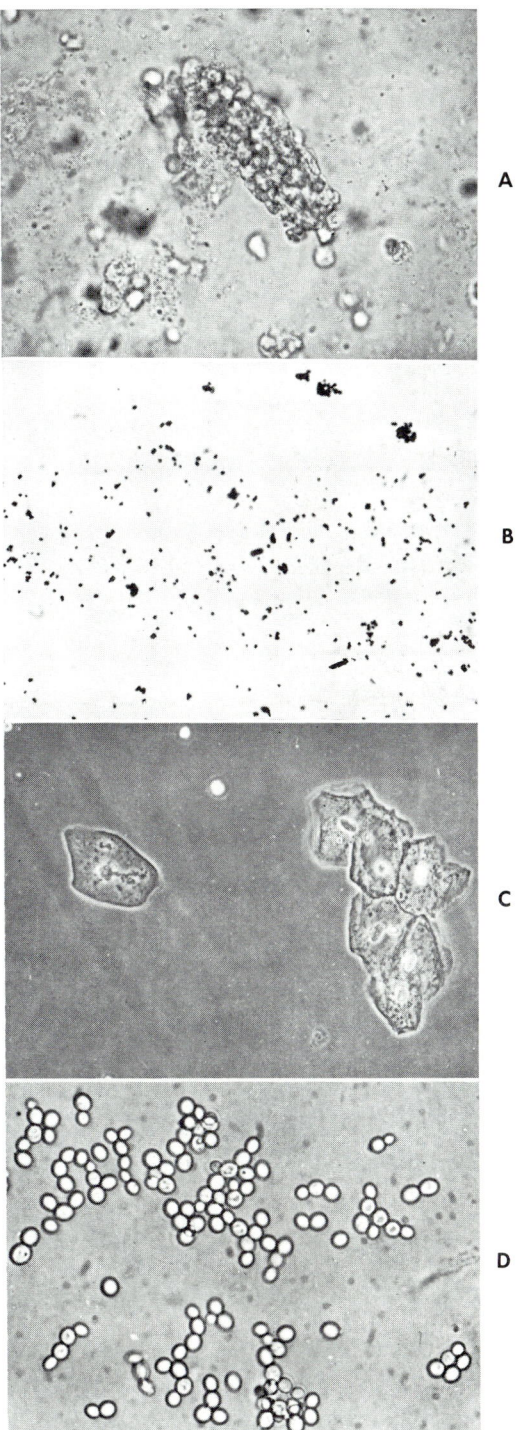

Fig. 27-17. A, Pus cast. **B,** Cocci in urine. **C,** Epithelial cells in sediment. **D,** Budding yeast in urine. (Courtesy Ames Co., Elkhart, Ind.)

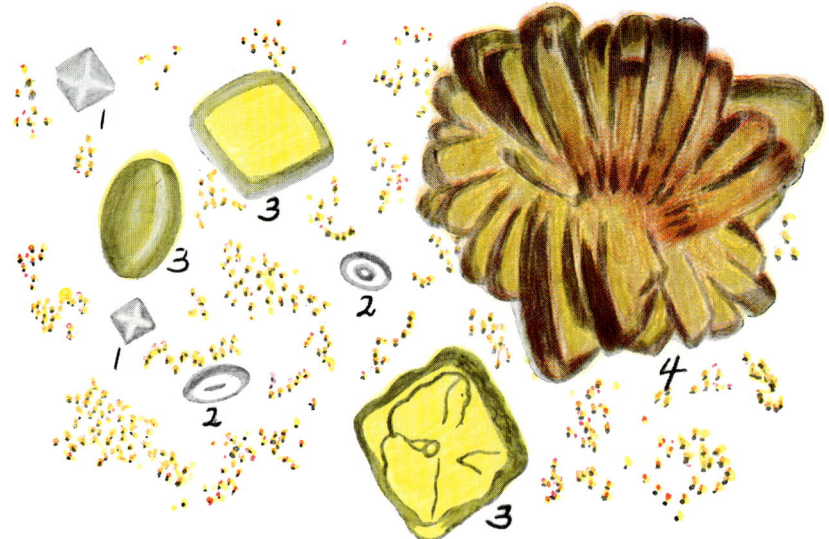

Plate 12. Crystalline and amorphous sediment in acid urine.

1 Calcium oxalate crystals, typical double envelope forms

2 Calcium oxalate crystals, unusual oval forms

Amorphous material is urates.

3 Uric acid crystals

4 Rosette of uric acid crystals

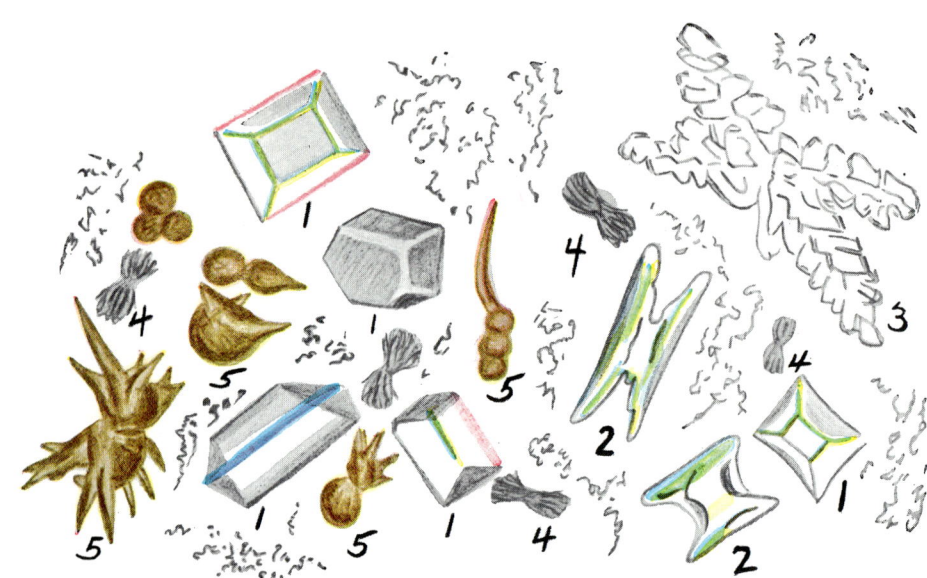

Plate 13. High-power field showing crystalline and amorphous sediment in alkaline urine.

1 Triple phosphate crystals, usual forms

2 Triple phosphate crystals, dissolving or poorly formed

3 Triple phosphate crystal, feathery form produced by rapid precipitation artificially

Amorphous material is amorphous phosphates.

4 Calcium carbonate crystals, dumbbell forms

5 Ammonium biurate crystals

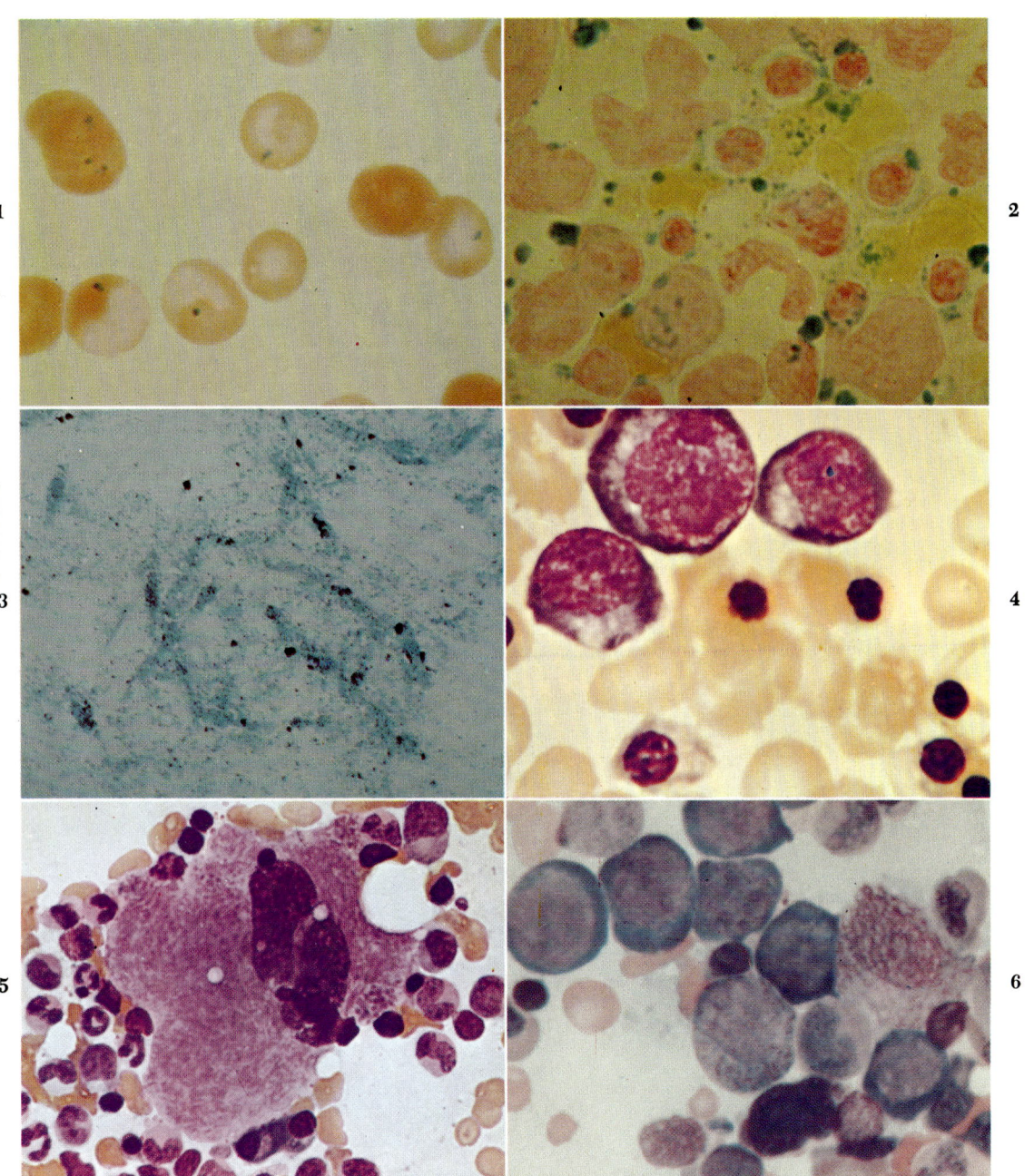

Plate 14. Peripheral blood, bone marrow, and urinary sediment in some anemias.

1 Siderocytes in peripheral blood in sideroachrestic anemia, Prussian blue stain (Courtesy V. Minnich.)

2 Ring sideroblasts in bone marrow in sideroachrestic anemia, Prussian blue stain

3 Hemosiderin casts in urinary sediment in paroxysmal nocturnal hemoglobinuria, Prussian blue stain (Courtesy V. Minnich.)

4 Hemolytic disease of the newborn (erythroblastosis fetalis), normoblasts and erythroblasts in peripheral blood, Wright stain

5 Platelet-producing megakaryocyte, Wright stain

6 Megaloblasts in bone marrow in pernicious anemia, Wright stain

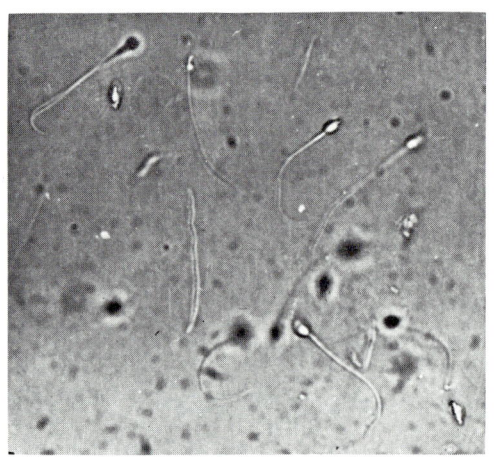

Fig. 27-18. Spermatozoa in urine. (Courtesy Ames Co., Elkhart, Ind.)

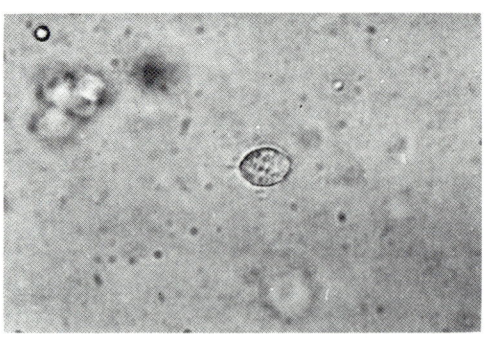

Fig. 27-19. *Trichomonas vaginalis* in urine. (Courtesy Ames Co., Elkhart, Ind.)

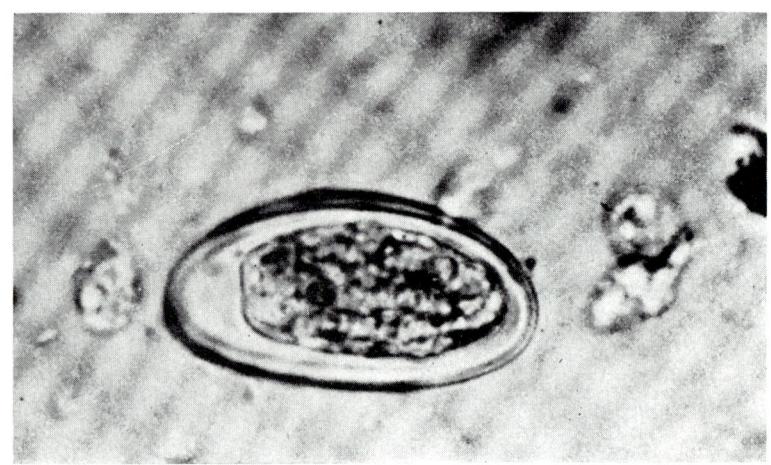

Fig. 27-20. Ovum of *Enterobius vermicularis* in urine. (Courtesy Ames Co., Elkhart, Ind.)

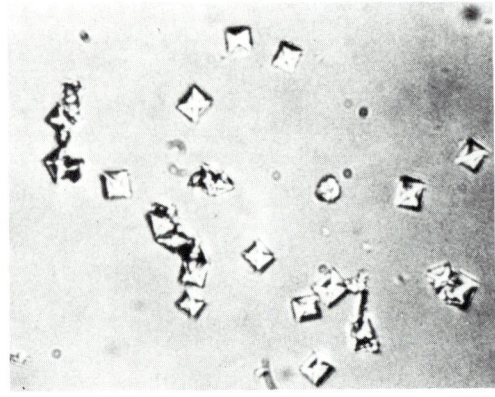

Fig. 27-21. Calcium oxalate crystals in urinary sediment.

Uric acid crystals are rhombic, usually whetstone-shaped, six-sided plates, often arranged in rosettelike clusters. Those occurring naturally are stained with urinary pigments and are yellowish or brownish, and in larger clusters they are grossly red like pepper granules. Large numbers of such crystals are often precipitated in the collecting tubules and in the calices of the kidney during the first week of life, and when passed in the urine, they may be mistaken for blood. Crystals precipitated artificially are colorless. They are soluble in sodium hydroxide and not in acid (Fig. 27-22).

Cystine crystals are colorless, flat, hexagonal plates with unequal sides. They are not soluble in acetic acid but are soluble in hydrochloric acid or alkali (Fig. 27-7). (See discussion of cystinuria, p. 689.)

Tyrosine and leucine: Tyrosine and leucine crystals are rare and indicate serious liver damage. **Tyrosine crystals** appear as fine needles arranged in radiating sheaves. They are soluble in hydrochloric acid or alkali (ammonia) but not in acetic acid (Fig. 27-23). **Leucine crystals** appear as oily yellowish or brownish refractive spheroids. They are soluble in alkali but not in dilute acetic acid or in hydrochloric acid. Leucine is soluble in boiling acetic acid, whereas tyrosine is not (Fig. 27-24).

Demonstration of crystals of tyrosine or leucine:

Procedure: Remove albumin by heat or acetic acid method; filter and evaporate to a smaller volume. Adjust one portion of the filtrate to a pH of 5.8 for leucine and another to a pH of 6.8-7.0 for tyrosine. Cool the filtrates in the refrigerator and examine for crystals.

Test for tyrosine:

Reagent: Morner reagent consists of formalin (1 part), water (45 parts), and concentrated sulfuric acid (55 parts).

Procedure: To 3 ml Morner reagent add the crystalline precipitate and bring to boil.

Result: Tyrosine gives a green color.

Test for leucine (Salkowski test):

Reagent: Aqueous copper sulfate, 10%.

Procedure: Dissolve crystals in 1 ml water. Add 1 drop of reagent.

Result: Leucine gives a blue color, which does not disappear on heating.

Crystals in alkaline urine (Fig. 27-25 and Plate 13, p. 720): **Ammonium magnesium phosphate (triple phosphate) crystals** are colorless, highly refractive prisms varying in size and presenting three, four, or six sides, giving the typical coffin-lid and hip-roof forms. They diffract the light, so that the edges often appear colored. When the crystals are precipitated artificially, they appear as feathery, star-shaped crystals. Dicalcium phosphate crystallizes out when the reaction is near the neutral point, forming slender colorless prisms with one pointed end, often arranged as rosettes, stars (stellar phosphates), or needles. Rarely, in alkaline urine, phosphate forms large, irregular, flat plates, usually granular, which float on the surface as an iridescent scum. They are soluble in 10% acetic acid without effervescence.

Calcium carbonate crystals are small and dumbbell shaped. They dissolve in 10% acetic acid with effervescence.

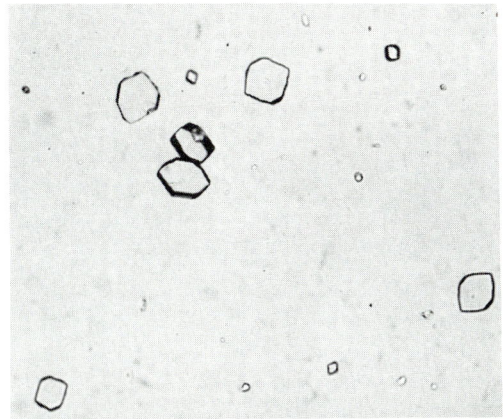

Fig. 27-22. Uric acid crystals in urinary sediment. (Courtesy Ames Co., Elkhart, Ind.)

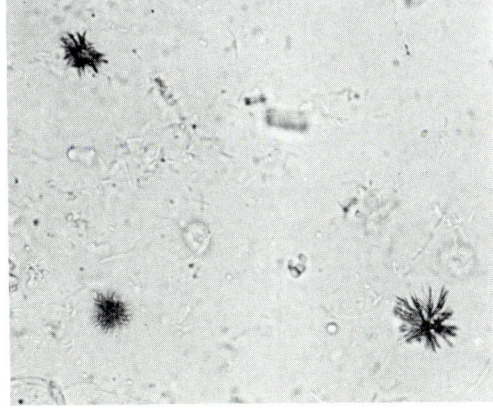

Fig. 27-23. Tyrosine crystals in urinary sediment. (Courtesy Ames Co., Elkhart, Ind.)

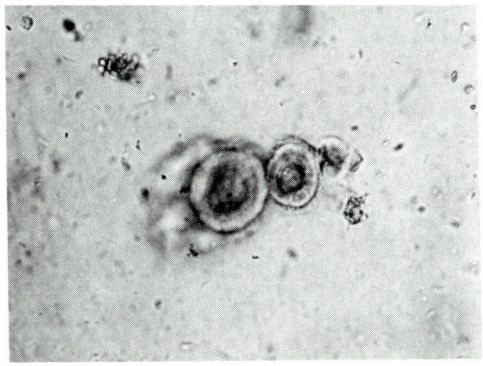

Fig. 27-24. Leucine crystals in urinary sediment. (Courtesy Ames Co., Elkhart, Ind.)

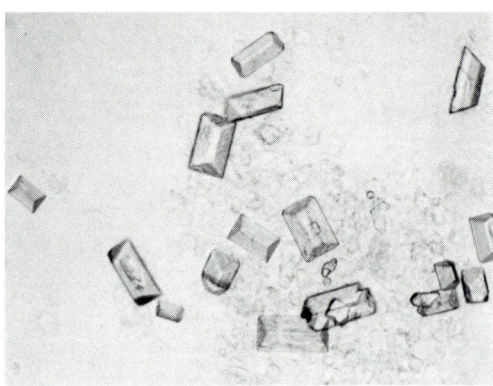

Fig. 27-25. Triple phosphate crystals in urinary sediment. (Courtesy Ames Co., Elkhart, Ind.)

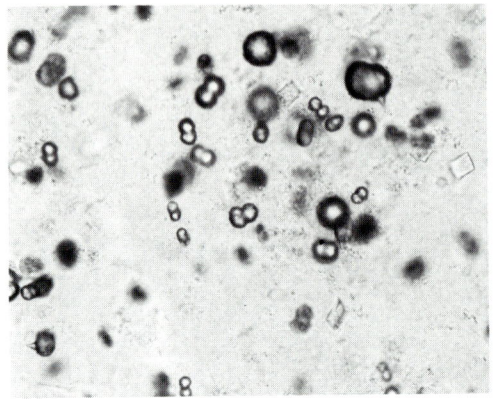

Fig. 27-26. Ammonium urate crystals in urinary sediment. (Courtesy Ames Co., Elkhart, Ind.)

Ammonium biurate crystals (Fig. 27-26), so-called thorn apple crystals, are yellowish, opaque, spheroidal bodies with irregular spines. They dissolve by warming and are soluble in acetic acid, with the formation of colorless uric acid crystals after standing. When sodium hydroxide is added, ammonia is liberated.

Hemosiderin

Hemosiderin is an iron-containing storage form of ferritin (see discussion of hemoglobin metabolism, p. 83) and can be demonstrated by the Prussian blue reaction (p. 113). Characteristically, in paroxysmal nocturnal hemoglobinuria (PNH) the urinary sediment contains hemosiderin either free as brown granular pigment or within shed epithelial cells or casts. The native hemosiderin is brown and stains blue with Prussian blue (Plate 14, p. 721).

Metachromatic granules[162,163]

There are a number of rare brain diseases, occurring mainly during childhood, in which there is diffuse demyelination of the white matter of the cerebral hemispheres. One subgroup of these diseases, called metachromatic leukodystrophy, also shows kidney involve-ment and metachromatic granules in the urinary sediment, which can be stained with toluidine blue.

Stain:

Reagent: Toluidine blue, 2% in water.

Procedure: Centrifuge 10 ml fresh urine for 5 min. Decant supernatant and add 2 drops of toluidine blue and mix. Transfer a small quantity to a microscope slide, cover with a coverslip, and examine for brownish granules that are 3-5 μm in diameter.

Result: Golden brown granules are found free, in casts, within cells, or in clusters in the sediment of patients with the metachromatic form of diffuse cerebral sclerosis. The technic should be checked by "running" a normal control urine specimen and by the use of polarized light, because the metachromatic granules are doubly refractile.

Austin et al.,[164] who described the aforementioned test for the diagnosis of metachromatic leukodystrophy, also noted that the urine of these patients was deficient in arylsulfatase A activity and developed a rapid urine test for this substance.

Foreign material

Foreign material may include powder or starch granules, hair, etc.

KIDNEY FUNCTION TESTS

Kidney function tests are indicated when urinalysis and/or blood chemistry tests point to kidney involvement but fail to reflect the extent of the renal lesion. Rarely, abnormal kidney function tests are the first indication of renal pathologic conditions. Kidney function tests are useful in following the clinical course of kidney disease and its response to treatment. A number of tests are available, some of which can be classified as **screening tests,** e.g., renal concentration test, phenolsulfonphthalein excretion test (PSP test), and endogenous creatinine clearance; others are **research**-type reference **methods,** e.g., inulin and *p*-aminohippurate clearance. Some of these tests measure **tubular-interstitial** function (concentration test and PSP test); others measure **glomerular** filtration rate (inulin clearance and endogenous creatinine clearance) or renal **plasma flow** (*p*-aminohippurate clearance).

Potential sources of error in renal function tests[165]

1. The timing of all function tests must be accurate to the minute.
2. The initial emptying of the bladder must be complete.
3. At urine collection time the bladder must be emptied completely, but catheterization should be avoided. Large amounts of residual urine invalidate most renal function tests.

These three points are so important that they must be supervised.

4. Adequate hydration of the patient is essential to guarantee adequate urine flow. Concentration tests are exempted.
5. Urinary volumes must be accurately measured.
6. For some tests the patient's weight, sex, and age must be known.
7. All specimens must be adequately identified.

Tests of tubular interstitial function

Concentration test (Fishberg):

Principle: The patient is placed on a water-restricted diet, and the urinary specific gravity, osmolality, and volume are measured to evaluate the renal concentrating power. The test measures primarily the ability of the distal tubules to concentrate urine solutes in excess of their plasma concentration. Despite the simplicity of the test, it affords an accurate measure of all kidney functions.

Preparation of patient: The patient should not receive any diuretics or other medication that may affect the urinary specific gravity. The specific gravity, osmolality, and composition of several first morning specimens should be known before the test to see whether (1) the specific gravity is increased because of the presence of protein or sugar, in which case the necessary corrections will have to be made (p. 683), (2) the concentration of a morning specimen is adequate, thus rendering the concentration test unnecessary, and (3) there is evidence of chronic kidney disease, which is a contraindication to the concentration test.

Procedure: At 6:00 PM the patient is served a supper that contains not more than 2 dl fluid. Allow no other fluid or food until the test is completed, although longer periods of fluid deprivation, e.g., 24 hr, may be necessary to achieve maximal concentration of the urine specimen.[166] Have the patient empty the bladder at bedtime and discard the urine. Allow the patient to sleep, and collect urine specimens at 7:00 AM and, if possible, at 8:00 AM and 9:00 AM, and see that he completely empties the bladder each time. Measure the volume, specific gravity, and osmolality of each specimen.

Normal values: Normally the specific gravity of at least one of the specimens will be 1.023-1.035, and the osmolality will be from 800-1300 mOsm/L. The minimal obtainable dehydration falls with age. While 20-year-old individuals achieve a maximal osmolality of 1109 ± 22 mOsm/L after 12 hr of water deprivation, individuals over 60 years attain an osmolality of only 882 ± 49 mOsm/L.[167]

Interpretation[168,169]: Urinary concentration depends on many factors:

1. Water deprivation stimulates the release of ADH by the pituitary gland, increasing the water absorption by the distal tubules.
2. Aldosterone has to do with the reabsorption of sodium by the distal tubules.
3. The amount of urea excreted by the kidney contributes significantly to the specific gravity and osmolality of the urine, establishing an important link between diet and urine concentration. Infants on breast milk, which is low in protein, appear to have a low concentrating power, which apparently rapidly improves when cow's milk is substituted.

The urine concentration is best measured by the refractometer and by obtaining the osmolality by freezing point determination.

The specific gravity decreases with increasing kidney impairment, approaching 1.010, the specific gravity of the glomerular filtrate. Absorption of edema fluid lowers the specific gravity but does not indicate decreased function. In progressive renal insufficiency the urinary specific gravity or osmolality is low. Decreased concentrating power may precede overt kidney disease. If the glomerular filtration rate is normal, decreased urinary concentration may be caused by tubular involvement, as seen in potassium deficiency, Fanconi's syndrome, hypercalcemia, sickle cell trait, interstitial nephritis, chronic pyelonephritis, hydronephrosis, and polycystic kidney.

Various modifications of the concentration test have been described, such as one using intramuscular Pitressin tannate in oil to concentrate the urine.[170]

Phenolsulfonphthalein test:

Principle: A small amount (6 mg) of phenolsulfonphthalein (PSP) is administered intravenously. Ninety-four percent of the injected dye is combined with plasma proteins and secreted by the proximal tubules into the urine. The remaining unbound dye (6%) is excreted by the glomeruli, but under the conditions of the test this amount can be disregarded. The rate of excretion of the dye in a fixed period is measured. The test is based on the assumption that the dye is excreted by the tubules at such a rapid rate at low plasma concentrations that the blood leaving the kidney in the renal vein is almost free of the dye.[171] The test is not ordered as frequently as in the past, because a number of circumstances and substances interfere significantly. The tubular secretion is a limiting factor only if the plasma dye concentration is 1 mg/dl or above. Since the plasma dye concentration after the injection of 6 mg/dl is only 0.2 mg/dl, the limiting factor is not the tubular secretion but the renal blood flow, so that the test becomes a measure of the effective renal plasma flow,[171] which can be measured equally well by the endogenous creatinine clearance without dye injection.

Reagents:
1. Sodium hydroxide, 10% (10 g/dl)
2. Glacial acetic acid
3. Sodium carbonate, anhydrous, 10% (10 g/dl)
4. Phenolsulfonphthalein, 6 mg/ml, sterile, two ampules, one for injection and one for standard.)

Preparation of patient: The patient should not have taken any medication for 24 hr (including diuretics) and should be well hydrated.

Procedure: Thirty minutes before beginning the test ask the patient to drink 5 dl water to ensure adequate secretion of urine. Have the patient empty the bladder and discard the specimen. Administer 1 ml dye (6 mg) intravenously and record the exact time. Make sure that there is no extravasation of the dye. Have the patient empty the bladder exactly 15, 30, 60, and 120 min after injection of the dye and collect it in separate, labeled containers. Record the exact time of each collection.

Estimation of dye:
1. Measure the volume of each specimen; it should be at least 40 ml.
2. Filter each urine sample into a 5 dl volumetric flask, wash the filter with 20-30 ml water, and add the washings to the flask.
3. Dilute to about 4 dl, add 10 ml of 10% sodium hydroxide, mix, and dilute to 5 dl.
4. After mixing, add 7 ml aliquots of each sample

dilution to two 19 mm cuvets. To one cuvet add 1 drop of glacial acetic acid. If a red color does not disappear, add a second drop.

5. Read each colored sample against the acidified aliquot as a blank at 560 nm.

6. Obtain the percent of excretion from a calibration curve. If the reading on any sample is less than 15% T (transmission) (0.08 absorbance), dilute both blank and sample with 7 ml water, mix, and read again. Multiply the value obtained from the calibration curve by 2.

Standards for calibration of spectrophotometer:

1. Add 0.50 ml dye from an ampule used for injection to a 5 dl volumetric flask.

2. Add about 4 dl water and 10 ml of 10% sodium hydroxide and dilute to 5 dl. Since variations have been found in different lots of the dye, it is preferable to use as a standard an ampule having the same lot number as the dye used for injection.

3. Add to a series of pairs of tubes, 1, 2, 3, 4, 5, 6, and 7 ml of dye solution and add water to make 10 ml.

4. To one tube of each pair add 1 drop of glacial acetic acid. For each pair read the colored solution against the acidified solution at 560 nm. These standards then correspond to 5%, 10%, 15%, 20%, 30%, and 35% excretion when the urine is made up to 5 dl.

Interfering substances: Bile and blood in the urine interfere with the PSP test. If the urine is bloody, centrifuge the entire portion, decant the supernatant, add one half of the original volume to a 250 ml volumetric flask, followed by 5 ml of 10% sodium hydroxide, and proceed as above. If centrifugation does not clear the urine (hemoglobinuria), to the half volume in the 250 ml flask add 10 ml of 10% anhydrous sodium carbonate instead of the sodium hydroxide and dilute to volume. In preparing the blank, add just the minimal amount of glacial acetic acid to discharge the color (0.1-0.5 ml).

Drugs other than diuretics that may interfere with the PSP test include probenecid, sufinpyrazone, and radiographic contrast media, which inhibit PSP excretion, and penicillin, salicylates, and sulfonamides, which compete with PSP for renal tubular excretion.[99] In addition, drugs or other ingested substances that give a marked color to the urine (e.g., phenazopyrine) (p. 681) may interfere with the colorimetric determination. At 560 nm wavelength even 10 mg bilirubin/dl urine will cause only a negligibly higher reading (5%).

Since the liver normally removes some of the dye from the bloodstream and excretes it into the bile, higher than normal PSP excretion has been reported in liver disease, because the liver is unable to excrete its ''fraction,'' but the 15 min excretion value is not usually affected.

Normal values: The normal kidney excretes about 35% of the dye within 15 min, an additional 15% at 30 min, and an additional 10% at 60 min, so that about 55-60% of dye is excreted in the first hour and 75% in the second hour. The critical measurement is the 15 min dye excretion.

Interpretation: If the 15 min dye excretion is 25% or less, kidney function is impaired. Under the clinical conditions of the test the PSP excretion is not so much a test of tubular function (since the small amount of dye injected is no challenge to even diseased tubules) but is rather a test of plasma flow. It is therefore decreased in a wide variety of renal diseases[172] from congenital polycystic kidney to chronic glomerulonephritis and chronic pyelonephritis. The PSP excretion is also lowered in lower nephron nephrosis, amyloidosis, and advanced essential hypertension. In most of the conditions mentioned the PSP test is more sensitive than or equally as sensitive as the endogenous creatinine clearance test.[173]

Nitrogen retention in the blood begins when the dye excretion is less than 40% in 2 hr, and the excretion of dye practically stops when the BUN reaches 80 mg/dl. In chronic passive congestion, excretion of the dye is decreased without an increase in urea nitrogen.

An important use of the PSP test lies in the fact that it allows testing of **each kidney separately** when the specimens are collected for 15 min by means of ureteral catheters. There should be no leak around the catheters into the bladder.

Contraindications: In acute renal insufficiency the test should not be performed; the large amount of residual urine seen in prostatic hypertrophy interferes with the test because of dilution effect. The test cannot be performed on children because of the required rapid succession of urine samples.

Tests of glomerular filtration rate

Ideally the glomerular filtration rate (GFR) is determined by measuring the clearance of a completely filterable substance that is neither absorbed nor excreted by the renal tubules. The research type of reference method is inulin clearance; the clinically acceptable method is endogenous creatinine clearance (C_{cr}). Urea clearance is of no value as a measure of GFR, because it is influenced by too many variables (see below).

Concept of clearance: As a means of quantitatively expressing the rate of excretion of a given substance by the kidney glomeruli, clearance of the substance is measured. Clearance is the volume of plasma that contains the amount of a given substance excreted in the urine in 1 min. Alternatively, the clearance of a substance may be defined as that volume of plasma cleared of the amount of that substance found in the urine in 1 min.

Clearance can be mathematically expressed by the following formula, which shows clearance to be the amount of excreted substance divided by its plasma concentration: $C = UV/P$. C = clearance in milliliters per minute, V = urine flow in milliliters per minute, U = urinary concentration of test substance in milligrams per milliliter, and P = plasma concentration of test substance in milligrams per milliliter.

If a substance is not affected by the tubules at all (neither secreted nor absorbed), the amount found in the urine will equal the amount filtered by the glomerulus per minute. The clearance of such a substance, e.g., inulin (which has no threshold), is a measure of GFR (123 ml/min). The clearance of a substance completely reabsorbed by the tubules, e.g., glucose, is zero. Substances having clearances greater than that of glucose but less than that of inulin are in part reabsorbed by tubules (these include most urinary constituents). Substances having higher clearances than that of inulin are added to the urine by tubular cell secretion, e.g., *p*-aminohippurate (PAH), and ammonia. The highest clearance is the PAH clearance, the plasma being cleared almost entirely by tubular secretion (about 650 ml/min). The plasma flow through the kidneys (about 7 dl/min) represents the highest possible clearance.

All clearance tests have some difficulties:

1. They measure two renal functions (although not equally well): plasma flow and GFR.
2. The handling of the test substance by the normal and abnormal kidney may differ.
3. The chemical assay method may not be sensitive enough.
4. A complete, timed urine collection without catheterization may be hard to obtain.

Inulin clearance: Inulin clearance is a research tool of little value in routine clinical practice, but because of its accuracy and precision it serves as a reference method. It has the disadvantage of being time-consuming, of requiring infusion pumps, of utilizing a foreign substance, and of requiring complicated biochemical assay methods.

Principle: A priming infusion of inulin, given at a rapid rate, is followed by a sustaining infusion at a slow constant rate. The urine specimen should be obtained by catheterization. The difficulties associated with the calculation, preparation, and administration of the inulin solution weigh against the clinical use of this test. The average inulin clearance of normal adults is 123 ml/1.73 m^2 of body surface.

Endogenous creatinine clearance: Because of the innate difficulties associated with clearance tests employing exogenous substances (inulin and PAH), for clinical purposes the clearance of endogenous substances such as creatinine and urea is utilized. Creatinine is freely filtered by the glomerulus, and, even though some of it is secreted by the tubules, clinically, it can be accepted as a measure of GFR. Creatinine clearance is not completely independent of the flow rate of urine.

Procedure: Perform the test in the morning. Give the patient three glasses of water to drink to guarantee adequate urine flow during the test period. Have the patient empty the bladder completely, and note the exact time (including minutes). Exactly 5 hr later have the patient void again to completely empty the bladder, and immediately afterward obtain a blood sample for the determination of the creatinine level. Send both specimens (urine and blood) to the laboratory, where the urine volume is accurately measured and the creatinine level of serum and urine is determined by the methods given in the chemistry section.

Calculation: The previously mentioned clearance formula (C = UV/P) is used.

Normal values: The endogenous creatinine clearance in men is 140.0 ± 27.2 ml/min; in women it is 112.0 ± 20.2 ml/min.

Discussion: In the normal individual, endogenous creatinine clearance comes close to the GFR, but in advanced renal disease it exceeds the GFR because of tubular secretion, so that the true GFR is below the creatinine clearance value. Corrections for body surface and urine flow rate are not necessary. Increasing age produces a progressive fall in the creatinine clearance, even though the plasma creatinine concentration remains essentially unaltered.[174] In infants the clearance is also markedly reduced.[175] Creatinine clearance is a sensitive indicator of renal allograft rejection.

Urea clearance:

Definition: Urea clearance is the number of milliliters of plasma cleared of urea per minute.

Principle: Urea is produced by the liver and is freely filtered through the glomeruli but is partially absorbed by the tubules. The passive absorption is dependent on (1) the rate of urine flow in milliliters per minute, (2) the amount of urea present, and (3) the state of the tubular epithelium.

1. At a low rate of urine flow, up to 60-80% of urea may be absorbed and the clearance is therefore low. At a high rate of urine flow, only 30-40% of urea is absorbed and the clearance rate is therefore high.
2. The amount of urea present in the plasma is dependent on the protein content of the diet. A high protein content results in an increased urea level. The metabolism of 1 g protein produces 0.3 g excreted urea.[171] The amount of urea excreted is also influenced by catabolic metabolism, which may be increased in infections, leukemia, etc.

Since urea clearance is influenced by so many variables, it is neither a test of GFR nor of tubular absorption and should therefore not be used in clinical practice.

Radionuclides in kidney function tests

Because of the disadvantages of the reference methods, radionuclides have been introduced to measure GFR and other kidney functions. The most commonly used radioactive reagents include ^{51}Cr-EDTA, ^{197}Hg-chlormerodrin, and ^{131}I-orthoiodohippurate. The use of ^{131}I-orthoiodohippurate and ^{197}Hg-chlormerodrin in combination has been suggested to evaluate renal allografts. The normal renogram, after injection of radio-

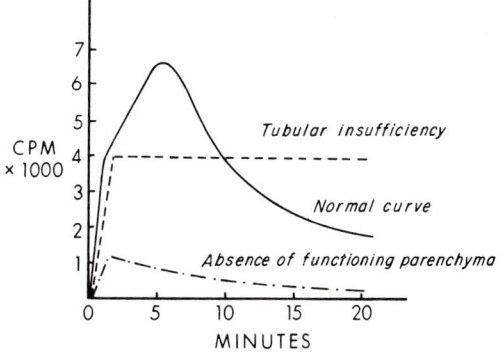

Fig. 27-27. Renogram patterns after intravenous injection of radioactive iodinated hippurate.

Table 27-13. Classification and manifestations of kidney diseases

Type	Urine	Blood	Function	Systemic changes	Prognosis
Acute glomerulonephritis					
Focal glomerulonephritis	Hematuria Moderate albuminuria (trace) Casts: hyaline and granular, possibly blood Pus, variable amount Normal specific gravity	Normal unless very slight increase in nitrogen	Normal	None	Good
Diffuse glomerulo-nephritis	Oliguria Dark red and cloudy Acid, unless blood makes alkaline High specific gravity (1.020-1.030) Albuminuria (1-1.5 g/dl) Casts: hyaline, granular, brown granular, and cellular, including blood and epithelial cells Blood	Nitrogen retention Urea to 120 mg/dl Uric acid 3-6 mg/dl Creatinine 1-7 mg/dl Anemia	Impairment in proportion to severity	Blood pressure increased Edema present Eyeground changes absent or only slight Anemia	Most recover May be fatal May progress to subacute or chronic form
Subacute glomerulo-nephritis	Intermediate, between diffuse and chronic forms Late in disease: may be polyuria with low fixed specific gravity and small amount of fat and lipids in epithelial cells	Nitrogen retention increases	More and more impairment	Blood pressure becomes higher Edema present or absent Eyeground changes more marked Moderate to severe anemia	Poor Fatal usually within 2 yr
Chronic glomerulonephritis					
Without edema (diffuse glomerulonephritis with hypertension)	Polyuria; nocturia Pale yellow Clear; no gross sediment Acid reaction Low fixed specific gravity (1.005-1.015) Albuminuria (trace) Casts: hyaline and granular Blood present at times Late in disease: oliguria with low fixed specific gravity Doubly refractive substances in sediment	Nitrogen retention Albumin/globulin ratio reversed	Impaired Slight at first (dye 40%) Second stage: moderate (dye 10-20%) Third stage: severe (dye 0 to trace) Absolute insufficiency	Blood pressure increased Edema absent Eyeground changes absent or present Moderate to severe anemia Heart enlarged Chronic uremia, late	Fatal in 2-25 yr
With edema (nephrotic phase of chronic glomerulonephritis)	In general, similar to chronic form, but usually smaller amount, with somewhat higher specific gravity, with more albumin and casts, and sometimes with fat and lipids in epithelial cells and casts Doubly refractive substances in sediment	Similar to chronic form, but when edema prominent, blood may show findings similar to those in lipoid nephrosis Hypoproteinemia; increase in α_2- and β-globulins; hypoalbuminemia	Similar to chronic form unless edema interferes with tests	Similar to chronic form except for presence of edema Edema resulting from: Recurrent acute attacks Cardiac failure Combination with lipoid nephrosis	Similar to chronic form

Nephrosis					
Lipoid	Oliguria in proportion to edema Normal color Normal to very high specific gravity Marked albuminuria (5-20 or 60 g/L) Albumin much greater than globulin Casts: hyaline, granular, and fatty Leukocytes and epithelial cells, both containing fat and lipids Free lipid granules Occasional blood cell Doubly refractile crystals	Nitrogen *not* increased Chlorides *not* increased Lipids increased and plasma may appear milky Cholesterol increased Total protein decreased $1/3$-$1/2$ (normal, 6.5-8.2%) Albumin/globulin ratio changed from 1.5:1.0 (normal) because albumin decreased and globulin increased, with ratio 1:2 or 1:6	Normal unless edema interferes with tests	Edema marked No increase in blood pressure No eyeground changes Sedimentation velocity of red cells greatly increased Faulty protein metabolism More marked in young persons	May recover Condition may last from months to many years Some finally develop insufficiency (See chronic glomerulonephritis, with edema)
Kidney of toxemia of pregnancy	Lipoid nephrosis but less marked	Nitrogen usually normal or slightly increased Urea low Uric acid slightly increased	Normal or slightly impaired	Blood pressure usually increased Edema present or absent Eyeground changes present or absent May have very severe anemia	Usually good Some progress to chronic nephritis
Amyloid disease	Varies from normal to that of lipoid nephrosis	BUN increased; Congo red test may be positive; plasma protein changes	Insufficiency	Generalized amyloidosis	Death due to primary disease
Hemoglobinuric or myoglobinuric nephrosis	Oliguria to anuria Acid Low and fixed specific gravity Albuminuria Hemoglobinuria (or myohemoglobinuria) Casts: hyaline and granular Heme casts (breakdown products of hemoglobin) Hemosiderin	Urea and creatinine increased Phosphorus increased CO_2-combining power of plasma, serum sodium, and chloride decreased	Impaired as in chronic form	Blood pressure elevated after second day Edema, especially pulmonary Uremia	Poor if oliguria and hypertension persist

Continued.

Table 27-13. Classification and manifestations of kidney diseases—cont'd

Type	Urine	Blood	
Arteriosclerotic glomerulonephritis			
Glomerulosclerosis, benign hypertension	May be normal (early) Later shows trace of albumin with a few hyaline and granular casts With cardiac failure, findings same as in chronic passive congestion	Normal unless cardiac failure present	Blood pressure increased Edema absent unless cardiac failure present Eyeground changes absent or very slight Cardiac dilation, hypertrophy, and failure rare	Good unless complicated by cardiac failure
Glomerulonephritis, malignant hypertension	Early, like arteriosclerotic form Late, like chronic form Blood pressure higher Very small amount of albumin	Like chronic form	Blood pressure high, usually over 200 mm Hg Edema absent unless cardiac failure present Eyeground changes marked Cardiac hypertrophy, dilatation, and failure common Apoplexy common Chronic uremia, late Anemia marked	Bad, but condition may last from few years to decade Fatal about 6 mo after absolute insufficiency occurs
Pyelonephritis	Trace of albumin White cells Red cells Bacteria	Urea normal or increased	Impaired	Pyelitis Cardiac edema	Depends on circulation Uremia

active iodinated hippurate, consists of three segments: (1) a steep initial inflow segment produced by the inflow of blood containing the radioactive tracer, (2) a less steep, still rising second segment representing the glomerular filtration and tubular secretion of the tracer, and (3) a decreasing segment representing the urinary outflow (Fig. 27-27).

The use of radioisotopes eliminates difficult biochemical assay methods and allows detection of unilateral kidney impairment as seen in renal allograft rejection or in hypertension resulting from unilateral kidney disease.

Kidney function tests as indicators of renal allograft rejection

Incipient allograft rejection can frequently be reversed if it is diagnosed early.[176] This diagnosis is often difficult because of the interplay of such factors as immunosuppression, operative ischemia, infection, and surgical technic, all of which may mask the rejection.

Based on the time of occurrence after transplantation, the **immunologic rejection** is classified as hyperacute (within minutes to hours), acute (12 hr to 12 days), delayed (12 days to 18 months), or chronic (6 months to 6 years).

In **hyperacute rejection,** anuria or oliguria rapidly follow initial adequate creatinine clearance and immediate diuresis. In **acute renal rejection,** decreased urinary output and kidney function are usually the most outstanding laboratory findings. Diminished creatinine clearance (or ^{131}I-orthoiodohippurate clearance) is a reliable sign of a beginning rejection. It is accompanied by reduced osmolar (sodium) excretion. A characteristic **urinary sediment pattern** has been described[177] using a membrane filter and a modified Papanicolaou technic.[178] The presence of five of the following seven features suggests acute rejection: (1) increased nuclear cytoplasmic ratio characterized by increased nucleoli and abnormal nuclear shapes, (2) casts, (3) red cells, (4) dirty amorphous background, (5) bacteria, (6) mixed cell clusters consisting of a mixture of mononuclear cells and tubular cells, and (7) polymorphs. In **delayed rejection,** proteinuria in excess of 2.5 g/day develops, coupled with a decrease in the previously stable creatinine clearance. **Chronic rejection** is characterized by steroid-resistant proteinuria and by progressive decline of the creatinine clearance. Refractive fat bodies are found in the urinary sediment similar to the ones seen in nephrotic syndrome. Serum biochemical analysis reveals hyperlipidemia and hypoproteinemia.[179]

Laboratory findings in selected kidney disorders

See Table 27-13.

URINARY CALCULI (UROLITHIASIS)

Small calculi are often difficult to detect; it is therefore suggested that the urine of patients with a history of renal colic be filtered through double-thickness gauze.

Urinary calculi are crystalloids embedded in a binding substance of mucus and protein and also contain inclusions of bacteria and epithelial cells. Although the cause of calculi (stones) formation in the urinary tract is unknown, it is hoped that knowledge of the composition of calculi will aid the physician in preventing future stone formation and in diagnosing the underlying disease. Of prime importance is the prevention of calcium oxalate or phosphate stones (seen in hyperparathyroidism), cystine stones (found in cystinuria), and/or uric acid stones (accompanying gout).

Present methods of examining urinary calculi by x-ray diffraction or by infrared spectroscopy identify the crystalline compounds present rather than enumerate the elemental components, which can only be detected by chemical analysis.[180] The first two methods allow the examination of minute calculi (measuring only angstrom sizes). Infrared absorption identifies crystalline as well as noncrystalline compounds, whereas x-ray diffraction allows the study of crystalline material only.

The most commonly found crystalline components are calcium oxalate monohydrate, calcium oxalate dihydrate, hydroxyapatite, magnesium ammonium phosphate hexahydrate, uric acid dihydrate, L-cystine, and ammonium acid urate. The most commonly found chemical compounds are calcium oxalate, phosphate, magnesium, ammonium, and uric acid.

Because of the inadequacy of chemical analysis, it is suggested that calculi be sent to laboratories specializing in the above-mentioned physical methods of stone analysis.

A detailed discussion of kidney stone analysis is presented by Freeman and Beeler.[181]

GLOSSARY

albuminuria Increased albumin in urine.

alkalosis Clinical term commonly employed to indicate increased pH of blood or increased blood bicarbonate with a tendency toward increased blood pH.

aminoaciduria Excess of one or more amino acids in urine.

amorphous Having no difinite form.

anhydrous Without water.

anuria Total lack of urine excretion.

calculus Abnormal inorganic mass occurring within animal body and usually composed of mineral salts.

catheter Tubular surgical instrument used to withdraw fluids from a cavity of the body, especially one for insertion into the bladder via the urethra for the removal of urine.

cholestasis Suppression of the flow of bile.

chromatography (paper) Method of chemical analysis whereby certain components of a mixture may be separated by employing solubility and absorptive properties.

chromogen Any substance that produces color.

crenation Abnormal notched appearance, as of the margins of red cells after exposure to excessively high solute concentrations.

cystitis Inflammation of bladder.

diuretic Substance that, when taken into the body, promotes the secretion of urine.

diurnal Occurring during the day.

electrophoresis Migration of colloidal particles, e.g., protein, under the influence of an electric field. Velocity and extent of migration are dependent on the molecular weight and electric charge of the colloidal particles. A colloidal mixture, therefore, can be effectively separated into its component parts by means of the differential migration of these parts.

empiric Based on experience or observation.

erythrocyte Red blood cell.

glomeruli Coils of blood vessels projecting into the expanded end of capsule of each of the uriniferous tubules of the kidney.

glycogenesis Formation of synthesis of glycogen.

glycogenolysis Splitting up of glycogen in body tissues.

glycosuria Presence of glucose in the urine.

hematuria Presence of blood in the urine.

hemoglobinuria Presence of hemoglobin in the urine.

hepatic Pertaining to the liver.

hepatocellular Pertaining to the liver cells.

hyaline Glassy or transparent.

hydrometer Instrument used for determining the specific gravity of a fluid.

hypouricemia Decreased uric acid levels in the blood.

iatrogenic Pertaining to any condition in a patient occurring as a result of treatment by a physician.

in vitro Within glass, e.g., a test tube or a flask.

in vivo Within the living body.

ion An atom or group of atoms possessing a charge of negative or positive electricity.

isosthenuria Maintenance of constant osmolality of urine.

isotonic Pertaining to solutions having the same osmotic pressure as the system to which they are compared. For example, isotonic saline has the same solute concentration as the body fluids from human beings.

jaundice Condition characterized by increased bilirubin levels in the blood and a deposition of bile pigment in the skin and mucous membranes with a resulting yellow appearance of the patient.

ketonemia Presence of ketone bodies in the blood.

ketonuria Presence of ketone bodies in the urine.

lesion Any pathologic or traumatic discontinuity of tissue.

leukocyte White blood cell.

lipid Any one of a group of organic compounds consisting of fats and other substances with similar properties. They are insoluble in water, soluble in fat solvents and alcohol, and greasy to the touch.

melanin Dark amorphous pigment of the skin, hair, and certain tumors. It is a product of cell activity and contains sulfur and iron.

moiety A part or portion.

monoclonal Of one kind.

mucoprotein An amino compound of undetermined action.

nephritis Inflammation of the kidney.

nephrosis Disease of the kidney.

oliguria Reduced daily excretion of urine.

pathogenic Pertains to giving origin to disease.

penicillamine An amino acid obtained from penicillin by treatment with hot mineral acids.

pH Symbol used to express hydrogen ion concentration. It signifies the logarithm of the reciprocal of the hydrogen ion concentration in gram-molecules per liter of solution.

phosphatemia Elevated blood phosphorus levels.

phosphaturia Elevated urine phosphorus levels.

polyuria Passage of abnormally large volumes of urine.

porphyrins Group of iron-free or magnesium-free pyrrole derivatives that occur universally in protoplasm. They constitute the basis of the respiratory pigments in animals and plants.

postprandial Occurring after a meal.

protein Any one of a group of complex organic nitrogen-containing compounds found widely distributed in plants and animals. Proteins form the principal constituents of the cell protoplasm. Structurally, they are primarily combinations of α-amino acids and their derivatives.

proteinuria Increased protein in urine.

PSP Phenolsulfonphthalein.

qualitative Pertaining to quality or qualities. In chemistry,

qualitative refers to determinations of the mere presence or absence of a substance.

quantitative Pertaining to quantity. In chemistry, quantitative refers to determinations of the exact quantity of a particular substance present in another substance.

renal Pertains to kidney.

saturated Unable to hold in solution any more of a given substance.

soluble Capable of being dissolved.

solute Substance dissolved in a solution.

solvent Liquid that dissolves or is capable of dissolving solutes.

specific gravity Weight of a substance compared with that of an equal volume of another substance taken as a standard.

splenomegaly Enlarged spleen.

supernatant Layer of a substance situated above or on top of another substance.

urinometer Instrument used to determine the specific gravity of urine.

REFERENCES

1. Ganong, W.F.: Reveiw of medical physiology, Los Altos, Calif., 1979, Lange Medical Publications.
2. Harper, H.A., Rodwell, V.W., and Mayes, P.A.: Review of physiological chemistry, ed. 16, Los Altos, Calif., 1977, Lange Medical Publications.
3. Gottschalk, C.W.: Am. J. Med. **36**:670, 1964.
4. Wirz, H., Hargitay, B., and Kuhn, W.: Helv. Physiol. Acta **9**:196, 1951.
5. Ohren, D.E.: In Schreiner, G.E., editor: Urinalysis in the 70's, Elkhart, Ind., 1973, Ames Co.
6. Goodman, D.A.: In Schreiner, G.E., editor: Urinalysis in the 70's, Elkhart, Ind., 1973, Ames Co.
7. Lawler, D.P.: Aldosterone, New York, 1969, Medical Communications, Inc.
8. von Hofstetter, A.: Z. Allg. Mikrobiol. **52**:333, 1976.
9. Roberts, A.: Nurs. Times **73**:25, 1977.
10. Sahu, S.: J. Iowa Med. Soc. **66**:11, 1976.
11. Free, A.H., and Free, H.M.: Urinalysis in clinical laboratory practice, Cleveland, 1975, CRC Press.
12. Crim, M.C., et al.: J. Nutr. **105**:428, 1975.
13. Edwards, O.M., et al.: Lancet **2**:1165, 1969.
14. Greenblatt, D.J., et al.: J. Clin. Pharmacol. **16**:321, 1976.
15. Rao, L.G.S.: Br. Med. J. **2**:874, 1977.
16. Banda, P.W., et al.: Clin. Chem. **26**:535, 1980.
17. Walker, M.S.: Ann. Clin. Biochem. **14**:203, 1977.
18. Segal, M.A., and Fox, A.L., Jr.: Minn. Med. **58**:196, 1975.
19. Mitchell, G., Field, B., and Kerr, C.: Br. Med. J. **1**:811, 1977.
20. Assa, S.: Clin. Chem. **23**:126, 1977.
21. Free, A.H., and Free, H.M.: CRC Crit. Rev. Clin. Lab. Sci. **3**:481, 1972.
22. Simpson, E., and Thompson, D.: Lancet **2**:361, 1977.
23. Hoeltge, G.A., and Ersts, A.: Am. J. Clin. Pathol. **73**:403, 1980.
24. Rosenbloom, A.L., and Malone, J.I.: J.A.M.A. **240**:2462, 1978.
25. Bush, C.L., and Hagen, C.H.: Lab. Med. **5**:34, 1974.
26. Bradley, M., et al.: In Henry, J.B., editor: Clinical diagnosis and management by laboratory methods, ed. 16, Philadelphia, 1979, W.B. Saunders Co.
27. Modern urine chemistry, a guide to the diagnosis of urinary tract diseases and metabolic disorders, Elkhart, Ind., 1977, Ames Co.
28. Wert, E.B.: In Sunderman, F.W., and Sunderman, F.W., Jr., editors: Laboratory diagnosis of kidney diseases, St. Louis, 1970, Warren H. Green, Inc.
29. Pfohl, R.A.: Arch. Intern. Med. **116**:681, 1965.

30. Jacobson, M.H., et al.: Arch. Intern. Med. **110**:83, 1962.
31. Boyd, D.R., et al.: Arch Surg. **102**:363, 1971.
32. Weisberg H.: Osmolality. Check sample program, Chicago, 1972, Committee on Continuing Education, American Society of Clinical Pathologists.
33. Gyure, W.L.: Clin. Chem. **23**:876, 1977.
34. Bowie, L., Smith, S., and Gochman, N.: Clin. Chem. **23**:128, 1977.
35. Newell, J.E., and Duke, E.: Workshop on urinalysis and renal function studies, the routine examination of urine in the laboratory, Chicago, 1961, American Society of Clinical Pathologists.
36. Kosta, M.J., and Glenn, G.C.: Clin Chem. **25**:1335, 1979.
37. Lindstedt, G.: J. Pediatr. **91**:170, 1977.
38. Karlsson, F.A., and Hellsing, K.: J. Pediatr. **89**:89, 1976.
39. Waldmann, T.A., Strober, W., and Mogielnicki, R.P.: J. Clin. Invest. **51**:2162, 1972.
40. Virella, G., and Lopes-Virella M.F.L.: Clin. Chem. **23**:1793, 1977.
41. Peele, J.D., Gadsden, R.H., and Loadholt, C.B.: Clin. Chem. **23**:86, 1977.
42. Pesce, A.J., et al.: Clin. Chem. **22**:667, 1976.
43. Webb, T., Rose, B., and Sehon, A.H.: Can. J. Biochem. **36**:1159, 1958.
44. Rayner, H., et al.: J. Lab. Clin. Med. **74**:586, 1969.
45. Tamm, I., and Horsfall, L.: J. Exp. Med. **95**:71, 1952.
46. Blainey, J.D., et al.: Q. J. Med. **29**:235, 1960.
47. Keogh, J.B., et al.: Invest. Urol. **14**:446, 1977.
48. Balant, L.P., and Fabre, J.: Compr. Ther. **4**(10):54, 1978.
49. Butler, E.A., and Flynn. F.V.: Lancet **2**:978, 1958.
50. Rochefort, M.J., et al.: Am. J. Clin. Pathol. **62**: 373, 1974.
51. Quittner, H., Quittner, C.W., and Morges, W.: In Sunderman, F.W., editor: Manual for procedures for the applied seminars on laboratory diagnosis and monitoring of disorders of the kidney, Philadelphia, 1980, Institute for Clinical Science, Inc.
52. Dent, C.E., and Walshe, J.M.: Br. Med. Bull. **10**:247, 1954.
53. Hill, A., Casey, R., and Zaleski, W.A.: Clin. Chim. Acta **72**:1, 1976.
54. Efron, M.L., et al.: Engl. J. Med. **270**:1378, 1964.
55. Gerritsen, T., and Niederwieser, A.: In Curtius, H. Ch., and Roth, M., editors: Clinical biochemistry, principles and methods, Berlin, 1974, Walter de Gruyter & Co., vol. II.
56. Hsia, D. Y-Y.: In Stefanini, M., editor: Progress in clinical pathology, New York, 1966, Grune & Stratton, Inc.
57. Free, A.H., and Free, H.M.: In Sunderman, F.W., and Sunderman, F.W., Jr., editors: Laboratory diagnosis of kidney diseases, St. Louis, 1970, Warren H. Green, Inc.
58. Efron, M.L.: In Sunderman, F.W., and Sunderman, F.W., Jr., editors: The clinical pathology of infancy, Springfield, Ill., 1967, Charles C Thomas, Publisher.
59. Pasieka, A.E., et al.: Clin. Biochem. **2**:41, 1968.
60. Mabry, C.C.: CRC Crit, Rev. Clin. Lab. Sci. **1**:135, 1970.
61. Bickel, H., et al.: Acta Paediatr. Scand. **42**(suppl. 90):1, 1952.
62. Asatoor, A.M., et al.: Clin. Sci. Mol. Med. **23**:285, 1962.
63. Lewis, H.B.: Ann. Intern. Med. **6**:183, 1932.
64. Fischl, J., Sason, I., and Segal, S.: Clin. Chem. **7**:674, 1961.
65. Humbel, R., and Kutter, D.: Helv. Paediatr. Acta **22**:390, 1967.
66. Cheuk, Y.H., Free, H.M., and Free, A.H.: In Proceedings of the Division of Biological Chemistry, One-hundred Forth-third Meeting of American Chemical Society, Cincinnati, 1963, p. 43A (abstracts).
67. Tu, J.B., et al.: In Bergsma, D., et al., editors: Immunologic deficiency diseases in man; Wilson's disease. Birth defects original article series, New York, 1968, National Foundation, March of Dimes, vol. IV.
68. Efron, M.L.: In Sunderman, F.W., and Sunderman, F.W., Jr., editors: The clinical pathology of infancy, Springfield, Ill., 1967, Charles C Thomas, Publisher.
69. Hsia, D. Y-Y.: Inborn errors of metabolism, ed. 2, Chicago, 1966, Year Book Medical Publishers, Inc.
70. Menkes, J.H.: In Proceedings of the international conference on inborn errors of metabolism, Washington, D.C., 1967, Children's Bureau, U.S. Department of Health and Human Services.
71. Carpenter, G.C., Auerbach, V.H., and DiGeorge, A.M.: Pediatr. Clin. North Am. **15**:313, 1968.
72. Hsia, D. Y-Y.: Deve. Med. Child Neurol. **9**:531, 1967.
73. Cunningham, G.C.: CRC Crit. Rev. Clin. Lab. Sci. **2**:45, 1971.
74. Mitoma, C., Auld, R.M., and Udenfriend. S.: Proc. Soc. Exp. Biol. Med. **94**:634, 1957.
75. Berry, J.P., and Woolf, L.I.: Nature **169**:202, 1952.
76. Centerwall, W.R., Chinnock, R.F., and Pusavat, A.: Am. J. Public Health **50**:1667, 1960.
77. Berry, H.K., et al.: J. Nerv. Ment. Dis. **137**:577, 1963.
78. Lancaster, R.G., and Marsh, H.H.: Urinalysis workshop, New Orleans, 1968, American Society of Clinical Pathologists.
79. Gibbs, N.K., and Woolf, L.I.: Br. Med. J. **2**:532, 1959.
80. Guthrie, R.: J.A.M.A. **178**:863, 1961.
81. McCaman, M.W., and Robins, E.: J. Lab. Clin. Med. **59**:885, 1962.
82. Wong, P.W., O'Flynn, M.E., and Inouye, T.: Clin. Chem. **10**:1098, 1964.
83. Berry, H.K., Sutherland, B.S., and Umbarger, B.: Pediatrics **37**:102, 1966.
84. Anderson, J.A., et al.: J. Pediatr. **68**:351, 1966.
84a. Griffin, R.F., and Elsas, L.T.: J. Pediatr. **86**:512, 1975.
85. Kaufman, S., and Milstien, S.: Ann. Clin. Lab. Med. **7**:178, 1977.
86. Pediatrics **60**(suppl.):396, 1977. (Prepared by N.A. Holtzman for Health Services Administration, U.S. Department of Health and Human Serices, Washington, D.C.)
87. Levy, H.L., et al.: N. Engl. J. Med. **285**:424, 1971.
88. Holtzman, N.A., et al.: J. Pediatr. **85**:175, 1974.
89. Milstien, S., et al.: Pediatrics **60**(suppl.):396, 1977 (quotation).
90. Watson, B.M., Schlesinger, P., and Cotton, R.G.H.: Clin. Chim. Acta **78**:417, 1977.
91. Brenton, D.P., Cusworth, D.C., and Gaull, G.E.: J. Pediatr. **67**:58, 1965.
92. Neufeld, E.F.: Hosp. Pract. **7**:107, 1972.
93. McKusick, V.A., et al.: Medicine (Baltimore) **44**:445, 1965.
94. Berman, E.R., Vered, J., and Bach, G.: Clin. Chem. **17**:886, 1971.
95. Diferrante, N.: Anal. Biochem. **21**:98, 1967.
96. Berman, E.R., and Bach, G.: Biochem. J. **108**:75, 1968.
97. Fratantoni, J.C., et al.: N. Engl. J. Med. **280**:686, 1969.
98. Renuart, A.W.: N. Engl. J. Med. **274**:384, 1966.
99. Garb, S.: Clinical guide to undesirable drug reactions and interferences, New York, 1971, Springer-Verlag New York Inc.
100. Benedict, S.R.: J.A.M.A. **57**:1194, 1911.

101. Walford, S., et al.: Lancet **1:**732, 1978.
102. Griffin, N.K., et al.: Arch. Dis. Child. **54:**371, 1979.
103. Smith, B.C., Peake, M.J., and Fraser, C.G.: Clin. Chem. **23:**2337, 1977.
104. James, G.P., and Bee, D.E.: Clin. Chem. **25:**996, 1979.
105. Wilson, D.M.: Minn. Med. **58:**9, 1975.
106. Dyerberg, J., Pedersen, L., and Aagaard, O.: Clin. Chem. **22:**205, 1976.
107. Berry, H.K., et al.: Clin. Chem. **14:**1033, 1968.
108. Haer, F.C.: An introduction to chromatography on impregnated glass fiber, Ann Arbor, Mich., 1969, Ann Arbor Science Publishers, Inc.
109. Young, D.S., and Jackson, A.J.: Clin. Chem. **16:**954, 1970.
110. Burman, D., Holton, J.B., and Pennock, C.A.: Inherited disorders of carbohydrate metabolism, Lancaster, England, 1979, Medical and Technical Publishing Co., Ltd.
111. Wang, Y.M., and van Eys, J.: N. Engl. J. Med. **282:**892, 1970.
112. Beutler, E., and Baluda, M.: J. Lab. Clin. Med. **68:**137, 1966.
113. Beutler, E., et al.: Lancet **1:**353, 1965.
114. Ganong, W.F.: Review of medical physiology, ed. 9, Los Altos, Calif., 1979, Lange Medical Publications.
115. Young, D.S., Pestaner, L.C., and Gibberman, V.: Clin. Chem. **21:**1D, 1975.
116. Orten, J.M.: Ann. Clin. Lab. Sci. **1:**113, 1970.
117. Robinson, S.H.: Semin. Hematol. **9:**43, 1972.
118. Robinson, S.H., et al.: J. Clin. Invest. **45:**1569, 1966.
119. Muller-Eberhard, U., and Bashore, R.: N. Engl. J. Med. **282:**1163, 1970.
120. McNeely, M.D.D.: In Sonnenwirth, A.C., and Jarett, L., editors: Gradwohl's clinical laboratory methods and diagnosis, ed. 8, St. Louis, 1980, The C.V. Mosby Co.
121. Nyman, M.: Scand. J. Clin. Lab. Invest. **11**(suppl. 39):1, 1959.
122. Adams, E.C.: Ann. Clin. Lab. Sci. **1:**208, 1971.
123. Adams, E.C., Jr., and Layman, J.M.: In Sunderman, F.W., editor: Applied seminar on the laboratory diagnosis of cancer, Philadelphia, 1973, Association of Clinical Scientists.
124. Levere, R.D., and Kappas, A.: Hosp. Pract. **5**(3):61, 1970.
125. Pindyck, J., Kappas, A., and Levere, R.D.: CRC Crit. Rev. Clin. Lab. Sci. **2:**639, 1971.
126. Levere, R.D., and Pindyck, J.: Ann. Clin. Lab. Sci. **1:**101, 1971.
127. Watson, C.J.: N. Engl. J. Med. **263:**1205, 1960.
128. Dean, G.: S. Afr. Med. J. **34:**745, 1960.
129. Fernandez, A.A., and Jacobs, S.L.: Stand. Meth. Clin. Chem. **6:**57, 1970.
130. Fuhrop, J.-H., and Smith, K.M.: Laboratory methods in porphyrin and metalloporphyrin research, Amsterdam, 1975, Elsevier Publishing Co.
131. Ford, R.E., Ou, C-N., and Ellefson, R.D.: Clin. Chem. **26:**964, 1980.
132. Mauzerall, D., and Granick, S.: J. Biol. Chem. **219:**435, 1956.
133. Wilkinson, J.H.: In Sunderman, F.W., Jr., editor: Applied seminar on the laboratory diagnosis of diseases caused by toxic agents, St. Louis, 1970, Warren H. Green, Inc.
134. Davis, J.R., and Andelman, S.L.: Arch. Environ. Health **15:**53, 1967.
135. Roels, H., et al.: Clin. Chem. **20:**753, 1974.
136. Weissberg, B.A., Lipschutz, F., and Oski, F.A.: N. Engl. J. Med. **284:**565, 1971.
137. Burch, H.B., and Siegal, A.L.: Clin. Chem. **17:**1038, 1971.
138. Tschudy, D.P.: In Brown, S.S., Mitchell, F.L., and Young, D.S., editors: Amsterdam, 1979, Elsevier Publishing Co.
139. Bottomly, S.S., Tanaka, M., and Everett, M.A.: J. Lab. Clin. Med. **86:**126, 1975.
140. Beeler, M.F., and Henry, J.B.: J.A.M.A. **176:**52, 1961.
141. Agrup, G., et al.: Acta Derm. Venereol. (Stockh.) **55:**337, 1975.
142. Winkel, P., Statland, B.E., and Jørgensen, K.: Clin. Chem. **20:**436, 1974.
143. Lindquist, B., and Wahlin, A.: Acta Med. Scand. **198:**505, 1975.
144. De Voogt, H.J., Beyer-Boon, M.E., and Brussee, J.M.: Acta Cytol. **19:**542, 1975.
145. Kark, R.M., Lawrence, J.R., Pollak, V.E.: A primer of urinalysis, ed. 2, Philadelphia, 1963, J.B. Lippincott Co.
146. Haber, M.H.: Am. J. Clin. Pathol. **57:**316, 1972.
147. Schumann, G.B., and Henry, J.B.: Lab. Manage. **15:**18, 1977.
148. Sternheimer, R., and Malbin, B.: Am. J. Med. **11:**312, 1951.
149. Schumann, G.B., Harris, S., and Henry, J.B.: Am. J. Clin. Pathol. **69:**18, 1978.
150. Wilson, D.M.: Minn. Med. **58:**9, 1975.
151. Schreiner, G.E.: Arch. Intern. Med. **99:**356, 1957.
152. Taft, P.D., and Flax, M.H.: Transplantation **4:**194, 1966.
153. Haber, M.H.: Urine casts: their microscopy and clinical significance, Chicago, 1976, American Society of Clinical Pathologists.
154. Kurtzman, N.A., and Rogers, P.W.: A handbook of urinalysis and urinary sediment, Springfield, Ill., 1974, Charles C Thomas, Publisher.
155. McQueen, E.G.: Lancet **1:**397, 1966.
156. Haber, M.H., and Lindner, L.E.: Am. J. Clin. Pathol. **68:**547, 1977.
157. Lippman, R.W.L.: Urine and the urinary sediment, ed. 2, Springfield, Ill., 1957, Charles C Thomas, Publisher.
158. Puchtler, H., and Sweat, F.: Arch. Pathol. **75:**588, 1963.
159. Daysog, A., Jr., and Dobson, H.L.: Am. J. Clin. Pathol. **39:**419, 1963.
160. Schumann, G.B., Palmieri, L.J., and Jones, D.B.: Am. J. Clin. Pathol. **67:**580, 1977.
161. Bolande, R.P.: Pediatrics **24:**7, 1959.
162. Austin, J.H.: Neurology **7:**415, 1957.
163. Castleman, B., and Kibbee, B.U.: N. Engl. J. Med. **267:**1198, 1962.
164. Austin, J., et al.: Arch. Neurol. **14:**259, 1966.
165. Wesson, L.G.: Med. Clin. North Am. **47:**861, 1963.
166. Miles, B.E., Paton, A., and De Wardener, H.E.: Br. Med. J. **2:**901, 1954.
167. Rowe, J.W., Schock, N.W., and De Fronzo, R.A.: Nephron **17:**270, 1976.
168. Volini, F., De La Huerga, J., and Madera-Orsini, F.: In Sunderman, F.W., and Sunderman, F.W., Jr., editors: Laboratory diagnosis of kidney diseases, St. Louis, 1970, Warren H. Green, Inc.
169. De Wardener, H.E.: Lancet **1:**1037, 1956.
170. Pillay, V.K.G.: Med. Clin. North Am. **55**(1):231, 1971.
171. Black, D.A.K., and Cameron, J.S.: In Brown, S.S., Mitchell, F.L., and Young, D.S., editors: Chemical diagnosis of disease, Amsterdam, 1979, Elsevier Publishing Co.
172. Chapman, E.M., and Halsted, J.A.: Am. J. Med. Sci. **186:**223, 1933.
173. Lapides, J., and Bobbitt, J.M.: J.A.M.A. 166:866, 1958.
174. Kampmann, J., et al.: Acta Med. Scand. **196:**517, 1974.

175. Barratt, T.M., and Chantler, C.: In Rubin, M.I., and Barrett, T.M., editors: Paediatric nephrology, Baltimore, 1975, The Williams and Wilkins Co.

176. Flanigan, W.J., et al.: Ann. Surg. **173:**733, 1971.

177. Bossen, E.H., et al.: Acta Cytol. **14:**176, 1970.

178. Johnston, W.W., et al.: Acta Cytol. **13:**605, 1969.

179. Harlan, W.R., Jr., et al.: N. Engl. J. Med. **277:**769, 1967.

180. Pollack, S.S., and Carlson G.L.: Am. J. Clin. Pathol. **52:**656, 1969.

181. Freeman, J.A., and Beeler, M.F.: In Laboratory medicine—clinical microscopy, Philadelphia, 1974, Lea & Febiger.

CHAPTER 28

Semen analysis and infertility investigations, pregnancy tests, and placental hormones

EXAMINATION OF SEMEN

Semen[1,2] (correctly called ejaculate or seminal fluid, since it may not contain spermatozoa) is a milky liquid that contains secretions of the prostate, seminal vesicles, epididymides, and urethral glands, spermatozoa and some of their precursor cells (spermatocytes), and Sertoli cells.

Evaluation of spermatozoa is only one step in the investigation of male infertility. Other suggested procedures include chemical analysis of seminal plasma, e.g., determination of fructose level; hormonal evaluation of the patient, e.g., assay of luteinizing hormone, follicle-stimulating hormone, testosterone, prolactin, thyroxine, and corticosteroids.[3] Other investigations are the evaluation of cervical mucus, the Sims-Huhner test, the sperm–cervical mucus contact test, the antisperm antibody titer, chromosomal studies, basic biochemical investigations such as blood sugar, blood urea, liver function tests and, lastly, testicular biopsy.

Semen analysis and infertility investigations
Collection

Collection of semen should follow a period of sexual abstinence of 3 days. The specimen is collected by masturbation or by coitus interruptus into a prewarmed (21° C), sterile, wide-mouthed glass or plastic container. Condoms, even when thoroughly washed and rinsed, contain spermicidal agents and must not be used. It is best to obtain the specimen in the laboratory so that coagulation and liquefaction of the ejaculate can be observed and timed. Exposure of spermatozoa to cold (and to heat) should be avoided, since cold markedly decreases motility of spermatozoa (cold shock).[4] Note the date and exact time when the specimen was obtained. The material should be examined within 1-3 hr.

At least three specimens should be examined if any abnormality is noted in the first specimen. The examination should include the following:

1. Macroscopic (gross) examination: amount, color and turbidity, viscosity, and pH
2. Microscopic examination: motility, number, and morphology of spermatozoa
3. Chemical examination: fructose level

Characteristics of normal semen are listed below. It must be pointed out that a single deficiency cannot be equated with sterility.

Average normal values

Volume: The average volume is 3-3.5 ml ± 0.84 ml.

Number: The average number is 60-130 million/ml (sperm density).

Mean percentage of motile spermatozoa: The average normal value for mean percentage of motile spermatozoa is 63% ± 16%; 70-90% are motile in the first hour, 70-60% in the second to fourth hour, 60-50% in the fourth to seventh hour, 50-35% in the seventh to tenth hour, and 35-25% in the tenth to fifteenth hour.

Morphology: There are an average of 79-90% normal forms (oval heads).

Lower limits of normal

Volume: The lower limit of normal volume is 0.5 ml.

Number: The lower limit of normal for number of spermatozoa is 10 million/ml.*

Motility: The lower limit of normal is 40% motile in first hour.

Morphology: The lower limit of normal is 60% normal forms.

Gross examination

Volume: The average volume is 3-3.5 ml. A volume of less than 1 ml or greater than 4 ml is associated with infertility.[5]

Color and turbidity: In humans color and turbidity have no relation to sperm contents.

Viscosity: Fresh ejaculate gels, but it then liquefies after 10-20 min. Failure of the ejaculate to coagulate or persistence of the gel is associated with infertility. Examination of the semen should not be undertaken until it is liquefied, since only then do the spermatozoa attain full mobility.

pH: The pH ranges from 7.2-7.6. The alkaline pH protects the semen from the acid environment of the vagina. An ejaculate that consists mainly of prostatic secretions has a pH below 7 and is usually poor in spermatozoa.[6]

Microscopic examination

When the specimen has liquefied, place 1 drop of semen on a microscope slide to determine whether spermatozoa are present and, if present, to judge their motility. If no spermatozoa are seen, centrifuge specimen and examine sediment.

In addition to the spermatozoa, the type and number of other cells in the ejaculate should be noted. Polymorphonuclear leukocytes are indicative of prostatitis, which is responsible for one form of infertility.[7] Bacteriologic confirmation of the diagnosis of prostatitis may be indicated since *Escherichia coli* interferes with normal sperm motility.[8] Diagnosis of prostatitis may also be confirmed by a low semen zinc concentration.[9]

Motility

Mount 1 drop of semen on a microscope slide, cover with cover slip, and seal with petrolatum. Under the high-power dry lens, count the motile and nonmotile spermatozoa in several fields, reporting the percent of motile forms. Only those spermatozoa that move forward actively are considered motile. Examine at 1, 3, 6, and 24 hr.

Motility depends on the temperature and the number of cells. At 37° C in a normal ejaculate, only 50% of the spermatozoa are motile after 3 hr; at 21° C, 50% are still motile after 7 hr.

Interpretation of motility: Fewer than 70% spermatozoa motile in the first hour points toward some semen abnormality but not necessarily to infertility.

Type of movement: The type of movement can be classified as quick, sluggish, etc. The degree of activity is important, since more active spermatozoa lose their motility faster than sluggish cells.

Revitalization test: If spermatozoa are immobile and appear to be dead, allow 1 drop of glucose Ringer solution to flow under the coverslip and observe whether some of the spermatozoa recover and become motile again.

Eosin test[10]:

Principle: Because lack of motility is not synonymous with mortality, eosin stain is used to differentiate live (unstained) and dead (stained) spermatozoa.

Procedure: Mix 1 drop of semen with 0.5% yellow aqueous eosin and examine under the microscope. Living spermatozoa will not accept the dye, whereas dead spermatozoa stain pink-yellow.

Sperm count

Reagent: Prepare formalin solution by mixing 5 g sodium bicarbonate, 1 ml 40% formalin, and 1 dl distilled water.

Procedure: In a white cell diluting pipet, draw semen to mark 0.5 and formalin solution to mark 11 to obtain a 1:20 solution. Let mixture stand until mucus dissolves, shake thoroughly, and fill a blood-counting chamber. Count spermatozoa in a 1 mm^2 area (one large square) and multiply result by 200,000 to obtain number of spermatozoa per milliliter.

Normal values: Normal values for the sperm count by this method are 60-130 million/ml.

Lower limit of normal: The lower limit of normal is 10 million/ml.

Disappearance of spermatozoa from ejaculate after vasectomy

Sperm counts are the only objective method available to evaluate the result of vasectomy. Within 6 months of vasectomy 48% of men are azoospermic, at 12 months 88% are cleared, and at 18 months 95% are free of spermatozoa in the ejaculate.[11] Men over 50 years of age clear much slower than younger men, a phenomenon that may be related to the frequency of intercourse following the operation. It is suggested that for vasectomy patients monthly sperm counts be taken until two consecutive azoospermic specimens are obtained.[12] Motile spermatozoa disappear more rapidly than nonmotile spermatozoa. The nonmotile forms are not fertile, and they can be disregarded in a postvasectomy seminal assay if motile spermatozoa are absent.[13]

Morphology

Morphologic appearance is best studied in stained smears, which can be prepared from the specimen diluted for the sperm count. Make smears as described for blood, and stain with one of the following: Wright-Giemsa stain, hematoxylin-eosin stain, or Papanicolaou stain. Count several hundred spermatozoa and spermatocytes under the oil-immersion lens and report the percent of normal cells.

---

*There is a large variability in sperm counting, and multiple specimens should be analyzed in order to obtain a reliable count. There is a large overlap between fertile and infertile sperm counts, indicating the participation of other factors determining fertility of sperm. Thus the minimal number of 10 million/ml should be recognized as a guide only.

Normal morphology

Of the spermatozoa counted, 80-85% should have normal morphology, accompanied by 0.5-2% normal spermatogenic cells.

The normal smear of semen contains spermatozoa, spermatocytes (cells that have to do with spermatogenesis), Sertoli cells, macrophages containing sperm heads in the cytoplasm, epithelial cells, and occasionally white and red cells and crystals (Figs. 28-1 and 28-2).

For descriptive purposes, spermatozoa are divided into head, neck, and tail, but variations of the head are most important (Fig. 28-3). Normal spermatozoa may show slight variations in the shape and size of the head, e.g., small, round, pointed, or enlarged. They may also show some variation in staining, either absence of staining or diffuse staining (senile forms).

Joel[14] suggested the preparation of a "tissue button" of formalin-fixed ejaculate that is prepared, fixed, stained, and handled exactly like any "fluid button" in the tissue laboratory.

Abnormal morphology

The lower the number of spermatozoa, the more abnormal forms usually occur. The abnormality may be morphologic or tinctorial.

Sperm abnormalities include juvenile forms with cytoplasmic appendages, senile forms with diffuse or absent staining of the head, and pathologic variations in the configuration and number of heads.

Clumping of spermatozoa in the ejaculate associated with a low sperm count and decreased motility should make the observer suspicious that there may be an antibody problem.[15]

Chemical examination: determination of fructose

Fructose is the main sugar of semen,[16] and diminished levels have been shown to parallel androgen deficiency.[17] There is an inverse relationship between fructose level and sperm count.[18] A low fructose concentration is the result of a low testosterone level or seminal vesicle insufficiency.[19]

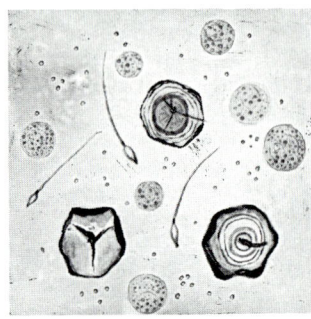

Fig. 28-1. Spermatic fluid showing spermatozoa, corpora amylacea, and lecithin granules. (From Gershenfeld, L.: Urine and urinalysis, Philadelphia, 1948, Lea & Febiger.)

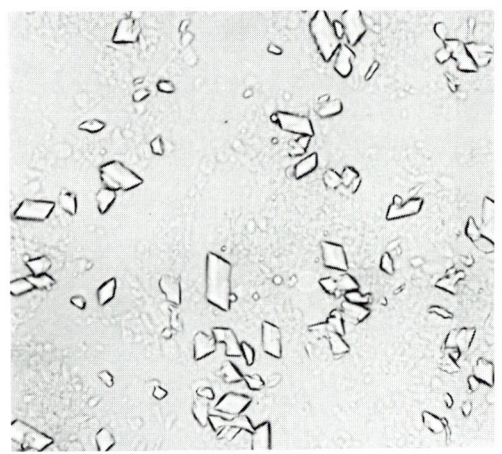

Fig. 28-2. Spermine hydrochloride crystals in normal spermatic fluid.

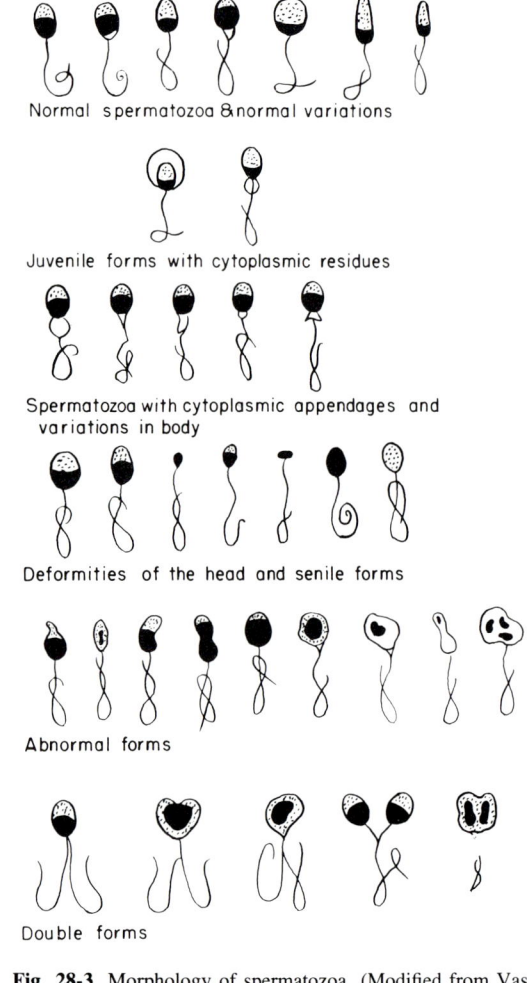

Fig. 28-3. Morphology of spermatozoa. (Modified from Vasterling, H.W.: Praktische Spermatologie, Stuttgart, West Germany, 1960, Georg Thieme Verlag.)

There are several methods available for the quantitation of fructose. These include colorimetric analysis with resorcinol, enzymatic determination, and condensation with indole-3-acetic acid.[20] The latter procedure, also used for determination of inulin, is presented below.[21]

Principle: An aliquot of a trichloroacetic acid protein-free filtrate from semen is treated with indole-3-acetic acid and concentrated hydrochloric acid. A purple color is developed by the reagent in the presence of fructose. The color is compared with that of a sample similarly treated.

Reagents:

1. Trichloroacetic acid, 0.6 mole/L
   Dissolve 10 g trichloroacetic acid in water to make 1 dl, or dilute a 1.8 moles/L solution 1:3.
2. Serum
   Any control or other serum of low bilirubin and glucose levels that is not lipemic or markedly hemolyzed may be used. The serum is added in the preparation of the protein-free filtrate since some semen specimens by themselves do not give a clear supernatant. The small amount of glucose present will not interfere.
3. Indole-3-acetic acid, 30 mmole/L
   Dissolve 525 mg indole-3-acetic acid in 1 dl 95% ethanol. Store in the refrigerator and discard if discoloration develops.
4. Hydrochloric acid, concentrated
5. Fructose standard, 225 mg/dl (12.5 mmole/L)
   Dissolve 225 mg fructose in saturated benzoic acid solution to make 1 dl. This solution is stable for several months at room temperature.

Procedure: To 5 ml centrifuge tubes labeled sample, blank, and standard add 1.0 ml trichloroacetic acid solution. To each tube add 0.1 ml serum. To sample tube add 0.1 ml semen, to standard tube add 1.0 ml standard, and to the blank tube add 0.1 ml water. Cover tops with Parafilm and mix well. Allow to stand for 10 min; then centrifuge strongly and transfer 0.25 ml supernatant to appropriately labeled tubes. To each tube add 0.25 ml water, mix, and add 4 ml concentrated hydrochloric acid. Mix by inversion and place in a 37° C water bath for 75 min. Remove the tubes and read the sample and the standard against the blank at 520 nm.

Calculation: Since sample and standard are treated similarly,

$$\frac{\text{Absorbance of sample} \times \text{Conc. of standard}}{\text{Absorbance of standard}} = \frac{\text{Conc.}}{\text{of sample}}$$

Normal values: The mean fructose level of normospermic men is 246.9 mg/dl ± 12.46 mg.

Discussion: Seminal fructose levels in necrospermic men (198.4 mg/dl ± 14.72 mg) are significantly lower than those in normospermic men. Phadke et al.[22] state that the fructose level in semen is inversely related to germinal cell activity irrespective of whether spermatozoa are present or absent in the semen or whether they are dead or motile.

CERVICAL MUCUS

In fertility studies the nature of the cervical mucus plays an important role, since at or near the time of ovulation it allows spermatozoa to ascend into the uterine cavity but at all other times it prevents their entry. In different phases of the ovarian cycle the cervical mucus undergoes cyclic, physical, and chemical changes.

As part of an assessment of fertility, the cervical mucus should be examined at its peak of maximal sperm receptivity. Since this time interval is normally at or near the time of ovulation, the day of ovulation has to be established with a considerable degree of confidence. Several tests that are used to estimate the time of ovulation are given below and are followed by tests of cervical mucus for sperm receptivity.

Determinants of ovulation

As pictured in Fig. 28-4 there are a number of physical and biochemical parameters that change in parallel during the ovulatory cycle.[23,24] Serum luteinizing hormone (LH) and certain physical characteristics of cervical mucus all peak at or right before ovulation.

Daily serum LH levels determined by radioimmunoassay show a characteristic midcycle surge, preceding ovulation by about 24 hr.[25] Because the LH assay is expensive and the turnaround time exceeds 24 hr, the test is clinically impractical for the determination of ovulation. There are a number of other indicators of ovulation that can be utilized.[26] The serum LH surge is accompanied by a sudden marked decreased in cervical mucus viscosity, an increase in leukocyte alkaline phosphatase activity, the lowest value of basal body temperature, and changes in the fern test pattern.

Evaluation of the viscoelastic properties of ovulatory cervical mucus: the stretchability (spinnbarkeit) test

During the midcycle week the cervical mucus is tested daily for viscosity either by a viscometer[27] or by the simple stretchability test.

Procedure: Expose the cervical surface using a nonlubricated speculum and clean the cervical surface, using a disposable 1 ml tuberculin syringe without a needle, aspirate the endocevical mucus. Record physical properties such as amount, color, clarity, and pH. Place 0.1 ml mucus on a slide and cover with a coverslip. Pull the coverslip away from the slide and measure in centimeters the spinnbarkeit, i.e., the ability of the mucus to be drawn into a thread, the length of which is measured before it breaks.

Results: The cervical mucus at ovulation is somewhat watery as compared to the mucus found before and after ovulation. At ovulation, mucus threads up to 9 cm and over can be obtained by this method. However, since the stretchability test is only qualitative and relatively inaccurate, the results should be confirmed by the more accurate and reliable fern test.

Fern test

The fern test is considered to have a direct relationship to sperm receptivity and to be a sensitive indicator of hormonal changes.[28,29] The midcycle ferning pattern

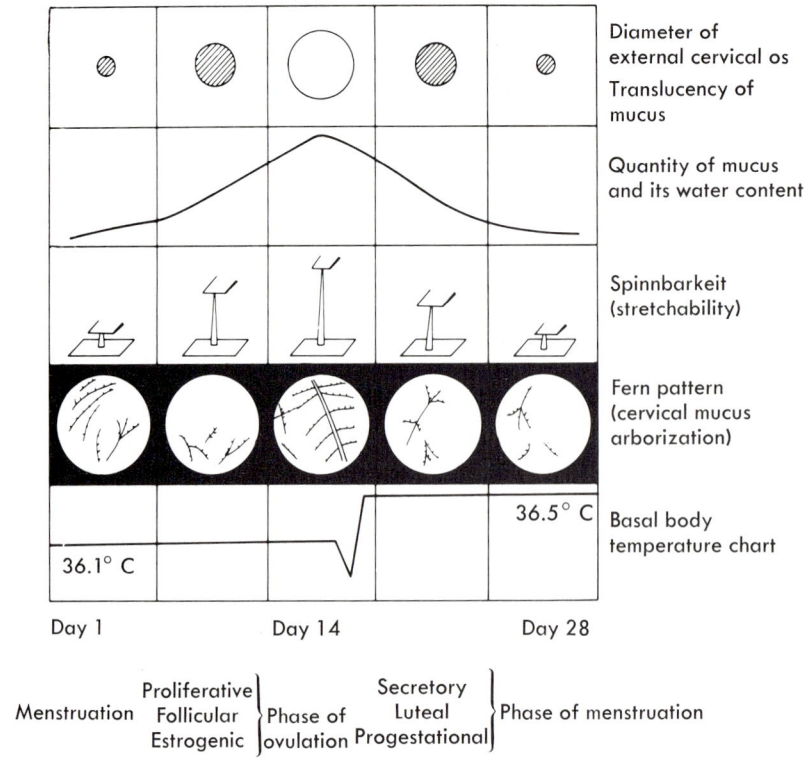

Day 1   Day 14   Day 28

	Proliferative		Secretory	
Menstruation	Follicular	Phase of	Luteal	Phase of menstruation
	Estrogenic	ovulation	Progestational	

Fig. 28-4. Outline of cervical mucus function tests and their relationship to menstrual cycle. (From Elstein, M.: In Cohen, J., and Hendry, W.F., editors: Spermatozoa antibodies and infertility, Oxford, England, 1978, Blackwell Scientific Publications Ltd.)

depends on the presence of both protein and electrolytes in the appropriate mucous milieu.

Principle: The cervical mucus is spread thinly on a slide and allowed to dry and to produce the "ferning" or arborization pattern of the electrolytes crystallized in the presence of protein.[30] The fern test pattern is a good indicator of the midcycle elevation of LH and of ovulation.

Procedure: Obtain cervical mucus with a cotton swab introduced into the cervical canal. Smear mucus on a coverslip and allow to air dry. Observe crystallization pattern under low power (4×) of the microscope. Report degree of ferning as follows[31]: 1+, linear ferning only (minimal degree of estrogen effect); 2+, arborization of leaves at 90 degrees to each other producing some palm leaf appearance; 3+, moderate degree of arborization when palm leaf appearance involves angulation at three right angles; and 4+, maximal arborization with palm leaves appearing at four right angles to each other.

Tests evaluating relationship of cervical mucus to spermatozoa
Postcoital (Sims-Huhner) test

Procedure: Perform the test as close to the time of ovulation as possible (see determinants of ovulation above). Instruct the patient to abstain from sexual intercourse for 2 days before the test.

Perform the test $2^{1}/_{2}$ hr after intercourse.[32] If the test is not performed at the specified time, record the inter-val between intercourse and test. Obtain mucus from the ectocervix and low endocervix by means of a sterile tuberculin syringe without needle. Place mucus on slide, cover with coverslip, and examine under 40× power.

Interpretation (Figs. 28-4 and 28-5): If exocervical or low endocervical samples are aspirated 2-3 hr after intercourse 25 or more progressively motile spermatozoa per high-power field (hpf) will be observed if conditions are within normal limits. Ten or more spermatozoa per hpf with directional motility are considered satisfactory. Less than five spermatozoa per hpf when associated with "localized motility" is an indication of oligoasthenospermia or an abnormality of cervical mucus.[33]

Beginning at 4 hr after coitus the number of spermatozoa in the mucus gradually decreases.[33]

An abnormal postcoital test must be repeated several times to substantiate the diagnosis of oligoasthenospermia or abnormal cervical mucus.

Sperm–cervical mucus contact test

The sperm–cervical mucus contact test (SCMCT) evaluates the penetration and migration in cervical mucus of nonagglutinated spermatozoa in ejaculates with partial autoagglutinins. Kremer and Jager[34] observed that spermatazoa in ejaculates with partial autoagglutinins changed their progressive motility into quick, shaking, and jerkinglike movements as soon as they came in contact with cervical mucus and were therefore un-

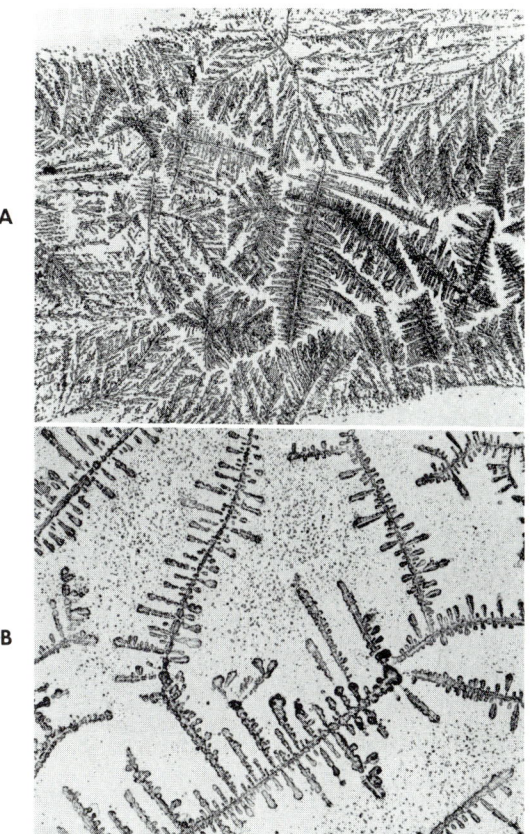

Fig. 28-5. Fern test. **A,** Typical fern pattern of cervical mucus obtained in midcycle. **B,** Atypical pattern observed in amniotic fluid close to term.

able to penetrate the mucoid barrier. The same movement is seen when the ejaculate is normal but the mucus contains agglutinating antisperm antibodies.[35]

Procedure: Mix 1 drop of semen and 1 drop of cervical mucus on a microscope slide. Cover with a coverslip and observe behavior of spermatozoa after 15-20 min.

Interpretation: In the presence of significant antisperm antibodies in the male or female, spermatozoa do not progress normally in the cervical mucus, a phenomenon depending on IgA in the genital secretions.[31] The attachment of the spermatozoa to the glycoprotein of the cervical mucus is responsible for the jerking, nonprogressive movement. To decide whether the antibodies are located in the ejaculate or in the cervical mucus the SCMCT can be performed in a cross system, the Miller-Kurzrok test.[35]

Tests for antisperm antibodies

Spermagglutinating antibodies (SAA)[1,36,37] may occur as autoantibodies in the male as the result of sensitization by his own spermatozoa, which are allowed to escape into the tissues after trauma, inflammation, testicular infarction, etc. These autoantibodies may be responsible for damage to spermatogenesis and for infertility in the male, because they specifically destroy the germinal cells of the testis.[38] More commonly the

SAA react with mature spermatozoa in the seminal fluid,[36] interfering with their motility and their relationship to cervical mucus.

In the female, immunization with sperm antigens leads to the production of antibodies that agglutinate spermatozoa to kill or immobilize them in the presence of complement,[39] or inhibit the sperm enzyme hyaluronidase required for entry into the ovary.[40]

The antisperm antibody methods can be divided into the following[41,42]:

1. Agglutination methods
   a. Tube-slide agglutination test (TSAT): see below
   b. Gelatin agglutination test (GAT): see reference 15
   c. Tray agglutination test (TAT): see reference 15
2. Immobilization method: sperm immobilization test (SIT)
3. Sperm–cervical mucus methods
   a. Sperm–cervical mucus penetration test (SCMPT): see reference 31
   b. Sperm–cervical mucus contact test (SCMCT): see above
4. Radiolabeled antiglobulin test

Tube-slide agglutination test (TSAT)

Principle: The method given here is Boettcher's modification of the Franklin-Dukes microscopic agglutination test.[43] Semen is added to a dilution of test serum in a culture tube and incubated at 37° C for 1-2 hr. One drop is removed from the bottom of the tube and is placed on a slide; the agglutination pattern is viewed under the microscope.

Reagents:
1. Baker's buffer, pH 8.1
   a. Glucose, 3.00 g
   b. $Na_2HPO_4.7H_2O$, 0.46 g
   c. Sodium chloride, 0.20 g
   d. KH_2PO_4, 0.01 g
   e. Water to 1 dl
2. Human serum inactivated at 56° C for 30 min
3. Semen suspension in Baker's buffer, 50×10^6 70% motile spermatozoa/ml

Procedure: Place 10 drops of inactivated serum in a test tube and add 1 drop of semen suspension. Incubate at 37° C. At intervals of 1-4 hr remove 1 drop from the bottom of the tube, place on a microscope slide, and cover with a coverslip. Examine microscopically and count the number of agglutinates seen per 100 motile nonagglutinated spermatozoa. Score only head-to-head agglutinates (Fig. 28-6).

Result: A score of 8/100 or greater is considered to be positive for the presence of antisperm antibodies. A positive test should be confirmed by a quantitative procedure as suggested below.

Radiolabeled antiglobulin test for antisperm antibodies[44]

The assay is a modification of the radiolabeled Coombs antiglobulin test used to measure antiplatelet IgG antibodies.[45]

Principle: Two million donor spermatozoa, negative for antisperm antibodies, are incubated with undiluted

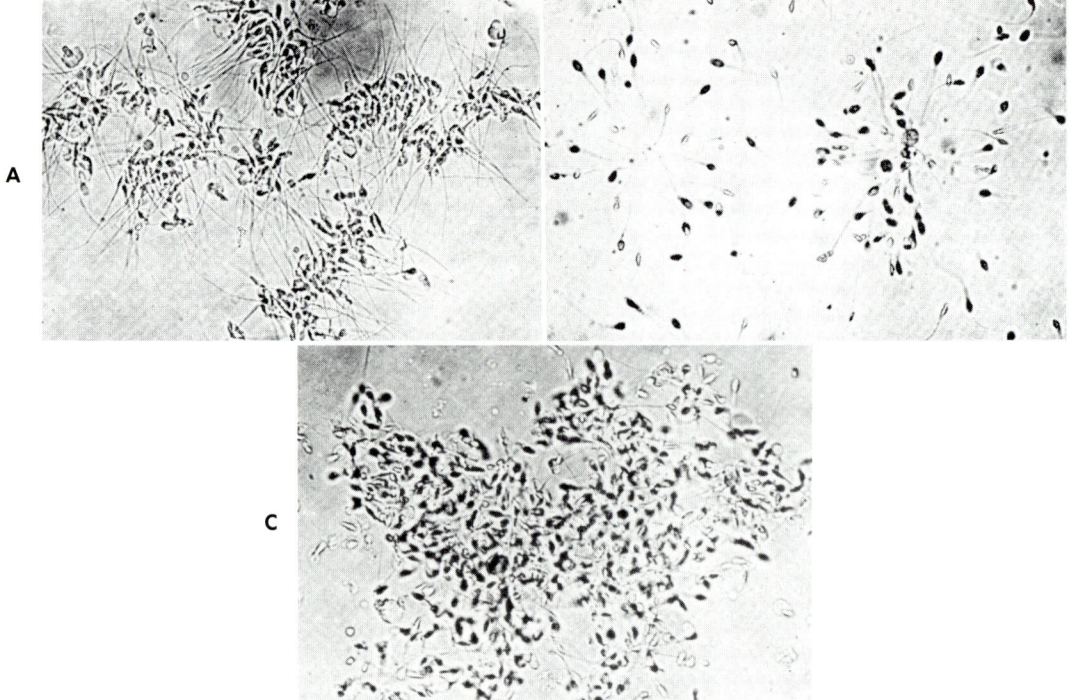

Fig. 28-6. A, Head-to-head agglutination of normal spermatozoa. **B,** Tail-to-tail (tip of tail) agglutination of normal spermatozoa. **C,** Tail-to-tail (main part of tail) agglutination of normal spermatozoa. (From Rümke, P., and Hellinga, G.: Am. J. Clin. Pathol. **32:**361, 1959.)

plasma from each patient (male and female). The specimen is then centrifuged, the sperm button washed, and the spermatozoa resuspended and incubated with radiolabeled rabbit anti-IgG. The spermatozoa are then washed, and the sperm-associated radioactivity is determined in a γ-counter. It is expressed as the percentage of the total ^{125}I anti-IgG radioactivity incubated with each aliquot of sperm.

Normal values: Normal values are 1.15 ± 0.68.

PREGNANCY TESTS AND PLACENTAL HORMONES

Almost from its earliest stage of development, the placenta produces hormones either on its own or in collaboration with the fetus (**fetoplacental unit**).[46] The very young (9-day-old) placental trophoblast produces appreciable amounts of **human chorionic gonadotropin (HCG),** a hormone that is excreted into the urine and that is not found in the urine of normal young nonpregnant women. Because of its association with the growing placental trophoblast, increased levels of HCG form the basis of most tests for pregnancy and for trophoblastic tumors in men and women.

At about age 6 weeks, the fetoplacental unit produces, in addition to HCG, detectable levels of a growth-type hormone called **human placental lactogen (HPL),** the level of which rises during the first and second trimester, reaches a plateau during the third trimester, and rapidly (within minutes) falls after delivery.[47] Because of its association with human trophoblasts, the plasma or urine levels of HPL can be used

to monitor a growing trophoblast. Low and falling concentrations indicate danger of immediate abortion, but it must be stressed that placental function may be normal even if the fetus is dead. Radioimmunoassay is the method of choice.

At about the time HPL can be detected in the urine of the pregnant patient, the fetoplacental unit begins to synthesize increasing quantities of **estrogen,** which are excreted into the urine mainly in the form of **estriol.** In the third trimester the production of estrogen can be used to monitor the status of the fetoplacental unit. Fetal distress or death diminishes the estriol excretion, since fetal precursor substances are apparently needed by the placenta to produce estrogens.

Placental hormones can be assayed in plasma or urine samples. The plasma assays evaluate production and catabolism of a substance over a relatively short period of time whereas a 24 hr urinary assay mirrors the production over a much longer time period. Current trends indicate a preference for serum analysis because of the difficulty of obtaining a proper 24 hr urine collection and in order to more closely monitor acute, short-term changes in the fetoplacental unit. Such changes can often indicate the necessity for clinical intervention in a pregnancy.

Pregnancy tests

All pregnancy tests are designed to detect HCG, a hormone produced by placental trophoblasts. HCG is present in blood and urine whenever there is living placental (chorionic) tissue and can be demonstrated in the

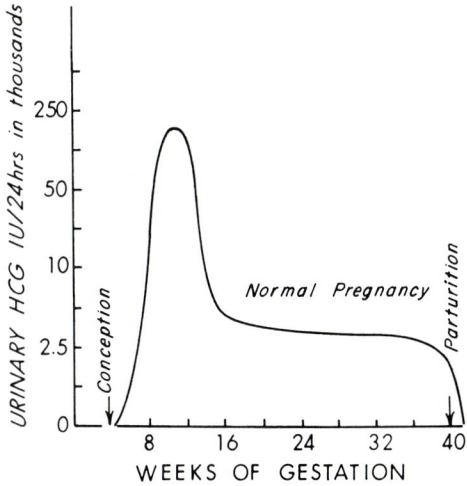

Fig. 28-7. Typical curve of HCG excretion levels throughout normal pregnancy.

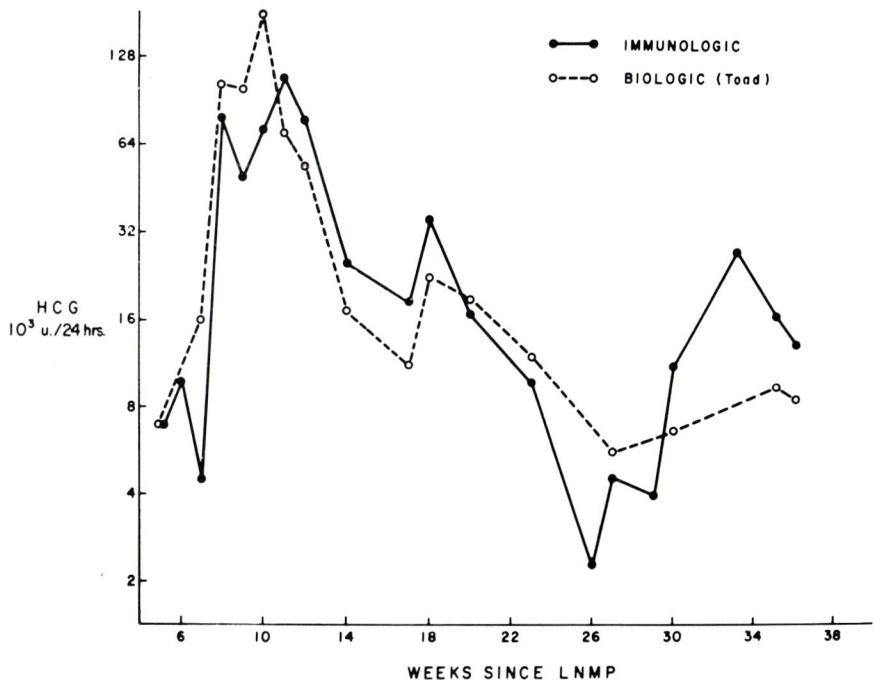

Fig. 28-8. Mean excretion levels of HCG by immunologic and biologic assay in four normal patients throughout pregnancy. LNMP, Last normal menstrual period. (From Taymor, M.L.: Clin. Obstet. Gynecol. **10:**309, 1967.)

urine of pregnant women as early as 7 days after ovulation (see assay of HCG β-chain below). About 2 weeks after conception the chorionic tissue begins to produce HCG, the concentration of which rises rapidly after the sixth week and reaches a peak level at about the tenth to twelfth week. After the twelfth week the HCG level falls abruptly and at the eighteenth to twentieth week levels off at a low plateau until delivery. The HCG levels during normal pregnancy vary widely, so that the

peak level between the tenth and twelfth weeks of gestation may fall between 7000 and 220,000 IU/24 hr (Figs. 28-7 and 28-8).

Pregnancy tests should be negative 3-4 days after delivery. Of 15 patients with normal deliveries, all had positive pregnancy tests 1 hr post partum, 10 had negative tests after 24 hr, and the remaining five patients had negative tests after 48 hr.[48]

To be clinically acceptable a pregnancy test must be

(1) sensitive to increased amounts of HCG, (2) accurate, (3) fast, and (4) reproducible. The most sensitive reference method is the radioimmunoassay of HCG,[49] which is based on the competition between unlabeled and radioactive-labeled HCG for a small amount of specific antibody (see assay of HCG β-chain below).

Immunoassay systems

Because the immunologic methods are available in kit form a description of their technic is omitted, but the manufacturer's instructions must be carefully followed. The principle of the methods, the sensitivity, the false positive and false negative results, and the controls need to be discussed.

The immunoassays are either hemagglutination inhibition or latex particle inhibition procedures (Fig. 28-9). It must be emphasized that they test HCG elevations from whatever cause and not ''pregnancy'' per se. The tests may be employed as qualitative as well as quantitative assays.

Hemagglutination (latex) inhibition tube test:

Principle: An antigen-antibody system is utilized. Red cells or latex particles coated with HCG are used as antigen. In the presence of anti-HCG antiserum, the HCG-coated red cells or latex particles agglutinate and settle out. The red cells and the latex particles are the visible markers of the antigen-antibody reaction. When the urine of a pregnant woman containing HCG is added to the antiHCG antiserum before the addition of the HCG-coated red cells or latex particles, the HCG present in the urine neutralizes the antiserum so that it fails to agglutinate the HCG-coated cells or latex particles that are subsequently added. Absence of agglutination therefore indicates pregnancy. If red cells are used as a marker, they will settle to the bottom of the tube in the form of a ''doughnut,'' similar to the one seen in the positive control in Fig. 28-10. The urine of a nonpregnant woman containing no HCG does not inhibit agglutination of the red cells or latex particles by the antiserum. Agglutination of the marker material therefore represents a negative test for pregnancy. If red cells are used as the marker, a mat of red cells with or without a faint ring develops at the bottom of the tube, indicating a negative test (Fig. 28-10).

If the end point is not clear, the test should be repeated using the original specimen and, if necessary,

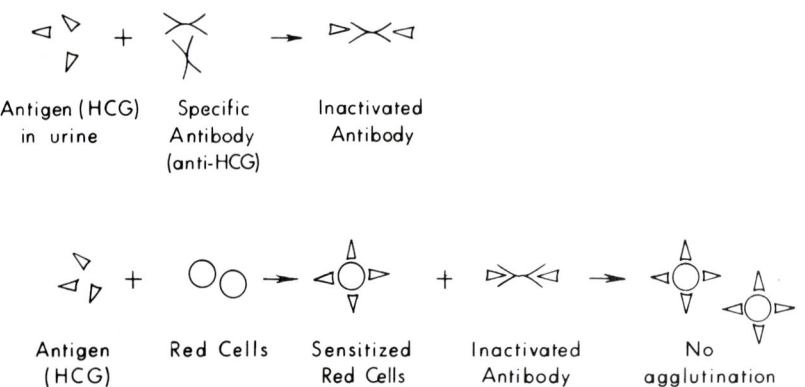

Fig. 28-9. Scheme of hemagglutination inhibition test.

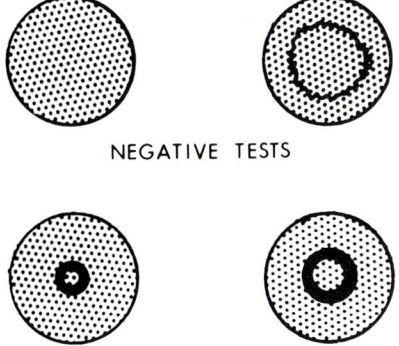

NEGATIVE TESTS

Fig. 28-10. End points of immunodiagnostic pregnancy tube test. Positive: clear-cut brown ring at bottom of test tube. Negative: diffuse yellow-brown sediment, or if there is an ill-defined irregular broken line at bottom of tube, repeat test since sedimentation has been disturbed.

repeated again in 1-2 weeks with a fresh specimen.

Direct agglutination slide tests: Also available are direct agglutination slide tests, e.g., DAP Test (Wampole Laboratories, Cranbury, N.J.), the principle of which is as follows (Fig. 28-11). Latex particles coated with anti-HCG antiserum will agglutinate if urine containing HCG, the specific antigen, is added. Agglutination therefore is indicative of a positive pregnancy test. Absence of agglutination is interpreted as a negative test.

Interpretation of immunologic tests: The accuracy of immunologic tests is influenced by many factors,[50] so that erroneous results may be expected in about 2% of normal pregnancies. In general, it may be stated that tube tests are more sensitive than slide tests.[51] For further discussion, see interpretation of quantitative pregnancy tests below.

Quantitative tests

The quantitative test[52,53] is subject to the same limitations as the qualitative test, but certain factors, e.g., glass absorption by HCG, are more significant.

The concentrated early morning urine specimen is preferred, since random urine specimens are often diluted (check specific gravity) and may therefore give false negative results. Cloudy and bloody urine samples tend to interfere with the reading of the test and should be cleared by centrifugation rather than by filtration, because HCG adheres to filter paper and glass, although some manufacturers specifically require filtration.

HCG in urine is stable for 4 months in the freezer ($-18°C$), but at room or refrigerator temperature it is stable for 72 hr only.[54]

Normal values: It must be noted that in normal preg-

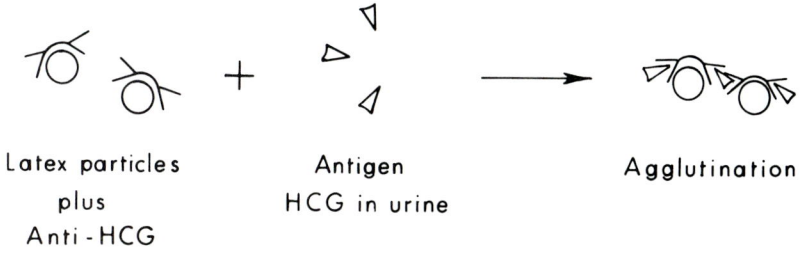

Latex particles
plus
Anti-HCG

Antigen
HCG in urine

Agglutination

Fig. 28-11. Scheme of direct agglutination test.

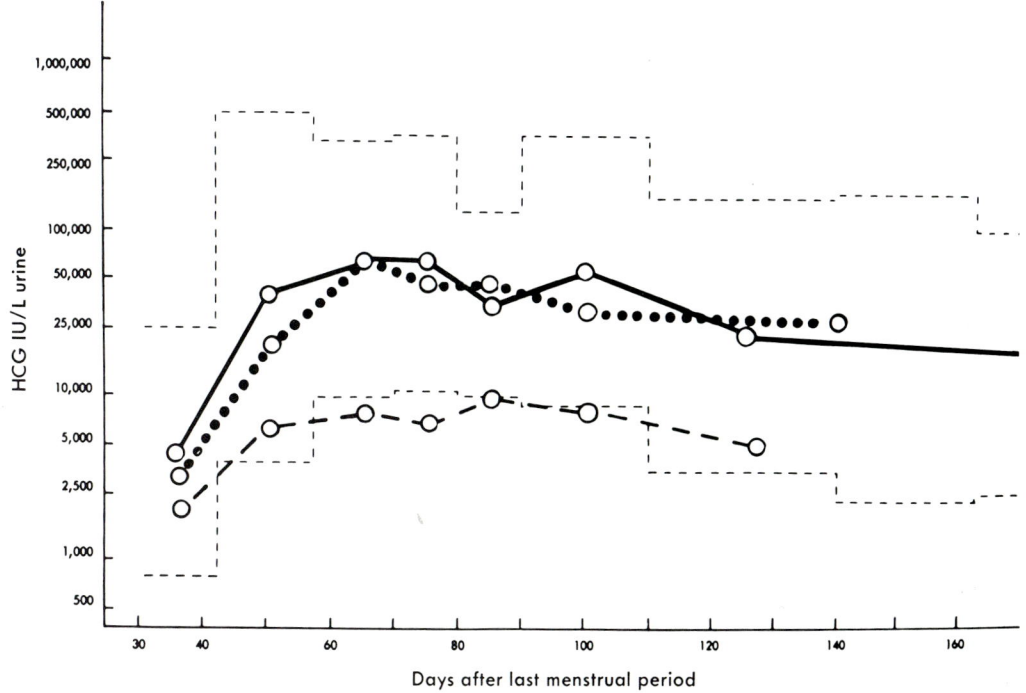

Fig. 28-12. Mean values of HCG excretion in morning. Solid line: normal pregnancy. Hatched line: threatened abortion, terminating in abortion. Dotted line: threatened abortion terminating in delivery of normal infant. Upper and lower broken lines: upper and lower limits of normal. (From Mishell, D.R., and Davajan, V.: Am. J. Obstet. Gynecol. **96:**231, 1966.)

nancy there may be wide variations in the HCG level, e.g., from 6000-500,000 IU/24 hr in the period from the eighth to twelfth week, although the average level in this period varies from 32,000-120,000 IU/24 hr. In general, titers greater than 1000 IU/L can be considered positive for pregnancy and titers less than 600 IU/L are considered negative. The average titers throughout the first one and one-half trimesters of normal pregnancy may vary between 5000 and 350,000 IU/L and in the third trimester from 2500-150,000 IU/L. During the second trimester a second short rise in the titer may occur (Figs. 28-7 and 28-12).

Interpretation:

Low HCG values: In patients about to abort or in ectopic pregnancies[55] the mean levels of HCG concentration are usually lower than in normal pregnancy.

False low levels: False low levels or negative tests may result from a low specific gravity (dilute) urine specimen or from a specimen that was obtained too early in pregnancy.

High HCG values: In patients with choriocarcinoma, hydatidiform mole, teratomas containing chorionic elements, or gonadotropin-producing tumors, e.g., carcinoma of lung, the HCG excretion is usually increased, but the variations of the HCG excretion are such that the HCG titer is not a reliable test for cancer detection. Titers varying by several millions from the normal range have been recorded in trophoblastic disorders. Titration of HCG may be used to monitor the results of surgery or of chemotherapy in the conditions mentioned, as the original high titer will fall rapidly after removal or destruction of the tumor (Fig. 28-13).

False positive results: False positive results may be seen in proteinuria, hematuria, excessive excretion of pituitary gonadotropin, and after administration of psychotropic drugs,[56] e.g., anticonvulsant, antiparkinsonian, and hypnotic drugs. The list of drugs includes phenothiazine derivatives, chlorpromazine derivatives, and thioridazine.

Assay of specific human chorionic gonadotropin (HCG β-chain)

The cross-reaction of HCG with LH results from the fact that they share α-subunits. β-subunits (β-glycoprotein), on the other hand, are specific for HCG, are produced by the trophoblast, and provide the basis for a highly specific and sensitive radioimmunoassay for trophoblastic activity, allowing early diagnosis of pregnancy (7 days after ovulation) and careful follow-up and diagnosis of patients with trophoblastic tumors.[57,58]

Newer slide tests, utilizing HCG β-chain—specific antibodies, are available with detection limits less than 1 IU/ml. Newer tube tests have reported sensitivities of 0.2 IU/ml. At the latter sensitivity, normal pregnancies can be detected at about 4 weeks after menses.

Quality control of pregnancy tests

Follow the manufacturer's instructions carefully and eliminate outdated reagents. Always use negative and positive controls with each test. Keep aliquots of frozen negative and positive urine samples available. Have a second immunologic test kit from a different commerical source available to repeat doubtful tests in parallel. Check slide test methods by the tube test method, as the latter is more sensitive. The technologist must be familiar with the technic and the variables influencing the test result.

Assessment of fetal age and well-being

Many attempts have been made to assess fetoplacental function by means of laboratory tests. HCG is a product of placental activity not influenced to any degree by the fetus. Although there is some evidence that fetal death lowers the HCG values somewhat, HCG assay is not a test of fetal viability. **Heat-stable serum alkaline phosphatase** apparently reflects fetoplacental function with a high degree of accuracy. **Urinary estriol** is another compound that has attracted attention because of its ability to monitor fetoplacental function.

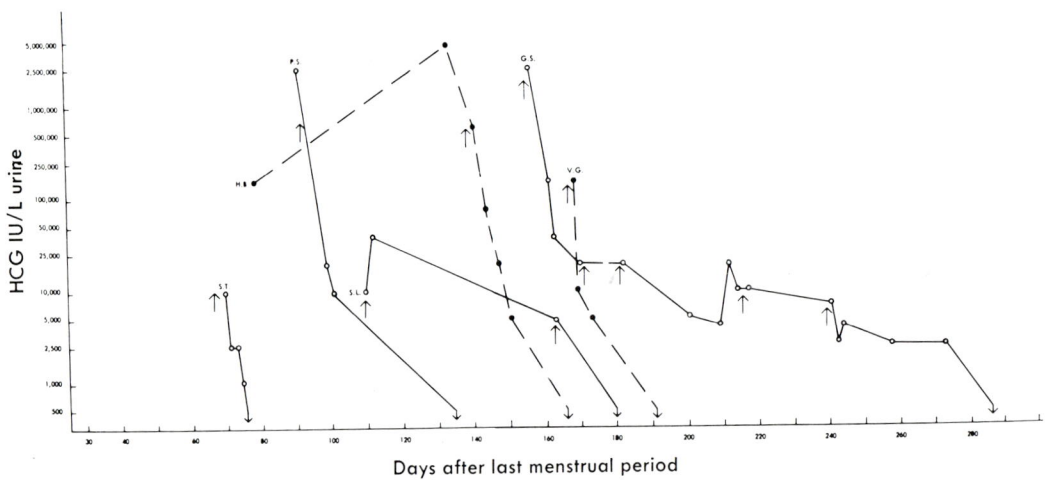

Fig. 28-13. Immunoassays of HCG in urine from six women with hydatidiform moles. First upward arrows indicate day of expulsion of mole. Any further upward arrows indicate uterine curettage on subsequent days. Downward arrows indicate first day that no urinary HCG was detected. (From Mishell, D.R., and Davajan, V.: Am. J. Obstet. Gynecol. **96:**231, 1966.)

Urinary estriol and estrogen assays

In the nonpregnant woman, urinary estriol is a metabolic end product of ovarian estrone and estradiol excretion. In the pregnant woman, estriol is excreted by the placenta and reflects mainly fetal sources (liver and adrenal) rather than maternal contributions.[59] The fetus excretes large amounts of 16-α-hydroxyepiandosterone sulfate, which is converted by placental enzymes to estriol, which enters the maternal circulation. This process results in a 1000-fold rise in maternal serum estriol concentration during an average pregnancy. The estriol can then be conjugated in the maternal liver as either the glucuronide or sulfate derivatives, which are then excreted into urine.

In the first trimester the maternal ovary is primarily responsible for the estriol excreted, but in the second and third trimesters, it is mainly the fetus who accounts for the high estriol level, thus establishing a relationship between estriol level and fetal viability.[60,61] Death of the fetus diminishes estriol excretion. The levels of estriol in maternal serum or urine (Fig. 28-14) thus reflect the interaction and integrity of fetus and placenta during gestation. Failure of the fetoplacental unit to grow or function properly will be reflected by either a decrease in estriol accumulation or a decrease in concentration.

In normal pregnancy the average urinary estriol excretion rises from 1-2 mg/24 hr at 8-12 weeks' gestation to 12-25 mg/24 hr at term[62,63] (Fig. 28-14). Although wide daily variations of the estriol level have been reported, the overall pattern in normal pregnancy is that shown in Fig. 28-14. In general, rising urinary estriol values indicate normal fetal growth and a sudden 4 mg/24 hr fall or a declining curve indicates fetal distress. In certain diseases known to portend danger to the fetus, e.g., diabetes, hypertension, and preeclampsia, serial estriol determinations two or three times a week should be performed after 33 weeks' gestation. Experience has shown that values of 4-7 mg/24 hr point toward fetal distress, and values of 4 mg/24 hr or less herald fetal death.

The measurement of either total urinary estrogens per 24 hr or estriol per 24 hr has diminished in recent years. One major reason has been the difficulty in obtaining an accurate 24 hr urine collection. This problem can be obviated by using an estriol/creatinine value on random urine samples.[65] This ratio has been shown to correlate well with the results for estriol excretion per 24 hr and has similar clinical relationships.

However, in cases of high-risk pregnancies where the monitoring of the fetoplacental unit is closely followed, changes in estriol synthesis over short periods of time are important in assessing acute change in the condition of the fetus. A decrease in estriol synthesis may be detected in serum as much as 24 hr earlier than in urine. Also, measurement of the unconjugated estriol fraction in serum gives a value independent of maternal renal and hepatic function, which can often be impaired in pregnancy. To increase the specificity even further, it has been suggested that it might be desirable to monitor serum estetrol, a tetrahydroxy estrogen produced by the fetoplacental unit.[65] For these reasons, plus the more ready availability of sensitive radioimmunoassays, the measurement of serum estriol has become a widely accepted procedure.[66]

The use of radioimmunoassays is discussed in Chapter 25, and the assay of total urinary estrogens is discussed on p. 615.

Heat-stable serum placental alkaline phosphatase

Because of the considerable variations of HCG produced by the placenta, HCG assay is not a satisfactory placental function test. Heat-stable serum placental alkaline phosphatase (HSAP) is an enzyme produced by the placenta that appears to reflect placental function better than HCG. For a number of years physical means such as heating of the serum have been used to distinguish alkaline phosphatase isoenzymes from each other, e.g., isoenzymes of hepatic, osseous, and placental origin. To separate hepatic and osseous isoenzymes, incubation at 56°C is satisfactory; but to separate placental from nonplacental alkaline phosphatases, incubation for 30 min at 65°C is necessary.[67] Serial determinations of HSAP can be used to monitor placental

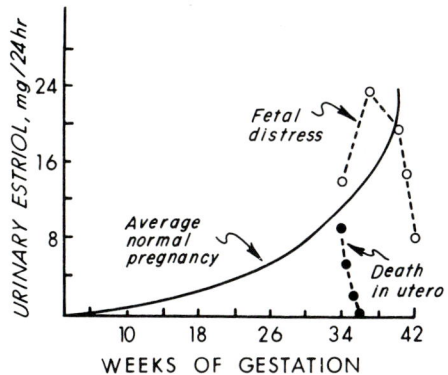

Fig. 28-14. Urinary estriol patterns in normal pregnancy, fetal distress, and fetal death in utero. (Based on Greene, J.W., Jr., and Duhring, J.L.: Hosp. Pract. **2:**74, 1967.)

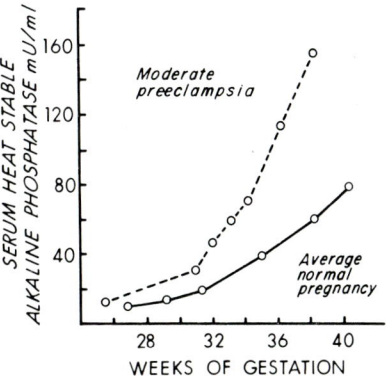

Fig. 28-15. Serum heat-stable alkaline phosphatase patterns in normal pregnancy and in moderate preeclampsia. (Based on Hunter, R.J., Pinkerton, J.H.M., and Johnston, H.: Obstet. Gynecol. **36:**536, 1970.)

function. In the course of a normal pregnancy the HSAP output increases gradually throughout the pregnancy, the largest increase occurring during the second half. The curve is smooth and curvilinear. In eclamptic patients the HSAP level is significantly higher than in normal patients, the rise depending on the degree of eclampsia, because the eclamptic placenta apparently excretes more HSAP than the normal placenta does. Furthermore, the increased production precedes fetal distress by 2-3 weeks, allowing adequate time to institute treatment. Placental failure is indicated by a sudden fall of the previously high HSAP level. A similar fall may indicate a satisfactory response to treatment, if such has been instituted (Fig. 28-15).

Although HSAP does increase with the time of gestation, this test is not considered to be especially valuable, and its use has decreased in recent years.[68] This procedure certainly does not provide more information than does the measurement of human **placental lactogen.** Like any test being used to monitor pregnancy, serial analysis is needed.

Assessment of fetal development

α-Fetoprotein concentration and the lecithin/sphingomyelin (L/S) ratio have an important bearing on perinatal morbidity and are discussed under the section on amniotic fluid in Chapter 29.

GLOSSARY

androgen Any substance that possesses masculinizing activities, e.g., testicular hormone.

choriocarcinoma Epithelial malignant tumor composed of trophoblast. It may accompnay or follow any type of pregnancy.

chorion Outermost envelope of the growing fertilized ovum.

corpora amylacea Small hyaline masses of degenerate cells found in the prostate in the prostatic component of the ejaculate.

eclampsia Convulsions and coma occurring in a pregnant or puerperal woman that are associated with hypertension, edema, or proteninuria.

estrogen Generic term for estrus-producing compounds.

hormone Chemical substance produced in the body that has a specific effect on the activity of a certain organ.

hydatidiform mole Placenta with large grapelike hydropic villi and variable trophoblastic proliferation.

lecithin A monoaminomonophosphatide found in animal tissues, especially nerve tissue, semen, and yolk of egg and in smaller amounts in bile, blood, and amniotic fluid.

macrophage A large mononuclear wandering phagocytic cell.

preeclampsia Toxemia of late pregnancy characterized by hypertension, albuminuria, and edema.

prostate Gland in the male that surrounds the neck of the bladder and the urethra. Its secretion is part of the seminal fluid.

psychotropic Exerting an effect on the mind.

Sertoli cell Elongated cell in the tubules of the testes to the ends of which the spermatids become attached, apparently for the purpose of nutrition until they become transormed into mature spermatozoa.

spermatogenesis Process of formation of spermatozoa.

teratoma Neoplasm made up of a number of different types of tissue, none of which is native to the area in which it occurs.

testosterone Hormone produced by the testes in the male that functions in the induction and maintenance of male secondary sex characteristics.

trophoblast Layer of extraembryonic ectodermal tissue on the outside of the blastodermic vesicle.

REFERENCES

1. Joel, C.A.: Fertility disturbances in men and women, a textbook with special references to etiology, diagnosis and treatment, Basel, Switzerland, 1971, S. Karger A.G.
2. Vasterling, H.W.: Praktische Spermatologie, Stuttgart, West Germany, 1960, Georg Thieme Verlag.
3. Hendry, W.F.: Br. J. Hosp. Med. **22:**47, 1979.
4. Watson, A.A., and Robertson, C.M.G.: J. Med. Lab. Tech. **23:**1, 1966.
5. Milne, J.A.: Scott. Med. J. **21:**218, 1976.
6. Raboch, J., and Skachova, J.: Fertil. Steril. **16:**252, 1965.
7. Caldamone, A.A., and Cockett, A.T.K.: Urology **12:**304, 1978.
8. Paulson, J.D., Polakoski, K.L.: Fertil. Steril. **28:**182, 1977.
9. Marmar, J.L., Katz, S., and Praiss, D.E.: Fertil. Steril. **26:**1057, 1975.
10. Joel, C.A., and Kwiat, S.: Schweiz. Med. Wochenschr. **85:**428, 1955.
11. Marwood, R.P., and Beral, V.: Br. Med. J. **1:**87, 1979.
12. Jackson, L.N.: Br. Med. J. **3:**589, 1973.
13. Edwards, I.S., and Farlow, J.L.: Br. Med. J. **1:**87, 1979.
14. Joel, K.: J. Lab. Clin. Med. **24:**970, 1939.
15. Shulman, S.: In Cohen, J., and Hendry, W.F., editors: Spermatozoa antibodies and infertility, Oxford, England, 1978, Blackwell Scientific Publications.
16. Mann, T.: The biochemistry of semen and of the male reproductive tract, London, 1964, Methuen & Co., Ltd.
17. Landau, R.L., and Loughead, R.: J. Clin. Endocrinol. **11:**1411, 1951.
18. Phadke, A.M., Samant, N.R., and Dewal, S.D.: Fertil. Steril. **24:**894, 1973.
19. Mauss, J., Börsch, G., and Tórók, L.: Fertil. Steril. **25:**411, 1974.
20. Davis, J., and Gander, J.: Anal. Biochem. **19:**72, 1967.
21. Anderson, R.A., et al.: Clin. Chem. **25:**1780-1782, 1979.
22. Phadke, A.M., Samant, N.R., and Dewal, S.D.: Fertil. Steril. **26:**1021, 1975.
23. Elstein, M., Moghissi, K.S., and Borth, R., editors: Cervical mucus in human reproduction, Copenhagen, 1977, Scriptor.
24. Ludwig, H., and Tauber, P.F., editors: Human fertilization, Littleton, Mass., 1978, PSG Publishing Co., Inc.
25. Yussman, M.A., et al.: Fertil. Steril. **21:**119, 1970.
26. Lotan, Y., and Diamant, Y.Z.: Int. J. Gynaecol. Obstet. **16:**309, 1976.
27. Karni, Z., et al.: Int. J. Fertil. **16:**185, 1971.
28. Rolan, M.: Clin. Obstet. Gynecol. **5:**218, 1962.
29. Kesseru, E.: Fertil. Steril. **24:**584-591, 1972.
30. Wolf, D.P., et al.: Fertil. Steril. **28:**41, 1977.
31. Elstein, M.: In Cohen, J., and Hendry, W.F., editors: Spermatozoa antibodies and infertility, Oxford, England, 1978, Blackwell Scientific Publications.
32. Tredway, D.R., et al.: Am. J. Obstet. Gynecol. **121:**387, 1975.
33. Moghissi, K.S.: Clin. Obstet. Gynecol. **22:**27, 1979.
34. Kremer, J., and Jager, S.: Fertil. Steril. **27:**335, 1976.
35. Kremer, J., et al.: In Cohen, J., and Hendry, W.F., editors: Spermatozoa antibodies and infertility, Oxford, England, 1978, Blackwell Scientific Publications.
36. Rumke, P., and Hellinga, G.: Am. J. Clin. Pathol. **32:**357, 1959.

37. Shulman, S.: CRC Crit. Rev. Clin. Lab. Sci. **2:**393, 1971.
38. El-Alfi, O.S., and Bassili, F.J.: Reprod. Fertil. **21:**23, 1970.
39. Menge, A.C.: Proc. Soc. Exp. Biol. Med. **135:**108, 1970.
40. Metz, C.B., Seiguer, A.C., and Castro, A.E.: Proc. Soc. Exp. Biol. Med. **140:**776, 1972.
41. Menge, A.C., and Behrman, S.J.: Clin. Obstet. Gynecol. **22:**231, 1979.
42. Rose, N.R., et al.: Clin. Exp. Immunol. **23:**175, 1976.
43. Franklin, R.R., and Dukes, C.D.: Am. J. Obstet. Gynecol. **89:**6, 1964.
44. Haas, G.G., Jr., Cines, D.B., and Schreiber, A.D.: N. Engl. J. Med. **303:**722, 1980.
45. Cines, D.B., and Schreiber, A.D.: N. Engl. J. Med. **300:**106, 1979.
46. Villee, D.B.: N. Engl. J. Med. **281:**473, 533, 1969.
47. Samaan, N. et al.: J. Clin. Endocrinol. **26:**1303, 1966.
48. Mullins, D.F., Jr., Collins, L.R., and Clark, J.R.: J. Med. Assoc. Ga. **54:**16, 1965.
49. Midgley, A.R., Jr.: Endocrinology **79:**10, 1966.
50. Noto, T.A., and Polt, S.S.: Technical improvement service, no. 7, Chicago, 1971, Commission on Continuing Education, American Society of Clinical Pathologists.
51. Driscoll, S.G., et al.: Am. J. Obstet. Gynecol. **110:**1083, 1971.
52. Mishell, D.R., and Davajan, V.: Am. J. Obstet. Gynecol. **96:**231, 1966.
53. Taymor, M.L.: Clin. Obstet. Gynecol. **10:**303, 1967.
54. Noto, T.A., and Miale, J.B.: Am. J. Clin. Pathol. **43:**311, 1965.
55. Glass, R.H., and Jesurun, H.M.: Obstet. Gynecol. **27:**66, 1966.
56. Paoletti, F., et al.: Am. J. Med. Sci. **252:**570, 1966.
57. Bagshawe, K.D.: J. Clin. Pathol. [Suppl.] **10:**140, 1976.
58. Grudzinskas, J.G., et al.: Lancet **1:**333, 1977.
59. Bolte, E.: Clin. Obstet. Gynecol. **10:**60, 1967.
60. Greene, J.W., Jr., and Touchstone, J.C.: Am. J. Obstet. Gynecol. **85:**1, 1963.
61. Watson, D., et al.: J. Clin. Pathol. **26:**249, 1973.
62. Greene, J.W., Jr., and Duhring, J.L.: Hosp. Pract. **2:**74, 1967.
63. Greene, J.W., Jr., and Tweeddale, D.N.: Clin. Obstet. Gynecol. **11:**1106, 1968.
64. Dickey, R.P., et al.: Am. J. Obstet. Gynecol. **113:**880-886, 1972.
65. Shore, J.M., and Suzuki, K.: Obstet. Gynecol. Surv. **29**(2):97-103, 1974.
66. Kirkish, L.S., et al.: Clin. Chem. **24:**1830-1832, 1978.
67. Hunter, R.J., Pinkerton, J.H.M., and Johnston, H.: Obstet. Gynecol. **36:**536, 1970.
68. Korday, A.R., et al.: Br. J. Obstet. Gynaecol. **82:**882, 1973.

CHAPTER 29

Examination of biologic fluids, sputum, and pus

PLEURAL, PERICARDIAL, AND PERITONEAL EFFUSIONS

In health the spaces surrounding the lungs, heart, and abdominal organs are compressed into slitlike compartments because parietal and visceral mesothelial linings almost touch each other, being separated only by a minute amount of clear lubricating fluid. The potential space surrounding the lungs is the pleural cavity, the one surrounding the heart is the pericardial cavity, and the one surrounding the abdominal organs is the peritoneal cavity. Physiologically the fluid flow in the body cavities is controlled by (1) the osmotic and hydrostatic pressures of the plasma and (2) the permeability of blood vessels, lymphatics, and mesothelium. An imbalance in these factors may lead to a pathologic accumulation of fluid, or effusions, in these cavities. All effusions, irrespective of their anatomic location, have much in common, so that one diagnostic approach applies to all.

Collection of specimen

The specimen is obtained by a physician, who must tap the cavity involved with a sterile syringe and needle and should collect about 20 ml fluid in a sterile flask containing 2 ml sterile 4% sodium citrate or a few drops of sterile heparin. Also a small amount of fluid without citrate or heparin is collected in order to observe clot formation. A separate heparinized syringe (3 ml) should be used for pH measurements.

Laboratory investigation: The results of the following investigations should be recorded[1]:

1. Physical examination
   a. Amount
   b. Color and transparency
   c. pH
   d. Specific gravity
2. Biochemical examination
   a. Protein
   b. Cholesterol
   c. Glucose
   d. Lactic acid dehydrogenase
3. Bacteriologic examination
   a. Gram stain
   b. Acid-fast stain
   c. Culture (routine and acid fast)
4. Cytologic examination
   a. Cell count and differential count
   b. Papanicolaou smear for malignant cells

Characteristics of normal serous fluid: The normal fluid of body cavities is present in such small amounts that it cannot be aspirated. It is believed that it is similar to interstitial fluid.[2]

Amount: about 1 ml (just moistens mesothelium of serous cavities)
Color: straw colored
Transparency: clear
pH: 7.4
Specific gravity: less than 1.016

Total protein: 1-2 g/dl
Noncolloidal solutes: sodium, potassium, chloride, glucose, etc. (same level as in plasma)
Clot formation: none
Sediment: few scattered lymphocytes and mesothelial cells

Physical examination

Amount: The amount of the effusion is measured in graduated cylinder.

Color: Fluid color may indicate the origin of the effusion: red (blood, fresh or changed), green (bile from gallbladder, duodenal ulcer, or pancreatitis), and milky (chyle from a possible lymphatic obstruction).

Transparency and general appearance: Fluids may be serous, fibrinous, purulent, milky (chylous), putrid, sanguineous, or combinations of these.

If the fluid is milky, make it alkaline with a few drops of sodium hydroxide and shake with ether. Fat dissolves in ether; thus the fluid clears if fat causes the turbidity.

pH: The pH must be measured anaerobically as for arterial blood without undue delay. The pH of the effusion is of some diagnostic importance since acidosis of the fluid is encountered in leakage of gastric fluid through a perforated esophagus or peptic ulcer, rheumatoid pleurisy[3,4] (pH less than 7.2), empyema,[5] and tuberculosis,[6] whereas the pH in malignancy and systemic lupus erythematosus exceeds 7.35.

Generally, a pH of an effusion below 7.3 indicates a poor prognosis in parapneumonic processes, requiring surgical intervention.[7]

Specific gravity: Use a hydrometer to measure specific gravity. The specific gravity reflects the protein content of the fluid.

Clot formation: Record the presence or absence of clots and state whether clot formation is slight, weblike, or en masse.

Clot formation reflects fibrinogen content. Fibrinogen is a large molecular protein and does not escape unless there is much damage to the mesothelium.

Biochemical examination

Proteins

Screening test: Use a **refractometer** (TS meter, American Optical Corp., Buffalo, N.Y.) calibrated for protein.

Quantitative test: Use the method given in Chapter 21.

Interpretation: See the later discussion of transudates and exudates.

Glucose

Screening test: Use reagent strip (Ames Co., Elkhart, Ind.) as for urine.

Quantitative test: Use the method given in Chapter 21.

Interpretation: The concentration of glucose in effusions is the same as in plasma, the level of which should be determined at the same time the sugar level of the serous fluid is measured. The equilibration of plasma and serous fluid is not immediate and requires several hours. In bacterial (including tuberculous) in-

fections, rheumatoid arthritis, and malignancies the sugar level is depressed. In systemic lupus erythematosus the glucose level is normal, a phenomenon that may help to distinguish systemic lupus erythematosus from rheumatoid arthritis.[8]

Lactic dehydrogenase

The serum and serous fluid levels of lactic dehydrogenase (LDH) must be determined simultaneously. The method given in Chapter 24 should be used.

Interpretation: Primary and metastatic tumors involving the mesothelium produce elevated LDH levels in serous fluids. The LDH level aids in the differentiation of transudates from exudates (see below).[9] In inflammatory and malignant effusion, pleural fluid LDH levels are above 550 units; in transudates, they are below 550 units. In ascitic fluid a maximal LDH elevation (as compared to serum) is seen in patients with malignancy.[10] The LDH concentration in rheumatoid arthritis exceeds 700 units/L, whereas in systemic lupus erythematosus it is below 500 units/L.

Amylase

In acute pancreatitis the amylase level of abdominal and pleural fluid is higher than the serum amylase level and remains elevated longer.[11] The amylase level is also elevated in perforated peptic ulcer and necrosis of the intestines.

Microscopic examination

White cell count: If fluid is slightly cloudy or bloody, moisten a small pipet with glacial acetic acid; blow out excess. Mix specimen thoroughly and draw 1-3 drops of fluid into a pipet. Mix by rotating the pipet and transfer to a blood counting chamber, filling both sides. If there are few cells, count 10 fields, 1 mm^2 each. In this case the number of cells counted equals the number of cells per cubic millimeter. When there are many cells, count as for leukocytes in blood.

Interpretation: See the later discussion of transudates and exudates.

Differential count: Centrifuge citrated specimen, pour off supernatant, smear sediment on slide, allow to dry, and stain with Wright stain. Proceed with differential count as described in Chapter 7.

Interpretation: See the later discussion of transudates and exudates.

Culture

For a discussion of culture technics for effusions see Chapter 32.

Papanicolaou technic for malignant cells

Prevent clotting by the addition of heparin or EDTA. Use the Cytocentrifuge (Shandon Southern Instruments, Sewickley, Pa.) technic and prepare smears as soon as the fluid is delivered to the laboratory. If delay is unavoidable, mix well, and store in a refrigerator until the material can be centrifuged and smeared.

Tissue sections

Pack the sediment by centrifuging, carefully decant supernatant fluid, and fix by overlaying the sediment with 10% formalin. With a fine capillary glass rod, carefully loosen the sediment from the sides of the centrifuge tube and allow to harden. Use paraffin method as for tissue specimen.

Rheumatoid factor

In seropositive rheumatoid patients the effusion is positive for rheumatoid factor with a titer greater than in the serum. In lupus erythematosus effusion the factor is not present. Unfortunately the rheumatoid factor is present also in effusions accompanying bacterial pneumonia (41%), carcinoma (21%), and tuberculosis (14%).[12] Rheumatoid effusions are also rich in immune complexes, which can be detected by monoclonal rheumatoid factor radioimmunoassay (RIA), Clq binding assay, and Raji cell RIA.[3] The immune complexes are not found in systemic lupus erythematosus, since the latter is an expression of intravascular immune complexes[3] rather than of extravascular complexes as seen in rheumatoid arthritis. (See Chapters 35 and 36.)

Transudates and exudates

Clinically, effusions are divided into transudates and exudates (Table 29-1). A transudate occurs when there is an increase in the osmotic or hydrostatic pressure of the capillaries of the body cavities, whereas an exudate is the result of inflammation and injury of the mesothelial lining, which becomes increasingly permeable.

Transudates

Transudates (noninflammatory serous fluids)[13] are generally clear, serous, light yellow fluids, usually resulting from cardiac failure, venous obstruction, or hypoproteinemia (caused by renal or hepatic disease). While the specific gravity of these fluids is often below 1.015, it can vary from 1.010-1.020. Although the total protein concentration is usually below 3 g/dl, the absolute protein concentration is less useful in distinguishing exudates from transudates than the ratio of fluid protein to serum protein. The transudate does not clot because of its low fibrinogen content. The sugar content is approximately the same as in blood. The sediment reveals a few white cells, red cells, and mesothelial cells after centrifugation. A predominance of mesothelial cells suggests neoplastic involvement of the pleura.

Exudates

Exudates (inflammatory serous fluids)[13] may be clear, cloudy, serous, fibrinous, purulent, hemorrhagic, chylous, or a combination of these. In pulmonary tuberculosis, the pleural effusion is usually serofibrinous; in pyogenic infections (pneumococcal and staphylococcal) it is usually purulent; it is serosanguinopurulent in streptococcal infections; and it is often hemorrhagic in malignancy.

In mild inflammation the fluid resembles serous fluid. In chronic or severe inflammatory processes the fluid composition changes.

The most consistent biochemical characteristics of exudates are a fluid/serum protein ratio greater than 0.5, a fluid/serum LDH activity ratio greater than 0.6, and an absolute fluid LDH activity greater than 200 IU/L. The presence of at least one of these factors has been reported by Light et al.[14] to give a diagnostic sensitivity and specificity of greater than 98%. The specific gravity is usually 1.018 but may be as high as 1.02. The protein content of exudates more closely resembles that of plasma than does the protein profile of transudates. As the fibrinogen content is increased to about 7% of the total protein, the fluid may clot spontaneously.

Cultures frequently grow the causative organisms.

Examination of the sediment after centrifugation reveals a predominance of polymorphonuclear cells in pyogenic infections and predominance of lymphocytes in tuberculous infections, chronic pyogenic infections, viral infections, and lymphoproliferative disorders. The predominance of mesothelial cells mixed with red cells suggests malignant disease. The predominance of eosinophils suggests a hypersensitivity reaction.

Although exudates tend to have more red cells and white cells than do transudates, the diagnostic accuracy of these criteria is relatively poor unless the numbers of cells present are quite large (over 100,000 red cells or 2500 white cells).[14,15]

The sugar content is decreased[16] (less than 60 mg/dl) except in exudates from patients with lupus erythematosus, in which the sugar level reflects the plasma level.[17] In exudates from patients with rheumatoid arthritis the sugar level is decreased as in most exudates.[8] In some types of fluids, cholesterol crystals are associated with an increased cholesterol content. The crystals

Table 29-1. Differentiation of transudate (noninflammatory) and exudate (inflammatory) serous fluids

	Transudate	**Exudate**
Color	Clear, straw colored	Clear, turbid, bloody, purulent
Total proteins	Less than 50% of serum levels	Greater than 50% of serum levels
LDH	Less than 60% of serum levels	Greater than 60% of serum levels
Fibrinogen	0.3%-4%	4-6% or greater
Clot formation	None	Usually
Red cells	Usually few to none	Often present in high numbers
White cells	Usually few to none	Often present in high numbers
Glucose	As in plasma	Often less than in plasma, especially in lupus erythematosus, empyema, malignancy, and tuberculosis
Differential count	Few lymphocytes or mesothelial cells	Lymphocytes, neutrophils, and polymorphonuclear cells
Amylase	—	Usually less than half of serum value unless pancreatitis is present

are flat, transparent, and rhombic, with one corner notched (Fig. 29-1).

Clinical correlation of transudates and exudates[18]

Serous pleural effusions (transudates): Serous effusions (with a fluid protein/serum protein ratio below 0.5) may develop in the course of cardiac insufficiency, hypoalbuminemia (nephrosis, cirrhosis of liver), obstruction to venous flow, constrictive pericarditis, and Meigs' syndrome (benign uterine and ovarian tumors).

Serofibrinous pleural effusions (exudates): Serous effusions (with fluid protein/serum protein ratios above 0.5) may accompany pulmonary tuberculosis, bacterial and viral pneumonias, pulmonary infarcts, metastatic pleural involvement, mesothelioma, rheumatoid pneumonia, trauma to chest wall and pleura, uremia, acute pancreatitis, periarteritis nodosa, and sarcoidosis.

Purulent effusion: Purulent effusion (with a fluid protein/serum ratio above 0.5) is seen in empyema, pleural extension of subdiaphragmatic abscess, trauma, and actinomycosis.

Hemorrhagic effusion: Hemorrhagic effusion follows trauma, pulmonary infarct, and tumor involvement (primary or secondary) (Fig. 29-2).

Chylous effusion: Traumatic injury to the thoracic duct and involvement of the duct by tumor or by scarring may cause chylous effusion. The latter is milky and creamy and can be cleared with ether extraction and stained with Sudan III. Lipoprotein electrophoresis demonstrates a wide chylomicron band. For differentiation from cholesterol effusion see below.

Cholesterol effusion: Cholesterol effusion[19] is usually caused by tuberculosis, malignancy, hypothyroidism, or rheumatoid arthritis. The fluid contains choles-

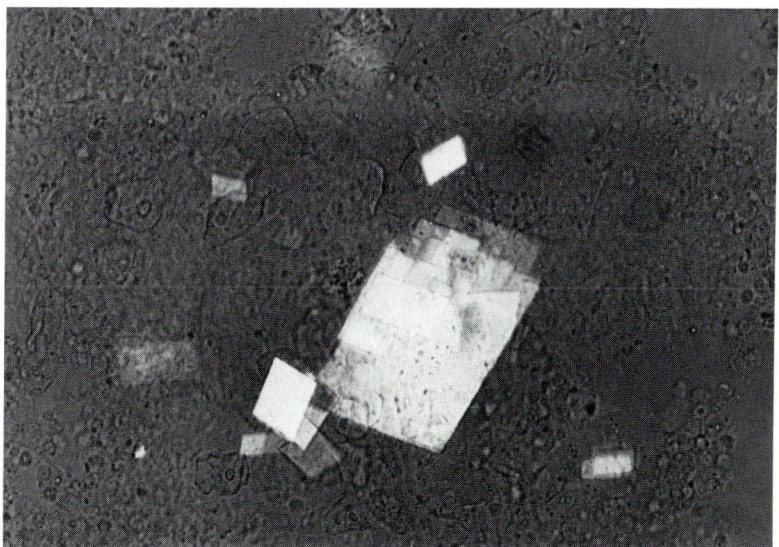

Fig. 29-1. Cholesterol crystals in biologic fluid (polarized light).

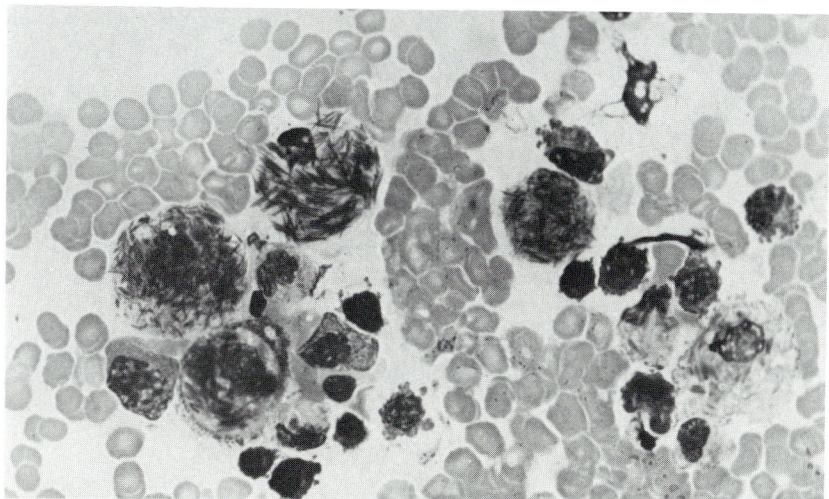

Fig. 29-2. Hemorrhagic effusion in multiple myeloma; paraprotein crystals in tumor cells.

terol crystals, does not stain with Sudan III, does not clear with ether, and does not reveal a chylomicron band on the lipoprotein electrophoretogram. The cholesterol concentration may reach several thousand milligrams per deciliter.

CEREBROSPINAL FLUID

Cerebrospinal fluid (CSF) is the product of continuous secretory activity of choroidal and extrachoroidal sites of the brain.[20,21] It fills the ventricles and the subarachnoid space surrounding the brain and the spinal cord. Fifty percent of the fluid is formed in the choroid plexuses, and the remainder escapes from the vessels lining the ventricles (choroidal and extrachoroidal origin of CSF).[22] Each choroid plexus is the result of the invagination of the ependyma (the transparent delicate lining of the ventricles) by the blood vessels of the pia mater. The choroid plexus of the fourth ventricle protrudes through the foramina of Luschka and Magendie into the subarachnoid space (Fig. 29-3) allowing the CSF to leave the ventricular system, fill the subarachnoid space, and be absorbed through the arachnoid villi into the cerebral sinuses. The production of CSF is the result of two separate processes: (1) filtration across the choroidal capillary wall and (2) secretion by choroidal epithelium.

Collection of specimen

The CSF sample is obtained by a physician, usually by lumbar puncture and occasionally by the suboccipi-

tal route. During radiologic or surgical procedures, CSF may be obtained directly from the ventricles of the brain. The specimen should be collected in three sterile, labeled, capped tubes that are numbered 1, 2, and 3 in the order in which they are filled. Each tube should contain 2-4 ml CSF. Tube 1 may be contaminated with blood and may have to be discarded. Tube 2 should contain enough spinal fluid for all tests requested. Tube 3 is reserved for the bacteriologic investigation.

If **tuberculous meningitis** is suspected, a fourth specimen should be collected and placed in the refrigerator without being shaken in order to observe clot formation. If the fluid is very cloudy or highly colored, one specimen should be collected in a test tube containing 0.5 ml sterile 4% sodium citrate/5 ml CSF to prevent clotting.

Characteristics of normal spinal fluid[23-25]

Total volume: 150 ml
Color: colorless, like water
Transparency: clear, like water
Osmolality at 37°C: 281 mOsm/L
Specific gravity: 1.006-1.008
Acid-base balance:

pH	7.31
Pco_2	47.9 mm Hg
HCO_3^-	22.9 mEq/L

Sodium: 138-150 mEq/L
Potassium: 2.7-3.9 mEq/L
Chloride: 116-127 mEq/L

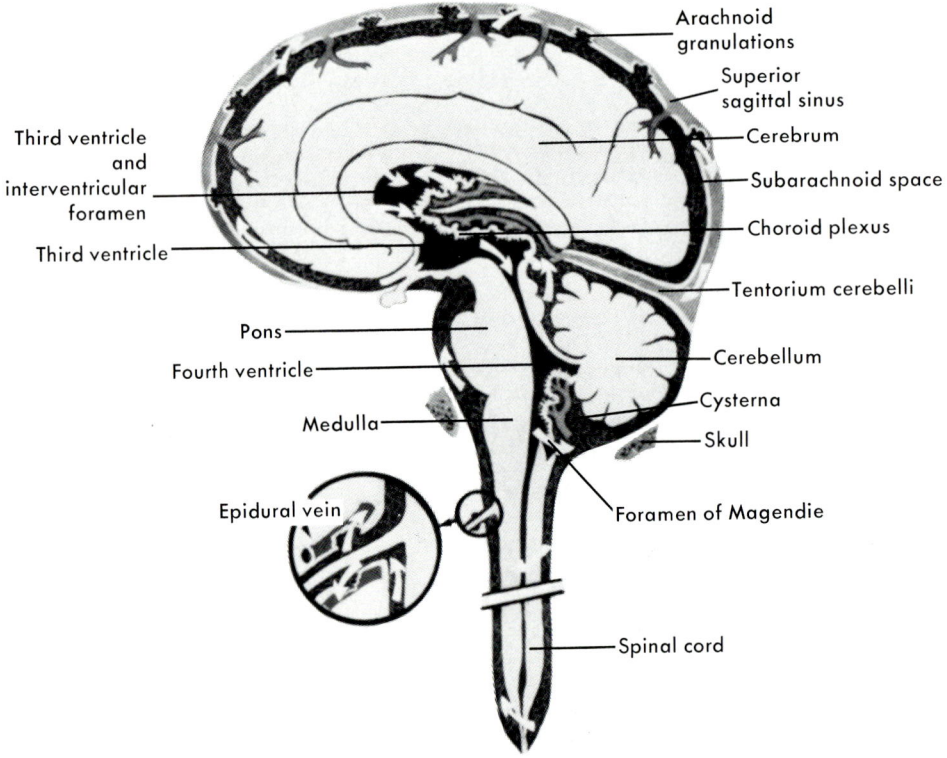

Fig. 29-3. Circulation of cerebrospinal fluid (black areas). (Modified from Fishman, R.A.: Cerebrospinal fluid in diseases of the nervous system, Philadelphia, 1980, W.B. Saunders Co.)

Calcium: 2.0-2.5 mEq/L
Magnesium: 2.0-2.5 mEq/L
Lactic acid: 1.1-2.8 mmole/L
Lactic acid dehydrogenase: Absolute activity depends on method, approximately 10% of serum value
Creatinine: 0.4-1.5 mg/dl
Glucose: 45-60 mg/dl
Glutamic oxalacetic transaminase: 0-19 units
Urea: 8-28 mg/dl
Uric acid: 0.07-2.8 mg/dl
Phosphorus, inorganic: 1.2-2.1 mg/dl
Proteins: 20-40 mg/dl

Lumbar	20-40 mg/dl
Cisternal	15-25 mg/dl
Ventricular	5-10 mg/dl

Normal values in children:

Up to 6 days of age	70.0 mg/dl
Up to 4 years	24.4 mg/dl

Electrophoretic separation of spinal fluid proteins:

Prealbumin	2-7%
Albumin	56-76%
α_1-Globulin	2-7%
α_2-Globulin	3.5-12%
β- and τ-Globulin	8-18%
γ-Globulin	7-12%
IgG	1-4 mg/dl
IgA	0-0.2 mg/dl
IgM	0-0.06 mg/dl
κ/λ ratio	1.0

Erythrocyte count:

Newborn	0-675/mm^3
Adult	0-10/mm^3

Leukocyte count:

< 1 year	0-30/mm^3
1-4 years	0-20/mm^3
5 years to puberty	0-10/mm^3
Adult	0-5/mm^3

Identification of cerebrospinal fluid: To differentiate CSF from other biologic fluids see Table 27-1.

Characteristics of cerebrospinal fluid from different levels: The composition varies somewhat with the level from which the specimen is obtained. The protein varies from about 5-10 mg/dl in the ventricles to about 40 mg/dl in the lumbar area. The chlorides show no variation, and the reducing substances are only slightly decreased from above downward.

Physical examination[26]

Spinal fluid should be examined at once.

Color: Normal CSF fluid is clear and colorless. Abnormal colors may be produced by blood, bile, yellow pigments (xanthochromia), or pus.

Blood: If gross inspection reveals much blood, omit the CSF examination except for the culture, but examine a wet preparation of the bloody fluid microscopically for presence or absence of crenated red cells.

If moderate amounts of blood are present, the CSF cell count and the protein determination can roughly be corrected for the presence of blood. See discussion of method of counting mixture of white and red cells on p. 759. Blood contributes 1 mg protein/dl CSF for each 700 RBCs/mm^3 provided the blood chemistry measurements are within normal limits. The fluid is cloudy, xanthochromic, or slightly pink if there are 500-6000 erythrocytes/mm^3.

Bloody tap and the three-tube test[27]: When the CSF is bloody it becomes necessary to decide whether the blood is caused by a traumatic spinal puncture or a preexisting subarachnoid hemorrhage. At the time of the spinal puncture the fluid should be collected in three separate test tubes. Blood resulting from injury to blood vessels in the course of the puncture is not evenly distributed in the three specimens; there is more blood in the first tube and little or none in the last tube. In doubtful cases the cell counts of the fluid in the first and the last tubes should be compared. Bilirubin is absent. After centrifugation, the supernatant fluid should be clear and colorless. The CSF tends to clear in 2-5 days after a bloody tap.

In subarachnoid and cerebral hemorrhage the blood is evenly mixed in all three tubes, and if the specimen is centrifuged, the supernatant fluid is yellowish a few hours after the hemorrhage. Crenated red cells are observed in the sediment when examined microscopically in wet preparation; they do not clot. The CSF remains discolored for several weeks. Bilirubin is increased after 2 days. The supernatant can be red following in vivo lysis of red cells. In vivo lysis can occur within 4-10 hr of a subarachnoid hemorrhage. The peroxidase test for blood can be positive unless hemoglobin metabolism has progressed to the bilirubin stage. Oxidation of hemoglobin to methemoglobin can result in a brownish coloration to CSF. The sedimented blood has a tendency to clot. If wet preparations of the bloody sediment are examined microscopically, the red cells are recognized as normal biconcave disks.

Clear spinal fluid does not rule out intracranial hemorrhage, since fewer than 360 RBCs/mm^3 cannot be seen with the naked eye. Traumatic bleeding and subarachnoid hemorrhage may occur together.[28]

Xanthochromia: Xanthochromia refers to a yellowish discoloration of the spinal fluid. Its presence is indicative of past subarachnoid and cerebral bleeding with subsequent degradation of released hemoglobin to bilirubin and other hemoglobin metabolites. Destruction of brain tissue can also result in yellowish lipidlike substances in CSF.[29] A yellow CSF containing a large amount of protein and tending to clot en masse (Froin's syndrome) indicates the formation of a cul-de-sac below some obstruction, e.g., a tumor, but is also seen in polyneuritis and meningitis. The tests for blood and for bile pigment are usually negative.

In jaundice the CSF is not usually yellow, except in severe and chronic icterus (bilirubin level above 6 mg/dl). The van den Bergh test is positive for nonconjugated bilirubin in cases of chronic hemolytic anemias. Xanthochromia can also occur in normal full-term and premature infants and may persist for several weeks even in the absence of jaundice. It has not been determined whether this xanthochromia is physiologic or pathologic.[30] Peripheral blood carotenemia can also impart a yellow tinge to CSF.

Usually yellow CSF is caused by disintegrated blood, as seen after subarachnoid and cerebral hemorrhage or after hemorrhage caused by previous lumbar puncture. Xanthochromic fluid with protein levels below 150 mg/dl usually indicates subarachnoid or intracerebral hemorrhage.[31]

Transparency: Normal spinal fluid is clear. Turbidity is usually caused by an increase in cellular elements. Fewer than 200 WBCs/mm[3] do not give rise to macroscopic clouding of the fluid. Haziness is produced by 200-500 WBCs/mm[3] and over 500 WBCs/mm[3] causes turbidity. Lower concentrations of cells (either leukocytes or erythrocytes) can be detected by the Tyndall effect, which is based on the scattering of light by small particles. The tube is held into a beam of daylight against a black background and the CSF is agitated by flicking the tube with one finger. A cell-free control must be observed under similar circumstances.[32] In acute meningitis the fluid may vary from slight cloudiness to almost pure pus. It is clear in tuberculous meningitis and in encephalitis.

Clot and pellicle formation: Clot formation indicates the presence of fibrinogen. Normally a clot does not form, since normal CSF does not contain fibrinogen. Clot formation is enhanced by refrigeration. Record the presence or absence of a clot and also the type of cot. In paresis there may be small clots; in tuberculous meningitis, a weblike clot; in purulent meningitis, a large clot; and in blockage of spinal fluid circulation, a tendency to clot en masse because of the high protein (fibrinogen) content. In suppurative meningitis the pellicle forms in a short time; in tuberculous meningitis it may take up to 12-24 hr. Microscopically the pellicle consists of white cells against a fibrinous background and should be examined for bacteria by culture, Gram stain, and acid-fast stains. Bloody CSF will also clot if the red cell count exceeds 1 million RBCs/ml CSF.[31]

Biochemical examination[23]

The methods of qualitative and quantitative analysis of the various components are discussed in Unit IV unless some features are specific for CSF.

Calcium

Because calcium is not affected by central nervous system diseases, there is no clinical justification for its assay in CSF.[31]

Chlorides

The normal CSF chloride level is higher than the serum level. In hypochloremia and hyperchloremia it reflects the serum changes, and there is therefore no reason for its assay in CSF.[31]

Proteins

The CSF protein concentration is less than 1% of the serum protein concentration and depends on the sampling site. The protein concentration is highest in the lumbar spinal fluid (20-40 mg/dl). It is lowest in the ventricular fluid, varying from 5-10 mg/dl, and in cisternal fluid it is between 15 and 25 mg/dl. The latter value tends to be even lower in children (10-20 mg/dl). The normal ratio of albumin to total globulin comes close to 1:1.

Quantitative protein assay: The method based on the principle of the protein-dye complex formation[33,34] is four times more sensitive than the trichloroacetic acid method. Both methods are described on pp. 501 and 502. It requires only one reagent, Coomassie brilliant blue, and is available in kit form (Environmental Clinical Specialties, Anaheim, Calif.).

Interpretation: Under pathologic conditions the spinal fluid may show an increase in the total protein level and an alteration in the albumin/globulin (A/G) ratio. Marked elevations of protein in the range of 500 mg to a few thousand milligrams per deciliter occur in Froin's syndrome (complete spinal block), meningitis, and Guillain-Barré syndrome. In Froin's syndrome it is the fluid entrapped below the block that contains the elevated protein concentration. The etiology of the block is quite varied and includes such conditions as spinal cord tumors, arachnoiditis, extramedullary abscesses, and systemic tumors (multiple myeloma, metastatic carcinoma).

A rise in CSF protein is seen in various diseases as a result of three primary mechanisms. These are (1) decreased absorption, (2) increased local synthesis of immunoglobulins, and (3) increased capillary permeability.

The increase in CSF protein seen in a number of disease entities is a relatively nonspecific indicator of the etiology of the disease. The usefulness of CSF protein measurements can be increased by comparing CSF protein and albumin to the concentration of these proteins in serum. A useful index[35-37] combining these factors has been proposed:

$$\text{IgG-albumin index} = \frac{\text{CSF IgG/serum IgG}}{\text{CSF albumin/serum albumin}}$$

The **IgG-albumin index** can be used to distinguish diseases affecting permeability (meningitis, cerebral infarctions, neoplastic infiltration of the spinal cord, tumors of the brain or spine, and polyneuropathies) from diseases resulting in increased immunoglobulin (usually IgG) synthesis (i.e., multiple sclerosis and other demyelinating diseases) and some inflammatory diseases (e.g., idiopathic polyneuropathies). A normal range for this index has been proposed to be 0.34-0.58. In diseases associated with increased IgG production, the ratio is elevated, whereas in diseases affecting CSF permeability the ratio is decreased because of increased CSF albumin concentration. Of course, some disorders can affect both CSF IgG concentration and blood permeability.

Low spinal fluid protein concentrations (3-20 mg/dl) may be encountered in infants, in increased intracranial pressure,[38] and after removal of large volumes of spinal fluid.

Fractionation of cerebrospinal fluid protein: The fractionation of CSF proteins is accomplished by cellulose acetate electrophoresis, immunoelectrophoresis, immunodiffusion, and radioimmunoassay.

Protein electrophoresis: The CSF electrophoretogram differs from that of serum not only in the quantitative distribution of the fractions but also in the quality of some of the proteins.[39,40]

In CSF the percentage of albumin is increased compared to the corresponding serum value, while the percentage of CSF γ-globulin is less than the serum value.

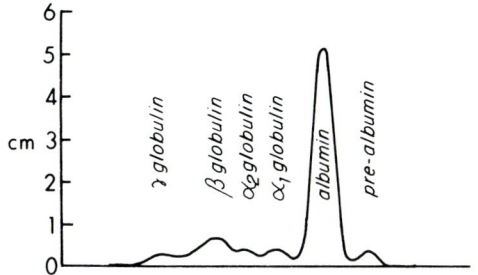

Fig. 29-4. Normal CSF electrophoretogram. Note prealbumin and elevation of β-globulin.

In addition, CSF electrophoresis shows a characteristic "prealbumin" band whose percentage of total (CSF) protein is much higher than in serum (Fig. 29-4). An additional band is found between γ and β, the τ-fraction, which resembles a slow β and is not found in serum. It probably represents modified transferrin.[41,42] The A/G ratio is usually close to 1:1.

Normal range: The following are normal values for CSF protein fractions (percent of total CSF protein)[24,43]:

Prealbumin: 2-7%
Albumin: 56-76%
α-Globulin: 2-7%
$α_2$-Globulin: 3.5-12%
β- and τ-Globulins: 8-18%
γ-Globulin: 5-12%

Interpretation: γ-Globulin elevations are seen in multiple sclerosis, brain tumors, neurosyphilis, and subacute sclerosing leukoencephalitis.[44] The elevation of γ-globulin produces a change in the A/G ratio but may not materially influence the total protein level, because the albumin fraction will either be normal or decreased. γ-Globulin levels exceeding 15% are considered increased.

Oligoclonal bands: In inflammatory diseases of the CNS not only is there a quantitative increase in γ-globulins, but there is also a qualitative change. The latter change can be demonstrated by agarose electrophoresis of CSF in multiple sclerosis and other inflammatory brain diseases in which the γ-globulin does not migrate toward the negative pole (cathode) as a homogeneous band but breaks up into several discrete bands, which can be demonstrated in the gel by staining with amido black or Coomassie blue[45,46] (Fig. 29-5).

Interpretation: The presence of oligoclonal bands has been reported to have a sensitivity of 77% for multiple sclerosis but a specificity of 99%.[47] Other diseases demonstrating CSF oligoclonal bands are neurosyphilis, subacute sclerosing panencephalitis, and polyneuropathy. In these conditions oligoclonal bands may be detected even if the CSF γ-globulin concentration is normal. Since these bands are not found in serum, they may represent antibodies produced in the central nervous system. These bands are not seen in vascular diseases, brain tumors, or other nonimunologic brain diseases.

Myelin basic protein: Myelin basic protein is a my-

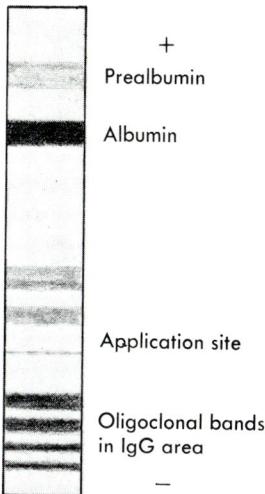

Fig. 29-5. Agarose electrophoresis pattern in multiple sclerosis. (Data from Johnson, K.P., et al.: Neurology [Minneap.] 27:273, 1977.)

elin protein that is found in the CSF of patients in the acute phase of multiple sclerosis. It is demonstrated by radioimmunoassay methods and is not found in normal CSF,[48,49] but its relationship to the oligoclonal bands of agarose electrophoresis awaits further research.

Immunoelectrophoresis: The immunoelectrophoretic technic permits identification of immunologically distinct proteins, e.g., IgG, IgA, IgM, IgD, and IgE, lipoproteins, haptoglobulins, and transferrin.[50-52]

Procedure: The immunoelectrophoresis is performed on the spinal fluid, which is concentrated 100 times by the Minicon multiple ultrafilter technic (Amicon Corp., Lexington, Mass.).

Interpretation: Immunoelectrophoretic abnormalities may be found in the γ-globulins even though they appear to be normal in the conventional CSF electrophoretogram. IgM is increased in meningitis, tumors, and multiple sclerosis. Increases in IgG are seen in inflammatory diseases of the brain, subacute sclerosing leukoencephalitis, brain tumor, neurosyphilis, rubella encephalopathy, and, strikingly, in multiple sclerosis. A small percentage of patients with multiple sclerosis also show some IgA elevation. The normal κ-λ **ratio** in CSF is about 1.0, but in multiple sclerosis and inflammatory brain diseases the ratio is elevated to 2.6 ± 1.3.[53]

Radial immunodiffusion: Radial immunodiffusion is a sensitive (1 mg IgG/dl CSF) method of quantitating immunoglobulins.[54-56] In the diagnosis of multiple sclerosis and many other brain diseases the elevation of IgG is a most valuable diagnostic feature and IgG is the only immunoglobulin requiring quantitation.

Principle: See Chapter 35.

Reagents: Use commercially available low-level human IgG immunoplates that contain antihuman IgG antiserum in buffered agar gel interrupted by 12 prepunched wells. Purchase IgG standards of 4, 10, and 30 mg/dl and prepare lower standards of 1 and 2 mg/dl by diluting the commercial standards with saline.

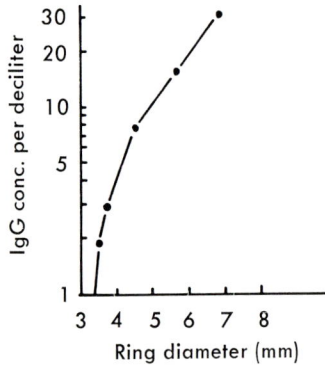

Fig. 29-6. Calibration curve. Quantitation of IgG in CSF by radial immunodiffusion. Ring diameter is directly proportional to logarithm of IgG concentration in agar.

Procedure: Fill wells exactly with refrigerated CSF; reserve five wells for the above-mentioned standards (1, 2, 4, 10, and 30 mg/dl). Cover the plates and incubate for 4 hr at 37° C. After incubation, measure the diameter of precipitin rings to the nearest 0.1 mm, using a precision magnifier with a 15 × 0.1 mm division reticle. Measure the diameter of the rings of the standards. Plot the concentrations of the standards on the vertical axis and the ring diameter in 0.1 mm units on the horizontal axis of semilog graph paper (Fig. 29-6). Draw a line or curve connecting these points. Read the concentration of the unknown immnoglobulin from the standard curve.

Normal values: The normal values with radial immunodiffusion are 1-4 mg/dl. The IgG values may be reported as follows[35,36]:
1. Absolute concentration of IgG
2. IgG/total protein (%) (normal range: 5-12%)
3. IgG/albumin ratio (normal range: 0.10-0.18)
4. IgG index (see above)

Glucose

The spinal fluid glucose concentration varies with the blood sugar level, normally remaining between 50-80% of the latter. A blood specimen for glucose determination should therefore be obtained immediately before performing the spinal puncture. The spinal fluid sugar elevation lags 2-4 hr behind any rise in blood glucose content.

Normal range: Since approximately 4 hr is required for CSF glucose to equilibrate with serum glucose, a fasting CSF glucose value must be compared with the corresponding postprandial serum value. The CSF glucose concentration varies at different levels of the spinal canal. The highest level is found in the ventricular fluid (100 mg/dl) and the lowest in the lumbar fluid. CSF glucose levels in premature newborns are lower than for full-term infants (24-63 mg/dl vs. 34-119 mg/dl).[24]

Low levels of spinal glucose (below 40 mg/dl) are associated with hypoglycemia and are also encountered in pyogenic, tuberculous, and fungal meningitides, toxoplasmosis, sarcoidosis, subarachnoid hemorrhage, primary and secondary tumors of the brain and choroid plexus, lymphomas, leukemias, meningeal carcinomatosis, and melanomatosis. The depressed sugar levels are explained on the basis of (1) increased utilization of glucose in anaerobic glycolysis and by polymorphonuclear leukocytes and (2) inhibition of entry of glucose because of membrane changes.[31]

The CSF sugar levels remain normal in some viral infections of the brain and meninges.

High levels of CSF glucose are found in diabetes, in some cases of encephalitis, e.g., postinfectious encephalitis (mumps), and in some conditions associated with increased intracranial pressure, e.g., after cerebral trauma, brain tumors, and hypothalamic lesions. Increased glucose levels are of no diagnostic significance except for the fact that the presence of hyperglycemia may mask a reduction in CSF glucose concentration.

Lactic acid: Since CNS glucose levels depend on serum levels, the measurement of CSF lactic acid has been recommended. Independent of serum lactic acid concentrations, an increase in CSF lactic acid accurately reflects increased glucose utilization in this fluid. CSF lactic acid levels above 35 mg/dl (3.9 mEq/L) have been reported in bacterial, fungal, and mycobacterial infections but not in viral infections of the spine.[57,58] A fall in CSF lactic acid levels is also indicative of effective therapy in such purulent infections.[59]

Acid-base balance

Because of the blood-brain–CSF barrier, the changes in the blood acid-base balance (pH, P_{CO_2}, HCO_3^-) are not necessarily reflected in the CSF; at times they actually move in opposite directions.[60–62] In general the lumbar fluid can be accepted as representing the steady state of the CSF, whereas the cisternal fluid is subject to frequent changes.

The normal CSF values are pH, 7.31; P_{CO_2}, 47.9 mm Hg; and HCO_3^-, 22.9 mEq/L. The CSF pH of 7.31 is slightly more acid than the blood pH. The P_{CO_2} and pH are measured directly with a P_{CO_2} electrode and pH electrode, respectively. The HCO_3^- value is calculated on the basis of a nomogram (see Chapter 22). The higher the P_{CO_2} or the lower the HCO_3^- in the fluid, the more acid is the pH. In normal CSF both these conditions apply; the P_{CO_2} exceeds that of blood (arterial P_{CO_2}, 38.3 mm Hg), and the HCO_3^- concentration is lower than that of the blood (arterial HCO_3^-, 23.4 mEq/L).

Spinal fluid lacks many of the buffering systems available to blood to maintain a constant pH; **pH deviations** in either the acid or alkaline direction interfere with the metabolism of nervous tissue and lead to the clinical picture of encephalopathy. The homeostatic mechanisms available to the protein-poor CSF are (1) change in the rate of cerebral blood flow, (2) active transport of H^+ or HCO_3^- ions across the blood-CSF barrier, and (3) change in ventilation and thus in CO_2 excretion.

Under pathologic conditions, because of the blood-brain barrier and the absence of an internal buffering system, the pH change in the CSF in acute respiratory acidosis is different from the change produced by metabolic acidosis. In the former the CSF is unable to provide any compensatory protective mechanism, whereas in the latter, adequate compensation can be established.

In **metabolic acidosis,** blood pH and CSF move discordantly, so that the patient remains conscious even though the blood pH is lowered. In **respiratory acidosis,** blood pH and CSF pH move parallel, so that the acidotic patient may become comatose. In **respiratory** or **metabolic alkalosis** the compensation in the CSF is less adequate than that for metabolic acidosis.

Enzymes

The normal blood-CSF barrier results in CSF enzyme concentrations that are relatively independent of their serum levels.[63,64] Under pathologic conditions the blood-CSF barrier may show increased permeability, but the CSF enzyme concentrations, although changed, remain independent of the serum concentrations. The increased enzyme levels appear to depend on the degree of cell destruction, cell membrane damage, tumor growth, necrosis, and infection. Nevertheless, whenever CSF enzymes are assayed, the corresponding serum enzymes should be ascertained. In general CSF enzyme assays have proven of little clinical value.

Glutamic oxalacetic transaminase: The normal value for CSF glutamic oxalacetic (GOT) activity ranges from 0-19 units,[65-67] whereas the serum value ranges from 0-50 units.

Elevated GOT values have been reported in cerebral infarction (traumatic or vascular) and after convulsions. This increase is primarily caused by escape of cellular GOT rather than a defect of the blood-brain barrier.

Lactic dehydrogenase: The normal CSF LDH activity is about one tenth that of serum[68] and shows marked variations from 8-50 units, with an average value of 23.3 units. In necrotic lesions such as infarcts and cerebrovascular accidents and in demyelinating diseases the LDH value rises to an average of 33.7 units.[61,69] Low LDH values are seen in multiple sclerosis.

The relative proportions of the LDH isoenzymes have been investigated by the use of various forms of electrophoresis. LDH_2 and LDH_3 are significantly increased in organic brain diseases such as multiple sclerosis, tumor, head injury, cerebrovascular disease, and hydrocephalus and are normal in nonorganic brain diseases such as idiopathic epilepsy and neuroses.

Phosphohexose isomerase[70]: In general phosphohexose isomerase (PHI) is more frequently elevated in the CSF than is LDH. The assay procedure is that of Bodansky, based on the colorimetric determination of fructose-6-phophate formed under the conditions of the test. The normal range is 0-4.2 Bodansky units, with an average value of 1.85 ± 1.15 units. In two thirds of patients with brain tumors, elevations of PHI occur. This correlation is more sensitive than the association of brain tumors and increased levels of GOT, LDH, and proteins or decreased levels of glucose. PHI elevations are also seen in infectious processes of the CNS caused by bacteria, fungi, and viruses. PHI values are normal in benign tumors of the brain and in chronic and subacute processes involving the CNS.

Microscopic examination
Total cell count

The cells should be counted as soon as the specimen is received, since they rapidly deteriorate and become enmeshed in fibrin or clumped. The method of counting varies with the number of cells expected.

Technic if spinal fluid appears clear—low cell count

Procedure: Transfer 1 drop of well-mixed undiluted fluid to a counting chamber. Count all the cells in nine large squares (see Chapter 7). Since this number represents a volume of $^9/_{10}$ mm^3, the result is multiplied by $^{10}/_9$ to obtain the number of cells per cubic millimeter. For practical purposes the multiplication may be omitted.

Technic for moderate cell count

Diluting fluid:
1. Crystal violet, 0.2 g
2. Glacial acetic acid, 10 ml
3. Distilled water, 1 dl

Procedure: Mix specimen thoroughly. If it is not very cloudy or bloody, draw spinal fluid to mark 1 in a white cell counting pipet and add diluting fluid to mark 11, producing a dilution of 1:10. Mix, discard one third, and place 1 drop on each side of the blood counting chamber as in the method for leukocyte counting. Count the cells in five squares, 1 mm^2 each (four corner squares and the central square), in each of the 2 drops. Add the result of all 10 squares counted. Multiply by 10 to obtain the number of cells in 1 mm^3.

Technic for high white cell count

The white cell count in purulent CSF is made as outlined for white cells in the peripheral blood (see p. 198).

Technic for counting mixture of white and red cells

To find the true white cell count when the CSF is bloody, perform red and white cell counts on the patient's blood as well as on the CSF specimen. Multiply the ratio of the red cell count of the fluid to the red cell count of the blood by the blood leukocyte count and subtract this product from the white cell count of the spinal fluid.

$$1. \quad \frac{\text{WBCs (blood)} \times \text{RBCs (CSF)}}{\text{RBCs (blood)}} = x$$

$$2. \quad \text{WBCs (CSF)} - x = \text{True WBCs (CSF)}$$

EXAMPLE: If RBCs of blood = 5,000,000 and RBCs of spinal fluid = 25,000, WBCs of blood = 12,000 and WBCs of spinal fluid = 70.

$$\frac{25,000 \times 12,000}{5,000,000} = 60$$

$$70 - 60 = 10 \text{ WBCs/mm}^3$$

Normal blood will add one leukocyte for each 700 red cells.

Normal values

Normal spinal fluid is essentially free of cells, containing only 0-5 mononuclear cells/mm^3, chiefly small lymphocytes or mononuclear cells. Infants at the age of a few weeks may have as many as 30 lymphocytes/mm^3 in CSF.

Variations of total cell count

A total cell count of 5-10 cells is considered borderline; one of over 10 is elevated. An increase in the number of cells in CSF is called **pleocytosis.** It may be classified according to number of cells into slight pleocytosis (5-10 cells), moderate pleocytosis (25-50 cells), and severe pleocytosis (over 50 cells). It may also be classified according to the predominant cell involved, e.g., polymorphonuclear pleocytosis, lymphocytic pleocytosis, and mixed pleocytosis. See following discussion of differential count.

Differential count

Various methods of cell concentration have been described.[71,72] Centrifugation is the easiest but least satisfactory, since cells may be damaged. Sedimentation technics are probably best, but the necessary equipment is not commercially available at this time. Sedimentation of cells directly onto the slide appears to be superior to the Millipore technic. If centrifugation is used as the method of concentration, the sediment is smeared similar to blood in the preparation of a blood film. The Cytocentrifuge offers a satisfactory method for the concentration of CSF cells. Whatever concentration method is used, the cells are stained with Wright or Papanicolaou stain and a differential count is made.

Significance

Normal pattern: The spun normal sediment shows from 60-100% lymphocytes. If other cells are present,

they are ependymal cells, monocytes, and plexus cells that can be recognized by their lighter staining and cytoplasmic vacuoles. A normal sediment does not exclude CNS pathologic conditions.

Pathologic pattern: Pathologic processes may lead to (1) a shift to the right or left of otherwise normal cells and (2) the appearance of cells not usually found in the CSF.

Abnormal cell distribution: A predominantly **polymorphonuclear pleocytosis** occurs in acute pyogenic meningitis. A slight to moderate increase of polymorphonuclear cells accompanies brain abscesses, early stages of tuberculous meningitis, syphilitic meningitis, and poliomyelitis. A predominantly **lymphocytic pleocytosis** is seen in aseptic meningitis, postinfectious encephalitis (mumps), lymphocytic choriomeningitis, and later stages of neurosyphilis. A predominantly **monocytic pleocytosis** of 40% or over is indicative of a reactive process. It may be seen, for instance, in the CSF after subarachnoid hemorrhage.

Presence of abnormal cells:

Neoplastic cells: Malignant cells of both primary and metastatic brain tumors may be recovered.

Lymphocytoid and plasmacytoid cells: Lymphocytoid and plasmacytoid cells are seen in subacute and chronic inflammatory processes and in demyelinating diseases such as multiple sclerosis, subacute sclerosing leukoencephalitis, delayed hypersensitivity–type responses, subacute viral encephalitis, and some brain tumors. The lymphocytoid and plasmacytoid cells are re-

Table 29-2. CSF findings in various conditions*

Disease	Appearance	Cells/mm³ and type	Protein (mg/dl)	Chlorides (mEq/L)	Glucose (mg/dl)
Normal	Clear, colorless	0-5 lymphocytes	20-40	112-127	45-80
Brain abscess (submeningeal)	Clear or turbid	+ chiefly polymorphonuclear cells	+ to 2 +	N to slightly decreased	N to slightly decreased
Encephalitis	Clear, colorless	N to + lymphocytes	±	N	N
Hemorrhage					
Cerebral	N to bloody to xanthochromic	N to many RBCs	N to 3 +	N	N
Subarachnoid	Bloody to xanthochromic	Many RBCs	N to 2 +	N	N
Subdural	N	N	N	N	N
Meningitis					
Choriomeningitis	N, slightly turbid	2 + lymphocytes	+	N	N
Purulent	Purulent	3 + chiefly polymorphonuclear cells	3 +	N	—
Tuberculous	Opalescent	2 + chiefly lymphocytes	2 +	—	—
Multiple sclerosis	N	N to ± lymphocytes	N to + IgG +	N	N
Neurosyphilis					
Meningovascular	N	+	N to +	N	N
Paresis	N	N to ± lymphocytes	+ to 2 +	N	N
Tabes dorsalis	N	N to ± lymphocytes	N to +	N	N
Polyneuritis	N to xanthochromic	N	N to 3 +	N	N
Thrombosis	N	N to ± lymphocytes	N to +	N	N
Tumor					
Brain	N to xanthochromic	N to + lymphocytes	± to 2 +	N	N
Cord	N to xanthochromic	N to + lymphocytes	3 +	N	N

*N, Normal; +, increased; —, decreased; ±, slightly increased.

sponsible for the increase in IgG (7S) and for the patterns described in the section on immunoelectrophoresis.

Macrophages: Macrophages may contain hemosiderin, phagocytosed bacteria, or white and red cells. In parenchymatous destruction, as seen in traumatic or ischemic infarcts, the macrophages may contain lipid material.

Cells of nervous tissue: After trauma or surgical procedures, groups of glial, ependymal, and plexus cells may be found.

Bacterial stains: Examination of the sediment should also include **Gram** and **Ziehl-Neelsen stains** and an **India ink preparation** for cryptococci. The latter is a must before the diagnosis of lymphocytic pleocytosis is reported.

Cerebrospinal fluid in disease

For CSF findings in various diseases see Table 29-2.

SYNOVIAL FLUID

Synovial fluid[73,74] is a modified connective tissue fluid found in joints and tendon spaces. It is a dialysate of plasma to which a characteristic mucoid substance (hyaluronic acid) is added that is responsible for the viscid nature of joint fluid. The hyaluronic acid is a product of the secretory activity of synovial lining.[75] Other components of the fluid, e.g., electrolytes and most nonelectrolytes, show the same concentration in synovial fluid as in plasma. Small amounts of synovial fluid normally lubricate all of the joints. Analysis of the synovial fluid is indicated whenever there is an accumulation of fluid (effusion) in a joint or other evidence of joint disease.

Collection of specimen

The fluid is collected by a physician by means of needle aspiration of the joint space. The specimen should be distributed into three sterile test tubes; 2-5 ml into each tube for chemical, cytologic, and microbiologic analysis. Two tubes should contain heparin for cytologic and microbiologic assays, and a third tube should be free of any anticoagulant, so that clot formation can be observed. Analysis of the fluid for complement should be performed in the absence of anticoagulant.

Characteristics of normal synovial fluid

Amount: 1 ml
Transparency: clear
Color: Colorless to straw colored
Viscosity: high
pH: 7.1
Total cell count:
  <200 WBCs/mm^3
  RBCs usually present in very low numbers but may be present because of trauma of aspiration[74]
Differential count:

Polymorphonuclear cells	0-25% (mean = 6%)
Lymphocytes	0-78% (mean = 25%)
Monocytes	0-71% (mean = 48%)
Macrophages	0-26% (mean = 10%)

Mucin clot: firm

Glucose: serum level
Total protein: 1.07-2.13 g/dl
  Albumin   1.02 g/dl
  Globulin   0.5 g/dl
Wet preparation:
  No crystals
  No rheumatoid arthritis cells
  No cartilage fibers
  No bacteria

Physical examination[76,77]

Volume: The normal amount of joint fluid can hardly be aspirated, since it usually does not exceed 1-3 ml (knee joint) and some of it may be hidden in synovial folds and pockets. If an effusion is present, the amount of fluid aspirated is an indicator of the severity of the joint involvement.

Transparency: Normal fluid is clear and transparent. In septic joint disease it becomes cloudy to purulent; in inflammatory disease it may be cloudy, and in noninflammatory disease it remains clear or is only slightly turbid. If newsprint cannot be read through a glass tube containing the synovial fluid, it is described as cloudy. The cloudiness may be caused by inflammatory cells, suspended crystals, or floating synovial and cartilaginous fragments. If ochronosis is present the fluid may contain black particles,[78,79] and metallic particles may be present after prosthetic knee arthroplasty.[80]

Color: Normal fluid is colorless to straw colored. In hemarthrosis (hemophilia, etc.) the joint fluid is bloody; the blood is evenly mixed throughout all specimens and does not clot. After centrifugation the supernatant fluid is xanthochromic (p. 755). Hemarthrosis must be distinguished from a "bloody" tap. Following a traumatic bloody tap, the blood is unevenly distributed in the three specimens and may form clots. The synovial fluid has a blood-streaked appearance.

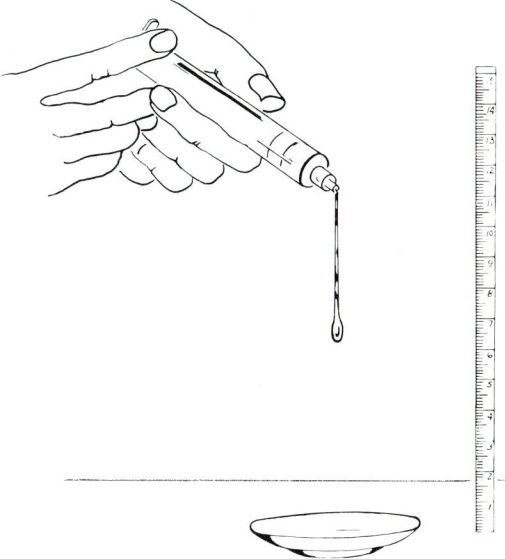

Fig. 29-7. Ability of normal synovial fluid to form a long tenacious string. (Drawn from Schmid, F.R., and Ogata, R.I.: Med. Clin. North Am. **49:**165, 1965.)

Viscosity: The viscosity of the joint fluid is a reflection of its hyaluronic acid content. Two tests are available to assess viscosity: (1) the falling drop or string test and (2) the mucin clot formation test.

Falling drop test:

Procedure: Joint fluid is aspirated into a pipet and then released. If the falling drop of joint fluid is drawn out into a 5 cm long or longer tenacious band, the viscosity is normal (Fig. 29-7). If the drop falls like water, the viscosity is low.

Interpretation: In inflammatory effusions as seen in rheumatoid arthritis, septic arthritis, and gout,[81] the viscosity is markedly decreased, indicating the presence of a thin watery fluid containing degraded small molecular hyaluronidase particles.[82]

Mucin clot formation test[83]:

Principle: Mucin (a hyaluronic acid–protein complex) is precipitated by acetic acid. The morphology of the precipitate is a reflection of the hyaluronic acid content and quality of the joint fluid.

Reagent: Acetic acid, 7N: Mix 408 ml glacial acetic acid and 1 L distilled water.

Procedure: Add 1 ml joint fluid to 4 ml distilled water in a test tube. Then add 0.14 ml of 7N acetic acid and stir briskly with a glass rod. Examine immediately and after 2 hr.

Interpretation: If hyaluronic acid is normal, a tight ropy mass forms in a clear solution, indicating "good" mucin. "Fair" mucin is indicated by a softer precipitate that shreds into the solution; "poor" precipitate consists of shreds in a turbid solution (Fig. 29-8).

In noninflammatory effusion the clot is good, in rheumatoid arthritis it is fair, and in infectious inflammatory effusions it is poor.

Clotting is also seen in hemorrhagic fluids and in septic arthritis.

Clot formation: Because of lack of fibrinogen and other clotting factors, normal joint fluid does not clot.[84] Inflammatory processes allow the plasma clotting factors to escape into the joint fluid, which then clots. The size of the clot is graded from 1-3+ and is directly proportional to the severity of the inflammation. The clot forms spontaneously when the untreated joint fluid is allowed to stand. A 3+ clot occupies three fourths of the joint fluid volume and forms rather rapidly, a 2+ clot occupies one half of the volume, and a 1+ clot occupies one fourth of the volume and takes several hours to form.[85]

Microscopic examination
Total cell count

The white cell counting technic is used, but isotonic saline solution is substituted for the usual acetic acid white cell diluting fluid since the latter precipitates the hyaluronic acid–protein complex. The cell count should be completed without delay to prevent spontaneous clumping of leukocytes.

Reagent: Normal saline solution (may be colored

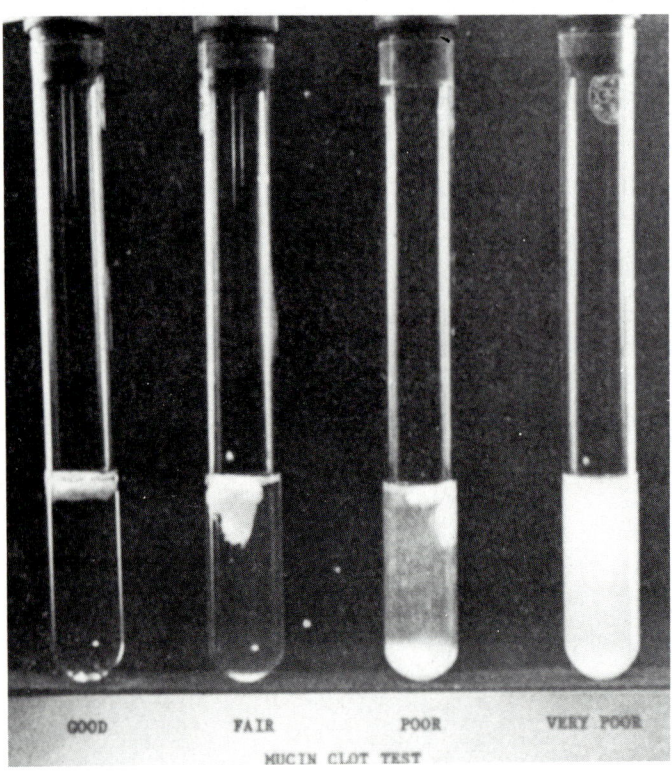

GOOD   FAIR   POOR   VERY POOR

MUCIN CLOT TEST

Fig. 29-8. Various types of mucin precipitates formed in synovial fluids with increasing severity of inflammation. (From Schmid, F.R., and Ogata, R.I.: Med. Clin. North Am. **49:**165, 1965.)

with methylene blue). Saline, 0.3%, should be used as the diluting fluid if the effusion is bloody in order to lyse the red cells.[86]

Procedure: The synovial fluid, anticoagulated with heparin, is mixed well in a rotator before it is drawn up in a white cell pipet to mark 0.5. For further details of the technic, see CSF counting technic for moderate numbers of white cells on p. 759.

Differential count

Centrifuge the anticoagulated specimen at about 2000 rpm for 10 min and decant the supernatant, except for 0.5 ml in which the sediment is resuspended. Prepare coverslip preparation as described in Chapter 10, and when smear is dry stain it with Wright-Giemsa stain. The smears must be thin, so that the hyaluronic acid does not precipitate and interfere with the recognition of the cells present.

Normal values: Synovial fluid is almost acellular, containing only 200 WBCs/mm³. Of these cells, fewer than 25% are polymorphonuclear cells. The remainder are mononuclear cells.

Interpretation of total white cell count and differential count

On the basis of the total white cell and differential counts Schumacher[87] divides the synovial effusions and arthritides into groups I, II, and III (Table 29-3).

The noninflammatory joint effusions (less than 2000 WBCs/mm³) are seen in osteoarthritis and other degenerative joint diseases, Charcot's joint, traumatic arthritis, Paget's disease, mechanical derangement, villonodular synovitis, aseptic necrosis, sickle cell disease, hypertrophic pulmonary osteoarthropathy, osteochondritis dissecans, epiphyseal dysplasia, amyloidosis, and hemochromatosis.[86]

Inflammatory joint effusions (over 2000 WBCs/mm³) are seen in rheumatoid arthritis, connective tissue diseases (i.e., polymyositis, scleroderma, systemic lupus erythematosus), Reiter's disease, psoriasis, ulcerative colitis, regional enteritis, rheumatic fever, postileal bypass state, sarcoidosis, subacute bacterial endocarditis, and crystal-induced arthritis (i.e., gout and hydroxyapatite joint disease).[86]

Septic effusions (100,000 or more WBCs/mm³) are encountered in bacterial and fungal infections. If the septic arthritides are treated the synovial leukocytosis drops.

Examination of the dried, stained smear reveals not only the already discussed percentage of polymorphonuclear cells but also lymphocytes and monocytes. The latter cells must be distinguished from synovial lining cells and other large cells, e.g., stimulated lymphocytes, that are seen in rheumatoid arthritis and not in crystal-induced arthritides.[88]

Wet preparations

Microscopic examination of wet preparations of synovial fluid (either untreated or sedimented) for crystals and other components is an important diagnostic procedure.

Crystals:

Procedure: Use synovial fluid that has not been collected in lithium heparin or oxalate, since both may produce crystals,[89] but the fluid must not be clotted. Place 1 drop of uncentrifuged fluid on a microscope slide, apply coverslip immediately, and seal with fingernail polish. Examine the preparation by regular light microscopy under high magnification and also by polarized light and phase microscopy.

In about 90% of fluids from acutely inflamed joints, two kinds of birefringent crystals are found: monosodium urate crystals are found in gouty fluids and calcium pyrophosphate dihydrate crystals are found in chondrocalcinosis. The **urate crystals** are needle shaped, doubly refractive under polarized light, and found free as well as within neutrophils. The crystals vary in length from 3-20 µm, and when a first-order red compensation is used they are strongly negatively birefringent and appear yellow when their long axes are aligned parallel to the direction of the slow ray of the compensator (Fig. 29-9).[90] The majority of crystals are intracellular during the active phase of the disease (Figs. 29-10 to 29-13). The **pyrophosphate crystals** are only weakly birefringent, rhomboid, and shorter than the uric acid crystals. When their long axes are aligned parallel to the direction of the slow ray of the compensator, they exhibit positive birefringence and appear blue. Other crystals that may be encountered are **cholesterol crystals,** which are seen in rheumatoid arthritis (Fig. 29-1). They are flat, rectangular plates with one notched corner. Depot **corticosteroid** preparations injected into the joint space may at some later date be discovered in the synovial fluid as phagocytosed, doubly refractile crystals within the mononuclear cells.[91] As mentioned above anticoagulants such as lithium heparin[89] and sodium oxalate[92] may form intracellular, positively birefringent crystals. Other positively birefringent crystals are composed of **dihydrate calcium hydrogen phosphate.**[93]

Noncrystalline material found in the sediment includes red and white cells, fragments of cartilage and synovia, collagen fibrils, fibrin, and phagocytic cells containing hemosiderin (hemochromatosis, pigmented

Table 29-3. Classification of synovial effusions

	Normal	Noninflammatory (group I)	Inflammatory (group II)	Septic (group III)
Total white cell count (WBCs/mm³)	<200	200-2000	2000-100,000	≥100,000
Polymorphonuclear cells (%)	<25	<25	>25	>75

USE OF FIRST-ORDER RED COMPENSATOR
(RETARDATION PLATE)

*Long axis of monosodium
urate crystals aligned
parallel to direction of
slow ray of compensator*

*Long axis of calcium
pyrophosphate crystals
aligned parallel to direction
of slow ray of compensator*

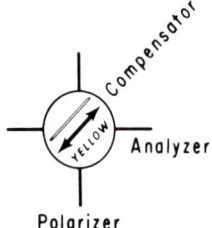

*Color: yellow
(negative birefringence)*

*Color: blue
(positive birefringence)*

Fig. 29-9. Polarization microscopy in synovial fluid analysis. (Table 1 from Cohen, A.S., editor: Laboratory diagnostic procedures in the rheumatic diseases, ed. 2, Boston, 1975, Little, Brown & Co. Copyright © 1975 Little, Brown & Co.)

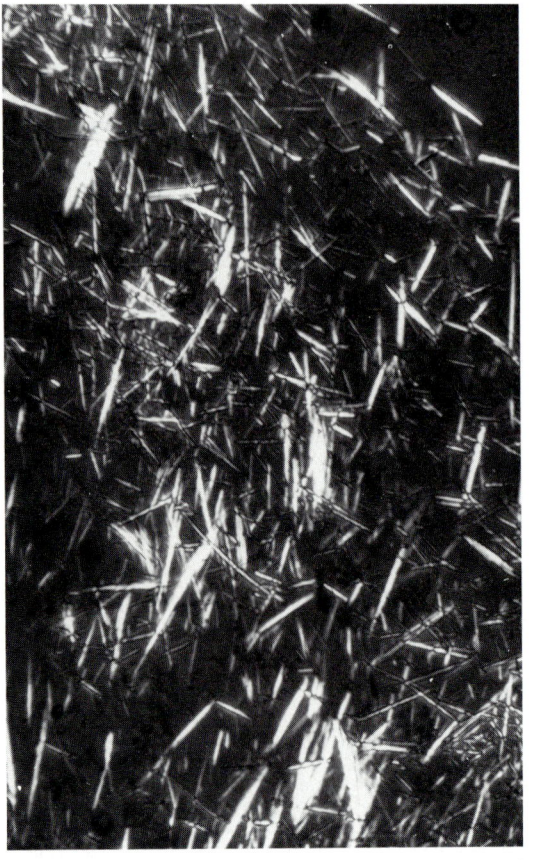

Fig. 29-10. Uric acid crystals in joint fluid as seen under polarized light.

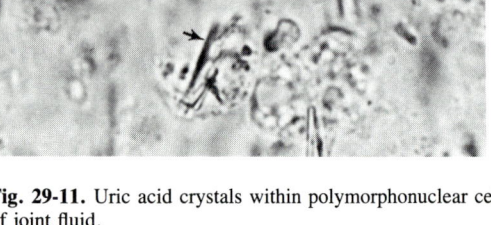

Fig. 29-11. Uric acid crystals within polymorphonuclear cell of joint fluid.

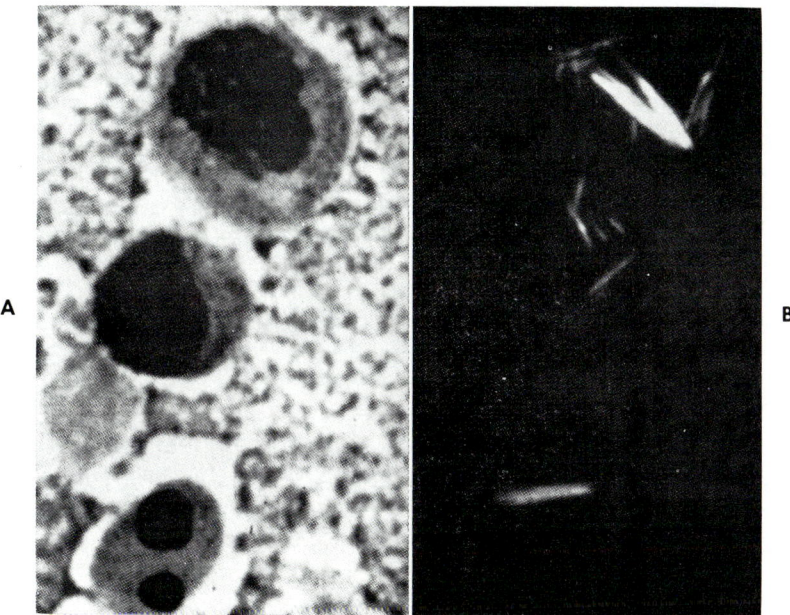

Fig. 29-12. Synovial fluid from knee involved with acute gout. **A,** Inflammatory cells viewed with ordinary light. **B,** Same cells viewed with polarized light show birefringent intracellular sodium urate crystals. (From Good, A.E., and Frishette, W.A.: J.A.M.A. **198:**80 1966.)

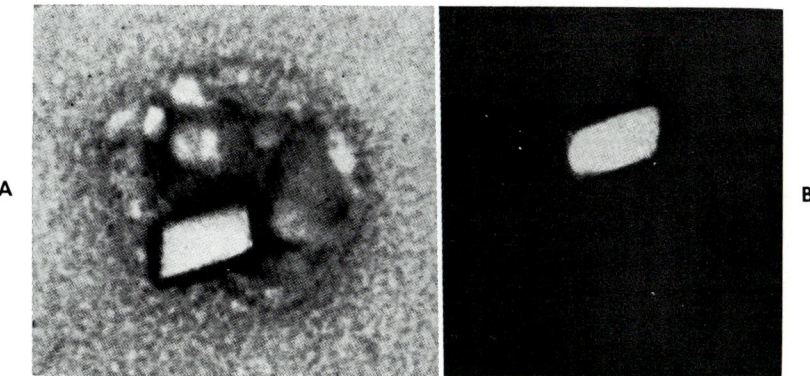

Fig. 29-13. Synovial fluid obtained from knee involved with acute pseudogout. **A,** Mononuclear leukocyte containing rhomboid-shaped calcium pyrophosphate crystals viewed with ordinary light. **B,** Same cell viewed with polarized light shows birefringence of crystals. (Wright stain; ×2000.) (From Good, A.E., and Frishette, W.A.: J.A.M.A. **198:**80, 1966.)

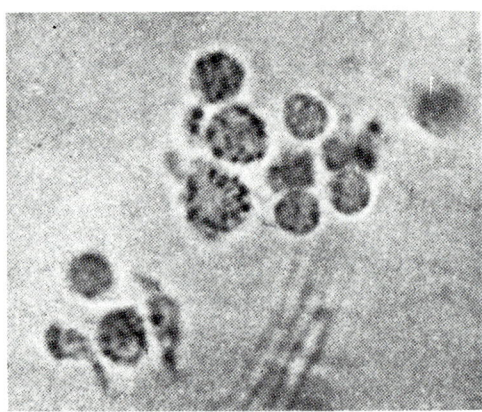

Fig. 29-14. Polymorphonuclear leukocytes containing typical cytoplasmic inclusions in wet preparation of synovial fluid from patient with rheumatoid arthritis. (Courtesy G.B. Backer; from Hollander, J.L., et al.: Med. Clin. North Am. **50:**1281, 1966.)

villonodular synovitis) or intracytoplasmic vacuoles (rheumatoid arthritis).[94] In multiple myeloma the sediment may contain fragmented amyloid, and in ochronosis the already mentioned black-pigmented synovial or cartilaginous chips may be encountered. It should be noted that collagen fibrils are doubly refractile.

Rheumatoid arthritis cell: Under ordinary light microscopy, wet preparations of synovial fluid from patients with rheumatoid arthritis (RA) show small, dark, multiple nodular inclusions within polymorphonuclear cells and macrophages; these inclusions can be visualized even better by phase microscopy. They are immunoglobulin deposits (Fig 29-14) that contain the rheumatoid factor, hence, the name *RA cell*. Neither the demonstration of the rheumatoid factor nor of the RA cell is diagnostic of rheumatoid arthritis. The test for rheumatoid factor is described in Chapter 35.

Rheumatoid factor

The serum and synovia of about 80% of patients suffering from rheumatoid arthritis contain a macroglobu-

Table 29-4. Synovial analysis in arthritis

Disease	Appearance	Viscosity	Mucin clot	White cell count	Crystals	Cartilage debris	Special features
Normal	Straw colored, clear	High (normal)	Good	200-600, 25% PMNs*	0	0	0
Traumatic arthritis	Cloudy, bloody	Normal	Good	2000 ± (many RBCs)	0	0 or +	0
Osteoarthritis	Yellow, clear	Normal	Good	1000 ±, 20% PMNs	0	Fragments, fibrils	0
Rheumatic fever	Yellow, slightly cloudy	Low	Fair	10,000 ±, 50% PMNs	0	0	Antistreptolysin O antibodies in serum
Systemic lupus erythematosus	Yellow, slightly cloudy	Normal	Good	3000 ±, 10% PMNs	0	0	LE† cells, antinuclear antibodies in serum
Gouty arthritis	Yellow, cloudy	Low	Poor	10,000 +, 75% PMNs	Many (urate)	0	Crystals in cells or free; negative birefringence
Pseudogout	Yellow, slightly cloudy	Normal or low	Good	6000 +, 75% PMNs	Few to many (calcium pyrophosphate)	0 to many	Crystals in cells or free, or in cartilage fragments (weakly positive birefringence)
Rheumatoid arthritis and variants	Yellow to greenish, cloudy	Low	Poor	8000-40,000, 70% PMNs	Rare (cholesterol)	0	5-95% of PMNs show inclusions (RA cells), RF positive
Tuberculous arthritis	Yellow, cloudy	Low	Poor	25,000 ±, 40-50% PMNs	0	0	Glucose low, acid-fast bacterial culture
Septic arthritis	Grayish to bloody, turbid	Low	Poor	80,000 ±, 90% PMNs	0	0	Culture positive, negative for RF, decreased glucose

From Hollander, J.L., et al.: Med. Clin. North Am. **50:**1281, 1966.
*Polymorphonuclear nentrophil leukocytes.
†Lupus erythematosus.

lin antibody (IgM) called rehumatoid factor (RF). It is directed against an antibody, IgG, and is therefore better designated as anti-γ-globulin factor. The RF is thus an anti-antibody, which in vitro is detected by its ability to agglutinate latex particles or red cells coated with IgG. The red cells may be human or sheep. In all tests an indicator material is coated with IgG, which then reacts with the RF in the patient's serum and causes the indicator (red cells or latex particles) to agglutinate or precipitate.

The RF is not causally related to rheumatoid arthritis, which is probably a disease caused by a virus or by *Mycoplasma.*

Screening test: The latex fixation test for RF, which is commerically available in kit form (Difco Laboratories, Detroit), is based on the work of Singer and Plotz.[95] The latex-globulin reagent agglutinates in the presence of diluted serum containing RF. Follow the manufacturer's instructions in performing the test. Positive and negative controls must be included.

Watson[96] suggests heating the test serum at 56° C for 30 min to destroy a serum antiglobulin factor normally present that may lead to false positive tests by agglutinating the globulin-coated latex particles.

Biochemical examination
Glucose

Because the joint fluid glucose equilibrates with blood glucose, whenever the joint fluid glucose is assayed the blood glucose level should also be determined.[97] To allow complete equilibration of joint fluid with plasma, a fasting (8 hr) sampling is desirable. The glucose concentration in the normal synovial fluids equals that of plasma. In degenerative joint diseases the same relationship holds true, whereas in inflammatory joint disease, i.e., rheumatoid arthritis, the synovial glucose level is about 60% of that in plasma and in septic arthritis it drops to 40% of the plasma concentration.[98]

Proteins

The total protein concentration is determined by the usual serum protein method and amounts to approximately one fourth the total serum protein value (1.07-2.13 g/dl). In infalmmatory joint diseases the protein level increases to about 4.5 g/dl. Cohen[76] states that a synovial fluid content of 2.5 g protein/dl indicates some joint fluid abnormality.

Electrophoresis

The **hyaluronic acid** must first be removed by treatment with hyaluronidase. Instead of treating the fluid with hyaluronidase, the joint fluid may be kept in the refrigerator for 2-3 days after aspiration, at which time reproducible patterns resembling those in serum protein are obtainable.[99]

Normal synovial fluid shows an α_2-depression as compared with the α_2-value in serum. In inflammatory joint disease the effusion is rich in γ-globulin, which forms 30-50% of the synovial protein.

Immunodiffusion: Haptoglobin is almost absent in joint fluid; and in rheumatoid effusion complement is decreased (to approximately 10% of serum values).

Enzymes: The **alkaline phosphatase** level in synovial fluid is lower than it is in serum. The synovial **acid phosphatase** concentration is higher in specimens obtained from patients with rheumatoid and inflammatory arthritis than it is in normal joint fluid.[100]

Culture

One of the anticoagulated sterile specimens should be centrifuged and the sediment used to inoculate appropriate media for the culture of *Neisseria,* tubercle bacilli, anaerobes, and aerobes.

If gonorrhea is considered the etiologic agent, a serum specimen should be obtained to determine the gonococcal **antibody level** by complement fixation. The sediment should also be used to prepare smears to be stained with Gram stain and Ziehl-Neelsen stain. Precipitated hyaluronic acid–protein complexes may interfere with the interpretation of the smear.

AMNIOTIC FLUID

The relative ease with which, in experienced hands, transabdominal amniocentesis can be performed focuses interest on amniotic fluid analysis as a means of assessing the condition of the fetus.

Amniocentesis is usually performed at 16 weeks' gestation when the volume of amniotic fluid should have reached 2 dl[101] and a sample can be obtained without difficulty at a site previously established by ultrasound. The risk of fetal injury is well below 1%.[102] There are numerous indications for amniocentesis[103]:

1. To predict the severity of hemolytic disease of the newborn in Rh erythroblastosis fetalis[104,105]
2. To assess intrauterine fetal maturity before cesarean section to assure the delivery of an infant with a good chance of survival[106]
3. To detect fetal sex in pregnant women heterozygous for X-linked recessive disorders such as hemophilia and muscular dystrophy[107]
4. To discover genetic fetal disorders in genetic high-risk patients, e.g., with chromosomal translocations (Down's syndrome) or congenital metabolic disorders,[108] e.g., Pompe's and Tay-Sach's diseases and Lesch-Nyhan syndrome
5. To assess pulmonary maturity[109]
6. To predict spontaneous onset of labor[110]
7. To determine fetal jeopardy, i.e., Rh isosensitization, diabetes mellitus, preeclampsia, and eclampsia[106]

Identification

Identification of amniotic fluid in the vagina or its differentiation from urine may be necessary in premature rupture of membranes[112] or rarely in amniocentesis. Amniotic fluid is diagnosed on the basis of the alkaline pH, the presence of fat-laden fetal surface cells, and the fern test (see Table 27-1).[112] Urine is identified on the basis of the urea nitrogen and the creatinine concentration.

Characteristics of normal amniotic fluid

Amniotic fluid is composed of materials from fetal lungs and urine and placental membranes.[111] The origin of amniotic fluid is not completely understood. The lung secretion of the fetus is probably its major component, a fact that is important in assessing fetal pulmonary maturation.

Amniotic fluid resembles extracellular fluid in which undissolved material is suspended.[113]

Volume: varies markedly; at term about 15 dl[114]
Color: straw colored or colorless
Calcium: 4 mEq/L
Chloride: 102 mEq/L
CO_2: 16 mEq/L
Creatinine: 1.8 mg/dl
Glucose: 29.8 mg/dl
pH: 7.04
Potassium: 4.9 mEq/L
Sodium: 133 mEq/L
Total protein: 25 g/dl

Albumin	56.5%	1.42 g
α_1-Globulin	7.3%	0.19 g
α_2-Globulin	6.5% ·	0.17 g
β-Globulin	15.5%	0.40 g
γ-Globulin	12.2%	0.32 g

Urea: 31 mg/dl
Uric acid: 4.9 mg/dl

Gross examination

Visual examination must be undertaken as soon as the specimen is received. Record color, transparency, and the presence of blood.

Color: Normal fluid is colorless or a pale straw color. Bilirubin imparts a yellow-orange color, and if bilirubin is to be assayed the specimen must be wrapped in aluminum foil to prevent photodecomposition. If the fluid is bloody it should be spun immediately to remove the red cells and prevent hemolysis. It should also be ascertained whether the blood is fetal or maternal (Kleihauer stain on the smear of the sedimented red cells). Severe hemolysis is reponsible for a brown-colored amniotic fluid. Contamination with meconium produces a green color, which prevents spectral analysis.

Turbidity: Normal amniotic fluid contains vernix, which renders it turbid. If the specimen is clear it must be ascertained that it is indeed amniotic fluid and not urine (see above). Before spectral analysis is performed the specimen should be cleared by centrifugation. The optical density of amniotic fluid provides a rapid test for the assessment of fetal lung maturity.[115]

Biochemical examination
Pigment analysis in erythroblastosis fetalis (hemolytic disease of newborn, HDN)

If the anti-Rh_0 antibody titer in a pregnant Rh_0-negative patient steadily increases until it reaches a level frequently associated with fetal or neonatal death, pigment analysis is the only available method to monitor the condition of the fetus.[116] The extensive use of hyperimmune anti-D (Rh_0) globulin has dramatically reduced the incidence of RH_0 erythroblastosis fetalis but has left untouched the instances of maternal isosensitization with other blood groups such as Kell, Duffy, and c.

Bevis[117] and Walker and Jenimson[118] reported increased bilirubin pigment in the amniotic fluid of erythroblastotic fetuses, which reflected the intravascular fetal hemolysis and correlated well with the level of cord hemoglobin. The pigment, which is not excreted by the mother (as is the fetal serum bilirubin), is apparently acquired by the amniotic fluid during its circulation through the fetal gastrointestinal tract. On spectrophotometric analysis of the amniotic fluid, the pigment shows a distinct peak at 450 nm.

About 10 ml of amniotic fluid should be collected, if possible, and placed at once in a brown bottle, which in turn should be placed in a light-proof container. The fluid should be sent to the laboratory as soon as possible. It may then be inspected visually (see below) and immediately centrifuged for 30 min at high speed. If, after centrifugation, it is still turbid, it may be filtered through Whatman no. 40 filter paper. The filtration should be carried out in subdued light. The specimen may be kept for up to 24 hr in the refrigerator before analysis. If a longer time is to elapse before analysis, the specimen should be frozen. If frozen, it remains stable for several months when protected from light.

Care should be taken to minimize the inclusion of any blood in the specimen. If initial aspiration produces a bloody fluid, the needle should be repositioned to obtain a specimen free of red cells. Bloody fluid must be centrifuged at once before any of the cells have hemolyzed. If the centrifuged specimen has more packed cells than about 5% by volume, the specimen will usually be unsatisfactory for spectral analysis.

Spectrophotometric analysis

1. A spectral absorption curve is obtained by reading against a water blank, preferably on a recording spectrophotometer from 350-700 nm. If a recording instrument is not available, readings may be taken at 350, 365, 380, 390, 400, 410, 415, 420, 430, 440, 450, 460, 470, 485, 500, 515, 530, 540, 555, 570, 585, 600, 620, 640, 670, and 700 nm.

2. The absorbance is then plotted against the wavelength, as shown in Fig. 29-15. If the fluid is still too turbid after filtration to make accurate readings, it may be diluted with distilled water to allow light transmission in an acceptable range. An appropriate correction for the dilution is made in the calculation of the actual absorbance difference.

3. Normally a straight line can be drawn through several of the points. The bilirubin pigment produces a "hump" in the curve (Fig. 29-13). The hump is maximal at 450 nm. The amount of deviation is measured and reported as the difference between the expected and plotted curves at 450 nm (**Δ450**). If the specimen has been diluted, a correction must be made for the dilution. The deviation of the abnormal curve (Δ450) is graded by Freda[119] according to optical density at 450 nm from 1-4+ (Table 29-5). Grades of 3+ and 4+ indicate severe fetal distress and imminent death, respectively.

A linear amniotic absorption curve is only obtained in the later months of pregnancy (thirty-fourth week).

Dissolved hemoglobin (fetal or maternal) produces a peak at 415 nm (oxyhemoglobin), thus increasing the apparent deviation at 450 nm (Δ450). If both bilirubin

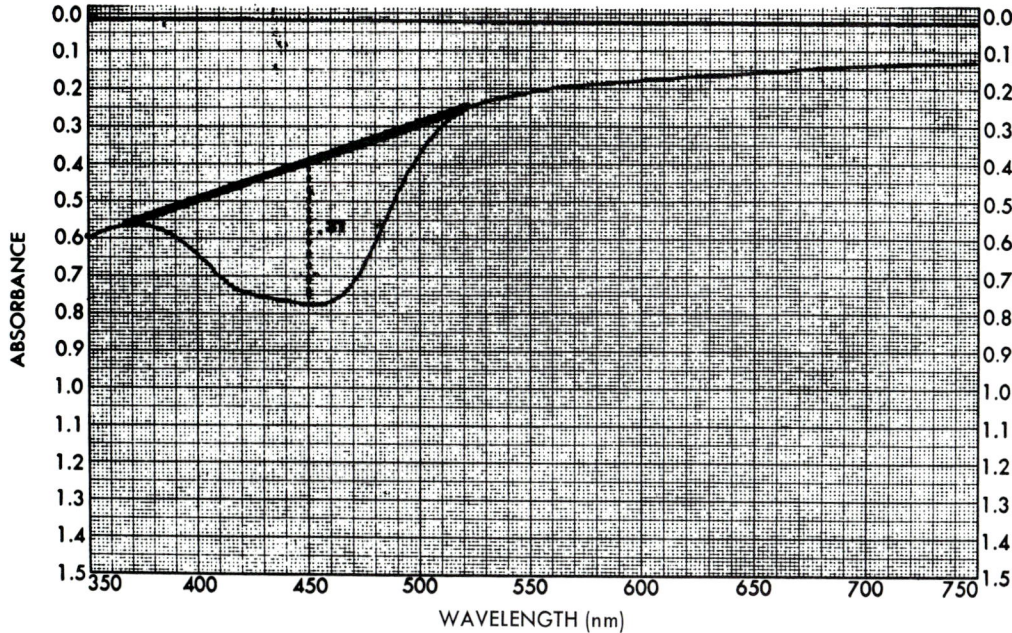

Fig. 29-15. Amniotic fluid spectrophotometric scan on a linear scale demonstrating a typical "bilirubin hump." Heavy line projected from 375-525 nm demonstrates approximate course of amniotic fluid scan in absence of bilirubin. Upright (broken) line drawn at 450 nm shows deviation of this bilirubin peak from normal, in this case 0.37. (From Queenan, J.T.: Clin. Obstet. Gynecol. **9:**491, 1966.)

Table 29-5. Freda's classification of clinical condition of fetus based on Δ450 of amniotic fluid

Freda's classification	Clinical status	Total bilirubin (mg/dl)	Net absorbance (OD) at 450 nm (Δ450)
1+	Normal or slightly affected	<0.28	0.0-0.20
2+	Affected but not in danger	0.28-0.46	0.20-0.35
3+	Greatly affected and in danger	0.47-0.95	0.3-0.70
4+	Impending fetal death	>0.95	>0.70

and oxyhemoglobin are present, Liley[120] uses a correction factor that is 5% of the deviation at 415 nm.

Amniotic fluid bilirubin assay

In the course of a normal pregnancy the bilirubin pigment in the amniotic fluid decreases, but if fetal red cells are destroyed by maternal antibodies that cross the placenta the bilirubin concentration fails to decline and may even increase. The degree of fetal involvement and the severity of the anemia can be judged on the basis of the bilirubin concentration.

The Gambino modification[121] of the Jendrassik and Graf[113] method[122] of bilirubin assay is given below.

Principle: See Jendrassik and Graf method (see p. 537).

Reagents: Regents 1-4 are found in the original Jendrassik and Graf method (see p. 537).
1. Caffeine solution
2. Diazo I
3. Diazo II
4. Alkali mixture
   a. Sodium hydroxide, 100 g
   b. Potassium sodium tartrate, 350 g
   c. Water to 10 dl
   Mixture is stable for 6 months at room temperature.

Standardization: Lyophilized bilirubin standard in serum is commerically available.

Procedure: Prepare two tubes, an unknown and a blank. Add 2.0 ml caffeine mixture to each tube. Add 1.0 ml amniotic fluid to each tube and mix. Add 0.5 ml diazo I reagent to the unknown and mix. Add 0.5 ml diazo I to the blank and mix. Allow both tubes to stand at room temperature for 10 min. Add 1.5 ml alkaline mixture to both tubes and mix. Read absorbance of unknown at 600 nm with blank at zero.

Normal values: Normal values are below 0.10 mg/dl.

Interpretation: Levels between 0.10 and 0.27 mg/dl suggest fetal involvement. Fetal distress is indicated by values exceeding 0.47 mg/dl, and fetal death is inevitable if the total bilirubin value exceeds 0.95 mg/dl.

Assessment of maturity of fetus and of its lungs

Perinatal mortality is related to fetal prematurity at time of birth. If pregnancy needs to be terminated by induction or cesaren section because of complications resulting from erythroblastosis fetalis, diabetes, placental insufficiency, etc., a reliable method for assessing fetal maturity may help to decrease perinatal mortality. Parameters used for assessing fetal maturity are optical density of amniotic fluid, creatinine concentration of amniotic fluid, cytologic study of amniotic fluid, quantitation of amniotic lipids, and amniotic microviscosity.

Optical density of bilirubin in amniotic fluid: Close to term the concentration of bilirubin pigments in the amniotic fluid decreases progressively as determined by ΔOD at 450 nm,[123] but the measurement of the decreasing bilirubin values has not proved to be a good test for fetal maturity because of the wide range of variation.[111]

Optical density of amniotic fluid at 650 nm: Hill et al.[115] describe a rapid screening procedure for assessment of fetal lung maturity. The optical density determined at 650 nm correlates well with the lecithin/sphingomyelin (L/S) ratio.

Procedure: Exclude bloody or meconium-stained samples. Centrifuge sample for 10 min at 900 g. Determine optical density at 650 nm using appropriate red filter and a 1 cm light path and water as blank.

Interpretation: An optical density below 0.15 corresponds to an L/S ratio below 2 and indicates immaturity. An optical density above 0.15 corresponds to an L/S ratio above 2 and indicates maturity.

The technic reported by Hill et al. produced a false negative rate of 7% and a much smaller false positive rate of 1.3%. The use of a slightly higher optical density cutoff (0.2-0.5) would reduce the false positive results even further. In any case, any negative values by this procedure would require confirmation by a thin-layer chromatography L/S ratio.

Creatinine concentration: The creatinine concentration of the amniotic fluid rises close to term.[124] It is measured by the serum creatinine method described in Chapter 21. Amniotic fluid creatinine concentrations of 1.0 mg/dl or less are indicative of prematurity, while concentrations of 1.5 mg/dl and greater indicate fetal maturity. A value of 2.0 mg/dl is accepted as indicative that the pregnancy is over 35 weeks. The renal function of the mother must be adequate (serum creatinine level should be known) before the amniotic fluid creatinine value is interpreted. In abnormal fetal growth the creatinine concentration may not rise appropriate to maturation, since it primarily reflects the increasing fetal muscle mass.[111]

Cytologic study

The cells present in amniotic fluid originate in the fetal skin, respiratory and urinary tracts, and amniotic membrane and can be used for fetal sex chromatin determination, enzymatic studies, cell culture, and karyotyping.

Cells are obtained for cytologic examination from uncentrifuged specimens or from the **junction** of supernatant and sediment of centrifuged specimens.[125,126]

Nile blue sulfate stain: Nile blue is a two-color stain, staining keratin yellow and nonkeratinizing cells blue. The uptake of Nile blue sulfate results in orange or blue staining and correlates well with fetal maturity.

Procedure: Mix 1 drop of aqueous Nile blue sulfate (0.2 g/dl) and 1 drop of amniotic fluid on a microscope slide. Warm slide gently, apply cover slip, and examine microscopically. Count the percentages of orange and blue cells.

Interpretation: The most superficial anucleated fetal squamous cells stain orange, whereas the nucleated squamous cells and the deeper parabasal-like cells stain blue. During the last 4 or 5 weeks of pregnancy the number of orange-staining anucleated squamous cells increases rapidly. A count of 20 or more orange-staining cells indicates fetal maturity or pregnancy of 36 weeks or longer and a fetal weight of over 2500 g.[127-129] A low count of orange-staining cells does not necessarily indicate prematurity (Fig. 29-16).

Amniotic fluid analysis to predict spontaneous onset of labor

The combination of the three above-mentioned tests performed on amniotic fluid can be used to predict that labor will or will not occur within a specified period of time. The selected tests are creatinine assay, cytologic study, and the optical density of amniotic fluid. If all three tests are negative, labor will not occur for 3 weeks; if two or all three tests are positive, labor will occur within 3 weeks. If only one test is positive and two are negative, only 24% of the patients will go into labor within 3 weeks.[110]

Prenatal sex determination

As previously stated, amniotic cells are of fetal origin and prenatal sex determination is indicated in **X-linked recessive disorders.**[107] The **sex chromatin** (see Chapter 6) can be studied in cultured amniotic cells and in uncultured amniotic cells, provided the latter prepa-

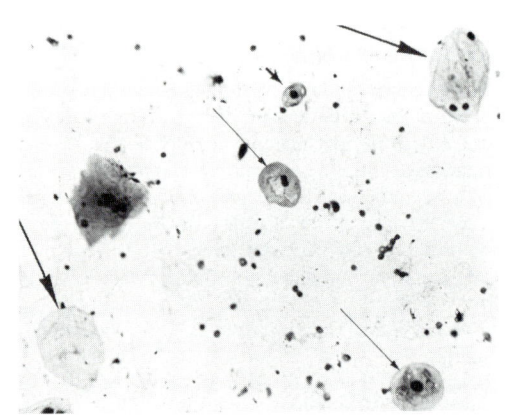

Fig. 29-16. Cytologic findings in amniotic fluid of term infant. (Papanicolaou technic.) Small arrow indicates parabasal type of cell; thin arrows, nucleated squamous cells; and heavy arrows, anucleated squamous cells.

ration is satisfactory, which it is not in one third of the cases.

Sex chromatin study

Reagents:
1. Fixative (chilled)
   a. Methanol, 3 parts
   b. Acetic acid, 1 part
2. Methyl violet, 1%

Procedure: Centrifuge 1-2 ml amniotic fluid at 2500 rpm for 30 min. Decant supernatant and suspend cell button in 2 ml chilled fixative. Allow mixture to incubate at room temperature for 30 min. Spin again for 10 min. Decant fixative and resuspend cells in 0.25 ml fixative. Prepare smears using the final suspension. Stain with 1% methyl violet. Examine microscopically for sex chromatin bodies.

An accurate diagnosis based on examination of the sex chromatin is not possible in all cases, e.g., in XO or XXY fetuses. Chromosomal analysis of cultured amniotic fluid (**karyotyping**) should be utilized to determine the sex of the fetus. This method allows not only the diagnosis of multiple X and Y chromosomes[130] but also the intrauterine diagnosis of Down's syndrome.[130]

Prenatal detection of familial metabolic disorders

A number of familial metabolic disorders have been detected in utero. The cellular components of the amniotic fluid can be evaluated cytochemically either cultured or uncultured and the supernatant can be assayed biochemically. Cultured amniotic cells can be used to diagnose[106,131,132] galactosemia (galactose-1-phosphate uridyl transferase deficiency), Pompe's disease (1,4-glucosidase deficiency), Tay-Sachs disease (hexosaminidase A deficiency), Hurler's disease (α-L-iduronidase), Lesch-Nyhand disease (hypoxanthine quanine phosphoribosyl transferase deficiency), Fabry's disease (α-galactoside deficiency), and others.

Pulmonary phospholipids in amniotic fluid— a measure of fetal lung maturity

The amniotic fluid phospholipid profile measures surfactant production by the fetus and is at present the best predictor of fetal maturity. Surfactant is a generic term for a complex that lowers the surface tension of the water that lines the alveoli.[111] It is composed of phospholipids (90%), the most important of which is lecithin. Sphingomyelin, another phospholipid, is also highly surface active and is secreted by the lung.

Premature birth is frequently associated with breathing difficulty of the delivered infant resulting from lack of alveolar stability because of developmental immaturity of the lungs. The alveolar stability is related to a deficiency of a surface-active material composed of phospholipids, the lecithin component of which is primarily deficient.[133]

Amniotic fluid, being primarily a product of fetal pulmonary secretion, can be used to measure the relationship of **lecithin** to **sphingomyelin (L/S ratio)**, as an index of fetal pulmonary maturity.

During gestation the pulmonary phospholipids present a characteristic pattern. Up to about the twenty-sixth week of gestation the amount of lecithin in amniotic fluid is less than the amount of sphingomyelin (L/S ratio less than unity). The amount of lecithin then gradually increases, so that at about the thirty-sixth week the amounts of the two phospholipids are approximately equal. After this time the amount of lecithin increases markedly, while the amount of sphingomyelin remains relatively constant or may decrease somewhat. When the fetal lung is mature, the L/S ratio in amniotic fluid is greater than 2. An infant delivered when the L/S ratio is close to unity will almost certainly develop **respiratory distress syndrome** (RDS) and very probably fatal **hyaline membrane disease** (HMD). If the L/S ratio is about 1.5, the infant will develop some degree of RDS but will usually survive with adequate treatment. If the L/S ratio is over 2, the fetal lung is relatively mature and RDS should not develop except under extremely adverse conditions. If early delivery seems indicated (because of diabetes, erythroblastosis, or other conditions), a determination of the L/S ratio in the amniotic fluid will indicate if the fetal lung is sufficiently matured to function properly. If the L/S ratio is less than about 1.2, it is preferable to delay the induced delivery, if possible, until the lung has become more mature.

Two tests for lung maturity are presented: thin-layer chromatography and amniotic fluid microviscosity.

Thin-layer chromatography method to separate and quantitate lecithin and sphingomyelin lipids

Principle: The phospholipids are extracted from the amniotic fluid with a mixture of chloroform and methanol. The extract is evaporated and the phospholipids are dissolved in a small amount of chloroform and applied to a thin-layer chromatography (TLC) plate. After chromatographic development and visualization of the spots by charring or other means, the lecithin and sphingomyelin spots are identified by their R_f values in comparison with known standards of the two compounds similarly applied to the plate. A visual comparison of the relative size and intensity of the two spots will give an estimate of the relative amounts of the two phospholipids present, although it is preferable to scan the plates with a recording densitometer to obtain more quantitative data (Fig. 29-17).

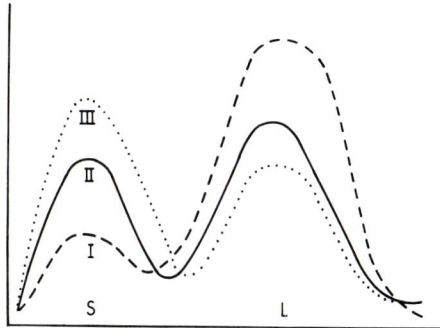

Fig. 29-17. Thin-layer chromatography of amniotic fluid. Phospholipids show changing relationship of lecithin *(L)* to sphingomyelin *(S)* as fetal pulmonary maturation nears. *I*, Maturity, L/S ratio 4:1; *II*, slight immaturity, L/S ratio 1.5:1; *III*, immaturity, L/S ratio 0.8:1.

There are several potential sources of error. The amniotic fluid should be centrifuged to remove cells and debris immediately after collection, and, if not analyzed at once, kept frozen to prevent hydrolysis of the phospholipids by enzymes that may be present. Since the actual amount of the phospholipids is not great, contamination of the fluid by even small amounts of blood will introduce a sufficient quantity of blood phospholipids to give erroneous results. The fluid should not contain more than 1 or 2 vol% of packed red cells after centrifugation. The centrifugal force must be carefully controlled, since it will cause sedimentation of phospholipids.[134] Samples collected by the vaginal route may be contaminated with bacteria or other material containing lipids as well as enzymes capable of hydrolyzing the phospholipids. The presence of meconium will interfere with the extraction of the phospholipids.

Reagents:
1. Methanol
2. Chloroform
3. Developing solution
   Mix together just before use 170 ml chloroform, 20 ml methanol, and 3 ml concentrated ammonium hydroxide.
4. Iodine crystals
5. Modified Dragendorff reagent
   A. Dissolve 1.7 g bismuth subnitrate in 80 ml water and 20 ml glacial acetic acid.
   B. Dissolve 20 g potassium iodide in 50 ml water. Just before use, mix together 20 ml of solution A, 5 ml of solution B, and 70 ml of 20% acetic acid.
6. Sulfuric acid, 50%
   Cautiously add 50 ml concentrated sulfuric acid to 50 ml water. Mix and cool to room temperature.
7. Standards
   Dissolve lecithin (dipalmitoyl) and sphingomyelin (General Biochemical, Chagrin Falls, Ohio) in separate chloroform solutions to give concentrations of 5 mg/ml (e.g., 50 mg in 10 ml chloroform). Store in freezer.

Procedure[135-137]: Centrifuge the amniotic fluid to remove cells and use the supernatant. See precautions listed previously regarding collection and storage of fluid. Add a convenient volume (preferably 4 or 5 ml if available) to a centrifuge tube. Then add a volume of chloroform equal to that of the amniotic fluid plus methanol (e.g., 5 ml of amniotic fluid, 5 ml of methanol, and 10 ml of chloroform), and shake the mixture vigorously. Then centrifuge the tube if necessary to break any emulsion formed and carefully remove the upper aqueous layer by suction and discard.

Filter the chloroform layer through Whatman no. 1 paper into an evaporating dish and evaporate the filtrate to about 0.5 ml on a steam bath. Then transfer this solution to a small test tube with the aid of 1 or 2 ml chloroform and further evaporate to 40-50 μl.

Apply the residual solution along with standards to the TLC sheets. Use Gelman glass-fiber impregnated sheets, type SG (Gelman Instrument Co., Ann Arbor, Mich.). (See p. 688 for the general directions concerning the TLC technic.) At separate positions on each of two 5 × 20 sheets, apply 5 μl each of the two standards and one half of the evaporated extract. The extract is applied in 5 μl portions to keep the size of the spot small. Then develop both sheets in the same chamber with the chloroform-methanol-ammonia developing solution. Allow the development to proceed for about 20 min until the solvent front has traveled about 15 cm. Then remove and air dry the sheets. Exercise care in handling the sheets, since lipids or other material from the fingers may cause spurious spots.

Place one sheet in a closed container containing iodine crystals. Yellow or brown spots will develop in the presence of the lipids. Outline the position and size of the spots with a pencil, because the spots will fade on standing. Lipids other than lecithin and sphingomyelin extracted from the amniotic fluid may also appear as spots on this sheet, but the two desired spots can be identified by comparison with the standard spots. Spray the other sheet with the modified Dragendorff reagent. Air dry the sheet somewhat and then place in a pan containing 20% acetic acid until most of the background color is removed. Lecithin and sphingomyelin should appear as bright orange on a light background.

Outline these spots with a pencil, since they may fade on standing. Only lecithin and sphingomyelin should show up with this reagent. Lecithin should have an R_f value of about 0.56 and sphingomyelin about 0.45. Slight variations in the composition of the developing solution may cause some changes in the R_f values but that for sphingomyelin should be about 80% of that for lecithin, and spots from the sample are always compared with those from the standards. With iodine treatment, other spots may show up with higher and lower R_f values, but these may be disregarded. The relative amounts of the two phospholipids may be estimated from the relative sizes and intensity of the spots. The sheet that has been treated with iodine may be heated in a stream of warm air for a few minutes and then sprayed with 50% sulfuric acid. It is heated to about 200° C on a hot plate to char the lipids. The resulting black spots may be quantitated in a densitometer after sandwiching the sheet between two layers of cellophane or similar material to avoid contact of the acid sheet with the apparatus. If the charring technic is used, great care must be taken to prevent contamination of the sheet with dust or other organic material that will also give black spots on heating.

A TLC method for determining the L/S ratio that includes controls and standards is commercially available in a kit form (Helena Laboratories, Beaumont, Tex.).

Analysis of lecithin in amniotic fluid by TLC, for use in the L/S ratio, measures all species of lecithins. Recently it had been suggested that a more significant and specific risk factor for RDS and HMD is the concentration of disaturated phosphatidylcholine in amniotic fluid, especially dipalmitoyl phosphatidylcholine.[138] The measurement of other specific phospholipids, e.g., phosphatidylglycerol (PG) and phosphatidylinisitol (PI) has also been put forward as an additional correlate of fetal maturity to be used with the traditional L/S ratio.[139,140] Measurement of the saturated lecithins and PG plus PI is also performed using

TLC technic combined with fluorescent or colorimetric analysis.[139-141]

Amniotic fluid microviscosity

Amniotic fluid microviscosity as measured by 1,6-diphenylhexatriene (DPH) fluorescence polarization shows an excellent correlation with the L/S ratio,[142] and predicts the risk of newborn respiratory distress syndrome as well as the L/S ratio.[142]

Principle: DPH becomes fluorescent in the hydrocarbon region of lipid aggregates. The degree of polarization of its fluorescence (P value) is a reflection of the DPH molecule and depends on the viscosity of its microenvironment (or microviscosity) in the lipids. Each P value has a corresponding numeric microviscosity value.[143] In amniotic fluid the relative quantities of lecithin and sphingomyelin greatly influence the microviscosity. During gestation the pattern of change of amniotic fluid microviscosity parallels the expected development of the surfactant system. Microviscosity is high during early gestation and decreases between weeks 28 and 36 of gestation, reflecting the process of fetal maturation.

Reagents and equipment:
1. DPH
2. Fluorescence polarimeter (Microviscosimeter, Model MV-1, Elscint, Inc., Hackensack, N.J.)

The fluorescence polarimeter provides monochromatic excitation at a wavelength of 365 nm and determines the fluorescence polarization of emitted light at a wavelength of 418 nm.

Procedure[144]: Vigorously mix 100 μl of DPH (2 mmole/L) in tetrahydrofuran with 2 dl of the phosphate buffered saline. Add 2 ml of this mixture to 0.5 ml amniotic fluid and incubate at 37° C for 30 min. Determine the fluorescence polarization (p) with a fluorescence polarimeter. Place a thermometer in the cuvet; measure the temperature of the solutions after each p value is determined.

The microviscosity in poise (η) is calculated from the fluorescence polarization (p) by using the approximate relation: $\eta = 2p/(0.46 - p)$.

Foam stability (shake) test

Laboratory methods for quantitating amniotic phospholipids are all relatively difficult technics requiring highly trained technologists. These assays are often not routinely available throughout the entire day. In 1972 a technically simple procedure was introduced to serve as a screen for fetal maturity.[145] This test simply requires shaking a sample of amniotic fluid with alcohol. Phospholipids in amniotic fluid act as a foaming agent, while the alcohol inhibits bubble formation. The more phospholipid present in amniotic fluid, the more bubbles will remain after shaking, i.e., a positive test. Positive foam tests correlate very well with L/S ratios greater than 2, indicating fetal maturity. However, this test can result in false negative results.

Modifications of the original foam test include the use of 100% ethanol[146] and the use of a foam stability index.[147] The latter foam test attempts to semiquantitate the levels of phospholipid present in amniotic fluid. The following method, incorporating the use of abso-

lute ethanol, was reported to give no false positive results.[148]

Procedure: Add 1 ml uncentrifuged amniotic fluid to a 1.3 × 5.0 cm screwcap test tube to which 1 ml absolute (100%) ethanol has been added. Cap immediately with an air-tight screw cap and vigorously shake for 30 sec. Evaluate test 15 sec after completion of shaking.

Interpretation: A scale of 0-4 is used:

0	No bubbles seen at meniscus
1+	Incomplete layer of bubbles, but ring of bubbles surrounds meniscus
2+	One complete layer of bubbles
3+	Two complete layers of bubbles
4+	Entire surface covered with two or more layers of bubbles

To avoid problems related to the hydroscopic nature of the 100% ethanol, the reagent can be prepipetted into the screw-cap test tubes, capped, and taped shut. The tubes can then be stored in a box dessicator ($CaCl_2$) until the time of analysis.

Determination of amniotic fluid volume by spectrophotometric assay of injected para-aminohippuric acid

In the assessment of the risks of erythroblastosis the measurement of bilirubin-type pigments ($\Delta 450$) or bilirubin in the amniotic fluid have proved to be of value. In the assessment of fetal maturity the $\Delta 450$ or the concentration of creatinine has been used, and for measurement of the risk of respiratory distress syndrome, the amount of surface-active agents in amniotic fluid has been employed. In all instances, serial measurements are of much greater value than single determinations. In most cases the predictive value of these measurements has been quite high. In some instances these results do not agree too well with the clinical picture.[149] This may be due to the fact that one is usually measuring the concentration of these substances in the amniotic fluid, whereas the actual total amount is of importance. Thus marked changes in the volume of amniotic fluid would decrease the predictive value of serial concentration measurements. Thus it has been suggested that measurements of the total volume of amniotic fluid would be helpful in estimating the changes in total amounts of these substances. The fluid volume can be conveniently measured by injecting a small known amount of para-aminohippuric acid (PAH) into the fluid and, after allowing time for mixing, determining the concentration of PAH in the fluid. A simple method has been devised for this determination by the direct measurement of the absorption at 272 nm.[150,151]

If the volume of amniotic fluid shows appreciable change during the course of the pregnancy, the comparison may be made in terms of the total amount of substance, i.e., 450 × volume in liters for each sample, or milligrams per deciliter × volume in liters per deciliter; or the values obtained may be corrected to an assumed average volume. For purposes of comparison, the average volumes may be approximated as 350 ml at 15 weeks, 450 ml at 20 weeks, 750 ml at 25 weeks, 1500 ml at 30 and 35 weeks, and then decreasing to 1250 ml at term. These are only rough values, but they can serve for comparative purposes. One would then have the following:

$$\text{Measured level} \times \frac{\text{Actual volume}}{\text{Average volume}} = \text{Corrected level}$$

where the measured level might be 450 mg/dl bilirubin or some other determination. With large variations in fluid volume for a given patient, these corrected values might be more indicative of the actual trend than the measured values.

Procedure: Obtain a sample of amniotic fluid and inject exactly 0.5 ml of a 20% solution of PAH. Add the same amount of PAH (preferably measured with the same syringe as used for injection) to a 1 L volumetric flask and dilute to the mark with water (diluted standard). After the injection, mobilize the patient and 30 min later obtain a second sample of amniotic fluid. Centrifuge the two samples at 3000 rpm for 10 min.

Set up standard, sample, and blank tubes as follows: a blank containing 0.4 ml preinjection sample and 4.6 ml water; a standard containing 0.4 ml preinjection sample, 0.4 ml diluted standard, and 4.2 ml water; and a sample tube containing 0.4 ml postinjection sample and 4.6 ml water. Mix the tubes by gentle inversion and read the standard and sample against the blank at 272 nm.

Calculation: Since the same amount of PAH as injected is diluted 1:1000 and the diluted standard is treated the same as the sample:

$$\frac{\text{Absorbance of sample}}{\text{Absorbance of standard}} \times 1000 = \text{Amniotic fluid vol. (ml)}$$

If the reading of the sample is too high for accurate results, the sample tube and blank may be diluted equally with water (a 1:2 dilution is usually sufficient) and the diluted sample read against the diluted blank. The volume obtained in the calculation above is then divided by the dilution factor (factor of 2 for a 1:2 dilution, etc.).

α-Fetoprotein

High α-fetoprotein (AFP) concentrations in amniotic fluid and maternal serum are associated with neural tube defects (NTDs), e.g., anencephaly, spina bifida, and encephalocele.[152-154] Extensive studies of maternal sera make it clear that AFP levels from pregnancies with or without fetal NTDs overlap, so that serum AFP levels are not diagnostic but serve well as screening tests. The markedly elevated AFP value in amniotic fluid is considered to be a diagnostic test for NTDs. Elevated serum AFP values are recorded in such pregnancy complications as toxemia, diabetes, and fetal death. To separate the "unimportant" elevations from elevations associated with NTDs the test should be repeated in 1-2 weeks. Sporadic elevations are also reported in Turner's syndrome, esophageal and duodenal atresia, hydrocephalus, and other congenital conditions.[155] AFP is the principal fetal protein during the first weeks of life following conception.[94] It is synthesized first in the yolk sac and then in the fetal liver,[94] and fetal urine discharges it into the amniotic fluid. As the normal pregnancy progresses, the AFP concentration in the serum and in the amniotic fluid decreases.[156]

Table 29-6. AFP values in amniotic fluid and serum of women with normal pregnancies

Gestation	AFP (ng/ml) in amniotic fluid	AFP (ng/ml) in serum*
First trimester	<43,000	<119
Second trimester	<14,000	<550
Third trimester	<5,000	<400

*Normal (not pregnant) serum value is 25 ng/ml.

Smith, Kline & French Co. (St. Louis) publishes the values in Table 29-6 for AFP in amniotic fluid and serum of women with normal pregnancies.

The assay methods for AFP include radioimmunoassay, rocket immunoelectrophoresis, and other immunologic methods. Contamination with fetal blood that contains high levels of AFP is the most likely cause of false positive values of amniotic AFP.

SPUTUM

Sputum is the secretion of the goblet cells of the bronchial lining and of the mucus-secreting glands of the bronchial tree. It should therefore be obtained from the lower respiratory tract (bronchi and lungs). Saliva produced by the salivary glands in the mouth is not sputum but is frequently and mistakenly sent to the laboratory instead of sputum. Sputum can be identified on microscopic examination by the presence of carbon dust–laden macrophages (dust cells).

Sputum is a mixture of water, electrolytes, proteins, lipids, hormones, and enzymes mixed with exfoliated epithelial cells and a large number of hematologic cells.

Collection of specimen

Sputum is obtained by expectoration or by bronchoalveolar lavage and should contain only lower respiratory tract secretions. The patient should be carefully instructed as to the type of specimen required. It must be "coughed up from deep down in the chest." If the patient is unable to produce the required specimen, aerosol technics must be used. Heated aerosol technics have been developed (1) to produce sputum not mixed with other secretions and (2) to induce patients whose pulmonary lesion is not cough producing to expectorate.[157]

An early-morning specimen is the preferred material. The patient is instructed to first brush his teeth, rinse his mouth well, and then cough the specimen directly into a wide-mouthed sterile container, which is then closed with a tight-fitting sterile lid.

Physical examination

Amount: The amount of sputum depends on the number of active mucus-secreting cells present in the bronchial mucosa at a given time. Acute bronchial irritation (acute bronchopneumonia) leads to diminished sputum production, whereas chronic irritation (bronchiectasis, chronic bronchitis) causes increased sputum secretion.

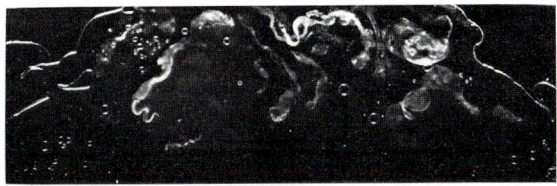

Fig. 29-18. Curschmann's spirals in sputum from patient with asthma. Specimen of sputum is pressed between slides over a black background. (Natural size.)

Copious amounts of sputum are seen in pulmonary adenomatosis, alveolar cell carcinoma of the lung, bronchiectasis, and abscesses and cavities (tuberculosis) that open into bronchi. The sputum from abscesses and bronchiectasis separates into three layers on standing.

Color: Normal sputum is colorless. Inflammatory processes impart a greenish gray color, while increasing numbers of white cells are responsible for a thick purulent appearance. "Cheesy" particles may be seen in cavitary tuberculosis. Acute heart failure is responsible for blood-tinged sputum, while chronic passive congestion of the lungs produces rust-colored sputum. Pyogenic organisms are responsible for purulent sputum that may at times be rust colored *(Pneumococcus)*.

Consistency: Normal sputum is watery. In pulmonary edema it is frothy and may be blood tinged. Pus renders the sputum opaque and often foul smelling. In *Klebsiella pneumoniae* infections and in asthma the secretion is tenacious, while it may be caseous in tuberculosis.

Odor: Normal sputum is odorless, but as indicated above, suppurative, cavitary, necrotizing lesions may be responsible for a foul, even fecal, odor.

Macroscopic examination

Place sputum in a sterile Petri dish and examine macroscopically or with a hand lens against a black background.

Cheesy masses: Cheesy masses are fragments of necrotic lung tissue.

Dittrich's plugs: Dittrich's plugs are plugs from bronchi or bronchioles consisting of cellular detritus, fat, and bacteria. They are seen in chronic lung disease, e.g., bronchiectasis.

Curschmann's spirals: Curschmann's spirals are spirally twisted mucoid strands (Fig. 29-18) enclosing epithelial cells, leukocytes, chiefly eosinophils, and sometimes Charcot-Leyden crystals.

Casts: Bronchial casts are molded in the bronchi and consist of fibrin and mucus. They are usually grayish white, but they may be reddish brown because of blood pigment. They are frequently so tangled that they cannot be recognized until they are floated in water over a black background.

Pneumoliths: Pneumoliths (broncholiths, lung stones) are calcium carbonate and phosphate concretions and are seen in chronic lung disease (tuberculosis).

Parasites: Only a limited number of parasites can be seen grossly; they are *Echinococcus granulosus* (hyda-tid sand in sputum), *Toxocara canis* (visceral larva migrans), *Paragonimus westermani,* and *Ascaris lumbricoides.*

Mycetomas: Patients on long-term antibiotic or steroid therapy may expectorate rounded masses (fungus balls) of so-called opportunistic fungi such as masses of *Aspergillus,* called **aspergilloma.**[158]

Microscopic examination
Unstained preparation

Microscopic examination of the unstained sputum preparation has lost much of its importance since there are better methods of diagnosing lung disease now available, but it is still the most rapid method for differentiating saliva from sputum (carbon-pigmented macrophages).

Procedure: Place 1 drop of sputum on a slide under a coverslip. Examine under bright-field (lowered condensor), phase-contrast, or interference-contrast microscope for epithelial cells, inflammatory cells, red cells, Curschmann's spirals, elastic tissue fibers, crystals, parasites, phagocytic cells containing pigment, dust particles, mineral oil, fat, or fungi.

Stained preparations

Smears are air dried and stained with Wright-Giemsa stain for hematologic cells, with Gram stain for bacteria, with India ink or Gomori methenamine silver stain for fungi, and with carbol-fuchsin stain for acid-fast organisms. For cytologic examination (Papanicolaou technic), smears are quickly fixed with a cytologic fixative, e.g., Fix-Rite (Richard-Allan Medical Industries, Richland, Mich.).

Cell types in sputum

The cells contained in the sputum arise from the bronchial epithelium or enter the bronchus from the circulating blood.

Bronchial epithelial cells: The sloughed-off bronchial cells reflect the pathologic state of the bronchi and lungs. Most of these cells are columnar and ciliated in type.[159] Degenerated bizarre-shaped cells are referred to as showing **"myelin degeneration."** Differential counts are used to (1) estimate the number of basal cells and ciliated bronchial epithelial cells, (2) evaluate their degenerative changes, and (3) establish the number of associated histiocytes and other blood-borne cells (polymorphonuclear cells, lymphocytes, etc.) In chronic bronchitis the differential count may be as follows: monocytes, 1-2%; polymorphonuclear cells, up to 75%; histiocytes, 5-20%; and bronchial epithelial cells, 5-15%.

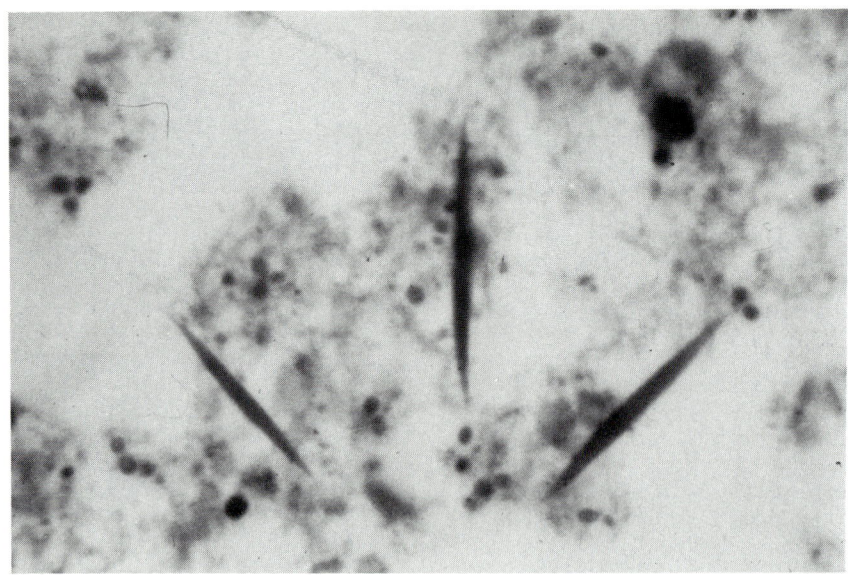

Fig. 29-19. Charcot-Leyden crystals.

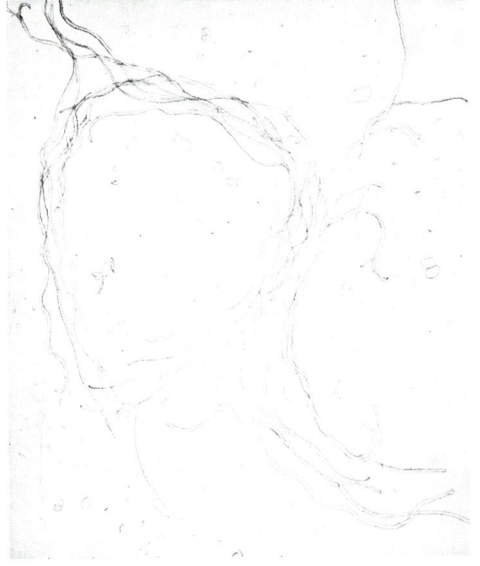

Fig. 29-20. High-power field showing elastic tissue fibers in sputum of patient with lung abscess. (Sodium hydroxide preparation.)

Hematologic cells: Lymphocytes and monocytes are common in sputum. Leukocytes reflect an inflammatory process, and **macrophages** reflect the patient's resistance. Macrophages are the microscopic hallmark of sputum. They contain dust and carbon particles, fat droplets in lipid pneumonia, and hemosiderin in chronic heart failure (**heart failure cells**).

In **pneumoconiosis** there are a large number of phagocytic leukocytes containing various **dust particles,** e.g., silicosis (silica or sand); anthracosis (coal);

siderosis (iron); calicosis (marble or lime); and asbestosis (asbestos).

The **asbestos bodies** are extracellular, highly refractile bodies with a central needlelike crystal (greenish tinge) around which is deposited a yellowish homogeneous substance. The bodies often have clubbed ends and show segmentation. They give the Prussian blue reaction for iron.

In bagassosis the sputum contains silica-impregnated fibers.

In **lipid pneumonia,** macrophages contain liquid petrolatum or vegetable and animal oils. Animal and vegetable oils stain both with Sudan IV (scarlet red) and osmic acid; mineral oil stains with Sudan IV but not with osmic acid.

Pus cells: Attempts have been made to grade the purulence of sputum on the basis of the number of pus cells to evaluate therapeutic results in chronic lung disease.[160]

Eosinophils: Eosinophilia (number of eosinophils in sputum) has been used to observe patients with asthma and chronic bronchitis. The sputum is stained with an eosin-formalin solution and examined wet. An increased number of eosinophils (exceeding the number in the peripheral blood) are found in chronic bronchitis and aspergillosis and with increasing age.

Eosin-formalin solution:
Eosin, aqueous   0.5 g
Formalin, 10%   1 dl

Erythrocytes: Small numbers of erythrocytes are normally present in sputum, but large numbers indicate hemorrhage or severe infections (viral or bacterial).

Charcot-Leyden crystals

Charcot-Leyden crystals are believed to be derived from eosinophils. They are hexagonal, slender crystals with pointed ends (Fig. 29-19).

Elastic fibers

Elastic fibers are highly refractive and curlylike springs. The ends are often split (Fig. 29-20).

Chemical investigation
Neuramic acid assay

The glands in the bronchial tree produce **acid gly-coproteins** that form the bulk of sputum, to which is added saliva and a transudate that originates in the tissue spaces.[161] The glycoprotein is a large molecule that consists of several amino acids (serine, glycine, proline, etc.) and sialic and neuramic acids. It is interesting that the influenza virus contains an enzyme (neuramidase) that destroys sialic acid in the epithelial mucin. The viscosity of the sputum is related to its glycoprotein content, which can be monitored by neuramic acid assays. In **asthma** the neuramic acid content is high and so is the viscosity of the sputum. In saliva, the neuramic acid content is almost zero and so is the viscosity. Between these two extremes lies the viscosity and the neuramic acid content of the sputum of individuals with chronic bronchitis and of normal individuals. It is possible that analysis of the neuramic acid content of sputum will provide a method for evaluating the effectiveness of treatment for asthma and chronic bronchitis.

α-Antitrypsin

α-Antitrypsin is a serum protein, the absence or low level of which has a direct relationship to pulmonary disease in adulthood and liver disease in childhood. In the adult pulmonary emphysema appears at an unusually early age,[162] while in the infant and child (rarely in the adult) the deficiency leads to neonatal hepatitis and cirrhosis, which in the young may be responsible for the development of hepatocellular carcinoma.

The enzyme has a trimodal distribution in the serum; there is the normal level on one end of the scale and severe α_1-antitrypsin deficiency on the other end. The latter occurs in individuals **homozygous** for the genetic defect of low levels of α_1-antitrypsin. Individuals homozygous for the defect develop pulmonary emphysema in early middle age. Intermediate levels indicate **heterozygosity** for the gene controlling α_1-antitrypsin levels. Heterozygotes appear to carry no increased risk. By starch electrophoresis, several genetic variants of α_1-antitrypsin deficiency have been demonstrated that collectively constitute the **Pi system.**

Quantitative test: radial immunodiffusion assay of α_1-antitrypsin: The radial immunodiffusion test is commercially available (ICL Scientific, Fountain Valley, Calif.).

Principle: The buffered agar medium of the plate contains a specific α_1-antitrypsin antibody. Known controls and the patient's serum containing the α_1-antitrypsin are placed in wells located in the immunodiffusion plate. The controls contain three known levels of α_1-antitrypsin.

At the end of the "run," which takes 18-20 hr, the reference serum results are plotted and the resulting curve is used to "read off" the concentration of the unknown α_1-antitrypsin level.

Results: The normal values of α_1-antitrypsin are 180-400 mg/dl. Homozygous deficient individuals have levels of 19-31 mg/dl, while the level for heterozygotus individuals is 79-171 mg/dl.

PUS

Pus is a yellow to yellow-green liquid that contains many polymorphonuclear cells in all stages of degeneration, much granular and fatty debris from disintegrated pus cells and tissue, and the causative organisms as well as secondary invaders at times. Some pus contains many eosinophils (gonorrheal pus, purulent pleuritic fluids, and asthmatic sputum). Pus from old abscesses may show numerous fatty acid and cholesterol crystals, and when there has been hemorrhage, hematoidin crystals are also present. In some liver abscesses, bilirubin crystals and amebae are found.

REFERENCES

1. Hoeprich, P.D., and Ward, J.R.: The fluids of body cavities, New York, 1959, Grune & Stratton, Inc.
2. Agostoni, E.: Physiol. Rev. **52:**57, 1972.
3. Halla, J.T., Schohenloher, R.E., and Volanakis, J.E.: Ann. Intern. Med. **92:**748, 1980.
4. Editorial: Br. Med. J. **281:**763, 1980.
5. Lowell, J.R.: Diagnosis: fluid and tissue examination in pleural effusions, Baltimore, 1977, University Park Press.
6. Light, R.W., et al.: Chest **64:**591, 1973.
7. Potts, D.E., Taryle, D.A., and Sahn, S.A.: Arch. Intern. Med. **138:**1378, 1978.
8. Carr, D.T., and Mayne, J.G.: Am. Rev. Respir. Dis. **85:**345, 1962.
9. Chandrasekhar, A.J., et al.: Arch. Intern. Med. **123:**48, 1969.
10. Fleisher, G.A., et al.: Gastroenterology **37:**325, 1959.
11. Hammarstein, J.F., Houska, W.L., Jr., and Limes, B.J.: Am. Rev. Respir. Dis. **79:**606, 1959.
12. Levine, H., et al.: Ann. Intern. Med. **69:**487, 1968.
13. Black, L.F.: Mayo Clin. Proc. **47:**493, 1972.
14. Light, R.W., et al.: Ann. Intern. Med. **77:**507, 1972.
15. Glasser, L.: Diagn. Med., pp. 79-80, Sept.-Oct. 1980.
16. Berger, H.W., and Maher, G.: Am. Rev. Respir. Dis. **103:**427, 1971.
17. Carr, D.T., Lillington, G.A., and Mayne, J.G.: Mayo Clin. Proc. **45:**409, 1970.
18. Hain, E., and Engel, J.: Pneumonologie **145:**175, 1971.
19. Matsuura, C., et al.: Hiroshima J. Med. Sci. **20:**195, 1971.
20. Crosby, R.M.N., and Weiland, G.L.: Arch. Neurol. Psychiatr. **69:**732, 1953.
21. Logothetis, J., and Bovis, M.: World Neurol. **2:**747, 1961.
22. Hammock, M.K., and Milhorat, T.H.: Ann. Clin. Lab. Sci. **6:**22, 1976.
23. Davson, H.: Physiology of the cerebrospinal fluid, Boston, 1967, Little, Brown & Co.
24. Glasser, L.: Diagn. Med., pp. 23-33, Jan.-Feb. 1981.
25. Savory, J., and Heintges, M.G.: Neurologia **23:**953-958, 1973.
26. Bronnestam, R., Dencker, S.J., and Swahn, B.: Arch. Neurol. **4:**288, 1961.
27. Cole, M.: Hosp. Pract. **4:**47, 1969.
28. Ivers, R.R., McKenzie, B.F., and McGuckin, W.F.: J.A.M.A. **176:**515, 1961.
29. Fleisher, G.A., Wakim, K.G., and Goldstein, N.P.: Clin. Proc. **32:**188, 1957.
30. Naidoo, B.T.: S. Afr. Med. J. **42:**933, 1968.

31. Fishmann, R.A.: Cerebrospinal fluid in diseases of the nervous system, Philadelphia, 1980, W.B. Saunders Co.
32. Simon, R.P., and Abele, J.S.: Ann. Intern. Med. **89:**75, 1978.
33. Bradford, M.M.: Anal. Biochem. **72:**248, 1976.
34. Spector, T.: Anal. Biochem. **86:**142, 1978.
35. Tibbling, G., Link, H., and Ohman, S.: Scand. J. Clin. Lab. Invest. **37:**385-390, 1977.
36. Ganrot, K., and Laurell, C.-B.: Clin. Chem. **20:**571-573, 1974.
37. Killingsworth, L.M., et al.: Diagn. Med., pp. 23-29, March-April 1980.
38. Greer, M.: Clin. Neurosurg. **15:**161, 1968.
39. Landes, R., Reich, J.P., and Perlow, S.: J.A.M.A. **116:**2482, 1941.
40. Lyons, H.A., and Harrison, J.G.: Blood **4:**734, 1949.
41. Epstein, E., et al.: Ann. Clin. Lab. Sci. **6:**27, 1976.
42. Verheecke, P.: J. Neurol. Sci. **26:**277, 1975.
43. Good, A.E., and Frishette, W.A.: J.A.M.A. **198:**80, 1966.
44. Greenhouse, A.H., and Speck, L.B.: Am. J. Med. Sci. **248:**333, 1964.
45. Johnson, K.P., and Nelson, B.J.: Ann. Neurol. **2:**425, 1977.
46. Johnson, K.P., et al.: Neurology (Minneap.) **27:**273, 1977.
47. Gerson, B., and Orr, J.M.: Am. J. Clin. Pathol. **73:**87-91, 1980.
48. Panitch, A.S., Hooper, C.J., and Johnson, K.P.: Arch. Neurol. **37:**206, 1980.
49. Whitaker, J.N.: Neurology (Minneap.) **27:**911, 1977.
50. Fuchs, F., editor: Clin. Obstet. Gynecol. **9**(entire issue), 1966.
51. Barach, A.L., et al.: Can. Med. Assoc. J. **83:**211, 1960.
52. Pons, E.R.: Arch. Intern. Med. **106:**230, 1960.
53. Eickhoff, K., and Heipertz, R.: Ann. Neurol. **3:**509, 1978.
54. Berner, J.J., Ciemins, V.A., and Schroeder, E.F., Jr.: Am. J. Clin. Pathol. **58:**145, 1972.
55. Link, H., and Müller, R.: Arch. Neurol. **25:**326, 1971.
56. Tourtellotte, W.W., et al.: Arch. Neurol. **25:**345, 1971.
57. Brook, I., et al.: J. Infect. Dis. **137:**384-390, 1978.
58. Knight, J.A., Dudek, S.M., and Haymond, R.E.: Clin. Chem. **25:**809-810, 1979.
59. Bland, R.D., Lister, R.C., and Ries, J.P.: Am. J. Dis. Child. **128:**151-156, 1974.
60. Posner, J.B., Swanson, A.G., and Plum, F.: Arch. Neurol. **12:**479, 1965.
61. Fencl, V., Miller, T.B., and Papenheimer, J.R.: Am. J. Physiol. **210:**459, 1966.
62. Bradley, R.D., and Semple, S.J.: J. Physiol. **160:**381, 1962.
63. Chutorian, A., et al.: Trans. Am. Neurol. Assoc. **91:**206, 1966.
64. Jefferson, M.: Clin. Sci. Mol. Med. **13:**599, 1954.
65. Spalter, H., and Hartwell, G.L.: Neurology (Minneap.) **12:**53, 1962.
66. Reitman, S., and Frankel, S.: Am. J. Clin. Pathol. **28:**56, 1957.
67. Myerson, R.M., Hurwitz, J.K., and Sall, T.: N. Engl. J. Med. **257:**273, 1957.
68. Lowenthal, A., van Sande, M., and Karcher, D.: J. Neurochem. **7:**135, 1961.
69. Wroblewski, F., and La Due, J.S.: Proc. Soc. Exp. Biol. Med. **90:**210, 1955.
70. Bodansky, O.: Cancer **7:**1191, 1954.
71. Enestrom, S.: Acta Neurol. Scand. **41**(suppl. 13):153, 1965.
72. Sayk, J.: Arztl. Wochenschr. **9:**1042, 1954.
73. Hollander, J.L., Reginato, A., and Torralba, T.P.: Med. Clin. North Am. **50:**1281, 1966.
74. Glasser, L.: Diagn. Med. pp. 35-50, Nov.-Dec. 1980.
75. Ropes, M.W., Bennett, G.A., and Bauer, W.: J. Clin. Invest. **18:**351, 1939.
76. Cohen, A.S.: Laboratory diagnostic procedures in the rheumatic diseases, Boston, 1975, Little, Brown & Co.
77. Gottlieb, N.: J. Fl. Med. Assoc. **56:**323, 1969.
78. Hunter, T., Gordon, D.A., and Ogryzlo, M.A.: J. Rheumatol. **1:**45, 1974.
79. Schumacher, H.R., and Holdsworth, D.E.: Semin. Arthritis Rheum. **6:**207, 1977.
80. Kitridou, R., et al.: Arthritis Rheum. **12:**520, 1969.
81. Perez, J.S., and Russel, A.S.: Can. Med. Assoc. J. **112:**1320, 1975.
82. Cracchiolo, A., III: Am. Fam. Physician **4:**87, 1971.
83. Ropes, M.W., and Bauer, W.: Synovial fluid changes in joint diseases, Cambridge, Mass., 1953, Harvard University Press.
84. Cho, M.H., and Neuhaus, O.W.: Thromb. Haemost. **5:**108, 1960.
85. Ropes, M.W., Muller, A.F., and Bauer, W.: Arthritis Rheum. **3:**496, 1960.
86. Schumacher, H.R., Jr.: In Kelley, W.N., et al., editors: Textbook of rheumatology, Philadelphia, 1981, W.B. Saunders Co.
87. Schumacher, H.R., Jr.: Ann. Clin. Lab. Sci. **5:**242, 1975.
88. Traycoff, R.B., Pascual, E., and Schumacher, H.R.: Arthritis Rheum. **19:**743, 1976.
89. Schumacher, H.R.: N. Engl. J. Med. **274:**1372, 1966.
90. McCarty, D.J., Jr., and Hollander, J.L.: Ann. Intern. Med. **54:**452, 1961.
91. Kahn, C.B., Hollander, J.L., and Schumacher, H.R.: J.A.M.A. **211:**807, 1970.
92. Tanphaichitr, K., Spilberg, I., and Hahn, B.: Arthritis Rheum. **19:**966, 1976.
93. Moskowitz, R.W., et al.: Arthritis Rheum. **14:**109, 1971.
94. Borer, W.Z.: In Brown, S.S., Mitchell, F.L., and Young, D.S., editors: Chemical diagnosis of disease, Amsterdam, 1979, Elsevier Publishing Co.
95. Singer, J.M., and Plotz, C.M.: J.A.M.A. **168:**180, 1959.
96. Watson, R.G.: Am. J. Clin. Pathol. **43:**152, 1965.
97. Cohen, A.S., Brandt, K.D., and Krey, P.R.: In Cohen, A.S., editor: Laboratory diagnostic procedures in rheumatic diseases, ed. 2, Boston, 1975, Little, Brown & Co.
98. Rodman, G.P.: J.A.M.A. **224:**661, 1973.
99. Kindler, H.: Ger. Med. Mon. **5:**62, 1960.
100. Lehman, M.A., Kream, J., and Brogna, D.: J. Bone Joint Surg. [Am.] **46:**1732, 1964.
101. Fuchs, F.: Clin. Obstet. Gynecol. **9:**449, 1966.
102. NICHD Amniocentesis Registry Symposium: J.A.M.A. **236:**1471, 1976.
103. Bergsma, D., editor: Birth Defects **7**(entire issue), 1971.
104. Whitfield, C.R.: Am. J. Obstet. Gynecol. **108:**1239, 1970.
105. Whitfield, C.R.: Clin. Obstet. Gynecol. **14:**537, 1971.
106. Dito W.R., Patrick, C.W., and Shelly, J.: Clinical pathologic correlations in amniotic fluid, Chicago, 1975, American Society of Clinical Pathologists.
107. Nadler, H.L., and Gerbie A.B.: N. Engl. J. Med. **282:**596, 1970.
108. Nadler, H.L., and Gerbie, A.: Obstet. Gyneco.. **38:**789, 1971.
109. Gluck, L., et al.: Am. J. Obstet. Gynecol. **109:**440, 1971.

110. Moltz, A., Pomerance, W., and Wechsler, R.: Obstet. Gynecol. **39:**107, 1972.
111. Gluck, L.: Clin. Obstet. Gynecol. **21:**547, 1978.
112. Steinman, G., Kleiner, G.J., and Greston, W.M.: N.Y. State J. Med. **79:**1849, 1979.
113. Bonsnes, R.W.: Clin. Obstet. Gynecol. **9:**440, 1966.
114. Whitfield, C.R.: Clin. Obstet. Gynecol. **14:**537, 1971.
115. Hill, C.M., et al.: Br. J. Obstet. Gynaecol. **86:**773, 1979.
116. Queenan, J.T.: Clin. Obstet. Gynecol. **14:**505, 1971.
117. Bevis, D.C.A.: Br. J. Obstet. Gynaecol. **63:**68, 1956.
118. Walker, A.H.C., and Jenimson, R.F.: Br. Med. J. **2:**1152, 1962.
119. Freda, V.J.: Am. J. Obstet. Gynecol. **92:**341, 1965.
120. Liley, A.W.: Am. J. Obstet. Gynecol. **86:**485, 1963.
121. Gambino, S.R., and Freda, V.J.: Am. J. Clin. Pathol. **46:**198, 1966.
122. Jendrassik, L., and Grof, P.: Biochem. Ztsche. **297:**81, 1938.
123. Nelson, G.H., and Talldeo, O.E.: Am. J. Clin. Pathol. **52:**363, 1969.
124. Woyton, J.: Zentralbl. Gynaekol. **85:**552, 1963.
125. Nelson, M.M., and Emery, A.E.H.: Br. Med. J. **1:**523, 1970.
126. Nelson, G.H., et al.: South, Med. J. **64:**1, 1971.
127. Parmley, T., and Miller, E.: Am. J. Obstet. Gynecol. **105:**354, 1969.
128. Horger, E.O.: South. Med. J. **65:**299, 1972.
129. Lind, T., and Billewicz, W.Z.: Br. J. Hosp. Med. **5:**681, 1971.
130. Gertner, M., Hsu, L.Y., and Hirschhorn, K.: Paper presented at the Fortieth Annual Meeting of the Society of Pediatric Research, Atlantic City, N.J., 1970.
131. Butterworth, J.: J. Inher. Metab. Dis. **1:**25, 1978.
132. Nyhan, W.L.: Clin. Symp. **32**(5), 1980.
133. Gluck, L.: Hosp. Pract. **6:**45, 1971.
134. Olson, E.B. Jr., Graven, S.N., and Zachman, R.D.: Pediatr. Res. **9:**65, 1975.
135. Gluck, L., Kulovich, M., and Brody, S.: J. Lipid Res. **1:**570, 1966.
136. Foreman, D.T., and Balis, J.N.: In Sunderman, F.W., editor: Manual of procedures for applied seminar on the clinical pathology of the lipids, Washington, D.C., 1971, Association of Clinical Scientists.
137. Coch, E.H., and Kessler, G.: Clin. Chem. **18:**490, 1972.
138. Shelley, S.A., et al.: N. Engl. J. Med. **300:**112-116, 1979.
139. Gotelli, G.R., et al.: Clin. Chem. **24:**1144-1146, 1978.
140. Freer, D.E., Statland, B.E., and Sher, G.: Clin. Chem. **25:**960-968, 1979.
141. Mitnick, M.A., DeMarco, B., and Gibbons, J.M.: Clin. Chem. **26:**277-281, 1980.
142. Cheskin, H.S., et al.: Clin. Chem. **26:**301, 1980.
143. Blumenfeld, T.A., Cheskin, H.S., and Stark, R.I.: Diagn. Dialog., vol., 2, September 1980.
144. Blumenfeld, T.A., Cheskin, H.S., and Shinitzky, M.: Clin. Chem. **25:**64, 1979.
145. Clements, J.A., et al.: N. Engl. J. Med. **286:**1077-1081, 1972.
146. Edwards J., and Baillie, P.: S. Afr. Med. J. **47:**2070-2075, 1973.
147. Statland, B.E., and Freer, D.E.: Diagn. Med. pp. 73-86, Nov.-Dec. 1979.
148. Statland, B.E., et al.: Am. J. Clin. Pathol. **69:**514-519, 1978.
149. Whitfield, C.R.: Clin. Obstet. Gynecol. **14:**537, 1971.
150. Abramovich, D.R.: Br. J. Obstet. Gynaecol. **77:**865, 1970.
151. Thompson, W., Lappin, T.R.J., and Elder, G.E.: Br. J. Obstet. Gynaecol. **78:**341, 1971.
152. U.K. collaborative study on alpha-fetoprotein in relation to neural-tube defects: Lancet **1:**1323, 1977.
153. Henry, G.P., and Robinson, A.: Clin. Obstet. Gynecol. **21:**329, 1978.
154. Cowchock, F.S.: Clin Obstet. Gynecol. **19:**871, 1976.
155. Brock, D.J.II.: Biochem. Soc. Trans. **7:**1179, 1979
156. Hay, D.M., et al.: Br. J. Obstet. Gynaecol. **83:**534, 1976.
157. Paez, P.N., and Miller, W.F.: Chest **60:**312, 1971.
158. O'Neill, R.P., and Penman, R.W.B.: South, Med. J. **64:**392, 1971.
159. Chodosh, S.: N. Engl. J. Med. **282:**854, 1970.
160. Miller, D.L.: Am. Rev. Respir. Dis. **88:**473, 1963.
161. Keal, E., and Reid, L.: Internist **12:**416, 1971.
162. Sharp, H.L.: Gastroenterology **70:**611, 1976.

CHAPTER 30

Gastric, duodenal, and pancreatic juice analysis

Gastric analysis
    Intubation method
    Other methods for measuring gastric acidity
    Gross examination of gastric juice
    Chemical investigation of gastric juice
    Microscopic examination of gastric juice
Pancreatic juice analysis
    Gross examination of pancreatic juice
    Microscopic examination of pancreatic juice
Fibrocystic disease of the pancreas
    Laboratory investigation

Gastric secretion: Gastric secretion contains hydrochloric acid secreted by the parietal cells of the fundus and upper body of the stomach and an alkaline enzyme–mucoprotein complex secreted by the superficial mucosal cells (antral, pyloric, and fundal glands). The alkaline component contains enzymes such as pepsin and lipase and electrolytes such as sodium, potassium, calcium, chloride, hydrogen, and phosphorus. The secretion is under central (vagal), chemical (intestinal), and hormonal (gastric) control.

GASTRIC ANALYSIS
Intubation method
Measurement of gastric acid[1-3]

The most useful information is obtained by a single test that measures basal secretion and maximal (pentagastrin-histamine–stimulated) secretion.

Procedure for intubation

Intubation of patient: Although this is now rarely done in the laboratory, particularly since fluoroscopic examination is needed for best results, the directions are included here. The patient should be fasting (12 hr [overnight]) and should have received no medication in the previous 24 hr period. Place the stomach tube in ice water and slightly lubricate the tip with petrolatum. Seat the patient and instruct him to take deep breaths through his mouth while a radiopaque 16-18 French gauge Levine tube is inserted into the floor of the nose and then slowly and gradually passed into the pharynx and esophagus. The tube has distance markers. The distance between the teeth and the cardia of the stomach is about 45 cm, whereas the distance from a well-positioned tube tip to the teeth is about 60 cm. Fluoroscopic control is necessary to ensure proper tube placement. The tip of the tube should lie in the lower-

most part of the body of the stomach. When correctly in position fasten the tube securely to the patient's nose and forehead to ensure that there is no displacement during subsequent aspirations. Place the patient on his back and slightly to his left and allow him to relax before the gastric residue is collected. Then apply suction at 3-5 mm Hg and interrupt at 3 min intervals. Aspirate completely the gastric juice present at the start of the procedure. (It is termed the residual juice.) The fasting, resting, or basal secretion is assessed by aspiration and collection for the next 1 hr period. This is usually collected at two consecutive periods of 30 min each. To determine the capacity of the stomach to secrete acid, a stimulation test is carried out by using one of a number of agents, including histamine, Histalog (bentazole), insulin, and pentagastrin. Although histamine (0.01-0.04 mg/kg) and Histalog (0.5 mg/kg) have been used for a number of years, they are rapidly being replaced by pentagastrin. Pentagastrin or pentapeptide is a synthetic peptide related to the active portion of the gastrin molecule. It produces a highly reproducible stimulus to gastric secretion that is more potent than the histamine or Histalog and is both safe and virtually free of side effects.[4] Pentagastrin is administered at a dose of 6 μg/kg body weight, and gastric juice is aspirated in 15 min aliquots for 1 hr with acid secretion determined by one of the methods described below.

Basal secretion: Basal secretion is the amount of gastric juice obtained in the absence of any stimuli. It may be obtained by continuous aspiration during a 12 hr period overnight. It has been found that a 1 hr morning collection of basal secretion is equivalent to a 12 hr overnight collection.

Maximal secretion[5,6]: Maximal secretion is measured after subcutaneous administration of an augmented dose of 0.05 mg/kg histamine dihydrochloride or 2 mg/kg Histalog. After the injection the gastric secretion is collected by continuous aspiration for 60 min in four 15 min specimens.

Titration of acid with 0.1N sodium hydroxide, using Töpfer reagent and phenolphthalein

Procedure: Although the titration method is still used and is given here, the preferred method is the one using the pH meter as given below.

In either method filter the contents of the sample through two thicknesses of gauze, if necessary, to remove most of the food residue and mucus. In a small graduated cylinder, measure 10 ml and transfer to a porcelain evaporating dish. Add 1 or 2 drops Töpfer reagent (dimethylaminoazobenzene, 0.5% alcoholic solution) and 1 or 2 drops of phenolphthalein (1% alcoholic solution) and titrate with 0.1N sodium hydroxide from a buret until the last trace of red color disappears. Take this reading for free hydrochloric acid. Continue the titration until the red color of phenolphthalein appears, titrating to the point at which further addition of alkali does not deepen the color. Take the buret reading for the total acidity, counting from the original reading.

The total acidity equals the hydrochloric acid plus the combined acidity. The latter is produced by organic acids (lactic, butyric, acetic, and carbonic), phosphates, and proteins.

Calculation: Since 10 ml of gastric contents are titrated with 0.1N (0.1 mEq/L) alkali, the concentration of acid (hydrogen ions) in the contents equals $10 \times 0.1 \times V_1 = V_1$, where V_1 is the number of milliliters of alkali used in the titration.

If the sodium hydroxide solution is not exactly 0.1N or if an amount other than 10 ml of gastric contents is used, the value obtained above is multiplied by the factor 100 N/V, where N is the actual normality of the sodium hydroxide solution used and V is the actual volume in milliliters of the gastric contents used.

Units of measurement: The acidity is expressed now in milliequivalents per liter of hydrogen ions. Formerly the term *degree of acidity* was used. This is numerically equivalent to the value in milliequivalents per liter, but the former term is now obsolete. The total amount of acid secreted may be of more diagnostic value than the concentration of acid in the contents. This may be readily calculated as

Total milliequivalents secreted =
Sample vol. (L) × Conc. in milliequivalents per liter

The rate of secretion in milliequivalents per hour may be calculated by dividing the total amount secreted by the collection time in hours. One recommended method is to calculate the maximal acid output per hour by adding the amounts of acid secreted in the two highest consecutive 15 min aliquots and multiplying by 2.

Values of gastric analysis expressed in milliequivalents secreted[7]:

One-hour basal acid output:

<2 mEq	Normal, gastric ulcer, or gastric cancer
2-5 mEq	Normal, gastric ulcer, or duodenal ulcer
>5 mEq	Duodenal ulcer
>20 mEq	Zollinger-Ellison syndrome

One-hour maximal acid output:

0 mEq	True achlorhydria, gastritis, or gastric cancer
1-20 mEq	Normal, gastric ulcer, or gastric cancer
20-35 mEq	Duodenal ulcer
35-60 mEq	Duodenal ulcer, high normal secretion, or Zollinger-Ellison syndrome
>60 mEq	Zollinger-Ellison syndrome

Ratio of basal acid output to maximal acid output:

20%	Normal, gastric ulcer, or gastric cancer
20-40%	Gastric ulcer or duodenal ulcer
40-60%	Duodenal ulcer or Zollinger-Ellison syndrome
>60%	Zollinger-Ellison syndrome

Other methods for measuring gastric acidity

Various other methods of measuring gastric acidity and reporting the results have been suggested. Bock[8] suggested discontinuing the terms *free acid* and *total acid* and recording acidity obtained by titration to pH 7.0 with a glass electrode in milliequivalents of hydrochloric acid per liter. Baron[9] suggested the discontinuation of the titration of free acid to pH 3.5 with Töpfer reagent and of total acidity with phenolphthalein to pH 8.0-10.0. He replaced both titrations with measurements of the concentration of the acid, the titratable acidity (in milliequivalents per liter) obtained by titration with sodium hydroxide to neutrality (pH 7.0-7.4) electrometrically or colorimetrically with phenol red. Lubran[10] offered theoretic reasons and experimental data in favor of titrating gastric acid to a pH of 3.5 with Töpfer reagent or with a glass electrode.

Moore and Scarlata[11] determine the acidity by direct measurement of the pH with a **glass electrode.** In theory this is the most accurate method. Accurate titrations can be made with pure hydrochloric acid solutions, but with gastric contents the titration curve does not have a sharp inflection point and any choice of a particular pH for the end point is somewhat arbitrary. The collection of specimens as outlined by Burke[13] is essentially the same as already presented. The gastric tube is positioned fluoroscopically, so that the tip is just distal to the junction of the antrum and the body of the stomach. Four 15 min specimens are collected in the basal state. After the adminstration of Histalog, six 15 min specimens are collected. The volume of each specimen is measured and, after the determination of the pH and the calculation of the acidity in milliequivalents as described below, the milliequivalent of the four basal 15 min specimens are added to give the total basal output in milliequivalents. If only three specimens are available, the sum of these three is multiplied by $^4/_3$ to give a 1 hr output. For the output after stimulation, the four consecutive 15 min periods giving the highest total output are used to calculate the 1 hr output after stimulation. The results by this method are similar to those given earlier, with an average normal basal output of 1.5 mEq/hr and an upper limit of 2.5 mEq/hr. The mean value for the output after histamine is taken as 11 mEq/hr, with an upper limit of 21 mEq/hr.

Determination of gastric acidity by glass electrode

This requires a high-quality glass electrode and a pH meter that can read to 0.001 pH unit. Two calibrating buffers are required. One, of pH 7.0, may be obtained commercially from the manufacturers of the pH instruments or various supply houses. The other buffer, of pH 1.68, is prepared from potassium tetraoxalate obtained from the National Bureau of Standards (NBS Standard Sample 189, National Bureau of Standards,

Washington, D.C.). Dissolve 12.61 of this material in distilled water and dilute to exactly 1 L. This solution will have a pH of 1.675 at 20° C, 1.679 at 25° C, and 1.683 at 30° C.

Calibration of pH meter: Rinse off electrodes and place in pH 7.0 buffer. Allow to stand for several minutes with occasional swirling; then adjust the meter to read exactly 7.0. Remove electrodes from this buffer, rinse well with water, wipe off gently, and place in a beaker containing the pH 1.679 buffer. Allow to stand for several minutes to attain equilibrium; then adjust the meter to read 1.679 by using the temperature-compensating knob or scale-expansion dial if the instrument has one. If a number of samples are being measured, the electrodes and meter should be checked occasionally at this pH.

Measurement of gastric secretion: Measure the volume of the specimen and mix well. Transfer a portion to a small beaker, rinse off the electrodes, and insert in the beaker. Swirl gently for several minutes for equilibrium and take a pH reading. Several readings should be taken after further swirling until a constant reading is obtained. The acidity (hydrogen ion concentration) is obtained from the pH reading as outlined below. Readings are taken similarly on all the specimens, rinsing the electrodes well with water between determinations.

Calculation of hydrogen ion concentration from pH reading: The actual pH is related not to the hydrogen ion concentration directly but to the thermodynamic activity of the hydrogen ions. This will differ somewhat from the actual concentration, depending on the presence of other ions (principally Na^+ and K^+). Moore[12] gives a complete table showing the relationship for different concentrations of the other ions. Since these ions are not ordinarily determined in gastric contents, a simplified calculation is presented that assumes an average concentration of 50 mEq/L for Na^+ plus K^+. Express $-$pH as a positive number minus 10 in the usual logarithm convention. Add to this the factor log F obtained from Table 30-1 (by interpolation if necessary) for the pH measured. The antilog of the resulting number is the hydrogen ion concentration in milliequivalents per liter. The examples given with Table 30-1 should make this method clear.

Gross examination of gastric juice

Amount: The overnight secretion of gastric juice after 1 hr of aspiration amounts to 50-80 ml. Over 80 ml is pathologic. The fasting volume is increased in gastric hypomotility, pyloric obstruction, and Zollinger-Ellison syndrome. The volume is decreased, at times to almost zero, by gastric hypermotility.

Color: Normal gastric juice is almost colorless. Bile will stain it yellow-green and blood will produce a red to coffee-ground brown color.

Odor: Note pathologic fecal or rancid odor.

Character: Gastric juice usually separates into three layers: mucus is found in the top layer, opalescent fluid in the center, and sediment at the bottom. Mucus which increases the viscosity of gastric juice, is increased in gastritis and pyloric obstruction.

Sediment: Note amount of undigested food.

pH: Add 2 drops of Töpfer reagent. Free acid will produce a pink color.

Chemical investigation of gastric juice
Determination of acidity (hydrogen ion concentration)

See previous pages.

Lactic acid

Procedure: Add about 2 drops of 10% ferric chloride solution to a test tube full of water and mix. The mixture should appear colorless when held before the light but should present a faint yellow color when examined vertically over a white surface. Divide the mixture and put it into two test tubes, and to one add a small amount of gastric contents. Lactic acid gives a charac-

Table 30-1. Calculation of milliequivalents per liter of hydrogen ion concentration from pH*

pH	log F	pH	log F	pH	log F
3.5	3.082	1.90	3.089	1.30	3.104
3.0	3.083	1.80	3.090	1.25	3.105
2.8	3.084	1.70	3.093	1.20	3.107
2.6	3.084	1.60	3.095	1.15	3.109
2.4	3.085	1.50	3.097	1.10	3.110
2.2	3.086	1.45	3.099	1.05	3.111
2.0	3.087	1.40	3.100	1.00	3.113
		1.35	3.102	0.95	3.115
				0.90	3.117

Examples of calculations

A pH	B $-$ pH as log	C log F from table	D B + C	E antilog D = mEq/L†
3.26	6.740 − 10	3.082	9.822 − 10	0.66
2.51	7.490 − 10	3.085	10.575 − 10 = 0.575	3.76
1.65	8.350 − 10	3.096	11.446 − 10 = 1.446	27.9

*For pH values numerically greater than 3.5, use the factor for pH 3.5.
†Refer to any available antilog table.

teristic greenish yellow (canary yellow) color. Compare with other test tube as control.

This method is not specific. Lactic acid associated with Boas-Oppler bacilli and with achlorhydria is seen in carcinoma of the stomach.

Blood

Hydrochloric acid transforms hemoglobin into brown acid hematin.

Procedure: Neutralize the gastric juice by adding 10% sodium bicarbonate so that the pH is 7.0 (use nitrazine paper) and shake with ether. Treat the aqueous extract just like urine when testing for blood.

Hormones and enzymes

Gastrin: Although Bayliss and Starling hypothesized in 1902 that gastrin exists, it was not until 1964 that gastrin was isolated in a pure state and soon after that synthesized. Chemically, gastrin exists in a number of forms. The active form of gastrin known as G-17 consists of 17 amino acids, and this is the form most commonly found in the circulation. Other forms of circulating gastrin include big gastrin (G-34), with 34 amino acids, and big-big gastrin, which is considered the preprohormone and is degraded to active gastrin and thought to occur only in the G cell. In addition ,there is minigastrin (G-13), which consists of 13 amino acids and is thought to be a fragment from big gastrin. The C-terminal is active in minigastrin, gastrin, and big gastrin. The distribution is predominantly within the G cells, which are found in the pyloric glands of the antrum of the stomach. Gastrin is also found in the proximal duodenum and has been reported to be produced by the D cell of the pancreas.

Determination by radioimmunoassay: The measurement of gastrin is made by radioimmunoassay. However, there are numerous difficulties with the standardization and measurement of serum gastrins. A number of commerical kits are available (e.g., Radioassay System Laboratories, Carson, Calif.; Pantex, Santa Monica, Calif). The normal range is usually 20-100 pg/ml, although values of under 200 are considered by some to be within the normal range. Because of the numerous circulating forms of gastrin, it has been suggested that chromatographic separation before radioimmunoassay would yield more meaningful results.

Gastrin release mechanism: Gastrin release is stimulated by three mechanisms: (1) luminal stimulation by mechanical distention as well as peptides and amino acids within the diet, (2) neural stimulation mainly through vagal adrenergic stimulation associated with the cephalic phase of digestion, and (3) the humoral mechanism associated with circulating calcium and epinephrine. There appear to be inhibitors of gastrin release via two mechanisms—the first being the luminal acid content, which exhibits a negative feedback on gastrin, and the second being humoral, with negative feedback caused by secretin, vasoactive intestinal polypeptide (VIP), gastrin inhibitory polypeptide (GIP), glucagon, and calcitonin. The effects of gastrin secretion are seen throughout the bowel and affect secretion, absorption, and smooth muscle activity. Gastrin secretion increases water and electrolyte secretion from the stomach, pancreas, liver, and small intestine. In addition, it causes enzyme release from the stomach and pancreas. It stimulates smooth muscle activity in the lower esophagus, stomach, and small intestine. It inhibits the sphincter of Oddi and the pyloric and ileocecal valves. It also causes increased blood flow through the superior mesenteric artery to the stomach, pancreas, and small intestine. It has a trophic action on the gastric mucosa as well as on the mucosa of the small bowel and pancreas. In physiologic doses its most important actions are probably acid release, pepsin secretion, and the increase of gastric blood flow. The trophic action is one of the most important and striking actions, as seen especially with gastrinomas. Here there is significant hyperplasia of the gastric mucosa with an increase of up to six times in the number of gastrin-secreting cells. This may result from a stimulation of DNA and RNA synthesis within the cell. This increase in cell mass may be reversed by antrectomy and removal of gastrin secretion. Gastrin is believed to be catabolized and removed in the kidneys by peptidase activity.

Clinical implications: The role of gastrin in human disease is predominantly that of hypersecretion, which is found in Zollinger-Ellison syndrome, gastrinomas, antral G cell hyperplasia, gastric outlet obstruction, and isolated retained antrum. These disorders should be distinguished from other causes of elevated blood levels of gastrin that are not associated with gastrin hypersecretion. These latter disorders include pernicious anemia with atrophic gastritis, gastric carcinoma, pheochromocytoma, and vitiligo associated with achlorhydria.

Gastric inhibitory polypeptides: Gastric inhibitory polypeptide was first isolated from cholecystokinin in 1969 and is now known to consist of 43 amino acids. Fifteen of the first 26 amino acids are the same as secretin; however, the terminal 17 amino acids are not common to any other known hormones. GIP is found predominantly in the D_1 cells of the stomach, duodenum, and jejunum. It is believed that GIP plays a major role in causing insulin release as well as in having an inhibitory effect on both gastric secretion and pepsin release.

Measurement: GIP can be measured in serum by radioimmunoassay with normal levels of approximately 250 pg/ml. Its release can be seen in two phases following the ingestion of food. An early peak, which is thought to be caused by glucose, is seen at approximately 45 min, and a late response is seen at 3 hr and is thought to be caused by dietary fat.

Vasoactive intestinal polypeptides: Vasoactive intestinal polypeptide (VIP) consists of 28 amino acids and is of the glucagon-secretin family. It is found in the pancreatic D_1 cell and in the intestine. It has a powerful action in causing vasodilation and hypotensive episodes. In smooth muscle VIP produces relaxation and abolishes all constrictive actions in the gut. It inhibits histamine, pentagastrin, and food stimulation of gastrin release and produces an increase in the bicarbonate and water production of the pancreas. In the small bowel VIP induces bile flow and stimulates secretions and contractions of the small intestine.

Clinical implications: Clinically VIP has been implicated in the pancreatic cholera syndrome described by Krejis et al.[13a] In one series of 30 patients, 28 were found to have elevated VIP levels.

Measurement: VIP can be measured by radioimmunoassay, although no commercial kits are available yet.

Pepsin and pepsinogen[14]: Pepsin, an enzyme, is preformed as pepsinogen in the chief cells of the stomach mucosa and is activated by hydrochloric acid. About 1% of the predominantly exocrine secretion is discharged into the bloodstream (like a hormone) and excreted in the urine as uropepsinogen. The serum and urine pepsinogen levels reflect the rate of gastric pepsin production.

Pepsin test: Mix a portion of stomach contents with an equal amount of 0.1N hydrochloric acid. Divide this among three test tubes. To one add a small amount of pepsin for positive control; boil one tube to kill enzymes and cool for negative control. Place a small gelatin square into each test tube and incubate at 37° C for 12 hr. Examine for evidence of digestion. Digestion of the gelatin by the sample similar to that by the control indicates the presence of pepsin in the sample, whereas an appearance after digestion similar to that of the negative control indicates lack of pepsin.

Insulin:

Insulin test[15] (Hollander test): The hypoglycemia produced by insulin causes increased gastric secretion by acting through the vagus nerves. Insulin is therefore used as a test to see whether vagotomy would be of value and to determine whether vagotomy has been complete.

Procedure: The stomach tube should be in place. Obtain fasting blood sugar specimen and fasting gastric juice. Inject 15 units of regular insulin intravenously. Obtain blood sugar specimens every 30 min for 2 hr and gastric aspirations every 15 min for the same period. (At least one of these samples should demonstrate a blood sugar level less than 40 mg/dl.)

Interpretation: Hypoglycemia associated with hyperacidity and an increased volume of gastric juice indicates intact vagal pathways.

Microscopic examination of gastric juice

Mount 1 drop of sediment, including any particles suspected of being food residue, on a slide and cover with coverslip. Report all structures seen.

Add 1 drop of iodine solution used in Gram stain and 1 drop of Sudan III or IV to the microscopic preparation to differentiate more easily between **fat, yeast,** and particles of **starch.** Fat stains red, yeast yellow, and starch lilac-purple or black.

Starch, yeast, mouth organisms, and a small amount of mucus are normally found. Food taken previously, pus, blood, Boas-Oppler bacilli, sarcinae, fat droplets, increased mucus, protozoa or other parasites, and occasionally tissue fragments are abnormal findings.

Boas-Oppler bacilli are large nonmotile bacilli that are present as chains in large numbers in gastric contents containing little or no free hydrochloric acid. They stain brown with Gram iodine solution, which distinguishes them from mouth organisms that have been swallowed, because the mouth organisms stain blue or black. Boas-Oppler bacilli are lactic acid bacilli

and indicate stasis with fermentation in the absence of free hydrochloric acid.

Sarcinae are large coccoid organisms that divide in three planes, forming packets that are often compared to bales of cotton. They stain brown with iodine. They are found in conditions associated with stasis and high acidity, e.g., gastric ulcers.

Lugol's iodine stains **yeast** organisms slightly yellow. They are found in the same conditions as sarcinae.

Special methods must be utilized to obtain a satisfactory specimen for screening for **cancer cells.**

• • •

Duodenal secretion

Duodenal juice consists of (1) the duodenal excretion of Brunner's glands, (2) bile (of hepatic origin), and (3) pancreatic juice (trypsin, lipase, and amylase).

PANCREATIC JUICE ANALYSIS

Have the patient fast for 12 hr. Introduce a stomach tube as for gastric analysis and aspirate the fasting stomach contents. Have the patient lie on the right side with knees flexed and hips elevated 15 or 20 cm on cushions and swallow the tube to about 75 cm. Usually within $1/2$-1 hr the tip will be in the duodenum and the contents will siphon off.

The tip is in the duodenum when a colorless or yellow viscid alkaline fluid is obtained. The entire procedure must be fluoroscopically controlled.

To drain the biliary tract by the Meltzer-Lyon method, introduce 50-100 ml of 25% magnesium sulfate through the tube. Whereas originally three specimens were obtained separately, it is usually sufficient, after drainage is well started, to collect all in one bottle. Use a dark amber bottle and examine promptly (within 30 min).

Gross examination of pancreatic juice[16,17]

Volume: 7-20 dl/24 hr.

Character: Clear and watery.

Viscosity: Varies from thin, watery secretion during periods of activity to a thick, more viscid secretion in the basal state.

Specific gravity: 1.007-1.042.

pH: 7.0-8.7.

Pancreatic enzymes

Pancreatic enzymes are digestive enzymes: trypsin hydrolyzes proteins, amylase hydrolyzes carbohydrates, and lipase hydrolyzes fats.

Trypsin:

Screening test: Make duodenal contents slightly alkaline (faint pink with phenolphthalein) with 2% sodium carbonate. Place a small amount in three tubes. Boil one tube and cool for negative control and add a small amount of trypsin to another tube for positive control. Place a small gelatin square into each tube and incubate overnight at 35° C.

Interpretation: Digestion of gelatin by sample as compared with positive and negative controls indicates the presence of trypsin in contents.

Determination of trypsin in duodenal aspirate (quantitative)[18,19]:

Principle: The method uses the substrate benzoyl-arginine-*p*-nitroanilide. The nitroaniline is split off by the enzyme and determined by its absorption at 410 nm. The trypsin is largely present in the inactive form, trypsinogen, and must first be activated. This is done by adding a small amount of free trypsin.

Reagents:

1. Buffer, tris–hydrochloric acid, 0.1 mole/L, pH 7.6, with 0.02 mole/L calcium chloride
   A. Tris, 0.5 mole/L. Dissolve 60.6 g tris–(hydroxymethyl)aminomethane in water and dilute to 5 dl.
   B. Hydrochloric acid, 0.2 mole/L. Dilute 8.3 ml concentrated hydrochloric acid to 5 dl with water.
   C. Calcium chloride, 0.2 mole/L. Dissolve 14.7 g calcium chloride dihydrate in water to make 5 dl.
   Add 20 ml 0.5 mole/L tris solution, 39 ml of 0.2 mole/L hydrochloric acid, and 10 ml calcium chloride solution to a volumetric flask and dilute to 1 dl.
2. Buffer, tris–hydrochloric acid, 0.05 mole/L, pH 8.2, with 0.02 mole/L calcium chloride
   Mix 1 dl solution A, 114 ml solution B, and 50 ml solution C; check pH, adjust to 8.2 if necessary, and dilute to 5 dl.
3. Substrate solution
   Dissolve 43.5 mg benzoyl-arginine-*p*-nitroanilide (Item no. B4875, Sigma Chemical Co., St. Louis) in 1 ml dimethylsulfoxide at 37° C and dilute to 1 dl with buffer 2.
4. Standards
   Prepare fresh daily a standard containing 1 mg crystalline trypsin per milliliter of 1 mmole/L hydrochloric acid (above hydrochloric acid solution B diluted 1:200). Dilutions are made from this with the hydrochloric acid to give concentrations of 50, 100, 150, and 200 μg/ml.

Procedure: For the activation of the enzyme add 20 μl of 1 mg/ml standard to 1 ml of buffer 1, mix 0.8 ml of this with 0.2 ml sample, and incubate at 37° C for 20 min.

Determination: Add two 1 ml aliquots of the substrate to a number of cuvets and incubate at 25° C. At timed intervals add 100 μl of the activated solution to the cuvets and measure the absorbance at 410 nm at timed intervals. The samples are read against a blank containing 2 ml of the substrate and 100 μl of plain buffer. Treat the standards similarly, without the preliminary incubation. Read the results for the samples from a calibration curve, remembering that the samples were diluted 1:5 in the original activation step. If necessary other aliquots may be used depending on the cuvets and spectrophotometer used.

The normal range has been set at 150-600 μg/ml. Fat malabsorption has been noted at levels below 50 μg/ml.

Amylase (diastase):

Screening test: Prepare a 1:10 dilution of the duodenal contents. Add 2 ml of the dilution to 2 ml of a starch solution (0.5 g soluble starch dissolved in 50 ml water), and incubate at 37° C for 30 min. Add 1 drop of iodine solution (that used for Gram stain is satisfactory). A blue color indicates an amylase deficiency.

Quantitative test: See Chapter 24.

Urinary amylase[20]: The urine often shows a prolonged elevation of amylase in patients with acute pancreatitis as compared to the short-lived serum peak. The 2 hr amylase excretion in the urine is a more sensitive test than either the serum amylase or lipase test. (For technic, see Chapter 24.)

Normal value: 200 units/hr.

Lipase (Steapsin):

Screening test[21]: Place 1 ml duodenal contents in two large test tubes; boil one tube to destroy the lipase and cool. To each tube, add 1 ml ethyl butyrate, 10 ml water, and 1 ml toluol. Mix and incubate at 37° C for 24 hr, shaking several times. Titrate each tube with 0.1N sodium hydroxide, using 2 drops phenolphthalein. Subtract the amount used to neutralize the boiled specimen (blank) from the amount used in the other. The difference represents the amount of digestion caused by the lipase, expressed in terms of the number of milliliters of 0.1N sodium hydroxide required to neutralize the fatty acids formed in the unheated specimen as a result of lipase activity. The normal amount required is 0.2-2 ml.

Serum enzyme measurements: Serum amylase and lipase are elevated in acute pancreatitis (see Chapter 24).

Secretin and pancreozymin stimulation test of pancreatic function[22]

Principle: Pancreatic secretion is measured after intravenous injection of secretin and pancreozymin. Serum amylase and lipase measurements are made at the same time, since the levels may rise in the presence of pancreatic duct obstruction.

Procedure: Give the patient a skin test with 0.1 ml of an isotonic saline solution of secretin and pancreozymin containing 1 unit/ml. Under fluoroscopic observation insert a Dreiling double-lumen gastroduodenal tube and connect each tube to a suction pump, providing continuous aspiration. Samples are collected for 20 min before stimulation and for 10 min after pancreozymin administration (100 units intravenously), followed by 10 and 20 min fractions after secretin administration (75 units).

Blood samples for serum amylase are taken before pancreozymin administration and at 1, 2, and 4 hr after secretin stimulation.

The duodenal aspirate is examined for amount, color, pH, bicarbonate concentration, and amylase output.

Normal values of duodenal aspirate[23]:

Postpancreozymin (10 min period)
  Volume: 16-72 ml
  Bicarbonate concentration: 8-24 mEq/L
  Amylase: 28.000-182.000 IU/L at 37° C
Postsecretin (60 min period)
  Volume: 99-377 ml
  Maximal bicarbonate concentration: 69-126 mEq/L

Interpretation: A reduction in bicarbonate concentration is a reliable index of pancreatic dysfunction. A rise in serum enzymes above the normal limit is indicative of ductal obstruction. Bile staining should be intermittent. Absence of bile indicates obstruction of the duct.

Titration of bicarbonate in duodenal aspirate[24,25]

Principle: An excess of acid is added to liberate carbon dioxide from bicarbonate, and the equivalent amount of hydrogen is used for the formation of water.

Reagents:

1. Hydrochloric acid, 0.05N
   Prepare from 1N solution by 1:20 dilution.
2. Sodium hydroxide, 0.01N
   Prepare fresh from 1N solution by 1:100 dilution.

Procedure: Measure pH value as soon as specimen is obtained. Add 1 ml duodenal aspirate to 1 ml of 0.05N acid and mix well. Add water so that fluid level reaches the electrodes. Back-titrate with 0.01N sodium hydroxide to original pH value.

Calculation:

Bicarbonate (mEq/L) =
$$50 - (\text{sodium hydroxide [ml]} \times 10)$$

Interpretation: Reduction in the bicarbonate level is indicative of pancreatic damage.

Tolerance tests in investigation of pancreatic function

Glucose tolerance test: Destruction of the islets by chronic pancreatitis or by a tumor produces a diabetic type of curve. (For technic, see Chapter 21.)

Starch tolerance test: The starch tolerance test is similar to the oral glucose tolerance test, but the patient receives 100 g starch instead of 100 g glucose.

The test represents an attempt to measure the amylolytic activity of the pancreatic juice. It requires 2 days. On the first day a 3 hr glucose tolerance test is performed (100 g glucose), and on the second day 100 g soluble starch is administered. The maximal rise in blood sugar after the glucose tolerance test is compared with that after ingestion of starch. The result is expressed in percent and ranges from -39% to $+83\%$, with an average of $+19\%$. It is calculated on the basis of the following formula:

$$\frac{(P^1 - F^1) - (P - F)}{P - F} \times 100 = \%$$

In the formula, P^1 is the peak and F^1 the fasting blood sugar levels of the glucose tolerance test; P and F are the peak and fasting blood sugar levels of the starch tolerance curve.

Tests for malabsorption

Radioactive iodine (^{131}I) triolein test: Fecal fat studies are important in the investigation of fat metabolism in all forms of steatorrhea, but they are time consuming. ^{131}I triolein is a fat consisting of oleic acid groups esterified with 1 mole of glyceryl. In the process of absorption of this fat there is no appreciable loss of iodine, and therefore the amount of ^{131}I in the blood or feces can be accepted as evidence of absorption or lack

of it. The maximal total blood level of 8-12% of the original dose should be reached rapidly in 3-4 hr under normal circumstances. In steatorrhea the maximal absorption of 3-5% is reached only slowly. In poor absorption it may be caused by absence of pancreatic enzymes or by mucosal inadequacy. These two conditions can be distinguished by administration of ^{131}I oleic acid, which requires no hydrolysis and is absorbed normally in the absence of enzymes, but not if there is a mucosal block. (See discussion of steatorrhea, Chapter 31.)

Microscopic examination of pancreatic juice

Examine pancreatic juice within 30 min. Mix specimen and centrifuge a portion for 15 min at highest speed. Pour off supernatant fluid and mount sediment on a slide under a coverslip.

Record whatever is found, but note especially the presence or absence of bile-stained columnar epithelial cells, bile-stained pus cells (give approximate number per high-power field when present), increased cholesterin crystals, increased calcium bilirubinate crystals, other crystals, and parasites.

Bile-stained cells and increased numbers of crystals indicate stasis. An occasional cholesterin or calcium bilirubinate crystal is normal. Amebas, hookworms, *Ascaris,* flagellates, and *Strongyloides* have been reported.

Special double-lumen gastrointestinal tubes allow the aspiration of neoplastic cells from lesions of the duodenum, pancreas, and biliary tract following stimulation with secretin.

FIBROCYSTIC DISEASE OF THE PANCREAS

Fibrocystic disease of the pancreas (mucoviscidiosis) is a congenital, probably enzymatic disorder that clinically can be classified into three groups, depending on the age of onset. In newborn infants it is called **meconium ileus.** In children it is called **fibrocystic disease** and is characterized by repeated pneumonia, failure to gain weight, and large foul stools, producing a clinical picture similar to that of celiac disease. In adults it manifests itself as a tendency to **repeated** pulmonary **infections.**

Laboratory investigation
Changes in exocrine secretions

Duodenal fluid: The outstanding feature is an increase in viscosity associated with a decrease in pancreatic enzymes. (See discussion of tests for fecal trypsin.) The increased viscosity, which is readily measured by the Ostwald viscosimeter, is caused partly by changes in the mucopolysaccharide composition, e.g., low sialic acid and high fucose content.

Bronchial secretion: The bronchial secretion is unusually viscid and forms a good culture medium for coagulase-positive staphylococci (*Staphylococcus aureus*) and *Pseudomonas aeruginosa*.

Saliva: The sodium and chloride concentrations are increased.

Sweat: In sweat the concentrations of **sodium** and **chloride** are two to five times the normal values. The rise in the concentrations of these two electrolytes may not be equal.

There are a few other conditions in which chloride concentration in the sweat is elevated, e.g., in adrenal insufficiency and in some cases of nephrosis. Parents or siblings of patients with fibrocystic disease may also have increased concentrations.

Normal values: The level of chlorides varies from 5-35 mEq/L and average 25 mEq/L.

Pathologic values: Chloride values in the range of 35-60 mEq/L indicate possible fibrocystic disease but are not definite. Values above 60 mEq/L are definite indications of the disease.

Tests for chloride in sweat

The tests for chloride in sweat include (1) the pilocarpine iontophoresis technic using the chloridometer, (2) the cystic fibrosis analyzer using a conductivity bridge, and (3) the chloride electrode method.

Pilocarpine Iontophoresis technic[26,27]:

Principle: Sweating is induced in a local area by the action of the drug pilocarpine, which is introduced into the skin by means of an electric current (**iontophoresis**). Two electrodes are placed on the opposite sides of an arm or leg. The positive electrode is moistened with a pilocarpine solution and the negative one with a sodium nitrate solution. A current of about 1.5 mamp is passed between the electrodes. Some of the pilocarpine is carried into the skin, where it stimulates the eccrine sweat glands. After stimulation and removal of the electrodes, the sweat is collected on a filter paper pad. The amount of sweat collected in the pad is measured by the pad's increase in weight. The sweat is eluted from the pad with water and the solution analyzed for chloride.

Iontophoresis procedure:
Equipment:
1. Iontophoresis current supply and electrodes
2. Sweat collection pads
   These circular disks of thick filter paper are about 33 mm in diameter.
3. Weighing bottles for sweat collection pads. Plastic bottles are preferred, because they are lighter and not subject to breakage.

Reagents:
1. Pilocarpine solution, 0.5%
   Dissolve 0.5 g pilocarpine nitrate in distilled water to make 1 dl. This solution is stable for 1 month when kept in a brown bottle in a refrigerator.
2. Sodium nitrate, 1%
   Dissolve 1 g sodium nitrate in water to make 1 dl. It is stable for several months at room temperature.

Both of the above solutions may be purchased.

Iontophoresis and sweat collection: The details of the electrodes may vary somewhat from instrument to instrument, but in general cotton pads are moistened with the two reagents and placed over the electrodes. Moisten the positive electrode (red) with the pilocarpine solution and the negative electrode with the sodium nitrate solution. Place the two electrodes on the opposite sides of the forearm with the positive electrode on the inner (flexor) surface. Fasten the electrodes in place with a strap. They should be fitted snugly against the skin, but the strap should not be so tight as to impede circulation. The metallic portion of the electrode should not touch the skin, only the moistened pad. Turn the current on and gradually increase it to 1.5 mamp over a period of 1-2 min. The patient may feel a slight tingling or prickling but should feel no pain or shock.

Procedure: Continue the iontophoresis for 5-7 min. Then turn the current off, remove the strap and electrodes, and allow about 5 min for the sweat glands to flush out the accumulated salt secretion. Wash the area that was under the pilocarpine electrode with distilled water and blot dry with a clean gauze sponge. Using a forceps remove the sweat collection pad, which has been previously weighed in the weighing bottle to the nearest milligram, from the weighing bottle and place it over the stimulated area. Cover the pad with a 6 cm square of Parafilm, and then tape tightly to the skin on all sides. Also place strips of tape across the top of the Parafilm to hold the pad firmly in place. Leave the pad on for 1 hr. Then lift one edge of the Parafilm, remove the pad with a forceps, and replace it into the weighing bottle. Reweigh it at once. The increase in weight of the pad plus weighing bottle represents the amount of sweat collected.

Care must be taken not to contaminate the sweat collection pad or site with sweat from the operator's fingers. It has been found that if the collection site has been recently washed with a detergent containing hexachlorophene, erratic results may be obtained in the analysis. There may be difficulty in obtaining an appreciable amount of sweat from premature, very young, or dehydrated infants. Keeping the infant quite warm and forcing fluids for several hours will often aid in the production of sweat. In other instances one must wait until the infant is a few weeks older.

Determination of sweat chloride: The chloride content of the sweat may be measured with the Cotlove chloridometer (see Chapter 22) on the "low" range, or it may also be determined by microtitration with mercuric nitrate (Schales and Schales method, Chapter 22).

Titration with chloridometer: The diluting fluid and gelatin solution are the same as used for serum analysis. A 5 mEq/L standard is prepared by diluting 5 ml of the 100 mEq/L standard to 1 dl with water. To the weighing bottle containing the pad and absorbed sweat, add exactly 2, 3, or 4 ml distilled water, depending on the amount of sweat obtained. For 0.15 g or less, use 2 ml water; for 0.15-0.30 g sweat, use 3 ml water; and for larger amounts of sweat, use 4 ml water. Stopper the weighing bottle and extract the pad by gentle swirling of the contents. Allow to stand for 20 min with frequent gentle swirling. Titrate 0.1 ml aliquots of the extract in the chloridometer, as described in Chapter 22, using the "low" range and the "piggyback" method after conditioning the electrodes. Also titrate several 0.1 ml aliquots of the 5 mEq/L standard. If the titration of the sample is more than twice that of the standard, then 0.05 ml of the sample may be titrated, multiplying the reading obtained by 2 for the calculations.

Calculation:

$$\text{Chloride in extract (mEq/L)} = \frac{\text{Titration of sample}}{\text{Titration of standard}} \times 5$$

Chloride in sweat (mEq/L) =

$$\text{Chloride in extract (mEq/L)} \times \frac{V + S}{S}$$

where V is the milliliters of water added and S is the grams of sweat obtained.

Titration with mercuric nitrate (Schales and Schales method, Chapter 22): Titration with mercuric nitrate requires the use of an ultramicroburet of about 0.5 ml capacity that can be read to 0.0001 ml. Dilute the 0.01N mercuric nitrate solution used in the serum method 1:2 with water containing 6 ml nitric acid per liter to give a 0.005N solution. The indicator is the same as in the regular titration. Using the ultramicroburet and titrating vessel, titrate 0.1 ml aliquots of the standard and samples obtained exactly as in the previous method after the addition of 0.1 ml diluted nitric acid (6 ml concentrated nitric acid to 1 L with water). Also titrate a blank using the diluted nitric acid alone, and subtract any titration reading for the blank from that of the standard and sample titrations. The calculations are exactly the same as given above when the corrected milliliters of titration are used instead of the seconds as measured on the chloridometer.

Cystic fibrosis analyzer: The cystic fibrosis analyzer (Advanced Instruments, Needham Heights, Mass.) estimates the chloride content of the sweat by measuring the electrical conductivity. The main contribution to the electrical conductivity in sweat is the sodium chloride present, although small amounts of other ions also contribute. The method gives a fair estimate of the chloride content and is suitable as a screening procedure. The sweating is induced by pilocarpine iontophoresis and the sweat collected in a small plastic cup taped over the stimulated site. The small amount of sweat collected is transferred to a capillary for conductivity measurement. The apparatus is used both for furnishing the iontophoresis current and for the conductivity measurements. About 50 mg sweat is needed to properly fill the capillary, so that difficulty may be experienced with infants who yield only small amounts of sweat.

Chloride electrode method[28,29]: A specific ion electrode that measures directly the concentration of chloride ions in solution together with the required electric measuring instrument (essentially an expanded-scale pH meter) is available from a number of manufacturers (e.g., Orion Research, Cambridge, Mass.).[30] The sweating is induced by iontophoresis or by applying a heating block at about 42° C to the skin for a short time. In the latter instance the interscapular region of the back is often used in small infants. When the proper sweating has been induced, the chloride electrode is placed on the moist skin and the reading taken on the meter. The electrode is calibrated by dipping in solutions of known chloride concentration such as 1, 10, and 100 mEq/L. If the reading is in millivolts, the cal-

ibration points are plotted on semilog paper for the calibration curve. Some instruments have a logarithmic scale on which the concentrations can be read directly. The use of the chloride electrode is much more rapid than other methods for sweat chloride and is thus well suited for screening purposes.

Estimation of fecal fat and enzymes

In pancreatic fibrosis the pancreatic ferments in the stool are markedly depressed. Small amounts of lipase and amylase are sometimes present, but trypsin is never present in significant amounts. The stool is bulky, the fat content is very high, and most of the fat is unsplit (neutral fat), producing the so-called butter stool. (See discussion of fecal fat, Chapter 31.)

GLOSSARY

cystic fibrosis A generalized hereditary disorder in which there is widespread dysfunction of the exocrine glands characterized by signs of chronic pulmonary disease, pancreatic deficiency, and abnormally high levels of electrolytes in the sweat.

gastric Pertaining to the stomach.

pancreatitis Inflammation of the pancreas.

pylorus The opening of the stomach leading into the duodenum.

Zollinger-Ellison syndrome A triad comprising (1) intractable, sometimes fulminating, atypical peptic ulcers; (2) extreme gastric hyperacidity; and (3) non-β- cell, non-insulin-secreting islet cell tumors.

REFERENCES

1. Rovelstad, R.A.: Gastroenterology **45:**90, 1963.
2. Barow, J.H.: Scand. J. Gastroenterol. **5:**9, 1970.
3. Barow, J.H., and Williams, A.J.: In Taylor, S., editor: Recent advances in surgery, London, 1973, Churchhill Livingstone.
4. Konturek, S.J., and Lankosz, J.: Scand. J. Gastroenterol. **2:**112, 1967.
5. Laudano, O.M.: Gastroenterology **50:**653, 1966.
6. Zaterka, S., and Neves, D.P.: Gastroenterology **47:**3, 1964.
7. Segal, H.L.: J.A.M.A. **196:**655, 1966.
8. Bock, O.A.: Lancet **2:**1101, 1962.
9. Baron, J.H.: Gastroenterology **45:**1, 1963.
10. Lubran, M.: Lancet **2:**1070, 1966.
11. Moore, E.W., and Scarlata, R.W.: Gastroenterology **49:**178, 1965.
12. Moore, E.W.: Gastroenterology **54:**501, 1968.
13. Burke, E.L.: U.S. Navy Medical Newsletter **55:**32, 1970.
13a. Krejis, G.J., et al.: Am. J. Dig. Dis. **22:**280, 1977.
14. Seljffers, M.J., et al.: Gastroenterology **48:**122, 1965.
15. Ross, B., and Kay, A.W.: Gastroenterology **46:**379, 1964.
16. Rosenberg, I.R., and Jonowitz, H.D.: Gastroenterology **48:**350, 1965.
17. Haverback, B.J.: J.A.M.A. **193:**279, 1965.
18. Bergström, K., and Lundh, G.: Scand. J. Gastroenterol. **5:**553, 1970.
19. Barns, R.J., and Elmslie, R.G.: Clin. Chim. Acta **58:**165, 1975.
20. Kirshen, R., Gambill, E.E., and Mason, H.L.: Gastroenterology **46:**746, 1964.
21. Roe, J.H., and Golstein, N.P.: J. Lab. Clin. Med. **28:**1334, 1943.
22. Fitzgerald, O., et al.: Gut **4:**193, 1963.
23. Sun, D.C.: Gastroenterology **44:**602, 1963.

24. Jacobs, W.H., Chaudhuri, T., and Pickering, L.I.: Mo. Med. **69:**33, 1972.

25. Van Slyke, D.D., and Cullen, G.E.: J. Biol. Chem. **30:**289, 1917.

26. Gibson, L.E., and Cooke, R.E.: Pediatrics **23:**545, 1959.

27. Hansen, L., et al: Minn. Med. **50:**1191, 1967.

28. Jirka, M.: Clin. Chim. Acta **11:**78, 1965.

29. Kopito, L., and Schwachman, H.: Pediatrics **43:**794, 1969.

30. Hansen, L., et al.: Am. J. Clin. Pathol. **49:**834, 1968.

CHAPTER 31

Stool analysis

Physical examination
  Macroscopic examination
  Microscopic examination
Chemical examination
  pH
  Tests for blood
  Tests for bilirubin (bile pigment) and some of its derivatives
Malabsorption and steatorrhea
Analysis of stool electrolytes

PHYSICAL EXAMINATION
Macroscopic examination[1]

Color: The substance that is reponsible for the brown color of stool is stercobilin, which is the result of the action of reducing bacteria on bilirubin. Stool darkens on standing. Color is influenced by diet, various food dyes, certain foods, drugs, and blood.

Many drugs can produce abnormal color changes in feces. Antacids and barium enemas can produce a white discoloration, whereas the anthraquinones can produce a light brownish color. Strongly colored drugs containing azo groups can impart an orange color. Unexplained unusual fecal coloring should be correlated with the drug history of the patient.

Yellow to yellow-green: The stool of breast-fed infants who lack normal intestinal flora contains bilirubin but no stercobilin. Severe diarrhea and sterilization of the bowel by antibiotics produce similar results.

Green: Chlorophyll-rich vegetables, severe diarrhea, and calomel produce a green stool.

Black: Black stool results from bleeding into the upper gastrointestinal tract or it may be caused by drugs such as iron, charcoal, and bismuth or by foods such as cherries. Bleeding into the lower segments of the large bowel leads to blood-streaked stools.

Tan: Blockage of the common bile duct as well as pancreatic insufficiency produces pale, greasy, "acholic" stool.

Red: Red stool results from bleeding into the lower segments of the large bowel or from massive bleeding in the upper gastrointestinal area accompanied by a rapid transit time through the distal segments of the large bowel.

Odor: Substances called indole and skatole, the results of intestinal putrefaction and fermentation, are primarily responsible for the odor of normal stools. The odor varies with the PH of the stool, since it is dependent on bacterial fermentation and putrefaction.

Consistency:

1. *Diarrhea mixed with mucus and blood* is caused by typhus, typhoid, cholera, large bowel carcinoma, and amebiasis.

2. *Diarrhea mixed with pus and mucus* is caused by ulcerative colitis, shigellosis, salmonellosis, and regional enteritis.

3. *Pasty stool* is caused by high fat content as in sprue, pancreatic insufficiency, etc. (p. 793). A significant increase of fat is usually detected grossly. In obstruction of the common bile duct the fat gives a puttylike appearance to the stool **(acholic stool).** In sprue and celiac disease the appearance of the feces often suggests aluminum radiator paint because of the fatty acid crystals. In cystic fibrosis of the pancreas the increase of neutral fat gives the greasy "butter-stool" appearance.

Concretions: Gallstones and fecaliths may be present.

Extraneous material: The gross examination should be directed at finding parasites (whole worms or their fragments) and undigested food and evaluating the amount of blood, pus, mucus, and fat present.

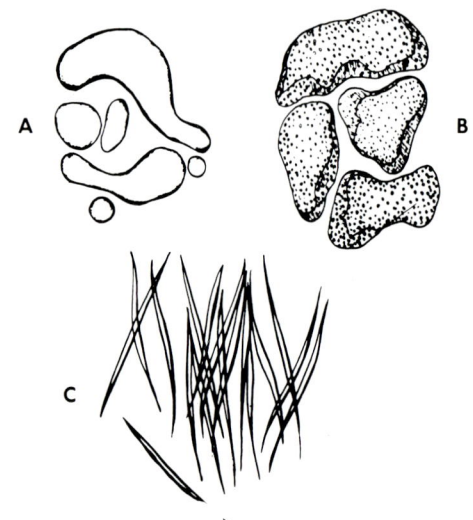

Fig. 31-1. Microscopic appearance of neutral fat, **A;** fatty acid salts as soaps, **B;** and fatty acid crystals, **C.** (From Searcy, R.L.: In Stefanini, M., editor: Progress in clinical pathology, New York, 1970, Grune & Stratton, Inc., vol. 2.)

Microscopic examination

The purpose of microscopic examination is to find undigested food particles (starch, muscle fibers, elastic fibers, etc.), eggs and segments of parasites, fats, and yeasts.

Procedures: See discussion of stool examination in Chapter 34.

Interpretation: Skeletal muscle fibers consist of cylinders with clear-cut outlines and prominent cross striations (see Fig. 34-8). Elastic fibers appear as refractile springs (see Fig. 34-8). Starch granules stain light blue with diluted iodine such as D'Antoni or Gram iodine solutions.

Fat: Alcoholic Sudan III solutions stain only neutral fats pale orange to red. Fatty acid crystals and fatty acid salts (soaps), normally present in stool, are not stained by the Sudan stain but can be detected by microscopic observation (Fig. 31-1). The presence of free fat is indicative of interference with normal fat absorption and with bile or pancreatic excretion.

CHEMICAL EXAMINATION
pH

The normal pH of stool is neutral or weakly alkaline. Carbohydrate fermentation changes the PH to acid, and protein breakdown changes the pH to the alkaline side. The pH measurements do not correlate well with the presence of sugar.

Tests for blood

The tests for detecting blood in feces employ substances that are oxidized to colored compounds by oxygen liberated from hydrogen peroxide through the action of the peroxidase activity of the heme portion of hemoglobin. Substances that have been used for this purpose include the naturally occurring gum resin guaiac; reduced forms of colored compounds such as phenolphthalein, dichlorophenol-indophenol, or malachite green; or aromatic diamines such as benzidine, *o*-tolidine, or diethyl-*p*-phenylenediamine. The problem with these tests is that if they are sufficiently sensitive to detect small amounts of blood in feces, they may give false positive reactions because of other substances found in the feces. The interfering substances include iron salts, traces of heme compounds from myoglobin from meat in the diet, and chlorophyll and plant peroxidases from leafy vegetables (particularly when eaten uncooked). It is usually recommended that the patient be given a diet free of meat and fish for 2 days before a test is made. Not all iron compounds give the same amount of reaction in the test. This may be one cause of the differences in opinion as to the effect of oral iron ingestion on the test for fecal blood. It is often suggested that the patient stop taking iron for 2 days before the test is made. If the presence of iron is suspected, it may be detected by the test given below.[1]

Vitamin C, when taken in large doses (2-4 g/day), can cause a negative interference by interfering in the oxidation reaction with guaiac.[1]

According to Deadman[2] and Woodson,[3] it is difficult to control the sensitivity of the test using reduced compounds such as reduced phenolphthalein or leukomalachite green, because they tend to give erratic results.

Tests using guaiac give a low percentage of false positive results, but the substance supposedly is difficult to secure. However, a modified guaiac test using guaiac-impregnated paper is available commercially. (Hemoccult slides, Smith, Kline & French Laboratories, Philadelphia.), and this has proved generally satisfactory, particularly as a screening test for blood in feces. It has the advantage that the small amount of feces may be smeared on the special filter paper in a holder at the bedside or nursing station, and the dried paper in the holder can be sent to the laboratory. Here the supplied reagent is added and the result noted.

The American Cancer Society[4] has recommended the use of guaiac-impregnated paper for the screening of high-risk populations or people older than 50 years. They recommend that these tests be used under the following conditions:

1. Patients must be placed on a meat-free, vitamin C–free diet for at least 2 days before the sampling.
2. Two separate stool specimens must be collected on each of 3 consecutive days.
3. Samples may be stored for no more than 4 days before testing.
4. No rehydration of slides before testing is permitted, because this will lead to a large number of false positive results.
5. Results must be recorded as positive or negative.

Care should be taken to avoid using stool samples contaminated by toilet water. Oxidizing cleaning reagents in the toilet water could cause false positive results. When performing the filter paper guaiac test the technologist should closely observe the test strip. A positive color can fade quickly within a short period of time, giving an apparently negative result.[1]

In the past, the most commonly used of the diamines for detecting blood in feces was benzidine. This compound was found to be carcinogenic and has been replaced in many tests by *o*-tolidine, which is also somewhat more sensitive. In view of the close chemical similarity of benzidine and *o*-tolidine, it is probable that *o*-tolidine is also carcinogenic. Commercial tablets are available that use *o*-tolidine (Hematest, Ames Co., Elkhart, Ind.). Huntsman and Liddell[5] found that these tablets were too sensitive for use with feces, since they often gave false positive results in normal subjects on a meat-free diet and that the use of guaiac was more satisfactory.

There are also some test procedures in which a sample of the feces is added to a solution in a test tube and the reaction noted. These tests may be somewhat more sensitive, but many also use benzidine or *o*-tolidine. A test has been developed for plasma hemoglobin using the noncarcinogeneic compound 3,3′,5,5′-tetramethylbenzidine but this has not yet been applied to the detection of blood in feces. For a tube test the following procedure is recommended.

Tube test for fecal blood[3]:

Principle: The tube test for fecal blood uses the noncarcinogenic compound diphenylamine. A chelating agent is added to bind any iron present that might interfere, and the sample is heated in solution to boiling to destroy any peroxidases present.

Reagents:
1. Glacial acetic acid
2. Acetic acid, approximately 8 moles/L
   Dilute glacial acetic acid with an equal volume of water.
3. Diphenylamine solution, 1% in glacial acetic acid
   Dissolve 1 g diphenyamine in 1 dl glacial acetic acid.
4. *N*,*N*-bis (2-hydroxyethyl)glycine, sodium salt, 2 moles/L
   The free acid is obtainable under the name of bicine for use as a buffer. To prepare the solution, dissolve 16 g of the free acid and 4 g sodium hydroxide in 50 ml water.
5. Hydrogen peroxide, 3% solution
   This is comerically available or may be prepared by dilution of a 30% solution.

Procedure: Add a specimen of feces about 10 mm in diameter to 10 ml of 8 moles/L acetic acid and heat to boiling; then cool to room temperature.

In a small test tube mix together 0.5 ml diphenylamine solution, 0.1 ml of 3% hydrogen peroxide and 0.3 ml bicine solution. Allow to stand for 1 min to ensure that no color develops because of contamination of tubes or reagents. Then add 0.2 ml of the fecal suspension and mix.

Interpretation: A distinct green color that develops within 90 sec indicates a positive reaction; color developing betwen 90 and 120 sec indicates a weak reaction; and color developing after 120 sec is not considered a positive reaction.

The test is fairly sensitive—it is said to give a positive reaction when 5 ml blood is administered directly into the stomach of an adult. This represents about 1 ml blood for each 20-50 g feces. When first using the test, one may wish to check the method by adding varying amounts of diluted blood to small amounts of feces.

Quality control: Tests for blood in feces are often checked by noting whether a positive reaction can be obtained by the addition of a minute amount of blood to a negative feces sample or by the addition of a few drops of diluted blood to the reagents. Inhibitory substances are present in feces, so that more blood is required to give a positive reaction in the presence of feces than in a simple aqueous dilution. Using diphenylamine in a tube test. Woodson[3] found that a 1:3000 dilution of blood in water gave a strong positive reacton. When the dilution was made with a fecal suspension, the reaction was strongly positive only in a 1:500 or 1:750 dilution. Furthermore, in the passage of blood through the gastrointestinal tract, further degradation to inactive substances occurs; thus an even greater amount of blood is required to give a positive reaction. Usually the ingestion of 5-10 ml blood is sufficient to give a positive reaction. This corresponds to a dilution of fresh blood in the stool of about 1:100.

Interfering substances[6]:
1. *Drugs:* iron, bromides, iodides
2. *Food:* rare meats, blood sausage

Influence of iron on occult blood tests: Ferrous fumarate and ferrous carbonate may produce false positive results with the *o*-tolidine test tablets and with the guaiac filter paper procedure. Other iron preparatons do not interfere.

Test for ingested iron[8]:
Principle: Iron plus potassium ferricyanide produces ferrous ferricyanide (Turnbull's blue). The presence of blood does not interfere with the test.

Reagents:
1. Hydrochloric acid, 2N
   Dilute 168 ml concentrated with distilled water to make 10 dl.
2. Potassium ferricyanide, 0.25%
   Dissolve 0.25 g in 1 dl distilled water.

Procedure: Emulsify a small amount of stool in 2N hydrochloric acid with two orange sticks. Using the sticks again, transfer 1 drop of emulsion to Whatman no. 1 filter paper. The consistency of the specimen must be such that after 1 or 2 min a 3-4 mm halo of fluid surrounds the fecal drop. Place 1 drop of 0.25% potassium ferricyanide close to the fecal specimen so that the two fluids meet. A positive result is evidenced by the immediate appearance of a blue color at the interface of the liquids.

Tests for bilirubin (bile pigment) and some of its derivatives
Oxidation tests

Principle: Bilirubin is oxidized to blue cholecyanin and to green biliverdin by nitric acid (as in the Gmelin test) or by ferric chloride (as in the Fouchet reagent).

Gmelin test:
Reagent: Yellow concentrated nitric acid (concentrated nitric acid containing a couple of wooden applicator sticks).

Procedure: Make a thin fecal smear on filter paper and add 1 drop of nitric acid.

Results: In the presence of bilirubin a blue or green color is produced.

Fouchet test:
Reagents:
1. Trichloroacetic acid, 25 g
2. Distilled water, 1 dl
3. Ferric chloride, 10%, 10 ml
Dissolve 10 g ferric chloride in 1 dl distilled water.

Procedure: Prepare fecal emulsion in a test tube containing about 3 ml distilled water. Add drop by drop 3 ml Fouchet reagent.

Results: Same as in Gmelin test.

Interpretation of tests for bilirubin: Under normal conditions, bilirubin is present only in the stool of newborn babies. Pathologically it may be found in severe cases of diarrhea because of the accelerated fecal transport, and it may also be found pathologically after antibiotic therapy.

Qualitative screening procedure for fecal urobilin and urobilinogen (Watson)[9]

Principle: Urobilin and urobilinogen are extracted with a saturated alcoholic (95% ethyl alcohol) solution of zinc acetate. Urobilin gives a green fluorescence, and, after the addition of Ehrlich aldehyde reagent, urobilinogen imparts a pink color to the mixture.

Reagents:
1. Saturated solution of zinc acetate
   Dissolve 50 g zinc acetate ($2H_2O$) in 1 L of 95% ethyl alcohol. Heat in water bath to 50° C, stirring frequently. The cooled solution must show crystals at the bottom of the container.
2. Saturated solution of sodium acetate
   Dissolve 140 g sodium acetate ($3H_2O$) in 1 dl distilled water. Heat to 60° C and allow to cool. There must always be crystals at the bottom of the container.
3. Ehrlich aldehyde reagent
   Combine 0.7 g *p*-dimethylaminobenzaldehyde (colorless) and 150 ml concentrated hydrochloric acid in 1 dl distilled water. Store in a brown bottle with a glass stopper.

Procedure: Emulsify about 2 g stool in 10 ml saturated alcoholic solution of zinc acetate and filter. If urobilin is present, the solution will show green fluorescence. To 2.5 ml filtrate, add 2.5 ml Ehrlich aldehyde (Watson modification) and after 15 sec add 5 ml saturated aqueous solution of sodium acetate.

Results: A pink color indicates urobilinogen. Green fluorescence of the untreated zinc acetate filtrate in transmitted light is a rough quantitative measurement of urobilin in the filtrate. To determine urobilinogen, the stool specimen must be fresh; however, any stool specimen can be used to test for urobilin.

Interpretation: **Urobilin (stercobilin)** is normally present in stool and absent as a result of complete obstruction to bile flow.

Urobilinogen is normally present in stool, although in somewhat decreased amounts in infants. The amount is increased in hemolytic anemia and decreased as the result of partial obstruction to the flow of bile, the administration of antibiotics, and diminished blood production (aplastic anemia).

Urobilinogen may be absent if all of it is converted to urobilin, the test for which should be positive. The absence of urobilinogen and of urobilin is evidence of complete obstruction of the common bile duct (see Table 27-7 and Fig. 27-10).

Test for trypsin

X-ray film method:

Principle: As a screening test in infants, the x-ray film method for fecal trypsin is of value in detecting pancreatic insufficiency, especially when it results from cystic pancreatic fibrosis. This test is usually run as part of a workup for malabsorption syndrome in infants or children below 4 years of age. In older children the test is unreliable because of protease inactivation by intestinal flora. Trypsin can be demonstrated in 95% or more of the stools of normal infants. Absence of trypsin is presumptive evidence of pancreatic deficiency and is usually accompanied by the absence of the other ferments, lipase and amylase.

Procedure: Make a suspension of feces in distilled water in dilutions of 1:5, 1:10, 1:20, and 1:40. Place a large drop of each dilution on the surface of an unexposed, unfixed gelatin (x-ray) film and incubate at 37° C for 1 hr or at room temperature for 2 hr. The drops should be large enough to prevent drying or caking during the test. Wash in cold running water with gentle rubbing. Complete digestion (clearing) is read as 4 + and a slight clearing only at the periphery of the drop as 1 + .

Run a control with the feces of a normal infant. Run the test on three separate fresh stools. Tests positive for trypsin should be checked once or more at intervals of a week to rule out the possibility that the positive reaction might be caused by proteolytic bacteria of the intestines. For older children, test stools following the administration of a cathartic.

MALABSORPTION AND STEATORRHEA[10,11]

Malabsorption is a general term describing a failure to absorb one or more of the body's dietary nutrients. **Malabsorption syndrome** is a general type of malabsorption involving lipids and a wide range of other dietary components. **Steatorrhea**, or the presence of increased fats in stool, is usually a major clinical presentation of the malabsorption syndrome. The etiologies of the syndromes follow:

1. Genetic atrophy of intestinal mucosa: celiac disease, idiopathic steatorrhea, tropical sprue
2. Failure to digest fat: obstructive jaundice, chronic pancreatitis, fibrocystic disease of pancreas
3. Abnormal intestinal flora: blind loop syndrome, fistulas
4. Blockage of intestinal lymphatics: Whipple's disease, scleroderma, lymphoma
5. Iatrogenic steatorrhea: therapy using irradiation and antibiotics, surgical resection of segments of small bowel or of stomach
6. Miscellaneous: pneumatosis intestinalis
7. Parasitic diseases: *Giardia lamblia* and hookworm infestation
8. Carcinoid syndrome
9. Inadequate mesenteric blood supply: arteritis, atherosclerosis

Laboratory investigation of steatorrhea[12,13]

The laboratory can play an important role in the diagnosis of malabsorption problems. Laboratory tests used in making such a diagnosis are listed in Table 31-1.[10]

Steatorrhea may be determined by gross examination of feces, microscopic examination for fat, and measurement of total fat in feces.

To determine the cause of steatorrhea, test for pancreatic competence (secretin-pancreozymin test, p. 785), plasma protein leakage into the bowel (rate of degradation of injected ^{131}I-labeled albumin), disaccharidase deficiency (lactose tolerance test), small bowel competence (D-xylose excretion test), and small bowel morphology (transoral biopsy of intestinal mucosa).

Gross examination of feces: Typically the feces are foamy, greasy, soft, and foul smelling.

Microscopic examination for fat[14]:

Principle: The fecal fats are stained with Sudan III. By preliminary treatment with acetic acid and heating with the stain, the fatty acids are stained. By using ethanol with the stain, the neutral fats are stained.

Table 31-1. Laboratory tests commonly employed to study malabsorption

	Normal values*	Malabsorption syndrome
Serum		
Albumin	4.0-5.2 g/dl	Diminished
Carotene	0.06-0.4 mg/dl	Diminished, particularly in small bowel disease
Calcium	9.0-10.5 mg/dl	Diminished, particularly in small bowel disease
Cholesterol	150-250 mg/dl	Diminished
Potassium	3.5-4.7 mEq/L	Diminished
Magnesium	1.7-2.0 mEq/L	Diminished
Vitamin B_{12}	100-700 pg/ml	Diminished, particularly in tropical sprue and bacterial overgrowth
Folic acid	5-21 ng/ml	Diminished, particularly in small bowel disease
Plasma		
Prothrombin time	Control value	Elevated
Tolerance tests		
D-Xylose (25 g orally)	Urinary excretion of 4.5 g or greater per 5 hr	Diminished in diseases of the mucosa, particularly celiac disease, and in intestinal stasis; normal in pancreatic insufficiency
Glucose (100 g orally)	35 mg over fasting plasma level	Flat curve in celiac disease and diseases of intestinal wall and in monosaccharide malabsorption
Lactose (50-100 g orally; 2.0 g/kg in children)	Rise in blood glucose of 20 mg/dl	Low to flat curve in primary lactose deficiency, celiac disease, and diseases of the intestinal wall
Sucrose (100 g orally)	Rise in blood glucose of 20 mg/dl	Low to flat curve in celiac disease and disease of intestinal wall
Vitamin B_{12} (μCi ^{60}CO B_{12})	> 7% urine excretion/24 hr	Decreased with intestinal stasis, ileal dysfunction, or resection
Stool fat		
Chemical determination (80-100 g fat daily)	> 6 g/24 hr	Increased
Miscellaneous		
5-Hydroxyindoleacetic acid (urinary excretion)	1.7-8.0 mg/24 hr	9-20 mg in adult celiac disease; 30-600 mg in metastatic carcinoid syndrome
Indole-3-acetic acid (urinary excretion)	< 18 mg/24 hr	
Indican (urinary excretion)	10-20 mg/24 hr	Elevated in bacterial overgrowth and ileal dysfunction
Bile acid breath test	Minute amounts of $^{14}CO_2$/4-8 hr	

From Sleisenger, M.H.: In Beeson, P.B., and McDermott, W., editors: Textbook of medicine, ed. 14, Philadelphia, 1975, W.B. Saunders Co.
*Usual findings. Some values for serum tests may be normal in some patients, e.g., carotene, calcium, and vitamin B_{12} in pancreatic insufficiency and calcium in tropical sprue.

Reagents:
1. Acetic acid, 36%
   Dilute 36 ml glacial acetic acid to 1 dl with water.
2. Sudan III, saturated solution in 95% alcohol

Procedure: To test for fatty acids, mix a few drops of a stool suspension with a few drops of 36% acetic acid on a slide. Add several drops of Sudan III solution and heat to boiling for a few seconds. Examine the slide while still warm with a high dry lens. To determine the neutral fats, mix 2 drops of fecal suspension with 2 drops of 95% ethanol on a slide. Add several drops of Sudan III solution and examine microscopically.

Interpretation: The **fatty acids** will appear as deep orange globules that become spiked on cooling. Normal stool may exhibit as many as 100 small fatty acid globules per high-power field, ranging from 1-4μm in di-

ameter. In steatorrhea a large number of fat globules, ranging from 6-75 μm in diameter, may be seen. When the fat globules are predominantly the larger sizes (>30 μm), the probability of significant stool fat loss increases. Positive or borderline results can be confirmed by the measurement of total fecal fat.

Neutral fats form yellow to pale orange refractile globules. Normal stool shows only occasional neutral fat globules, but many such globules are seen in specimens from patients with pancreatic insufficiency.

Measurement of total fat in feces[15-18]: See also Microanalysis of fecal fat.

Principle: Fecal fat may be determined by extracting the fat from the stool and either weighing the amount of extracted material or titrating the fatty acids extracted after hydrolysis. In the gravimetric methods any mineral oil or other nonfat material soluble in ether or petroleum ether is included in the weight of fat. In the titration methods one must assume an average molecular weight for the titrated fatty acids to calculate their actual amount. Although there is some variation with the type of diet, the differences are rarely large enough to influence the clinical interpretation. The method chosen for presentation is a wet-extraction method, with titration of the extracted fatty acids.

Collection: Collection of the specimen presents some problems. The determination of fat on a random specimen is of little value. It is generally agreed that, if possible, all the stool excreted over a 3-5 day period should be collected for analysis. Also it is preferable that the patient be on a fairly constant diet, one in which the fat content is at least approximately known, for 2 or 3 days before and throughout the collection period. The samples should be preserved in the refrigerator until analyzed. If more than an occasional determination is made, it is helpful to collect the specimens in new preweighed 1 gal metal paint cans. These have tight-fitting covers, and after the entire specimen has been collected it can be well mixed in the original can by adding some water if necessary and shaking on a paint-shaking machine. This usually gives a homogeneous sample. Subtract the weight of the can from the weight of the can plus contents to obtain the weight of the specimen. The addition of water makes no difference since one is determining the fat in an aliquot from an entire 3-day specimen. If the feces are collected in other containers, the entire specimen must be well mixed. This is best accomplished with a Waring blender or similar machine and with the addition of a small amount of water. The weight of the total homogenized specimen must then be obtained.

Reagents:
1. Ethyl alcohol containing 0.4% amyl alcohol
   Add 0.4 ml amyl alcohol to 1 dl of 95% ethyl alcohol.
2. Potassium hydroxide, 33%
   Dissolve 33 g potassium hydroxide in water, cool, and dilute to 1 dl.
3. Hydrochloric acid, 25% (w/v)
   Mix together 250 ml concentrated hydrochloric acid and 125 ml water.
4. Thymol blue indicator solution
   Dissolve 0.2 g thymol blue in 1 dl of 50% alcohol.
5. Sodium hydroxide, 0.1N, standardized, or dilute from standardized 1N solution
6. Hydrochloric acid, 2.5%, with 25% sodium chloride
   Add 10 ml 25% hydrochloric acid and about 60 ml water to a flask. Add 25 g sodium chloride, dissolve, and dilute to 1 dl.

Procedure: Weigh out to the nearest 10 mg 5-7 g feces into an Erlenmeyer flask. Add 10 ml of 33% potassium hydroxide and 40 ml ethyl alcohol containing 0.4% amyl alcohol. A simple way of determining the weight is to use small screw-capped vials of about 10 ml capacity. These are first weighed, the stool is then added, and they are weighed again. The material is then rinsed into the flask with the potassium hydroxide and alcohol solutions.

Boil the solution gently under a reflux condenser for 20 min. Cool, add 17 ml of 25% hydrochloric acid and cool again. Add exactly 50 ml petroleum ether, stopper, and shake for 1 min. Allow the layers to separate. Since the petroleum ether is rather volatile, separation is best accomplished by allowing the flask to stand in a refrigerator to avoid loss of the petroleum ether.

Remove exactly 25 ml of the petroleum ether layer, taking care not to include any of the aqueous layer. Transfer this to a flask and evaporate to dryness on a steam bath. (CAUTION: Flammable!) Add about 20 drops of thymol blue indicator to 1 dl ethyl alcohol. Then add 0.1N sodium hydroxide by drops until the color changes to green; avoid any excess. Add 10 ml of this neutralized alcohol to the flask containing the residue from the petroleum ether evaporation. Warm slightly to dissolve and titrate with 0.1N sodium hydroxide. The color changes of the indicator is from yellow to blue, but the end point may not be pure blue in the yellow material usually extracted from the feces.

Calculation:

Fatty acids (g) per 100 g stool =

$$\frac{n \times 284 \times 1.04 \times 2 \times 100}{10,000 \text{ W}} = \frac{5.91 \text{ n}}{\text{W}}$$

where n is the milliliters of 0.1N sodium hydroxide required for the titration, W is the weight of the stool taken, 284 is the average molecular weight of the fatty acids, and 1.04 is a factor to compensate for incomplete extraction.

This gives the total amount of fatty acids. If one wishes to determine the split fat, weigh another sample, add 22 ml of 2.5% hydrochloric acid with sodium chloride, boil under a reflux condenser for exactly 1 min, cool well, and add 40 ml ethyl alcohol containing 0.4% amyl alcohol and 50 ml petroleum ether. Proceed with the extraction and titration as for total fat. The calculations are the same.

Normal values and interpretation: The amount of fat in the stool depends on the dietary intake. With the usual diet the normal excretion is 1-7 g/day for adults, which is usually less than 10% of the intake. The normal value has been given as 1-9% of the intake. In steatorrhea the fat excretion is increased; in some cases as much as 40% of the ingested fat may be excreted. This increase in fat in the stool is indicative of malabsorption, but for accurate results one must at least know the approximate fat intake.

Formerly it was considered of value to determine the amount of fat in the split and unsplit forms, the former being the fats hydrolyzed to fatty acids. Impaired absorption or pancreatic dysfunction would increase the amount of unsplit fat. It has been found that even at refrigerator temperature some fats will still be slowly hydrolyzed, and the value of the determination has been doubted on theoretic grounds. Usually one can consider that the ratio of split fat to unsplit fat is about 3:1, so that about 75% of the fat is in the split form.

Microanalysis of fecal fat[19]: The method requires only a small amount of stool and is suitable for determinations on newborns.

Principle: The stool is dried on a small segment of

glass fiber paper. The fats are then extracted from the dried specimen with alcohol-ether. The solvent is then evaporated and the fat in the residue determined by a turbidimetric method.

Reagents:
1. Bloor solvent
   Mix together 3 volumes of absolute ethyl alcohol and 1 volume of ether.
2. Hydrochloric acid, 4N
   Mix 34 ml concentrated hydrochloric acid in distilled water to make 1 dl.
3. Sulfuric acid, 1.4N
   Add 4.0 ml concentrated sulfuric acid to about 50 ml water, cool, and dilute to 1 dl.
4. Dioxane
   Histologic grade is satisfactory.
5. Glass fiber paper, type E (Gelman Instrument Co., Ann Arbor Mich.)
6. Standard
   Triolein could be used as a standard, but since the fecal fats are a mixture of different compounds, an extract obtained from a serum sample with a known total lipid content determined gravimetrically or a control serum having a known value for total lipids can be used. An extract is prepared from the serum as follows: Place about 35 ml Bloor solvent in a 50 ml volumetric flask. Heat nearly to boiling on a steam bath, remove from the heat, and cautiously add with swirling exactly 1 ml of the serum. Allow to cool to room temperature; then dilute to the mark with solvent. Mix well and filter, placing a watch glass over the top of the funnel to prevent evaporation. The extract is stable for several weeks if kept tightly stoppered in the refrigerator. If the original serum contained 600 mg/dl total lipids or 6 mg/ml, then the extract would contain $6/50 = 0.12$ mg/ml. The exact value depends on the serum used, but one giving a value in this range is preferable.

Procedure: Apply an aliquot of stool containing about 1-5 mg of total solids (usually 1 or 2 drops of a 1:2 mixture of the stool and water) to a small preweighed strip of the glass fiber paper. Dry the strip in an oven at 50° C for at least 30 min and then reweigh. Until some experience is gained in judging how much stool suspension to add, it is important to prepare several strips containing different amounts of stool. If the total fat is desired, cover the material on the strips with a few drops of 4N hydrochloric acid to convert any soaps to free fatty acids. For estimation of free fatty acids and neutral fats, use strips without hydrochloric acid treatment. Transfer the strips to test tubes containing 5 ml Bloor solvent. Then incubate at 60° C for at least half an hour. Drain the strips against the side of the tube, remove, and discard. Then evaporate the solvent to dryness in a boiling water bath. Similarly evaporate 1, 3, and 5 ml aliquots of the standard extract in test tubes. When the solvent has been completely evaporated, dissolve the residue in 1.5 ml dioxane with the aid of gentle warming. After cooling to room temperature, add 5 ml of 1.4N sulfuric acid to each tube and mix well. Allow the tubes to stand for 1 hr; then read

at 650 nm against a reagent blank (1.5 ml dioxane plus 5 ml 1.4N sulfuric acid).

Calculation:

Percent by weight of fat in dry stool =

$$\frac{\text{Absorbance of sample}}{\text{Absorbance of standard}} \times \frac{S}{W} \times 100$$

where S is the weight in milligrams of total lipid in the standard having a reading closest to that of the sample, and W is the weight in milligrams of the dried stool on the original strip. The fecal soaps (split fat) are estimated by the difference in percentage of fat obtained from strips treated with hydrochloric acid and from those that were not so treated.

Interpretation: In normal infants not more than 25-30% of the dry weight should be total fats. The result is influenced somewhat by diet, but values above 35% are indicative of steatorrhea. The amount of split fat is apparently relatively lower in infants than the ratio given under the macromethod.

[131]I triolein adsorption test: See p. 786.

Vitamin A and carotene absorption tests: The suspicion of steatorrhea can be investigated or confirmed by other complementary procedures. The decrease in lipid absorption resulting in steatorrhea can also cause a decrease of intestinal absorption of lipid soluble nutrients, e.g., vitamin A and its precursor, carotene. The oral challenge test for vitamin A is less readily performed in most laboratories, and serum carotene levels are generally more easily measured as a screening procedure for lipid malabsorption.

Vitamin A absorption test[20]: The absorption of lipids may be studied by means of the vitamin A absorption test. The patient is given a large dose of vitamin A followed by a meal containing 50 g fat. A blood sample is taken before the ingestion of the vitamin and 3 and 5 hr later. The levels of vitamin A and fatty acids are determined. In patients with malabsorption there will be a minimal rise in these levels as compared to normal individuals.

Procedure: The patient should receive only liquids on the morning of the test. After a fasting blood sample has been taken, give the patient 250,000 IU vitamin A alcohol or vitamin A acetate in a glass of milk. One hour later have the patient ingest a mixed meal containing 50 g fat. Take blood samples 3 and 5 hr after the administration of the vitamin A. Then analyze the serum samples for vitamin A (p. 555) and triglycerides.

Interpretation: Normal subjects will have a fasting level of vitamin A of 100-300 IU/dl. This will rise to more than 800 IU/dl after the test. Malabsorption is indicated if the vitamin level fails to rise above about 600 IU/dl with only a slight or no increase in the triglycerides.

Serum carotene absorption test[21]:
Principle: The major precursor of vitamin A in humans is β-carotene. Carotene is extracted into petroleum ether to remove it from interfering substances in the serum. Because of its hydrophobic properties, carotene usually binds to serum proteins. Ethanol is added to the serum to break these complexes and release the

carotene. The resultant orange-yellow color is read at 450 nm.

Specimen: 10 ml blood in a foil-wrapped, red-topped tube (minimum: 2 ml serum).

Reagents:

1. Ethyl alcohol, 95%
2. Petroleum ether (benzin) (E-139, Fisher Scientific Co., Pittsburgh)
3. β-carotene (Sigma Chemical Co., St. Louis)
   CAUTION: Decomposes on exposure to light and air; keep refrigerated.
4. Reagent-grade chloroform
5. Pooled serum (in freezer)

Procedure: Label one round-bottom centrifuge tube for blank, patient, and control. Wrap the tubes in foil. Run duplicates whenever possible. Add 2 ml water to the blank and 2.0 ml serum or control to their respective tubes. Add 2.0 ml ethanol to each tube by drops while mixing on a vortex mixer. Add 4.0 ml petroleum ether to each tube. Cap the tubes. Mix each tube for 2 min on a vortex mixer. Allow the layers to separate. Carefully pipet off the petroleum ether (top) layer into a cuvet. Read the absorbance at 450 nm against the blank. Convert the absorbance to concentration by using the standard curve. Multiply *all* concentration values by 2 to account for the extraction of 2.0 ml serum into 4.0 ml ether.

Standard curve: Transfer 100 mg β-carotene to a 5 dl volumetric flask. Dissolve in about 20 ml chloroform and dilute to volume in petroleum ether. This yields a stock standard of 20,000 μg/dl. Pipet 10 ml stock standard into a 1 dl volumetric flask and dilute to volume with petroleum ether; this will yield 2000 μg/dl. Pipet 2.5, 5.0, 10.0, 15.0, and 20.0 ml of the 2000 μg/dl standard into respective 1 dl volumetric flasks. Dilute to volume with petroleum ether. These will yield working standards of 50, 100, 200, 300, and 400 μg/dl, respectively. (These standards are only stable for a few hours at 25° C and should be used as soon as possible. All standards must be protected from direct light because of the lability of carotene.) Place the standards into cuvets and read the absorbance at 450 nm against a petroleum ether blank. Plot absorbance vs. concentration on linear graph paper.

Normal value: 50-250 μg/dl.

Clinical significance[21]: Carotene or provitamin A determination in serum or plasma is the most useful single screening method for detecting malabsorption of fat. Carotene is a fat-soluble pigment that is slowly absorbed. It is found in leafy vegetables, fruits, and liver. The absorption of carotene requires the presence of dietary lipids; limited amounts of these lipids are stored in the liver. When malabsorption of fats is the problem, serum carotene is markedly decreased.

Carotene levels are lowest in primary malabsorption. Levels may increase to normal during successful steroid therapy. Carotene levels may also be low in enteritis and many diseases associated with steatorrhea. High fever, hepatic disease, and deficient diet may also cause low carotene levels. Low dietary intake of carotene as a cause of lowered serum carotene values can be determined by repetition of the serum analysis after 15,000

units of carotene in oil is given by mouth for 5 days. If the cause is low dietary intake, a twofold or threefold increase in serum values will occur.

Carotene values are increased in diabetes, hyperlipemia, carotenemia, and hypothyroidism.

Lactose and D-xylose absorption tests: Malabsorption of dietary sugars from the intestines can result in diarrhea because of the water-retaining properties of the unabsorbed compounds. These two challenge tests are used to diagnose a carbohydrate malabsorption as the cause of a diarrhea. The carbohydrate intolerance leading to diarrhea can be caused by a disaccharidase deficiency, as in lactose, sucrose-isomaltose, or glucose-galactose malabsorption, or can be caused by a general defect in the absorption of monosaccharides.

Lactase deficiency is most commonly seen during childhood in blacks, Orientals, Jews, Arabs, Eskimos, and Indians. The enzyme deficiency becomes most apparent with an increase in lactose (milk) consumption. Secondary lactase deficiency can occur as a result of other diseases of the small intestine, primarily celiac sprue, protein malabsorption, and infection.

Monosaccharide malabsorption is most easily diagnosed by use of the D-xylose absorption test. D-xylose is a pentose not normally present in blood. When absorbed the sugar is excreted by the kidney after passing unchanged through the liver. A rise in blood and urinary D-xylose concentrations following an oral challenge is used as a measure of the functional integrity of the jejunum.

Lactose tolerance test: See Chapter 21, p. 481.

D-Xylose excretion test[22-25]:

Principle: The D-xylose excretion test is used as an indirect measure of intestinal absorption. A definite amount of the pentose xylose, which is not metabolized by the body, is administered, and the amount excreted in the urine during the next 5 hr is measured. In the absence of severely impaired kidney function the amount excreted is dependent on the amount absorbed in the intestines. In the presence of significant renal dysfunction, excretion of D-xylose is decreased, giving an impression of malabsorption. To reduce the error caused by renal dysfunction, a blood determination of D-xylose should be carried out along with the urinalysis.

The D-xylose test is a simplified colorimetric procedure using phloroglucinol (Trinder and Tollen application). D-Xylose is heated in strong acid to form furfural. Furfural reacts with phloroglucinol to produce a pink-colored compound, with high molar absorptivity at 554 nm.

Collection: Have the patient ingest 5 g xylose* dissolved in about 250 ml water. Collect all the urine voided during the next 5 hr. Give additional water to drink during this period, if necessary, since a very low urine volume may lead to unreliable results.

Specimen: Serum plasma (50 μl); urine (5 μl).

Reagent: The working reagent consists of 0.5 g

---

*Xylo-Pfan (D-Xylose), Pfanstiel Labs., Waukegan, Ill. NOTE: This is the only brand of D-xylose that meets the requirements for diagnostic use in humans.

phloroglucinol (Sigma product P-3502, Sigma Chemical Co., St. Louis), 1 dl glacial acetic acid, and 10 ml concentrated hydrochloric acid. Keep it in a dark bottle. It is stable for only 4 days. (CAUTION: Do *not* pipet by mouth. Use gloves in handling the reagent. Perform the test under the hood.)

Standard: D-Xylose dissolved in saturated benzoic acid. (Do not refrigerate standards.) It is stable for 3 months.

Stock standard: 0.3755 g xylose/50 ml saturated benzoic acid = 50 mmole/L standard. To prepare different standards see following chart:

Standard					Saturated benzoic acid
15.0 mmole/L	=	3 ml stock standard	+		7 ml
10.0 mmole/L	=	1 ml stock standard	+		4 ml
7.5 mmole/L	=	2 ml of mmole/L standard	+		2 ml
5.0 mmole/L	=	1 ml of stock standard	+		9 ml
2.5 mmole/L	=	2 ml of 5 mmole/L standard	+		2 ml
1.0 mmole/L	=	1 ml of 5 mmole/L standard	+		4 ml

Routinely run the 5 and 1 mmole/L standards in the assay and select the one with the optical density (OD) closest to the OD of the patient's sample. For calculation see below.

Procedure: Set the Dow heat block to 105° C (under hood). Run standards and patients' samples in duplicate. Label 13 × 100 mm disposable tubes as follows: one serum blank, one standard blank, two for each standard, and two for each patient.

Pipet 5 ml working reagent into each tube. Add 50 μl water to the standard blank (zero the *standards* against this). Add 50 μl of any normal (xylose-free) serum to the serum blank (zero all *patients' samples* against this). Add 50 μl plasma, serum, or standard to respective tubes. In addition, add 5 μl urine if running a urine sample.

Mix well on a vortex mixer. Immediately before putting the tubes in the heat block, add several drops of water to each hole to be used. Then *simultaneously* add *all* tubes to the heat block and set the clock for 4 min. (NOTE: Do not add tubes at intervals, because the temperature will drop during incubation and different tubes will be affected differently.)

After incubation immediately cool the tubes under the tap. Mix again. Read absorbance on a Coleman spectrophotometer at 550 nm.

Using a 250 μl pipet, pipet the standard blank into a clean cuvet, rotate to the reading position, and set zero. Pipet the standards into clean cuvets and read the absorbance. Read patients' samples likewise, setting zero with serum blank. It is important to add the sample to the cuvet and read the absorbance *immediately* before adding the next sample. (The OD will change on sitting.)

Calculation:

$$\frac{\text{OD of patient's sample}}{\text{OD of standard}} \times \frac{\text{Standard}}{\text{(mmole/L)}} = \frac{\text{Millimoles}}{\text{per liter}}$$

Urine:
1. Multiply urine results by 10 (use only 5 μl urine but 50 μl standard). This is measured in millimoles per liter.
2. Convert millimoles per liter to milligrams per deciliter: Millimoles per liter × 15 = Milligrams per deciliter.
3. Calculate for 5 hr: Milligrams per deciliter × Total volume/100.
4. Divide by 1000 and report as grams per 5 hr urine.

NOTE: Run a glucose test on the patient's specimen. Record on a slip.

Linearity: Color reaction linear to 10.0 mmole/L.

Interfering substances: There is a slight interference in patients' specimens with high glucose (>500 mg/dl), but all specimens should be checked for glucose and this factor accounted for.

Normal values:
Blood: Adult (after 25 g dose): >25 mg/dl (>1.66 mmole/L)
Child (after 25 g dose): >30 mg/dl (>2.0 mmole/L)
Urine: Adult (after 25 g dose): >4 g/5 hr urine
Child (16-33% of given dose)

Interpretation: Some workers have administered 25 g xylose instead of 5 g, but this occasionally causes nausea or diarrhea, which interferes with the test. Five grams is sufficient for good results. When 5 g xylose is given in the absence of impaired kidney function, an excretion of more than 1.2 g is indicative of satisfactory intestinal absorption. Excretion of 0.9-1.2 g would be a doubtful result but may indicate some degree of malabsorption. If less than 0.9 g is excreted, malabsorption is present, providing kidney function is near normal.

A normal increase in blood D-xylose in the presence of a low urine xylose output can be seen in renal retention or myxedema or as a result of an improper urine collection. In such cases, the results are invalid. A decreased blood D-xylose level accompanying low urine D-xylose concentrations is seen in 80% of those patients with a malabsorption syndrome.

ANALYSIS OF STOOL ELECTROLYTES

In select cases of diarrhea, it may be necessary to quantitate the loss of body sodium and other electrolytes.[11,26] The amounts of fecal sodium or potassium excreted over a 24 hr period should be compared to the amount ingested over the same time period to determine the net intestinal loss. The measurement of intestinal electrolyte loss can be used to correct for systemic electrolyte disturbances secondary to the severe diarrhea, e.g., dehydration or acid-base disorders.

The diarrheic stools should be collected over a 72 hr period (see collection procedure for fecal fat above). An aliquot of stool water should be removed and centrifuged and/or filtered to remove solid particulate matter. If necessary, the stool water can be diluted with distilled water to facilitate this process. The particle-free fluid can then be analyzed for electrolytes by standard methods.

Interpretation: Normally, the concentration of potas-

Table 31-2. Comparison of approximate daily water and electrolytes delivered to and from the normal colon

	Fluid delivered to colon		Fluid delivered to stool	
	Amount	Concentration (mEq/L)	Amount	Concentration (mEq/L)
Water	600 ml		100 ml	
Sodium	75 mEq	125	4 mEq	40
Potassium	5 mEq	9	9 mEq	90
Chloride	36 mEq	60	2 mEq	15
Bicarbonate	44 mEq	74	3 mEq	30

From Fordtran, S.S.: Fed. Proc. **26**:1405-1414, 1967.

sium in stool water is greater than that of sodium (Table 31-2). As the diarrheic disease becomes more severe and the volume of stool border increases, the loss of sodium and chloride increases and exceeds the loss of potassium. In most intestinal disorders the loss of sodium plus potassium exceeds that of chloride. However, in congenital chloridorrhea the reverse is true.

Although the osmolality of stool water can be measured, the clinical utility of this measurement is undetermined (Table 31-2).

GLOSSARY

amebiasis Disease caused by infection with *Entamoeba histolytica*.

bilirubin Bile pigment.

blind loop syndrome Malabsorption and megaloblastic anemia occurring in patients whose fecal stream stagnates in a loop of bowel (usually congenital or postoperative).

cholera Disease caused by infection with *Vibrio cholerae*.

cystic fibrosis Generalized hereditary disorder in which there is widespread dysfunction of exocrine glands characterized by signs of chronic pulmonary disease, pancreatic deficiency, and abnormally high levels of electrolytes in sweat.

enteritis Inflammation of intestines.

fecalith Calcified feces.

fistula Abnormal passage between two internal organs or leading from an internal organ to the outside.

indole Product from decomposition of tryptophan in intestines.

malabsorption Disorder of normal nutritive absorption of food from bowel.

peroxidase Enzyme that catalyzes transfer of oxygen from hydrogen peroxide.

pneumatosis intestinalis Condition characterized by gas-containing cysts in wall of intestines.

regional enteritis Granulomatous inflammation of bowel.

salmonellosis Disease caused by infection with organisms of the genus *Salmonella*.

scleroderma Systemic disease that involves connective tissues of body; skin is thickened, hard, and rigid.

shigellosis Disease caused by infection with organisms of the genus *Shigella*.

skatole Product from feces.

sprue Chronic disease marked by sore mouth, raw-looking tongue, and gastrointestinal catarrh with periodic diarrhea in which the stools are frothy, fatty (steatorrhea), and fetid.

steatorrhea Fatty stool.

typhoid fever Disease caused by infection with *Salmonella typhi*.

typhus Disease caused by infection with a species of *Rickettsia*.

Whipple's disease Intestinal lipodystrophy; a disease marked by diarrhea with fatty stools, arthritis, emaciation, and loss of strength.

REFERENCES

1. Bradley, G.M.: Diagn. Med. **3**(2):64-74, 1980.
2. Deadman, N.M.: Clin. Chim. Acta **35**:273, 1971.
3. Woodson, D.D.: Clin. Chim. Acta **29**:249, 1970.
4. Cancer **30**(4):194-240, 1980.
5. Huntsman, R.G., and Liddell, I.J.: J. Clin. Pathol. **14**:436, 1961.
6. Garb, S.: Clinical guide to undesirable drug interactions and interferences, New York, 1971, Springer Publishing Co., Inc.
7. Illingworth, D.C.: J. Clin. Pathol. **18**:103, 1965.
8. Afifi, A.M., et al.: Br. Med. J. **1**:1021, 1966.
9. Watson, E.J., and Hawkinson, V.: Am. J. Clin. Pathol. **17**:108, 1947.
10. Sleisenger, M.H., and Lloyd, L.B.: In Smith, L.H., Jr., editor: Major problems in internal medicine, Philadelphia, 1977, W.B. Saunders Co., vol. 13.
11. Sleisenger, M.H., and Fordtran, J.S., editors: Gastrointestinal disease, Philadelphia, 1973, W.B. Saunders Co.
12. Jefferies, G.H., Weser, E., and Sleisenger, M.H.: Gastroenterology **46**:434, 1964.
13. Kalser, M.H.: J.A.M.A. **188**:37, 1964.
14. Drummey, G.D., Benson, J.A., Jr., and Jones, C.N.: N. Engl. J. Med. **264**:85, 1961.
15. van de Kamer, J.H., ten Bokkel Huinink, H., and Weyers, H.A.: J. Biol. Chem. **177**:34, 1949.
16. Cooke, W.T., et al.: Q. J. Med. **15**:141, 1946.
17. van de Kamer, J.H.: In Seligson, D., editor: Standard methods of clinical chemistry, New York, 1958, Academic Press, Inc., vol. 2, p. 347.
18. Jover, A., and Gordon, R.S., Jr.: J. Lab. Clin. Med. **59**:878, 1962.
19. Searcy, R.L., et al.: Am. J. Clin. Pathol. **41**:477, 1964.
20. Fitzgerald, O., Fennelly, J.J., and Hingerty, J.J.: Gut **3**:74, 1962.
21. Levinson, S.A., and MacFate, R.P., editors: Clinical laboratory diagnosis, ed. 6, Philadelphia, 1961, Lea & Febiger.
22. Eberts, T.J., et al.: Clin. Chem. **25**(8):1440-1443, 1979.
23. Roe, J.H., and Rice, E.W.: J. Biol. Chem. **173**:507, 1948.
24. Kerstell, J.: Scand. J. Clin. Lab. Invest. **13**:637, 1961.
25. Santini, R., Jr., Sheehy, T.W., and Martinez-De Jesue, J.: Gastroenterology **40**:772, 1961.

MICROBIOLOGY

CHAPTER 32

Bacteriology, virology, and rickettsial diseases

Pseudomonas
Achromobacter
Acinetobacter
Moraxella
Aeromonas
Flavobacterium
Alcaligenes faecalis
Brucella
Yersinia
Pasteurella
Francisella
Haemophilus
Actinobacillus
Bordetella
Calymmatobacterium
Legionella
Gram-negative anaerobic non-spore-forming bacilli
Bacteroidaceae
Bacteroides
Fusobacterium
Gram-positive non-spore-forming bacilli
Lactobacillaceae
Lactobacillus
Listeria
Corynebacterium
Erysipelothrix
Mycobacteriaceae
Mycobacterium
Nocardiaceae
Nocardia
Actinomycetaceae
Actinomyces
Streptomycetaceae
Gram-positive spore-forming bacilli
Bacillaceae
Gram-positive aerobic spore-forming bacilli (Bacillus)
Gram-positive anaerobic spore-forming bacilli (Clostridium)
Vibrionaceae
Vibrio
Spirillaceae
Spirillum
Streptobacillus
Spirochaetaceae
Treponema
Leptospira
Borrelia
Hospital environmental cultures and hospital-acquired infections
Rickettsiaceae
Rickettsia
Methods in virology
Adenoviruses
Enteroviruses
Human enteroviruses
Animal enteroviruses
Arboviruses
Herpes virus group
Epstein-Barr virus
Cytomegaloviruses
Varicella–herpes zoster virus
Rabies virus

Myxoviruses
Measles virus
Serology of rubella: evaluation of immune status
Chlamydiae-Psittacosis-Lymphogranuloma-Trachoma group
Lymphogranuloma venereum
Trachoma
Inclusion conjunctivitis
Psittacosis
Viral hepatitis
Hepatitis A
Hepatitis B
Hepatitis virus non A–non B
Variola and vaccinia viruses
Mycoplasmataceae
Mycoplasma

Microbiology includes the study of bacteria, rickettsiae, viruses, parasites, and fungi. Some serologic investigations are also performed in the bacteriology laboratory. Fungi and parasites are discussed in Chapters 33 and 34, respectively.

INTRODUCTION TO CLINICAL BACTERIOLOGY[1-7]

The clinical bacteriologist's main concern is the rapid and precise identification of pathogenic bacteria. To render this service the bacteriologist must know (1) the origin of the specimen, (2) the nature of the investigation the clinician wants, and (3) the normal flora of the area from which the specimen is taken. For clinical purposes the identification of the genus of a microorganism and the antimicrobial susceptibility should be sufficient in many instances, so that treatment is not delayed. Rapid examination of a direct smear may allow a preliminary report within a few minutes after the specimen has been received. The final identification of an organism must be based on all methods available: smears, cultures on routine and special media, biochemical tests, and serologic analysis. Accurate records must be kept that indicate not only the identity of the specimen but also the steps taken in the identification of the organism such as the media employed, the biochemical and serologic tests performed, and the results of these tests.

Bacteria are minute microorganisms that vary in length from 0.2-10 μm with an average length of 1.5 μm. The average diameter is less than 1 μm. Clinical bacteriology is concerned with the bacteria that may injure the host, depending on such factors as host resistance and defense, bacterial toxicity, virulence, and invasive power.

The classification of bacteria is based on morphologic, cultural, physiologic, immunologic, and biochemical characteristics.

Morphologic classification of bacteria

Morphologically, bacteria are classified into the following types: **cocci,** which are oval or round; **bacilli,** which are rod shaped; and **vibrios** and **spirochetes,**

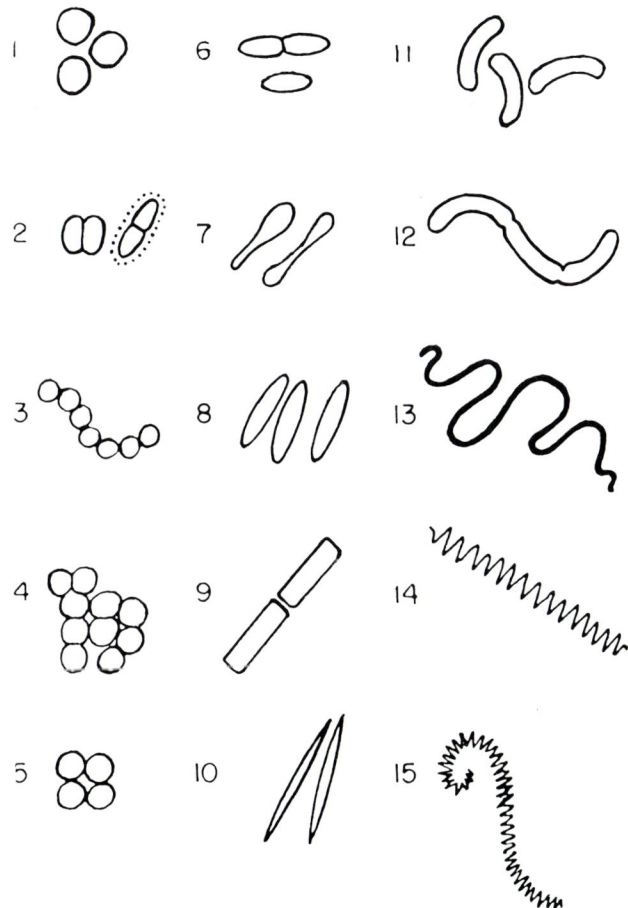

Fig. 32-1. Morphology of bacteria. *1,* Single cocci; *2,* cocci in pairs; *3,* cocci in chains; *4,* cocci in clusters; *5,* cocci in tetrads; *6,* coccobacilli; *7,* club-shaped bacilli; *8,* bacilli with rounded ends; *9,* bacilli with square ends; *10,* fusiform bacilli; *11,* vibrios; *12,* spirilla; *13, Borrelia; 14, Treponema;* and *15, Leptospira.* (From Smith, D.T., et al., editors: In Zinsser, H.: Microbiology, ed. 12, New York, 1960, Appleton-Century-Crofts Co., Inc.)

Table 32-1. Examples of morphologic types of some bacteria

Cocci (spheric)	Bacilli (rod shaped)		Vibrios (comma shaped) and spirochetes (spiral shaped)
	Non-spore-forming	Spore forming	
Staphylococci	*Escherichia coli*	*Clostridum*	*Treponema*
Streptococci	Corynebacteria	*Bacillus*	*Leptospira*
Gonococci	*Brucella*		*Borrelia*
Meningococci	*Shigella*		*Vibrio*
			Spirillum

which are curved or spiral shaped (Fig. 32-1 and Table 32-1).

Division of bacteria

Bacteria divide by transverse binary fission. Cocci form characteristic groups, depending on the direction of splitting and the number of planes (diplococci, chains, clusters, etc.). The average rate of reproduction varies from every 16-20 min *(Escherichia coli)* to once a day *(Mycobacterium tuberculosis)*. Some species do not remain in a single form and are described as pleomorphic. This type of regularly encountered irregularity is one of the diagnostic criteria of some bacteria, e.g., corynebacteria.

Structure of bacteria

Structurally, bacteria possess a nucleoid structure containing DNA, cytoplasm containing RNA, cell membranes, and a cell wall. Surrounding the cell wall is an outer slime layer that is called a capsule (Fig. 32-2). The motile bacteria possess appendages called flagella that are responsible for their motility and are antigenically different from the somatic (body) antigen. The position and number of flagella can also be used to classify bacteria. The capsule, which consists of mucopolysaccharides, is related to the virulence of the organisms. In cultures the composition of the medium determines capsule production. Encapsulated forms produce smoother or more mucoid colonies than nonencapsulated cells.

Gram stain: The Gram stain is the most widely used staining procedure in bacteriology. Bacteria fall into two categories: gram positive (blue) and gram negative (pink). During the staining process, gram-positive bacteria retain the crystal violet-iodine complex whereas gram-negative bacteria readily lose it after alcohol or acetone treatment and are counterstained with safranin, a red dye. The basis of the Gram stain reaction is a function of the basic biochemical and physiologic differences between these two groups of organisms. In addition to Gram stain reactions, gram-negative and -positive bacteria vary as to the structural complexity of the cell envelope, amount of lipid and amino acids in the cell wall, antibiotic susceptibility, lysozyme sensitivity, etc. Table 32-2 shows some typical staining reactions.

Spores: Two clinically significant genera, *Bacillus* and *Clostridium,* form spores, one cell producing only one spore, which may be located centrally, terminally, or subterminally according to the species. Spores represent resistant dormant bacterial forms that can survive extremely unfavorable conditions.

Pigments: Some bacteria produce pigments or fluorescing material. Some pigments are water soluble, e.g., that of *Pseudomonas;* others are not, e.g., that of *Staphylococcus aureus.*

Bacterial enzymes and toxins

Bacteria produce various enzymes that are able to split food elements and are responsible for the fermentation reactions of bacteria, i.e., the formation of acid or acid and gas as a result of carbohydrate metabolism, as well as for putrefaction and decay, resulting in production of hydrogen sulfide (H_2S), amines, and ammonia. Some enzymes are characteristic of certain organisms, e.g., coagulase production by staphylococci, or streptokinase synthesis by streptococci. The energy for these metabolic activities is derived from light (photosynthesis) or from oxidation of chemical substances (chemosynthesis). All bacteria associated with human beings are chemosynthetic.

Bacteria produce toxins that are subdivided into **exotoxins** and **endotoxins.** Exotoxins are excreted by the living bacterial cells into their surroundings; they are heat (60° C) labile, highly toxic, and antigenic. Endotoxins are liberated by bacterial cell walls when they disintegrate; they are relatively heat (60° C) stable, weakly toxic, and weakly antigenic.

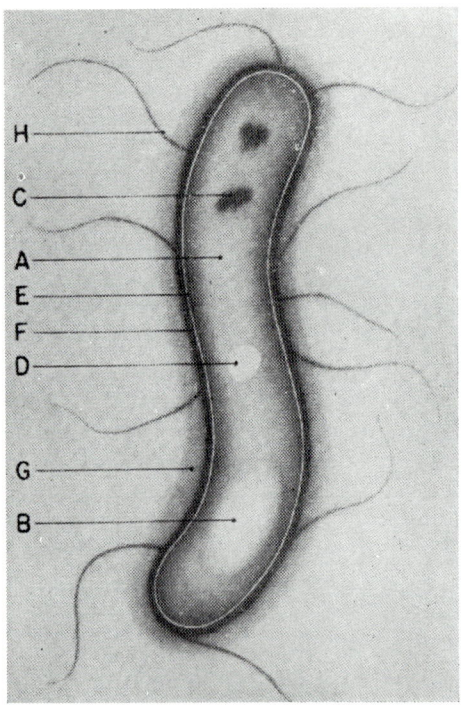

Fig. 32-2. Morphologic structure of a bacillus. *A,* Cytoplasm; *B,* nucleus; *C,* cytoplasmic granules; *D,* vacuole; *E,* cytoplasmic membrane; *F,* cell wall; *G,* slime layer or capsule; *H,* flagellum. (From Smith, D.T., et al.: In Zinsser, H.: Microbiology, ed. 12, New York, 1960, Appleton-Century-Crofts Co., Inc.)

Table 32-2. Gram stain reaction of some important bacteria

Gram negative	Gram positive
Gonococci	Staphylococci
Meningococci	Streptococci
Coliform bacteria	*Streptococcus pneumoniae*
Proteus vulgaris	Clostridia
Yersinia pestis	*Actinomyces*
	Diphtheria bacilli
	Bacillus subtilis

Factors affecting bacterial growth

The chemical composition of bacteria varies according to the species and the media on which they are grown. The **growth** of bacteria in culture media is determined by environmental factors such as moisture, composition of air, pH, temperature, salt, availability of carbon and nitrogen, and growth factors such as the presence of thiamine. The gas requirements vary; **obligate aerobes** grow only in free oxygen and **obligate anaerobes** grow only in an oxygen-free atmosphere. Aerobes and anaerobes that do not clearly belong to either group are called **facultative** aerobes or anaerobes. Most bacteria grow better with the addition of carbon dioxide. The optimal pH is close to neutral or is slightly alkaline. The optimal temperature for most pathogens is 35° C, and the optimal salt concentration is below 1%. Media may produce temporary chemical and/or morphologic changes in bacteria called **adaptations,** or they may reveal **transmissible** permanent changes called **mutations.**

L-phase variants of bacteria

Cell wall–deficient bacterial variants (CWD) are called spheroplasts, protoplasts, or L forms.[8-10] They are involution forms produced by nongenetic adaptations caused by changes in culture media factors such as pH, nutrients, and salt content. Penicillin in the nutrient media can produce L forms from such organisms as *Salmonella, Shigella, E. coli, Proteus,* and *Corynebacterium diphtheriae.* The L form possesses no rigid bacterial shape but is a mass of protoplasm lacking a rigid cell wall; it is surrounded by an electron-dense layer and can be maintained in pure culture. The L forms of certain bacteria have few characteristics in common with *Mycoplasma* except that both lack cell walls. In the absence of penicillin in the medium the L forms revert to the parent bacterial form. *Mycoplasma* fails to do so. The "fried-egg" colony is common to both. There is no good evidence to substantiate a major role for CWDs in disease.

Colonies

Groups of bacteria forming on solid media as a result of repeated division of one or a few organisms are called colonies; features of these colonies may vary according to the genus or species they represent.

Normal flora

Following is a list of flora normally present in human beings. These organisms are usually commensal but may become opportunistic pathogens.

1. **Ear:** Coagulase-negative staphylococci and diphtheroids.
2. **Intestinal tract:** Stomach—sterile if acid, Boas-Oppler bacilli if achlorhydric; duodenum—sterile; jejunum and ileum—lactobacilli; cecum and colon (feces)—*Escherichia coli, Bacteroides,* and smaller numbers of *Proteus, Streptococcus faecalis,* lactobacilli, *Pseudomonas,* clostridia, *Enterobacter,* and yeast. These bacteria appear gradually within the first 24-48 hr after birth. If any one group predominates, a pathologic condition may be produced.
3. **Male genitourinary tract:** Mycobacteria, diphtheroids, and micrococci.
4. **Mouth:** Lactobacilli, streptococci (γ and α), micrococci, spirochetes, fusiform bacteria, yeast *Branhamella, Streptococci pneumoniae,* diphtheroids, anaerobic streptococci and micrococci, *Candida, Geotrichum,* and actinomycetes.
5. **Nose and nasopharynx:** Streptococci, staphylococci, micrococci, *Streptococcus pneumoniae,* and intestinal organisms such as *Escherichia coli, Proteus,* and *Pseudomonas.*
6. **Skin:** Yeast, *Staphylococcus epidermidis,* streptococci (γ), *Bacillus subtilis,* diphtheroids, *Escherichia coli* in some areas, *Proteus,* mycobacteria, and *Candida albicans.*
7. **Sputum:** Streptococci (α and γ), *Branhamella,* diphtheroids, pneumococci, *Candida,* spirochetes, fusiform bacilli, *Haemophilus,* and *Staphylococcus.* Any of these organisms may cause disease when present in large numbers in a susceptible host.
8. **Throat:** Streptococci (α and γ hemolytic), *Neisseria catarrhalis,* staphylococci (coagulase negative), *Haemophilus haemolyticus, H. influenzae, Streptococcus pneumoniae,* diphtheroids, coliform bacteria, and yeasts, including *Candida albicans.*
9. **Urine (contaminants):** Staphylococci (coagulase negative), diphtheroids, and *Bacillus* species.
10. **Vagina:** Sterile at birth, later contains micrococci, enterococci, diphtheroids, and lactobacilli (Döderlein's bacillus). At puberty, *Escherichia coli,* yeasts, lactobacilli, diphtheroids, streptococci, and micrococci are present. After menopause, the flora is as before puberty.

Sterilization

Sterilization[11] is complete destruction of living microbial forms (bacteria, spores, viruses, and fungi).

Dry heat: All glassware should be absolutely dry when placed in the sterilizer; if it is not dry, keep the temperature low and leave the door ajar until drying is complete. Sterilize at 170° C for 1½ hr. Dry heat is not an efficient method of sterilization since it is slow and destroys such materials as rubber and plastics. Dry heat must be used for materials that are damaged by steam, e.g., dehydrated substances, dry chemicals, and oils. See also the following discussion of ethylene oxide gas sterilization.

Moist heat (steam)—autoclaving: Sterilize at 15 pounds pressure (121.6° C) for 15 min after the temperature and pressure both reach the proper levels. Media and other material for sterilization must not be more than 5 cm thick. Autoclave culture media, vaccine bottles, discarded blood culture bottles, and any dangerous spore-forming organisms as well as other infected material handled in the bacteriology laboratory before disposal. Steaming under pressure is an effective method of sterilization since steam rapidly penetrates the material to be sterilized when air is removed from the autoclave.

Filtration: Filtration through special filters is useful for removing bacteria from materials that are coagulated or broken down by heat, e.g., serum, ascitic fluid, and sugars. Several kinds of such filters are available. Seitz filters are made of asbestos; other filters are made of cellulose, porcelain, etc. Millipore (Millipore Corp., Bedford, Mass.) membrane filters of 0.22 μm (GS) effectively remove all bacteria from liquids being filtered. The membrane filters are not only used for sterilization but also for isolation and counting of bacteria, because the bacteria retained by the filter can be grown on the filter surface provided the filter is brought into contact with a suitable culture medium.

Chemical sterilization

Chemical sterilization[12] is accomplished by high concentrations of liquid or gaseous germicides and is used for heat-sensitive items. Formaldehyde and glutaraldehyde solutions are used as liquid chemical sterilizing agents.

Ethylene oxide[13] is an effective, safe agent for sterilization of objects that may be injured by steam. It is usually slower than other methods. Depending on the material sterilized, periods up to 12 hr in an aeration chamber are required to remove accumulated residues.

Disinfection

Disinfection is partial destruction of living agents, since vegetative microorganisms only are killed, reducing, nevertheless, the bacterial population to subinfective levels. Spores, resistant bacteria, and viruses are relatively unaffected. The effectiveness of disinfection is directly proportional to the concentration of the germicidal agent and the length of contact and is indirectly proportional to the amount of organic material contaminating the area to be disinfected. Thorough cleaning before disinfection is thus essential.

Several types of disinfectants are available:

1. **Quarternary ammonium compounds:** Quaternary ammonium disinfectants are primarily effective against vegetative cells. They are rendered ineffective by soaps and organic matter and must therefore be used on clean surfaces. They are antibacterial but not effective against tubercle bacilli.
2. **Heavy metals:** Mercurials are poor hospital disinfectants but are used as clinical antiseptics, topically applied.
3. **Iodophors:** The disinfecting property of iodophors, which are combinations of iodine and detergents, depends on the release of iodine. They are active against vegetative microorganisms and tubercle bacilli. If present in adequate concentration, they are not inactivated by organic material.
4. **Chlorine germicides** (hypochlorite salts): Although extensively used as germicidal agents in the food industry, chlorine germicides are irritating to the tissues and damaging to various materials. They are inactivated by organic compounds.
5. **Phenols:** Synthetic phenols, often combined with detergents, are good germicidal agents, active against vegetative bacterial forms and tubercle bacilli. They are not effective against spores, are not inactivated by organic matter, and form a bacteriostatic layer.
6. **Alcohol:** The 70% aqueous solutions of ethyl and isopropyl alcohol are effective against vegetative forms and tubercle bacilli. They are not effective against spores.

Autoclave sterility testing

Steam sterilizers: Use *Bacillus stearothermophilus* spore strips (Barnstead Co., Boston). Inoculate exposed strips into 10 ml trypticase soy broth. Include both a positive and a negative control. Incubate the tubes at 55° C for 7 days. Observe daily for the presence of growth.

Dry heat and ethylene oxide gas sterilizers: Use *Bacillus subtilis* spore strips (Barnstead Co., Boston). Inoculate exposed strips into 10 ml trypticase soy broth. Include both a positive and a negative control. Incubate the tubes for 7 days at 37° C. Observe daily for the presence of growth.

Control: A positive control is an unexposed spore strip. A negative control may consist of one or two tubes of the trypticase soy broth.

Quality control in bacteriology laboratory

See Chapter 1.

Safety in bacteriology laboratory[14]

The bacteriology laboratory shares with other laboratories the dangers of unsafe electrical equipment, volatile, explosive materials, and substances that are toxic when swallowed. There are, however, a few dangerous areas characteristic of the bacteriology laboratory, e.g., the fire hazard of the Bunsen burner and the contact with dangerous bacteria and fungi. Special safety devices are necessary when handling *Mycobacterium tuberculosis*, meningococci, and some fungi. The airflow in the laboratory should be unidirectional, an exhaust fan should draw at least 50-75 linear feet of air per minute, and ultraviolet lights should be mounted in strategic areas. A supply of 5% phenol must be available to periodically wipe the work area and the outside of specimen containers and to immerse contaminated equipment and material. Discarded material must be autoclaved before it is removed to the disposal area.

BACTERIOLOGIC METHODS
Handling of specimens

Specimens for culture should be sent to the laboratory without delay. They should be labeled with the patient's name and age, the date, the time of collection, and the clinical impression. Also included should be the type of specimen (sputum, feces, etc.), how it was obtained (scrapings, biopsy, bronchoscopy, etc.), information regarding antibiotic therapy, and the physician's name. The correct choice of primary media depends on this information.

Specimens should be cultured and smeared as soon as they are received because some bacteria are sensitive to air and to standing at room temperature. Delays may change the relative number of bacteria by enhancing the growth of some and suppressing others.

All containers and cups must be sterile and suitable in size and shape, so that the submitted material can be received without danger of contamination. All containers must be closed and labeled.

Scanty material should be submitted on swabs moistened with transfer medium, e.g., Culturettes (Marion Scientific Co., Kansas City, Mo.). The addition of the holding medium prevents drying of the specimens and maintains the bacterial status quo.

When the specimen is received in the laboratory, it is entered in an accession book (see discussion of quality control in bacteriology) and given a number, and then a work sheet is made out that indicates date and type of each investigative step, result of each procedure, and final diagnosis. The work sheet must be filed in the laboratory for easy reference should any questions arise about handling or diagnosis of the specimen.

Make a direct smear from each material cultured and stain by the Gram method and any additional applicable method. This will often help in the choice of primary culture media and in the handling of the specimen.

If the material is from a patient receiving antibiotic therapy, several approaches may be used. Blood or other fluids may be treated with penicillinase. This procedure must be performed with caution using a negative control, e.g., sterile broth and penicillinase, since contamination may result. A new product, the Antibiotic Removal Device (ARD) (Marion Scientific Co., Kansas City, Mo.), may be used to remove by ion exchange a variety of antibiotics from blood and body fluids. Simpel dilution of part of the specimen by inoculation into broths, e.g., thioglycollate, is effective in negating the effect of antibiotics. This is one of the reasons for using thioglycollate broth routinely.

Examine cultures daily; subculture to special media as indicated on the basis of cultural appearance and gram-stained smear. Disinfect hands after handling cultures and infectious material. Disinfect and clean up if cultures and infectious material are spilled. Autoclave discarded cultures. Dispose of specimens safely, e.g., by autoclaving. Keep stock and reagent bottles clean, properly labeled, and in their proper places.

Swabs

In general, aspirated material is preferable to material collected on swabs. The swab must not be allowed to dry. If delay is unavoidable, the swab should be inserted in a transport medium and kept at room temperature. Rayon-tipped swabs are commercially available; these come in a tube that contains an ampule of **Stuart transport medium.**[15] After the specimen has been obtained, the swab is returned to the tube and the transport medium is squeezed out of the ampule to prevent drying of the swab and to maintain the status quo of the bacterial population.

At the time of culturing the swab is twirled in the desired broth and then rubbed on the desired solid medium with a rotating motion. After inoculation the broth is rolled between the palms of both hands to distribute the material evenly so that levels of subsequent growth may be meaningful (aerobic vs. anaerobic bacteria). Because the amount of material on most swabs is small, smears are made last.

Transport media

If swabs cannot be cultured immediately, they should be placed in transport media. Some organisms, e.g., *Bordetella pertussis, Shigella* species, and *Neisseria*

gonorrhoeae, survive poorly over a period of several hours on dry swabs. They survive for 24 hr or longer in Stuart transport medium,[15] which is a semisolid nonnutrient agar gel that prevents oxidation and enzymatic changes of bacteria, thus preserving the original bacterial flora. The medium should be used with calcium alginate–tipped swabs. For stool specimens **Amies** (Difco Laboratories, Detroit)[16] and **Cary-Blair** (BBL, BioQuest Div., Becton-Dickinson & Co., Cockeysville, Md.)[17] **transport media** are suggested.

Several transport media are available for material to be processed anaerobically. The use of these should be actively encouraged. Aspiration material delivered in a syringe can be protected from oxygen if the residual air is expelled from the syringe and the needle capped with a rubber Vacutainer (BBL, BioQuest Div., Becton-Dickinson & Co., Cockeysville, Md.) stopper.

EXAMINATION OF BACTERIOLOGIC MATERIAL
Macroscopic examination

It is wise to quickly scan the specimen to ascertain whether it really is what it is labeled to be, e.g., sputum rather than saliva, and to locate the best area to culture, e.g., purulent hemorrhagic particles. Actinomycotic granules may also be discovered.

Motility

Hanging drop method: Prepare a saline suspension of young culture and place 1 drop in center of a coverslip that is inverted over the well in a depression slide. Examine for motility, as evidenced by the organisms moving away from each other. Brownian movement, which is not an expression of motility, is a constant to-and-fro movement. Examine with bright-field or darkfield microscope.

Semisolid motility medium technic: Motility is evidenced by growth away from the line of inoculation. Nonmotile organisms grow only along the line of inoculation. The motility medium technic is the method of choice to evaluate motility (Fig. 32-3).

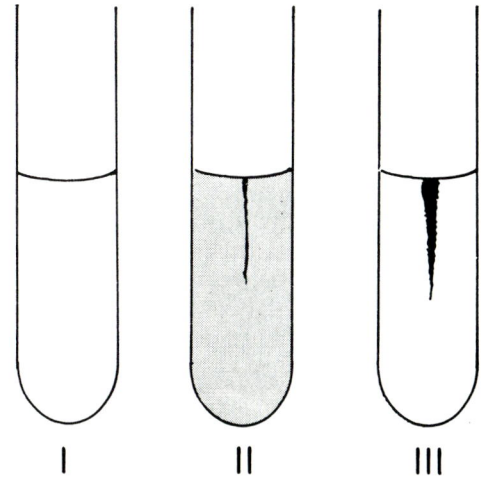

Fig. 32-3. Motility test. **I,** Uninoculated tube. **II,** Motile organism. **III,** Nonmotile organism.

Wet preparation

Wet mounts are prepared for examination for fungi and for darkfield microscopy.

Microscopic examination
Smears

Direct, gram-stained smears are prepared before culture as a check on the culture results and as a guide to the selection of culture media. Any discrepancy between smear and culture must be investigated. The direct smear (smear of original material before culture) gives some indication of the type of bacteria (gram positive or negative, cocci or rods, etc.) present, their quantity, and the predominance of one organism. The gram-stained smear of a culture may confirm purity. Smears are also helpful in the diagnosis of tuberculosis (Kinyoun stain) and diphtheria (Albert stain).

Prepare the **smear** as follows: With forceps, remove a clean slide that has been stored in 70% ethyl alcohol and flame. Identify the slide, and if several preparations need to be made, divide into sections with wax pencil. Then draw a key to the slide on a 3 × 4 in. card, indicating which cultures are in which spaces. Using a flame-sterilized loop, transfer a loopful of well-shaken liquid medium or emulsify a segment of colony on solid medium in a loopful of sterile water. Spread over an area of about 1 cm. Make heavy smears of broth cultures and thin smears of emulsified colonies taken from solid media. Allow to air dry and fix by passing the slide quickly through the top of a Bunsen flame. Allow to cool and then stain. The stained preparation should be examined for size and shape, arrangement and grouping of bacteria (e.g., singly, in clusters, or in pairs), special morphologic features such as spores and capsules, and Gram stain reaction.

STAINING METHODS
Gram staining method

Cultures 24-48 hr old are used in the differential staining method described by Gram. The gram-staining property may not be characteristic in exudates, pus, or in very young, old, dead, or degenerating cultures. It is also not dependable when the organisms have been grown on sugar media. Acids in media or staining solutions interfere with the Gram stain.

Reagents:
1. Hucker crystal violet
   a. Solution A: crystal violet, 2 g, and ethyl alcohol, 95%, 20 ml
   b. Solution B: ammonium oxalate, 0.8 g, and distilled water, 80 ml
   Mix solutions A and B and allow to mature for 24 hr.
2. Burke iodine
   a. Potassium iodide, 2 g
   b. Iodine crystals, 1 g
   c. Distilled water, 1 dl
   Grind iodine crystals and potassium iodide together in a mortar with a pestle, adding only a little water. The iodine is readily soluble in strong potassium iodide solution. As soon as the iodine is dissolved, add the balance of water and mix thoroughly.

3. Hucker counterstain
   a. Solution A: safranin O, 2.5 g, and ethyl alcohol (95%), 1 dl
   b. Solution B: solution A, 10 ml, and distilled water, 1 dl
4. Mixture of acetone and 95% alcohol, equal parts
Procedure: Make a thin smear, dry in air, and fix in flame. Apply crystal violet for 1 min. Wash and apply iodine solution for about 1 min. Wash and decolorize with 50:50 mixture of 95% alcohol and acetone until no further violet washes off. Wash and counterstain with solution B for about 30 sec. Wash with water and dry by blotting.

Procedure for feces: Fat interferes with the stain and must be removed. Make smear and let dry. Fix with methyl alcohol for 5 min. Wash with xylene and dry. Apply the gram stain as usual.

Results: **Gram-positive** organisms stain dark blue. They retain the violet stain with the iodine acting as mordant. **Gram-negative** organisms stain red. They are decolorized and restained by the red counterstain.

The stain is satisfactory if pus cell nuclei stain deeply with the counterstain and if control spots of gram-negative and gram-positive bacteria stain correctly. Use carbolfuchsin as the counterstain when searching for small gram-negative organisms such as *Bordetella pertussis, Haemophilus influenzae,* or Koch-Weeks bacilli.

Albert stain

Albert stain is used for detection of diphtheria bacilli.

Reagents:
1. Solution 1
   Dissolve 0.15 g toluidine blue and 0.2 malachite green in 2 ml of 95% ethyl alcohol and then add 1 dl distilled water and 1 ml glacial acetic acid. Mix well, let stand for 24 hr, and filter.
2. Solution 2
   Grind 2 g iodine crystals and 3 g potassium iodide in about 10 ml distilled water and then add 2% ml distilled water. The usual Gram iodine solution may be substituted for solution 2.
Procedure: Allow smear to dry and fix with heat. Stain with solution 1 for 2 min. Rinse with water and blot dry. Apply solution 2 for 1 min. Rinse with water, blot dry, and examine.

Results: The granules of diphtheria bacilli stain black; the cytoplasm stains light green.

Capsule stain

The following is the capsule stain method of Howie and Kirkpatrick.

Reagents:
1. Water-soluble eosin, 1 g
2. Serum (any), 25 ml
3. Water, 1 dl
4. Thymol, 1 crystal
   Allow mixture to stand 3 days, centrifuge, and harvest supernatant.
5. Ziehl-Neelsen carbolfuchsin stain diluted 1:5
Procedure: Mix 1 drop broth culture with 1 drop carbolfuchsin and allow to stand 30 sec. Add 1 drop eosin and allow to stand 1 min. Spread out the prepa-

ration as for blood film, air dry, and examine with oil-immersion lens.

The background and bacterial cells will stain deep red. Capsules, if present, will stain lightly or not at all, leaving a light halo around bacteria.

Kinyoun acid-fast stain for mycobacteria

The Kinyoun acid-fast stain is used for the detection of mycobacteria, which are surrounded by a waxy envelope that is resistant to staining, but which, once stained, retains the stain, whereas other bacteria are decolorized by acid alcohol and accept the blue counterstain. Acid-fast bacilli are stained red.

Reagents:
1. Carbolfuchsin-Kinyoun
   a. Basic fuchsin, 4 g
   b. Phenol crystals, 8 g
   c. Alcohol, 95%, 20 ml
   d. Water, 1 dl
   Dissolve fuchsin in alcohol and add to phenol crystals that have been melted in a hot water bath; then add the water. To increase the rapidity of staining, add a detergent (Tergitol no. 7 or Aerosol), 1 drop for each 30-40 ml stain. Since the rapid staining property is lost after a few days, the detergent must be renewed accordingly.
2. Acid alcohol
   a. Ethyl alcohol, 95%, 97 ml
   b. Concentrated hydrochloric acid, 3 ml
   Add the acid to the alcohol.

Procedure: Fix the dried smear with heat. Stain with carbolfuchsin for 5 min. Wash and decolorize with acid alcohol. Wash well and counterstain 1 min with 1% methylene blue or 1% malachite green.

Results: Acid-fast bacteria are red against blue or green background.

Ziehl-Neelsen staining method for acid-fast organisms

Reagents:
1. Carbolfuchsin (mordant and dye)
   a. Saturated solution of basic fuchsin (10 g basic fuchsin in 1 dl 95% ethyl alcohol), 10 ml
   b. Aqueous solution of crystalline phenol, 5%, 90 ml
2. Acid alcohol (decolorizing agent)
   a. Concentrated hydrochloric acid, 3 ml
   b. Ethyl alcohol, 95%, 97 ml
3. Counterstain
   a. Methylene blue, 0.3 g
   b. Distilled water, 1 dl

Procedure: Fix the smear by heating on a slide warmer for 2 hr at 65° C or overnight at room temperature. Place a piece of filter paper (cut slightly smaller than the slide) over the smear. Cover smear with carbolfuchsin. Steam for 5 min. **Do not boil and do not allow slide to dry.** (If an electric staining rack is used, allow up to 15 min.) Wash with distilled water. Decolorize with acid alcohol for 2 min. Wash with distilled water. Counterstain with methylene blue for 30-60 sec. Wash in distilled water, dry, and examine.

Results: Mycobacteria stain red against a blue background (Plate 15, below).

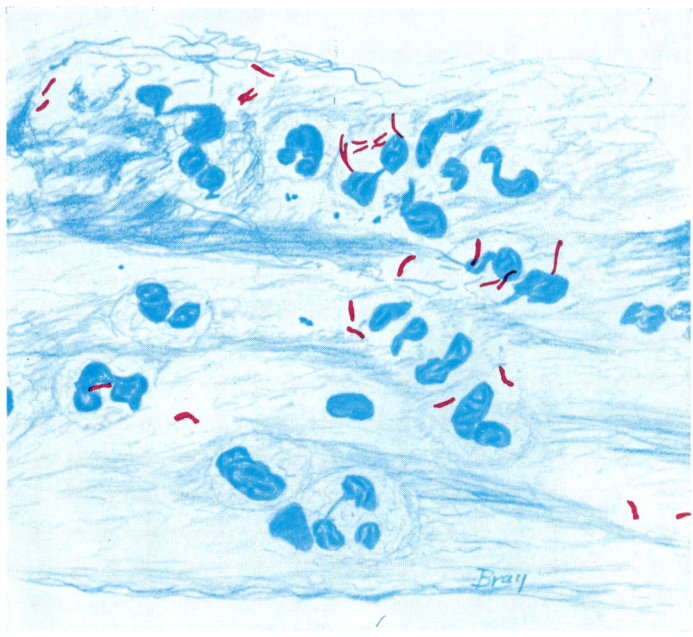

Plate 15. Tubercle bacilli in sputum. (Acid-fast stain.)

Fluorescent dye method for acid-fast organisms
Truant fluorescent dye[18]

Reagents:
1. Stain
   a. Auramine, 1.5 g
   b. Rhodamine, 0.75 g
   c. Glycerol, 75 ml
   d. Phenol, 10 ml
   e. Distilled water, 50 ml
   Filter through glass wool to clarify. Solutions keep several months at 4° C or at room temperature. Store in dark bottle.
2. Decolorant solution (acid alcohol): hydrochloric acid (0.5%) in ethanol (70%)
3. Counterstain (potassium permanganate): 0.5 g potassium permanganate in 1 dl distilled water
   Store in dark bottle.

Procedure: Prepare smear using new slides. Fix smears by heating on slide warmer for 2 hr at 65° C or overnight at room temperature. Cover smear with auramine-rhodamine dye. Stain for 15 min at room temperature or at 37° C. Rinse off stain with distilled water. Decolorize for 2-3 min with acid alcohol. Wash with distilled water. Flood smear for 2-4 min with 0.5% potassium permanganate. Rinse, dry, and examine.

Confirm all positive smears by restaining the original smear using one of the acid-fast methods.

Results: The reagent is a fluorescent dye that stains mycobacteria selectively. No antigen-antibody reaction is involved in this procedure.

The fluorescent dye method allows rapid scanning of smears magnified 100 times. Positive smears can be confirmed by overstaining with acid-fast stain. Patients receiving drug therapy may discharge organisms that stain by fluorescent methods but not by the conventional acid-fast stains.

Loeffler methylene blue stain

The Loeffler methylene blue stain is used for the identification of diphtheria bacilli since it differentiates the deeply staining metachromatic granules from the pale blue-staining cytoplasm. This stain is also an excellent stain for bacterial morphology and may demonstrate bacteria in spinal fluid preparations that are negative by Gram's method.

Reagents:
1. Methylene blue, certified, 0.3 g
2. Ethyl alcohol, 95%, 30 ml
3. Distilled water, 1 dl
Dissolve stain completely before adding water.

Procedure: Apply the stain for 1 min to the heat-fixed smear. Wash and blot dry.

Results: See above.

Fluorescent antibody technic[19]

Fluorescein-labeled antibodies are potentially applicable to the detection of all bacteria. The fluorescent technic allows the detection and localization of organisms or substances because of their ability to fluoresce under certain conditions. Fluorescence is the property of converting invisible light rays of short wavelengths into visible rays of longer wavelengths. The fluorescence may be primary (natural) or secondary (only after treatment with certain dyes). The light source is usually a high-pressure mercury arc lamp. The microscope is equipped with a darkfield condenser and with filters that determine the wavelengths and color mixture of the light. Between the lamp and the object is the primary or exciter filter, which allows only the fluorescence-exciting waves of the light source to reach the stained object. Between the object and the eye of the observer there is placed the secondary or excluding filter, so that the eye is protected and only the light characteristic of the fluorescent dye in use is seen. Nonfluorescing oil is applied to the undersurface of the slide beneath the area of the specimen and also to the surface of the specimen.

The following fluorescent methods are given in detail in the appropriate sections: identification of group A streptococci, *Neisseria gonorrhoeae*, enteropathogenic *Escherichia coli,* and rabies virus.

Spore stain (Wirtz-Conklin)

Reagents:
1. Malachite green, 5 g, and water, 1 dl
2. Safranin, 0.5 g, and water, 1 dl

Procedure: Prepare slide, heat, and fix. Cover with malachite green. Steam over burner for 5 min. Wash and counterstain with safranin for 30 sec.

Results: The negative cell will stain red. Spores, if present, will remain green. Spores may be intracellular or free of cell debris.

Wayson stain for bipolar staining

Reagent:
1. Solution A: basic fuchsin, 0.2 g, methylene blue, 0.75 g, and absolute ethyl alcohol, 20.9 ml
2. Solution B: 5% phenol in water, 2 dl

Procedure: Add solution A to solution B. Stain for a few seconds, wash, and dry.

Results: The polar bodies stain dark blue, and the remainder of the cell stains light blue to reddish.

Hanging drop method

Prepare a saline suspension of young culture and place 1 drop in the center of a coverslip that is inverted over the depression in a well slide. Examine for motility, as evidenced by the organisms moving away from each other. Motility is best seen at lower temperatures: 15-5° C. Brownian movement, which is not an expression of motility, is a constant to-and-fro movement. Examine with bright-field or darkfield microscope.

Semisolid motility medium technic

Motility is evidenced by growth away from the line of inoculation. Nonmotile organisms grow only along the line of inoculation. The motility medium technic is the method of choice to evaluate motility (Fig. 32-3).

Wet preparation

Wet mounts are prepared for examination for fungi and for darkfield microscopy.

SELECTION OF MEDIA

Most media are available in dry powder form or as already prepared culture media. For details, consult catalogs such as the BBL *Manual of Products and Laboratory Procedures* and Difco's *Supplementary Literature.* They list many kinds of culture media for various purposes. No laboratory ever employs all these media, but each laboratory uses certain combinations, which are mentioned in the discussion of the various organisms and their isolation.

Primary culture media

Primary culture media are used for the immediate culture of clinical material, since they support the growth of most organisms. They include blood agar (for aerobic and anaerobic incubation), brain-heart infusion agar, brain-heart infusion broth, chocolate agar, and thioglycollate broth.

Differential media

Differential media contain a substance and often an indicator system that indicate utilization or nonutilization of the substance by bacteria, allowing a presumptive identification of bacterial species. Blood agar, which contains 5-10% sterile defibrinated sheep blood, is not only an excellent primary medium but also substitutes as a differential medium because it can detect types of hemolysis. The most widely used differential media contain carbohydrate and a pH indicator to distinguish carbohydrate fermenters from nonfermenters.

MacConkey agar prevents *Proteus* from spreading. *Salmonella, Shigella, Escherichia coli,* and most members of the Enterobacteriaceae family grow well on this medium. *Salmonella* and *Shigella* (SS) agar, xylose-lysine-deoxycholate (XLD) agar, Hektoen agar, and deoxycholate-citrate agar also suppress *Escherichia coli* and other coliform bacteria but allow *Salmonella* and *Shigella* to grow.

Selective media

Selective media, while supporting the growth of some bacteria, contain inhibitors that suppress the growth of other organisms. Among these inhibitor substances (dyes, chemicals, etc.) are phenylethyl alcohol and chloral hydrate; dyes such as crystal violet, brilliant green, and basic fuchsin; and substances such as sodium deoxycholate and potassium tellurite. Some selective media contain antibiotics such as colistin and nalidixic acid. Strains isolated on inhibitory media must be checked carefully for purity and should be transferred by touching the dome of a colony only, since the base may contain suppressed contaminants. *Neisseria gonorrhoeae* and *Neisseria meningitidis* grow well on a modified Thayer-Martin medium. This selective agar medium is incorporated into plates, bottles (Transgrow), or small plastic rectangular dishes and functions also as an effective transport medium. *Haemophilus influenzae* requires both $NADH_2$ (V factor) and hemin (X factor) for growth. These cofactors may be found in chocolate agar, impregnated disks, or a culture of *Staphylococcus aureus* streaked on sheep blood agar.

Special media

Some organisms require special media, e.g., Lowenstein-Jensen medium, 7H-10 agar medium, and 7H-9 broth medium for *Mycobacterium tuberculosis,* Fletcher medium for *Leptospira,* and W medium for *Brucella.* Bordet-Gengou agar base enriched with 20% blood is recommended for the isolation of *Bordetella pertussis.* Selective media for clostridia contain neomycin and sodium azide. Mannitol salt agar is a selective medium for staphylococci. For fungi, selective media are Sabouraud dextrose agar and media containing cycloheximide and chloramphenicol. Some special media identify enzymes that are characteristic for certain bacteria. Such enzymes include urease *(Proteus),* lysine decarboxylase *(Arizona),* carbohydrases (enteric gram-negative rods), and deoxyribonuclease (staphylococci).

Enrichment media

Additional nutriments in some media selectively support the growth of certain organisms; e.g., selenite broth, GN broth, and tetrathionate broth stimulate the growth of *Salmonella* and suppress other gram-negative bacteria.

Inoculation of media

All specimens should be cultured as soon as possible on suitable primary isolation media, the choice of which depends on (1) the nature (origin) of the specimen, (2) the result of a Gram stain, and (3) the physician's request, e.g., for fungal culture. At least one liquid medium, e.g., thioglycollate broth, and one nonselective plating medium, e.g., blood agar, should be employed. All media must be at room temperature or at 37° C before they are inoculated.

Inoculation of liquid media

If the inoculum is liquid, use a sterile Pasteur pipet for inoculation, although a loop may also be employed. In general, liquid media are used to (1) foster the growth of a small number of bacteria, (2) dilute antibacterial agents in the specimen (antibiotics, antibodies, etc.), and (3) depending on the choice of the liquid medium, stimulate the growth of certain bacteria (e.g., anaerobes in thioglycollate broth).

Hold all tubes almost horizontally. Loosen cap (or cotton plug) and hold between fingers to avoid contamination. Sterilize loop by heating it until it is red hot; allow it to cool, obtain inoculum, and transfer it into liquid. It is important to flame the entire length of the loop before inoculation of a liquid medium. Replace cap or cotton and mix by tapping on tube.

Incubate liquid medium at 35-37° C under 3-5% CO_2 until growth occurs. Check for growth every 12 hr with Gram stain. If growth occurs, subculture to solid medium. If no growth occurs after 1 week, the medium may be discarded and "no growth" should be reported.

Liquid media are examined for turbidity, sediment, arrangement of colonies (floating, floccules, chains, etc.), pellicle formation, color development, and gas and odor production.

Inoculation of solid media

Four technics are used for inoculation of solid media: (1) streak plate, (2) pour plate, (3) streak-pour plate, and (4) slant.

Streak plate: The purpose of the streak plate (Fig. 32-4) is to isolate organisms in pure culture. Collect specimen in sterile (flamed) loop that is slightly bent so that it will glide smoothly over the surface of the medium. Deposit inoculum at one edge and streak back and forth over the area, progressing across the agar until one fourth of the plate surface is covered. Flame the loop, streak at right angles to the originally inoculated agar, and cover the second quarter of the plate. Flame loop again and repeat procedure until third and fourth quadrants are covered. Instead of flaming the loop, which is time consuming, two loops may be used alternately or the loop may be used to cut deeply twice into the agar before progressing from one quadrant to the next. Whichever method is used, a small area of the agar should be undercut with the loop to streak the undersurface of the agar. Turn plate upside down to prevent contamination by water condensation. Incubate at 35-37° C under 3-5% CO_2. Examine for growth every 12 hr. Keep medium for 1 week before reporting "no growth."

Examine solid media for size, shape, color, outline, and consistency of colonies, changes in the medium, and odor.

Aerosol contamination of the plates must be minimized by holding the plates vertically when streaking. If the medium is accidentally cut into with the streaking loop, interrupt the streak and start anew, using material from the starting area.

For subculture and bacterial identification choose well-isolated colonies only. Prepare a Gram stain of each morphologically different colony and subculture to a suitable differential medium. Touch only the dome of the center of a colony with the end of a straight wire (after flaming and cooling) and transfer the inoculum to a suitable differential medium (see below). If colonies are not adequately isolated after overnight incubation, transfer a small amount of the entire growth with a loop to a second nonselective plate. Streak out the inoculum to obtain adequate isolation of colonies.

Pour plate: The pour plate is used to determine the approximate number of viable organisms in a liquid medium. They are reported as number of colonies per milliliter of inoculum. Blood agar pour plates are also excellent for determining the type of hemolysis produced by streptococci.

Melt a tube of 10 ml agar in water bath, cool to 45° C, and inoculate tubes with measured volume of suitably diluted inoculum. Pour inoculated agar into sterile Petri dish. Distribute evenly by tilting plate and cool, leaving the top half of the Petri dish partially open for a few minutes to allow vapor to escape. Incubate plate at 35-37° C and increase CO_2 tension to 3-5%.

Streak-pour plate: Streak a blood agar plate as described for a streak plate and cover streaked surface with melted blood agar. This is a good method for studying hemolysis.

Slant: Slants are tubes containing media gelled in such a way that the upper surface is slanted. Handle and hold slant as described for liquid media. Heat entire length of inoculating loop until red hot and allow to cool inside the tube holding the inoculum. Pick up inoculum with loop and transfer the material to the bottom of the slant, which is inoculated by zig-zagging across the entire surface toward the mouth of the tube. Flame mouth of tube and replace cap or cotton plug.

If the slant consists of a butt and a slanted portion, handle as above but inoculate the butt first by stabbing the needle to the bottom of the medium and then streak the surface.

Incubation
Aerobic cultures

All aerobic cultures should be incubated at 35-37° C under 3-5% CO_2 tension, since most organisms grow better when the CO_2 tension is slightly increased. Some organisms require increased CO_2 tension for their growth in culture, e.g., *Haemophilus influenzae*, *Brucella abortus*, and *Neisseria gonorrhoeae*.

Cultures under increased carbon dioxide tension

If a CO_2 incubator is not available, a candle jar or Gaspak with CO_2 generator may be used.

Candle jar: Place the culture plates and tubes into a large-mouthed jar with a well-fitting ground-glass lid or any other well-fitting top. Pull one of the Petri dishes close to the top of the stack about halfway out and place on it a medicine glass containing a short, thick candle. The candle should be in the upper half of the jar rather than on the bottom. Light candle. Close jar airtight, using Plasticine if necessary. The candle flame will die when the atmosphere contains 2-3% CO_2, which accumulates at the bottom. Do not move jar until flame dies, since the movement may extinguish the flame.

Gaspak with carbon dioxide generator: The candle jar has certain disadvantages. The CO_2 tension is about 2%, while the ideal level is from 5-10%, and a small amount of carbon monoxide is generated by the flame, which may be injurious to some organisms. The Gaspak jar used for anaerobic cultures can be coupled with

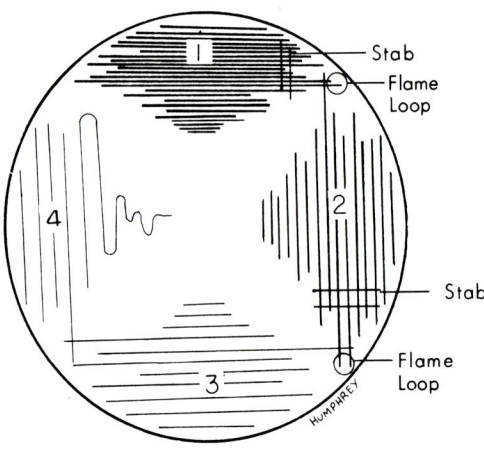

Fig. 32-4. Method of streaking agar plates for isolation.

a commercially available CO_2 generator (BBL, Bio-Quest Div., Becton-Dickinson & Co., Cockeysville, Md.) to provide a 5% CO_2 atmosphere and obviate the disadvantages of the CO_2 jar.[20]

Anaerobic cultures

Oxygen requirements of bacteria: Aerobes grow in the normal atmosphere. Microaerophils require reduced O_2 tension. Anaerobes require a relative or absolute absence of O_2. Obligate anaerobes require the complete absence of O_2, whereas facultative organisms grow either anaerobically or aerobically.

The recommended methods of anaerobic culture are the use of thioglycollate broth and simultaneous cultivation of specimens in an anaerobic jar using prereduced media.

Thioglycollate broth: Thioglycollate broth contains a reducing agent, sodium thioglycollate (0.3-0.5%), and methylene blue as an indicator of degree of oxidation. Thioglycollate broth is stored at room temperature in the dark, since, at refrigerator temperature, it absorbs more O_2. Oxidation of the medium, which starts on the surface, is seen by a blue-green color change. If the color change involves 20% of the column, the medium should be boiled not more than once, cooled, and used. Repeated boiling destroys the medium. Tubes boiled and not used must be discarded.

Gaspak anaerobic jar[20]: In the Gaspak anaerobic jar (BBL, BioQuest Div., Becton-Dickinson & Co., Cockeysville, Md.) a Pyrex glass jar is fitted tightly with a lid that carries a small basket in which a catalyst is housed; the catalyst is active at room temperature and consists of aluminum pellets coated with palladium. The system uses a disposable hydrogen and CO_2 generator that is activated by adding water. A disposable methylene blue indicator of anaerobiosis (it turns blue if O_2 is present) must be included whenever the jar is used (Fig. 32-5).

Use of prereduced media: See discussion of antibiotic susceptibility testing of anaerobic bacteria.

Newer anaerobic methods:

Roll tube technic: Commercially available rubber-stoppered prereduced media are inoculated with material collected by means of sterile syringe and needle, keeping free air space to a minimum. Transfers are made under a stream of sterile inert gas (N_2, CO_2, and H_2) to isolate organisms. They are transferred under exclusion of oxygen into roll tubes that have prereduced media solidified on their walls.[21]

Glove box procedure: The anaerobic glove box[22] is made of clear plastic and heated to 37° C. The atmosphere is a mixture of CO_2, H_2, and N_2 and is closely monitored for free oxygen. The bacteria are identified by differential tests using special prereduced media and also by gas-liquid chromatography.

The two methods mentioned above have been compared to the Gaspak method.[23]

Reports

Save material and cultures from which transfers are made until satisfactory growth is obtained and the final diagnosis is made.

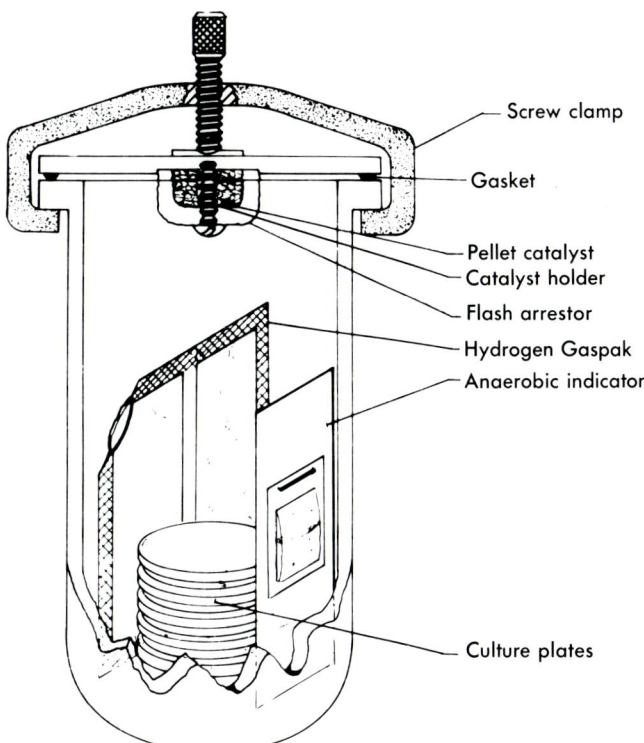

Fig. 32-5. Schematic cutaway view of cold-catalyst anaerobic jar (Brewer type) using Gaspak hydrogen and CO_2 generator. (Courtesy BBL, BioQuest Div., Becton-Dickinson & Co., Cockeysville, Md.)

Some cultures must be held for several weeks before the final report is made, e.g., blood cultures for 3 weeks, cultures for *Brucella* and tubercle bacilli for 4 weeks, and cultures for *Listeria monocytogenes* for 4 months.

Reports should be issued as soon as clinically significant data are obtained. The report of the Gram stain must be issued the same day the specimen is received. Interim reports will assure the physician that the laboratory is still working on his case.

MEDIA AND PROCEDURES

Some media and procedures used in microbiology are as follows:

Alkaline peptone water medium
Blood agar
Bordet-Gengou medium
Brain-heart infusion (BHI) agar
Carbohydrate fermentation medium (bromcresol purple)
Chapman stone agar
Chocolate (heated blood) agar
Cystine trypticase agar (semisolid)
Cytochrome oxidase (*p*-aminodimethylaniline oxalate) test
Decarboxylase test
Ehrlich reagent (see indole test)
Fletcher medium
FLO agar
Gelatin liquefaction
Gluconate oxidation test
GN broth
Indicators used in bacteriology
Indole production test
KCN (potassium cyanide) broth
Kovac reagent (see indole test)
Loeffler medium
Lowenstein-Jensen (L-J) medium (Gruft modification)
MacConkey agar
Malonate broth
Mannitol salt agar
Methyl red (MR) test
Methylene blue reductase medium
Middlebrook-Cohn 7H-11 agar
Motility agar
Mueller-Hinton agar or broth
Mycoplasma (PPLO) agar
Mycoplasma (PPLO) broth
Nitrate reduction test
O-F (oxidation-fermentation) medium
ONPG test (β-D-galactosidase)
Oxidase test
Phenylalanine agar
Phenylethyl alcohol agar
Salmonella-Shigella (SS) agar
Selenite F broth
Sellers agar
SIM medium
Simmons citrate agar (citrate utilization)
Stuart transport medium
TCBS agar
Thayer-Martin medium
Thioglycollate broth
Thiol broth
Tinsdale medium
Transfrow medium
Triple sugar iron (TSI) agar
Trypticase soy agar and broth
Tween-albumin (Dubos) broth

Urea agar–Christensen (urease) test
Voges-Proskauer (VP) test
XLD (xylose-lysine-deoxycholate) agar

All media except thioglycollate broth should be stored in the refrigerator. Plates should be stacked with the agar surface up so that the water of condensation does not drip onto the agar surface. The number of media stored should not exceed a 2-3 week supply. All media must be checked for sterility and specificity before use. (See quality control in bacteriology, p. 15.) Almost all media mentioned in this section are commercially available as powder or as prepared media (Difco Laboratories, Detroit; BBL, BioQuest Div., Becton-Dickinson & Co., Cockeysville, Md.). If not available, the formula is given.

Alkaline peptone water medium

Alkaline peptone water medium supports the growth of *Vibrio*.
Peptone, 10 g
Sodium chloride, 5 g
Distilled water, 10 dl
Adjust to pH 8.4-8.5 with 1N NaOH. Dispense in 10 ml tubes. Autoclave at 121° C for 15 min.

Blood agar

Blood agar is the most commonly used nonselective medium, since it supports the growth of a wide range of bacteria. It consists of trypticase soy agar and 5-10% sterile defibrinated sheep blood for enrichment. Sheep blood is preferred for the study of hemolysis (see discussion of streptococcal hemolysis.) Blood bank blood (human) should be avoided because of the adverse effect of possible antibiotics, antibodies, and anticoagulants. The agar layer should not exceed a 3-4 mm thickness. The plates may be incubated aerobically, anaerobically, or under increased CO_2 tension.

Bordet-Gengou medium

A potato glycerin agar, the Bordet-Gengou medium contains 20% fresh blood (human, horse, sheep, etc.). The addition of 0.5 unit penicillin/ml just before pouring is advisable. The medium is used for culture of *Bordetella pertussis* and *B. parapertussis*.

Brain-heart infusion agar

Brain-heart infusion (BHI) agar is a suitable medium for many types of pathogenic bacteria. With the addition of blood, it supports *Histoplasma capsulatum;* with the addition of antibiotics, it can be used for the isolation of fungi from materials with mixed flora. The medium should not be used to study hemolysis.

Carbohydrate fermentation medium (bromcresol purple)

The carbohydrate fermentation medium is a liquid or semisolid meat extract broth to which an indicator and a carbohydrate are added. The most commonly used carbohydrates are glucose, lactose, sucrose, and mannitol. Carbohydrate tablets may also be used.
Principle: Organisms that ferment the carbohydrate added to the broth produce acid, thus changing the in-

dicator color to yellow. When the carbohydrate is not fermented but growth is observed, the indicator remains purple.

Inoculation: Inoculate the broth lightly. Using sterile technic, add commercially prepared filter paper tabs that are impregnated with the appropriate carbohydrates. Incubate overnight.

Reaction: The pH indicator used is bromcresol purple; its range is 5.2 (yellow) to 6.8 (purple). Record the reaction after overnight incubation. Yellow indicates positive (fermentation); purple (must be turbid, indicating growth) signifies negative (no fermentation).

Chapman stone agar

Because of its high salt content, Chapman stone agar is a selective medium suppressing most organisms except *Staphylococcus aureus,* which produces pigmented colonies surrounded by a clear zone (gelatinase activity). The medium contains mannitol, the fermentation of which can be detected by dropping 1 drop bromcresol purple on the agar surface from which colonies have been removed. The yellow color indicates fermentation (acid pH).

Chocolate agar

Chocolate (heated blood) agar is made by enriching proteose agar (rich in the peptones, minerals, etc. necessary for growth of pathogenic bacteria) with hemoglobin (factor X) and yeast extract (factor V). The resultant medium is suitable for culture of fastidious organisms such as *Neisseria gonorrhoeae, Neisseria meningitidis,* and *Haemophilus influenzae.*

Cystine trypticase agar (semisolid)

Cystine trypticase medium supports most fastidious organisms (see discussion of trypticase soy agar below) and can be used as a motility agar and for the study of fermentation reactions of *Neisseria.*

Carbohydrates may be added in the form of disks (sterile forceps). Only the surface of the medium is inoculated. Phenol red is the indicator, which turns yellow in response to fermentation of carbohydrates. If fermentation does not occur, the pH is alkaline in response to the growth of bacteria and the indicator color remains red.

Cytochrome oxidase (*p*-aminodimethylaniline oxalate) test

Reagent:
1. α-Naphthol, 1%, in ethyl alcohol, 96%
2. Aqueous solution of *p*-aminodimethylaniline hydrochloride or oxalate, 1%

Mix equal volumes by gently tapping.

Procedure: Ewing and Johnson suggest the following procedure: Spread 2-3 drops of reagent over an 18 hr culture.

Results: Within 30 sec (time is critical) *Pseudomonas* colonies take on a blue color. *Alcaligenes* and *Aeromonas* may also be positive.

One drop of reagent may also be applied to filter paper. One colony is rubbed into the reagent spot, and if the organism is *Pseudomonas,* an immediate blue color develops.

Decarboxylase test

Principle: The basic decarboxylase medium is a glucose broth to which the various amino acids and an indicator are added. The purpose of this test is to detect the presence of enzymes (decarboxylases and dihydrolases) that break down specific amino acids.

All of the gram-negative bacilli of the Enterobacteriaceae group ferment glucose with resultant production of acid; thus all of these organisms will produce a yellow color in the glucose broth used for the decarboxylase tests when no amino acid is added to the broth; such a tube would serve as a control. If the organism is producing an enzyme that decarboxylates a specific amino acid in the medium, the products of such enzymatic action are alkaline, thus changing the color of the broth to purple.

Inoculation: Inoculate each of four tubes (lysine, arginine, ornithine, and control) lightly and then overlay the broth with $1/4$ in. of sterile mineral oil. Without the addition of the oil, the reactions are invalid after 24 hr of incubation. Incubate up to 4 days.

Reactions: Acid reaction is yellow; alkaline reaction is purple. Always read the control tube first. If it is not yellow, disregard all reactions in the set of tubes.

Purple color in the amino acid tube indicates a positive test. Make sure that these tubes have growth in them, since uninoculated broth is purple also. Yellow color indicates a negative reaction.

The decarboxylase reactions of Enterobacteriaceae are given in Table 32-18. The reactions of *Pseudomonas, Alcaligenes,* and *Flavobacterium* species are given in Table 32-3.

Fletcher medium

Fletcher medium is a serum-enriched gelatin medium used for isolation, cultivation, and maintenance of *Leptospira* species.

FLO agar

The magnesium sulfate and potassium phosphate contained in FLO agar promote the formation of fluorescein by *Pseudomonas.* Under ultraviolet light, bright greenish yellow colors are seen. Slants are inoculated and incubated at 35° C. They should be kept under observation for 6 days.

Gelatin liquefaction

Gelatin strips (Key Scientific Products, Los Angeles) are used in the rapid test for gelatin liquefaction. A strip is dropped into a test tube containing 1 ml of heavy suspension of the organism being tested and is incubated at 35° C. Liquefaction can often be observed in 30-60 min, appearing first along the surface of the

Table 32-3. Decarboxylase reactions of certain oxidative organisms

Bacteria	Lysine	Arginine	Ornithine
Pseudomonas	−	+	−
Alcaligenes	−	−	−
Flavobacterium sp.	−	−	−

liquid. As the gelatin is removed, the blue color of the supporting base appears. Among the *Proteus* species, *P. morganii* and *P. rettgeri* are unable to liquefy gelatin. Other *Proteus* species and some *Aerobacter* and *Pseudomonas* strains are positive, whereas *Salmonella* and *Shigella* are uniformly negative.

Gluconate oxidation test

See p. 859.

GN broth

Incorporated salts and carbohydrates make GN broth a selective enrichment medium for *Salmonella*, but it also supports the growth of *Shigella* and suppresses all other Enterobacteriaceae, including *Proteus* and *Pseudomonas*. The deoxycholate and citrate contents inhibit the growth of gram-positive organisms. After inoculation the medium should be incubated for not longer than 16 hr at 35° C so that pathogens will not be overgrown by nonpathogens.

Indicators used in bacteriology

See Table 32-4.

Indole production test

Principle: In the presence of oxygen some bacteria are able to split tryptophan into indole and α-aminoproprionic acid. The presence of indole can be proved by the addition of **Ehrlich** or **Kovac reagents** (*p*-dimethylaminobenzaldehyde), which produce a red color soluble in ether, chloroform, and alcohol.

Kovac reagent:
1. *p*-Dimethylaminobenzaldehyde, 5 g
2. Amyl alcohol, 75 ml
3. Concentrated hydrochloric acid, 25 ml

Mix alcohol and aldehyde and heat in water bath at 50° or 60° C until aldehyde is dissolved. Cool and slowly add the hydrochloric acid. Store in stoppered brown bottle in the dark.

Procedure: Add 0.5 ml Kovac reagent to 3 ml of a 2-day-old peptone water culture (must contain tryptophan). Use as controls one uninoculated broth tube, one inoculated with *Escherichia coli*, and one inoculated with *Salmonella typhosa*.

Results: A red color indicates indole positive; no change indicates indole negative.

Salmonella and *Klebsiella* are indole negative, while most *Proteus* species and *Escherichia coli* are indole positive.

Table 32-4. Indicators used in bacteriology

Dye	pH range	Change of color	
		Acid	Alkaline
Bromphenol blue	3.0-4.6	Yellow	Blue
Methyl red	4.2-6.3	Red	Yellow
Bromthymol blue	6.0-7.6	Yellow	Blue
Litmus	4.5-8.3	Red	Blue
Cresol red	7.2-8.8	Yellow	Red
Phenol red	6.8-8.4	Yellow	Red
Bromcresol purple	5.2-6.8	Yellow	Purple

KCN broth

Media containing KCN (potassium cyanide) permit differential growth of some members of the Enterobacteriaceae family. *Escherichia coli, Salmonella,* and *Shigella* are inhibited in the medium, while *Klebsiella, Citrobacter,* and *Proteus* grow freely. The media must be stored in the refrigerator in tightly capped tubes for not longer than 2 weeks.

Inoculate the media very lightly with a straight wire and stopper tubes quickly. Incubate for 48 hr at 35° C or until growth is observed.

Results: Cloudy growth at any time up to 48 hr after inoculation constitutes a positive reaction. No growth or minimal growth after 48 hr incubation is considered a negative reaction.

Control cultures: Positive: *Klebsiella, Enterobacter,* and *Proteus;* negative: *Escherichia coli.*

Loeffler medium

Loeffler medium is an inspissated serum medium useful for the demonstration of chromogenesis (e.g., *Staphylococcus aureus*) and for the detection of *Corynebacterium*. Cultures should be examined after 24 hr of incubation. The media may also be used to study proteolysis of the coagulated serum, e.g., by enterococci. The white background of the medium is excellent to study color production of bacterial colonies.

Lowenstein-Jensen medium (Gruft modification)

The Lowenstein-Jensen (L-J) medium contains eggs and a partially inhibitory dye, malachite green. Gruft[24, 25] added ribonucleic acid, penicillin, and nalidixic acid. Penicillin inhibits the growth of gram-positive bacteria; nalidixic acid inhibits the growth of gram-negative bacteria. This medium allows the use of a less concentrated sodium hydroxide solution (2% vs. 4%) in the concentration and decontamination procedure. Despite its penicillin content, the medium supports the growth of penicillin-sensitive *Nocardia*. Its primary use is the culture of mycobacteria.

Slants are inoculated and incubated at 35° C, the tubes being kept tightly closed. They should be examined at weekly intervals. The cultures are used to test for light sensitivity and for niacin production.

MacConkey agar

MacConkey agar is used for isolation and differentiation of gram-negative bacilli. It is considered both a selective and a differential medium. It is selective in that it inhibits the growth of gram-positive organisms. This inhibition is due to the presence of bile salts and crystal violet in the medium. It is differential in that gram-negative bacilli that ferment lactose (sometimes referred to as coliform bacilli) produce red colonies and nonlactose fermenters produce colorless colonies. The basis for this differentiation is that the coliforms ferment the lactose, which is the only carbohydrate in the medium. This results in the production of acid in the area of colonial formation. This acid changes the color of the pH indicator included in the medium (neutral red, pH range 6.8 [red] to 8.0 [yellow]) from its unnoticed color to red. The nonlactose fermenters do not ferment the sugar; thus they produce no acid and do not change the color of the indicator.

Malonate broth

Enteric organisms can be differentiated on the basis of their ability to utilize malonate. The broth contains malonate and bromthymol blue as indicator in a slightly acid pH (green color). After inoculation incubate malonate broth at 35° C overnight.

Results: Some bacteria (*Enterobacter, Klebsiella,* and most *Arizona*) utilize malonate as their energy source, rendering the medium alkaline, so that the color of the medium changes from green to blue. *Escherichia, Salmonella,* and *Serratia* are unable to utilize malonate, so that the color of the medium remains green.

Mannitol salt agar

The mannitol salt medium is a selective medium for the isolation of pathogenic (coagulase-positive) staphylococci from contaminated sources such as feces. Collective inhibition of other organisms is obtained by means of a high salt (7.5%) content, which suppresses nonpathogenic cocci. Mannitol fermentation is indicated by phenol red in the medium. The medium is incubated at 35° C under increased (5-10%) CO_2 tension for 36 hr.

Interpretation: At the end of this period, colonies of nonpathogenic cocci are white, small, and surrounded by red or purple zones, whereas the mannitol-fermenting pathogenic organisms are yellow and surrounded by yellow zones. Other bacteria are usually inhibited.

Methyl red test

Principle: The broth used for the methyl red (MR) test is a delicately buffered glucose medium. In this medium a high degree of acidity is produced by some gram-negative bacilli, whereas others produce much less acid or even an alkaline reaction. The methyl red indicator is used to measure the degree of acidity to distinguish between some of these bacteria.

Broth: MR-VP medium (Difco Laboratories, Detroit) (may also be used for Voges-Proskauer reaction).

Indicator: Methyl red, pH range 4.5 (red) to 6.0 (yellow); 0.1 g methyl red in 3 dl 95% (yellow) ethyl alcohol. Dilute to 5 dl with distilled water.

Procedure: Inoculate the broth lightly and incubate overnight.

Results: After overnight incubation, add 2-3 drops MR indicator to the tube and record the immediate reaction: red indicates positive (pH 4.5); yellow indicates negative (pH over 4.5).

Interpretation: MR positive, *Escherichia coli;* MR negative, *Enterobacter aerogenes* and *Klebsiella.* (These organisms may also be used as positive or negative controls.)

Methylene blue reductase medium

The methylene blue reductase medium consists of skimmed milk, tryptone, and methylene blue thiocyanate. It is used to test bacteria for their ability to reduce the blue indicator to its colorless leukobase.

Middlebrook-Cohn 7H-11 agar[26]

Middlebrook-Cohn 7H-11 agar is a synthetic oleic acid–albumin agar for the cultivation, isolation, and sensitivity testing of mycobacteria. The incorporation of casein hydrolysate stimulates the growth of these organisms, so that even drug-resistant strains develop readily. The medium is used in biplates and Felsen plates with or without drugs.

Motility agar

Semisolid agar medium, e.g., SIM agar, is inoculated by stabbing the inoculating needle through the center of the agar to a depth of $1/4$-$1/2$ in. The agar is incubated for 14-24 hr at 35° C.

Results: Motile organisms grow away from the stab down into the medium. Growth only at the inoculation site indicates absence of motility. Reincubation may be necessary for slowly growing organisms.

Mueller-Hinton agar or broth

The Mueller-Hinton medium is specially suited to support the growth of *Neisseria*. In its semisolid form after the addition of a carbohydrate and of a fermentation indicator, the medium is used to monitor carbohydrate utilization by *Neisseria*. The medium is incubated at 35° C under 5-10% CO_2 tension.

Mycoplasma agar

The Mycoplasma (PPLO) medium is a peptone-rich beef heart infusion agar that must be enriched by the addition of horse serum, yeast extract, penicillin, and thallium acetate. It supports the growth of *Mycoplasma*. It is inoculated on the surface, incubated at 35° C under 10% CO_2 tension, and prevented from drying by Mylar bags. It is examined every 24 hr for 21 days. For method of examination and of subculture, see p. 904.

Mycoplasma broth

The Mycoplasma (PPLO) broth medium is a peptone–beef heart infusion enriched by 20% serum, penicillin, thallium acetate, and yeast extract. It is recommended for the cultivation and isolation of *Mycoplasma* species. As the *Mycoplasma* colonies are not visible to the naked eye, the broth must be subcultured after 1-5 days to PPLO agar.

Nitrate reduction test

Pseudomonas rapidly reduce nitrates to nitrites and gaseous nitrogen.

Principle: The reduction of nitrates (NO_3) leads to the formation of nitrites (NO_2) and may progress to liberation of nitrogen (N).

In test 1 below the medium is examined for the presence of nitrites. If none are present, test 2 is performed to discover residual nitrates. If none are found, it can be assumed that the reduction of the nitrates has proceeded beyond the nitrite stage.

Reagents:
1. Sulfanilic acid, 8 g, and acetic acid, 5N*, 10 dl
2. α-Naphthylamine, 5 g, and acetic acid, 5N*, 10 dl

---

*Glacial acetic acid, 290 ml; distilled water to 10 dl.

The reagents listed are commercially available (BBL, BioQuest Div., Becton-Dickinson & Co., Cockeysville, Md.).

Test 1: Inoculate nitrate reduction test broth (must be free of nitrites) with pure culture and incubate at 35° C for 12-24 hr. To 10 ml broth culture, add 0.2 ml sulfanilic acid and 0.2-0.3 ml α-naphthylamine in drops. A red color indicates nitrites. The pH of the medium must be acid. A control test must be performed on the uninoculated broth.

Test 2: Reduce residual nitrate to nitrite with a reducing agent such as zinc dust and repeat the nitrite test. The presence of nitrate can also be proved by the addition of 1 drop diphenylamine H_2SO_4 reagent (1 crystal diphenylamine in 1 drop H_2SO_4). Blue color development indicates nitrates. Pure nitrogen can sometimes be seen as gas bubbles.

Interpretation: Test 1 detects nitrate-positive organisms that reduce nitrate to nitrite but do not go any further; therefore no gas appears. Nitrate-negative organisms fail to reduce nitrate and therefore no red color or gas appears. Test 2 will confirm the presence of unreduced nitrate.

Nitrite-positive organisms reduce nitrate to nitrite and then progress to break down nitrite to liberate ammonia or nitrogen; thus gas bubbles may be seen. If the utilization of nitrate and nitrite is complete, tests 1 and 2 will be negative except for gas formation.

Pseudomonas is nitrate positive; *Achromobacter* is nitrate negative.

Oxidation-fermentation medium

The oxidation-fermentation (O-F) medium distinguishes oxidative acidity from fermentative acidity. It contains added carbohydrates (glucose, lactose, and sucrose—one tube for each) and an indicator of acid production (bromthymol blue).

Two tubes of each carbohydrate are inoculated from young blood agar cultures. Usually the dextrose medium only is used. Stab the medium once with a straight needle, stabbing almost to the bottom of the agar. Cover one tube of each pair with a 5 mm layer of melted petrolatum (preferred to mineral oil). Incubate at 35° C for 48 hr or longer. Record acid or acid and gas production or no change in color (pH), and record motility of organism. Nonmotile organisms grow only along the line of inoculation, whereas motile organisms grow away from the line of inoculation (Table 32-3).

Changes in covered agar are considered to be caused by true fermentation, whereas changes in the open tubes are caused by oxidative utilization of the carbohydrate present. If the carbohydrate is not utilized by either method, there is no acid production in either tube. Comparison with the uninoculated tube should be made.

Carbohydrate oxidizers (e.g., *Pseudomonas* species oxidize dextrose only) produce oxidative acidity on the surface of the medium in the open tube, indicating their oxygen need. In the sealed tube these organisms fail to grow or grow very poorly. Carbohydrate fermenters produce fermentative acidity throughout the medium in the aerobic as well as the anaerobic (sealed) tube. If the carbohydrate is not utilized by either method (fermen-

tative or oxidative), there is no acid production in either tube.

The O-F medium is helpful in the identification of *Pseudomonas, Acinetobacter,* and *Alcaligenes.*

Controls must be set up with each test, utilizing known bacterial cultures.

Oxidation: *Pseudomonas* (oxidizer, nonfermenter)
Fermentation: *Escherichia coli* (fermenter, aerogenic)
Inactive: *Alcaligenes faecalis* (nonoxidizer, nonfermenter)

ONPG test (β-D-galactosidase)[27]:

Principle: Lactose fermentation requires two enzymes: (1) a permease that allows lactose to enter the bacterium and (2) an intracellular enzyme, β-galactosidase, that splits lactose into its molecules, glucose and galactose. Organisms that lack permease, although potentially capable of fermenting lactose, are unable to do so since lactose cannot enter the cell. If these organisms are grown on lactose-containing media, some of the bacteria acquire permease and the colony will exhibit delayed lactose fermentation. The production of the β-galactosidase-permease enzymatic system is fostered by growth on lactose-containing media. The presence of β-galactosidase can be demonstrated by using *o*-nitrophenyl-β-D-galactopyranoside (ONPG), which, when acted on by the galactosidase, produces yellow *o*-nitrophenol.

Procedure: Add 1 ONPG tablet (Key Scientific Products, Los Angeles) to 1 ml distilled water. Suspend entire surface growth of organisms in 1.5-2.0 ml distilled water and use 2 drops of the suspension to inoculate ONPG medium. Incubate at 35° C for 6 hr or less and examine for yellow color, which indicates the presence of β-galactosidase.

Interpretation: Late lactose-fermenting *Escherichia coli, Klebsiella, Citrobacter, Shigella, Yersinia pestis,* etc. are ONPG positive, as are some nonlactose fermenters, e.g., *Vibrio, Aeromonas,* and *Serratia.* The nonlactose fermenters *Salmonella, Proteus,* and *Pseudomonas* are ONPG negative.

The prime indication for the test is the differentiation of *Salmonella* (ONPG negative) from *Citrobacter* and *Arizona* (both ONPG positive).

Oxidase test

Principle: The test detects oxidase-producing bacteria.

Kovacs test: Place a 6 cm² piece of Whatman no. 1 filter paper in a Petri dish and then place 2 or 3 drops 1% solution of tetramethyl-*p*-phenylenediamine dihydrochloride on the center of the paper. The test colony is removed with a platinum loop and streaked onto the reagent-impregnated paper. The colony turns dark purple in 5-10 sec if the reaction is positive. *Pseudomonas* and *Neisseria* are oxidase positive.

Phenylalanine agar

Principle: The *Proteus* and *Providencia* organisms produce an enzyme that breaks down phenylalanine to phenylpyruvic acid. Phenylpyruvic acid reacts with the ferric ion to produce a green color.

Inoculation: Streak the surface of the slant with a moderate amount of inoculum. Incubate overnight at 35° C.

Reagent: Ferric chloride, aqueous, 10%. Store in brown bottle in refrigerator.

Reaction: Allow 4-5 drops phenylalanine reagent (10% aqueous solution of ferric chloride) to run down over the growth of the slant. Dark green color on the surface of the slant and in the fluid on the slant indicates a positive test. No change in color of the reagent indicates the test is negative.

Phenylethyl alcohol agar

The phenylethyl alcohol contained in the medium suppresses the growth of gram-negative organisms, allowing identification of gram-positive cocci such as staphylococci and streptococci in autopsy material and in feces.

Phenylethyl alcohol agar is a selective medium for gram-positive cocci.

Salmonella-Shigella agar

The Salmonella-Shigella (SS) medium is used for the isolation of the enteric pathogens *Salmonella* and *Shigella*. It, like MacConkey agar, is both selective and differential. In addition to suppressing the gram-positive organisms because of its bile salts and crystal violet content, it suppresses the coliform bacilli (lactose fermenters that are predominant flora in feces) with brilliant green. Lactose and neutral red are included in the medium to allow differentiation of lactose-fermenting and non-lactose-fermenting organisms in the same way MacConkey agar does.

Selenite F broth

The selenite F broth is used as is GN broth to suppress coliform bacilli from feces in order to isolate enteric pathogens. Selenium salts are the inhibitory agents in this medium. After an 18-24 hr incubation period, a drop of this medium is transferred to a MacConkey plate. If the transfer is not made after this length of time, the coliform organisms begin to overgrow any enteric pathogens that are present.

SIM medium

Principle: SIM medium is a semisolid medium containing basic nutrients plus sodium thiosulfate, peptonized iron, and tryptophan. The name SIM is an acronym for sulfide production, indole production, and motility.

The sodium thiosulfate is broken down by some bacteria to produce hydrogen sulfide, which reacts with the peptonized iron in the medium to form FeS, a black compound.

Indole is a by-product of the breakdown of tryptophan carried out by some bacteria. Indole forms a pink-colored compound in the presence of *p*-dimethylaminobenzaldehyde, the main component of Ehrlich indole reagent.

This semisolid medium allows motile organisms to demonstrate their motility by producing cloudiness in the medium or by growing in brushlike patterns around the line of inoculation.

Inoculation: Use short ($^1/_2$-$^1/_4$ in.) stab with straight needle and overnight incubation at 35° C under 5-10% CO_2 tension.

Reactions:

S: Blackening of tube—sulfide production present (sulfide positive); no color change in tube—sulfide negative

I: Deep pink color development after addition of indole reagent—indole positive; no color development—indole negative

M: Cloudiness throughout medium or brushlike growth around line of inoculation—positive motility

Simmons citrate agar (citrate utilization)

Principle: Simmons citrate agar is a synthetic medium that incorporates citrate as the only form of carbon in the medium. Some of the gram-negative bacilli are able to utilize carbon in this form and can thus survive and grow well on this medium. As they grow, they break down the inorganic ammonium and citrate salts and produce alkaline products, thus giving the blue (alkaline) reaction in the medium. Other organisms that are unable to utilize carbon in the form of citrate do not survive on the medium and leave it unchanged (green).

Inoculation: Very lightly streak the surface of the slant from butt upward and incubate overnight at 35° C.

Reactions: The pH indicator used is bromthymol blue, range 6.0 (green) to 7.6 (blue). Blue color on slant with growth indicates positive test; no color change (green) together with no growth indicates negative test.

Stuart transport medium

The Stuart transport medium promotes viability of microorganisms while the specimen (swab) is in transit. The medium is nonnutrient and semisolid and it contains sodium thioglycollate to suppress oxidative changes.

TCBS agar

Thiosulfate citrate bile salt sucrose (TCBS) agar is used for selective isolation of **vibrios.** *Vibrio cholerae* produces yellow colonies in 18-24 hr. Nonpathogenic vibrios from colonies with blue to greenish centers.

Proteus and enterococci may produce small translucent colonies (except *Proteus mirabilis,* which ferments sucrose so that yellow colonies result). *Pseudomonas* and *Aeromonas* give rise to blue colonies.

Thayer-Martin medium[28, 29]

Thayer-Martin medium is recommended for primary isolation of *Neisseria gonorrhoeae* and *Neisseria meningitidis*. Overgrowth by gram-positive and other gram-negative bacteria and yeast is reduced by the antibiotics incorporated into the medium (vancomycin, colistin, and nystatin [VCN] inhibitors [BBL, BioQuest Div., Becton-Dickinson & Co., Cockeysville, Md.]). The base is a Mueller-Hinton agar with 5% chocolated sheep blood. The medium is dispensed in plates that are inoculated by rolling the swab on the surface in a large Z-shaped pattern, which is then cross streaked with a sterile wire loop. Incubate medium at 35° C under 10% CO_2 tension (Fig. 32-6).

Thioglycollate broth

Thioglycollate broth contains a reducing agent, sodium thioglycollate (0.3-0.5%), and methylene blue as an indicator of degree of oxidation. Thioglycollate broth is stored at room temperature in the dark, since, at refrigerator temperature, it absorbs more O_2. Oxidation of the medium, which starts on the surface, is seen by a blue-green color change. If the color change involves 20% of the column, the medium should be boiled not more than once, cooled, and used. Repeated boiling destroys the medium. Tubes boiled and not used must be discarded. It is often useful to supplement thioglycollate broth with hemin and menadione for optimal growth of anaerobic bacteria.

Thiol broth

Thiol broth (BBL, BioQuest Div., Becton-Dickinson & Co., Cockeysville, Md.) is a blood culture medium suitable for aerobic and anaerobic culturing of blood and other body fluids (e.g., CSF, synovial fluid, and pleural fluid) and exudates. The medium contains BHI agar, thioglycollate medium, and trypticase soy broth with CO_2 under vacuum. Thiol broth neutralizes the bacteriostatic or bactericidal properties of streptomycin and penicillin.

Tinsdale medium

See p. 871.

Transgrow medium[30]

Transgrow medium is a selective medium recommended for primary isolation of *Neisseria gonorrhoeae* and *Neisseria meningitidis*. It is an outgrowth of the Thayer-Martin medium (see above), from which it differs as follows: increased agar percentage from 1-2%, increased glucose from 0.1-0.25%, larger surface area obtained by placing medium into a flat bottle, and controlled 10% CO_2 tension.

Inoculation: Keep the neck of the bottle elevated and remove cap only when ready to inoculate. Roll swab from side to side across medium starting at the bottom of the bottle (Fig. 32-7). Incubate at 35° C under 10% CO_2 tension.

Triple sugar iron agar

Principle: The triple sugar iron (TSI) is used to characterize the various gram-negative bacilli by testing for acid and gas production from glucose (0.1%), lactose (1%), and sucrose (1%) in a single solid medium. The gram-negative bacilli of the Enterobacteriaceae group can react in various ways. In group I, fermentation of glucose, lactose, and sucrose results in acid and gas throughout the tube. The organisms that ferment only glucose can produce one of two reactions, depending on their ability or inability to produce gas from glucose fermentation. The reactions of groups II and III are similar except for the gas production.

From the time the organisms are placed on the slant and in the butt, they begin to ferment the glucose aerobically and anaerobically, respectively. While both types of fermentation are in progress, the tube is acid throughout. However, since the aerobic fermentation

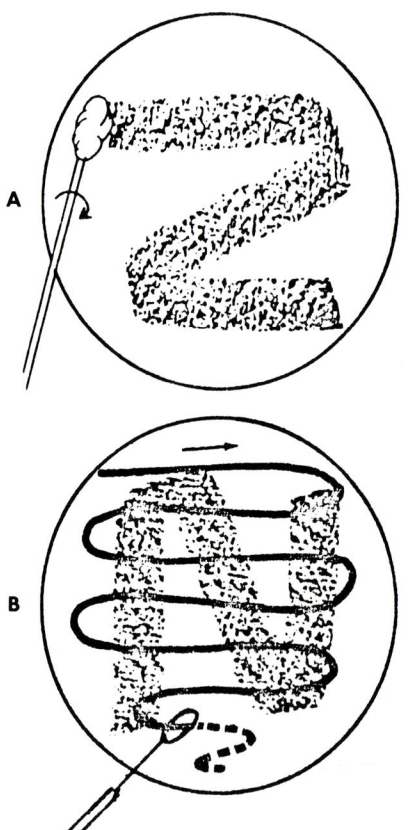

Fig. 32-6. Method of streaking Thayer-Martin plates. **A,** Roll swab on medium in a large Z-shaped pattern to provide maximal exposure of swab to plate for transfer of organisms. **B,** Cross streak with a sterile loop. (From Criteria and techniques for the diagnosis of gonorrhea, Atlanta, 1972, Centers for Disease Control.)

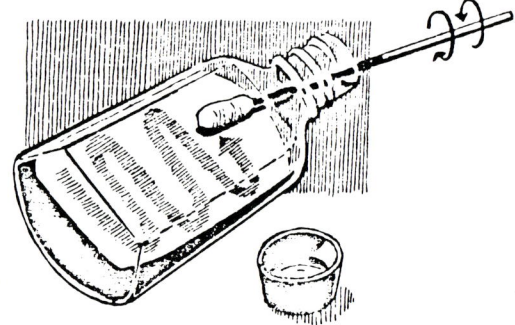

Fig. 32-7. Method of streaking Transgrow bottle. Keep neck of bottle elevated and roll swab from side to side across medium. Starting at bottom. (From Criteria and techniques for the diagnosis of gonorrhea, Atlanta, 1972, Centers for Disease Control.)

proceeds at a faster rate than the anaerobic fermentation, before the overnight incubation is complete, the supply of glucose is used up and the organisms begin breaking down the peptone in the medium. The products of this metabolism are alkaline in nature; thus the slant reverts to the alkaline state, whereas the butt remains acid because of the slower anaerobic breakdown of glucose (groups III and IV).

The nonfermentative gram-negative bacilli such as *Pseudomonas* species break down the peptones, producing an alkaline slant and butt without gas (group V).

Inoculation: Streak the surface of the slant and stab the butt. Incubate overnight.

Reactions: The pH indicator in the medium is phenol red, with a range of 6.8 (yellow) to 8.4 (red). The TSI reactions are classified as follows:

Group I	Acid slant/acid butt with gas, no H_2S
Group II	Acid slant/acid butt with gas and H_2S
Group III	Alkaline slant/acid butt with gas
Group IV	Alkaline slant/acid butt with no gas
Group V	Alkaline slant/alkaline butt with no gas

The TSI reactions are also discussed on p. 847.

Trypticase soy agar and broth

The trypticase soy agar and broth all-purpose media are made from a pancreatic digest of casein plus soybean peptone. They will support the growth of most ordinary bacteria encountered in medical microbiology.

Tween-albumin (Dubos) broth

The broth enriched with bovine albumin fraction V is used for the cultivation of mycobacteria. The broth may be used as the primary medium for specimens such as CSF or pleural fluid that are not contaminated by other bacteria.

Urea agar–Christensen (urease) test

Principle: The urease test is used to detect organisms that produce an enzyme, urease, that acts in the following way:

$$Urea \xrightarrow{Urease} CO_2 + NH_3$$

Reaction: The urea-splitting reaction liberates ammonia. This alkaline product raises the pH of the medium and causes the phenol red indicator to become pinkish red.

All the *Proteus* species are **rapid** urea splitters. Other organisms are also urease positive after **overnight** incubation. Among the latter are *Cryptococcus* species, *Brucella* species, and the following members of the family Enterobacteriaceae, which may give positive slant reactions: *Klebsiella, Citrobacter, Enterobacter cloacae, Serratia,* and *Yersinia enterocolitica.*

Inoculation: Streak the slant only. Incubate at 35° C. Urea agar satisfies all the basic nutritional requirements of most bacteria. In addition to the nutrients, it contains urea and phenol red as the pH indicator, range 6.8 (yellow) to 8.4 (pinkish red).

Results: A medium pinkish red color indicates urease positive; a medium yellow color indicates urease negative.

Record presence or absence of color after 4-6 hr and after overnight incubation. Indicate slant as either positive or negative and slant and butt as either positive or negative.

Voges-Proskauer (V-P) test[31]

Principle: Some bacteria have the ability to produce acetoin from glucose. In an alkaline pH, acetoin is oxidized to diacetyl, which reacts with the guanidine compound in the buffered deoxycholate glucose (BDG) broth. Creatine is added to prevent false negative results.

Reagents:
1. α-Naphthol, 5%, in 95% ethyl alcohol
2. KOH, 40%, in distilled water
3. Solution of creatine, 0.5%, in distilled water

Broth: Buffered deoxycholate glucose (BDG) broth or test tablets (Key Scientific Products, Los Angeles) are used.

The above reagents are stable for several months when stored in dark sealed containers and refrigerated.

Direct test (MacConkey agar): In 2 drops creatine solution, prepare a dense suspension of pink or red colonies from a MacConkey agar plate incubated overnight. To this suspension, add 3 drops α-naphthol, shake, add 2 drops KOH, shake, and observe for a pink to light red color, which appears within 15 min.

Rapid indirect test: Inoculate 0.2 ml MR-VP broth with no more than one colony and incubate for 4-6 hr at 37° C. Add 2 drops creatine solution, 3 drops α-naphthol, and then 2 drops KOH, shaking after the addition of each reagent. Observe for a pink to red color, which appears within 5 min.

Interpretation: *Escherichia* is V-P negative; *Enterobacter* and *Klebsiella* are V-P positive. These organisms may also be used as positive or negative controls.

Xylose-lysine-deoxycholate agar

Xylose-lysine-deoxycholate (XLD) agar is a selective and differential medium recommended for the isolation of enteric pathogens, especially *Shigella*. Phenol red is incorporated as a pH indicator, and sodium thiosulfate is incorporated as a sulfide indicator. The medium con-

Table 32-5. Differentiation of enteric bacteria—XLD agar

Group or genus	Colonies
Salmonella * *Arizona*	Red with black center
Shigella *Providencia*	Red
Some *Pseudomonas* and *Providenica rettgeri*	Red (falsely positive)
Escherichia	Yellow
Citrobacter	Yellow
Klebsiella	Yellow
Enterobacter	Yellow
Proteus	Yellow

*S. paratyphi A, *S. cholera-suis, S. pullorum,* and *S. gallinarum* may give red colonies without black centers.

Table 32-6. Quality control for commonly used microbiologic media*

	Blood agar (sheep blood)	EMB agar†	SS agar	XLD agar‡	Mycosel agar	CTA	Motility medium	Thayer-Martin medium	Chocolate agar with supplement A§ or B§	Chocolate agar without supplement	Mannitol salt agar	TSI agar
Penicillium sp.					−							
Escherichia coli	+, hemolysis	+		+				−			−	+, observe for proper reactions
Shigella sp.		+	+	+								
Salmonella sp.		+	+	+		+, motility positive	+, motility positive					+, observe for proper reactions
Listeria monocytogenes						+, motility negative	+, motility negative	−	−, with supplement A			
Streptococcus pyogenes	+, β-hemolysis											
Staphylococcus aureus	+, β-hemolysis	−			−						+, mannitol fermentation positive	
Candida albicans		−			+							
Trichophyton sp.					+							
Neisseria gonorrhoeae						+		+	+	±		
Neisseria meningitidis						+		+	+	±		
α-Hemolytic streptococci	+, α-hemolysis											
Enterococcus (group D)	+, β- or γ-hemolysis		−	−							±, mannitol fermentation slow	
Haemophilus influenzae	−							−	+	−		
Staphylococcus epidermidis	+										+, mannitol fermentation negative	
Haemophilus haemolyticus	−											
γ-Hemolytic streptococci	+, no hemolysis											

*+, Good growth; ±, minimal or slight growth or growth delayed; −, no growth.
†Endo and MacConkey agars may be used as alternatives.
‡Deoxycholate agar may be used as an alternative.
§Difco Laboratories, Detroit.

tains three carbohydrates—xylose, lactose, and sucrose. The amino acid lysine is present in the medium. The reactions of the organisms on this medium are based on their differential abilities to ferment the carbohydrates, decarboxylate lysine, and produce hydrogen sulfide (Table 32-5).

Special anaerobic media
Anaerobic blood agar

Anaerobic blood agar is a nonselective medium that supports the growth of all anaerobic organisms. The medium contains palladium chloride as a reducing agent. The medium should be prereduced by holding it in an anaerobic environment for 24 hr before use.

Columbia CNA agar

Columbia CNA agar is a medium that contains palladium chloride as a reducing agent plus colistin and nalidixic acid for the inhibition of gram-negative organisms. The medium is selective for gram-positive anaerobes.

Columbia neomycin agar

Because of the neomycin contained in Columbia neomycin agar, it is selective for *Clostridium* species.

Cooked meat glucose medium

Cooked meat glucose medium is an excellent medium for all anaerobes. It is also suitable for carrying anaerobic organisms in stock culture.

Egg yolk agar

Egg yolk agar is a medium used to isolate *Clostridium* species. Lecithinase and lipase production of organisms is indicated by clear zones developing around colonies producing these enzymes. Neomycin (100 μg/ml) may be added to make the medium selective for *Clostridium* species.

Kanamycin-vancomycin agar

Kanamycin-vancomycin (K-V) agar is designed to inhibit gram-positive organisms and is selective for *Bacteroides* species.

Quality control of media

See Table 32-6.

PRIMARY CULTURE OF VARIOUS SPECIMENS
Blood[32]

In the course of any bacterial infection there are transient phases of bacteremia. In some diseases the resulting bacteremia persists and becomes the dominant clinical feature. The primary focus may not be known, and the organisms involved may not be generally accepted as pathogenic.

Blood cultures should be obtained before antibacterial treatment is instituted. There are various ways that laboratories schedule blood cultures. In the author's laboratory both aerobic and anaerobic cultures are drawn immediately when an order is received. In 30 min this process is repeated, resulting in four culture bottles being inoculated for each culture ordered.

The culture medium is tryptic broth with the anticoagulant polyanethol added. Both aerobic and anaerobic bottles contain CO_2.

Procedure: Use aseptic technic. Paint site, usually over median basilic vein (Fig. 3-1, p. 27), with tincture of iodine or an iodophor such as Betadine. Place tourniquet over arm above elbow. Insert needle of sterile disposable transfer set into vein and add 5 ml blood to each blood culture bottle containing 50 ml of broth each (1:10 ratio). Remove tourniquet, clamp transfer set, withdraw needle, and place a sterile dry sponge over puncture site. Label cultures and send to laboratory. The use of sterile syringes and needles instead of the transfer sets increases the danger of contamination. Vacutainer (B-D Div., Becton-Dickinson & Co., Rutherford, N.J.) blood culture tubes further lessen the danger of contamination.

Incubate both blood culture bottles at 35° C for 18-24 hr. Examine cultures daily for evidence of visible growth. After a 24 hr period of incubation, handle the aerobic and anaerobic cultures alike except that anaerobic conditions should be maintained for the anaerobic culture. Shake each bottle well and, using a sterile syringe and needle, obtain enough material from each bottle to inoculate two chocolate agar plates and two blood agar plates. One trypticase soy broth receives material from the aerobic culture and one thioglycollate broth receives material from the anaerobic culture. Gram stains must be prepared from both bottles. Incubate subcultures from the aerobic blood culture bottle aerobically and from the anaerobic blood culture bottle anaerobically. If after 48 hr at 35° C no microorganisms are seen, repeat the Gram stain and subcultures after 13-14 days. If *Brucella* is suspected, incubate the culture bottles in CO_2 and keep for 30 days. Shake the bottle every third day, and make transfers by means of sterile syringes and needles in amounts of 0.2 ml. Keep the aerobic culture and subcultures under increased (5-10%) CO_2 tension.

If subcultures reveal organisms—they are usually present in pure culture—the Kirby-Bauer sensitivity test can be set up before the identification of the organism. A preliminary report, e.g., "gram-negative rod," should be given to the physician even if the organism is not completely identified. All blood cultures are kept 7-10 days unless growth occurs earlier.

Organisms that grow only anaerobically and not aerobically are anaerobic streptococci, *Bacteroides, Clostridium,* and *Actinomycetes.* The only organisms that at times do not grow in thioglycollate broth are *Pseudomonas, Neisseria, Haemophilus,* and aerobic diphtheroids. If only one bottle shows growth, it may be that the organism cannot adjust itself to the medium of the other bottle, or it may be a contaminant.

Radiometric detection of bacteria

There are some drawbacks to the above-mentioned visual and microscopic examinations of blood cultures. Usually bacteria are not detected until after 24 hr incubation, and the daily handling of culture carries with it the danger of contamination. The radiometric method of detection of bacteria[33] does not identify the organism but it records evidence of bacterial metabolism. ^{14}C

glucose and ^{14}C amino acids are incorporated into the medium. Bacterial metabolism leads to the formation of radioactive CO_2, the presence of which can be detected by a bacterial growth detector (Bactec, Johnston Laboratories, Cockeysville, Md.) that withdraws some of the atmosphere from the culture bottle and assays for $^{14}CO_2$ in a counting chamber. By using this method, positive blood cultures may be detected in as little as 4 hr. The radiometric method of blood culture needs further evaluation[34] before it can be universally recommended as the only method of culture, but at this time it can give an early result that may be very helpful in diagnosis.

There is some evidence that indicates bacterial growth may occur without the evolution of radioactive CO_2 and thus fail to be detected by this system.

Bile

The specimen is usually obtained at the time of operation or through a T tube. Essentially the methods outlined for feces also apply to bile. The possibility of *Salmonella* infection must be kept in mind. Bile is inoculated into a tube of thioglycollate and selenite F broth and plated on a blood agar and MacConkey agar plate. An anaerobic blood agar plate should be included. The media are incubated at 37° C. After overnight incubation, the selenite F broth is again subcultured onto MacConkey agar.

Bone marrow culture

Add 5 ml of the marrow and blood mixture to 50 ml trypticase soy broth and inoculate blood and chocolate agar plates. This method is superior to blood cultures for the isolation of *Brucella* species.

For the diagnosis of generalized histoplasmosis, bone marrow may be cultured on two blood agar and two Sabouraud agar plates, one set to be incubated at room temperature and the other at 37° C.

If tuberculosis is suspected, since there are no contaminating organisms, 5 ml bone marrow–blood mixture is added to 30 ml Middlebrook 7H-9 broth and incubated at 37° C under 5% CO_2 tension. It is examined weekly and, if positive, it is subcultured to 7H-10 agar and incubated at 37° C under 5% CO_2 tension.

If *Salmonella* infection is suspected, inject bone marrow into selenite F broth. After 16 hr subculture the broth onto MacConkey agar and blood agar, since the organism is usually present in pure culture.

Cerebrospinal fluid

If cerebrospinal fluid is submitted in two or three sterile, capped tubes, obtain culture from the second or third tube rather than from the first. If there is no plastic cap, be sure to anchor stopper or cotton plug with a pin before centrifuging. Centrifuge specimen at 3000 rpm for 15 min, decant supernatant into a sterile tube, and use sediment to inoculate one blood agar plate, one chocolate agar plate, one thioglycollate borth, and one MacConkey agar plate. Then prepare two smears, one to be stained with Gram stain and the other with methylene blue. An India ink preparation should be prepared to demonstrate *Cryptococcus* if the differential count reveals a predominance of lymphocytes, which may be confused with cryptococcal organisms.

Incubate all media at 37° C under 5% CO_2 tension.

If the Gram stain and the morphology of the organisms suggest *Streptococcus pneumoniae, Neisseria meningitidis, Haemophilus influenzae,* or *Klebsiella* species, institute appropriate immunologic procedures at once for rapid preliminary identification. If the Gram stain shows organisms, inform the physician immediately, even before identification of the organisms.

Any sediment remaining and the supernatant fluid should be saved in a sterile tube and deposited in the incubator for reexamination on the next day.

If *Haemophilus influenzae* is suspected, cross streak the blood agar plate with a staphylococcal culture or apply X-V strips (BBL, BioQuest Div., Becton-Dickinson & Co., Cockeysville, Md.).

If a yeast infection is suspected on the basis of the initial Gram stain or India ink preparation, inoculate two Sabouraud dextrose agar slants, one to be incubated at room temperature and one at 37° C.

If tuberculous meningitis is suspected—since there is usually no contamination—transfer sediment to Middlebrook 7H-9 broth and to 7H-10 agar, both incubated at 37° C under 5% CO_2 tension. Incubate the plate in CO_2-permeable polyethylene waterproof bags for 3-4 weeks. Use sediment also for preparation of smear to be stained by the Ziehl-Neelson or Kinyoun method.

Eye and ear culture

The material is usually submitted on a swab in holding medium. The following media should be employed: blood agar (to the surface of which should be added an X-V disk as an aid in the recognition of *Haemophilus influenzae),* chocolate agar, MacConkey agar, thioglycollate broth, phenylethyl alcohol medium with blood, two BHI agar slants, and two Sabouraud dextrose agar slants. All media are incubated at 37° C under 5% CO_2 tension with the exception of one BHI agar and one Sabouraud dextrose agar slant, which are incubated at room temperature. If an infection with *Moraxella lacunata* is considered, inoculate a Loeffler serum slant. The organism is proteolytic and forms pits on the surface of the slant.

Scrapings from the conjunctivae are stained by the Gram technic and with Wright-Giemsa stain for the presence of inclusion bodies and eosinophils.

Feces

Instruct the patient to collect the stool in a clean, preferably sterile bedpan and avoid contamination with urine. With a sterile spatula, transfer a small portion of fecal material into a disposable sterile plastic container with lid. Identify the specimen and send to the laboratory. Alternately, collect stool on a Culturette-type swab, either by blind insertion into the rectum after cleaning of the anal area or under proctoscopic guidance, using commercially available protected swabs (recommended if *Shigella* infection is suspected). Select purulent, mucoid, or bloody portions and inoculate into the following media: phenylethyl alcohol blood agar (staphylococci and yeast), blood agar (*Escherichia coli* and *Shigella dysenteriae*), MacConkey agar, SS agar, XLD agar, and selenite F broth. Inoculate the plates and broth in the order given with increasing amounts of material. Incubate all media at 35° C. After overnight incubation, examine for non-lactose-fermenting bacteria and other stool pathogens, and subculture selenite F broth onto SS agar, XLD agar, MacConkey agar, and bismuth sulfite agar.

Make a direct Gram-stained smear for staphylococci, yeast, vibrios, and *Campylobacter*.

Fluids from serous cavities (pleurae, pericardium, peritoneum, joints, etc.)

Since most of the fluids from serous cavities are exudates and have a tendency to clot (fibrinogen content), the laboratory should supply large, graduated, screw-topped, sterile centrifuge tubes containing sterile mixed oxalate, heparin, or sodium citrate (1 ml of 20% solution). Mix specimen well and centrifuge at 3000 rpm for 15-30 min. Use the sediment to make routine and acid-fast smears and to inoculate routine media and media for acid-fast organisms.

Inoculate two blood agar plates, one chocolate agar plate, one MacConkey plate, and one thioglycollate or BHI broth. Incubate all at 37° C aerobically except for one blood agar plate, which is incubated anaerobically.

Culture joint fluid on Thayer-Martin or Transgrow agar and incubate under 5% CO_2 tension at 37° C.

If tuberculosis is suspected and the material is free of contaminants, transfer 5 ml fluid directly into 30 ml Middlebrook 7H-9 broth and incubate at 37° C under 5% CO_2 tension. Examine weekly and, if positive, subculture it to 7H-11 agar and incubate at 37° C under 5% CO_2 tension.

Genital tract

Venereal infections require a special approach (see discussion of *Neisseria gonorrhoeae* and *Treponema pallidum*). Other infections can be handled the same way as urinary tract infections.

Pus, purulent exudates, and infected wounds

The preferred method is to aspirate the material into a sterile syringe. If this is not possible, at least two Culturette swabs should be inoculated with the material.

Inoculate one blood agar plate, one chocolate agar plate, one anaerobic blood agar plate, one MacConkey plate, and one thioglycollate broth. Incubate broth and plates at 37° C under 5% CO_2. Incubate the anaerobic blood agar plate anaerobically. Prepare at least two smears, one to be stained by Gram stain and the other stained by Kinyoun stain for tubercle bacilli.

If gonorrhea is suspected, inoculate chocolate agar and incubate at 35° C under 5% CO_2 tension.

Examine purulent material carefully for actinomycotic granules. Culture material under strict anaerobic conditions.

In cases of infected wounds, gram-positive and gram-negative aerobic and anaerobic bacteria may be involved; therefore selective agars containing antibiotics should be employed, e.g., Columbia CNA agar (BBL, BioQuest Div., Becton-Dickinson & Co., Cockeysville, Md.), which suppresses gram-negative organisms. If tuberculous or fungal infections are suspected, follow directions given in the appropriate sections. When Gram stains are examined, immediately inform the physician if gram-positive bacilli resembling

Clostridium are seen. These organisms may later be shown to be no more than aerobic contaminants; however, the physician should be informed even if clostridial infection is only suspected.

Clostridia will grow in thioglycollate broth and on the anaerobic blood agar plate.

Sputum

Sputum should be processed as soon as it is obtained so that it is suitable for the detection of predominant organisms. It should be obtained in the early morning and should be expectorated into disposable sterile plastic containers with lids. The patient should be instructed as to the purpose of the test and should brush his teeth and rinse his throat before the specimen is collected. Every attempt should be made to exclude saliva and nasal secretions.

Select hemorrhagic, purulent, or cheesy particles. Make routine bacterial and acid-fast smears and employ routine bacterial and acid-fast staining methods. Also employ routine smear and culture methods for fungi.

If acid-fast organisms are not suspected, the following media should be used: one MacConkey agar plate, one chocolate agar plate, two blood agar plates, one with phenylethyl alcohol, and one thioglycollate broth. Incubated all aerobically at 37° C under 5% CO_2 tension.

The bacteriology of sputum is difficult to interpret since there is often little correlation between Gram stain, culture, and clinical impression. Attempts should be made to determine which specimens are most appropriate for culture.

If nocardiosis or actinomycosis is suspected, three Sabouraud dextrose agar slants without antibiotics are plated as well as three BHI agar plates. One Sabouraud dextrose agar slant and one BHI agar plate are incubated anaerobically at 35-37° C if actinomycosis is suspected. Of the remaining two sets, one set is incubated aerobically at room temperature and one set at 37° C.

An Optochin disk for the detection of *Streptococcus pneumoniae* and an X-V strip for the detection of *Haemophilus influenzae* may be added to the blood agar plate to speed up recovery and identification of these organisms.

If pertussis is suspected, Bordet-Gengou medium should be used. If fungal or tuberculous infections are suspected, the usual culture method for fungi or tubercle bacilli should be employed. If *Histoplasma capsulatum* infection is a possibility, the blood agar plate should be kept for 3 weeks at room temperature tightly closed with a wide rubber band.

A Gram stain should be prepared, since it is sometimes helpful in staphylococcal or pneumococcal gram-negative pneumonia.

The Quellung reaction may be performed on the sputum for *Streptococcus pneumoniae* and *Haemophilus influenzae*.

Throat, nose, nasopharynx, and sinuses

The paranasal sinuses are normally sterile. Specimens from throat, nose, and nasopharynx are usually collected on swabs. Nasopharyngeal material is obtained by means of wire swabs protected from contamination by plastic tubing. Calcium alginate wool is suggested to take the place of absorbent cotton. The swabs should be inserted in holding media. The following primary culture media should be utilized: two blood agar plates (to the surface of one should be applied an X-V strip for *Haemophilus influenzae* and an Optochin disk for *Streptococcus pneumoniae*), one MacConkey plate, one chocolate agar plate, and one thioglycollate broth. If *Corynebacterium diphtheriae* is suspected, use Loeffler or Tinsdale medium. To best detect all streptococcal hemolysis, incubate the second blood agar plate anaerobically or use a blood agar pour plate. In the case of pertussis, Bordet-Gengou medium should be chosen. Since gram-negative organisms are frequently found in the throats of children, MacConkey agar is included. Include one plate of anaerobic blood agar.

Prepare two smears, one for Gram stain and one for Loeffler methylene blue stain.

Tissue (autopsy and surgical)

All material for bacteriologic cultures must be obtained by aseptic technic. Mince tissue specimens and then grind and homogenize in sterile saline solution. If a large amount of tissue is available, divide it with sterile instruments and store some of the tissue in the deep freeze ($-20°$ C). On the basis of history, gross examinations, Gram stain, or frozen section, choose the best culture methods. The following media should be employed: thioglycollate broth, blood agar, MacConkey agar, and phenylethyl alcohol medium. Stain one smear with Gram stain and a second smear for acid-fast bacteria. If blood culture is indicated, use the method described in the discussion of blood culture. If mycobacteria are suspected, the material should be handled according to the methods for acid-fast organisms. If fungi are considered, the material should be handled according to the outline for fungal cultures.

Urethral, prostatic, and cervical specimens

Inoculate one Transgrow medium or Thayer-Martin medium, two blood agar plates, one chocolate plate, and one thioglycollate broth. Incubate all at $37°$ C under 5% CO_2 tension except for one blood agar plate. Incubate one blood agar plate at $37°$ C anaerobically. Prepare a gram-stained smear and be alert for *Neisseria gonorrhoeae* and *Listeria monocytogenes*.

If the direct smear suggests *L. monocytogenes*, inoculate trypticase broth and store at $4°$ C. Subculture 0.2 ml from the trypticase broth into 5 ml potassium thiocyanate broth at weekly intervals for the first month and monthly for 4 months. Incubate potassium thiocyanate broth at room temperature for 48 hr and transfer to blood agar plate incubated at $35°$ C.

Because of the possibility of asymptomatic gonococcal infections, bacteria from the areas mentioned should always be plated on Transgrow or Thayer-Martin medium.

If fungal etiology is suspected, inoculate two Sabouraud dextrose slants and incubate one at room temperature and one at $35°$ C.

In the case of *Gardnerella vaginalis* infection, Gram stains may reveal epithelial cells covered and accompanied by large masses of gram-negative bacilli (**clue cells**) (Fig. 32-8).[35]

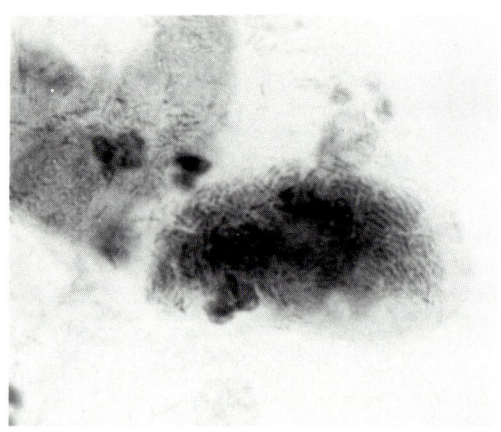

Fig. 32-8. ''Clue'' cell. (Vaginal smear, Papanicolaou technic.) Note intracellular concentration of *Gardnerella vaginalis*.

Urine
Collection of specimen

Male patient: Thoroughly clean glans penis and collect cleanly voided **midstream** portion of urinary stream in disposable sterile plastic container with lid.

Female patient: Catheterization may be avoided by placing the patient in the lithotomy position, cleaning the vulva from front to back, separating the labia, and collecting the urine specimen from midstream in a sterile container with lid.

• • •

Cleaning for both sexes consists of two separate washes with soap and water. Record collection time.

Urine specimens for culture should not be centrifuged and should not be allowed to stand at room temperature for more than 30 min. Urine is an excellent culture medium, so that rapid bacterial proliferation in the specimen will render a quantitative approach inaccurate. If the specimen cannot be handled immediately after it is received, it should be stored in the refrigerator for not longer than 2 hr or at $0°$ C for 24 hr. One of the quantitative or semiquantitative methods should be used to plate urine on blood and MacConkey agar. Thioglycollate broth is not necessary.

In most cases, quantitative bacterial cultures allow differentiation of true urinary tract infections from contamination of the urine by bacteria from the urethra and the external genitals. A concentration of 100,000 or more bacteria/ml urine is accepted as diagnostic of bacteriuria. A count of less than 1000 bacteria/ml urine is considered insignificant, probably because of contamination, while counts between 10,000 and 100,000/ml urine are suggestive of infection and require a repeat culture of a fresh specimen. Finding more than one kind of bacteria in large quantities suggests contamination. The urinary sediment should always be examined for the presence of pus cells in support of a urinary infection.

Methods for estimating number of bacteria in urine[36]

1. Screening tests: Griess nitrite test,[37] triphenyl tetrazolium chloride (TTC) test (Uroscreen, Pfizer, New York), Gram stain on undiluted urine
2. Semiquantitative test: standard loop method
3. Quantitative urine method: serial dilutions of urine

Screening tests: Since the screening tests discover only about 60% of the colony counts between 10,000 and 100,000 colonies/ml and since the quantitative methods are readily performed, the screening tests will not be discussed in detail.

A Gram-stained smear of the uncentrifuged urine is a fairly good screening test to distinguish between bacteriuria and contamination. A positive smear (indicating bacteriuria) is one that shows several bacteria in the majority of the oil-immersion fields.

Semiquantitative test:

Standard loop method[38]**:** Mix the specimen thoroughly and inoculate each side of a divided blood agar and MacConkey agar plate with a standard loopful (3 mm diameter equal to 0.01 ml) of urine. The loop is a platinum-rhodium fused loop that after flaming must be allowed to cool completely before the urine is picked up. Spread 1 loopful of urine (avoid air bubble) evenly over the blood agar area and spread a second loopful over the MacConkey agar area. Incubate biplate overnight at 37° C. After incubation use Gram stain and appropriate subcultures to identify all colony types. Report number of colonies present per milliliter of urine (colony count × 100). The small amount of material used reduces the accuracy of this method.

Quantitative urine method[39,40]**:** Prepare a hundredfold and a thousandfold dilution of urine in sterile distilled water. Transfer 1 ml urine to 9 ml sterile water, mix well, and with a sterile pipet, transfer 1 ml of the 1:10 dilution to 9 ml sterile water to obtain a 1:100 dilution. Transfer 1 ml of the 1:100 dilution to 9 ml sterile water to obtain a 1:1000 dilution.

Spread 0.1 ml (using a sterile disposable serologic pipet) of the 1:100 and of the 1:1000 dilutions on one blood and one MacConkey plate each. Altogether two blood agar plates and two MacConkey plates are needed. Immediately spread inoculum with sterile glass spreader evenly over the surfaces of the plates. Incubate plates overnight at 37° C, and on the next day count colonies and identify organisms by subculturing them to appropriate media. Multiply number of colonies by 10 (0.1 ml was used) and by dilution factors (100 and 1000) to obtain the number of bacteria per milliliter urine.

Antibody-coated bacteria: The detection of antibody-coated bacteria is helpful in determining the site of urinary tract infection.[41] Bacteria infecting only the bladder (cystitis) are usually not coated with antibody while bacteria infecting the upper urinary tract (pyelonephritis) are usually found to be antibody coated.

The bacteria are "stained" by the FA procedure using fluorescein-conjugated antihuman serum.[42] After staining, the slides are examined with the ultraviolet microscope. Bacteria that are antibody coated show bright green fluorescence while noncoated bacteria are not seen.

Collection, handling, and shipment of bacteriologic specimens

The Department of Health and Human Services publishes detailed instructions on the collection, handling, and shipment of diagnostic specimens.*

Pathogenic organisms most likely to be isolated from clinical material

Although the most common organisms are listed below, it must be remembered that any organism may be found in clinical material. For normal flora, see p. 807.

Blood cultures
Staphylococci (pathogenic and saprophytic)
Coliform bacilli and related organisms
α- and β-hemolytic streptococci
Streptococcus pneumoniae
Streptococcus faecalis
Clostridium perfringens
Proteus species
Bacteroides species and related anaerobes
Neisseria meningitidis
Salmonella species
Brucella species
Francisella tularensis
Listeria monocytogenes
Acinetobacter species
Streptobacillus moniliformis
Vibrio species
Pathogenic yeasts and molds
Cerebrospinal fluid cultures
Haemophilus influenzae, type b (infants and children)
Neisseria meningitidis
Streptococcus pneumoniae
Mycobacterium tuberculosis
Staphylococci and streptococci, including *Streptococcus faecalis*
Cryptococcus neoformans
Coliform bacilli, *Pseudomonas* and *Proteus* species
Bacteroides species
Listeria monocytogenes
Acinetobacter species
Leptospira species
Ear cultures
Pseudomonas aeruginosa
Staphylococcus aureus
Proteus species
β-Hemolytic streptococci
Streptococcus pneumoniae
Coliform bacilli
Aspergillus fumigatus
Eye cultures
Staphylococcus aureus
Neisseria gonorrhoeae
Streptococcus pneumoniae
β-Hemolytic streptococci
Moraxella lacunata
Haemophilus species
Acinetobacter species
Diphtheroids, including *Corynebacterium xerosis*
Pseudomonas species and other enteric rods
Fungi

---

*Collection, handling, and shipment of diagnostic specimens, Public Health Service Publication no. 976, Washington, D. C., 1962, U. S. Government Printing Office.

Gastrointestinal tract cultures (stool)
Salmonella species
Shigella species
Yersinia enterocolitica
Campylobacter fetus, ssp. *jejuni*
Various yeast forms, including *Candida albicans,* when in
  large numbers
Vibrio species
Escherichia coli
Genital tract cultures
Coliform bacilli, enterococci, and other intestinal commen-
  sals, including *Bacteroides* species
Lactobacilli
Haemophilus species
β-Hemolytic streptococci of groups B and D
Anaerobic streptococci
Neisseria gonorrhoeae
Haemophilus ducreyi
Mycobacterium tuberculosis
Cultures from newborn infants
Staphylococci
Group B streptococci
Enteric rods
Sinus tract cultures
Mycobacteria
Fungi
Bacteroides species
Proteus species
Streptococci
Staphylococci
Sputum cultures
Streptococcus pneumoniae
Klebsiella species
Haemophilus influenzae
Staphylococcus aureus
Streptococcus species
Cryptococcus or other fungi
Bordetella bronchiseptica
Throat cultures
β-Hemolytic streptococci of group A and occasionally
  groups B, C, and G
Corynebacterium diphtheriae
Bordetella pertussis
Meningococci
Predominance of *Staphylococcus aureus,* coliform bacilli,
  Streptococcus pneumoniae, Haemophilus influenzae,
  Candida albicans, etc.
Urinary tract cultures
Coliform bacilli
Streptococcus faecalis
Proteus species
Pseudomonas species
Staphylococci
Alcaligenes species
Haemophilus species
Candida albicans
β-Hemolytic streptococci, usually groups B and C
Gonococcus
Mycobacterium tuberculosis
Salmonella species
Candida species
Wound cultures
Staphylococcus aureus
Streptococcus pyogenes
Coliform bacilli
Proteus species
Pseudomonas species
Clostridium species
Anaerobic cocci
Streptococcus faecalis
Bacteroides species

ANTIBIOTIC SUSCEPTIBILITY

Since some microorganisms consistently respond to adequate and well-chosen antibiotic therapy, sensitivity testing may not be indicated. Sensitivity tests do not need to be performed if (1) the organisms have a predictable sensitivity pattern or (2) the culture reveals only a mixture of commensal organisms of doubtful relationship to the clinical picture.

Organisms with a predictable sensitivity pattern include the pyogenic streptococci and *Clostridium perfringens,* both of which are sensitive to all pencillins and cephalothin. Organisms that are known to be sensitive to penicillin G are most *Neisseria, Actinomyces,* and *Corynebacterium diphtheriae. Brucella* is sensitive to tetracycline.

Sensitivity testing is necessary under the following conditions:

1. The culture reveals organisms that are frequently resistant to antibiotics or have a variable sensitivity pattern, e.g., *Escherichia coli, Enterobacter, Klebsiella, Salmonella, Shigella, Listeria, Proteus, Pseudomonas, Streptococcus faecalis,* and *Staphylococcus.*
2. The clinical picture warrants the use of a rapid bactericidal drug (not merely bacteriostatic), e.g., in bacterial meningitis, endocarditis, and osteomyelitis.
3. In the course of therapy the bacteria become resistant in varying degrees to certain drugs or to the dosage used.
4. The patient's defense mechanism is impaired, as in hypogammaglobulinemia and lymphoproliferative disorders.

Disk diffusion tests and dilution tests are available to ascertain the sensitivity of bacteria to antibiotics. In vitro testing does not take into consideration the patient's own resistance factors and the variable antibiotic concentration in sites other than blood.

Disk diffusion antimicrobial susceptibility tests

Principle: Disk diffusion antimicrobial susceptibility tests[43,44] measure the inhibition of growth of a microorganism on the surface of an inoculated agar plate by an antimicrobial agent diffusing into the surrounding me-

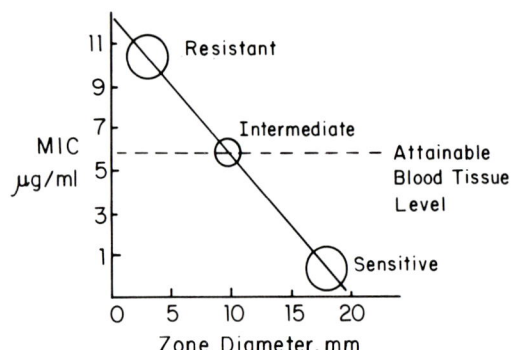

Fig. 32-9. Size of inhibition zone of a given bacterial strain is inversely proportional to the minimum inhibitory concentration (MIC) of a given antibiotic. (Tube dilution method.)

dium from an impregnated disk. The size of the inhibition zone of a given bacterial strain is inversely proportional to the minimum inhibitory concentration of a given antibiotic as determined by the tube dilution test, when the test conditions are constant (Fig. 32-9).

Definition of terms: **Susceptibility** of microorganisms is usually used synonymously with **sensitivity.** It means that in vitro tests indicate that the organism is killed or inhibited by a concentration of antibiotic obtainable in the blood by administering the standard therapeutic dosage.

The **minimum inhibitory concentration** (MIC), expressed in micrograms per milliliter, is the lowest concentration of the antibiotic that prevents visible growth of a cultured organism.

Susceptibility testing of pure culture (Kirby-Bauer method)[45-48]

Susceptibility testing should always be done on pure cultures and not on mixed cultures. If for any reason a mixed culture sensitivity test is performed, it should be followed by sensitivity testing on pure subcultures.

The Kirby-Bauer method has the advantage that it **standardizes** most of the factors that influence inhibition zone size except bacterial susceptibility. These factors are inoculum size, pH of medium, depth of medium, concentration of agar, rate of diffusion of drug (a function of the molecular weight of the antibiotic), concentration of antibiotic-impregnated disks, and incubation.

Procedure: Transfer with a wire loop five colonies of a pure culture of the organism to be tested from the original culture plate to a test tube containing 4 ml trypticase soy broth and 1% yeast extract. The trypticase soy broth will support the growth of the great majority of bacteria found in clinical infections with the exception of *Haemophilus influenzae*. The latter must be grown on chocolate agar and suspended in Mueller-Hinton broth. The Kirby-Bauer method is not recommended, however, for fastidious isolates such as *H. influenzae*.

Incubate broth 2-5 hr to produce a bacterial suspension of moderate cloudiness.

Dilute suspension, if necessary, with sterile water or saline solution to a density visually equivalent to that of a barium sulfate standard prepared by adding 0.5 ml of 1.17% barium chloride (BaCl$_2 \cdot$ 2H$_2$O) to 99.5 ml of 1% sulfuric acid (0.36N). The standard should be replaced monthly and be kept in the dark when not in use.

For sensitivity plates, use large (15 cm) Petri dishes with Mueller-Hinton agar, 4 mm in depth. Add 5% defibrinated sheep blood for enterococci. The large Petri dishes accommodate about nine disks in an outer ring and three to four more in the center. It is advantageous to place antibiotics that diffuse well in the outer circle and disks that produce smaller inhibition zones (such as vancomycin, polymyxin B, colistin, and kanamycin) in the central area of the plate.

Plates are inoculated within 15 min of dilution of broth culture so as not to alter the standardization of the broth. The bacterial broth suspension is streaked evenly (in three planes—horizontal, vertical, and diagonal—and once circularly around periphery) onto the surface of the medium with a cotton swab (not a wire loop or glass rod). Surplus suspension is removed from the swab by rotating it against the side of the tube before the plate is seeded.

After the inoculum has dried (3-5 min) the disks are placed on the agar with flamed forceps or a disk applicator and gently pressed down to ensure contact.

Plates are aerobically incubated within 15 min. Incubate overnight (optimal time: 14 hr) at 37° C in the absence of CO$_2$.

After overnight incubation, measure zone diameters (including the 6 mm disk) with a ruler or calipers from the back of the plate. Blood plates have to be read with calipers at the agar surface. A reading of 6 mm indicates no zone. Zone diameters may be read after incubation for 6-8 hr if they are needed but should be checked again after overnight incubation.

The end point is taken as complete inhibition of growth as determined by the unaided eye (Fig. 32-10). In the case of sulfonamides, organisms must grow through several generations before inhibition takes effect. Slight growth (80% or more inhibition) with sulfonamides is therefore disregarded; the margin of heavy growth is read to determine the zone size. Swarming of *Proteus* species is not inhibited by all antibiotics; a veil of swarming into an inhibition zone should also be ignored. With cephalosporins and penicillin, a ring of inner colonies at the periphery of the zone may be found.[49] Take reading within this zone. This is also found with *Serratia* and polymyxin, and the strain is regarded as resistant.

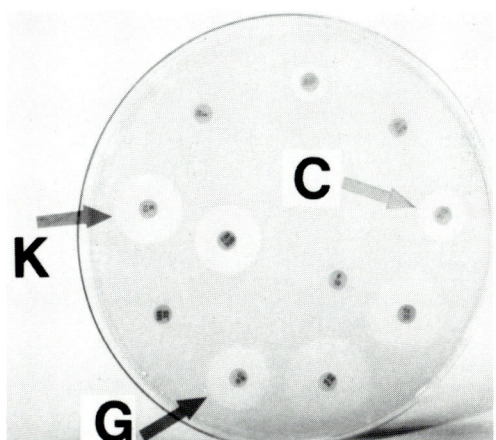

Fig. 32-10. Kirby-Bauer sensitivity plate. Each clear zone represents inhibition of growth by a specific antimicrobial. Zone size is significant: 30 μg cephalosporin, *C,* shows inhibition, but zone is smaller than prescribed for clinical effectiveness; the organism will therefore be reported as resistant to cephalothin. All other zones are equal to or greater than the zone size equivalent to a minimum inhibitory concentration (MIC) value. Note that kanamycin, *K,* has a larger zone than gentamicin, *G;* this reflects diffusion rates and does not indicate per se that kanamycin will be more effective than gentamicin. (From Blaker, R.G.: Condenser, February, 1972.)

Table 32-7. Kirby-Bauer zone diameter interpretive standards[50-53]

Antimicrobial agent	Disk potency	Inhibition zone diameter (mm)			Approximate MIC correlates	
		Resistant	Intermediate	Sensitive	Resistant	Susceptible
Amikacin[54]*	30 μg	≤14	15-16	≥17	≥16 μg/ml	≤8 μg/ml
Ampicillin†						
Enterobacteriaceae and enterococci	10 μg	≤11	12-13	≥14	≥32 μg/ml	≤8 μg/ml
Staphylococcus and penicillin-sensitive organisms	10 μg	≤20	21-28	≥29	≥2.0 μg/ml penicillinase‡	≤0.2 μg/ml
Haemophilus	10 μg	≤19	—	≥20	—	≤2.0 μg/ml
Carbenicillin						
Proteus and E. coli	100 μg	≤17	18-22	≥23	≥32 μg/ml	≤16 μg/ml
P. aeruginosa§	100 μg	≤11	12-14	≥15	≥250 μg/ml	≤125 μg/ml
Cefamandole	30 μg	≤14	15-17	≥18	>32 μg/ml	≤18 μg/ml
Cefoxitin	30 μg	≤14	15-17	≥18	>32 μg/ml	≤18 μg/ml
Cephalothin‖	30 μg	≤14	15-17	≥18	≥32 μg/ml	≤10 μg/ml
Chloramphenicol	30 μg	≤12	13-17	≥18	≥25 μg/ml	≤12.5 μg/ml
Clindamycin¶	2 μg	≤14	15-16	≥17	≥2 μg/ml	≤1 μg/ml
Colistin#	10 μg	≤8	9-10	≥11	—	—
Erythromycin	15 μg	≤13	14-17	≥18	≥8 μg/ml	≤2 μg/ml
Gentamicin	10 μg	≤12	13-14	≥15	≥6 μg/ml	≤6 μg/ml
Kanamycin	30 μg	≤13	14-17	≥18	≥25 μg/ml	≤6 μg/ml
Methicillin**	5 μg	≤9	10-13	≥14	—	≤3 μg/ml
Nafcillin	1 μg	≤10	11-12	≥13	—	≤3 μg/ml
Nalidixic acid††	30 μg	≤13	14-18	≥19	≥32 μg/ml	≤12 μg/ml
Neomycin	30 μg	≤12	13-16	≥17	—	≤10 μg/ml
Nitrofurantoin††	300 μg	≤14	15-16	≥17	≥100 μg/ml	≤25 μg/ml
Penicillin G‡‡						
Staphylococci	10 units	≤20	21-28	≥29	Penicillinase‡	≤0.1 μg/ml
Other organisms	10 units	≤11	12-21	≥22	≥32 μg/ml	≤1.5 μg/ml
Polymyxin B#	300 units	≤8	9-11	≥12	≥50 units/ml	
Streptomycin	10 μg	≤11	12-14	≥15	≥15 μg/ml	≤6 μg/ml
Sulfonamides						
N. meningitidis only	250-300 μg			≥40		
Other organisms††	250-300 μg	≤12	13-16	≥17	≥350 μg/ml	≤100 μg/ml
Tetracycline	30 μg	≤14	15-18	≥19	≥12 μg/ml	≤4 μg/ml
Tobramycin	10 μg	≤11	12-13	≥14	≥11 μg/ml	≤14 μg/ml
Trimethoprim-sulfamethoxazole[50]	1.25-23.75 μg	≤10	11-15	≥17 = S/ ≥23 = SS	≥200 μg/ml	≤ 35μg/ml
Vancomycin	30 μg	≤9	10-11	≥12	—	≤5 μg/ml

From Matsen, J.M.: In Sonnenwirth, A.C., and Jarett, L., editors: Gradwohl's clinical laboratory methods and diagnosis, vol. 2, ed. 8, St. Louis, 1980, The C.V. Mosby Co.

*Tentative standard from Bristol Laboratories, Syracuse, N.Y.

†Class disk for ampicillin, hetacillin, and amoxicillin.

‡Resistant strains of *S. aureus* produce penicillinase. There are significant reports of ampicillin-resistant *Haemophilus* strains that produce penicillinase.

§Tentative standards.

‖Class disks for cephalothin, cephaloridine, cephalexin, cefazolin, cephacetrile, cephradine, and cephapirin.

¶The clindamycin disk is used to test susceptibility to both clindamycin and lincomycin. Because of the greater activity of clindamycin, separate interpretative categories of zone diameters are recommended when reporting susceptibility to lincomycin as follows: ≤16 = R, 17-20 = I, ≥21 = S.

#Colistin and polymyxin B diffuse poorly in agar, and thus the accuracy of diffusion tests is less than that found with other antimicrobials; MIC correlates cannot be calculated reliably from regression analysis.

**Class disk for penicillinase-resistant penicillins (i.e., methicillin, cloxacillin, dicloxacillin, oxacillin, and nafcillin). Nafcillin and oxacillin disks are also available.

††Urinary tract infections only.

‡‡Class disk for penicillin G, phenoxymethylpenicillin, and phenethicillin.

If colonies are seen within a zone of inhibition, the strain should be checked for purity and retested.

Standard control organisms of known susceptibility should be employed at least once a week as a check on the activity of the disks and on the reproducibility of the test. They are *Staphylococcus aureus* ATCC (American Type Culture Collection, Rockville, Md.) 25923, *Escherichia coli* ATCC 25922, and *Pseudomonas aeruginosa* ATCC 27853. The diameter of the inhibition zone of the various antibiotics tested with the control organisms is plotted every week to see whether it remains in the acceptable range or to spot any abnormal values.

After measurement the zone diameters are recorded and interpreted according to Table 32-7.

The method should not be used for (1) organisms requiring longer than 24 hr to grow (see method for sensitivity testing of anaerobic bacteria below), (2) *Neisseria gonorrhoeae,* or (3) sulfonamide sensitivity testing of *Neisseria meningitidis* or group A streptococci (for these organisms, use agar dilution technic).

Choice of antibiotics: **Gram-negative** organisms and enterococci should be tested against ampicillin, cephalothin, chloramphenicol, kanamycin, nitrofurantoin (urine samples only), polymyxin B, streptomycin, tetracycline, and gentamicin. **Gram-positive** organisms should be tested against penicillin G, methicillin, chloramphenicol, tetracycline, cephalothin, kanamycin, erythromycin, streptomycin, and ampicillin.

Interpretation: Sensitivity (S) implies that the organism may be expected to be inhibited by therapeutic blood levels of a given antibiotic on the usual dosage schedule. R implies resistance.

Intermediate (I) falls between S and R and is relatively uncommon. If a particular drug is clinically desirable and gives an intermediate zone result, dilution tests should be performed. Clinically, an intermediate zone should be considered equal to resistance unless the tube dilution test is performed.

Dilution tests
Tube dilution susceptibility test (Cleveland Clinic Foundation method)

The tube dilution method determines by titration the least amount of drug (MIC in micrograms per milliliter) that will inhibit visible growth of an organism in pure culture in BHI broth[40] (Fig. 32-11).

The method must be standardized similar to the Kirby-Bauer method with regard to inoculum size, choice of medium, pH, incubation time, and temperature. The dilution technic is indicated whenever the Kirby-Bauer method cannot be used or gives intermediate results (p. 834).

Concentration of inoculum: An inoculum of a 1:1000 dilution of an 18 hr pure BHI broth culture is used.

Concentration of antibiotic:
1. Stock solution: A stock solution of 1000 μg/ml of active drug in BHI broth is prepared for each antibiotic to be tested. Reference standard antibiotic preparation must be obtained from the manufacturer of the antibiotic. Clinical preparations cannot be used. Prepare 1 ml aliquots, sterilize by filtration, and store at $-20°$ C.
2. Working solution: Before use, dilute stock solution 1:5 with BHI broth to obtain an antibiotic concentration of 200 μg/ml.

Procedure: Set up a rack with 12 sterile 13×75 mm test tubes for each antibiotic to be tested. Pipet 0.5 ml BHI (BBL, BioQuest Div., Becton-Dickinson & Co., Cockeysville, Md.) culture of the organism to be tested into tubes 1 to 12 (Table 32-8). Add 1 ml antibiotic working solution (200 μg/ml) to tube 1. Using a sterile 1 ml serologic pipet, transfer 0.5 ml from tube 1 to

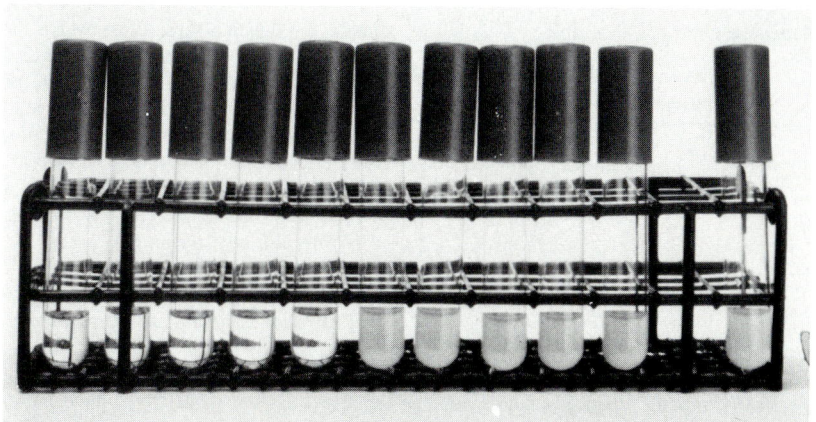

Fig 32-11. Tube dilution susceptibility test. Determination of minimum inhibitory concentration (MIC). Antibiotic concentration decreases from left to right. Fifth tube contains 16 μg/ml ampicillin; this is MIC for that strain of *Staphylococcus aureus*. Minimum bacterial concentration (MBC) would be derived by subculturing each of the five tubes showing no visible growth to differentiate suppression of growth from lethal effect. With ampicillin, MBC is usually significantly higher than MIC. Last tube in rack is a viability control containing no antibiotic to ensure that the bacteria being tested are capable of growing in the basic medium. (From Blaker, R.G.: Condenser, February, 1972.)

Table 32-8. Outline of tube dilution method

Tube no.	BHI (ml)	Antibiotic		Final concentration of antibiotic (μg/ml)
		Working solution (ml)	From previous tube (ml)	
1	0.5	1	0	100
2	0.5	0	0.5	50
3	0.5	0	0.5	25
4	0.5	0	0.5	12.5
5	0.5	0	0.5	6.25
6	0.5	0	0.5	3.12
7	0.5	0	0.5	1.56
8	0.5	0	0.5	0.78
9	0.5	0	0.5	0.39
10	0.5	0	0.5	0.19
11	0.5	0	0.5	0.095
12	0.5	0	0	0

Table 32-9. Antimicrobials and their test range in MIC determinations

Drug	Concentration (μg/ml)						
Ampicillin (gram-positive)	8	4	2	1	0.5	0.25	0.12
Carbenicillin	512	256	128	64	32	16	8
Cephalothin	64	32	16	8	4	2	1
Chloramphenicol	32	16	8	4	2	1	0.5
Clindamycin	16	8	4	2	1	0.5	0.25
Erythromycin	16	8	4	2	1	0.5	0.25
Gentamicin	16	8	4	2	1	0.5	0.25
Kanamycin	64	32	16	8	4	2	1
Methicillin	16	8	4	2	1	0.5	0.25
Penicillin G	4	2	1	0.5	0.25	0.12	0.06
Tetracycline	16	8	4	2	1	0.5	0.25
Nitrofurantoin	64	—	—	—	—	—	—
Trimethoprim	32	16	8	4	2	1	0.5
Sulfamethoxazole	608	304	152	76	38	19	9.5
Polymixins (colistin)	4	—	—	—	—	—	—

Table 32-10. Zone size chart for anaerobic susceptibility tests

Antibiotic	Resistant	Susceptible
Ampicillin	15	17
Carbenicillin	15	18
Cephalothin	15	18
Clindamycin	15	17
Penicillin	15	17
Tetracycline	15	16

tube 2 and mix well by drawing mixture up and expelling it several times. Transfer 0.5 ml from tube 2 to tube 3 and continue through tube 11; remove and discard 0.5 ml from this tube. Tube 12 is a culture control.

Prepare a control set (follow procedure thus far) using the same antibiotic and an organism of which the MIC of the antibiotic is known. Incubate tubes overnight at 37° C. On the next day perform gross examination for the first clear tube, which indicates the end point, i.e., the minimum concentration of antibiotic necessary to inhibit the growth of the organism tested. It indicates the sensitivity of that organism to the antibiotic. The control tube must show adequate growth.

The tube dilution method has been adapted to the microtiter system[55] and has also been automated.[56] A modification of this method has been suggested by the World Health Organization.[57]

Microquantitative susceptibility test

With the introduction of prediluted microdilution trays and inoculation equipment for them, the use of dilution sensitivity testing is becoming more widespread.[58] Trays of serially diluted antibiotics[59] are delivered frozen by the manufacturer and are available for gram-positive and gram-negative organisms and for urinary pathogens. Test results are expressed as the minimal inhibitory concentration (MIC) of a particular antibiotic for the organism being tested. This is similar to the result of the tube dilution test except that with the micro procedure a multiplicity of antibiotic determinations are made simultaneously on an 80-well disposable tray. The report form for the micro method is very helpful in that it includes information concerning the level of antibiotic expected in the various physiologic compartments of the body (blood, tissue, urine, and bile) according to the dosage selected and route of administration. With this information the physician can accurately select the best antibiotic for the patient. The range of dilutions for the various antibiotics is given in Table 32-9.

Agar plate dilution method

The method is similar to the tube dilution method except that a solid medium is used.[8]

Standardized single disk method for antibiotic susceptibility testing of anaerobic bacteria

Some question remains as to the validity of the results of any method of anaerobic sensitivity testing.

The standardized Kirby-Bauer method for sensitivity testing of aerobic bacteria cannot be used for anaerobic organisms because they grow too slowly. The method described by Wilkins et al.[60] can be used in the clinical laboratory since it requires only the already described Gaspak system and O_2-free CO_2. The media suggested are **prereduced** chopped (cooked) meat glucose (CMG) broth or prereduced chopped (cooked) meat carbohydrate (CMC) broth and supplemented BHI-S. The CMC broth is CM medium with 0.1% cellobiose, 0.1% soluble starch, and 0.4% glucose. The CMG is CM medium with 0.5% glucose added. The BHI-S broth is BBL BHI infusion broth supplemented with 0.0005% heme, 0.0002% menadione, and 0.5% yeast extract (BHI-S). For agar plates, 2.5% agar is added.

Prereduced media are media that are prepared under O_2-free CO_2 and are dispensed into tubes under O_2-free N_2 gas.[61] The prereduced media mentioned here are commercially available, ready for use from Robbin Laboratories, Chapel Hill, North Carolina. Colonies to be tested are picked and transferred under O_2-free CO_2 into CMC broth that is incubated anaerobically for 18 hr or until growth occurs and produces maximal turbidity. Then 1.5 ml CMC broth is added to 10 ml melted and cooled (50° C) BHI-S agar in rubber-stoppered tubes. The contents are mixed twice by inversion, poured into a plastic Petri dish (90 × 15 mm), and allowed to gel at room temperature.

The antibiotic disks used contain the following antibiotics: ampicillin, carbenicillin, cephalothin, clindamycin, penicillin, and tetracycline. They are applied by means of a commercial dispenser immediately before the plates are placed into a Gaspak jar fitted with a fresh catalyst. The plates are not inverted and are incubated for 18-24 hr at 37° C. The inhibition zone is measured as in the aerobic technic. Inhibition of 80% or more growth is considered a zone of inhibition. If more than one ring is formed, the most obvious zone of inhibition is measured.

Zone sizes given by Wilkins et al.[60] are listed in Table 32-10.

The anaerobic sensitivity testing method must be as carefully standardized as the Kirby-Bauer method for aerobic bacteria.

Sulfonamide sensitivity tests

Many of the commercially available 250 or 300 μg sulfonamide disks can be used with the Kirby-Bauer method, since the Mueller-Hinton medium contains only traces of *p*-aminobenzoic acid, not enough to neutralize sulfonamides.

Surveillance of use of antibiotics

Once a month the sensitivity pattern of the various bacteria should be tabulated and checked against the antibiotics used in the hospital. Antibiotic drugs should be carefully chosen, so that bacteriostatic drugs are not used when bactericidal drugs are indicated, or that potentially hazardous antibacterial drugs are administered in preference to less toxic but equally efficient drugs.

• • •

In the following discussion, bacteria are classified according to morphologic (cocci, rods, etc.) and tinctorial (Gram stain) characteristics.

GRAM-POSITIVE COCCI

Gram-positive cocci include *Streptococcus, Staphylococcus, and Sarcina*. Cocci are spheric bacteria.

STREPTOCOCCEAE

Streptococceae are gram-positive cocci occurring singly, in pairs, or in chains. They include the genera *Streptococcus* and a strict anaerobe, *Peptostreptococcus*. Normally, streptococci are found in the mouth, nasopharynx, and tonsils. Some groups inhabit the intestines. Pathologically, they are responsible for upper respiratory tract and wound infections, scarlet fever, acute glomerulonephritis, rheumatic fever, subacute bacterial endocarditis, and meningitis.

Streptococcus
Laboratory diagnosis

Specimen: The material submitted for culture usually consists of nasopharyngeal, tonsillar, or nasal swabs, sputum, blood, bone marrow, pus, exudate from infected wounds, pleural and peritoneal fluid, cerebrospinal fluid, urine, or feces.

For **handling of specimens,** see p. 808.

Morphology (Gram stain): Streptococci are gram-positive cocci that are spheric or elliptic in shape. They occur in pairs or in chains of varying lengths but not in packets. Some decolorize so easily that they may appear to be gram negative. Swollen, elongated, bizarre forms occur in old cultures or in response to antibiotic therapy. The cocci divide at right angles to their long axis. Most streptococci are nonmotile and show varying degrees of capsule formation, most marked in cocci of mucoid colonies.

Primary culture: Streptococci are able to grow in most media used for primary isolation of gram-positive organisms. These media are thioglycollate broth or trypticase soy broth and blood agar. For other media see "Isolation and identification of streptococci," published by the U.S. Department of Health and Human Services, Public Health Service.

Liquid media: Thioglycollate broth or trypticase soy broth is incubated at 35° C under 5-10% CO_2 tension. After overnight incubation, the liquid media are diffusely turbid if the streptococci form short chains, or they show snowflakelike accumulations or actual chains if the organisms form longer chains.

Solid media: Blood agar containing 5-10% defibrinated sheep blood is the solid medium of choice for primary isolation and classification of streptococci. The medium is incubated at 35° C under 5-10% CO_2 tension. Blood agar prepared with sheep blood is preferred because human blood may contain antistreptolysins, and sheep blood has the added advantage of inhibiting the hemolysis of *Haemophilus haemolyticus,* which macroscopically might be confused with streptococci. Defibrinated blood is used in the preparation of blood agar, since citrate-anticoagulated blood may inhibit streptococci.

On a solid medium the typical colony is small, discoid, and 1-2 mm in diameter. The colonies may be matte or glossy. Matte colonies are more likely to be virulent. On blood agar there may or may not be hemolysis. There are some strains that form minute, pinpoint-sized colonies surrounded by wide zones of hemolysis.

Hemolysis by streptococci

The hemolytic action of streptococci is due to two enzymes, streptolysin S and streptolysin O. Because streptolysin O is inactivated by atmospheric oxygen, colonies that produce only streptolysin O may on surface growth appear nonhemolytic. Methods that allow bacterial growth under reduced oxygen tension are best for studying this type of hemolysis. They are the pour plate method (p. 814) and undercutting the agar at the time of primary inoculation. Incubation under anaerobic conditions aids in the development of hemolysis.

Hemolysis is divided into three types—α, β, and γ. On the basis of the presence (or absence) and the type of hemolysis, streptococci are divided into three groups designated as (1) α-hemolytic streptococci (viridans), (2) β-hemolytic streptococci, and (3) nonhemolytic streptococci. To establish the type of hemolysis present, the blood agar immediately around and beneath the colonies is examined microscopically with the low-power lens under reduced light. The colonies should be about 24-48 hr old.

α-Hemolytic streptococci: The colony rests on and is surrounded by a greenish zone that microscopically reveals unhemolyzed, intact red cells. Outside this greenish zone there is a zone of hemolysis, the width of which varies. The α-hemolytic reaction can often be intensified by overnight refrigeration of the culture. Streptococci that, when cultured aerobically, develop α-hemolysis may, when grown anaerobically, produce β-hemolysis.

α-Hemolytic streptococci are often referred to as **viridans streptococci** or "green streps." They do not correspond to a specific serologic group. They grow at 45° C under 5-10% CO_2 tension, but they do not grow at a low temperature, at an alkaline pH (pH 9.6), in salt solution, or in 0.1% methylene blue dye solution. They are often associated with subacute bacterial endocarditis.

The α-hemolytic streptococci can be speciated[8]; however, the routine laboratory will usually not be required to differentiate between the multiple species of the "viridans" streptococci, e.g., *S. sanguis, S. mutans,* and *S. salivarius.*

α-Hemolysis is not restricted to streptococci; it is also produced by some *Escherichia coli, Streptococcus pneumoniae,* and micrococci.

Sensitivity to Optochin: α-Hemolytic streptococci can be distinguished from *Streptococcus pneumoniae* by the use of an Optochin disk. Streptococci are not sensitive to Optochin (Optochin differentiation disk), whereas pneumococci are inhibited.

β-Hemolytic streptococci: The colony rests on and is surrounded by a clear transparent zone of blood agar in which no intact red cells can be seen microscopically. The β-hemolytic zones of groups A and C streptococci are usually clear and wide, but not all group A, C, and G strains are β-hemolytic. Group B streptococci often produce a double zone of β-hemolysis. The first ring develops within 24-48 hr under incubation at 35° C and the second ring follows, separated from the first by a ring of intact red cells, when the culture, subsequent to 35° C incubation, is incubated at room or refrigerator temperature. β-Hemolysis is not diagnostic of streptococci or of group A streptococci, since some strains of group B and C (and others) are also β-hemolytic. In addition to the streptococci, *Haemophilus haemolyticus* and hemolytic staphylococci are also β-hemolytic. The Gram stain differentiates *H. haemolyticus* (a gram-negative small rod) from streptococci. Further, *H. haemolyticus* does not grow on sheep blood agar. Staphylococci can be differentiated from streptococci by the catalase test. Staphylococci are catalase positive, whereas streptococci are catalase negative (Table 32-11).

α-Hemolytic streptococci may at times be difficult to distinguish from β-hemolytic streptococci. In this case the culture should be repeated using the pour plate method and incubated under increased CO_2 tension or anaerobically.

• • •

Catalase test:

Principle: Some microorganisms contain the enzyme catalase, which liberates oxygen from hydrogen peroxide.

Procedure: Add 0.5 ml 3% hydrogen peroxide solution to bacterial growth transferred from a blood agar plate to a slide.

Results: Gas bubbles indicate the presence of catalase and are characteristic of staphylococci but do not occur with streptococci. In transferring the bacterial growth, care must be taken not to transfer any catalase-containing red cells. The test may also be performed on 0.5 ml broth culture, which must not include catalase-containing body fluids.

Control: Negative control streptococci and positive control staphylococci must be used to check on the activity of hydrogen peroxide. The latter must be kept in the refrigerator.

γ-Hemolytic streptococci: In γ-hemolytic studies the colonies are nonhemolytic. No macroscopic

Table 32-11. Identification of hemolytic streptococci*

Characteristics	Group A	Group B	Group C human	Group D (Streptococcus faecalis)
On blood agar				
Surface colonies	White to gray, opaque, hard, dry; 2 mm zones of β-hemolysis	Gray, translucent, soft; narrow β-hemolytic zone: a few RBCs may be observed microscopically under colonies	Similar to group A	Gray, translucent, soft; zone of hemolysis wider than colony; usually nonhemolytic
Subsurface colonies	2-2.5 mm zones of hemolysis, with sharply defined edges	0.5 mm zone of hemolysis after 24 hr; 1 mm zone of hemolysis after 48 hr; refrigeration produces double zones of hemolysis	Similar to group A	3-4 mm zones of hemolysis; usually nonhemolytic
Bacitracin susceptibility	Susceptible	Resistant	Resistant	Resistant
Sodium hippurate	Not hydrolyzed	Hydrolyzed	Not hydrolyzed	Not hydrolyzed
Growth at 10° C	−	−	−	+
Growth at 45° C	−	−	−	+
SF medium	No growth	No growth	No growth	Growth, acid
Bile-esculin agar	No growth	No growth	No growth	Growth; agar turns brown
6.5% NaCl broth	No growth	No growth	No growth	Growth
Source	Throat, blood, wounds, rarely spinal fluid	Urine, peritoneum, rarely blood, occasionally human throat	Throat, nose, vagina, intestinal tract	Urine, peritoneum, feces; milk and milk products
Pathogenicity	Septicemia, tonsillitis, scarlet fever, puerperal sepsis, pneumonia, erysipelas	Rare cases of endocarditis, meningitis, and female genital tract infections	Erysipelas, puerperal sepsis, throat infections; opportunistic pathogen	Subacute bacterial endocarditis; urinary tract infections

Modified from Finegold, S.M., Martin, W.J., and Scott, E.G.: Bailey and Scott's diagnostic microbiology, ed. 5, St. Louis, 1978, The C. V. Mosby Co.
*NOTE: Groups A, B, and C will not grow at pH 9.6 or in 0.1% methylene blue milk—two criteria that will distinguish them from group D (Streptococcus faecalis).

changes are seen in the red cells of the underlying and surrounding medium.

Serologic identification

On the basis of capsular group-specific carbohydrates (C-carbohydrate), streptococci are divided into serologic groups from A through T (Lancefield groups). Each Lancefield group is further subdivided by means of **M protein** (precipitation reaction) into M types and by means of **T antigens** (slide agglutination) into T types.[62]

Slide agglutination

An alternative to the precipitin test for streptococcal group identification is the slide agglutination test using latex particles (Streptex, Burroughs Wellcome and Co., Research Triangle Park, N.C.) or dead protein A−containing staphylococcal cells (Phadebact, Pharmacia Laboratories, Piscataway, N.J.) coated with group-spe-

cific antiserum. When sensitized latex particles are used, the C-carbohydrate is extracted enzymatically from a suspension of the streptococcal cells. When using the sensitized staphylococcal cell preparation, the streptococcal cells are used without extraction.

Group A streptococci (Streptococcus pyogenes)

Ninety percent of all human streptococcal infections are caused by group A streptococci, most of which are also β-hemolytic. Group A streptococci are characteristically sensitive to bacitracin, although 10% of groups B, C, and G may also be sensitive. Group C is usually resistant.

Group A streptococci do not usually grow on 10% bile agar, in 6.5% NaCl broth, at 45° C, or after heating at 70° C for 15 min, and they do not ferment mannitol or sorbitol.

Sensitivity to bacitracin: Place a **bacitracin differ-**

entiation disk (not sensitivity disk) on a heavily sur-
face-streaked segment of an agar plate. After 18-24 hr
of incubation, a clear zone will be seen around the disk
if the organisms are group A streptococci. Most other
streptococcal strains grow in the presence of the bacitracin differentiation disk.

Control: The activity of the disk should be assayed
with known resistant and sensitive streptococcal strains.

Lancefield grouping by precipitin test: Lancefield
grouping by the precipitin test has two phases: (1) preparation of streptococcal extract by acid heat extraction
of the C capsular antigen and (2) grouping by the precipitin test, using commercially available group A
streptococcus antiserum.

Preparation of streptococcal extract: Transfer a
pure culture of streptococci to 30 ml Todd-Hewitt broth
and incubate overnight at 37° C. Centrifuge broth culture for 30 min at 2000 rpm and discard supernatant
into disinfectant. Add to the sediment 1 drop 0.04%
metacresol purple (200 mg powder ground with 26.7
ml 0.2N sodium hydroxide, diluted to 5 dl with distilled water for working solution) and 0.3 ml 0.2N hydrochloric acid in physiologic saline solution. Mix with
capillary pipet and transfer to small tube. The suspension should be pink (pH 2.0-2.4). If necessary, add another drop or two of 0.2N hydrochloric acid.

Place suspension in a boiling water bath for 10 min.
Shake several times. Centrifuge for 30 min at 2000
rpm. Decant the supernatant, which is the extract, into
a clean tube. Discard the sediment into disinfectant.
Neutralize extract by adding 0.2N sodium hydroxide
carefully and slowly drop by drop until the color is lavender (pH 7.4-7.8). Avoid too alkaline a reaction, as
evidenced by a deep purple color. It may give rise to
false positive tests. Centrifuge for 10 min at 2000 rpm.
Decant the supernatant, which represents the extract,
into a small test tube. It can be stored in the refrigerator
in a small screw-capped vial.

Group precipitin test for group A streptococci:
Rehydrate commercial group A streptococcus antiserum. Dip sterile capillary tube (supplied by manufacturer of antiserum) into group A streptococcus antiserum and allow a 1 cm long column to rise in the tube
by capillary attraction. Remove tube and keep finger on
free end to prevent air from replacing serum. Wipe
capillary, insert into the prepared extract, and allow an
amount equal to the antiserum to enter the tube. Remove tube, keeping one finger on free end, and wipe
outside. Allow fluid column to rise to midportion of the
tube. There should be no air at the interface of extract
and antiserum, but there should be an air column at
either end of the tube. Invert capillary and insert gently
into soft Plasticine block. After 10 min, examine tube
against dark background for white ring at the center of
the column. Examine at frequent intervals between 10
and 30 min. False positive results may appear after
30 min.

Fluorescent antibody identification of group A streptococci

Direct smear method: The direct smear method for
fluorescent antibody (FA) identification of group A
streptococci[63] is similar to the one described below, but

the culture phase is eliminated. It may be used if a
duplicate gram-stained smear shows streptococci in
chains. Troublesome, interfering FA reactions of
groups C and G streptococci and *Staphylococcus aureus* may occur, so that this method should not be used.

**Method utilizing smears from cultured strepto-
cocci:**

Reagents:
1. Phosphate-buffered saline solution, pH 7.5 (Difco
   Laboratories, Detroit)
   a. NaCl, 8.77 g
   b. Na_2HPO_4, 1.42 g
   c. $NaH_2PO_4 \cdot H_2P$, 1.38 g
   d. Distilled water to 1 L
2. Fluorescein-labeled group A streptococcus antiserum (Difco Laboratories, Detroit)
3. Fluorescein-labeled group C streptococcus antiserum (Difco Laboratories, Detroit)

Procedure: Transfer β-hemolytic colonies as seen on
blood agar to 1 ml Todd-Hewitt broth. Incubate broth
for 4 hr at 37° C. Centrifuge for 5 min to pack the
bacteria. Pour off supernatant into disinfectant and resuspend bacteria in 1 ml phosphate-buffered saline solution, pH 7.2. Prepare duplicate smears of suspended
bacteria spreading 1 loopful throughout each etched circle on both FA microscopic slides. Air dry over lighted
microscope lamp. Fix with Bunsen burner flame. These
smears may be stored in the deep freeze as future controls and reference.

Cover smear nearest to the etched end of the slide
with a small drop of group A streptococcus antiserum
labeled with fluorescein. Cover second smear on slide
with mixture of labeled group A streptococcus antiserum (0.1 ml), labeled group C streptococcus antiserum
(0.15 ml), and buffered saline solution (2.75 ml).
Spread conjugate over entire smear with applicator
sticks held horizontally. Also stain previously prepared
known positive and negative controls that have been
stored in the deep freeze.

Cover slides with a large Petri dish lid fitted with
moist filter paper and allow to stand for 30 min in darkness at room temperature. Pour off excess conjugate
and rinse in free-flowing buffered saline solution. Continue rinsing in a container filled with buffered saline
solution for 10 min in darkness. Rinse quickly in distilled water. Blot slides very gently with new bibulous
paper and cover with small drops of **buffered glycerin-
saline solution** (1 part buffered saline solution and 9
parts glycerin) and cover with a no. 1 coverslip. The
completed preparations may be stored in the refrigerator. Examine smears with fluorescent microscope under
oil immersion with darkfield condenser.

Interpretation: If group A streptococci are present,
both smears on each slide will show fluorescing cocci
in chains. The fluorescence should be of grade 3+
(bright yellow-green).

Group B streptococci (Streptococcus agalactiae)

Group B streptococci together with groups C, G, and
F are found normally in material from the throat, vagina, and vulva. In blood agar pour plates they often
show a double zone of hemolysis. They hydrolyze so-

dium hippurate and do not grow at 45° C or in 6.5% NaCl broth. Serologic grouping is necessary for definitive identification.

Group C streptococci (Streptococcus dysgalactiae)

Group C streptococci produce mastitis in cows but are only occasionally found in human throat cultures and in puerperal sepsis. They are β-hemolytic and do not hydrolyze sodium hippurate nor do they grow on SF medium, but they are able to grow on 10% bile agar.

Group D streptococci (Streptococcus faecalis—enterococcus group)

The organism is found in the genitourinary and intestinal tracts and in throat cultures after treatment with antibiotics.

Most organisms show no hemolysis, but they may be β- or α-hemolytic. The organism is characterized by resistance to antibiotics and physical insults. It is bile-esculin positive and grows in 6.5% NaCl broth and on 40% bile-blood agar. It is a facultative anaerobe, able to grow at pH 9.6 and to resist heat, e.g., 60° C for 15 min. Enterococcus on blood agar may resemble staphylococcus, which may also grow in 6.5% NaCl broth but is **catalase** positive. The coagulase test does not distinguish between enterococcus and staphylococcus since both are coagulase positive. The enterococcus utilizes the citrate in the citrated plasma, which then clots.

Enterococci do not hydrolyze sodium hippurate, are able to grow in 0.1% methylene blue milk, liquefy gelatin, and grow on SF medium with acid reaction. They are able to ferment mannitol.

Heat resistance test: Plate a broth culture onto half of a blood agar plate. Heat the broth culture for 15 min at 60° C and plate it on the other half of the plate. If the organism has withstood the heating, equal growth will occur on both sides of the plate. *Streptococcus faecalis* resists heating.

Anaerobic streptococci (Peptostreptococcus)[64]

Anaeorbic streptococci are part of the normal flora of the mouth, skin, gastrointestinal tract, and genitourinary system. Pathologically they combine with *Bacteroides* and *Staphylococcus aureus* to produce necrosis. Fifty percent of anaerobic streptococci have a pungent odor, are chemically unreactive, and only liquefy gelatin.

Although the anaerobic streptococci are frequently not speciated, the genus *Peptostreptococcus* contains five species: *P. anaerobius, P. productus, P. lanceolatus, P. micros,* and *P. parvulus.* All of these species have been isolated from humans.

Streptococcal extracellular products of clinical importance

There are a number of streptococcal enzymes that are of clinical and laboratory significance. They include the following:

1. **Streptolysins O and S,** which are responsible for β-hemolysis of mainly group A streptococci but also of groups B and C
2. **α-Hemolysin,** which is responsible for α-hemolysis of viridans streptococci
3. **Streptokinase,** which activates plasminogen and lyses fibrin
4. **Deoxyribonuclease,** which destroys DNA of tissue cells
5. **Hyaluronidase** (spreading factor), which breaks down intracellular cementing substances

Antibodies to extracellular products of group A streptococci

In the course of streptococcal infections the extracellular products act as antigens to which the body responds by producing specific antibodies, which thus become indicators of streptococcal infection.

Antistreptolysin O titer: Almost 90% of patients with untreated streptococcal group A infection will show a rise in the antistreptolysin O (ASO) titer; i.e., there will be a rise in the concentration of the antibody directed against the streptococcal streptolysin O, which is oxygen labile (hence the name) and produces lysis of red cells. (Streptolysin S is not antigenic.) However, approximately 50% of patients with streptococcal-related acute glomerulonephritis will show a normal ASO titer but will elicit a rise to one of the other streptococcal antigens, e.g., NADase or DNAse B. Low titers of ASO antibody from 0-120 Todd units/ml may be found in normal individuals because of the frequency of subclinical streptococcal infections, but titers of 360 Todd units/ml and over are indicative of recent streptococcal infection. The titers begin to rise about 7 days after the onset of the infection and reach maximal levels after 4-6 weeks. A rise in titer of 50 Todd units in a 1-2 week period is of greater diagnostic significance than is a single titer level. A persistently low titer rules out group A streptococcal infection.

ASO titration[65]:

Principle: Streptolysin O, a streptococcal extracellular product, produces lysis of red cells unless it is inactivated. In the test procedure, streptolysin O is inactivated by the antistreptolysin antibody in the patient's serum. A constant quantity of commercially available streptolysin O antigen is added to progressively decreasing amounts of the patient's serum, which contains ASO. If the ASO level in the serum is sufficient to bind the added antigen, no hemolysis occurs when red cells are subsequently added. In the titration a point is reached when the antigen exceeds the antibody present in the serum, so that the excess streptolysin hemolyzes the added red cells.

The ASO titer is expressed as the reciprocal of the highest serum dilution that prevents hemolysis of red cells.

Procedure: The reagents and instructions are commercially available.

Normal values: 0-120 Todd units.

Interpretation: An elevated ASO titer is helpful in the diagnosis of recent group A streptococcal infections, acute rheumatic fever, and actue glomerulonephritis. The ASO titer is normal in rheumatoid arthritis.

Micro ASO test[66]: The micro serologic technic permits a considerable saving in reagents and time. The micro technic is rapid and reliable. It is thus indicated if there is much demand for ASO titrations.

Antistreptococcal hyaluronidase (ASH) titer: Most strains of group A streptococci produce hyaluronidase, which can be monitored by the appearance of antihyaluronidase in the patient's serum.

Mucin clot prevention test for quantitating antihyaluronidase:

Principle: A constant volume of hyaluronidase is added to serially diluted patient's serum, which contains antihyaluronidase. To determine whether the added hyaluronidase has been inactivated, a potassium hyaluronate solution and dilute acetic acid are added to each tube to form a clot. The free hyaluronidase dissolves the clot; the inactivated hyaluronidase does not. Beyond the level at which the antihyaluronidase is neutralized by the added hyaluronidase, the free hyaluronidase dissolves the clots.

Interpretation: The normal level is about 250 units. In streptococcal infections the titer exceeds 1042 units. A rising titer is more significant than a single titer level. The clinical interpretation is similar to the interpretation of the ASO titer.

Streptococcus pneumoniae

Physiologically, *Streptococcus pneumoniae* is found in the upper respiratory tract (nasopharynx) of 40-70% of normal individuals. Pathologically, it may invade the organs that drain into the nasopharynx and thus become the etiologic agent of lobar pneumonia, otitis media, sinusitis, tonsillitis, meningitis, and conjunctivitis.

Laboratory diagnosis

Specimen: Nasopharyngeal swabs, cerebrospinal fluid, sputum, vaginal excretion, pus, and synovial, pleural, and abdominal fluid are the material submitted.

Morphology (Gram stain):

Smear: Smears show pairs and short chains of gram-positive lanceolate diplococci. The free ends of the cocci are pointed, whereas the opposite ends, which are facing each other, are round.

The strongly gram-positive staining reaction of the young colonies is quickly lost as the culture ages. After 6 hr the organisms may become gram negative.

Other streptococci and enterococci that form gram-positive lanceolate diplococci may mimic *S. pneumoniae*. *Klebsiella*, which may occur as gram-negative lanceolate diplococci, may be confused with overdecolorized *S. pneumoniae*.

Quellung test: Although the Quellung test is not needed for the indentification of pneumococci, it provides a rapid method of determining capsular types and may be useful in the rapid diagnosis of pneumococcal disease. Knowing the antigenic type of the pneumococcus is not important in treatment with antibiotics but was important when therapeutic antiserum was used.

When viewed microscopically, the capsule of pneumococcus appears much larger in the presence of specific capsular antiserum. The method given below can be used on pure cultures as well as on organisms in clinical specimens.

Procedure: Place 1 drop of fresh sputum or 1 loopful of culture suspension or broth on a microscope slide.

Add 1 loopful of Loeffler methylene blue and mix with applicator stick. Then add 1 drop antiserum pool, mix again, apply coverslip, and examine under oil-immersion lens. A positive reaction should occur within 3-5 min up to 1 hr and is indicated by a definite increase in capsular size.

Prepare a control to which 0.95% saline solution is added instead of the antiserum pool. Examine this slide first to establish the normal size of the capsule.

The Quellung reaction is superior to the FA test, which is also available for rapid identification of *S. pneumoniae*. The FA test cannot be used on mixed cultures and materials, e.g., sputum, because of possible cross-reactions with other organisms.

Primary isolation:

Media: Blood agar and thioglycollate broth are incubated at 35° C under 3-5% CO_2 tension overnight.

Small, round, translucent, α-hemolytic, glistening colonies appear on blood agar. They are dome shaped when young but later develop central depressions (autolysis). Colonies of type 3 are larger and have the appearance of drops of water. The organisms grow diffusely in thioglycollate broth, forming a faint cloud.

Identification

For identification the following procedures are carried out: Optochin test or bile solubility test, and inulin fermentation.

Optochin test[67]: Optochin (ethylhydrocupreine hydrochloride, 1:4000) inhibits *S. pneumoniae* and is available in filter paper disks.

Procedure: Place a filter paper disk in heavily streaked blood agar plate and incubate for 17 hr at 35° C. *S. pneumoniae* in the vicinity of the disk may be lysed, so that a 15-18 mm zone of inhibition appears around the disk. α-Hemolytic streptococci, which closely resemble *S. pneumoniae* on blood agar, are not inhibited.

Controls: Use known *S. pneumoniae* and α-hemolytic streptococci as controls.

The Optochin disk can be applied on primary cultures of *S. pneumoniae* is suspected and can then be read after overnight incubation.

Bile solubility test[68]:

Reagent: Sodium deoxycholate, 2% solution, in sterile water.

Procedure: Place 1 drop of sterile 2% aqueous sodium deoxycholate directly over a pneumococcus-like colony on solid medium and then observe the colony for lysis using a hand lens. If the colony is a pneumococcus colony it will completely disappear in 3-5 min. The method can be applied to a turbid broth culture. A few drops of the solution will clear the turbid broth in a few minutes.

Inulin fermentation: *Streptococcus pneumoniae* is the only α-hemolytic streptococcus that ferments inulin. Inoculate 0.5% inulin fermentation medium with a pure culture. Pneumococci will give an acid reaction after overnight incubation.

Micrococcaceae

Micrococcaceae are gram-positive cocci that divide in more than one plane. They may occur as single cells or clusters. They are catalase positive, grow in 5%

NaCl broth, and are aerobic or facultatively anaerobic. There are three genera in this family: *Micrococcus, Staphylococcus,* and *Peptococcus.* Human pathogens are found in the genera *Staphylococcus* and *Peptococcus.*

Staphylococcus

On the basis of cultural and chemical characteristics, at least three species are recognized that are associated with human infection: (1) *S. aureus,* which is aerobic, hemolytic, and coagulase and mannitol positive; (2) *S. epidermidis,* which is aerobic, coagulase negative, and ferments glucose but not mannitol (*S. epidermidis* leads a saprophytic existence on normal skin and mucosa [nasopharnx]. It can also be demonstrated in air and dust.); and (3) *S. saprophyticus,* which is aerobic, coagulase negative, does not ferment mannitol, and is resistant to novobiocin.

S. saprophyticus is a causative agent of urinary tract infection.

S. aureus is responsible for skin infections (carbuncles, abscesses, and furuncles), impetigo, osteomyelitis, bronchopneumonia, and bacteremia. Some strains produce a heat-stable enterotoxin that is responsible for staphylococcal food poisoning.

Toxic shock syndrome[69, 70]

Staphylococcus aureus has been associated with a recently recognized syndrome most frequently seen in young women which appears to be associated with the use of vaginal tampons. The illness appears shortly after menstruation and is characterized by high fever, diarrhea, headache, conjunctivitis, abdominal tenderness, and erythematous rash. *S. aureus* is frequently isolated from the vagina, mouth, stool, and nose but not from blood cultures. The etiology of this disease remains unclear.

• • •

Antibiotic-resistant staphylococci are responsible for hospital-acquired infections and rare cases of enterocolitis following antibiotic therapy.

Laboratory diagnosis

Specimen: The material submitted for culture may be pus, drainage from fistulas and wounds, sputum, urine, feces, cerebrospinal fluid, fluid from serous cavities, and nasopharyngeal swabs. For **handling of specimens** and primary culture, see p. 808.

Morphology (Gram stain): Staphylococci are gram-positive spheres that characteristically appear in grapelike clusters but also appear singly, in pairs, and occasionally in chains of three or four that are morphologically difficult to distinguish from streptococci.

Primary culture: The primary isolation media are blood agar and thioglycollate broth incubated at 35° C under 3-5% CO_2 tension.

If the specimen is known to contain a variety of organisms (feces, sputum), the following media should be inoculated in addition: mannitol salt agar and phenylethyl alcohol agar.

Appearance on solid media: After 12-18 hr on blood agar, large, round, opaque, slightly convex colonies appear that have a smooth edge and may be white, yellow, or cream colored. They may be surrounded by zones of hemolysis. In some strains, hemolysis does not appear until later. Pigment production may also take several days; it is improved by exposure to sunlight and room temperature. It appears earlier if the material is subcultured to special media such as Loeffler agar or Chapman-Stone agar. If several colonies are scraped together on the agar surface, it is sometimes easier to appreciate pigment production. The color of the colonies bears little relationship to pathogenicity.

Laboratory methods to determine pathogenicity and virulence of staphylococci

Pathogenic staphylococci tend to be coagulase positive, hemolytic, pigment producing, mannitol fermenting, and gelatin liquefying.

Coagulase test:

Principle: Free coagulase released by staphylococci into the medium interacts with a plasma factor to produce clotting of plasma fibrinogen.

Procedure: In a small test tube, mix a loopful of organisms or 2 drops of an 18 hr broth culture with 0.5 ml reconstituted commercial desiccated coagulase plasma. Let stand up to 3 hr in the incubator and examine for clotting. Any clotting (firm clot, flocculi, or gelatinous globule) is positive. The earlier the clotting, the more coagulase is present. This test is critical for the diagnosis of pathogenic staphylococci.

Untested human or rabbit plasma may be unsatisfactory for the test; therefore pretested commercial plasma is preferable. Stock cultures of coagulase-positive staphylococci suitable for pretesting plasma may in time become coagulase negative. The plasma must contain adequate supplies of coagulase reacting factor (CRF) and fibrinogen and must lack inhibitors. Commercial plasma is not sterile, and incubation for over 3 hr is not recommended.

All staphylococcal colonies, irrespective of presence or absence of hemolysis or of pigmentation, must be tested for coagulase activity.

Slide test for clumping factor of staphylococci: The clumping factor, or bound coagulase, is different from free coagulase and the slide test must be used to demonstrate its presence. The bound coagulase does not require the presence of a plasma factor. A negative slide test must be checked with a coagulase tube test.

Procedure: Emulsify a single colony in 1 small drop of 0.85% sodium chloride on a slide. Add 1 small drop of coagulase plasma and mix. Read within 5 sec. Agglutinated strains are almost all coagulase positive. If there is no clumping, perform the coagulase tube test because a few coagulase-positive staphylococci are negative with the slide test. The slide coagulase test is a good screening test for coagulase.

Erroneous coagulase test results: False positive clotting results are produced by some gram-negative rods (*Serratia* and *Pseudomonas*) and by *Streptococcus faecalis,* since they utilize the citrate anticoagulant of the plasma so that the plasma clots.

False negative clotting results may be caused by small amounts of coagulase, which may require overnight incubation to be detected.

Staphylococcus epidermidis

Morphologically, tinctorially, and culturally, *Staphylococcus epidermidis* and *Staphylococcus saprophyticus* are similar to *Staphylococcus aureus* except that the colonies are usually white and the organism is coagulase and mannitol negative and nonhemolytic on blood agar. *S. epidermidis* is rarely pathogenic, but *S. saprophyticus* is.

Micrococcus

Micrococci are gram-positive, coagulase-negative, catalase-positive, nonmotile cocci occurring in pairs, irregular clusters, and tetrads. They only utilize glucose aerobically. They are often isolated from fomites, air, and dairy products.

Peptococcus

The genus *Peptococcus* is made up of the anaerobic staphylococci that are usually found in mixed infections. These organisms are rarely isolated as the only cause of infection and their significance is difficult to assess. The eighth edition of *Bergey's Manual of Determinative Biology*[9] describes five species: *P. niger, P. asaccharolyticus, P. aerogenes, P. activus,* and *P. anaerobius.* All of these species have at one time or another been isolated from humans.

GRAM-NEGATIVE COCCI

NEISSERIACEAE
Neisseria

Neisseria are gram-negative, bean-shaped diplococci that embrace *N. gonorrhoeae, N. meningitidis, N. lactamicus,* and *N. sicca,* among other species.

Neisseria can be divided into two groups, group I consisting of the pathogens *N. gonorrhoeae* and *N. meningitidis,* and group II consisting of bacteria that are usually classified as nonpathogens, e.g., *N. sicca* and *N. lactamicus.*

Neisseria gonorrhoeae

Neisseria gonorrhoeae is the cause of urethritis, cervicitis, salpingitis in adults (gonorrhea), vulvovaginitis in children, and ophthalmia in newborns.

Laboratory diagnosis

Specimen: Material is usually submitted on swabs taken from the urethra, cervix, rectum, vagina, and Skene's and Bartholin's glands.

Morphology (Gram stain):

Smear: Intracellular gram-negative diplococci may appear singly or in groups within the cytoplasm of pus (polymorphonuclear) cells; also, some extracellular organisms may be present. The contiguous sides are flattened or slightly concave, while the lateral contour is convex, so that the organisms resemble paired kidney beans. They measure 0.6-1.0 μm in diameter (Plate 16, opposite).

It is not wise to make a diagnosis of *N. gonorrhoeae* without a culture, since some gram-negative coccobacilli, e.g., *Acinetobacter* species and *N. (Branhamella) catarrhalis,* and coliform bacteria have shapes suggesting *N. gonorrhoeae*. Decolorized diphtheroids, streptococci, and staphylococci may also resemble *Neisseria*. The report of the smears should read "intracellular gram-negative diplococci resembling *N. gonorrhoeae* are (are not) found." If only extracellular organisms are seen after adequate search, a repeat specimen should be examined and cultured. A statement as to the number of pus cells should also be included in the report, i.e., few or many.

The diagnosis of gonorrhea in men is frequently made on the basis of the Gram stain but is best confirmed by culture. In women with chronic infection the smear is usually negative and cultures **must** be obtained.

Primary culture and isolation: The medium of choice is Transgrow medium[30] (Tg bottles) or Thayer-Martin medium[30] (TM plates). Chocolate agar may be used, but the first two media are preferred because they are specific, selective, and sensitive, and they suppress organisms other than *N. gonorrhoeae* and *N. meningitidis.*

Immediate culture is necessary. Culture should be made directly onto Tg (transport and growth) medium or TM medium, in which the organisms survive 48 hr or longer without incubation. If it is not possible to make the culture promptly, place the swab in Stuart transport medium, in which the organisms survive 24 hr. In the laboratory the swab is used to streak Tg medium in a Z pattern from base to top. For a description of the application of Tg and TM media, see p. 822. If a swab is submitted in Amies or Stuart transport media, roll swab on TM plate in a Z pattern and cross streak before incubation. The culture must be incubated at 35-36° C under 3-10% CO_2 tension. The latter may be provided by a candle jar (p. 814), the atmosphere of which is kept moist by inserting wet filter paper into the screw top. The above-mentioned media may be ob-

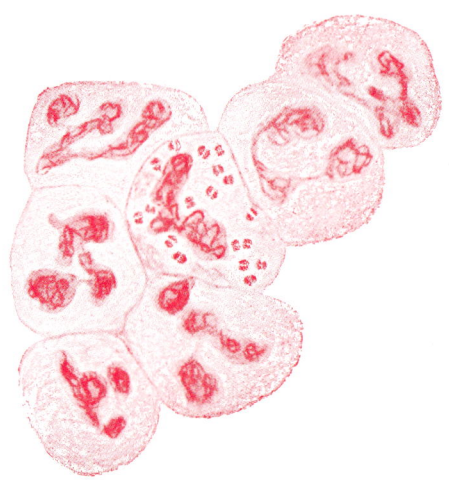

Plate 16. Gonococci in a cervical smear showing well-preserved pus cells and characteristic clear spaces around organisms.

tained in a JEMBEC (John E. Martin Biological Environmental Container, Centers for Disease Control) plate. This plate is used with a small capsule that produces CO_2 when wetted, which assures an increased CO_2 supply for early growth and eliminates the need for a candle jar.

Since the colonies are small (1-3 mm in diameter), slightly elevated, grayish, and rubbery mucoid, a portion of a colony cannot be easily separated. They are transparent and have lobate margins.

Prepare gram-stained smears from selected colonies. Because of the rapid autolysis, many atypical forms may be seen.

Presumptive diagnosis

Oxidase test: *Neisseria* produces an oxidizing enzyme that, in the presence of air, acts on some aromatic amines to produce colored compounds. The test is not diagnostic for *N. gonorrhoeae* since other species of *Neisseria,* some yeasts, and *Pseudomonas* are also oxidase positive, but these organisms are suppressed on Tg and TM media and are culturally different from *Neisseria.* Gram-negative diplococci grown on Tg and TM media, which are oxidase positive, allow a presumptive diagnosis of gonorrhea. The diagnosis must be confirmed by sugar fermentation or by a positive FA test.

The oxidase test can be used to detect colonies of *Neisseria* in mixed cultures or to confirm their presence in pure culture.

Procedure: Small amounts (0.5 ml) of 1% aqueous solution of dimethyl-*p*-phenylenediamine are kept frozen in the deep freeze. After thawing, the solution is either dropped onto the colony on a solid medium or 1 drop is added to filter paper and the colony to be tested is spread onto the impregnated paper. In a positive reaction the colonies become pink, then red, and finally purple-black. On solid agar the colonies usually remain viable through the pink stage, in which they may be subcultured, but they are killed by the reagent on longer contact. The reagent does not interfere with the Gram stain or the FA technic.

Definitive identification

Definitive identification is based on possible FA staining or on typical carbohydrate fermentation.

Direct fluorescent antibody identification: The fluorescent antibody (FA) procedure may be performed as an immediate direct test or as a delayed direct test on an 18 hr culture that is oxidase positive on Tg or TM media. The delayed method will be described, since the immediate method is not recommended because of its lack of specificity.

Procedure[71]: Prepare a thin smear on a slide having an etched circle 6 mm in diameter. Place a loopful of distilled water in the area of the circle, lightly touch a loop or needle to the suspected colony, emulsify the material in the water, and spread as thinly as possible over the etched circle and the surrounding area. Air dry the smear. (Smears may be prepared from a colony and stained with fluorescein-labeled conjugate up to 15 min after the colony has been treated with oxidase reagent.)

The FA **staining technic** proceeds as follows: Thoroughly air dry and gently heat fix the smear. Place a full 3 mm loopful of GC conjugate evenly over the specimen **within the 6 mm circle** and incubate at room temperature for 5 min. Prevent drying.

Gently rinse smears in running distilled water. Air dry or blot gently with clean bibulous paper. Mount with a coverslip, using a mounting medium of 9 parts glycerin and 1 part carbonate-bicarbonate buffer, pH 9.0. Examine the smears with a fluorescence microscope fitted with a $10\times$ ocular, a $100\times$ oil-immersion objective, a BG-12 primary filter, and a Corning 3-72 (3387) or equivalent secondary filter (GG9). The gonococci appear as yellow-green diplococci.

With this method, use a positive urethral smear or a smear prepared from a known fresh isolate of gonococci as a positive staining **control.** Use a smear of a boiled suspension of *Enterobacter cloacae* as a nonspecific staining control.

Carbohydrate fermentation (oxidation): A presumptive identification of a culture as *N. gonorrhoeae* can be confirmed by carbohydrate fermentation. *N. gonorrhoeae* ferments only glucose, producing acid and no gas. A semisolid medium such as cystine trypticase agar (BBL, BioQuest Div., Becton-Dickinson & Co., Cockeysville, Md.) containing phenol red as an indicator of acid production is used as the basic medium. Glucose, maltose, sucrose, and lactose are added to individual tubes to make 1% carbohydrate solutions.

Inoculation of medium: In order to have a more uniform inoculum in **all** carbohydrate tubes, prepare a heavy suspension of organisms from a chocolate agar plate in 0.5 ml sterile trypticase soy broth (TSB) or sterile distilled water. With a sterile bacteriologic loop, transfer a loopful of the heavy suspension of organisms to the surface and area just below the surface of the

Table 32-12. Differentiation of *Neisseria**

Species	Sugar fermentation				Oxidase reaction
	Glucose	**Maltose**	**Sucrose**	**Lactose**	
N. meningitidis	+	+	−	−	+
N. gonorrhoeae	+	−	−	−	+
N. (Branhamella) catarrhalis	−	−	−	−	+
N. sicca	+	+	+	−	+
N. lactamicus	+	+	−	+	+

* +, Acid (Yellow); −, no reaction.

carbohydrate medium, or using a sterile, plugged, disposable capillary pipet, add 2-3 drops of the heavy suspension to the surface of the medium. Replace cap and tighten; incubate at 35-36° C without added CO_2 tension. The culture must be pure; otherwise, contaminants will cause erroneous fermentation reactions.

Examine tubes at 24, 48, and 72 hr for growth and production of acid (indicator changes from red to yellow) (Table 32-12). Prepare a gram-stained smear of the growth from tubes giving an acid reaction and examine for purity of culture.

Acinetobacter species are also oxidase positive, but none of the sugars (glucose, maltose, and sucrose) are fermented.

Coagglutination test: A rapid slide test is available that is best done on pure cultures grown on TM medium or chocolate agar (Phadebact Gonococcus Test, Pharmacia Laboratories, Piscataway, N.J.). Although not a replacement for carbohydrate fermentation tests, the coagglutination test may be helpful when *Neisseria* organisms grow poorly or produce little acid.

Neisseria meningitidis

Physiologically, *Neisseria meningitidis* is found in the nasopharynx of normal carriers (3% of the population). During the winter season, carriage may increase to 30-40%. Pathologically, *N. meningitidis* is responsible for such diseases as meningitis, septicemia, bacteremia, endocarditis, and pneumonia.

N. lactamicus is found in normal throats and will be identified as *N. meningiditis* unless lactose is added to the fermentable carbohydrates. *N. lactamicus* is lactose positive, whereas the meningicoccus is lactose negative. Both organisms ferment maltose and glucose.

Veillonella parvula and *Veillonella alcalescens* are anaerobic organisms found in the mouth that may be confused with *Neisseria,* since these organisms appear as gram-negative diplococci. Neither specimen is pathogenic.

Laboratory diagnosis

Specimen: Spinal fluid, blood culture, nasopharyngeal swabs, swabs from petechial skin lesions, and sputum are the material used. For handling of specimen and primary culture, see also p. 841.

The organism is very susceptible to drying and must therefore be plated immediately or kept in transport medium.

Morphology (Gram stain):

Smear: Spinal fluid is centrifuged in sterile containers, and a smear is made from the sediment or from cultures of spinal fluid, sputum, and material from the throat. Prepare spinal fluid smear as soon as the specimen is received. The organism is an intracellular and extracellular gram-negative diplococcus with flattened adjacent sides and curved lateral borders. The physician should be informed as soon as meningococci are suspected. In the case of spinal fluid, supportive evidence must be provided by other spinal fluid findings, e.g., pleocytosis and low sugar and high protein levels.

Primary culture and isolation: All specimens are plated on inhibitory media such as TM and Tg media[72] and on chocolate agar only if TM and Tg media are not

available. Mueller-Hinton broth is the suggested liquid medium. Incubate at 35° C under 5-10% CO_2 tension. A candle jar with inserted moistened filter paper may be used. After 24-48 hr, smooth, 2-3 mm, moist, gray, mucoid colonies appear. They are translucent and have a musty odor.

Spinal fluid itself is a good culture medium, and the remaining sediment and supernatant should be incubated at 35° C under increased CO_2 tension.[73]

Presumptive identification

Oxidase test: The oxidative test is the same as for *N. gonorrhoeae.*

Definitive identification

Definitive identification is established by a characteristic carbohydrate fermentation (oxidation) pattern and by a positive FA test.

Carbohydrate fermentation: Table 32-12 shows differentiating fermentation reactions of gram-negative diplococci. Inoculate semisolid cystine trypticase agar (CTA) containing 1% solutions of glucose, maltose, lactose, and sucrose. See discussion of *N. gonorrhoeae* for further information.

Direct fluorescent antibody technic: The direct FA method for *N. meningitidis* is similar to the FA method for *N. gonorrhoeae.*

Serologic identification

Polyvalent antisera are available and should be used to confirm the diagnosis of meningococci by means of a slide test. The organisms are emulsified in a small amount of 0.1% potassium cyanide saline solution to which the polyvalent serum is added. If agglutination occurs in the polyvalent serum, repeat the test with meningococcal groups A to D antisera. Slide agglutination serum may also be used for typing by capsular swelling. This procedure can be done directly on spinal fluid. There is some importance to the typing of meningococci because group A is usually associated with epidemics, while groups B and C are linked to sporadic cases. Serogroups X, Y, and Z are associated with upper respiratory tract infection and meningitis in adults.

Diagnosis of bacterial meningitis by counterimmunoelectrophoresis

Counterimmunoelectrophoresis (CIE), which was established as a method for the detection of Australia antigen (see p. 1032), is now used for the identification of meningococcal,[74] pneumococcal,[75] and *Haemophilus*[76] antigens in biologic fluids, including cerebrospinal fluid. The CIE method is specific and highly sensitive, allowing the three most common bacterial agents associated with meningitis to be identified within 30 min.

GRAM-NEGATIVE AEROBIC NON-SPORE-FORMING BACILLI
ENTEROBACTERIACEAE

Physiologically, certain genera of the family Enterobacteriaceae—the coliform enteric bacteria—are found in the intestinal tract. *Escherichia coli* is the most com-

Table 32-13. Classification of Enterobacteriaceae*

Edwards and Ewing	Bergey's Manual (ed. 8)
Family: Enterobacteriaceae	Family: Enterobacteriaceae
Tribe I: Escherichieae	Genus I: Escherichia
Genus I: Escherichia	Species: *E. coli*
Species: *E. coli*	Genus II: Edwardsiella
Genus II: Shigella	Species: *E. tarda*
Species: *S. dysenteriae*	Genus III: Citrobacter
S. flexneri	Species: *C. freundii*
S. boydii	*C. intermedius*
S. sonnei	Genus IV: Salmonella
Tribe II: Edwardsielleae	Species: *S. cholerae-suis*
Genus I: Edwardsiella	*S. typhi*
Sepcies: *E. tarda*	*S. enteritidis*
Tribe III: Salmonelleae	Genus V: Shigella
Genus I: Salmonella	Species: *S. dysenteriae*
Species: *S. cholerae-suis*	*S. flexneri*
S. typhi	*S. boydii*
S. enteritidis	*S. sonnei*
Genus II: Arizona	Genus VI: Klebsiella
Species: *A. hinshawii*	Species: *K. pneumoniae*
Genus III: Citrobacter	*K. ozaenae*
Sepcies: *C. freundii*	*K. rhinoscleromatis*
C. diversus	Genus VII: Enterobacter
Tribe IV: Klebsielleae	Species: *E. cloacae*
Genus I: Klebsiella	*E. aerogenes*
Species: *K. pneumoniae*	Genus VIII: Hafnia
K. ozaenae	Species: *H. alvei*
K. rhinoscleromatis	Genus IX: Serratia
Genus II: Enterobacter	Species: *S. marcescens*
Species: *E. cloacae*	Genus X: Proteus
E. aerogenes	Species: *P. vulgaris*
E. hafnia	*P. mirabilis*
E. agglomerans	*P. morganii*
Genus III: Serratia	*P. rettgeri*
Species: *S. marcescens*	*P. inconstans*
S. liquefaciens	Genus XI: Yersinia
S. rubidaea	Species: *Y. enterocolitica*
Tribe V: Proteeae	*Y. pseudotuberculosis*
Genus I: Proteus	*Y. pestis*
Species: *P. vulgaris*	Genus XII: Erwinia (plant pathogens)
P. mirabilis	Species: *E. herbicola* (has been considered
P. morganii	a human pathogen)
P. rettgeri	
Genus II: Providencia	
Species: *P. stuartii*	
P. alcalifaciens	
Tribe VI: Yersineae	
Genus I: Yersinia	
Species: *Y. enterocolitica*	
Y. pseudotuberculosis	
Y. pestis	
Tribe VII: Erwinieae (plant pathogens)	
Genus I: Erwinia	
Genus II: Pectobacterium	

From Finegold, S.M., Martin, W.J., and Scott, E.G.: Bailey and Scott's diagnostic microbiology, ed. 5, St. Louis, 1978, The C. V. Mosby Co.
*Recent taxonomic changes have established a new genus, *Morganella,* and a new species, *M. morganii,* to replace *P. morganii.* Similarly, *P. rettgeri* is now *Providencia rettgeri.*

mon coliform organism in the intestines, whereas *Enterobacter, Klebsiella, Citrobacter, Proteus,* and *Providencia* are found in small numbers.

Pathologically, all genera may be responsible for sporadic or epidemic diarrheal diseases, acute gallbladder infections, genitourinary tract infections, appendicitis, peritonitis, septicemia, and bacteremia. The latter may lead to irreversible shock and diffuse intravascular coagulation (DIC). Some genera are mainly plant parasites; others are pathogens.

Classification

There are two major classification schemes in use today: *Bergey's Manual of Determinative Bacteriology,* ed. 8,[9] and Edwards' and Ewing's *Identification of the Enterobacteriaceae.*[77] The latter will be used throughout this writing (Table 32-13).

Enterobacteriaceae are divided into seven tribes, and each tribe is divided into several genera.[78-80]

Antigens

The coliform bacteria possess a **somatic antigen (O),** a **capsular antigen (K),** and, if motile, a **flagellar antigen (H).**

The O antigen is heat stable and is not inactivated by heating (100° C for 1 hr), whereas most K antigens are inactivated by heating (100° C for 1 hr). The K antigen inhibits the agglutination of the O antigen of the living organism. Some organisms have specific K antigens, e.g., the Vi antigen of *Salmonella typhi* and the L, A, and B antigens of *Escherichia coli.* The H antigen is also inactivated by heating (100° C for 1 hr). It determines the serotype of a specific somatic group.

Laboratory diagnosis

Specimen: The material submitted for culture usually consists of feces, but it may be blood, spinal fluid, bile, material from wounds and abscesses, urine, throat swabs, etc. For collection and handling of specimens, see p. 841.

Morphology (Gram stain):

Direct smear: Prepare a Gram stain from all liquid stools (hemorrhagic and mucoid particles) and from material submitted in preservative solution or in enrichment medium. Enteric bacteria are gram-negative, nonspore-forming, straight, plump, small rods. If the material is old, long filamentous forms may appear. Usually *Escherichia coli* does not have a well-developed capsule. The appearance of the smear cannot be relied on for distinction of enteric gram-negative rods, but the smear allows recognition of staphylococci, yeast, and **pus.** The presence of much pus indicates shigellosis and contraindicates the diagnosis of amebiasis (wet saline preparation). Candidiasis is suggested by large numbers of budding yeast cells and pseudohyphae.

If the Gram stain suggests gram-positive cocci, inoculate one phenylethyl alcohol plate to suppress the growth of enteric gram-negative rods and to support the growth of staphylococci and streptococci.

Primary isolation: A battery of **noninhibitory** and only slightly **inhibitory** plating media are used along with enrichment media for primary culture of feces, urine, and bile. Gram-negative bacteria found in the course of culture of nonfecal specimens are subcultured onto the same media. The media mentioned are discussed in more detail on p. 813.

Primary media: Blood agar, MacConkey agar (or Endo agar), xylose-lysine-deoxycholate (XLD) agar (or Salmonella-Shigella [SS] agar), and bismuth sulfite (BS) agar serve as primary media. Since blood agar is noninhibitory and MacConkey and XlD agar are only slightly inhibitory, they should be lightly inoculated. The selective media SS and BS should be inoculated more heavily.

Table 32-14. Composition of suggested enteric differential media

Medium	Gram-positive bacteriostatic agent	Fermentable carbohydrate	Indicator	Colony color	
				Fermenters	Nonfermenters
MacConkey agar	Crystal violet, bile salts	Lactose	Neutral red	Pink	Colorless
XLD agar	Bile salts	Xylose, lactose, sucrose	Phenol red and H$_2$S indicators	Yellow	Pink-red

Table 32-15. Composition of suggested enteric selective media

Medium	Gram-positive bacteriostatic agent	Fermentable carbohydrate	Indicator	Colony color	
				Fermenters	Nonfermenters
Salmonella-Shigella (SS) agar	Bile salts	Lactose	Neutral red	Pink	Colorless
Bismuth sulfite (BS) agar	Brilliant green	Glucose	Bismuth sulfite	Salmonellae produce black colonies	

Enrichment media: Inoculate GN broth (or tetrathionate or selenite broth). Emulsify 1 g feces (2-3 ml liquid material) in 8-10 ml broth and mix well. Incubate solid media overnight at 35° C. The broth tubes should be incubated no longer than 12-16 hr. This is best accomplished by leaving them at room temperature until evening and then incubating them overnight. After incubation, subculture the GN broth onto MacConkey agar, XLD agar, SS agar, and BS agar. GN broth enriches the growth of *Salmonella* but only supports the growth of *Shigella*.

After overnight incubation, examine the solid media for colony identification.

Blood agar: Blood agar allows the recognition of staphylococci, yeast, and enteric gram-negative organisms. The latter produce shiny, convex, opaque colonies, some of which may be α-hemolytic. The pattern of growth is suggestive at times of a particular family, e.g., some *Proteus* species "swarm"; *Klebsiella* and *Enterobacter* are mucoid and may "string"; and *Serratia* species may be pigmented. *Pseudomonas* species and *Flavobacterium,* which do not belong to the Enterobacteriaceae family, produce pigmented colonies. *Pseudomonas* species are responsible for a "fruity" odor.

Enteric differential and selective media: The suggested media (MacConkey, XLD, SS, and BS agars) contain gram-positive bacteriostatic agents and a fermentable carbohydrate, usually lactose, as well as an indicator dye to differentiate lactose-fermenting from non-lactose-fermenting organisms. For composition, see Tables 32-14 and 32-15.

Incubation: All media are incubated at 35° C for 18 hr (overnight).

Biochemical identification

After overnight incubation, lactose-fermenting and non-lactose-fermenting colonies are subcultured, **each** to a series of biochemical media. The GN broth culture lags 1 day behind, since its biochemical identification must await the results of its growth on the inhibitory and selective media. If the subculture of GN broth on MacConkey and XLD agars reveals a "new" type of colony, a third biochemical set is inoculated. If it does not reveal "new" colonies, the GN broth procedure is not carried any further.

Lactose-fermenting colonies from MacConkey and XLD agars are used to inoculate a "short" biochemical set, which consists of the following:

TSI agar
Christensen urea agar slant
SIM agar
Methyl red broth
Simmons citrate agar
Decarboxylase broth
  Lysine
  Ornithine
  Arginine
  Control
ONPG for slow lactose fermenters

Non-lactose-fermenting colonies from MacConkey and XLD agars are subcultured to the following "long" set of media:

TSI agar slant
Christensen urea agar slant
Simmons citrate agar
Phenylalanine agar
SIM agar
MR-VP broth
Decarboxylase broth
  Lysine
  Ornithine
  Arginine
  Control
Bismuth sulfite agar, if typhoid fever is suspected

The main components, purpose, and method of inoculation of the media mentioned are discussed on p. 813.

Triple sugar iron (TSI) agar slant: After 18 hr incubation, representative colonies from MacConkey and

Table 32-16. Triple sugar iron agar reactions

	Reaction		Products		Carbohydrates fermented			
Group	Slant	Butt	Gas in butt	H$_2$S	Glucose	Lactose	Sucrose	Possible organisms
1	Acid	Acid	+	−	+	+	+	*Escherichia coli, Klebsiella, Enterobacter, Proteus, Providencia, Enterobacter hafniae*
2	Acid	Acid	+	+	+	+	+	*Arizona, Citrobacter*
3	Alkaline	Acid	+	+	+	−	−	*Proteus, Salmonella, Arizona, Citrobacter, Edwardsiella*
4	Alkaline	Acid	−	−	+	−	−	*Shigella, Salmonella typhi, Proteus, Providencia, Salmonella, Serratia, Escherichia,* late fermenters
5	Alkaline	Alkaline	−	−	−	−	−	*Alcaligenes, Pseudomonas, Flavobacterium, Acinetobacter**

*These organisms do not belong to the family Enterobacteriaceae.

XLD (or SS) agars are subcultured to TSI medium. Pink (from SS) or yellow (from OXD) pure colonies are subcultured to TSI tubes. Colorless or black (from SS) or pink (from XLD) colonies are subcultured to another set of TSI tubes. Use a heated and cooled staight wire to touch only the dome of the colonies on MacConkey and XLD agars and do not penetrate to the level of the agar (see discussion of selective media, p. 813). Stab the entire length of the butt of the TSI agar first and then streak the slant from the butt up.

Incubate TSI agar slants at 35° C and examine after 18-24 hr. The screw caps of the TSI tubes must allow air to enter so as to prevent erroneous results.[81]

TSI agar contains 1% lactose, 1% sucrose, 0.1% glucose, ferrous sulfate, and phenol red as indicator. All Enterobacteriaceae ferment glucose, but not all ferment lactose or sucrose, and some ferment lactose only gradually.

Reactions on TSI agar (Table 32-16):

1. Fermentation of glucose only (by non-lactose- and non-sucrose-fermenting organisms) produces acid throughout the medium (yellow) at first (12 hr); but as soon as the small amount of glucose (0.1% is used up, oxidation at the surface of the slant leads to neutralization of the acid so that the final results, after about 24 hr, are an acid butt (yellow) and an alkaline slant (red).

2. Fermentation of lactose and sucrose produces enough acid throughout the medium to maintain butt and slant yellow. Some bacteria that ferment lactose

slowly can metabolize sucrose readily so that they still produce enough acid to maintain butt and slant yellow.

3. Fermentation of sucrose only usually does not produce enough acid to change the pH of the entire medium, so that the butt turns yellow but the slant changes to red.

4. If none of the three sugars is fermented, the butt and slant become alkaline (red).

5. Gas-forming organisms produce gas bubbles in the butt, which are evident on inspection if the butt has been carefully stabbed.

6. H_2S production leads to blackening of the butt.

TSI is a poor medium by which to judge H_2S production because the medium is deficient in sulfhydryl groups and contains ferrous sulfate as indicator, which is less sensitive than lead acetate of SIM agar. See also the discussion of TSI agar on p. 847.

Identification of lactose-fermenting Enterobacteriaceae

See also discussion of individual genera and Tables 32-17 to 32-22. On the basis of the first four tests of the "short" biochemical set, *E. coli* can be confirmed as seen in Table 32-17. The majority of lactose fermenters other than *E. coli* can be identified on the basis of the "short" biochemical set, as shown in Table 32-18.

The remaining species of *Enterobacter* (also *Serratia*) may be identified by subculture onto arabinose, raffinose, and rhamnose. The use of **TSI** and **urea agar combination** allows the recognition of *E. coli*, *Klebsiella*, *Enterobacter*, and *Proteus* (Table 32-19).

Identification of non-lactose-fermenting Enterobacteriaceae

See also discussion of individual genera and Tables 32-20 to 32-22. The combination of **TSI, SIM,** and **urea agars** allows quick identification of *Proteus* species (Table 32-29).

Table 32-17. Biochemical identification of *Escherichia coli*

	TSI reaction group	SIM	MR	Citrate
E. coli	1	− + +	+	−

Table 32-18. Biochemical identification of majority of lactose fermenters other than *Escherichia coli*

	TSI reaction group	SIM	MR	Citrate	Lysine	Ornithine	Arginine
Citrobacter	2 or 1	+ − +	+	+	−	+ / −	+ , late
Arizona	2 or 1	+ − +	+	+	+	+	+ , late
Klebsiella	1	− − −	−	+	+	−	−
Enterobacter cloacae	1	− − +	−	+	−	+	+

Table 32-19. Presumptive identification of Enterobacteriaceae on basis of combined TSI and urea agar reactions

	TSI reaction group	Urea agar
Escherichia coli	1	−
Klebsiella, Enterobacter	1	± , slant only
Proteus	3 or 4	+ , throughout agar column

Table 32-20. Identification of *Salmonella* and *Arizona*

	Dulcitol	Malonate
Salmonella	+	−
Arizona	−	+

Table 32-21. Reactions of Enterobacteriaceae using "long" biochemical set*

| | TSI | | | | Urea | Indole | MR | VP | Citrate | PPA | Motility | KCN | Decarboxylases | | |
	Slant	Butt	Gas	H₂S									Lysine	Arginine	Ornithine
Shigella	K	A	–	–	–	+ or –	+	–	–	–	–	–	–	– or (+)	– or +
Escherichia	A or K	A	+ or –	–	–	+	+	–	–	–	+ or –	–	+ or –	+ or –	+ or –
Salmonella (general)	K	A	+	2-4+, rare –	–	–	+	–	+	–	+	–	+	(+)	+
S. typhi	K	A	–	+ or –	–	–	+	–	–	–	+	–	+	– or (+)	–
Arizona	K or A	A	+	2-4+	–	–	+	–	+	–	+	–	+	(+)	+
Citrobacter	K or A	A	+	2-4+	– or + s	–	+	–	+	–	+	+	–	(+)	– or +
Klebsiella	A	A	+	–	– or + s	–	– or +	+	+	–	–	+	+	–	–
E. cloacae	A	A	+	–	– or + s	–	–	+	+	–	+	+	–	+	+
E. aerogenes	A	A	+	–	– or + s	–	–	+	+	–	+	+	+	–	+
E. hafniae															
37° C	K	A	+	–	–	–	+	+ or –	+ or –	–	+ or –	+	+	–	+
22° C	K	A	+	–	–	–	–	+	+	–	+	+	+	–	+
Serratia	K	A	– or + w	–	– or + s	–	–	+	+	–	+	+	+	–	+
P. vulgaris	A or K	A	+	2-4+	+	+	+	–	+ or –	+	+	+	–	–	–
P. mirabilis	K or A	A	+	4+	+	–	+	+ or –	+	+	+	+	–	–	+
P. morganii	K	A	–	–	+ or ½ +	+	+	–	–	+	+	+	–	–	+
P. rettgeri	K	A	– or +	–	+	+	+	–	+	+	+	+	–	–	–
Providencia	K	A	– or +	–	–	+	+	–	+	+	+	+	–	–	–
Edwardsiella	K	A	+	3+	–	+	+	–	–	–	+	–	+	–	+

From Douglas, G.W., and Washington, J.A.: Identification of Enterobacteriaceae in the clinical laboratory, Atlanta, 1972, Bacterial Reference Unit, Centers for Disease Control.
*PPA, Phenylalanine; s, slant; E, *Enterobacter*; p, *Proteus*; w, weak positive reaction.

Table 32-22. Differentiation of Enterobacteriaceae by biochemical tests*

	Escherichieae		Edwardsielleae	Salmonelleae				Klebsielleae								Proteae						Yersinieae			Erwinieae	
						Citrobacter			Enterobacter				Serratia			Proteus				Providencia		Yersinia				
	Escherichia	Shigella	Edwardsiella	Salmonella	Arizona	freundii	diversus	Klebsiella pneumoniae	cloacae	aerogenes	hafniae	agglomerans	marcescens	liquefaciens	rubidaea	vulgaris	mirabilis	morganii	rettgeri	alcalifaciens	stuartii	pestis†	pseudotuberculosis‡	enterocolitica‡	Erwinia§	Pectobacterium†
Indole	+	− or +	+	−	−	−	+	−	−	−	−	− or +	−	−	−	+	−	+	+	+	+	−	−	−	−	− or +
Methyl red	+	+	+	+	+	+	+	− or +	−	−	− or +	− or +	− or +	+ or −	− or +	+	+	+	+	+	+	+	+ 35°C + 25°C	+	−	+ or −
Voges-Proskauer	−	−	−	−	−	−	−	+	+	+	+ or −	+ or −	+	− or +	+	−	− or +	−	−	−	−	− 35°C − 25°C	− 35°C − 25°C	− 35°C + or − 25°C	+	+ or −
Simmons citrate	−	−	−	d	+	+	+	+	+	+	d	d	+	+	+ or (+)	d	+ or (+)	−	+	+	+	−	−	−	+	d 35°C + + or (+) 25°C
Hydrogen sulfide (TSI)	−	−	+	+	+	+	−	−	−	−	−	−	−	−	−	+	+	−	−	−	−	−	−	−	−	−
Urease	−	−	−	−	−	d	d	+	+	+	+	d	d	d	d	+	+	+	+	−	−	−	+	+	−	d
KCN	−	−	−	−	−	+	+	+	+	+	+	− or +	+	+	− or +	+	+	+	+	+	+	−	−	−	−	− or +
Motility	+ or −	−	+	+	+	+	+	−	+	+	+	d	+ or (+)	+ or (+)	+ or −	+	+	+ or −	+	+	+	− 35°C − 25°C	− 35°C (+) or + 25°C	− 35°C + 25°C	+	+ or (+)
Gelatin (22° C)	−	−	−	−	−	−	−	−	− or (+)	−	−	d	+	+	+ or (+)	+	+	−	−	−	−	−	−	−	+	+ or (+)
Lysine decarboxylase	d	−	+	+	+	−	−	+	−	+	+	−	+	+	+	−	−	−	−	−	−	−	−	−	−	−
Arginine dihydrolase	d	d	−	+ or (+)	+ or (+)	d	d	−	+	−	−	−	−	−	−	−	−	−	−	−	−	−	−	−	−	−
Ornithine decarboxylase	d	d#	+	+	+	d	+	−	+	+	+	−	+	+	−	−	+	+	−	−	−	−	−	+	−	−
Phenylalanine deaminase	−	−	−	−	−	−	−	−	−	−	−	− or +	−	−	−	+	+	+	+	+	+	−	−	−	−	−
Malonate	−	−	−	−	+	− or +	− or +	+	+ or −	+ or −	+ or −	+ or −	−	−	+ or −	−	−	−	−	−	−	−	−	−	−	− or +

Gas from glucose	+	−#	+	+	+	+	+	+	d	d	+	+	−	− or + 35°C / d 25°C
Lactose	+	−#	−	+	d	+	+	d	d	+	+	−	−	d 35°C / + or (+) 25°C
Sucrose	d	−#	−	(+) or +	d	+	+	d	−	d	+	+	+	+ or − 35°C / + 25°C
Mannitol	+	+ or −	+	+	+	+	+	+	+	+	+	−	−	+ or −
Dulcitol	d	d	d††	+ or +	d	−	d	−	−	−	−	−	−	−
Salicin	d	−	−	+ or +	d	+	+	d	d	d	+	d	+	d 35°C / + 25°C
Adonitol	−	−	−	− or +	+	−	−	−	−	−	−	−	−	w
Inositol	−	−	d	+	d	+	−	d	d	d	+	d	d	−
Sorbitol	d	d	+	+	+	+	+	d	d	+	+	−	+ or +	−
Arabinose	+	d	+††	+	+	+	+	−	−	d	+	+	+	+ or − 35°C / + or (+) 25°C
Raffinose	d	d	−	+	d	+	+	d	−	d	+	−	− or +	d 35°C / + or + 25°C
Rhamnose	d	d	−	+	+	+	d	d	d	+	+	−	+	d

From Finegold, S.M., Martin, W.J., and Scott, E.G.: Bailey and Scott's diagnostic microbiology, ed. 5, St. Louis, 1978, The C. V. Mosby Co.
*Adapted from Edwards, P.R., and Ewing, W.H.: Identification of Enterobacteriaceae, ed. 3, Minneapolis, 1972, Burgess Publishing Co.
†Adapted from Sonnenwirth, A.C.: In Lennette, E.H., Spaulding, E.H., and Truant, J.P., editors: Manual of clinical microbiology, ed. 2, Washington, D.C., 1974, American Society for Microbiology.
‡Adapted from Darland, G., Ewing, W.H., and Davis, B.R.: The biochemical characteristics of *Yersinia enerocolitica* and *Yersinia pseudotuberculosis*, DHEW Publ. no. (CDC) 75-8294, Washington, D.C., 1974, Department of Health and Human Services.
§Adapted from Buchanan, R.E., and Gibbons, N.E., editors: Bergey's manual of determinative bacteriology, ed. 8, Baltimore, 1974, The Williams & Wilkins Co.
‖Majority of strains isolated in the United States are indole positive, whereas most of the strains isolated in Europe have been indole negative.
¶Rare exceptions.
#Certain biotypes of *S. flexneri* produce gas; cultures of *S. sonnei* ferment lactose and sucrose slowly and decarboxylate ornithine.
**Gas volumes produced by cultures of *Serratia, Proteus,* and *Providencia* are small.
††*S. typhi, S. cholerae-suis, S. enteritidis* bioser, *paratyphi-A* and *pullorum* and a few others ordinarily do not ferment dulcitol promptly. *S. cholerae-suis* does not ferment arabinose. +, 90% or more positive in 1 or 2 days; −, 90% or more negative; d, different biochemical types [+, (+), −]; (+), delayed positive (decarboxylase reactions, 3 or 4 days); + or −, majority of cultures positive; − or +, majority negative; w, weakly positive reaction.
NOTE: This chart is simply a guide. Users are urged to consult other publications, such as CDC publications entitled "Biochemical Reactions Given by Enterobacteriaceae in Commonly Used Tests" and "Differentiation of Enterobacteriaceae by Biochemical Reactions," for percentage data, additional tests, and references.

Identification of Shigella

All shigella are nonmotile and the vast majority do not produce gas or ferment lactose (Table 32-21). Test all TSI group 4 urea-negative cultures with *Shigella*-grouping antisera.

Identification of Salmonella-Arizona-Citrobacter group

Test all TSI group 3 bacteria that are urea-negative, nonlactose fermenters, and produce H_2S with **Salmonella antisera.**

Arizona can be differentiated from *Salmonella* using dulcitol and malonate, producing the reactions shown in Table 32-20.

Citrobacter is KCN positive and lysine negative and may give a positive urea slant after overnight incubation (Table 32-22).

• • •

TSI group 5 organisms do not ferment carbohydrates of the TSI medium (including lactose) and are not in the Enterobacteriaceae family *Pseudomonas aeruginosa* can be identified on the basis of its metallic sheen and its fruitlike odor.

Escherichia and Shigella

Escherichia and *Shigella* are assigned to the same division because they share many biochemical and serologic reactions. They are both methyl red positive; they are both Voges-Proskauer, Simmons citrate, urease, KCN, gelatin liquefaction, and phenylalanine deaminase negative; and both lack H_2S production on TSI.

Escherichia coli

Escherichia coli organisms occur in the gastrointestinal tract of humans and in sewage and soil and may be responsible for infections in the genitourinary tract, wounds, lungs, skin, etc.

E. coli are gram-negative rods. The most useful clue to this genus is the characteristic IMViC pattern of + + − − . *E. coli* are indole and methyl red positive and Voges-Proskauer and citrate negative. Most strains are motile, and the motility improves at lower temperatures. On blood agar some strains are α-hemolytic and mucoid. They grow well in thioglycollate broth but are inhibited by enrichment media; 80% are lysine decarboxylase positive (Table 32-22). Most strains ferment lactose, producing acid and gas promptly, and must be differentiated from *Klebsiella* and *Enterobacter* by the use of malonate broth and the IMViC reaction. *E. coli* leaves malonate broth unchanged (green), whereas *Klebsiella* and *Enterobacter* turn it blue. Some strains ferment lactose slowly, and some do not ferment it at all. Slow lactose fermenters may produce an acid butt and alkaline slant, no gas, and no H_2S on TSI and thus may be confused with *Proteus* and *Shigella*. *Proteus* is urea and phenylalanine deaminase positive, while *E. coli* is urea and phenylalanine deaminase negative.

Escherichia can be differentiated from *Shigella* by the fact that *Shigella* is always nonmotile, whereas *Escherichia* is usually motile (70%). The lysine decarboxylase test is always negative in *Shigella* and usually positive in *Escherichia*. *Shigella* is agglutinable with *Shigella* antisera.

IMViC reactions

When it is necessary to differentiate *Escherichia* from other coliform organisms, the use of four tests designated by the mnemonic formula IMViC is indicated. These tests are **indole production, methyl red reaction, Voges-Proskauer reaction,** and **citrate reaction.** In practice, the performance of only two tests (indole and methyl red) may be sufficient. Test tablets for all these procedures are commercially available (Key Scientific Products, Los Angeles). The tablets are handled with sterile forceps, dissolved in sterile distilled water, and the resulting solution is inoculated.

Some typical IMViC formulas are *E. coli* + + − − and *Klebsiella* − − + + . The usefulness of the IMViC formula as a diagnostic tool is diminished by the fact that some *Enterobacter* and *Serratia* have a − − + + formula and some *Shigella* have a + + − − formula. Other organisms give intermediate reactions, e.g., + − + − or − + − + .

Antigens

Escherichia coli possesses a **somatic O antigen,** a **flagellar H antigen,** and a **capsular K antigen,** which is divided into three varieties—L, A, and B. The O antigen consists of several groups (about 150), and in addition to the groups, serotypes are determined on the basis of the K and H antigens. The most important K antigen is the B variety. K antigens inhibit the agglutination of living *E. coli* by O antisera, so that O antisera do not agglutinate live bacterial suspension. OB sera are able to agglutinate live bacteria containing O and B antigens. If B antigen (like most K antigens) is destroyed by heating, the live cells become agglutinable by O antisera. The antigenic composition (serotype) of one strain of *E. coli* may thus be expressed as O26:B6.

Enteropathogenic Escherichia coli

E. coli has been shown to be the cause of enterocolitis in newborns and infants. The disease may occur as an isolated case or in epidemic form. The strains causing this disease have been serotyped according to their somatic antigens (O antigens) and one of their capsular antigens (B antigen). This group of serotypes of the pathogenic organism is classified as enteropathogenic *E. coli* (EPEC). Typing sera (Lederle Diagnostics, American Cyanimide Co., Pearl River, N.Y.) are available to identify these organisms. However, recently many pathogenic strains have been isolated from adults with diarrhea ("travellers' diarrhea")[82] that were not of the EPEC serotypes. Furthermore, since no close correlation betwee serotype and toxin production can be demonstrated,[83] serotyping to identify pathogenic *E. coli* has generally been discontinued.

Two types of toxin have been demonstrated in pathogenic *E. coli*. A heat-labile enterotoxin (LT) is produced that is detected by injecting the ligated rabbit ileum with a culture filtrate. If present, the ileum will become dilated after 18 hr. This heat-labile toxin is antigenic, and in the future a serologic procedure may be expected to provide the clinical laboratory with a means of identifying toxigenic strains. These stains are called enterotoxigenic *E. coli* (ETEC).[84]

A second and probably less important toxin is produced by some strains of *E. coli*. This toxin is heat stable (ST), nonantigenic, and has a smaller molecular weight than the heat-labile enterotoxin. This toxin is demonstrated by the use of newborn mice. There are other tests of toxin production but all are technically difficult and expensive and consequently have not found widespread application.

Shigella

Shigella is the causative organism of bacillary dysentery. The identification of *Shigella* is based on cultural, biochemical, and serologic findings.

Laboboratory diagnosis

Specimen: Dysenteric bacilli are difficult to isolate, especially after the first few days of the disease. Hemorrhagic and purulent particles in liquid stool should be cultured immediately on receipt of the specimen. Specimens obtained from the rectum on a swab and plated immediately or sent to the laboratory in transport medium give best results.

Culture: For handling of specimen and primary inoculations, see p. 841. Organisms that produce acid (but not gas) in butt, alkaline slant, and no H_2S on TSI and that are nonmotile should be tested with *Shigella* group antisera A to D.

Serologic identification

Macroscopic slide test: Divide a microscope slide into two sections by marking with a wax pencil. Place 1 drop *Shigella* antiserum onto one section and 1 drop 0.5% saline solution onto the other section. This will serve as a negative control. Transfer 1 loopful of the culture taken from a solid medium to the saline solution and 1 loopful to the antiserum. Mix well to emulsify the mixtures. Tilt the slide back and forth for 1-2 min to enhance agglutination. Positive agglutination will be rapid and complete. Perform this procedure with group A antiserum; if no reaction occurs, proceed to groups B, C, and D.

A positive reaction with a polyvalent group antiserum identifies the organism as a member of that *Shigella* group. Final identification of the specific type within a group is accomplished by using individual type-sepecific sera (Difco Laboratories, Detroit).

Cultures that show the characteristics of *Shigella* but fail to react with antisera should be suspended in saline solution and heated at 100° C for 30 min and then retested with *Shigella* group antisera A to D, since heat-labile K antigen may inhibit O agglutination; this testing should be performed in a reference laboratory.

Biochemical identification

Shigella fails to grow on Simmons citrate or on KCN medium and does not hydrolyze urea. It does not contain phenylalanine deaminase or lysine decarboxylase.

Edwardsiella[85]

Edwardsiella tarda is a motile gram-negative rod that grows well on MacConkey or SS agar and is non-lactose-fermenting. It shares the following biochemical reactions with *E. coli:* indole and methyl red tests are positive; Voges-Proskauer. Simmons citrate, KCN, urease, phenylalanine deaminase, and gelatin tests are negative. It differs from *E. coli* in that it does not ferment lactose, sucrose, and mannitol.

Since it ferments glucose (not lactose or sucrose) with gas formation, and since it produces H_2S (3 +), its TSI pattern is group 3, suggesting *Salmonella*. It differs from *Salmonella* in that the latter ferments mannitol and is indole negative. It shares with *Salmonella* a positive reaction to the lysine decarboxylase test.

If *E. tarda* is suspected, mannitol agar should be inoculated.

Salmonella-Arizona-Citrobacter

The entire division of *Salmonella, Arizona,* and *Citrobacter* shares the following reactions: they are indole, Voges-Proskauer, urease (except some *Citrobacter*), and phenylalanine negative; methyl red and Simmons citrate tests are usually positive. H_2S is usually produced on TSI agar.

The species within the genera are differentiated on the basis of carbohydrate reactions, as listed in Table 32-22.

Salmonella

Salmonella[86] organisms are pathogens that can be isolated from feces, urine, and blood. They may also be found in bile, bone marrow, or sputum. Their habitat is the gastrointestinal tract of humans and wild and domestic animals. The organism has also been found in food products, water, milk, fish, and organic fertilizers.

Salmonella infections are responsible for gastroenteritis and bacteremia (enteric fever) and may lead to a carrier state.

Laboratory diagnosis

Specimen: Blood, stool, and urine are the specimens used. Bacteremia occurs usually during the first 7-10 days when blood cultures are positive. Stool cultures become positive after the first week and remain positive during the course of the disease. Urine cultures are often positive after the first 7-10 days.

Culture and isolation: The majority of *Salmonella* fall into TSI group 3, producing an acid butt, alkaline slant, gas, and H_2S. Some produce gas but no H_2S. *S. typhi* produces little H_2S and no gas. Any organism that produces a group 3 pattern on TSI agar and is urease negative should be considered to be a possible *Salmonella* strain and must be serologically confirmed (or not confirmed) as *Salmonella* by the use of polyvalent *Salmonella* O antiserum.

Antigenic structure

Salmonella species are divided into groups on the basis of their thermostable **O (somatic) antigen** and are subdivided into serotypes on the basis of their thermolabile **H antigen, the flagellar antigen.** The groups are denoted by capital Roman letters (A, B, C, etc.). Each group is serologically subdivided into factors denoted by Arabic numerals (1, 2, 3, etc.). The H antigen is divided into serogroups denoted by small Roman letters

Table 32-23. Antigenic formulas of four common *Salmonella* species

Species	Group	Somatic O antigens	Flagellar H antigens Phase 1	Phase 2
S. paratyphi A	A	1, 2, 12	a	—
S. paratyphi B	B	1, 4, 5, 12	b	1, 2
S. paratyphi C	C	6, 7, Vi	c	1, 5
S. typhi	D	9, 12, Vi	d	—

(a, b, c, etc.) for phase 1 and Arabic numerals (1, 2, 3, etc.) for phase 2. Occasionally a third antigen, the Vi antigen, which is a capsular surface antigen, is present in some *Salmonella* strains. It is thermolabile and prevents the agglutination of O antigen by anti-O sera. It must therefore be heat inactivated before proceeding with the serologic typing of organisms containing Vi antigen (Table 32-23).

Serologic identification

Principle: The heat-stable O antigen is identified first by the use of polyvalent *Salmonella* O antiserum. If screening with polyvalent *Salmonella* O antiserum is positive, the somatic group is identified by using *Salmonella* O group A, B, C_1, C_2, D, and E antisera. If the first two screenings are positive, report *Salmonella* O group A or B or C, etc. Further serologic identification should be performed in a reference laboratory.

Technic of serologic O grouping: The same technic is used for typing *Shigella* except that the antisera are different.

Macroscopic slide test:

Procedure: Use commercially available antisera (BBL, BioQuest Div., Becton-Dickinson & Co., Cockeysville. Md.; Difco Laboratories, Detroit). Prepare a dense suspension of the organism to be tested in normal saline solution, using an 18 hr growth on TSI agar. Using a wax pencil, mark off a microslide into two rectangular sections. Place 1 drop of polyvalent *Salmonella* O antiserum into one square. Transfer 1 loopful of bacterial suspension to the antiserum and mix serum and antigen with the loop, producing an oblong pattern. Continue mixing by tilting the slide back and forth for 1-2 min. Place 1 drop of saline solution into the second square of the slide and add 1 loopful of bacterial suspension; mix, tilt as before, and observe as control of roughness of bacterial suspension. Saline control should be run simultaneously with each test.

Results: Positive agglutination must be rapid and complete. No agglutination or delayed agglutination is considered negative.

Antigenic formulas of four common *Salmonella* species are given in Table 32-23.

If agglutination occurs with polyvalent *Salmonella* O antiserum, proceed further to identify the group O (A, B, C, etc.) to which the organism belongs, using *Salmonella* O group antisera and the technic described above for the polyvalent serum.

If the culture reacts with *Salmonella* polyvalent O antiserum but does not react with the specific *Salmonella* O antisera groups, it should be checked with *Sal-*

monella Vi antiserum. If there is no agglutination with the *Salmonella* Viantiserum at this point, the culture may be regarded as not of the *Salmonella* genus. If the culture reacts with the *Salmonella* Vi antiserum, the culture suspension in saline solution should be heated to 100° C in a boiling water bath for 30 min and cooled. After cooling, the heated culture should be retested with the individual *Salmonella* O antisera groups A, B, C, etc., and with *Salmonella* Vi antiserum. If the organism does not react with the Vi antiserum after heating, but, for instance, does react with *Salmonella* O antiserum group D, it is most likely *S. typhi* and the diagnosis should be confirmed by testing an unheated saline suspension of the culture with *Salmonella* H antiserum group d. If the heated culture continues to react with Vi antiserum and does not react with any of the *Salmonella* O antisera, the organism may be *Citrobacter* and should be tested in KCN broth.

Salmonella typhi

If typhoid fever is suspected, **bismuth sulfite agar** should be added to the list of differential and selective media. *Salmonella typhi* produces black colonies with a metallic sheen on this medium whereas other *Salmonella* species are usually dark green with black centers.

The biochemical reactions of *S. typhi* are at variance with the great majority of *Salmonella*. *S. typhi* produces little H_2S and no gas. It does not utilize Simmons citrate (Tables 32-20 and 32-21).

Serologic identification

If *S. typhi* lacks the capsular Vi antigen, the *Salmonella* typing procedure will identify *S. typhi* as *Salmonella* O group D. If the biochemical findings support the diagnosis of *Salmonella*, the organism can be diagnosed presumptively as *S. typhi*.

If the Vi antigen is present, it will interfere with the agglutination of the organism by polyvalent *Salmonella* O antiserum (Difco Laboratories, Detroit). If, despite a negative polyvalent *Salmonella* O antiserum test, *S. typhi* is suspected, test a saline suspension of the organisms against the following three antisera: polyvalent *Salmonella* O antiserum, *Salmonella* O antiserum group D, and *Salmonella* Vi antiserum. Do not omit a saline control to judge the roughness of the live bacteria.

Results (Table 32-24)**:** No agglutination with any of the three *Salmonella* antisera indicates that the organism is not a *Salmonella* species. Agglutination with polyvalent serum only suggests that the organism may be a *Salmonella* species other than group D. Repeat the test using *Salmonella* O antisera of other groups (A, B, C_1, etc.). If there is agglutination with Vi antiserum only, or with Vi antiserum strongly and weakly with polyvalent *Salmonella* O serum, *S. typhi* is the presumptive diagnosis.

If the culture reacts with the Vi antiserum, the culture suspension should be heated in boiling water for 15 min. After cooling, the heated culture should be retested with the above three *Salmonella* antisera (polyvalent, group &, and Vi) and with a saline control to judge the degree of roughness of the heated culture. If the organism does not react with the Vi antiserum after heating but does react with polyvalent *Salmonella* O

Table 32-24. Reactions of *S. typhi* with three *Salmonella* antisera

Salmonella antiserum	Antigen	
	Live bacteria	Heated bacteria
Polyvalent O	± or −	+
O group D	−	+
Vi	+	−

Table 32-25. *Salmonella-Arizona-Citrobacter* division*

Substrate or test	*Salmonella*	*Arizona*	*Citrobacter*
Lactose	−	+ or ×	+ or ×
Dulcitol	+	−	d
Gelatin	−	(+)	−
KCN	−	−	+
Lysine decarboxylase	+	−	−
Arginine dihydrolase	− or (+)	− or (+)	(+)
Ornithine decarboxylase	+	−	− or +
Malonate	−	+	−

From Ewing, W.H., and Edwards, P.R.: The principal divisions and groups of Enterobacteriaceae and their differentiation, Atlanta, 1962. Communicable Disease Centers.

*+ Positive in 1 or 2 days: − negative; (+), delayed positive; ×, late and irregularly positive; d, different biochemical types; − or +, majority of strains negative but positive varieties occur.

NOTE: The majority of salmonellae ferment dulcitol promptly, but *S. typhi*, *S. pullorum*, *S. paratyphi* A, *S. cholerae-suis*, and a few others do not do so. Members of *Arizona* group are uniformly negative on this substrate. *S. paratyphi* A is lysine negative. *S. typhi* is ornithine negative.

antiserum and the *Salmonella* O group D antiserum, the diagnosis is *S. typhi* (Table 32-24).

If the heated culture reacts with Vi antiserum and does not react with the other *Salmonella* antisera, the organism may be *Citrobacter*. Confirm the identification with the lysine decarboxylase reaction (negative) and with the KCN test (positive).

Agglutination test for enteric fever: Agglutination tests are used to detect antibodies in the patient's serum against *Salmonella* antigens, e.g., the antigens of *S. paratyphi* A, *S. paratyphi* B, *S. paratyphi* C, and *S. typhi* O and H. This collective group of tests, called **febrile agglutination tests,** is used also to diagnose brucellosis, tularemia, and rickettsial diseases, depending on the nature of the homologous antigen.

Principle: The patient's serum is titrated for the presence of antibodies to homologous, commercially obtainable suspensions of bacterial antigens. If the homologous antibody is present, the patient's serum will agglutinate the antigen.

Procedure: Add the patient's serum in varying dilutions to a constant amount of antigen in a slide test. With a 0.2 ml pipet, deliver 0.08, 0.04, 0.02, 0.01, and 0.005 ml quantities of the patient's serum to the rings or squares of a glass slide from left to right. Mix the contents of the antigen vial, and by means of the dropper provided, place 1 drop of antigen on each quantity of serum in one row. Mix the serum-antigen mixture in the row with a wooden applicator stick, moving from right to left. Rotate the slide for 3 min.

The highest dilution producing agglutination represents the serum titer. The dilutions are 1:20, 1:40, 1:80, 1:160, and 1:320. If the titer is greater than 1:320, dilute the serum 1:10 with saline solution and repeat the test. The dilutions will then be 1:200, 1:400, 1:800, etc.

Interpretation: A single agglutination titer is of little value. A rising titer (fourfold) 3-5 days apart is significant.

Low titers (1:20 to 1:80) may be caused by immunization or an anamnestic reaction, or they may be normal for some individuals. A rise in titer usually occurs in the first 8-15 days of enteric fever. A high O titer (over 1:160) is indicative of active infection even if the H titer remains low. A normal titer does not rule out an infection, since there may not have been enough time for the titer to develop.

Arizona

Members of the genus *Arizona* are pathogenic organisms that are gram-negative, short, motile rods closely related to salmonellae. On MacConkey agar they pro-

duce colorless colonies. On TSI agar they produce a *Salmonella*-like pattern (alkaline slant, acid butt, H$_2$S). *Arizona* differs from *Salmonella* by liquefying gelatin slowly in 7-20 days and by slowly utilizing malonate and lactose. If *Arizona* does not form H$_2$S, it has to be distinguished from *E. coli* and *Citrobacter*. *Arizona* will grow on Simmons citrate; *E. coli* will not. *Arizona* is lysine decarboxylase positive and KCN negative, while *Citrobacter* gives opposit reactions (Table 32-25).

Occasionally *Arizona* strains will agglutinate *Salmonella* antisera and vice versa. In human material, *Salmonella* is the more likely diagnosis. The organism should be sent to a reference laboratory for confirmation of identification.

Citrobacter

The organisms called *Citrobacter*, which were formerly called *Escherichia freundii*, are gram-negative motile rods that generally ferment lactose slowly. There are two species in the genus, *C. freundii* and *C. diversus*. They may be separated by ornithine decarboxylase and adonitol fermentation. *C. freundii* is positive for both reactions and *C. diversus* is negative for both reactions. The colonies on MacConkey agar may be colorless to pale pink. On TSI agar they produce group 2 or rarely group 3 reactions with H$_2$S. They give a positive urea agar test after 18-24 hr of incubation, grow on Simmons citrate, and are indole and Voges-Proskauer negative and methyl red positive. They may have to be distinguished from *Arizona*, *Salmonella*, and possibly *Proteus*. The negative lysine decarboxylase reaction and growth in KCN broth distinguish these organisms from *Arizona* and *Salmonella*. The delayed urease test distinguishes them from *Proteus* (Table 32-22).

Klebsiella-Enterobacter-Serratia

Typical cultures of these three genera (Table 32-22) are indole, methyl red, phenylalanine deaminase, and H₂S negative. Urease is not present or gives a delayed reaction. The organisms are KCN and Voges-Proskauer positive. They ferment lactose rapidly, except for *Serratia*.

Klebsiella

The *Klebsiella* organism is, at times, responsible for a severe form of pneumonia (Friedländer's pneumonia).

Laboratory diagnosis

Specimen: Stool, sputum, urine, and blood are used.
Morphology (Gram stain): The organisms are encapsulated, gram-negative, short rods.
Culture: On MacConkey agar they produce large, pink, mucoid colonies that may "string" when touched with the inoculating loop. The organism is nonmotile.

Biochemical reactions

Klebsiella species are active fermenters of lactose and other sugars with production of acid and gas (TSI reaction group 1). They are indole, methyl red, phenylalanine, H₂S, and ornithine decarboxylase negative. *Klebsiella* are Voges-Proskauer, urease, and lysine decarboxylase positive. The urease reaction is delayed and involves only the slant. The IMViC formula is usually $- - + +$ (p. 850) but may be $- + - +$.

Klebsiella does not liquefy gelatin at 22°C.

Two other species of *Klebsiella* are *K. ozaenae* and *K. rhinoschleromatis*. Both of these organisms cause chronic disease of the respiratory tract. The three species may be separated by the biochemical reactions shown in Table 32-26.

Table 32-26. Separation of the *Klebsiella* species

	M-R	V-P	Malonate
K. pneumoniae	−	+	+
K. ozaenae	+	−	−
K. rhinoschleromatis	+	−	+

Enterobacter

The organisms are found wherever *E. coli* is encountered: intestinal tract, soil, contaminated water, etc. The species of this genera are very similar to *Klebsiella* but differ in that they are motile and ornithine decarboxylase positive (Table 32-22).

Four species are identified: *E. cloacae*, which is the most common form, *E. aerogenes*, *E. hafniae*, and *E. liquefaciens* (Table 32-27). The remaining species of *Enterobacter* and *Serratia* can be identified by subculture onto arabinose, raffinose, and rhamnose.

Serratia

Serratia species are isolated with increasing frequency from patients on steroid and antibiotic therapy, in whom they are responsible for a great variety of infections.[87,88]

Serratia consists of three species: *S. marcescens*, *S. liquefaciens*, and *S. rubidaea*, with *S. marcescans* one of the more recognized or important hospital pathogens. These species are differentiated by the reactions shown in Table 32-28.

Laboratory diagnosis

Specimen: Sputum, urine, and stool are the material used.
Morphology (Gram stain): The organisms are gram-negative motile rods.
Culture: *Serratia* ferments lactose slowly or not at all. About 40% of the species form a red pigment, which is more pronounced when the organism is grown at 22° C and in the dark. Some strains are hemolytic. They share most of the biochemical reactions with *Enterobacter* but liquefy gelatin rapidly at 22° C, are arabinose negative, and have a different sensitivity pattern.

Nonpigmented *Serratia* must be differentiated from late lactose-fermenting *Escherichia coli*, *Shigella*, *Proteus-Providencia*, and possibly *Salmonella typhi*. *Serratia* can be differentiated from *Proteus* by the absence of the prompt urease reaction and from *Providencia* by the absence of phenylalanine deaminase. It can be differentiated from *Shigella* and *Escherichia coli* by growth in KCN broth, a positive Voges-Proskauer re-

Table 32-27. Identification of *Enterobacter* species and *Serratia*

Species	TSI reaction group	Arabinose	Raffinose	Rhamnose	Arginine dihydrolase
E. cloacae	1	+	+	+	+
E. aerogenes	1	+	+	+	−
E. hafniae	2	+	−	+	−
Serratia	2 or 1	−	−	−	−

Table 32-28. Differentiation of *Serratia* species

	Ornithine decarboxylase	Lactose	Raffinose
S. marcescens	+	−	−
S. liquefaciens	+	+ or −	+
S. rubidaea	−	+	+

action, and a usually negative methyl red test. *Serratia* can be differentiated from *Salmonella typhi* by citrate utilization of Simmons citrate. *Salmonella typhi* and *S. paratyphi* A are Simmons citrate negative, in contradistinction to other *Salmonella*.

Proteus-Providencia
Proteus
Laboratory diagnosis

Specimen: *Proteus* is infrequently found in normal stool but in debilitated patients and in patients on antibiotic therapy, it may be responsible for septicemia and for infections of the urinary tract and wounds.

Morphology (Gram stain): *Proteus* organisms are motile, gram-negative rods that vary somewhat in size and thickness (hence the name*). On blood agar *P. vulgaris* and *P. mirabilis* swarm, forming a thin transparent veil with an undulating periphery. They produce an ammoniac odor and at times hemolysis. Strains lacking the H antigen do not swarm and are not motile. The swarming or wavelike spreading on solid media of the motile forms can be inhibited by increasing the agar concentration to 5-8%, by incorporating chloral hy-

---

*Proteus was a sea god who could change his shape at will.

drate, bile salts, or phenylethyl alcohol. Because of their bile salt content, MacConkey agar, SS agar, and XLD agar suppress swarming.

Biochemical reactions

Proteus species are nonlactose fermenters and are urease (rapidly, 2-4 hr) and phenylalanine deaminase positive. *P. vulgaris* and *P. mirabilis* produce H_2S on TSI, swarm on solid media that lack bile salts, and liquefy gelatin. The majority produce gas. The strains that produce gas and H_2S may be confused with *Salmonella* on TSI agar. All species produce an enzyme called urease that hydroyzes urea in urea agar in 4 hr. *Salmonella* is urease negative (Table 32-29). For other reactions, see Table 32-22.

The ***Proteus*** species are *P. mirabilis, P. vulgaris, P. morganii,* and *P. rettgeri*. They can readily be identified on the basis of their reactions on TSI and SIM agars (Table 32-30).

Most *Proteus* species are resistant to antibiotic therapy with the exception of *P. mirabilis*, which responds to penicillin. Recently *Proteus rettgeri* has been reassigned to the genus ***Providencia*** and is known as *Providencia rettgeri*.

Table 32-29. *Proteus-Providencia* division*

	Proteus group				*Providencia* group	
Substrate or test	*vulgaris*	*mirabilis*	*morganii*	*rettgeri*	*alcalifaciens*	*stuartii*
Indole	+	−	+	+	+	+
Voges-Proskauer						
37° C	−	−	−	−	−	−
22° C	− or +	+ or −	−	−	−	−
Simmons citrate	d	d	−	+	+	+
Hydrogen sulfide (TSI)	+	+	−	−	−	−
Urease	+	+	+	+	−	−
Gelatin—22° C	+	+	−	−	−	−
Lysine decarboxylase	−	−	−	−	−	−
Arginine dihydrolase	−	−	−	−	−	−
Ornithine decarboxylase	−	+	+	−	−	−
Gas from glucose	+	+	+	− or +	+ or −	−
Mannitol	−	−	−	+	−	d
Adonitol	−	−	−	+	+	−
Inositol	−	−	−	+	−	+
Maltose	+	−	−	−	−	− or +

Modified from Ewing, W.H., and Edwards, P.R.: The principal divisions and groups of Enterobacteriaceae and their differentiation, Atlanta, 1962, Communicable Disease Centers.
*+, Positive in 1 or 2 days; −, negative, no reaction; d, different biochemical types; − or +, majority of strains negative but positive varieties occur; + or −, majority of cultures positive but negative varieties occur.
NOTE: Gas volumes formed from glucose are relatively small (a bubble to about 15%).

Table 32-30. Identification of *Proteus* species

Species	TSI group	SIM	Urea (2-4 hr)	Indole	Remarks
P. mirabilis	1 or 2	+ − +	+	−	Ampicillin sensitive, swarm
P. vulgaris	1 or 2	+ + +	+	+	
P. morganii	2	− + +	+	+	
P. rettgeri	3	− + +	+	+	Swarm

Providencia

Providencia organisms are gram-negative motile rods that do not ferment lactose on TSI agar and fail to produce H₂S. If they do not produce gas, they resemble *Shigella* on TSI *Providencia* is urease negative as is *Shigella*, but it differs from *Shigella* by growing on Simmons citrate, by being motile, and by being phenylalanine deaminase and indole positive. *Providencia* does not liquefy gelatin, and lysine, arginine, and ornithine are not decarboxylated.

Erwineae
Pectobacterium

Ewing suggested the term *pectobacterium* for a gram-negative rod that liquefies sodium pectate medium and reduces nitrates. It does not decarboxylate arginine, lysine, or ornithine. It grows well at 25° C but poorly, if at all, at 37° C. The organism is very rarely found in human material.

Comparison of conventional methods with multitest systems for identification of enteric gram-negative bacteria

The large number of media required for the identification of Enterobacteriaceae, the time and cost involved in their preparation, and the storage space needed have been the stimulating factors in the development of multitest systems that either employ paper reagent strips or tubes containing several culture media. In general these systems employ the established methods of identification of the members of the family Enterobacteriaceae and show a high degree of accuracy (90-97%), provided the organisms give characteristic reactions. The bacteria must first be isolated on such differential media as MacConkey or SS agars. For each unit of enteric gram-negative rod present, one multitest unit must be used.

The use of API strips (Other systems are PathoTec rapid 1-D system, General Diagnostics, Morris Plains, N.J.; Analytab system [API Profile recognition system, Analytab Products, New York]) has a high degree of accuracy.[89] The Enterotube System (Roche Diagnostics, Nutley, N.J.) not only identifies Enterobacteriaceae but also *Pseudomonas,* using one single tube containing eight compartments. The r/b Enteric Differential System[90,91] (Diagnostic Research, Roslyn, N.Y.) employs two tubes of culture media and a reagent for detection of indole.

The Minitek System (BBL, Baltimore) employs reagent-impregnated paper disks in small disposable wells and a disk-dispensing aparatus. The Minitek System (General Diagnostics, Morris Plains, N.J.) is a rapid identification system that is reported to give results after 4 hr of incubation.

There are several good reasons why these systems are finding wider application.[92,93] These methods save time in setting up cultures. Some of them require only a 4 hr incubation time. More importantly, the level of accuracy that these methods can bring to a laboratory, particularly one that handles few cultures, is probably superior to that attained by older methods.

Gram-negative bacteremia, endotoxemia, and the Limulus test

A number of factors account for an increase in gram-negative septicemia in hospital populations. They are the increased incidence of chronic disease in older population groups and the increased use of multiple antibiotics, steroids, and antimetabolites. Some of these infections are community acquired, whereas others are **nosocomial infections,** i.e., they are acquired in the hospital. Among the latter, infections by *Escherichia coli, Klebsiella, Proteus,* and *Pseudomonas* are the most common ones and are important for the following reasons: (1) they often follow instrumentation and the modalities of treatment mentioned above and (2) compared to the **community-acquired** infections they are more resistant to antibiotic therapy.[94,95]

Patients with **gram-negative septicemia** may have **bacteremia, endotoxemia,** or both. Bacteremia, the presence of organisms in the bloodstream, is diagnosed by positive blood culture and is not synonymous with endotoxemia. The latter is responsible for many of the clinical manifestations of gram-negative septicemia, e.g., hypofibrinogenemia, diffuse intravascular coagulation (DIC), elevated serum triglyceride levels, lowered complement levels, and death in about 60% of cases.

Until very recently the laboratory diagnosis of gram-negative sepsis depended on a positive blood culture, which is diagnostic of bacteremia but not of endotoxemia, since the latter does not necessarily occur simultaneously with bacteremia. **Gram-negative endotoxemia** could not be diagnosed until the development of the *Limulus* test, which detects gram-negative endotoxins in the serum of patients independent of the presence or absence of bacteremia..

Principle of Limulus test[96,97]: The *Limulus* test is based on the reaction of lysates derived from blood cells (amebocytes) of the horseshoe crab *(Limulus)* with endotoxin. Plasma (heparinized) is extracted with chloroform and the extract is mixed with the amebocyte lysate. The mixture is incubated at 37° C for 4 hr and at room temperature (25° C) for 24 hr. The presence of endotoxins is evidenced by a definite increase in viscosity.

Interpretation: The *Limulus* test is theoretically negative in patients who have gram-positive bacteremia only. It is theoretically positive in patients who have gram-negative or *Candida* endotoxemia. A microdilution method[96] is available that results in a saving of reagents and time. Recent evidence sheds doubt on the usefulness of the *Limulus* test for endotoxemia, although it is widely used to detect pyrogens in pharmaceutical preparations.

PSEUDOMONADACEAE
Pseudomonas

The genus *Pseudomonas* includes bacteria found in soil, water, plants, and sewage. Some species are pathogenic for humans and have taken the place formally held by *Staphylococcus aureus* as the most important hospital-acquired, antibiotic-resistant microorganism. It can be found in water faucets, soap dishes, whirlpool baths, etc. Ulcers, wounds, and burns after treatment with antibiotics often become secondarily invaded by *Pseudomonas*.

Fluorescein-producing Pseudomonas—Pseudomonas aeruginosa

Pseudomonas aeruginosa may be found in small numbers in the normal intestinal flora, but it may assume pathogenic proportions in patients on antibiotic therapy. It may be cultured from wounds (blue-green pus), ears, bile, diarrheic stool in children, and urine. It is important because of its resistance to treatment and its tendency to attack debilitated patients.

Laboratory diagnosis

Specimen: Material submitted includes urine, blood, material from wounds, burns, abscesses, and sinus tracts. As already mentioned, hospital cultures may be a rich source of *Pseudomonas*.

Morphology (Gram stain): *Pseudomonas* species are gram-negative motile (polar flagella) rods.

Culture: The organism grows well on primary culture media incubated at 35° C with or without increased CO_2 tension.

On blood agar the colonies are spreading, moist, flat, gray, and shiny with scalloped edges. They produce a sweetish grapelike aromatic odor and a greenish pigment that extends into the surrounding agar. β-Hemolysis is also seen. The water-soluble greenish pigment develops better at room temperature and on exposure to sunlight.

Two types of pigment are important: **fluorescein**, which is greenish yellow, fluorescent, and soluble in water but not in chloroform, and **pyocyanin**, which is bluish and soluble in water and chloroform. **Pyorubin,** a third pigment, is infrequently produced. Pyomelanin is a brown-black water-soluble pigment that may be rarely produced by *P. aeruginosa*.[8]

Pseudomonas grows on MacConkey agar and also on SS agar, although it is somewhat inhibited on the latter. In broth, diffuse turbidity is produced. On TSI agar no changes occur in slant or butt (group 5 TSI reaction). *Pseudomonas* shares the biochemical inactivity with the genera *Alcaligenes, Achromobacter,* and *Flavobacterium* (Table 32-31).

Biochemical identification

Pseudomonas is catalase and oxidase positive. It does not ferment sugar (glucose) but produces carbo-

hydrate breakdown by oxidation, thus producing **gluconic acid** but no gas.[99] To determine whether the carbohydrate is broken down by oxidation (O) or fermentation (F), O-F medium should be used.

Malonate and citrate are utilized, and growth occurs in KCN broth and on cetrimide medium. Catalase and urease tests are positive and gelatin is liquefied.

Differential tests

The tests to identify *Pseudomonas* include the gluconate oxidation test[100] (see below), oxidase test[101] (p. 843), cytochrome oxidase test[102] (p. 817), nitrate reduction test (p. 819), and acid production from glucose (O-F medium) (p. 820).

Gluconate oxidation test:

Principle: Gluconate is converted by *P. aeruginosa* to 2-ketogluconate, which is a reducing substance and can be tested for with Clinitest tablets (Ames Co., Elkhart, Ind.).

Procedure: The use of substrate tablets (Key Scientific Products, Los Angeles) is suggested. One gluconate tablet is added to 1 ml distilled water, which is then heavily inoculated. After 18-24 hr a Clinitest tablet is added to the test system. Reducing substances change the color of the Clinitest tablet from blue to yellow.

Results: *P. aeruginosa* is gluconate positive; *P. fluorescens* and *P. putida* may or may not be positive. Some strains of *Klebsiella, Enterobacter,* and *Serratia* are also gluconate positive.

Oxidase and urease tests: *Pseudomonas* is **rapidly** oxidase and cytochrome oxidase positive. Many strains are urease positive after 18-24 hr.

Differential diagnosis

The differential diagnosis involves all organisms that give a group 5 TSI reaction, i.e., alkaline slant and alkaline butt.

Nonpigmented *Pseudomonas* must be differentiated from *Alcaligenes, Acinetobacter, Achromobacter, Flavobacterium,* and *Aeromonas* (Tables 32-31 and 32-32).

Identification is based mainly on the following **criteria:**

1. Pigment production
2. O-F medium
3. Motility
4. Sellers agar
5. 10% glucose oxidation
6. 10% lactose oxidation
7. Nitrate reduction
8. Gelatin liquefaction
9. Citrate utilization

Table 32-31. Differentiation of cultures giving group 5 TSI reactions

	Pseudomonas	*Flavobacterium*	*Alcaligenes faecalis*	*Achromobacter*	*Acinetobacter calcoaceticus*
Pigment	Blue-green	Tan	−	−	−
Motility	+	−	+	−	−
10% glucose oxidation	+	+	−	−	(±)
10% lactose oxidation	−	+	−	−	(±)
Nitrate reduction	+	−	Variable	−	−
Oxidase	+	+	Delayed	−	−
Citrate utilization	+	−	+	+	+

Table 32-32. Some differential characteristics of aerobic pseudomonads and certain other oxidative or nonoxidative organisms*

Reactions	Fluorescein produced			Fluorescein not produced					A. calcoaceticus	Flavobacterium species	Alcaligenes faecalis
	P. aeruginosa	P. fluorescens	P. putida	P. pseudomallei	P. alcaligenes	P. acidovorans	P. stutzeri	P. maltophilia			
O-F medium	O	O	O	O	N	N	O	O	O	O/H	N
MacConkey	+	+	+	+	?	?	+	+	+	+/−	+
Motility	+	+	+	+	+	+	+	+	−	−	+
Oxidase	+	+	+−	w+	+	+	+	−	−	+	+
Growth at 42° C	+	−	+/−	+	+	−	+ (−)	+/−	+/−	−	+/−
Growth at 4° C	−	+	+/−	−	−	−	−	−	−	−	?
Gluconate oxidation	+	+/−	+	−	−	−	−	−	−	−	−
Glucose (O-F)	+	+	−	+	−	−	−	−	+	+/−	−
Gelatin	+	+	+	+	−	−	−/+	+	−	+	−
Arginine dihydrolase	+	+		+	+	−	−	−	−	−	−

Modified from Sonnenwirth, A.C.: In Frankel, S., Reitman, S., and Sonnenwirth, A.C.: Gradwohl's clinical laboratory methods and diagnosis, ed. 7. St. Louis, 1970. The C. V. Mosby Co.
*O, oxidizer; F, fermenter; N, nonoxidizer, inactive; ?, not determined; +/−, variable; +, positive; −, negative; w, weakly positive.

Table 32-33. Reactions in O-F basal medium

	Open	Covered	Motility
Pseudomonas	Acid*	−	+
Alcaligenes	−	−	+
Acinetobacter calcoaceticus	−	−	−
Shigella	Acid	Acid	−
Salmonella	Acid	Acid	+
	+, Gas	+, Gas	

*Yellow.

Pigment production: The pigment production of *Pseudomonas,* which is often absent on routine media, can be stimulated by Tech (BBL, BioQuest Div., Becton-Dickinson & Co., Cockeysville, Md.) medium to enhance pyocyanin production and by FLO (BBL, BioQuest Div., Becton-Dickinson & Co., Cockeysville, Md.) medium to enhance fluorescein production.[95] The addition of cetrimide[96] (cetyltrimethyl ammonium bromide) to Tech medium (Pseudosel agar [BBL, BioQuest Div., Becton-Dickinson & Co., Cockeysville, Md.]) renders this medium selective for *P. aeruginosa* by inhibiting other organisms. Five percent of *Pseudomonas* species are not pigment producing.

O-F basal medium: *P. aeruginosa* can be differentiated from the other genera mentioned by the production of an oxidative reaction in O-F basal medium of Hugh and Leifson.

Technic of inoculation: See p. 820.

Pseudomonas mallei

Pseudomonas mallei is the causative organism of **glanders,** an infectious disease of horses.

Laboratory diagnosis

Pseudomonas mallei is a dangerous organism to handle in the laboratory.

Specimen: Examine pus from one of the discharging lesions or material from an incised nodule.

Morphology (Gram stain):

Smear: The organism is a gram-negative, slender, long, often beaded rod, which at times is slightly curved and varies from 0.4-0.8 μm in length. In older cultures long filaments are found. The ends are clubbed. It stains poorly with Gram stain and stains best with methylene blue.

Culture: For primary isolation the medium must contain glycerol. On Loeffler agar, small, opaque, slimy colonies appear slowly, while on blood agar, methemoglobin formation produces brownish-colored colonies. As the culture ages, the colonies tend to flow together, so that a heavy, shiny, brownish mass is produced. On glycerin agar slants the colonies appear slowly; they are yellowish at first and then become brownish. In broth the organism grows slowly, producing diffuse clouding, which in older cultures settles to the bottom of the tube as a mucoid viscid ring.

Serologic identification

An antigen is available that is precipitated by immune serum that contains complement-fixing antibodies before cutaneous ulcerating lesions appear, thus eliminating dangerous bacteriologic procedures. An extract, **mallein,** is available for diagnostic cutaneous and conjunctival tests.

Animal inoculation

The organism is pathogenic to guinea pigs. Exudate or pure culture material is injected subcutaneously and in 4-5 days an abscess forms. The **Straus reaction** involves the appearance of caseating testicular necrosis 1-2 weeks after intraperitoneal injection of the *Actinobacillus* into guinea pigs. *Brucella* may produce a similar reaction.

Non-fluorescein-producing Pseudomonas— Pseudomonas pseudomallei

Pseudomonas pseudomallei is the causative organism of melioidosis, a disease of Southeast Asia, including Vietnam.

Laboratory diagnosis[103]

Morphology (Gram stain): The organism is a gram-negative rod.

Culture: The organism is motile and grows well on primary culture media. After 48-72 hr of incubation the colonies wrinkle.

Biochemical characteristics

The organism is oxidative, producing acid from glucose in O-F medium. It is catalase, oxidase, Simmons citrate, and gelatinase positive, does not grow on SS agar, and is H_2S and indole negative. It does not fluoresce.

• • •

Because the taxonomy is undergoing a period of transition and in the absence of any generally accepted nomenclature, the following bacteria are classified by genera only.

ACHROMOBACTER

Achromobacter species are nonmotile, non-pigment-forming, aerobic to faculatively anaerobic, biochemically inactive, gram-negative rods that may assume diplococcal shapes. They are saprophytic soil and water organisms. The classification of these organisms is questionable at this time. In the eighth edition of *Bergey's Manual of Determinative Biology* they are incorporated with *Alcaligenes*.

ACINETOBACTER
Acinetobacter calcoaceticus

Acinetobacter calcoaceticus has been responsible for a variety of human infections, e.g., bacterial endocarditis, meningitis, abscesses, and vaginal and skin infections. *A. calcoaceticus* grows well on primary isolation media, as rods in liquid media, and as blunt-ended diplococci on solid media. The diplococci may resemble *Neisseria gonorrhoeae* but are oxidase negative.

On blood agar the colonies are white, smooth, moist, viscid, and foul smelling.

The organism is biochemically inactive, although some strains ferment carbohydrates. It is catalase positive and on TSI agar produces a neutral or alkaline slant and a neutral butt (Tables 32-32 and 32-33).

MORAXELLA

Moraxella is a nonmotile, short, gram-negative diplococcus that is oxidase positive and does not ferment carbohydrates. *Moraxella* species are mainly parasites of mammals. A large group of *Moraxella* organisms is called *M. osloensis;* others are *M. bovis, M. phenylpyruvica, M. nonliquefaciens,* and *M. lacunata.*

Moraxella lacunata

Moraxella lacunata is the cause of a form of conjunctivitis in humans (Morax-Axenfeld's conjunctivitis). It is a gram-negative, plump, short bacillus measuring about 2-3 μm in length and up to 1.5 μm in diameter. It is frequently paired. It grows slowly on blood agar and after 5-6 days the colonies measure 2-3 mm in diameter. It thrives on Loeffler medium, which is liquefied by the organism so that pitted areas appear around the colonies.

AEROMONAS

Aeromonas species are motile gram-negative organisms that are parasites, primarily of cold-blooded animals,[104] but they may often be found in humans associated with septicemia and wound infections after aquatic exposure.

FLAVOBACTERIUM

Flavobacterium species are soil and water organisms. They are gram-negative, aerobic, oxidase-positive, nonmotile rods. Carbohydrates are slowly oxidized with weak acid production (Table 32-32). On solid media, yellow-tan colonies are formed.

F. meningosepticum is occasionally isolated from blood and spinal fluid.

ALCALIGENES FAECALIS

Alcaligenes faecalis, although found in stool, does not belong to the Enterobacteriaceae. It is a sometimes motile gram-negative rod that is chemically inactive on routine media. On MacConkey agar it produces small colorless colonies that may be mistaken for those of a pathogen. On TSI agar it gives an alkaline reaction throughout the medium.

The organism is aerobic and fails to utilize carbohydrates (Table 32-31).

BRUCELLA

Brucella is a small nonmotile, aerobic, gram-negative coccobacillus that grows poorly on ordinary media, requiring special media and often additional CO_2 tension. The species are *B. abortus, B. melitensis, B. suis, B. neotomae, B. ovis,* and *B. canis.*

Brucellosis is a disease of animals that is transmitted to humans. Infections may occur from contact with infected animals or from ingestion of infected dairy products. During the first week of the disease, and often during the febrile stage of recurrence, the organism may be found in blood culture. Culture of the urine and feces is usually not successful. After the second week, specific agglutinins may be demonstrated, possibly remaining in the blood for several months or for many years but sometimes disappearing after a few months.

Laboratory diagnosis[105]

The diagnosis of brucellosis depends on (1) culture of *Brucella* from blood or other specimens, (2) detection of antibodies against *Brucella* in the patient's serum, and (3) animal inoculation.

Specimen: Best results are obtained with blood cultures. However, urine, pus, bone marrow, and lymph nodes may also be cultured.

Morphology (Gram stain): The organism varies in length from 0.3-2.3 μm and has an average diameter of 0.4 μm. It is difficult to counterstain, so that the staining time of safranin should be increased from 30 sed to 4 min. The organism is a gram-negative coccobacillus that may be found intracellularly within the cytoplasm of polymorphonuclear leukocytes.

Culture: The medium of choice is trypticase soy broth or agar incubated at 35° C in an atmosphere of 10% CO_2 (candle jar).

Blood culture: Place 5-10 ml blood into 50 ml trypticase soy broth with 10% CO_2 and incubate at 35° C for 4-7 days. After 7 days of incubation, mix the culture and transfer 1 loopful of blood culture to a trypticase soy agar plate and incubate for 4 days at 35° C in a CO_2 jar. Reincubate blood culture for another 7 days, replenishing the CO_2 if necessary. After 7 days, streak the blood culture again; this process may have to be repeated a third time before the culture can be reported as negative. After 4 days, examine the agar plate for small (2-3 mm), transparent, smooth, well-defined, soft, spheroid colonies that later become opalescent because of a brownish tinge. **Smooth colonies** can be differentiated from rough ones by tilting the plate 45 degrees and examining it under transmitted light with the low-power objective of the microscope. The rough colonies appear darker than the smooth ones. Make a Gram stain of suspicious colonies and perform a **slide agglutination test** with polyvalent antiserum, using smooth colonies only. If the test with polyvalent antiserum is positive, use the dye plate method for species differentiation.

Presumptive identification can also be accomplished by the **FA technic.**

If *B. suis* is suspected, urea agar should be heavily inoculated. It will rapidly turn pink if the organism is *B. suis*.

A negative blood culture does not exclude brucellosis.

Slide agglutination test:

Procedure: See technic of slide agglutination for *Salmonella* and *Shigella*, p. 854. Mix polyvalent *Brucella* antiserum, diluted 1:10 with saline solution, with a saline suspension of suspected colonies. A saline control of saline-suspended organisms must be used in parallel with the test to judge the roughness of the bacterial suspension in saline solution.

Differentiation of species

The differential diagnosis is based on the following characteristics of a pure culture (Table 32-34):

1. Growth-inhibiting action of thionine and basic fuchsin (dye sensitivity)
2. H_2S production
3. CO_2 requirements
4. Agglutination by monospecific sera
5. Urease test for *B. suis*

Dye sensitivity test: Species differentiation is made according to characteristic sensitivity to thionine and basic fuchsin. Seed a trypticase soy agar plate with the suspected pure culture and place commercially available filter paper strips impregnated with thionine (1:100,000) and basic fuchsin (1:100,000) on the inoculated agar surface. Incubate the plate at 35° C under increased CO_2 tension (10%) for a period of up to 6 days. Examine daily for presence or absence of distinct growth close to the filter paper strips.

Tests for H_2S production and CO_2 requirement: Using a pure culture, inoculate two trypticase agar slants. Suspend strip of lead acetate paper over one slant so that it does not touch the medium. Incubate this culture at 35° C under 10% CO_2 tension for 7 days. Examine daily for black discoloration of the strip and replace negative strips daily. Record H_2S production as 0-1 + and 2 +.

Incubate the second slant aerobically (without added CO_2) at 35° C for 4 days and examine daily for growth.

Serologic investigation of antibody formation in patients with brucellosis

Agglutination tests: The test tube method is recommended, using an antigen prepared with avirulent National Institutes of Health *B. abortus* strain no. 256. One antigen is used for the diagnosis of all three forms of brucellosis. Cross-reaction with *Francisella tularensis* may occur.

Tube dilution method:

Procedure: Use fresh (not inactivated) serum, free from hemolysis.

Set up 11 small tubes and add 0.9 ml saline solution to the first tube and 0.5 ml to the others. To the first

Table 32-34. Characteristics of *Brucella* species

| Species | CO_2 requirements on initial isolation | Growth in presence of | | Serologic typing | | H_2S production |
		Thionine (1:100,000)	Basic fuchsin (1:100,000)	*B. abortus* sera	*B. melitensis* sera	
B. abortus	+	−	+	+	−	+ for 4 days
B. suis	−	+	−	+	−	+ for 5 days
B. melitensis	−	+	+	−	+	0 throughout 4 days
B. neotomae	−	−	−	+	−	+
B. ovis	+	+	+	−	−	−
B. canis	−	+	−	−	−	−

tube, add 0.1 ml serum, mix by drawing it in and out of the pipet seven or eight times, and transfer 0.5 ml to the second tube. Continue in like manner through the tenth tube, discarding 0.5 ml and leaving tube 11 for a negative control.

To all tubes, add 0.5 ml diluted antigen (National Institutes of Health strain no. 256) and mix. The dilutions of the serum are 1:20, 1:40, 1:80, 1:160, 1:320, 1:640, 1:1280, 1:2560, 1:5120, and 1:10,240.

Incubate for 48 hr in a water bath at 37° C before making the final reading. The titer is the highest dilution showing complete (4+) agglutination. Do not use serum when hemolysis is present. Hemolysis causes nonspecific clumping.

Rapid slide method:

Procedure: Use slides that contain six rows of rings painted with alkyl resin paint, five or six to the row. Serum and antigen must be at room temperature.

Shake the antigen thoroughly. Place 0.08, 0.04, 0.02, 0.01, and 0.005 ml amounts of serum in a row of circles. Place 1 drop of antigen on each quantity of serum. Mix the serum and antigen in each circle in the row with a wooden applicator, working from the smallest quantity of serum to the largest. Lift the plate and tilt it back and forth for no more than 3 min. Read in indirect light against a dark background and determine the highest serum dilution that still gives agglutination of the antigen.

Interpretation of agglutination tests[106]:

Acute brucellosis: After about 10 days of illness a rising titer is noted that persists for up to 6 weeks before it declines. It may never return to zero. As in all agglutination tests, a rising titer is more significant than one single titer value.

Repeated negative cultures and repeated absence of a titer of 1:20 may be significant. Titers of 1:160 or higher are considered diagnostic.

Animal inoculation

Guinea pigs (300-600 g), which must be tested for the absence of *Brucella* agglutinins, are injected subcutaneously (if culture is pure) with 2 ml material. After 8 weeks, test for *Brucella* agglutinins. If present, kill the animal and look for granulomatous lesions in the spleen, liver, and testes.

YERSINIA

Three species of *Yersinia* are human pathogens: *Y. pestis, Y. pseudotuberculosis,* and *Y. enterocolitica.*[107] They are short, at times elliptic, gram-negative rods that show bipolar staining, are nonmotile (with the exception of *Y. pseudotuberculosis,* which shows some motility at 20° C), grow aerobically on most media, and do not produce hemolysis. *Yersinia* organisms are catalase-positive, aerobic, gram-negative coccobacilli or rods that ferment carbohydrates without gas production.

Yersinia pestis[108]

Plague, caused by *Yersinia pestis,* was once the most devastating of all human infectious diseases. It is primarily a disease of rats and is transmitted by the rat flea to other rats and to humans. In the southwestern United States plague is endemic in the wild rodent population. Human cases of plague in these areas develop following bites from rodent fleas.

Laboratory diagnosis

Specimen: Material consists of fluid aspirated from infected skin lesions (fleabites), lymph nodes (buboes), blood, and autopsy material such as spleen, lymph nodes, bone marrow, and blood. All material is highly infectious and should only be handled in reference laboratories.

Morphology (Gram stain): *Y. pestis* is a short, thick, straight, gram-negative bacillus[109] with rounded ends that sometimes occurs in pairs or in very short chains. Bipolar staining ("safety pin" appearance) and the presence of swollen vacuolated involution forms in older cultures or after antibiotic treatment are characteristic for the organism. *Y. pestis* is encapsulated.

Smears: Smears are fixed in methyl alcohol (absolute) for 3-5 min instead of with heat, which interferes with bipolar staining. Stain one smear with Gram stain and another with Loeffler methylene blue stain. Bipolar staining is characteristic and is best seen with Wayson stain.

Culture: On blood agar at 28-35° C after 48 hr the colonies are 1-2 mm in size, grayish white, and convex. Before 48 hr the colonies are not visible to the naked eye. The slow growth is characteristic for the organism; after 7 days' incubation the colonies measure about 4 mm in diameter. In BHI agar the organisms form floccules that adhere to the side of the tube until handling of the tube shakes them loose, so that they settle at the bottom of the tube, leaving the supernatant clear. The organism is able to grow in the presence of bile salts (MacConkey agar). It is aerobic and nonmotile at 35° C and at 20° C (room temperature).

Biochemical characteristics

The organism does not grow on Simmons citrate and does not produce acid from lactose or sucrose. It does, however, ferment glucose with acid but not gas production. Indole, Voges-Proskauer, urease, and decarboxylase tests are negative. The test for catalase is positive. Biochemical investigations are used to differentiate *Y. pestis* from other *Yersinia* and from *Pasteurella, Enterobacteriaceae,* and vibrios (Table 32-22).

Serologic identification

Antiplague serum for agglutination of suspected *Y. pestis* is available from public health laboratories. Agglutinins present in the patient's serum are demonstrated by using a known strain of formalin-killed *Y. pestis.*

Bacteriophage typing: Lysis of colonies by specific bacteriophage is a rapid method of identification. Filter paper strips containing lyophilized virus are available from certain centers, e.g., U. S. Public Health Service, Department of Health and Human Services, San Francisco.

Virulence: The organisms are pathogenic to mice and guinea pigs (danger to laboratory personnel). Inoculate a white mouse or guinea pig subcutaneously or intraperitoneally with 24 hr broth culture. Death occurs in 2-4 days. Autopsy will reveal multiple abscesses.

Fluorescent microscopy: Staining with fluorescent antibodies can be utilized.

Yersinia pseudotuberculosis

Yersinia pseudotuberculosis produces tuberculosis-like lesions in many wild animals and in animals kept as pets (cats, canaries, etc.). Human infections produce a picture of gastroenteritis or acute appendicitis.

Laboratory diagnosis

Specimen: Bile, blood, feces, macerated lymph nodes, liver, or spleen is the specimen used.

Morphology (Gram stain): The organism is a pleomorphic, gram-negative rod that may exhibit coccoid and ovoid forms.

Culture: The organism will grow on all selective and enrichment media used routinely to isolate non-lactose-fermenting Enterobacteriaceae at 22-35° C and after 24 hr will form minute 1-2 mm colonies.

Biochemical reactions are shown in Tables 32-22 and 32-34.

This species can be differentiated from *Pasteurella* biochemically and on the basis of motility (motile at 20° C), phage typing, agglutination, and FA technic (Table 32-35).

Yersinia enterocolitica

Yersinia enterocolitica is responsible for enteric diseases[110,111] with or without septicemia in humans and animals and produces such clinical manifestations as mesenteric lymphadenitis, appendicitis, enteritis, ileitis, and even meningitis in the septicemic phase. *Y. enterocolitica* infections seem to be increasing. Small local epidemics associated with contaminated food or drink are reported where the disease resembles appendicitis. The organisms are isolated on blood or MacConkey agar. Cold temperature enrichment enhances recovery of the organisms.[112] The reactions are listed in Table 32-36.

Pasteurella

Pasteurella species are aerobic coccobacilli and occur in pairs. They are nonhemolytic and require blood-enriched media for primary isolation. Four species are primarily of veterinary importance: *P. multocida, P. pneumotropica, P. haemolytica,* and *P. ureae. P. multocida* is the only species of importance in human medicine.

Pasteurella multocida

Pasteurella multocida produces severe gastroenteritis in fowl, birds, and domestic animals and may be transmitted from animals to humans by bites.[113] Virtually any infected animal bite must be suspicious for *P. multocida* infection.

Laboratory diagnosis

Specimen: Clinical material includes sputum, saliva, pus, blood, urine, and macerated tissue.

Morphology (Gram stain): Blood smears and imprints are stained with Wright-Giemsa stain or Wayson stain and examined for organisms that are oval to coccoid short rods measuring 0.3-1.25 μm. The organism is gram negative and usually encapsulated. The individual cell shows polar staining, the middle remaining almost unstained ("safety pin" appearance).

Culture: Primary isolation is obtained on cystine trypticase agar or BHI agar. Blood added to the medium may inhibit the growth of *P. multocida*. Incubate cultures at 35° C. On cystine trypticase agar the organism grows in the form of transparent, droplike colonies. It does not grow on media containing bile, e.g., MacConkey agar. In broth it forms wooly masses.

Biochemical reactions

The reactions used to differentiate *P. multocida* from other *Pasteurella* species are as follows: indole production, no growth on MacConkey agar, oxidase and catalase positivity, negative urease test, and fermentation of glucose and sucrose with no gas formation. H_2S production may be demonstrable with lead acetate paper.

Table 32-35. Differentiation of *Yersinia* and *Pasteurella*

	Pasteurella multocida	*Yersinia pseudotuberculosis*	*Yersinia pestis*	*Yersinia enterocolitica*
Optimal temperature	35° C	30° C	28° C	35° C
Motility at 20° C	−	+	−	+
Motility at 35° C	−	−	−	−
Sucrose utilization (acid, no gas)	+	−	−	+
Lactose	−	−	−	−
Indole production	+	−	−	Variable
Pathogenicity for mice	+	−	+	−
Urease	−	+	−	+
Growth in the presence of bile (MacConkey)	−	+	+	+
Methyl red test	−	+	+	+
H_2S production (TSI)	+	+	−	−
β-D-Galactosidase	−	+	+	+
Oxidase	+	−	−	−

Differentiation of Yersinia and Pasteurella

See Table 32-35.

Serologic identification

Antiserum for the slide agglutination of *P. multocida* is available in specialized laboratories.

FRANCISELLA

Francisella species are gram-negative coccobacilli that are sometimes paired. They are mainly parasites of mammals. *F. tularensis* is the most important species.

Francisella tularensis

Francisella tularensis is a small, nonmotile, gram-negative, pleomorphic, coccoid, strictly aerobic organism that produces a fatal septicemia (**tularemia**) in rodents and especially in rabbits. It is transmitted to humans by handling infected animals or material and by the bite of insects such as ticks, lice, and fleas. The wood tick *(Dermacentor andersoni)* is an intermediate host that transmits the organism through the egg stage.

Laboratory diagnosis

The following laboratory methods are available for the diagnosis of tularemia: (1) culture, (2) agglutination tests, and (3) animal inoculation. The organism occurs in two varieties, var. *tularensis* and var. *palaearetica,* which may be distinguished by their degrees of virulence. The first is found only in North America, the latter in Europe and Asia.

Specimen: Material from primary skin lesions, lymph nodes, sputum, pleural fluid, or conjunctival scrapings is submitted.

Morphology (Gram stain): The organism occurs as a gram-negative rod or as a small coccus. It varies from 0.3-07 μm in length, the smallest organisms being slightly larger than rickettsiae. Giemsa and Wayson stains reveal bipolar staining.

Culture: The organism does not grow on plain blood agar. Blood glucose cystine agar is the preferred medium. It is a differential point that the organism will not grow on blood glucose agar without cystine. Cystine heart agar enriched with 5-10% defibrinated blood to form a chocolate agar is a suitable culture medium. Small, viscid, transparent to milky colonies appear slowly in 2-7 days.

Biochemical reactions

Biochemical reactions are of little value in the diagnosis of *F. tularensis* except for the fermentation of 1% glycerol in cystine heart agar (without blood) with bromthymol blue as the indicator (green). Virulent *F. tularensis* ferments glycerol (yellow color).[114]

Serologic identification

Agglutination tests:

Identification of organism: A commercially available *F. tularensis* antiserum (American Type Culture Collection, Rockville, Md.) can be used for direct serologic identification on pure cultures. This serum can also serve as a positive control for the slide agglutination test.

Identification of antibody in patient's serum: By slide or tube technic the patient's serum will agglutinate *F. tularensis.* Because of the danger involved in handling the organisms from the patient, strain no. 38 (American Type Culture Collection, Rockville, Md.) should be used as antigen and tested with patient's serum. It is avirulent, smooth, easily cultured, and highly agglutinable. An *F. tularensis* slide test antigen is commercially available (Difco Laboratories, Detroit).

Test tube agglutination test: Because of frequent cross-agglutination between *F. tularensis* and *Brucella melitensis* and *Brucella abortus,* sera from suspected persons should be set up with both *F. tularensis* and *B. melitensis* (or *B. abortus*) organisms in dilutions from 1:10 to 1:2560.

Sera from the acute and convalescent phases should be tested simultaneously, and known positive and negative control sera should be included. The commercially available *F. tularensis* antiserum may be used as positive control.

Procedure: Mark tubes from 1-10. Add 0.8 ml saline solution to the first tube and 0.5 ml to the others. Pipet 0.2 ml test serum into first tube, mix (dilution 1:5), and transfer 0.5 ml of mixture of first tube to second tube, mix, and repeat. Discard 0.5 ml from ninth tube. Add 0.5 ml antigen to each tube and shake. The tenth tube is the antigen control. The final serum dilutions are 1:10, 1:20, 1:40, 1:80, 1:160, 1:320, 1:640, 1:1280, and 1:2560.

Incubate test tubes in a water bath at 56° C for 2 hr, and after incubation place them in a refrigerator overnight. Record the result of each tube as 4-1+ agglutination or as negative.

4+ = Compact sediment, clear supernatant
3+ = Compact sediment, slightly turbid supernatant
2+ = Floccular sediment, turbid supernatant
1+ = Floccular turbidity only

Results: If the homogeneous mixture is similar to the antigen control mixture, the test is negative. A positive test is indicated by the highest dilution of the patient's serum that gives a 3-4+ agglutination. If the serum is from a patient with tularemia, the *F. tularensis* antigen will be agglutinated in higher dilution and earlier than the *Brucella* antigen. If the serum is from a patient with undulant fever, the reverse will be true. Should the serum agglutinate tularemia and undulant fever organisms to the same titer, agglutination absorption tests will have to be performed. Cross-reaction with *Proteus* OX-19 has also been reported. The antigen is commercially available.

Repeated agglutination tests are necessary to appreciate the fall or rise of a given titer. After the first week, agglutination of the organism with the patient's serum is usually positive. Positive reactions persist for many years or life.

Skin test: The intracutaneous test[115] with bacterial protein (detoxified) is highly specific and will be positive as early as the third day of symptoms.

Guinea pig inoculation

The suspected material should be ground in a mortar and suspended in saline solution, and penicillin should be added. Inject the material subcutaneously into the abdomen of the guinea pig. The animal dies within 1 week, presenting gray, granular caseation of enlarged lymph glands of the groin and a great number of white areas of necrosis in the enlarged spleen and liver. Obtain smears and imprints from the organs and culture blood, spleen, heart, and liver.

CAUTION: Laboratory infection with *F. tularensis* is common. Animals should not be inoculated unless technicians are immune to tularemia.

HAEMOPHILUS

Haemophilus species are gram-negative coccobacilli that are facultatively anaerobic. They are parasites of mammals. The organisms affect the respiratory tract, meninges, conjunctivae, and genitourinary tract.

Haemophilus species can be differentiated on the basis of (1) cultural characteristics, e.g., the requirement of growth **factor X,** which is considered to be hemin, a thermostable substance present in blood, and/or of **factor V,** which is nicotinamide adenine dinucleotide (NAD), a coenzyme that is thermostable and supplied by blood, bacteria, and yeast (blood also contains an enzyme that counteracts factor V) and (2) the presence or absence of hemolysis on blood agar.

Classification on basis of growth factors and hemolysis

Factors X and V are required by *H. influenzae* (non-hemolytic) and *H. haemolyticus* (β-hemolytic). Factor X only is required by *H. ducreyi* (weakly hemolytic) and *H. aphrophilus* (nonhemolytic). Factor V only is required by *H. parainfluenzae* (nonhemolytic) and *H. parahaemolyticus* (hemolytic).

Haemophilus influenzae

The *Haemophilus influenzae* organism is a small gram-negative rod that may or may not be encapsulated. Six types of encapsulated *H. influenzae* (a to f) are distinguished serologically. The most important one is type b, which causes most of the serious infections in infants and children, e.g., septicemia, endocarditis, and meningitis.[117] The nonencapsulated forms are not type specific and are part of the normal laryngeal flora.

Haemophilus species can be rapidly identified by the aminolevulenic acid (ALA) test of Kilian.[116] Haemophilus stains that do not require factor X can use ALA for protoporphyrin IX production. This compound produces a red fluorescence under the Wood lamp.

ALA (2 mM) in Sörenson's buffer (Sigma Chemical Co., St. Louis), pH 6.9 with magnesium sulfate (0.8 mM) is used as the test medium. Tubes containing 0.5 ml are inoculated heavily with the isolate and then incubated for 4-5 hr at 37° C. At this time the tubes are examined under the Wood lamp for fluorescence.

H. influenzae is the only species demonstrating the satellite phenomenon that is nonhemolytic and negative for the ALA test.

H. influenzae is one of the agents of infectious conjunctivitis. For growth it requires factors X and V.

Laboratory diagnosis

Specimen: Spinal fluid, throat swabs, sputum, and exudates.

Morphology (Gram stain): The organism is a small, nonmotile, gram-negative, pleomorphic coccobacillus that sometimes appears as long filaments called thread forms. The average length is 1-1.5 μm, and the average thickness is 0.3 μm. The form of the organism is dependent on the age of the culture.

Smears reveal lightly staining, slightly elongated rods.

Culture: For culture the organism requires growth factors X and V and is best isolated on chocolate agar under increased CO_2 tension. The organism grows best around colonies of other bacteria, particularly staphylococci, a behavior pattern that is called the **satellite phenomenon.**

The staphylococci provide NAD (factor V). Instead of streaking the plate with *Staphylococcus aureus,* one may paint the plate with a swab dipped in a mixture of 1 mg NAD added to 2 ml of 0.01% sodium thioglycollate in sterile water. The plate is allowed to dry and is then inoculated. Strips and disks impregnated with factors V and X are commercially available (BBL, Bio-Quest Div., Becton-Dickinson & Co., Cockeysville, Md.). For best recovery both chocolate and blood agar plates should be used.

Incubate both plates at 35° C under 10% CO_2. The colonies are small, clear, colorless, and nonhemolytic, with a dewdrop appearance and a mousy odor. The capsule of pathogens is best developed in an 8 hr culture; older colonies may lose it.

Chocolate agar is superior to blood agar, which may contain substances that are bactericidal and depress factor V.

H. influenzae may not grow on blood agar prepared with human or sheep blood. Rabbit and horse blood are able to support its growth.

Identification of species with X, V, and X-V factor strips

Inoculate trypticase soy agar plate with a pure culture of *Haemophilus* and aseptically place strips X, V, and X-V on the inoculated agar about 2 cm apart. Incubate at 35° C under increased CO_2 tension (10%) and observe growth around strips. Growth indicates requirement for adjacent factor. For growth requirements, see above.

β-Lactamase production

Although most strains of *H. influenzae* are sensitive to ampicillin, the number of resistant isolates appears to be increasing. A rapid method to determine β-lactamase (penicillinase) production has been developed[118] whereby a suspension of test organisms is mixed with penicillin. Bromcresol purple is added as an indicator. The indicator is purple at a neutral pH but rapidly turns yellow when the substrate (penicillin) is hydrolyzed.

A more convenient approach is to use Beta-Lactam (Remel Co., Lenexa, Kan.) disks that are impregnated with benzyl pencillin and an indicator. The disk is wetted with 1 drop of water before applying a loop of test organisms to the surface. The test is read in 30 min.

Biochemical reactions

Carbohydrate fermentation is weak and glucose is fermented by all strains.

Bile solubility: All *Haemophilus* species are **soluble** in 1-2% **sodium deoxycholate.**

Procedure: See bile solubility test of *Streptococcus pneumoniae.*

Quellung (capsular swelling) test: The Quellung test should be used for rapid identification of *H. influenzae* in spinal fluid. The technic is the same as used in typing *Streptococcus pneumoniae.*

Direct fluorescent antibody test: If conjugated antisera are available, they allow a rapid identification of *H. influenzae* in the spinal fluid.

Serologic identification

Agglutination slide test and Quellung slide test antisera are available for serologic identification. If positive results are obtained with polyvalent serum, typing with specific antisera follows. The counterimmunoelectrophoresis (CIE) procedure may be used to rapidly identify *H. influenzae* antigen in spinal fluid. Antiserum types a, b, c, and d are used. Type b is most frequently found in cases of *H. influenzae* meningitis.

Gardnerella vaginalis

Gardnerella vaginalis requires only factor X for growth (not factor V, and therefore the satellite phenomenon is negative). It is a short gram-negative rod that does not grow on EMB. It grows best in 10% CO_2 on sheep blood (not human blood) and in thioglycollate medium without methylene blue, the indicator of oxidation-reduction.

This organism has been isolated from the human genitourinary tract (prostate, vagina, and urine). *G. vaginalis* concentrates in certain vaginal and cervical squamous cells, so that all cellular details are obliterated by bacterial masses, called **clue cells** (Fig. 32-8).

Haemophilus ducreyi

Haemophilus ducreyi is the causative organism of an ulcerative venereal disease: chancroid or ''soft chancre.''

Laboratory diagnosis

Direct smear: The ulcer base is cleaned, and material from the growing edge is smeared on a slide. The organism is a gram-negative, ovoid to cylindric bacillus occurring singly, in clumps, or in chains of two to four. It varies in length from 1.1-1.5 μm and has an average diameter of 0.6 μm. It may be intracellular or extracellular and is accompanied by polymorphonuclear cells. It may be plentiful or very scarce, and the smear may only help to exclude granuloma inguinale. Smears of aspirated material from abscessed inguinal lymph nodes may also show only a very few organisms.

Culture: The organism requires blood (growth factor X, but not V). On 30% rabbit blood agar at 35° C, very small (0.5-1 mm in diameter), smooth, glistening colonies appear after 24 hr. Defibrinated rabbit blood that has been stored in the refrigerator for 3-4 days before use is an excellent medium if after inoculation it is incubated in 10% CO_2 at 35° C.

Haemophilus aegyptius (Koch-Weeks bacillus)

Haemophilus aegyptius is the same organism as *H. influenzae* (see *Haemophilus influenzae*).

Haemophilus haemolyticus and Haemophilus parahaemolyticus

These two hemolytic species may be mistaken for hemolytic streptococci on blood agar. *Haemophilus haemolyticus* is hemolytic and requires growth factors X and V. *Haemophilus parahaemolyticus* requires only factor V.

The diagnosis of *H. parahaemolyticus* can be suggested by the Gram stain, which reveals pleomorphic, tangled, threadlike, gram-negative structures with globoid expansions.

Haemophilus parainfluenzae

Haemophilus parainfluenzae is a nonhemolytic species and requires only factor V. It is normally found in the upper respiratory tract. The organism is slightly longer than *H. influenzae*, is gram negative, and has pointed ends.

ACTINOBACILLUS[119]

Actinobacillus is a nonmotile aerobic or facultatively anaerobic gram-negative rod that ferments carbohydrates without gas production and grows best under 5-10% CO_2. The organisms are β-galactosidase positive, MR negative, indole negative, and urease positive. Nitrates are reduced to nitrites. On some media it produces pleomorphic coccobacilli that may give rise to filamentous forms. Two species are of importance: *Actinobacillus lignieresii*[120] and *Actinobacillus equuli*.[121] The organisms must be distinguished from *Pseudomonas (P. pseudomallei)*, which is motile.

Actinobacillus produces ulcerating, granulomatous to purulent lesions in the subcutaneous and deep tissues of cattle and horses. The superficial lesions contaminate the drinking water, which, when consumed by humans, allows the bacteria to cause human infection.

Culture: The organism grows well on primary isolation media, in which it forms moist to mucoid colonies.

BORDETELLA

The genus *Bordetella* consists of three species that have an absolute requirement for nicotinic acid and are associated with respiratory infections. They are gram-negative coccobacilli and include *B. pertussis, B. parapertussis,* and *B. bronchiseptica.*

Bordetella pertussis

Bordetella pertussis is the causative organism of whooping cough.

Laboratory diagnosis

Specimen: Secretions from bronchi, nasopharynx, and nasal passages are collected by means of long swabs, and they must be cultured immediately. The use of **cough plates** to collect the specimen is not as good a method as the **nasopharyngeal swab,** which can also be used to prepare smears for immediate identification of *B. pertussis* by the direct FA technic.

Cough plate: Hold an uncovered plate of **Bordet-Gengou medium** 4-6 in. in front of the patient's mouth during several expulsive coughs.

Nasopharyngeal swab: Pass a sterile swab of Dacron on a soft wire through the nose and into the nasopharynx, leave it in place for about 30 sec, and then remove and streak the plate with a swab. This method is superior to the cough plate method.[122]

Morphology (Gram stain): The organism is a small gram-negative coccoid bacillus that stains faintly with Gram stain. It occurs singly or in pairs and shows short chains. Old colonies show degenerated filamentous forms.

Culture: Culture is only successful in the early stages (first 2 weeks) of the disease. The specimens must be streaked immediately onto Bordet-Gengou medium. Smears for the FA technic may also be prepared.

For primary culture the organism requires blood agar containing potato infusion and 20% sheep blood (Bordet-Gengou medium). The growth is slow, requiring 2-4 days to become visible. Since penicillin suppresses the growth of gram-positive organisms, the use of two plates is suggested, one without penicillin and one containing 1 unit of penicillin per milliliter of medium.

Incubate at 35° C under increased CO_2 tension. Examine several times during the first 48 hr, and with a sterile scalpel cut out any molds or spreading contaminants. Then examine twice daily for *B. pertussis.* using a hand lens and placing the plates (uncovered) over a substage lamp. Do not discard as negative for 1 week. The colonies are smooth, raised, glistening, pearly, and nearly transparent. They are surrounded by a small zone of hemolysis that is not sharply defined. This hemolysis is more a darkening of the medium than overt hemolysis. At times the colony must be removed to reveal this discoloration.

Cultures are positive for about 1 month after the onset of whooping cough if untreated. During the first 2 weeks of the disease the culture is positive in over 90% of cases.

If antipertussis serum is available, the colonies may be identified without further delay.

Serologic identification

Slide agglutination test (identification of organism by antiserum): Divide the microscope slide into two rectangular areas with a wax pencil. Suspend suspected colonies in saline and add 1 drop of suspension to each rectangular area. To one area, add 1 drop of antipertussis serum (1:10 dilution), which should produce immediate agglutination of bacteria. The saline suspension serves as a roughness control.

The **FA technic** may also be utilized to identify direct smears and young cultures.

Fluorescent antibody technic: Nasopharyngeal smears may be stained with *B. pertussis* antiserum conjugated with fluorescein isothiocyanate.[123]

Biochemical reaction

B. pertussis organisms are inert (Table 32-36).

Differential diagnosis

B. pertussis should be differentiated from *Haemophilus influenzae*, which is also a gram-negative rod found in sputum and morphologically similar to *B. pertussis*. *B. pertussis* must also be distinguished from *B. parapertussis* and *B. bronchiseptica*. These organisms are morphologically indistinguishable but can be separated biochemically and serologically.

Bordetella bronchiseptica

Bordetella bronchiseptica shows all the characteristics of the species except that it is motile. It reduces nitrates to nitrites. It grows more rapidly than *B. pertussis* on Bordet-Gengou medium (2-3 days), and the colonies are larger.

B. parapertussis and *B. bronchiseptica* are morphologically indistinguishable from *B. pertussis*. They are occasionally isolated from human sputum and must be differentiated from *B. pertussis* by biochemical and serologic characteristics.

CALYMMATOBACTERIUM
Calymmatobacterium granulomatis

Granuloma inguinale is a venereal disease which, in the United States, is almost totally confined to blacks. It is characterized by granulomatous lesions involving the external genitals, the anal area, and at times the face.

The cause of the disease is the bacterial organism *Calymmatobacterium granulomatis*. It can be cultured in the yolk sac of the chick embryo and is seen in direct smears of the lesions.

Laboratory diagnosis
Donovan bodies:

Smears: Scrape the lesions and crush the material between two slides. Dry the resulting two smears and stain with Wright stain. Large mononuclear cells are seen that contain many **Donovan bodies.** These are straight to slightly curved rods that stain purple and are surrounded by a pink-staining ovoid capsule.

Table 32-36. Differential characteristics of *Bordetella* and *Haemophilus*

	B. pertussis	*B. bronchiseptica*	*B. parapertussis*	*H. influenzae*
Motility	−	+	−	−
Growth on Bordet-Gengou medium	+	+	+	−
Reduction of nitrates	−	+	+	−
Hemolysis on 20% blood agar	+	+	+	− or +
Factors X and V needed	−	−	−	+
Indole production	−	−	−	+ (80%)
Urease production	−	4 hr	+	−

Tissue sections

Biopsy specimens of the lesion stained with hematoxylin and eosin show the previously mentioned mononuclear cells containing Donovan bodies.

LEGIONELLA

Legionella pneumophila is the etiologic agent of Legionnaires' disease. The disease most frequently presents as pneumonia, in isolated cases or in epidemic fashion. At present, there are six serotypes of *L. pneumophila* (I-VI). In addition, there have been *Legionella*-like organisms isolated and named, e.g., WIGA, the Pittsburgh agent, and Tatlock. These isolates form the bases for additional species of *Legionella*, e.g., *L. bozemanii*, *L. micdadei*, and *L. dumoffi*.

Laboratory diagnosis[124,125]

Specimen: Sputum or tissue from the lungs, spleen, or other organs.

Morphology (Gram stain): These organisms are small gram-negative bacilli 0.3-0.4 μm in width by 2-3 μm in length. Longer forms may be seen.[126] The Dieterle stain may reveal the organisms in tissue, but they must be confirmed with direct fluorescent antibody (FA) staining.

Culture: The organism has been grown on Mueller-Hinton agar containing 2% Isovitalex (Baltimore Biological Laboratories, Baltimore, Md.) and 1% hemoglobin. An alternate medium is charcoal yeast extract (CYE) medium.[127] Increased CO_2 enhances isolation. The organism has also been isolated in embryonated hens' eggs.

Serologic identification: Antibodies to Legionnaires' disease are detected by the microagglutination test and by the indirect fluorescent antibody (IFA) test. Since at this time there are no reagents commercially available, the tests are only performed in reference laboratories. An IFA single titer of $\geq$ 1:256 or paired sera showing a fourfold increase to $\geq$ 1:128 are considered diagnostic.

• • •

The diagnostic approach to the patient suspected of legionellosis is multifaceted. Blood should be drawn every 2-3 weeks for IFA titers. If tissue or respiratory secretions are available, then a direct FA stain for *Legionella* can be done. Culture of the organism should be attempted, although it is rarely positive on sputum specimens and may take at least a week to grow. Tests such as radioimmunoassay, enzyme-linked immunosorbent assay, latex agglutination, and coagglutination are being developed, which will detect soluble antigens in body fluids.

GRAM-NEGATIVE ANAEROBIC NON-SPORE-FORMING BACILLI
BACTEROIDACEAE

Organisms of the Bacteroidaceae family are gram-negative, generally nonmotile, nonencapsulated, and non-spore-forming rods. They are **obligate anaerobes,** and all pathogens within the group produce gas to a greater or lesser degree.

They are commonly found in the mouth and in the intestinal and urogenital tracts. Pathologically, they may be responsible for lung and brain abscesses, peritonitis, tonsillitis, bartholinitis, septicemia, and appendicitis. These organisms often occur in combination with aerobic pyogenic bacteria.[128].

The most commonly identified genera in this group are *Bacteroides* and *Fusobacterium*.

Bacteroides
Bacteroides fragilis
Laboratory diagnosis[129,130]

Specimen: Material from wounds and abscesses, serous fluids, cerebrospinal fluid, joint fluid, etc. is submitted. Aspirated material is preferred, but if aspiration is not feasible, swabs suffice. They should immediately be placed in thioglycollate broth or into prereduced media.

Morphology (Gram stain): Gram-negative, slender, pleomorphic rods with rounded ends are seen. Some species produce filamentous forms and have round, swollen bodies. Pseudobranching and irregular and bipolar staining may also be seen.

Culture: The organism grows slowly in thioglycollate broth and may require 2 weeks before it can be recovered. It produces diffuse turbidity.

Primary isolation: The media should be fresh, and exposure to oxygen should be held to a minimum. It is best to keep a working supply of plated media in the anaerobic jar or transfer chamber to have completely reduced media for culture. Thioglycollate broth and anaerobic Columbia CNA agar and anaerobic kanamycin-vancomycin agar (KV agar) should be inoculated. CNA contains colistin and nalidixic acid to inhibit overgrowth of gram-negative aerobes. The KV agar contains kanamycin and vancomycin and inhibits gram-positive organisms. *B. fragilis* grows well on these media. One blood agar plate should be inoculated. All plates should be incubated anerobically at 35° C. On blood agar the organism forms semitranslucent, small, almost clear, colorless colonies without hemolysis.

The organisms are often "lost" on routine culture since they are obligate anaerobes. No growth appears on the plates, and the thioglycollate, which may show growth of gram-negative rods, is routinely plated on aerobic culture plates. Thus another day elapses and by this time the organisms in thioglycollate may have died.

The organism is difficult to culture even under complete anaerobiosis. Subculture should be made on several tubes of media to ensure survival of the organism. Most species require blood. Hemolysis is rarely seen. The various species can be differentiated on the basis of biochemical reactions, but they are difficult to perform because of the requirement of strict anaerobiosis. Some stains produce pigment. See newer methods of culture of anaerobic organisms, p. 825.

Bacteroides melaninogenicus

Bacteroides melaninogenicus is isolated from wounds less frequently than *B. fragilis*. The organism grows well on anaerobic media. On solid media the colonies are dark colored. After continued incubation they turn black. As with most anaerobic pathogens *B. melaninogenicus* occurs as part of the flora of mixed infections and rarely is found to be the single pathogen in an infectious process.

Fusobacterium

Two species are normal inhabitants of the mouth and upper respiratory tract, *F. necrophorus* and *F. fusiforme*.

Fusobacterium necrophorus
Laboratory diagnosis

Morphology (Gram stain): The organism forms gram-negative filamentous structures with large, round bodies characterized by irregular staining.

Culture: The organism grows diffusely in thioglycollate broth at 35° C. On blood agar at 35° C under anaerobic conditions the colonies are flat with a central dome-shaped elevation (fried-egg appearance). They are often surrounded by a thin zone of hemolysis.

Fusobacterium fusiforme

Fusobacterium fusiforme is a gram-negative nonmotile rod with pointed ends. It is associated with Vincent's angina (trench mouth), an ulcerative infection of the mouth and larynx.

Laboratory diagnosis

Smear: Smears are stained with crystal violet. The organism is a somewhat pleomorphic gram-negative rod with pointed to rounded ends. It is slightly bent at times and often occurs in pairs, the blunt ends touching. It is nonmotile and varies from 8-16 μm in length and 0.5-1.0 μm in diameter.

Culture: The organism is an anaerobe that grows on blood agar with a narrow zone of hemolysis and produces a foul odor (H_2S). The colonies are yellowish green. In thioglycollate broth the organism forms floccules.

GRAM-POSITIVE NON-SPORE-FORMING BACILLI
LACTOBACILLACEAE

Genera collected in the family Lactobacillaceae are *Lactobacillus, Listeria, Corynebacterium, Erysipelothrix*, etc.

Lactobacillus

Lactobacillus acidophilus occurs in the stool of newborn infants and in adults in the mouth, gastrointestinal tract, and vagina (**Döderlein's bacillus**) as well as in the stomach (**Boas-Oppler bacillus**) during pyloric obstruction. It may be found along with yeast in sputum specimens. Some relationship exists between *Lactobacillus* counts in saliva and dental caries.

Laboratory diagnosis

Morphology (Gram stain): Lactobacilli are gram-positive non-spore-forming rods. *L. casei* is characterized by curved rods in curling chains. *L. fermentum*

and *L. acidophilus* produce long straight rods. Morphologically, lactobacilli may resemble *Actinomyces* and diphtheroids.

Culture: Lactobacilli are microaerophilic to anaerobic organisms that ferment glucose. They grow on thioglycollate broth at 35° C, requiring several days and a pH of 6.1-6.8 for growth. The organism grows better when CO_2 is added.

Lactobacilli are the test organisms in the turbidimetric assay of folic acid and vitamin B_{12}; however, these vitamin assays are best performed by radioimmunoassay. Cultures of lactobacilli are used clinically to normalize the intestinal and vaginal flora. These organisms are usually ignored in clinical specimens.

Listeria

Listeria organisms cause disease in humans and domestic animals.

Listeria monocytogenes[131-133]

Listeria monocytogenes is the cause of listeriosis, a purulent meningitis and septicemia of the newborn. The focus of infection lies in the pregnant mother who transfers the infection transplacentally to the fetus, which leads to abortion, or to the newborn infant via the infected genital tract. The name of the organism is derived from the monocytic reaction to infection, which may not often occur.

Laboratory diagnosis

Specimen: Blood, spinal fluid, and sputum are the materials used.

Morphology (Gram stain): The organism is a small, motile (tumbling motion), gram-positive rod measuring 0.5-2.0 μm in length and 0.4 μm in diameter. The rods may be single, parallel, or at angles to each other. They may be somewhat pleomorphic, with coccoid forms appearing in smears of cultures. Because of these coccoid forms, *Listeria* may be mistaken for *Streptococcus* or *Corynebacterium*. *Listeria* stains uniformly, lacking the granularity of *Corynebacterium*. The degenerate forms may show long filamentous structures.

Culture: One blood agar and two thioglycollate broths are used as primary media. The blood agar plate and one broth are inoculated and then incubated at 35° C, while the second thioglycollate broth is refrigerated after inoculation. This is called "cold enrichment" and frequently enhances recovery of the organism, particularly from tissues.

In the case of blood cultures, one blood culture bottle should be refrigerated and the other incubated at 35° C. The broth cultures incubated at 35° C are subcultured to blood agar plates at suitable intervals for up to 2 weeks, and the refrigerated broth cultures for up to 3 months.

Tissue must be left in the refrigerator for at least 24 hr before it is ground and cultured. Round, soft, transparent colonies that produce β-hemolysis are seen on blood agar at 35° C after 24 hr. **Smooth** and **rough forms** occur together. The smooth forms appear as previously described and have a smooth surface. Under the oblique light of the scanning microscope they have a bluish green opalescence. In a mixed culture this process may allow the identification of *Listeria* colonies.

Table 32-37. Characteristic properties of *Listeria* and *Corynebacterium*

	Listeria monocytogenes	*Corynebacterium*
Catalase	+	+
	+ at 20° C	−
Motility	± at 37° C	−
Glucose (acid only)	+	+
Hemolysis	+(β)	−
Indole	−	−
Salicin (acid only)	+	−
Nitrate reduction	−	+
Methyl red	+	−

The rough forms have irregular edges and folds on the surface that radiate from a central elevation. Hemolysis is only poorly developed. Many transitions between smooth and rough forms can be found. The organisms characteristically survive 8 weeks when placed in 20% sodium chloride and stored in the refrigerator; this is helpful in culturing *Listeria* from contaminated autopsy and surgical material because other organisms fail to survive.

Motility: Use motility agar incubated at 20-25° C. *Listeria* organisms are motile, but they are less motile at 37° C.

Biochemical reactions: The biochemical reactions of *Listeria* are as follows:

Glucose, maltose, fructose: acid
Sucrose, sorbitol, xylose: acid, delayed, longer than 3 days
Mannitol, inulin, starch: no utilization or fermentation
Indole, H_2S, urease, oxidase: negative
Nitrates: not reduced
Methyl red, catalase: positive

Listera species can be differentiated from diphtheroids by β-hemolysis on blood agar and by motility, both characteristic of *Listeria*. They are differentiated from *Cornyebacterium* according to Table 32-37.

Animal inoculation: Inject 1 loopful of saline-suspended culture into the conjunctival sac of a rabbit or guinea pig. Purulent conjunctivitis will sometimes result after about 8 hr, but usually a period of 2-5 days should be allowed. The conjunctivitis will heal spontaneously.

Listeriosis is a common disease of animals, and therefore the usual inoculation routes cannot be used.

Serologic identification: Antisera to **Listeria** are commercially available but are not usually required.

Corynebacterium

Corynebacteria are pleomorphic organisms causing disease in humans, animals, and plants.

Corynebacterium diphtheriae

Corynebacterium diphtheriae is a small, slender, nonmotile, gram-positive rod that is the etiologic agent of human diphtheria. It produces a powerful exotoxin that is responsible for local tissue necrosis and gener-

alized toxemia. The local toxicity leads to pseudomembranous inflammation that may involve the tonsils, pharynx, larynx, and nose.

Classification: Three types of *C. diphtheriae* are distinguishable on the basis of their gross cultural characteristics on blood tellurite medium: gravis, mitis, and intermedius. This classification has little value since all types produce the same toxin and therefore are not further discussed.

Laboratory diagnosis

Specimen: Prior to antibody therapy, material from the nasopharynx and throat is collected on swabs, which, after collection of the specimen, are moistened with transport medium.

Morphology (Gram stain): The organism is a gram-positive, straight, or slightly bent rod that may vary in length from 0.8-5 μm. The ends are usually rounded but at times may be nodular or pointed. The organisms form V- and L-shaped patterns as well as packages of parallel forms and "Chinese-letter" arrangements. Older cultures may be pleomorphic. The smears may be stained with methylene blue or Gram stain. **Albert stain** reveals metachromatic granules. The direct smear is not an adequate tool for the diagnosis of diphtheria because diphtheroids and actinomycetes resemble *C. diphtheriae*.

Culture: *C. diphtheriae* is a nonmotile aerobic organism. It grows well on media containing coagulated serum and eggs. Culture swab on blood agar and on Loeffler medium. Examine both, especially the **Loeffler slant,** after 18 hr, when grayish white, soft, 1 mm colonies that can be easily emulsified in water may be seen on the slant. It is often possible to harvest diphtheria bacilli from Loeffler medium in 4-6 hr. The colonies are smeared and stained. If suspicious on the basis of the Gram stain, the colonies are transferred from Loeffler slant to a serum-cystine-thiosulfate-tellurite agar (**Tinsdale medium**) plate for the production of characteristic colonies. This medium is stabbed as well as streaked, because the brown to black halo is first noted around the stabs.

Tinsdale medium: On serum-cystine-thiosulfate-tellurite agar, *C. diphtheriae* forms smooth, shiny, black to grayish colonies with (very important) black halos. H_2S is produced by the action on cystine and it then reacts with the tellurite in the medium. The halo is best seen after 48 hr, but it may appear after 24 hr. *C. ulcerans* gives a similar picture. It may be isolated from skin ulcers or throat lesions. Most bacteria form black colonies on Tinsdale medium, but they are devoid of the brown to black halo. Included in the list of bacteria that produce black colonies are the following: diphtheroids (nonpathogenic corynebacteria), streptococci, staphylococci, *Neisseria,* pneumococci, *Klebsiella, Haemophilus,* and *Escherichia coli.* Included in the group of **nonpathogenic diphtheroids** are *C. xerosis* and *C. ulcerans. Propionibacterium acnes,* the anerobic diphtheroid, will grow on Tinsdale medium but only when incubated anerobically.

If black colonies with black halos appear on the Tindsale medium, the organism is transferred again to Loeffler medium or to **Pai egg medium** to confirm the characteristic morphology. Smears should not be made directly from Tinsdale medium. If the smears from Loeffler medium again suggest *C. diphtheriae*, send a report to the physician and to the hospital ward stating that the organisms morphologically resemble *C. diphtheriae*.

Chemical reactions: Chemical reactions are not reliable, although characteristically *C. diphtheriae* ferments dextrose without gas and fails to ferment sucrose.

Definitive diagnosis

Demonstration of toxicity (virulence tests): Virulence tests include animal inoculations or the agar diffusion test. One of these tests must be performed on all suspicious cultures.

Animal inoculation (in vivo method): Guinea pigs are usually used. The hair of the animal is shaved with an electric clipper so that the skin of the back and flanks is exposed. Inject 0.1 ml of 2-3 ml broth suspension of an 18 hr growth of bacteria on Loeffler slant intracutaneously into the nonimmune animal. Give 500 units of diphtheria antitoxin intraperitoneally 5 hr later and at the same time inject 0.1 ml bacterial suspension intracutaneously into a different site. A virulent toxogenic strain may be used as a control. If the test is positive, 48 hr after the injection into the guinea pig a necrotic area will appear on the skin. This necrotic response is not found in the area injected after the administration of diphtheria antitoxin.

Agar diffusion test: Prepare Petri plates using a special agar media, which is prepared as follows:
1. Proteose-peptone agar (Difco Laboratories, Detroit), 20 g
2. Lactic acid, 0.7 ml in 5 dl distilled water
3. Sodium hydroxide, 4%, 1.5 ml

Bring to boil, filter, adjust to pH 7.8 with 1N hydrochloric acid, and refilter through fluted filter paper.

Prepare filter paper strips saturated with 50 units of diphtheria toxin and place on top of freshly prepared and just-gelled agar plate. Allow to dry completely in an incubator (3 hr). Streak saline emulsion of unknown *C. diphtheriae* and of known positive and negative diphtheria control bacteria at right angles to the centrally placed impregnated filter strip. Incubate the plate at 35° C. If the diphtheria bacilli are toxin producing, a precipitation line will form between the impregnated filter paper and the bacterial streak (Fig. 32-12).

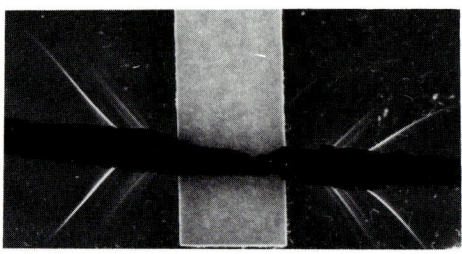

Fig. 32-12. Agar diffusion test for toxicity of *Corynebacterium diphtheriae*. White precipitation lines at a 45-degree angle are seen between filter paper strip (gray) and bacterial streak (black–potassium tellurite effect).

NOTE: After 48 hr, secondary lines may form that are not related to toxin production.

Erysipelothrix
Erysipelothrix rhusiopathiae

Erysipelothrix rhusiopathiae is widely distributed in animals and is important as the cause of an infectious disease in swine and other animals. It causes skin lesions (erysipeloid) in humans.

Laboratory diagnosis

Specimen: Use a biopsy of skin, including the advancing edge of erysipeloid.

Morphology (Gram stain): The organism is a gram-positive, nonmotile, beaded rod that is slender, straight, and often paired. It may be curved (S shaped) and may give rise to long, slender, tangled filaments. It becomes decolorized easily and may appear gram negative.

Culture: The organism is anaerobic or microaerophilic. Place the specimen in thioglycollate broth, incubate at 35° C, subculture to blood agar after 24 hr, and incubate at 35° C. The organism grows well at 35° C on blood agar. Cystine-glucose-blood agar (see discussion of *Pasteurella*) is also a good primary medium.

The organism is catalase negative (*Listeria* and *Corynebacterium* are catalase positive) and reduces nitrates. It is weakly saccharolytic and may produce H_2S. It is indole negative.

Animal inoculation

Intraperitoneal injection of 0.25 ml bacterial suspension will kill mice in 2-4 days.

MYCOBACTERIACEAE
Mycobacterium

Mycobacterium comprises a large group of strictly aerobic, acid-fast organisms, some of which cause disease in humans and animals, whereas others lead a saprophytic existence in water, fruits, vegetables, manure, and humans. Of greatest clinical importance is *M. tuberculosis*, the etiologic agent of tuberculosis, but other mycobacteria are also able to cause disease in humans.

Classification: See Table 32-38.

Laboratory diagnosis[134-137]

Laboratory diagnosis and differentiation of mycobacteria include special methods of collection, concentration, staining (acid-fast), culture, pigment production, biochemical reactions, and other differentiating tests as well as methods for detecting drug susceptibility patterns, animal pathogenicity, and antibodies to *M. tuberculosis*.

Special methods of collection and concentration: Contaminated specimens:

Sputum: If the specimen is not processed immediately, store it in the refrigerator. Sputum of children may have to be obtained by gastric lavage, which in general should be avoided. Special plastic, sterile, wide-mouthed, screw-capped centrifuge tubes for the collection of sputum are available in which the concentration procedure can be carried out, thus minimizing the handling of infectious material.

The first morning expectoration provides the best specimen; it is superior to a large pooled specimen, which may be heavily contaminated and toxic to tubercle bacilli and may also dilute a single positive contribution. A minimum of three single specimens should be collected on successive days; each specimen should not exceed 10 ml. Methods employing **heated aerosols** are successful in stimulating sputum production if expectoration is difficult.

Other methods of sputum collection may be the hypopharyngeal swab (especially useful in children) and bronchoscopy.

Gastric contents: Gastric contents should be collected directly into 5 ml of 10% trisodium phosphate or 1 ml of 10% anhydrous sodium bicarbonate to reach pH 7.0-8.0 (use indicator).

The normal acidity and enzymatic activity of the gastric juice are detrimental to tubercle bacilli. Since saprophytic tubercle bacilli on smears are indistinguishable from pathogenic forms, the gastric material should only be cultured, not smeared. Digest with *N*-acetyl-L-cysteine-sodium hydroxide (see below). Positive cultures must be carefully identified before reporting them as *M. tuberculosis*. The use of gastric aspiration should be avoided. It should only be used when the physician is confronted with a highly suspicious chest x-ray film and a patient who is unable to produce sputum.

Urine: The specimen of choice is the first morning specimen, which represents an overnight collection of urine. Other types of specimens may be utilized, such as a pooled 24 hr specimen, a clean-voided midstream specimen, or a specimen obtained by ureteral catheterization of one kidney.

During the collection period all urine specimens must be kept in the refrigerator.

If a large amount of urine is received in the laboratory, the specimen is transferred to a clean Erlenmeyer flask, the mouth of which is covered. The specimen is allowed to sediment overnight in the refrigerator. Next morning the upper portion is discarded and the sediment and the lower 200-300 ml of urine are centrifuged in multiple centrifuge tubes. The supernatants are discarded and the sediments are combined. For purposes of concentration, the specimen is handled as is sputum.

A first morning specimen is preferred since it is less contaminated than a 24 hr specimen. Cleaning of the genitals will prevent contamination with smegma bacilli. Positive smears must be interpreted with caution, and positive cultures must be carefully identified before reporting them as *M. tuberculosis*.

Tissues: Tissues from surgical or autopsy specimens should be homogenized by using a mortar and pestle or a glass tissue homogenizer.

Skin: Acid-fast organisms of skin lesions should be cultured at 30° C, since *M. ulcerans* and *M. balnei* fail to grow at 35° C.

Feces: Examination of feces for tubercle bacilli is not encouraged, because any tubercle bacilli present most likely result from swallowed pulmonary material.

The specimen is concentrated as is sputum.

Noncontaminated specimens: Noncontaminated specimens include catheterized urine specimens, clear body fluids, e.g., pleural, pericardial, and peritoneal fluids, and cerebrospinal fluid. Do not use a digestion method, because it unavoidably leads to loss of vital bacteria. Centrifuge specimens at high speed and use sediment for smear, culture, and rarely for animal inoculation.

Cerebrospinal fluid: Spinal fluid examination should be done promptly. If there is a pellicle, it should be

Table 32-38. Classification of *Mycobacterium*

Runyon group	Usually produces disease in humans	Usually saprophytic	Cultural (on 7H-11)[137-140] and other characteristics of pathogens
	M. tuberculosis (human tubercle bacillus)		Tightly corded texture; rough colonies; slow growth; positive niacin test; nitrate reduction; negative catalast after heating at 68° C
	M. bovis		Tightly corded texture; rough to smooth colonies; variable rate of growth; niacin negative
I (photochromogens)	*M. kansasii*		Yellow to orange to red pigment when exposed to light; carotene crystals; no pigment in dark; colonies smooth to rough; strong catalase activity
	M. marinum		Optimal temperature 25° C; similar to *M. kansassi* but smoother; nitrate not reduced
II (scotochromogens)	"Tap water bacillus"		Yellow pigment when grown in light or dark; slow growth; colonies tend to be smooth; loose cording; never in sputum; from superficial lesions; medium growth rate
III (nonphotochromogens)	*M. intracellulare* (Battey bacillus)	*M. terrae, M. gastri*	Slow growers; no pigment; colonies thin, transparent, and circular; Tween hydrolysis positive
	M. xenopi		Yellowish pigment; raised colonies with branching filaments
IV (rapid growers)	*M. fortuitum*[141]	*M. smegmatis, M. phlei*	Nonpigmented, branching filaments; rapid growth at 25° C (3-4 days); pigmented

spread on a slide, fixed, and stained for acid-fast bacteria. If no pellicle is found, centrifuge the specimen, decant the supernatant, and use the sediment for smears, culture, and rarely for animal inoculation.

Methods of concentration and decontamination: The purpose of concentration and methods is to destroy contaminating organisms while allowing tubercle bacilli to survive, so that they can be concentrated, cultured, stained, and, if necessary, injected into animals.

N-acetyl-L-cysteine–sodium hydroxide (NALC-NaOH) digestion method:

Reagents:

1. *N*-Acetyl-L-cysteine–sodium hydroxide digestant, 50 ml

   Combine 25 ml of 4% 1N sodium hydroxide, 25 ml of 2.94% 0.1M. trisodium citrate, and 0.25 g *N*-acetyl-L-cysteine powder.

Sterilize the sodium hydroxide and the trisodium citrate separately by autoclaving; mix and store in the refrigerator. The mixture is stable for several weeks. Add the *N*-acetyl-L-cysteine powder within 24 hr of use.

2. Phosphate buffer, 0.067M, pH7.0
   a. Stock solution. Combine 9.48 g/L of 0.067M Na_2HPO_4 and 9.07 g/L of 0.067M KH_2PO_4.
   b. Working solution, pH 7.0. Combine 61.1 ml stock Na_2HPO_4 and 38.9 ml stock HH_2PO_4. Check the pH with a pH meter.

3. Bovine albumin (Sigma Chemical Co., St. Louis), fraction V, 0.2%, in saline solution (Adjust pH to 6.8 with 10% sodium hydroxide. Sterilize by Seitz filtration. For use, prepare 1:10 albumin solution in sterile 0.067M phosphate buffer (solution 2).

Procedure: To 10 ml sputum specimen collected in a 50 ml sterile, disposable, plastic, screw-capped centrifuge tube, add an equal volume of *N*-acetyl-L-cysteine–sodium hydroxide solution. (The volume of sputum should not exceed one fifth the volume of the tube.) Mix in a vortex mixer for 5-30 sec, or until digested. Let stand at room temperature for 15 min to decontaminate. Fill tube to within $1/2$-$3/4$ in. of the top with sterile 0.067M phosphate buffer, pH 6.8. Centrifuge at (or near) 3000 rpm for 30 min. Carefully decant supernatant fluid. Retain sediment.

Prepare a smear from the sediment. If direct drug susceptibility tests are to be done, it is necessary to roughly quantitate the number of acid-fast organisms in the sediment. For this purpose use a sterile (flamed) inoculating loop 3 mm in diameter, and spread the material over an area approximately 1 × 2 cm. Stain by the acid-fast or fluorescent method and determine the number of acid-fast bacilli per oil-immersion field. Add 1 ml of 0.2% bovine albumin fraction V in 0.85% saline solution to the remaining sediment (concentrated specimen). Using 1 ml of this sediment, make a 1:10 dilution with sterile water (diluted specimen).

Inoculate the concentrated and the diluted specimens onto two plastic biplates, half containing Middlebrook-Cohn 7H-11 agar and half Lowenstein-Jensen egg medium. If the acid-fast smear is negative, 3 drops of the suspected material are spread over each half of the biplate onto drug-free media. If the acid-fast smear is positive, the material is spread directly onto drug susceptibility test plates using quadrant plates containing 7H-10 agar with isoniazid, streptomycin, *p*-aminosalicylic acid (PAS), and a drug-free control.

After inoculation place all media into CO_2-permeable Mylar bags to prevent drying and incubate at 35° C under 5-10% CO_2 tension.

Sodium hydroxide digestion method: Transfer the specimen into a heavy, round-bottomed, screw-capped tube and add an equal amount of autoclaved 4% sodium hydroxide. Mix and then shake forcefully for 15 min in a paint shaker; centrifuge at 3000 rpm for 20 min. Decant the supernatant and add 1 drop of bromthymol blue to sediment (bromthymol blue: acid—yellow; alkaline—blue). Neutralize sediment accurately with sterile 2N hydrochloric acid until yellow color is obtained. Back titrate with sterile 4% sodium hydroxide until the first persistent blue color appears.

Inoculate sediment onto Middlebrook-Cohn 7H-11 agar and Lowenstein-Jensen egg medium using sterile pipets. Prepare smears for acid-fast stains.

Gruft procedure for processing sputum specimen for Gruft modification of Lowenstein-Jensen medium: Add an equal amount of 2% sodium hydroxide to the sputum specimen and shake for 15 min in a paint shaker. Centrifuge the specimen at 3000 rpm for 30 min. Discard the supernatant.

Add 20 ml of 0.067M phosphate buffer, pH 6.5, containing bromthymol blue to the sediment and adjust to pH 6.5, if necessary, with normal hydrochloric acid. Centrifuge the specimen again at 3000 rpm for 30 min, and discard most of the supernatant. Inoculate the neutralized sediment on duplicate tubes of Gruft-modified Lowenstein-Jensen medium and incubate in an atmosphere of 8% CO_2 in a slant position for 1 week and upright for 7 weeks.

Trisodium phosphate–Zephiran procedure:

Reagent: The reagent consists of 1000 g trisodium phosphate ($Na_3PO_4 \cdot 12H_2O$), 40 dl hot distilled water, and 7.5 ml Zephiran.

An equal volume of 10% trisodium phosphate is added to the specimen. The mixture is shaken in a paint shaker for 30 min and centrifuged at 3000 rpm for 30 min. Decant the supernatant and neutralize with 1N hydrochloric acid containing bromthymol blue. Inoculate the sediment onto egg medium and onto 7H-11 medium after the addition of 10 mg/dl mixture lecithin to neutralize Zephiran, since without neutralization it has a bacteriostatic effect on mycobacteria.

Clorox (5.25% sodium hypochlorite) digestion method: The Clorox concentration method can be used only for the preparation of smears because it kills the organisms. Mix one half to equal parts of Clorox with specimen. Allow to stand for 15 min. Centrifuge at 3000 rpm for 30 min. Decant the supernatant and prepare the smear from the sediment.

Acid-fast stained smear: The **purpose** of the acid-fast stained smear is to accomplish the following:

1. Allow presumptive diagnosis of acid-fast infection
2. Evaluate progress of treatment
3. Confirm cultural growth
4. Demonstrate acid-fast bacteria in tissue

5. Evaluate morphology of acid-fast organisms
6. Evaluate the degree of acid fastness of bacteria, e.g., weakly acid fast
7. Arrive at a rough estimate of the number of acid-fast organisms per oil-immersion field or per slide
8. Standardize inoculum size for drug susceptibility testing of acid-fast organisms
9. Standardize inoculum for direct drug susceptibility testing

The **number** of **organisms (Gaffky number)** found in concentrated smears is reported as follows:

3-9 organisms per slide: rare acid-fast organisms
10 or more organisms per slide: few acid-fast organisms
More than 1 organism per oil-immersion field: numerous acid-fast organisms

Stains for acid-fast organisms: The three methods of staining are (1) the Kinyoun acid-fast staining method, (2) the Ziehl-Neelsen acid-fast staining method, and (3) the fluorescent dye method using the Truant fluorescent dye[142] (see staining methods).

General morphology

Mycobacteria are straight or slightly curved, thin rods that require special staining because of their lipid content. Once stained, they are not readily decolorized **(acid fast).** In cultures the bacteria are often coccoid, filamentous, and branching (hence mycobacteria). Staining is not uniform; it is accentuated by granules and interrupted by poorly stained segments. Acid-fast bacteria are difficult to stain with Gram stain, but they are gram positive. The number of bacilli in the direct smear is not a good index of the severity of the disease but rather of the infectivity of the patient.

Primary isolation of acid-fast organisms

Liquid media: Liquid media are not suitable for primary isolation, because clouding of the medium is produced by *M. tuberculosis* as well as by atypical tubercle bacilli.

If it is necessary to employ liquid media, **Middlebrook 7H-9 medium** and **Middlebrook-Tween-albumin broth** are used and incubated at 35° C. After 7-10 days' incubation they are subcultured onto **Middlebrook-Cohn 7H-11** and **Lowenstein-Jensen egg media.**

Synthetic media: Middlebrook-Cohn 7H-11 agar is a synthetic medium that, because of its agar base, is transparent. It is a modification of the Middlebrook 7H-10 medium, to which casein hydrolyzate has been added. It allows recognition of early (3 weeks) growth and of microcolonial characteristics of various types of mycobacteria. Because of the transparency of the medium, it is possible to "read through" contaminations. The medium permits more accurate drug susceptibility testing, because drugs are not subject to potential inactivation by inspissation, since they can be added after sterilization of the medium.

Incubate Middlebrook-Cohn 7H-11 plates in CO_2-permeable polyethylene bags at 35° C under 5-10% CO_2 tension for 3 weeks in the dark or in Mylar CO_2-impermeable bags containing heavily seeded plates of growing *M. phlei.* Examine plates both macroscopi-

cally and microscopically only once at the end of 3 weeks, using a dissecting microscope.

Egg media: Lowenstein-Jensen and Petragnani media are the most commonly used egg media. They are opaque; therefore early colonies may be missed. Drug-resistant organisms frequently fail to grow on these media. Drugs incorporated into egg media may lose some of their potency during the process of inspissation.

Gruft modification of Lowenstein-Jensen medium: The Gruft modification of Lowenstein-Jensen medium inhibits the growth of gram-positive and gram-negative bacteria and thus allows the use of a lesser concentration of sodium hydroxide in the sodium hydroxide concentration and decontamination procedure.

Inoculate the neutralized sediment on duplicate tubes of Gruft-modified Lowenstein-Jensen medium and incubate at 35° C in an atmosphere of 10% CO_2 tension in a slant position for 1 week and upright for 7 weeks. Examine and aerate the tubes once a week.

Methods for differentiation of mycobacteria

The differentiation of mycobacteria is based on a number of criteria, which should all be evaluated before the final diagnosis is made (Table 32-39).
1. Source of specimen (location of lesion)
2. Morphology of acid-fast stained organisms
3. Cultural characteristics: rate of growth, optimal temperature of growth, and shape and texture of colonies
4. Pigment production and effect of light on color
5. Drug susceptibility pattern
6. Biochemical tests

Source of specimen: *M. marinum* is never found in sputum but always originates from a superficial lesion. *M. ulcerans* also usually comes from a superficial lesion of an individual who has been in the tropics.

Morphology: The average tubercle bacilli may vary in size from 0.8-5.0 μm in length and from 0.2-0.6 μm in width. They vary from a coccobacillus to an elongated rod. Longer bacilli may be stained unevenly in a beaded or bipolar fashion. Cross-banded cells are characteristic of *M. kansasii.* Pleomorphic, at times branching forms point toward Runyon group III organisms.

Cultural characteristics:
Rate of growth:
Slow growers: The organisms require over 10 days to form visible colonies on solid media inoculated from a diluted 7- to 10-day-old broth culture. Slow growers include *M. tuberculosis, M. bovis, M. kansasii, M. ulcerans,* and *M. intracellulare.*

Rapid growers: The organisms require less than 7 days to fully mature on solid media inoculated from a diluted 7- to 10-day-old broth culture. Rapid growers include Runyon group IV organisms, e.g., *M. fortuitum* and, seldom, *M. marinum* of group I.

Optimal temperature of growth: The optimal temperature for growth of *M. marinum* is 32-33° C; it grows poorly at temperatures over 33° C. *M. kansasii* is able to grow at 22° C. *M. tuberculosis* is unable to grow at 22° C. *M. xenopei* grows well at 45° C. Most mycobacteria grow at 35-37° C.

Table 32-39. Characteristics of some *Mycobacterium**

Species	Culture				Drug pattern (INH)	Niacin test	Nitrate reduction	Semiquantitative catalase activity (mm)	Tween 80 hydrolysis (days)	Tellurite reduction in 3 days	Arylsulfatase in 3 days	Growth on MacConkey agar
	Growth rate	Pigment		Morphology (711-10)								
		Dark	Light									
M. tuberculosis	Slow	—	—	R	R	S	+	+	<40	10	—	—	—
M. bovis	Slow	—	—	R	R	S	—	—	<40	—	—	—	—
M. kansasii	Slow	—	Y	S	S	R or S	—	+	>50	5	—	—	—
"Tap water bacillus"	Slow	Y	O	Often S	R or S	—	—	>50	—	—	—	—
M. intracellulare (Battey bacillus)	Slow	—	—	Often S	R	—	—	<40	—	+	—	— or +
M. fortuitum	Rapid	—	—	R or S	R	—	— to +	>50	—	+	+	+

Based on data from Runyon[138] Wayne and Doubek[139] Vestal and Kubica[140] and Canilang and Armstrong.[141]
*Y, Yellow; O, orange; R, rough; S, smooth or sensitive; INH, isoniazid.

Shape and texture of colonies: Microscopic examination of mycobacterial colonies on 7H-11 medium under the low-power objective permits the earliest possible diagnosis of *Mycobacterium*.

For microcolonial characteristics of mycobacteria, see Table 32-38.

Pigment production: Mycobacteria can be classified according to whether pigment appears during growth when light is present or excluded or if it appears regardless of light exposure. Exclusion of air interferes with pigment production; thus caps on the culture tubes must be loosened. Pigment is best seen in well-isolated young cultures. Group II scotochromogens are characterized by a deep yellow to orange color that appears even if the organisms are grown in the dark. Exposure to light for 2 weeks may change the color from orange to red. Group III nonphotochromogens are pale yellow whether exposed to light or not. After exposure to light for 1 hr, group I photochromogens turn light yellow when reincubated for 6-24 hr in the dark.

Exposure to light for 1 hr:

Light source: Use a 30- to 60-watt lamp. The culture tubes should be 8-10 in. from the light source.

Procedure: Select cultures with well-isolated colonies (grown in dark). Loosen cap on culture tube. Remove whole shield from culture and cover half of slant with one half of the shield. Expose to light for 1 hr as directed. Replace whole shield and incubate at 35° C in the dark for 6-12 hr or overnight. Check for pigmentation by comparing pigment of colonies on both exposed and shielded portions of the tube.

If results are not clear cut, compare with other tube of same specimen that has remained in the dark.

NOTE: Tests must be made with actively growing cultures. (Up to 5 or 6 days **after** colonies have appeared is usually satisfactory. Older cultures should not be used.)

Interpretation: *M. kansasii* and *M. marinum* will develop yellow pigment within 1 hr.

Exposure to continuous light for 2 weeks[143]:

Light source: Use a 36 in., cool white, 30-watt light bulb (General Electric fluorescent bulb). Place cultures approximately 8 in. from the light source. The light intensity should be 150 candles/sq. ft. Measure with a Weston Master no. 3 light meter.

Procedure: Prepare two Lowenstein-Jensen slants so as to have well-isolated colonies. Treat tubes as follows: For the light tube (1 tube), shield from light and incubate for 2 weeks in dark. Remove shield and expose to light for 2 weeks. For the dark tube (1 tube), incubate for 4 weeks and shield from light.

Compare pigmentation of colonies on both sets of cultures at the end of 4 weeks.

Interpretation: All colonies of photochromogens may require 2 weeks of exposure before developing orange pigments.

Drug susceptibility pattern: The drug susceptibility pattern is helpful in the identification of mycobacteria. *M. tuberculosis* is susceptible to primary antituberculous drugs, e.g., isoniazid, streptomycin, and *p*-aminosalicylic acid (PAS). Most other mycobacteria are somewhat resistant to isoniazid and streptomycin. See discussion on p. 878.

Biochemical procedures (Table 32-38)

Semiquantitative catalase test:

Principle: All acid-fast bacteria contain catalase, an enzyme that liberates oxygen from hydrogen peroxide.

Reagents: Mix in equal parts 10% Tween 80 in distilled water and 30% hydrogen peroxide. Prepare fresh mixture for each day's use.

Media:

Lowenstein-Jensen (L-J) butt tubes: Dispense 5 ml L-J medium in 20 × 150 mm screw-capped tubes. Inspissate with tubes in upright position in water bath at 85° C for 60 min. Remove tubes and incubate at 35° C overnight to check for sterility of medium.

Inoculation of media: Add 0.2 ml of a 7-day Tween-albumin broth (TAB) culture to L-J butt tube. Incubate "rapid growers" for 1 week with caps loose at 35-37° C. Incubate "slow growers" for 2 weeks with caps loose at 35-37° C. Perform test on "rapid growers" after 1 week's incubation, and on "slow growers" after 2 weeks' incubation.

Procedure: Add 1.0 ml Tween-peroxide mixture to L-J culture. Let culture stand in upright position for 5 min at room temperature. Measure column of bubbles in millimeters. Record as <40 mm or >50 mm.

Controls: Set up two positive culture controls, one with 40 mm bubbles *(M. tuberculosis)* and the other with 50 mm bubbles (group II). Also set up a negative control on uninoculated medium.

Interpretation: Mycobacteria of groups IV, II, and I *(M. kansasii)* produce more than 50 mm bubbles; *M. tuberculosis, M. bovis, M. avium*, and some group III organisms produce less than 40 mm bubbles.

Catalase test at 68° C in pH 7.0 buffer:

Principle: Catalase activity of human and bovine tubercle bacilli ceases at 68° C in buffered solution, pH 7.0. All other mycobacteria (and *Nocardia*) maintain catalase activity at this pH and temperature.

Reagents:

1. Tween-peroxide mixture.
   Mix in equal parts 10% Tween 80 in distilled water and 30% hydrogen peroxide. Prepare fresh mixture for each day's use.
2. Phosphate buffer. 0.067M, pH 7.0.
   Mix together 61.1 ml of 0.067M (9.47 g/L) of disodium phosphate (Na_2HPO_4) and 38.9 ml of 0.067M (9.07 g/L) postassium acid phosphate (KH_2PO_4).

Procedure: Scrape several spadesful of growth from the slant of organism to be tested. Suspend growth in 0.5 ml of pH 7.0 phosphate buffer (0.067M) in a 16 × 125 mm screw-capped tube. Place the tube in a 68° C water bath for 20 min. Cool the suspension to room temperature.

Add 0.5 ml of the Tween-peroxide mixture. Observe for bubbling and record as + or −. Hold tubes for 20 min before discarding as negative.

Controls: At 68° C the negative control is a known negative organism *(M. tuberculosis)*. The positive control is a known positive organism *(M. kansasii)*.

Interpretation: See discussion of principle.

Niacin test:

Principle: The large amount of niacin produced by *M. tuberculosis* forms a yellow color compound with cyanogen bromide and aniline. (Cyanogen bromide forms tear gas when vaporized and must be used under a well-ventilated fume hood.)

Reagents:

1. Sterile water or saline solution
2. Aniline, 4%, in ethyl alcohol
3. Cyanogen bromide, 10% aqueous

Procedure: Add 1 ml sterile water or saline solution to the culture slant (L-J) of the test organism. Colonies should be present at least 3 weeks before the test is performed and may require 8-9 weeks after colonies have appeared before yielding a positive test. Slant the culture so that the fluid covers the colonies and let it remain in this position for 15 min. Remove 0.5 ml of this aqueous extract and transfer to a 16 × 125 mm screw-capped test tube. The technic for removing the extract is as follows: Rotate the culture tube so that the slant faces downward, insert a pipet along the glass side, and remove the extract without touching the slant. Culture tube may be used again since the colonies have not been disturbed (Fig. 32-13).

Add 0.5 ml aniline and 0.5 ml cyanogen bromide to the extract. Mix and observe for the formation of a yellow color. If niacin is present, the color appears almost immediately throughout the solution.

Controls: Prepare a niacin-positive culture (known *M. tuberculosis*), a niacin-negative culture (e.g., known group III nonphotochromogen), and a saline control on the uninoculated tube of medium.

Results: The test is positive when the development of a yellow color indicates the presence of niacin. No color change indicates absence of niacin; therefore the test is negative.

Interpretation: *M. tuberculosis* is the only niacin-positive *Mycobacterium*.

NOTE: Stock solutions of aniline and cyanogen bromide may be prepared and stored in brown bottles in the refrigerator. If either solution changes color or precipitates, it should be discarded and a fresh solution prepared. The 10% cyanogen bromide solution is close to saturation and therefore storage in the refrigerator may cause precipitation. However, warming to room temperature will bring about solution of most of the compound.

Nitrate reduction test:

Principle: Some mycobacteria contain a nitrate reductase that converts nitrates into nitrites. Nitrites give a red color with the color reagent.

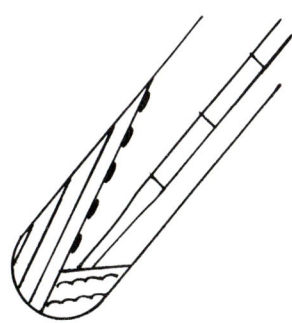

Fig. 32-13. Technic of niacin test (see text).

Reagents:
1. NaNO$_3$, 0.01M, in 0.022M phosphate buffer, pH 7.0
   Combine 0.85g NaNO$_3$, 0.117g KH$_2$PO$_4$, 0.485 g Na$_2$HPO$_4$ · 12H$_2$O, and 1 dl distilled water.
2. Concentrated hydrochloric acid, 1:2 dilution (reagent 1)
3. Sulfanilamide, 0.2% aqueous (reagent 2)
4. *N*-Naphthylethylenediamine dihydrochloride, 0.1% aqueous (reagent 3)

Store solutions at room temperature. They remain stable for approximately 2 weeks. If either reagent 3 or 4 changes in color, discard and prepare a fresh solution.

Procedure: Place a few drops of sterile distilled water in a 16 × 125 mm screw-capped tube. Add in 1 loopful or 1 spadeful of growth from an L-J slant that is 3-4 weeks old. Add 2 ml NaNO$_3$ solution. Shake and incubate in a 37° C water bath for 2 hr. Add 1 drop of reagent 1, 2 drops of reagent 2, and 2 drops of reagent 3. Examine immediately for development of a pink to red color.

To all negative tubes add a small amount of powdered zinc. Unreacted nitrate will be reduced to nitrite. Hence formation of a red color after addition of zinc indicates that the negative reading was valid.

Controls: Prepare a nitrate-positive culture *(M. tuberculosis)* and a reagent control without organisms.

The test may also be quantiated.

Interpretation: *M. tuberculosis* and *M. kansasii* are strongly positive.

Tween 80 degradation (hydrolysis) test:

Reagent: The substrate consists of 1 dl of 0.067M (ph 7.0) phosphate buffer, 0.5 ml Tween 80, and 2.0 ml of 0.1% aqueous neutral red stock solution.

Dispense in 4 ml amounts in 16 × 125 mm screw-capped tubes and autoclave at 121° C for 15 min. Incubate at 35-37° C overnight to check for sterility. Store in refrigerator.

The substrate is stable for 2 weeks at 4°-10° C.

Procedure: From an actively growing culture on L-J medium, emulsify a 3 mm loopful of growth in a tube of substrate. Incubate at 35-37° C. Observe tubes for a color change from the original amber (straw) to red at 4 hr and daily for 21 days. Compare results with that of an uninoculated control.

Controls: Prepare a Tween 80 degradation-positive culture *(M. kansasi)* and a reagent control of unioculated substrate.

Interpretation: *M. kansasii* is usually positive within 5 days, *M. tuberculosis* is usually positive in from 5-10 days, and the other pathogens remain negative for 3 weeks.

MacConkey agar:

Medium: Prepare plates of MacConkey agar from commercial dehydrated base using approximately 15 ml medium in each plastic Petri dish.

Procedure: Inoculate each plate with one 3 mm loopful of a 7-day Tween-albumin broth culture. Incubate plates at 35-37° C. Record results on the basis of growth or no growth after 5 and 11 days' incubation.

Controls: Prepare a MacConkey agar–positive culture *(M. fortuitum)*, a MacConkey agar–negative culture *(M. phlei)*, and an uninoculated MacConkey agar plate.

Interpretation: *M. fortuitum* grows on MacConkey agar.

Tellurite reduction test:

Principle: Battey bacillus is able to reduce colorless tellurite salt to the black metal tellurium.

Medium: Middlebrook 7H-9 liquid medium.

Reagent: Sterilized potassium tellurite, 0.2% aqueous.

Procedure: Transfer culture to 7H-9 medium and incubate at 37° C for 10 days. Add 2 drops of reagent to bacterial growth. Incubate at 37° C and examine daily for reduction of colorless tellurite salt to black metallic tellurium.

Interpretation: *M. intracellulare* reduces tellurite within 3-4 days.

Three-day arysulfatase test:

Principle: *M. fortuitum* is able to attack phenolphthalein sulfate contained in the medium so that phenolphthalein is released.

Medium: Wayne sulfatase agar.

Reagent: Sodium carbonate, 1M.

Procedure: Inoculate the surface of the medium with actively growing culture. Incubate the tubes in an upright position for 3 days. Add 6 drops of reagent to the culture and examine for pink to red color, which fades on standing.

Interpretation: *M. fortuitum* is positive.

Drug susceptibility testing[144]

Untreated *M. tuberculosis* is usually susceptible to isoniazid, *p*-aminosalicylic acid (PAS), and streptomycin. Runyon groups III and IV are resistant.

There are many variables in drug susceptibility testing, e.g. (1) the type of test done (direct or indirect), (2) the choice of drugs and their concentrations, and (3) the choice of medium.

Types of tests:

Direct tests: Undiluted or diluted sputum is used as inoculum of drug-containing media. Results may be reported in 3 weeks. Direct tests should be performed on all specimens with positive smears.

Indirect tests: Growth from primary cultures is used as inoculum of drug-containing media, and the results are therefore delayed for 6 weeks.

Choice of drugs and their concentrations: Streptomycin (2 µg), isoniazid (0.2 µg), and PAS (2 µg) are the drugs that are used per milliliter 7H-10 medium.

Choice of medium: Use Middlebrook 7H-10 agar with oleic acid–albumin–dextrose–catalase (OADC) enrichment.

Preparation of medium for drug susceptibility testing: A **Felsen plate** is used. The first quadrant contains dyed medium without any drug, the second quadrant contains isoniazid, the third contains streptomycin, and the fourth contains PAS.

The amount of drug or dye stock solution to be added to 2 dl Middlebrook 7H-10 agar with OADC enrichment is as follows:
1. 1 ml 5 µg/ml Congo red as control
2. 0.4 ml 100 µg/ml isoniazid
3. 0.4 ml 1000 µg/ml streptomycin

4. 0.4 ml 1000 μg/ml PAS (Add enough dilute sodium hydroxide to dissolve.)

Solutions 1, 2, and 4 are sterilized by autoclaving; solution 3 is prepared from sterile vials.

Direct drug susceptibility testing[145]: Two inocula are recommended in setting up the sensitivity plates. One is inoculated with the undiluted concentrate, while the other is inoculated with the diluted concentrate. Standardization of the inocula is necessary for reliable test results, since overinoculation may exaggerate the incidence of primary resistance due to spontaneous drug-resistant mutants.

Procedure: Stain and read smears of digested sputa. Dilute the concentrates of positive specimens with sterile distilled water on the basis of smear results as follows:

No. of AFB per oil-immersion field	Dilutions of concentrate for use as inocula
Less than 1	Undiluted and 10^{-1}
1-10	10^{-1} and 10^{-2}
More than 10	10^{-2} and 10^{-3}

Inoculate drug media in Felson quadrant plates with each of the two dilutions selected. Use 3 drops from a Pasteur capillary pipet for each quadrant. Incubate at 35° C for 3 weeks in Mylar bags with *M. phlei*. Examine the plates for growth, both macroscopically and microscopically, with a dissecting microscope fitted with a $10\times$ ocular lens. Record bacterial growth **per quadrant** as follows:

Confluent	$+ + + +$
Almost confluent	$+ + +$
Approximately 100 colonies	$+ +$
50-100 colonies	$+$
Below 50	Actual count

Report results obtained with both dilutions of inocula.

NOTE: Since spontaneous drug-resistant mutants may appear in heavily inoculated media, readings on specimens giving 4+ growth in the control quadrants may not be valid.

Animal pathogenicity

Culture of repeated specimens is superior to animal inoculation. Some mycobacteria are not pathogenic to guinea pigs, the laboratory animal most frequently used.

Guinea pig inoculation should be considered if repeated cultures are contaminated or are negative in the face of strong clinical suspicion of active tuberculosis.

Guinea pig inoculation: Use two guinea pigs that are negative to intracutaneous injections of 0.1 ml of 5% old tuberculin. The concentrated neutralized specimen is injected subcutaneously into the animal's groin and at 6 weeks the animals are killed. At autopsy examine for tubercles in the inguinal lymph nodes, liver, and spleen. Smears of these tubercles must contain acid-fast organisms, and tissue sections should confirm the diagnosis of tuberculosis. Involvement of the lymph nodes alone is not enough; the spleen and liver must be involved to prove invasion by the organism. Involvement of the lung only indicates spontaneous tuberculosis and nullifies the test. If the guinea pig dies within 21 days, the test should be repeated.

Isoniazid-resistant tubercle bacilli may fail to produce disease in guinea pigs.

Rabbits are injected intravenously with cultures of bovine or avian myobacteria.

Immunologic methods for detecting antibodies to Mycobacterium tuberculosis[146-148]

The suggested test for detecting antibodies to *M. tuberculosis* is the gel double-diffusion technic, which is based on the Ouchterlony precipitin reaction in gels. This test may lend itself to rapid screening of large groups of individuals for active cases of tuberculosis.

Mycobacterium leprae (Hansen's bacillus)[149,150]

The causative organism of leprosy is *Mycobacterium leprae*. The organism is a straight or slightly curved rod that is 1-8 μm long and 0.3-0.5μm in diameter. It is strongly acid fast and stains evenly.

Laboratory diagnosis

The only procedure available for laboratory diagnosis is the acid-fast smear.

Acid-fast smear: Obtain smears from nasal secretion, skin nodules, or ulcers on nasal septum and stain by acid-fast or fluorescent (auramine) methods.

In lepromatous leprosy the bacilli are present in large numbers in rounded masses, but in tuberculoid leprosy even serial sections reveal only a few fragmented organisms.

Scraping the entire thickness of the skin by the **Wayson technic** is recommended.[151] Pinch an area of the skin between the thumb and forefinger, using sufficient pressure to blanch the skin. Make an incision about 5 mm in length, going through the full thickness of the skin but not into the fatty tissue. Scrape the cut surfaces and make smears for staining.

NOCARDIACEAE
Nocardia

Nocardia organisms are slender, gram-positive, **aerobic** filaments or coccoid and bacillary fragments of filaments, some of which are branched or swollen. Mycelium formation is not conspicuous. Some species are weakly acid fast and may resemble mycobacteria.

There are several species of *Nocardia,* two of which are of clinical importance: *N. asteroides* and *N. brasiliensis.* They are soil saprophytes that are able to produce disease in humans and animals. **Nocardiosis** may be systemic, disseminated, subcutaneous, or localized. The systemic form leads to disseminated abscesses and granulomas in the lungs and parenchymal organs of the body, the subcutaneous form leads to multiple abscesses, and the localized form is responsible for **mycetomas.**

Laboratory diagnosis

Specimen: Pus, sputum, and tissue are used.

Gross examination: No granules are found in material from systemic nocardiosis, but in mycetomas the pus may contain small granules that may be white, cream, yellow, or red.

Morphology (Gram stain): Material should be stained with Gram and acid-fast stains. The Gram stain reveals gram-positive, slender, long, branched mycelial filaments that stain irregularly, resembling chains of granules. They break up into coccoid and bacillary forms. The acid-fast stain also reveals an irregular, weakly acid-fast staining pattern. Any acid-fast stain may be used, but 1% sulfuric acid in water should be employed as a decolorizing agent so as not to decolorize the weakly acid-fast organism too much.

Culture: Sputum should be cultured before and after digestion (p. 874). Digestion eliminates some of the contaminating organisms.

Use one thioglycollate broth, two blood agar, and two Sabouraud dextrose agar plates. The thioglycollate and one set of inoculated solid media are incubated aerobically at 35° C, while the second set of solid media is incubated at room temperature. Media containing antibiotics should not be used.

Surface growth occurs in broth, with a pellicle often growing upward on the wall of the tube.

Growth is relatively rapid on blood agar, appearing in as little as 2 days. The colonies are similar to those on Sabouraud agar.

On Sabouraud dextrose agar, 5-10 mm colonies develop slowly in 4-5 days. They are folded, elevated, and tan to yellow. They may produce aerial hyphae, which distinguish them from the otherwise similar colonies of some species of mycobacteria. This distinction is important since *Nocardia* survives concentration methods, grows on acid-fast culture media in 1-2 weeks (earlier than most pigmented mycobacteria), and is acid fast. Substrate hyphae, which are not observed in mycobacteria, may be seen in *Nocardia* cultures.

Slide culture technic: Fill the concavities of culture slides with heated chlamydospore agar, using a quantity sufficient to bring the surface of the medium to a level just higher than the surrounding surface of the slide. Inoculate the surface of the medium. Place a cover glass over the inoculum, so that it is in contact with the medium and the surrounding slide. Place the slide culture in a sterile Petri dish, which is lowered into a jar containing a moist paper towel. Incubate at 35° C.

Slide or cover glass cultures show slowly branching mycelia.

The slide culture technic may be used to distinguish yellow colonies of *Nocardia* from rapidly growing yellow group IV mycobacteria *(M. phlei)*.

Biochemical reactions: *Nocardia* is catalase positive and nonmotile, utilizing carbohydrates by oxidation.

Differential tests (Table 32-40)

The following tests can be used to distinguish *N. asteroides* from *N. brasiliensis* and to distinguish both from *Streptomyces* species.

Casein hydrolysis test: Suspend 5 g skimmed milk powder (Difco Laboratories, Detroit) in 15 ml distilled water. Dissolve 1 g agar in 50 ml water. Autoclave separately and cool to 47° C. Mix milk and agar and pour into five sterile Petri dishes. Each culture is heavily streaked once across, incubated at 28° C, and observed for 7-14 days for clearing of the opaque casein underneath and around the colonies.

N. asteroides is incapable of hydrolyzing casein, whereas *Streptomyces* species and other *Nocardia* can hydrolyze this protein.

Growth on gelatin:

Medium: Use 4 g gelatin in 1000 ml distilled water. Adjust to pH 7.0. Dispense 5 ml into tubes and autoclave at 121° C for 5 min. Inoculate with organism from Sabouraud dextrose agar. It may take over 3 weeks of incubation at room temperature before growth appears.

Interpretation: *N. asteroides* will not grow, *Streptomyces* species will grow poorly, and *N. brasiliensis* shows good growth.

Decomposition of L-tyrosine and xanthine: Suspend 0.5 g L-tryosine or 0.4 g xanthine (both are insoluble) in 100 ml nutrient agar; then autoclave, mix, and pour into Petri dishes. Heavily streak each plate once across, incubate at 28° C, and examine at 14 and 21 days for the disappearance of the crystals underneath and around the growth.

N. asteroides does not decompose tyrosine or xanthine, *N. brasiliensis* decomposes tyrosine only, and *Streptomyces* decomposes both.

Animal toxicity

N. asteroides is the only species pathogenic to humans and laboratory animals, e.g., guinea pigs and mice. Mix the growth of several slants with 5% hog gastric mucin and inject 1 ml of this mixture intraperitoneally into at least two guinea pigs. At autopsy after spontaneous death or after killing one guinea pig after 2 weeks and the other after 4 weeks, examine for lesions containing mycelia.

ACTINOMYCETACEAE
Actinomyces

Actinomyces organisms are anaerobic, catalase-negative, nonmotile, non-acid-fast, gram-positive rods and

Table 32-40. Laboratory identification and differentiation of pathogenic *Nocardia* and *Streptomyces*

Characteristics	*N. asteroides*	*N. brasiliensis*	*Streptomyces* species
Acid fast	±	±	−
Casein hydrolysis	−	+	+
Growth on gelatin	− or ±	+	− or ±
Decomposition of L-tyrosine	−	+	+
Decomposition of xanthine	−	−	+
Pathogenicity to guinea pig	+	−	−

filaments that may break up into bacillary forms. Five species are found in humans: *A. israelii, A. bovis, A. naeslundii,* and *A. odontolyticus.*

A. israelii, A. naeslundii, A. eriksonii, and *A. odontolyticus* are part of the normal flora of the human mouth, throat, pharynx, and intestines but are also found in lesions of actinomycosis. **Actinomycosis** is characterized by granulomatous suppurative lesions that are usually localized to the face, abdomen, and chest. They tend to form sinus tracts that discharge pus containing masses of *Actinomyces* collected into colonies called **granules (sulfur granules).**

Actinomyces israelii and bovis

Actinomyces israelii and *Actinomyces bovis* are the causative organisms of actinomycosis. *A. israelii* is usually isolated from human sources and *A. bovis* from cattle.

Laboratory diagnosis

Material: Pus, sputum, and scrapings are used.

Examination for sulfur granules: Sulfur granules measure about 0.5-2.0 mm in diameter and are just vis-

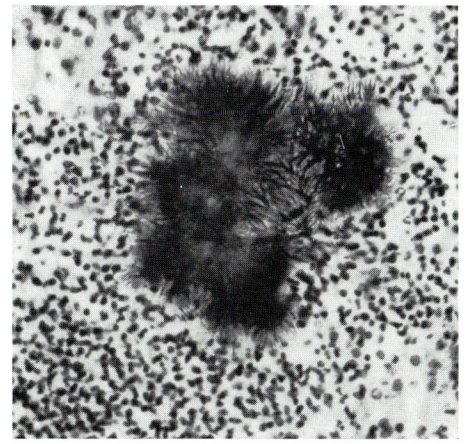

Fig. 32-14. Sulfur granules in pus. (Hematoxylin-eosin stain.)

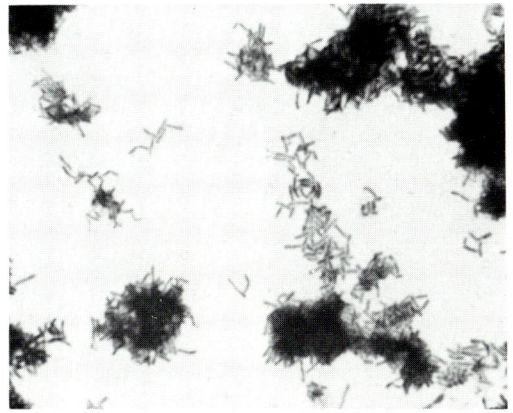

Fig. 32-15. *Actinomyces israelii* in thioglycollate broth.

ible with the naked eye, but a hand lens is usually helpful. Pour the material into a Petri dish, spread thinly, and examine for the so-called sulfur granules, which are colonies of the fungus and are often pearly gray and translucent instead of yellow. When placed on a slide, they are not easily mashed (distinguishing them from caseous particles). The sulfur granules appear typically in serosanguineous pus, often containing mucoid material. Study a granule in 10-20% potassium or sodium hydroxide. Make an impression preparation of a granule by mashing it between two slides; lift the slides apart and stain with Gram and acid-fast stains.

In the pus the unstained granule (Fig. 32-14) is a tangled mass of small, branching septate filaments that tend to be arranged radially at the periphery of the granule. In granules from tissue the tips of the filaments are sometimes surrounded by hyaline or gelatinous material, giving the appearance of clubbed ends.

Gram stain: The bacterium is gram positive, and the tips of the filaments tend to break up into bacillary and coccoid forms. The gelatinous material forming the clubbed end is gram negative. If granules are not found, smear the pus or sputum and examine for gram-positive, fine, short rods and filaments that break up into bacillary and coccoid forms. True branching is rarely seen (Fig. 32-15).

Culture: The material is cultured aerobically and anaerobically, and both liquid and solid media are employed.

Liquid media: Use thioglycollate broth, freshly boiled and cooled. For best results it should be enriched with trypticase soy broth or tryptose broth.

Solid media: Use BHI agar. Inoculate one thioglycollate broth and three BHI agar plates. Incubate the thioglycollate broth and one BHI plate in the anaerobic jar at 35° C. The use of prereduced media is suggested.

Most strains of *A. israelii,* which are isolated from human sources, produce rough colonies on BHI agar. After 7-10 days these rough colonies are a dull white and have irregular surfaces and edges. They feel dry and crumbly and do not adhere to the agar surface. Suspicious colonies are subcultured to thioglycollate broth. In this broth they produce large lobulated "bread-crumb" type colonies as well as discrete granules. Gram stains of the cultures show gram-positive, branched elements (Fig. 32-15).

A. bovis produces smooth colonies that after 7-10 days on BHI agar are large, convex, round, dull white, glistening, and smooth. They vary in consistency from soft to firm. In thioglycollate broth they vary from "bread-crumb" type growth to diffuse growth at the bottom of the tube to mucoid ropes. Gram stain shows gram-positive diphtheroid forms.

Biochemical reactions

Actinomyces is catalase and indole negative and fails to liquefy gelatin. The catalase reaction is most useful in separating *Actinomyces* from anaerobic diphtheroids (corynebacteria).

A. israelii differs from *A. bovis* in that it does not reduce nitrate and does not hydrolyze starch. *A. bovis* reactions are the opposite.

Table 32-41. Characteristics of some *Actinomyces* and anaerobic diphtheroids

Tests	*A. israelii*	*A. bovis*	*A. naeslundii*	**Diphtheroids**
Catalase production	−	−	−	+
Nitrate reduction	+ (a few −)	−	+	+
Starch hydrolysis	−	+	−	−
Gelatin liquefaction	−	−	−	+ slow
Acid production from:				
Glucose	+	+	+	+
Xylose	+ (a few −)	−	−	−
Mannitol	+ (a few −)	−	−	+

Differential diagnosis

A. israelii and *A. bovis* must be differentiated from (1) *A. naeslundii*, a common, catalase-negative inhabitant of the mouth that grows aerobically and tolerates 10% bile salts and (2) anaerobic diphtheroids *(Propionibacterium acnes)*, which are catalase positive (Table 32-41).

STREPTOMYCETACEAE

The family of Streptomycetaceae embraces over 500 species that are widely distributed in nature (soil). Some are used for the production of antibiotics (tetracycline, actinomycin, erythromycin, neomycin, streptomycin, amphotericin B, nystatin, and chloramphenicol). Only a few species are pathogenic to humans, causing mycetomas.

Laboratory diagnosis

Material: Pus and sulfur granules (grains), which are large and vary from red to pink depending on the species, are the material submitted.

Gross examination: Examine as for *Actinomyces*.

Morphology (Gram stain): Streptomycetaceae are gram-positive, filamentous, branching bacteria that break up into coccoid forms.

Culture: They are aerobic to microaerophilic organisms that grow on blood agar. In thioglycollate broth at 35° C they form a loosely bound mycelium.

Biochemical reactions: The pathogenic species liquefy gelatin and decompose casein and tyrosine. They ferment glucose to form acid.

For differentiation from *Nocardia* see Table 32-41.

GRAM-POSITIVE SPORE-FORMING BACILLI

All bacilli in this group are able to form spores under unfavorable circumstances. Their normal habitat is soil and the intestine of humans and animals. Outside the bowel some species are disease producing. Spores are resistant to the usual disinfectants and to some extent to heat. These bacilli can therefore be used in sterilization control **(bacterial spore strips).**

BACILLACEAE

The family Bacillaceae includes the genera *Bacillus* and *Clostridium*. The first is aerobic, the latter anaerobic.

Gram-positive aerobic spore-forming bacilli (Bacillus)

Bacillus organisms are rod-shaped aerobic bacteria that form endospores. They are widely distributed in nature. Although *B. anthracis* is the primary pathogen for humans (the causative agent of anthrax), other *Bacillus* species, e.g., *B. cereus*, cause food poisoning, septicemia, and wound infections.

Bacillus anthracis

Bacillus anthracis (anthrax bacillus) is the etiologic agent of anthrax, which is primarily a disease of animals. If transmitted to humans, it occurs in cutaneous, pulmonary, or intestinal forms. The cutaneous form consists of a necrotizing, vesicular, carbuncle-like lesion that may be accompanied by bacteremia and septicemia. The pulmonary form leads to death because of the ensuing septicemia. The intestinal form, resulting from eating raw contaminated meat, also leads to bacteremia and septicemia.

Laboratory diagnosis

Specimen: Material from a previously unopened vesicle, sputum, blood, and stool are used.

Morphology (Gram stain): *B. anthracis* is a gram-positive, spore-forming, rectangular, large rod (4-8 μm in length and 1-2 μm in diameter) occurring in chains of two or more organisms. The bacillus is nonmotile and in culture produces oval spores that hardly distend the cell body and are centrally or subterminally located. Organisms in tissue are encapsulated.

Culture: The organism grows well on blood (sheep) agar and forms rough, flat, granular, white colonies with irregular margins and no hemolysis. The colonies are grayish white and opaque when viewed by transmitted light and are tough and stringy, so that they adhere to the touching loop. When examined under the dissecting microscope, the periphery of the colony appears to be composed of filaments resmelbing wavy

Table 32-42. Differentiation of *B. anthracis* and *B. cereus*

Test	*B. anthracis*	*B. cereus*
Motility	−	+
Hemolysis (sheep blood)	−	+
Colonies	Rough	Smooth
Salicin fermentation at 45° C	−	+
Methylene blue reduction	−	+ (within 24 hr)
Growth on penicillin agar (10 units/ml)	− or ±	+
Gelatin hydrolysis (within 7 days)	−	+
Antianthrax FA	+	−
Growth on:		
PEA medium	−	+
CH medium	−	+

hair (caput medusae). This picture is characteristic for pathogenic forms of *B. anthracis*.

Bacillus cereus produces moist, nonviscid, nonadherent colonies that are often strongly β-hemolytic.

Apart from the differences in microcolonial appearance, features that distinguish virulent forms, from nonpathogenic anthraxlike organisms *(b. cereus)* are as follows: *B. anthracis* lacks motility, fails to reduce methylene blue broth in 24 hr, is pathogenic for guinea pigs, and is sensitive to penicillin (10 units of penicillin per milliliter of agar will suppress the growth of anthrax bacilli). Almost all nonpathogenic anthraxlike organisms are motile, reduce methylene blue broth in 48 hr, and are not pathogenic to laboratory animals. *B. anthracis* fails to lyse gelatin strips within 7 days, whereas *B. cereus* does lyse gelatin (Table 32-42).

In thioglycollate broth, *B. anthracis* concentrates close to the surface, producing a stringy mass below a layer of clear broth.

Fluorescent antibody technic: The technic of direct identification of *B. anthracis* depends on the staining of the capsule of the bacillus by anthrax fluorescent antibody conjugate. It is therefore restricted to imprints of fresh tissues and to smears of vesicular fluids, because the organism is only encapsulated when found in tissue. The FA staining is not specific, since *B. subtilis* shows similar capsular staining.

Differential media: Two differential media are available to distinguish *B. anthracis* from *B. cereus*.[152] They are phenylethanol (PEA) medium and chloral hydrate (CH) medium. These media, in combination with the differential tests mentioned above, are adequate to distinguish the pathogenic *B. anthracis* from the nonpathogenic form.

Animal inoculation: Animal inoculation is dangerous and should only be performed in reference laboratories. Any organism suspected to be *B. anthracis* should be submitted to the state laboratory.

Bacillus subtilis (Hay bacillus)

Bacillus subtilis may be found as a contaminant of wounds. It is motile, catalase and $H_2 S$ positive, and able to curdle milk and to reduce nitrates. Gram stain shows a slender gram-positive rod. Ovoid spores are seen that do not distend the bacillary body. Rough, wrinkled colonies are formed on blood agar. The organism is insensitive to penicillin.

Gram-positive anaerobic spore-forming bacilli (Clostridium)

Clostridium organisms are anaerobic gram-positive (at least when young) rods that form spores. Older organisms are easily decolorized and may appear to be gram negative. The natural habitats are soil and the intestinal tracts of animals and humans. Most are saprophytic soil bacteria that decompose proteins.

Clostridium species are divided into the following groups:

1. Neurotoxin-producing organisms: *C. botulinum* and *C. tetani*
2. Gas gangrene–producing organisms: *C. histolyticum, C. novyi, C. perfringens, C. septicum,* and *C. sordellii*
3. Associated clostridia: *C. bifermentans, C. sporogenes,* etc.

Characteristics that aid in the identification of clostridia include Gram stain reaction; spore formation (size, shape, and location); motility; presence of capsule; hemolysis; microcolonial features on blood agar; liquefaction of gelatin; fermentation of glucose, lactose, and sucrose; formation of H_2S, indole, and catalase; and reduction of nitrates.

Some species of *Clostridium, Bacteroides,* and the gram-positive, non-spore-forming bacilli may be identified only by the use of recently developed technics of **gas chromatographic analysis,**[130] whereby profiles of culture extracts are compared to those published in the V.P.I. laboratory manual.[129] Numerous selective media are used in conjunction with gassed-out tubes and prereduced media. These procedures require maximal efforts to protect sensitive stains from toxic atmospheric oxygen from the time the culture is collected until species identification is made. Relatively few laboratories are equipped to use this method of identification.

Laboratory diagnosis

Specimen: Debrided wound tissue and aspirated fluid from wounds, abscesses, and swabs are used, but the swabs are least satisfactory. The tissue and swabs should be cultured immediately, preferably in the operating room.

Morphology (Gram stain): Clostridia are large, cylindric, straight rods, although curved and irregular forms appear in cultures. *C. perfringens* is encapsulated, although most other species are not. Young cultures are strongly gram positive. Capsules may be visualized by the India ink method (p. 919).

Spores: Location may vary even in a given species, and several days of growth in an alkaline medium may be required to produce spores. The medium should be sugar free, so that acid production does not lower the pH. Spores are highly refractive, so they can easily be visualized by phase microscopy.

Culture: Primary isolation media are thioglycollate broth with dextrose (plus 10% rabbit serum), chopped meat dextrose medium, and three blood agar plates. The thioglycollate broth, chopped meat dextrose medium, and one blood agar plate are incubated anaerobically. Of the remaining two blood agar plates, one is incubated in a candle jar and the other aerobically. All cultures are incubated at 35° C for 24-48 hr. It should be noted that *C. perfringens* grows best at about 45° C[153] See newer methods of culture of anaerobic organisms, p. 825.

Selective media: The use of selective inhibitory media is indicated because many of the organisms infecting wounds are facultative anaerobes capable of overgrowing clostridia colonies. The most frequently used inhibitory media are **chloral hydrate–sodium azide blood agar** and **sorbic acid–polymyxin broth.** Because all inhibitory media may also restrict the organisms that they are designed to select, parallel cultures on routine media must not be omitted.

Chloral hydrate–sodium azide blood agar: To liquid and cooled blood agar (5 dl), add 1 ml of 1% solution of chloral hydrate and 2 ml of 1% solution sodium azide. Both solutions should be sterilized by Seitz filtration.

Sorbic acid–polymyxin broth: To 1 dl thioglycollate broth add 0.12 g sorbic acid. After autoclaving add 1.5 mg polymyxin.

The inhibitory media will tend to prevent spreading of contaminating organisms *(Proteus* and *Pseudomonas).* As a further step to prevent spreading, keep the agar surface dry by including calcium chloride in the anaerobic jar.

Hemolysis: Blood agar (anaerobic) is the medium of choice. Most clostridia are hemolytic.

Fermentation of carbohydrates: Add 1% sterile carbohydrate solution to thioglycollate broth without carbohydrates of its own and without indicators (Table 32-43).

Add 10% carbohydrate solution sterilized by Seitz filtration to thioglycollate medium without glucose to form a final concentration of 1%. Acid production as an index of carbohydrate fermentation is detected by adding 0.05% aqueous solution of bromthymol blue (acid—yellow) to a small portion of medium removed with a sterile pipet.

On the basis of fermentation reaction the following three main groups can be established: (1) glucose negative *(C. tetani),* (2) glucose positive and lactose negative *(C. sporogenes, C. botulinum,* and *C. novyi),* and (3) glucose and lactose positive *(C. perfringens* and *C. septicum).*

H₂S formation: Lead acetate paper strips are suspended over a growing culture.

Motility: Most species, with the exception of *C. perfringens,* are slowly motile (peritrichic flagella). One drop of a 12 hr culture of clostridia in thioglycollate broth **without sugar** is examined on a slide for motility (p. 809).

Indole test: Culture the organism for 3 days in thioglycollate medium without glucose. Then test the medium with Ehrlich reagent. Clostridia are indole negative.

Nitrate reduction: To thioglycollate medium without glucose, add 0.1% sodium nitrate and 0.1% glucose. This medium is inoculated with pure culture and incubated from 12-24 hr at 35° C. It is then tested with sulfanilic acid and α-naphthylamine reagents (Table 32-43).

Gelatin liquefaction: Use Thiogel medium (BBL, BioQuest Div., Becton-Dickinson & Co., Cockeysville, Md.), a thioglycollate medium plus 5% gelatin. Most clostridia liquefy gelatin.

Virulence test: Inject 0.5 ml of equal parts of an 18 hr chopped meat dextrose culture and 10% sterile calcium chloride into the thigh muscle of a guinea pig. Hemorrhagic necrosis of the muscle may follow the injection in 4-5 days.

Catalase test: For method see p. 836. All clostridia are catalase negative.

Iron milk: Add whole milk to culture tubes, add a few iron filings, and autoclave tubes. Allow to cool and inoculate iron milk with organisms. Clostridia that ferment lactose coagulate milk rapidly and disrupt the co-

Table 32-43. Characteristics of some *Clostridium**

Species	Meat	Spores	Fermentation of		
			Glucose	**Lactose**	**Sucrose**
C. bifermentans	D (late)	OST	A	–	–
C. botulinum	D (some)	OST	A	–	v
C. histolyticum	D	OST	–	–	–
C. novyi	–	OST	A	–	–
C. perfringens	–	OST	A	+	+
C. septicum	–	OST	A	+	–
C. sordellii	D	OST	A	–	–
C. sporogenes	D	OST	A	–	v
C. tetani	v	RT	–	–	–

*A, Acid; C, clot; G, gas; D, digested; – , negative; + , positive; v, variable; O, oval; R, round; T, terminal; ST, subterminal.

agulant with gas *(C. perfringens)*. Proteolytic clostridia blacken and digest meat particles in chopped meat medium and digest and blacken milk (and liquefy Loeffler medium).

Lecithinase and lipase production: On egg yolk agar lecithinase produces an opaque zone in the agar surrounding the colony, and lipase activity leads to an iridescent zone around the colony. Clearing of the medium results from proteolytic activity.[154]

Fluorescent antibody technic: The FA technic has been employed in the diagnosis of many clostridia.[155]

Clostridium perfringens

Clostridium perfringens is commonly found in the intestinal tract of humans and animals. It is the most important contributor to the production of **gas gangrene.** Serologically, types A to S can be distinguished.

Laboratory diagnosis

Gram stain: *C. perfringens* is a short, thick, gram-positive rod, 0.8-1.2 μm in diameter and 4 μm in length. The parallel sides are straight and the ends are rounded. Spores are seldom seen, but if present (in alkaline pH) they are ovoid, central, or terminal. The organism is nonmotile and encapsulated.

Culture: In 24 hr under anaerobic conditions, opaque, smooth 2-4 mm colonies with translucent edges appear on blood agar. At times the periphery of the colony is striated and the medium beneath and around the colonies shows β-hemolysis. Growth in cooked meat broth is seen in a few hours and is evidenced by gas production and the pink color of meat. Stormy fermentation is rapidly produced in milk. The organisms ferment glucose, maltose, lactose, and sucrose and liquefy gelatin (Table 32-43).

Clostridium novyi

Clostridium novyi is primarily a soil organism.

Laboratory diagnosis

Gram stain: Gram stain reveals gram-positive rods measuring 2-5 μm in length and up to 1.2 μm in di-

ameter. The organism is motile and nonencapsulated. It readily forms ovoid, central, or preterminal spores that have a wider diameter than the bacillus. They may be found free.

Culture: The organism is a strict anaerobe and is very sensitive to free oxygen. Cooked meat medium produces moderate growth only, even if all oxygen is carefully removed by heating of the medium before inoculation. Rounded, 2-3 mm, shiny, uneven, hemolytic colonies appear on blood agar in 48 hr, provided contact with oxygen is prevented. They have irregular edges and may have some tendency to spread.

Biochemical reactions: All types liquefy gelatin and are indole negative. Most types ferment glucose (Table 32-43).

Clostridium septicum

Clostridium septicum is a gram-positive, motile rod that is 2-6 μm long, and up to 0.6 μm in diameter. The rods have parallel sides and rounded ends. Filamentous forms are common. Young colonies are gram positive, whereas older ones are frequently gram negative. The ovoid spores are subterminal and distend the organism. Under strict anaerobiasis at 35° C there appear on blood agar rounded, hemolytic (α to β), transparent, somewhat spreading colonies with irregular edges. For biochemical reactions see Table 32-43.

Clostridium sporogenes

Clostridium sporogenes is a thin, gram-positive rod with rounded edges. It is not encapsulated and forms subterminal ovoid spores that are frequently found free. It is aerobic and naturally nonpathogenic, but it enhances the pathogenicity of other clostridia. Glistening to yellow-gray-white, rounded, hemolytic colonies with rhizoid projections are formed on blood agar. The colonies are soft and have a tendency to flow. For biochemical reactions see Table 32-43.

Clostridium tetani

Tetanus is a disease characterized by severe toxemia and absence of bacteremia. Cultivated soil is rich in

			Fermentation of				
Gelatin	**Motility**	**Milk**	**Nitrate reduction**	**Indole**	**Lecithinase**	**Hemolysis**	**Catalase**
D	+	D	−	+	+	+	−
D	+	D (some)	−	−	±	+	−
D	+	CD (late)	−	−	−	+	−
D	+	ACG (late)	+	−	+	+	−
D	−	ACG	+	−	+	+	−
D	+	ACG (late)	v	−	−	+	−
D	+	D	−	+	+	+	−
D	+	D	−	−	+	+	−
D	+	−	−	+	−	+	−

Clostridium tetani, which is also found in the intestinal tract of humans and animals.

Laboratory diagnosis

Material: Use excised wound tissue.

Smear: The organism is a slender rod that frequently gives rise to filamentous forms. The cells are not encapsulated; they are motile, and are strongly gram positive when young. They have terminal globoid spores that distend the organisms and do not stain with Gram stain (**drumstick appearance**).

Culture: The organism is a strict anaerobe. It grows well on blood agar, where it forms shiny, granular, 2-5 mm, hemoltyic, transparent colonies that give rise to spreading pseudopods and to swarming. There are, however, nonmotile (nonspreading) forms of *C. tetani.* The colonies have a burnt-flesh odor.

Biochemical reactions: *C. tetani* does not ferment sugars or liquefy gelatin.

Animal inoculation and protection: Inject 0.25 ml supernatant of cooked meat broth culture or emulsified fresh wound material intramuscularly into the thigh muscles of two mice, one of which has been protected by subcutaneous injection of 0.5 ml (1500 units) of tetanus antitoxin 1 hr before the inoculation. If the material is solid, a pocket has to be formed that must be closed airtight with collodion. Calcium chloride (2.5%) in the inoculum may be necessary to initiate necrosis. If the test is positive, after a few hours the hind leg of the unprotected mouse will be first to show the characteristic rigid spasms of tetanus that later, at the slightest provocation, involve the whole animal.

Determination of toxin production: To prove the presence of toxin in the patient's serum, inject mice subcutaneously as follows:

Mouse 1: 0.5 ml serum

Mouse 2: 0.5 ml serum + 0.5 ml tetanus antitoxin (1:10)

Mouse 3: 0.5 ml serum + 0.5 ml diphtheria antitoxin (1:10)

Mouse 4: 0.5 ml serum previously heated to 100° C for 30 min

If toxins are present in the serum, mice 2 and 4 will live, and mice 1 and 3 will die.

Clostridium botulinum

Clostridium botulinum[156] usually does not multiply in the living body of human beings but grows in inadequately preserved meat, vegetables, and fruit. It is widely distributed in soil and causes **botulism** by the ingestion of preformed toxins formed under anaerobic conditions. The toxins are extremely dangerous, and any suspected material must be handled with great care, so that not even the smallest amounts come in contact with the skin or mucous membrane. The toxins are rapidly destroyed by boiling. Six types of the organism (A to F), each with its specific toxin, have been described, but only two types of toxin, A and B, are important as the etiology of botulism in the United States. Recently, infant botulism[157, 158] has been encountered that appears to be related to colonization of the infant gut by *C. botulinum.* In one investigation[159] honey was implicated as the source of the organism.

Laboratory diagnosis

Smear: The organism is a gram-positive rod that is 4-8 μm long and 1 μm in diameter. It is often paired, at times in chains. The spores are ovoid, short, terminal, or subterminal. The organism is motile, strictly anaerobic, and nonencapsulated.

Culture:

Material: Use ground suspected food.

Media: The organism is cultured on blood agar and cooked meat medium. At 35° C under strict anaerobiasis. 2-3 mm slightly hemolytic colonies appear on blood agar. These colonies appear slightly brown under transmitted light.

Determination of toxin production: The test is made on suspected food. Filter 10 ml fluid or extract, boil one portion 30 min to destroy the toxin, and inoculate two mice intraperitoneally with 0.5 ml, one with the unheated and the other with the heated portion (negative control). If positive, the mouse inoculated with the unheated portion will show dyspnea and a decrease of respiration from 120-160 to 20-30 per minute with costal breathing and will die in 3 or 4 hr. The control mouse will not be affected. Protection tests with mice immunized with specific antitoxins may be used to determine the type.

Clostridium difficile

Clostridium difficile is a toxigenic organism isolated from the gut of humans and lower animals. This organism is recently reported to cause pseudomembranous colitis (PMC) following antibiotic therapy.[160]

C. difficile can be isolated from the feces on cycloserine–cefoxitin–egg yolk–fructose agar.[161]

The colonies are large, 4-8 mm, and yellow on this medium. Other bacterial colonies are never more than 1.5 mm in diameter. *C. difficile* ferments only glucose and mannose, is indole negative, and is not proteolytic. The organism is motile by means of peritrichous flagella and forms spores that are subterminal. The organism is a strict anaerobe.

In suspected cases of PMC, fecal samples should be sent to a reference laboratory for tissue culture analysis of *C. difficile* toxin present. Alternatively, *C. difficile* may be isolated from the feces, but this procedure is tedious and time consuming.

VIBRIONACEAE
Vibrio

Vibrios are short, motile, curved or straight rods, most of which are parasitic. Only a few are pathogenic for humans and animals. They are gram-negative and frequently isolated from water. They can be differentiated from *Spirillum* by the latter's bipolar flagella and spiral shape. The vibrios have a single polar flagellum. The differentiation from *Pseudomonas* can be accomplished by the use of O-F medium. *Pseudomonas* are oxidative, whereas vibrios are fermentative (Table 32-44), producing acid without gas formation from carbohydrates.

Vibrio cholerae

Vibrio cholerae[162] causes cholera, an epidemic form of severe enteritis, recent outbreaks of which have been reported in India, Indonesia, and the Philippines. The organism is a curved, motile, non-spore-forming, gram-negative, aerobic rod with a single polar flagellum.

A variant of *V. cholerae* designated as *V. cholerae* biotype El Tor[163] is similar in almost every respect to *V. cholerae* and is the organism found in some acute outbreaks and in cholera carriers.

V. cholerae must be distinguished from a group of noncholera vibrios that may also be found in diarrheal stool.

Laboratory diagnosis[164]

Specimen: Liquid stool, vomit, foods, and rectal swabs in transport medium or in alkaline peptone water.

Morphology (Gram stain): The organisms vary in length from 2-4 μm and measure about 0.5 μm in diameter. They appear singly or are arranged end to end, producing S curves. The Gram stain may fail to show curved forms; thus the organisms may appear as straight rods. A 1:10 carbolfuchsin solution should be used as counterstain in place of the safranin in the gram stain.

Primary media: Two solid media are inoculated—one uninhibitory agar plate and one inhibitory **thiosul-**

fate citrate–bile salts–sucrose agar (TCBS)—and one enrichment broth should be utilized, e.g., **alkaline peptone water** (APW) (pH 8.4). Inoculate nutrient agar lightly and TCBS agar heavily. Incubate plates at 35° C for 18-24 hr and the enrichment broth for 6-8 hr (not longer), after which time the broth is subcultured to a second set of nutrient and TCBS plates.

V. cholerae forms small (3 mm), yellow, flattened colonies with opaque centers on TCBS agar. Noncholera vibrios form colonies with greenish blue centers. On nutrient agar *V. cholerae* produces flattened, transparent colonies with opaque halos and evidence of liquefaction of the gelatin base of the medium.

Suspicious colonies on nutrient agar should be tested with **cholera polyvalent O antiserum** by the slide agglutination technic (p.854). The colonies should also be transferred to TSI agar (or preferably to Kligler iron agar, since it does not contain sucrose), on which they produce an acid slant and butt, no gas, and no H_2S. Motility of the cultured organism is characteristically dartlike and should be confirmed by the wet preparation technic. Movement ceases after the addition of cholera polyvalent O antiserum (saline control needed).

Fermentation reaction: *V. cholerae* ferments glucose and sucrose, producing acid and no gas. Lactose fermentation is delayed.

Table 32-44. Comparison of biochemical reactions of *V. cholerae*, *V. parahaemolyticus*, *V. alginolyticus*, and lactose-positive *Vibrio* species*

Test or substrate†	V. cholerae			V. parahae-molyticus		V. alginolyticus			Vibrio species (lactose positive, lac +)		
	Sign	% + ‡	(% +)§	Sign	% +	Sign	% +	(% +)	Sign	% +	(% +)
Indole	+	100		+	99	+	87		+	97	(3)
Methyl red	+ʷ	95		+	99.5	−	0			NR	
Voges-Proskauer	− or +	47.3		−	0	+	100		−	0	
Citrate (Simmons')	(+ʷ) or −	0	(74ʷ)	+	98	d	20	(47)	d	76	(11)
Lysine decarboxylase	+	100		+	96.5	+	100		+	97	(3)
Arginine dihydrolase	−	0		−	0	−	0		−	0	
Ornithine decarboxylase	+	95.5		+	95.5	− or +	40		+ or (+)	66	(26)
Phenylalanine deaminase	−	0		−	0	−	0			NR	
Gelatin (22° C)	+	96		+	100	+	100		+	(1-7 days)	
Gas from glucose	−	0		−	0	−	0		−	0	
Lactose	(+)	0	(100)	−	0	−	0		+ or (+)	81	
Sucrose	+	96		−	5	+	100		−	3	
Arabinose	− or +	10.1		+ or −	81	−	6		−	0	
Mannose	+	99		+	100	+	100		+	100	
Mannitol	+	100		+	100	+	100		+ or −	66	
Salicin	−	0		−	0	d	12.5	(41.7)	+	100	
Esculin	−	0		+	99.5	−	0			NR	
Melibiose	−	0		− or +	15	−	0		d	26	(52)
Motility	+	96		+	99	+	98	(2)	+	97	

From Ewing, W.H., Tomfohrde, K.M., and Naudo, P.J.: API Species **(2):**10, 1979.

*+, 90% or more positive within 1 or 2 days; (+), positive reaction after 3 or more days (decarboxylase tests: 3 or 4 days); −, no reaction (90% or more); + or −, most cultures positive, some strains negative; − or +, most strains negative, some cultures positive; + or (+), most reactions occur within 1 or 2 days, some are delayed; d, different reactions: +, (+), or −; w, weakly positive reactions; NR, not recorded.

†All cultures included oxidase positive, β-galactosidase positive, and reduced nitrate to nitrite. Nitrite not reduced. Detectable H_2S not produced in Kligler's iron or triple sugar iron agar. Urease not produced. None ferment dulcitol, inositol, adonitol, xylose, rhamnose, or melezitose.

‡Percent positive within 1 or 2 days.

§Percent positive after 3 or more days (decarboxylase test: 3 or 4 days).

Differential tests

A number of tests are available to distinguish *V. cholerae* from its biotype El Tor. These include the string test[165] and the polymyxin B disk susceptibility test.[166]

String test: On a glass slide emulsify a pure culture of vibrios in 0.5% deoxycholate, using the inoculating loop to string out the suspension.

Results: An initial string is seen in most vibrios. Use the loop again 45-60 sec later to string out the suspension a second time. This attempt fails in most vibrios except *V. cholerae*.

Polymyxin B disk susceptibility test: Use the Mueller-Hinton technic (p. 831), culture (pH 8.4), and a 50 IU polymyxin B disk.

Results: *V. cholerae* shows an inhibition zone of 12-15 mm, whereas the inhibition zone of the El Tor variant is not more than 1-2 mm.

Serologic identification

The H antigen is nonspecific. Vibrios are divided into six groups (I to VI) by means of the O antigen. All known pathogens belong to group I. In addition, each comma bacillus contains A, B, and C antigens, which form the basis for two specific antisera: anti-AB (Ogawa) and anti-AC (Inoba) antisera, or a mixture of both. Rough forms are agglutinated by saline solution, which therefore must be used as a control.

Vibrio parahaemolyticus is associated with various kinds of seafood and is found in seawater throughout the world. The organism causes gastroenteritis in human beings when contaminated seafood is consumed raw or incompletely cooked. Most outbreaks occur in Japan, but several incidents of infection in humans have been detected in the United States. The organism resembles *V. cholerae* with the exceptions of requiring 3% sodium chloride for growth and being able to utilize citrate as its sole energy source. *Vibrio alginolyticus* is similar to *V. parahaemolyticus* but does not cause gastroenteritis.

Table 32-44 presents the biochemical differentiation of the important *Vibrio* species.

SPIRILLACEAE
Spirillum

Spirillum includes motile (bipolar flagella), aerobic or microaerophilic, crescent-shaped to spiral bacteria collected into long or short spirals; they grow well on routine media. The parasitic forms are found in water and food, and only a few species are pathogenic for humans.

Spirillum minor

Spirillum minor is a rigid, corkscrewlike organism that usually displays two or three (sometimes up to six) undulations and bipolar flagella. It measures 3-5 μm in length and 0.3 μm in width. In the process of motion, which is dartlike, it rotates around its long axis. It is gram negative, but Giemsa stain is preferred for smears and tissue imprints.

The organism causes sodoku, or **rat-bite fever,** which may follow the bite of a rat, mouse, or other rodent.[167] An ulcer forms at the site of the bite, followed by generalized symptoms such as lymphadenitis, fever, and rash.

Laboratory diagnosis

Laboratory diagnosis is based on demonstration of the organism in the exudate of the primary or secondary skin lesion, in blood, and in smears of regional lymph nodes. The blood smears and tissue imprints are stained with Giemsa stain.

The **darkfield technic** is excellent for the examination of wet preparations.

Animal inoculation: Since the direct examination of human material is usually unsatisfactory and since the organism cannot be cultured, the clinical material should be injected subcutaneously or intraperitoneally into guinea pigs or white mice. Blood smears or heart imprints are examined by the darkfield technic or by the Giemsa staining method 14-17 days after inoculation. White mice must be examined for *S. minor* before inoculation, since they may normally harbor these organisms.

Campylobacter fetus

Campylobacter fetus is associated with infection in cattle, sheep, goats, and other livestock. Recently, human infections have been diagnosed in scattered areas of the United States.[168,169]

C. fetus ssp. *jejuni* is a small, gram-negative, curved rod that is motile with a corkscrew motion. There is one flagellum at one end. The organism is catalase positive and negative for nitrate reduction and

Table 32-45. Characteristics of the subspecies of *Campylobacter fetus*[171]

Characteristic	Subspecies		
	fetus	*intestinalis*	*jejuni*
H₂S (TSI)	−	−	−
H₂S (lead acetate)	−	+	+
Growth in Brucella broth + 1% glycine	−	+	+
Growth in Brucella broth + 3.5% NaCl	−	−	−
Growth at 25° C (Brucella broth)	+	+	−
Growth at 42° C (Brucella broth)	−	−	+

From Sonnenwirth, A.C.: In Sonnenwirth, A.C., and Jarett, L., editors: Gradwohl's clinical laboratory methods and diagnosis, ed. 8, St. Louis, 1980, The C.V. Mosby Co., vol. 2.

H_2S production. The organism will not grow at 25° C. The organism is anaerobic to microaerophilic. *C. fetus* causes gastroenteritis in humans and is isolated from the feces.

Skirrow's isolation medium contains vancomycin, polymyxin, and trimethoprim. The organisms are best isolated under microaerophilic conditions. This is achieved by using the Campy Pak 11 (cat. no. 71033, BBL, BioQuest Div., Becton-Dickinson & Co., Cockeysville, Md.), which establishes a microaerophilic environment within a Brewer jar or other suitable closed container.

The characteristics of the subspecies of *Campylobacter* are given in Table 32-45.

STREPTOBACILLUS

Streptobacillus organisms are pleomorphic, facultatively anaerobic rods that may give rise to long, curved filaments and that require enriched media.

Streptobacillus moniliformis

Nonspirillar rat-bite fever (**Haverhill fever**) is caused by *Streptobacillus moniliformis,* which laboratory and wild rats harbor in the nasopharynx.

Laboratory diagnosis

Specimen: Pus, joint fluid, and blood are submitted.
Morphology (Gram stain): The organism is a pleomorphic, gram-negative rod that is nonmotile and measures 2-3 μm in length. On culture the organism gives rise to long, branching filaments, often exhibiting spindle-shaped swellings. Giemsa and Wayson stains are preferred to Gram stain.
Culture: Thioglycollate broth, blood agar, and trypticase soy broth are inoculated. All media must be enriched with ascitic fluid (20%) or serum (10-30%). The media are incubated at 35° C in 10% CO_2-enriched atmosphere.

The thioglycollate broth should be inoculated with 1 ml of the patient's blood. After 48 hr on blood agar, small, round, colorless, hemolytic colonies appear. Under the dissecting microscope the colonies reveal peripheral filaments. After 4 days, accompanying **L colonies** between the original colonies or in the center of the original colonies may be found by microscopic examination.

In broth the bacteria form floccules that rest on the surface of the sedimented red cells of the inoculum, leaving the supernatant clear.
Animal inoculation: Mice are susceptible to intraperitoneal injection of 0.5 ml citrated infected blood. It must be ascertained first that the mice do not harbor the organism.

SPIROCHAETACEAE

Spirochetes are elongated, motile, flexible, corkscrewlike organisms that divide transversely. They vary in length from 4-16 μm, and most forms cannot be stained by the usual dyes. They can be detected by **darkfield microscopy** and **silver impregnation** methods. Most are difficult to culture or cannot be propagated on artificial media.

Included in the family of Spirochaetaceae are the genera *Treponema, Leptospira,* and *Borrelia.*

Treponema
Treponema pallidum

Treponema pallidum is a delicate spirochete 6-14 μm long and 0.2 μm thick. It is the causative organism of **syphilis.**

Laboratory diagnosis

Laboratory diagnosis includes darkfield examination and serologic tests for syphilis (STS). The usual methods of smear and culture are not satisfactory.
Darkfield examination: Clinically, syphilis is divided into three stages. *T. pallidum* may be demonstrated by darkfield microscopy in the ulcer of the **primary chancre** or in the aspirate of enlarged inguinal lymph nodes in primary syphilis. It may also be found in the cutaneous and mucosal lesions in **secondary** and **congenital syphilis.**
Procedure: Squeeze or scrape the ulcer base to stimulate the release of serum. Press the slide against moist ulcer base, add 1 drop of saline, and cover immediately with cover glass. Examine with darkfield illumination (Figs. 32-16 to 32-18).

T. pallidum is a slender spiral with close regular curves like a corkscrew (Fig. 32-17). It is motile, moving forward and backward and rotating on its long axis but still retaining its rigid curves. In ulcerated lesions and on mucous membranes it is often found with other spiral forms, especially *T. macrodentium, T. microdentium,* and *T. vincentii.*

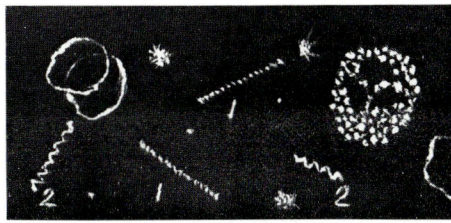

Fig. 32-16. Darkfield microscopy showing, *1, Treponema pallidum* and, *2,* other spirals (contaminating organisms).

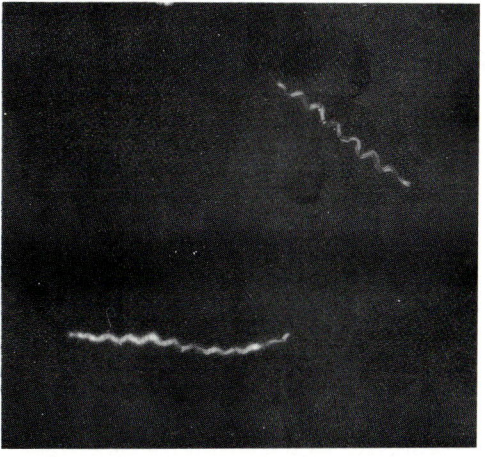

Fig. 32-17. *Treponema pallidum.* (Darkfield microscopy.) (Courtesy Centers for Disease Control, Atlanta.)

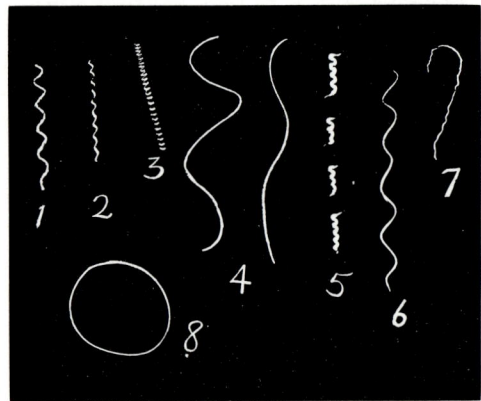

Fig. 32-18. Darkfield microscopy showing spiral organisms. Diagram showing comparative morphology of the following: *1, Treponema macrodentium; 2, Treponema microdentium; 3, Treponema pallidum; 4, Treponema vincentii; 5, Spirillum minus; 6, Borrelia recurrentis; 7, Leptospira icterohaemorrhagiae;* and *8,* erythrocyte (7.5μm) for comparison.

Serologic tests for syphilis: Two types of antibodies are formed in response to the invasion of the human body by *T. pallidum* One group of antibodies is directed against the treponeme and its components, and therefore they are classified as **treponemal antibodies.** These antibodies are tested for with treponemal antigens such as the **Reiter treponema strain** or its protein. The other group of antibodies forms in response to the tissue damaged by the action of the spirochetes, and they are classified as **nontreponemal antibodies** or **reagins.** These antibodies are measured by the use of **nontreponemal antigens** e.g., cardiolipin-lecithin-cholesterol antigens.

Nontreponemal tests: VDRL and its various modifications, e.g., Rapid Plasma Reagin (RPR), Plasmacrit, and Rapid Plasma Reagin Card, are nontreponemal tests.

Interpretation: The nontreponemal tests are not specific but rather indicate the presence of a chronic disease that may be syphilis. This lack of specificity is offset by the fact that they are well standardized, reproducible, and easily performed with a small amount of equipment and skill. When determined quantitatively they can be used to follow treatment and cure.

Treponemal tests: In recent years many treponemal tests have been described. The test of choice is the **fluorescent treponemal antibody absorption** (FTA-ABS) test.

Indications for using FTA-ABS test: The main indications are (1) to distinguish biologic false positive reactions, which usually consist of reactive reagin tests, from the truly specific reactions, and (2) to establish the diagnosis of **late syphilis** in which nontreponemal tests are usually nonreactive. Many laboratories use the RPR test merely as a screening device and confirm all reactive sera with the FTA-ABS test.

Although the FTA-ABS test is highly sensitive, false positive results do occur, primarily in patients with autoimmune disease. In such cases, the infrequently performed treponema immobilization test (TPI) may resolve the conflict.

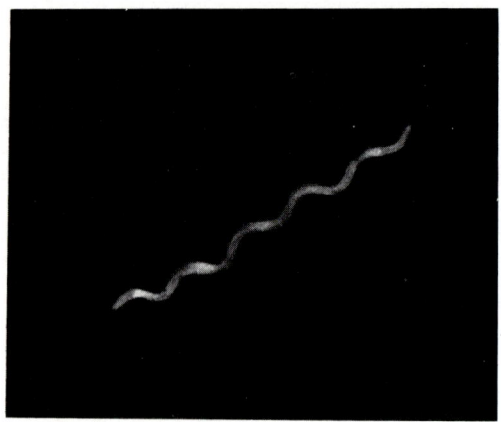

Fig. 32-19. *Treponema vincentii.* (Darkfield microscopy.) (Courtesy Centers for Disease Control, Atlanta.)

Treponema pallidum identification by immunofluorescent stain: The immunofluorescent staining technic is specific for *T. pallidum* and is used on air-dried unfixed smears, so that after the darkfield examination the smear may be allowed to dry and then be stained by the FA technic to confirm the diagnosis of the darkfield examination.

Identification of other treponemes: Other treponemes morphologically indistinguishable from *T. pallidum* are found in yaws *(T. pertenue)* and pinta *(T. carateum).* Pinta occurs chiefly in Central and South America and is nonvenereal. The comparative morphology of the spiral organisms of chief interest in medical diagnosis may be seen in Fig. 32-18.

Treponema vincentii

Treponema vincentii, 3-10 μm long, is a microaerophilic or anaerobic spirochete with flat, irregular loops. It occurs with fusiform bacilli, mainly in neglected oral mucosa and in Vincent's angina, an ulcerative lesion of the mouth, pharynx, and tonsils.

Laboratory diagnosis

The Gram-stained smear is used for the laboratory diagnosis of *T. vincentii* (Fig. 32-19). Gram-negative, loosely wound spiral organisms with tapered ends are seen with fusiform organisms *(Fusobacterium fusiforme).*

The material is obtained by swabbing the areas involved and immediately spreading it on a slide, which is allowed to dry and is then Gram stained.

Leptospira

Leptospires are aerobic, tightly coiled, thin spirochetes. Some are saprophytic, whereas others are pathogenic for humans. Two species are identified: *L. interrogans,* the pathogenic form, and *L. biflexa,* the saprophytic form.

Leptospira interrogans

Leptospira interrogans is the etiologic agent of **leptospirosis (Weil's disease),** a febrile systemic disease of humans and animals characterized by kidney and liver involvement.

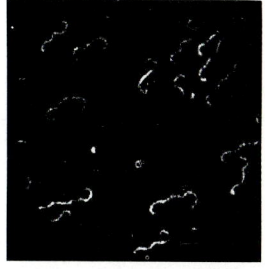

Fig. 32-20. *Leptospira interrogans.* (×950.) (From Handbuch der path. Mikro-organismen. Band VII.)

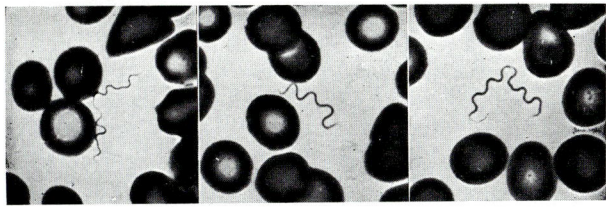

Fig. 32-21. *Borrelia recurrentis* in blood. (From Todd, J.C., and Sanford A.H.: Clinical diagnosis, ed. 9, Philadelphia, 1939, W.B. Saunders Co.)

Laboratory diagnosis[172,173]

Specimen: Blood, spinal fluid, and tissues (kidney and liver) are used.

Morphology: Leptospires in smears of body fluids can be demonstrated by using the Giemsa stain. The FA technic may also be used.

These organisms are tightly coiled, thin spirochetes, the ends of which may be turned at a sharp angle to form a hook. The organisms measure 5-15 μm in length and about 1 μm in diameter (Figs. 32-18 and 32-20).

Darkfield examination: Darkfield examination is useful for the examination of urine, but positive findings must be confirmed by culture and animal inoculation.

Care must be taken in interpretation of darkfield results of urine containing red cells and blood, because red cell fibrils may be mistaken for leptospires.

Culture: Fletcher medium (Difco Laboratories, Detroit) is the medium of choice for isolation of leptospires from blood, urine, and various tissues such as kidneys. Inoculate four to six tubes with 1 or 2 drops of specimen or tissue emulsion and incubate at 26-30° C.

Small inocula are preferred to minimize the influence of inhibitors. Blood and spinal fluid are usually positive in the first week of the disease. Fletcher medium should be inoculated at the bedside. After the first week the organisms disappear from the blood but may be recovered from the urine.

Incubate all tubes for at least 6 weeks. In semisolid media a disk of leptospiral growth forms below the surface. When the growth appears, remove 1 drop with a sterile pipet and examine under darkfield illumination.

Animal inoculation: Because cultures are frequently contaminated, animal inoculation is a necessary diagnostic step. Four young guinea pigs (less than 150 g) or young hamsters are injected intraperitoneally with 0.5 ml of specimen, e.g., as urine and tissue emulsion.

Heart blood and intraperitoneal fluid of the test animals should be cultured every sixth day unless death occurs, at which time the autopsy will reveal hemorrhagic spots in the lungs and other organs. Occasionally, heart blood drawn by cardiac puncture 15 min after intraperitoneal injection will contain leptospires. These can easily be demonstrated by darkfield examination of a drop of blood.

Serologic identification:

Detection of antibodies: The serologic tests include complement-fixation, microagglutination, and agglutination-lysis tests. The antigens and control antisera are commercially available. As in all serologic tests, positive findings in a single specimen are of limited value, but a fourfold rise in titer is significant.

Identification of organisms: The pure cultures are tested with serogroup antisera to establish the serotype.

Fluorescent antibody technic: Fluorescein-labeled antispiral globulins are available for identification of the more commonly encountered leptospires. The most common serogroups of *L. interrogans* are *icterohaemorrhagiae, javanica, canicola,* and *pomona.*

Borrelia

Borrelia are spirochetes that are 8-10 μm long with flat spirals of various sizes and thin, tapered ends. They are easily stained with aniline dyes.

Borrelia recurrentis

Borrelia recurrentis is one of the causative agents of **relapsing fever** in humans.

The disease is characterized by a febrile stage of 3-10 days' duration, ending by crisis and recurring at intervals of about a week. There are several types of the disease, varying in different localities and transmitted by different vectors, but the organisms are practically alike. The European type and the Central African type are chiefly louse borne, whereas the types in northern Africa, in Central and South America, in Spain,[174] and in the United States (Texas, California, Colorado, and Kansas) are transmitted by a tick (some species of *Ornithodorus*). Infection is caused by contamination of the bite lesion with the body fluids of the crushed louse or with the excretory wastes of the tick.

Laboratory diagnosis

Specimen: During the febrile stage the organisms are found in the blood and can be demonstrated in the wet specimen by darkfield microscopy and in the dried blood film by Wright-Giemsa stain.

Morphology: The spirochete is a motile spiral with a flexible body and three to seven loose, irregular coils that are inconstant. The organism measures 15-40 μm in length. The ends are pointed. The stain of choice is Wright-Giemsa stain (Figs. 32-18 and 32-21).

Animal inoculation: When the organisms disappear from the bloodstream, mouse inoculation is the diagnostic test of choice. A mouse is inoculated with 0.2-0.5 ml of blood, and the blood obtained from the tail of the mouse is examined 2 days later and thereafter daily for 5-10 days.

HOSPITAL ENVIRONMENTAL CULTURES AND HOSPITAL-ACQUIRED INFECTIONS[88,175-178]

Hospital-acquired (**nosocomial**) infections and the bacterial milieu of the hospital environment are related to the extent that it is theoretically beneficial to reduce the patient's exposure to bacteria present in the hospital environment. It is well established that contact with nonsterile surfaces, air, and fomites plays only a minor role in hospital-acquired infections, most of which are directly related to droplet (coughing and sneezing) and hand contact between individuals and to breakdowns in sterile technics.[5,6]

Notwithstanding, routine surveillance of the hospital environment is neither recommended nor desirable. Time used in the past to determine carriage rates of *Staphylococcus aureus*, (numbers of organisms on floors, on walls, in the air, and on knives and forks) can be more effectively spent in employee education and episodic surveillance. Hospital infection control programs should stress (1) an active infection control committee, (2) a well-trained hospital epidemiologist, (3) an ongoing program to detect infection trends in the environment, and (4) a competent microbiology laboratory that can effectively work with the epidemiologist to provide intensive surveillance services when the need arises. Table 32-46 summarizes those critical areas to be monitored and the frequency of sampling.

If environmental sampling becomes necessary, the media and methods discussed below may be used.

Primary culture media

The primary solid medium used is trypticase soy agar (TSA) overlaid by a thin layer of TSA enriched with 2% blood. The exposed plates are incubated for 24 hr

Table 32-46. Infection control procedures

Activity	Program	Frequency
Item or area		
Air conditioning		As needed
Anesthesiology	Random items	As needed
Dairy products	Bacterial counts on milk, cream, and ice cream	Monthly
Dietary items	Utensils, glasses, plates, etc. randomly checked	Monthly
Hemodialysis unit	Deionized water and dialysis fluid as sent by unit	Monthly
Ice machines	Bacterial counts on all ice machines in use	Bimonthly
Nursery	Incubator reservoirs	Monthly
	Sink traps and faucets	As needed
	Infant formulas	As needed
Pharmacy	Laminar flow hood	Monthly
	Hyperalimentation fluid	Monthly
Physical therapy	All whirlpools in use cultured by department	Monthly
Respiratory therapy	Culture of swabs sent by department	Monthly
Sterilized products	Selected at random from central supply, clinics, operating room, etc. divided between gas and steam	As needed
Sterilizers	Spore strips run in all sterilizing equipment	Weekly
Surgical soaps	Operating room, emergency room, etc.	As needed
Any area of hospital		As needed
Personnel		
Food handlers	Stool culture, parasite examination	On employment and as needed thereafter
Home care	Nose, throat, and stool culture and parasite examination	On employment (if required by state)
Any personnel	Nose, throat, and stool culture and parasite examination	As needed

From Weissfeld, A.S.: In Sonnenwirth, A.C., and Jarett, L., editors: Gradwohl's clinical laboratory methods and diagnosis, ed. 8, St. Louis, 1980, The C.V. Mosby Co., vol. 2.

at 35° C. The colonies are then counted and identified. The plates should be kept at room temperature for 1 week to allow fungi and slow-growing colonies to develop.

The primary liquid medium is trypticase soy broth, known amounts of which are dispensed into sterile tubes and sterile polyethylene plastic bags. After inoculation, aliquots are quantitatively cultured (see below).

Sampling technics

The following five sampling technics are available:
1. Settling plates
2. Volumetric agar impaction samples (Reyniers slit sampler)
3. Swab sampling
4. Use of liquid media
5. Rodac contact plates

Settling plates: TSA plates overlaid with 2% blood-enriched agar are exposed to air for 2 hr and cultured after exposure for 24 hr at 35° C. The colonies are then counted and identified. This form of bacterial collection is subject to humidity (particle size) and air currents. Under average circumstances, 1 colony/15 min exposure may be expected.

Reyniers slit sampler: Reyniers slit sampler (Reyniers and Son, Chicago) is used for sampling air and aerosols. An agar plate (TSA agar as described above) rotating at a constant rate is exposed for a set time (usually 2 hr) to a known quantity of air. A calibrated flowmeter must be furnished with the instrument. After exposure the plate is incubated for 24 hr at 35° C. The colonies are counted and identified. Bartlett et al.[178] give an average acceptable value of 12 colonies/cu. ft. of air.

If aerosols of inhalation equipment are monitored, Reinarz et al.[179] considers 50 colonies/cu. ft. aerosol as evidence of contamination.

Swab sampling: Swabs are used to monitor drains, faucets, hoses, drinking fountains, valves, aerators, etc. To obtain quantitative results use swabs to cover a specified area (10 sq. in.) outlined by a template. First cover the entire area by longitudinal back and forth strokes and then a second time by vertical strokes. Place the swab into 10 ml trypticase soy broth, so that 1 ml trypticase broth corresponds to 1 sq. in. Break off the segment of the stick that was handled, close the tube, and mix well by inversion for a specified period of time. Keep in ice until cultured. With a sterile pipet, transfer 0.1 and 1.0 ml each into one sterile Petri dish and prepare pour plates with TSA (20 ml).

Calculation:

No. of colonies/10 sq. in. =

No. of colonies × 10 (1 ml cultured)
No. of colonies × 100 (0.1 ml cultured)

Use of liquid media: With a sterile pipet, transfer known amounts of liquids to be tested, e.g., water and sterile fluids, to a known quantity of trypticase soy broth, which is then quantitatively cultured (see above).

Rodac contact plates: Rodac plates (Mono-Flex Contact Plates, Hyland Div., Travenol Laboratories, Costa Mesa, Calif.) are overfilled standardized plates containing TSA enriched with lecithin and Tween 80.

It forms a convex contact area that is pressed firmly against the surface to be tested.

Rodac plates are used to monitor floors, sinks, and other surfaces. After exposure, the plates are incubated for 24 hr at 35° C.

It is suggested to use at least 10 Rodac plates for any given designated floor area and to average the results.

RICKETTSIACEAE

The family Rickettsiaceae embraces the tribe Rickettsieae, which contains the genera *Rickettsia*, *Rochalimaea*, and *Coxiella*.

RICKETTSIA

Rickettsiae are obligate, intracellular, gram-negative organisms that, like most bacteria, can be stained with aniline dyes and appear as small pleomorphic rods or cocci that measure 0.3-1 μm in length and can therefore just be seen under the light microscope. The organisms contain RNA and DNA, and the electron microscope reveals an electron-dense nucleus and a cell membrane. They also differ from viruses by maintaining their own, although limited, enzyme systems. They cannot be Seitz filtered. They stain best with Giemsa stain.

The tribe Rickettsiae, with the exception of *Rochalimaea*, can only be propagated in laboratory animals, tissue cultures, and yolk sacs of fertile eggs. For a more detailed discussion see the following section on viruses, because the laboratory investigation of both infectious agents is similar.

Insects (lice, fleas, ticks, and mites) are the natural reservoir of these organisms. Rickettsiae do not produce disease in the arthropods that transmit the organisms to humans, but in humans they cause diseases characterized by fever and rash (Table 32-47).

Table 32-47. Rickettsiaceae that produce diseases in humans

Disease	Species	Vector
Typhus group		
Epidemic typhus	*Rickettsia prowazeki*	Louse
Brill-Zinsser disease	*Rickettsia prowazeki*	Tick
Endemic typhus	*Rickettsia typhi*	Flea
Spotted fever group		
Rocky Mountain spotted fever	*Rickettsia rickettsii*	Tick
Siberian tick typhus	*Rickettsia sibirica*	Tick
Mediterranean fever (boutonneuse fever), South African tick-bite fever	*Rickettsia conorii*	Tick
Rickettsialpox	*Rickettsia akari*	Mite
North Queensland tick typhus	*Rickettsia australis*	Tick
Scrub typhus	*Rickettsia tsutsugamushi*	Mite
Q fever	*Coxiella burnetii*	Tick
Trench fever	*Rochalimaea quintana*	Louse

Laboratory diagnosis of rickettsial infections

Fertile egg cultures: Rickettsiae grow readily in the yolk sac of the developing chick embryo (chickens must not have been on antibiotics).

Tissue culture: Intracellular localization of rickettsiae is a diagnostic feature.

Animal inoculation

Susceptible laboratory animals are the guinea pig and the white mouse. Inject 3 ml ground clotted blood intraperitoneally into several guinea pigs or white mice. The clinical and pathologic anatomic changes of rickettsial infections are the same in humans and animals.

R. prowazeki in the guinea pig produces fever, vascular lesions, and encephalitis within 4-8 days. *R. typhi* in the male guinea pig leads to fever and scrotal edema and in mice to peritonitis within 4-6 days. *R. rickettsii* in the guinea pig is responsible for fever for 14 days, edema of the scrotum, and hemorrhagic necrosis of various parts of the body. *R. conorii* produces changes similar to the changes produced by *R. rickettsii*.

Coxiella burnetii is responsible for chronic enlargement of the spleen in the guinea pig and for peritonitis in the mouse. *R. tsutsugamushi* in the albino mouse produces pleurisy and peritonitis.

Serologic identification

Almost all rickettsial infections lead to the development of specific antibodies which may be utilized in the diagnosis and identification of rickettsial infections.

Heterogenous antibodies (Weil-Felix reaction):
Principle: Convalescent serum of epidemic and endemic typhus *(R. prowazeki* and *R. mooseri)* agglutinates nonmotile strains of Proteus OX-19. Convalescent serum of scrub typhus *(R. orientalis)* agglutinates Proteus OX-K.

For method of titration see discussion of febrile agglutination, p. 854.

Specificity of antibodies: Different rickettsial species are cultivated in the yolk sac and are then used as antigens in the complement-fixation technic to identify specific antirickettsial antibodies in the patient's serum.

METHODS IN VIROLOGY

Viruses are ultramicroscopically sized, intracellular infectious biochemical units (nucleic acid) resembling genes, varying in size from about 20 nm (poliovirus and parvovirus) to 300 nm (poxvirus). Viruses are able to penetrate the cells of the host and genetically alter the cell metabolism to produce viral particles rather than normal cell products. The viral nucleic acid is not only able to produce identical viral units but also to induce the host cell to form new similar viruses. The clinical manifestations of viral disease are caused by the cellular damage resulting from viral penetration, duplication, and regeneration.

Classification of viruses: On the basis of their nucleic acid content, viruses are divided into two large groups, RNA viruses and DNA viruses. Whereas bacteria contain both RNA and DNA, viruses contain either one or the other.

Viruses are further subdivided on the basis of presence or absence of a lipid envelope, architectural symmetry, number of capsomeres (protein capsules), and thus size.

Major groups of viruses:

RNA viruses
  Picornaviruses
    Enteroviruses
      Polioviruses
      Coxsackie viruses
      Echoviruses
    Rhinoviruses
    Encephalomyocarditis virus
  Reoviruses
    Reoviruses (3 types)
  Arboviruses
    Group A: western encephalitis, eastern encephalitis
    Group B: St. Louis encephalitis virus
    Group C: viruses found in Panama, Brazil, etc.
  Myxoviruses
    Subgroup 1: influenza viruses, respiratory syncytial viruses
    Subgroup 2: mumps virus, parainfluenza virus
  Myxovirus-like viruses: measles virus
DNA viruses
  Adenoviruses: human and animal adenoviruses
  Papovaviruses (tumor viruses): polyoma virus, wart virus, etc.
  Herpes viruses
    Herpes simplex
    Herpes B
    Varicella-zoster
    Cytomegalovirus
  Poxviruses
    Variola
    Vaccinia
    Molluscum contagiosum

Laboratory diagnosis of viral diseases[180]

Laboratory diagnosis includes (1) virus isolation, i.e., isolation of the causative agent; (2) serologic tests, i.e., demonstration of a rise in the specific antibody titer in the course of the disease; and (3) examination of tissue for characteristic pathologic changes (Table 32-48).

Collection and handling of clinical material: Label and identify each specimen separately. Do not use water-soluble ink.

Types of specimen: Use stool (walnut size), rectal swabs, throat washings (15 ml sterile nutrient broth) or throat swabs, cerebrospinal fluid, clotted blood (15-20 ml), and tissue specimens. Other specimens may consist of pleural fluid, contents of vesicles, urine, scrapings of skin lesions, etc. The material should be obtained fresh when the patient is admitted, and a similar specimen should then be collected about 2 weeks after the onset of symptoms. All material—even if contaminated—should be collected in sterile containers using sterile technic, frozen, and kept frozen. Freeze-drying technics may also be used. To prevent drying out, swabs should be placed in 1 ml nutrient broth or in **Hanks balanced salt solution** (Becton-Dickinson & Co., Rutherford, N.J.).

If shipping is required, the material should be packed and shipped on dry ice. If facilities for freezing are not available, the material may be placed in 50% buffered glycerin.

Table 32-48. Practical diagnostic tests for viral disease of humans

Virus	Clinical presentation	Specimens for isolation	Available tests
Respiratory			
Influenza	Acute respiratory disease	Throat washings or swabs, nasal excretions	CF, EE, FA, HI
Parainfluenza	Pharyngitis, croup, bronchiolitis	Sputum, throat washings	CF, CPE, HI
Adenovirus	Acute respiratory illness, pneumonia, pharyngitis, coryza, conjunctivitis	Throat swab, rectal swab, stool, CSF, conjunctival secretion	CF, CPE, HI, N
RS	Bronchiolitis, pneumonia, coryza	Throat swab, nasal swab	CF, CPE, HI, N
Psittacosis (nonviral)	Pneumonia	Throat washings, sputum, blood	CF, EE, FA, I, IA, N
Central nervous system			
Poliovirus	Paralysis, aseptic meningitis, undifferentiated respiratory illness	Throat washings and swabs, rectal swabs, CSF, blood, urine	CF, CPE, FA, IA, N
ECHO	Aseptic meningitis, paralysis, exanthem, respiratory disease, diarrhea	Throat washings and swabs, rectal swabs, CSF, blood urine	CF, CPE, FA, HI, N
Insect-borne encephalitis	Acute febrile disease, encephalitis, aseptic meningitis	Blood, throat washings, CSF, urine, brain and other tissues (if fatal)	CF, CPE, HI, IA, N
Herpes	Encephalitis, aseptic meningitis	Blood, CSF, brain tissue (if fatal)	CF, CPE, EE, FA, I, IA, N
Mumps	Encephalitis	Saliva, blood, urine, milk, brain tissue (if fatal)	CF, CPE, EE, HI, IA, N, skin test
Lymphocytic choriomeningitis	Aspetic meningitis	Blood, CSF, brain tissue (if fatal)	CF, CPE, HI, IA, N
Rabies	Fatal systemic disease	Saliva, throat and eye swabs, CSF	CF, FA, IA, N, NB
Aseptic meningitis	Meningitis	CSF	CF, CPE, N
Exanthems			
Variola-vaccinia	Smallpox, eczema vaccinatum	Vesicle, pustular or scab material	CF, CPE, EE, FA, HI, I, N, precipitin test
Varicella–herpes zoster	Chickenpox, herpes zoster	Vesicle, pustular or scab material	CF, CPE, FA, I, N, Ouchterlony gel reaction
Rubeola	Measles, pneumonitis, encephalomyelitis	Blood, urine, throat swabs, conjunctival secretion	CF, CPE, HI, N
Rubella	Rubella, neonatal defects	Blood, urine, throat washings and swabs	CF, EE, FA, IA, N, interference test
Miscellaneous			
Colorado tick fever	Acute febrile disease	Blood, throat washings, stool	CF, CPE, EE, HI, IA, N
Obscure febrile diseases	Acute fever	Throat washings, stool, CSF	CF, N

CF, Complement fixation; CPE, cytopathogenic effect in tissue culture; EE, embryonated eggs; FA, fluorescent antibodies; HI, hemagglutination inhibition; I, inclusion bodies; IA, inoculation into animals; N, neutralization; NB, Negri bodies.

Collection of specimens for serologic tests: Two or three specimens of blood (15-20 ml) are drawn at suitable intervals with sterile syringes and discharged into sterile screw-capped test tubes. The blood is allowed to clot and the serum separated by sterile technic. The serum is then stored in the deep freezer, but it must be prevented from absorbing CO_2, which renders it anticomplementary. All sera are examined at the same time with identical antigen and reagents.

Handling of autopsy specimens: Specimens should be collected under sterile conditions and immediately deposited in the deep freezer.

Methods of virus isolation: Before isolation is attempted it is necessary to remove bacteria and particles

from the material. This is accomplished by the use of bacterial filters of progressively decreasing porosity, e.g., Berkfeld filters and Seitz filters.

Further preparation of the specimen includes the addition of antibiotics that will not harm the virus, e.g., penicillin and streptomycin or gentamicin, and, finally, differential centrifugation. In the routine clinical virology laboratory, antibiotics are added to transport media and tissue cultures to minimize bacterial contamination.

Tissue culture: The virus can be cultivated in growing tissue suspended in nutrient medium. Not all viruses grow on all cells; **monolayer cell cultures** and **permanent cell strain cultures** of various tissues are commercially available. They include tissue cultures

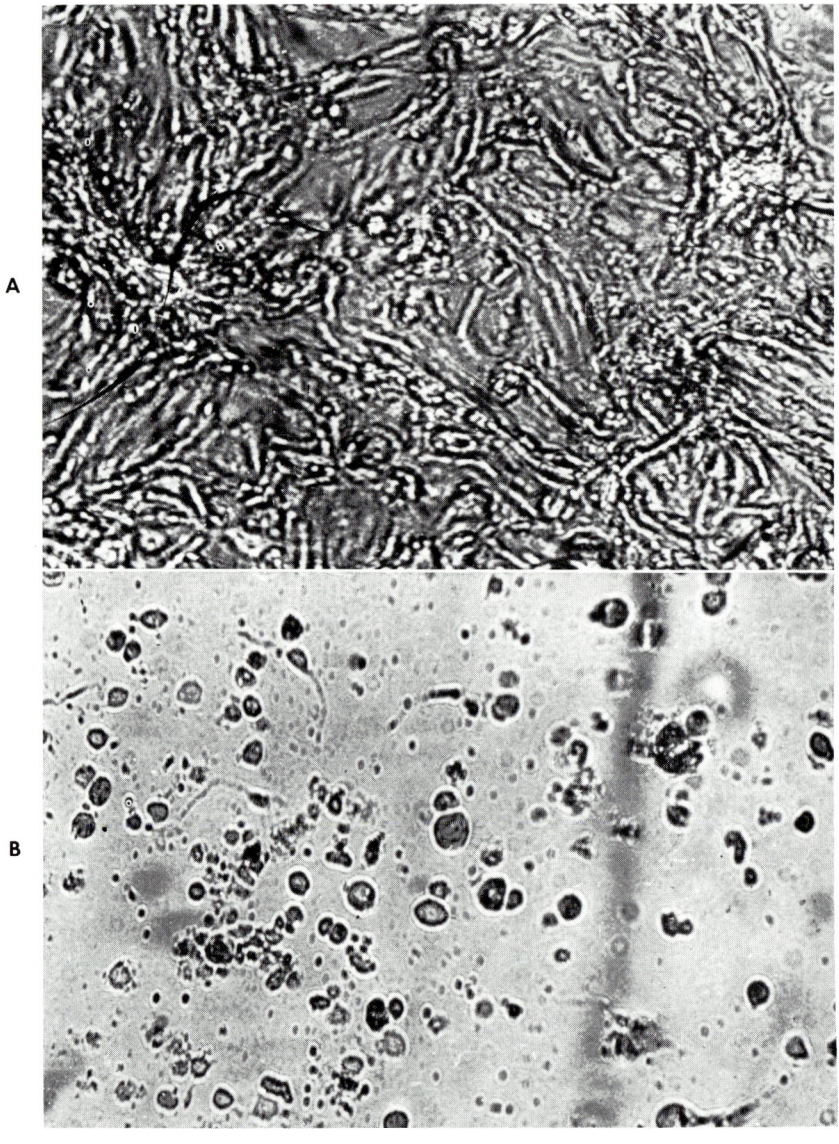

Fig. 32-22. Effect of poliovirus on monkey kidney tissue culture. **A,** Before infection there is a continuous layer of polygonal cells. **B,** After inoculation the cells degenerate, demonstrating viral cytopathogenic effect. Two days after infection most cells have died; survivors are swollen or shrunken and show pyknotic nuclei. (From Schaeffer, M.: Hosp. Pract. **1:**51, 1966.)

sensitive to a wide range of viruses, e.g., **human amnion** and **HeLa cells.** These cultures are inoculated, and, as viral growth develops **cytopathogenic changes** of individual cells may be produced (Fig. 32-22). These are visualized when fragments of the culture are removed, stained on a cover glass, and examined microscopically. The affected cells become granular, round up, shrivel, and finally disappear. The following viruses produce **cytopathogenic changes** or **effects (CPE):** Coxsackie, ECHO, herpesvirus, adenovirus, vaccinia, influenza, etc. The destroyed cells form areas of necrosis within the sheets of cultured cells called **plaques.** The morphology of these plaques is characteristic for certain viruses and can be brought out as areas of decolorization by staining the living cells with vital dyes. Specific immune sera will inhibit the cytopathogenic effect.

Cultivation of virus in chick embryo: In most cases the fertile eggs are incubated for 10-12 days at 37°-38° C before they are inoculated. Several different locations may be chosen for the inoculation, depending on the nature of the virus.

Egg inoculation (Fig. 32-23): **Chorioallantoic inoculation** of vaccinia, variola, and herpes simplex viruses produces characteristic pocks.

Allantoic inoculation is used for influenza. Newcastle disease, and mumps viruses.

Amniotic sac inoculation is used for the isolation of influenza virus from throat washings.

Yolk sac inoculation is adopted for primary isolation of members of the psittacosis–lymphogranuloma venereum group and for neurotropic viruses.

Inoculation of laboratory animals: The tissue culture and the embryonated egg inoculation have largely replaced the laboratory animal in the virus laboratory. Nevertheless, intracerebral inoculation of the suckling mouse is necessary for the cultivation of Coxsackie viruses, arboviruses, and the virus of lymphocytic choriomeningitis.

Serologic tests

Serologic tests are retrospective methods employing acute and convalescent sera that contain antibodies, the nature of which can be elicited by in vitro antigen-antibody reactions. In response to the infection, various antibodies, e.g., neutralizing and complement fixing, appear, all at the same time or at various times, and of varying titers. Two sepecimens must be obtained, one on admission and one at a later date, the time interval varying from a few days to 2 weeks. A fourfold increase in antibody titer is considered diagnostic. The serologic tests include neutralization, hemagglutination inhibition, complement fixation, precipitation, agglutination, and immunofluorescence.

Neutralization: When a specific immune serum is added to the corresponding virus, the virus is rendered noninfective or is neutralized. Any one of the methods of virus propagation discussed lends itself to neutralization. The immune serum and the virus are mixed and kept in contact for a short period of time and then the virus is inoculated into the original system. Under the influence of the immune serum the expected viral effect must be prevented. This expected effect will vary according to the system used; e.g., in cell cultures the CPE will be absent, plaques will fail to form, or hemadsorption will not take place.

Hemagglutination and hemagglutination inhibition tests: Hemagglutination and hemagglutination inhibition tests are based on the principle that the suspensions of certain viruses will cause agglutination of red cells. If specific immune serum is introduced into this system, it will inhibit the agglutination of the red cells in proportion to the amount of antibody in the serum.

These tests are useful for the identification of myxoviruses, poxviruses, some groups of arboviruses and adenoviruses, and measles virus.

Complement-fixation test: In viral and rickettsial diseases, complement-fixing specific immune antibodies appear at various times, some in 2 weeks, others in 3 or 4 weeks. They are usually not found in the wake of vaccinations with virus. The test follows the principle of all complement-fixation tests and is of value only if performed as a quantitative procedure. Phase 1 combines the antigen with the inactivated immune serum and complement; in phase 2 the hemolytic system of sheep cells and hemolysin is added as an indicator of complement fixation. The binding of the complement to the antigen-antibody complex is evidenced by the absence of hemolysis. Many of the viral antigens are commercially available.

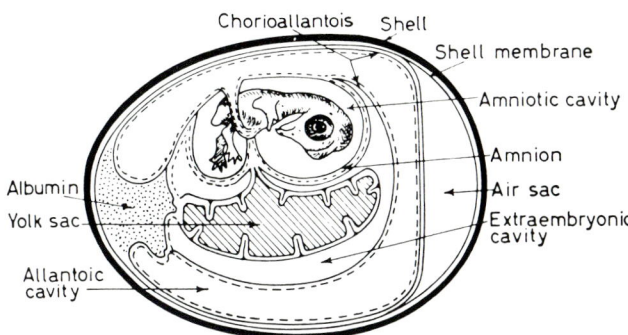

Fig. 32-23. Diagram of developing chick embryo. (From Baker, F.J.: Handbook of bacteriological technique, London, 1962, Butterworth & Co.)

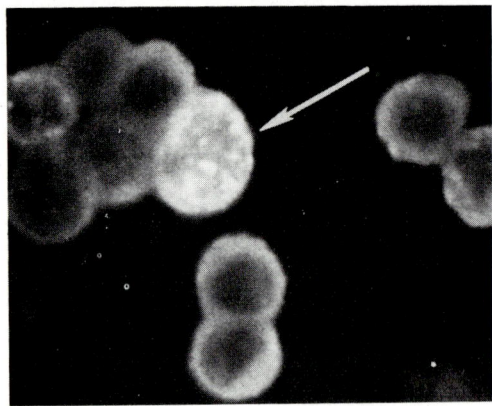

Fig. 32-24. Visualization of viral antigens by means of immunofluorescence. Cells are infected with herpes simplex virus and are allowed to react with herpes virus antibody conjugated with fluorescein isothiocyanate. One cell shows fluorescence in nuclear patches. (From Nahmias, A.J.: Hosp. Pract. **5**:53, 1970.)

Agglutination, precipitation, and flocculation tests: Agglutination, precipitation, and flocculation all describe similar phenomena of clumping of antigen by the action of antibodies. If the antigen is large, the term **agglutination** is used; if it is small, it is **precipitated** out of suspension. If both phenomena occur, the process is called **flocculation.** The **agar diffusion** method of Oudin-Ouchterlony can also be used as a **precipitation** method.

Fluorescent antibody technic: The FA technic is used primarily for the diagnosis of rabies and influenza but may be used for the diagnosis of most viral diseases.[181]

Direct method: The fluorescein-labeled antiserum is directly applied to the smear (the antigen) (Fig. 32-24).

Indirect method: The antigen is first treated with unlabeled specific immune serum, which may be the patient's serum. The homologous antigen in a smear or tissue slide will fix the antibodies of the immune serum in situ. The excess immune serum is washed off. The fixed γ-globulin is detected by fluorescent anti-γ-globulin of the same species that produced the unlabeled immune globulin.

Tissue examination

The diagnosis of some viral diseases can be made on the basis of pathologic anatomic tissue patterns and/or the presence of **inclusion bodies,** which may be found in the nucleus, the cytoplasm, or both. Inclusion bodies are either pure viral particles, as is the case in adenoviruses, or they are virus-directed cell proteins or viral by-products. They are acidophilic solid structures surrounded by a clear zone. The involved cells or nuclei are usually enlarged. Inclusion bodies are helpful in the diagnosis of cytomegalic inclusion disease, molluscum contagiosum, verruca vulgaris, herpes infections, inclusion encephalitis, and rabies.

Electron microscopy: The initial phase of virus-cell interaction and the final phase of virus release are usually discovered by electron microscopy. RNA viruses may appear as groups of viral particles surrounded by a membrane or may form intracytoplasmic crystals. DNA viruses are usually produced within the nucleus, where virus-synthesizing centers are formed.

Viral antigens in leukocytes

In the viremic stage of a large number of viral infections, viral antigens are carried by polymorphonuclear leukocytes. These antigens can be visualized by immunofluorescent staining. The antigen-carrying cells vary from 5-80% of the total number of polymorphonuclear leukocytes and disappear at the end of the viremic phase of the infection. Leukocytic viral antigens have been demonstrated in buffy coats of the following viral diseases: Coxsackie B virus, herpes zoster, adenoviruses, echoviruses, measles, mumps, and influenza.

ADENOVIRUSES
Laboratory diagnosis[182]

Clinically, adenoviruses produce upper respiratory and eye infections.

Cytologic examination of sputum: The ciliated respiratory cells show evidence of degeneration, which is not specific for adenoviral infections, because it is also seen in influenza.

Fluorescent microscopy: Fluorescent microscopy is a sensitive test for detecting adenovirus in infected cells.

Serologic identification: The complement-fixation test is the most useful procedure for diagnosis. The type- and group-specific antigens are produced in tissue culture. Adenoviruses are easily cultured in tissue culture in which typical CPE and intranuclear inclusions are produced. The antibodies produced by adenoviruses are of the hemagglutinating type.

Cat-scratch disease

The etiology of cat-scratch disease is unknown, although the histologic response in excised lymph nodes is consistent with a viral infection.

ENTEROVIRUSES[183]
Human enteroviruses

Polioviruses, Coxsackie viruses, or echoviruses may produce no symptoms or may lead to an upper respiratory infection, myocarditis, meningitis, encephalitis, pleurodynia, and herpangina.

Laboratory diagnosis

Laboratory diagnosis includes isolation of the virus from pharyngeal washings and stool in tissue culture, detection and titer of neutralizing antibodies in the patient's serum, and detection and titer of complement-fixing antibodies.

Poliomyelitis virus

The poliomyelitis virus is found in stool and in cerebrospinal fluid. It readily grows in tissue culture, in which it produces necrosis of the cells, a characteristic CPE that can be neutralized by type-specific immune serum.

Coxsackie virus

Coxsackie viruses occur in the human gastrointestinal tract and are responsible for one type of abacterial meningitis and for epidemic myalgia. Coxsackie viruses are pathogenic for suckling mice, producing a degenerative myositis (type A) or paralysis (type B).

Echovirus

Echoviruses are not pathogenic for mice or only slightly so, but they produce a characteristic CPE in tissue culture.

Rhinovirus

Rhinoviruses are responsible for catarrhal inflammation of the nose, pharynx, and larynx. Rhinoviruses can be cultured in tissue culture and produce a characteristic CPE (diploid fibroblasts). They are not transmissible to laboratory animals and vary in their antigenicity, so that convalescent antisera show varying degrees of avidity. Antisera of sufficient titer are able to neutralize the CPE.

Animal enteroviruses
Enterovirus

The enteroviruses are found in the intestinal tract usually of children, infants, and domestic animals. They are responsible for epidemic or sporadic diarrhea in infants.

Laboratory diagnosis

Diagnosis involves virus isolation by means of the CPE in tissue cultures or by the plaque method and demonstration of compelement-fixing antibodies.

ARBOVIRUSES[184]

The name *arbovirus* is derived from "arthropod borne." Arboviruses have an arthropod-vertebrate cycle—the arthropod is the vector and the vertebrate is the reservoir. Human's are an incidental host. The vector is frequently a mosquito *(Culex, Anopheles,* or *Aedes)* or a tick, and the disease in humans may be a form of encephalitis (St. Louis, eastern equine, Japanese), yellow fever, or dengue.

Laboratory diagnosis

For virus isolation, blood or autopsy material is needed. The clinical diagnosis is therefore usually based on serologic methods.

Serologic identification

The neutralization test is used. The virus grows readily in the cerebrum of baby mice. This growth can be inhibited (neutralized) by immune serum.

After adaptation, arboviruses grow well in tissue cultures of HeLa cells, chicken embryonic cells, and hamster kidney cells.

HERPES VIRUS GROUP[185]

Depending on its localization, this virus group produces a variety of clinical pictures, most of them harmless diseases or infections, although some may lead to death. If localized in the skin, the virus produces herpes simplex; in the mouth or vagina it leads to stomatitis and vaginitis; in the eye, to conjunctivitis; and in the central nervous system, to meningoencephalitis.

Laboratory diagnosis

Tissue examination: Intranuclear inclusions are found in giant cells. Herpes elementary bodies can be seen by electron microscopy in the fluid of vesicles. The FA technic offers a rapid method of diagnosis.

Culture: Herpes virus grows best in the chick embryo, but it also grows in HeLa cells, monkey kidney, and human amniotic cell cultures, where it produces a CPE.

Animal inoculation: Intracerebral or intraperitoneal injection into suckling mice provides a rapid method (3 days) of identification.

Serologic identification: Rising titers of neutralizing and complement-fixing antibodies should be seen.

Fluorescent antibody technic

The direct method (fluorescein-conjugated antiherpes virus antibody) may be used to rapidly identify the virus in clinical specimens (Fig. 32-24).

Epstein-Barr virus

The Epstein Barr (EB) virus is a herpeslike virus associated with one form of lymphoma called **Burkitt's lymphoma (BL).**[186] The virus is directly related to **infectious mononucleosis (IM).** Patients with BL develop EB virus antibodies and so do patients with IM. In IM this antibody persists for many years and by immunofluorescent staining methods can be shown to act on virus-infected Burkitt cells and on cultured IM cells.[187,188] The role of the virus in IM is still unknown. Because the clinical course and the geographic and age distribution of BL and IM are different, it appears to be somewhat unlikely that there is a direct relationship between the virus that causes BL and the EB virus that causes IM, unless it is stipulated that there are several species of the EB virus or that the host's resistance or both account for the differences in clinical behavior. Burkitt first described the lymphoma that bears his name in areas in tropical Africa where malaria is endemic, suggesting that the factor that determines the outcome of EB viral infections is the chronic reticuloendothelial stimulation caused by malaria. According to Burkitt the interaction of EB virus and a chronically stimulated reticuloendothelial system leads to lymphoma, whereas the EB virus infection without reticuloendothelial proliferation produces IM.[189] See also discussion of etiology of IM, pp. 260 and 1059.

CYTOMEGALOVIRUSES

Cytomegaloviruses[190,191] include the virus formerly called **salivary gland virus,** which only locally involves the parotid gland, and **cytomegalic inclusion disease virus,** which produces generalized **cytomegalic inclusion disease.** An increasing number of infections with this virus has been reported in adults with neoplastic diseases, leukemia, or tissue transplants.

Laboratory diagnosis

Histopathology: It must be noted that the characteristic inclusions may be very few and may be missed when only a single section is examined. The involved cell is enlarged, at times to four times its normal size. The nucleus, which is also enlarged, is pushed to the cell base and contains an acidophilic inclusion that is surrounded by a clear ring, giving rise to the characteristic owl-eye appearance.

Exfoliative cytology: Cells bearing inclusions have been found in urine, saliva, and gastric washings.

Virus isolation: Human embryonic skin and muscle cell cultures support the virus. The cultured virus is suited for neutralization and complement-fixation tests.

VARICELLA–HERPES ZOSTER VIRUS

Varicella virus is the etiologic agent of varicella and of herpes zoster. **Chickenpox** is a very contagious, generalized exanthematous disease, whereas herpes zoster is a localized skin disease of very low infectivity that occurs in individuals with limited immunity.

Laboratory diagnosis

Smears of the scrapings of the base of the vesicles reveal intranuclear inclusions and multinucleated giant cells. (Poxviruses also show intracytoplasmic inclusions.)

The contents of the vesicle may show elementary bodies (see **Gutstein method,** p. 904) that can be differentiated from the elementary bodies of smallpox by **electron microscopy.**

The virus is isolated in tissue culture using blood, spinal fluid, vesicular contents, and pharyngeal and nasal washings.

The complement-fixation test is used for the detection of antibodies.

RABIES VIRUS

Rabies virus infects mainly the central nervous system, but it also multiplies in the salivary glands, lacrimal glands, and lungs and therefore may be secreted in saliva, tears, and upper respiratory excretions.

Human rabies follows the bite of a rabid animal, which injects his virus-containing saliva into the wound. A large number of wild and domesticated animals may carry the virus, including foxes, bats, skunks, raccoons, coyotes, wolves, cats, and dogs. In humans and animals the virus produces an encephalitis characterized by inclusion bodies, called **Negri bodies,** which are found in nerve cells of the midbrain and medulla. Negri bodies are pathognomonic for rabies.

Laboratory diagnosis

Laboratory diagnosis is based on staining of impressions and of smears for Negri bodies using Sellers stain, the examination of stained tissue sections, the rabies FA test, and the complement-fixation test.

Material: Use the salivary gland and brain of the animal. The head should be shipped in dry ice. Small animals such as bats may be fixed in 10% formalin. Ship spinal fluid, saliva, and throat swabs in dry ice in sealed ampules.

Animal inoculation: Inoculate infant white mice intracerebrally.

Sellers staining method: This method was first published in 1927 and has largely been replaced by the FA method in most laboratories.

Without previous fixation and while the impression preparation or smear is still moist, dip it into the stain and remove it at once. Rinse in tap water and dry without blotting. When properly stained, the smear by transmitted light appears reddish violet in thin areas and purplish in thicker areas.

Sellers stain: Make a saturated solution of basic fuchsin and also a saturated solution of methylene blue in absolute methyl alcohol (acetone free). Prepare the stain as follows, using first only 2 ml of the basic fuchsin solution.
1. Basic fuchsin solution, 2-4 ml
2. Methylene blue solution, 15 ml
3. Methyl alcohol, absolute (acetone free), 25 ml

Mix and make a trial stain. If too bluish, add 0.5 ml more fuchsin solution and make another trial stain. Repeat until satisfactory. Usually not more than 3 ml fuchsin solution will be necessary.

The stain improves after standing 24 hr and keeps indefinitely if evaporation is prevented. It may be made in larger quantities and stored.

Under the low-power objective locate thin areas containing large nerve cells and examine with the oil-immersion lens.

The **Negri bodies,** located in the cytoplasm of the large nerve cells and often extracellularly, are round or oval, stain cherry red, and contain **blue-staining granules** or **masses** that are usually clearly visible. The cytoplasm of the nerve cells stains somewhat purplish blue and the nucleus more deeply blue. The background (stroma) is rose pink. Nerve fibers are deeper pink, bacteria are deep blue, and erythrocytes are copper colored.

Procedure for rabies fluorescent antibody test:
Materials:
1. Normal mouse brain suspension stored in 1 ml amounts in freezer
2. Rabid mouse brain suspension stored in 1 ml amounts in freezer
3. Antirabies conjugate stored in 0.2 ml amounts in freezer
4. Positive control slides that are already fixed in acetone and stored in freezer

Preparation of smears: Remove a 1 mm thick cross section of Ammon's horn with a scissors or scalpel and place on a wooden tongue depressor. Touch a special double-ringed slide very lightly to the brain cross section. Make duplicate impression smears on the same microscope slide. Make at least two slides per animal. Allow slides to air dry for about 30 min.

Drop the slide into a Coplin jar containing acetone at freezer temperature. Store the Coplin jar and a supply of acetone permanently in the freezer; a temperature of $-20°$ C is sufficient. Allow at least 4 hr for fixation (overnight preferable). Remove slide from acetone and allow to drain dry while still in the freezer.

Staining: Remove slide from freezer and allow to warm to room temperature. Prepare two portions of antirabies conjugate and dilute each with an equal volume of mouse brain suspension or follow the directions enclosed with the conjugate. Use normal brain suspension for the first dilution and infected brain suspension for the second. CAUTION! The infected brain suspension contains live rabies virus!

Cover one smear with a small drop of the first dilution and cover the other smear with a drop of the second solution. Place in humid chamber at 35° C for 30 min. Use large Petri dishes with wet toweling in top. Rinse slides with buffered saline solution and place in staining rack. Then immerse staining rack in buffered saline solution for 10 min. Rinse slide in distilled water to prevent formation of salt crystals.

Blot dry with bibulous paper. (When the slides are drained dry, the fluorescence seems to fade.) Mount in glycerin medium (90% glycerol and 10% buffer at pH 7.0). Carefully apply cover glass to omit air bubbles.

Interpretation: First examine the positive control smear stained with the **first** dilution. Since only normal mouse brain was contained in the suspension, the labeled antirabies antibody should stain any rabies antigen that was present in the smear. The stained particles will appear as Negri bodies, as fine, dustlike, green material, or usually as both.

Next, the positive control smear stained with the **second** dilution must be examined. Since rabies antigen was present in this suspension, the labeled antirabies antibody should have been absorbed; hence it is not available for staining. Therefore no stained particles should be seen in this smear. If any green staining material is seen, the test is not conclusive.

A positive interpretation can be made only when staining is seen in the smear treated with the first dilution but **not** seen in the smear treated with the second.

Examine test slides and compare with controls.

MYXOVIRUSES

Myxoviruses include influenza viruses (types A and B), mumps virus (myxovirus parotidis), parainfluenza virus, Newcastle disease virus (myxovirus multiforme), and RS virus (respiratory syncytial virus). All myxoviruses have an affinity for mucoproteins and agglutinate red cells.

Laboratory diagnosis

Hemagglutination: Myxoviruses agglutinate the red cells of guinea pigs, chickens, sheep, and human group O cells. The agglutination is produced by adsorption of the virus onto the red cells, from which it can be eluted again.

Hemadsorption: Infected tissue culture cells adsorb red cells added to the culture. This hemadsorption can be prevented by immune serum.

Sensitivity to ether: Ether inactivates myxoviruses.

Fluorescent antibody technic: The FA technic used on nasal smears or on bronchial-laryngopharyngeal washings allows a rapid diagnosis of influenza type A.

MEASLES VIRUS

The measles virus is the etiologic agent of measles, a mild disease of childhood but a somewhat more serious infection in adults. If it occurs in pregnant women during the first trimester of pregnancy, it may seriously affect the fetus. Rubella in the **first trimester of pregnancy** is associated with an increased incidence of abortions, stillbirths, and congenital malformations.[194,195] **Congenital rubella**[196] is responsible for such **self-limiting** conditions as thrombocytopenic purpura, hepatosplenomegaly, and skeletal changes and for

such **non-self-limiting** conditions as patent ductus arteriosus, pulmonary artery stenosis, cataracts, and deafness. As a group, children born to these mothers have a high mortality. Since one attack of rubella is followed by lifelong immunity and since the childhood disease is mild, childhood exposure to rubella is of distinct advantage. Similar immunity to rubella can be produced by the administration of an attenuated-life virus vaccine, which, at the present time, is given to all children irrespective of their immune status. Women of childbearing age who by laboratory tests are shown to be susceptible to rubella should also receive the vaccine, provided they are not already pregnant and are willing not to become pregnant for 2-3 months after the vaccination.

Serology of rubella: evaluation of immune status

Laboratory diagnosis[197]

The laboratory diagnosis of rubella relies on serologic tests and virus isolation. Antibodies to rubella can be detected by complement fixation, neutralization, passive hemagglutination, ELISA, and other procedures. The most widely used test is the **hemagglutination inhibition test.**

Virus recovery is only attempted in congenital rubella and in abortions performed therapeutically because of rubella or rubella vaccination.

Hemagglutination inhibition test: The hemagglutination inhibition (III) test is specific and sensitive.[198] Its principle is described on p. 897. The antigen (rubella virus hemagglutinin) is derived from rubella-infected hamsters, the indicator cells are sheep cells, and the patient's serum, when mixed with the antigen, will prevent hemagglutination if it contains antirubella antibody. The use of the microtiter method is suggested. It is commercially available in kit form (Abbott Scientific Products Div., Abbott Laboratories, South Pasadena, Calif.).

The HI test may be used to identify the etiology of the rash and evaluate the immune status.

1. **Etiology of viral rash.** Obtain one serum specimen within 3 days of the onset of the rash and the second specimen 3 weeks later. A fourfold increase in the HI titer from the first to the second specimen indicates that the rash resulted from measles.
2. **Evaluation of immune status.** One single serum specimen is required. A titer of 1:20 or over is indicative of immunity. Titers of 1:10 or lower point to lack of immunity.

CHLAMYDIA-PSITTACOSIS-LYMPHOGRANULOMA-TRACHOMA GROUP

Chlamydiae at one time were classified as large viruses (0.2-0.35 μm in diameter), but they differ from viruses in that they contain RNA as well as DNA, have their own metabolic system, are able to grow and multiply, are surrounded by a cell membrane, and respond to antibiotic therapy. They are basophilic staining, oval, small, intracellular, gram-negative microorganisms.

The following species are recognized: *C. trachomatis* and *C. psittaci. C. trachomatis* is the cause of infections in humans that occur on the oral, conjunctival, and genital mucous membranes. Both *C. trachomatis* and *C. psittaci* cause respiratory disease.

Lymphogranuloma venereum

Lymphogranuloma venereum is a venereal disease caused by a strain of *C. trachomatis* and characterized by involvement of the regional lymph nodes, which become enlarged, break down, and tend to form sinuses. This glandular enlargement may follow a primary skin lesion (papule, pustule, or vesicle), usually unobserved, or urethritis and is accompanied by systemic symptoms of an infection.

Laboratory diagnosis

Smears: Make a smear of pus from infected lymph nodes and stain with Giemsa stain for intracellular **elementary bodies.** (See discussion of trachoma below.)

Tissue sections: The lymph nodes have a characteristic, although not diagnostic, appearance.

Frei skin test: The Frei test is a delayed skin sensitivity reaction to an inactivated antigen **(Lygranum).** A positive reaction indicates past or previous infection. The Frei test has limited usefulness and is not widely available.

Complement-fixation test: A commercial antigen, Lygranum, may be used. Once sero positive, the individual may remain so for years. Any previous chlamydial infection may result in a positive titer. Thus a fourfold increase in titer shown in poured sera drawn 10-14 days apart is necessary for a serologic diagnosis.

Trachoma

Trachoma is a disease of the conjunctiva and cornea, producing a chronic keratoconjunctivitis. The strains of *C. trachomatis* causing trachoma and inclusion conjunctivitis are called the TRIC agents.

Urethritis caused by *C. trachomatis* may be the most widespread venereal disease in the United States. More than 50% of patients with nongonococcal or postgonococcal urethritis may be infected with *C. trachomatis.* This organism causes pelvic inflammatory disease and anterior urethral syndrome in females. It can also be transmitted from mother to infant and cause a newborn pneumonitis.

Laboratory diagnosis

Specimen: Preferred specimens are urethral scrapings containing epithelial cells, conjunctival epithelial scrapings, and nasopharyngeal aspirates for infant pneumonitis.

Conjunctival epithelial scrapings: Allow scraped material to dry on a microscope slide, fix with absolute methyl alcohol (acetone free) for 5 min, and stain with dilute Giemsa stain.

The organisms appear as small, coccoid bodies, called **elementary bodies,** grouped in clusters, in pairs, singly, or as intracellular inclusions. To identify the bodies with certainty a specific FA technic is available.

Isolation procedures: Originally, chlamydiae were isolated by yolk-sac inoculation. Tissue culture methods are now available that have an advantage over earlier chick embryo methods. Cell lines such as McCoy,

BHK 24, and HeLa are successfully used after they are treated with antimetabolites to enhance susceptibility to chlamydial infection. Two to three days after inoculation the cells are stained with Giemsa stain or iodine or by the FA procedure.[199,200]

Inclusion conjunctivitis

Inclusion conjunctivitis is a mucopurulent conjunctivitis that the newborn acquires from the mother during the passage through the birth canal. It appears on the fifth to the fourteenth day of life and heals spontaneously after 3-6 months.

Laboratory diagnosis

Conjunctival scrapings of the infant and cervical scrapings of the mother are examined for inclusion bodies as described for trachoma. See the discussion of the **Gutstein method** below. When available, isolation procedures are more productive.

Psittacosis

Psittacosis is a respiratory disease of humans acquired from contact with infected birds, which excrete the *Chlamydia psittaci* organisms in the stool. The clinical picture varies from an upper respiratory infection to pneumonia. Humans are infected via the respiratory system.

Laboratory diagnosis

Material: Use sputum and blood.

Isolation: *Chlamydia psittaci* can be isolated by inoculation of the yolk sac of 6-day-old chick embryos or by intracerebral, intranasal, or intraperitoneal injection into mice and by inoculation of tissue culture cells.

Serologic identification: Complement-fixation and agglutination tests are done using yolk sac antigen.

VIRAL HEPATITIS

Acute viral hepatitis occurs in three forms: hepatitis A, formerly infectious hepatitis or long incubation hepatitis, hepatitis B, formerly serum hepatitis or short incubation hepatitis, and hepatitis non A−non B.

Hepatitis A

Hepatitis A virus (HAV) is usually transmitted to humans via the fecal-oral route. Contaminated water, milk, and shellfish frequently are found to be the cause of epidemic or sporadic disease. Childhood hepatitis results from HAV. Hepatitis A is characterized by jaundice, nausea, abdominal pain, anorexia, and fever. The incubation period is 15-50 days.

Laboratory diagnosis

Laboratory diagnosis includes the urinary, hematologic, serum enzymatic, and biochemical findings of hepatitis. During the course of the disease HAV can be found in the stool and the blood. However, HAV is present in such low titers and for such a short time that virus isolation is not a reliable method of diagnosis. Antibody to HAV (anti-HAV) is detected early in the disease.[201] Both IgG and IgM classes of antibody are detected, with IgM being the most useful. The methods for detecting anti-HAV (IgM) and anti-HAV (IgG) include complement fixation, immune adherence hemagglutination, radioimmunoassay and enzyme-linked immunosorbent methodologies.[202,203] Both acute and convalescent sera are helpful in establishing the diagnosis.

Hepatitis B[204,205]

Hepatitis B virus (HBV) is the etiologic agent of hepatitis B. The virus was formerly called the Dane particle and more recently Australian antigen or HAA. The present terminology uses HBsAg to indicate the large 42 nm double-shelled particle and HBcAg for the smaller 27 nm inner core.[206] Both antigens elicit specific antibody responses (anti-HBs and anti-HBc).[206a] The virus is transmitted by parenteral inoculation of infected blood or blood derivatives and by unsterilized needles and syringes. The virus is also transmitted orally (dental work and toothbrushes). It is partially responsible for hepatitis in multitransfused patients and

in drug addicts and accounts for sporadic cases of hepatitis. The virus is probably not present in stool but may be found in urine and menstrual blood.

Hepatitis B antigen (HBsAg) is only found in association with hepatitis B (Table 32-49). It can be detected in 85% of patients within the first 12 days of their illness. It usually disappears from the serum within 4-6 weeks of the onset of symptoms, but there are instances in which the antigen persists. If the antigen is cleared from the patient's serum, permanent immunity to HBV follows. Patients who have some defect in their immune mechanism are more likely to become chronic carriers, e.g., patients with leukemia and patients with previous liver disease. Down's syndrome is also characterized by an increased incidence of chronic carriers. HBsAg has also been demonstrated in apparently healthy carriers. For methodology and further discussion of HBsAg see p. 1060.

The incubation period of hepatitis B lasts 50-160

Table 32-49. Serologic technics for detecting hepatitis B antigens and antibodies

Technic	Relative sensitivity for detection					Cost	Time required (hr)
	HBsAg	Anti-HBs	HBcAg	Anti-HBc	HBeAg and anti-HBe		
Agar gel immunodiffusion	1	1	—	—	1	Inexpensive	24-72
Counterimmuno-electrophoresis	5-15	5-10	1-5	1-5	—	Moderate	2
Complement fixation	15-20	5-10	1-5	1-5	—	Inexpensive	2-24
Immune adherence hemagglutination	20-2000	50-150	50-150	20-2000	—	Inexpensive	2
Reverse passive latex agglutination	15-100	—	—	—	—	Inexpensive	0.1-0.2
Reverse passive hemagglutination	20-1000	10,000	—	—	—	Expensive	2
Solid phase radio-immunoassay	2000-10,000	10,000-1,000,000	20-2000	2000-10,000	—	Expensive	3-24
Enzyme immuno-assay	2000-10,000	—	—	—	—	Moderate	0.5-1.0

From Ladd, D.J.: In Sonnenwirth, A.C.: Gradwohl's clinical laboratory methods and diagnosis, ed. 8, St. Louis, 1980, The C.V. Mosby Co., vol. 1.

Table 32-50. Detection of hepatitis A virus (HAV), hepatitis A antibody (anti-HAV) with IgM/IgG differentiation, hepatitis B surface antigen (HBsAg), hepatitis B surface antibody (anti-HBs), and hepatitis B core antibody (anti-HBc) during type A or B infection*

Type A infection	HAV	Anti-HAV (IgM)	Anti-HAV (IgG)
Late incubation period	+	−	−
Onset of acute hepatitis	+ or −	+	−
1-4 wk postonset	−	+	+
5-9 wk postonset	−	+ or −	+
9 wk or longer	−	−	+

Type B infection	HBsAg	Anti-HBs	Anti-HBc
Late incubation period	+	−	−
Onset of acute hepatitis	+	−	+
1-4 wk postonset	+ or −	+ or −	+
5-9 wk postonset	+ or −	+ or −	+
9 wk or longer	−	+	+

From Osterholm, M.T.: Clin. Microb. Newsletter, vol. 1, no. 21, 1979.
*+, Detected; −, undetected.

days, after which time a disease is produced that is similar to hepatitis A.

Table 32-49 summarizes serologic technics for the detection of HBsAg and antibodies. As can be seen in Table 32-49, RIA is the most sensitive but also the most costly.

Hepatitis virus non A–non B

At present there are no commercially available diagnostic tests for non A–non B hepatitis. Recent investigations have indicated that most cases of transfusion-induced hepatitis may be non A–non B.

Table 32-50 describes the sequence of antigen and antibody detection in both hepatitis A and B infections.

VARIOLA AND VACCINIA VIRUSES

The variola and vaccinia viruses are poxvirus variolae (**smallpox**), poxvirus officinalis (**vaccinia virus**), poxvirus bovis (**cowpox**), and poxvirus mollusci (**molluscum contagiosum virus**).

Laboratory diagnosis

Laboratory diagnosis involves **microscopic examination** of the contents of the pustule and of scrapings obtained from its floor and sides. The material can be stained for **elementary bodies** by the Gutstein method or examined unstained with the electron microscope.

Gutstein method[207]

Stain:
1. Methyl violet, 1% aqueous, equal parts
2. Sodium bicarbonate, 2% aqueous, equal parts

Procedure: Allow smear to air dry. Fix in methyl alcohol for 30 min and filter stain onto slide. Cover slide and incubate at 37° C for 20-30 min. Rinse in distilled water, air dry, and examine under oil-immersion lens.

Interpretation: Elementary bodies stain light violet.

Virus isolation: Use blood in the preeruption stage and saliva and pustular material in the later stages. The virus may be isolated by inoculation of the chorioallantoic membrane of the embryonated egg and by inoculation of tissue culture.

Serologic identification: Antibodies in the patient's serum may be detected by the hemagglutination inhibition, neutralization, and complement-fixation tests.

MYCOPLASMATACEAE

Mycoplasmas are minute, gram-negative, nonmotile, pleomorphic organisms varying in shape from spheres to filaments. The spheres measure from 125-250 nm in diameter. Numerous genera are included in the family of Mycoplasmataceae; one of the clinically more important organisms is *Mycoplasma pneumoniae*.

Mycoplasma

Mycoplasmas[208-210] are bacteria-like organisms that are surrounded by a cell membrane and not by a well-defined cell wall. Mycoplasmas are not L forms, which have nonexistent or defective cell membranes and are devoid of any constant shape. Mycoplasmas do not revert to bacterial forms. These organisms have long been known in veterinary medicine as etiologic agents of pneumonia. In human pathology two species are of importance: *M. pneumoniae,* the cause of primary atyp-

ical pneumonia, and *M. hominis,* the cause of a nongonococcal urethritis. Mycoplasmas may also be involved in the etiology of some forms of arthritis and upper respiratory infections.

A well-defined group of mycoplasmas that has not as yet been named is the T (tiny) mycoplasma. These T strains are distinct from other mycoplasmas in that they are urease positive. They are associated with infections of the urogenital tract of humans and lower animals. *Ureaplasma urealyticum* is the proposed name for this group. *U. urealyticum* colonies can be detected on solid medium by flooding the surface with a solution of 0.3 g urea and 0.24 g $MnCl_2$ in 30 ml distilled water. *U. urealyticum* colonies will become stained within 5 min.[211]

Laboratory diagnosis

Morphology: The organisms vary in shape because of their plasticity, which is the result of the absence of a rigid cell wall. They have been described as coccoid, occurring singly or in chains, as vesicular, or as filamentous. The shape may depend on the culture medium used.

Specimen: Sputum, throat washings (normal saline solution), and pharyngeal swabs are used. Other specimens may be urethral discharge, joint fluid, urine, and serous fluid.

Gram stain: Because mycoplasmas stain poorly and are usually very small, microscopic examination of the so-called colony-forming unit (CFU) is not recommended. Culture is the method of choice and even on agar the colonies are difficult to find under the low-power objective of the microscope.

Primary culture: *Mycoplasma* survives in transport medium. The specimen is cultured in one enriched PPLO broth (Difco Laboratories, Detroit) medium and transferred onto two enriched PPLO agar (Difco Laboratories, Detroit) plates.[212] The enrichment consists of horse serum, yeast extract, penicillin, and thalium acetate. The plates are sealed with Parafilm, placed in CO_2-permeable plastic bags, and incubated aerobically at 37° C under 5% CO_2 tension. It usually takes 7-15 days before the colonies appear. Do not discard plates as negative until 3 weeks have elapsed. The same medium is used for T-strain growth, but thalium acetate must be omitted, because it inhibits the growth of T strains. A subculture is made weekly for 3 weeks. Colonies are observed by oblique transillumination under the dissecting microscope, focusing through the medium onto its surface. *M. pneumoniae* colonies appear slowly within 5-10 days, are small (10-250 μm in diameter), have a ground-glass, somewhat granular appearance, and are deeply submerged in agar. They are β-hemolytic in 24-48 hr, and the appearance of some organisms can be likened to fried eggs, the yolk being embedded in the agar while the base rests on the agar surface.

Since the colonies are deeply embedded in agar, transfer of colonies is accomplished by cutting out a square agar block containing the colony, using a sterile thin spatula as used in mycologic procedures. The block is then inverted and either simply placed on the new agar surface or it is held with sterile forceps and used to "streak" the plate.

Colonies on the agar blocks can be visualized easily by the use of Dienes staining procedure.[212a] Small spheres that cannot be seen grossly are formed in broth.

Identification

Identification[213,214] of *Mycoplasma* depends on the appearance of the colonies, β-hemolysis, glucose fermentation, inhibition by specific antisera, and serologic procedures.

Serologic methods are used for the following purposes:

1. To identify the organism, e.g., complement-fixation test, agar gel diffusion, and growth inhibition. The latter is accomplished by using **immune serum–saturated disks.**
2. To demonstrate nonspecific and specific antibodies in the patient's blood. (Nonspecific antibodies include cold agglutinins and agglutinins for *Streptococcus* MG.)

Tests for nonspecific antibodies: Cold agglutinins develop during the second week of *M. pneumoniae* infections and are found in almost 90% of atypical pneumonia cases.

Titration of cold agglutinins:

Procedure: Obtain patient's serum from clot that has not been refrigerated. Make a 2% saline suspension of washed group O blood cells (0.1 ml blood added to 4.9 ml saline solution). Set up a series of 12 small tubes in a rack. Place 1.5 ml saline solution in the first tube and 1 ml saline solution in each of the following tubes. Add 0.5 ml of the patient's serum to the first tube and mix. Transfer 1 ml from the first tube to the second tube and mix. Continue on through the eleventh tube, from which 1 ml is discarded. The twelfth tube is the control.

Add 0.1 ml of the cell suspension to each tube. Mix and place in the refrigerator at 0-4° C overnight. Examine for agglutination immediately after taking from the refrigerator and inverting each tube against Parafilm. The highest dilution of the serum giving a 3-4 + agglutination represents the cold agglutinin titer. If positive, allow tubes to stand at room temperature for several hours, and then read again to ascertain whether the reaction is reversible at room temperature and therefore represents true cold agglutination.

Tube	Titer	Tube	Titer
1	1:4	6	1:128
2	1:8	7	1:256
3	1:16	8	1:512
4	1:32	9	1:1024
5	1:64	10	1:2048
		11	1:4096

Interpretation: See interpretation of *Streptococcus* MG agglutination test.

Agglutinins for Streptococcus MG: *Streptococcus* MG is a strain of hemolytic streptococci. Agglutinins to *Streptococcus* MG are present in 20-75% of cases of *M. pneumoniae* infections (atypical pneumonia).

Streptococcus MG agglutination test: *Streptococcus* MG antigen is commercially available (Difco Laboratories, Detroit).

Procedure: Set up a twofold serial dilution of the serum, from 1:5 to 1:1280, with saline solution. The serum is not inactivated, since heating decreases the tier. Add an equal amount of the streptococcus suspension (antigen). Final dilutions are 1:10 to 1:2560.

Set up 10 tubes and number from 1-10. To tube 1 add 0.8 ml normal saline solution; add 0.5 ml to the remaining 9 tubes. To tube 1 add 0.2 ml serum, mix, and transfer 0.5 ml of tube 1 mixture to tube 2; mix and continue to transfer, discarding 0.5 ml from tube 9. Tube 10 is the saline solution control. The initial serum dilutions are 1:5, 1:10, 1:20, 1:40, 1:80, 1:160, 1:320, 1:640, and 1:1280.

Add 0.5 ml antigen to each tube, giving final serum dilutions of 1:10, 1:20, 1:40, 1:80, 1:160, 1:320, 1:640, 1:1280, and 1:2560. Place in water bath at 35° C for 2 hr and then refrigerate (4° C) for 18 hr. Place again in water bath at 35° C for 2 hr to rule out nonspecific agglutination. Shake and read.

Interpretation: *Streptococcus* MG agglutinin titer is the highest dilution of the patient's serum that produces agglutination. Acute and convalescent sera are tested.

Cold and *Streptococcus* MG agglutinins may be demonstrated after the second week, reaching a peak in the fourth or fifth week. The agglutinins are found in **low** titers (under 1:20) in normal individuals and in patients suffering from acute respiratory diseases and streptococcal infections. A fourfold increase in titer in the course of the disease is significant. Absence of agglutinins does not rule out primary atypical pneumonia. A single titer of 1:80 is indicative of disease.

Tests for specific antibodies:

Complement-fixation test: The cultured organisms provide a satisfactory antigen.

Fluorescent antibody technic: Sections of the thorax of a chick embryo infected with PPLO are treated with fluorescein-tagged antibody (direct method), or fluorescein-tagged antiglobulin if the indirect method is used.

Convalescent sera usually show a variety of immunologic reactions such as false positive serologic tests for syphilis, cold hemagglutinins, and agglutinins for *Streptococcus* MG.

GLOSSARY

abscess Localized collection of pus in a cavity formed as a result of an infectious process.

acute stage That phase during the course of a disease that is most severe and generally of short duration in patients who recover.

aerobe Organism whose growth and reproduction are favored by the presence of air or free oxygen.

aerosol Suspension of small particles in a gas, e.g., distribution of small particles into the air when coughing or sneezing.

allergy Sensitivity to a specific substance that in similar amounts is harmless to most people.

amorphous Without visible differentiation in structure.

anaerobe Organism whose growth and reproduction are favored by the absence of air or free oxygen.

anoxia Condition in which the cells of the body do not have or cannot utilize sufficient oxygen.

antigen Any substance that, when introduced into the blood or tissues, incites the formation of antibody and that, when mixed with the antibody, reacts with it in some observable way.

antiserum Serum that contains antibody.

aseptic technic Technic used in an attempt to prevent the introducion or access of microorganisms.

bacteremia Presence of bacteria in the blood.

biochemical test Bacteriologic test in which chemicals are employed as indicators of biologic activity.

bipolar At both poles or ends of the bacterial cell.

bronchitis Inflammation of the bronchial tubes.

bubo Inflamed swelling of a lymph gland, usually in the armpit or groin.

capsule Gelatin-like envelope surrounding bacteria.

catheterize To remove urine from patient by use of a sterile tube (catheter).

cervicitis Inflammation of that portion of female genitourinary tract known as the cervix.

chain Four or more bacterial cells attached end to end.

chancre Venereal sore or ulcer.

chemotherapy Use of chemical agents in the treatment of disease.

chromogen Any organic coloring matter.

coagulate To curdle or clot by chemical action or fermentation.

concave Curving in.

confluent growth Bacterial growth in which colonies overlap each other and cannot be successfully picked out individually for subculture.

conjunctivitis Inflammation of inner lining of membranes that surround the eye.

contaminant Any substance or biologic agent whose presence results in other substances or biologic agents being impure, i.e., foreign organisms developing accidentally in a pure culture.

convalescent stage Stage of disease in which the patient is on the way to recovery.

convex Curving out.

cutaneous At surface of skin.

cystitis Inflammation of bladder.

defibrinate Removal of fibrin from blood.

detergent Purifying or cleansing agent.

dextrose Grape sugar or glucose.

diplococci Cocci that occur in pairs.

disinfectant Agent used to destroy vegetative stage of pathogenic microorganisms.

dissemination Scattering or distribution; herein applied to microorganisms.

edema Swelling, usually resulting from the presence of abnormally large amounts of fluid in the intercellular spaces of the body.

endotoxin Toxic substance that is retained within bacterial cell until cell disintegrates.

enterotoxin Exotoxin excreted by certain bacteria.

enzyme Protein capable of influencing a chemical reaction without being structurally changed in the reaction.

erythema Redness of skin.

etiologic agent Specific causative organism of a disease.

exotoxin Toxin secreted into surrounding medium or tissue by intact, living organism.

extracellular Outside a cell body.

exudate Substance that oozes out.

facultative anaerobe Organism that prefers to live as an anaerobe but will adapt to aerobic conditions of growth.

fermentation Decomposition of organic matter by enzymes secreted by microorganisms or other cells.

filamentous Growth composed of long, irregularly placed or interwoven threads.

flagella Fine hairlike extensions on certain bacteria that are used to propel them through liquids.

flocculent Containing small adherent masses of various shapes floating in culture fluid (usually groups of bacteria).

fluorescent Having one color by transmitted light and another by reflected light.

friable Easily pulverized or crumbled; as applied to cultures, growth that is dry and brittle when touched with an inoculating needle.

gatroenteritis Inflammation of any portion of the intestinal tract.

granular Composed of small discrete particles.

granulomatous Composed of granulation tissue, a tissue formed in wounds and composed of small, rounded, fleshy masses.

heat labile Destructible by heat.

heat stable Indestructible by heat.

hemolysin Substance that liberates hemoglobin from red cells.

hemolysis Presence of zone of hemolyzed red cells around colony grown on blood agar plate.

homogenize To subject a specimen to physical processes that result in a mixture of uniform consistency.

hyaline Glassy in appearance and transparent or nearly so.

hydrolysis Chemical reaction in which a compound reacts with water.

hypersensitivity Stateo of reactivity in which the body reacts to a foreign agent more strongly than normal.

inhibitory Substances that either prevent or greatly reduce the capabilities of a microorganism to grow or reproduce.

involution forms Retrograde and abnormal forms assumed by microorganisms under certain conditions.

isolation Obtaining bacteria in pure culture by subculturing discrete colonies.

lactose Milk sugar.

laryngotracheitis Inflammation involving both the larynx and trachea.

liquefaction Change of a solid into a liquid.

lyse Process of cell destruction that results from action of specific substances.

membranous Growth that is thin and filmlike.

meningitis Inflammation of membranes covering the brain and/or spinal cord.

microaerophilic Preferring low concentrations of oxygen.

morphology Form and structure, including principally size and shape, of an organism.

motile Having the power of motion.

mucoid Resembling gummy, watery liquid that covers mucous membranes.

mucopurulent Containing both mucus and pus.

nasopharynx That part of the pharynx that lies above the level of the soft palate.

necrosis Death of a cell or group of cells that is in contact with living tissue.

nephritis Inflammation of kidney.

neurotoxin Toxin that affects nerve tissue.

nonchromogenic Lacking chromogens or coloring matter.

normal flora Those living forms that normally occur in a given type of habitat or environment.

obligate aerobe Organism having the ability to grow only in the presence of air or free oxygen.

obligate anaerobe Organism having the ability to grow only in the absence of air or free oxygen.

opaque Impervious to light.

optimal temperature Temperature at which growth is most rapid.

osteomyelitis Inflammation of bone caused by a microorganism, usually pyogenic.

otitis externa Inflammation of external ear.

otitis interna Inflammation of internal ear.

papule Small and clearly defined elevated area of the skin.

parenchymatous Pertaining to that portion of an organ that performs its essential functions.

pathogen Microorganism capable of causing disease.

pellicle Bacterial growth forming either a continuous or interrupted film at the surface of a liquid medium.

pericarditis Inflammation of the membranous sac that contains the heart

peritoneum Glistening and smooth inner lining of the abdominal cavity of the body.

peritonitis Inflammation of peritoneum; a condition usually accompanied by exudation of serum, fibrin, cells, and pus into the peritoneal cavity.

phagocyte Cell capable of ingesting bacteria.

pharynx Area of body between the mouth nares, and esophagus.

pleomorphic Different forms within the same species.

pneumonia, bronchial Pneumonia characterized by associated inflammation of the bronchial tubes.

pneumonia, lobar Pneumonia characterized by inflammation of lung tissue of one or more lobes of the lung.

pneumonitis Localized acute inflammation of lung.

presumptive diagnosis Initial tentative diagnosis of a disease based on clinical evidence and without other evidence, e.g., laboratory findings.

primary isolation Initial isolation of microorganisms from a specimen.

proteolysis Hydrolysis or decomposition of proteins.

pseudomembrane False membrane; more specifically membrane produced as a result of activity of the organism that causes diphtheria.

pustule Small pus-filled elevation at surface of skin.

putrefaction Decomposition of animal or vegetable proteins by microorganisms.

pyogenic organism Organism characterized principally by the fact that it produces pus.

reduction Removal of oxygen from a compound, addition of hydrogen to a compound, or a gain of electrons or loss in positive valence.

reticuloendothelial system System of the body that produces and removes blood cells.

rhizoid Growth of an irregularly branched or rootlike character.

saprophyte Organism that normally inhabits certain areas of the body, particularly the gastrointestinal tract, without invading tissue and producing disease.

sensitize To render more reactive.

sepsis Poisoning that is caused by the products of pathogenic microorganism activity.

septicemia Morbid condition resulting from presence of pathogenic bacteria and their associated toxins in the blood.

serologic test Laboratory test performed on blood serum of a patient.

sinusitis Inflammation within sinus cavity.

subterminal Situated toward, but not at, the end.

sucrose Cane sugar.

suppurative Pus producing.

systemic Involving the entire body.

tenacious Holding fast or adhesive.

terminal Situated at the extreme end.

therapeutic agent Substance administered in treatment of a disease.

transient Lasting only a brief period.

translucent Semitransparent.

transparent As applied to cultures, growth that is water clear.

true motility Moving voluntarily.

turbid Cloudy; turbidity may be uniform, flocculent, or granular.

ulcer Loss of substance on a cutaneous or mucous surface, with gradual disintegration and necrosis of the tissues.

urethritis Inflammation of membranous lining of the canal (urethra) that conveys urine from the bladder to the exterior.

vaginitis Inflammation of that portion of female genital tract known as the vagina.

viable Capable of living: specifically, alive and capable of reproducing.

virulent Unusually capable of producing disease.

viscous Thick substance that adheres to the inoculating needle when touched: sediment that arises as a coherent swirl when liquid media are shaken.

viscus Any large internal organ within the three great cavities of the body, especially the abdomen.

REFERENCES

1. Koneman, E.W., et al.: Color atlas and textbook of diagnostic microbiology, Philadelphia, 1979, J.B. Lippincott Co.
2. Bondi, A., Bartola, J.T., and Prier, J.E.: The clinical laboratory as an aid in chemotherapy of infectious disease, Baltimore, 1977, University Park Press.
3. Joklik, W.K., Willett, H.P., and Amos, D.B.: Zinsser microbiology, ed. 17, New York, 1980, Appleton-Century-Crofts.
4. Bartlett, R.C.: In Lorian, V.L., editor: Significance of medical microbiology in the care of patients, Baltimore, 1977, The Williams & Wilkins Co.
5. Sonnenwirth, A.C.: In Sonnenwirth, A.C., and Jarett, L., editors: Gradwohl's clinical laboratory methods and diagnosis, St. Louis, 1980, The C.V. Mosby Co., vol. 2.
6. Bodily, H.L., Updike, E.L., and Mason, J.O., editors: Diagnostic procedures for bacterial, mycotic and parasitic infections, ed. 5, New York, 1970, American Public Health Association, Inc.
7. Cowan, S.T., and Steel, K.J.: Identification of medical bacteria, New York, 1966, Cambridge University Press.
8. Lennette, E.H., et al.: Manual of clinical microbiology, ed. 3, Washington, D.C., 1980, American Society for Clinical Microbiology.
9. Buchanan, R.E., and Gibbons, N.E., editors: Bergey's manual of determinative bacteriology, ed. 8, Baltimore, 1974, The Williams & Wilkins Co.
10. Kenny, G.E.: In Barile, M.F., and Razin, S., editors: The mycoplasmas, New York, 1979, Academic Press, Inc., vol. 1.
11. Phillips, C.R.: In Block, S.S., editor: Disinfection, sterilization and preservation, ed. 2, Philadelphia, 1977, Lea & Febiger.
12. Spaulding, E.H.: J. Hosp. Res. **1**:5, 1965.
13. Kereluk, K., and Lloyd, R.: J. Hosp. Res. **7**:7, 1969.
14. Lab safety, Atlanta, 1974, Centers for Disease Control.
15. Stuart, R.D.: Public Health Rep. **74**:431, 1959.
16. Amies, C.R., and Douglas, J.I.: Can. J. Public Health **56**:27, 1965.
17. Cary, S.G., and Blair, E.B.: J. Bacteriol. **88**:96, 1964.
18. Truant, J.P., Brett, W.A., and Thomas, W.: Henry Ford Hosp. Med. Bull. **10**:287, 1962.
19. Johnson, G.D., and Holborrow, E.J.: In Weir, D., editor: Immunochemistry, Handbook of experimental immunology, Oxford, England, 1973, Blackwell Scientific Publications, vol. 1.
20. Brewer, J.H., and Allgeier, D.L.: Appl. Environ. Microbiol. **14**:985, 1966.
21. Moore, W.E.C.: Int. J. System. Bacteriol. **16**:174, 1966.
22. Aranbri, A., et al.: Appl. Environ. Microbiol. **17**:568, 1969.
23. Killgorf, G.E., et al.: Am. J. Clin. Pathol. **59**:552, 1973.
24. Gruft, H.: Health Lab. Sci. **8**:79, 1971.
25. Gruft, H.: J. Bacteriol. **90**:829, 1965.
26. Cohn, M.L., Waggoner, R.F., and McClatchy, J.K.: Am. Rev. Respir. Dis. **98**:295, 1968.

27. Lubin, A.H., and Ewing, W.H.: Public Health Lab. **22:**83, 1964.
28. Kellog, D.S., Holms, K.K., and Hill, G.A.: In Marcus, S., and Sherris, J.C., coordinating editors: Cumitec 4: laboratory diagnosis of gonorrhea, Washington, D.C., 1976, American Society for Microbiology.
29. Thayer, J.D., and Martin, J.E.: Public Health Rep. **81:**559, 1966.
30. Martin, J.E., and Lester, A.: HSMHA Health Rep. **86:**1, 1971.
31. Barry, A.L., et al.: Appl. Environ. Microbiol. **20:**866, 1970.
32. Washington, J.A.: Appl. Environ. Microbiol. **23:**956, 1972.
33. DeBlanc, H.J., Jr., Deland, R., and Wagner, H.N.: Appl. Environ. Microbiol. **22:**846, 1971.
34. Renner, E.D., Gatheridge, L.A., and Washington, J.A., II: Appl. Environ. Microbiol. **26:**368, 1973.
35. Dunkelberg, W.E., Jr.: Am. J. Obstet. Gynecol. **91:**998, 1965.
36. Kunin, C.M.: Detection, prevention and management of urinary tract infections: a manual for the physician, nurse and allied health worker, Philadelphia, 1972, Lea & Febiger.
37. Smith, L.G., et al.: Ann. Intern. Med. **54:**66, 1961.
38. Hoeprich, P.D.: J. Lab. Clin. Med. **56:**899, 1960.
39. Simmons, N.A., and Williams, J.D.: Lancet **1:**1377, 1962.
40. Dalton, H.P.: Am. J. Med. Technol. **29:**247, 1963.
41. Jones, R.S., et al.: N. Engl. J. Med. **290:**11, 1974.
42. Thomas, V., and Shelokov, A.: N. Engl. J. Med. **290:**588-590, 1974.
43. Fed. Register **37:**20527, 1972.
44. National Committee on Clinical Laboratory Standards: Performance standards for antimicrobic disc susceptibility tests, approved standard ASM-2, ed. 2, Villanova, Pa., 1979, The Committee.
45. Bauer, A.W., et al.: Am. J. Clin. Pathol. **45:**493, 1966.
46. Neff, J.: Antimicrobial susceptibility testing, MT-26, Telephone lectures for medical technologists, Columbia, Mo., 1971, University of Missouri–Columbia Medical Center and Extension Division.
47. Ryan, K.J., Schoenkencht, F.D., and Kirby, W.M.M.: Hosp. Pract. **55:**991, 1970.
48. Gavan, T., Cheatle, E.L., and McFadden, H.W.: Antimicrobial susceptibility testing, Chicago, 1971, Committee on Continuing Education, Council on Microbiology, American Society of Clinical Pathologists.
49. Sherris, J.C., Raskad, A.L., and Lighthart, G.A.: Ann. N.Y. Acad. Sci. **145:**248, 1967.
50. National Committee on Clinical Laboratory Standards: Performance standards for antimicrobial disc susceptibility tests, approved standard ASM-2, Villanova, Pa., 1975, The Committee.
51. Bauer, A.W., et al.: Am. J. Clin. Pathol. **45:**493, 1966.
52. Fed. Register **37:**20525, 1972.
53. Fed. Register **38:**276, 1973.
54. Kelly, M.T., and Matsen, J.M.: Antimicrob. Agents Chemother. **9:**440, 1975.
55. Marymont, J.H., Jr., and Wentz, R.M.: Am. J. Clin. Pathol. **45:**548, 1966.
56. MacLowry, J.D., and Marsh, H.H.: J. Lab. Clin. Med. **72:**685, 1968.
57. Ericsson, H.M., and Sherris, J.C.: Acta Pathol. Microbiol. Scand. [B] **217**(suppl.): entire issue, 1971.
58. Mertens, B.F.: Microdilution methodology, Potomac, Md., 1980, Micro-Media Systems, Inc.
59. Advanced microbiology: recent developments and new frontiers, Williamsburg, Va., 1980, American Society of Clinical Pathologists Educational Center Program.
60. Wilkins, T.D., et al.: Antimicrob. Agents Chemother. **1:**451, 1972.
61. McMinn, M.T., and Crawford, J.J.: Appl. Environ. Microbiol. **19:**207, 1970.
62. Moody, M.D., et al.: Health Lab. Sci. **2:**149, 1965.
63. Petran, E.I.: Am. J. Clin. Pathol. **41:**224, 1964.
64. Pien, F.D., Thompson, R.L., and Martin, W.J.: Mayo Clin. Proc. **47:**251, 1972.
65. Rantz, L.A., and Randall, E.: Proc. Soc. Exp. Biol. Med. **59:**22, 1945.
66. Klein, D.C., et al.: Appl. Environ. Microbiol. **16:**184, 1968.
67. Lund, E.: Acta Pathol. Microbiol. Scand. **47:**308, 1959.
68. Hawn, C.D.Z., and Beebe, E.: J. Bacteriol. **90:**519, 1965.
69. Todd, J., Fishaut, M., and Welch, T.: Lancet **2:**1116-1118, 1978.
70. McKenna, U.G., et al.: Mayo Clin. Proc. **55:**663-672, 1980.
71. Kellog, D.S., Jr., and Deacon, W.E.: Proc. Soc. Exp. Biol. Med. **115:**963, 1964.
72. Creitz, J.R., et al.: HASMHA Health Rep. **86:**270, 1971.
73. Sayeed, Z., et al.: J.A.M.A. **210:**312, 1972.
74. Edwards, E.A.: J. Immunol. **106:**314, 1970.
75. Dorff, G.J., Coonrad, J.D., and Rytel, M.W.: Lancet **1:**578, 1971.
76. Edwards, E.A., Muehl, P.M., and Peckinpaugh, R.O.: J. Lab. Clin. Med. **80:**449, 1972.
77. Edwards, P.R., and Ewing, W.H.: Identification of the Enterobacteriaceae, ed. 3, Minneapolis, 1972, Burgess Publishing Co.
78. Ewing, W.H.: Revised definitions for the family Enterobacteriaceae, its tribes and genera, Atlanta, 1972, Centers for Disease Control.
79. Douglas, G.W., and Washington, J.A.: Identification of Enterobacteriaceae in the clinical laboratory, Atlanta, 1970, Centers for Disease Control.
80. Ewing, W.H.: Differentiation of Enterobacteriaceae by biochemical reactions, Atlanta, 1973, Centers for Disease Control.
81. Smith, H.H., and Anderson-Langmuir, C.: Am. J. Clin. Pathol. **45:**218, 1966.
82. Rowe, B., et al.: Lancet **1:**1-5, 1970.
83. Goldschmidt, M., and DoPont, H.L.: J. Infect. Dis. **133:**153-156, 1976.
84. Clin. Microb. Newsletter **1**(11), 1979.
85. Schneierson, S.S., and Bottone, E.J.: CRC Crit. Rev. Clin. Lab. Sci. **4:**341, 1973.
86. Ewing, W.H.: Isolation and identification of *Salmonella* and *Shigella*, Atlanta, 1972, Centers for Disease Control.
87. Fields, B.N., et al.: Am. J. Med. **42:**89, 1967.
88. National nosocomial infections study quarterly report, second quarter 1972, Atlanta, 1973, Centers for Disease Control.
89. Washington, J.A., II, Yu, P.K.W., and Martin, W.J.: Appl. Environ. Microbiol. **22:**267, 1971.
90. Isenberg, H.D., and Painter, B.G.: Appl. Environ. Microbiol. **22:**1126, 1971.
91. Smith, P.B., et al.: Appl. Environ. Microbiol. **22:**928, 1971.
92. Isenberg, H.D.: Clinical Microbiology Newsletter **1**(14), July 5, 1979.
93. Oberhofen, T.R.: J. Clin. Microbiol. **9**(2):220, 1979.
94. Lorian, V., and Topf, B.: Arch. Intern. Med. **130:**104, 1972.
95. Maiztegui, J.I., et al.: N. Engl. J. Med. **272:**222, 1965.
96. Levin, J., et al.: Ann. Intern. Med. **76:**1, 1972.
97. Levin, J., et al.: N. Engl. J. Med. **283:**1313, 1970.

80. Prion, R.B., and Spagna, V.A.: J. Clin. Microbiol. **10:**394, 1979.
99. Hugh, R., and Leifson, E.: J. Bacteriol. **66:**24, 1953.
100. Hayes, W.C.: J. Gen. Microbiol. **5:**939, 1951.
101. Kovacs, N.: Nature **178:**703, 1956.
102. Gaby, W.L., and Hadley, C.: J. Bacteriol. **74:**356, 1957.
103. Weaver, R.E.: Public Health Lab. **25:**202, 1967.
104. Ewing, W.H., Hugh, R., and Johnson, J.G.: Studies on the *Aeromonas* group, Atlanta, 1961, Centers for Disease Control.
105. McAllister, T.A.: Scott, Med. J. **21:**129-131, 1976.
106. McCullough, N.B.: In Rose, N.R., and Freeman, H., editors: Manual of clinical immunology, Washington, D.C., 1976, American Society for Microbiology.
107. Gutman, L.T., et al.: N. Engl. J. Med. **288:**1372, 1973.
108. Sonnenwirth, A.C.: In Lennette, E.H., et al., editors: Manual of clinical microbiology, Washington, D.C., 1980, American Society for Microbiology.
109. Kartman, L., Goldenberg, M.I., and Hubbert, W.T.: Am. J. Public Health **56:**1554, 1966.
110. Sonnenwirth, A.C., and Weaver, R.: N. Engl. J. Med. **283:**1468, 1970.
111. Sedgwick, A.K., and Tilton, R.C.: Appl. Environ. Microbiol. **21:**383, 1971.
112. Pai, C.H., et al.: J. Clin. Microbiol. **9:**712-715, 1979.
113. Bain, R.V.S., Rountree, P.M., and Walker-Smith, J.: Med. J. Aust. **48:**395, 1961.
114. Marchette, N.J., and Nicholes, P.R.: J. Bacteriol. **82:**26, 1961.
115. Forshay, L.: J. Infect. Dis. **51:**286, 1932.
116. Kilian, M.A.: Acta Pathol. Microbiol. Scand. [B] **82:**835-842, 1974.
117. Robbins, B., et al.: Ann. Intern. Med. **78:**259, 1973.
118. Thornsberry, C., and Kirven, L.A.: Antimicrob. Agents Chemother. **6:**653, 1974.
119. Gaby, W.L., and Free, E.: J. Bacteriol. **76:**442, 1958.
120. Phillips, J.E.: J. Pathol. **79:**331, 1960.
121. Maguire, L.C.: Vet. Rec. **70:**989, 1958.
122. Brooks, A.M., Bradford, W.L., and Berry, G.P.: J.A.M.A. **120:**883, 1942.
123. Holwerda, J., and Eldering, G.: J. Bacteriol. **86:**449, 1963.
124. Jones, G.L., and Herbert, G.A., editors: "Legionnaires' disease," the disease, the bacterium, and methodology, Atlanta, 1978, Centers for Disease Control.
125. Edelstein, P.H., Meyer, R.D., and Finegold, S.M.: Am. Rev. Respir. Dis. **121:**317-327, 1980.
126. McDade, J.E., et al.: N. Engl. J. Med. **297:**22, 1977.
127. Feeley, J.C., et al.: In Jones, G.L., and Herbert G.A., editors: "Legionnaires' disease," the disease, the bacterium, and methodology, Atlanta, 1978, Centers for Disease Control.
128. Bornstein, D.L., et al.: Medicine **43:**207, 1964.
129. Holdeman, L.V., Cato, E.P., and Moore, W.E., editors: Anaerobic laboratory manual, ed. 4, Blacksburg, Va., 1977, Virginia Polytechnic Institute and State University.
130. Sutter, V.L., Vargo, V.L., and Finegold, S.M.: Wadsworth anaerobic bacteriology manual, ed. 2, Los Angeles, 1975, Wadsworth Hospital Center.
131. Barber, M., and Okubadejo, O.A.: Br. Med. J. **2:**735, 1965.
132. Gray, M.L., Seeliger, H.P.R., and Patel, J.: Clin. Pediatr. **2:**614, 1963.
133. Gray, M.L.: Ann. N.Y. Acad. Sci. **98:**686, 1962.
134. Laboratory methods in medical mycobacteriology, course 8550-C, Technique section, Atlanta, 1965, Centers for Disease Control.
135. Recommended safety measures for mycobacteriology, Atlanta, 1965, Centers for Disease Control.
136. David, H.L.: The bacteriology of the mycobacterioses, Atlanta, 1975, Centers for Disease Control.
137. Kubica, G.P.: Current concepts in the isolation and identification of clinically significant mycobacteria, Atlanta, 1967, Centers for Disease Control.
138. Runyon, E.H.: Am. J. Clin. Pathol. **54:**578, 1970.
139. Wayne, L.G., and Doubek, J.R.: Appl. Environ. Microbiol. **16:**925, 1968.
140. Vestal, A.L., and Kubica, G.P.: Am. Rev. Respir. Dis. **94:**247, 1966.
141. Canilang, B., and Armstrong, D.: Am. Rev. Respir. Dis. **97:**451, 1968.
142. Truant, J.P., Brett, W.A., and Thomas, W.: Henry Ford Hosp. Med. Bull. **10:**287, 1962.
143. Wayne, L.G., and Doubek, J.R.: Am. J. Clin. Pathol. **42:**431, 1964.
144. Weyer, E.M.: Ann. N.Y. Acad. Sci. **130:**681, 1966.
145. Cannetti, G., et al.: Bull. WHO **29:**565, 1963.
146. Froman, S., et al.: Am. J. Clin. Pathol. **42:**340, 1964.
147. DeGroat, A., Anastassiadis-Aries, U.E., and White, M.F.: Am. J. Clin. Pathol. **41:**441, 1964.
148. Parlett, R.C.: Ann. N.Y. Acad. Sci. **98:**637, 1962.
149. Soule, M.H.: Ann. N.Y. Acad. Sci. **54:**34, 1951.
150. Soule, M.H.: Int. J. Lepr. **32:**195, 1964.
151. Maddock, P.K.: J.A.M.A. **148:**44, 1952.
152. Knisely, R.F.: J. Bacteriol. **92:**784, 1966.
153. Hobbs, B.C.: J. Appl. Bacteriol. **28:**74, 1965.
154. Holdeman, L.V., Cato, E.P., and Moore, W.E.C.: Int. J. System. Bacteriol. **17:**323, 1967.
155. Batty, I., and Walker, P.D.: J. Appl. Bacteriol. **28:**112, 1965.
156. Eadie, G.A., et al.: J.A.M.A. **187:**134, 1964.
157. Arnou, S.S., et al.: J.A.M.A. **237:**1946-1951, 1977.
158. Pickett, J., et al.: N. Engl. J. Med. **295:**770-772, 1976.
159. Midura, T.F., et al.: J. Clin. Microbiol. **9:**281-284, 1979.
160. Bartlett, J.G.: Rev. Infect. Dis. **1:**530-539, 1979.
161. George, W.L., et al.: J. Clin. Microbiol. **9:**214-219, 1979.
162. Mukerjee, S.: Br. Med. J. **2:**546, 1964.
163. Feeley, J.C.: Bacteriol. **89:**665, 1965.
164. Balows, A., Hermann, G.J., and DeWitt, W.E.: Health Lab. Sci. **8:**167, 1971.
165. Smith, H.L.: Bull. W.H.O. **42:**817, 1970.
166. Gangarosa, E.J., Bennett, J.V., and Boring, J.R.: Bull. W.H.O. **35:**987, 1967.
167. Farquar, J.W., Edmunds, P.N., and Tilley, J.B.: Lancet **2:**1211, 1958.
168. Morbidity and Mortality Weekly Report **27:**207, 1978.
169. Morbidity and Mortality Weekly Report **2:**226-227, 1978.
170. Skirrow, M.B.: Br. Med. J. **2:**o-11, 1977.
171. Director, Bureau of Laboratories, Identical Memorandum. Centers for Disease Control: Diarrheal disease caused by *Campylobacter fetus* subspecies *jejuni,* Atlanta, Aug. 7, 1978, Centers for Disease Control.
172. Edwards, G.A., and Domm, B.M.: Medicine **39:**117, 1960.
173. Galton, M.M.: Ann. N.Y. Acad. Sci. **98:**675, 1962.
174. Ferron, E.D.: Rev. Clin. Esp. **20:**283, 1946.
175. LeFrock, J.L., and Klainer, A.S.: Nosocomial infections, Scope monograph series, Kalamazoo, Mich., 1976, The Upjohn Co.
176. National Nosocomial Infections Study, Report, annual summary, pub. no. 78:8257, Washington, D.C., 1976, Centers for Disease Control.
177. American Hospital Association: Infection control in the hospital, ed. 3, Chicago, 1974, The Association.

178. Bartlett, R.C., Hammond, J.B., and Wickersham, V.: Hospital associated infections, Chicago, 1971, Commission on Continuing Education, American Society of Clinical Pathologists.
179. Reinarz, J.A., et al.: J. Clin. Invest. **44**:831, 1965.
180. Lennette, E.H.: Am. J. Clin. Pathol. **57**:737, 1972.
181. Sommerville, R.G.: Prog. Med. Virol. **22**:165, 1971.
182. Ginsberg, H.S.: Am. J. Clin. Pathol. **57**:771, 1972.
183. Werner, H.A.: Am. J. Clin. Pathol. **57**:751, 1972.
184. Casals, J.: Am. J. Clin. Pathol. **57**:762, 1972.
185. Kaplan, A.S.: Am. J. Clin. Pathol. **57**:783, 1972.
186. Burkitt, D.P.: Int. Rev. Exp. Pathol. **2**:67, 1963.
187. Henle, G., Henle, W., and Diehl, V.: Proc. Natl. Acad. Sci. U.S.A. **59**:94, 1968.
188. Klein, G., et al.: J. Exp. Med. **129**:697, 1969.
189. Burkitt, D.P.: J. Natl. Cancer Inst. **42**:19, 1969.
190. Carlstrom, G.: Acta Paediatr. Scand. **54**:17, 1965.
191. Duvall, C.P., et al.: Ann. Intern. Med. **64**:531, 1966.
192. Cox, H.R.: Am. J. Clin. Pathol. **57**:794, 1972.
193. Laboratory methods for the detection of rabies, course 8260-C, Atlanta, 1972, Centers for Disease Control.
194. Siegel, M., and Greenberg, M.: Am. J. Obstet. Gynecol. **77**:620, 1959.
195. Siegel, M., Fuerst, H.T., and Peress, N.S.: Am. J. Obstet. Gynecol. **96**:247, 1966.
196. Baylor Rubella Study Group: Hosp. Pract. **2**:27, 1967.
197. Meyer, H.M., Parkman, P.D., and Hopps, H.E.: Am. J. Clin. Pathol. **57**:803, 1972.
198. Auletta, A.E., et al.: Appl. Environ. Microbiol. **16**:691, 1968.
199. Grayston, J.T., and Wang, S.P.: J. Infect. Dis. **132**:87-105, 1975.
200. Wentworth, B.B., and Alexander, M.: Appl. Environ. Microbiol. **27**:912-916, 1974.
201. Zuckerman, A.J.: Br. Med. J. **7**:84, 1979.
202. Zuckerman, A.J.: J. Med. Virol. **3**:1-8, 1978.
203. Bradley, D.W., et al.: J. Clin. Microbiol. **5**:521, 1977.
204. Sherlock, S.: Am. J. Med. Technol. **38**:333, 1972.
205. Blumberg, B.S.: Am. J. Med. Technol. **38**:321, 1972.
206. Koff, R.S.: Viral hepatitis, New York, 1978, John Wiley & Sons, Inc.
206a. Ladd, D.J.: In Sonnenwirth, A.C., and Jarett, L., editors: Gradwohl's clinical laboratory methods and diagnosis, ed. 8, St. Louis, 1980, The C.V. Mosby Co.
207. Gutstein, M.: J. Pathol. **45**:313, 1937.
208. Hayflick, L.: Ann. N.Y. Acad. Sci. **143**:5, 1967.
209. Symposium on mycoplasma, January 1967, Pathological Society of Great Britain and Ireland.
210. Editorial: Br. Med. J. **5477**:1499, 1965.
211. Smith, T.F.: Virology laboratory procedure manual, Rochester, Minn., 1978, Mayo Foundation.
212. Allen, V. Sueltman, S., and Lawson, C.: Health Lab. Sci. **4**:90, 1967.
212a. Joseph, J.M.: In Sonnenwirth, A.C., and Jarett, L., editors: Gradwohl's clinical laboratory methods and diagnosis, ed. 8, St. Louis, 1980, The C.V. Mosby Co.
213. Clyde, W.A., Jr.: Immunology **92**:958, 1964.
214. Chanock, R.M.: N. Engl. J. Med. **273**:1199, 1965.

MYCOLOGY

CLASSIFICATION OF PATHOGENIC FUNGI

The identification of fungi is based primarily on the observation of gross colonial characteristics, e.g., color, size, texture, and rate of growth. Microscopic examination of morphologic characteristics, e.g., the visualization of conidia, is essential. Some fungi, e.g., yeasts, may be identified on the basis of their biochemical activity. Clinical mycology must determine whether a fungus exists as a yeast exclusively, as a mold, or as both as a function of environmental conditions.

There are four main groups of fungi distinguished by the mode of reproduction, sexual or asexual: Zygomycetes, Ascomycetes, Basidiomycetes, and Deuteromycetes. No sexual reproductive cycle has yet been discovered for Deuteromycetes (imperfect fungi).

A simplified classification scheme based on that presented by Lennette et al.* follows:

Kingdom Myceteae (fungi)
Division Amastigomycota
Subdivision Zygomycotina (division Zygomycota)
Class Zygomycetes
  Order Mucorales
  1. Representative genera: *Rhizopus, Mucor, Absidia, Cunninghamella, Saksenaea*
  2. Human disease: opportunistic pathogens in patients having diabetes, leukemia, severe burns, or malnutrition
  Order Entomophthorales
  1. Representative genera: *Basidiobolus, Conidiobolus*
  2. Human disease: cause subcutaneous zygomycosis and rhinoenteromophthoromycosis
Subdivision Ascomycotina (Division Ascomycota)
Class Ascomycetes
  Subclass Hemiascomycetidae
  1. Representative genera: *Saccharomyces, Pichia*
  2. Human disease: very rare; important in baking and brewing industries; some *Candida* species related to this
  Subclass Plectomycetidae
  Order Onygenales
  Family Gymnoascaceae
  1. Representative genera: *Arthroderma*, perfect state of *Trichophyton, Nannizzia*, perfect state of *Microsporum; Ajellomyces*, perfect state of *Blastomyces; Emmonsiella*, perfect state of *Histoplasma*
  2. Human disease: perfect states of important human pathogens
  Order Eurotiales
  Family Eurotiaceae
  1. Representative genera: perfect states of some human pathogenic *Aspergillus* and *Penicillium* species
  2. Human disease: perfect states of some human pathogenic *Aspergillus* species
Subdivision Basidiomycotina (division Basidiomycota)
Class Basidiomycetes
  Subclass Holobasidiomycetidae
  Order Agaricales
  1. Representative genera: *Amanita* (poisonous) and *Agaricus* (edible)
  2. Human disease: poisonous and edible mushrooms
  Subclass Teliomycetidae
  Order Ustilagenales
  Family Ustilagenaceae
  1. Representative genus: *Filobasidiella*, perfect state of *Cryptococcus*

---

*From Cooper, B.H.: In Lennette, E.H., et al.: Manual of clinical microbiology, ed.3, Washington, D.C., 1980, American Society for Microbiology. Modified from Alexopoulos, C.J., and Mims, C.W.: Introductory mycology, ed. 3, New York, 1979, John Wiley & Sons, Inc.

2. Human disease: *Cryptococcus neoformans* (important human pathogen)
Subdivision Deuteromycotina (division Deuteromycota)
Class Deuteromycetes
  Subclass Blastomycetidae: imperfect yeasts
    1. Representative genera: *Candida, Cryptococcus*
    2. Human disease: imperfect forms of human pathogenic yeasts
  Subclass Hyphomycetidae
    Family Moniliaceae
      1. Representative genera: *Epidermophyton, Cocidioides, Sporothrix, Paracoccidioides*
      2. Human disease: imperfect forms of major human pathogens
    Family Dematiaceae
      1. Representative genera: *Phialophora, Fonsecaea, Exophiala, Wangiella, Cladosporium;* molds with darkly pigmented hyphae
      2. Human disease: fungi cause chromomycosis, phaeohyphomycosis, tinea nigra, and mycetoma

STRUCTURE AND REPRODUCTION[1-5]

Fungi are nonphotosynthetic microorganisms that lack chlorophyll, feed on organic material, and possess nuclei, cytoplasm, a cell membrane, and often a capsule. The cytoplasm may contain pigment and is usually rich in glycogen, which is stained histochemically by some of the fungal stains.

The cell walls of fungi, unlike bacteria, contain polysaccharides such as mannan, glucan, chitin, and cellulose. On gross inspection some fungi are pigmented. Pigments may be cell associated or diffusible.

Capsules are found external to the cell wall in some fungi, e.g., cryptococci. Fungi are mucopolysaccharides and will stain readily with PAS or mucicarmine.

Fungi reproduce by spores that are formed sexually or asexually. When the spore germinates, it enlarges and sends out a tubelike projection, the **germ tube.** The germ tube elongates into filamentous structures that eventually branch. The branching tubelike structures are called **hyphae** (Fig. 33-1). If they are divided by cross walls, they are **septate hyphae.** If the septa are absent, they are **nonseptate hyphae.** The terminal growing cell of a hypha is often swollen and refractive and does not branch.

On artificial culture media the fungi form colonies that consist of masses of hyphae collectively called a **mycelium.** The part of the mycelium that penetrates the culture medium is the **vegetative mycelium,** which absorbs nutrients. The part that projects above the surface of the medium is the **reproductive mycelium.** The aerial mycelium produces specialized branches, **conidiophores,** on which **conidia (asexual spores)** are produced (Fig. 33-2). In some fungi the hyphae break up into separate cells, the **arthrospores** (Fig. 33-2). When spores are formed without previous fusion of nuclei, they are called **asexual spores.** If nuclear fusion precedes spore formation, the spores are **sexual spores.**

Not all spores produce germ tubes and hyphae; some produce cells like the mother cell, e.g., **buds** or **blastospores.**

IMPERFECT FUNGI

Many fungi of medical importance are called imperfect fungi or Deuteromycetes, because sexual reproduc-

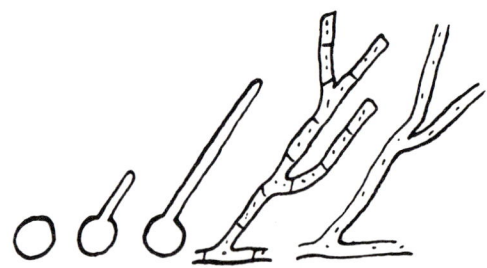

Fig. 33-1. Fungal spore gives rise to germ tube that elongates into hyphae (one septate and the other nonseptate). (From Moss, E.S., and McQuown, A.L.: Atlas of medical mycology, Baltimore, 1969, The Williams & Wilkins Co.)

tion is not observed (Figs. 33-3 and 33-4). The organisms can be distinguished morphologically as yeasts or as dimorphic fungi.

Yeasts: Some yeasts (e.g., *Cryptococcus*) reproduce by budding and give rise to asexual blastospores, which leave the mother cell and form daughter cells. No mycelium is formed under any environmental conditions. Other yeasts, e.g., *Candida albicans,* produce yeastlike surface colonies at 20° C and 35° C and reproduce by budding but also undergo exvaginations of the cell wall (germ tubes or pseudohyphae) (Fig. 33-3).

Dimorphic fungi: Dimorphic fungi (e.g., *Blastomyces*) form yeastlike colonies at 35° C and a septate mycelium and spores at 20° C (Fig. 33-3). In clinical material, however, only yeasts are observed.

NOMENCLATURE OF SPORES
Sexual spores

Sexually formed spores are oospores, zygospores, ascospores, and basidiospores (Figs. 33-2 and 33-5 to 33-8).

Oospores: Oospores are the result of the fertilization of the female sex structure by a male nucleus or sperm, forming a thick-walled body.

Zygospores: Zygospores are the result of the union of the tips of special copulation branches that fuse to form a thick-walled body, a **zygote.**

Ascospores: Ascospores result from the fusion of two special ascus-forming hyphae. The ascus (sac) contains eight ascospores.

Basidiospores: Basidiospores are exogenous sexual spores, usually four in number, resting on a club-shaped structure called a basidium.

Asexual spores

Asexual spores are divided into thallospores and conidiospores. (A thallus is a septate mycelium.)

Thallospores (Figs. 33-2 and 33-4)

Blastospores: Blastospores are asexual spores that arise by budding from yeast, e.g., *Cryptococcus* species and *Candida* species.

Chlamydospores: Chlamydospores (*Candida albicans*) are thick-walled asexual spores that arise from hyphae and are usually intercalary (between septa of hyphae), but they may be terminal (end of hypha) or

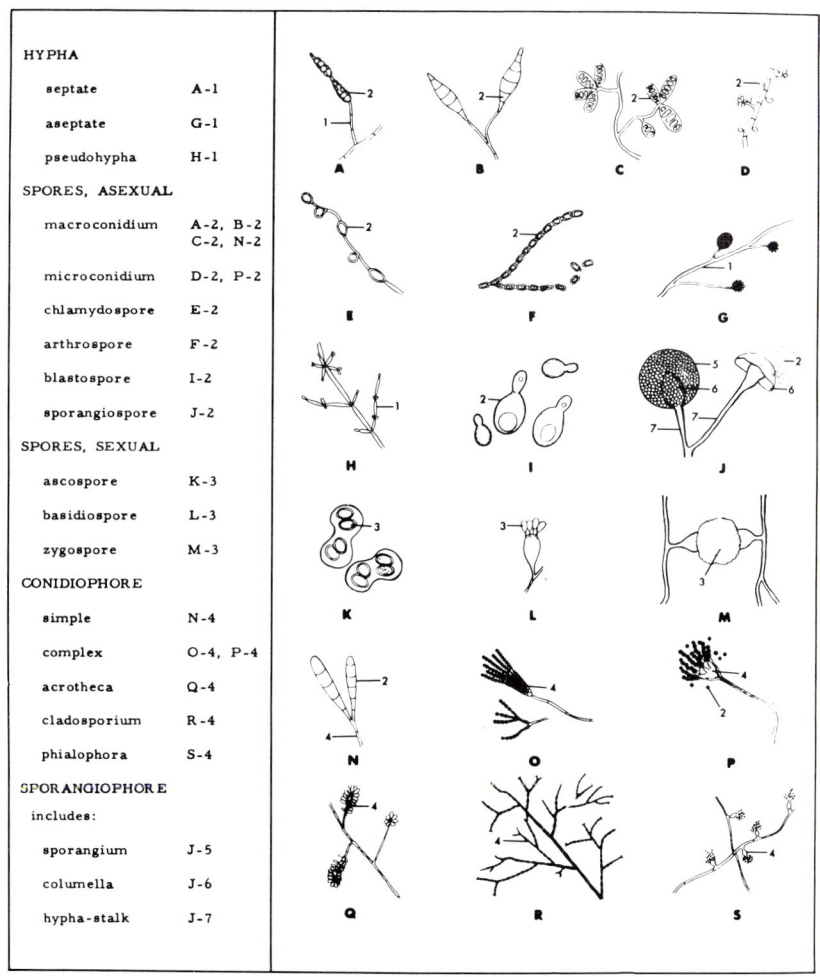

Fig. 33-2. Schematic microscopic morphologic findings of fungal components. (From Laboratory procedures in clinical mycology, Technical manual TM8-227-8, Washington, D.C., 1964, U.S. Department of the Army.)

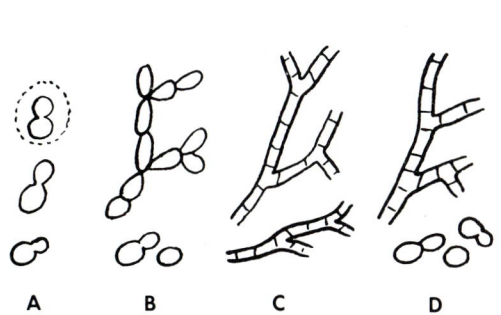

Fig. 33-3. Reproduction of imperfect fungi, true yeasts, and yeastlike fungi. **A,** Blastospores (*Cryptococcus* species). **B,** Pseudohyphae (*Candida* species). **C,** Septate hyphae (*Tricho-phyton* species). **D,** Dimorphism (*Blastomyces* species), yeast phase and mold phase. (From Moss, E.S., and McQuown, A.L.: Atlas of medical mycology, Baltimore, 1969, The Williams & Wilkins Co.)

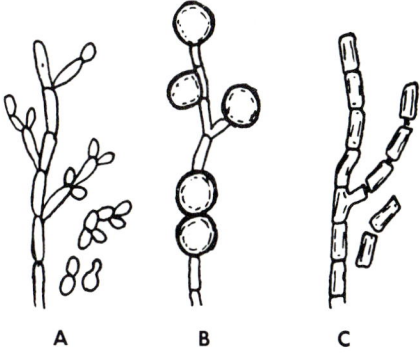

Fig. 33-4. Reproduction of imperfect fungi, spores formed by septate mycelium (thallospores). **A,** Blastospores (*Cryptococcus* species and *Candida* species) formed at swollen end of a hypha. **B,** Chlamydospores (*Candida albicans*), thicker walled spore developed from a hypha. **C,** Arthrospores (*Geotrichum* species) resulting from fragmentation of a hypha. (From Moss, E.S., and McQuown, A.L.: Atlas of medical mycology, Baltimore, 1969, The Williams & Wilkins Co.)

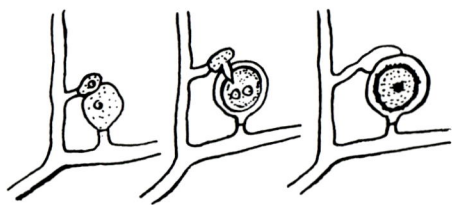

Fig. 33-5. Formation of oospore. (From Moss, E.S., and McQuown, A.L.: Atlas of medical mycology, Baltimore, 1969, The Williams & Wilkins Co.)

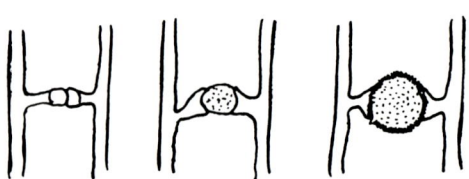

Fig. 33-6. Formation of zygospore. (From Moss, E.S., and McQuown, A.L.: Atlas of medical mycology, Baltimore, 1969, The Williams & Wilkins Co.)

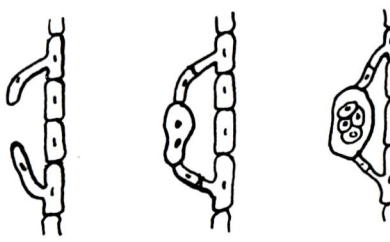

Fig. 33-7. Formation of ascospores. (From Moss, E.S., and McQuown, A.L.: Atlas of medical mycology, Baltimore, 1969, The Williams & Wilkins Co.)

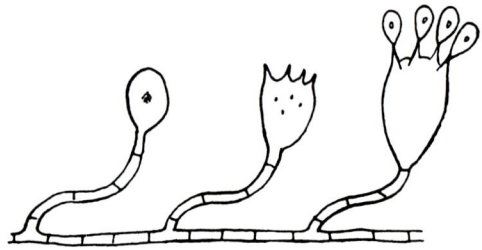

Fig. 33-8. Formation of basidiospores. (From Moss, E.S., and McQuown, A.L.: Atlas of medical mycology, Baltimore, 1969, The Williams & Wilkins Co.)

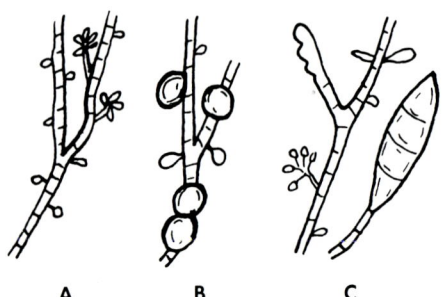

Fig. 33-9. Types of conidiospores. **A,** Microconidia. **B,** Sessile conidia. **C,** Macroconidia. (From Moss, E.S., and McQuown, A.L.: Atlas of medical mycology, Baltimore, 1969, The Williams & Wilkins Co.)

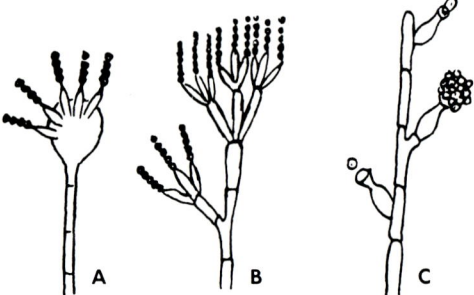

Fig. 33-10. Types of conidiospores of imperfect fungi. **A,** *Aspergillus* species. **B,** *Penicillium* species. **C,** *Hormodendrum* species. (From Moss, E.S., and McQuown, A.L.: Atlas of medical mycology, Baltimore, 1969, The Williams & Wilkins Co.)

lateral (attached to side of hypha). They are the result of physicochemical factors of the culture medium.

Arthrospores: Arthrospores result from fragmentation of a hypha into thick-walled rectangular or ovoid spores (e.g., *Geotrichum* species).

Conidiospores (conidia) (Figs. 33-2 and 33-9)

Conidiospores are terminal spores attached to specialized hyphae, **conidiophores.** They are pinched off from the tip of the conidiophore. The spores vary in size, shape, number of septa, etc.

Microconidia: Microconidia are small single-celled spores that vary in shape from round to ovoid to pyriform and may be arranged in chains or clusters or singly attached to the side of the hypha.

Macroconidia: Macroconidia are large multicellular conidia.

• • •

Conidiophores and conidia may assume shapes that are characteristic for certain fungi. Characteristic conidiophores are produced by *Aspergillus* species, which are typified by a swollen end of the conidiophore called a **vesicle.** From it arise flask-shaped ''sterigmata,'' which give rise to chains of spores (Fig. 33-10, *A*, and 33-41). *Penicillium* has sterigmata and chains of spores, but the vesicle is replaced by branches (Fig. 33-42).

In *Hormodendrum* species the conidiophores produce buds, which in turn give rise to additional buds that fail to leave the parent organism (Fig. 33-10, *C*).

IDENTIFICATION OF FUNGI

The identification of fungi is based on direct examination of wet material, staining (usually not necessary), culture, animal inoculation, serologic methods, and biochemical studies.

Collection of specimens

Every effort should be made to collect specimens for fungus examination as free from bacterial contamination as possible. It requires less time to collect a specimen properly than to identify contaminants.

Hair: The scalp should be examined under ultraviolet light (Wood's light) in a dark room, since certain dermatophytes *(Microsporum audouini, M. canis, M. ferrugineum,* and *M. distortum)* produce yellow-green fluorescence of infected hair. Under normal lighting, infected hairs have a twisted appearance, often break off easily, and may fall out. Infected or suspicious hairs should be epilated with sterile forceps and collected in a sterile Petri dish. Both the hair shaft and the hair root should be obtained.

Most **tinea capitis** infections *(Trichophyton* species and *Microsporum gypseum),* black *(Piedraia hortae)* and white *(Trichosporon beigelii)* piedra, do not cause fluorescence of the involved hair; thus it is essential that nonfluorescing hair also be examined and cultured if a fungus is suspected clinically.

Skin: The skin lesion should be cleansed with 70% alcohol and sterile water. Using a sterile scalpel, obtain scrapings from several sites of the spreading edge of the lesion. Collect scrapings in a sterile Petri dish. Skin infected with *Malassezia furfur* (tinea versicolor) **fluoresces** under ultraviolet light. The fluorescing areas should be scraped and examined (see also discussion of cellophane tape preparation).

Nails: After cleaning the nail with 70% alcohol the nail surface should be scraped with a sterile scalpel. The most superficial shavings are discarded. The deeper shavings are collected in a sterile Petri dish. If necessary, obtain small nail clippings with sterile scissors.

Pus: Pus should be obtained before the abscesses rupture. The surface of the fluctuant abscess is cleansed with 70% alcohol, povidone-iodine, and sterile water. By aseptic technic, pus is collected with a sterile needle and syringe before the incision is made. From draining sinuses collect as much pus as possible by aspirating with a sterile pipet after cleansing the sinus opening with 70% alcohol, povidone-iodine, and sterile water. Gentle pressure or massage over the sinus tract (when not contraindicated) may be helpful. Segments of the sinus tract may have to be removed surgically, ground, and then cultured. When only a small amount of pus can be obtained, it should be left in the pipet and delivered to the laboratory promptly. More material is needed for mycologic examination than for bacteriologic examination. The use of cotton swabs for specimens is seldom satisfactory.

Sputum: Fresh specimens of sputum should be collected after the patient has brushed his teeth and rinsed his mouth thoroughly. The specimen should be collected directly in a sterile container equipped with a tight-fitting lid. Aerosol technics may also be employed to obtain bronchial secretions.

Urine: Urine collected by the midstream, clean-catch method is satisfactory.

Cerebrospinal fluid: Cerebrospinal fluid (CSF) should be centrifuged at $3000 \times g$ for 15 min and the sediment used for microscopic examination and culture. The supernatant may still be used for the detection of *Cryptococcus* capsular polysaccharide.

Blood: The utility of blood culture for all but a few of the pathogenic yeasts is questionable. Most fungi of clinical significance will eventually grow in commercially available aerated blood culture media. The provision of an agar surface within the broth media (biphasic culture) will often speed up fungal growth and enable visualization of colonial morphologic characteristics within 3 or 4 days. Membrane filtration procedures have been used for fungal isolation from blood. They consist of rupturing the cellular components of blood and then filtration of the liquid phase. The filter is then placed on an agar plate such as brain-heart infusion (BHI), which supports growth of the organism, and incubated. Advantages include (1) the ability to remove the fungus from cellular components and antibiotics and (2) concentration of the organisms probably present in small numbers. Disadvantages include the likelihood of contamination caused by excessive manipulation.

Concentration of sputum for fungus culture

Sputum specimens often are processed for both mycobacteria and systemic fungi. In general the same concentration methods should not be used for both organisms, because the fungi may not survive mycobacterial digestion. One method of sputum concentration is described.

Pancreatin method: The method suggested by Sanford[6] is as follows. Mix a fresh early morning specimen with equal parts of a 1% pancreatin solution in phosphate buffer, pH 7.5. Shake well and incubate at 35° C for 1-1½ hr or until liquefied, shaking occasionally. Centrifuge the liquefied specimen at 3000 rpm for 20 min and decant the supernatant. Mix the small amount of sediment (0.1-0.2 ml) well and use for inoculation of culture plates and for direct microscopy.

4% Sodium hydroxide concentration method: See p. 872.

METHODS OF EXAMINATION

Ultraviolet examination of hair and skin: The fluorescence of hair infected with *Microsporum audouini, M. canis,* or *M. distortum* has already been mentioned. Skin infected with *Malassezia furfur* also fluoresces. *Trichophyton*- infected hairs usually do not fluoresce, but a dull whitish glow may occur with *T. tonsurans.* In some instances *T. schoenleini* may fluoresce a bright yellow-green.

Wet preparations and mounting fluids:
Potassium hydroxide wet mounts:

Principle: Potassium hydroxide (KOH) acts as a clearing agent, and by suppressing debris, potassium hydroxide allows fungal elements to become more prominent.

Specimen: Segments of hairs and scrapings of skin and nails.

Reagent: Dissolve 10 g potassium hydroxide in distilled water to make 1 dl.

Procedure: Place 1 drop of 10% KOH in the center of a clean glass slide. Wet the teasing needle in KOH. Pick up material with needle, using several pieces of material if available. Tease material into a thin preparation. Mount the cover glass over the material and gently heat the preparation by passing it through a Bunsen burner flame two or three times. Spread material by gently pressing with the butt end of the teasing needle on the cover glass. Let it stand for 5 min, and, if material is not flat, press again.

If the preparation is not clear, allow it to stand for 15 min and then examine it. It may be necessary to wait two or three hours for nail scrapings to soften sufficiently to spread them out for microscopic examination.

Results: Fungal elements appear as clear hyaline structures. Examine the preparation microscopically under low power and confirm the observation by using the high-power objective (Fig. 33-13).

KOH preparation of hair: Examine for hyphae and spores. In *Microsporum* infections the small spores tend to be arranged in a sheath surrounding the hair shaft, producing a mosaic-like pattern or **ectothrix** (Fig. 33-11) type of involvement. The large-spore type *(T. verrucosum)* produces large (3-5 μm) arthrospores; the small-spore type *(T. mentagrophytes)* produces arthrospores that are 2-3 μm. *T. rubrum* also produces an ectothrix pattern.

In most *Trichophyton* infections the arthrospores tend to be arranged in chains within the substance of the hair, producing parallel rows of arthrospores in the inside and no recognizable growth on the outside. This is an **endothrix** pattern of involvement (Table 33-1 and Fig. 33-12).

In **piedra** infections, white or black nodules are located along the hair shaft.

KOH preparation of skin: Examine for mycelial elements and spores. Most hyphae are septate, have a uniform diameter, and form straight or wavy lines (Figs. 33-13 to 33-15).

Artifacts: Cotton fibers, cellulose fibers, cholesterol deposits, and debris may be mistaken for hyphae (Figs. 33-16 and 33-17). Do not confuse elastic tissue fibers, which are not segmented, and cotton fibers, which are irregular and flat, with fungal hyphae.

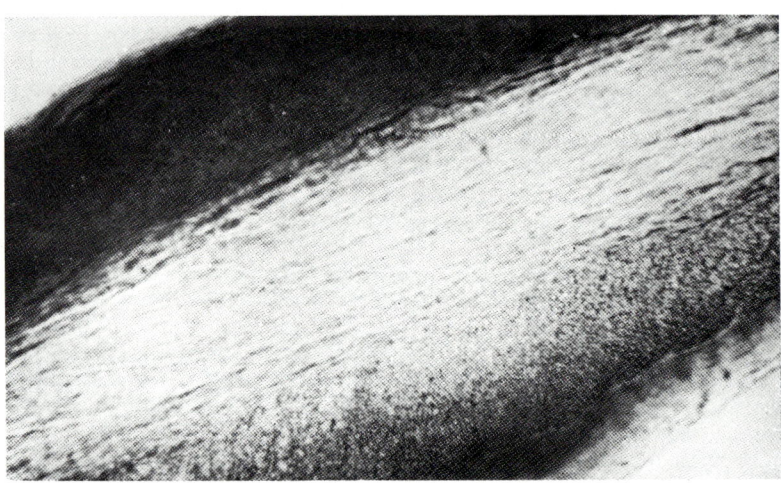

Fig. 33-11. Hair infected with *Microsporum audouini.* Arthrospores are in outer portion of hair along both sides (ectothrix pattern). (Courtesy McNeil Laboratories, Inc., Fort Washington, Pa.)

Table 33-1. Type of hair involvement by dermatophytes

Ectothrix	Endothrix
Microsporum audouini	*Trichophyton violaceum*
Microsporum canis	*Trichophyton tonsurans*
Microsporum gypseum	*Trichophyton schoenleini*
Trichophyton mentagrophytes	
Trichophyton rubrum	

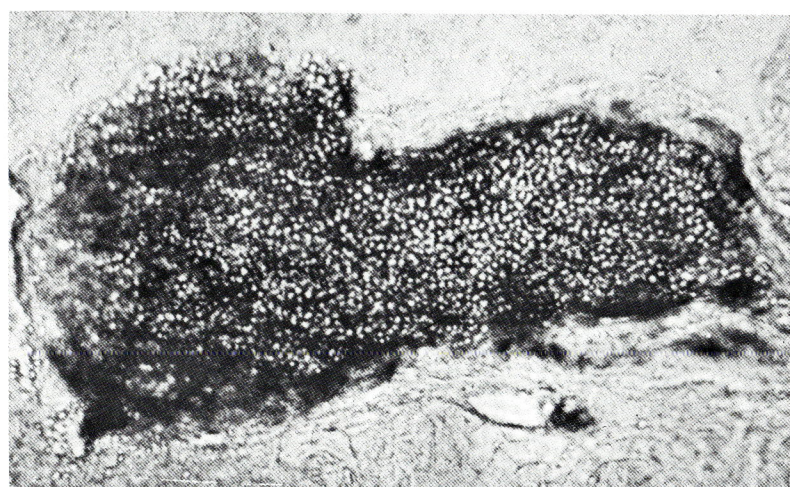

Fig. 33-12. Hair stump infected with *Trichophyton tonsurans*. Arthrospores are within substance of hair (endothrix pattern). (Courtesy McNeil Laboratories, Inc., Fort Washington, Pa.)

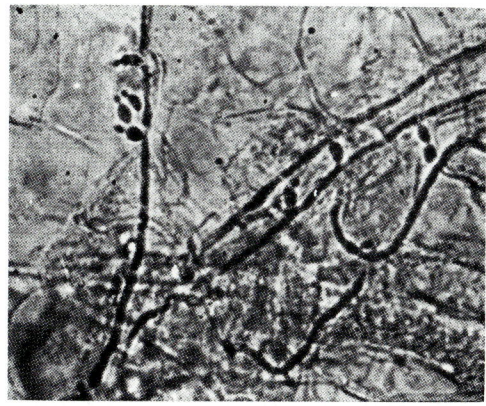

Fig. 33-13. Hyphae and budding cells of *Candida albicans* in epidermal scale. (Courtesy McNeil Laboratories, Inc., Fort Washington, Pa.)

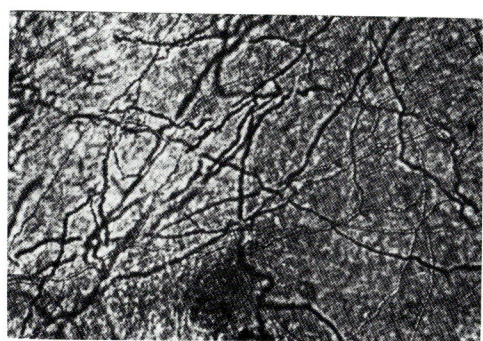

Fig. 33-14. Young hyphae of *Trichophyton* in epidermal scale. They appear as dark or light lines, depending on whether they are sharply in focus. (Courtesy McNeil Laboratories, Inc., Fort Washington, Pa.)

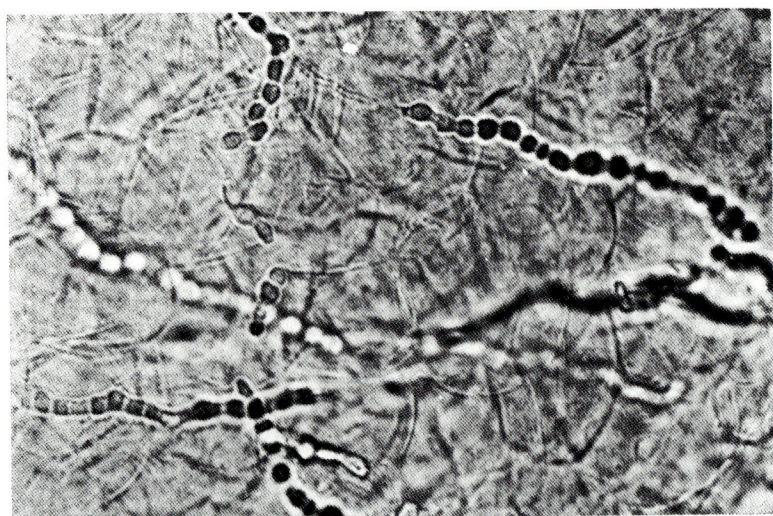

Fig. 33-15. Old hyphae of *Trichophyton* in epidermal scale, broken up into chains of arthrospores. (Courtesy McNeil Laboratories, Inc., Fort Washington, Pa.)

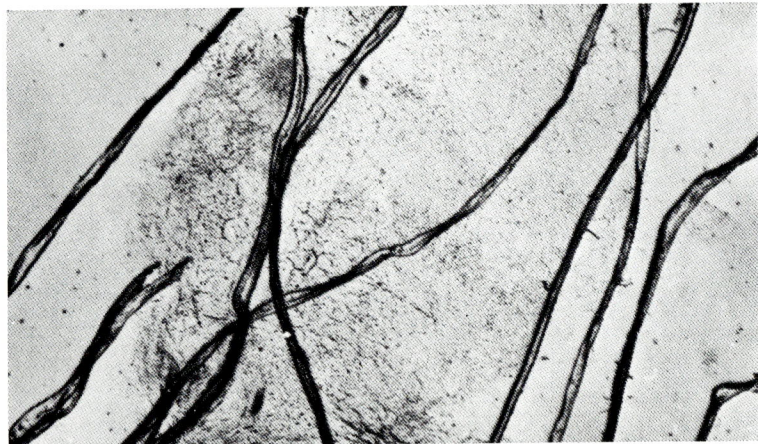

Fig. 33-16. Cotton fibers in potassium hydroxide. (Courtesy McNeil Laboratories, Inc., Fort Washington, Pa.)

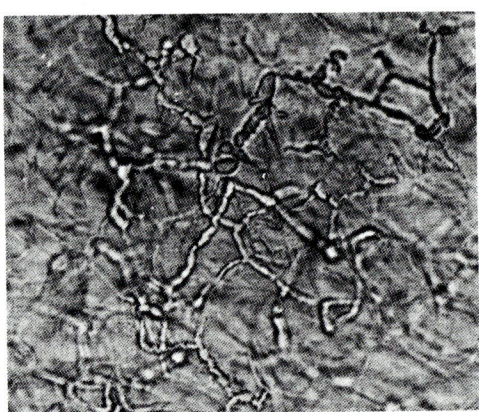

Fig. 33-17. Mosaic artifact showing deposits of cholesterol and debris among epithelial cells. It is differentiated from fungal hyphae by (1) arrangement in spaces between cells, (2) abrupt changes in diameter, (3) tapering and indefinite terminations, and (4) characteristic reentrant angles at points of abrupt change in width.

Lactophenol cotton blue preparation:

Principle: Lactic acid preserves fungal structures that are killed by phenol and stained by cotton blue.

Reagent: The reagent consists of 20 g phenol crystals (melted in water bath and then weighed), 20 g lactic acid, 40 g glycerin, 0.05 g cotton blue (Poirrier blue), and 20 ml distilled water.

Procedure: Clean microscope slide with silicone-coated paper and add a few drops of lactophenol cotton blue. Add a small drop of 95% alcohol separately. With a rigid, sterile inoculating needle, remove a segment of aerial mycelium, dip it quickly into the alcohol drop, and transfer to the mounting fluid. Tease the segment apart by using two needles, apply cover glass, and examine under the low- and high-power objectives of the microscope with reduced illumination or lowered condenser. The preparation may be sealed with nail polish.

Results: Fungal elements appear pale to dark blue.

India ink preparation (capsule stain):

Principle: India ink fails to stain fungal or bacterial cells or their capsule and results in a black background.

Reagent: The reagent consists of 15 ml india ink, 30 ml aqueous (1:1000) thimerosal (Merthiolate), and 0.1 ml aqueous (1:1000) Tween 80. Filter before use.

Procedure: Place two 3 mm loopfuls of india ink in the center of a clean glass slide. Mix a small amount of the yeast culture that has been picked up on a 22-gauge Nichrome wire in the ink drop. Place a clean cover glass over the preparation, taking care to prevent air bubbles from being trapped.

If the preparation is too dark, a new preparation must be made by adding 1 loopful of sterile distilled water to the ink before adding the specimen.

Results: *Cryptococcus neoformans* appears as a clear disk against a black background. The faintly visible unstained cell is surrounded by a wide, clear, capsular space (Fig. 33-18).

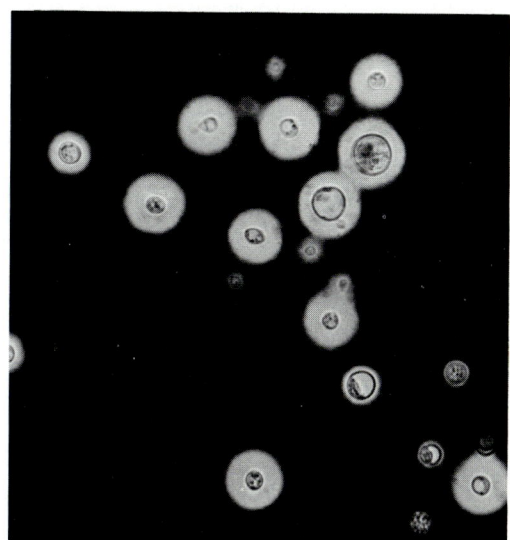

Fig. 33-18. *Cryptococcus neoformans*. (India ink preparation; culture.)

Although the india ink stain for capsules of *Cryptococcus neoformans* is a valuable identification tool, commercial latex agglutination kits are now available for the detection of soluble capsular polysaccharide in cerebrospinal fluid and serum. Controls must be employed, because rheumatoid factor cross-reacts with antibody to cryptococcal antigen.

Wet mounts in water:

Procedure: With a sterile 3 mm loop, place 1 drop of water on a clean slide. Touch the center of the suspected yeast colony with a sterile 22-gauge Nichrome inoculating wire and make a light suspension of the yeast in the water. Mount with a 22 mm cover glass and examine microscopically.

Results: The thin aqueous preparation permits examination of the cells for size, shape, and purity as well as for the presence of ascospores.

Parker's superchrome blue-black ink preparation:

Principle: This mixture serves as a staining as well as a clearing solution.[7, 8]

Reagent: The reagent consists of equal parts of blue-black ink and 20% potassium hydroxide.

Stains: Staining of fungal elements is usually not necessary. The methods described above using lactophenol cotton blue and superchrome blue-black ink as well as methylene blue may be used.

Methylene blue stain:

Reagent: The reagent consists of 2.5% methylene blue and 95% alcohol.

Other stains that should be available are Wright-Giemsa stain for **intracellular** forms of **fungi** (e.g., *Histoplasma capsulatum*, some forms of *Penicillium*, and *Torulopsis glabrata*), PAS stain, and acid-fast stain for acid-fast bacteria (e.g., *Nocardia*).

Culture of fungi

The purpose of culture media is to support the growth of medically important fungi and to suppress the accompanying bacterial flora and saprophytic contaminating fungi.

Occasionally what are thought to be contaminants may be the etiologic or co-etiologic agent or agents, because under certain circumstances (diabetes, suppression of normal immune mechanisms by corticosteriods and other drugs, lymphoproliferative disorders, etc.) opportunistic fungi are pathogenic.

Several media should be inoculated with clinical material. The type of medium used will somewhat depend on the specimen and on the degree of bacterial contamination.

Media for primary isolation

All media are commercially available as a powder or in prepared form.*

Sabouraud dextrose agar: Sabouraud dextrose agar is a dextrose peptone medium that supports the growth of most fungi pathogenic to humans. Its acid pH (6.5) retards the growth of most bacterial contaminants.

Emmons-Sabouraud dextrose agar is a modifica-

*Supplement literature, Detroit, 1972, Difco Laboratories; BBL manual of products and laboratory procedures. Cockeysville, Md., 1968, BioQuest Div., Becton-Dickinson & Co.

tion of the original Sabouraud formula that reduces the dextrose content from 4-2% and raises the pH from 6.5-7.0. The higher pH and the lower sugar content are better for the growth of some fungi. If bacterial suppression is desired, antibiotics are added.

Sabouraud dextrose agar with antibiotics: If the specimen is contaminated (sputum, pus, stool, exudates, etc.), antibiotics such as cycloheximide (0.5 mg/ml) and chloramphenicol (0.04 mg/ml) or penicillin (20 μm/ml) and streptomycin (40 mg/ml) should be incorporated in the medium. Antibiotic-containing Sabouraud dextrose agar is commercially available as Mycosel agar (BBL, BioQuest Div., Becton-Dickinson & Co., Cockeysville, Md.) and Mycobiotic agar (Difco Laboratories, Detroit).

Cycloheximide suppresses the growth of many bacteria and of saprophytic fungi but also of *Allescheria (Petriellidium) boydii, Aspergillus fumigatus, Cryptococcus neoformans, Torulopsis, Trichosporon cutaneum, Rhizopus* species, *Mucor* species, and some species of *Candida* (*C. krusei* and *C. tropicalis;* not *C. albicans*). It also inhibits the growth of the yeast phase of dimorphic fungi incubated at 35° C. Media containing cycloheximide are therefore incubated at room temperature only.

Chloramphenicol inhibits *Nocardia* and other actinomycetes as well as other bacteria.

Sabouraud dextrose agar with antibiotics may be used exclusively in the isolation of dermatophytes, since none of them are sensitive to the antibiotics. In the isolation of systemic fungi it must be used in parallel with media not containing antibiotics.

Littman oxgall agar: Bacteria are inhibited by the crystal violet and bile contained in Littman medium. Streptomycin may also be added. The medium is superior to Sabouraud dextrose agar for isolating fungi in mixed infections. Since fungal colonies tend to remain small and do not spread, they are easier to subculture.

Plates should be inoculated in duplicate, one incubated at 22° C and the other at 35° C; the plate with antibiotic should be incubated at 22° C only.

Brain-heart infusion agar with or without antibiotics and with or without sheep blood: Brain-heart infusion agar (BHI) is a good medium for systemic fungi because of its higher nutrient content. Incubate at room temperature only if antibiotic activity is desired.

Special media: Most special media stimulate **sporulation,** since they suppress vegetative growth because of their low nutrient content.

Potato dextrose agar: Potato dextrose agar contains dextrose and potato infusion. It is used for slide culture of yeasts and fungi; it stimulates spore production and thus aids in the study of sporulation.

Cornmeal agar plus 1% Tween 80: Cornmeal agar plus 1% Tween 80 consists of an infusion of cornmeal and aids in the differentiation and the identification of yeasts, mainly *Candida albicans.* Tween 80 stimulates chlamydospore formation.

Rice agar plus 1% Tween 80: Rice agar plus 1% Tween 80 aids in the differentiation and identification of yeasts, mainly *Candida albicans.* It consists of an infusion of rice dried on agar. Tween 80 enhances the formation of chlamydospores.

Yeast extract agar: Yeast extract agar is used to stimulate spore production, especially of macroconidia of *Trichophyton,* and to study morphologic characteristics and carbon and nitrogen assimilation of yeasts.

Inoculation of media: Inoculate 4-6 slants (do not use plates) using a straight 22-gauge Nichrome wire, the terminal 1 cm of which has been flattened. Pick up a small amount of material to be cultured and make two or three deep cuts into the surface of the medium. Incubate half the tubes at 22° C (room temperature) and half at 30-35° C. Apply screw caps loosely. Examine cultures every 24 hr for young colonies. Subculture colonies if they are in danger of being contaminated. Examine colony microscopically as soon as sporulation begins and again a few days later.

Since the colonies are often tough and embedded in agar, transfer of colonies is accomplished by using a sterile thin spatula to cut out a square block containing the colony. The block is then inverted and either simply placed on the new agar surface or held with sterile forceps and used to "streak" the plate.

Method of inoculation of special media: Pick up a small amount of the suspected colony with the tip of a 22-gauge inoculating needle (sterile). Make three parallel slits in the surface of the agar plate. With an inoculating loop, streak across the three slits. Flame an alcohol-dipped cover glass and, after it has cooled, place it over the center area of the inoculated slits. Include a positive control, e.g., a known chlamydospore-producing colony of *Candida albicans.*

Incubate the plates at 22-25° C. Read plates at 24, 48, and 72 hr. Remove the top of the Petri dish and observe microscopically the growth under and around the cover glass.

Results: Chlamydospores are thick-walled spores, variable in size, that develop from hyphae (not on conidiophores) and are often intercalary. Almost all fungi parasitic to humans form chlamydospores. If the medium contains crystal violet, the chlamydospores take up the dye (Figs. 33-24 and 33-27).

Slide culture (Fig. 33-19)

Purpose: The culture of fungi on glass slides in a moist chamber allows observation of the undisturbed relationship between the reproductive and vegetative mycelia.

Procedure: Place a slide on a bent glass rod in the bottom of a Petri dish. Cover and sterilize. Prepare Sabouraud dextrose agar plates with about 15 ml agar per plate. Permit to solidify. Use agar blocks about 1 cm square and 2-3 mm deep.

Using sterile technic, place block of agar on slide in Petri dish. Inoculate centers of four sides of agar block with fungus to be studied. Cover inoculated block with sterile cover glass. With sterile technic, add 8 ml sterile water to bottom of Petri dish. Incubate at 25° C until sporulation occurs.

When spores appear, carefully lift off cover glass and lay aside, with fungus growth upward. Lift agar square from slide and discard. Place 1 drop of lactophenol cotton blue on this slide and cover with a clean cover glass. Obtain clean slide, place 1 drop of lactophenol cotton blue near one end, and cover with origi-

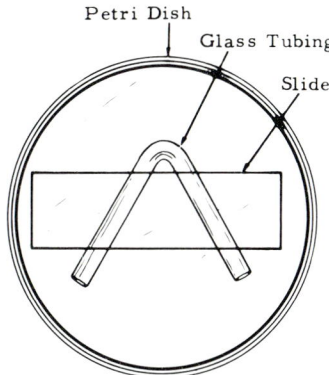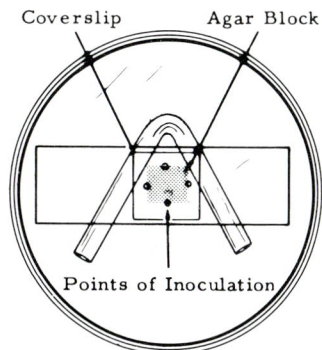

Fig. 33-19. Slide culture technic (four points of inoculation). (From Laboratory procedures in clinical mycology, Technical manual TM8-227-8, Washington, D.C., 1964, U.S. Department of the Army.)

nal cover glass, placing mycelial surface down. Blot away excess mounting fluid from cover glasses of the two preparations. When dry, seal edges with nail polish.

Animal inoculation[9]

Purpose: Animal inoculation is done to evaluate pathogenicity and to study the tissue phase of fungi. The skin of guinea pigs, white mice, and rabbits can be infected with dermatophytes. *Histoplasma, Cryptococcus,* and *Coccidiodes* are pathogenic to mice. Guinea pigs and mice can be infected with *Nocardia* and *Blastomyces*. Care must be taken with these fungi, and animal inoculation should be reserved for reference laboratories.

Fluorescent antibody technic

The fluorescent antibody method has many advantages over conventional methods. The technic is more rapid, the organisms do not need to be viable and are easily spotted even if there are only a few, and the morphologic characteristics of the fluorescent cell can be appreciated.

Fluorescent methods have been used for the identification of *Cryptococcus neoformans, Candida albicans, Sporothrix schenkii, Histoplasma capsulatum,* and *Blastomyces dermatitidis;* however, they are not widely used.

Histopathologic procedures

Tissue slides made from surgical and autopsy specimens and from experimentally injected animals are stained with hematoxylin-eosin stain, MacCallum-Goodpasture stain, periodic acid–Schiff stain (PAS), mucicarmine stain, Gomori methenamine silver nitrate stain, and Gridley stain. The Schneidan modification of the Gram stain[10] and the Alcian blue stain may also be used.

Serologic tests[11]

The following tests are employed in the diagnosis of coccidioidomycosis, histoplasmosis, and cryptococcosis: complement fixation, tube precipitin, immunodiffusion, latex particle agglutination, and fluorescent antibody (FA) inhibition. Cross-reactions, skin tests,

and weak reactions sometimes make these tests difficult to interpret. Two serum samples should be obtained, one in the first few days **(acute serum)** of the disease and one 2-3 weeks later **(convalescent serum).** A fourfold or greater rise in the titer followed by a fall is usually diagnostic.

MONOMORPHIC PATHOGENIC YEASTS

Monomorphic pathogenic yeasts grow in the yeast phase at room temperature (22° C) and at 37° C (although some species fail to grow at 37° C). The fungi in this group are *Candida* species, *Cryptococcus* species, *Geotrichum* species, *Trichosporon* species, *Torulopsis* species, and *Rhodotorula*. Recent evidence suggests that *Torulopsis glabrata* is similar, if not identical, to *Candida*.[12]

Differential diagnosis

The differential diagnosis[13-15] is based on the following tests:
1. Direct examination (potassium hydroxide or 10% sodium hydroxide wet mounts)
2. Capsule detection (india ink preparation, latex agglutination)
3. Germ tube test
4. Culture and chlamydospore formation
5. Urease test
6. Temperature tolerance test
7. Utilization of carbohydrates
   a. Carbon assimilation test
   b. Oxidation-fermentation (O-F) medium
   c. Fermentation test
8. Nitrate assimilation test

Germ tube test:

Principle: The germ tube test is a screening procedure for *Candida albicans* and *C. stellatoidea*. A germ tube, or pseudohypha, is a nonseptate tubular process produced by a germinating spore, which if allowed to grow becomes a hypha (Fig. 33-1).

Reagent: Serum.

Procedure: Add a yeast cell colony to 0.5 ml serum in a 10 × 75 mm test tube. Incubate at 37° C for 2-4 hr. Transfer 1 drop of culture onto a microscope slide and examine with a high-dry lens under subdued light for germ tubes.

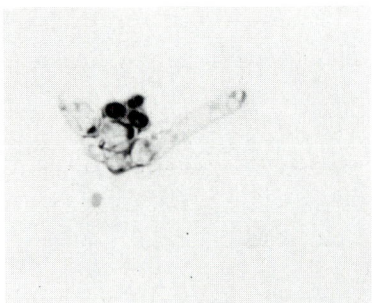

Fig. 33-20. *Candida albicans* producing single germ tube.

Results: *C. albicans* and *C. stellatoidea* form germ tubes within 2-4 hr (Fig. 33-20). These two *Candida* species are easily separated on the basis of sucrose assimilation and sensitivity to cycloheximide.

Urease test:
Procedure: Inoculate the slant of Christensen urea agar with material from the top of a yeast colony. Incubate at 25-30° C for 5 days. Examine daily. *Cryptococcus, Rhodotorula*, some species of *Candida*, and *Trichosporon* are urease positive. *Cryptococcus* is urease positive in 24 hr.

Temperature tolerance test:
Procedure: Inoculate two Sabouraud dextrose agar slants. Incubate one at 35° C and the other at room temperature for 24-72 hr. Pathogenic *Cryptococcus neoformans* grows at 37° C, whereas saprophytic strains of *Cryptococcus* do not grow at 37° C.

Utilization of carbohydrates:
Carbon assimilation test (Wickerham method)[16-18]:
Principle: Various carbohydrates are added to vitamin-enriched yeast broth to study the assimilation of carbon by various yeasts.

Media:
1. A dilute, "starved" fungal suspension is prepared by transferring growth from a 24-48 hr Sabouraud dextrose agar culture into 5 ml sterile distilled water. Use a 2 mm sterile loop to accomplish the transfer.
2. Stock yeast nitrogen base–carbohydrate mixture. Combine 6.7 g yeast nitrogen base for carbon assimilation tests (Difco Laboratories, Detroit) and 5.0 g carbohydrate (e.g., dextrose or other) in distilled water to make 1 dl. Sterilize this 10× strength medium by filtration and keep in refrigerator.
3. Working solution of yeast nitrogen base–carbohydrate mixture
   Combine 0.5 ml stock yeast nitrogen base–carbohydrate mixture and 4.5 ml sterile distilled water.

Procedure: Set up one tube (16 × 150 mm) for each carbohydrate: dextrose, maltose, sucrose, lactose, galactose, melibiose, cellobiose, inositol, xylose, raffinose, trehalose, and dulcitol. Stopper tubes with cotton. Add 0.1 ml dilute yeast inoculum to each tube. Incubate at 22° C and examine for growth after 48 hr and after 6 and 20 days.

Results: Growth clouds the tubes, and the degree of turbidity is read against a white card that shows three india ink lines, each 0.75 mm wide. This "Wickerham card" is similar to the card used in the dithionite (solubility) test for Hb S.

Method of recording:

Growth in tube obliterates lines	3+
Growth in tube renders lines indistinct	2+
Growth in tube just allows recognition of lines	1+

The density of the fungal suspension used for the inoculation of the yeast nitrogen base should read ±.

The test is considered to be more critical than the oxidation-fermentation test, the results of which vary somewhat with the inoculum, the temperature, and the purity of the carbohydrate. Table 33-2 gives some of the characteristics of yeast isolates.

Controls: Both positive *(C. albicans)* and negative *(C. tropicalis)* controls should be used for every assay.

Fermentation reactions:
Procedure: Add filter-sterilized carbohydrates to each medium tube to a final concentration of 1%. The same 12 carbohydrates that are used in the Wickerham assimilation test should be used in the fermentation test. Inoculate the medium with a yeast culture by using a straight wire.

Interpretation: Acid production in the medium produces a bright yellow color. Weak acid production is responsible for hues of orange to yellow. The uninoculated medium is orange-red. Incubate the medium at 25° C for 10 days. Most patterns of carbohydrate utilization are complete in 5 days.

Fermentation test: The inoculum used for the assimilation test is also used for the fermentation test. Table 33-2 gives some of the characteristics of yeast isolates.

Medium: To make the basal fermentation broth, combine 0.55% yeast extract, 0.75% peptone, and 1 ml of 1.6% bromcresol purple (aqueous solution) in distilled water to make 1 L. Dispense fermentation base into 16 × 125 mm screw-capped test tubes that contain Durham tubes for gas collection. Sterilize by autoclaving.

Procedure: Carbohydrates to be tested for fermentation are glucose, lactose, galactose, maltose, sucrose, and trehalose in a concentration of 6% and raffinose in a concentration of 12%.

Sterilize the carbohydrates separately by filtration and add 2 ml aseptically to each broth tube. Inoculate each tube with 0.1-0.2 ml yeast suspension (see discussion of carbon assimilation test). Incubate at 25° C and read at 48-72 hr intervals over a period of 14 days.

Results: Oxidative fermentation produces minimal acid (yellow) or acid and gas. The latter collects in the inverted Durham tube.

Nitrate (KNO₃) assimilation test (Wickerham tube broth method):
Media:
1. Stock broth solution
   Combine 11.20 g yeast carbon base and 0.78 g KNO₃ in distilled water to make 1 dl. Sterilize by filtration.
2. Working broth solution
   Add 0.5 ml stock broth (sterile) to 4.5 ml sterile water (final pH 5.6).

Procedure: Add 0.1 ml inoculum (see discussion of

Table 33-2. Characteristics of *Candida* species*

	Assimilation of:												Fermentation of:						Other				
	Dextrose	Maltose	Sucrose	Lactose	Galactose	Melibiose	Cellobiose	Inositol	Xylose	Raffinose	Trehalose	Dulcitol	Dextrose	Maltose	Sucrose	Lactose	Galactose	Trehalose	Urease	KNO₃	Pseudo-hyphae	Growth at 37°C	Germ tubes
C. albicans	+	+	+	-	+	-	-	-	+	-	+	-	AG	AG	A†	-	AG or A†	AG or A†	-	-	+	+	+
C. stellatoidea	+	+	-	-	+	-	-	-	+	-	+	-	AG	AG	-	-	A†	-	-	-	+	+	+
C. parapsilosis	+	+	+	-	+	-	-	-	+	-	+	-	AG or A	A†	A†	-	AG or A	AG or A†	-	-	+	+	-
C. tropicalis	+	+	+	-	+	-	+	-	+	-	+	-	AG	AG	AG	-	AG	AG	-	-	+	+	-
C. pseudotropicalis	+	-	+	-	+	-	+	-	+	+	-	-	AG	-	AG	AG	AG	AG or A†	-	-	+	+	-
C. krusei	+	-	-	-	-	-	-	-	-	-	-	-	AG	-	-	-	-	-	+†	-	+	+	-
C. guilliermondii	+	+	+	-	+	+	+	-	+	+	+	+	AG	-	AG or A†	-	AG	AG or A†	-	-	+	+	-
C. rugosa	+	-	-	-	+	-	-	-	+	-	-	-	-	-	-	-	A†	-	-	-	+	-	-
C. pseudotropicalis	+	-	+	+	+	-	+	-	+	+	-	-	A	-	A	A	A	-	-	-	+	+‡	-

Modified from Webb, C.D., Papageorge, C., and Hall, C.T.: Identification of yeasts, Atlanta, 1973, Centers for Disease Control.
*+ = Assimilation, growth density greater than 1 + turbidity (see text) or on O-F medium; AG = acid and gas: A = acid only: – = negative.
†Strain variation.
‡Growth at 40-42° C.

carbon assimilation test) to each tube. Incubate at 25°
C for 7 days. When growth is obtained in KNO_3 tube,
subculture this tube to a second KNO_3 assimilation tube
and observe for growth for 7 days.

Results: If growth is obtained in the second KNO_3
tube, the organism can assimilate KNO_3. If there is no
growth or only 1+ growth (see Wickerham chart), the
test is negative.

Controls:

Nitrate positive	*Candida utilis*
Nitrate negative	*Candida pseudotropicalis*

Yeast identification systems

Several yeast identification systems are available.
These systems or kits make yeast identification convenient for laboratories that are requested to identify yeast
isolates. The API 20C (Analytab Products Inc. [API],
Plainview, N.Y.) is a paper strip containing a number
of cupules that provide both fermentation and assimilation determinations. The Uni-Yeast-Tec (Corning
Glass Works, Corning, N.Y.) is a plastic dish with 12
wells that contain various substrates. Both systems are
accurate and time saving when compared to conventional tube methods.

YEASTS
Candida

Candida is responsible for acute and chronic superficial infections (thrush, paronychia, and vulvovaginitis
[susceptibility increased by use of birth control pills])
and for a disseminated mycosis (endocarditis and candidiasis) in patients whose immune mechanisms are impaired or who have been receiving extensive antibiotic
therapy for a period of time. Under these circumstances
Candida septicemia is about half as common as septicemia resulting from gram-negative organisms.

Laboratory diagnosis

Specimen: Scrapings of skin, mucosal surfaces, sputum, pus, urine, blood, cerebrospinal fluid, and vaginal
and cervical secretions are used. Since *Candida* species
are commonly found in sputum and in the mouth, isolation from a single specimen and in small and moderate numbers may or may not be of etiologic significance. The sputum must be fresh (do not allow to stand
for any length of time), and the mouth and teeth must
be cleaned before the sputum specimen is obtained.
Candida species must be cultured repeatedly to be etiologically significant, and cultures from multiple sites
are more reliable for the diagnosis of candidiasis.

The laboratory diagnosis of *Candida* species is based
on the tests enumerated in Table 33-2.

Smear and wet preparation: Hyphae and oval, budding, yeastlike cells can be seen in skin and nails. In
stool, urine, etc. the oval budding cells predominate.
The hyphae are characteristically constricted at the
level of the septa (Figs. 33-13 and 33-21).

The approximate number of organisms per field
should be included in the report, since finding only a
few organisms may lack clinical significance. On the
basis of the wet preparation the organisms can be reported as *Candida* species.

Culture: The organisms grow well on most media at
room temperature and at 35° C. Most grow in the pres-

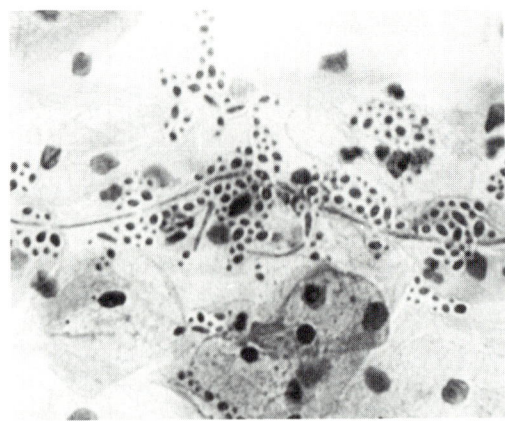

Fig. 33-21. *Candida* species in cervical smear. (Papanicolaou
technic.)

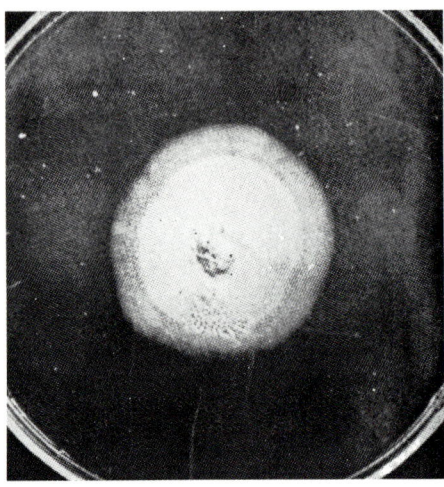

Fig. 33-22. *Candida albicans.* Colony 5 weeks old showing
pasty appearance with honeycombed edge. (From Dobes,
W.L.: South. Med. J. **36:**614, 1943.)

ence of chloramphenicol and cycloheximide, a characteristic that can be used effectively for isolation of the
yeast from contaminated specimens, but strains of *C.
krusei, C. parapsilosis, C. tropicalis,* and *C. stellatoidea* are inhibited by cycloheximide.

Inoculate two sets of Sabouraud dextrose agar with
and without antibiotics and one set of Sabouraud dextrose broth. Incubate one set at 22° C and one at 30-35°
C. Examine every 24 hr for fungus colonies, which
may grow at either temperature.

Soft, white to tan, smooth colonies will appear on
both plates (Fig. 33-22), and microscopic examination
will reveal thin-walled budding cells accompanied by
mycelia and **pseudomycelia** in the deeper and peripheral portions of the colony. The term *pseudomycelium*
is applied to a tubular cell (germ tube or pseudohypha)
originating from a blastospore that elongates and remains in contact with the mother cell (Fig. 33-1). The
term *blastospore* connotes a spore produced by a budding process along the mycelium (Fig. 33-3, *A*).

Suppression of contaminants: If the solid media

are too contaminated to isolate the fungi, inoculate the yeast-bacteria mixture from the solid medium into four tubes of Sabouraud dextrose broth to which 1, 2, 3, and 4 drops of 1N hydrochloric acid have been added to suppress bacterial growth. Incubate the four tubes at room temperature for 24 hr, after which time one of the tubes should be relatively free of bacterial contamination.

Differential diagnosis

The finding of yeast cells in cultures incubated at room temperature and at 35° C is suggestive of any one of the following species of fungi: *Candida, Cryptococcus, Geotrichum, Torulopsis, Rhodotorula,* and *Trichosporon.*

If the culture is pure, the differential diagnosis may be made on the basis of a wet preparation, although biochemical differentiation is preferable.

Candida species give rise to budding cells, with pseudomycelia and mycelia penetrating the deeper portions of the agar. If *Candida* is suggested by the morphologic characteristics, transfer a segment of culture to **cornmeal** or **chlamydospore agar.**

Cryptococcus fails to produce a mycelium and can be differentiated from *Candida* species and from true yeast by the single-budding cells surrounded by a wide capsule (india ink preparation).

If a mycelium is present, the yeast may be either *Geotrichum* or *Trichosporon.*

Geotrichum species give rise to septate hyphae and rectangular arthrospores.

Torulopsis is a pure budding yeast that does not produce hyphae or pseudohyphae.

Trichosporon produces arthrospores as well as blastospores.

Rhodotorula has a characteristic carotenoid pigment.

Production of chlamydospores: Chlamydospores are formed terminally on enlarged hyphae and are thick-walled macroconidia, 8-12 μm in diameter (Fig. 33-23).

For technic of inoculation of chlamydospore agar, see p. 920. Incubate plates at room temperature for 7 days and examine daily for chlamydospores. Chlamydospores and pseudohyphae of *C. albicans* may be seen in 24-48 hr.

All species of *Candida* have mycelia with blastospores, the name given to budding spores (Fig. 33-24). *C. albicans* blastospores occur in large ball-like groups at the junction of the mycelial segments, distinguishing it from other species except *C. stellatoidea,* which can be distinguished by star-shaped colonies on blood agar. The blastospores of *C. tropicalis* are irregularly distributed, occurring both between and at the joints, whereas those of *C. parakrusei* and *C. krusei* appear chiefly at the joints. The blastospores of *C. krusei* are arranged in characteristic whorls. *C. albicans,* in addition to mycelia and blastospores, also shows chlamydospores.

Temperature tolerance test: *Candida* species retain the yeast form at 22° and 35° C.

Biochemical findings: For results of carbon assimilation, fermentation, and nitrate assimilation tests, see Table 33-2.

Animal inoculation: Only *C. albicans* is lethal to rabbits; death occurs within 1 week after intravenous

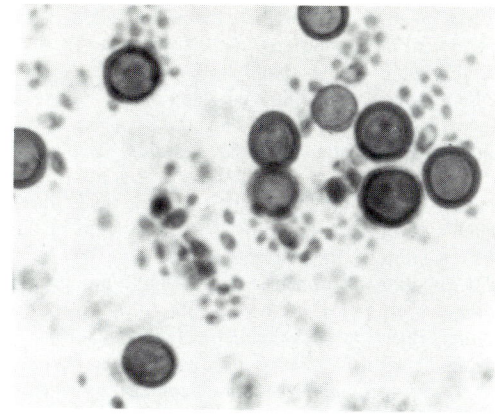

Fig. 33-23. Chlamydospores of *Candida albicans* accompanied by masses of spores.

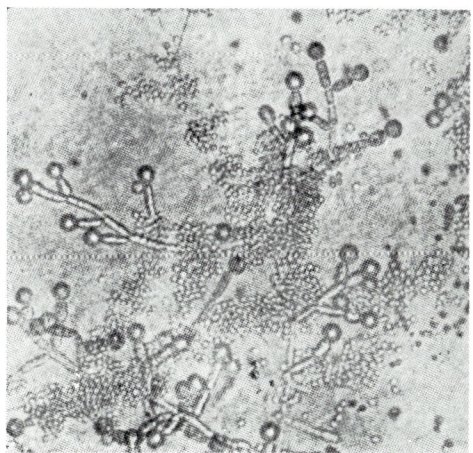

Fig. 33-24. *Candida albicans* showing mycelium and characteristic masses of spores and terminal chlamydospores. (From Dobes, W.L.: South. Med. J. **36:**614, 1943.)

inoculation of 1 ml of a 1% suspension of the organisms in sterile saline solution.

Histopathologic findings: In tissue preparations *Candida* produces mainly mycelia, which are difficult to see in sections stained with hematoxylin-eosin but can be visualized well with PAS stain.

Cryptococcus neoformans

Infection resulting from the yeast *Cryptococcus neoformans* is known as cryptococcosis. Although it is sometimes called European blastomycosis, it is not an infection caused by *Blastomyces.* Since the organism has a tendency to invade the central nervous system, one of the common clinical manifestations is cryptococcal meningitis.

Laboratory diagnosis[19, 20]

Material: Respiratory secretions, spinal fluid, urine, blood, and serous exudates.

Smear and wet preparation: In 10% potassium hydroxide, unicellular, large budding yeast cells are seen, and no mycelia are formed. **India ink** preparations show a well-developed capsule. The addition of 0.1% **toluidine blue** to the spinal fluid differentiates pink-staining cryptococcal cells from deep blue-staining leukocytes. Red cells remain unstained.

Stained smears are not of much value, because the nucleus is gram positive, and the capsule is not stained. **Wright stain** colors the organism deep blue; thus it resembles lymphocytes. (This should be remembered when examining spinal fluid sediments.)

The organism is a spheric fungus that reproduces by budding at any point of the wall. The buds break off at varying stages of development; thus organisms of varying diameter (4-20 μm) are found in the specimen. The cell is surrounded by a wide mucopolysaccharide capsule and may produce occasional short hyphae.

Culture: Large amounts of the original specimen (5 ml spinal fluid, 20 ml pleural fluid, etc.) may have to be concentrated by centrifugation or ultrafiltration to yield positive findings in early cases of cryptococcosis.

Blood agar: In 2-10 days, mucoid, yeastlike, white to cream colonies grow at 35° C and at room temperature after 3-4 days.

Temperature tolerance test: The ability to grow at 35° C differentiates pathogenic from nonpathogenic forms of *Cryptococcus,* because saprophytic strains usually grow at room temperature only.

BHI agar: The organism may require an enriched medium, and therefore BHI agar should be included among the media used. *C. neoformans* is sensitive to **cycloheximide;** isolation should not be attempted on media containing this antibiotic.

Differential diagnosis

C. neoformans must be differentiated from other yeastlike fungi that grow at 35° C and at room temperature. *C. neoformans* does not produce mycelia on cornmeal agar, but *Candida* species do (see discussion of identification of *C. albicans*). Septate hyphae and barrel-shaped spores differentiate *Geotrichum.*

Birdseed agar: *Cryptococcus neoformans* produces a reddish brown pigment on birdseed agar. The agar is inoculated heavily with the test organism and incubated at 37° C. *C. neoformans* will produce pigment within 1 week. The caffeic acid medium of Hopfer[21] is a more rapid test, with pigmentation being developed by *C. neoformans* after as early as 6 hr.

Urease test: For principle and chemical reaction see p. 922.

Touch top of fungal colony to be tested with sterile loop and inoculate slant surface of Christensen urease agar. Incubate slant at room temperature for 5 days and examine daily for pink color. *Cryptococcus* will produce a positive reaction in 24 hr. Some *Candida* species and *Rhodotorula* are also urease positive, but it takes longer than 24 hr for the color to develop.

Biochemical findings: The results of typical carbon and nitrate assimilation tests and of the fermentation tests are seen in Table 33-3. The table also shows the distinguishing criteria of pathogenic *C. neoformans* and of saprophytic cryptococci.

Animal inoculation: *C. neoformans* is pathogenic to mice, whereas saprophytic cryptococci are not. Mice injected intravenously with a 2-day-old culture of *C.*

Table 33-3. Characteristic reaction of *Cryptococcus neoformans* and of a saprophytic strain*

	Assimilation of:												Fermentation of:						Other						
	Dextrose	Maltose	Sucrose	Lactose	Galactose	Melibiose	Cellobiose	Inositol	Xylose	Raffinose	Trehalose	Dulcitol	Dextrose	Maltose	Sucrose	Lactose	Galactose	Trehalose	Urease	KNO₃	Pseudohyphae	Growth at 37° C	Germ tubes	India ink capsule	Mouse toxicity
C. neoformans	+	+	+	-	+†	-	+	+	+	+†	+	+	A	A†	A†	-	-†	A†	+	-	R	+†	-	+	+
Saprophytic strain	+	+	+	-	-	-	-	+	+	+	+	-	A	A	A	-	-	-	+	-	-	-	-	+	-

Based on data from Webb, C.D., Papageorge, C., and Hall, C.T.: Identification of yeasts, Atlanta, 1973, Centers for Disease Control.
* + = Positive; R = occasional to rare hyphae; — = negative; A = acid only produced in fermentation broth.
†Strain variation in assimilation.

neoformans develop cryptococcosis. The animal inoculation procedure is seldom indicated.

Serologic identification: A slide latex agglutination kit for the detection of cryptococcal antigen is commercially available. Other serologic methods that allow identification of antigen or detection of antibodies in the patient's serum are available, e.g., the fluorescent antibody technic and the hemagglutination test.[22]

Histopathologic findings[23,24]: *Cryptococcus* is the only yeastlike fungus in which the capsule contains acidic polysaccharides. The capsule may be overlooked in sections stained with hematoxylin-eosin and may stain poorly with PAS. The capsules of cryptococci stain metachromatically with toluidine blue and are colored by mucicarmine, colloidal iron, and Alcian blue. The latter two are the more sensitive methods.

Geotrichum candidum

Geotrichum candidum is a yeast that reproduces by **arthrospores.** It is saprophytic but may cause an infection of the mouth and of the respiratory and gastrointestinal tracts called geotrichosis.

Laboratory diagnosis

Specimen: Sputum, feces, and scrapings of oral mucosa are used. The organism is common in soil, on tomatoes and fruits, and in milk. Because the fungus is so widespread in nature, it must be grown repeatedly from sputum or feces before it can be considered etiologically involved in the patient's condition.

Wet preparation: Oval, barrel-shaped to round cells are seen on smears in wet preparations in association with septate hyphae that break into rectangular arthrospores. In wet preparations *Geotrichum* can be differentiated from *Trichosporon* since the arthrospores of *Trichosporon* are spheric.

Culture: The organism grows readily at 22° C on Sabouraud dextrose agar with and without antibiotics. Most species do not grow at 37° C. The surface growth is white to gray and flat with spreading, undulated edges. The center of the colony develops aerial hyphae and a wrinkled appearance. Microscopic examination reveals that the mycelium consists of hyphae containing rectangular arthrospores that show little tendency to round up (Fig. 33-25).

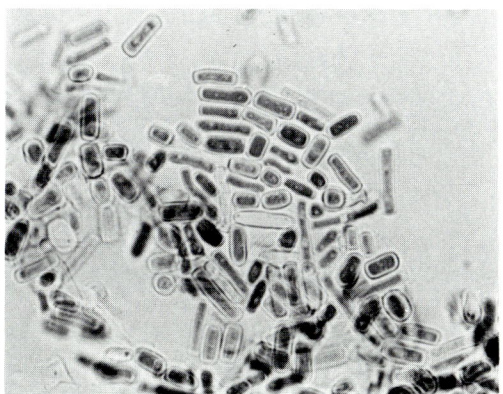

Fig. 33-25. *Geotrichum candidum.* Elongated arthrospores from Sabouraud dextrose agar.

Table 33-4. Characteristics of *Trichosporon biegelii* and *Geotrichum candidum**

	Assimilation of:												Fermentation of:						Other				
	Dextrose	Maltose	Sucrose	Lactose	Galactose	Melibiose	Cellobiose	Inositol	Xylose	Raffinose	Trehalose	Dulcitol	Dextrose	Maltose	Sucrose	Lactose	Galactose	Trehalose	Urease	KNO₃	Pseudohyphae	Growth at 37° C	Growth in malt extract broth‡
T. biegelii	+	++	++	+	+	++	+	++	+	++	++	++	A or −	A or −	A or −	A or −	A or −	A or −	++	−	+	++	Pellicle or ring blastospores
G. candidum	+	−	−	−	+	−	−	−	+	−	−	−	−	−	−	−	−	−	−	−	−	−	Pellicle or white islets

* + = Assimilation, growth density greater than or equal to 1 + turbidity by the Wickerham card method. O-F, and oxidative production of acid; A = acid production with no gas in fermentation broth; − = negative reaction.
† BBL, BioQuest Div., Becton-Dickinson & Co., Cockeysville, Md.
‡ Strain variation.

Biochemical findings: For results of assimilation and fermentation tests see Table 33-4.

Trichosporon biegelii

Trichosporon produces soft, white mycelial nodules on hair shafts (scalp, axilla, groin, or beard [piedra]). The fungus not only produces nodules outside the hair but also grows within the hair shaft, causing the hair to be brittle and to break easily.

Laboratory diagnosis

Specimen: Hair.

Wet preparation: A 10% potassium hydroxide preparation shows mycelia that form nodules loosely attached to the surface of the hair. The hyphae are seen to produce arthrospores and blastospores.

Culture: The organism grows readily on Sabouraud dextrose agar at 37° C, producing cream-colored yeast-like colonies that are smooth at first but soon become wrinkled. Many arthrospores and hyphae and some blastospores are seen microscopically.

Biochemical findings: For results of assimilation and fermentation tests see Table 33-4.

Torulopsis

Torulopsis (Candida) glabrata[25-27] is an important secondary parasitic yeast that causes pulmonary, renal, and cardiac infections in patients whose resistance is lowered by steroid and other immunosuppressive drugs. *T. glabrata* is also important, because it may mimic *Histoplasma capsulatum*, exhibiting at times intracytoplasmic location.

Laboratory diagnosis

Specimen: Urine, sputum, and blood.

Culture: On Sabouraud dextrose agar the organisms produce cream-colored, smooth, yeast-like colonies. Lactophenol blue preparation reveals budding, oval fungal cells, the bud originating at the pointed end of the yeast cell.

DIMORPHIC FUNGI

Dimorphic fungi are characterized by their ability to produce a yeast form when growing at 35° C or in vivo and a mycelial (mold) form when grown in culture at 22° C.

Histoplasma capsulatum

Histoplasma capsulatum is the causative organism of histoplasmosis, a disease that has a widespread, self-limiting asymptomatic pulmonary form, a rare systemic fatal form, and an equally rare chronic stage. The fungus may involve every organ of the body but is usually found in macrophages and in reticulum cells of organs of the reticuloendothelial system (liver, spleen, bone marrow, blood monocytes, and histiocytes).

H. capsulatum is a soil saprophyte that grows well in chicken and pigeon droppings deposited on the ground.

Laboratory diagnosis

Smear and touch preparations: In the systemic form, bone marrow smears, peripheral blood buffy coat films, and touch preparations of lymph nodes, spleen, and liver are searched for the tissue-yeast phase of the organism. In Wright-Giemsa–stained preparations the organism is found singly or in large numbers within macrophages and free, since some macrophages rupture. The individual yeast cell is a small, oval to pear-shaped structure measuring 2-4 μm in diameter. Budding occurs at the more pointed end of the cell, and the bud easily breaks off. The more rounded segment of the yeast cell contains a crescentic mass that is separated from the distinct cell wall by a clear space. The organisms resemble *Leishmania* but lack the kinetoplast. The organism is gram positive. Culture of the organism is necessary to differentiate it from *Blastomyces dermatitidis,* which may be intracellular (Fig. 33-26).

Specimen for culture: In the asymptomatic pulmonary form, sputum should be cultured, but since these patients are usually unable to produce sputum, aerosol technics may have to be used to obtain a specimen. Materials suitable for culture in the systemic form besides sputum are urine, pus, peripheral blood, bone marrow, and biopsy specimens of lymph node, spleen, liver, ulcer base, etc.

The clinical material should not be allowed to stand at room temperature for any length of time and should be cultured as soon as possible. The following media should be inoculated: BHI agar (or glucose-cystine-heart blood agar) with and without antibiotics (penicillin or chloramphenicol and streptomycin) and also Sabouraud dextrose agar with and without antibiotics. Neutral Emmons-Sabouraud dextrose agar is preferred.

Media: Inoculate two plates of BHI blood agar and two plates of Sabouraud agar without antibiotics and one plate each of BHI agar and Sabouraud dextrose agar with antibiotics. Incubate one set of plates at 35° C and one set at room temperature.

Although antibiotic-containing agar plates may be used for the isolation of systemic fungi, care must be taken, because some fungi and many bacteria are susceptible to the commonly used antimicrobial agents; e.g., *C. neoformans* is susceptible to cycloheximide, *H. capsulatum* and *Aspergillus* are inhibited by high doses of chloramphenicol, and *Nocardia* and *Actinomyces* are susceptible to penicillin.

H. capsulatum forms the mycelial phase at room temperature, whereas it grows in the yeast phase at 35° C.

Mycelial phase: After 10-14 days of incubation at 25° C (room temperature) on Sabouraud dextrose agar or on BHI agar, white, fluffy colonies with fine aerial mycelia form. As the culture ages, it acquires a tan color. The first spores that appear and can be seen on wet preparations are **microconidia,** which are round to pyriform, sessile or stalked structures measuring 2-3 μm in diameter. They are borne on lateral **conidiophores** arising at right angles from **septate hyphae.** Large **macroconidia** called **chlamydospores,** which are **tuberculated** and measure 8-25 μm in diameter, develop later (Fig. 33-27). The tuberculate appearance results from rounded projections attached to the surface of the macroconidia.

To obtain the characteristic chlamydospores it may

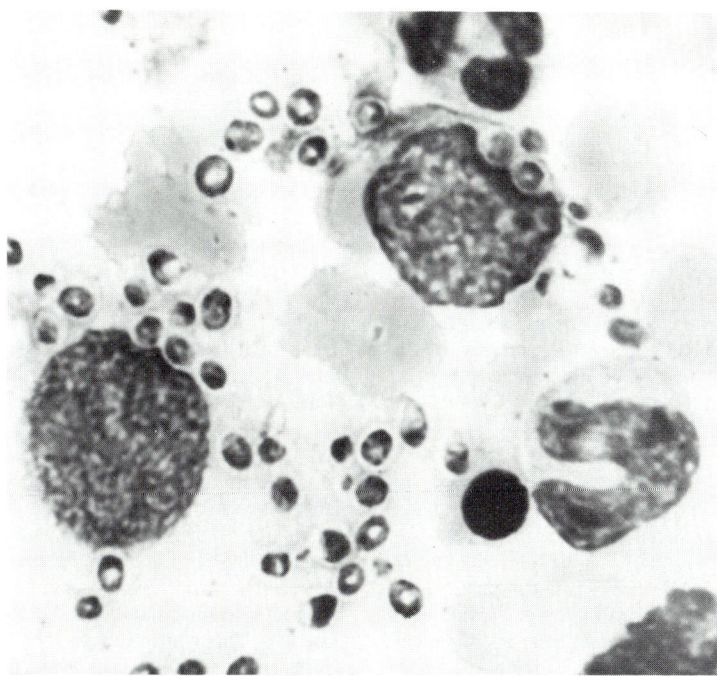

Fig. 33-26. *Histoplasma capsulatum* in bone marrow.

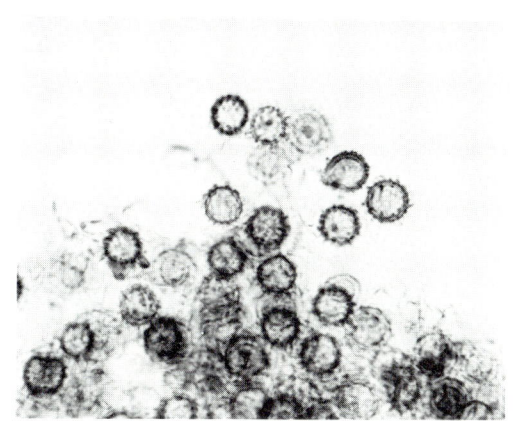

Fig. 33-27. Culture showing diagnostic tuberculate chlamy-dospores of *Histoplasma capsulatum.*

be necessary to transplant the culture to sporulation me-dia such as **chlamydospore** or **cornmeal agars.**

Yeast phase: The mycelial phase can be converted to the yeast phase by subculturing a colony to BHI agar and incubating it at 35° C. To avoid drying of the me-dium the Petri dishes should be sealed with Parafilm. After 2-3 days, small, white to cream-colored, moist, convex colonies will appear at the periphery of the original inoculum. Wet preparations will show small, oval, thin-walled yeast cells that exhibit budding and measure 2-4 μm. This is particularly important to dif-ferentiate *H. capsulatum* from the saprophytic fungus *Sepedonium.*

Tissue phase, animal inoculation, and histopath-ologic findings: The tissue phase is similar to the yeast phase.

*Procedure***:** The original clinical material or the cul-ture may be injected intraperitoneally into mice. Mix sputum, gastric washings, or ground tissue with equal parts of sterile saline solution until liquefied. Add 10,000 units of penicillin and 1000 units of streptomy-cin per milliliter of specimen. (If the specimen is not contaminated, this procedure is not necessary.) Inject 1 ml of the mixtures **intraperitoneally** into two or three mice. Kill the mice after 4 weeks and examine the spleen and liver, which contain the yeast phase. On slides stained with hematoxylin-eosin it is difficult to discover the unstained outlines of the organisms within the cytoplasm of macrophages. The PAS stain is not reliable for the detection of histoplasmosis. Other stains give better results, e.g., **Gomori methenamine silver stain** and **Gridley stain.**

Serologic identification: A **complement fixation test** with yeast-phase and tissue-phase antigens is avail-able. To be diagnostic the titer of the complement fix-ation test must be over 1:32 and should rise within a period of about 6 weeks. The titer may persist for sev-eral weeks or months and then fall rapidly, or it may remain elevated for as long as 1 year, even in the event of clinical recovery. Pulmonary cavitation is usually accompanied by a rise in titer, whereas in single pul-monary nodules the serologic methods are of no value.

Although a skin test for histoplasmosis is available, it is not a reliable diagnostic tool, because it does not differentiate between past and recent infection. A pos-itive histoplasmin skin test preceded by a documented negative result may be useful. When skin tests are used, multiple antigens should be used, since these fungi *(Histoplasma, Coccidioides,* and *Blastomyces)* share common antigens.

Newer serologic methods include the fluorescent antibody technic[28] and agar gel precipitin reaction[29] and are used in addition to such serologic tests as histoplasmin-latex agglutination[30] and histoplasmin-collodion agglutination.[31]

Blastomyces dermatitidis

North American blastomycosis, or **Gilchrist's disease,** is caused by *Blastomyces dermatitidis.* Blastomycosis is a granulomatous disease primarily of the lung that may also involve the skin and other organs in the disseminated form.

Laboratory diagnosis

Specimen: Pus, sputum, biopsy specimens of tissues, cerebrospinal fluid, body fluids, and scrapings from the periphery of cutaneous lesions.

Wet preparation: A 10% potassium hydroxide (KOH) preparation reveals thick-walled, spheric bodies, some of which will be seen budding. A wide neck connects the single bud to the parent cell. The organism measures 7-15 μm in diameter and is devoid of a capsule. The protoplasm of the fungus shows marked granulation that is best seen in the Wright-stained smear. It is pulled away from the cell wall, leaving a clear space between it and the capsule; it contains several nuclei. The single bud is thin walled, and its attachment area is as wide as its greatest diameter. The attachment of the bud to the parent cell is difficult to break; thus free buds are not plentiful. The picture of the KOH preparation of sputum is characteristic (Figs. 33-28 and 33-29).

Unstained wet preparations may be ringed with nail polish. After a few hours examine for **single germ tubes** (Fig. 33-20) originating from the spheroid cell bodies.

Blastomyces may vary in size; thus it may be difficult to distinguish them from *Histoplasma capsulatum.* One of the distinguishing features is that *H. capsulatum* has only one nucleus, whereas *Blastomyces* species have several. Cells without buds must be differentiated from *Coccidioides immitis,* which shows endosporulation.

Culture: The fungus is **biphasic;** there is a **yeast**

phase at 35° C, which is similar to the **tissue phase,** and a **mycelial phase** at room temperature.

Media: BHI blood agar and Sabouraud agar should be inoculated in duplicate; incubate one set at room temperature and one at 35° C. The cultures should be held for 4 weeks before being considered negative and must therefore be sealed with Parafilm to prevent drying.

On Sabouraud agar at room temperature the mycelial phase produces woolly colonies with white aerial hyphae and a central, small elevation, which later turns buff and brown. On microscopic examination the colonies reveal septate hyphae and round to pyriform, thick-walled microconidia, varying in size from 3-8 μm, borne on short lateral conidiophores.

On BHI blood agar at 35° C the yeast phase leads to wrinkled, waxy, gray to tan colonies, which on microscopic examination are seen to be composed of spheric cells 7-15 μm in diameter that show single budding, although occasional multiple buds may be seen. The absence of a capsule is one feature that distinguishes *B. dermatitidis* from *Cryptococcus neoformans.*

Serologic identification: The **complement fixation test** is valuable in following the course of the disease, since the titer usually rises gradually as the disease progresses and disappears on recovery. Its use in diagnosis of blastomycosis is limited because of its insensitivity. The immunodiffusion test is specific and is the preferred test for serologic diagnosis.

Tissue phase and histopathologic findings: PAS, Gomori methenamine silver, or Gridley stains will reveal the yeastlike, thick-walled, single-budding organisms in **giant cells** or macrophages.

Paracoccidioides brasiliensis (Blastomyces brasiliensis)

Paracoccidioidomycosis (South American blastomycosis) is a chronic fungal disease caused by *Paracoccidioides brasiliensis* that usually affects the lungs first and then disseminates to other organs, mainly skin and nasal and buccal mucosa.

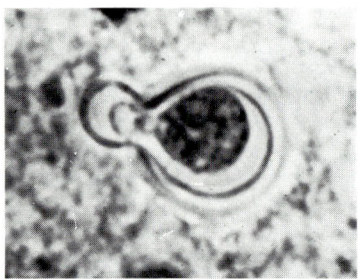

Fig. 33-28. Blastospore of *Blastomyces dermatitidis.* (Oil-immersion lens; ×1200.)

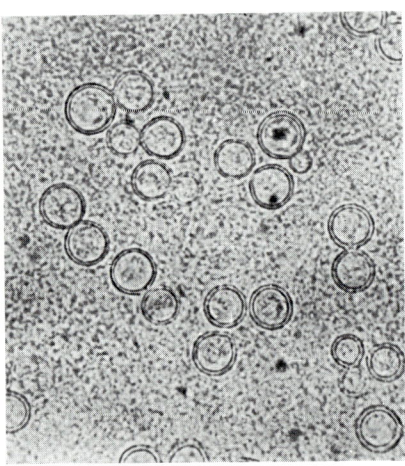

Fig. 33-29. *Blastomyces dermatitidis.* Budding forms in exudate. (×500.) (Courtesy Dr. Francis D. Smith.)

Laboratory diagnosis

Specimen: Pus, blood, sputum, and tissue from sinuses, lymph nodes, and ulcers.

Wet preparation: Unstained 10% potassium hydroxide preparations reveal organisms with thick (not as thick as *Blastomyces dermatitidis*), refractive walls. The cells measure 10-30 μm in diameter and give rise to a single or to several thin-walled buds that are fairly uniform in size. Multiple buds are arranged in a circle around the mother-cell wall and, because of their uniform size, give rise to a characteristic picture (Fig. 33-30). Single buds often reach the size of the mother cell. The buds vary in size according to age from 2-10 μm and are pinched off at their attachment site. This pinched-off attachment differentiates *P. brasiliensis* from *B. dermatitidis,* the buds of which have a wide attachment area. The buds of *P. brasiliensis* are round or oval, and the younger they are, the thinner are their walls.

Culture: The organism is biphasic. Inoculate two sets of BHI blood agar and two sets of neutral Sabouraud dextrose agar with antibiotics. To isolate the organism in the mycelial phase, incubate two sets of plates (with and without antibiotics) at room temperature. To isolate the organism in the yeast phase, incubate one plate each at 30-35° C. It may take up to 15-20 days for the colonies to appear at 22° or 35° C.

Mycelial phase: On Sabouraud dextrose agar at room temperature, irregularly folded or flat white colonies slowly appear. The surface is velvety because of short, aerial hyphae. Wet preparations reveal septate, branching hyphae and a few pyriform chlamydospores without conidia. The mycelial phase is not diagnostic.

Yeast (tissue) phase: On BHI blood agar at 35° C the colonies are yeastlike, wrinkled, waxy, and white to gray and grow slowly. Wet preparations reveal thick-walled, round spheres 6-30 μm in diameter with multiple budding, as described in the discussion of the wet preparation.

Histopathologic findings: The yeast or tissue phase can also be produced by injection of the fungus into the testes of guinea pigs, which after several weeks de-velop an orchitis accompanied by draining sinuses. The thick-walled structures can be demonstrated by PAS, Gomori methenamine silver, and Gridley stains.

The organism is chemically inert.

Coccidioides immitis

Coccidioidomycosis (coccidioidal granuloma, San Joaquin fever, or valley fever) can be a relatively mild, granulomatous lung disease that is usually self-limiting or a progressive and frequently fatal disease. The etiologic agent is *Coccidioides immitis*. The fungus occurs in the soil of only a few areas in America, primarily the southwestern United States. The spores, which are carried by wind and air, enter the human body through the respiratory tract.

Laboratory diagnosis

Specimen: Sputum, tissue, pus, and pleural fluid.

Wet preparation: Large, thick-walled, spheric bodies called **spherules** (sporangia) that vary from 10-200 μm in diameter are seen. They contain small, spheric or irregular **endospores** varying from 2-5 μm in diameter. Some spherules are tightly filled with spores, whereas others show spores that are peripherally arranged. Other spherules are empty and broken, and the spores are free (Fig. 33-31). The slide may be sealed with fingernail polish. **Multiple** germ tubes (mycelial filaments) will be seen projecting from spherules within 3-4 hr at room temperature.

Culture: The organism is **biphasic** and grows readily on Sabouraud agar. Since it is resistant to the action of cycloheximide and chloramphenicol, Sabouraud agar containing these antibiotics can be used as the primary isolation medium.

Inoculate several slants of Sabouraud dextrose agar with and without antibiotics with the clinical material.

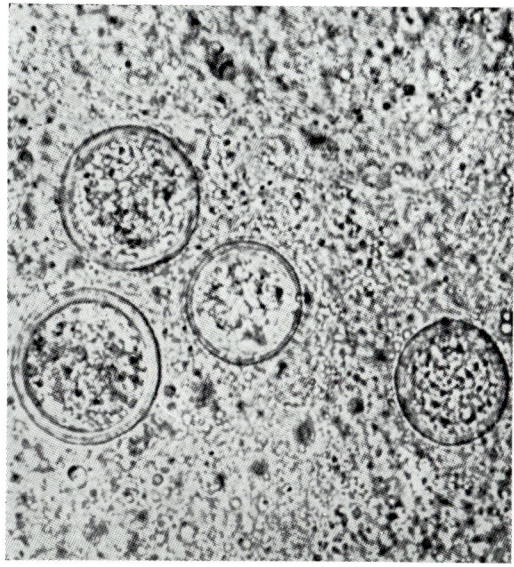

Fig. 33-31. *Coccidioides immitis* in pus from lymph node. (×600.) (From Stiles, G.W., and Davis, C.L.: J.A.M.A. **119:**765, 1942.)

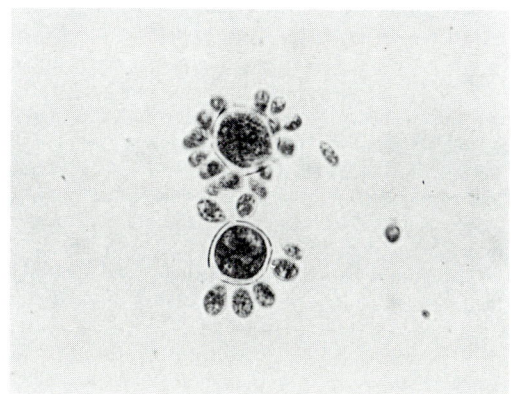

Fig. 33-30. *Paracoccidioides brasiliensis.* Multiple budding cells surround periphery of parent cell.

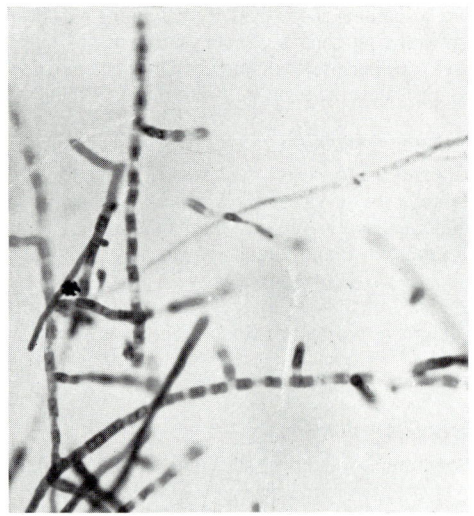

Fig. 33-32. *Coccidioides immitis.* Hyphae showing segmentation into arthrospores with characteristic light areas. (Lactophenol cotton blue stain.)

Do not use plates! If plates are used because coccidioidomycosis was not suspected, suspicious colonies should be subcultured onto slants as soon as discovered, and the plates should then be autoclaved. At room temperature and at 35° C the organism produces mycelia. The Sabouraud dextrose agar slants with and without antibiotics are incubated at 35° C, and within a few days a white aerial mycelium develops that imparts a white, cottony look to the originally smooth, gray, flat, moist colony. The growth may develop a brownish pigment on the reverse side; thus the entire colony appears tan. Sporulation occurs in 7-14 days.

On microscopic examination the aerial mycelium shows hyaline septate hyphae, which, as they mature, segment into cylindric or barrel-shaped arthrospores measuring about 3-4 μm in length (Fig. 33-32). They are separated by empty cells. When the hyphae rupture, many of these spores are set free, thus making handling of cultures dangerous. Before wet preparations are prepared, the culture should be flooded with sterile normal saline solution that is injected into the culture tube through the unopened top to prevent escape of spores.

C. immitis must be differentiated from other fungi such as *Arthroderma* and *Geotrichum.* Careful evaluation of colonial morphologic characteristics and microscopic appearance may help in the differentiation, but animal inoculation may be necessary.

Animal inoculation: The material used may be a culture of clinical material without the benefit of prior culture.

A 0.2 ml saline suspension of spores or mycelium is injected into the testes of a guinea pig or into the peritoneum of a mouse. After 1-2 weeks the animal should be killed and the tissues examined for the tissue (yeast) phase of the organism.

For animal inoculation with clinical material, cover the material with 10,000 units of penicillin per milliliter of specimen and 1000 units streptomycin per milliliter

of specimen. Shake for 1 hr, and centrifuge at 2500 rpm for 15 min. The sediment is suspended in sterile saline solution. Use the inoculation technic that was just given.

Histopathologic findings: The spherules are visible in hematoxylin-eosin preparations, but they and their endospores are better visualized by the use of Gridley or PAS stains. Immature spherules are devoid of endospores.

Skin tests: Skin tests with coccidioidin may be helpful in assessing the prognosis of the disease.

Serologic identification: Precipitins appear early in the disease (1-4 weeks) and then disappear. The immunodiffusion test[32] can be used as a screening test for precipitating antibodies. Complement-fixing antibodies do not appear at all in some cases, whereas in others they remain low, appear late, and persist longer.

SUBCUTANEOUS MYCOSES

Subcutaneous mycoses are a group of fungi that usually involve skin and subcutaneous tissue but may spread to internal organs.

Sporotrichosis
Sporothrix schenckii

Sporothrix schenckii produces a subacute and chronic subcutaneous lymphatic mycosis (**sporotrichosis**) characterized by abscesses, granulomatous nodules, and, rarely, late dissemination.

Laboratory diagnosis

Specimen: Pus or exudate from an ulcerated lesion or aspirated material from a fluctuant nodule is used. The latter material is preferred, although at best pus contains only a few fungal elements.

Wet preparation: Because of the paucity of fungal elements in clinical material, direct microscopic examination is of little value.

Culture: The organism is biphasic, demonstrating a mycelial phase in cultures at room temperature and a yeast phase in tissues and cultures at 35° C. Inoculate two sets of Sabouraud dextrose agar and of BHI blood agar with and without antibiotics.

Mycelial form: After 3-7 days on Sabouraud dextrose agar at room temperature, moist, white, smooth, leathery colonies appear that soon develop wrinkled or folded areas. They lack cottony aerial mycelia and after 1 week or so turn brown and finally black.

Wet preparations reveal delicate septate hyphae 1-1.5 μm in diameter and small pyriform conidia arranged in clusters on the ends of lateral conidiophores. The lateral conidiophores project at a 45- to 90-degree angle from the supporting hyphae. In older cultures a second set of conidiophores appears on the sides of conidiophores and hyphae (Fig. 33-33).

Yeast form: The culture incubated at 35° C develops small, glistening, moist, cream-colored, yeastlike colonies in 3-5 days. Wet preparation of the colonies reveals nonencapsulated 2 × 6 μm **fusiform** yeast cells that resemble sperm heads in shape and reproduce by budding.

Animal inoculation: The yeast phase may also be demonstrated by injecting a saline suspension of the

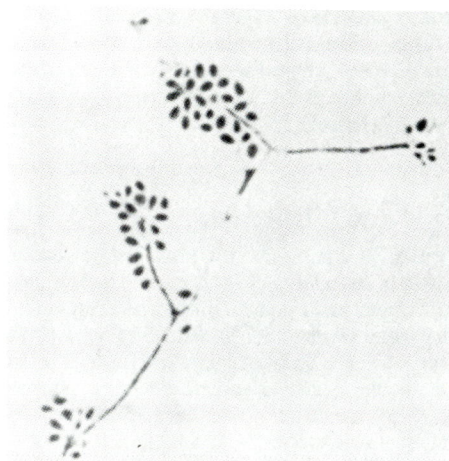

Fig. 33-33. *Sporothrix schenckii*. Mycelial form showing delicate hyphae and conidiophores bearing spores at the tips and sides. (From Lennette, E.H., et al., editors: Manual of clinical microbiology, ed. 3, Washington, D.C., 1980, American Society of Microbiology.)

Table 33-5. Morphology of grains of agents of maduromycosis

Fungus	Color	Size (μm)	Texture	Composition
Petriellidium boydii	White-gray	1-2	Soft	Hyaline hyphae and chlamydospores
Madurella mycetomatis	Black	0.5	Hard	Light brown hyphae and chlamydospores (peripheral)
Madurella grisea	Black	0.5-1	Soft	Colorless central hyphae and peripheral brown "cement" hyphae
Exophiala jeanselmei	Brown	0.5-1	Soft	Brown chlamydospores

mycelial form intraperitoneally into several mice. Some mice will develop peritonitis, orchitis, and bone involvement.

Histopathologic findings: The organisms are difficult to find in sections stained with hematoxylin and eosin. PAS and Gomori methenamine silver stains are required to bring out the elongated oval yeast cells.

Serologic identification: Antibodies develop during the course of sporotrichosis. Two tests, tube agglutination and latex agglutination, are available at the Centers for Disease Control in Atlanta, and may be useful for diagnosis.

Maduromycosis

Maduromycosis is a chronic granulomatous infection **(mycetoma)** usually involving the soft tissues and bones of the feet **(Madura foot)** and rarely other parts of the body.

There are two types of mycetomas: (1) **actinomycetic mycetoma,** resulting from infection by the aerobic actinomycetes and (2) **maduromycotic mycetoma,** caused by a variety of fungi.

These fungi, of which there are 17 common species, have been placed in two groups[1]: the Ascomycota and the Deuteromycota. Representative genera of the Ascomycota include *Petriellidium boydii (Allescheria boydii)* and *Aspergillus nidulans*. Genera of the Deuteromycota are *Exophiala jeanselmei (Phialophora jeanselmei)* and *Madurella mycetomati*. Most of these organisms are identified by their gross and microscopic morphologic characteristics. Each species produces characteristic **granules** (color, size, shape, and texture listed in Table 33-5), characteristic **colonies,** reproductive mycelia, and spores. **Grains** or granules are dense collections of hyphae with or without spores.

Petriellidium boydii

Petriellidium boydii is the most common causative agent of maduromycosis in the United States.

Laboratory diagnosis

Specimen: Pus and curettings should be examined grossly for **grains** or **granules** that are small, irregularly shaped, white to gray masses of fungus (0.5-5 mm). The most suitable material is obtained by aspiration from a fluctuant lesion. If granules are found, they should be washed several times in sterile saline solution to reduce the number of contaminants.

Wet preparation: Examine granules in 10% potassium hydroxide, and flatten under a cover glass. The granules are light colored, are composed of white septate hyphae, are 2-3 μm in diameter, and contain numerous chlamydospores. The granules of *P. boydii* must be distinguished from those of *Actinomyces,* which have a delicate mycelium (1 μm or less wide), show peripheral clubs that break up into diphtheroid-like, short, branching segments, and do not form chlamydospores.

Culture: Inoculate Sabouraud dextrose agar with penicillin and streptomycin with aspirated granules and incubate at 35° C. Prior to culture the granules should be washed as stated above. The rapidly growing colonies are filamentous and cottony, at first white and later becoming a dark brownish gray. The reverse side is gray to **black.**

The wet preparation reveals hyaline hyphae and brownish, single, ovoid conidia that are borne singly or are aggregated into lateral clusters. They are attached to conidiophores that may collect into bundles called **coremia.** Many strains produce perithecia, spheric ascocarps that are black and thick walled and measure 100-200 μm in diameter. Elliptic ascospores (4-8 μm escape from the ruptured mature ascocarp.

Histopathologic findings: The grains stain well with hematoxylin-eosin and PAS stains.

Madurella mycetomatis
Laboratory diagnosis

Specimen: Firm, large (5 mm) grains that may collect into large fungal masses are found within pus.

Wet preparation: The grains are composed of septate hyphae and chlamydospores, both containing black to reddish brown pigment granules.

Culture: The organism grows on Sabouraud dextrose agar, but sporulation is only seen on cornmeal agar at 37° C. At this temperature the organism forms a slow-growing, smooth or folded, velvety, powdery, white to yellow-brown colony, the brown pigment of which diffuses into the agar. On cornmeal agar, branched conical conidiophores are seen; these give rise to clusters of ovoid and round conidia on their tips.

Madurella grisea
Laboratory diagnosis

Specimen: The pus contains granules 1-2 mm in size that are black with unpigmented pale areas.

Wet preparation: The grains are composed of colorless hyaline hyphae surrounded by a peripheral brown substance containing brown hyphae.

Culture: The organism grows better at 30° than at 35° C. On Sabouraud dextrose agar it forms folded, grayish colonies that darken with age and produce a diffusible brown pigment.

Macroscopic examination reveals thin septate (1-3 μm) as well as wider (3-5 μm) hyphae that appear to be sterile.

Biochemical findings: *M. grisea* utilizes sucrose, whereas *M. mycetomatis* (which resembles *M. grisea*) does not.

Exophiala jeanselmei
Laboratory diagnosis

Specimen: The granules found in pus are brown, irregular, and elongated.

Wet preparation: The granules are composed of brown chlamydospores and occasional brown hyphae.

Culture: On neutral Sabouraud dextrose agar at 30° C, colonies develop that are at first yeastlike and greenish black but later develop a grayish black aerial mycelium that renders the colony dome shaped and velvety.

In wet preparation septate hyphae are seen to produce septate conidiophores arising at 45-degree angles from the main hyphal segments. The conical terminal segments of the conidiophores produce clusters of oval, elongated conidia.

Chromoblastomycosis (chromomycosis)

Chromblastomycosis is a chronic mycosis of skin characterized by ulcerated verruciform lesions. Chromomycosis is a clinical entity produced by a number of fungi such as *Phialophora verrucosa, Fonsecaea pedrosoi, F. compacta,* and *Cladosporium carrionii.*

The tissue form of all chromoblastomycosis-producing fungi is characterized by yellowish brown, spheric septate bodies found in abscesses within giant cells or free. They do not allow identification of the etiologic fungal genus or species (Fig. 33-34).

The fungi responsible for chromoblastomycosis produce dark colonies with black reverse sides and short, gray aerial mycelia. The different species are distinguished by the **types of conidiophores** they form. There are three types of sporulation (Fig. 33-35).

1. *Cladosporium (Hormodendrum)*-type sporulation. Ovoid spores in branching chains arise from the terminal cells of conidiophores that vary in length (*Cladosporium carrionii*).
2. *Phialophora*-type sporulation. Spores escape from the bottom of cup-shaped openings of flask-shaped structures (phialides) (*Phialophora verrucosa*).
3. *Acrotheca*-type sporulation. Spores arise from the sides of conidiophores (*Fonsecaea pedrosoi* and *F. compacta*).

Laboratory diagnosis

Material: Scrapings and biopsy tissue.

Culture: Use Sabouraud agar with cycloheximide and chloramphenicol and incubate at room temperature. On Sabouraud agar, brown to black, flat to dome-shaped colonies that have a short aerial mycelium are formed. The fungi are identified, as previously mentioned, by the type of sporulation seen in wet preparations. The fungi causing chromblastomycosis do not liquefy gelatin and do not hydrolyze Loeffler medium. Saprophytic *Cladosporium* does both.

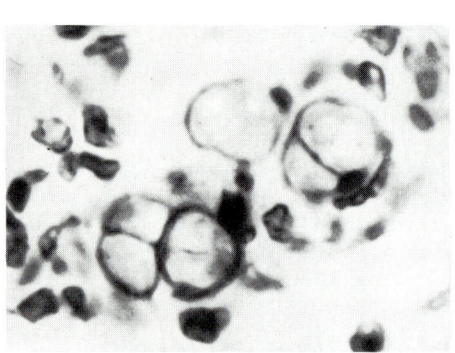

Fig. 33-34. Chromoblastomycosis organisms. Dark brown septate cells in tissue section of granuloma (Hematoxylin-eosin stain.)

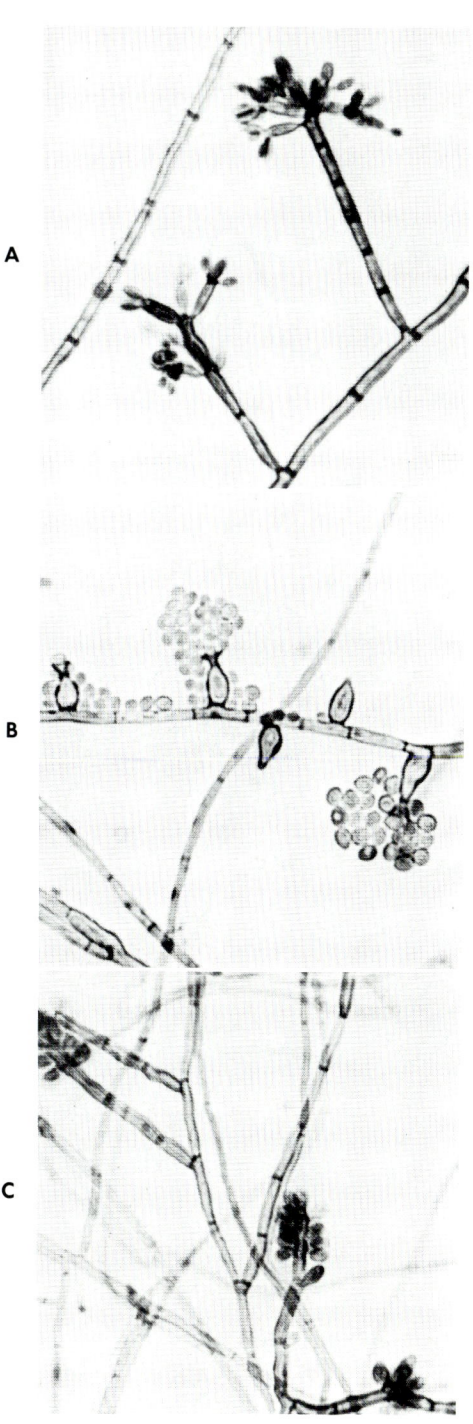

Phialophora verrucosa

The colony of *Phialophora verrucosa* grows slowly and is dark, black to olive gray, and velvety. Sporulation is best seen on cornmeal agar. Microscopic examination reveals that septate hyphae give rise to single, 90-degree, flask-shaped conidiophores (phialides), producing small (1-4 μm), oval to round terminal conidia collected in groups (*Phialophora*-type conidiophores).

Fonsecaea pedrosoi

The colony of *Fonsecaea pedrosoi* is slow growing, olive to black, smooth, and heaped. Sporulation is best seen on cornmeal agar. Microscopic examination reveals that septate hyphae produce short branching chains of conidia borne by conidiophores (*Cladosporium* [*Hormodendrum*]-type conidiophores). Detached conidia are elongated to oval.

Other hyphae reproduce by the *Acrotheca* type, in which terminal or lateral conidiophores bear lateral strings of conidia. A third type of reproduction is of the *Phialophora* type, which is described above.

Fonsecaea compacta

Fonsecaea compacta is slow growing and produces dark, greenish black, heaped, brittle colonies. Microscopic examination reveals that septate hyphae produce conidiophores of *Cladosporium*, *Acrotheca*, and *Phialophora* types, similar to *F. pedrosoi*.

Cladosporium carrionii

The colony of *Cladosporium carrionii* is dark, olive green, smooth, or irregular. Microscopic examination reveals that septate hyphae give rise to conidiophores, which produce long chains of progressively smaller conidia (*Cladosporium* type of conidiophores).

CUTANEOUS MYCOSES
Dermatomycoses (fungi [ringworm] of skin, nails, and hair)

The dermatomycoses are known as **tinea infections,** or **ringworm.** They are caused by dermatophytes, fungi that specifically involve skin, hair, and nails and produce athlete's foot (tinea pedis), ringworm of the body (tinea corporis) or of the scalp (tinea capitis), and jock itch (tinea cruris). Fungus infection of the nails is called onychomycosis.

The three most important agents of dermatomycosis are *Trichophyton* (21 species), *Epidermophyton* (2 species), and *Microsporum* (16 species). The dermatophytes are differentiated primarily by the morphologic characteristics of their microconidia and macroconidia, although cultural growth patterns are also considered (Figs. 33-36 and 33-37).

Laboratory diagnosis

Specimen: Segments of hair, including roots, and scrapings of skin are used. For collection of hair and skin samples see p. 915.

Wet preparation: Examine hair, skin, and nail scrapings in 10% potassium hydroxide. The hair preparation may show an ectothrix or endothrix pattern of spore growth, and the skin scrapings may show branching septate hyphae.

Fig. 33-35. A, *Cladosporium*-type conidiophores of *Fonsecaea pedrosoi*. **B,** *Phialophora*-type conidiophores of *Phialophora verrucosa*. **C,** *Acrotheca*-type conidiophores of *Fonsecaea pedrosoi*. (From Lennette, E.H., et al., editors: Manual of clinical microbiology, ed. 3, Washington, D.C., 1980, American Society of Microbiology.)

Trichophyton Epidermophyton Microsporum

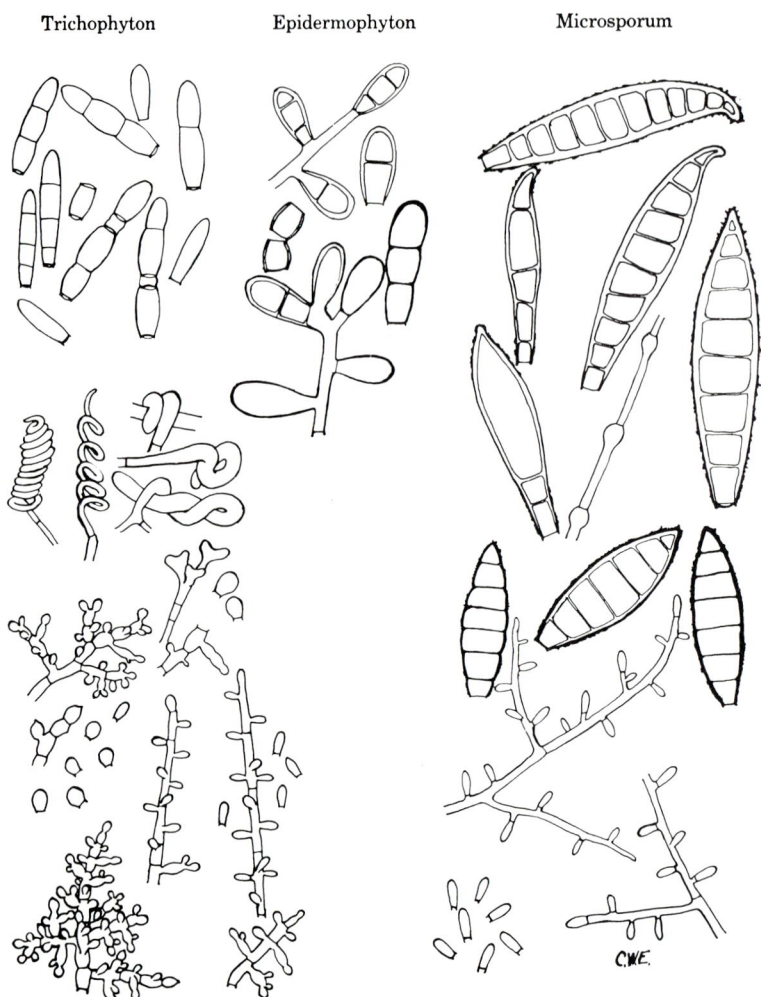

Fig. 33-36. Spore types and other organs in three genera of dermatophytes. *Trichophyton*—Lower third: Branching conidiophores (left); *T. mentagrophytes*-type conidiophores (right). Middle third: Spiral hyphae (left); ascogonia (female cells), antlerlike hyphae, and later development of antlerlike hyphae (right). Upper third: Macroconidia. *Epidermophyton*—Lower third: Sporulation (conidia); racket mycelium. Middle and upper thirds: Macroconidia. *Microsporum*—Lower third: Sporulation (conidia). Middle and upper thirds: Macroconidia.

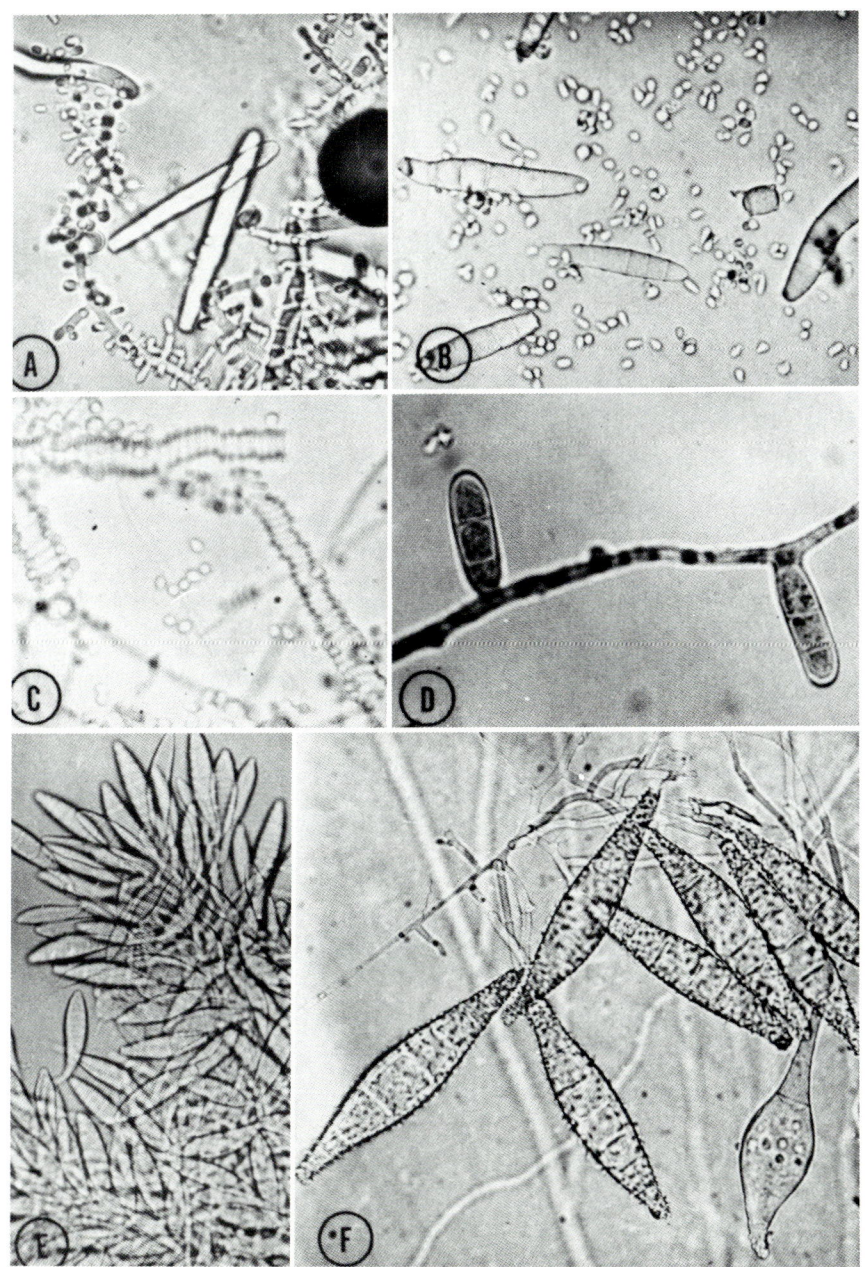

Fig. 33-37. Spores of dermatophytes. **A** to **C,** Conidia and spirally coiled hyphae of *Trichophyton mentagrophytes.* **D,** Macroconidia of *Epidermophyton floccosum.* **E,** Macroconidia of *Microsporum gypseum.* **F,** Macroconidia of *Microsporum canis.* (From Emmons, C.W., Binford, C.H., and Utz, J.P.: Medical mycology, Philadelphia, 1970, Lea & Febiger.)

Culture: Transfer material onto two plates of Sabouraud dextrose agar, one with cycloheximide and chloramphenicol and one without antibiotics. Incubate both plates at room temperature. Incubation at 37°C inhibits most dermatophytes except *Trichophyton verrucosum,* which requires 37° C for growth. The specimens should be pressed into the agar and examined for growth every week.

Trichophyton

Most species of the genus *Trichophyton* invade hair. The genus *Trichophyton* is characterized by a few (0-4) clavate, smooth-walled, septate macroconidia and by many spheric (2 μm) and clavate microconidia. The growth pattern in and on hair divides *Trichophyton* into the endothrix and ectothrix groups (Table 33-1).

Trichophyton mentagrophytes

Trichophyton mentagrophytes involves hair, producing a small-spored ectothrix pattern; skin and nails may also be involved.

Laboratory diagnosis

Culture: On Sabouraud dextrose agar the colonies grow rapidly and are cottony or granular to powdery. The surface mycelium is white to beige. The reverse side is yellow at first and then brownish to red.

Wet preparation: Wet preparations of culture show numerous microconidia that are small and slender or somewhat spheric. They develop on lateral, terminal, simple, or branched conidiophores or along hyphae. Macroconidia are rarely seen; they are thin walled, septate (2-5 cells), and spindle or club shaped (Figs. 33-36 and 33-37). In some strains numerous coiled hyphae, nodular bodies, and racket hyphae are seen.

Trichophyton rubrum

Trichophyton rubrum rarely involves hair; if it does, it produces an ectothrix pattern. The fungus usually involves nails and the skin of feet, groin, and perianal area.

Laboratory diagnosis

Culture: On Sabouraud dextrose agar the colony usually grows slowly and develops a white aerial mycelium. The margins may be glabrous. Some strains are velvety and change in color from white to cream to red. The reverse sides of most strains are deep red.

Wet preparation: Wet preparations may reveal only a few or many microconidia arising from the sides of hyphae on short conidiophores. Macroconidia are rare; they are thin walled, elongated with blunt ends, and contain 3-8 cells.

Trichophyton violaceum
Laboratory diagnosis

Wet preparation: Infected hair reveals an endothrix pattern (epidemic tinea capitis). The scrapings of skin and nails may reveal septate hyphae of *Trichophyton violaceum,* occasional conidiospores, and rare microconidia. Macroconidia are absent.

Culture: On Sabouraud dextrose agar the colony grows slowly and is deep violet in color. Sometimes

white aerial hyphae develop in subcultures (Fig. 33-38). Microscopic examination reveals septate hyphae, occasional chlamydospores, and rare microconidia. Macroconidia are absent.

Trichophyton tonsurans
Laboratory diagnosis

Wet preparation: The fungus shows an endothrix growth pattern within hair, in which it produces large spores. *Trichophyton tonsurans* may also be found in scrapings of skin and nails.

Culture: On Sabouraud dextrose agar the colony develops slowly into a flat structure that later becomes heaped, folded, and even cerebriform with a depressed center. The aerial mycelium is fine and powdery and is yellow to reddish brown. The reverse side is yellowish to mahogany red.

Wet preparations of the culture show numerous microconidia on short lateral conidiophores. They are elongated and delicate but later become large and irregular. Macroconidia are rare and clavate.

Trichophyton schoenleini
Laboratory diagnosis

Wet preparation: *Trichophyton schoenleini* shows an endothrix pattern within the hair. The hair is invaded by septate hyphae that produce arthrospores. Scrapings from skin and nails may also contain *T. schoenleini.*

Culture: On Sabouraud dextrose agar the fungus grows slowly, producing folded, heaped, glabrous, waxy, leathery colonies that grow into and split the agar. The surface is white to tan and may be powdery (Fig. 33-38).

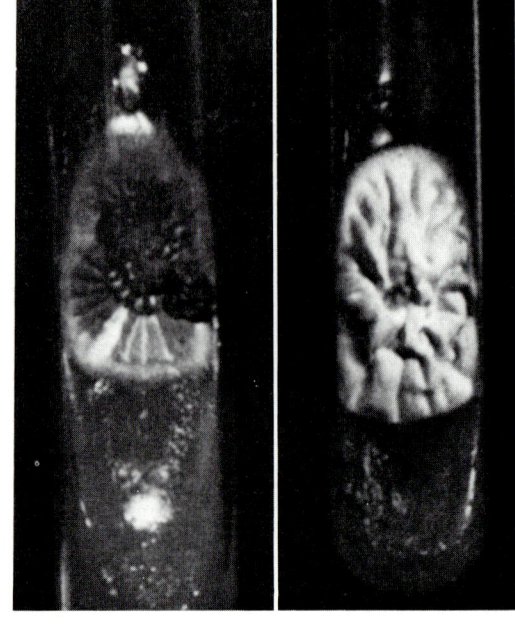

Fig. 33-38. Culture of *Trichophyton* species. **A,** *T. schoenleini.* **B,** *T. violaceum.* (Courtesy Merck Sharp & Dohme Div., Merck & Co., Inc., West Point, Pa.)

Table 33-6. Growth patterns of some *Trichophyton* species on *Trichophyton* agar

Dermatophyte	Trichophyton agar*			
	1 **Casein†**	**2** **Casein†** **and inositol**	**3** **Casein,† inosital,** **and thiamine**	**4** **Casein† and** **thiamine**
T. rubrum	4+	4+	4+	4+
T. mentagrophytes	4+	4+	4+	4+
T. tonsurans	1+	1+	4+	4+
T. violaceum	1+	1+	4+	4+
T. verrucosum (some strains)	±	±	4+	4+
T. verrucosum (most strains)	±	±	4+	±
T. schoenleini	4+	4+	4+	4+

*4+ = Rich abundant growth; 1+ = submerged growth of approximately 10 mm; ± = no growth or growth around 2 mm.
†Difco Laboratories, Detroit.

Table 33-7. Characteristics of more commonly isolated dermatophytes

Dermatophyte	Microscopic characteristics of clinical material in KOH or PAS	Colonial morphologic characteristics	Characteristic colonial features for microscopic identification	Growth on rice grains	Growth rate
Trichophyton rubrum	Skin: hyphae either segmented or branching Hair: large spored ectothrix and endothrix	White, cottony to downy, occasionally pink, powdery, and folded; reverse: wine red to yellow	Hyphae usually with teardrop microconidia that are usually laterally borne from hyphae; macroconidia usually absent, but when present are smooth, thin walled, and pencil shaped	Not applicable for identification	Slow growing; in 2 weeks a white, cottony colony with red pigment just starting to develop
Trichophyton tonsurans	Skin: branching hyphae or fragments Hair: large spores in parallel rows within hair shaft (endothrix)	White, cream-yellow to red, velvety or powdery colonies with heaped or sunken center; reverse: yellow to tan or red	Microconidia are teardrop- or club-shaped and larger than those of other dermatophytes; rare macroconidia	Not applicable for identification	Fairly fast growing; in 2 weeks an irregularly folded or heaped colony
Trichophyton schoenleini	Skin: scutula shows profuse growth of fungus; few hyphae in lesions Hair: large-spored endothrix	Irregularly heaped, glabrous, white to tan colony with radiating grooves; reverse: white to brown	Branching, antlerlike hyphae ending in swollen tips ("favic chandeliers")	Not applicable for identification	Slow growing; 2-3 weeks for typical heaped colony
Trichophyton violaceum	Skin: hyphae and arthrospores Hair: large-spored endothrix	Heaped, irregular, deep violet colony; may become more downy and lose pigment on subculture	Branched hyphae with thickened ends; macroconidia and microconidia may be produced on thiamine	Not applicable for identification	Slow growing; in 2 weeks grayish aerial mycelium forming with purple pigment developing
Trichophyton verrucosum	Skin: hyphae Hair: large-spored ectothrix may form sheath	Glabrous to velvety white colonies; rare strains produce yellow colonies	Microconidia on fresh isolation and on thiamine; branching hyphae and many chlamydospores, often seen in rows at 37° C	Not applicable for identification	Slow growing; growth enhanced at 37° C; requires thiamine

From Webb, C.D., and Hall, C.T.: Summary analysis of results for the proficiency testing survey in mycology, Atlanta, 1971, Centers for Disease Control.

Wet preparations of culture show irregular hyphae with clubbed ends (''favic chandeliers'') and numerous chlamydospores. Microconidia are very rare, and macroconidia are absent.

Use of Trichophyton agars: *Trichophyton* agars are commercially available. Their composition is based on the nutritional requirements of the various *Trichophyton* species. Agar 1 contains casein; agar 2, casein and inositol; agar 3, casein, inositol, and thiamine; and agar 4, casein and thiamine.

Procedure: Transfer a 2 mm segment of colony grown on thiamine-free agar to each *Trichophyton* agar. Incubate at room temperature for 1 week.

Results: The growth pattern of different species are given in Table 33-6.

The growth patterns of *T. violaceum* and of *T. tonsurans* are similar, but their colonial characteristics differ (Table 33-7). *T. mentagrophytes* and *T. rubrum* also have identical growth patterns but can be differentiated by their rate of growth at 22° C (*T. mentagrophytes* is faster) and by urease production within 5 days by *T. mentagrophytes*.

Epidermophyton

Epidermophyton invades the skin and nails, but not hair. It usually has broad filaments with rectangular segments that tend to disintegrate in 10% potassium hydroxide. In culture it is characterized by numerous clavate macroconidia and the absence of microconidia. *Epidermophyton* does not fluoresce.

Epidermophyton floccosum
Laboratory diagnosis

Specimen: Scrapings of skin of feet, groin, and nails are used. Hair is not involved.

Wet preparation: Hyphae and arthrospores are seen in 10% potassium hydroxide.

Culture: The colony is first powdery and greenish yellow and later becomes white and cottony (Fig. 33-39).

Microscopic characteristics: No microconidia are formed. The numerous clavate, snowshoelike macroconidia contain 2-4 cells and have thin walls. They occur in groups of two or three (Figs. 33-36 and 33-37). Chlamydospores are numerous in old cultures.

Microsporum

Members of *Microsporum* invade hair and skin but not nails. They occur primarily in children (Table 33-8).

Microsporum audouini
Laboratory diagnosis

Specimen: Hair clippings and scrapings of skin are used. Areas affected by *Microsporum audouini* and *M. canis* show greenish fluorescence under Wood's light.

Wet preparation: Wet preparations of hair reveal a sheath of spores that measure 2-3 μm each in diameter and form a mosaic pattern. The spores surround the hairs, whereas the hyphae grow down the hair shaft but stop short of the bulb (Fig. 33-11). Shavings of the skin in 10% potassium hydroxide reveal septate hyphae and chains of arthrospores.

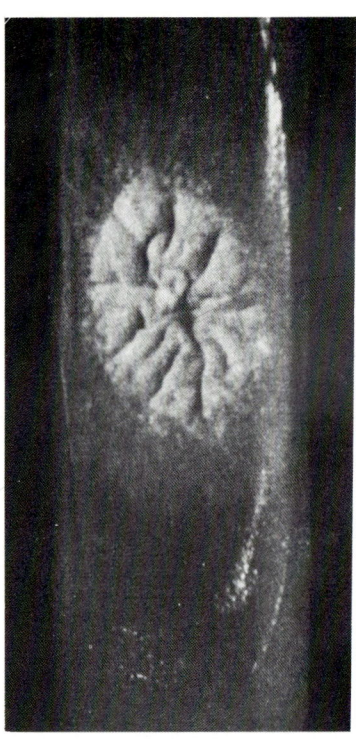

Fig. 33-39. Culture of *Epidermophyton floccosum*. (Courtesy Merck Sharp & Dohme Div., Merck & Co., Inc., West Point, Pa.)

Culture: Inoculate two tubes of Sabouraud dextrose agar containing cycloheximide and chloramphenicol and incubate at room temperature. Within 2 weeks, flat, velvety colonies appear slowly; they are covered by short aerial hyphae. Old cultures sometimes show grooves. The reverse side is salmon pink and the fringes of the colony may also show a pink tinge. The surface of older colonies is tan (Fig. 33-40, *A*). Microscopic examination reveals septate hyphae and chlamydospores. The latter vary in number from many to just occasional forms. Macroconidia are usually absent, and microconidia are quite rare. The macroconidia, when present, are large, thick walled, and spindle shaped, with few or no septa, and are commonly imperfectly formed, producing bizarre shapes. The mycelia may contain racket hyphae (Fig. 33-36).

Microsporum canis
Laboratory diagnosis

Specimen: Scrapings of skin, nails, and segments of hair are used. The organism is not frequently seen in humans.

Wet preparation: In 10% potassium hydroxidate (KOH), hyphae and occasional arthrospores are seen on **skin.** KOH preparations of **hair** reveal a small-spored ectothrix pattern.

Culture: On Sabouraud dextrose agar with antibiotics the colonies grow rapidly (within 1 week), producing woolly, white aerial mycelia and yellow-brown pigmentation of the periphery of the colony and in the

Table 33-8. Characteristics of more commonly isolated dermatophytes

Dermatophyte	Microscopic characteristics of clinical material in KOH or PAS	Colonial morphologic characteristics	Characteristic colonial features for microscopic identification	Growth on rice grains	Growth rate
Microsporum audouini	Skin: mycelium and chains of arthrospores Hair: sheath of small spores in mosaic	Downy white to salmon pink colony; reverse: tan to salmon pink	Mycelium and chlamydospores; macroconidia rarely seen, usually bizarre shaped; microconidia usually rare	No growth	In 2 weeks downy white colony with pink to reddish fringe; reverse: salmon pink
Microsporum canis	Skin: hyphae and occasional arthrospores Hair: mosaic hair, small spores	Center of colony white over orange-yellow; reverse: yellow-orange	Thick-walled, spindle-shaped, multiseptate, echinulate macroconidia; few microconidia laterally attached to hyphae	White, fluffy growth	In 1 week center of colony shows white downy mycelia over yellow-orange colony with yellow periphery; reverse: yellow
Microsporum gypseum	Skin: hyphae Hair: mosaic sheath of spores	Cinnamon colored, powdery colony; reverse: light tan	Thick-walled, elliptic multiseptate echinulate macroconidia; few microconidia	Cinnamon-colored, powdery growth	Rapid growth; in 1 week cinnamon-buff, powdery colony
Epidermophyton floccosum	Skin: hyphae and arthrospores Hair: not attacked	Folded center of colony khaki green, periphery yellow; reverse: yellowish brown with observable folds	Macroconidia large, smooth, multiseptate, clavate, borne in clusters; no microconidia	Yellowish olive green, velvety growth	In 1 week olive green center of colony folded and periphery yellow; reverse: brown
Trichophyton mentagrophytes	Skin: chains of spores or nonsegmented hyphae Hair: small-spored ecthothrix	White to pinkish, granular to powdery to cottony; reverse: buff to reddish brown with occasional light yellow periphery	Many globose microconidia either in pine-tree or engrappe form; spiral hyphae; thin-walled, club-shaped macroconidia, rare or numerous according to strain	Not applicable for identification	Fast growing; in 7-10 days mature colony as described under colonial morphologic characteristics

From Webb, C.D., and Hall, C.T.: Summary analysis of results for the proficiency testing survey of mycology, Atlanta, 1971, Centers for Disease Control.

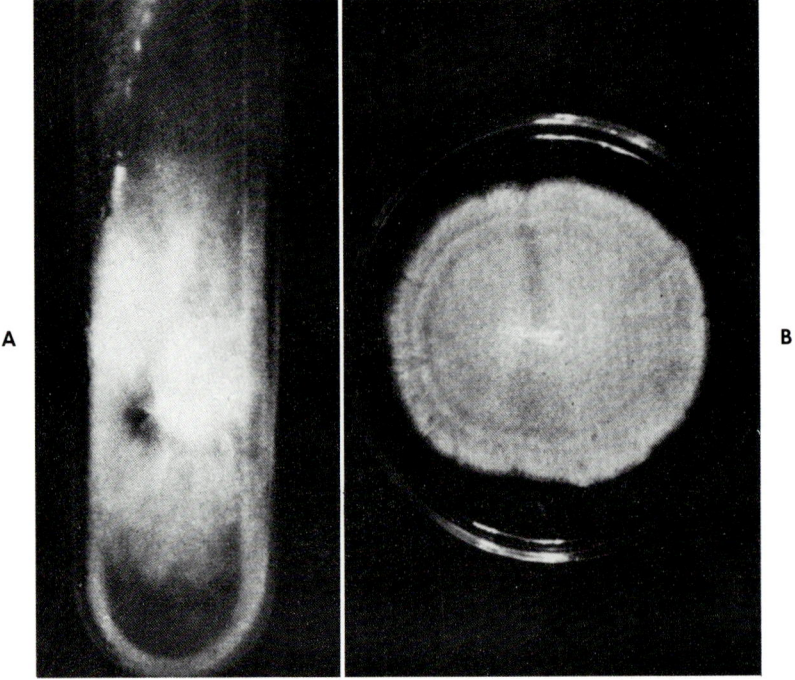

Fig. 33-40. Culture of *Microsporum* species. **A,** *M. audouini.* **B,** *M. canis.*

agar. The reverse side of the colony is yellow; thus the colony may appear orange. After 2-4 weeks concentric rings appear on the colony, and the reverse side becomes brown (Fig 33-40, *B*). Microscopic examination reveals that numerous spindle-shaped microconidia have 8-15 cells, thick and roughened walls, and a terminal knob (Figs. 33-36 and 33-37). A few sessile lateral microconidia can be detected that are pear shaped.

Microsporum gypseum
Laboratory diagnosis

Specimen: Hair and scrapings of skin are used. The organism rarely infects humans.

Wet preparation: A potassium hydroxide (KOH) preparation of skin shows hyphae, and a KOH preparation of hair shows an ectothrix pattern of spores.

Culture: On Sabouraud dextrose agar with antibiotics the organism grows rapidly (within 1 week) and forms flat, coarse, powdery colonies with irregular borders and dull orange to light brown pigmentation. The reverse side of the colony is dull yellow to tan. Microscopic examination reveals numerous spindle-shaped, multicelled (3-6), slightly thickened, echinulate, prickly macroconidia. They are shorter and broader than those of *M. canis.* Microconidia are rare; when present, they are sessile and pear shaped.

SUPERFICIAL MYCOSES

Superficial mycotic infections involve the outermost layers of the skin and hair. Three genera are responsible for superficial infections: *Piedraia hortae, Trichosporon beigelii,* and *Malassezia furfur.*

Piedraia hortae
Laboratory diagnosis

Specimen: Segments of involved hair are used. The organism produces nodules on hair and is not usually seen in the United States.

Wet preparation: A potassium hydroxide preparation of hair reveals septate hyphae, chlamydospores, asci, and ascospores.

Culture: The organism grows slowly on Sabouraud dextrose medium without antibiotics. Cycloheximide inhibits growth. The colonies are raised, black, glabrous, and partially velvety because of grayish, short aerial hyphae. The organism does not form spores on culture media.

Trichosporum beigelii
Laboratory diagnosis

Specimen: Light brown nodules along hair shafts.

Wet preparation: A potassium hydroxide preparation reveals a mycelium consisting of hyaline hyphae and rectangular arthrospores alternating with blastospores.

Cultures: The organism grows on Sabouraud dextrose agar and is inhibited by cycloheximide. The colonies are cream colored and soft but become leathery as they age. On microscopic examination the culture shows the same picture as that found in the wet preparation. Cornmeal agar is the preferred medium for sporulation.

Malassezia furfur (Pityrosporum)

Malassezia furfur is the cause of tinea versicolor, a superficial skin infection.

Laboratory diagnosis

Specimen: Skin scales from periphery of lesions as determined by ultraviolet light are used. Affected skin areas fluoresce under ultraviolet light, varying in color from yellow to brown.

Wet preparation: In 10% potassium hydroxide *M. furfur* is easily demonstrated, because it forms abundant mycelia and many groups or clusters of spheric or ovoid conidia in scrapings of the advancing edge of the lesion.

Tape test: Transparent adhesive tape may be used in the same way as it is used in the diagnosis of enterobiasis. Apply the tape to the affected skin area, remove it, place adhesive side of tape on a drop of Gram iodine on a glass slide, and examine for hyphae and spores under the microscope.

Culture: The organism can be cultured on Sabouraud dextrose agar overlaid with sterile olive oil. Incubate culture at 37° C. The organism grows as a white- to tan-colored yeast. Microscopic examination reveals groups or clusters of spheric or ovoid conida.

SAPROPHYTIC FUNGI

Saprophytic fungi, which are not usually disease producing, are widely disseminated in nature and can be found as molds on decaying food articles. They are also responsible for focal human infections (otomycosis) and for generalized infections, mainly in debilitated patients.

Saprophytic fungi are important because (1) they exceed in number the fungi pathogenic to humans, (2) they are common laboratory contaminants and must therefore be identified, and (3) they are **opportunist invaders** that attack individuals whose resistance is lowered by disease or forms of treatment.

Aspergillus[33]

Aspergilli are frequently found in cultures and may represent the causative organisms of a disease process, or they may be contaminants.

A. fumigatus is most commonly associated with pathologic lung conditions, either with granulomatous lesions or with cavity formation. It may complicate preexisting lung disease, e.g., tuberculosis or silicosis.

A. niger, which is usually associated with fungal otitis externa, may lead, in the lung, to the formation of a **fungus ball,** a compact rounded mass of mycelia and debris.

Laboratory diagnosis

Specimen: Sputum, bronchial washings, and shavings of cornea or external ear canal.

Wet preparation: The white septate hyphae of *Aspergillus* can be seen in potassium hydroxide (KOH) preparations. If *A. fumigatus* is present in sputum, characteristic conidiophores and conidia may be seen. In *A. niger* infections of the ear canal, characteristic conidiophores are seen in the KOH preparations of the canal material.

Culture: Most aspergilli are sensitive to cycloheximide. The preferred medium is Sabouraud dextrose agar without antibiotics, incubated at 22-37° C. The

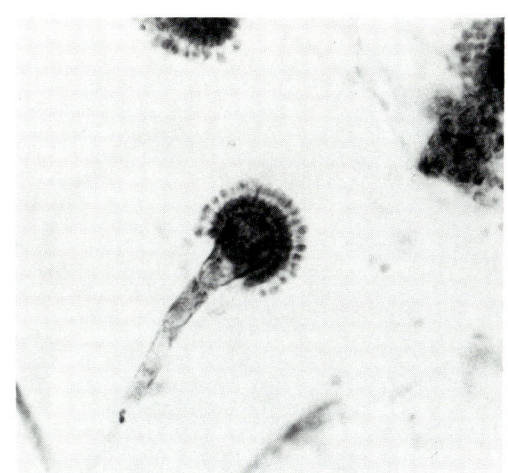

Fig. 33-41. *Aspergillus* species. Note vesicle and sterigmata with microconidia.

latter temperature is preferable, since it will eliminate many other contaminating fungi. A flat colony appears rapidly (48 hr), is white at first, and then becomes bluish green and powdery. Microscopic examination reveals septate hyphae that give rise to conidiophores, which have a stalk and a bulbous end called the vesicle. The vesicle is partially hidden by rows of sterigmata, which in turn give rise to chains of globose green conidia (Fig. 33-41).

Penicillium

Because of the ubiquity of *Penicillium* in our environment and the likelihood of insignificant contamination of specimens by it, the etiologic significance of this fungus, when discovered in a specimen, is difficult to evaluate.

Penicillium notatum
Laboratory diagnosis

Specimen: Sputum.

Wet preparation: In 10% potassium hydroxide fragments of septate hyphae and possibly small conidiophores are revealed.

Culture: The organism grows readily on Sabouraud dextrose agar at room temperature, in about 48 hr forming heaped, wrinkled, gray colonies with a white periphery. White aerial hyphae give the colony a soft appearance. Microscopic examination reveals branching septate hyphae with terminal brushlike spores (Fig. 33-42).

Zygomycosis (phycomycosis)

Zygomycosis includes infections by the genera *Mucor, Rhizopus,* and *Absidia,* among others. The organisms are found in soil, manure, and vegetables. In humans they are often secondary invaders of debilitated patients, producing infections of the orbital tissues, brain, and lungs.

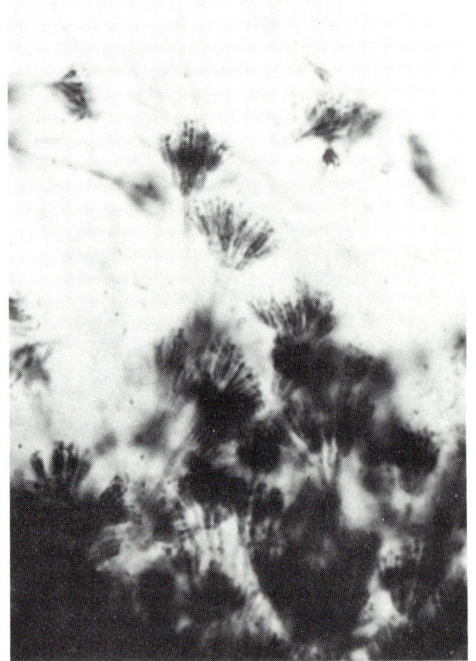

Fig. 33-42. *Penicillium* species. Note terminal brushlike spores.

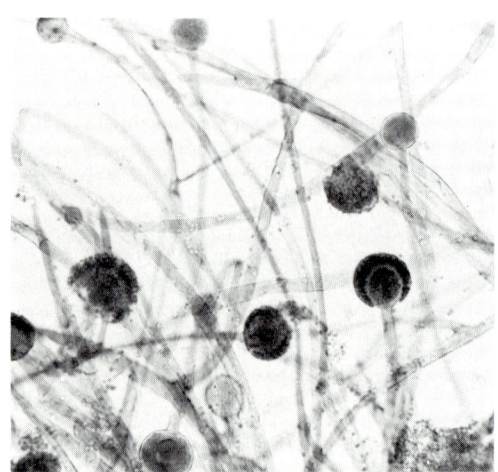

Fig. 33-43. *Mucor* species. Nonseptate hyphae give rise to sporangiophores that bear spore-filled, globose sporangia that break easily.

Mucor

Mucor grows rapidly on Sabouraud agar, producing an aerial mycelium that is soft and white at first but later becomes gray to brown. Microscopic examination reveals nonseptate hyphae that lack rhizoids (roots) and give rise to tall, single, erect sporangiophores with terminal **sporangia** (Fig. 33-43).

Rhizopus

Rhizopus grows rapidly on Sabouraud agar, producing a rich woolly mycelium that is white at first and later becomes gray with black and brown dots. Microscopic examination shows that the hyphae are **nonseptate** and give rise to long sporangiophores capped by spheric **sporangia** that contain spheric spores and a **columella.** The sporangiophores arise from nodes opposite **rhizoids** (rootlike structures) (Fig. 33-44).

CONTAMINANTS

Some of the fungi mentioned in the preceding pages are frequent contaminants, although under certain circumstances they may be pathogens. *Saprophytic fungi* appear early, grow rapidly, and are heavily pigmented. Some common contaminants are *Alternaria* species (Fig. 33-45, *A*), *Aspergillus* species (Fig. 33-41), *Cryptococcus* species (Fig. 33-18), *Fusarium* species (Fig. 33-45, *B*), *Geotrichum* species (Fig. 33-24), *Helminthosporium* species (Fig. 33-45, *C*), *Mucor* species (Fig. 33-43), *Penicillium* species (Fig. 33-42), *Rhizopus* species (Fig. 33-44), *Scopulariopsis* species (Fig. 33-45, *D*), and *Syncephalastrum* (Fig. 33-45, *E*).

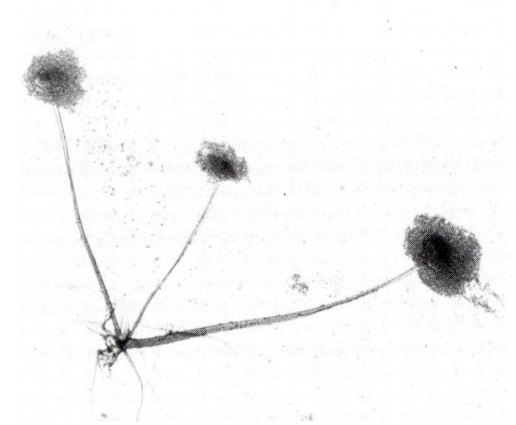

Fig. 33-44. *Rhizopus* species. Unbranched, nonseptate sporangiophores arise from rootlike hyphae or rhizoids. Sporangiophores support spore-filled sporangia arranged around columella, the swollen tip of the sporangiophore.

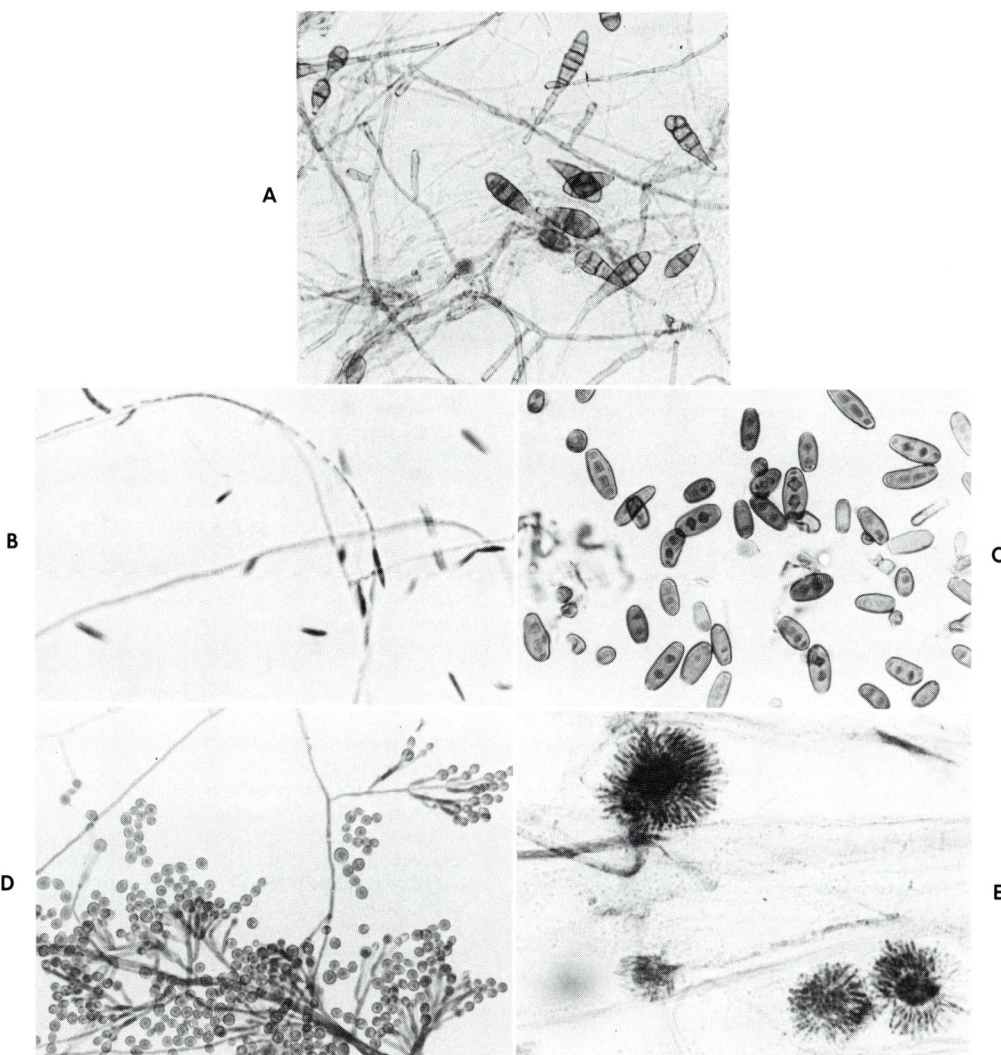

Fig. 33-45. A, *Alternaria* species. Club-shaped, longitudinally and vertically septate conidia are produced from ends of conidiophores. **B,** *Fusarium* species. Short conidiophores give rise to sickle-shaped, pointed, sometimes septate conidia. **C,** *Helminthosporium* species. Large, oval, septate conidia are attached to knotted conidiophores. **D,** *Scopulariopsis* species. Conidia-bearing hyphae are arranged in branched clusters to resemble *Penicillium* species. Conidia are oval and often come off directly from hyphae. **E,** *Syncephalastrum* species. End of sporangiophores is distended and gives rise to ovoid endospores.

GLOSSARY

acrotheca Type of spore formation characteristic of genus *Fonsecaea* in which conidia are formed along sides of irregular club-shaped conidiophores.

Actidione Trade name for cycloheximide.

aerobe Organism whose growth and reproduction are favored by presence of air or free atmospheric oxygen.

anaerobe Organism whose growth and reproduction are favored by absence of air or free atmospheric oxygen.

antibody Substance formed in blood (circulating) or tissues (fixed) in response to presence of an antigen.

antigen Substance that when introduced into the body of an animal induces formation of antibodies.

arthrospore Asexual spore formed by disarticulation of mycelium.

ascocarp Structure of varying complexity that bears asci and ascospores.

ascospore Spore formed within an ascus.

ascus Specialized saclike structure characteristic of Ascomycetes in which ascospores are produced.

aseptate Refers to absence of cross walls in hyphal filament or spore.

basidiospore Spore borne on basidium.

basidium Structure (usually single clavate cell) that bears basidiospores.

basipetal Development in direction of the base, e.g., spore chain in which apical spore is oldest.

blastospore Spore produced by budding process along mycelium or by single spore.

budding Asexual reproductive process characteristic of unicellular fungi or spores involving formation of lateral outgrowth from parent cell that is pinched off to form a new cell.

capsule Hyaline, mucopolysaccharide sheath on wall of cell or spore.

chlamydospore Thick-walled resistant spore formed by direct differentiation of mycelium in which there is concentration of protoplasm and nutrient material.

chloramphenicol Antibiotic (Chloromycetin) produced by *Streptomyces*.

cladosporium Type of spore formation characteristic of genera *Cladosporium* and *Fonsecaea* in which conidia are formed in branched chains by conidiophore of various lengths.

clavate Club shaped.

columella Persistent dome-shaped apex of the sporangiophore in some Phycomycetes.

conidophore Specialized stalklike branch of mycelium on which conidia are developed singly or in groups.

conidium Asexual spore that may have one or many cells and may be of any size and shape.

coremium Bundle of conidiophores.

cycloheximide Antibiotic (Actidione) produced by *Streptomyces griseus*.

dichotomous Type of branching, often repetitious, in which two branches are approximately equal.

dimorphic Refers to fungi that can grow and reproduce in either mold or yeast form.

diploid Having the 2n number of chromosomes.

echinulate Covered with small spines.

ectothrix Outside hair shaft.

endogenous Derived from internal source.

endospore Spore formed within special spore case.

endothrix Within hair shaft.

exogeneous Derived from external source.

facultative Refers to the ability of an organism to grow and reproduce as an aerobe or an anaerobe.

favic chandeliers Specialized hyphae that are curved, freely branching, and antlerlike in appearance. They are found in certain dermatophytes, especially *Trichophyton schoenleini*.

floccose Woolly.

fungus Chlorophyll-lacking saprophytic or parasitic member of plant kingdom whose plant body is not differentiated into roots, stems, or leaves; in most species, fundamental structural unit is mycelium.

fusiform Spindle shaped.

germ tube Tubelike process produced by germinating spore that develops into mycelium.

glabrous Smooth.

granulomatous Composed of granulation tissue.

hyaline Glassy.

hypha One of branching, usually septate tubular structures that constitute vegetative portion of mycelium of fungi.

imperfect fungi Former term for fungi that apparently lack sexual means of reproduction. They are now known to reproduce sexually and asexually.

intercalary Refers to spores produced between two hyphal segments.

kerion Pustular infection of hair follicles of the scalp characterized by raised, boggy lesion.

lateral Refers to spores produced on side of hypha.

macroconidium Large, often multicellular spore.

macroscopic Refers to gross, cultural morphologic characteristics that can be observed and studied with naked eye.

microconidium Small, single-celled spore.

micrometer One thousandth of a millimeter; represented by Greek letter μ (pronounced "mew"), e.g., 10μ.

microscopic Refers to minute morphologic characteristics that can only be observed and studied under lens of microscope.

mold Macroscopic: filamentous or mycelial form of fungus growth. Microscopic: predominance of hyphae.

monomorphic Refers to fungi that grow and reproduce in only the mold or yeast form.

mycelium Mat of intertwined and branching hyphae.

mycetoma Fungus tumor.

mycosis Fungus disease.

nodes Those points on stolon where rhizoids are suspended.

nodular organ Knot of closely knit hyphae considered to represent abortive attempts toward sexual reproduction.

onychomycosis General term for fungal infection of nails.

oogonium Female cell of Oomycetes.

oospore Sexual spore produced through fusion of two unlike gametangia; found in class Phycomycetes.

pectinate Comblike.

pectinate hyphae Vegetative hyphal branches with unilateral digitate projections resembling teeth of comb.

perfect fungi Fungi that possess sexual and asexual means of reproduction.

perithecium Special round, oval, or beaked structure in which asci are formed.

phaeo Prefix meaning dark.

phialide Cell (either sporophore or terminal or lateral cell of sporophore) that bears succession of phialospores at its tip.

phialophora Type of spore formation characteristic of genus *Phialophora* in which conidia are formed endogenously in flasklike conidiophores called phialides.

pseudohypha Fragile chain of cells with characteristics intermediate between chain of budding cells and a hypha.

pyriform Pear shaped.

racket hyphae Vegetative hyphae showing terminal swelling of segments suggesting a tennis racket in shape.

rhizoid Branched and rootlike radiating hyphae extending into culture medium.

ringworm Superficial fungus infection; word derived from ancient belief that these infections were caused by wormlike organisms and from fact that lesions are often circinate or circular in form.

saprophyte Any organism living on decaying or dead organic matter.

sclerotic Hardened, thick walled.

septate Refers to presence of cross walls in hyphal filament or spore.

septum A wall, usually a cross wall in a hypha.

spirals Specialized tightly coiled branches of mycelia found in many fungi; their function is unknown.

sporangiophore Specialized mycelial branch bearing a sporangium.

sporangiospore Spore that is borne within a sporangium.

sporangium Closed structure within which asexual spores are produced by cleavage.

spore Generally, reproductive body of a fungus.

sporophore Specialized mycelial branch on which spores are produced.

sterigmata Short or elongate specialized projections from sporophores on which spores are developed.

stolon A runner; horizontal hypha that sprouts where it touches culture medium and forms rhizoids in culture medium.

suppurative Producing pus.

synonym Another name for species or taxonomic group.

thallospore A sexual spore produced by septation of hypha, e.g., arthrospore.

thallus Term used for fungus plant.

tinea (ringworm) Term used to designate various types of superficial fungus infections, e.g., tinea capitis, ringworm of scalp; tinea pedis, ringworm of foot.

tuberculate Having knobby projections.

uncinate With tip bent to form a hook.

verrucose Warty in appearance.

virulence Degree of pathogenicity; disease-producing ability of microorganism.

yeast Macroscopic: pasty or mucoid form of fungus growth. Microscopic: predominance of budding cells.

zygospore Thick-walled sexual spore found in Phycomycetes that is produced through fusion of two similar gametangia.

REFERENCES

1. Lennette, E.H., et al.: Manual of clinical microbiology, ed. 3, Washington, D.C., 1980, American Society for Microbiology.
2. Emmons, C.W., Binford, C.H., and Utz, J.P.: Medical mycology, ed. 2, Philadelphia, 1977, Lea Febiger.
3. Laboratory procedures in clinical mycology, Technical manual TM8-227-8, Washington, D.C., 1964, U.S. Department of the Army.
4. Moss, E.S., and McQuown, A.L.: Atlas of medical mycology, Baltimore, 1969, The Williams & Wilkins Co.
5. Snell, W.H., and Dick, A.E.: A glossary of mycology, ed. 2, Cambridge, Mass., 1971, Harvard University Press.
6. Sanford, L.U., Mason, K.N., and Hathaway, B.M.: Am. J. Clin. Pathol. **44:**172, 1965.
7. Swartz, J.H., and Lamkins, B.E.: Arch. Dermatol. **89:**89, 1964.
8. Cohen, M.M.: J. Invest. Dermatol. **22:**9, 1954.
9. Strauss, R., and Klingman, A.: J. Infect. Dis. **88:**151, 1951.
10. Schneidan, J.D., Jr.: Am. J. Clin. Pathol. **40:**659, 1963.
11. Buechner, H.A., et al.: Chest **63:**259, 1973.
12. Yarrow, D., and Heyer, S.A.: Int. J. Sys. Bacteriol. **28:**611-615, 1978.
13. Hall, T., Papageorge, C., and Webb, C.D., Jr.: Identification of yeasts, Atlanta, 1973, Centers for Disease Control.
14. Dolan, T.C.: Am. J. Clin. Pathol. **55:**580, 1971.
15. Dolan, T.C.: Am. J. Clin. Pathol. **55:**632, 1971.
16. Wickerham, L.J.: Taxonomy of yeasts, Technical bulletin no. 1029, Washington, D.C., 1951, U.S. Department of Agriculture.
17. Wickerham, L.J.: J. Trop. Med. Hyg. **42:**176, 1939.
18. Wickerham, L.J.: J. Bacteriol. **52:**293, 1946.
19. Dolan, T.C., and Woodward, M.R.: Am. J. Clin. Pathol. **55:**591, 1971.
20. Jennings, A., Bennett, J.E., and Young, V.: Mycopathologia **35:**256, 1968.
21. Hopfer, R.L., and Grochel, D.: J. Clin. Microbiol. **2:**96-98, 1975.
22. Bindschadler, D.D., and Bennett, J.E.: Ann. Intern. Med. **69:**45, 1968.
23. Oxford, A.E., Raistrick, H., and Simonart, P.: Biochem. J. **33:**240, 1939.
24. Brown, C., Jr., et al.: J.A.M.A. **152:**206, 1953.
25. Grimley, P.M., Wright, L.D., and Jennings, A.E.: Am. J. Clin. Pathol. **43:**216, 1965.
26. Wickerham, L.J.: J.A.M.A. **165:**47, 1957.
27. English, M.T.: Rev. Med. Vet. Mycol. **6:**103, 1967.
28. Shamiyeh, B., and Shipe, E.L.: Public Health Lab. **22:**198, 1964.
29. Klite, P.D.: J. Lab. Clin. Med. **66:**770, 1965.
30. Carlisle, H.N., and Saslaw, S.: J. Lab. Clin. Med. **51:**793, 1958.
31. Saslaw, S., and Campbell, C.C.: J. Lab. Clin. Med. **35:**780, 1950.
32. Huppert, M., and Bailey, J.W.: Am. J. Clin. Pathol. **44:**369, 1965.
33. Seabury, J.H., and Samuels, M.: Am. J. Clin. Pathol. **40:**21, 1963.

Parasitology

The methods employed for the investigation of parasitic infections depend on the biologic behavior of the parasite, the organ or organs it involves, and where and by what method it reproduces and is transmitted. In some cases the laboratory investigation searches for the adult form of the parasite; other cases involve examination for ova and larvae, scrutiny of imprints of lymph nodes or of smears of blood, and examination of biopsy (bladder, muscle, skin, rectum, or duodenum) or autopsy (liver or spleen) specimens. Culture of parasites is not a routine diagnostic approach at the present time, but certain serologic and immunologic methods—based on antigens obtained by culture—provide a high degree of diagnostic accuracy. Materials to be examined include stool, bile, sputum, urine, blood, tissues,

anal or vaginal swabs, or spinal fluid, depending on the characteristics of the parasite. The third edition of *Medical Parasitology* by Beck and Davies[1] and the second edition of *Diagnostic Parasitology: a Clinical Laboratory Manual* by Garcia and Ash,[2] as well as the third edition of *The Manual of Clinical Microbiology* by Lennette et al.,[3] may be referred to for expanded information and practical procedures.

Quality control in parasitology

Quality control in parasitology, as in the rest of the clinical laboratory, is based on a multiplicity of practice procedures, all of which ensure that the final report to the physician is as error free as possible. The following are but a few principles that broadly apply (see p. 16):

1. A current methods manual with detailed procedures on specimen collection, transport, processing, and reporting
2. An adequate library consisting of reference texts in both basic and clinical parasitology
3. Well-trained, motivated personnel
4. Continuing education program
5. Proficiency test program
6. A stock culture collection and/or a slide transparency collection
7. A program to ensure the reactivity of reagents
8. Preventive maintenance records for microscopes, centrifuges, and water baths
9. Daily check of refrigerators and water bath for desired temperature

Most errors in parasitology are caused by the following:

1. Lack of familiarity with parasite
2. Cursory examination
3. Confusion of parasite and artifact

LABORATORY PROCEDURES FOR DIAGNOSIS OF INTESTINAL PARASITES

The laboratory examination for ova and parasites involves the following steps: obtaining the specimen, transport of the specimen, preparation and preservation of the specimen, macroscopic examination of the material, and microscopic examination of temporary and permanent preparations.

Specimen collection

Use a clean, wide-mouthed container that allows ready access to and visualization of the specimen. The lid should be tight fitting. The specimens must be ade-

Table 34-1. Most important parasitic infections of humans[1,4-6]

Protozoa	Helminths
Amebae	**Nematodes (roundworms)**
Entamoeba histolytica	Intestinal nematodes
Entamoeba hartmanni	*Trichuris trichiura*
Entamoeba coli	*Enterobius vermicularis*
Entamoeba gingivalis	*Necator americanus*
Endolimax nana	*Ancylostoma duodenale*
Iodamoeba buetschlii	*Ancylostoma braziliense*
Flagellates	(cutaneous larva migrans)
Intestinal and atrial (body cavities) flagellates	*Ancylostoma caninum*
Chilomastix mesnili	*Ascaris lumbricoides*
Trichomonas hominis	*Toxocara canis* and *cati*
Trichomonas vaginalis	(visceral larva migrans)
Trichomonas tenax	*Strongyloides stercoralis*
Giardia lamblia	*Trichostrongylus* species
Retortamonas intestinalis	*Angiostrongylus cantonensis*
Enteromonas hominis	*Capillaria philippinensis*
Dientamoeba fragilis	Blood and soft tissue nematodes
Blood and subcutaneous flagellates	*Wuchereria bancrofti*
Leishmania donovani	*Brugia malayi*
Leishmania tropica	*Loa loa*
Leishmania braziliensis	*Dipetalonema perstans*
Trypanosoma gambiense	*Mansonella ozzardi*
Trypanosoma rhodesiense	*Onchocerca volvulus*
Trypanosoma cruzi	*Dracunculus medinensis*
Trypanosoma rangeli	*Trichinella spiralis*
Ciliates	**Trematodes (flukes)**
Balantidium coli	*Fasciola hepatica*
Sporozoa	*Clonorchis sinensis*
Isospora belli	*Opisthorchis* species
Plasmodium vivax	*Fasciolopsis buski*
Plasmodium falciparum	*Metagonimus yokogawai*
Plasmodium malariae	*Heterophyes heterophyes*
Plasmodium ovale	*Paragonimus westermani*
Toxoplasma gondii	*Schistosoma japonicum*
Pneumocystis carinii	*Schistosoma haematobium*
Babesia	*Schistosoma mansoni*
	Cestodes (tapeworms)
	Taenia saginata
	Taenia solium
	Diphyllobothrium latum
	Echinococcus granulosus
	Echinococcus multilocularis
	Hymenolepis nana
	Hymenolepis diminuta
	Dipylidium caninum

quately identified and the labels should list patient's name, source of specimen, physician, etc., as well as the time the specimen was obtained, since unpreserved fecal specimens should be examined within 1 hr after passage, especially if the specimen is loose and may contain trophozoites. The specimen should be passed directly into the container or transferred into the container from commercially available special collection devices, which are inserted into the toilet bowl and allow separate collection of feces or urine. The specimen should not be contaminated with urine or water and should be obtained before any type of therapy is initiated, since antibiotics, anthelmintics, antidiarrheal drugs, antacids, laxatives, soap, and hypertonic salt enemas suppress parasites. At least 1 week should be allowed to elapse after treatment before reexamination of the stool for parasites. Saline cathartics or Epsom

salt may be used to obtain purged specimens. Good results may be obtained by the examination of three daily consecutive specimens obtained after the administration of $1/2$ oz. Epsom salt, which the patient should take on arising followed by a liquid breakfast.[7] The multiple stool examinations are necessitated by the fact that some parasites are passed irregularly (protozoa) or shed their eggs irregularly (helminths). Purged specimens have the advantage that they are loose and often contain whole parasites or portions of them.

Specimens should be examined as soon as possible. Living trophozoites of protozoa become nonmotile or die after about 6 hr at room temperature and such specimens may then be falsely reported as negative. If immediate examination is not possible, store the specimen in the refrigerator or at room temperature not longer than a few hours.

Macroscopic (gross) examination

Note the following characteristics of the specimen.
1. Consistency of stool
   a. Formed: may contain cysts, eggs, and larvae
   b. Soft: may contain trophozoites, cysts, eggs, and larvae
   c. Liquid or loose: may contain mainly trophozoites, a few cysts, eggs, and larvae
2. Character of stool: may be bloody, mucoid, watery, or pussy
3. Presence or absence of whole worms or of parts of worms in strained specimen, e.g., proglottids, scolices, or adult organisms such as pinworms, roundworms, tapeworms, or hookworms

Methods: Using a hand lens pick up small organisms with an applicator stick and transfer them to 1 drop of saline placed on a microscopic slide. Protect the specimen with a coverslip and examine under the low-power objective (10X) of the microscope.

Wire sieve method to collect parasites or parts of parasites: Liquefy the specimen with water and strain through a wide-mesh sieve (10-20 mesh) that allows medium-sized worms to pass through but retains bulky fecal components. Then strain the sieved material through a finer sieve (40-50 mesh) to retain scolices and smaller worms.

Microscopic examination

Summary of procedure:
1. Direct examination of fresh specimens
   a. Saline wet mounts: trophozoites (motility), cysts, eggs, and larvae
   b. Eosin in saline: trophozoites (motility), cysts, eggs, and larvae—an optional technic
   c. Iodine wet mounts: cysts, eggs, and larvae
   d. Buffered methylene blue
2. Concentration method (formalin–ethyl acetate)
   a. Saline wet mounts: cysts, eggs, and larvae
   b. Iodine wet mounts: cysts, eggs, and larvae
3. Preservation of specimens
   a. Formalin
   b. Polyvinyl alcohol (PVA) fixative
4. Permanent stains

If the stool is liquid, several small samples should be examined within 1 hr. If the stool is formed, several preparations should be prepared from surface scrapings, making quite certain not to omit bloody or mucoid areas. Three direct temporary slide preparations should be employed: (1) a temporary stain, e.g., buffered methylene blue, for trophozoites, (2) saline, and (3) iodine. All stool specimens must be handled as potentially infectious to prevent hand-to-mouth transmission. NOTE: Although direct microscopic methods are described, it is recommended that all specimens be concentrated.

Buffered methylene blue stain for trophozoites: Dissolve 0.06% methylene blue dye in acetate buffer with the pH range of 3.6-4.8. Several commercial buffers are available. Mix a small quantity of stool and the staining reagent on a glass slide. Apply a coverslip and let stand 5-10 min. Read within 30 min. Trophozoite nuclei stain deep blue against a pale blue cytoplasm.

Combination of saline and iodine wet mounts:
Reagents:
1. Normal saline
2. Lugol's iodine *or* D'Antoni's iodine
   a. Lugol's iodine. For stock solution dissolve 10 g potassium iodide in distilled water to 1 dl, slowly add 5 g powdered iodine crystals, and shake until dissolved. Filter and store in a tightly stoppered brown bottle. For working solution prepare a 1.5 dilution in distilled water every 2 weeks.
   b. D'Antoni's iodine. Grind 1 g potassium iodide and 1.5 g powdered iodine crystals in a mortar with about 5 ml distilled water before adding the remaining portion of water (to 1 dl). Any excess iodine should remain at the bottom. Transfer solution into a glass-stoppered dark brown bottle. Prepare fresh every 3 weeks since it deteriorates on standing (the color lightens).

Procedure: Place 1 drop saline solution on one end of a glass slide and 1 drop iodine solution on the other. Emulsify 1-2 mm^3 of fecal material with an applicator stick, first in the saline solution and then in the iodine solution. Choose mucoid hemorrhagic particles to look for amebae and schistosome eggs. Remove fibers and large particles and cover each emulsion with a 22 × 22 mm coverslip. The emulsion should be just thin enough to allow reading of print. Seal mounts with nail polish or with paraffin-petrolatum (1:1) mixture kept liquid in a heated water bath.

Interpretation: In the saline preparation, trophozoites are characterized by their motility, whereas cysts, which are somewhat refractile, can be recognized as glistening, round to ovoid objects when the objective is moved up and down for a short distance. They are usually about two to four times as large as red cells. Saline preparations also allow recognition of endoplasmic inclusions, e.g., chromatoid bodies and red cells, and they may reveal larvae, pus cells, macrophages, eosinophils, red cells, yeast, Charcot-Leyden crystals, undigested material, and artifacts. They are inadequate for the demonstration of nuclei or glycogen. The preparation must be examined within 30 min[8] and should not be allowed to dry or to be disturbed by air bubbles.

Iodine preparations are of value in demonstrating protozoan cysts and complement the saline preparation. Chromatoid bodies are poorly seen as compared to the eosin stain, but nuclei (membrane and karyosome) and glycogen masses stain dark brown. Trophozoites are killed by iodine. The iodine concentration must not be too strong, since overstaining with a too concentrated iodine solution coagulates fecal particles and renders the protozoan cysts less refractile, while too weak an iodine solution understains the organisms.

To obtain a suitable transparency of wet mounts, they may be diluted with saline solution. If a thin formalin suspension is used, no additional saline solution is needed. Formalized specimens must be well mixed before examination and, when mounted in saline solution, usually allow recognition of nuclei without the addition of iodine.

Concentration methods

Sedimentation and flotation methods are available. The formalin–ethyl acetate technic is the sedimentation method of choice while the preferred flotation technic utilizes zinc sulfate.

Formalin–ethyl acetate concentration method[9]:
Reagents:
1. Saline
2. Ethyl acetate[10]
3. Formalin, 10%

Fresh, PVA-fixed, or formalin-fixed specimens may be concentrated.

Procedure:
1. Comminute 2 ml stool in 3 ml saline solution in a 15 ml conical centrifuge tube.
2. Add saline solution to mark 15 and strain about 10 ml of the emulsion through two layers of wet gauze into a second 15 ml pointed centrifuge tube.
3. Centrifuge at 1500 rpm for 2 min and decant the supernatant fluid.
4. Resuspend the sediment in fresh saline solution, centrifuge, and decant as before. This step may be repeated if a cleaner sediment is desired.
5. Add about 10 ml 10% formalin to the sediment, mix thoroughly, and allow to stand for 5 min.
6. Add 3 ml ethyl acetate, stopper the tube, and shake vigorously; remove the stopper carefully.
7. Centrifuge at 2500 rpm for about 2 min.
8. Four layers should result; a small amount of sediment containing most of the parasites, a layer of formalin, a plug of fecal debris on top of the formalin, and a topmost layer of ethyl acetate.
9. Free the plug of fecal debris from the sides of the tube by ringing with an applicator stick and carefully decant the top three layers.
10. Mix the remaining sediment with the small amount of fluid that drains back from the sides of the tube.
11. Prepare iodine and unstained saline mounts of the sediment in the usual manner for microscopic examination.

The formalin–ethyl acetate sedimentation method is excellent for the recovery of protozoan cysts and of ova and larvae of most intestinal helminths. The method does not concentrate trophozoites of fresh material, but if PVA-preserved material is used trophozoites can be seen but must be confirmed by permanent (trichrome) stain technic.

Zinc sulfate centrifugal flotation*:
Reagents and equipment:
1. Zinc sulfate, 331 g, and water to 10 dl
   Check specific gravity with hydrometer and adjust to 1.180 with water or additional zinc sulfate. Store in stoppered bottle and check specific gravity weekly.
2. Conical, calibrated, 15 ml centrifuge tube
3. Wire loop, 5-7 mm, the loop bent at 90 degrees to the long axis of the wire and handle

Procedure: Emulsify 0.5-1 ml stool in about 5 ml water and then add water to the 15 ml level. Centrifuge

*Modified from reference 2.

1 min at 2000 rpm and discard supernatant fluid. Mix sediment with zinc sulfate solution to 15 ml mark and strain through funnel lined with two layers of gauze into a second 15 ml conical centrifuge tube. Add zinc sulfate to 15 ml mark. Centrifuge for 1 min at 2000 rpm and allow centrifuge to come to a stop without any vibration. Do not remove centrifuge tube and touch surface only of the fluid meniscus with flamed and cooled wire loop, but so that it is parallel to the fluid surface, and transfer film of fluid to previously prepared saline and iodine drops on a microscope slide. Protect with coverslip and examine immediately microscopically. Decant fluid and examine sediment.

The zinc sulfate method concentrates protozoan cysts and helminth eggs but also shrinks them if left in contact too long. Large nematode, tapeworm, and infertile *Ascaris* ova fail to be concentrated by the zinc sulfate technic. A large amount of fatty material in the stool interferes with the concentration of the diagnostic stages of the parasite on the fluid meniscus.

Bartlett et al.[11] describe a modified zinc sulfate flotation concentration technic that compares favorably with the formalin–ethyl acetate concentration method but is not satisfactory for schistosome eggs.

A modification of the formalin–ethyl acetate method, which is capable of concentrating ova up to 300 times, is suggested by Zierdt[12] who describes his approach as a quick, clean, and efficient procedure and less distasteful than the standard formalin–ethyl acetate method.

Concentration methods for certain larvae, helminths, and helminth eggs are mentioned in the sections dealing with the particular parasites.

Preservation of fecal specimens

If a specimen cannot be examined immediately, or if it is delayed before reaching the laboratory, it should be divided into three portions: one is left unpreserved, one is mixed with PVA fixative, and one is mixed with formalin. If specimens are sent to specialty laboratories for consultation, PVA-fixed material should be submitted.

Formalin method:
Reagents:
1. Formalin, 10%
   Mix well 10 ml of formalin (40% commercial formaldehyde) and 90 ml of water.
2. Formalin, 5%
   Mix well 5 ml of formalin and 95 ml of water.

Directions for use: For routine purposes, 5% formalin is preferred; 10% formalin is superior for helminths. Mix 1 volume of feces with 3 volumes of formalin.

Polyvinyl alcohol fixative solution: Polyvinyl alcohol (PVA) is suitable for the preservation of trophozoites and cysts and is commercially available (PVA Fixative, Regional Media Laboratories, Lenexa, Kan.). Its main advantage is the fact that permanent (stained) slides can be prepared from the PVA-feces mixture.

Directions for use: If only a small amount of fecal material is available or if it is very liquid or mucoid the glass slide method is employed. The vial-mix technic is suggested for the "routine" specimen.

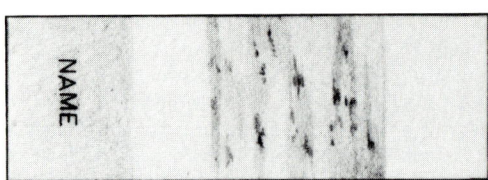

Fig. 34-1. Appearance of smear of PVA-fixed feces.

Glass slide method: Mix 1 part fresh feces with 3 parts preservative and place a small amount on a glass slide. Saline wet mounts on slides may also be fixed by removing the coverslip and adding a few drops of fixative. Spread stool fixative mixture with an applicator stick over one third of the slide's surface, extending across entire width of slide, by rolling the applicator stick back and forth creating alternating slightly thicker and thinner areas. If smear is too thin it will destain too rapidly and if too thick it is difficult to examine. Allow it to dry overnight at 37° C and stain as above. Preparation is stable for 2 months (Fig. 34-1).

Vial-mix technic: Vial fixation may be preferred if sufficient material is received. Use 1 part feces to 3 parts fixative. Mix thoroughly. Prepare films (as described above) using 2 or 3 drops of the mixture smeared over approximately one third of the slide, extending material to edge of the slide.

Merthiolate-iodine-formaldehyde fixative stain: Merthiolate-iodine-formaldehyde (MIF), which is commercially available, may be used as a fixative stain in place of PVA. PVA preserves trophozoites better than cysts, but MIF fixes and preserves trophozoites and cysts equally well.

Permanent staining procedure

Permanent stained preparations should be prepared especially from all diarrheal stools and from all stools showing trophozoites or cysts in wet preparations. Stained smears not only confirm the diagnosis of wet preparations but also supply a lasting record. The trichrome stain may be used on fresh stool specimens fixed with Schaudinn solution or on PVA-preserved material. Formalin-fixed stool is not suitable.

Trichrome stain[13]:
Reagents:
1. Schaudinn solution (fixative)
    a. Saturated aqueous solution of mercuric chloride, 2 parts: 13-14 g mercuric chloride and 1 dl distilled water. Dissolve crystals with the aid of heat. On cooling, excess mercuric chloride crystallizes out. Filter and store in glass-stoppered bottle.
    b. Ethyl alcohol, 95%, 1 part
    c. Glacial acetic acid, 5 ml/dl solution, to be added before use
2. Iodinated alcohol
    Add enough iodine crystals to 70% ethyl alcohol to prepare a dark brown solution. Prepare the working solution by adding sufficient 70% ethyl alcohol to produce a tea-colored solution. The exact concentration is not as important as is the color. Too dark a solution will interfere with the trichrome stain and too light a solution will fail to prevent mercuric chloride crystals from forming during the staining procedure.

3. Trichrome stain
    a. Chromotrope 2R, 0.60 g
    b. Light green SF, 0.15 g
    c. Fast green FCF, 0.15 g
    d. Phosphotungstic acid, 0.70 g
    e. Glacial acetic acid, 1.00 ml
    f. Distilled water, 1 dl
    To the dry powder mix, add glacial acetic acid, mix, and allow to stand for 30 min. Add distilled water and mix well. The stain is deep purple to black.
4. Acid alcohol (destaining and differentiation solution)
    a. Acetic acid, 0.45 ml
    b. Ethyl alcohol (90%), 99.55 ml
5. Alcohol (95%) in two separate containers
6. Carbolxylene
    a. Phenol crystals liquefied by heating in hot water, 1 volume
    b. Xylene, 3 volumes
    Add phenol to xylene and mix.
Procedure: See Table 34-2.
The preparation of PVA-fixed smears is described above. Fresh stool specimens are smeared in the same way as PVA-fixed material, but the smear must be inserted into the Schaudinn fixative as soon as it is prepared, since during the entire process of staining the smear must never be allowed to dry. This statement also applies to the staining of PVA-fixed material.
Examine smear under oil-immersion lens after locating suspicious areas under low power.

Result: Trophozoites usually stain lighter than cysts. Some cysts *(Endolimax nana, Entamoeba hartmanni, Giardia,* and *Chilomastix)* usually stain light. Variation in staining result from PVA fixation (red cysts), from degeneration (green cysts), and from normal variations.
Cytoplasm: Blue-green with pink tinge.
Chromatoid bodies: Red.
Nuclei: Dark red.
Yeast and mold: Green.
Background: Green.
Ingested red cells: Red to green, depending on degree of digestion.

Report: Report organisms in descending order of frequency or order of importance (pathogenicity) if preferred.

Cultivation procedures

A number of media are available that support the growth of amebae and flagellates. Cultivation acts as an augmentation process provided the specimen is less than 8 hr old, is watery, and is known to contain amebae other than *Entamoeba histolytica*. The disadvantages of cultivation are that it is time consuming, requires experience, and still necessitates identification of the cultured amebae since the media are not selective.
Media for culturing amebae:
1. Balamuth egg yolk infusion medium (Difco Laboratories, Detroit)[14]
2. Liver infusion agar
3. Diphasic charcoal medium of McQuay
Media for culturing flagellates (except *Giardia*):
1. Feinberg medium[15]
2. Trypticase serum medium

Table 34-2. Outline of trichrome staining technic of smears of PVA-fixed and unfixed specimens

Reagents	Fresh specimens	PVA-fixed film
Schaudinn solution (fixative)	1 hr at room temperature or 5 min at 50° C	Fixation not required
Iodinated alcohol, 70%	1 min	10 min
Alcohol, 70%	1 min	3-5 min
Alcohol, 70%	1 min	3-5 min
Trichrome stain	2-8 min	4-8 min
Acid alcohol, 90%	10-20 sec (one brief dip usually suffices)	10-20 sec (one brief dip usually suffices)
Alcohol, 95%	Rinse	Rinse 5 min
Alcohol 95%	Rinse	Rinse 5 min
Alcohol, 100%	1 min	Carbolxylene, 5-10 min
Xylene	1 min	10 min
	Apply Permount* and coverslip	Apply Permount* and coverslip

*Fisher Scientific Co., Pittsburgh.
Keep all jars (Coplin jars with screw tops) covered at all times, even when the slides are staining. Remember that destaining with acid alcohol continues until it is washed off in 95% alcohol. After completion of the trichrome step remove the excess stain by touching the slide onto filter paper before destaining it in acid alcohol.

Examination of specimens other than feces

Bile: Examine wet fresh preparation. Centrifuge specimen at 2000 rpm for 10 min and examine sediment unstained for *Echinococcus* hooklets, ova of *Fasciola hepatica, Clonorchis sinensis,* and *Giardia lamblia.*

Blood: Fresh preparations and fixed smears may be examined for microscopic filariae, trypanosomes, and malarial plasmodia as well as other parasites that are intraerythrocytic. Concentration by centrifugation may be necessary in order to find trypanosomes.

Duodenal contents: Duodenal aspiration (and mucosal biopsy) is best performed by endoscopy by a gastroenterologist, since the Enterotest (HEDECO Co., Palo Alto, Calif.) may require frequent exposure to x-rays. The sediment of the centrifuged specimen may contain larvae and trophozoites of *Strongyloides* and cysts and trophozoites of *Giardia lamblia.* Examine drops of sediment and mucus on a glass slide as soon as they are obtained.

Spinal fluid: Wet fresh and fixed preparations are examined for *Acanthamoeba* and *Naegleria.* Centrifuge at 2000 rpm for 10 min and examine sediment. The amebae may attach to the sides of the container; therefore the tube should be gently shaken before centrifugation.

Sputum: The sputum is digested in 4% sodium hydroxide (see discussion of method for tubercle bacilli), centrifuged, and the sediment is examined for *Paragonimus westermani* eggs and possibly for roundworm larvae (hookworm, ascaris, and *Strongyloides*), *Entamoeba histolytica* (cysts), and *Echinococcus.* Direct wet preparation allow the discovery of *Entamoeba histolytica* trophozoites.

Urine: The sediment of the centrifuged specimen may contain *Trichomonas vaginalis* and *Schistosoma haematobium* eggs. Examine drops of sediment on a glass slide.

Vaginal swab: Place several drops of saline on a glass slide and twirl a swab in them to obtain a wet preparation to be examined microscopically for *Trichomonas vaginalis.*

Biopsy specimen (skeletal muscle, rectal, duodenal, and bladder specimen): Place part of specimen on a glass slide and add drops of saline. Tease gently with teasing needle.

Apply coverslip and examine the muscle biopsy specimen for *Trichinella* larvae, the rectal biopsy specimen for schistosome ova and *Entamoeba histolytica* trophozoites, the duodenal biopsy specimen for *Giardia lamblia* and larvae of *Strongyloides stercolaris,* and the bladder biopsy specimen for *Schistosoma haematobium* ova. Send any remaining specimen to the surgical pathology department.

Preservation of specimens for teaching or quality control

Preserve specimens of feces containing ova and larvae by emulsifying the feces in 10% formalin. Add about 5% glycerin to prevent loss by drying. Store at room temperature.

Wash nematodes with water or physiologic saline solution and drop into hot 70% alcohol (heated to bubbling). Store in 70% alcohol, adding glycerin to make 5% solution.

Wash trematodes with water or saline solution and drop into hot 10% formalin (heated to bubbling). Store in 70% alcohol containing glycerin to make 5% solution.

Wash cestodes with water and leave in water until they are dead (a few hours for small specimens; overnight for large ones). Fix in 10% formalin. Store in 70% alcohol containing glycerin to make 5% solution.

Place spiders, ticks, mites, fleas, lice, or other arthropods in a mixture of 97 parts 20% alcohol and 3 parts ether (room temperature) until dead.[16] Store in 70% alcohol containing glycerin to make 5% solution.

Drop fly larvae or mosquito larvae into boiling water. Store in 70% alcohol containing glycerin to make 5% solution.

Mount small insects and parasites directly without previous dehydration and clearing in Turtox (General Biological Supply House, Chicago) nonresinous mounting medium.

PROTOZOA
Classification

See Table 34-1. With few exceptions protozoa occur in two stages—as infective cysts and as motile, noninfective trophozoites (vegetative forms). The exceptions are *Dientamoeba fragilis* and *Trichomonas*, which occur as trophozoites only. The cysts offer protection from an unfavorable environment and are associated with multiplication and propagation.

Amebae

Seven species of amebae are found in the human intestines, only one of which is pathogenic, i.e., *Entamoeba histolytica,* a tissue invader. The other amebae are the entamebae (*Entamoeba hartmanni, Entamoeba coli, Entamoeba gingivalis, Entamoeba polecki*) and the ''other'' amebae (*Endolimax nana* and *Iodamoeba buetschlii*). All these amebae except *Entamoeba histolytica* are collectively called commensal amebae in that their presence is generally nonsymptomatic and they are nontissue invaders. Some investigators claim that saprophytic amebae may indicate pathogenic organisms.

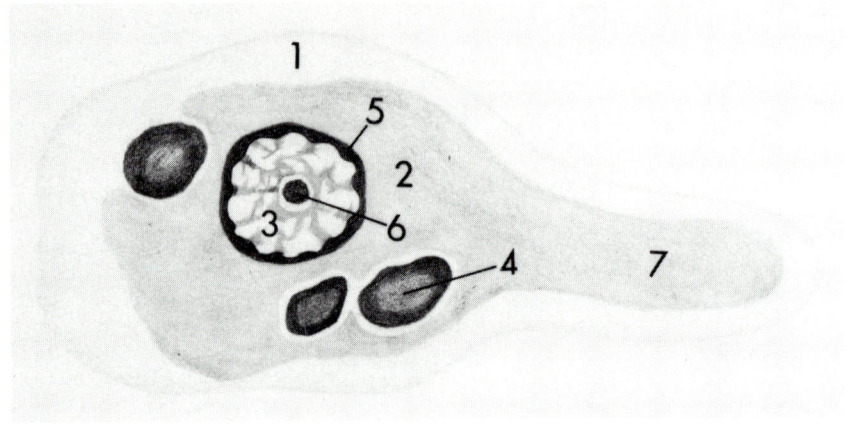

Fig. 34-2. Schematic drawing of *Entamoeba histolytica.*

1 Ectoplasm	**5** Peripheral chromatin
2 Endoplasm	**6** Karyosome
3 Nucleus	**7** Pseudopod
4 Red cell inclusion	

Amoebae						
Entamoeba histolytica	*Entamoeba hartmanni*	*Entamoeba coli*	*Entamoeba polecki**	*Endolimax nana*	*Iodamoeba bütschlii*	*Dientamoeba fragilis*
Trophozoite						
Cyst						No cyst

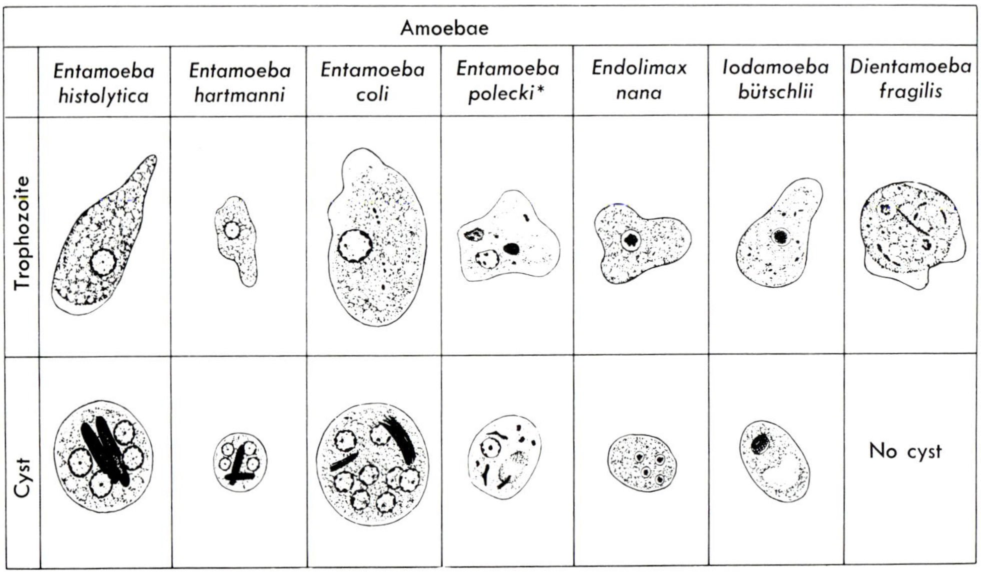

Fig. 34-3. Morphology of amebae found in human stool. (From Brooke, M.M., and Melvin, D.M.: Morphology of diagnostic stages of intestinal parasites of man, Public Health Service Publication no. 1966, Atlanta, 1969, Centers for Disease Control.) *Rare; of animal origin.

Descriptive terminology

The morphologic terminology used in describing the distinguishing criteria of the different species is summarized below (Figs. 34-2 and 34-3).

Trophozoite:

Size: The size of the organism may be compared with the size of red cells (7.5 μm or less in stool) but where size is critical, a calibrated micrometer disk placed in the ocular of the microscope must be used. *Entamoeba histolytica* and *Entamoeba hartmanni* are distinguishable only by size.

Motility: The movement may be progressive or nonprogressive, explosive or slow, and the pseudopods may be blunt or slug shaped.

Nucleus: Only one, with the exception of *Dientamoeba fragilis*.

Peripheral chromatin: Present or absent, with or without a characteristic pattern.

Karyosome: Size and location.

Cytoplasm: Ectoplasm differentiated or undifferentiated; endoplasm granular, coarse, or vacuolated.

Inclusions: Red cells, bacteria, and vacuoles.

Cyst:

Motility: None.

Nucleus: Number, peripheral chromatin, and karyosome.

Size: Varies with organism.

Shape: Ovoid or spheric.

Cytoplasm: Chromatoid bodies (best seen in saline mounts) present or absent.

Glycogen masses: Present or absent.

• • •

NOTE: When confronted with amebic organisms it must first be established whether the organisms are entamebae or other types of amebae. All entamebae are characterized by their "entameba nucleus," which displays a karyosome and peripheral chromatin deposited immediately below the nuclear membrane. This nuclear configuration is not seen in the other amebae, the nuclei of which exhibit mainly karyosomal material of varying shapes, sizes, and location within the nucleus. The nuclear membrane is usually so indistinct that the karyosome appears to be surrounded by a halo.

The cysts of entamebae are often strikingly refractile in saline preparations and are usually round, while the cysts of the other species are less refractile and often ovoid or irregular. The nuclei of the entameba cyst exhibit the characteristics of the nuclei of the entamebic trophozoites.

Once the diagnosis of entameba has been established, *Entamoeba histolytica* must be differentiated from the other species of entamebae.

Entamoeba histolytica

Entamoeba histolytica (Table 34-3 and Figs. 34-2 to 34-5) is the only ameba clearly pathogenic to humans.

Life cycle (Fig. 34-5): The trophozoites produce deep irregular mucosal ulcers in the colon, where they feed on red cells escaping from injured capillaries. The amebic ulcers are responsible for the production of acute amebic dysentery, a form of severe bloody diarrhea. When trophozoites are passed with the diarrheic stool

and are exposed to the outside temperature they die and do not encyst. They are not infective when accidentally ingested but they are the diagnostic criterion of the acute dysenteric form of amebiasis. If they are dislodged from the ulcer bed into the fecal stream they round up and extrude any ingested material to form a precyst. As the precyst matures it forms a cyst wall, the number of nuclei doubles, and inclusions such as glycogen and chromatoid bodies appear in the cytoplasm. The fully mature cyst characterized by four nuclei lacks these inclusions. Cysts form only within the bowel lumen, are infective when passed and ingested, and are diagnostic of the chronic form of amebiasis, which presents a variable clinical picture and may be asymptomatic as in the carrier stage. If the mature cyst is ingested (drinking water contaminated with fecal material), it excysts in the lower small bowel of the new host and finds its way into the colon where it invades the mucosa and multiplies by binary fission. If the amebae break into a blood vessel at the ulcer base, the bloodstream may carry them to the liver or lung where they may form amebic abscesses (amebic hepatitis, amebic hepatic abscess, pleuropulmonary amebiasis).[17]

Habitat: Cecum, large bowel, liver, and rarely lung.

Trophozoite:

Size: 20-60 μm in length. The lower limit of the invasive form is 12 μm. A trophozoite smaller than 10 μm is considered to be a nonpathogenic commensal form referred to as *Entamoeba hartmanni*. This distinction based on size cannot be made on the basis of a single organism but is probably correct if the majority of organisms found measure less than 10 μm in diameter.

Motility: Explosive (sluglike) expulsion of pseudopodia.

Nucleus: One, with fine and even peripheral chromatin and a usually small but not necessarily central karyosome.

Cytoplasm: Finely granular.

Inclusions: Red cells (diagnostic), seldom bacteria.

Cyst:

Size: The cysts measure 10-20 μm. Cysts measuring less than 10 μm are considered to belong to the nonpathogenic genus *Entamoeba hartmanni*.

Nucleus: One to four nuclei are present, similar to the trophozoite nucleus; there are four nuclei in the diagnostic mature stage.

Inclusions: Inclusions include an inconspicuous glycogen vacuole and rodlike chromatoid bodies with rounded, blunt ends. Both inclusions are usually not visualized in the four-nucleated mature cyst.

Remarks: *E. histolytica* shows a distinct periodicity, so that repeated stool examinations are necessary to exclude amebiasis. In proven cases one stool examination is successful in only 30% of cases while three to six examinations are successful in 98% of cases. One proctoscopic examination will detect about 30% of cases.[18] In the acute phase of amebiasis trophozoites predominate and represent the diagnostic feature. In chronic amebiasis both trophozoites and cysts may be passed. The chronic asymptomatic carrier is epidemiologically most important since he excretes mainly infective cysts. Diagnostic difficulties arise when an *E. histolytica*

Table 34-3. Differential diagnosis of human intestinal amebae

	Entamoeba histolytica	*Entamoeba hartmanni*	*Entamoeba coli*	*Endolimax nana*	*Iodamoeba buetschlii*
Trophozoite					
Unstained (saline solution)					
Diameter (μm)	10-60 (15-20)†	5-12* (8-10)	15-50 (20-25)	6-12 (8-10)	9-20 (12-15)
Motility	Active, directional explosive extension of pseudopods	Progressive and sluggish or nonprogressive	Slow; nondirectional pseudopods flow out slowly	Very slow; several blunt pseudopods at one time, nondirectional	Slow; nondirectional blunt pseudopods
Nucleus					
Number	1	1	1	1	1
Visibility	Faint or invisible	Faint or invisible	Visible	Faintly visible	Usually not visible
Cytoplasm	Endoplasm finely granular; vacuolated in degenerated specimens; ectoplasm sharply differentiated	Endoplasm finely granular, ectoplasm sharply differentiated	Endoplasm coarse, granular, vacuolated; ectoplasm not sharply differentiated	Endoplasm granular, vacuolated; ectoplasm not sharply differentiated	Endoplasm granular, vacuolated; ectoplasm not sharply differentiated
Inclusions	Red cells; seldom bacteria	Bacteria	Bacteria, debris	Bacteria, debris	Bacteria, debris, yeast
Nucleus stained with iodine or trichrome					
Karyosome	Small, central, at times eccentric	Small, central	Small, eccentric	One large, irregular, lobulated, central or semicircular	Large, central, surrounded by refractile granules
Peripheral chromatin	Thin, finely granular; uniform in size and distribution	Thin, finely granular; uniform in size and distribution	Heavy, thick, granular; irregular in size and distribution; coarse on one side, fine on the other	None; nuclear membrane dimly stained	None, nuclear membrane dimly stained
Cyst					
Unstained (saline solution)					
Diameter (μ)	10-20 (12-15)	5-10* (6-8)	10-35 (15-25)	5-10 (6-8)	8-20 (10-12)
Shape	Spheroid	Spheroid	Spheroid	Ellipsoid or spheroid	Irregularly ovoid, spheroidal, or triangular
Cytoplasm stained with iodine	Diffuse brown staining in old cysts; well-defined brown glycogen mass in young cysts; chromatoid bodies do not stain	Diffuse brown staining in old cysts; well-defined brown glycogen mass in young cysts; chromatoid bodies do not stain	Diffuse brown staining in old cysts; well-defined brown glycogen mass in young cysts; chromatoid bodies do not stain	Glycogen sometimes present in young cysts	Large distinct mass, dark brown
Nucleus unstained	Faint or invisible	Faint or invisible	Distinct	Faint	Faint or invisible
Nucleus stained with iodine or trichrome	Like trophozoite nucleus	Like trophozoite nucleus	Like trophozoite nucleus	Like trophozoite nucleus	Large eccentric karyosome on one side; achromatic granules on opposite side
Number	4 in mature cyst; 2 in precyst	4 in mature cyst; 2 in precyst	8 in mature cyst; 2 in precyst (seldom found)	4 in mature cyst; 2 in precyst (seldom found)	1 in mature cyst
Chromatoid bodies	Usually 1 or more rodlike with rounded ends; often absent in mature cysts	Usually 1 or more rodlike with rounded ends; often absent in mature cysts	Splinterlike; often absent in mature cysts	None; sometimes small dots or minute rods; often in vacuoles	None

*There may be exceptional size variations.
†Numbers in parentheses indicate usual range.

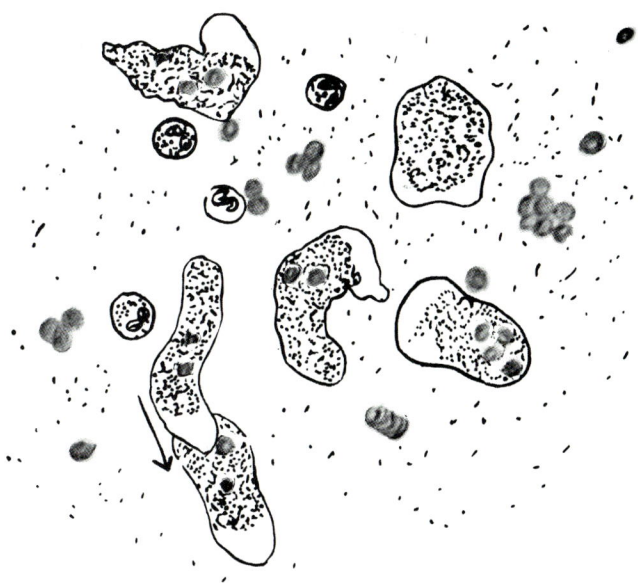

Fig. 34-4. *Entamoeba histolytica* showing ameboid activity and phagocytosis of red cells.

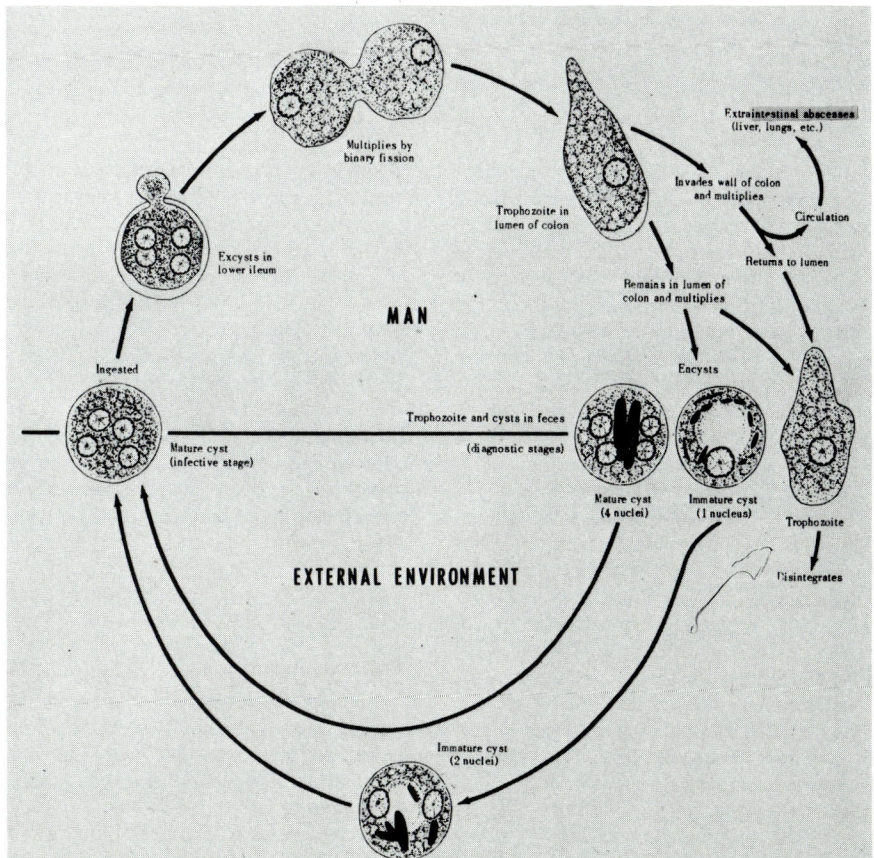

Fig. 34-5. Life cycle of *Entamoeba histolytica*. (From Brooke, M.M., and Melvin, D.M.: Common intestinal protozoa of man, Public Health Service Publication, no. 1140, Atlanta, 1964, Centers for Disease Control.)

Table 34-4. Immunodiagnostic tests for parasitic diseases*

Parasitic diseases	Complement fixation	Agglutination tests			
		Bentonite flocculation	Indirect hemagglutination	Latex	Special agglutination
Amebiasis	1	2	1	2	3†
Chagas' disease	1		1	2	2†
African trypanosomiasis	2		3		3–
Viscereal leishmaniasis	1		1	3	3†
Malaria	2		1	2	
Pneumocystosis	1			3	
Toxoplasmosis	1		1	3	
Ancylostomiasis	3		1	2	
Ascariasis	3	1	1		
Clonorchiasis	1		1		
Cysticercosis	2		2	2	
Echinococcosis	1	1	1	2	
Fascioliasis	1	3	1	2	
Filariasis	2	1	1	3	
Paragonimiasis	1	3	3		
Strongyloidiasis			1		
Schistosomiasis	1	2	1	3	1–
Toxocariasis	3	1	1		
Trichinellosis	1	1	1	1	1§

Modified from Walls, K.W.: In Friedman, H., Linna, T.J., and Prier, J.E., editors: Immunoserology in the diagnosis of infectious diseases.
*1, Evaluated test; 2, experimental test; 3, reported in the literature.
†Direct agglutination.
‡Charcoal agglutination.
§Cholesterol agglutination.

strain is encountered with atypical nuclei that exhibit an eccentric karyosome or uneven peripheral chromatin or with cytoplasm that contains bacteria and vacuoles but no red cells. These morphologic features suggest *Entamoeba coli* and a careful prolonged search for typical organisms must be undertaken. Seldom are both nuclei and cytoplasm atypical. The presence of a mixed infection compounds the problem of identification.

Culture of E. histolytica and other protozoa: All the amebae and flagellates (except *Giardia lamblia*) grow in the initial culture, but only *E. histolytica* grows vigorously in subcultures. Culture of stool specimens for *E. histolytica* is not a practical diagnostic procedure because of the organism's uncertain bacterial requirements, but it is a useful teaching tool that allows the study of live amebae. Several media are available commercially, e.g., the diphasic charcoal medium of McQuay (Dr. R.M. McQuay, Mt. Sinai Hospital, Chicago). This tube medium contains charcoal, glycerine, cholesterol, and acetone. Other media available include Endameese medium (Difco Laboratories, Detroit) and modified Hirsch-Charrod medium (BBL, Microbiology Systems, Cockeysville, Md.)

Inoculation: Emulsify several small stool samples obtained from bloody and mucoid areas in the sterile buffered saline overlay. Incubate the inoculated tubes at 37° C for 48 hr and examine sediment for protozoa.

Serodiagnosis of amebiasis: A number of serologic methods (Table 34-4) are specific, sensitive, and useful for the diagnosis of invasive amebiasis but are relatively insensitive for the detection of the carrier or of the acute or chronic forms of intestinal amebiasis since the latter exhibit minimal tissue invasion or none at all. The traditional complement fixation test is now replaced by the indirect hemagglutination test (IHA),[19] which may be up to 100% positive in cases of amebic liver abscesses and up to 98% positive in acute amebic dysentery.[20-22] A titer of 128 or above is considered positive. The ready availability of antigen prepared from cultured *E. histolytica* has led to the development of several immunodiagnostic tests that are not as time consuming as the IHA test but are equally sensitive and specific. Tests that compare favorable with the IHA test are the indirect fluorescent antibody test,[23-26] the gel diffusion precipitin test,[27,28] and the bentonite flocculation test (see Chapter 35).[29]

Table 34-5 shows the specificity and sensitivity of three serologic tests for amebiasis.

Entamoeba hartmanni

Entamoeba hartmanni is a nonpathogenic commensal organism that closely resembles *Entamoeba histolytica* except in size and nonprogressive movement. Size is **the** differential diagnostic criterion. The correct evaluation of size requires the use of a **calibrated ocular micrometer.** The upper limits of the size of the trophozoite and of the cyst of *E. hartmanni* are below the lower limits of the dimensions of *E. histolytica*. Since the trophozoite survives on bacteria no red cell inclusions are seen within its cytoplasm. The diagnostic features are found in Table 34-3.

		Agglutination tests			
Indirect immuno-fluorescence	Immuno-diffusion	Immunoelectro-phoresis	Countercurrent electrophoresis	Enzyme linked immuno-sorbent assay	Intradermal
1	1	1	2	3	2
1	3	2	3	2	3
2	2			3	
2	3	3			1
1	1	3	3	3	
1					
1	3			3	1
3		3			2
2	2	3		3	2
		3			1
2	2	3	3		3
1	2	1	3	3	1
2	3	3	3		2
1		3			2
	3	3			1
2					
1	2	3		3	1
2	3	3		3	2
1	2	2	3	2	1

Baltimore, 1979, University Park Press.

Table 34-5. Sensitivity and specificity of three serologic tests in amebiasis as compiled from reports in the literature

Human serum	Indirect hem-agglutination		Double diffusion		Indirect immuno-fluorescence	
	No. tested	% Positive	No. tested	% Positive	No. tested	% Positive
Amebic abscesses	314	91	622	92	484	98
Amebic dysentery	514	84	595	72	257	58
Asymptomatic cyst carriers	191	9	19	55	74	23
Patients with other diseases* and healthy people	658	2	198	10	1667	1

From Kagan, I.G.: In Lennette, E.H., et al., editors: Manual of clinical microbiology, ed. 3, Washington, D.C., 1980, American Society for Microbiology.
*Including inflammatory bowel disease.

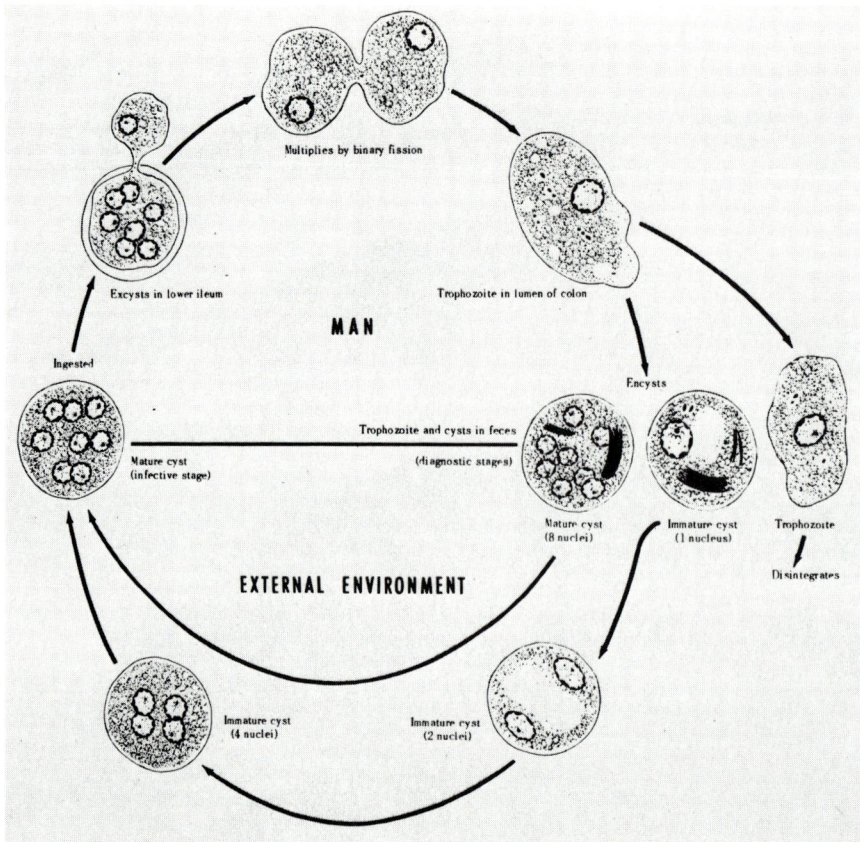

Fig. 34-6. Life cycle of *Entamoeba coli*. (From Brooke, M.M., and Melvin, D.M.: Common intestinal protozoa of man, Public Health Service Publication, no. 1140, Atlanta, 1964, Centers for Disease Control.)

Entamoeba coli

The importance of *Entamoeba coli* (Table 34-3 and Fig. 34-6) lies in the fact that it closely resembles *Entamoeba histolytica* but is a nonpathogenic commensal organism that must carefully and correctly be differentiated from its pathogenic counterpart. The differential diagnosis is presented in Table 34-3. The life cycle (Fig. 34-6) of *E. coli* is similar to that of *E. histolytica*, but it does not invade the mucosa of the colon, which therefore remains intact. It is essentially an intraluminal organism that feeds on bacteria.

Since the organism is not disease producing, trophozoites may be found in normal formed stool.

Trophozoite:

Size: 15-50 μm in length.

Characteristics:

1. Protrusion of pseudopodia not explosive
2. Ingestion of bacteria but not of red cells
3. Considerable chromatin in nucleus, with a distinct peripheral layer and an eccentric karyosome

Cyst:

Size: 10-35 μm in diameter.

Characteristics:

1. Eight or more nuclei, similar to trophozoite nucleus
2. Distinct glycogen mass
3. Usually no chromatid bodies, but when present, the chromatid bodies resemble bars with splintered ends

Since the nuclei of the cyst are distributed at various levels of the globe, it is necessary to move the objective up and down to count them. If only four nuclei are encountered, the organism should **not** be diagnosed as *E. coli*, but rather as *E. histolytica* provided the diagnosis is supported by the other amebae found.

Generally *E. coli* stains heavier and coarser than *E. histolytica*. Since atypical forms of *E. coli* may resemble *E. histolytica*, as many organisms as possible should be examined before a conclusion is reached.

Entamoeba gingivalis

Entamoeba gingivalis may be found in periodontal pockets in some instances of pyorrhea. The trophozoite resembles *Entamoeba histolytica* and when present in sputum may be confused with *E. histolytica* of pulmonary amebiasis. Stained preparations reveal polymorphonuclear cells or fragments thereof in the cytoplasm of *E. gingivalis*. *E. histolytica* trophozoites do not ingest white cells.

Entamoeba polecki

Entamoeba polecki, primarily a parasite of pigs and monkeys, is seldom found in humans but must be distinguished from *Entamoeba histolytica*.[30]

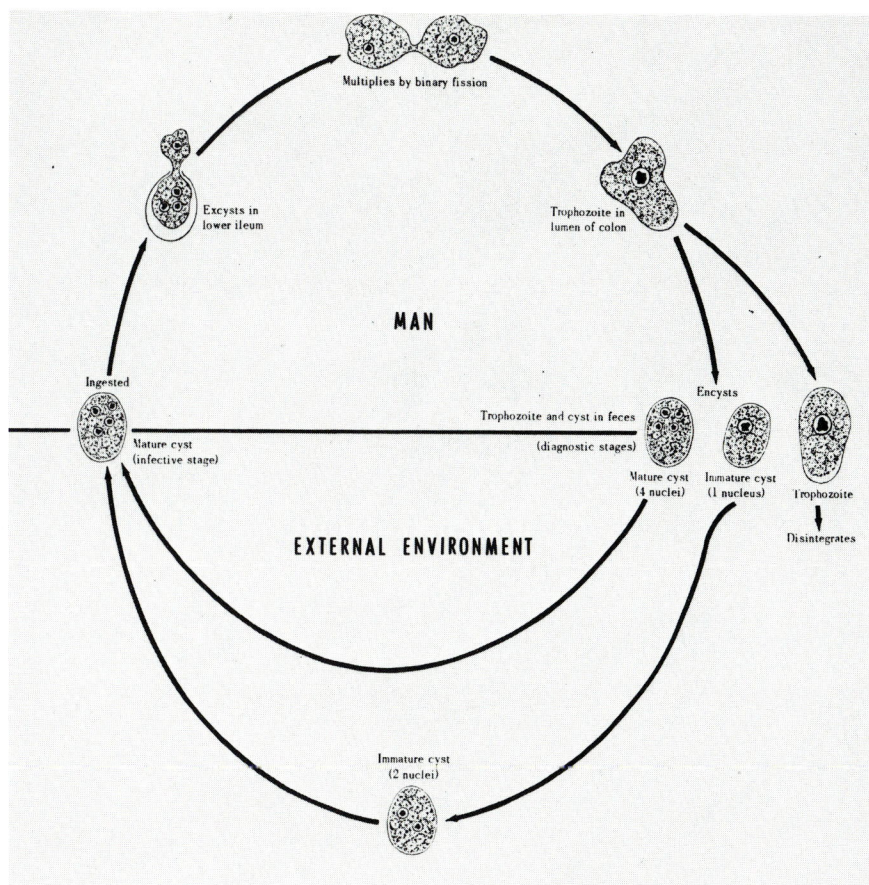

Fig. 34-7. Life cycle of *Endolimax nana*. (From Brooke, M.M., and Melvin, D.M.: Common intestinal protozoa of man, Public Health Service Publication, no. 1140, Atlanta 1964, Centers for Disease Control.)

Endolimax nana

Endolimax nana (Table 34-3 and Fig. 34-7) and *Entamoeba coli* are encountered about twice as frequently as *Entamoeba histolytica*. The trophozoites resemble *Entamoeba hartmanni* in size and in the rapidity with which they produce hyaline pseudopods, but the movement is nondirectional, slow, and sluggish. The cytoplasm is finely granular and contains bacteria. The stained nucleus shows a large central or eccentric or peripheral (semicircular) karyosome, but there is no peripheral chromatin. The cyst is oval (occasionally round) and is of the size of the trophozoite. It contains four nuclei, each showing the above characteristics.

Habitat: Colon.

Trophozoite:

Size: 6-12 μm in length.

Characteristics:
1. Trophozoite is sluggish and shows only minimal locomotion.
2. Blunt hyaline pseudopodia project from the trophozoite.
3. The large karyosome is only seen well in the iodine preparation.
4. Nucleus is spheroid; when stained with trichrome, it shows a thick nuclear membrane that lacks

chromatin beading. The karyosome is large, irregular, and lobulated.

Cyst:

Size: 5-10 μm in diameter.

Characteristics:
1. It is thin walled and oval or spheric.
2. Nucleus is similar to trophozoite nucleus.

Iodamoeba buetschlii

The ameba *Iodamoeba buetschlii* (Table 34-3 and Fig. 34-3) owes its name to the large smooth glycogen vacuole that is always seen in its cyst stage. Glycogen vacuoles are also seen in young cysts of other amebae, but theirs are usually smaller and often irregular in outline. In the saline preparation the trophozoite's movement is nondirectional with blunt pseudopods. The cytoplasm is coarsely granular and loaded with bacteria. The nucleus of the trophozoite is not seen in saline preparations but the addition of iodine reveals a large, irregular, more or less central karyosome. The permanently stained nucleus shows the karyosome surrounded by a halo since the nuclear membrane is not visible or is indistinct. Fine chromatin granules may surround the nucleus. The cyst is ovoid and irregular and in the unstained preparation the cyst wall and the glycogen mass

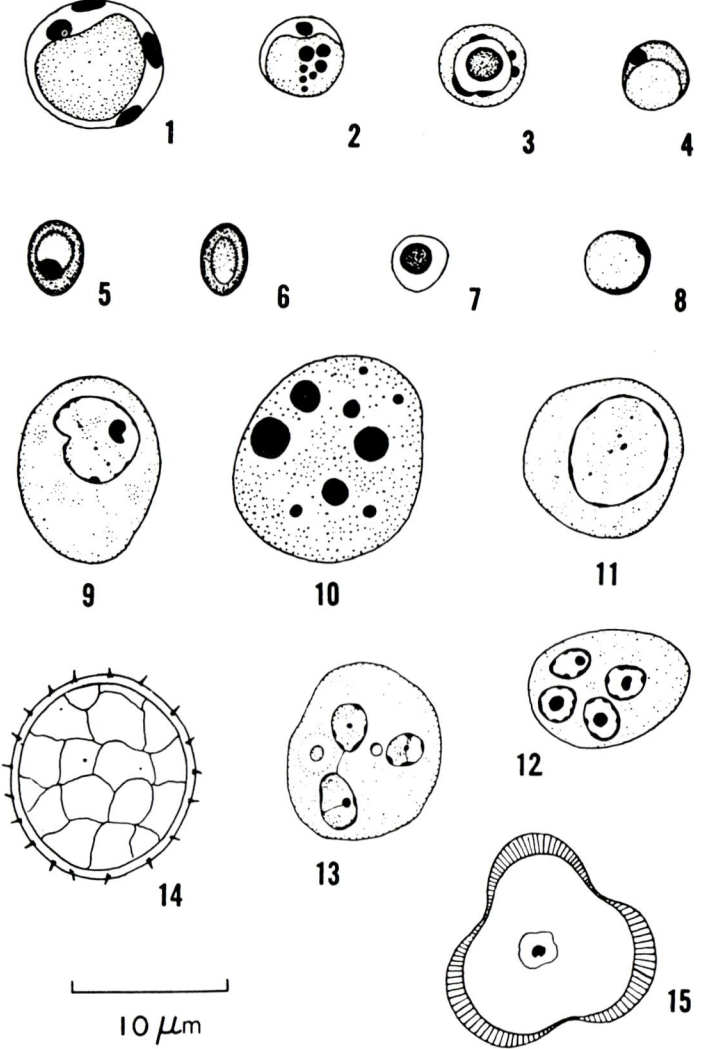

Fig. 34-8. Various structures that may be seen in stool preparations. **1, 2,** and **4,** *Blastocystis hominis*. **3, 5, 6, 7,** and **8,** Various yeasts. **9** and **11,** Squamous cells from rectal mucosa. **10,** Deteriorated macrophages without nucleus. **12** and **13,** Polymorphonuclear leukocytes. **14** and **15,** ''Pollen grains.'' (From Markell, E.K., and Voge, M.: Medical parasitology, ed. 3, Philadelphia, 1971, W.B. Saunders Co.)

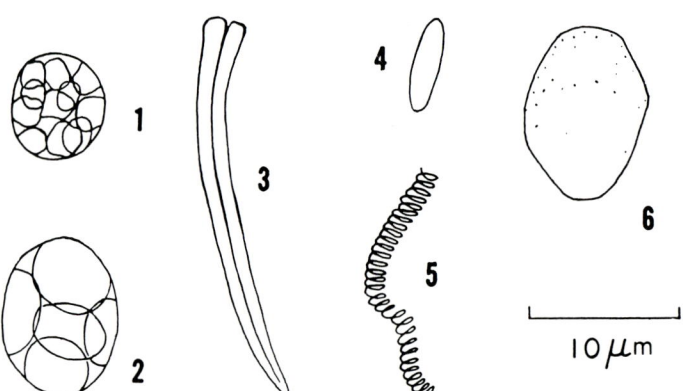

Fig. 34-9. Plant structures seen in stool. **1** and **2,** Aggregates of starch granules. **3,** Plant hair. **4** and **6,** Amorphous vegetable materials, superficially resembling ova or protozoan cysts. **5,** Vegetable spiral. (From Markell, E.K., and Voge, M.: Medical parasitology, ed. 3, Philadelphia, 1971, W.B. Saunders Co.)

light up because of their refractility. Iodine stains the glycogen mass brown but in the trichrome preparation a vacuole indicates the location from which the glycogen has been dissolved out. The cyst has only one nucleus, which in the trichrome preparation exhibits a nuclear membrane often hugging a large eccentric round to irregular karyosome. The chromatin granules may form a half-moon around the karyosome. There is no peripheral chromatin.

Habitat: Colon.

Trophozoite:

Size: 9-20 μm in length.

Characteristics:

1. Trophozoite is rarely seen; it is a sluggish organism that produces broad hyaline pseudopodia.
2. Nucleus is not seen in the unstained preparation. In the stained preparation the nucleus is large with an achromatic nuclear membrane and a large centrally placed karyosome.

Cyst:

Size: 8-20 μm in diameter.

Characteristics:

1. Cyst is thick walled, irregular in shape, and characteristically contains a large round or oval glycogen mass.
2. Stained nucleus shows an unbeaded, thin membrane and a large, often eccentric karyosome in contact with the nuclear membrane.
3. The nucleus is not visible in the unstained preparation and the glycogen mass appears as a vacuole. In the stained preparation (iodine) the glycogen mass is well delineated and dark brown.

Structures resembling intestinal protozoa

There are fecal components that may be mistaken for protozoa when temporary stains are used. In permanent preparations these mistakes are less likely to occur. The following structures may be mistaken for protozoa (Figs. 34-8 and 34-9).

Yeast: The organism is small, ovoid to spheric, and may be mistaken for *Endolimax nana* cysts.

Pollen grains: Pollen grains may resemble protozoan cysts.

Blastocystis hominis: *Blastocystis hominis* is a yeast that is often found in feces and is sometimes mistaken for a cyst of some intestinal parasite.

It is ovoid or spheric, 10-15 μm in diameter, and surrounded by a cyst wall–like membrane (Fig. 34-10).

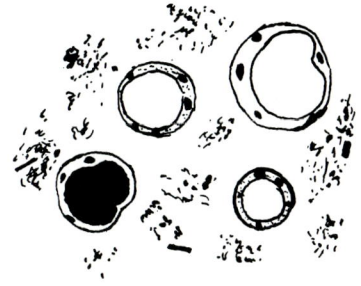

Fig. 34-10. *Blastocystis hominis* from human feces. (Oil-immersion lens.)

The cytoplasm is hyaline and refractive. The outer layer of the cytoplasm contains refractive granules. One or more nuclei are often seen in unstained as well as in iodine-stained preparations. The entire cytoplasm stains brownish with iodine.

Macrophages: The cytoplasm is hyaline, uninucleate, vacuolated, and may contain red cells. Macrophages lack mobility, but they send out pseudopodia. They are usually accompanied by polymorphonuclear cells (which themselves may be found confusing), and the nucleus is more prominent than it would be in the unstained trophozoite.

Free-living amebae

Numerous groups of free-living amebae can be found in stagnant water and in decaying vegetation. Organisms belonging to the genera *Acanthamoeba* and *Naegleria* were considered harmless free-living organisms until Culbertson et al.[31] described pathogenic forms. *Naegleria* species are the etiologic agent of primary **acute amebic meningoencephalitis** and *Acanthamoeba* species cause **chronic granulomatous amebic meningoencephalitis**[32,22] and have also been identified as the causative agent of eye infections.[34] The pathogenic free-living amebae secrete cytolytic enzymes.[35]

Diagnosis: The diagnostic procedures for both organisms are similar. **Wet mounts** of the fresh spinal fluid reveal the unstained actively moving living amebae among a mixture of pus and red cells. The use of phase-contrast microscopy aids in the diagnosis of the amebae in their native forms. In gram-stained preparations the amebae are easily missed since they resemble degenerated white cells, but on **Wright-stained films** of the cerebrospinal fluid sediment the amebae can be recognized. **Hematoxylin stains,** e.g., phosphotungstic acid and hematoxylin (PTAH), allow recognition of nuclear details. Refrigeration is fatal to the organisms, and centrifugation is followed by locomotion paralysis. The amebae can be **cultured** on nonnutrient agar plates that are streaked with live *Entamoeba coli* bacteria. The differentiation of the two species of free-living amebae is outlined below. Intracerebral inoculation of mice with spinal fluid sediment or a tissue emulsion will produce infection, allowing demonstration of the organisms in the animal brain and spinal fluid.

Naegleria species

Naegleria (Fig. 34-11) produces an **acute, fulminating, necrotizing, hemorrhagic meningoencephalitis** by gaining entrance to the base of the brain via the nasal passages and the olfactory bulbs. The infection is acquired by **immunologically normal healthy individuals** from sewage water in man-made lakes and from infected heated swimming pools. Affected tissues contain the trophozoites but no cysts.[31,36,37] *Naegleria* organisms are **triphasic,** having amebic, flagellate, and cystic forms. The cysts are not infective for humans.[38]

Amebic form:

Size: Sluglike shape; 22 × 7 μm.

Motility: Progressive, directional, wavelike motion of pseudopods, explosive.

Nucleus: There is a single nucleus, which is indistinct in fresh and saline preparations. When stained by

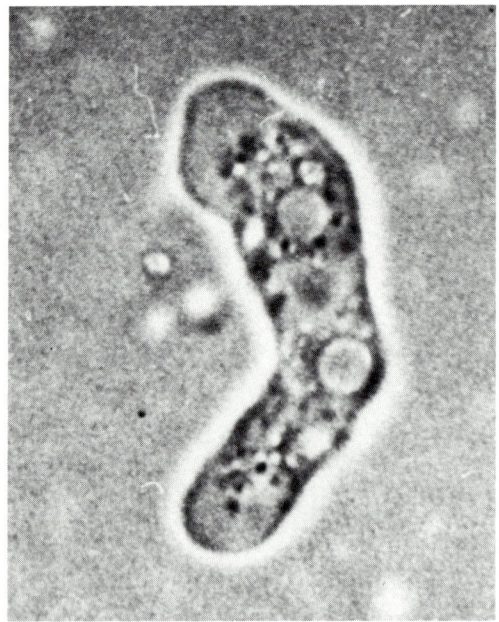

Fig. 34-11. *Naegleria fowleri* (trophozoite) in spinal fluid of patient with primary amebic meningoencephalitis. (Courtesy R.F. Carter, North Adelaide, South Australia.)

the addition of 1 drop of 1% cresyl fast violet, a fine nuclear membrane with fine sparse peripheral chromatin and a central karyosome can be differentiated.

Cytoplasm: Contractile vacuoles, bacteria, and red cells are present; when stained as above, granular **endoplasm** can be differentiated from clear **ectoplasm.**

Flagellate form: Temporary flagellate forms occur in agar culture and when warm, sterile water is added to spinal fluid. The appearance of flagellate forms within 1-2 hr is a diagnostic feature of *Naegleria* organisms.

Cyst form:

Size: 7-10 μm in diameter.

Shape: Spheroid.

Nucleus: There is a single nucleus, which is not seen in saline mounts. Stained preparations show it to be very small, 1.5 μm in diameter, with no peripheral chromatin but with a tiny central karyosome.

Cytoplasm: In stained preparations the cytoplasm contains eosinophilic granules.

Culture: Naegleria grows well on plain nonnutrient agar covered with live *Escherichia coli* at 37° C. The growing amebae form a sharply defined advancing demarcation line, separating them from the bacteria-smeared agar. Pathogenic strains can be differentiated from nonpathogenic strains by the use of isolation media and animal inoculation.

Acanthamoeba species

Amebic meningoencephalitis is a **chronic granulomatous,** opportunistic infection caused by *Acanthamoeba* species in immunologically compromised or chronically ill patients. The portal of entry of the organism is the respiratory system and the parasite reaches the brain via the bloodstream. Because of the

hematogenous dissemination other organs are involved as well.

Trophozoite:

Size: 25-35 μm in length.

Motility: Pseudopods are tapering projections, with active directional locomotion.

Nucleus: Single nucleus with delicate membrane and no peripheral chromatin, karyosome central and round.

Cytoplasm: Bacteria, spongy, vacuoles.

Cyst: 10-15 μm round or stellate, accompany trophozoites within lesions.

Culture: The method described above for *Naegleria* is also used for acanthamoebae, but the latter do not metamorphose into flagellate forms.

Intestinal flagellates

The most important intestinal flagellates are *Dientamoeba fragilis,*[39] *Giardia lamblia, Trichomonas hominis,* and *Chilomastix mesnili.* The incidence varies greatly, but the distribution is cosmopolitan. Smaller flagellates, *Retortamonas intestinalis* and *Enteromonas hominis,* are less frequently found but may be confusing. Reproduction is by longitudinal division. Resistant forms (cysts) occur, except in *Dientamoeba fragilis* and *Trichomonas* (Table 34-6). *Dientamoeba fragilis, Giardia lamblia,* and *Trichomonas vaginalis* are the only organisms of clinical importance; *Giardia* and *Dientamoeba* are important because they may cause gastrointestinal symptoms and *T. vaginalis* because it causes vaginitis and cervical dysplastic epithelial changes. In the living state, flagellates—except *Dientamoeba*—can be identified by their characteristic body and flagellar movements while on stained smear preparations the trichrome stain brings out their morphologic details.

The diagnostic procedures for flagellates include direct wet film preparations with saline solutions and hanging drop preparations. Permanently stained preparations are also useful.

The differential diagnosis takes into account the following characteristics of trophozoite and cyst.

Trophozoite: Type of movement, shape, size, and number of nuclei, flagella, and undulating membrane.

Cyst: Shape, size, and number of nuclei and fibrils.

Dientamoeba fragilis

In past years *Dientamoeba* (Table 34-3 and Fig. 34-3) was classified as an ameba, but because of its two nuclei, absence of a cyst phase, and electron-microscopic evidence of flagellar rudiments,[40] it is now classified among the trichomonads despite the missing flagellum. The organism is responsible for attacks of acute gastroenteritis.

The trophozoite in saline preparations has blunt, broad, hyaline pseudopods but lacks locomotion. The nuclei (or nucleus) are not visible in saline preparations, but in stained smears the nuclei are characteristic. There is no peripheral chromatin and the nuclear membrane is faint, but the karyosome is seen to consist of four to six blocks of chromatin that are quite distinct in hematoxylin stains but appear to fuse in trichrome stains. Eighty percent of the organisms are binucleated. The cytoplasm is smooth to finely granular and contains bacteria. **The cyst stage is not known.** If small binucleated cysts are encountered they may be *Enteromonas hominis* cysts, i.e., cysts of an uncommon small flagellate.

Habitat: Colon.

Trophozoite:

Size: 5-15 μm in length.

Characteristics:

1. Trophozoite is characteristically binucleated. With trichrome stain the delicate nuclear membrane is hardly visible and only the large lobulated central karyosome stands out. The karyosome is composed of groups of chromatin granules. The nuclei may be connected by a dark-staining thread. Nuclear outline cannot be seen in the fresh preparation.
2. Pseudopodia are clear and indented, often leading to a cloverleaf-like appearance of the organism.

Cyst: Encysted stage has not been identified.

Chilomastix mesnili

The trophozoite of *Chilomastix mesnili* (Table 34-6 and Fig. 34-12) is pear shaped and the anterior broad end gives rise to three flagella that curve posteriorly in a shepherd's crook curve. In fresh preparations a spiral groove is seen to run the length of the body. The movement has been described as twisting and corkscrew like.

Habitat: Intestine, chiefly colon.

Trophozoite:

Size: 6-24 (10-15) μm in length.

Characteristics:

1. The trophozoite is pear shaped, rounded anteriorly and pointed posteriorly, with a characteristic oblique spiral groove across the ventral surface.
2. Motility is stiff—boring type of rotary movement.
3. Three flagella arise from the anterior end and a fourth (not usually seen) arises within the large mouthlike cavity or cytostome and extends across the body.
4. There is a large oval nucleus near the anterior end.

Cyst:

Size: 6-9 μm in diameter.

Characteristics:

1. The cyst is pyriform or spheroid (lemon shaped), extremely small, and hyaline. The lemon shape is caused by a characteristic nipplelike elevation that is separated from the cytoplasm by a clear area.
2. There is a single nucleus, invisible in saline solution.
3. Cytostome and fibrils extend across the cyst.

Diagnosis: The salient feature of the unstained living organism is its method of locomotion. It moves with a spiraling counterclockwise rotation of the body (Table 34-6 and Fig. 34-12).

Trichomonas hominis

Trichomonas hominis (Table 34-6 and Figs. 34-12 and 34-13) is a nonpathogenic organism found in feces, which by its habitat and morphologic details can be distinguished from the other two species of *Trichomonas*, *Trichomonas vaginalis* and *Trichomonas tenax*. The morphologic details are summarized below.

Diagnosis: Diagnosis is based on the observation of the living unstained organism in a saline suspension of a stool specimen in which its rapidly darting, jerky movement draws attention to its existence. The organism is characterized by an undulating membrane and is difficult to recognize when dead or in a stained preparation.

Habitat: Colon.

Trophozoite:

Size: 5-15 μm in length.

Characteristics:

1. The trophozoite is pear shaped, rounded anteriorly and pointed posteriorly, with a central axostyle that projects beyond the posterior end.
2. There is an undulating membrane on one side terminating in a flagellum posteriorly.
3. There are four flagella from anterior end; number varies with the species. The posterior flagellum arises anteriorly, runs posteriorly incorporated in the free edge of the undulating membrane, and projects beyond the posterior end of the organism as a free flagellum.
4. The nucleus is near the anterior end.
5. Motility is jerky, rapid, and darting.

Cyst: The cyst stage is unknown.

Trichomonas vaginalis

The morphologic characteristics of *Trichomonas vaginalis* are summarized below. It differs from *Trichomonas hominis* by the fact that the undulating membrane is short and the recurrent flagellum does not extend beyond the body of the organism (Table 34-6 and Fig. 34-14).

Habitat: Urogenital apparatus. The organism may be present in vaginal or urethral exudate, in urine, or in prostatic secretion, the result of prostatic massage.

Trophozoite:

Size: 7-23 μm in length.

Characteristics:

1. Pear shaped, rounded anteriorly, and pointed posteriorly with a central axostyle projecting beyond the posterior end
2. Undulating membrane extends three fourths of the length of the body and is not continued into a free flagellum
3. Four flagella from the anterior end
4. Nucleus near anterior end
5. Motility: jerky, rapid, darting

Diagnosis:

Vaginal and urethral swabs: The swabs (Culturette [Scientific Products, McGaw Park, Ill.]) must not be allowed to dry and must be moistened with a small amount of saline. Immediately after the receipt of the swab, several drops of saline are placed on the microscope slide and the swab is dipped into the saline and whirled so as to enlarge the area of the drop slightly. Since the tip of the swab may absorb some of the saline, additional saline drops may be required. A coverslip is then applied over the drop, and the specimen is examined under the high dry objective of the micro-

Table 34-6. Morphologic differentiation of flagellates

	Dientamoeba fragilis	*Chilomastix mesnili*	*Trichomonas hominis*
Trophozoite			
Shape	Amebic	Pear shaped	Pear shaped
Size (μm)	5-15 (9-12)*	10-20 (10-15)	5-15 (7-9)
Flagella	Not visible	3 anterior; 1 in cytostome	4 anterior; 1 posterior
Nucleus	1-2 not visible in saline	1, not visible in saline	1, not visible in saline
Movement	Pseudopodia nonprogressive	Stiff, rotary	Jerky, rapid
Other characteristics	Cytoplasm granular	Spiral grooves; cytostome	Undulating membrane; axostyle
Cyst			
Size (μm)	No cyst stage	6-10	No cyst stage
Shape		Anterior hook; lemon shaped	

*Numbers in parentheses indicate usual length.

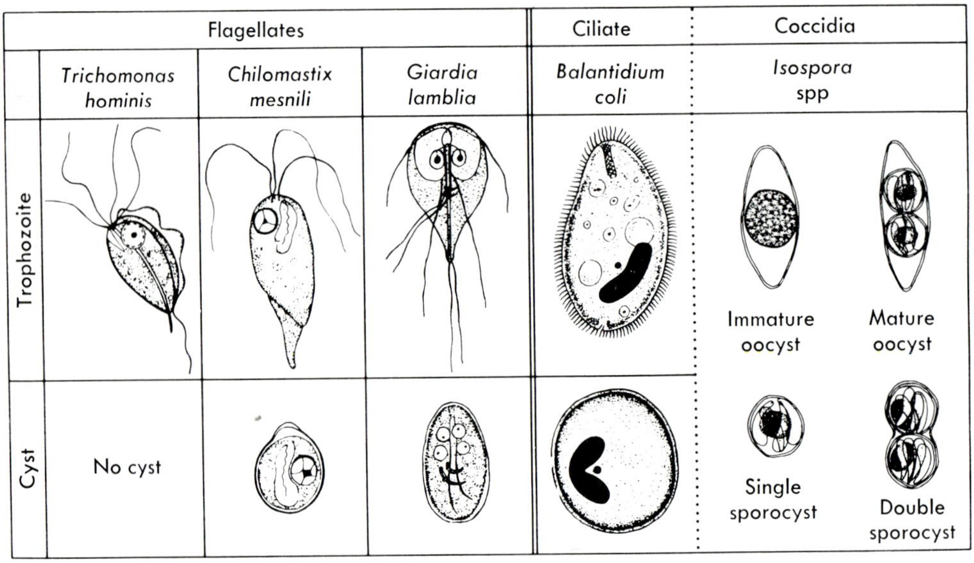

Fig. 34-12. Morphology of flagellates, ciliates, and coccidia found in human stool. (From Brooke, M.M., and Melvin, D.M.: Morphology of diagnostic stages of intestinal parasites of man, Public Health Service Publication no. 1966, Atlanta, 1969, Centers for Disease Control.)

Trichomonas vaginalis	*Trichomonas tenax*	*Giardia lamblia*	*Retortamonas intestinalis*	*Enteromonas hominis*
Pear shaped	Pear shaped	Pear shaped	Ovoid	Oval
7-23 (5-15)	6-12 (6-7)	4-20 (5-15)	4-10 (6-7)	4-10 (8-9)
4 anterior	4 anterior; 1 posterior	4 anterior; 2 ventral; 2 caudal	1 anterior; 1 posterior	3 anterior; 1 posterior
1, not visible in saline	1, not visible in saline	2, not visible in saline	1, not visible in saline	1, not visible in saline
Jerky, rapid	Jerky, rapid	Kitelike; falling leaf; tumbling	Jerky	Jerky
No posterior flagellum; short, undulating membrane	No posterior flagellum	Sucking disk; pear shaped front view; spoon shaped side view	Cytostome	Pointed short tail attached to oval body
No cyst stage	No cyst stage	7-19 Oval	4-7 Pear shaped	6-8 Resemble *E. nana* cysts

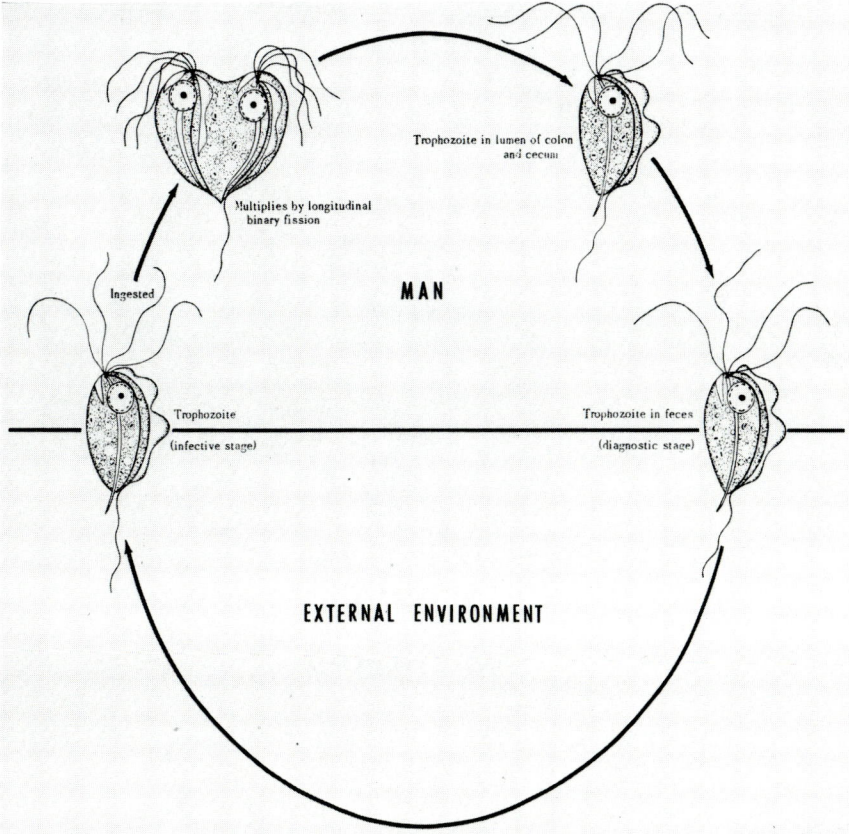

Fig. 34-13. Life cycle of *Trichomonas hominis*. (From Brooke, M.M., and Melvin, D.M.: Common intestinal protozoa of man, Public Health Service Publication, no. 1140, Atlanta, 1964, Centers for Disease Control.)

scope for living, rapidly moving *Trichomonas* organisms. The flagella and the undulating membrane can easily be identified. The dead or stained organisms are difficult to identify.

Urine: The sediment of a spun specimen is placed on a microscope slide and is covered by a coverslip. Again, living *Trichomonas* organisms are looked for. Chilling the specimen must be prevented since the chilled organisms lose their motility.

Trichomonas tenax

Trichomonas tenax may be found in pyorrheic pockets in conjunction with *Entamoeba gingivalis*. Morphologic characteristics are summarized below and in Table 34-6.

Habitat: Mouth, tonsils.

Trophozoite:

Size: 6-12 μm in length.

Characteristics:

1. Pear shaped, oval, similar to *Trichomonas vaginalis*
2. Four anterior flagella
3. Single anterior nucleus not seen in saline preparations
4. No free flagellum, but axostyle extends beyond body
5. Undulating membrane extending length of body

Cyst: Not known.

Diagnosis: A swab is used to scrape the periodontal area and is not allowed to dry. On receipt it is immediately dipped into a drop of saline placed on a microscope slide. The swab is used to spread the drop; a coverslip is then applied and the drop is examined under the high dry objective of the microscope. The organism is recognized by its jerky motility and by its flagellar arrangement.

Giardia lamblia

Giardia lamblia is a pathogenic flagellate found in the duodenal contents and bile. In the duodenum it can be demonstrated in the mucosal crypts where it attaches itself to the mucosal cells producing a form of gastroenteritis (giardiasis). When swept into the fecal stream the trophozoites encyst, so that most stool specimens contain the encysted parasite rather than the flagellate form, which is only found in severe diarrhea. The symmetric appearance of the trophozoite and of the cyst allows easy recognition (Fig. 34-12). Ventrally the trophozoite has one large sucking disk, and it has two nuclei and several pairs of flagella. One pair of chromatoid bodies called *parabasal bodies* crosses the central segment of the double midline axostyles. The cyst contains four nuclei, which may be difficult to see (Table 34-6).

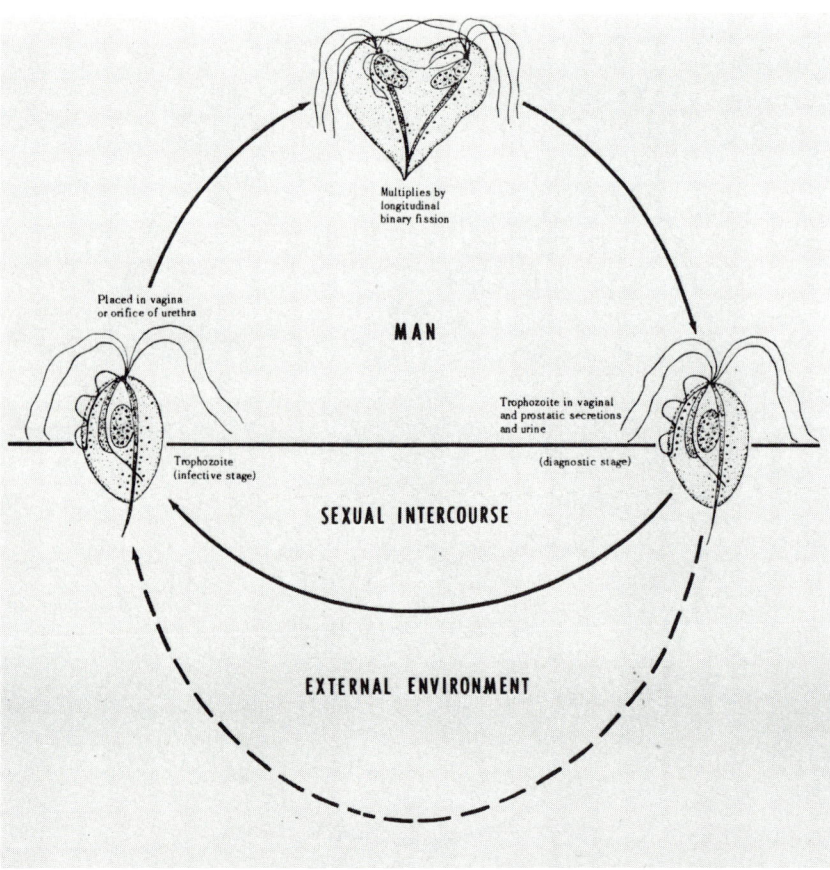

Fig. 34-14. Life cycle of *Trichomonas vaginalis*. (From Brooke, M.M., and Melvin, D.M.: Common intestinal protzoa of man, Public Health Service Publication, no. 1140, Atlanta, 1964, Centers for Disease Control.)

Habitat: Duodenum chiefly; gallbladder.
Trophozoite:
Size: 10 × 20 μm in length.
Characteristics:
1. Pear shaped, pointed posterior end
2. Sucking disk on ventral side of blunt end
3. Two nuclei
4. Eight pairs of flagella
5. Motility: spinning movement; "falling leaf"
Cyst:
Size: 7 × 19 μm.
Characteristics:
1. Oval and refractile
2. Four nuclei, usually at one end
3. Two curved longitudinal axostyles in center
4. Cytoplasm: shrunk away from cell membrane
Diagnosis: Saline and iodine-stained wet preparations as well as stained films of feces or bile are suitable. The unstained organism is shaped like a top, has a suction cup, and resembles the face of a tennis racket. The organism has a spinning and flip-flop movement. Stool is foul, steatorrheic, and foamy. In chronic diarrhea duodenal aspiration may be necessary to find the organism. It may also be encountered in the T-tube drainage of the common bile duct. Iodine staining of

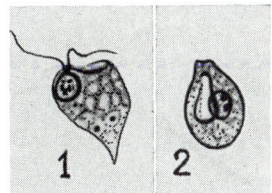

Fig. 34-15. *Embadomonas intestinalis.* **1,** Trophozoite. **2,** Cyst. (From Kourí, P., and Basnuevo, J.G.: Lecciónes de parasitología y medicina tropical, Havana, 1941, El Siglo XX. Adapted from Dobell, C., and O'Connor, F.W.: Intestinal protozoa in man, London, 1921, John Bale, Sons, and Danielsson.)

the cyst with its diffuse brown-staining glycogen may obscure the structural details. So characteristic is the appearance of the organism that only unstained saline wet films may be necessary for the diagnosis. The periodicity of the organism may make several stool examinations necessary and since saline laxatives act in the colon they are ineffective in aiding the diagnosis of giardiasis. The trichrome-stained organism shows all the details described above.

Retortamonas (Embadomonas) intestinalis

Retortamonas intestinalis (Fig. 34-15 and Table 34-6) is a rare nonpathogenic flagellate of humans that is probably acquired from contact with insects, frogs, and turtles.
Trophozoite:
Size: 4-10 μm in length.
Motility: Two anterior flagella.
Nucleus: If the nucleus is unstained it is not visible; stained, it is seen to be close to the anterior end. It shows fairly heavy peripheral chromatin and an eccentric karyosome.
Cytoplasm: Granular.
Inclusions: Bacteria.
Cyst:
Size: 4-7 μm.
Characteristics: Pear shaped; nucleus flanked laterally by fibrils.

Enteromonas hominis

Enteromonas hominis (Fig. 34-16 and Table 34-6) is a rare nonpathogenic flagellate that only temporarily inhabits the large bowel contents.
Trophozoite:
Size: 4-10 μm in length.
Motility: Three anterior flagella; one posterior flagellum that skirts the body and projects posteriorly as a free flagellum.
Nucleus: The nucleus is not visible in unstained wet films. In stained preparations there is a large karyosome in the center and a well-stained nuclear membrane.

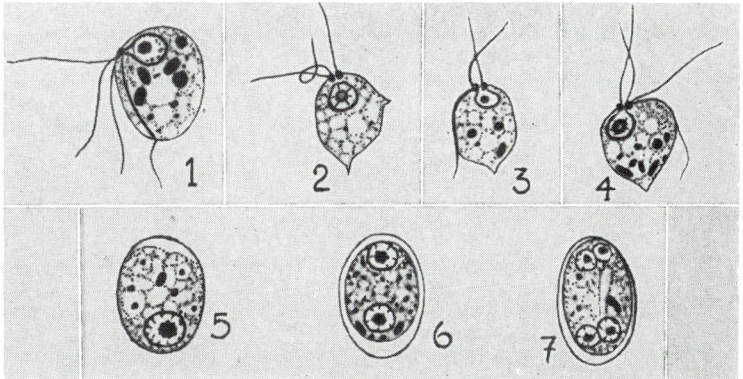

Fig. 34-16. *Enteromonas hominis.* **1,** Typical form of trophozoite with four flagella, three free and one recurrent. **2,** Recurrent flagellum is not clearly visible. **3,** Only two anterior flagella are visible. **4,** Typical form showing two blepharoplasts. **5-7,** Cysts uninucleate, binucleate, and quadrinucleate (mature), respectively. (From Kourí, P., and Basnuevo, J.G.: Lecciónes de parasitología y medicina tropical, Havana, 1941, El Siglo XX. Adapted from Dobell, C., and O'Connor, F.W.: Intestinal protozoa in man, London, 1921, John Bale, Sons, and Danielsson.)

Cytoplasm: Granular.
Inclusions: Bacteria and vacuoles.
Cyst:
Size: Ovoid, 6-8 μm in length.
Nucleus: Two to four, usually two at opposite ends of the cyst; structure as in trophozoite.

Blood and subcutaneous flagellates: hemoflagellates

Hemoflagellates are blood and tissue flagellates, two forms (genera) of which are of medical importance: *Leishmania* and *Trypanosoma*. Each has a vertebrate and an invertebrate host. They produce seven important diseases in humans; four are produced by *Leishmania* and three are produced by *Trypanosoma*. *Leishmania* produces kala-azar, oriental sore, mucocutaneous leishmaniasis, and Chiclero ulcer. *Trypanosoma* produces West African trypanosomiasis, East African trypanosomiasis, and Chagas' disease.

Morphologic forms

There are four developmental stages of hemoflagellates: leishmanial, leptomonad, crithidial, and trypanosomal (Fig. 34-17), which have been renamed amastigote (leishmonad form), promastigote (leptomonad form), epimastigote (crithidial form), and trypomastigote (trypanosomal form). The word "mastic" stands for lip or flagellum (Tables 34-7 and 34-8).

Each developmental stage contains a nucleus with a karyosome, a cytoplasmic kinetoplast consisting of a rodlike parabasal body and a dotlike blepharoplast, and a rhizoplast (flagellum). The latter may extend from the blepharoplast beyond the anterior (flagellar) end as a free flagellum. An undulating membrane may also be present. The characteristics of the four stages are as given in Table 34-8.

Leishmanial or amastigote form (Leishman-Donovan or L-D bodies): The parasite is intracellular in the reticuloendothelial system. It is ovoid, measures 1.5-5 μm, and contains the previously mentioned structures but no undulating membrane or free flagellum (Fig. 34-18).

In tissue sections and imprints, two diseases must be differentiated from visceral leishmaniasis. They are (1) histoplasmosis, a fungus disease caused by *Histoplasma capsulatum*, and (2) toxoplasmosis, a protozoan disease caused by *Toxoplasma gondii*. *Toxoplasma* lacks the kinetoplast and is not found in large numbers in phagocytic cells but rather in mesenchymal cells. *H. capsulatum* also lacks the kinetoplast and is also found in phagocytic histiocytes but stains with PAS and Gomori methenamine silver stains, which fail to stain L-D bodies.

Leptomonad or promastigote form: In the leptomonad stage the parasite is a slender, elongated spindle-shaped organism (14-20 × 1.5-3.5 μm) that exhibits the previously mentioned structures except for an undulating membrane. The kinetoplast is situated close to the anterior (flagellar) end and gives rise to a single flagellum.

Crithidial or epimastigote form: A spindle-shaped organism (10-20 × 1-3 μm), the crithidial form exhibits all the structures mentioned, including an undulating membrane, a flagellum, and a kinetoplast.

Trypanosomal or trypomastigote form: The trypanosomal form is a spindle-shaped organism exhibit-

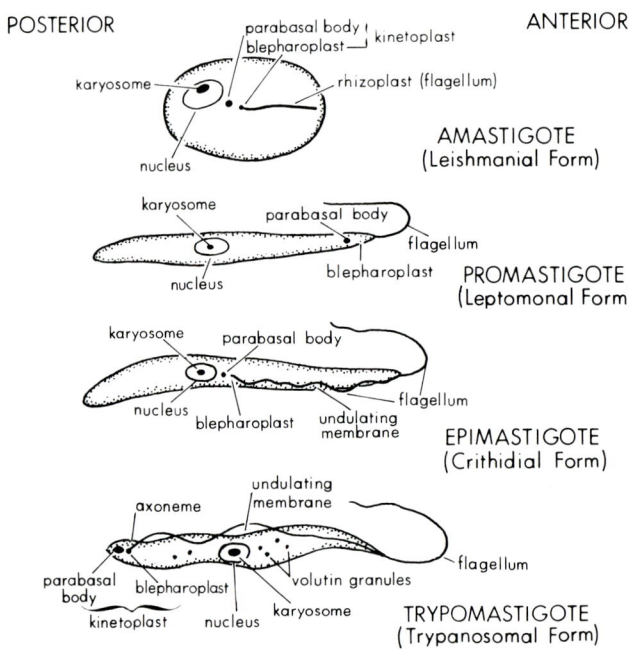

Fig. 34-17. Amastigote, promastigote, epimastigote, and trypomastigote forms of *Trypanosoma*. (Modified from Hunter, G., et al.: Manual of tropical medicine, ed. 4, Philadelphia, 1966, W.B. Saunders Co.)

ing all the structures mentioned, including a flagellum and an undulating membrane. The kinetoplast is posterior to the nucleus.

Not all species exhibit all four forms. *Leishmania* usually exists in the leishmanial form in humans and in the leptomonad form in the insect host and in culture. *Trypanosoma* exists in the trypanosomal form in humans and in the crithidial form in the insect host; *T. cruzi* and *T. rangeli* show all four forms.

Leishmania

The clinical manifestations of leishmaniasis depend on the infecting species. The three species found in humans are morphologically identical but can be differentiated serologically. They also differ in cultural characteristics, clinical manifestations, and species of vector. *Leishmania donovani* (the cause of visceral leishmaniasis, or kala-azar), *Leishmania tropica* (the cause of oriental sore, or cutaneous leishmaniasis of the Old World), and *Leishmania braziliensis* (the cause of mucocutaneous leishmaniasis of the New World) are closely related strains.

Life cycle: The basic life cycle is the same for all three *Leishmania* species. The vector (various species of sandflies) ingests the parasites in their amastigote form at the time of a blood meal. The amastigotes (leishmanial forms) parasitize monocytes, polymorphonuclear cells, and capillary endothelial cells. In the sandfly they are liberated from the aspirated cells and transform into the promastigotes, which mutiply and are introduced into a new victim at the site of the next blood meal. From the site of the bite the parasite makes its way to the organs of the reticuloendothelial system (liver, spleen, bone marrow) or to the macrophages and monocytes of the skin. The reservoirs of infection are usually humans, dogs, or wild rodents. The parasite occurs in the leishmanial and the leptomonad forms only, the first in humans and the second in sandflies.

Diagnosis of Leishmania donovani

In endemic areas the clinical combination of hepatosplenomegaly and leukopenia is highly suggestive of visceral leishmaniasis (kala-azar), but the definitive diagnosis requires demonstration of the parasite in tissues.

Blood smear: A thick and thin peripheral blood smear prepared as for the diagnosis of malaria should be examined first. Better results are obtained from the examination of a buffy coat smear since the patients are usually leukopenic with an absolute monocytosis. The Wright-Giemsa stain reveals the parasite within monocytes.

Bone marrow and splenic aspiration smears and imprints are stained with Giemsa stain and examined for reticulum cells containing L-D bodies.

Liver biopsy: Examine tissue sections for L-D bodies.

Animal inoculation: Hamsters, mice, and guinea pigs are susceptible to intraperitoneal injection of infected blood and splenic or lymph node material.

Culture: Leptomonad forms are produced in the condensation water of rabbit blood culture medium (NNN medium), which is not difficult to prepare.

NNN medium for Leishmania:

1. Bacto-agar (Difco Laboratories, Detroit), 14 g
2. Sodium chloride, 6 g
3. Distilled water, 9 dl

Bring mixture to boil and neutralize with 0.1N NaOH. Distribute 9 dl of media into six flasks (150 ml each) and sterilize in autoclave for $^1\!/_2$ hr at 12 pounds. Store in refrigerator. Using one 150 ml flask at a time, melt medium in boiling water. Cool to 50-55° C, and, using sterile technic, add 10 ml sterile defibrinated rabbit blood. Mix and distribute 5 ml into tubes to produce long slants.

Inoculum: Obtain cultures from blood and from splenic, hepatic, and lymph node material. Antibiotics

Table 34-7. Location of developmental stages of blood and tissue flagellates of humans

Species	Amastigote	Promastigote	Epimastigote	Trypomastigote
Leishmania				
L. donovani	Within cells of the reticuloendothelial system	Vector (sandfly) Culture		
L. tropica and *L. braziliensis*	Within cells of skin and mucous membranes	Vector (sandfly) Culture		
Trypanosoma				
T. gambiense			Vector (tsetse fly); culture	Blood, CSF, lymph nodes of humans; vector (tsetse fly)
T. rhodesiense			Vector (tsetse fly); culture	Blood, CSF, lymph nodes of humans; vector (tsetse fly)
T. cruzi	Within cells of heart, brain, intestines of humans	Within cells of humans	Vector (reduviid bug); culture	Blood of humans; feces of insect vector (tsetse fly); culture
T. rangeli			Vector (reduviid bug)	Blood of humans; vector (reduviid bug); culture

Table 34-8. Morphologic forms of hemoflagellates in humans

Forms of parasite	Leishmania		
	L. donovani	*L. trophica*	*L. braziliensis*
Leishmanial form (amastigote)	RES,* monocytes in peripheral blood	RES of skin, monocytes and polymorphonuclear cells	RES of skin and mucous membrane
Leptomonad form (promastigote) Crithidial form (epimastigote)	Culture; insect host (sandfly)	Culture; insect host (sandfly)	Culture; insect host (sandfly)
Trypanosomal form (trypomastigote)			

*RES, Reticuloendothelial system (spleen, liver, lymph nodes, macrophages, monocytes).

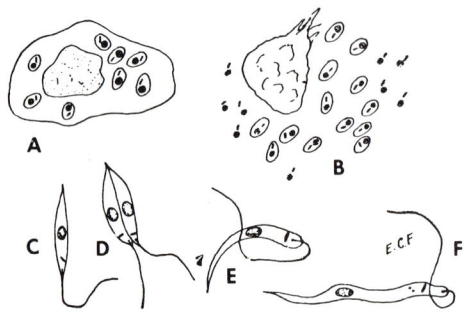

Fig. 34-18. *Leishmania donovani.* **A** and **B,** Leishmanial form from endothelial cells of spleen. **C** to **F,** Flagellate stage from culture. (×1000.) (From Faust, E.C.: J. Lab. Clin. Med. **17:**639, 1932.)

such as 20 units of penicillin/ml and 40 units of streptomycin/ml may be added to the inoculum to prevent bacterial contamination during the 4 or more weeks' incubation period. A positive culture yields leptomonad forms.

Schneider Drosophila medium: Schneider medium (Grand Island Biological Co., Grand Island, N.Y.), enriched with 39% v/v fetal calf serum (Grand Island Biological Co, Grand Island, N.Y.) allows rapid cultivation of *Leishmania* and *Trypanosoma.*

Formalin-gel test: To 1 ml serum add 2 drops of 40% formalin. If the test is positive, the serum will become opalescent and opaque within a few minutes and will finally solidify. This test is basically for increased γ-globulins and is therefore not diagnostic of leishmaniasis.

Serodiagnosis (Table 34-4): Visceral leishmaniasis can be diagnosed by the following serologic tests (Kagan and Norman)[21,22]: complement fixation, indirect hemagglutination, and indirect immunofluorescence.

Leishmania tropica

The term *Leishmania tropica* (cutaneous leishmaniasis, oriental sore) embraces a number of leishmanial species that invade the skin, i.e., they are dermatotrophic and do not involve the viscera, thus differing from the viscerotrophic forms such as *Leishmania donovani.*

Diagnosis: To arrive at a diagnosis the base of the skin ulcer is scraped and some of the material is cultured, while the remainder of the material is spread on slides and stained with Giemsa stain for the amastigote forms within macrophages. Serum aspirated from below the base of the ulcerative lesion or biopsy specimen may also be cultured on NNN or Schneider media and smeared and stained for parasitized white cells. Another approach is to inject about 0.5 ml sterile saline below the ulcer bed and then to aspirate the liquid and treat it like serum. The amastigote form of the parasite is indistinguishable from the corresponding form of *L. donovani.* It can be demonstrated as intracytoplasmic inclusions in monocytes, polymorphonuclear cells, and endothelial cells of dermal capillaries.

Serodiagnosis: The immunofluorescence test using amastigote antigen is the preferred method.[22,41]

Leishmania braziliensis

Clinically the disease caused by *Leishmania braziliensis* is characterized by ulcers of the mucosa of the nose and mouth (espundia) and by rather large cutaneous ulcers similar but often larger and more numerous than the ulcers of cutaneous leishmaniasis.

Diagnosis: The same procedures are used as for cutaneous leishmaniasis.

Serodiagnosis: The direct agglutination test using type-specific trypsinized formalin-fixed promastigotes is a sensitive diagnostic procedure.

Trypanosomes

There are three species of trypanosomes[42] pathogenic to humans: *Trypanosoma gambiense, Trypanosoma rhodesiense,* and *Trypanosoma cruzi.* The first two are the cause of African sleeping sickness and are transmitted by the bite of the tsetse fly. *T. cruzi* is the cause of Chagas' disease in Central and South America and is transmitted by the reduviid bug. A fourth species, *Trypanosoma rangeli,* is also transmitted by the reduviid bug but does not produce disease in humans.

Trypanosoma gambiense and Trypanosoma rhodesiense

Trypanosoma gambiense causes **West African** sleeping sickness while *Trypanosoma rhodesiense* causes

Trypanosoma			
T. gambiense	*T. rhodesiense*	*T. cruzi*	*T. rangeli*
		Heart, lymph nodes	Insect (reduviid bug)
		Brain	Insect (reduviid bug)
Insect host (tsetse fly)	Culture; insect host (tsetse fly)	Culture; insect host (reduviid bug) Tissue	Insect (reduviid bug)
Blood, lymph nodes, CSF, brain; tsetse fly	Blood, lymph nodes, CSF brain; tsetse fly	Blood	Blood; insect (reduviid bug)

East African sleeping sickness. Both parasites are similar in morphology and transmission; they produce similar diseases characterized by a febrile acute stage with lymphadenopathy and splenomegaly in which the parasites can be demonstrated in the peripheral blood and in the fluid aspirated from lymph nodes. In the chronic comatose stage of sleeping sickness the parasites can be demonstrated in the cerebrospinal fluid but not in the blood.

Life cycle: The tsetse fly (both sexes) acquires **trypomastigotes** at the time of its blood meal and after several reproductive and developmental stages in the fly's gut the parasites reach the salivary glands and render the fly infective. At the time of the next blood meal the fly transfers metacyclic trypomastigotes to the new host. In humans the trypanosomes divide by binary longitudinal fission. *T. rhodesiense* produces a more acute and severe infection, with death occurring usually within 1 year. *T. gambiense* produces a more chronic disease with a longer sleeping stage.

Diagnosis: The diagnosis is based on the demonstration of the trypanosomes, and, depending on the stage of the disease, trypanosomes may be demonstrated in fluid aspirated from lymph nodes, in blood, and/or in spinal fluid.

Blood smear: During the febrile stage, examine the peripheral blood, wet unstained and stained with Wright-Giemsa stain. In the unstained preparation the motility of the trypanosomes draws attention to their presence even if only a few parasites are in the specimen. A small drop of blood should be used for the wet film so as not to obscure the live organisms. Thick and thin stained blood smears are prepared as for malaria diagnosis and are examined for stained flagellate organisms. If the organisms are scarce, the buffy coat of centrifuged citrated blood should be examined by the thick and thin smear methods. In all suspected cases the cerebrospinal fluid should be centrifuged and the sediment examined using wet unstained and dried stained preparations. The trypomastigote forms are encountered in the bloodstream and cerebrospinal fluid.

In the acute phase, smears may also be prepared from aspirates of enlarged lymph nodes. A small amount of saline is injected into the lymph node and is then aspirated and examined as wet unstained and as dry stained preparation. In the lymph node the amastigote forms can be demonstrated.

Animal inoculation: Inoculate hamsters, mice, or guinea pigs intraperitoneally and examine blood for trypanosomes. The material used for injection may be blood or macerated lymph nodes. When inoculated into mice, *T. rhodesiense* is rapidly fatal; smears of blood and organs may reveal posterior nucleated forms, the nucleus being behind the kinetoplast. *T. gambiense* produces a chronic infection, and posterior nucleated forms are scarce (Figs. 34-19 and 34-20).

Culture: The organism will grow on NNN medium (see discussion of leishmania).

Serodiagnosis: Markedly increased IgM levels demonstrated by immunodiffusion in blood or spinal fluid are almost pathognomonic of African trypanosomiasis in endemic areas. Indirect immunodiffusion is most sensitive when the serum is tested with homologous trypanosomes.[21,22,43]

Trypanosoma cruzi

Trypanosoma cruzi is transmitted by the **reduviid bug,** the **feces** of which, containing the infectious parasites, are rubbed into the itching bite by the scratching victim. This trypanosome does not divide in the blood, but, losing its flagellum and undulating membrane, it invades endothelial and other tissue cells (especially heart muscle). It divides by binary fission, producing numerous amastigote forms within a cystlike cavity. The amastigote forms develop into trypomastigotes in the blood when the cyst ruptures.

T. cruzi is the causative agent of Chagas' disease.

T. cruzi exhibits four forms in humans: the amastigote forms in the heart, lymph nodes, and other tissues; the promastigote forms in the brain; the trypomastigote forms in the blood; and the epimastigote forms in human tissues and in the reduviid bug.

Diagnosis: The diagnosis is based on the demonstration of the parasites. *T. cruzi* is morphologically distinct from *T. rhodesiense* and *T. gambiense* by the large posterior kinetoplast, the large central nucleus, and the many U- and C-shaped organisms of variable length and thickness found in the peripheral blood. The blood examination involves thin fresh wet unstained preparations as well as thin and thick smears as for ma-

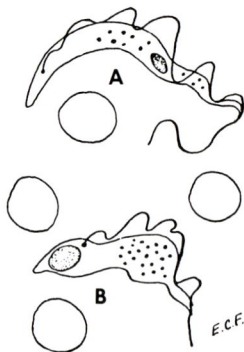

Fig. 34-19. *Trypanosoma rhodesiense* in blood. **A,** Usual form. **B,** Posterior nucleate type from rodent host. (× 1000.) (From Faust, E.C.: J. Lab. Clin. Med. **17:**639, 1932.)

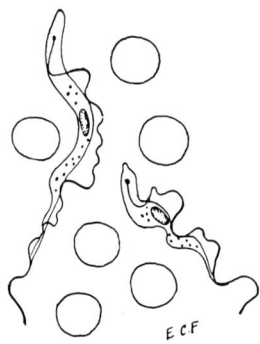

Fig. 34-20. *Trypanosoma gambiense* in blood. (× 1000.) (From Faust, E.C.: J. Lab. Clin. Med. **17:**639, 1932.)

laria investigation. In the acute phase of the disease, blood examination may prove to be diagnostic. In the later phases of the disease the organism is more difficult to find. Lymph node and liver biopsy specimens, imprints, or aspirates may show the amastigote form, which may be cultured on NNN medium. At autopsy the amastigote phase may be found in almost any organ, including the brain.

Other diagnostic investigations include a complement fixation test using *T. cruzi* as antigen (Machado-Guerreiro test) and xenodiagnosis.

Xenodiagnosis: Uninfected laboratory-bred reduviid bugs are allowed to feed on suspected patients. After about 2 weeks the epimastigote forms are found in the gut of the bugs if the patient has Chagas' disease.

Serodiagnosis: According to Kagan[21] and Cerisola,[44] Chagas' disease can be diagnosed serologically with a high degree of specificity and sensitivity provided that three tests are used: complement fixation, indirect hemagglutination, and immunofluorescence. The already-mentioned direct agglutination test[45] using trypsinized formalin-fixed epimastigotes obtained from culture provides a sensitive approach to the diagnosis of Chagas' disease.[22]

Trypanosoma rangeli

Trypanosoma rangeli infects humans but is not disease producing. It is transmitted by the bite of a species of reduviid bug as is *Trypanosoma cruzi* but it lacks the latter's amastigote phase. The kinetoplast of its trypomastigote form is far posterior and small compared to that of *T. cruzi*.

Ciliates
Balantidium coli

Balantidium coli, a parasite found in hogs, is the only ciliate that involves humans and it does so rarely and only after close hog-human contact. It survives in the large bowel subsisting on bacteria and may cause ulcerative colitis by penetrating the intestinal mucosa.

Diagnosis: Saline wet mounts of fecal specimens are diagnostic, revealing live, cilia-covered, large organisms. Stained preparations reveal the features enumerated below.

Incidence: Rare in humans; common in pigs.

Trophozoite:

Size: Varies greatly, 40-120 × 30-80 μm.

Characteristics:
1. Oval and covered with short cilia in parallel rows
2. Anterior end somewhat pointed; presents a deep cytostome
3. Food and contractile vacuoles present
4. Ingests blood, tissue, and bacteria
5. One large kidney-shaped nucleus (macronucleus) and a small micronucleus usually lying in the concavity of the macronucleus visible in stained preparations
6. Reproduction by binary transverse division
7. Rotary motility

Cyst:

Size: 45-65 μm.

Characteristics:
1. The cyst is spheroid and greenish or yellowish with a doubly outlined cyst wall.
2. The cyst contains a macronucleus and a micronucleus as in the trophozoite; the macronucleus is visible in saline solution.
3. In young cysts, cilia may be seen; in older cysts, the internal structure is granular and details of the organism are obscured.

Diagnosis: The unstained organism is large, it shows rapid rotary motility, and it has a rim of moving cilia.

Sporozoa

The name of the subphylum, i.e., Sporozoa, draws attention to the fact that these organisms produce spores at one stage in their life cycle that involves an intermediate host. The intermediate host harbors the asexual forms while the definitive host harbors the sexual forms. Humans may be both the definitive and the intermediate host. In lower animals (rabbits, chickens, etc.) sporozoa may produce fatal forms of enteritides (coccidiosis). Most sporozoa are intracellular organisms of worldwide distribution and of considerable economic and social importance.

Isospora

The life cycle of *Isospora* is not completely known. Of the three species that used to be described *(Isospora hominis, Isospora belli,* and *Isospora matalensis)* only *Isospora belli* is now recognized as a true parasite of humans.

Isospora belli

Isospora belli is difficult to diagnose and easily missed in stool specimens. It is thought to be responsible for a giardiasis-like form of enteritis.[46]

***Habitat and life cycle*:** All developmental stages of the organism are not known. It probably matures in the mucosal cells of the small intestine. The trophozoites are found in the epithelial cells of intestine and bile ducts, where they enlarge (schizonts) and undergo multiple division producing merozoites that rupture the cells. Some of the merozoites enter other cells and repeat the cycle; some develop into gametocytes and ultimately form **oocysts** that appear in the feces.

Characteristics:

Oocyst:

1. The oocyst is ovoid and 28 × 15 μm in diameter.
2. There is a colorless shell-like wall with a micropyle at the narrow end.
3. The protoplasm is unsegmented in a fresh specimen but soon divides into two parts **(sporoblasts)** that become surrounded by a thin wall, forming **sporocysts,** within each of which develop four **vermiform sporozoites** (Fig. 34-21). When liberated in the intestine, the sporozoites invade the epithelial cells of the intestine and bile ducts, becoming trophozoites.

Diagnosis: Diagnosis is based on detection of the oocyst in the stool. In saline preparations the oocysts are not visible but iodine staining brings out the diagnostic criteria—the two sporocysts within the oocyst.

Plasmodium and malaria

Malaria is caused by protozoa of the genus *Plasmodium,* which by parasitizing and destroying red cells produce the signs and symptoms of malaria. Similar parasites are found in animals, e.g., monkeys and birds. The number of cells parasitized varies from 10-40%, depending on the species.

Malaria induced accidentally or therapeutically (contaminated needles and syringes and blood transfusions) differs from natural malaria in the absence of relapses (no tissue phase), in irregular brood formation, and in smaller numbers of gametocytes.

Species

In humans, four *Plasmodium* species occur: *P. vivax* of tertian malaria, *P. malariae* of quartan malaria, *P. falciparum* of malignant tertian malaria, and rarely *P. ovale* of ovale malaria.

Life cycle

The life cycle includes the **asexual cycle in humans** and the **sexual cycle in the female *Anopheles* mosquito.** The cycle in humans is called **schizogony** and

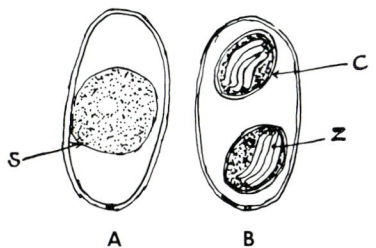

Fig. 34-21. Oocysts of *Isospora belli* (schematic). **A,** Immature: *S,* sporoblast. **B,** Mature: *C,* sporocyst; *Z,* sporozoites.

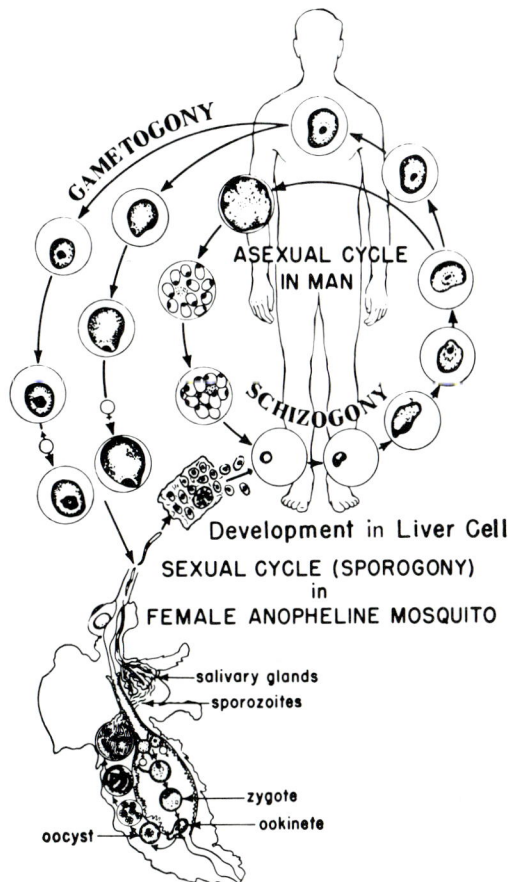

Fig. 34-22. Malarial parasite. (Modified from Ash, J.E., and Spitz, S.: Pathology of tropical diseases: an atlas, Philadelphia, 1945, W.B. Saunders Co.)

that in the mosquito **sporogony.** Humans are the intermediate host, and the mosquito is the definitive host (Fig. 34-22).

Cycle in humans:

Asexual cycle (schizogony):

***Exoerythrocytic schizogony (tissue phase)*:** The form of the parasite introduced into the blood of the bitten victim with the salivary secretion of the infected female mosquito is elongated, narrow, and spindle shaped and is called the sporozoite. The sporozoites soon disappear from the blood and enter liver cells, where they mature to tissue schizonts filled with thousands of merozoites. When the schizonts rupture, the liver cell is destroyed and the **merozoites** are free to attack red cells.

Erythrocytic schizogony (peripheral blood phase): When the merozoite enters a red cell, it assumes a spheroid shape and is then called a **ring trophozoite.** Growth and development occur in the red cell, the hemoglobin of which is used by the parasite. Each parasite consists of a nuclear mass called chromatin, which stains red with Wright stain, and of cytoplasm, which stains blue. A few hours after the merozoites enter the red cells, a ring of cytoplasm appears, indicating the young trophozoites. The parasite becomes actively ameboid, and in 8-10 hr, pigment granules representing the product of its catabolism are seen in the pseudopodia or in the periphery of the parasite. As the trophozoite enlarges, it grows more rapidly and become less active.

Most of the parasites undergo internal changes during the last 8-12 hr of this cycle in preparation for sporulation. The chromatin is distributed in fine granules throughout the parasite, the pigment begins to collect in masses that tend to assume a radial distribution, and the periphery tends to become scalloped or regularly notched (**presegmenters** or **immature schizonts**). Then the organism becomes divided into a definite number of spores (**merozoites**), each of which contains a small chromatin mass or dot, whereas the pigment between the merozoites becomes arranged in masses near the center. These forms are called **segmenters** or **mature schizonts.** Finally, the infected red cell ruptures, and the merozoites, the future young trophozoites, and pigment are set free in the plasma. The parasites enter new red cells, and the pigment is taken up by phagocytic cells and by the reticuloendothelial tissues. A number of merozoites are destroyed, chiefly by leukocytes.

Sexual cycle: After the infection has become established, some of the merozoites, apparently because of an unfavorable environment developing in the body about 12 days after the infection, will not continue the asexual cycle but will differentiate into **sexual forms** called **gametocytes,** of which there are males (**microgametocytes**) and females (**macrogametocytes**). They develop slowly, requiring about twice as long for maturing as the asexual forms, and persist in the blood (free in the plasma after rupture of the red cell membrane) for a very long time or until taken by a mosquito in feeding. These resistant forms are responsible for the preservation of the species and go through the developmental cycle in the female *Anopheles* mosquito described below.

All of the asexual and sexual forms described in the cycle in humans appear in the peripheral blood, except in *P. falciparum* infection, where only ring forms and crescents (gametocytes) are found. The older asexual forms of this species remain in the capillaries of the internal organs, where sporulation occurs. The red cells infected with *P. falciparum* tend to adhere to the cap-

illary walls and to block the vessels, giving rise to the special clinical forms of this type of malaria.

To complete the cycle, *P. vivax* requires 45 hr, *P. ovale* 48 hr, *P. malariae* 72 hr, and *P. falciparum* 48 hr. In the case of *P. vivax,* for instance, the cycle is calculated from the rupture of schizonts and the release of merozoites on day 1, maturation of trophozoites in red cells on day 2, and rupture of the new schizonts and release of merozoites on day 3.

The chill occurs at the time of sporulation and is considered to be caused by the liberation of the pigment, which is a neurotoxin. It is estimated that at least 1 billion parasites, or 200/mm^3, sporulating at the same time are necessary to produce a chill. This is about one parasite per 100 oil-immersion fields in thin blood smears. After the infection is established, there is a tendency, except in falciparum infection, for the parasites to become grouped into one or more broods so that all the same brood will sporulate about the same time. When more than one brood is formed, the broods usually sporulate on different days, often producing a chill each day. This is called a **multiple infection,** e.g., double tertian. If more than one species are present, the condition is called a **mixed infection,** e.g., tertian and quartan, or falciparum and tertian. The gametocytes in the peripheral bloodstream of humans are ingested by the female mosquito at the time of the blood meal. The female mosquito requires blood for reproduction; the male mosquito does not bite.

Cycle in mosquito: In the stomach of the mosquito the **macrogametocyte** casts off the polar body (becoming a **macrogamete**) and the **microgametocyte** throws out four to six very motile threadlike filaments (**microgametes**). The macrogamete fertilized by a microgamete is called a **zygote** and, becoming actively motile (**ookinete**), penetrates the stomach mucosa and forms a cyst (**oocyst**).

The cyst enlarges as numerous minute, slender, spindle-shaped **sporozoites** are formed by multiple division of the parasite, and when mature, it ruptures into the body cavity. The sporozoites invade the body of the mosquito, including the salivary glands from which they are injected into the next host on which the mosquito feeds.

This cycle requires about 1-3 weeks, depending on the species of *Plasmodium* and of mosquito. The mosquito remains infectious.

Laboratory diagnosis of malaria[47]

The diagnosis of malaria is based on the demonstration of the parasite in blood. The thick smear is used as a screening test to establish the presence of malaria, and the thin smear is used to speciate the organism.

Timing of blood smear: Blood smears should be obtained at the time of admission of the patient, irrespective of the periodicity of the fever. If these smears are negative, new smears should be made at various times midway between 6-12 hr after the next chill, since the blood will then contain the larger trophozoites and more mature forms. The chill accompanies either the release of merozoites from the schizonts or the parasitization of new red cells by merozoites. Merozoites and

Fig. 34-23. Thin and thick blood film (stained).

young ring forms are small and difficult to find, because they closely resemble platelets. When only ring forms are present in a smear, repeat the examination in about 8 hr to look for species-specific trophozoites and older forms. If only ring forms are present again, the species is *P. falciparum*.

Technic of thin smears: Use fresh nonanticoagulated or EDTA-anticoagulated blood and clean slides. Follow the method described for blood smear on p. 32. The smears should be very thin, dried rapidly under a fan to prevent drying artifacts, and fixed in absolute methyl alcohol before staining to prevent staining artifacts.

Technic of thick smears: The purpose of the thick smear is to concentrate a relatively large drop of blood in a small area. Before the blood is taken for the smear, all traces of alcohol must be removed from the puncture site by drying it carefully with sterile gauze, since alcohol-fixed red cells resist lysis. A large drop of blood is placed on a clean microscope slide and spread with the corner of a second slide to cover an area the size of a dime. The spread drop is allowed to dry overnight at room temperature. A drying fan may be used but heat fixation must be avoided because it prevents adequate lysis. The spread must not be too thick or it will flake off. Thick and thin smears may be prepared on the same slide by placing the drop at one end of the slide, but two separate slides are preferred since the staining procedure for thick and thin smears differs. Satisfactory smears may also be obtained using EDTA-anticoagulated blood (Fig. 34-23).

• • •

Reagents:
1. Stock Giemsa stain
   a. Giemsa stain powder, certified, 600 mg
   b. Methanol, absolute and certified, neutral, acetone free, 50 ml
   c. Glycerin (neutral), certified, 50 ml
   Grind well small portions of stain and glycerin in mortar and collect mixtures in a 5 or 10 dl flask until all measured material is mixed. Stopper flask with cotton plug, cover with heavy paper, and place in 55-60° C water bath for 2 hr, making sure that the water reaches the level of the stain. Shake gently at $1/2$ hr intervals. Allow to cool and add alcohol. Use a portion of the measured alcohol to wash out the mortar and add to the flask. Store in brown bottle. Allow to stand for 2-3 weeks. Filter before use.
2. Stock buffers

   a. Alkaline disodium phosphate buffer: 9.5 g anhydrous 0.67M Na_2HPO_4 and 1 L distilled water
   b. Sodium acid phosphate buffer: 9.2 g 0.67M $NaH_2PO_4H_2O$ and 1 L distilled water
3. Buffered water
   a. Disodium phosphate buffer, 61 ml
   b. Sodium acid phosphate buffer, 39 ml
   c. Distilled water, 9 dl
   The pH range should be 7.0-7.2; check with a pH meter before use.

Staining technics:

Thin smears: Air dry the slide and fix in absolute methyl alcohol for 30 sec. Allow to dry and stain in 1:20 Giemsa solution for 20 min. (Add 1 ml stock Giemsa to 20 ml buffered water.)

Dip a few times in buffered water to wash, and allow to dry in vertical position.

Thick smears: Dry slide overnight at room temperature. Do not expose slide to heat and do not fix in alcohol. Stain in a 1:50 Giemsa-buffered water solution for 45 min. (Add 1 ml stock Giemsa solution to 50 ml buffered water.)

Wash in buffered water for 2-3 min and allow to dry in a vertical position.

Combined thin and thick films: Fix the thin section of the film in a Coplin jar containing absolute methyl alcohol for 30 sec. Allow to dry in a vertical position. Lyse the thick blood film area in buffered water for 4 min and stain both thin and thick areas using a 1:50 Giemsa solution for 45 min. Rinse in buffered water, rinsing thin part briefly and thick part for 5 min. Allow to dry.

Wright stain: The Wright-Giemsa stain described in the hematology section (see p. 111) very adequately stains thin and thick malarial smears and appears to be preferable to a pure Wright stain. Rahimi[47a] suggests the following modification of the Wright stain.

Stock Wright stain:
1. Wright stain powder (Harleco 376 [Harleco, Gibbstown, N.J.]), 6.0 g
2. Glycerin (Harleco 811 [Harleco, Gibbstown, N.J.]), 60 ml
3. Absolute methyl alcohol (acetone free) (Mallinckrodt 3016 [Mallinckrodt, St. Louis]), 2 L

Mix powder with glycerin in mortar until smooth, add alcohol, and mix. Allow to ripen for 1 month at room temperature or 24 hr at 37° C. Store in dark bottle and shake frequently to dissolve crystals.

Buffer:
1. Potassium phosphate, monobasic (KH_2PO_4; Mallinckrodt 7100 [Mallinckrodt, St. Louis]), 13.26 g
2. Sodium phosphate, dibasic (anhydrous Na_2HPO_4), 5.13 g
3. Distilled water to 2 L

Staining: For thin smears allow slides to air dry. Apply 20 drops stock stain per slide. Add 20 drops buffer. Mix buffer and stain by blowing on slide and stain for 8 min. Wash in three rinses of distilled water. Dry immediately with bibulous paper and apply coverslip using Permount (Fisher Scientific Co., Pittsburgh). Examine slide under oil immersion.

For thick smears allow slides to dry overnight at room temperature. Hemolyze red cells by flooding slide with distilled water for 4 min. Allow slide to dry and stain as for thin smears.

Saponin hemolysis technic[48]:

Procedure: Obtain EDTA-anticoagulated venous blood and add 1.5 ml 1% solution of saponin in normal saline solution to 2 ml blood. Lysis is complete in 30 sec. Centrifuge in Sero-Fuge for 1 min at 3500 rpm. Save supernatant and prepare smears, using the bottom portion of the sediment.

Centrifuge the supernatant for 10 min at 3500 rpm and smear sediment again. Stain both smears with Wright or Giemsa stain.

This method preserves the morphology of the parasites and allows a higher concentration of parasites than the thick smear method.

General morphology and terminology of malarial parasites

The plasmodia in the peripheral blood stain well with Romanowsky stains. The chromatin dot, which is the nucleus, stains red, the cytoplasm blue, and the intraparasitic pigment brown, greenish brown, or black. The earliest intraerythrocytic form is referred to as a "ring" or "signet ring," since it consists of a ring of blue cytoplasm with one or two dots of red chromatin. Within hours the ring form develops into the ameboid, uninu-

Table 34-9. Microscopic identification of plasmodia of humans in Giemsa-stained thin blood smears

	Plasmodium vivax	*Plasmodium malariae*	*Plasmodium falciparum*	*Plasmodium ovale*
Appearance of parasitized red cells				
Size and shape	1.5-2 times larger than normal; oval to round	Both normal	Both normal	60% of cells larger than normal and oval; 20% have irregular, frayed edges
Schüffner dots (eosinophilic stippling)	Present in all cells except youngest ring forms	None	None; occasionally commalike red dots are present, (Maurer dots)	Present in all stages, including young ring form
Color of cytoplasm	Decolorized, pale	Normal	Normal, bluish tinge at times	Decolorized, pale
Multiple infections	Occasional	Rare	Common	Occasional
All developmental stages present in peripheral blood	All stages present	Ring forms few as ring stage brief; mostly growing and mature trophozoites and schizonts	Young ring forms and no older stages; few gametocytes	All stages present
Appearance of parasite				
Young trophozoite (early ring form)	Ring is one third the diameter of cell; cytoplasmic circle around vacuole; heavy chromatin dot	Ring often smaller than *P. vivax,* occupying one sixth of cell; heavy chromatin dot; vacuole at times "filled in''; pigment forms early	Delicate small ring with small chromatin dot (frequently 2); scanty cytoplasm around small vacuoles; sometimes at edge of red cell (appliqué form) or filamentous stretched out into slender form	Ring is larger and more ameboid than *P. vivax;* otherwise similar to *P. vivax*
Growing trophozoite	Multishaped irregular ameboid parasite; streamers of cytoplasm close to large chromatin dot; vacuole retained until close to maturity; increasing amounts of brown pigment; most characteristic of *P. vivax*	Nonameboid rounded or band-shaped solid forms; chromatin may be hidden by coarse dark brown pigment	Heavy ring forms fine pigment grains	Ring shape maintained until late in development

Table 34-9. Microscopic identification of plasmodia of humans in Giemsa-stained thin blood smears—cont'd

	Plasmodium vivax	*Plasmodium malariae*	*Plasmodium falciparum*	*Plasmodium ovale*
Mature trophozoite	Irregular ameboid mass; 1 or more small vacuoles retained until schizont stage; fills almost entire cell; fine brown pigment	Vacuoles disappear early; cytoplasm compact, oval, band shaped, or nearly round almost filling cell; chromatin may be hidden by mainly peripheral coarse dark brown pigment	Not seen in peripheral blood (except in severe infections); development of all phases following ring form occurs in capillaries of viscera	Compact; vacuoles disappear; pigment dark brown, less than *P. malariae*
Schizont (presegmenter)	Progressive chromatin division; cytoplasmic bands containing clumps of brown pigment	Similar to *P. vivax* except smaller, darker, larger pigment granules peripheral or central	Not seen in peripheral blood (see above)	Smaller and more compact than *P. vivax*
Mature schizont	16 (12-24) merozoites, each with chromatin and cytoplasm, filling entire red cell, which can hardly be seen	8 (6-12) merozoites in rosettes or irregular clusters filling normal-sized cells, which can hardly be seen; central arrangement of brown-green pigment	Not seen in peripheral blood	Three fourths of cells occupied by 8(6-12) merozoites in rosettes or irregular clusters
Macrogametocyte	Rounded or oval homogeneous cytoplasm; diffuse delicate light brown pigment throughout parasite; eccentric compact chromatin	Similar to *P. vivax*, but fewer in number, pigment coarser and darker	Sex differentiation difficult; "crescent" or "sausage" shapes characteristic; may appear in "showers"; black pigment near chromatin dot, which is often central	Smaller than *P. vivax*
Microgametocyte	Large pink to purple chromatin mass surrounded by pale or colorless halo; evenly distributed pigment	Similar to *P. vivax* but fewer in number pigment coarser and darker	See above	Smaller than *P. vivax*
Main criteria	Large pale red cell; trophozoite irregular, firm; pigment usually present; Schüffner dots not always present; several phases of growth seen in one smear; gametocytes appear early	Red cell normal in size and color; trophozoites compact, intensely stained; band forms not always seen; coarse pigment; no stippling of red cells; gametocytes appear late	Development following ring stage takes place in blood vessels of internal organs; characteristic delicate ring forms found not accompanied by other phases except crescent-shaped gametocytes	Red cell enlarged, oval, and frayed; Schüffner dots seen in all stages

cleated, more solid form—the **trophozoite.** As long as the organism retains its one nucleus, it continues to be referred to as a trophozoite. Nuclear division and multiplication precede cytoplasmic division. The organism containing two or more nuclei (chromatin dots) but a nonsegmented cytoplasm is a **presegmenting schizont.** It becomes a **mature schizont** when both nuclei and cytoplasm are completely segmented. Each segment represents a **merozoite** that will give rise to a new generation of plasmodia. The sexual forms are called **gametocytes** and consist of larger female **macrogametocytes** and smaller male **microgametocytes.**

Identification of plasmodia

For the identification of plasmodia in thin smears, see Table 34-9 and Plate 17 (p. 981). The characteristics in thick smears may be found in Table 34-11 and Plate 18 (p. 984).

Serodiagnosis of malaria

The indirect immunofluorescence[21,22,49] and the indirect hemagglutination tests[21,50] have a sensitivity of about 95% and a false positive rate of less than 1%. To maintain the degree of specificity, a sensitive homologous malarial antigen must be used.

Other laboratory findings in malaria

In addition to the diagnostic parasites, examination of the peripheral blood smear may, depending on the severity of the infection, reveal varying degrees of **anemia** with anisocytosis, poikilocytosis, often leukopenia with relative monocytosis, and, in chronic cases, malarial pigment within phagocytic cells. The recovery phase after treatment may be accompanied by **reticulocytosis.** Examination of the bone marrow may reveal intraerythrocytic parasites and pigment in macrophages, even if the peripheral blood is negative for parasites. Urine examination may reveal **proteinuria.** The hemolytic component of malaria accounts for the reduction in serum **haptoglobin.**

Hemoglobinopathies and malaria

The tropical areas where *P. falciparum* predominates are also the regions in which there is maximal concentration of Hb S, thalassemia, and G-6-PD deficiency. It is now generally accepted that the young heterozygous carrier of Hb S has some protection against *P. falciparum* infections.[51] A similar protection is not provided by Hb E or Hb C. There is also good evidence that G-6-PD deficiency[52] and thalassemia[53] are associated with increased resistance to malaria.

Plate 17. Malarial parasites—thin smears.

A, *Plasmodium vivax:* **1,** Normal-sized red cell with marginal ring form trophozoite. **2,** Young signet-ring form trophozoite in a macrocyte. **3,** Slightly older ring form trophozoite in red cell showing basophilic stippling. **4,** Polychromatophilic red cell containing young tertian parasite with pseudopodia. **5,** Ring form trophozoite showing pigment in cytoplasm, in an enlarged cell containing Schüffner stippling. (Schüffner stippling does not appear in all cells containing the growing and older forms of *P. vivax* as would be indicated by these photographs, but it can be found with any stage from the fairly young ring form onward.) **6** and **7,** Very tenuous medium trophozoite forms. **8,** Three ameboid trophozoites with fused cytoplasm. **9, 11, 12,** and **13,** Older ameboid trophozoites in process of development. **10,** Two ameboid trophozoites in one cell. **14,** Mature trophozoite. **15,** Mature trophozoite with chromatin apparently in process of division. **16, 17, 18,** and **19,** Schizonts showing progressive steps in divison (presegmenting schizonts). **20,** Mature schizont. **21** and **22,** Developing gametocytes. **23,** Mature microgametocyte. **24,** Mature macrogametocyte.

B, *Plasmodium malariae:* **1,** Young ring form trophozoite of quartan malaria. **2, 3,** and **4,** Young trophozoite forms of the parasite showing gradual increase of chromatin and cytoplasm. **5,** Developing ring form trophozoite showing pigment granule. **6,** Early band form trophozoite—elongated chromatin, some pigment apparent. **7, 8, 9, 10, 11,** and **12,** Some forms that developing trophozoite of quartan may take. **13,** and **14,** Mature trophozoites—one a band form. **15, 16, 17, 18,** and **19,** Phases in the development of the schizont (presegmenting schizonts). **20,** Mature schizont. **21,** Immature microgametocyte. **22,** Immature macrogametocyte. **23,** Mature microgametocyte. **24,** Mature macrogametocyte.

C, *Plasmodium ovale:* **1,** Young ring-shaped trophozoite. **2, 3, 4,** and **5,** Older ring-shaped trophozoites. **6, 7,** and **8,** Older ameboid trophozoites. **9, 11,** and **12,** Doubly infected cells, trophozoites. **10,** Doubly infected cell, young gametocytes. **13,** First stage of schizont. **14, 15, 16, 17, 18,** and **19,** Schizonts, progressive stages. **20,** Mature gametocyte.

D, *Plasmodium falciparum:* **1,** Very young ring form trophozoite. **2,** Double infection of single cell with young trophozoites, one a "marginal form," the other "signet-ring" form. **3** and **4** Young trophozoites showing double chromatin dots. **5, 6,** and **7,** Developing trophozoite forms. **8,** Three medium trophozoites in one cell. **9,** Trophozoite showing pigment, in a cell containing Maurer dots. **10** and **11,** Two trophozoites in each of two cells, showing variation of forms that parasites may assume. **12,** Almost mature trophozoite showing haze of pigment throughout cytoplasm. Maurer dots in the cell. **1,** Estivoautumnal "slender forms." **14,** Mature trophozoite, showing clumped pigment. **15,** Parasite in the process of initial chromatin division. **16, 17, 18,** and **19,** Various phases of development of schizont (presegmenting schizonts). **20,** Mature schizont. **21, 22, 23,** and **24,** Successive forms in development of gametocyte—usually not found in peripheral circulation. **25,** Immature macrogametocyte. **26,** Mature macrogametocyte. **27,** Immature microgametocyte. **28,** Mature microgametocyte.

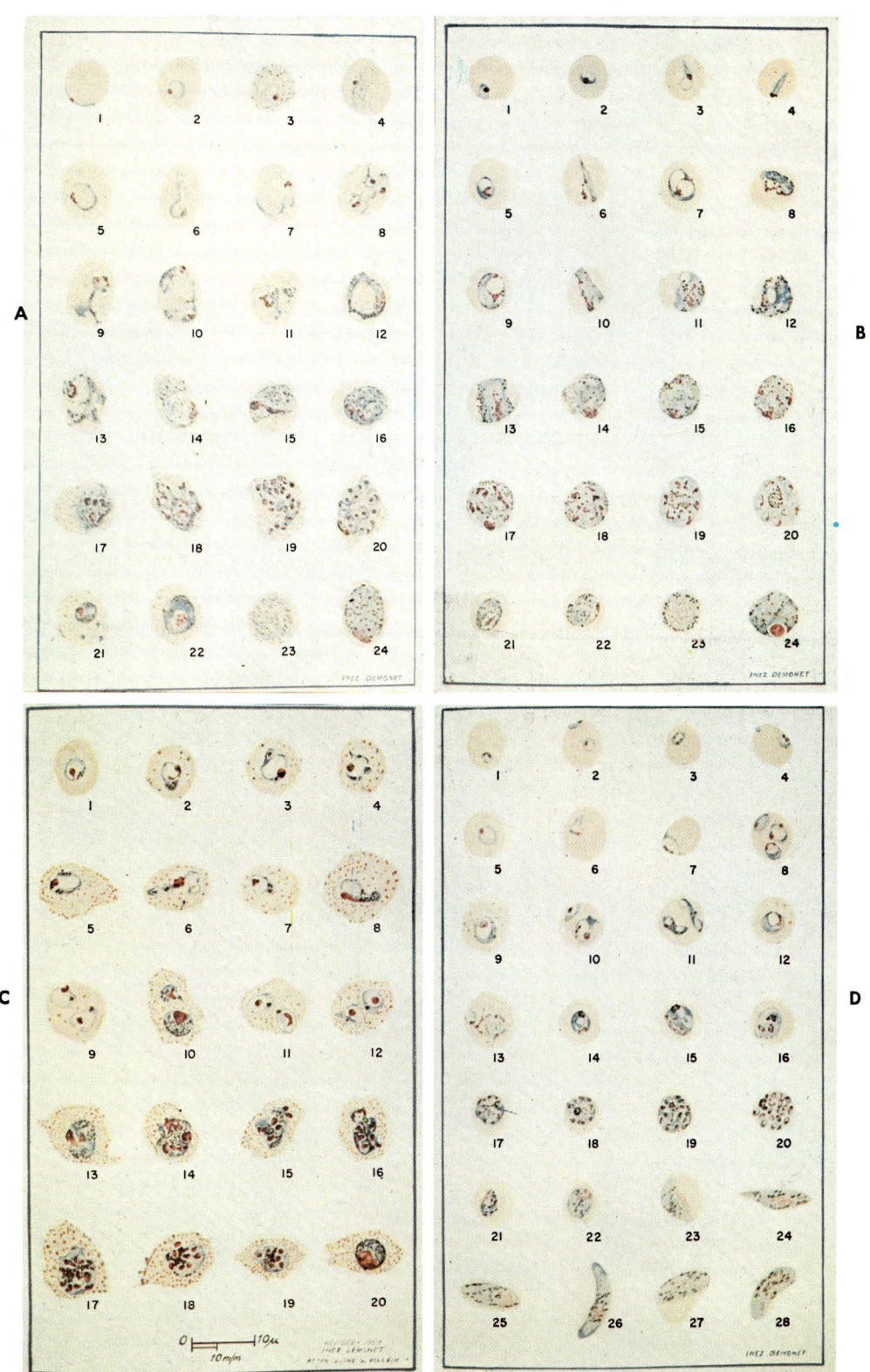

Plate 17. For legend see opposite page.

Table 34-10. Summary of differential characteristics of plasmodia of humans in stained thin film

Characteristics	Plasmodium falciparum	Plasmodium vivax	Plasmodium ovale	Plasmodium malariae
Infected erythrocyte enlarged	−	+	±	−
Infected erythrocyte, fimbriated and/or oval	Rare	Rare	Frequent	Rare
Infected erythrocyte decolorized	−	+	+	−
Infected erythrocyte, Schüffner dots*	−	+	+	−
Infected erythrocyte, Maurer dots*	+	−	−	−
Multiple infections in erythrocytest*	+	Rare	−	−
Parasite, all forms in peripheral blood	Rare	+	+	+
Parasite, large coarse rings	±	+	+	+
Parasite, double chromatin dots*	+	Rare	−	−
Parasite, accolé forms*	+	Rare	−	−
Parasite, band forms*	−	−	+	+
Parasite, sausage-shaped gametocytes	+	−	−	−
Number of merozoites	8-24	12-24	8-12	6-12

From Hunter, G.W., Frye, W.W., and Swartzwelder, J.C.: A manual of tropical medicine, ed. 4, Philadelphia, 1966, W. B. Saunders Co.
*Not invariable but suggestive when seen.

Table 34-11. Microscopic identification of plasmodia of humans in Giemsa-stained thick blood smears

	Plasmodium vivax	Plasmodium malariae	Plasmodium falciparum	Plasmodium ovale
Young trophozoite	Ring forms with irregular cytoplasmic borders; fine pigment; older forms also present	Ring forms with prominent chromatin; often solid cytoplasm; older forms also present; rings may be infrequent	Many small delicate ring forms with small chromatin dots; no older stages seen; forms may resemble exclamation marks, commas, or swallows and may show open rings	Resembles *P. vivax* and *P. malariae* and cannot be differentiated on thick smears
Mature trophozoite	Irregular dark-staining mass of cytoplasm; 1 or 2 vacuoles; fine brown pigment	Dark, heavily pigmented mass; band forms may become rounded	Not seen in peripheral blood unless there is severe infection	See above
Mature schizont	16 merozoites clustered around central pigment	Rosette of 8 merozoites, each with large chromatin dots; compact or separated; central black pigment	Not seen in peripheral blood	See above
Mature gametocyte	Large parasite with diffuse, light pigment; dense cytoplasm; resembles mature trophozoite	Similar to *P. vivax,* but smaller and more compact; much pigment present; may resemble rounded *P. falciparum* gametocyte	Crescent or sausage-shaped forms with pigment near center; may become rounded	See above

Toxoplasma

The taxonomy of *Toxoplasma* is somewhat in doubt but *Toxoplasma* is generally known as *Toxoplasma gondii,* a widespread parasite of domestic cats and other animals. Almost 50% of Americans over the age of 50 are serologically positive for toxoplasmosis.

The parasite was first observed in the gundi (North African rodent) and in the rabbit (Brazil) and has since been found in a large number of wild and domestic animals such as rabbits, guinea pigs, mice, rats, squirrels, dogs, cats, monkeys, and pigeons, as well as in humans. The parasite occurs in two forms, the vegetative form and the encysted form.

T. gondii is an obligate intracellular parasite found in tissue cells (brain, heart, muscle, and lung), leukocytes, and endothelial cells where they multiply. In tissue cells the parasite appears in closely packed colonies of trophozoites from which it can be freed by the rupture of the involved cells. It may then be found free in body fluids, but in the free form it does not survive.

In chronic infections the parasite often appears surrounded by a cyst wall. The parasites are not easily liberated even if the cyst is ruptured. In brain tissue in a schizogony type of development, a single parasite develops up to several thousand nuclei with an enlarging cytoplasmic mass each surrounding itself by a limiting membrane. The resulting cyst varies in diameter from 50-500 μm.

Life cycle: Cats and other domestic animals acquire the infection by eating uncooked meat scraps contaminated with oocysts or other developmental stages of the parasite. Sporozoites escape from the cyst and undergo a sexual plasmodium-like cycle (see discussion of malaria) within intestinal epithelial cells. **Oocysts** are shed in the feces and are acquired by herbivorous animals that eat grass contaminated by feces. Humans acquire the infection by eating poorly cooked meat (pork, lamb, beef, poultry). The cycle may also involve insects such as flies that may transport the infected feces.

Clinical classification: Toxoplasmosis occurs in two forms that differ markedly in their clinical expression: the congenital disease and the acquired disease.

Congenital toxoplasmosis: The acutely infected mother transmits the disease transplacentally to the fetus. Congenital toxoplasmosis may lead to fetal death or, if a viable infant is born, it may lead to the development of chorioretinitis, hydrocephalus, and diffuse cerebral calcification. In adults, chorioretinitis is also the most common severe manifestation, although serologic evidence suggests that most adults have been exposed to *Toxoplasma.*

Acquired toxoplasmosis: Acquired toxoplasmosis usually results in a subclinical presentation or nonspecific illness, although mononucleosis, aseptic meningitis, encephalitis, hepatitis, myocarditis, pneumonitis, and a lymphadenopathic form of intermediate severity have been reported.

Laboratory diagnosis: Laboratory diagnosis is based on the demonstration of neutralizing antibodies,[54-56] although the organisms can be cultured.

Stained smears: Imprints of tissue specimens (liver or lung) and smears of sputum, blood, bone marrow, and the sediment of centrifuged cerebrospinal, pleural,

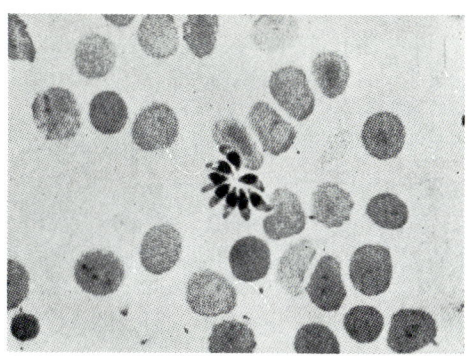

Fig. 34-24. *Toxoplasma* in Giemsa-stained smear from omentum of guinea pig. (From Pinkerton, H., and Henderson, R.G.: J.A.M.A. **116:**807, 1941.)

and peritoneal fluids are air dried, stained with Wright-Giemsa stain, and examined for toxoplasma (Fig. 34-24). In these specimens the parasite may be found free, within broken cysts, or in the tissue cells. The vegetative form is crescentic, pyriform, oval, or round and about 6-7 μm long and 2-4 μm wide. With Wright-Giemsa stain the cytoplasm is pale blue, and the **large nucleus,** which occupies the **whole width** of the **posterior portion** of the parasite, is deep purple. The yield of this method is poor and it is therefore not a suggested diagnostic approach.

Animal inoculation: Advances in serologic testing restrict animal inoculation (and the Sabin-Feldman test) to reference laboratories. After centrifugation (30 min at 3000 rpm), inject cerebrospinal fluid or other suspect fluid intracerebrally and intraperitoneally into six laboratory-bred mice. If the mice remain well after 14 days, aseptically remove the brain and spleen from two, and effect passage to another group of six mice. If tissue (brain, spleen, etc.) is available, it is prepared by grinding it with Hank's balanced salt solution mixed with 10% agammaglobulin calf serum and with penicillin and streptomycin. Young mice that are free of toxoplasmosis are injected intracerebrally (0.03 ml) and intraperitoneally (1 ml). If mice die in 2-3 weeks, imprints and sections of brain, lungs, liver, and lymph nodes are examined. The imprints are stained with Wright-Giemsa stain and the sections with hematoxylin and eosin. The cysts are PAS positive.

Serodiagnosis[21,22,57]**:** Since large segments of the population have antitoxoplasma antibodies, the level of a single titer may be of little significance, but a rising titer if interpreted against the background of clinical information may be indicative of toxoplasmosis. The methylene blue dye test[58] of Sabin and Feldman has firmly established the serologic diagnosis of toxoplasmosis, but for technical reasons the indirect immunofluorescence (IF)[59] and the indirect hemagglutination (IHA)[60] tests are preferred since they are as sensitive as the dye test.[59] They utilize killed antigen that does not endanger the laboratory workers. IHA titers over 256 may be of clinical significance, indicating recent infection. The IF test performed on sera of newborns with

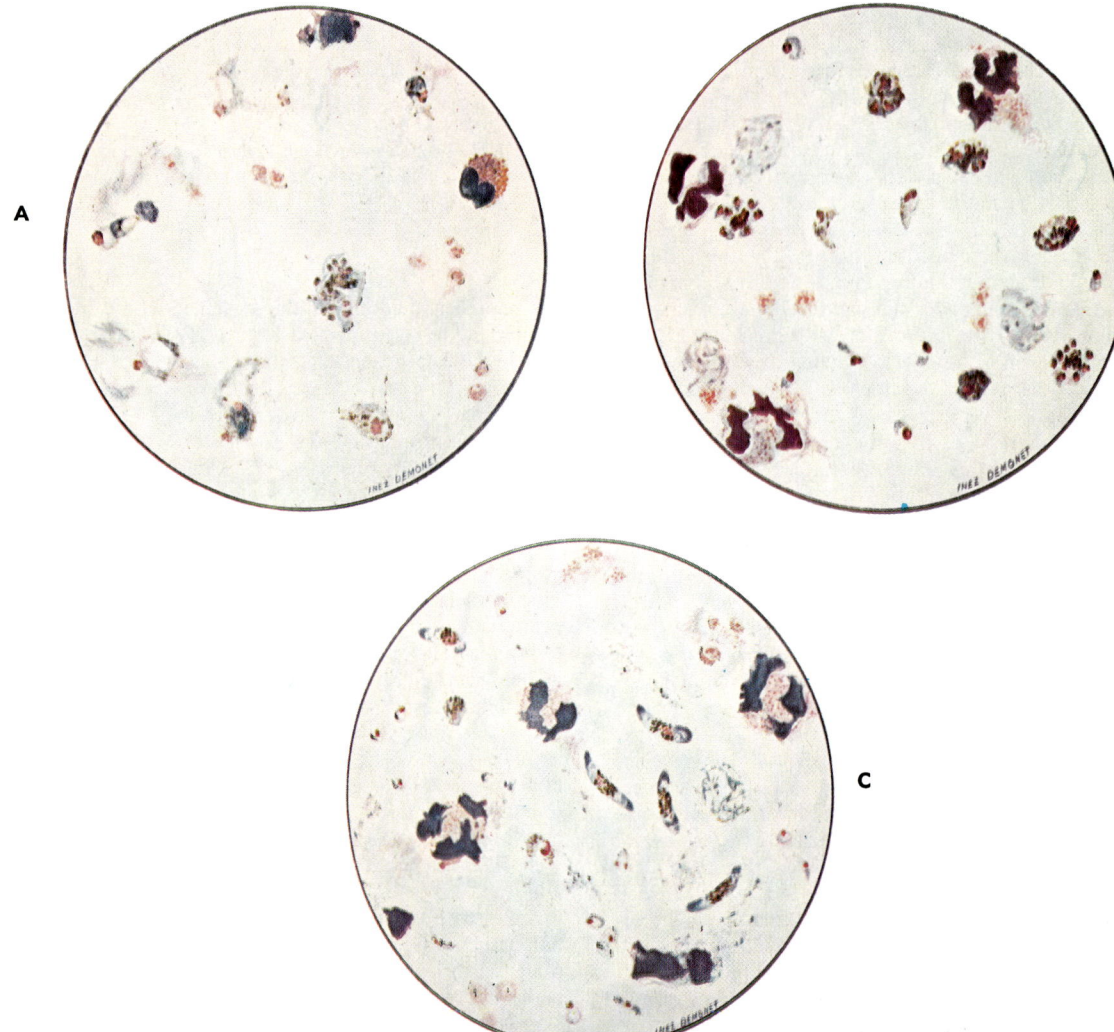

Plate 18. Malarial parasites—thick smears. **A,** *Plasmodium vivax.* Smear shows ameboid trophozoites, schizonts, one microgametocyte, and elements of peripheral blood. **B,** *Plasmodium malariae.* Smear shows several trophozoites and schizonts of varying ages and elements of peripheral blood. **C,** *Plasmodium falciparum.* Smear shows several small trophozoites and gametocytes and elements of peripheral blood. (From Brooke, M.M., and Melvin, D.M.: Morphology of diagnostic stages of intestinal parasites of man, Public Health Service Publication no. 1966, Atlanta, 1969, Centers for Disease Control.)

IgM conjugates may, if positive, point to congenital infections.[21]

Methylene blue dye test of Sabin and Feldman:

Principle: Living *Toxoplasma* organisms killed by antibodies in the patient's serum are not stained by alkaline methylene blue, whereas organisms not in contact with antibodies are stained by the dye.

Results: Dye test titer of "normal" sera rarely exceeds 1:64. The titer is the point at which 50% of the organisms stain. If the dye test titer is 1:256 or higher, a positive diagnosis can be made provided the patient is over 4 months old and the same or a higher titer is obtained on a repeat test 4 months after the first test. A newborn infant may have a high titer because of passive transfer of antibodies from the mother and therefore a repeat test after 4 months is necessary, since the passively transferred antibodies will have disappeared by then. As mentioned above the dye test should be limited to reference laboratories because it utilizes live organisms, is difficult to perform, and does not detect early IgM antibodies when IgG antibodies are present.

Indirect fluorescent antibody: Commercial kits are available for the indirect fluorescent antibody (IFA) test for *Toxoplasma* and include glass slides with fixed organisms. Generally single titers ≥ 1:256 are diagnostic, although a rising titer is preferred. In most laboratories, indirect hemagglutination (IHA) and IFA tests have replaced the Sabin-Feldman dye test.

• • •

Pneumocystis carinii [60,61]

Pneumocystis carinii, a parasite, is thought to be a protozoan that occurs in two forms: the vegetative trophozoite and the encysted organism.

Morphology:
1. The trophozoite varies from 5-12 μm in diameter and has a central nucleus measuring 0.5 μm that is surrounded by a clear zone (Fig. 34-25).
2. The cyst is round, 5-8 μm in diameter, and has a prominent cyst wall. The lumen contains eight

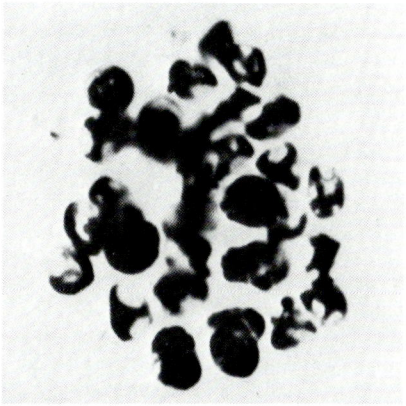

Fig. 34-25. Typical cluster of *Pneumocystitis carinii* cysts in an imprint of a lung biopsy specimen stained with Gram-Weigert. Note that cysts do not stain uniformly. (Original magnification × 760.) (From Rosen, P.P.: Am. J. Med. **58**:794, 1975.)

sporelike inner bodies measuring about 2-4 μm in diameter containing one 1 μm nucleus each.

Life cycle: Adults are carriers of the organism and appear to be able to transmit it to infants and debilitated individuals. The common denominator appears to be a lack of resistance because of absence or diminution of immune globulins.

The infants affected are usually 2-3 months old, a time when their antibodies are lowest since the transplacentally transmitted maternal antibodies have almost disappeared and the infant's own antibodies are just beginning to appear. In affected adults the immune mechanisms are depressed by such diseases as plasma-lymphocytic proliferative disorders or by therapeutic procedures such as the administration of antimetabolites, cortisone, or radiation.

Disease production[62-64]: The organism is an opportunistic invader able to produce interstitial plasma cell pneumonia in infants and a hyaline membrane and pulmonary proteinosis–like condition in adults. The organism is endemic in some areas of Europe.

Diagnosis: Lung biopsy specimens obtained by percutaneous needle biopsy or aspiration or by thoracotomy provide the best opportunity to arrive at a diagnosis. The thrombocytopenia that often accompanies *Pneumocystis carinii* renders any invasive blind procedure somewhat dangerous because of potential hemorrhage. Tissue sections are stained with hematoxylin-eosin, PAS, and methenamine silver stains while imprints of fresh tissue specimens are treated with toluidine blue O, Gram, Gram-Weigert,[63] and methenamine silver stains. Since these stains complement each other, all the staining procedures mentioned must be performed on each specimen.

Smears of sputum, of transtracheal aspirates, and of bronchial brushings and washings are handled like the lung tissue imprints but their diagnostic yield is low and unreliable.[65] The stains mentioned usually demonstrate the cyst form of the organism.

Gram-Wiegert stain[62]: Gram-Weigert stain is useful in demonstrating pneumocystis in tissue sections, smears, and imprints. The latter two are air dried and fixed in ether-alcohol.

Control slides must be stained at the same time as the unknown is handled.

Reagents:
1. Fixative: 50:50 concentration of 95% ethyl alcohol–ether
2. Eosin stain: 1 g eosin and 1 dl distilled water
3. Crystal (gentian) violet
   a. Aniline oil, 2 ml, and distilled water, 88 ml. Shake and filter.
   b. Crystal violet, 5 g, and absolute ethyl alcohol, 10 ml.
   c. Combine a and b and filter; solution is stable for 3 months.
4. Gram iodine
   Dissolve 2 g potassium iodide in 1 dl distilled water. Add 1 g iodine crystals.
5. Decolorizing agent
   Combine aniline oil and xylene 50:50 until no purple color comes off.

Procedure: Stain air-dried smears or imprints in

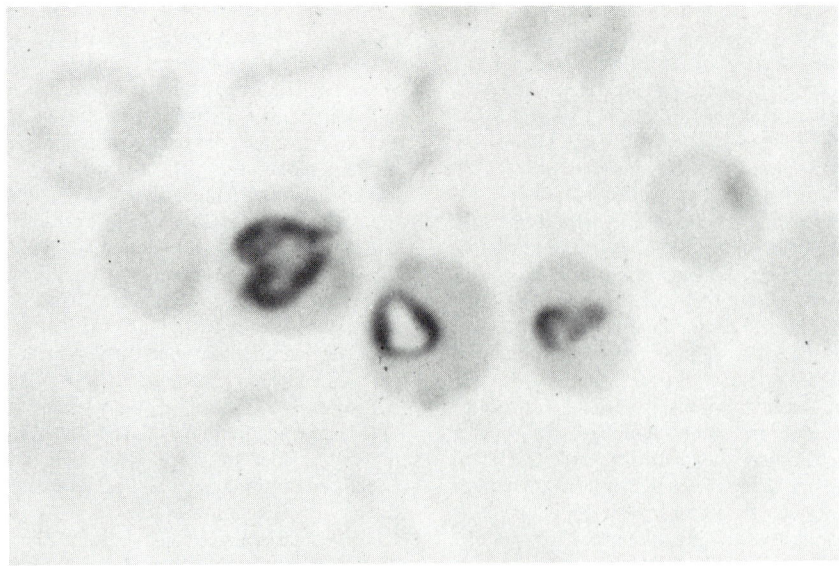

Fig. 34-26. Babesiosis.

eosin for 3-5 min. Rinse in water. Stain in gentian violet for 5-10 min. Rinse in Gram iodine for 5-10 min. Rinse in water and blot dry. Decolorize in aniline oil in xylene. Rinse in xylene.

Result: *Pneumocystis* is blue to deep purple against a pink background.

Serodiagnosis: Serologic methods are limited by the facts that most patients with pneumocystosis are immune suppressed and lack adequate antibodies, but these methods are useful for epidemiologic investigations. Recent culture methods[66] provide the antigen for the sensitive indirect immunofluorescence test.

Babesiosis

Babesiosis (piroplasmosis)[67,68] is a tick-transmitted protozoan infection (Fig. 34-26) that affects the red cells of cattle, horses, hogs, sheep, dogs, and many other animals including humans, although few human cases have been reported.[68-70] Earlier human infections have occurred in splenectomized individuals suggesting the importance of an intact spleen in defense against the organism. In contradiction, however, splenectomy had not been a factor in a number of more recent cases. The agent is a plasmodium-like organism, the sexual cycle of which takes place in the tick while the asexual cycle occurs in domestic or wild animals and in humans. There may also be an exoerythrocytic cycle in gut epithelium. In the red cells the trophozoites first appear as ring forms with small chromatin dots not unlike those of *Plasmodium falciparum*.

In the process of schizogony the organism produces a characteristic four–daughter cell formation in a red cell that is not enlarged, does not show Schüffner dots, and contains no malarial pigment. The latter three features aid in the differentiation from malaria. Other differential tests include serologic investigation, electron microscopy, and animal inoculation.

Diagnosis: The diagnosis is based on the demonstra-

tion of the organism in Wright-Giemsa–stained blood films. Two ovoid trophozoites, attached at one end, are often found within a red cell.

HELMINTHS
NEMATODES

Nematodes (roundworms) are parasites with a complete intestinal tract and a body cavity (without epithelial lining) into which project four longitudinal cords. They have nervous, excretory, and reproductive systems, and the sexes are separate.

In cross section, as sometimes found in sections of the surgically removed appendix, the type of musculature aids in distinguishing the species (Fig. 34-27).

There are two large groups of nematodes: intestinal nematodes and tissue-inhabiting nematodes.

Intestinal nematodes
Trichuris trichiura (whipworm) (Fig. 34-28 and Plate 19 [p. 988])

Habitat: Large intestine, usually cecum or appendix of humans.

Size: 3-5 cm long.

Characteristics: Anterior three fifths is slender and threadlike; posterior two fifths is thicker and bulbous, so that the entire organism is whiplike. The worm is white. The coiled posterior end of the male resembles a watch spring. The posterior end of the female is blunt and rounded.

Ova: Ovoid, yellow brown, and about 50-54 × 23 μm in diameter. There is a characteristic clear refractive plug at each end. They are barrel shaped and have a thick double wall; the inner wall is lighter than the outer. The unsegmented immature embryo fills the entire egg (Plate 19 [p. 988]).

Life cycle: The fertilized ova are passed unsegmented and require about 3 weeks in moist soil to develop to the mature embryo stage, at which time they

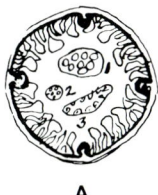 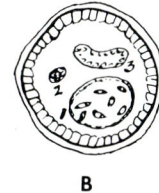 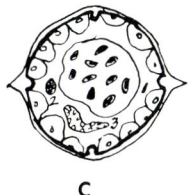

A   B   C

Fig. 34-27. Cross sections of female nematodes (schematic). **A,** Polymyarian type (*Ascaris* and *Toxocara*). **B,** Holomyarian type *(Trichuris).* **C,** Meromyarian type *(Enterobius, Ancylostoma,* and *Necator).* *1,* Uterus; *2,* ovary; *3,* digestive tract.

are infectious. When they reach the digestive tract of humans, usually in contaminated food and water, they release the larvae in the small intestines, where they mature and then migrate into the cecum where they attach themselves to the mucosa and mate, and the gravid female releases thousands of the brown eggs that can be detected in the stool.

Diagnosis: The characteristic ova are found in the feces by direct wet saline, iodine-stained slides, and concentration methods.

Enterobius vermicularis, formerly called Oxyuris vermicularis (pinworm) (Fig. 34-29)

Habitat: Humans are the only host; the organisms are found in the large intestine and appendix and may be found in the urinary bladder or the female genital tract.

Size: The female measures 5-10 × 0.5 mm. The male is almost microscopic in size, 2-5 mm long.

Characteristics: Both worms are white. The posterior end of the female is drawn out into a long, pointed clear tail. The vulva opens at the junction of the anterior and middle third of the body. The anterior end has cuticular expansions resembling lips, but there is no true buccal cavity (Fig. 34-29). The esophagus ends in a bulb. The gravid uterus of the mature female is distended with eggs. In tissue sections the cross section of *Enterobius vermicularis* is characterized by two lateral spines (Fig. 34-27). The male has a curved pointed tail and is hardly ever found in stool specimens.

Ova: The ova are asymmetrically ovoid, colorless, and about 50 × 20 μm in diameter. One side is characteristically flattened. The shell is thick and double contoured. The mature larva is coiled inside (Fig. 34-28).

Life cycle: The gravid female leaves the cecum at night to deposit the ova in the rugae of the anal margin. The ova contain embryos that are infectious. The migration of the gravid female is erratic and does not occur every night. Therefore up to seven successive cellophane tape or other preparations must be examined before a negative diagnosis can be accepted. Eggs are seldom found in fecal specimens, since they are not usually liberated within the intestines. Scratching of the pruritic anal area transfers ova to the fingers, so that eventually the ova reach the mouth and digestive tract, where they hatch into larvae, which molt twice, and, when mature, mate in the large intestine. The complete life cycle requires about 2-4 weeks.

Diagnosis: Ova are recovered from the anal margin by a number of methods. Preparations should be obtained in the morning before the patient has had a bath or has urinated (female) and may have to be repeated six times on six different days before pinworm infection can be ruled out.

Cellophane tape preparation (Fig. 34-30): Over one end of a tongue depressor, curve a 3 in. long strip of ³/₄ in. wide cellophane tape, sticky side out. Spread the anal folds apart and firmly touch all four quadrants of the mucocutaneous junction with the sticky tape. Spread the sticky surface of the tape on a microscope slide and examine microscopically for *Enterobius* ova. If none are found, lift the tape off the slide, place 1 drop toluene on the slide, and replace the tape. The toluene will clear the extraneous matter on the slide but will not harm the ova. Reexamine slide (Fig. 34-31).

Petrolatum-paraffin–coated swab method: There are commercial adhesive tape kits available for pinworm recovery (Ortho Pharmaceutical Corp., Raritan, N.J.).

Preparation of swab: Dip cotton swab in 1:1 mixture of hot paraffin and petrolatum until completely coated and allow to cool. Store each coated swab in a suitable test tube plugged with cotton and place in refrigerator.

The specimen is obtained as in the cellophane tape technic and the swab is placed back in the test tube. In the laboratory the tube containing the swab is filled with just enough xylene to cover the cotton tip of the swab. After 3-5 min the swab is removed and the xylene is centrifuged for about 1 min at slow speed. The supernatant is removed with a pipet and the sediment is transferred to a microscope slide and examined for ova.

Swube method: Swube (Scientific Products, McGaw Park, Ill.) is a commercially available plastic paddle suspended in a plastic tube. The patient is instructed to touch the stretched and flattened anal folds with the sticky surface of the paddle and to return it to the tube.

In the laboratory the nonsticky surface is placed lengthwise on a microscope slide and the sticky surface is examined like a cellophane tape preparation.

HOOKWORMS

The common name **hookworm** includes the following parasites: *Necator americanus, Ancylostoma duodenale, Ancylostoma braziliense,* and *Ancylostoma caninum.* **The life cycles of these parasites are similar.** Humans are the host of *A. duodenale* and *N. amer-*

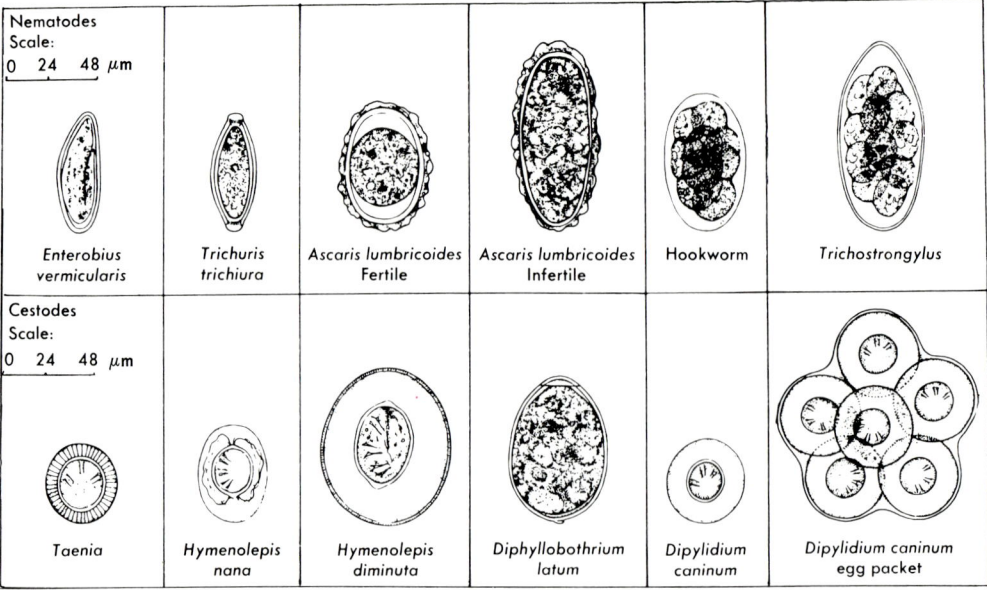

Fig. 34-28. Nematode and cestode eggs found in human stool specimens. (From Brooke, M.M., and Melvin, D.M.: Morphology of diagnostic stages of intestinal parasites of man, Public Health Service Publication no. 1966, Atlanta, 1969, Centers for Disease Control.)

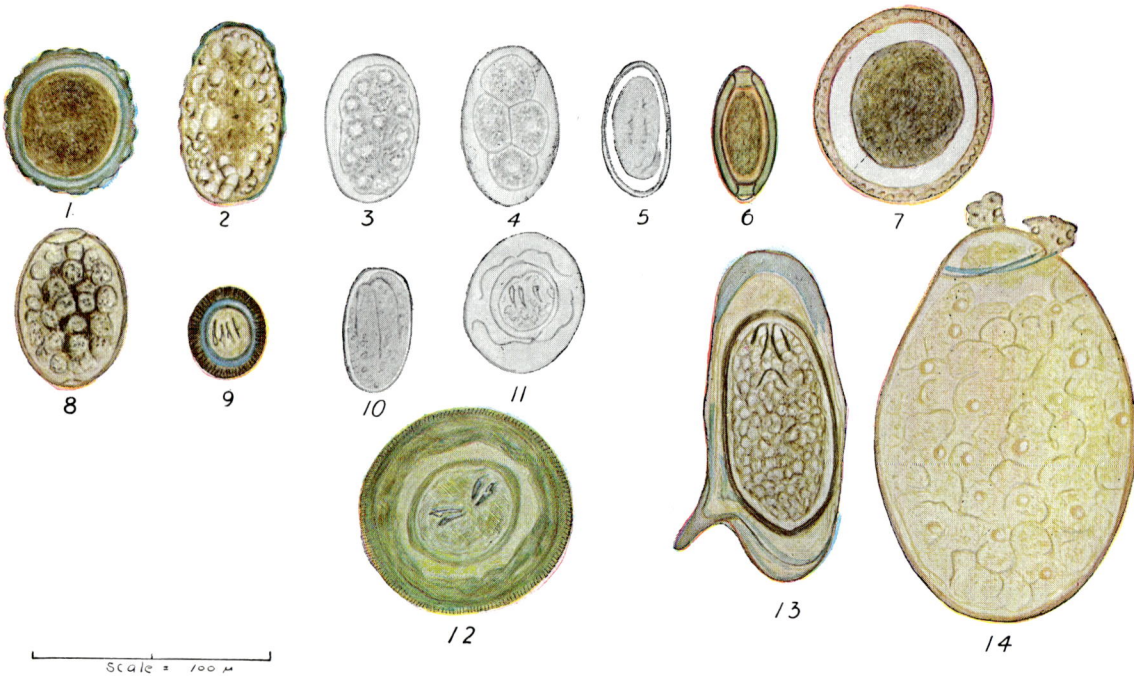

Plate 19. Ova of intestinal parasites.

1 *Ascaris lumbricoides* (fertilized egg)
2 *Ascaris lumbricoides* (unfertilized egg)
3 *Necator americanus* (late segmentation)
4 *Necator americanus* (four-cell stage)
5 *Enterobius vermicularis*
6 *Trichuris trichiura*
7 *Toxocara canis*

8 *Diphyllobothrium latum*
9 *Taenia saginata* or *T. solium*
10 *Rhabditis hominis*
11 *Hymenolepis nana*
12 *Hymenolepis diminuta*
13 *Schistosoma mansoni*
14 *Fasciolopsis buski*

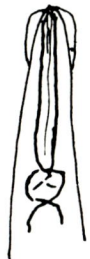

Fig. 34-29. Head of *Enterobius vermicularis* showing cuticular expansion.

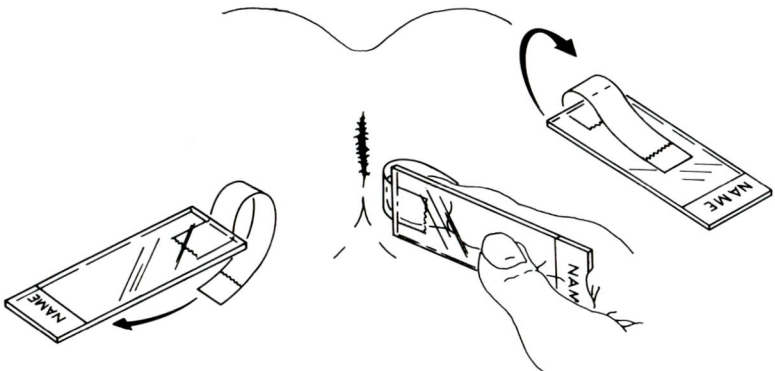

Fig. 34-30. Cellophane tape slide preparation. Attach 3 in. piece of cellophane tape to undersurface of clear end of microscope slide, which has previously been identified (ground-glass end). Press sticky surface of tape against perianal skin. Then roll back tape onto slide, sticky surface down. Wash hands and nails well.

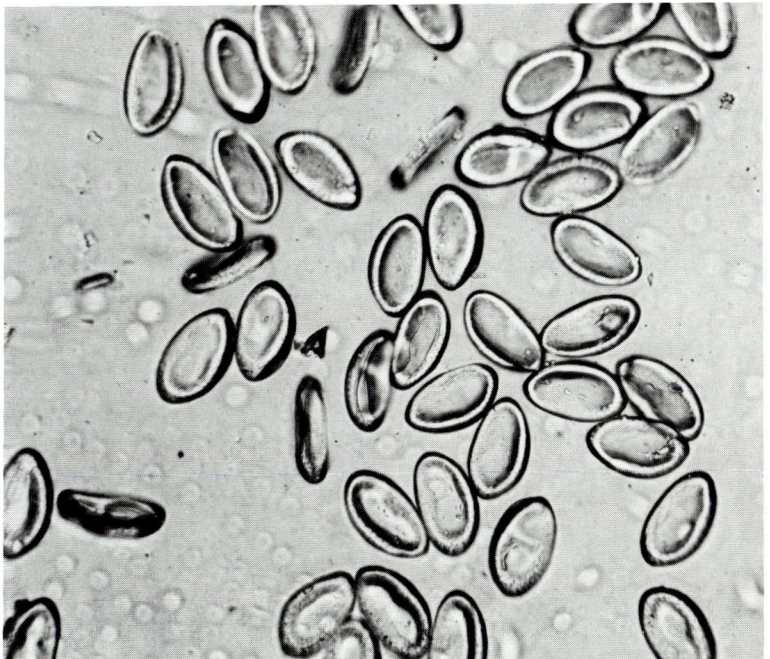

Fig. 34-31. Cellophane tape preparation of *Enterobius vermicularis* ova.

HOOKWORM

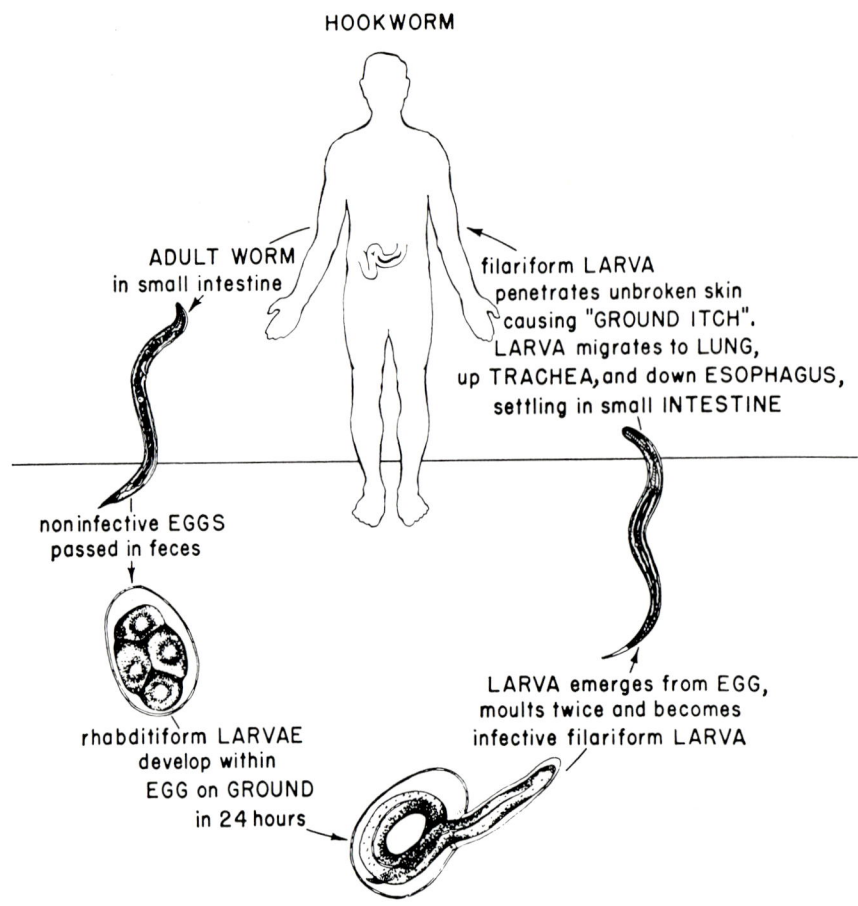

ADULT WORM
in small intestine

filariform LARVA
penetrates unbroken skin
causing "GROUND ITCH".
LARVA migrates to LUNG,
up TRACHEA, and down ESOPHAGUS,
settling in small INTESTINE

noninfective EGGS
passed in feces

rhabditiform LARVAE
develop within
EGG on GROUND
in 24 hours

LARVA emerges from EGG,
moults twice and becomes
infective filariform LARVA

Fig. 34-32. *Necator americanus.* (From Ash, J.E., and Spitz, S.: Pathology of tropical diseases: an atlas, Philadelphia, 1945, W.B. Saunders Co.)

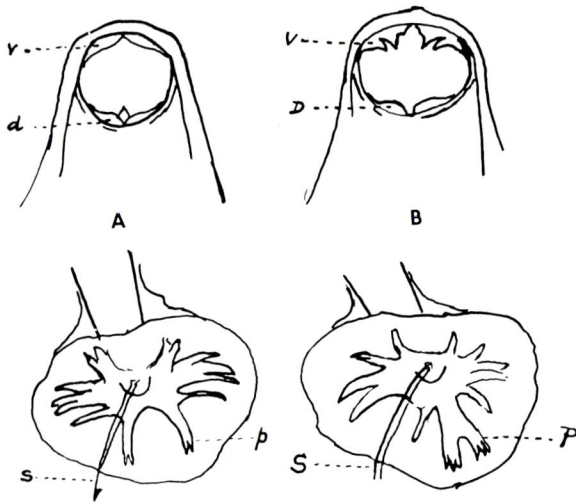

Fig. 34-33. Mouths and caudal bursae of hookworms. **A,** *Necator americanus: v,* ventral cutting plates; *d,* dorsal cutting plates and median tooth; *s,* pair of copulatory spicules, fused distally and ending in a barbed tip; *p,* characteristic posterior muscle ray. **B,** *Ancylostoma duodenale: V,* two pairs of ventral teeth; *D,* dorsal cutting plates; *S,* pair of copulatory spicules, not fused and without barbs; *P,* characteristic posterior muscle ray.

icanus. A. braziliense and *A. caninum* occur in cats and dogs.

Necator americanus (New World hookworm) (Figs. 34-32 and 34-33 and Plate 19 [p. 988])

Habitat: Small intestine of humans.

Size: Female is 9-11 mm long and 0.35 mm in diameter. Male is 5-9 mm long and 0.30 mm in diameter.

Characteristics: The anterior end, the head, of the adult hookworm is curved sharply into a dorsal hook (hence the name) which in *Necator* is much more pronounced than in *Ancylostoma*. The mouth cavity has one pair of broad semilunar chitinous plates anteriorly, one pair of smaller ones posteriorly, and a prominent dorsal toothlike structure projecting into the cavity from the posterior wall. The cutting **plates** differentiate *Necator* from *Ancylostoma*, which has teeth. The vulva of the female is anterior, and the caudal end of the female lacks the short spine that adorns the caudal end of the female *Ancylostoma duodenale*. The male **bursa,** a cuticular expansion over the caudal end, attaches itself to the female during copulation. It contains a number of **muscular groups** or **rays,** the two posterior ones of which are characteristic. They are small, and their **tips are divided** into two **fingerlike** projections. The **two** spicules (long bristlelike structures extending from the caudal end of the male parasite) are fused at their distal end and terminate into one single **barbed tip** (Fig. 34-33). The copulatory spicules of *Ancylostoma* are not fused and are not barbed.

Ova: The ova are ovoid, colorless, 40 × 70 μm, and hyaline. The shell is thin and transparent. When passed, the ovum contains an uncleaved **yolk mass** or a **cleaved embryo** in the early 2-4-8 cell stages. The cleaved cell mass is surrounded by a clear outer zone that separates it from the shell. The eggs resemble those of *Ancylostoma* but are slightly larger. If the stool specimen is allowed to stand, the embryonated eggs may mature into the **larval stage** and the **rhabditiform larvae** may eventually hatch.

Life cycle: The ova develop in warm moist soil, and the young worms, the noninfective **rhabditiform larvae,** hatch out in a few days. The larvae grow and molt twice, being transformed into the infective **filariform type** in about 3-6 weeks. The usual mode of infection is through the skin, although the larvae may reach the digestive tract directly with food or water from polluted soil. When infected earth comes in contact with the skin, the larvae may enter through the skin within 5 min. This produces **dermatitis,** the so-called **ground itch.** The larvae migrate by blood and lymph vessels to the lungs, enter the air sacs, make their way to the bronchi and pharynx, and are swallowed. They attach themselves to the mucosa of the small intestine by means of the buccal cavity and mature to adult forms. The ova are found in the feces within 7-10 weeks after the infection.

Diagnosis: Ova and larvae are found in the feces and are diagnostic of hookworms but not of the species. The characteristic features of the ova are described above. The eggs can be identified only as "hookworm eggs" (Fig. 34-28) and cannot be speciated. If the stool specimen is allowed to stand, the embryos may mature

into the larval stage and may hatch. In this case the stool specimen contains the larvae in the company of cleaved ova. These noninfective rhabditiform larvae of hookworms (the first larvae to be hatched) must be distinguished from the rhabditiform larvae of *Strongyloides stercoralis* and *Trichostrongylus,* from *Rhabditis hominis,* and from the infective filariform larvae. The differential diagnosis may also be accomplished when stained smears are examined. The differential diagnostic criteria are mentioned below. The most important one is the length of the buccal cavity, the space between the opening of the mouth and of the esophagus.

The hookworm egg count may be important in determining parasite load. The Stoll egg count technic is used. Detailed instructions as well as interpretive data can be found on p. 996.

Differential diagnosis of rhabditiform larvae (Fig. 34-34):

Characteristics of rhabditiform larvae of hookworm:

1. The buccal cavity is relatively long. In the rhabditiform larva of the hookworm it is about as long as the diameter of the larva, while in the rhabditiform larva of *Strongyloides* it measures about one half the diameter of the larva.
2. There is writhing, snakelike motion.
3. The esophagus has one bulb.
4. The genital primordium is insignificant.
5. The rhabditiform larvae of hookworm are not found in fresh stool specimens but may be found in specimens that are 1 day old or older.

Characteristics of rhabditiform larvae of Strongyloides stercoralis:

1. The buccal cavity is short.
2. There is purposeless, lashing movement.
3. The esophagus has one bulb.
4. Genital primordium is a prominent structure in the middle of the body.
5. In fresh stool specimens, *Trichostrongylus* eggs and rhabditiform larvae of *Stronglyoides stercoralis* may be found together if the infection is multiple.

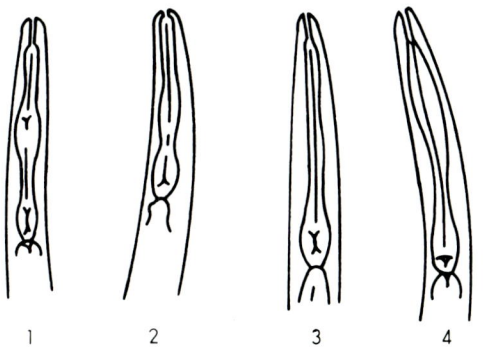

Fig. 34-34. Diagram of mouth and esophagus of rhabditiform larvae. **1,** *Rhabditis hominis.* **2,** *Strongyloides stercoralis.* **3,** *Necator americanus.* **4,** *Trichostrongylus.* (See text.)

Characteristics of rhabditiform larvae of Trichostrongylus:

1. The buccal cavity is long.
2. The esophagus has one bulb.
3. The genital primordium is small.

Trichostrongylus resembles hookworm in appearance and life cycle, but human infestation is often asymptomatic. The rhabditiform *Trichostrongylus* larvae cannot be differentiated from the corresponding hookworm larvae, but the *Trichostrongylus* ova differ from the hookworm ova inasmuch as they are larger and have pointed ends (Fig. 34-28).

Characteristics of Rhabditis hominis:

1. The buccal cavity is long.
2. The esophagus has two bulbs.
3. Adults and larvae are found in feces.

Rhabditis is a nematode found primarily in invertebrates or free living, and its presence in stool denotes soil contamination.

Diagnosis and differential diagnosis of infective filariform larvae (Fig. 34-35):

Characteristics of filariform larvae of hookworm:

1. The buccal cavity is relatively long.
2. The esophagus lacks a bulb and extends one fourth the length of the body.
3. The tail is pointed.

Characteristics of filariform larvae of Strongyloides: The *Strongyloides* rhabditiform larvae rarely

molt in the intestines, so that infective filariform larvae (Fig. 34-36) are hardly ever encountered in the stool specimen.

1. The buccal cavity is short.
2. The esophagus is straight, lacks a bulb, and extends one half the length of the body.
3. The tail is notched.

Additional laboratory findings: Since hookworms suck and hemolyse the victim's blood, a severe iron-deficiency anemia develops, depending on the duration and severity of the infestation.

Ancylostoma duodenale (Old World hookworm)
(Fig. 34-32)

Size: Female is 10-13 mm long; male measures 8-11 mm in length.

Characteristics: *Ancylostoma duodenale* is very similar to *Necator americanus,* but it is just slightly larger, and the head does not curve so sharply in a dorsal hook as that of the American type. The ova are somewhat more ovoid. The chief differences, however, are the mouthparts and in the male bursa. The **buccal cavity** of *A. duodenale* has two pairs of rather sharp curved teeth ventrally and one platelike pair posteriorly. The vulva of the female is just inferior to the middle of the body. The posterior rays of the **male bursa** are fused proximally, and each tip is divided into three fingerlike portions. The two spicules lack barbs and are not fused.

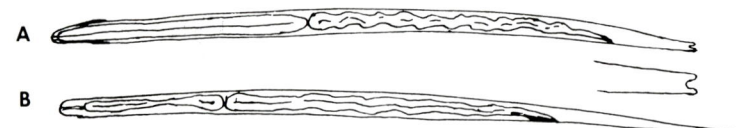

Fig. 34-35. Filariform larvae. **A,** *Strongyloides stercoralis* with notched tail (inset shows notch enlarged). **B,** *Necator americanus.*

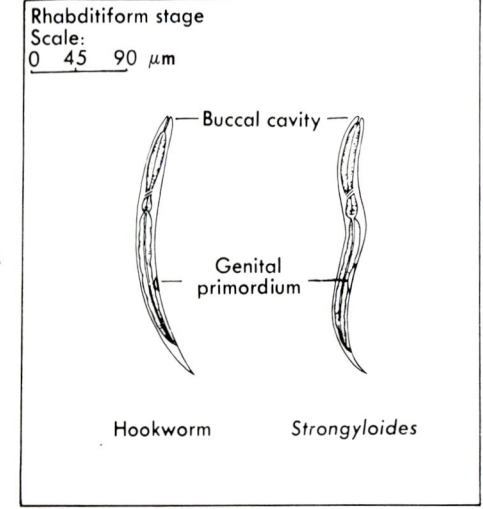
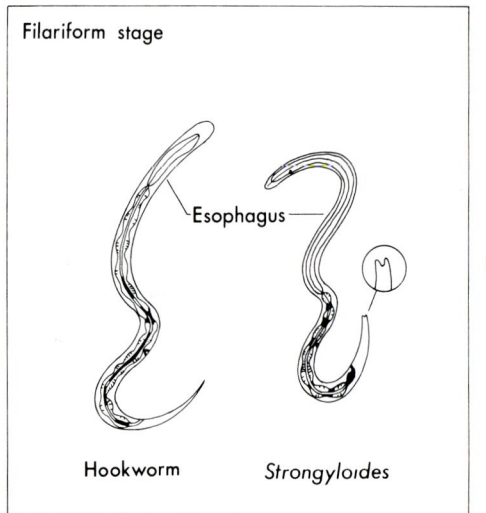

Fig. 34-36. Diagram of rhabditiform and filariform larvae of hookworm and of *Strongyloides.*

Life cycle: The life cycle of *Ancylostoma* is similar to that of *Necator*. When deposited in moist soil, the eggs hatch within 24 hr and the first larva, the noninfective rhabditiform larva, feeds on bacteria until it molts into the nonfeeding infective larva. The latter stays in the surface layer of the moist soil and in order to survive must penetrate human skin, usually of the foot between the toes or of the ankle. The larvae are carried in the bloodstream to the lungs and finally find their way via the pharynx into the esophagus. They mature in the intestines, attach themselves to the mucosa, and live on blood and tissue juices.

Diagnosis: See preceding discussion of *Necator*. The diagnostic approach is the same in all hookworm infestations.

Ancylostoma braziliense, Ancylostoma caninum, and cutaneous larva migrans

Cats and dogs are hosts to several species of hookworms. *Ancylostoma caninum* is found in dogs and *Ancylostoma braziliense* in cats and dogs. If humans come in contact with the filariform larvae of the dog or cat hookworms, they penetrate the skin but since humans are an unnatural host, the filariform larvae wander about in the skin, forming serpiginous tunnels, the course of which is outlined by redness and elevation of the skin followed by scaliness. This lesion is called **creeping eruption** or **cutaneous larva migrans** and must be differentiated from filarial involvement (p. 991) of the subcutaneous tissues. Itching is intense, and secondary infection often follows scratching. The cutaneous lesion may progress from a few millimeters to several centimeters a day, the larvae being in advance of the raised reddened portion of the tunnel. The larvae may continue the migration for weeks or months, apparently unable to penetrate through the skin in order to complete the life cycle.

Ancylostoma caninum (dog hookworm)

Dogs are host to several species of hookworms, e.g., *Ancylostoma braziliense* and *Ancylostoma caninum* (Fig. 34-37). The latter is the most common hookworm of the dog.

Size: The female is 14 mm long while the male is 10 mm long.

Characteristics: The buccal cavity has three pairs of ventral teeth.

• • •

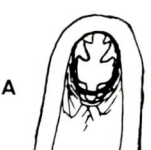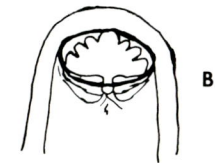

Fig. 34-37. Buccal cavities of dog hookworms. **A**, *Ancylostoma braziliense*. **B**, *Ancylostoma caninum*.

Ascaris lumbricoides (large roundworm)

The *Ascaris* roundworms (Figs. 34-38 and 34-39) are characterized by three lips surrounding the oral opening. *Ascaris lumbricoides* is the largest roundworm of humans. The name expresses its resemblance to the earthworm (*Lumbricus*).

Habitat: Humans are the definitive host. The adults are found in the small intestines.

Size: The female is 20-35 cm long (longer than the male) and 3-6 mm in diameter. The male is 15-25 cm long and 3-6 mm in diameter.

Characteristics: The adult worm is white or pink and has fine circular striations of the cuticle. The anterior end has three lips. The posterior ends of the male and female worms are pointed, but the male end is coiled.

Ova: The ova may be present in several different forms.

1. **Fertilized** eggs are ovoid and yellow to brown, measure 50-75 × 40-60 μm, and have a thick shell with a mammillated brown outer covering and a thick transparent hyaline **inner shell.** There is an inner crescentic clear space at either pole of the egg where the central **unsegmented protoplasmic** mass draws away from the shell.

2. **Unfertilized** eggs are usually larger than the fertilized eggs and measure about 50-90 μm in length. When only females are present in the intestines, the ova are elongated, have thinner shells, and are completely filled with a coarse granular or globular protoplasm. They are stained yellow or brown with bile, lack the crescentic clear space, and are often **misshapen and distorted.**

3. **Decorticated** eggs occur in old specimens. The outer mammillated shell is at times absent, leaving only the inner thick hyaline membrane. The eggs may or may not be fertile. If the brown outer coat is lost, the eggs may be confused with colorless hookworm eggs, although the shell of the decorticated *Ascaris* eggs is thicker. If the eggs are decorticated and unfertilized, they resemble *Trichostrongylus* eggs because of their longer and narrower shape (Fig. 34-28).

Life cycle: In feces the embryos in the eggs are unsegmented. To ensure further development, the eggs must reach soil. After 2-5 weeks in moist soil the fertilized eggs contain a wormlike embryo and are infectious. These eggs are highly resistant and can withstand winter temperatures without injury but not summer heat. They are viable for 5-6 years at least and can withstand 5% formalin for long periods of time. A person is usually infected after **eating soil-contaminated vegetables** or by other contact with contaminated soil; the ova reach the duodenum where the embryos leave the shell in about 15 hr, make their way through the intestinal wall into the bloodstream, and are carried to the liver and to the lungs. During this migration they grow to a length of 2 mm. From the lungs they make their way into the bronchi and are coughed up and swallowed. They develop in the duodenum to the familiar adult worm in about 1 month. In the intestines each female lays thousands of unsegmented ova, which are passed in the stool and must reach moist soil to mature.

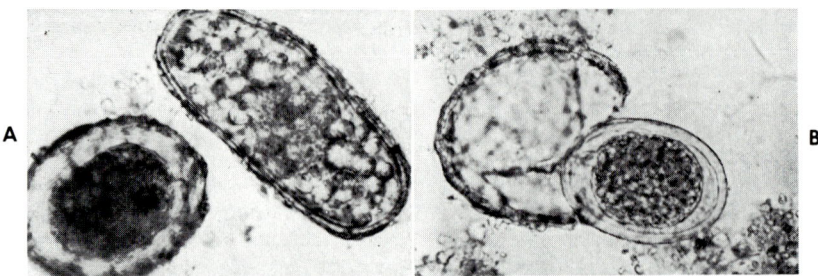

Fig. 34-38. Ova of *Ascaris lumbricoides*. **A,** Fertile and unfertile eggs. **B,** Fertile egg expressed from its ruptured outer mammillated membrane. (×400.)

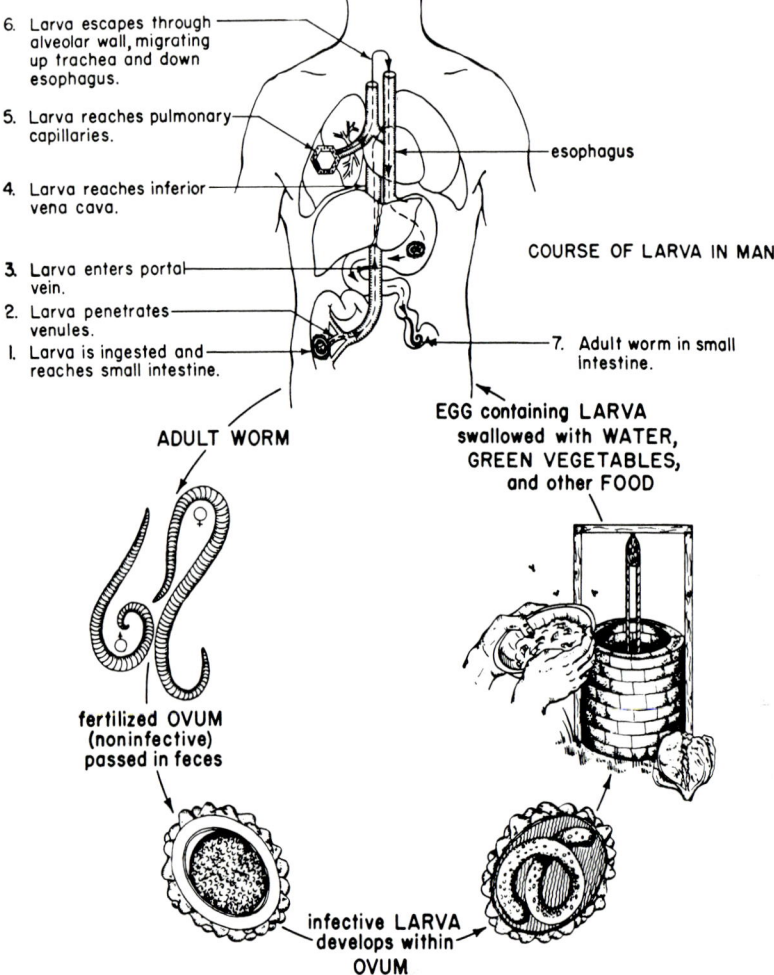

6. Larva escapes through alveolar wall, migrating up trachea and down esophagus.

5. Larva reaches pulmonary capillaries.

4. Larva reaches inferior vena cava.

3. Larva enters portal vein.

2. Larva penetrates venules.

1. Larva is ingested and reaches small intestine.

esophagus

COURSE OF LARVA IN MAN

7. Adult worm in small intestine.

EGG containing LARVA swallowed with WATER, GREEN VEGETABLES, and other FOOD

ADULT WORM

fertilized OVUM (noninfective) passed in feces

infective LARVA develops within OVUM

Fig. 34-39. *Ascaris lumbricoides*. (From Ash, J.E., and Spitz, S.: Pathology of tropical diseases: an atlas, Philadelphia, 1945, W.B. Saunders Co.)

Diagnosis: The diagnosis depends on finding eggs and adult worms in the stool. The adult worm is usually detected by the patient. Previously described methods of direct wet-film preparation and of concentration are employed on the fecal specimen. Because of the large number of ova usually present in the specimen, concentration methods are usually not necessary.

Other laboratory findings: Eosinophilia may accompany the pulmonary phase of parasitic infestation.

Toxocara

Toxocara canis and *Toxocara catis* are common intestinal roundworms of dogs and cats. Male and female worms are smaller than *Ascaris lumbricoides,* measuring up to 9 and 17 cm in length, respectively. As in *A. lumbricoides,* the female is longer.

Toxocara catis (roundworm of cat)

The adult form of *Toxocara catis* (Fig. 34-40) is characterized by the three *Ascaris* lips and a pair of lateral cervical alae, giving its head an arrowhead appearance. In other respects this parasite is similar to *T. canis.*

Life cycle: The life cycles of the dog and cat roundworms in the animals are similar to that of *A. lumbricoides* in humans. The animals are infected by eating the eggs, which then hatch in the duodenum from where the larvae start their journey via the bloodstream to the various organs, including the lung, from where they reach the pharynx and finally the esophagus and duodenum where they mate. The mature pregnant female lays eggs that are light brown, slightly mammillated, and have a prominent vitelline membrane. They need some time in moist soil for maturation before they are infective to dogs, cats, and humans.

Visceral larva migrans: If children eat the eggs of *Toxocara canis* or *Toxocara catis* the larvae escape in the duodenum and start their tour of the body, but since humans are an abnormal host the larvae are unable to mature and produce a granulomatous condition in liver and lungs referred to as **visceral larva migrans.** Clinically there is usually a pronounced **eosinophilia** associated with enlargement of the liver, hypergammaglobulinemia, and bronchopneumonia. A similar clinical picture may be produced by larvae of *Ascaris, Strongyloides,* and hookworm.

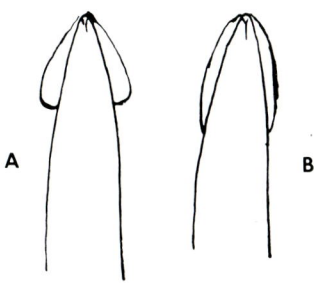

Fig. 34-40. Head showing cervical alae. **A,** *Toxocara cati.* **B,** *Toxocara canis.*

Toxocara canis (roundworm of dog) (Fig. 34-40)

Habitat: Small intestine.

Size: The female is 6-17 cm long; the male is 4-9 cm long. The head has narrow lateral cervical alae, the shape suggesting an arrowhead.

Ova: The ova are spheroid with a thick shell. They are not found in human feces since the parasite does not mature in human intestines.

Strongyloides stercoralis

Strongylos (Greek) means round, but taxonomically *Strongyloides* does not belong to the family of Strongyles. It is a parasitic worm of humans, dogs,[71] cats, and many other domestic and wild mammals, e.g., horses and monkeys. The incidence of strongyloidiasis[72] is much lower than that of hookworm.

Habitat: Duodenum of humans.

Size and morphology: The adult parasitic female worm is microscopic and filariform and measures about 2 mm in length. The cylindric eosphagus is one third the length of the body. The male worm is free living, rhabditiform, and seldom found in fecal specimens. It measures 0.7 mm in length.

Ova: The ova, which are similar to hookworm ova, are not found in feces except when diarrhea and hyperperistalsis exist. They can be differentiated from hookworm ova by the fact that they contain **well-developed larvae** when found in stool while hookworm ova contain a cleaved mass (embryo). The ova are confined to the small intestines where they hatch and liberate the **rhabditiform larvae,** which are found in the fecal specimens and which must be differentiated from the rhabditiform larvae of hookworm (p. 991).

Life cycle: The parasitic female bores deeply into the mucosa, chiefly that of the duodenum, and deposits eggs that hatch in situ and liberate the feeding but not infective **rhabditiform** larvae.

The parasite has three types of life cycle.

1. **Indirect cycle.** The actively motile **rhabditiform larvae** make their way into the lumen of the intestines and are voided with the feces. These larvae (Fig. 34-32) are rather short and thick; outside the body in the soil they develop into adult **free-living male** and **female forms.** These free-living forms resemble the filariform larvae of the hookworm but have a shorter mouth cavity, a longer esophagus, and a notch in the tail. After fertilization the free-living female produces eggs that develop into rhabditiform larvae, which develop into a second generation of free-living male and female adults, which produce the eggs to start the cycle over again. The free-living rhabditiform larvae may also choose a second type of life cycle and develop into free-living filariform larvae, the female of which penetrates human skin and initiates the direct cycle.

2. **Direct cycle.** The female filariform larvae penetrate human skin to enter the venous circulation and to be carried by the bloodstream to the heart and lungs. From the lungs the parasites ascend to the glottis, are swallowed, and reach the intestines, where they develop into adult females that reproduce parthenogenetically and lay eggs that hatch in the mucosa. The new generation of rhabditiform larvae finds its way into the lumen of the bowel and finally into the soil to start the indirect cycle.

3. **Autoinfection cycle.** The rhabditiform larvae develop into filariform larvae in the lumen of the intestines and penetrate the intestinal mucosa or the perianal skin to start a developmental cycle within the host by entering the venous circulation, which carries them to the lungs and back to the intestines where the female filariform larvae parthenogenetically produce ova that hatch and repeat the direct cycle.

Diagnosis: Rhabditiform larvae found in the feces are the diagnostic stage. They are microscopic, measuring 200-250 μm in length, and exhibit a characteristic lashing, purposeless motion. The buccal or mouth cavity is short, the length being less than half the diameter of the body. The genital primordium is prominent and is situated at about the middle of the body. As already stated they must be differentiated from the rhabditiform larvae of hookworm (p. 991).

Demonstration of rhabditiform larvae of Strongyloides: Wet saline mounts and formalin–ethyl acetate concentration method should be used to establish the fact that rhabditiform larvae are present in the stool specimen. The speciation of the larvae may be based on the examination of trichrome-stained fecal smears. If no larvae are found after several attempts, duodenal aspiration is advisable if the clinical picture suggests strongyloidiasis.

Duodenal aspiration: Rhabditiform larvae and the hookwormlike eggs may be found in mucus and bile-stained fragments. Duodenal aspirate may contain several parasites in addition to *Strongyloides*, e.g., the trophozoites of *Giardia lamblia* and the eggs of hookworms. *Strongyloides* rhabditiform larvae in their eggs will hatch at room temperature in 15-20 min.

For discussion of morphologic characteristics, see p. 995.

Culture of helminth larvae or eggs in feces:

Principle: Hookworm and *Strongyloides* rhabditiform larvae may be difficult to distinguish, but if allowed to mature to the filariform larval stage in a stool charcoal mixture, the differentiation may be easier since *Strongyloides* filariform larvae make their appearance in 2-3 days while hookworm filariform larvae require 5-6 days. Ova of hookworm, *Strongyloides*, and *Trichostrongylus* develop to the larval stage in the culture mixture.

Procedure: Mix fecal specimen with granular charcoal in equal amounts. Add chlorine-free water to produce a thick, moist, shiny, but not watery paste. Place mixture on filter paper in a Petri dish that is loosely covered. Incubate culture at room temperature and examine for larvae beginning with the second day. Culture must not be allowed to dry out. **Filariform larvae are infective. Take precautions.**

Concentration of larvae by Baermann technic[73]:

Principle: The tendency of larvae to migrate from feces into warm water provides a means to concentrate them.

Procedure: Arrange a ring stand so as to support a large funnel (15 cm diameter) and a 50 ml beaker located below the funnel. Attach short rubber tubing to stem of funnel and allow it to extend into the conical centrifuge tube or beaker. Attach pinch clamp to rubber tubing, close it tightly, and fill funnel with 370 ml wa-

ter. Place a sieve (20 mesh) on top of the funnel in contact with water and cover it with gauze, which must make contact with the warm water. The culture medium described above (stool-charcoal-water mixture) is then placed on the gauze.

After 1-2 hr release the clamp carefully, collect 5-6 ml water in a centrifuge tube or beaker, and close the clamp again. Cap the centrifuge tube and examine sediment for larvae. Repeat collection every 2 hr.

This cultural procedure is not routinely available but may reveal larvae when microscopic examinations are negative.

Additional laboratory findings in Strongyloides infestation: There is usually a marked eosinophilia in the peripheral blood in about one third of all patients. In immunosuppressed hosts (renal transplant patients, etc.) disseminated strongyloidiasis may occur. The larvae will be found in multiple body fluids. The mortality is very high.

Trichostrongylus

Habitat: Trichostrongylus organisms are found in the small intestine of humans. *Trichostrongylus* comprises many species that parasitize cattle, sheep, and many other mammals. The infection is worldwide but has a higher incidence in the Orient. The species resembles hookworms in appearance and life cycle.

Morphologic characteristics: The female measures 5-8 mm in length. The head is unarmed, there is no buccal dilation, and a notch indicates the excretory pore. The male is a small roundworm measuring 4-6 mm in length. It has a copulatory bursa with rays and spicules.

Ova: The ova resemble hookworm eggs but are much larger (85-115 μm). They are elongate and oval and have a transparent thin hyaline shell that is separated by a clear space from the embryo in the morula stage (Fig. 34-28). The ends are pointed, a morphologic feature that separates them form the hookworm eggs.

Life cycle: Adults live in the small intestines attached to the mucosa, which supplies them with blood. The eggs hidden in feces reach the ground, where they hatch. The rhabditiform larvae molt to develop into the infective filariform larvae, which usually fail to penetrate skin but are ingested when they contaminate food or water. They mature and mate in the small intestine and start the cycle anew.

Diagnosis: Macroscopic sieving (20 mesh) may be used to detect the adult worm. Microscopic methods include wet saline mounts and formalin–ethyl acetate concentration to detect the characteristic eggs in the stool specimen.

Stoll egg count[74]: The Stoll egg-counting technic, a procedure appropriate for certain investigations, provides an adequate measure of the worm burden of a patient and allows the evaluation of the effectiveness of therapy. It is not routinely performed.

Procedure: Weigh 4 g feces of a previously weighed 24 hr fecal specimen. Transfer the 4 g material into a graduated cylinder and add 0.1N sodium hydroxide to bring volume to 60 ml. Add several glass beads, stopper cylinder, and shake the emulsion until a uniform suspension is obtained. Transfer 0.15 ml suspension onto a microscope slide, do not apply coverslip, and count all eggs. Multiply egg count by 100 to obtain the number of eggs per gram of feces and by weight of 24 hr fecal specimen to arrive at the number of eggs per 24 hr specimen. Use correction factor to compensate for the consistency of the stool specimen:

Formed stool	× 1.5
Mushy stool	× 2.0
Diarrhea	× 3.0
Flowing diarrhea	× 4.0
Watery stool	× 5.0

Normal value: No ova.

• • •

There is a poor relationship of egg counts to the serologic methods.[75]

Angiostrongylus cantonensis

The adult worm of *Angiostrongylus cantonensis* is found in mesenteric and pulmonary arterioles of rodents. The eggs, deposited in the blood vessels, develop into larvae, which penetrate the vessel walls and ultimately find themselves in the intestinal tract. They are passed in the feces and develop into the infective filariform larvae in slugs and snails. Rats complete the cycle by eating infected snails. Humans acquire the infection, which has been reported from Hawaii, Taiwan, and Indonesia, by eating raw snails. Since the parasite is species specific it dies in the abnormal human host. *A. cantonensis* has been reported from Central America. Serologic investigations aid in the diagnosis.[76]

Capillaria philippinensis

The 4-5 mm long parasite is confined to a small area in the Philippines. Large numbers of worms invade the mucosa of the small intestine, where they produce eggs and larvae, which are passed in the diarrheic stool. The ovoid ova measure 65 × 21 μm and have clear plugs on either end.

Blood and soft-tissue nematodes

Nematodes that inhabit blood and soft tissues include the filariae, *Dracunculus medinensis,* and *Trichinella spiralis.*

Filariae[77]

Classification[78]: The following filarial worms parasitize humans: *Wuchereria bancrofti, Brugia malayi,*

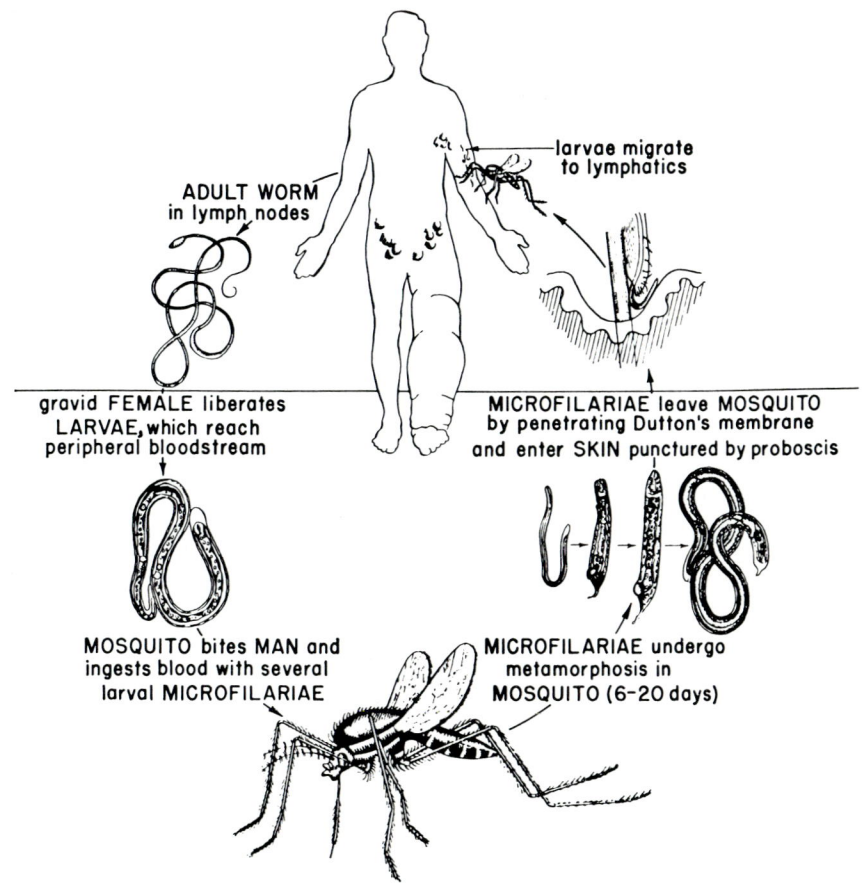

Fig. 34-41. *Wuchereria bancrofti.* (From Ash, J.E., and Spitz, S.: Pathology of tropical diseases: an atlas, Philadelphia, 1945, W.B. Saunders Co.)

Onchocerca volvulus, Loa loa, Dipetalonema perstans, Mansonella ozzardi, and *Dipetalonema stretpocerca.*[42]

Morphology: The threadlike adult worms vary in length from 19-60 cm. The female is twice as long as the male. The parasites are white and are covered with a smooth or patterned cuticle. There are no lips, and the esophagus has no bulb. The life cycle involves a blood-sucking insect vector.[79]

Microfilariae: The larvae produced by the female are called microfilariae and measure from 177-300 μm in length. Some retain their shells, or sheath, while others discard it and remain unsheathed. The sheath closely surrounds the organisms but can be detected where it projects beyond the tail or head. In addition to the presence or absence of a sheath, other morphologic criteria are (1) whether the nuclei extend to the tip of the tail and (2) the length of the cephalic space, the anuclear anterior end of the parasite.

The microfilariae migrate into the peripheral circulation, often periodically, or may be found in chylous urine, chylous exudate, or nodular swellings.

Life cycle: Humans are the definitive host. The microfilariae are ingested by a blood-sucking insect vector (mosquito, fly, or midge), in which they develop to the infective stage and migrate to the proboscis of the insect. When the insect feeds on humans, the parasites enter the body of the final host and migrate to their specific tissues where they develop into mature worms. After mating, the adult female gives birth to a new generation of microfilariae.

The adult threadlike worms, male and female, may be found in pairs in lymph vessels, lymph nodes, body cavities, or subcutaneous tissue, where they provoke a granulomatous and fibrous immune reaction that not only eventually kills them but may also obstruct the lymph flow, causing elephantiasis, chyluria, chylous exudates, or nodular swellings (Fig. 34-41). In *Wuchereria* and *Brugia* infections it is the adult worms that are responsible for the disease processes and not the microfilariae. In *Onchocerca* infections, adult worms are harmless and microfilariae do the damage.

Diagnosis:

Examination of blood[80]:

Wet mounts: Live microfilariae can be demonstrated in a thin wet preparation prepared from a small drop that is allowed to spread underneath a coverslip. *Onchocerca volvulus* has no hematogenous cycle, but the wet preparation can be prepared from tissue juice to demonstrate the microfilariae. In early infections microfilariae may be plentiful, but preparations from chronic cases are often negative.

Membrane filter technic[42,78,81]: Anticoagulated blood is passed through a membrane filter of 5 μm pore size for *Wuchereria* and *Brugia* species and of 3 μm pore size for *Dipetalonema* species. The microfilariae remain on the filter and are separated from red and white cells. The blood specimen should be obtained at the known time of the greatest concentration of microfilariae, which, in the case of *W. bancrofti,* is about midnight. If daytime collection is mandatory, microfilariae may be mobilized by the administration of 100 mg diethylcarbamazine 50 min before taking the blood sample.

Stained preparation: Thick and thin smears are stained with hematoxylin-eosin, a method especially good for staining the details of the microfilariae and their sheaths. The thick smears are prepared as outlined for malaria and the thin smears as detailed in the hematology section. Wright-Giemsa stain and the supravital methylene blue stain are also useful in demonstrating microfilariae.

Concentration methods:

Centrifugation: Anticoagulated blood is spun at 1000 rpm for 10 min, and the buffy coat is smeared and stained.[78] The blood may be lysed before centrifugation by saponin (see malaria technic).

Procedure[7]: Place 10 ml 4% aqueous acetic acid into a 15 ml centrifuge tube. Add 1 ml citrated blood. Centrifuge at 2000 rpm for 10 min. Decant supernatant fluid and examine sediment as wet preparation.

Serodiagnosis: The antigen most frequently used is prepared from the dog parasite *Dirofilaria immitis,* which may be transmitted to humans by mosquito bites, so that false positive reactions are fairly frequent. Adequate supplies of homologous antigen for species-specific tests are not available. The most frequently used tests are bentonite flocculation and indirect hemagglutination, but their sensitivity if heterologous antigen is used varies with different species and may show gross reactivity.

Differential diagnosis of microfilariae: Identification of the species is based on the presence or absence of a sheath, the distribution of nuclei in the tail (Fig. 34-42), and the length of the cephalic space (Tables 34-12 and 34-13).

Wuchereria bancrofti

General characteristics: The parasite *Wuchereria bancrofti* is widely distributed in tropic and subtropic zones and is at times responsible for the production of elephantiasis. The intermediate host is a mosquito *(Culex fatigans).* The microfilariae vary greatly in size (150-500 × 7.5 μm) and are enclosed in a sheath that extends beyond the tail and head. They show nocturnal periodicity, concentrating in the blood during the night, and collecting in the capillaries of the internal organs, especially the lungs (oxygen supply), during the day. The nuclei fail to extend to the tip of the pointed tail.

Brugia malayi

The microfilariae of *Brugia malayi* (found in the Dutch East Indies, New Guinea, and China) show nocturnal periodicity and are sheathed. The are characterized by two nuclei in the tip of the tail, which shows nodular swellings at the level of the nuclei.

Loa loa

General characteristics: The filarial worm is common in Africa and lives in the subcutaneous tissues where it causes fugitive swellings (Calabar swellings) as the parasite moves around the subcutaneous tissue. The intermediate host is a fly *(Chrysops).* The larvae measure about 250-300 × 7 μm, are enclosed in a sheath, and show a diurnal periodicity. The granules of the body cells extend to the tip of the tail, which is less sharply pointed than the tip of the tail of the microfi-

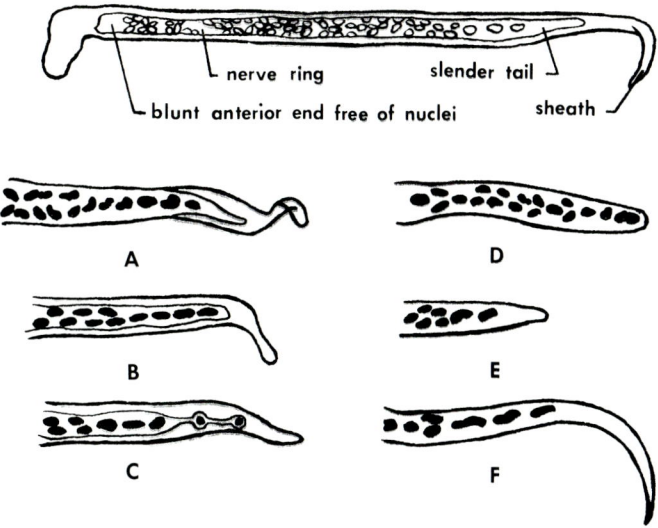

nerve ring   slender tail

blunt anterior end free of nuclei   sheath

A

B

C

D

E

F

Fig. 34-42. Microfilariae of humans: diagnostic characteristics. **A,** *Wuchereria bancrofti.* **B,** *Loa loa.* **C,** *Brugia malayi.* **D,** *Acanthocheilonema perstans.* **E,** *Mansonella ozzardi.* **F,** *Onchocerca volvulus.* (Modified from Brown, H.W., and Belding, D.L.: Basic clinical parasitology, ed. 3, New York, 1969, Appleton-Century-Crofts.)

Table 34-12. Key to microfilariae

	Sheathed	Unsheathed	Nuclei extending to tip	Nuclei not extending to tip	Length of cephalic space	Periodicity
Wuchereria bancrofti	Yes			Yes	As long as broad	Nocturnal
Brugia malayi	Yes		Yes (two)		Twice as long as broad	Nocturnal
Loa loa	Yes		Yes		As long as broad	Diurnal
Dipetalonema perstans		Yes	Yes		As long as broad	None
Mansonella ozzardi		Yes		Yes	As long as broad	None
Onchocerca volvulus		Yes		Yes	As long as broad	None

laria of *W. bancrofti.* The sheath extends beyond the tail and the head (Fig. 34-42).

Dipetalonema (Acanthocheilonema) perstans

General characteristics: The worm is prevalent in tropical Africa, coastal South America, and the West Indies. The adults live in the mesentery and retroperitoneal tissue, usually without causing symptoms. The intermediate host is a midge, a kind of gnat *(Culicoides).* The larvae (microfilariae) are small, 200 × 5 μm, are unsheathed, and do not show any periodicity, but usually they are more numerous in the peripheral blood at night. The nuclei extend to the tip of the blunt tail.

The microfilaria of *Mansonella ozzardi,* a very similar parasite, is distinguished by a rather blunt tail in which the nuclei do not extend to the tip.

Onchocerca volvulus[82]:

General characteristics: The parasite *Onchocerca volvulus* is widely distributed in Africa and is found also in Guatemala and southern Mexico. The intermediate host is a black fly *(Simulium damnosum).*

Life cycle: The bite of the vector injects microfilariae into the new host in whom they mature to adult filariae, which reside in the skin and subcutaneous tissues and are only indirectly responsible for the disease called onchocerciasis, which results from the inflammatory response provoked by masses of microfilariae flooding the soft tissues and dying after a few months of life. The disease is characterized by formation of hyalinized scars in the target organs, skin, and eyes. Blindness, cutaneous nodule formation, and dermatitis are evidence of microfilarial degeneration.

The larvae measure about 250 × 7.5 μm and are

Table 34-13. Filarial parasites

Characteristic	Wuchereria bancrofti	Brugia malayi	Loa loa	Dipetalonema perstans	Mansonella ozzardi	Dipetalonema streptocerca	Onchocerca volvulus
Geographic distribution	Asia, Pacific islands, tropical Africa and Americas	South and East Asia	West and Cental Africa	Africa, Central and South America	Central and South America	West Africa	Africa, Central and South America, Mexico
Location of adult worms	Lymphatic system	Lymphatic system	Subcutaneous tissues	Mesenteries, retroperitoneal tissues	Mesenteries, body cavities	Subcutaneous tissues	Subcutaneous tissues
Vector	Mosquitoes	Mosquitoes	Chrysops (deerfly)	Culicoides (biting midges)	Culicoides	Culicoides	Simulium (black fly)
Location of microfilariae	Blood	Blood	Blood	Blood	Blood and skin	Skin	Skin
Microfilarial periodicity	Nocturnal*	Nocturnal	Diurnal	None	None	None	None
Morphology of microfilariae Length (stained blood film) (μm)	244-296 (260)	177-230 (220)	250-300 (275)	190-200 (195)	163-203 (183)	180-240 (210)	Two sizes: 221-287 (254); 295-358 (332)
Width (stained blood film) (μm)	7.5-10	5-6	6-8.5	4-5	4-5	5-6	5-9
Length in formalin (μm)	275-317 (298)	240-298 (270)	257-313 (280)	183-225 (203)	203-245 (224)	—	—
Sheath	Present	Present	Present	Absent	Absent	Absent	Absent
Sheath staining reaction (Giemsa)	Does not stain	Pink	Does not stain	—	—	—	—
Tail and tail nuclei	Tapered to point; nuclei stop short of end of tail	Tapered with a constriction; last nucleus at end of tail and a nucleus at area of constriction	Tapered with nuclei extending to tip of tail	Tapered and bluntly rounded; nuclei to end of tail	Long slender tail; no nuclei in end of tail	Tail tapered and bent in hook shape; nuclei to end of tail	Tapered to point; no nuclei in end of tail

From Garcia, L.S., and Ash, L.R.: Diagnostic parasitology: clinical laboratory manual, St. Louis, 1979, The C.V. Mosby Co.
*Subperiodic in some Pacific islands.

unsheathed, and the nuclei do not extend to the tip of the pointed tail (Fig. 34-42). The microfilariae are found in the nodules with the adults or in the adjacent lymph vessels but not in the blood.

Diagnosis: *O. volvulus* is best diagnosed by the following method. Cleanse an area of skin, raise a fold, pinch slightly until it is blanched, and make several shallow punctures with a sterile needle to a depth of 2-3 mm to obtain tissue fluid without blood. Mount fluid on a microslide and examine stained or unstained. Microfilariae may be found in the skin even if it does not cover a nodule.

Dracunculus medinensis (guinea worm)

The guinea worm is a roundworm that does not belong to the filariae but to a group that possesses labial papillae (rather than lips) and an anterior muscular esophageal segment.

Distribution: The guinea worm is common in Asia, Africa, and Arabia and is less common in the West Indies and Brazil.

Size: The male is rarely found and is small, about 25-40 mm. The female measures about 80-120 cm × 1.6 mm and has been likened to a catgut thread.

Life cycle: The gravid female wanders through the subcutaneous tissues to the foot or the ankle and forms a nodule that ulcerates. The head of the parasite protrudes, and whenever the foot is in contact with fresh water, numerous larvae are discharged (through prolapse of uterus through the esophagus or head portion). The unsheathed larvae are 600 × 20 μm. A crustacean *(Cyclops)* is the intermediate host, and the infection is spread by swallowing the *Cyclops* in contaminated water. The parasite has been reported in North America in the fox, raccoon, and mink.

Diagnosis: Diagnosis is based on finding the pregnant adult female worm immediately below the skin in an ulcerated area. Washings of the ulcer will produce microfilariae discharged by the worm.

Trichinella spiralis[83]

The parasite *Trichinella spiralis* belongs to a family of nematodes that is characterized by a filamentous anterior portion and a wider and often shorter posterior portion. This family includes *Trichuris trichiura* (p. 986) and *Capillaria philippinensis,* a parasite restricted to a small area in the Philippines. *Trichinella* is responsible for the disease trichinosis,[84] and like all tissue nematodes it is larvaparous. Although trichinosis is not as prevalent as in the past, there are scattered reports of its presence. It is the larvae (rather than the adult form) that produce the disease, since the clinical manifestations are related to the muscle invasion by the larvae.[85] The most common symptoms are asthenia, fever, headaches, myalgia, and periorbital edema.

Habitat: Small intestine and skeletal muscle.

Size: The male is about 1.5 mm long; the female is 3 or 4 mm long. Larvae are about 100 μm in length soon after birth (in feces, blood, and cerebrospinal fluid) but grow rapidly to about 1 mm (encysted larvae).

Ova: There are no ova. The parasite is viviparous.

Life cycle: The infection is continuous in rats through cannibalism. Hogs are infected by eating scraps of infected slaughtered hogs and by feeding on infected rats. Humans become infected by eating raw or inadequately cooked infected pork. In the intestine the encysted larvae within the animal skeletal muscle are freed and penetrate the duodenal mucosa where they mature and mate. The male dies soon after copulation. Live larvae are discharged by the pregnant female within the intestinal wall, from which they reach the bloodstream. In heavy infections while in the bloodstream—a very rare occurrence—the larvae must be distinguished from parasites of the Filarioidea order, from which they differ morphologically. After reaching human muscle they grow to about 1 mm in size and become encysted. In humans the cysts usually become calcified and the larvae die. In animal infestations a second host is required to liberate the encysted larvae.

The parasite is killed by thorough cooking or by freezing at −30° C for 24 hr.

Diagnosis: Diagnosis is based on demonstration of the encysted larvae in biopsy specimens of the gastrocnemius or deltoid muscles.

Muscle teasing method: The muscle biopsy tissue should be teased out, pressed between two slides, and examined under the low-power lens.

Section method: The biopsy specimen may be fixed in formalin, sectioned in the surgical pathology laboratory, stained with hematoxylin-eosin, and examined under the microscope (Fig. 34-43).

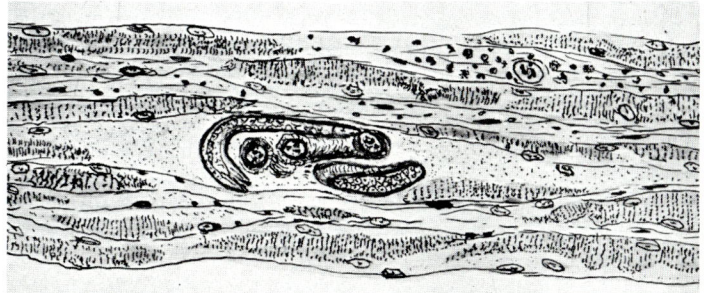

Fig. 34-43. Larva of *Trichinella spiralis* in striated muscle fiber at tendinous insertion. Low-power field showing myositis with infiltration of polymorphonuclear leukocytes and eosinophils. (Hematoxylin-eosin stain.)

Tissue press technic: The tissue press consists of two large, clear, heavy plastic plates (5 × 5 mm), each surrounded by a metal frame and connected by bolts controlled by wing nuts.

Procedure: Place muscle biopsy specimen in middle of bottom plastic plate and cover with top plate. Tighten the wing nuts so that the muscle biopsy specimen is flattened into a transparent thin layer that can be screened for *Trichinella* larvae under the dissection microscope.

Digestion technic[86]: The Baermann technic of demonstrating *Strongyloides* larvae can be used to concentrate *Trichinella* larvae. The specimen consists of a mixture of minced muscle and the digestion mixture.

Digestion mixture:
1. Pepsin, 5 g
2. Water, 1 L
3. Concentrated hydrochloric acid, 7 ml

Procedure: Mix minced muscle and digestion mixture and allow to interact overnight. The timing may need to be adjusted according to amount of muscle biopsy specimen available. Add 2-3 volumes of water at 37° C. Pour muscle digest mixture into Baermann's funnel. Let mixture stand for 1 hr or more. Maintain water at 37° C, draw off samples at suitable intervals, and examine wet preparation for larvae.

Animal inoculation: The muscle biopsy or autopsy material is fed to rats, which are killed after 4-6 weeks to allow examination of the skeletal muscles for *Trichinella* cysts.

Demonstration of larvae in blood or spinal fluid: During the period of migration the larvae may sometimes, although rarely, be found in the blood and spinal fluid. The blood is obtained from a vein, laked in 4% acetic acid solution, and centrifuged; the sediment is examined under a coverslip with the low-power lens.

Serodiagnosis: The intracutaneous test with larval extract is positive in most cases but not diagnostic because false positive reactions occur (5%).[7] The positive reaction is immediate and consists of a blanched raised weal surrounded by a red zone. The intracutaneous test becomes positive within 2-4 weeks after infection.

Bentonite flocculation test: The bentonite flocculation test is the most sensitive and specific procedure; it becomes positive (titer of 5) after the third week of clinical infection, rises rapidly for several weeks, and becomes negative 2-3 years after the initial infection.[87]

Countercurrent electrophoresis: Countercurrent electrophoresis[88] is an adequate procedure for diagnosis of *Trichinella spiralis* provided the antibody titer is high.

Eosinophilia: Except in the acute stage, the infection is accompanied by a marked increase in eosinophils.

TREMATODES OR FLUKES

Flukes (platyhelminthes) are parasitic worms that can be classified according to the preferred location of the adult worm in the definitive host:

Liver flukes
Fasciola hepatica
Clonorchis sinensis
Opisthorchis felineus

Intestinal flukes
Fasciolopsis buski
Metagonimus yokogawai
Heterophyes heterophyes
Lung flukes
Paragonimus westermani
Blood flukes
Schistosoma haematobium
Schistosoma mansoni
Schistosoma japonicum

They can also be classified according to whether they are hermaphroditic or diecious. The hermaphroditic flukes are *F. hepatica, O. Felineus, F. buski, C. sinensis,* and *P. westermani.* The diecious (two sexes in separate individual) flukes are the schistosomes.

Life cycle: The life cycle of all hemaphroditic trematodes is similar. It is complicated and depends on specific first and second intermediary hosts. The operculate eggs, which contain a larva in varying stages of development, are deposited by the adult fluke in the liver or other areas of the vertebrate host. The eggs finally make their way into the fecal stream or into the sputum. When the eggs reach shallow surface water, the ciliated mature larvae, the **miracidia,** escape through the opercula and swim about until they enter a specific intermediate host, a mollusk (snail or clam). Eggs of *Clonorchis* and *Opisthorchis* are ingested by a snail before the miracidia hatch. In the snail the miracidia develop into **sporocysts,** which produce rediae (**germ cells**). Finally, they become free-living cercariae and emerge. They are like the adult trematode, but with a tail or rudder for swimming. They swim about until they encyst and become infective **metacercariae** attached to water vegetation or to a specific second host. The metacercariae of *F. hepatica* are found attached to water vegetation. The metacercariae of *Paragonimus* enter a second host, the crayfish or crab, and cause infection when the host is eaten raw or is insufficiently cooked. The cercariae of the small liver flukes *(C. sinensis* and *O. felineus)* penetrate certain freshwater fish and become encysted. Humans acquire the infection by eating the encysted metacercariae. In humans the metacercariae escape from the cyst and develop into the adult worm.

H. heterophyes embryonated eggs are ingested by snails, in which they develop into cercariae that attach themselves to fish to form encysted metacercariae, which in turn are eaten by dogs or humans. The life cycle of *M. yokogawai* is essentially similar to that of *H. heterophyes.*

Diagnosis: The diagnosis (Tables 34-14 and 34-15 and Figs. 34-44 and 34-45) of the hermaphroditic flukes is based on the recognition of ova in feces or sputum or of the adult worm at autopsy. The adult hermaphroditic flukes vary in length from a few millimeters *(Heterophyes heterophyes)* to several centimeters *(Fasciolopsis buski).* They are ventrodorsally flattened, covered by a smooth or spiny cuticle, and have two suckers, the anterior one surrounding the mouth and the posterior one on the ventral surface. The larger flukes are fleshy and leaflike organisms. The esophagus gives way to the intestines, which end blindly. Most of the organism is occupied by the reproductive organs. There

Table 34-14. Morphologic characteristics of adult flukes of humans excluding schistosomes

Species	Size	Appearance	Definitive host
Fasciola hepatica (sheep liver fluke)	Length: 20-30 mm Width: 10 mm Thickness: 1 mm	Flat, thin, leaf-shaped organism; anterior pointed end with oral sucker; slightly larger ventral sucker close by; blunt posterior end; center of worm cream colored, periphery dark gray	Humans, sheep, rabbits, herbivorous animals
Fasciolopsis buski (large intestinal fluke)	Length: 30-70 mm Width: 15 mm Thickness: 2-3 mm	Flat, creamy, somewhat similar to *F. hepatica;* large ventral sucker; oral and ventral suckers close together	Humans, hogs
Clonorchis sinensis (Chinese liver fluke)	Length: 10-20 mm Width: 3-5 mm Thickness: 1-2 mm	Flat, very thin, almost transparent; reddish brown; oral sucker larger than ventral sucker	Humans, dogs, cats, hogs, rats
Paragonimus westermani (Oriental lung fluke)	Length: 8-20 mm Width: 4-9 mm Thickness: 2-5 mm	Plump, egg shaped; rust brown; subterminal oral sucker	Humans, dogs, cats, minks
Opisthorchis felineus (cat liver fluke)	Length: 7-12 mm Width: 2-3 mm	Transparent, lancet shaped; reddish	Humans, dogs, cats, hogs
Heterophyes heterophyes	Length: 1-2 mm Width: 0.5-0.7 mm	Oval, pear shaped; grayish; large ventral sucker in anterior half of body; small subterminal oral sucker; genital sucker at middle of body	Humans, fish-eating animals
Metagonimus yokogawai	Length: 1-2 mm Width: 0.6 mm	Pear shaped; brownish; small terminal anterior oral sucker; large lateral ventral sucker in anterior half of body	Humans, dogs, cats, hogs

are two testes leading to the ventral genital pore. The oviduct arising from the single ovary meets with the vasa from the testes and with the ducts from the vitelleria (which produce the egg shell) at the level of the uterus. The latter is filled with eggs and opens into the genital pore.

The ova are pigmented, hard shelled, and transparent (Table 34-15 and Fig. 34-45). They vary in size from about 30-150 μm and have an operculum, a hatch, through which the miracidium escapes. The edge of the operculum may fuse with the egg shell or it may be offset by a ridge (shoulder) or flare, which marks the cleavage line. The miracidia are ciliated.

The **methods of diagnosis** include the direct wet-film method, concentration method, and sieve method.

Concentration methods for trematodes[89]:

Acid-ether concentration: Emulsify 1 g feces in 5 ml 40% hydrochloric acid (40 ml concentrated hydrochloric acid diluted to 1 dl). Filter through two layers of moist gauze into a 15 ml centrifuge tube. Add equal quantity of ether and shake vigorously. Centrifuge at 1500 rpm for 1 min. Loosen debris at the interface with wooden applicator. Decant and examine sediment for eggs.

Efficiency is increased if 0.06 ml Triton NE (Rohm & Haas Co., Philadelphia) is added with the ether.

Sedimentation: Homogenize 10-100 g fecal specimen. Suspend in 20 volumes of 0.5% glycerin in tap water. Strain through four layers of gauze into a tall cylinder. Suspend sediment three times, decanting and resuspending in 20 volumes of 0.5% glycerin water, first settling, 1-2 hr; second settling, 45 min; third settling, 30 min. Examine sediment.

• • •

The formalin–ethyl acetate concentration method is quite satisfactory. The zine sulfate method is also satisfactory provided both the surface film and the sediment are examined.

Liver flukes
Fasciola hepatica

Fasciola hepatica,[90] the sheep liver fluke, is found in the liver, gallbladder, and bile ducts of sheep. Humans are seldom affected. For morphologic characteristics see Table 34-14.

Life cycle (Fig. 34-45): The adult fluke releases the eggs into the hepatic ducts of the host, which guide them into the intestines so that they are passed with the feces. The ova contain the motile embryo (miracidium). If the ova reach water the miracidia escape and soon penetrate a snail within which each miracidium forms a sporocyst filled with rediae, which after a few generations give rise to cercariae. The latter encyst on aquatic vegetations and are referred to as metacercariae. Humans acquire the cysts through drinking metacercariae-infected water or by eating freshwater plants to which the cysts are attached. The parasite excysts in

Table 34-15. Morphologic characteristics of eggs of flukes of humans excluding schistosomes

Species	Size (broadest diameter)	Shape	Color	Where found	Degree of maturation when passed
Fasciola hepatica (sheep liver fluke)	Large, 150 × 80 μm	Ovoid; small operculum	Yellow	Feces; duodenal contents; bile drainage	Immature; contains yolk cells, no embryo
Fasciolopsis buski (large intestinal fluke)	Large, 150 × 80 μm	Ovoid; small operculum	Yellow	Feces	Immature; contains yolk cells, no embryo (eggs cannot be distinguished from *F. hepatica* eggs)
Clonorchis sinensis (Chinese liver fluke)	Small, 30 × 16 μm	Flask-shaped operculum resting on a ring; small knob (often hook-like) on posterior end	Yellowish brown	Feces; biliary and duodenal drainage	Contains developed miracidium
Paragonimus westermani (Oriental lung fluke)	80 × 60 μm	Ovoid, widest portion anterior to center; distinct operculum with shoulders	Yellow	Sputum; feces only if sputum is swallowed	Immature; contains yolk cells, no embryo; resembles *D. latum* eggs (in *D. latum* eggs, widest area is centrally located and operculum is larger and more convex than operculum of *P. westermani*;
Opisthorchis felineus (cat liver fluke)	30 × 12 μm	Operculum; flask shaped; resembles *C. sinensis* eggs but more slender and with pointed terminal knob	Yellow	Feces; duodenal drainage	Contains developed miracidium
Heterophyes heterophyes	29 × 16 μm	Thick shelled; operculum with slight shoulders; small posterior nodule	Yellow to light brown	Feces	Contains developed miracidium; resembles *C. sinensis* eggs
Metagonimus yokogawai	28 × 17 μm	Thick shelled; operculum; posterior nodular thickening	Light yellow-brown	Feces	Contains mature miracidium; resembles *H. heterophyes* eggs

the intestines, and the metacercariae penetrate the intestinal wall to reach the peritoneal cavity and migrate to the liver where they mature in one of the major bile ducts. The ova follow the bile ducts into the duodenum and are then passed with the feces.

Diagnosis: Eggs in fecal specimen by direct smear or concentration methods (Table 34-15 and Fig. 34-45).

Serodiagnosis[21,22]: A number of antigens prepared from flukes or miracidia give fairly acceptable reactions with human sera by a number of technics, e.g., complement fixation, indirect hemagglutination, and indirect fluorescence. They become positive by the second or third week after exposure.[91]

Clonorchis sinensis

Clonorchis sinensis,[92] the Chinese liver fluke, is widespread in China and Southeast Asia. For morphologic details see Fig. 34-45. The ova have an electric bulb shape with the operculum at the base. The life cycle involves a snail (first intermediate host) that eats

the eggs or the miracidia. The cercariae leave the snail and enter a freshwater fish (second intermediate host) where they encyst. Humans acquire the infection by eating raw fish. The mature fluke resides in the liver, probably reaching it by climbing up the bile ducts from the small intestine. The eggs return to the small intestine by way of the common bile duct.

Diagnosis: Diagnosis is by eggs in fecal specimen by direct smear or concentration methods.

Serodiagnosis: Complement fixation and intradermal tests have been used, but the latter shows a cross-reaction with *Paragonimus.*[93]

Opisthorchis felineus

Opisthorchis felineus, the cat liver fluke, is about the size of *Clonorchis sinensis,* with which it shares its life cycle. It resides in the liver of humans, cats, and dogs in Europe and the Orient. The first intermediate host is a snail that feeds on the eggs. The second intermediate host is a fish, the flesh of which is penetrated by the

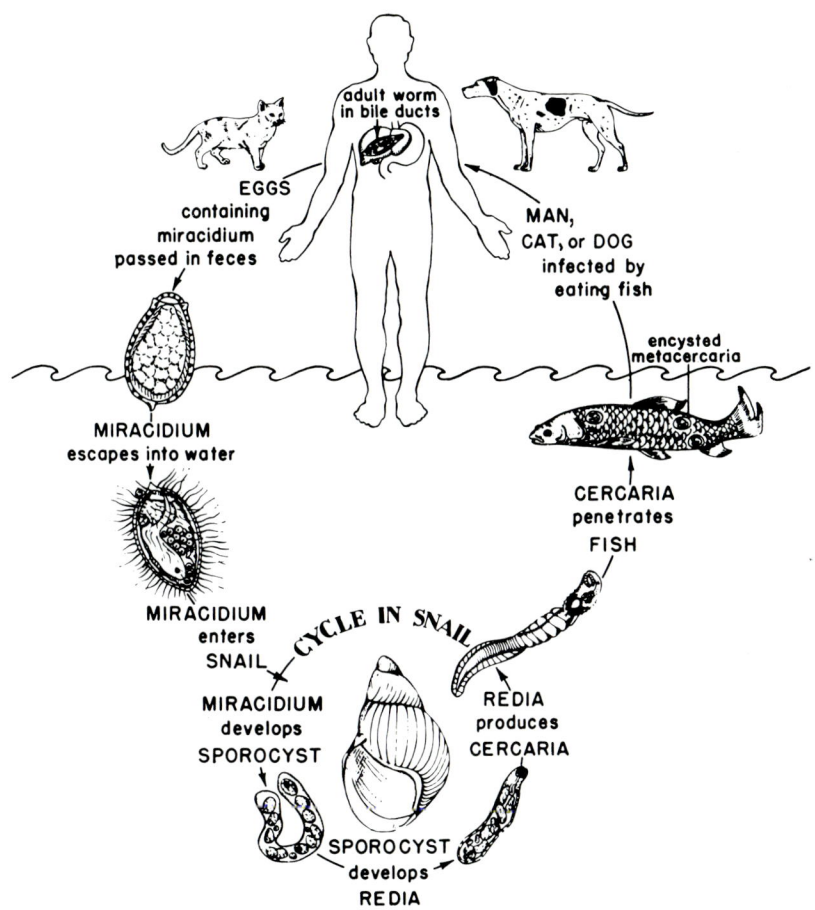

Fig. 34-44. *Clonorchis sinensis.* (From Ash, J.E., and Spitz, S.: Pathology of tropical diseases: an atlas, Philadelphia, 1945, W.B. Saunders Co.)

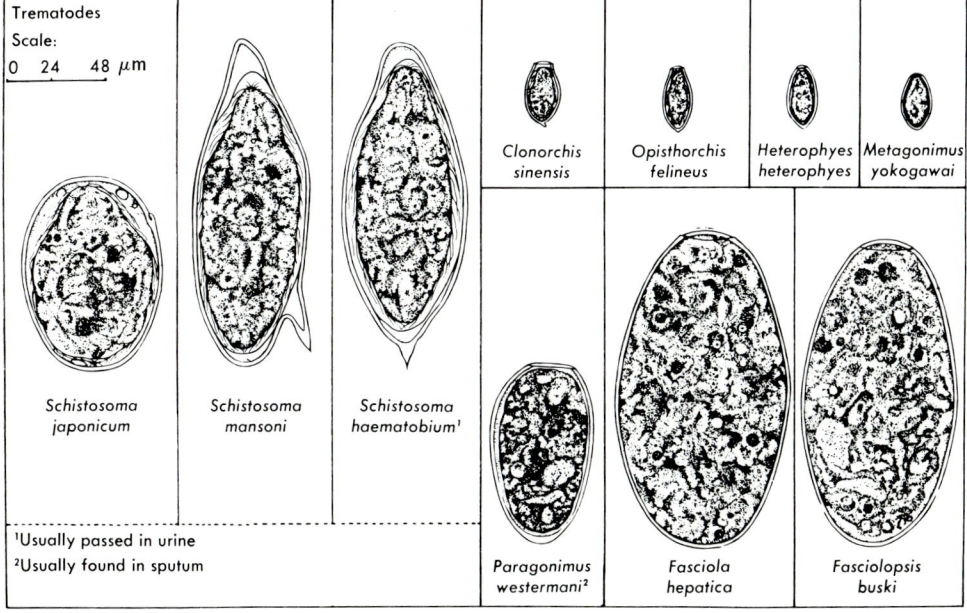

Fig. 34-45. Trematode eggs found in human stool specimens. (From Brooke, M.M., and Melvin, D.M.: Morphology of diagnostic stages of intestinal parasites of man, Public Health Service Publication no. 1966, Atlanta, 1969, Centers for Disease Control.)

cercariae. Humans become infested by eating the uncooked or inadequately cooked fish that hosts the metacercariae. In the human small intestine the metacercariae excyst and the flukes swim against the current up the bile duct into the liver. The eggs are returned to the duodenum by way of the common bile duct and are passed in the feces.

Diagnosis: The eggs are flask shaped and resemble *C. sinensis* ova. They can be demonstrated in feces by the wet saline preparation and by concentration methods.

Intestinal flukes
Fasciolopsis buski[90]

Fasciolopsis buski resembles *Fasciola hepatica* but lives in the small intestine of humans and pigs. The metacercariae are attached to water chestnuts or other water plants, which when eaten raw by humans allow the parasite to complete its cycle.

Diagnosis: Eggs (Fig. 34-45) are demonstrated in feces by wet saline preparations and by concentration methods.

Metagonimus yokogawai

Metagonimus yokogawai is a small intestinal fluke of humans, cats, and dogs. The life cycle is similar to that of *Heterophyes heterophyes*. The adult differs from the *Heterophyes* fluke by displacement of the ventral sucker to the posterior end of the organism.

Heterophyes heterophyes

Heterophyes heterophyes is a small intestinal fluke of humans, dogs, and cats (Table 34-14). The fluke is pear shaped, 1-2 mm long, and gives rise to eggs that are in the size range of some amebae (29 × 16 μm). The first intermediate host is a snail, and the second intermediate host is a fish. When humans eat raw fish they also ingest the metacercariae. The adult flukes survive in the intestines where they lay the eggs.

Diagnosis: Eggs (Fig. 34-45) are demonstrated in the fecal specimen by wet saline preparations and by concentration methods.

Lung fluke
Paragonimus westermani

Paragonimus westermani (Table 34-14) is an important fluke of humans in the Far East, hence the common name **oriental lung fluke.** The fluke is about 2 cm long, reddish, and plump and lives in the host lung, at times surrounded by a cyst wall. The operculated eggs can be found in the sputum or, if swallowed, they appear in the feces.

Life cycle[94]: The eggs reach water either within feces or coughed up in sputum. The miracidium enters the first intermediate host, a snail, and emerges as the cercaria, which infects the second intermediate host, a freshwater crab, and develops into the encysted metacercaria. If the crab is eaten uncooked, the metacercaria excysts in the human small intestine, and the escaping fluke penetrates the bowel wall, and via peritoneal and pleural cavities and diaphragm it reaches the lung where it lays its eggs.

Diagnosis: Eggs are present in sputum and may be present in feces. They are demonstrated by wet saline preparations and by concentration methods (Fig. 34-45).

Serodiagnosis[21, 22]: If purified antigen is available immunoelectrophoresis reveals precipitation bands if sera from infected patients are used.[88]

Blood flukes

From the public health point of view the blood flukes (schistosomes) are some of the most important disease-producing parasites, because they inflict their scourge on millions of people. Only the plasmodia of malaria top them in clinical and sociologic importance. Their activity may produce pathologic changes in liver, spleen, urinary bladder, kidney, intestines, etc. They are diecious, and the two sexes show marked morphologic dissimilarities. The female is thinner and longer than the male. She measures up to 2 cm in length and about 0.3 mm in diameter. On cross section she is circular, while her male counterpart is grooved by a gynecophoral canal that she usually occupies. It is the gynecophoral canal that led to the name of the parasite—schistosoma or split body. The male and female parasites have anterior (oral) and posterior (ventral) suckers. The male has testes and a genital pore while the female is equipped with a uterus, ovary, vitellaria, and the necessary ducts connecting these organs.

Life cycle: The flukes live in human blood vessels and when the eggs are ready to be deposited the female either completely or partially moves out of the gynecophoral canal and deposits the embryonated ova in the smallest venules and then retreats into the canal. Because of their spines and projections the ova remain wedged in the venules. The miracidium (motile embryo) releases an enzyme that diffuses through the eggshell and lyses the surrounding tissue so that the eggs escape into the lumen of the intestines or into the urinary bladder and leave the body with the feces or the urine. When they reach water the miracidium is released and enters a snail in which two sporocyst stages finally lead to the release of forked tailed cercariae, which penetrate human skin by releasing an enzyme (hyaluronidase?) at the site of their attachment to the skin. They finally enter small blood or lymph vessels and mature in the portal system where the cycle begins again.

There are three main species: *Schistosoma japonicum, Schistosoma haematobium,* and *Schistosoma mansoni* (Table 34-16).

Schistosoma japonicum

Schistosoma japonicum occurs in the Far East.

Adult fluke: The male is 15 × 0.5 mm. The female is 20 × 0.3 mm. The skin is smooth.

Life cycle: As described above except that the redial generation is omitted.

Ova: The ova (Table 34-16 and Fig. 34-46) are 90 × 60 μm, oval, yellow, with a very small lateral hook that is difficult to see. They contain the mature ciliated miracidium.

Diagnosis: The ova can be demonstrated in the feces by saline wet mounts and by ethyl acetate–formalin concentration. Since the eggs are passed in relatively

Table 34-16. Schistosomes

Parasite	Adult	Diagnostic eggs
Schistosoma mansoni (blood fluke)	Male: 6-10 mm, integument has tubercles; female: 7-16 mm	140 × 60 μm; elongated, oval, yellow-brown, lateral spine; contains miracidium, found in feces, rarely in urine
Schistosoma japonicum (oriental blood fluke)	Male: 15 mm, smooth integument; female: 20 mm	90 × 70 μm; broadly oval; yellow-brown; may have small lateral spine or knob; found in feces; contains miracidium
Schistosoma haematobium (vesical blood fluke)	Male: 10-15 mm, integument covered with small tubercles; female: 20 mm	140 × 15 μm; oval; yellow-brown; terminal spine; elongated, spindle shaped; contains miracidium; found in urine, seldom in feces

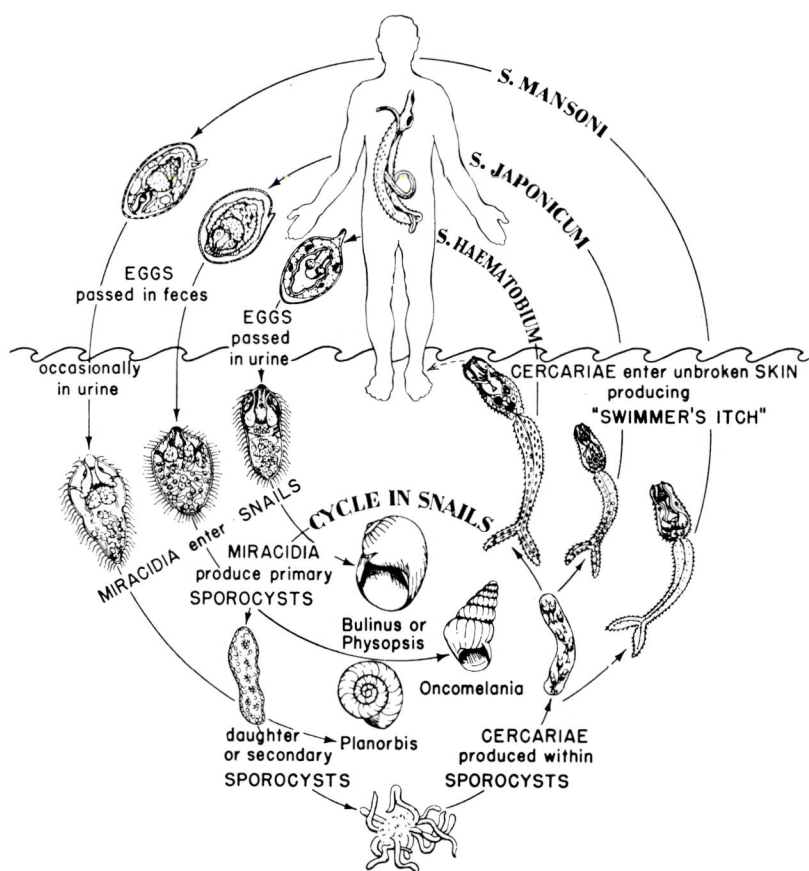

Fig. 34-46. *Schistosoma* (blood flukes). (From Ash, J.E., and Spitz, S.: Pathology of tropical diseases: an atlas, Philadelphia, 1945, W.B. Saunders Co.)

small numbers and at irregular intervals, the specimens should be obtained daily for 2 weeks, with a 1-week interval in which no specimens are taken. An entire stool specimen should be concentrated. In the chronic stage of the disease, ova may be difficult to find.

Rectal biopsy: Under sigmoidoscopic control a granulomatous mucosal lesion is taken for a biopsy specimen. Several bites of tissue should be obtained. One tissue specimen is fixed in formalin and embedded in paraffin, and hematoxylin-eosin–stained sections are examined for ova. The other specimen is handled fresh, squeezed between two microscope slides, and examined under the low power of the microscope for unstained ova surrounded by fibrous or vascular granulation tissue.

Viability of ova: Wet preparations are allowed to inspissate to such a degree that the high dry or oil-immersion lens can be focused on a *Schistosome* egg without dislodging it. If the egg is viable, the cells of the posterior third of the miracidia will be flickering like a lit candle (flame cells, solenocytes).[7]

Hatching test of schistosome eggs[95]

Principle: Schistosome eggs hatch rapidly when brought into contact with water, liberating miracidia, which rise to the surface attracted by light.

Reagent and equipment: Use a 1 L distillation flask with a vertical side arm (Fig. 34-47). Surround flask with foil but spare side arm.

Chlorine-free water: Boil water for 5-10 min and allow to cool.

Procedure: Suspend fecal material in a small amount of chlorine-free water in the bottom of the flask. Add water to the level of the side arm. After allowing the mixture to settle for a few minutes, slowly add water through the side arm to cover the junction of flask and arm; then rapidly add water to the side arm to fill the flask. The water in the side arm will remain clear. Place the flask near a light source (window) and watch for miracidia collecting in the side arm.

Serodiagnosis[21,22]: The complement fixation and indirect immunofluorescence tests are specific and sensitive provided adult worm antigens are used.[96]

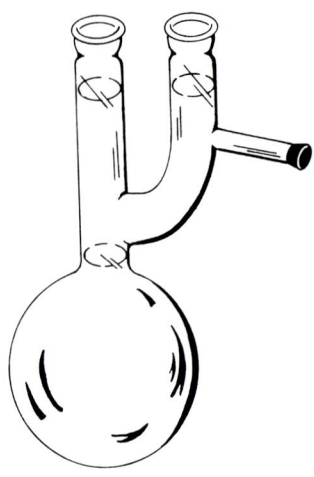

Fig. 34-47. Flask used for hatching schistosome eggs.

Schistosoma haematobium

The fluke *Schistosoma haematobium* is responsible for morbidity of millions of people in Africa and part of Asia. It involves primarily the urinary bladder and the genitourinary tract.

Adult fluke: The male is 10 × 1 mm. The female is 2 × 0.3 mm. The skin is tuberculated.

Life cycle: The life cycle is similar to that of all other schistosomes. The intermediate host is a snail in which sporocytes develop that give rise to cercariae without the benefit of the redial phase. The mature flukes mate in the perivesicular plexuses and the ova penetrate the bladder, causing mucosal ulcerations and the formation of papillomas.

Ova: The ova are 90-70 μm (Fig. 34-46). They are oval and yellow and have a terminal spine at the posterior end. The shell surrounds a mature miracidium.

Diagnosis: Ova are found in the urine and rarely in feces. They can be demonstrated by wet film and concentration methods. A biopsy specimen of the bladder lesion is handled in the same way as the rectal biopsy specimen is handled in the diagnosis of infestation by *Schistosoma japonicum*. Sediment from a 24 hr collection may be needed when ova are difficult to find.

Schistosoma mansoni

The intestinal fluke *Schistosoma mansoni* is smaller than the preceding two flukes and the surface sports numerous bosses. Its main domain is South America, where it is responsible for liver and spleen pathologic conditions accompanied by portal hypertension.

Adult fluke: The male is 10 × 0.5 mm. The female is 16 × 0.3 mm. The integument has bosses.

Life cycle: The life cycle of *Schistosoma mansoni* is similar to the life cycle of all schistosomes. The intermediate host is a snail from which the cercariae emerge to attack exposed human skin. No second intermediate host is required in the life cycle. The cercariae make their way to the liver where they mature in the venous spaces. They soon leave the liver via the portal vein and reach the sigmoid-rectal area where the ova penetrate the intestinal wall and are passed with the feces.

Ova: The ova are 60 × 140 μm, yellow, elongated and oval (Fig. 34-46). They have a prominent lateral spine and contain a live miracidium.

Diagnosis: Ova are demonstrated in feces, rarely in urine, by the wet film and concentration methods. Eggs are discharged at irregular intervals and may only be very few in number, so that daily stool examination for about 1 week is suggested. After 1 week's rest, daily examination for another week should be instituted.

It may be necessary to determine the egg load of patients in whom schistosomiasis has been diagnosed. The egg-counting technic applicable to *Necator* can be used for *Schistosoma mansoni*.

CESTODES (TAPEWORMS)[97]

Cestodes are flat tapelike or ribbonlike worms that consist of a series of segments (proglottids) that arise by a budding process from the smallest segment, the head or scolex, which is provided with sucking grooves or sucking disks. Its center is often adorned by a projecting structure, the **rostellum,** which, if it is ringed by hooklets, is referred to as armed. If no hooklets can be seen, it is unarmed. By means of the suckers and the hooklets, the parasite attaches itself to the mucosa (Figs. 34-48 and 34-49). The young immature segments are small, but as they are pushed distally by new ones, they increase in size and become sexually mature and gravid. The most immature small segments form the so-called neck. The tapeworm has no alimentary tract and derives its food by osmosis. It is a multiple parasite, like a chain of cocci or yeast cells, with each mature segment being a complete individual with nerves, excretory canals, and a reproductive system that includes organs of both sexes. The mature proglottid consists chiefly of a uterus dilated with ova (Fig. 34-48). The segmented portion of the worm (strobila) varies in length in the different species, from 3-8 mm *(Echinococcus granulosus)* to 10-12 m *(Diphyllobothrium latum)*.

The adults inhabit the intestinal tract of vertebrates, and the larvae inhabit the tissues of vertebrates and invertebrates.

There are two orders of cestodes that are important

medically. In the order Pseudophyllidea the scolex has grooves (or bothria) for attachment to the intestinal mucosa; the uterine pore is on the flat surface of the proglottid; the uterus has a saccular or rosettelike appearance; the vitellaria (yolk glands) are scattered; the ova are operculated; and the embryos, called oncopheres, which have six hooklets (hexacanth), are usually ciliated. In the order Cyclophyllidea the scolex has four cup-shaped suckers, with or without a rostellum and hooklets. There is no birth pore, but the ova are liberated when the gravid proglottid disintegrates; the vitellaria are concentrated; the ova do not have opercula; and the oncospheres, which have six hooklets, are not ciliated.

Diagnosis: The identification of all tapeworms (Figs. 34-28 and 34-48 to 34-50 and Plate 19 [p. 988]) is based on the recognition of taenia eggs in the stool and on finding the scolex and/or gravid proglottids, since specific identification cannot be made by the eggs alone. The diagnostic methods include macroscopic sieving of feces to find scolices and proglottids, which can be identified and speciated. It is usually not neces-

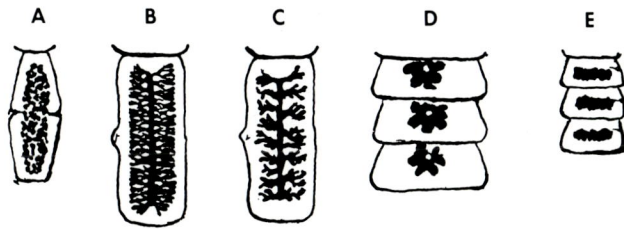

Fig. 34-48. Mature segments of tapeworms (schematic). **A,** *Dipylidium caninum.* **B,** *Taenia saginata.* **C,** *Taenia solium.* **D,** *Diphyllobothrium latum.* **E,** *Hymenolepis nana (Hymenolepis diminuta* is similar but larger).

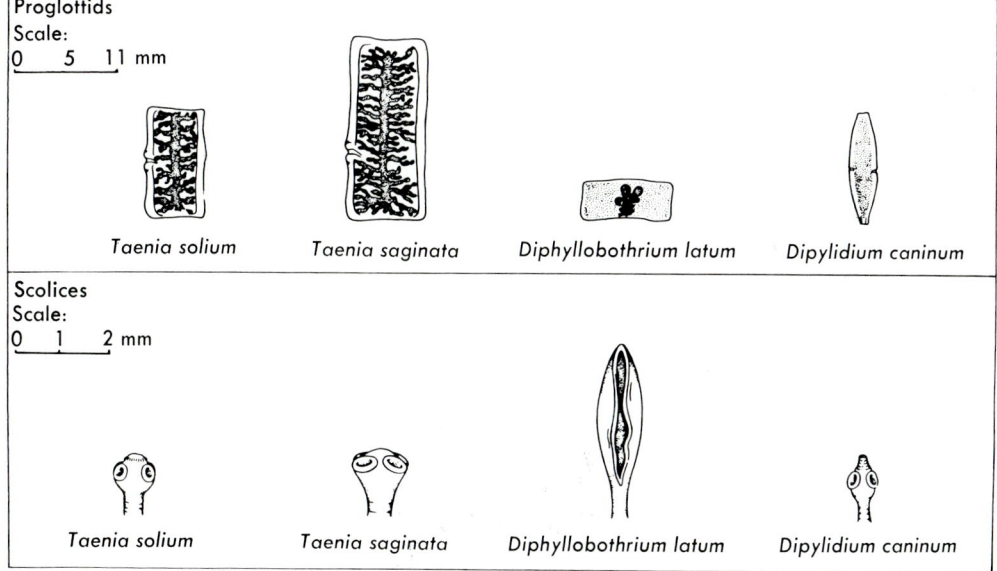

Fig. 34-49. Gravid proglottids and scolices of cestode parasites of humans. (From Brooke, M.M., and Melvin, D.M.: Morphology of diagnostic stages of intestinal parasites of man, Public Health Service Publication no. 1966, Atlanta, 1969, Centers of Disease Control.)

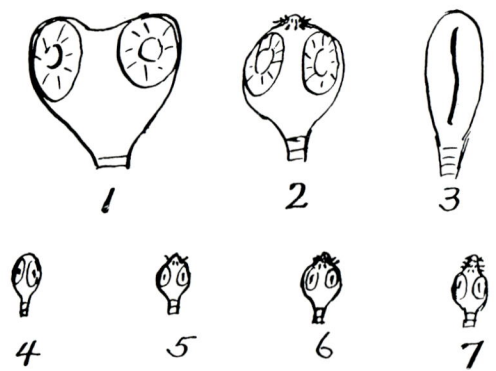

Fig. 34-50. Scolices of tapeworms. **1,** *Taenia saginata*. **2,** *Taenia solium*. **3,** *Diphyllobothrium latum*. **4,** *Hymenolepis diminuta*. **5,** *Hymenolepis nana* (one row of hooklets). **6,** *Echinococcus granulosus* (two rows of hooklets). **7,** *Dipylidium caninum* (three or more rows of hooklets).

sary to search for the minute scolices. Wet mounts of feces in saline and concentration methods are used to demonstrate the ova.

Cestodes (tapeworms) and trematodes (flukes) do not shed eggs as regularly as nematodes (roundworms). Therefore stool specimens must be examined for ova and proglottids over an **extended period of time,** e.g., 1-2 weeks.

Visualization of uterine pattern: The uterus of the proglottids can be injected with diluted India ink to outline its branches. A 25-gauge needle fits the birth pore. The proglottid is squashed between two slides and the uterine branches can be counted with a hand lens or a low-power microscope. The proglottids can be cleared in xylene or in lactophenol.

Taenia saginata (beef tapeworm, unarmed tapeworm)

Taenia saginata (Figs. 34-28 and 34-48 to 34-51 and Plate 19 [p. 988]) is more common than *Taenia solium* and exceeds it in length, having at times 1000-2000 proglottids.

Habitat: Upper part of human small intestine.

Size: *Taenia saginata* is 2.7-3.9 m long and 5-7 mm wide; the scolex (head) is about the size of a pinhead, 1-2 mm in diameter.

Ova (Fig. 34-28): The ova are spheroid, stained yel-

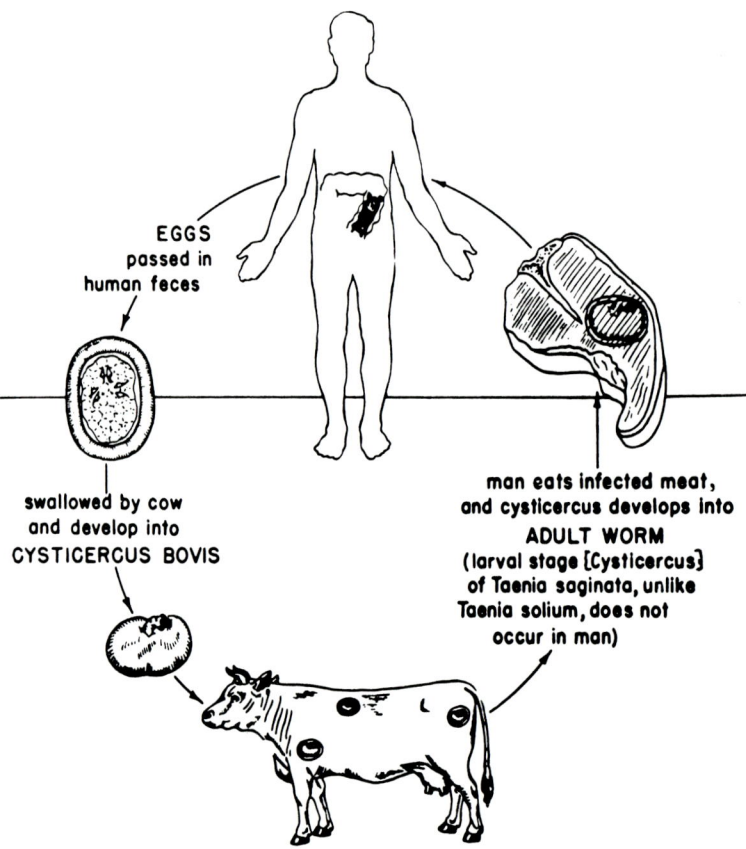

Fig. 34-51. *Taenia saginata*. (From Ash, J.E., and Spitz, S.: Pathology of tropical diseases: an atlas, Philadelphia, 1945, W.B. Saunders Co.)

low or brown with bile, and about 30-40 μm in diameter. They have a thick, radially striated shell surrounding a thin clear space, which in turn surrounds the embryo (hexacanth oncosphere) containing six characteristic hooklets. Ova of *T. solium* and *T. saginata* cannot be differentiated. Species identification must be based on morphology of the proglottid or scolex. Eggs should be identified as "taenia ova" without species identification.

Scolex: The scolex is tetragonal, without hooklets, and has four cup-shaped suckers.

Gravid proglottid: In mature segments the uterus branches dichotomously, with 15-30 branches on each side, and the genital pores are irregularly alternating. The mature segments are more long than broad and they are actively moving.

Life cycle[98]: The ova escape with the stool from detached proglottids and are deposited onto the grazing areas of cattle. The egg containing the embryo with the hooklets is swallowed by cattle, the shell is digested, and the embryo (hexacanth oncosphere) bores through the intestine, after which it loses its hooklets. It becomes encysted (*Cysticercus bovis;* "bladder worm") in the muscles and organs of the animal, where it lies dormant. Meat so infected is recognized on inspection and is called "measly meat." When this meat is eaten insufficiently cooked, the capsule is digested and the young parasite is set free in the human intestine, where it develops into the adult form in 2-3 months. Mature proglottids separate and are discharged in feces. They liberate the eggs, which may reach the ground on which cattle graze.

Diagnosis: Ova and segments of the parasite may be found in the feces.

The diagnostic methods employ macroscopic sieving of feces to find scolices and proglottids. There is rarely the need to look for the scolices. Wet mounts of feces in saline and concentration methods are used to demonstrate the ova.

Recovery of scolex following treatment: After treatment the patient takes magnesium citrate orally and from then on collects all stool specimens in a wide container. The material is then diluted with water, sieved (20 mesh), and diluted several times until the scolex is found. If unsuccessful, the procedure must be repeated in 24 hr.

Cellophane tape preparation: Eggs are sometimes found in the anal folds and can be demonstrated similar to the method for *Enterobius vermicularis* eggs.

NOTE: The most important differential criteria distinguishing *T. saginata* from *T. solium* are the presence or absence of a rostellum and the number of uterine branches.

Taenia solium (pork tapeworm, armed tapeworm)

As the common name implies, the infection with *Taenia solium* (Table 34-17, Figs. 34-28, 34-48 to 34-50, and 34-52, and Plate 19 [p. 988]) is caused by eating uncooked or inadequately cooked pork. The parasite is common in Europe and Mexico but uncommon

Table 34-17. Differential characteristics of some important tapeworms of humans

	Taenia saginata	*Taenia solium*	*Diphyllobothrium latum*	*Hymenolepis nana*
Length	2.7-3.9 m	1.8-3.1 m	2.7-4.6 m	1.5-2.5 cm
Scolex				
Shape	Quadrilateral	Globular	Almondlike	Pyramidal
Size	1 × 1.5 mm	1 × 1 mm	3 × 1 mm	1.3 × 0.5 mm
Rostellum and hooklets	−	+	−	
Suckers	4	4	2 grooves	4
Proglottids				
Number	2000	700-1000	3000-4000	150-200
Genital pore	Lateral border	Lateral border	Ventral surface	−
Uterine pore	−	−	+	−
Terminal segments (gravid)				
Size	19 × 7 mm, longer than wide	11 × 5 mm	3 × 11 mm, wider than long	3 × 12 mm, wider than long
Primary lateral uterine branches	15-30 on each side	6-12 on each side	Rosette shaped	Saccular
Color	Milky white	Milky white	Ivory	White
Appearance in feces	Usually appear singly	5 or 6 segments	Varies from a few inches to a few feet in length	None found
Ova				
Shape	Spheroid	Spheroid	Oval	Spheroid
Size	35 μm	35 μm	70 × 45 μm	30 × 40 μm
Color	Rusty brown	Rusty brown	Yellow-brown	Colorless
Embryo with hooklets	+	+	−	+
Operculum	−	−	+ (difficult to see)	−
Larvae	*Cysticercus bovis*	*Cysticercus cellulosae*	Plerocercoid (sparganum)	Cysticercoid
Size	5-9 mm	5-10 mm	2-15 mm	5 mm
Color	Milky white	Milky white	Chalky white	White
Multiple infections	−	−	+	−

−, Absent; +, present.

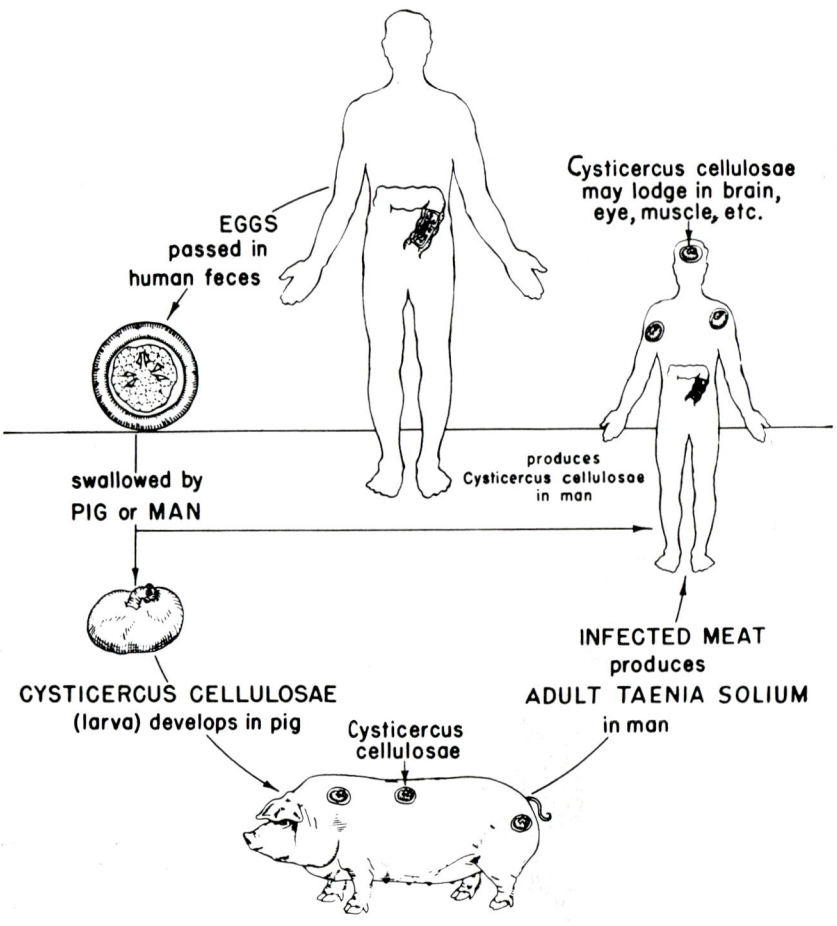

Fig. 34-52. *Taenia solium.* (From Ash, J.E., and Spitz, S.: Pathology of tropical diseases: an atlas, Philadelphia, 1945, W.B. Saunders Co.)

in the United States. The infection is often asymptomatic. The larval stage (cysticercus) is potentially more dangerous—depending on the location of the cyst—than the adult worm.

Habitat: Upper part of small intestine of humans.

Size: 1.8-3.1 m long and 5-6 mm wide.

Ova: The ova are similar to those of *T. saginata*. The freshly passed eggs consist of an external layer surrounding the embryosphere, which in turn consists of a radially patterned embryonic membrane surrounding the hexacanth oncosphere, the larva with three pairs of hooklets.

Cystic larva: The cysticercus is a thin-walled, plasma-filled cyst that contains the invaginated head of the larval worm.

Scolex: The scolex is 1 mm in diameter. It sports a rostellum with two rows of hooks and four suckers.

Gravid proglottid: It is sluggish, inactive, and the uterus has 5-10 lateral branches on each side. The proglottid is longer than wide.

Life cycle: The life cycle is similar to that of *T. saginata* except that the larval stage infects swine instead of cattle, and the scolex does not lose the hooklets.

Humans eliminate ova and five to six gravid segments at a time in the feces. The ova and segments may reach the feeding areas of the intermediate host, mainly hogs but also dogs and cats. Rarely, they reinfect humans, who then also become the intermediate host. The eggs mature in the intermediate host; the larvae (oncosphere) hatch in the small intestine and penetrate the intestinal wall, thus entering the bloodstream. The mature larvae leave the bloodstream and become encysted *(Cysticercus cellulosae)* in the organs, especially the muscles, of the intermediate hosts, usually pigs. If infected (measly) inadequately cooked pork is eaten by humans, the cyst wall is dissolved, the oncosphere is freed, and the mature worm develops in the jejunum.

Cysticercus cellulosae is sometimes found in humans, especially in the subcutaneous tissue and in the central nervous tissue (brain, eye), if they ingest infective ova and thus become the intermediate host.

Diagnosis: Ova and segments of the parasites may be found in the feces. After treatment, a search should be made for the scolex because the parasite will develop again unless this part is removed. The technics used are the same as for the diagnosis of *T. saginata*.

Serodiagnosis[21,22]: Human cases of cysticercus are

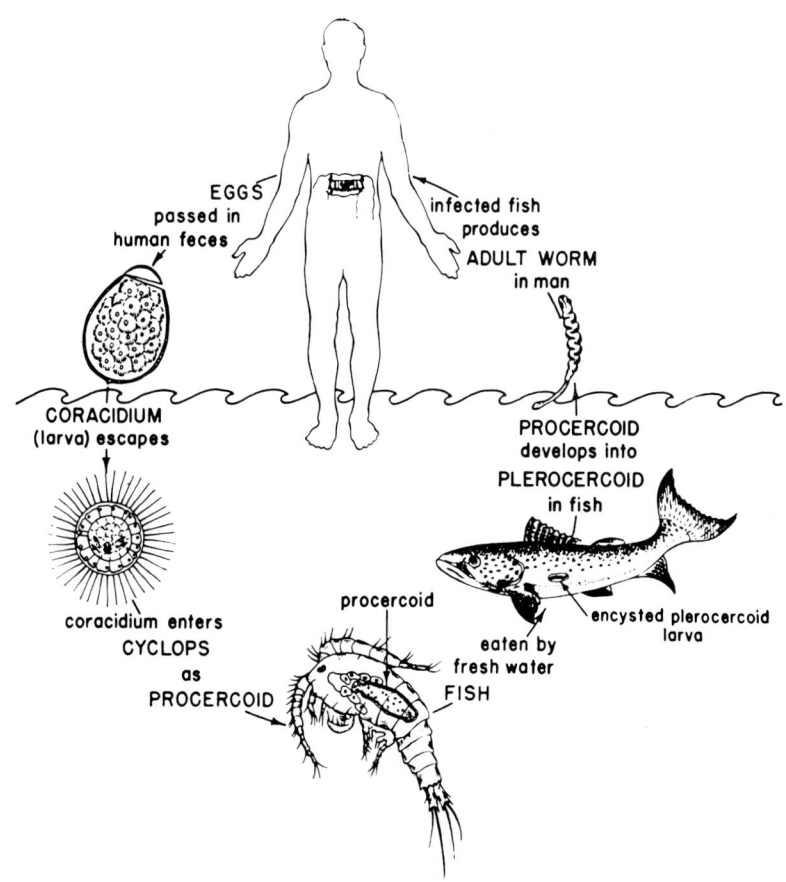

Fig. 34-53. *Diphyllobothrium latum.* (From Ash, J.E., and Spitz, S.: Pathology of tropical diseases: an atlas, Philadelphia, 1945, W.B. Saunders Co.)

rare, and it is therefore difficult to evaluate the various serologic reactions. The most sensitive and specific test is the indirect hemagglutination test when serum is the test material. The test is less sensitive with cerebrospinal fluid. The preferred antigen is extracts of whole worms of *T. solium* and *T. saginata*.

Diphyllobothrium latum (fish or broad tapeworm, Dibothriocephalus latus)

Diphyllobothrium latum (Figs. 34-28, 34-48 to 34-50 and 34-53 and Plate 19 [p. 988] is a common tapeworm of humans in the lake areas in Canada, Michigan, and Wisconsin.

Habitat: Small intestine of humans, dogs, cats, etc.

Size: Diphyllobothrium latum is 2.7-4.6 m long and 10-12 mm wide. The segments are short, about 3 mm.

Scolex: The scolex is almond shaped, with deep dorsal and ventral grooves and no hooklets.

Gravid proglottid: The gravid proglottid is more broad than long, creamy white, and motile. The terminal gravid segments may be longer than wide. The uterus is rosette shaped and centrally located.

Ova: The ova are about 45 × 70 μm, ovoid, yellowish brown, and operculate (with a lid), so that pressure on the coverslip may open them. The operculum is inconspicuous, but the peripheral break produced by

the rim can usually be seen. The posterior end is characterized by a small knob. The ovum contains a globular mass of yolk cells but no embryo. *D. latum* eggs must be differentiated from those of *Paragonimus westermani,* which are more ovoid, slender, and pointed at one end, which lack the terminal knob, and the operculum of which rests on a delicate ridge at the other end. *Paragonimus* eggs are usually found in sputum and seldom in feces. *D. latum* ova must also be differentiated from hookworm eggs, which have a thinner shell and no operculum. Unfertilized *Ascaris* eggs devoid of the outer brown mammillated coating also mimic *D. latum* eggs but lack the operculum.

Life cycle: The ova passed in human stool are not embryonated. They find their way to a body of water and develop ciliated embryos (ciliated hexacanth oncospheres), which hatch as free-swimming ciliated larvae **(coracidia).** The larvae are eaten by a crustacean *(Cyclops, Diaptomus),* the first intermediate host, and make their way through the stomach wall into the body cavity of the host, where they develop into **procercoid larvae.** The crustacean is eaten by a freshwater fish (pike, trout, salmon, etc.), the second intermediate host, in which the parasites migrate to the muscle tissue and are transformed into the **plerocercoid larvae.** When the infected fish is eaten without being sufficiently cooked, the larval forms develop in the human intestine into the adult worms, the eggs of which appear in the feces.

Diagnosis: The ova and sometimes segments of the parasite are found in the stool. After treatment a search should be made for one or more scolices, since infection is frequently multiple. Ova and proglottids are not shed regularly, so that frequent stool examinations over a period of 1-2 weeks are necessary.

The methods of diagnosis include macroscopic sieving of feces in search of proglottids and scolices, microscopic examination of saline wet preparations of stool, and complete blood count for "tapeworm anemia."

As mentioned in the discussion of macrocytic anemias, this tapeworm is responsible for a vitamin B_{12}–deficiency anemia. Investigations with ^{60}Co-labeled vitamin B_{12} show that this parasite selectively takes up significant amounts of vitamin B_{12}.[99]

Echinococcus granulosus (hydatid or Echinococcus cyst)

Echinococcus (Figs. 34-50 and 34-54 to 34-56) is widely distributed, being endemic to cattle and sheep growing areas in Europe, North and South America, and New Zealand. Humans become infected by the ingestion of eggs as the result of close contact with sheep and dogs. The disease is caused by the larval stage of the parasite rather than the activity of the mature worm, which is essentially asymptomatic.

Habitat: The adult worm is found in the intestine of dogs, sheep, cattle, and some wild animals, e.g., wolves; the larval stage (cyst) is found in the tissues of sheep and humans, the intermediate hosts. The cysts are found chiefly in the liver and lungs and sometimes in the brain or eye.

Size: The adult worm is very small, 0.5 cm long. It consists of four segments: one scolex, one immature, one mature, and one gravid proglottid.

Scolex: The scolex is pyriform and carries four suckers and a double row of hooklets on a prominent rostellum.

Gravid proglottid: The gravid proglottid has a median uterus with 12-15 primary lateral branches.

Ova: Ova are not found in human feces, but in feces of infected animals. They are spheroid, 30-50 μm in diameter, with thin, radially striated shells surrounding embryos with six hooklets **(oncosphere)**, resembling other **taenial eggs**.

Life cycle[100]: The worm resides in the small intestines of dogs, sheep, wolves, etc. The gravid proglottid, "when its time comes," detaches itself from the worm and bursts to liberate the taenia-type ova. The eggs reach the ground with the animal excreta and are

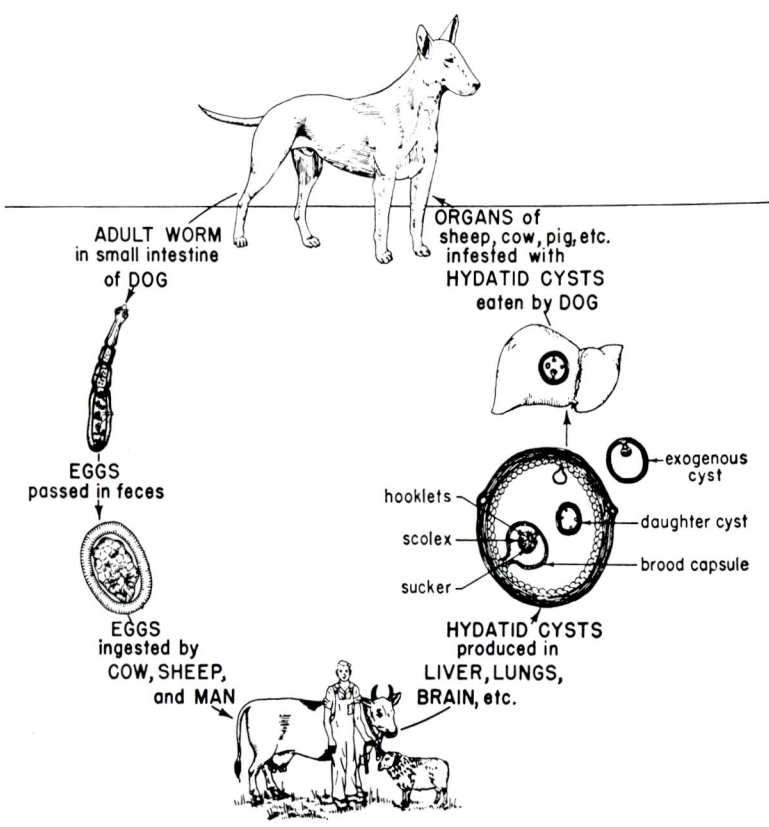

Fig. 34-54. *Echinococcus granulosus (Taenia echinococcus).* (From Ash, J.E., and Spitz, S.: Pathology of tropical diseases: an atlas, Philadelphia, 1945, W.B. Saunders Co.)

ingested by a variety of herbivorous intermediate hosts, e.g., sheep, dogs, horses, cattle, some wild animals such as giraffes and kangaroos, and by man. When the ova find their way into the digestive tract of the intermediate host, the oncospheres are liberated, penetrate the wall of the intestines, and find themselves in the mesenteric veins and ultimately in the systemic circulation, which guides them to the various organs, mainly liver, lung, spleen, heart, and brain. In these organs the oncospheres form cysts (hydatid cysts). The cyst walls are made up of two layers contributed by the parasite: an **outer lamellated** dense **hyaline** portion and an inner **granular** one, the **germinal** membrane, from which numerous **brood capsules, scolices,** and **daughter cysts** arise. The cyst is filled with a sterile colorless fluid containing **hooklets** from ruptured brood capsules and **daughter cysts** that have become detached. This material, which settles to the bottom of the cyst, is called **hydatid sand.** The cyst-infected organs of cattle, sheep, etc., may be eaten by dogs or other carnivorous animals in which the adult tapeworm develops. Humans are an intermediate host who interrupts the cycle.

Diagnosis: In humans the disease (presence of cysts) must be suspected on clinical grounds. Extreme care must be taken at surgery so as not to rupture the echinococcal cysts.

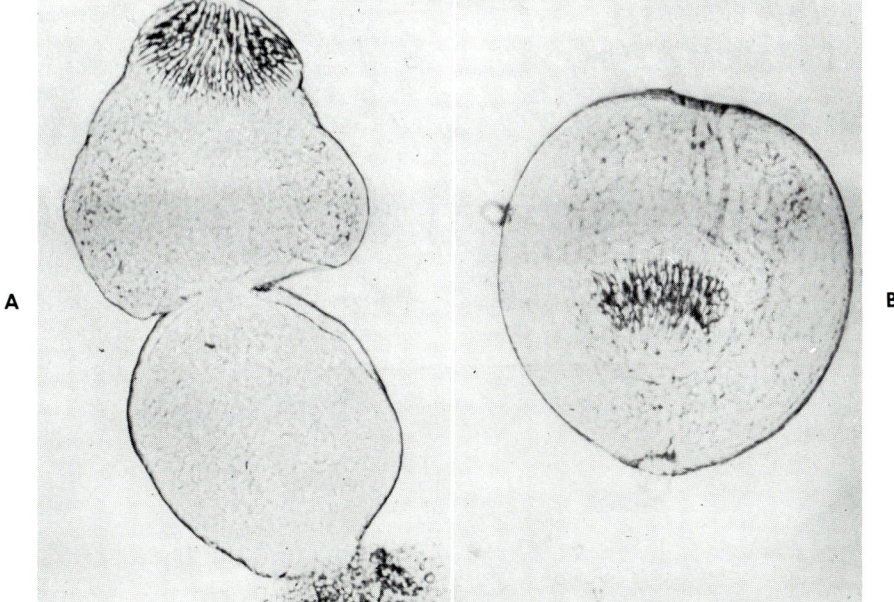

Fig. 34-55. Scolices of *Echinococcus granulosus*. **A,** Hooklets and suckers evaginated. **B,** Hooklets and suckers invaginated.

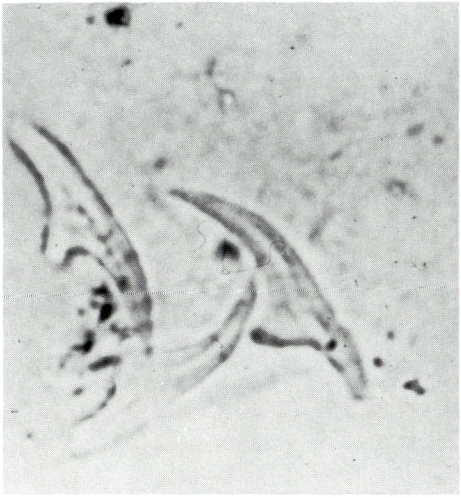

Fig. 34-56. Hooklets of *Echinococcus granulosus*.

Microscopic examination of the cyst fluid shows hydatid sand (Fig. 34-56), consisting of scolices, free hooklets, cholesterol crystals, and granular debris from the degenerated scolices and cyst wall (Figs. 34-55 and 34-56). The cyst contents are toxic and when released may produce severe allergic reactions.

Serodiagnosis[21,22]: The following tests are of particular value in the serologic diagnosis of echinococcosis: immunoelectrophoresis, immunofluorescence, and indirect hemagglutination. The latter test in combination with bentonite flocculation test is routinely performed at the Centers for Disease Control, Atlanta.

Hymenolepis nana (dwarf tapeworm)

Habitat: *Hymenolepis nana* (Figs. 34-28, 34-50, 34-51, and 34-57 and Plate 19 [p. 988]) is found in the small bowel of humans, mice, and rats. The dwarf tapeworm is the most common tapeworm in North America, since humans are both the intermediate and definitive host.

Size: *Hymenolepsis nana* is 1.5-2.5 cm long and 0.5 mm wide, hence the name "dwarf tapeworm." It has about 150-200 segments.

Scolex: The scolex bears four small suckers and a short retractable rostellum with 20-30 hooklets arranged in a single ring (Fig. 34-57).

Gravid proglottid: The gravid proglottid is about four times as wide as it is long and has a saccular uterus.

Ova (Fig. 34-28): The ova are nearly spheroid, colorless, transparent, and about 40 μm in diameter. There are two distinct walls, between which there is a gelatinous-appearing substance (space). At each pole of the inner wall there is a slight protuberance from which arise four to eight hairlike processes that are diagnostic and allow the differentiation from ova of *Hymenolepis diminuta*. The inner wall surrounds a fully developed embryo with three pairs of hooklets.

Life cycle: The ova are liberated in the small intestine by the disintegration of the proglottid and reach the outside hidden by feces. They may be ingested by grain beetles in which the hexacanth oncospheres develop into tailed cysticercoids. When the infected grain beetle is ingested by humans or mice, the larvae develop into the mature forms in the small intestine and produce eggs. If the eggs are swallowed directly by humans, the cysticercoids (minus tail) develop in the intestinal mucosa. When mature, they reach the intestinal lumen where they progress to develop into the mature worm, which lays eggs.

Diagnosis: The ova are found in the feces. See description above for diagnostic points. The diagnostic methods include the usual wet mounts and concentration technics.

Hymenolepis diminuta (rat tapeworm)

Habitat: *Hymenolepis diminuta* (Figs. 34-28, 34-48, and 34-50 and Plate 19 [p. 988]) is found in the intes-

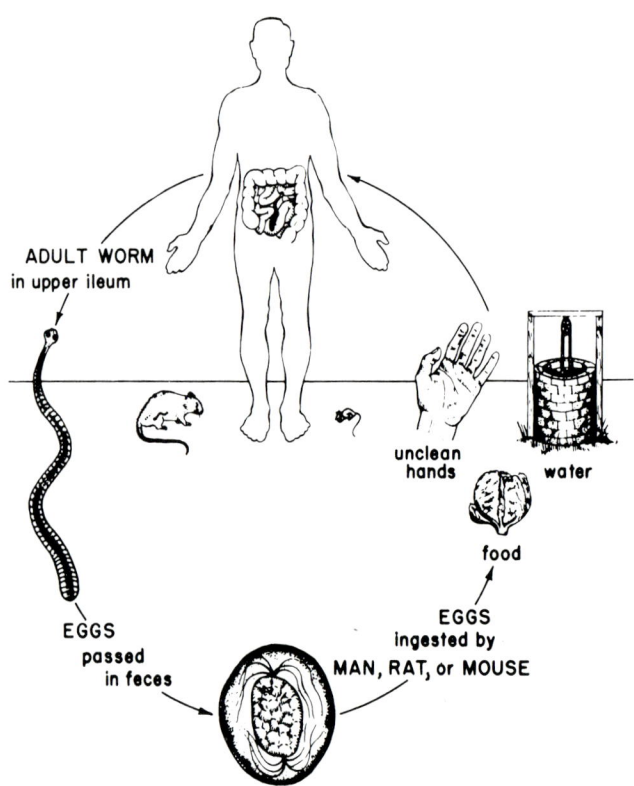

Fig. 34-57. *Hymenolepis nana.* (From Ash, J.E., and Spitz, S.: Pathology of tropical diseases: an atlas, Philadelphia, 1945, W.B. Saunders Co.)

tine of mice and rats. Humans (usually children) are infected accidentally and only occasionally. The infection usually does not produce any symptoms.

Size: Up to 10-60 cm long and 5 mm wide, up to 1000 proglottids.

Scolex: The club-shaped scolex has four suckers and an unarmed retractile rostellum.

Gravid proglottid: The gravid proglottid is wider than long and carries a central saccular uterus. The proglottid is seldom seen in stool.

Ova: The ova (Fig. 34-28) are spheric to ovoid and measure 50 × 70 μm. The distinct outer yellowish membrane is thick and has an irregular inner border. It is separated by a gelatinous layer (space) from the delicate inner membrane that surrounds the six-hooked oncosphere. There are no polar filaments, the absence of which differentiates the *Hymenolepis diminuta* ova from the ova of *Hymenolepis nana*.

Life cycle: Eggs are contained in the feces of the final host animals (rats and mice) and are acquired by various insects such as roaches, fleas, lice, and mealworms, in which the larvae (cercocystis) develop from the embryo. The insects in turn are ingested by various animals that act as final hosts and reservoirs, e.g., dogs, mice, and rats, in which the mature adult worm develops. Humans acquire infection through ingestion of parasitized insect hosts in grains and cereals.

Dipylidium caninum (dog tapeworm)

The infection caused by *Dipylidium caninum* (Figs. 34-28 and 34-48 to 34-49) is rare in humans but common in dogs and cats.

Habitat: Small intestine of dogs and cats.

Size: 10-50 cm.

Scolex: The rhomboid scolex has a conical retractile rostellum with rows of hooklets. Below the rostellum there are four suckers.

Gravid proglottid: The proglottids are longer than they are wide and contain a saccular uterus in which are collections of ova called egg packets.

Ova and life cycle: There are 5-30 eggs the size of taenia eggs (35 μm in diameter) collected in rounded egg packets. The oncosphere has three pairs of hooklets surrounded by a thick nonstriated shell. The gravid proglottid loses its grip on the strobila and when passed in the feces it reaches the outside where it ruptures to deliver the eggs. The eggs are ingested by fleas in which they develop into the cysticercoid stage. If the dog eats the infected flea, the larva matures into an adult worm in the small intestine.

Diagnosis: The proglottids are found in feces and are rarely accompanied by ova or egg packets.

ARTHROPODS OF MEDICAL IMPORTANCE
Dermacentor andersoni

Dermacentor andersoni[101] (Rocky Mountain wood tick) (Fig. 34-58) is a hard tick characterized in the male by a hard shield covering the entire dorsal surface. In the female the shield covers only the anterior one third to one half of the body. Both male and female are blood suckers, normally remaining attached to the host for a considerable length of time. They take only one blood meal in each of the developmental stages: larval, nymphal, and adult. They are usually found on the ground, infesting bushes and shrubs.

Members of this species can transmit Rocky Mountain spotted fever, Q fever, various forms of encephalitis, and tularemia. They can also cause a condition known as tick paralysis. Tick paralysis is not an actual disease but a series of symptoms caused by a toxic substance secreted by the tick's salivary gland. Since it results only from the bite of a female tick, it appears to be related to production of eggs. It is most commonly associated with the presence of the tick at the back of the neck or along the spinal column. Complete removal of the tick usually results in rapid termination of symptoms.

Ctenocephalides felix

Ctenocephalides felix[101] is the generic name for the cat flea (Fig. 34-58). Fleas come into close association with humans primarily as ectoparasites of domestic animals and rodents. Fleas display a marked preference for the blood of certain warm-blooded animals, but in the absence of the host of choice they readily accept substitute hosts. Fleas infesting rodents can transmit diseases such as plague, murine typhus, and tularemia. They also serve as intermediate hosts for two species of tapeworms transmissible to humans *(Hymenolepis diminuta* and *Dipylidium caninum).*

Pediculus humanus

Pediculus humanus[101] (human head and body louse) (Fig. 34-58) can be found throughout the world wherever the level of sanitation is low. Lice are true obligatory ectoparasites of humans, spending their whole life cycle on the human body or in clothing. An increased level of sanitation together with the development of more effective insecticides has reduced this pestilence.

Epidemic typhus, trench fever, and relapsing fever are transmitted by lice. Lice tend to leave individuals who have fever or who have died, thereby spreading louse-borne infections.

Phthirus pubis

Phthirus pubis[101] (human crab louse) (Fig. 34-58) is usually found on the hairs of the genital region but may occur on other parts of the body. It is readily recognized by the following characteristics: (1) its area of attachment; (2) its stout legs, which terminate in chitinous, curved, grasping claws; and (3) the square outline of the body.

Although *Phthirus pubis* is not involved in disease transmission, infestations cause considerable discomfort and may produce itching macular swellings.

Transmission is by contact with infested individuals, their clothing, or bedding or other objects with which they have come in contact, particularly toilet seats.

Musca domestica

Musca domestica[101] (house fly) (Fig. 34-58) is characterized principally by the occurrence of four longitudinal black stripes that extend the length of the dorsal side of the thorax.

House flies carry the etiologic agents of disease without playing an essential part in the cycle proper. When

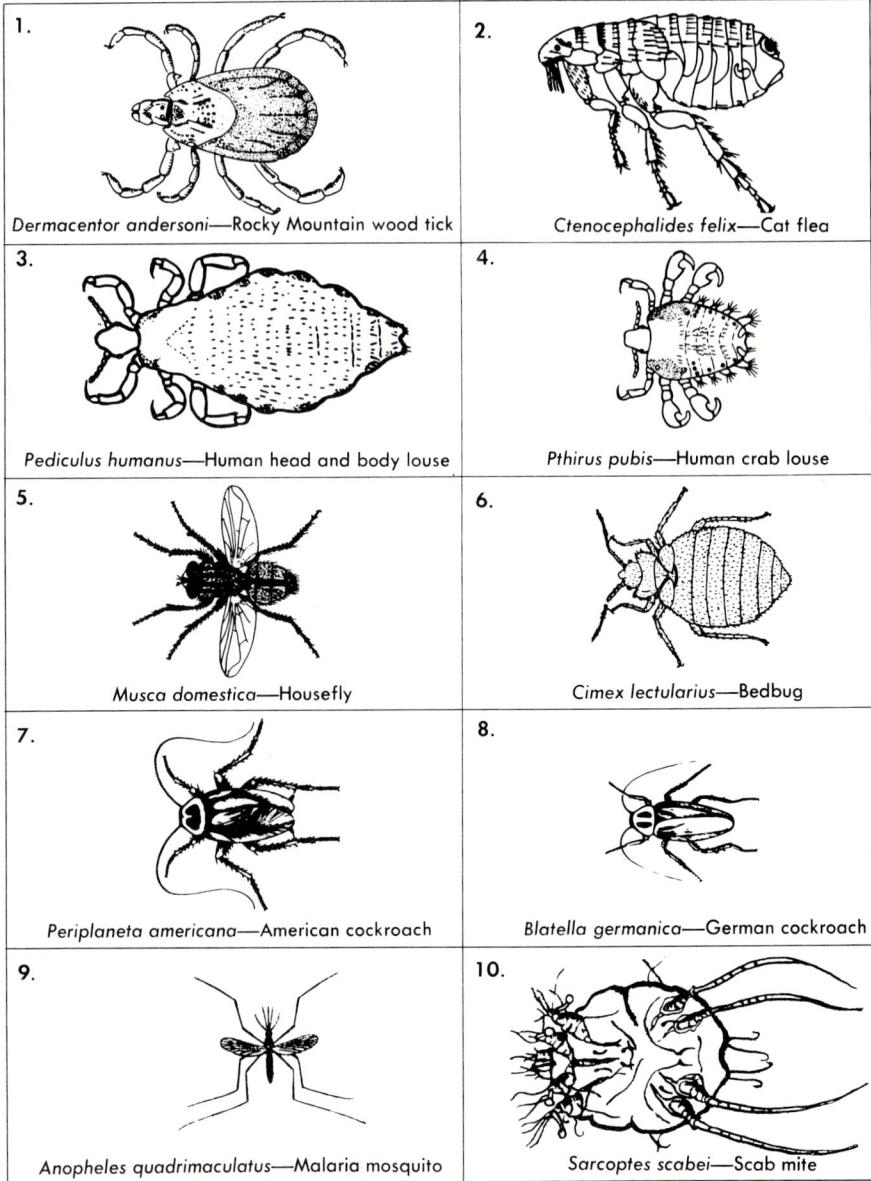

Fig. 34-58. Arthropods of medical importance. (Modified from Huffaker, R.H., editor: Collection, handling and shipment of microbiological specimens, Atlanta, 1974, Centers for Disease Control.)

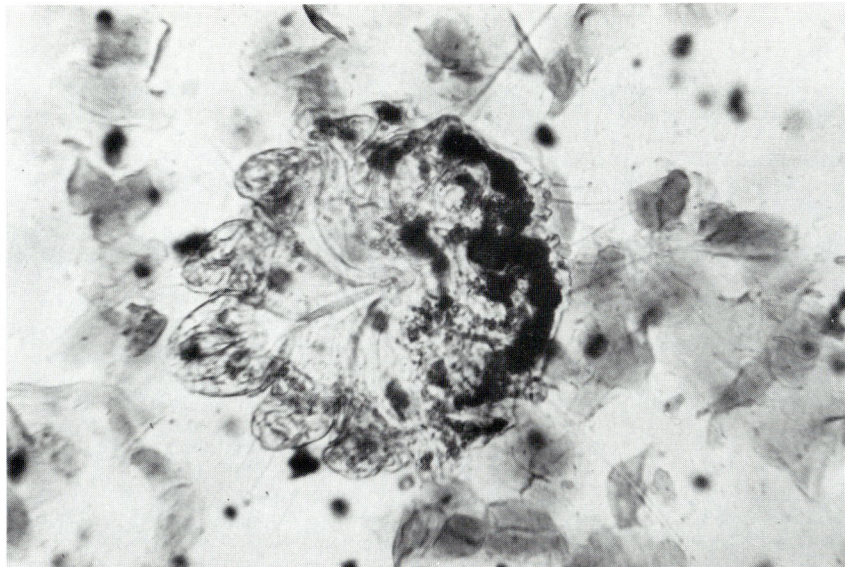

Fig. 34-59. *Sarcoptes scabei:* scab mite.

temperature, moisture, and food conditions are right, fly populations become excessive. Their breeding habits and preference for various foods, including the excrement of warm-blooded animals, explain the laboratory proof that flies transmit at least 30 different diseases. Cholera, typhoid, amebic and bacillary dysentery, various diarrheas, tetanus, anthrax, trachoma, yaws, leprosy, tuberculosis, and certain helminth infections (by eggs) are among those diseases spread by flies.

Cimex lectularius

Cimex lectularius[101] (bedbug) (Fig. 34-58) lives in close association with humans, in cracks and crevices of walls and flooring, or in the small tight areas in and on beds. Bedbugs are easily transported in clothing and baggage, and they will readily move from one house to another by way of walls, pipes, and electrical conduits.

They have never been proven to transmit any disease to humans naturally, although their bite produces intense itching that may persist for days or weeks.

Periplaneta americana

Periplaneta americana[101] (American cockroach) (Fig. 34-58) frequents filthy situations, readily feeding on both human excreta and sputum. Their favorite haunts are places where food is stored, prepared, or eaten. Their habits afford abundant opportunity to carry the etiologic agents of diseases on their hairy bodies and antennae.

Cockroaches can carry amebiasis, balantidiasis, cholera, bacillary dysentery, giardiasis, hymenolepiasis, poliomyelitis, paratyphoid fever, and typhoid fever.

Blatella germanica

Blatella germanica[101] is the generic name for the German cockroach (Fig. 34-58). For a discussion of this arthropod, see the discussion of the American cockroach.

Anopheles quadrimaculatus

Anopheles quadrimaculatus[101] is the generic name for the malaria mosquito (Fig. 34-58).

Mosquitoes constitute the most important single group of vectors of disease to humans. Mosquitoes are known vectors of filariasis, dengue, yellow fever, and a number of virus encephalitides. The *Anopheles quadrimaculatus,* as a transmitter of malaria, is of prime importance.

Sarcoptes scabiei

Sarcoptes scabiei[101] (scab mite) (Figs. 34-58 and 34-59) is a mite that burrows into the surface epithelium of the skin and causes inflammation, itching, and scab formation, hence the name "scab mites." The disease is called scabies. The mite deposits eggs within the burrows where the larvae hatch. The diagnosis is established by scraping the superficial skin layer to expose the mite. The scrapings are transferred to a slide and are examined under the low power of the microscope for mites. Clearing the specimen with 1-2 drops of 10% KOH aids in the discovery of mites and their eggs.

GLOSSARY

arthropods Animals belonging to the phylum Arthropoda, characterized by their many-jointed bodies.

autoinfection Reinfection by the progeny of a parasite while they are still within the host.

axenic Free from other organisms, such as occurs in a "pure" culture medium.

axostyle Rodlike organelles that function as internal structural support in certain protozoans.

bile duct An excretory duct of the liver containing bile.

biologic vector An arthropod vector in whose body the infecting organism develops before becoming infective to the recipient individual.

blepharoplast A minute oval or round granule forming a part of the complex known as the kinetoplast in blood and tissue flagellates belonging to the genera *Trypanosoma* and *Leishmania*.

cestode Common name applied to tapeworms as a group.

Charcot-Leyden crystals Crystals that are greatly flattened in the longitudinal axis and terminate in needlelike points at their opposite poles.

chitin The horny substance in the exoskeleton of beetles, crabs, and certain microorganisms; a polymer of *N*-acetyl-D-glucosamine, similar in structure to cellulose.

chitinous Of or relating to chitin.

chromatin Nuclear material that is Feulgen positive for DNA.

cilia Minute lashlike structures that serve as organelles of locomotion in protozoans belonging to the class Ciliata.

ciliate General term applied to protozoans of the class Ciliata, which are characterized by the presence of numerous fine hairlike fibrils on the surface of the body that serve as organelles of locomotion.

circadian rhythm Occurring approximately every 24 hr.

colon A part of the large intestine.

commensal An organism living in close association with another and benefiting therefrom without harming or benefiting the other.

cyst A parasite that is surrounded by a resistant wall or membrane.

cysticercosis A disease in which the developmental larval stage of the tapeworm invades body tissue.

cysticercus Larval form of tapeworm in which a single scolex is enclosed in a bladderlike cyst.

cytoplasm Protoplasm of cell outside the cell nucleus.

cytosome Opening within the outer wall of certain species of highly developed protozoans that serves as a primitive mouth through which solid food or waste material passes in or out of the cell.

definitive host The host in which the parasite undergoes sexual reproduction.

dichotomously Relating to dichotomy.

dichotomy Division into two parts.

diecious Having male reproduction organs in one organism and female in another.

disease A specific morbid process that has a characteristic set of symptoms and that may affect either the entire body or any part of the body.

diurnal Activity occurring during both daylight and darkness.

duodenum Segment of small bowel.

echinococcosis Disease that results from infection with *Echinococcus granulosis*.

ectoplasm Outer clear zone of cytoplasm on the immediate margin of a cell.

elephantiasis Disease caused by infection with *Wuchereria* species and characterized by inflammation and enlargement of various parts of the body.

embryophore Second eggshell formed by embryo after loss of first; seen in eggs of *Taenia* species since they are found in feces.

endoplasm Inner granular zone of cytoplasm within a cell.

epidemic A disease that affects a large number of organisms and spreads rapidly.

epidemiology The study of epidemics.

facultative parasite Parasite capable of living apart from a host, i.e., potentially free living.

fibrils Minute filaments that serve as organelles of locomotion in certain species of protozoans.

filariform larva Long, slender, nonfeeding, infective larva.

final host The host in which the parasite undergoes sexual reproduction.

flagellate General term applied to protozoans of the class Flagellata, which are characterized by the presence of whiplike fibrils (flagella) that serve as organelles of locomotion.

gamete Sexual cell that is the end product of gametogeny in the life cycle of the malaria parasite. In a process comparable to that of fertilization in higher forms, the macrogamete and microgamete combine to produce a zygote within the mosquito's body.

glycogen Chief carbohydrate form in which food is stored in an animal's body.

granuloma A mass or nodule composed of chronically inflamed tissue marked by the collection of macrophages, endothelial cells, and giant cells.

habitat The specific place where an organism usually lives.

helminth General term applicable to the various species of worms that may be parasitic in humans.

hemazoin The pigment found within malaria parasites; also the pigment deposited in body tissue as a result of the rupture of infected red cells at the completion of the schizogenous cycle of the malaria parasite.

hermaphrodite One individual that possesses both male and female reproductive organs.

hermaphroditic Of or pertaining to a hermaphrodite.

hexacanth Six-hooked embryo of certain species of tapeworms that is liberated from the egg when it hatches.

host Living animal or plant harboring or affording sustenance to a parasite; also a cell in which a parasite lodges (host cell).

host specificity Restriction of a parasite to one or more kinds of hosts.

hydatid Cyst stage of embryonic tapeworm in which cyst contains daughter cysts, each of which contains many scolices.

hyperplasia An increase in the number of tissue elements (excluding tumor formation), thereby increasing the mass of the part or organ involved.

hypertrophy An increase in the mass of tissue because of an increase in size but not an increase in the number of tissue elements; sometimes used to denote an increase in size to meet a demand for increased functional activity.

immunity Those natural processes that prevent infection, reinfection, or superinfection, that assist in destroying parasites or limiting their multiplication, or that reduce the clinical effects of infection.

incidence The number of cases of infection occurring during a given period of time in relation to the population unit in which they occur (a dynamic measurement).

infection Parasitic invasion of cells or tissues resulting in injury and reaction to the injury.

infestation Attack by parasites.

intermediate host Ordinarily, one that harbors the asexual or immature stages; note, however, that fertilization in *Plasmodia* occurs in the mosquito, usually considered to be an intermediate host.

karyosome One of the spheric masses of chromatin in the nucleus of a cell, generally situated at or near the center of the nucleus and more deeply staining with hematoxylin than the remaining nuclear chromatin.

larva A stage clearly different from the adult, requiring metamorphosis for further development.

Leishman-Donovan body Small oval-shaped nucleated organism that is the causative agent of all three forms of human leishmaniasis.

leishmaniasis Any of three diseases characterized by infection of skin or internal organs with Leishman-Donovan bodies.

leptomonad Simple flagellate developmental stage of members of the genera *Trypanosoma* and *Leishmania*.

lesion An abnormal change in structure of an organ or part because of injury or disease.

mammillated Having nipples or small protuberances like nipples.

merozoite Asexual forms in developmental cycle of malaria parasite that are liberated into bloodstream when schizont reaches maturity.

metacercaria Encysted resting stage of trematode either within tissues of a crustacean or fish or on surface of aquatic or semiaquatic vegetation.

mucosa Mucous membrane.

nocturnal Activity limited to the hours of darkness.

nucleus Spheric body made of chromatin (DNA) within cell that forms an essential and vital part that controls cell's activities.

obligatory parasite A parasite unable to live and multiply except as a parasite on or in a host.

onchocerciasis Disease that results from infection with the parasite *Onchocera volvulus*.

oocyst Swollen saclike structure that develops in the stomach wall of the mosquito as a result of invasion by the zygote of *Plasmodia*.

operculate Having an operculum.

operculum Cap that covers the opening through which embryos of certain species of flukes and tapeworms escape from eggs at time of hatching.

ova Eggs of parasites containing nutritive substances and germinal elements that give rise to developmental stage in life cycle of parasite.

papilloma Epithelial tumor that projects above the surface.

paragonimiasis Disease that results from infection with *Paragonimus westermani*.

parasite Organism that depends on its host for some essential metabolites and with which a reciprocal chemical relationship exists.

parasitism Association between two specifically distinct organisms in which the dependence of the parasite on its host is a metabolic one involving mutual exchange of substances.

parthenogenesis Reproduction by the development of an unfertilized egg.

parthenogenetically Of or pertaining to parthenogenesis.

pathogenic That which causes disease.

periodicity Regularly recurrent rhythmic changes in vital functions or recurrence of a parasite at regular intervals of time.

peritoneal cavity Abdominal cavity.

perivesicular Surrounding the urinary bladder.

portal vein Vein that carries blood from the intestines to the liver.

proglottids Individual segmentlike structures that make up the chain of tapeworms, exclusive of head and neck.

protozoa Single-celled animals characterized by a body composed of one or more nuclei surrounded by cytoplasm and contained within a limiting cell membrane.

pseudopod Temporary protrusion of outer margin of cell wall of an amoeba, serving locomotion and feeding.

rectum Terminal segment of the large intestine.

reservoir host Parasitized animals that may serve as a source of infection.

rhabditiform larva First-stage noninfective feeding larva liberated from ovum of nematode worm.

rostellum Hook-bearing portion of head of certain parasitic intestinal worms.

schistosome General term applied to blood flukes.

schistosomiasis Disease produced by blood flukes.

schizogeny Asexual cycle of sporozoa.

scolex Attachment end of tapeworm consisting of head and neck.

sigmoid colon Segment of colon.

sparaganosis Disease produced by the migration of larval tapeworms within body tissues.

sporocyst Cyst or sac that forms within snail as a result of entry of miracidial stage of fluke.

sporogony Formation of spores or sporozoites.

sporozoite Infective stage of the malarial parasite that migrates to the salivary gland of the mosquito.

strobila Entire adult tapeworm.

symbiosis The living together of different species of organisms.

tolerance In the immunologic sense, an induced state of unresponsiveness to a specific immunogen.

trematode Common name applied to flukes as a group.

trichinosis Disease caused by infection with "pork worm."

trophozoite Active vegetative feeding motile stage of a protozoan.

trypanosome Blood and tissue flagellate of genus *Trypanosoma*.

ulceration Process of forming an ulcer or of becoming ulcerated.

vacuole Membrane surrounded aggregations of material that float about in cytoplasm within protozoan cells.

vector Carrier, especially an animal that transfers an infective agent from one host to another.

venous plexus Network of interlacing veins.

viable In a living condition.

virulence Relative infectiousness of a parasite.

vitellarium Modified part of the ovary that produces yolk-filled cells serving to nourish the true eggs.

vitelline Relating to a yolk or an egg.

xenodiagnosis Method of diagnosis in which the vector is fed on a suspected host and later examined for the presence of parasites.

zoonosis Disease or infection that is naturally transferable between animals and humans.

zygote Cell resulting from fusion of two gametes.

REFERENCES

1. Beck, J., and Davies, J.: Medical parasitology, ed. 3, St. Louis, 1981, The C.V. Mosby Co.
2. Garcia, L.S., and Ash, L.R.: Diagnostic parasitology: clinical laboratory manual, ed. 2, St. Louis, 1979, The C.V. Mosby Co.
3. Lennette, E.H., et al., editors: Manual of clinical microbiology, ed. 3, Washington, D.C., 1980, American Society for Microbiology.
4. Hunter, G., Frye, W., and Swartzwelder, J.: A manual of tropical medicine, ed. 4, Philadelphia, 1966, W.B. Saunders Co.
5. Noble, E., and Noble, G.: Parasitology: the biology of animal parasites, ed. 4, Philadelphia, 1976, Lea & Febiger.
6. Markell, E., and Voge, M.: Medical parasitology, ed. 4, Philadelphia, 1976, W.B. Saunders Co.
7. Thompson, J.H.: Parasitology laboratory procedure manual, Mayo Clinic Foundation, Rochester, Minn., Boston, 1978, Little, Brown & Co.
8. Nair, C.P.: Nature **172:**1051, 1953.
9. Ridley, D., and Hawgood, B.: J. Clin. Pathol. **9:**74, 1956.
10. Clin. Microbiol. Newsletter **2:**6, 1980.
11. Bartlett, M., et al.: J. Clin. Microbiol. **7:**524, 1978.
12. Zierdt, W.S.: Am. J. Clin. Pathol. **70:**89, 1978.
13. Wheatley, W.B.: Am. J. Clin. Pathol. **21:**990, 1951.
14. Balamuth, W.: Am. J. Clin. Pathol. **16:**380, 1946.
15. Feinberg, J.G., and Whittington, M.J.: J. Clin. Pathol. **10:**327, 1957.
16. Boardman, E.T.: J. Parasitol. **30:**57, 1944.
17. Wilson, E.S.: J. Med. Soc. N.J. **72:**573, 1975.
18. Stamm, W.P.: Trans. R. Soc. Trop. Med. Hyg. **59:**712, 1965.
19. Kessel, J., et al.: Am. J. Trop. Med. Hyg. **14:**540, 1965.
20. Healy, G., Kagan, I.G., and Gleason, N.: Health Lab. Sci. **7:**109, 1970.

21. Kagan, I.G., and Norman, L.: In Friedman, H., editor: Manual of clinical immunology, Washington, D.C., 1976, American Society for Microbiology.
22. Walls, K., and Smith, J.: Lab. Med. **10**:329, 1979.
23. Cox, J., and Nairn, R.: J. Clin. Pathol. **27**:1018, 1974.
24. Ray, K., et al.: Indian J. Med. Res. **62**:1347, 1974.
25. Doxiades, T., and Candreviotis, N.: Br. Med. J. **1**:1810, 1962.
26. Jeanes, A.L.: Br. Med. J. **1**:1464, 1966.
27. Vinayak, V., et al.: Indian J. Med. Res. **62**:1317, 1974.
28. Powell, S., et al.: Lancet **1**:566, 1966.
29. Mahajan, R., et al.: Indian J. Med. Res. **62**:301, 1974.
30. Lawless, D.K., and Knight, V.: Am. J. Trop. Med. Hyg. **15**:701, 1966.
31. Culbertson, C., Ensminger, P., and Overton, W.: Am. J. Clin. Pathol. **43**:383, 1965.
32. Martinez, A., et al.: Acta Neuropathol. **37**:183, 1977.
33. Sotelo-Avila, C., Martinez, A., and Dos Santos Neto, J.: Anatomic pathology: "check sample" no. APII-23, Chicago, 1978, Commission on Continuing Education, American Society of Clinical Pathologists.
34. Nagington, J., et al.: Lancet **2**:1537, 1974.
35. Cursons, R., Brown, T., and Keys, E.: J. Parasitol. **64**:744, 1978.
36. Carter, R.F.: J. Pathol. **100**:217, 1970.
37. Weng, N., Wagner, W., and Parker, J.: South. Med. J. **64**:691, 1971.
38. De Jonckheere, J.: Appl. Environ. Microbiol. **33**:751, 1977.
39. Honigberg, B.M.: J. Protozool. **21**:79, 1974.
40. Camp, R.R., Mattern, C.F.T., and Honigberg, B.M.: J. Protozool. **21**:69, 1974.
41. Walton, B., Brooks, W., and Arjona, I.: Am. J. Trop. Med. Hyg. **21**:296, 1972.
42. Nelson, G.S.: N. Engl. J. Med. **300**:1136, 1979.
43. Latif, B., and Adam, K.: Bull WHO **48**:401, 1973.
44. Cerisola, J.A.: J. Parasitol. **56**:409, 1970.
45. Vattuone, N., and Yanovsky, J.: Exp. Parasitol. **30**:349, 1971.
46. Miller, F., Pizzuto, A., and McCauley, H.: Am. J. Trop. Med. Hyg. **20**:23, 1971.
47. Laboratory diagnosis of intestinal protozoa and malaria, Atlanta, 1972, Centers for Disease Control.
47a. Rahimi, A.: Parasitology procedure manual, St. Francis Hospital, La Crosse, Wisc., 1977.
48. Keffer, J.H.: Tech. Bull. Registered Med. Technol. **36**:153, 1966.
49. Sulzer, A., and Wilson, M.: Crit. Rev. Clin. Lab. Sci, **2**:601, 1971.
50. Farshy, D., and Kagan, I.G.: Infect. Immun. **7**:680, 1973.
51. Allison, A.C.: Ann. N.Y. Acad. Sci. **91**:710, 1961.
52. Allison, A.C., and Clyde, D.: Br. Med. J. **1**:1346, 1961.
53. Chatterjea, J., et al.: Blood **12**:585, 1957.
54. Harding, H.: Microbiology: "check sample" no. MB-25, Chicago, 1965, Commission on Continuing Education, American Society of Clinical Pathologists.
55. Wright, W.H.: Am. J. Clin. Pathol. **28**:1, 1957.
56. Jacobs, L., et al.: Bull. John Hopkins Hosp. **99**:1, 1956.
57. Lab Reports for Physicians, vol. 3, no. 9, 1981.
58. Sabin, A., and Feldman, H.: Science **108**:660, 1948.
59. Sulzer, A., and Hall, E.: Am. J. Epidemiol. **86**:401, 1967.
60. Callerame, M., and Nadel, M.: Am. J. Clin. Pathol. **45**:258, 1966.
61. Esterly, J., and Warner, N.: Arch. Pathol. **80**:433, 1965.
62. Rosen, P., Martini, N., and Armstrong, D.: Am. J. Med. **58**:794, 1975.
63. Kim, H., and Hughes, W.: Am. J. Clin. Pathol. **60**:462, 1973.
64. Repsher, L., Schröter, G., and Hammond, W.: N. Engl. J. Med. **287**:340, 1972.
65. Rosen, P., and Armstrong, D.: Microbiology: "check sample" no. MB-81, Chicago, 1976, Commission on Continuing Education, American Society of Clinical Pathologists.
66. Pifer, L.L., Hughes, W.T., and Murphy, M.J.: Am. J. Pathol. **86**:387, 1977.
67. Healy, G.: Microbiology: "check sample" no. MB-45, Chicago, 1970, Commission on Continuing Education, American Society of Clinical Pathologists.
68. Western, K., et al.: N. Engl. J. Med. **283**:854, 1970.
69. Garnham, P., et al.: Br. Med. J. **4**:768, 1969.
70. Healy, G.R.: Hosp. Pract. **14**:107, 1979.
71. Georgi, J., and Sprinkle, C.: Am. J. Trop. Med. Hyg. **23**:899, 1974.
72. Cruz, T., Reboucas, G., and Rocha, H.: N. Engl. J. Med. **275**:1093, 1966.
73. Baermann, G.: Meded. Geneesk. Lab., *Feestbundel*, p. 41, 1917.
74. Stoll, N.R.: Am. J. Hyg. **3**:59, 1923.
75. Ball, P., and Bartlett, A.: Trans. R. Soc. Trop. Med. Hyg. **63**:362, 1969.
76. Zuzuki, T., et al.: Am. J. Parasitol. **22**:187, 1973.
77. Harder, H., and Watson, D.: Am. J. Clin. Pathol. **42**:333, 1964.
78. O'Connell, J., and Kiandoli, L.: Advanced Microbiology: "check sample" no. AMB-8, Chicago, 1974, Commission on Continuing Education, American Society of Clinical Pathologists.
79. Hawking, F., and Worms, M.: Ann. Rev. Entomol. **6**:413, 1961.
80. Partono, F., et al.: Trop. Geogr. Med. **25**:286, 1973.
81. WHO Tech. Rep. Ser. no. 542, WHO Expert Committee on Filariasis, Geneva, 1974, World Health Organization.
82. Connor, D.H.: N. Engl. J. Med. **298**:379, 1978.
83. Gould, S., et al.: Am. J. Clin. Pathol. **40**:197, 1963.
84. Bourée, P., et al.: Br. Med. J. **1**:1047, 1979.
85. Beck, J., and Beverley-Burton, M.: Helminthol. Abstr. **37**:1, 1968.
86. Kohler, G., and Ruitenberg, E.: Bull WHO **50**:413, 1974.
87. Norman, L., and Kagan, I.G.: Public Health Rep. **78**:227, 1963.
88. Despommier, D., et al.: Am. J. Trop. Med. Hyg. **23**:41, 1974.
89. Hood, M.: Am. J. Clin. Pathol. **22**:396, 1952.
90. Dawes, B., and Hughes, D.: Adv. Parasitol. **8**:259, 1970.
91. Bénex, J., Guilhon, J., and Barnabé, R.: Bull. Soc. Pathol. Exot. Filiales **66**:116, 1973.
92. Komiya, Y.: Adv. Parasitol. **4**:53, 1966.
93. Sadun, E., et al.: J. Parasitol. **45**:129, 1959.
94. Yokogawa, M.: Adv. Parasitol. **7**:375, 1969.
95. McMullen, D., and Beaver, P.: Am. J. Hyg. **42**:128, 1945.
96. Wilson, M., Sulzer, A.J., and Walls, K.: Am. J. Trop. Med. Hyg. **23**:1072, 1974.
97. Gould, S., et al.: Am. J. Clin. Pathol. **40**:83, 1963.
98. Pawlowski, Z., and Schultz, M.: Adv. Parasitol. **10**:269, 1972.
99. von Bonsdorff, B.: Exp. Parasitol. **5**:207, 1956.
100. Smith, J.: Special topics: "check sample" no. ST-90, Chicago, 1976, Commission on Continuing Education, American Society of Clinical Pathologists.
101. Laboratory procedures in parasitology, Dept. of Army Technical Manual, no. TM8-227-2, Washington, D.C., 1961, U.S. Dept. of the Army.

SEROLOGY AND IMMUNOLOGY

CHAPTER 35

Clinical serology

INTRODUCTION TO SEROLOGIC REACTIONS AND METHODS[1-3]

Serology deals with the detection and quantitation of antibodies and antigens. In recent years the serologic armamentarium has been expanded to include immunochemical methods that employ labeled antigens such as radionuclides (as in radioimmunoassay), fluorescent dyes (as in fluoroimmunoassay), and enzymes (as in the enzyme multiplied immunoassay technic [EMIT] and in the enzyme-linked immunosorbent assay [ELISA]). Some of these investigative procedures are mentioned in other sections in this book, e.g., the chapters dealing with immunology, blood banking, biochemistry, toxicology, and coagulation.

Antigens and haptens

An antigen used to be defined as a foreign substance that, when introduced (usually parenterally) into a vertebrate organism, will induce its immune mechanism to produce antibodies that will specifically react with the antigen, an interaction that can be demonstrated by a number of laboratory methods. A more up-to-date definition characterizes an antigen as a "foreign" macromolecule that induces the animal to form immunoglobulins[1,2] (see discussion of B- and T-lymphocytes, Chapter 36). Proteins are antigens par excellence, but polysaccharides, polypeptides, lipoproteins, and nucleoproteins are also antigenic. Antigens have two characteristics: (1) antigenicity, i.e., they are capable of producing antibodies; and (2) specific reactivity, i.e., they specifically react with the antibodies, the formation of which they induce. The specificity of an antigen depends on its antigenic determinants, which are responsible for its uniqueness.

Haptens are substances (usually of low molecular weight) that are not antigenic by themselves when injected into an animal but coupled to an antigen lead to the formation of antibodies, which will react with the original antigen and with the hapten, even if the hapten is coupled to a new antigen different from the original one.

Antibodies

Antibodies are immunoglobulins that are formed by the body in response to contact with an antigen and specifically react with it. The structure of the antibody molecule is discussed in detail in Chapter 36. Antibodies in biologic fluids may be demonstrated by a number of serologic reactions, which depend on the physical state of the antigen. A soluble liquid antigen precipitates when it reacts with its specific antibody, whereas a cellular or particulate antigen clumps, agglutinates, and settles out after reacting with its antibody. Lysis is a type of reaction that occurs when blood or bacterial antigens are confronted with their antibodies. Neutralization occurs when an antigen has its toxic effect nullified as the result of contact with its antibody. The first three reactions can be directly observed, but special systems are required to detect neutralization.

Dilutions and titers

Titering is a semiquantitative technic used to assay the concentration of an antibody. It requires two to three steps: (1) serial dilution of the antibody solution (e.g., serum), (2) the addition of equal volumes of the

Portions of this chapter are taken from Part XI, "Serology of infectious diseases," in Sonnenwirth, A.C., and Jarett, L., editors: Gradwohl's clinical laboratory methods and diagnosis, ed. 8, St. Louis, 1980, The C.V. Mosby Co., vol. 2.

antigen, and (3) in various serologic procedures, the addition of standardized erythrocyte suspensions. In the usual serologic reaction, serial (twofold) dilutions of the serum are prepared based on the principle of progressively decreasing the volume of serum while maintaining a constant volume of fluid. Dilutions of serum are expressed as the ratio of the quantity of serum contained in the total volume of fluid to the total volume.

Preparation of red cell suspension

Principle: Suspensions are prepared by suspending the red cells in saline and washing them by centrifugation until the supernatant is clear. The packed red cells are then suspended in appropriate amounts of saline.

Equipment and reagent:
1. Gauze sponges, 3 × 3 in.
2. Graduated centrifuge tubes
3. Anticoagulated blood

Procedure: Add saline to blood; mix and centrifuge for 5 min at 1500 rpm. Remove supernatant fluid and buffy coat and resuspend red cells in 9-10 ml saline and recentrifuge. Repeat three times. The last supernatant must be colorless; if not, repeat with fresh blood. After removal of the last supernatant read the total packed cell volume and calculate the desired cell concentration of the suspension as follows:

$$\text{Total vol. (ml)} = \frac{\text{Packed cell vol.} \times 100}{\text{Desired cell concentration (\%)}}$$

EXAMPLE: A 2% cell suspension is desired, and the packed cell volume is 0.2 ml. Then

$$\text{Total vol. (ml)} = \frac{0.2 \times 100}{2} = \frac{20}{2} = 10$$

Total vol. − Packed cell vol. = Saline to be added (ml)
(For example: 10 − 0.2 = 9.8 ml saline to be added)

Spectrophotometric technic of standardization of erythrocyte suspensions

The spectrophotometric method as described by Palmer, Cavallaro, and Galt[4] is the preferred technic for the standardization of erythrocyte suspensions. A more rapid technic for preparation of sheep cell suspensions follows.

Reagents:
1. Sterile Alsever solution
2. Sheep cells in Alsever solution (commercially available)
   Store for 1 week at 40° C.
3. EDTA buffer, 0.01 M, 37.2 g in about 8 dl water
   Adjust pH to 7.65 ± .05 with 2N sodium hydroxide and add water to make 1 L. Store at 40° C.
4. Veronal buffered saline (VBS) (commercially available)

Procedure: Centrifuge 10 ml sheep cells in Alsever solution. After centrifugation discard supernatant and buffy coat. Suspend cells in EDTA buffer and incubate at 37° C for 10 min. Wash cells in EDTA buffer and then three times in VBS and discard supernatant after fourth spin.

Dilute packed cells 1:15 in VBS. Lyse 0.1 ml of dilute packed cells in 2.4 ml water. Measure optical density (OD) of lysate at 541 nm.

An OD of 0.420 corresponds to a cell concentration of 1×10^9 cells per milliliter. If indicated adjust cell suspension to obtain this value ± 0.02.

Serial dilutions

Macromethod:

Purpose: Serial dilutions provide a means of quantitating the antibody content of a serum specimen.

Principle: Suitable quantities of antigen are added to serial dilutions of the antiserum. Tubes lacking the antiserum or antigen serve as controls. After appropriate incubation at specified temperatures the tubes are examined for evidence of serologic reactions by comparing the test tubes with the control tubes.

Equipment and reagent:
1. Test tubes
2. Test tube rack
3. Gauze sponges, 3 × 3 in.
4. Serologic pipets, 5 ml
5. Serologic pipets, 10 ml
6. Normal saline

Procedure (Table 35-1): Number test tubes 1 to 10 and place them in a test tube rack. Pipet 8.0 ml normal saline into tube 1 and 5.0 ml into the remaining tubes. To tube 1 add 2.0 ml of the serum to be tested and mix. Transfer 5.0 ml of the contents from tube 1 to tube 2 and mix. Transfer 5.0 ml of the contents from tube 2 to tube 3 and mix. Continue this process through the last tube and after mixing the contents of tube 10 discard 5 ml from this tube.

Add 5 ml of red cell suspension to each tube if so indicated in the protocol. Stopper tubes to prevent evaporation and incubate at 37° C for 12-48 hr. Examine tubes for lysis or agglutination if so indicated in the protocol.

Results: The dilution of the serum in the last dilution tube to exhibit a positive reaction is the titer of the antiserum, usually reported as the reciprocal of the last dilution.

Discussion: The dilutions of the serum are expressed as the ratio of the quantity of serum contained in the total volume of fluid to the total volume. In tube 1, before the addition of the cell suspension, 2 volumes of serum are diluted in 10 volumes of total fluid (2 + 8), giving a dilution of 2:10 or 1:5. The first transfer of 5 ml of the 1:5 dilution transfers 1 ml of serum to 10 ml total fluid (before the addition of the cell suspension). The serum dilution in the second tube is therefore 1:10. The transfer from the second tube to the third tube transfers 0.5 ml serum. After transfer to the third tube there is 0.5 ml serum in 10 ml total fluid, giving a dilution of 1:20 before the addition of the cell suspension. This process is continued so that to each succeeding tube in the series the amount of serum transferred is half the amount present in the preceding tube. If the quantity of serum is halved but the total volume remains constant, then the dilution is doubled. When 5 ml red cell suspension is added to each tube (containing 5 ml liquid), the total volume and the serum dilutions are doubled again, so that the 1:5 dilution in tube 1 becomes a 1:10 dilution, etc.

Table 35-1. Outline of serial dilution procedure

	Tube no.									
	1	**2**	**3**	**4**	**5**	**6**	**7**	**8**	**9**	**10**
Saline (ml)	8	5	5	5	5	5	5	5	5	5
Serum (ml)	2	←			Transfer 5 ml from tube to tube and discard last 5 ml.					→
Dilution after serum transfer	1:5	1:10	1:20	1:40	1:80	1:160	1:320	1:640	1:1288	1:2560
Cell suspension (ml)	5	5	5	5	5	5	5	5	5	5
Total volume (ml)	10	10	10	10	10	10	10	10	10	10
Final dilution of serum	1:10	1:20	1:40	1:80	1:160	1:320	1:640	1:1280	1:2560	1:5120

When transferring from a low dilution to a higher dilution using a pipet, the outside of the pipet must be wiped off between each transfer.

The mixing of serum and saline can be accomplished by drawing up the diluted serum into the pipet and expelling it.

The macrotube dilution method has many disadvantages. It requires too much space, glassware, material, labor, cost, and technician's time. Microdilution technics eliminate many of these drawbacks.

Micromethod (microtitration): In the microtitration method the test tubes are replaced by plastic, multi-welled microtitration plates, each having eight rows of 12 wells, 6 mm in diameter with a working capacity of 125 μl. Specially designed wells are available for complement-fixation, hemagglutination inhibition, and hemagglutination tests. The pipets are replaced by calibrated microdiluters, which pick up and deliver 25 or 50 μl, and by pipet droppers, which deliver precalibrated volumes of fluid, e.g., antigen, buffer, or erythrocyte suspension. The microtiter technic is rapid and cost efficient.[5,6]

Equipment:
1. Microtiter plates (Dynatech, Dynatech Laboratories, Alexandria, Va.), with U- or V-shaped wells
2. Pipet droppers, 25 or 50 μl
3. Microdiluters (Dynatech)
4. Go-no-go delivery tester (Dynatech) (a blotter that determines the accuracy of the 25 or 50 μl delivery)
5. Plate sealing tape (Dynatech)
6. Test-reading mirror (Dynatech)

Procedure[6-8]: Flame the microdiluter; cool and prewet in saline. Dry on go-no-go delivery tester. Wet the microdiluter with water; touch marked center of one of the circles on the blotter. It should dampen the area immediately.

Fill pipet dropper with desired diluent, wipe with gauze, and place 1 drop (25 μl) into each well, leaving the first well empty. Fill the microdiluter by touching the surface of the fluid to be diluted, (e.g., serum) and transfer to desired well.

Mix by rotating the top of the microdiluter. Move microdiluter to successive wells and rotate. Avoid touching the sides of wells. Add appropriate antigen, complement, indicator red cells, etc., depending on the test.

Antigen-antibody reactions

Although the specificity of an antigen is mentioned above as one of its characteristics, this specificity is not absolute. Complex antigens may share antigenic determinants with other antigens, thus antibodies to one will cross-react with the other antigens. Shared antigens, for instance, are responsible for the numerous plant antibodies (phytoagglutinins or lectins) that cross-react with red cells of different animal species, including humans. Antigens that are apparently unrelated but stimulate cross-reacting antibodies (heteroantibodies) are called **heterophile** (heterogenetic) **antigens.** Heteroantibodies may be responsible for false positive antigen-antibody reactions. False negative antigen-antibody reactions may occur because of **zonal reactions.** In all serologic reactions there is an optimal serial dilution of the antiserum to which an optimal amount of antigen is added to give a clearly visible reaction in the shortest possible time. If, however, an excess of antibody or antigen is present, the resulting reactions may be weak or negative. In the first few tubes of a serum dilution the antibody concentration may be too high to give a positive reaction with the antigen of too low a concentration. This phenomenon is called a **prozone reaction.** A great excess of antigen may cause a **postzone reaction.** The first reaction is corrected by further dilution of the antiserum and the latter reaction by dilution of the antigen.

The methods by which antigen-antibody reactions may be detected may be classified under the headings of agglutination, precipitation, immunodiffusion, etc.

Agglutination

Agglutination is the visible clumping or aggregation of insoluble antigen (agglutinogen) when combined with a corresponding antibody (agglutinin). The reaction occurs in two phases. The first phase in which the reactants combine is extremely rapid and is followed by the second phase, the agglutination of the antigen-immunoglobulin complexes, a reaction influenced by such factors as electrolyte concentration, degree of ionization, and temperature. Agglutination can be enhanced by enzyme treatment of the antigen, centrifugation, temperature changes, and the addition of antiglobulin serum (Coombs serum), as in the case of incomplete antibodies (see discussion of blood grouping in Chapter 16). Complete antibodies (IgM) do not require the interaction with Coombs serum.

Soluble antigens may be adsorbed onto particles such as erythrocytes, bentonite, latex, and polystyrene (see discussion of titration of rheumatoid factor and of antistreptolysin O) and are then readily agglutinated by specific immunoglobulins.

Precipitation

Precipitation occurs when a soluble antigen in solution interacts with a specific antibody, a reaction that, like agglutination, occurs in two phases and requires optimal conditions regarding temperature, pH, and ion concentration. The precipitation tests may be performed in test tubes or capillaries in which the antiserum and the antigen are mixed to produce precipitation or flocculation, or the antiserum and antigen may be left unmixed to give rise to a ring at the interface of the two components. The widely used test for C-reactive protein is a precipitation test. Precipitation of antigen-immunoglobulin complexes may not only be studied in a liquid environment but also in gelled media (immunodiffusion) and can be modified for the identification of bacteria and of cellular markers. It also forms the basis of a very sensitive serologic reaction, the passive hemagglutination test.

Immunodiffusion

Systems are available in which precipitation tests are performed in a number of semisolid media, e.g., agar, agarose, polyacrylamide, and starch. Cellulose acetate, a nongel, can also be used as a support medium. Agar, prepared from seaweed, is composed of two polysaccharides, neutral agarose and acid agaropectin, which is responsible for its acid pH. Because of its interference with the migration of charged particles, agar, as a medium for immunodiffusion, is largely replaced by agarose. Agarose is a transparent, colorless neutral gel that allows the formation of sharp, precise precipitation lines, because proteins smaller than the large immune complexes are not retained and are washed off. The precipitated proteins can also be investigated histochemically. Polyacrylamide gel is clear, but the diffusion rate is slow, and starch gel is opaque.

Single diffusion in single- or one-dimensional system[9] (Fig. 35-1):

Principle: The antibody serum is added to a 0.7% agarose solution that has been melted and cooled to 50° C. The mixture is allowed to gel in a test tube and is then overlaid with fluid antigen. The test system is incubated at 37° C for 48 hr or longer. The antigen diffuses into the gel, and if the two reactants are present in proper proportions at the point of slight antigen excess, a stable precipitin band will form. The antigen-antibody may also be mixed on a slide or spot plate or in a capillary tube. An example of the direct precipitation method is the Lancefield grouping of streptococci.

A more accurate procedure is provided by the double diffusion system.

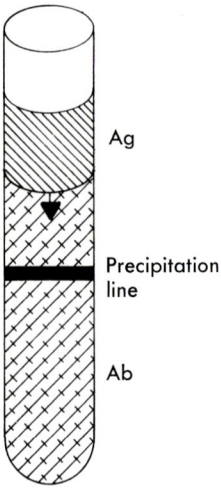

Fig. 35-1. Tube technics for double diffusion in gel without a middle layer of natural gel. *Ag,* antigen; *Ab,* antibody.

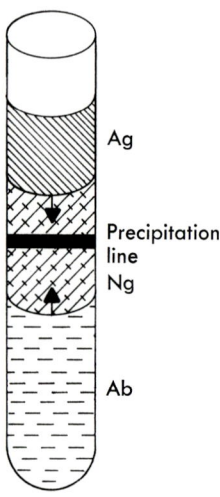

Fig. 35-2. Tube technics for double diffusion in gel with a middle layer of neutral gel. *Ag,* Antigen; *Ng,* netural gel; *Ab,* antibody.

Double diffusion system in single or one dimension (Fig. 35-2): Hayward and Augustin[10] introduced a middle layer of neutral agarose between the upper fluid antigen and the lower antibody gel. The antibody gradient is produced in the middle layer where the precipitation line forms. The one-dimensional methods are of historic interest only, since the two-dimensional systems of immunodiffusion and immunoelectrophoresis are more sensitive.

Double diffusion system in two dimensions[11]:

Principle: A square or round plexiglass dish about 3-9 cm in diameter is filled with 1% agarose 1.5 mm thick, and a suitable well pattern is cut with templates, which obtain reproducible sizes and designs of wells. The precut plates are commercially available (Behring Diagnostics, Somerville, N.J.). Antibody dilutions and specific antigens are placed in adjacent wells, covered to prevent evaporation, and allowed to diffuse into the agar. If the well size, well shape, distance between wells, temperature, and incubation time are optimal, precipitation lines will form at the point of equivalence perpendicular to the axis line between the wells. Their position will reflect the relative concentration of the reactants, so that in conditions of antibody excess they will be located nearer the antigen well.

***Reagents and equipment*:**
1. Immunodiffusion agarose plates (commercially available). If plates are to be prepared in the laboratory see "Preparation of gels," below.
2. Liquid antigen
3. Specific antiserum (commercially available) in 1:20 dilution
4. Known control antiserum dilutions and known antigen controls
   The dilutions of the antiserum vary from 1:1 to 1:640.
5. Micropipets

***Procedure*:** Remove commercial plate from envelope and allow to stand open for about 5 min so that any moisture that may have collected in the wells may evaporate. Number wells on bottom of plate with a permanent marker and on a reference card to identify sera, antigens, and controls.

Fill appropriate wells almost to the brim with 10 μg antigen and with diluted patient's serum and control antisera. (One-millimeter wells accept 1 μl quantities. See "Preparation of gels.") Tightly close plate. Put back in envelope and seal it. Incubate for 18-48 hr or longer at 37° C or for 2-3 days at room temperature.

Examine for precipitation lines and compare unknown with standard antigen, which has reacted with a known concentration of specific antibody in a companion setup. The immune precipitates are visible as white lines in the gel between the antigen well and the corresponding antibody well. The precise location depends on the concentration and rate of diffusion of antigen and antibody.

Preparation of gels:
***Equipment and reagents*:**
1. Glass plates, 80 × 80 mm
2. Horizontal table
3. Gel punch
4. Suction device
5. Phosphate buffer, 0.15M, pH 7.1
   a. Solution 1. Dissolve 26.7 g $Na_2HPO_4 \cdot 2H_2O$ in water to make 1 L.
   b. Solution 2. Dissolve 20.41 g KH_2PO_4 in water to make 1 L.
   Mix together 67 ml of solution 1 and 33 ml of solution 2.

***Procedure*:** Dissolve 4 g agarose in 1 dl buffer and 3 dl water. Heat in water bath to 100° C to dissolve the agar and allow to cool to 60° C. Pour onto glass slide and allow to cool to form a 1.5 mm thick gel. Using a template, cut 3 mm diameter wells into agar (Fig. 35-3). For micromethod cut 1 mm diameter wells and place them 4 mm apart. Using water suction pump, suck out agar plugs.

Discussion of Ouchterlony system: Ouchterlony[11]

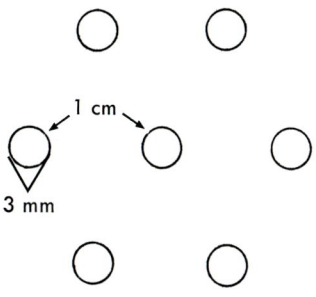

Fig. 35-3. Template for double diffusion.

describes four types of reaction patterns that may occur if two wells containing antigen are placed in opposition to one well containing antiserum. After diffusion two precipitation lines form, and the reaction patterns are the result of the relationships of these two lines to each other.

1. In the reaction of identity (type I) the two lines fuse completely into a single, smooth arc, indicating that the compared antigens are serologically identical and have an antigenic factor in common (Fig. 35-4, *A*).
2. In the reaction of nonidentity (type II) the antigens do not have any determinants in common, and the precipitation lines cross each other (Fig. 35-4, *B*).
3. In reactions of partial identity (type III), where the antigens carry nonidentical but serologically related determinants, a spur may appear in the pattern (Fig. 35-4, *C*).
4. In the type IV reaction the pattern is influenced by the inhibition of one of the reactants, so that the other determinant and its antibody occupy the leading edge during the diffusion (Fig. 35-4, *D*).

In general, the diffusion rate and the location and density of the precipitation line are influenced by the molecular weight and the amount of the reactants.

Single radial immunodiffusion: Radial immunodiffusion is a qualitative as well as a quantitative single diffusion–double dimensional system. The method was described in 1965 by Mancini, Carbonara, and Heremans[12] and modified by Fahey and McKelvey,[13] who reduced the completion time from days (in the Mancini method) to 18-24 hr. The protein is deposited into a well cut into the agar, which contains the specific antibody. Radial diffusion of the antigen produces a ring of precipitate, the diameter (area) of which is proportional to the concentration of the antigen, provided the antibody concentration and the gel thickness are uniform and constant. When the diameter of the ring (d^2) is plotted against the antigen concentration, a straight line results (Fig. 35-5). This is based on the following equation:

$$d^2 = K(Cag) + So$$

where K = constant, Cag = concentration of antigen, and So = intercept (function of antigen well diameter and of antigen volume).

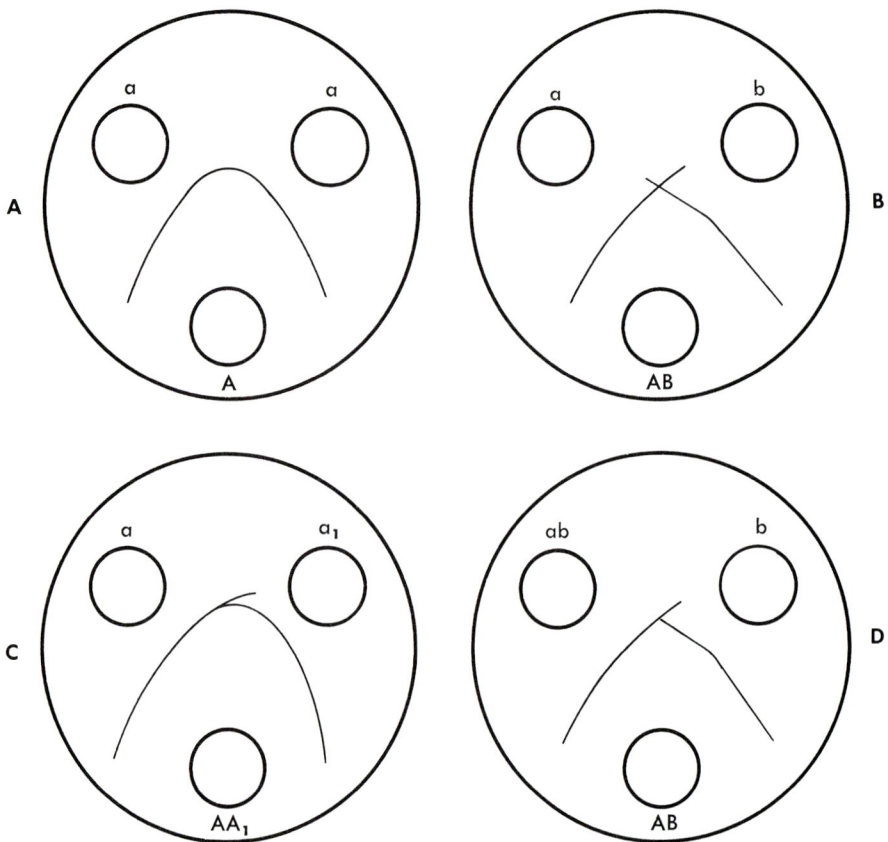

Fig. 35-4. Precipitation pattern of Ouchterlony type of immunodiffusion. **A,** Type I: reaction of identity. The antiserum cannot distinguish one antigen from the other. **B,** Type II: reaction of nonidentity. The two antigens react with different antibodies. **C,** Type III: reaction of partial identity. One antigen cross reacts with the other antigen to which it is serologically related but not identical. **D,** Type IV: reaction of inhibition. The antigens carry unrelated determinants, and the antibody contains separate antibody components.

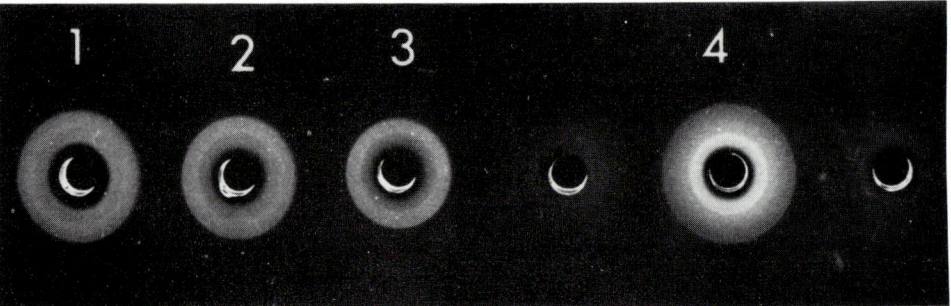

Fig. 35-5. Quantitation of IgG by radial immunodiffusion. Increasing diameters of precipitin rings reflect increasingly larger protein concentrations. *1* to *3,* Known IgG standards; *4,* unknown serum.

Procedure: The procedure is described in detail in Chapter 36.

The method is sensitive to 1.25 µl antigen per milliliter and is extensively used in laboratories to aid in the diagnosis of hypergammaglobulinemias, hypogammaglobulinemias, and complement disorders.

Reversed radial diffusion: If the antigen is incorporated into the gel, the titer of the antibody deposited in the wells can be calculated.

Immunoelectrophoresis

Immunoelectrophoresis successfully overcomes the main drawbacks of ordinary immunodiffusion: the long completion time and the formation of more than one precipitation line. Immunoelectrophoresis has two components: electrophoresis and an antigen-antibody (Ag-Ab) interaction. Electrophoresis separates protein into its constituents according to their different ionic properties. The various components migrate at different rates and exhibit different mobilities in an electric field created in various buffered support media such as agarose, agar, polyacrylamide gels, and cellulose acetate. Electrophoresis is described in detail in Chapter 23. It is based on protein migration, the interaction of the protein with the medium, the pH of the buffer, the voltage, the time the current is applied, and the distance between cathodic and anodic poles. In basic buffer, albumin moves farthest toward the anode, whereas γ-globulin stays closest to the cathode, followed toward the anode by β-, α_2-, and α_1-globulins. Wherever antigen and corresponding antibody meet at the point of equivalence, precipitation lines (Ag-Ab complexes) form. Like immunodiffusion tests, immunoelectrophoretic procedures are divided into one- or two-dimensional, single- or double-diffusion methods. The one-dimensional method with a single-component diffusion is known as the rocket immunoelectrophoresis method of Laurell.[14] The two-dimensional method is referred to as a crossed electrophoresis,[15] and the one-dimensional, double-diffusion method is known as counterimmunoelectrophoresis.

Rocket immunoelectrophoresis: Rocket immunoelectrophoresis (or electroimmunodiffusion) of Laurell[14] is similar to the radial immunodiffusion with the added features of electrophoresis.[16,17]

Principle: The antiserum is incorporated into a thin layer of agarose, the pH of which is adjusted to 8.6 by means of a veronal buffer. The antigen specific for the antiserum is placed into small wells along one edge of the antibody-containing gel (see Fig. 11-18). When an electric potential is applied, the protein migrates into the antibody-containing gel and antigen-antibody complexes form, which give rise to visual precipitates at the point of equivalence. Since the concentration gradient of the antigen diminishes as the distance from the starting line increases, the antigen-antibody precipitate dissolves and reprecipitates until there is no further migration of the sample with the highest antigen concentration. At the completion of the run, the length of the cone-shaped precipitate is directly proportional to the concentration of the antigen. On the basis of the distances traveled by a series of antigen solutions of known concentrations, a standard curve can be constructed, which allows the determination of the concentration of the antigen in an unknown sample (see Fig. 11-19).

Equipment and reagents:
1. Electrophoresis apparatus that can be cooled, power supply (10-12 V/cm in gel) and wicks
2. Agarose (SeaKem, MCI Biomedical, Rockland, Me).
3. Gel punch
4. Suction device
5. Template (see Fig. 11-18)
6. Barbital buffer, 0.2M, pH 8.6 (4.12 g sodium barbital and 0.8 g barbital; water to 100 ml)
7. Saline, 0.9%
8. Amido black stain
   Dissolve 6 g amido black in 405 ml water. Add 405 ml methanol and 90 ml glacial acetic acid, and strain through glass wool.
9. Destaining solution
   Combine 405 ml methanol, 405 ml water, and 90 ml glacial acetic acid.
10. Plastic film, Cronar clear base 0.004 in. thick, Dupont Graphic Arts film, or glass plates
11. Antiserum (Behring Diagnostics, Sommerville, N.J.)
12. Controls (e.g., Verify, General Diagnostics, Morris Plains, N.J.), undiluted and diluted 1:2 and 1:4 in 0.2M barbital buffer

Procedure: The method described is for factor VIII–associated antigen (see also discussion of electroimmunodiffusion in Chapters 11 and 36).

Prepare 20 ml of 1% agarose in 0.02M barbital (pH 8.6). Bring to boil with stirring to dissolve agarose (use automatic stirrer). Allow to cool to 56° C. Add antiserum to achieve 0.4% concentration (80 µl Behring antiserum added to 20 ml agarose). Mix well and pour onto clean plastic film placed on level stand to ensure uniform thickness of agarose gel. Allow to solidify. Keep in moisture chamber until used (not more than 2 hr).

Cut 3 mm wells (see Fig. 13-15). Use 10 µl Oxford pipet to put exactly 10 µl of each standard sample or patient sera (undiluted) into wells (wells should not be filled to top). Place slide in Brinkmann electrophoresis chamber with 400 ml of 0.02M barbital buffer (pH 8.6) in each buffer chamber. Place filter paper wicks on gel about 5 cm apart and cover chamber.

Perform electrophoresis for 16 hr at 1 V/cm across gel (actually, ends of wicks). After electrophoresis place film in saline for 24 hr. Dry film by compression between filter papers (903 grade; Schleicher & Schuell, Keene, N.H.). Stain with amido black and destain with 7% acetic acid.

Measure peak heights in millimeters and plot curve on logarithmic paper, using Verify as 100%, 50%, and 25% controls. Determine patient values from above and report as % Verify (100%) (see Fig. 13-19).

Results: A typical result is shown in Fig. 13-20. If immunoglobulins are quantitated by this method, the whole serum must first be carbamylated by a procedure described by Weeke.[18]

Immunoelectrophoresis: Immunoelectrophoresis[19] is a combination of zone electrophoretic separation of protein solutions in a gel and double-gel diffusion, so that the antigens in a mixture are separated by two methods. In the first phase the mixture to be analyzed is deposited in a circular well cut into a buffered gel film and is electrophoretically separated into its components along one axis of the agarose support medium. In the second phase these fractions act as antigens and interact with the corresponding antibodies deposited in an antibody trough (see Chapter 36). Diffusion of both the antigen and the antibodies toward each other results in antigen-antibody (Ag-Ab) complexes rendered visible by precipitation lines, each of which represents one specific serologically pure antigen fraction. The antibody diffuses as a uniform band parallel to the antibody trough, and the antigen diffuses in a circle if the protein is homogeneous (e.g., albumin) and in an ellipse if the protein is heterogeneous (e.g., globulins). The Ag-Ab precipitation line of the first albumin forms a markedly curved segment (arc) of a circle, whereas the precipitation line of the latter forms a slightly curved segment of an ellipse.

Procedure: The procedure is presented in detail in Chapter 36.

Interpretation: The shape and position of the precipitation bands of the unknown are compared with the bands produced by normal controls. Shape, density, and location of the bands are critically evaluated, and any deviation from the normal pattern is usually pathologic.

Two-dimensional immunoelectrophoresis (crossed immunoelectrophoresis): Two-dimensional immunoelectrophoresis is a combination of gel electrophoresis and immunoelectrophoresis, which results in a markedly increased power of resolution compared to the one-dimensional immunoelectrophoresis. The method utilizes zone electrophoresis in one direction, followed by electrophoresis in a second direction at right angles to the first into a gel containing antiserum.[20]

Microtechnic:

Equipment and reagents: Same as for rocket immunoelectrophoresis.

Procedure: Cover 50 × 75 mm glass slide with 1 mm thick gel of 1% agarose in Veronal immunoelectrophoresis buffer, pH 8.6 (Bioware, Wichita, Kan.). Cut a well 1.5 cm from cathodic end and 1 cm from edge of plate; fill with antigen.

Electrophorese in the first direction for 60 min at 10 V/cm at 4° C. Cut the gel 1 cm from the origin well with a razor blade and remove the excess agarose, which is replaced with antibody-containing gel.[21] Antiserum can also be added by diffusion into the gel surface by overlaying it with an antibody-charged gel slide[22] (see Fig. 11-21). A 1 cm strip of clear gel may be interpolated between the first and second electrophoresis gels.

Second-dimensional electrophoresis is carried out for 3 hr at 5-10 V/cm or overnight at 1-2 V/cm. View by darkfield lighting, or wash, dry, and stain. Precipitation peaks are outlined by converging precipitation lines indicative of Ag-Ab complexes (see Fig. 11-22).

Discussion: Crossed immunoelectrophoresis may be used for identification of complex antigens and antibodies.[23] A 50:50 mixture of carbamylated transferrin and

serum can be incorporated as an internal standard. A semiautomated method is described by Versey, Slater, and Hobbs.[24]

Counterimmunoelectrophoresis (immunoelectro-osmophoresis): The rapidity and sensitivity of counterimmunoelectrophoresis is responsible for its widespread use as a diagnostic tool in the serology, virology, bacteriology, and mycology laboratories.[25] This qualitative method can be used to identify antigens as well as antibodies. Liquid antigen and corresponding antibody (or antibody and corresponding liquid antigen) are deposited into wells cut into alkaline-buffered agarose gel, which is inserted into an electrophoresis chamber. When the electric circuit is switched on, the two reactants move toward each other, and where they meet a precipitation line forms. The antigen is deposited in the cathodic well, because at a pH of 8.2 antigens have a negative ionic charge and move toward the anode. The antibodies carry a slight positive charge at a gel pH of 8.2 and move toward the cathode. Numerous substances qualify as negatively charged antigens, e.g., bacterial polysaccharides, nucleoproteins, glycoproteins, and viruses. The anodic migration of many antigens can be improved by acetylation and carbamylation. The technical ease of the method belies the effort that is required to optimize the system. The antigen and antibody must be in exact proportions, so that the Ag-Ab precipitation lines that may form are not quickly dissolved. The pH must be alkaline, so that the antigens move toward the anode, and the agar itself must be near a neutral pH.

Equipment and reagents: Same as for immunoelectrophoresis.

Procedure[26]: Prepare 30 ml of 1% agarose in barbital buffer, pH 8.2, 0.05M. Use 0.3 g agarose in 30 ml buffer. Cover a Mylar sheet or glass slide with a 1 mm thick layer of agarose by using a 10 ml pipet, and allow agarose to gel. Cut 2-4 mm wells according to pattern (Fig. 35-6). They should be 5-10 mm apart. Remove the agar plugs with pipets attached to water vacuum pump.

Using a micropipet fill the wells with antigen and

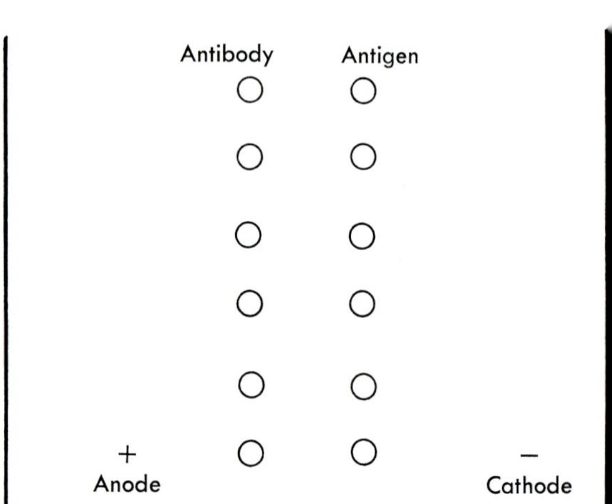

Fig. 35-6. Template for counterimmunoelectrophoresis.

antibody. Fill the electrophoresis trough with barbital buffer and adjust the wicks. Place the sheet or plate into the chamber, so that the antigen is on the cathodic side. Electrophorese at 100-130 V for 30 min.

Examine the gel for precipitation lines under a bright light. If no lines are visible, incubate the gel in the refrigerator for 30 min and reexamine. If it is still negative, stain the slide.

Complement-fixation tests

The complement-fixation (CF) tests make use of two properties of complement:
1. Complement is bound or fixed in antigen-antibody (Ag-Ab) reactions; thus free complement is removed from the test system.
2. Complement is required to hemolyze sensitized red cells.

The CF test consists of two Ag-Ab reactions: the nonhemolytic test system and the hemolytic indicator system. The first reaction is composed of the antigen and its corresponding (or probably corresponding) antibody, and the latter reaction consists of red cells and a lytic homologous antierythrocytic antibody (hemolysin). Complement takes part in both reactions. It is bound or fixed in the nonhemolytic test phase, the Ag-Ab reaction (hence the name of the test), which removes the complement from the system, so that it is unavailable to take part in the hemolytic indicator system. If complement is not fixed in the first phase, it is free to react in the hemolytic system to lyse the red cells sensitized by their homologous hemolysin. The test result is based on the extent of the hemolysis. The presence of hemolysis indicates that complement is not utilized in the test system in which no Ag-Ab reaction has taken place, and the test is therefore reported as negative. Absence of hemolysis indicates that the complement has been involved in the Ag-Ab reaction of the test system and is thus not available for the hemolytic system. The test is therefore reported as positive.

The CF test is more sensitive than the agglutination and precipitation tests described above but less sensitive than radioimmunoassay, immunofluorescence, or enzyme-linked immunosorbent assays.[3] The CF test is the preferred method for the serologic diagnosis of infections by *Mycoplasma pneumoniae, Blastomyces, Histoplasma, Coccidioides,* and most viruses.[3] The test, although straightforward in concept, in practice is delicate and difficult to perform, because almost all reagents must be titrated before use, and four controls must be run with each test. The reagents to be titrated are the sheep red cell suspension of the indicator system, the hemolysin to determine the dilution of the an-

tibody that causes 50% hemolysis (CH_{50}), the guinea pig complement to determine the CH_{50} value, and finally the antigen to obtain equivalence of antigen and antibody in the test system. The controls are used to detect anticomplementary factors, nonspecific hemolysis, red cell autolysis, strength of complement, and positive and negative reactions.

If the microtiter method is used, lysis of the sensitized sheep red cells is best measured by ^{51}Cr release from chromium-labeled cells, although spectrophotometric measurements may also be used (413 nm). The microtiter method is described in the references.[27-30]

Fluorescent antibody test

The fluorescent antibody (FA) technic represents a very successful attempt to demonstrate antigen-antibody (Ag-Ab) reactions at a microscopic level. It involves labeling of the antibody by fluorescein isothiocyanate (FITC), a fluorescent compound that has affinity for proteins.[31] When FITC is added to an antibody, a complex (**conjugate**) results that is able to react with the antigen to which the antibody was made.[32] Fluorescent conjugates are utilized in two basic methods. In the direct technic (Fig. 35-7, *A*) a conjugated antibody is used to detect the presence of the homologous antigen in tissue sections, in microorganisms, or in smears.[33] The indirect method (Fig. 35-7, *B*) is based on the fact that antibodies (immunoglobulins) not only react with the homologous antigens but also act as antigens in their own right and react with anti-immunoglobulins. This method is more economical and sensitive than the direct method and is used extensively in microbiology.

Direct method:
Equipment and reagents:
1. Diluted conjugate (commercially available)
2. Glycerol containing 10% phosphate buffered saline (PBS)
3. PBS
4. Magnetic stirrer
5. Fluorescent microscope

Procedure: Apply conjugate in 1:10 or 1:20 dilutions, and incubate in moist atmosphere at room temperature for 30 min. Wash off conjugate and place preparation on a carrier in a PBS bath agitated by a stirrer. Drain off fluid, mount in glycerol, and apply coverslip. Examine under fluorescent light.

Indirect method:
Equipment and reagents:
1. Dilutions of anti-immunoglobulin conjugate
2. Others as for direct method

Procedure: Apply 1:10 diluted antiserum to the

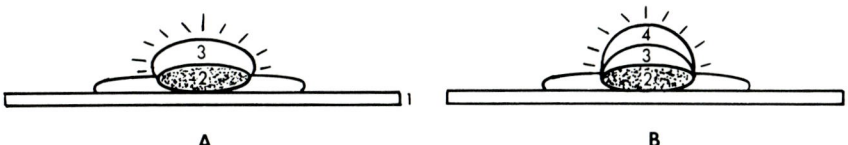

A	B

Fig. 35-7. Principles of direct and indirect FA technics. **A,** Direct fluorescent technic. **B,** Indirect fluorescent technic. *1,* Microslide; *2,* cell (cytoplasm and nucleus); *3,* antiserum, conjugated in **A** and unconjugated in **B**; *4,* conjugated antiglobulin serum.

preparation. Incubate at room temperature in a moist atmosphere for 30 min. Rinse with PBS and wash as for direct method for 10 min. Apply diluted conjugated anti-immunoglobulin. Incubate in a moist atmosphere for 30 min. Again rinse with PBS and wash as for direct method for 10 min. Blot, apply glycerol, and apply coverslip. Examine under fluorescent light.

Hemagglutination and hemagglutination inhibition tests

Hemagglutination and hemagglutination inhibition tests are used to detect antibodies to certain viruses and microorganisms. Their development is based on advances in the preservation of red cells[29,34] which may be stabilized by treatment with a number of chemicals, either alone or in sequence to render them resistant to lysis, to preserve their membrane integrity and surface adsorptive properties, and to extend their life span. Treatment of red cells with tannic acid and/or glutaraldehyde preserves the cells, improves the attachment of antigen and antibody, and transforms them into a sensitive agglutination test vehicle.[35] Microhemagglutination tests are now available for the diagnosis of syphilis, rubella, and toxoplasmosis. Soluble antigens attached to a carrier, such as red cells (or latex particles), are agglutinated if exposed to the appropriate antibody under controlled conditions. Inhibition of this reaction is often used to demonstrate the presence of an antigen in solution.[36] The diluted antibody is allowed to interact with the homologous antigen in solution for about 30 min. After incubation appropriate test cells are added to determine whether the antibody has been utilized or not. Absence of agglutination indicates an antigen-antibody reaction.

Summary of procedure of hemagglutination test[37]: Deposit serial twofold antibody dilutions in bovalbumin borate saline (BABS) in a microtiter plate. Add suspension of antigen-coated red cells. Seal plate with tape and mix. Incubate at 4° C for 1½-12 hr. Read agglutination with microtiter mirror as 1+ to 4+.

Summary of procedure of hemagglutination inhibition test: Deposit serial twofold dilutions of antibody containing serum in bovalbumin borate saline (BABS). Add antigen to diluted specimen. Incubate at room temperature for 1 hr. Add red cell suspension. Seal plate and mix. Incubate overnight at 4° C. Read test as for hemagglutination test.

Radioimmunoassays

Radioimmunoassay (RIA) is one of the most widely used technics in biology, physiology, and medicine. It is based on competition of a known excess amount of radiolabeled antigen (or hapten) and an unknown variable amount of the same antigen but unlabeled for binding sites of a constant amount of antibody.[38] Barrett[1] offers the following mathematical explanation of the reaction. One hundred molecules of IgG will bind 200 molecules of antigen, since each IgG molecule has two binding sites. If a mixture of 200 molecules of radiolabeled antigen and 200 molecules of unlabeled antigen is incubated with 100 molecules of IgG, half of the radiolabeled antigen will be displaced from the antibody, creating a bound/free ratio of 1:1. It can therefore be assumed that a 50% reduction in binding of the radiolabeled antigen occurs if the concentration of the unknown sample is exactly the same as that of the known radiolabeled sample. Other bound/free ratios of antigen can be used to determine other concentrations of the unknown antigen. The higher the initial concentration of unlabeled antigen, the lower will be the concentration of labeled antigen in the antigen-antibody complex at equilibrium.[39]

The critical step in RIA is the separation of the bound from the free portions of the labeled antigen. Numerous such methods are available. The most frequently used procedure is the **solid-phase RIA** in which the antibody to the substance being assayed is bound to polystyrene tubes. The coupled antibody is still able to interact with the antigen, and after equilibrium is reached centrifugation separates the bound from the free antigen.

The main advantage of the RIA method lies in its exquisite sensitivity and its ability to detect trace amounts of antigen (hapten). RIA is used extensively in hormone and peptide assays.

Enzyme immunoassay

The success of RIA methods is somewhat dampened by the intrinsic hazard and instability of the isotopes and by the deluge of governmental regulations that control their manufacture and use. The search for nonisotopic labels has produced the enzyme immunoassay (EIA), which shares with RIA the specificity, sensitivity, and rapidity and has the advantage of safety.[1]

The enzyme-labeled antibody (conjugate) is used to assay a variety of antigens. The enzyme with its substrate is instrumental in indicating the presence and quantity of antigen and in some tissue systems even its location.[40,41] The most commonly used enzymes are alkaline phosphatase[40,41] from *Escherichia coli* and horseradish peroxidase. The enzymes must fulfill a number of criteria: They must be stable, highly specific, absent from the antigen or antibody, and not affected by inhibitors within the system.[1] The enzyme activity is measured spectrophotometrically after the addition of the specific chromogenic substrate. Alkaline phosphatase cleaves its substrate, *p*-nitrophenylphosphate, leading to a color change, and peroxidase changes the color of *o*-dianisidine.

A number of variations of EIA have been developed[1]:

1. In the enzyme-linked immunosorbent assay (ELISA) the antigen or antibody is attached to a solid-phase support, the other immune reactant is linked to an enzyme, and the displaced enzyme label is quantitated.[38,42]

2. In the immunoenzymometric assay an unknown quantity of antigen is reacted with an excess of labeled antibody, and then the solid phase is added.[43]

3. The sandwich technic[44] requires that the antigen bind simultaneously with two molecules of antibody. The first antibody is a solid-phase reactant, whereas the second antibody is enzyme labeled and combines with the available determinants on the antigen.

4. The enzyme multiplied immunoassay technic (EMIT)[45] utilizes the ability of an antibody to directly inhibit enzyme activity when a homologous antigen is conjugated to the enzyme. Unlabeled antigen in the sample diminishes the degree of antibody binding to the enzyme-antigen and produces an increase in enzymatic activity.[46]

Laser nephelometry

Nephelometry measures the amount of light scattered or deflected from its path by macromolecules in solution. The technic utilizes an incidental light beam that passes through a test solution in a given direction. In dilute solution antigens and antibodies form complexes that scatter light. If the amount of antibody is kept constant, the number of complexes varies in direct proportion to the antigen concentration. The amount of scattered light of an unknown sample can therefore be compared with the amount of light scattered by dilutions of a reference serum of known antigen concentration, and the antigen concentration present in the unknown sample can then be determined. The use of polyethylene glycol (PEG)[47] enhances and stabilizes the precipitates, thus increasing the speed and sensitivity of the technic by controlling the particle size for optimal light angle deflection.[48] The method can be used to measure C3, C4, IgG, IgA, and IgM.

SEROLOGIC TESTS FOR SYPHILIS (STS)
General considerations

The causative organism of syphilis is *Treponema pallidum,* which naturally infects only humans and requires intimate contact for its transmission. After direct contact with an individual with a lesion containing *T. pallidum,* the organism is capable of penetrating small cutaneous breaks and intact mucous membranes. About 3 weeks after exposure, at the inoculation site there appears a usually solitary, firm, inflammatory, ulcerated lesion, the primary chancre, which is associated with enlarged regional lymph nodes. The chancre disappears spontaneously in 2-4 weeks, and, if untreated, weeks to months later it is followed by secondary syphilitic lesions, e.g., sore throat, skin rash, fever, and lymphadenopathy. In moist intertriginous areas, highly infectious condylomata may appear. The lesions of secondary syphilis also disappear spontaneously, and after years of a dormant existence the infection may be responsible for the neurologic and vascular manifestations of tertiary syphilis.

Congenital syphilis is the result of transplacental transmission of the treponemes to the fetus, who, if the mother is untreated, in 50% of cases is stillborn usually after the fourth month of pregnancy. Prenatal care of mothers and treatment with penicillin has almost eradicated congenital syphilis.[49]

The diagnosis of syphilis is based on the demonstration of the etiologic spirochete by darkfield microscopy and on the serologic demonstration of a number of antibodies. The first procedure utilizes the spirochete-rich serum and exudate expressed from the primary chancre, from the condylomata of the second stage, or from the parenchymatous organs of the stillborn child with congenital syphilis. The second method is based on the

appearance of a variety of antibodies in the patient's serum following the primary inoculation and is of major diagnostic significance in the long period of time that follows the primary infection, when the causative organism cannot be demonstrated any more in the syphilitic patient.

About 10 days after the development of the chancre a state of progressive antibody-based immunity develops, which peaks during the secondary phase and gradually diminishes in the course of the tertiary phase. The antibodies are qualitatively and quantitatively assayed by serologic methods, which are divided into two major groups based on the source of the antigen: (1) the nontreponemal tests, which employ crude lipoidal or cardiolipin-lecithin antigens, and (2) the treponemal tests, which employ *T. pallidum* (a Nichols' strain) as the antigen in either the viable, killed, or extracted forms.

Nontreponemal tests

Nontreponemal tests are also designated as **serologic tests for syphilis (STS).** In response to the tissue invasion by *T. pallidum,* an antibody complex, originally called **reagin,** appears in the serum of the syphilitic patient about 1-3 weeks after the primary chancre. Reagin combines with colloidal suspensions of lipoidal animal tissue extracts, which contain an antigen that is normally present in liver and many other mammalian tissues. It is isolated from beef heart muscle and given the name **cardiolipin.** Chemically it is diphosphatidyl glycerol. It is likely that the cardiolipin originates from the tissues in which the spirochetes grow and acting as hapten is incorporated into the spirochetes. In this combination it is immunogenic. To provide a multivalent hapten, cardiolipin is adsorbed onto cholesterol in the presence of lecithin. The reagin (antibody) clumps the antigen into visible floccules, a reaction that fixes complement.

There are two types of nontreponemal tests for syphilis, the complement-fixation test and the flocculation test. An example of the first procedure is the Wassermann reaction, which is of historic interest only. A multiplicity of flocculation tests has been described, but only three are still in vogue: the **VDRL** (Venereal Disease Research Laboratory) flocculation test, the **RPR** (rapid reagin test), and the **ART** (automated reagin test). They all use various cardiolipin-lecithin mixtures as antigens, which have some advantages over previously used crude lipoidal antigens, e.g., better standardization, reproducibility, and sensitivity.

Interpretation of serologic tests for syphilis

False positive reactions: Reagin is found in some patients who are not infected with treponemes. Of all positive serologic tests for syphilis (STS), 10-30% may be false positive. The concept that the genesis of reagin is related to the necrotizing effect of spirochetes on tissues[50] helps to explain some but not all biologic false positive (BFP) reactions. Acute BFP reactions occur in infectious diseases and revert to normal in about 6 months. They are found in 2-5% of patients with pneumococcal pneumonia, in 10% of patients with infectious hepatitis, in 90% of patients with malaria, and in 20% of patients who have infectious mononucleosis.

Chronic BFP reaction is often associated with autoimmune diseases, a finding that is not surprising, because reagin is an autoantibody. BFP reactions are encountered in 10-20% of patients with systemic lupus erythematosus, in 5-10% of patients with rheumatic fever, and in aging individuals. Other false positive reactions may result from diseases related to syphilis (yaws, pinta) or from technical errors.[51]

False negative reactions: False negative reactions occur in patients who have syphilis but in whom the reagin concentration is too low to give a reactive (positive) test. These seronegative patients may give a positive reaction with more sensitive treponemal tests such as the fluorescent treponemal antibody–absorption test (FTA-ABS). In addition to low antibody titers and insensitive test procedures, false negative test results may be caused by inhibitors in the patient's serum or by a prozone reaction.[51]

Indications for nontreponemal tests

Despite the existence of false positive and false negative test results, the nontreponemal tests are good screening procedures for syphilis, since they are usually reactive in the face of active disease, and they lend themselves to quantitation (titration), so that their rise in response to the acute disease and their fall in response to therapy may be observed.

Different tests use different proportions of cardiolipin, lecithin, and cholesterol and different volumes. The RPR test uses an antigen similar to that employed in the VDRL test, but it incorporates cholin, so that it can be used with untreated plasma, and it incorporates charcoal to aid in visualization.

Treponemal tests

In an attempt to avoid BFP reactions, tests have been devised that utilize specific antigens derived from treponemes. The treponemal tests are much more sensitive and specific for syphilis than are the nontreponemal tests. The treponemal tests include the Reiter protein complement-fixation test, the *Treponema pallidum* immobilization test, the fluorescent treponemal antibody–absorption test, the fluorescent treponemal antibody test, and the microhemagglutination assay for antibodies to *Treponema pallidum*.

Reiter protein complement-fixation test

The antigen is derived from cultured nonpathogenic Reiter treponemes. The procedure is not in use anymore because of poor specificity and sensitivity.[52]

Treponema pallidum immobilization test

The *Treponema pallidum* immobilization test (TPI) is a complement-dependent assay of the *Treponema*-immobilizing and treponemacidal properties of the antibodies in the serum of syphilitic patients. These antibodies are specific and not involved with reagin, which is removed from the serum by absorption. The antigen is the virulent Nichols' strain of *T. pallidum* grown in rabbits.[53] The theoretic excellence of the TPI is counterbalanced by a number of weaknesses, e.g., the virulent antigen, technical difficulties, and the relative lack of reproducibility. The test is performed in only a

few laboratories at the present time and is not available at the Centers for Disease Control.[54] It is surpassed in sensitivity by two tests, the **fluorescent treponemal antibody–absorption test (FTA-ABS)** and the *Treponema pallidum* **hemagglutination test (TPHA).**

Fluorescent treponemal antibody–absorption test and fluorescent treponemal antibody test

The fluorescent treponemal antibody–absorption test (FTA-ABS) is an outgrowth of the **fluorescent treponemal antibody** (FTA) test, which it exceeds in sensitivity. Both tests use the Nichols' strain of *T. pallidum* dried on a slide. In the FTA test the antibody (patient's serum) is diluted 1:5 and the antigen-antibody reaction is visualized by immunofluorescence by using a fluorochrome-labeled antihuman immunoglobulin. To increase the specificity of the test procedure, Hunter, Deacon, and Meyer[55] introduced an absorption-dilution step and created the FTA-ABS test. The FTA-ABS test is the most sensitive serologic procedure in primary syphilis (82%) compared to the VDRL test (73%), the TPI test (67%), and the microhemagglutination assay.[56] The antigen is the same as used in the FTA test, but the antibody (patient's serum) is adsorbed with ultrasonically disrupted Reiter treponemes or with a filtrate of heated Reiter treponeme cultures to remove group-specific antibodies. The false positive rate is very low and largely associated with autoimmune diseases,[57] e.g., systemic lupus erythematosus.[58] The Centers for Disease Control recommends the FTA-ABS test as a confirmatory procedure for syphilis and discourages its use as a screening test. Screening should be performed with reagin tests such as the VDRL.

False positive FTA-ABS tests occur in about 2% of patients who either suffer from other treponematoses such as pinta, yaws, or bejel or who have high titers of antinuclear antibodies (ANA) or rheumatoid factor (RF).[59] There is evidence that pregnant women occasionally have false positive FTA-ABS tests.[60] The FTA-ABS test is not readily quantitated, and neither the FTA-ABS nor the TPI can be performed in sufficient volume to be used as routine tests.

Microhemagglutination assay for antibodies to Treponema pallidum

In the microhemagglutination assay for antibodies to *Treponema pallidum* (TPMHA),[61,62] the antigen is derived from Nichols' strain of *T. pallidum* and is adsorbed onto red cells. The antibody is devoid of the group-specific component, which is removed by sorbent, an autoclaved extract of a culture of the Reiter strain, which is used as serum diluent. The TPMHA has some advantages over the other tests described, because it can be quantitated and automated and shares with the other treponemal tests the specificity and sensitivity. Its disadvantage is the fact that it is least sensitive in primary syphilis (Table 35-2).

Serology in congenital syphilis

An infant born with the stigmata of syphilis presents no diagnostic problem, but a normal appearing infant with a reactive STS poses the question whether the reactive test is caused by the passive transfer of maternal

Table 35-2. Comparison of TPHA and FTA-ABS reactivity in various stages of syphilis

Stage	TPHA positive	FTA-ABS positive
Primary syphilis		
Average	70%	90%
Range	50-92%	82-100%
Secondary syphilis		
Average	98%	100%
Range	97-100%	99-100%
Latent and late syphilis		
Average	96%	97%
Range	95-97%	96-100%

From Robertson, R.G., and Walsh, W.T.: In Friedman, H., Linna, T.J., and Prier, J.E., editors: Immunoserology in the diagnosis of infectious diseases, Baltimore, 1979, University Park Press. © 1979 University Park Press, Baltimore.

Table 35-3. Reactivity of VDRL, FTA-ABS, and TPI tests during various stages of syphilis

Category	No. tested	Percent reactive		
		FTA-ABS test	TPI test	VDRL test
Primary syphilis	191	85	56	78
Secondary syphilis	270	99	94	97
Late syphilis	117	95	92	77
Latent syphilis	954	95	94	74
Presumably normal	384	1	0	0

Reprinted by permission of the New England Journal of Medicine (**284:**642, 1971).

antibodies or by an active infection. If the antibody is passively transferred, its titer does not exceed the maternal titer, it will decline rapidly in 2-3 months, and it is an IgG, since only the latter crosses the placenta.[63] The presence of IgM in the cord, fetal, or infant blood correlates well with active syphilitic infection,[64] but since IgM is elevated in many other infectious diseases[64] the FTA-ABS test has been modified to use fluorescein-labeled antihuman IgM to detect specific antitreponemal IgM antibodies, which cannot cross the placenta and are therefore interpreted as evidence of congenital syphilis.[65,66] The modified test is called the IgM–FTA-ABS test.

Serology in neurosyphilis

Serum antibodies do not usually penetrate the blood-brain barrier; thus the presence of treponemal and nontreponemal antibodies in the cerebrospinal fluid (CSF) usually indicates central nervous system (CNS) syphilis. The VDRL test on CSF lacks sensitivity,[67,68] but false positive reactions are rare. The FTA-ABS test is too sensitive to be reliable; thus the Centers for Disease Control has warned against its use on CSF.[69]

Technics of serodiagnosis of syphilis
Procedure of VDRL slide test[70]

Principle: The patient's serum is mixed on a mechanical rotator with a buffered saline suspension of cardiolipin-lecithin-cholesterol antigen and examined microscopically for degrees of flocculation. Reactive sera are serially diluted and titrated.

Preparation of control sera:
Equipment and reagents:
1. Seitz filter
2. Deep freeze
3. Water bath, 56° C and 37° C
4. Erlenmeyer flask
5. Mechanical rotator
6. Vacutainers (BBL, BioQuest Div., Becton-Dickinson & Co., Cockeysville, Md.)
7. Antigen (commercially available, e.g., BBL)
8. Reactive and nonreactive sera

Control sera for nontreponemal antigen tests: Control sera of graded reactivity should be included each time serologic testing is performed. For the VDRL slide test with serum and spinal fluid the antigen suspension to be used each day is first examined with control sera of graded reactivity.

Collection and processing of sera:
1. Collect clear sera (free of hemolysis and lipemia) giving reactive (not weakly reactive) reactions in daily test runs in Pyrex bottles. Store in deep freezer for 60 days, in freezing compartment of the refrigerator for 30 days, or in liquid state in the refrigerator for 7-10 days.
2. Collect nonreactive sera in a similar manner.

3. When control sera are to be prepared, allow them to thaw at room temperature or in a 37° C water bath. Mix thoroughly.
4. Filter serum pools through Seitz filter, measure volume of each pool, and add 1 mg thimerosal (Merthiolate [Eli Lilly & Co., Indianapolis]) powder for each milliliter of serum.

Pretesting of serum dilutions:
1. Prepare preliminary dilutions of reactive serum in nonreactive serum according to Table 35-4 or use serial twofold dilutions (see p. 1026). Mix thoroughly.
2. Select for control sera a dilution that is 4+ reactive and one or more dilutions that show intermediate reactivity, e.g., as control no. 1 choose dilution 4 (Table 35-4), as control no. 2 choose dilution 6, and as control no. 3 choose dilution 10. Mix all dilutions thoroughly.
3. Heat serum dilutions for 30 min at 56° C.
4. Perform test on these serum dilutions with the antigen suspensions that reproduce reactivity patterns of standard control sera. Record results.
5. Select one dilution that is a clear-cut reactive dilution and at least one dilution that shows intermediate reactivity.
6. Calculate the amount of each serum dilution to be prepared. This will be determined by the quantity needed for each day's testing, the period of time during which the controls will be used, and the type of storage facility available. Control sera, properly stoppered, may be stored for 2-3 months in a freezer and for 1 month in the freezing compartment of a refrigerator.
7. Prepare the calculated volumes of each serum dilution and mix thoroughly by placing serum pool in wide-diameter bottle (Erlenmeyer flask) having a capacity three to five times the pool volume. Rotate the flask on the mechanical slide rotator for 30-60 min at about 100 rpm, or mix with a magnetic stirrer. Avoid foaming.
8. Test a sample of each serum mixture and if necessary adjust pools to higher or lower reactivity by the addition of small quantities of reactive or nonreactive sera. Mix well and retest.
9. Dispense aliquots of each dilution sufficient for one testing period into properly labeled tubes and

stopper lightly with paraffin-coated corks (small Vacutainers). Arrange in sets and store in freezer. After 24 hr reset the corks and return to freezer.

Establishing patterns of reactivity:
1. Remove one set of controls from storage, thaw at room temperature, and mix thoroughly.
2. New lots of control sera should be tested in parallel with the one currently in use. The pattern of reactivity is established by repeated testings with several antigen emulsions before being placed into routine use.

VDRL qualitative slide test with serum[71]

Equipment and glassware:
1. Rotating machine, adjustable to 180 rpm, circumscribing a circle $^3/_4$ in. in diameter on a horizontal plane
2. Slide holder for 2 × 3 in. microscope slides
3. Hypodermic needles, without bevels, 18-, 19-, and 23-gauge
4. Slides, 2 × 3 in., with 12 ceramic rings,* approximately 14 mm in diameter (When tests are performed in a dry climate, the slides may be covered with a box lid containing a moistened blotter during rotation to prevent evaporation.)
5. Syringe, Luer type, 1 or 2 ml
6. Bottles (Corning Glass Works, Corning, N.Y.) 30 ml, round, glass stoppered, with narrow mouth, approximately 35 mm in diameter, with flat inner-bottom surfaces (NOTE: Some of the bottles now available are unsatisfactory for preparing antigen suspension because of the convex inner-bottom surface that causes saline to be distributed only at periphery.)

Reagents:
1. VDRL antigen†
   a. The antigen is a colorless, alcoholic solution

---

*Rings must be high enough to prevent spillage when slides are rotated at prescribed speed. Slides must be cleaned, so that serum will spread to inner surfaces of ceramic rings. This type of slide should be discarded if or when ceramic rings begin to flake off.

†Available from BBL, Division of BioQuest, Becton-Dickinson & Co., Cockeysville, Md.; Difco Laboratories, Detroit; Hyland Laboratories, Costa Mesa, Calif.; Lederle Laboratories, Pearl River, N.Y.; The Sylvana Co., Millburn, N.J.; and Texas Biological Laboratories, Fort Worth, Tex.

Table 35-4. Results obtained with serum dilutions prepared for use as daily controls

Dilution no.	Reactive serum (ml)	Nonreactive serum (ml)	VDRL slide test*	RPR card test*
1	1.0	1.0	R	R
2	0.5	1.5	R	R
3	0.25	1.75	R	R
4	0.20	1.80	R	R
5	0.15	1.85	R_m	R
6	0.12	1.88	W	R
7	0.09	1.91	W_m	R_m
8	0.06	1.94	N	N
9	0.03	1.97	N	N
10	0.00	2.00	N	N

*R = Reactive; W = weakly reactive; N = nonreactive; m = minimal.

containing 0.03% cardiolipin, 0.9% cholesterol, and sufficient purified lecithin to produce standard reactivity. Each lot must be serologically standardized by proper comparison with an antigen of known reactivity.

b. Antigen is dispensed in screw-capped (Vinylite liners) bottles or hermetically sealed glass ampules and should be stored in the dark at either refrigerator (6-10° C) or room temperature. Components of this antigen remain in solution at these temperatures. Antigen that contains precipitate should be discarded.

c. A new lot of antigen should be compared with an antigen of standard reactivity before being placed in routine use.

2. VDRL buffered saline containing 1% sodium chloride, pH 6.0 ± 0.1, available commercially

a. Check pH of solution and store in screw-capped or glass-stoppered bottles. (When an unexplained change in test reactivity occurs, check pH of VDRL buffered saline to determine if this is a contributing factor. Saline outside the range of pH 6.0 ± 0.1 should be discarded.)

3. Saline, 0.9%

a. Add 900 mg dry sodium chloride (ACS) to each deciliter of distilled water.

Preparation of antigen suspension: Temperature of buffered saline and antigen should be in the range of 23-29° C (73-85° F) at the time the antigen suspension is prepared. Slide flocculation tests for syphilis are affected by room temperature. For reliable and reproducible results, tests should be performed within the temperature range of 23-29° C (73-85° F). At lower temperatures, test reactivity is decreased; at higher temperatures, test reactivity is increased.

1. Pipet 0.4 ml buffered saline to bottom of a 30 ml, round, glass-stoppered bottle.

2. Add 0.5 ml antigen (from lower half of 1.0 ml pipet graduated to tip) directly onto saline while continuously but gently rotating bottle on flat surface. (NOTE: Antigen is added drop by drop, but rapidly, so that approximately 6 sec are allowed for each 0.5 ml antigen. Pipet tip should remain in upper one third of bottle, and rotation should not be vigorous enough to splash saline onto pipet. Proper speed of rotation is obtained when center of bottle circumscribes a 2 in. diameter circle approximately three times per second.)

3. Blow last drop of antigen from pipet without touching pipet to saline.

4. Continue rotation of bottle for 10 sec.

5. Add 4.1 ml buffered saline from 5 ml pipet.

6. Place top on bottle and shake from bottom to top and back approximately 30 times in 10 sec.

7. Antigen suspension is ready for use and may be used during 1 day.

8. A double volume of antigen suspension may be prepared at one time by using doubled quantities of antigen and saline. A 10 ml pipet should be used for delivering the 8.2 ml volume of saline. If larger quantities are required, more than one antigen suspension should be prepared. Test these suspensions with control sera, and pool the ones with satisfactory reactivity.

9. Mix antigen suspension gently at each use. Do not mix suspension by forcing back and forth through syringe and needle, since this may cause breakdown of particles and loss of reactivity.

Testing accuracy of delivery needles:

1. Needles used each day should be checked. Practice will allow rapid delivery of antigen suspension and saline, but care should be exercised to obtain drops of uniform size.

2. For quantitative slide test on serum, dispense antigen suspension from syringe fitted with 18-gauge needle without bevel that will deliver 60 drops plus 2 drops of antigen suspension per milliliter when syringe and needle are held vertically.

Preparation and calibration of hypodermic needles for slide flocculation test:

1. File a deep nick in the needle just above bevel.

2. Break the point off of the needle with pliers.

3. Using a 1 or 2 ml syringe containing the material to be dispensed, check needle by counting the number of drops in 1 ml of reagent. Drops should be allowed to fall freely from the tip of the needle. Hold the needle and syringe perpendicular to the tabletop.

4. Needles not meeting the specifications (Table 35-5) should be adjusted to deliver the correct volumes before being used.

5. If too many drops per milliliter are delivered by the needle, the opening of the tip is too small; enlarge with a sharp-pointed instrument, e.g., the sharpened end of a triangular file.

6. If too few drops per milliliter are delivered by the needle, the opening of the tip is too large; adjust

Table 35-5. Specifications for hypodermic needles

Test	Reagent	Needle gauge	Size of drop required (ml)	No. of drops delivered per milliliter of reagent
USR*	Antigen suspension	18	0.22 or $^1/_{45}$	45 ± 1
VDRL	Antigen suspension	18	0.017 or $^1/_{60}$	60 ± 2
VDRL	Antigen suspension	19	0.013 or $^1/_{75}$	75 ± 2
VDRL	Saline, 0.9%	23	0.010 or $^1/_{100}$	100 ± 2
VDRL	Sensitized antigen	21 or 22	0.010 or $^1/_{100}$	100 ± 2

*For unheated serum reagin test, see p. 1042.

by squeezing together slightly or by filing the edges of the needle inward.

7. Once calibrated, protect the tips of needles against dropping to the floor, sink, or bottoms of bottles.

8. Check needles each day before use and adjust if necessary.

9. Clean needles and syringes by rinsing with water, alcohol, and acetone. Remove needle from syringe after cleaning.

Preliminary testing of antigen suspension:

1. Test control sera* of graded reactivity as described under "VDRL qualitative slide test with serum." Whole serum controls may be prepared as described under "Control sera for nontreponemal antigen tests."

2. Reactions with control sera should reproduce established reactivity pattern. Nonreactive serum should show complete dispersion of antigen particles.

3. Do not use an unsatisfactory antigen suspension or pool of antigen suspensions.

NOTE: Control sera of graded reactivity (reactive, weakly reactive, and nonreactive) are always included during testing period to ensure proper reactivity of antigen suspension at time tests are performed.

Preparation of serum:

1. Heat clear serum, obtained from centrifuged, clotted blood, in 56° C water bath for 30 min before testing.

2. Examine all sera when removed from water bath, and recentrifuge those found to contain particulate debris.

3. Reheat at 56° C for 10 min those sera to be tested more than 4 hr after original heating period.

4. When tested, sera must be at room temperature.

Procedure: Slide flocculation tests for syphilis are affected by room temperature. For reliable and reproducible results, tests should be performed within temperature range of 23-29° C (73-85° F). At lower temperatures, test reactivity is decreased; at higher temperatures, test reactivity is increased.

Pipet 0.05 ml heated serum into one ring of ceramic-ringed slide. (Glass slides with concavities, wells, or glass rings are not recommended for this test.) Add 1 drop ($\frac{1}{60}$ ml) of antigen suspension to each serum with 18-gauge needle and syringe. Rotate slides for 4 min. (Mechanical rotators that circumscribe a $\frac{3}{4}$ in. diameter circle should be set at 180 rpm.) When tests are performed in a dry climate, slides may be covered with box lid containing moistened blotter during rotation to prevent excessive evaporation.

Read tests microscopically with 10× ocular and 10× objective immediately after rotation. Report results as follows:

Reading	Report
Medium and large clumps	Reactive (R)
Small clumps	Weakly reactive (W)
No clumping or very slight roughness	Nonreactive (N)

*Available from BBL, Division of BioQuest, Becton-Dickinson & Co., Cockeysville, Md.; Dade Diagnostics, Miami, Fla.; Difco Laboratories, Detroit; and Hyland Laboratories, Costa Mesa, Calif.

A prozone reaction is encountered occasionally. This type of reaction is demonstrated when complete or partial inhibition of reactivity occurs with undiluted serum, and maximal reactivity is obtained only with diluted serum. This prozone phenomenon may be so pronounced that only a weakly reactive or "rough" nonreactive result is produced in the qualitative test by a serum that will be strongly reactive when diluted.

It is recommended that all sera producing weakly reactive or "rough" nonreactive results in qualitative tests be retested by using a quantitative procedure before a report of the VDRL slide test is submitted. When a reactive result is obtained on some dilution of a serum that produced only a weakly reactive or "rough" nonreactive result before dilution, report test as reactive and include quantitative titer (see "VDRL quantitative slide test with serum").

VDRL quantitative slide test with serum (safety pipettor method)

Additional equipment and reagent:

1. Eppendorf pipet (Brinkmann Instruments, Westbury, N.Y.) or Selectapette pipet (Clay-Adams, Parsippany, N.J.).

2. Saline, 0.9%

Retest quantitatively, to an end-point titer, all sera that produce reactive, weakly reactive, or "rough" nonreactive results in the qualitative VDRL slide test. The dilutions of the serum to be tested are undiluted (1:1), 1:2, 1:4, 1:8, 1:16, and 1:32. Three-serum quantitative tests through 1:8 dilution (Fig. 35-8) or two-serum quantitative tests through 1:32 dilution (Fig. 35-9) may be performed on one slide.

Procedure: Select tubes of serum for quantitation and place in rack. Measure 0.05 ml of 0.9% saline onto second, third, and fourth paraffin rings in row on slide. Do not spread saline. Saline may be delivered from 18-gauge needle without point (0.025 ml/drop; use 2 drops), or use large needle or calibrated dropper that delivers 0.05 ml in a single drop; these should be checked daily for accuracy of delivery.

Using safety pipettor device with disposable tip (it should deliver 0.05 ml or 50 μl), measure 0.05 ml serum to first and second rings. Avoid contamination of instrument with serum. Use same pipettor and tip to make serial twofold dilutions by drawing serum-saline mixture up and down in tip five or six times. Avoid excess bubbles. (Use clean tip for each serum tested.)

Mix serum and saline in ring 2 (1:2 dilution); transfer 0.05 ml of 1:2 dilution to ring 3 and mix (1:4 dilution); transfer 0.05 ml of 1:4 dilution to ring 4, mix (1:8 dilution), and discard 0.05 ml. Additional serial dilutions may be set up for strongly reactive sera. (If the 0.05 ml of serum dilution has not spread within entire area of paraffin ring, spread this with pipettor tip before proceeding to next ring.)

Add 1 drop ($\frac{1}{60}$ ml) of VDRL antigen suspension to each ring with 18-gauge needle and syringe (used for antigen suspension in qualitative test). Rotate slides for 4 min (mechanical rotators that circumscribe a $\frac{3}{4}$ in. diameter circle should be set at 180 rpm).

Read tests microscopically with 10× ocular and 10× objective immediately after rotation. Record reading for each dilution tested. Report titer in terms of

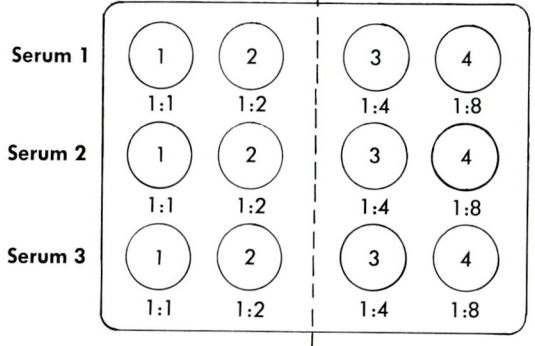

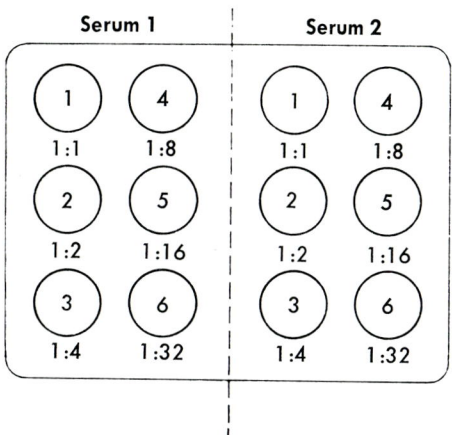

Fig. 35-8. Diagram of slide for quantitative, three-serum, VDRL slide test. (From 1975 Identical memorandum, Atlanta, 1975, Bureau of Laboratories, Centers for Disease Control.)

Fig. 35-9. Diagram of slide for quantitative, two-serum, VDRL slide test.

Table 35-6. Method of reporting VDRL quantitative slide test on serum

Undiluted serum (1:1)*	Serum dilutions*					Report
	1:2	1:4	1:8	1:16	1:32	
R	W	N	N	N	N	Reactive, undiluted only, or 1 dil†
R	R	W	N	N	N	Reactive, 1:2 dilution, or 2 dils
R	R	R	W	N	N	Reactive, 1:4 dilution, or 4 dils
W	W	R	R	W	N	Reactive, 1:8 dilution, or 8 dils
N (rough)	W	R	R	R	N	Reactive, 1:16 dilution, or 16 dils
W	N	N	N	N	N	Weakly reactive, undiluted only, or 0 dil

*R = Reactive; W = weakly reactive; N = nonreactive.
†A titer of 1:1 means that the serum was reactive in a dilution of 1 to 1. This may also be stated as "1 dil."

greatest serum dilution that produces a reactive (not weakly reactive) result, in accordance with the examples shown in Table 35-6.

VDRL qualitative slide test on spinal fluid

Additional equipment and reagent:
1. Hypodermic needles, without bevels, 23- or 22-gauge
2. Saline, 10% (10 g dry sodium chloride per deciliter of water)
3. Slides, agglutination, approximately 2 × 3 in. with concavities measuring 16 mm in diameter and 1.75 mm in depth
   When tests are performed in a dry climate, the slides may be covered with a box lid containing a moistened blotter during rotation to prevent evaporation.

Preparation of "sensitized antigen suspension":
1. Prepare antigen suspension as described for VDRL slide tests (see "Preparation of antigen suspension").
2. Add 1 part 10% saline to 1 part VDRL slide test suspension.

3. Mix by gently rotating bottle or inverting tube, and allow to stand at least 5 min but not more than 2 hr before use.

Testing of delivery needles:
1. It is of primary importance that the proper amount of reagent be used, and for this reason needles used each day should be checked. Practice will allow rapid delivery of antigen suspension, but care should be exercised to obtain drops of uniform size.
2. For qualitative and quantitative slide tests on spinal fluid, dispense sensitized antigen suspension from syringe fitted with a 21- or 22-gauge needle that will deliver 100 drops ± 2 drops sensitized antigen suspension per milliliter when syringe and needle are held vertically.
3. Adjust needles not meeting these specifications to deliver correct volume before being used (see "Preparation and calibration of hypodermic needles for slide flocculation tests").

Preliminary testing of sensitized antigen suspension:
1. Satisfactory control sera (BBL, Division of

BioQuest, Becton-Dickinson & Co., Cockeysville, Md.) for spinal fluid test are conveniently prepared by diluting serum in 0.9% saline (see "Control sera for serologic tests on spinal fluid specimens").

2. For daily use, remove one tube of reactive control serum from freezer, thaw, and mix thoroughly. Prepare designated serum dilutions in 0.9% saline. Controls are tested without preliminary heating in slide test.

3. Test control serum dilutions as described under "VDRL qualitative slide test on spinal fluid."

4. Reactions on control serum dilutions should reproduce established reactivity pattern, and nonreactive dilution should show complete dispersion of antigen particles.

5. Do not use an unsatisfactory sensitized antigen suspension.

NOTE: Control serum dilutions of graded reactivity (reactive, minimally reactive, and nonreactive) are always included during testing period to ensure proper reactivity of sensitized antigen suspension at the time tests are performed.

Control sera for serologic tests on spinal fluid specimens:

1. Select an individual serum or serum pool that is reactive in the spinal fluid test when diluted 1:80 or higher in 0.9% saline.

2. Dispense small quantities of the reactive serum, sufficient for one testing period, into labeled tubes and stopper tightly with paraffin-coated corks (small Vacutainers or equivalent may be used). Store in the freezer.

3. After 3 or more days' storage, thaw one tube of the reactive serum and mix thoroughly.

4. Prepare serial dilutions of the serum in 0.9% saline, starting at 1:80.

5. Test the serum dilutions in parallel with standard controls by using the spinal fluid technic.

6. Select three serum dilutions that produce reactive, minimally reactive, and nonreactive test results, respectively.

7. Confirm the reactivity pattern of these three dilutions by testing in parallel with standard controls on at least 3 testing days. Use a different tube of new control serum each test day.

Preparation of spinal fluid: Centrifuge and decant each spinal fluid. The spinal fluid is tested without preliminary heating. Spinal fluids that are visibly contaminated or contain gross blood are unsatisfactory for testing.

Procedure: Slide flocculation tests for syphilis are affected by room temperature. For reliable and reproducible results, tests should be performed within the temperature range of 23-29° C (73-85° F). At lower temperatures test reactivity is decreased; at higher temperatures test reactivity is increased.

Pipet 0.05 ml spinal fluid into one concavity of an agglutination slide. Add 1 drop (0.01 ml) of sensitized antigen suspension to each spinal fluid with 21- or 22-gauge needle. Rotate slides for 8 min on mechanical rotator at 180 rpm. When tests are performed in a dry climate, slides may be covered with a box lid containing a moistened blotter during rotation to prevent evaporation.

Read tests microscopically with a 10× ocular and a 10× objective immediately after rotation. Report results as follows:

Reading	Report
Definite clumping	Reactive (R)
No clumping or very slight roughness	Nonreactive (N)

VDRL quantitative slide test on spinal fluid

Quantitative tests are performed on all spinal fluids found to be reactive in the qualitative test.

Prepare spinal fluid dilutions as follows:

1. Pipet 0.2 ml of 0.9% saline into each of five or more tubes.

2. Add 0.2 ml unheated spinal fluid to tube 1, mix well, and transfer 0.2 ml to tube 2.

3. Continue mixing and transferring 0.2 ml from one tube to the next until the last tube is reached. The respective dilutions are 1:2, 1:4, 1:8, 1:16, 1:32, etc.

Test each spinal fluid dilution and undiluted spinal fluid as described under "VDRL qualitative slide test on spinal fluid." Report results in terms of the greatest spinal fluid dilution (dils)* that produces a reactive result.

Rapid reagin tests

The rapid reagin tests[72] are performed on unheated serum or plasma, thus simplifying the processing of specimens. The antigen used is a modified VDRL antigen suspension with choline chloride and EDTA added; the RPR card test antigen also contains charcoal for making macroscopic reading possible.

Rapid reagin tests include the following:

1. **Rapid plasma reagin (RPR) test.**[73] The original test used unmeasured amounts of plasma and was used as a field procedure for screening large numbers of persons. The test proved to be about 10% more reactive than the VDRL slide test.

2. **Unheated serum reagin (USR) test.**[74] The USR is a modification of the RPR test. It has a somewhat lower level of reactivity than the VDRL slide test. The test is performed on measured volumes of unheated serum.

3. **RPR (circle) card test.**[75] Testing is performed on unheated serum (less often on plasma). The card used for the test is rotated on a mechanical rotator, and the tests are read macroscopically (the antigen contains charcoal). The test is about as specific and sensitive as the VDRL slide test. In fact, there are indications that the test may be more sensitive than the VDRL slide test, as shown by retesting specimens that were VDRL nonreactive and RPR (circle) card test reactive with the FTA-ABS test. The RPR (circle) card test may detect more cases of syphilis than the VDRL test.[76]

---

*A titer of 1:8 means that the serum was reactive in a dilution of 1 to 8. This may also be stated as 8 dils.

4. **Automated reagin test (ART).**[77] This test uses modified AutoAnalyzer equipment (Technicon Instruments Corp., Tarrytown, N.Y.) and is not further described.

Rapid plasma reagin (RPR) (circle) card test with serum (qualitative)[78-80]

Equipment and reagents: All equipment and supplies necessary to perform the RPR (circle) card test are contained in a kit (Hynson, Westcott & Dunning, Baltimore), with the exception of the controls, the rotating machine, and the cover.

1. Test kit, which contains the following:
   a. RPR card test antigen. This antigen suspension is similiar to that prepared for the VDRL slide test (see "Preparation of antigen suspension," p. 1039). It also contains a suspension of specially prepared charcoal particles. Store antigen suspension in ampules or in the plastic dispensing bottle at 2-8° C. An unopened ampule has a shelf life of at least 12 months from the date of manufacture; antigen suspension in the plastic dispensing bottle (refrigerated) usually remains satisfactory for approximately 3 months. Do not use antigen suspension beyond the expiration date shown on the ampule. A new lot of antigen suspension should be compared with an antigen suspension of known reactivity before being placed in routine use.
   b. Needle, 20-gauge, without bevel
   c. Plastic dispensing bottle
   d. Plastic-coated cards, each with ten 18 mm circle spots
   e. Dispenstirs, 0.05 ml per drop
   f. Capillary pipets, 0.05 ml capacity
   g. Rubber bulbs
   h. Stirrers
2. Rotating machine, fixed speed or adjustable to 100 rpm, circumscribing a $^3/_4$ in. diameter circle on a horizontal plane
3. Humidifer cover (Hynson, Westcott & Dunning, Baltimore). Any convenient cover containing a moistened blotter may be used to cover the cards during rotation.
4. Pipets (optional). Any of these listed may be used instead of Dispenstirs or capillary pipets.
   a. 0.2 ml, graduated in 0.01 ml subdivisions
   b. 0.5 ml, graduated in 0.01 ml subdivisions
   c. 1.0 ml, graduated in 0.01 ml subdivisions

Testing accuracy of delivery needles:
1. It is of primary importance that the proper amount of reagents be used. For this reason, the needles used should be checked each day.
2. For the RPR card test, dispense antigen suspension from a plastic dispensing bottle with a 10-gauge disposable needle without bevel. These needles should deliver 60 drops ± 2 drops of antigen suspension per milliliter when held in a vertical position. Practice will allow rapid delivery of antigen suspension, but care should be exercised to obtain drops of uniform size.
3. To check accuracy of the needle, place needle on a 2 ml syringe or on a 1 ml pipet. Fill the syringe or pipet with the antigen suspension and, holding it in a vertical position, count the number of drops delivered from 0.5 ml. The needle is considered to be satisfactory if 30 drops ± 1 drop are obtained from 0.5 ml of suspension.
4. A needle not meeting this specification should be replaced with another needle that does meet this specification.

Preliminary testing of antigen suspension:
1. Attach needle hub to tapered fitting on plastic dispensing bottle. Shake antigen ampule to resuspend antigen particles, snap ampule neck at the break line, and withdraw all the RPR card antigen suspension into the dispensing bottle by suction, collapsing the bottle and using it as a bulb. Shake dispenser gently before each series of antigen drops is delivered.
2. Test control sera (Hynson, Westcott & Dunning, Baltimore) of graded reactivity each day as described under "Rapid plasma reagin (circle) card test with serum (qualitative)." Whole serum controls may be prepared as described under "Control sera for nontreponemal antigen tests" (p. 1037).
3. Use only those suspensions that have given the designated reactions with the controls.

Preparation of sera:
1. Centrifuge blood specimens at room temperature and at a force sufficient to separate the serum from the cells. Generally, 1500-2000 rpm for 5 min is satisfactory.
2. Specimens may be retained in the original collection tube.

NOTE: Sera are tested without heating and should be at 23-29° C (73-85° F) at the time of testing.

Slide flocculation tests for syphilis are affected by room temperature. For reliable and reproducible results, the controls, RPR card antigen suspension, and test specimens should be at room temperature (23-29° C [73-85° F]) when tests are performed.

Procedure: Place 0.05 ml of unheated serum onto an 18 mm circle of the test card, using a Dispenstir, a 0.05 ml capillary pipet with attached rubber bulb, or a serologic pipet. Spread serum with inverted Dispenstir (closed end) or a stirrer (broad end) to fill the entire circle. (The specimen may be spread with a serologic pipet if the tip is smooth and will not scratch the card surface.)

Add exactly 1 drop (1/60 ml) of RPR card test antigen suspension to each test area containing serum. Do not stir. Place card on rotator and cover with humidifier cover. Rotate 8 min at 100 rpm on mechanical rotating machine.

Read tests without magnification immediately after rotation. A brief rotating and tilting of the card by hand should be used to aid in differentiating nonreactive from minimally reactive results. Report results as follows:

Reading	Report
Small to large clumps	Reactive (R)
No clumping or very slight roughness	Nonreactive (N)

NOTE: Specimens giving any degree of clumping should be subjected to further serologic study, including quantitation.

On completion of the daily tests, remove needle, rinse in water, and air dry. (Avoid wiping needle, because this removes silicone coating.) Recap dispensing bottle and store in refrigerator.

Rapid plasma reagin (RPR) (circle) card test with serum (quantitative)

Quantitative testing with the RPR (circle) card test is described by Portnoy.[75,79] The quantitative test is not included in the *Manual of Tests for Syphilis, 1969,* but it is now an accepted standard test.

Procedure:
1. For each specimen to be tested, place 0.05 ml of 0.9% saline solution into rings 2-5. Use a serologic pipet, 1 ml or less, or an 18-gauge needle without point; the needle should deliver 0.025 ml/drop. Do not spread saline solution.
2. Using capillary pipet graduated at 0.05 ml (to tip) and rubber bulb, place 0.05 ml unheated serum or plasma in ring 1.

NOTE: Serum should not be drawn into rubber bulb, since this may cause incorrect results on subsequent tests.

3. Refill capillary and, holding in vertical position, prepare serial twofold dilutions by drawing mixture up and down capillary five or six times, transferring 0.05 ml from ring 2 to ring 3 to ring 4 to ring 5. Discard 0.05 ml after mixing contents in ring 5.
4. Place 1 drop (1/60 ml) of RPR card antigen suspension onto each ring.
5. Using broad end of clean stirrer for each specimen, start at highest dilution of serum (ring 5) and mix RPR card antigen suspension and serum, filling entire surface of ring. Then proceed to rings 4, 3, 2, and 1, and perform similar stirring.
6. Rotate for 8 min at 100 rpm on mechanical rotator.
7. Read tests and report in terms of highest dilution yielding reactive result.
8. If highest dilution tested (1:16) is reactive, proceed as follows:
   a. Prepare 1:50 dilution of nonreactive serum in 0.9% saline solution. (This is to be used for making 1:32 and higher dilutions of specimens to be quantitated.)
   b. Prepare 1:16 dilution of test specimen by adding 0.1 ml serum or plasma to 1.5 ml of 0.9% saline solution. Mix thoroughly.
   c. Place 0.05 ml of 1:50 nonreactive serum in rings 2, 3, 4, and 5.
   d. Using capillary pipet, place 0.05 ml of 1:16 dilution of test specimen in ring 1.
   e. Refill capillary, make serial twofold dilutions, and complete tests as described in steps 3 to 7.
9. Higher dilutions are prepared if necessary in 1:50 nonreactive serum.

Fluorescent treponemal antibody–absorption test on serum*

Principle: As discussed under "General considerations" (p. 1036), the specificity of the fluorescent treponemal antibody–absorption (FTA-ABS) test is increased by absorbing the patient's serum with an extract (sorbent) of the nonpathogenic Reiter treponemes to remove nonspecific reactants. The antitreponemal antibody present in the patient's serum is then allowed to combine with the antigen dried on a microscope slide. The latter consists of a suspension of *T. pallidum* (Nichols' strain) extracted from infected rabbit testicular tissue. The antigen-antibody reaction is detected by the indirect fluorescent antibody technic, using antihuman globulins labeled with fluorescein isothiocyanate.

Equipment:
1. Incubator, adjustable to 35-37° C
2. Darkfield fluorescence microscope assembly
3. Bibulous paper
4. Diamond point pencil (optional)
5. Template, used as a guide for cutting circles 1.0 cm in diameter on glass slides (optional)
6. Slide board or holder
7. Moist chamber (Place moistened paper inside a convenient cover fitting the slide board.)
8. Loop, bacteriologic, standard 2 mm, 26-gauge platinum
9. Oil, immersion, low fluorescence, nondrying
10. Microscope slides, 1 × 3 in., frosted end, approximately 1 mm thick†
11. Coverslips, no. 1, 22 mm square
12. Dish, staining, glass or plastic, with removable slide carriers
13. Glass rods, approximately 100 × 4 mm, both ends fire polished

Reagents:
1. *Treponema pallidum* antigen‡
   a. The antigen for the FTA-ABS test is a suspension of *T. pallidum* (Nichols' stain) extracted from rabbit testicular tissue. The extract should contain a minimum of 30 organisms per high-power dry field. The antigen may be stored at 6-10° C or processed by lyophilization.
   b. Store lyophilized antigen at 6-10° C and rehydrate for use according to the accompanying directions.
   c. Discard antigen suspension if it becomes bacterially contaminated or does not demonstrate the proper reactivity with control sera.
2. FTA-ABS test sorbent‡
   a. Sorbent is a standardized product prepared from cultures of Reiter treponemes. It may be purchased in lyophilized or liquid state.
   b. Store sorbent, and rehydrate, if lyophilized, according to accompanying directions.

---

*See references 55, 70, 71, and 81-83.
†Glass slides with two etched circles 1 cm in diameter are available from Clay-Adams, Parsippany, N.J.
‡Available from BBL, Divison of BioQuest, Becton-Dickinson & Co., Cockeysville, Md.; Difco Laboratories, Detroit; & The Sylvana Co. Millburn, N.J.

3. Fluorescein-labeled antihuman globulin* (conjugate)
   a. The conjugate should be of proven quality for the FTA-ABS test. Test each new lot of conjugate to determine its working titer and to verify that it meets the criteria for nonspecific staining and standard reactivity.
   b. Store lyophilized conjugate at 6-10° C. Dispense rehydrated conjugate in not less than 0.3 ml quantities and store at −20° C or lower. For practical purposes, a conjugate with a working titer of 1:400 or higher may be diluted 1:10 with sterile phosphate buffered saline (containing thimerosal [Merthiolate] in a concentration of 1:5000) before storage.
   c. When conjugate is thawed for use, do not refreeze but store at 6-10° C. It may be used as long as satisfactory reactivity is obtained with test controls.
   d. If a change in FTA-ABS test reactivity is noted in routine laboratory testing, the conjugate should be retitrated to determine whether it is the contributing factor.
4. Phosphate buffered saline (PBS), pH 7.2 ± 0.1. Formula per liter:
   a. NaCl, 7.65 g
   b. Na_2HPO_4, 0.724 g
   c. KH_2PO_4, 0.21 g
   Several liters may be prepared and stored in a large Pyrex (or equivalent) or polyethylene bottle. Determine the pH of each lot of PBS prepared for the FTA-ABS test. PBS outside the range of pH 7.2 ± 0.1 should be discarded.
5. Tween 80 (Hill Top Laboratories, Cincinnati)
   To prepare PBS containing 2% Tween 80, heat the two reagents in a 56° C water bath. To 98 ml of PBS, add 2 ml Tween 80 by measuring from the bottom of a pipet and rinse out the pipet. The 2% Tween 80 solution should have a pH of 7.0-8.2. Check the pH periodically, because the solution may become acid. This solution keeps well at refrigerator temperature; discard if a precipitate develops or if the pH changes.
6. Mounting medium
   The mouting medium consists of 1 part PBS at pH 7.2, plus 9 parts glycerin of reagent quality.
7. Acetone (ACS)

Check-testing of new lots of reagents: Each new lot of reagents should be tested in parallel with a standard reagent before being placed in routine use.
1. *T. pallidum* antigen
   a. A new lot of antigen should be compared with a standard antigen before being placed in routine use. Testing should be performed on more than one testing day with control sera, individual sera of graded reactivity, and nonreactive sera.
   b. A sufficient number of organisms should remain on the slide after staining so that tests may be read without difficulty.
   c. The antigen should not contain background material that stains to the extent that it interferes with the reading of the tests.
   d. The antigen should not stain nonspecifically with a standard conjugate at its working titer.
   e. Reportable test results on controls and individual sera should be comparable with those obtained with the standard antigen.
2. FTA-ABS test sorbent
   a. A new lot of sorbent should be compared with a standard sorbent before being placed in routine use. Testing should be performed on more than one testing day with control sera, individual sera of graded reactivity, and nonsyphilitic sera demonstrating nonspecific reactivity.
   b. The new sorbent should remove nonspecific reactivity of the nonspecific serum control.
   c. The new sorbent should not reduce intensity of fluorescence of the reactive (4+) control serum to less than 3+.
   d. The nonspecific staining control with the new sorbent should be nonreactive.
   e. Reportable test results on controls and individual sera should be comparable with those obtained with standard sorbent.
   f. The sorbent should be usable when rehydrated to the indicated volume on the label or according to accompanying directions.
3. Fluorescein-labeled antihuman globulin (conjugate)
   a. A satisfactory conjugate should not stain a standard antigen nonspecifically at three doubling dilutions below the working titer of the conjugate.
   b. Reportable test results on controls and individual sera should be comparable with those obtained with the standard conjugate. (NOTE: Most manufacturers designate on the label the working titer of the conjugate that was determined under the testing conditions and with the equipment in their laboratories. Since conditions and equipment vary from one laboratory to another, it is necessary to titer and to check-test a new lot of conjugate with the fluorescence microscope assembly that is available.)

Titration: Prepare serial doubling dilutions of the new conjugate in PBS containing 2% Tween 80 to include the titer indicated by the manufacturer. Examples are: (1) 1:2.5, 1:5, 1:10, 1:20, 1:40, 1:80, 1:160, and (2) 1:12.5, 1:25, 1:50, 1:100, 1:200, 1:400, 1:800. Prepare higher dilutions if necessary.

Test each conjugate dilution with the reactive (4+) control serum diluted 1:5 in PBS in accordance with the FTA-ABS procedure below. Include a nonspecific staining control with each conjugate dilution. A standard conjugate, at its titer, is set up at the same time with a reactive (4+) control serum, a minimally reactive (1+) control serum, and a nonspecific staining control with PBS for the purpose of controlling rea-

*Available from BBL, Divison of BioQuest, Becton-Dickinson & Co., Cockeysville, Md.; Difco Laboratories, Detroit; & The Sylvana Co. Millburn, N.J.

Table 35-7. Titration of a new conjugate

Conjugate	Nonspecific staining control (PBS)	Reactive (4+) control serum (1:5 in PBS)	Reactive (1+) control serum
Standard conjugate titer			
1:400	—	4+	1+
New conjugate titer			
1:12.5	1+	4+	
1:25	—	4+	
1:50	—	4+	
1:100	—	4+	
1:200	—	4+	
1:400	—	4+	
1:800	—	3+	

gents and test conditions. For an example of the titration of a new conjugate see Table 35-7.

Read slides in the following order: (1) Examine the three control slides to ensure that reagents and testing conditions are satisfactory. (2) Examine the slides with new conjugate; start with the lowest dilution of conjugate. Record readings in pluses.

The end point of the titration is the highest dilution giving maximal (4+) fluorescence. The working titer of the new conjugate is one doubling dilution below the end point. In Table 35-7, the dilution selected for the working titer is 1:200. The new conjugate should not stain nonspecifically at three doubling dilutions below the working titer of the conjugate. In Table 35-7 the conjugate would meet this criterion, since there is no nonspecific staining with the 1:25 dilution.

Dispense conjugate in not less than 0.3 ml quantities and store at −20° C or lower. (For practical purposes, a conjugate with a working titer of 1:400 or higher may be diluted 1:10 with sterile PBS containing thimerosal [Merthiolate] in a concentration of 1:5000 before storage in the freezer.) Verify titer of the conjugate after at least 3 days' storage in the freezer.

Check-testing: If the criterion of acceptability for the nonspecific staining has been met and a working titer has been determined, the new conjugate should be check-tested in parallel with a standard conjugate before being placed in routine use. Testing should be performed on more than one testing day with control sera, individual sera of graded reactivity, and nonreactive sera.

Individual sera tested in parallel with a standard and a new conjugate are read against the minimally reactive (1+) controls set up with the respective conjugates. A new conjugate is considered to be satisfactory when comparable test results are obtained with both conjugates.

Preparation of Treponema pallidum antigen smears:
1. Mix antigen suspension well with a disposable pipet and rubber bulb by drawing the suspension into and expelling it from the pipet at least 10 times to break the treponemal clumps and to ensure an even distribution of treponemes. Determine by darkfield examination that treponemes

are adequately dispersed before making slides for fluorescent treponemal antibody (FTA) test. Additional mixing may be required.
2. On clean slides, cut two circles 1 cm in diameter with a diamond point pencil. Wipe slides with clean gauze to remove loose glass particles. Slides with preetched circles may be used.
3. Smear one loopful of *T. pallidum* antigen evenly within each circle by using a standard 2 mm 26-gauge platinum wire loop. Experience with individual lots of antigen may indicate that a smaller or larger quantity should be spread in each circle. Allow to air dry at least 15 min.
4. Fix smears* in acetone for 10 min and allow to air dry thoroughly (not more than 60 slides should be fixed with 2 dl acetone). Store acetone-fixed smears at −20° C or lower. Fixed frozen smears are usable indefinitely, provided that satisfactory results are obtained with the controls. Do not thaw and refreeze antigen smears.

Preparation of sera: Heat test and control sera at 56° C for 30 min before testing. Reheat previously heated test sera for 10 min at 56° C on the day of testing. (NOTE: Bacterial contamination or excessive hemolysis may render specimens unsatisfactory for testing.)

Control sera: Store and use control sera from commercial sources† according to the accompanying directions. Include the following controls in each test run:
1. *Reactive (4+) control.* This consists of a reactive serum or a dilution of reactive serum demonstrating strong (4+) fluorescence when diluted 1:5 in PBS and only slightly reduced fluorescence‡ when diluted 1:5 in sorbent.
   a. Using a 0.2 ml pipet and measuring from the bottom, add 0.005 ml reactive control serum

---

*Smears may be fixed for 20 sec in a solution of 10% methyl alcohol in distilled water. (Not more than 20 slides should be fixed with 2 dl of 10% methyl alcohol; this solution should be prepared on the day of use.) Antigen smears to be fixed by this method should be prepared on the day of test.

†BBL, Division of BioQuest, Becton-Dickinson & Co., Cockeysville, Md.; Difco Laboratories, Detroit; Space Division, Aerojet-General Corp., El Monte, Calif.; and The Sylvana Co., Millburn, N.J.

‡A reduction of no more than 1+ fluorescence; e.g., 4+ changing to 3+.

into a tube containing 0.2 ml PBS. Mix well, at least eight times.

   b. Using a 0.2 ml pipet and measuring from the bottom, add 0.05 ml reactive control serum into a tube containing 0.2 ml sorbent. Mix well, at least eight times.

2. *Minimally reactive (1 +) control.* This consists of a dilution of reactive serum demonstrating the minimal degree of fluorescence reported as reactive for use as a reading standard. The reactive (4 +) control serum may be used for this control when it is diluted in PBS according to directions.

3. *Nonspecific serum controls.* This consists of a nonsyphilitic serum known to demonstrate at least 2 + nonspecific reactivity in the FTA test at a dilution in PBS of 1:5 or higher.

   a. Using a 0.2 ml pipet and measuring from the bottom, add 0.05 ml nonspecific control serum into a tube containing 0.2 ml PBS. Mix well, at least eight times.

   b. Using another 0.2 ml pipet and measuring from the bottom, add 0.05 ml nonspecific control serum into a tube containing 0.2 ml sorbent. Mix well, at least eight times.

4. *Nonspecific staining controls.* These consist of (1) antigen smear treated with 0.03 ml PBS, and (2) antigen smear treated with 0.03 ml sorbent.

NOTE: Controls 1, 3, and 4 are included for the purpose of controlling reagents and test conditions. Control 2 (minimally reactive [1 +] control serum) is included as the reading standard.

CONTROL PATTERN ILLUSTRATION

Control	Reaction
Reactive control	
1.5 PBS dilution	R (4 +)
1:5 sorbent dilution	R (4 + to 3 +)
Minimally reactive (1 +) control	R (1 +)
Nonspecific serum controls	
1:5 PBS dilution	R (2 + to 4 +)
1:5 sorbent dilution	N
Nonspecific staining controls	
Antigen, PBS, and conjugate	N
Antigen, sorbent, and conjugate	N

Test runs in which these control results are not obtained are considered unsatisfactory and should not be reported.

Procedure:

1. Identify previously prepared slides by numbering the frosted end with a lead pencil (see "Preparation of *Treponema pallidum* antigen smears").

2. Number the tubes to correspond to the sera and control sera being tested and place in racks.

3. Prepare reactive (4 +), minimally reactive (1 +), and nonspecific control serum dilutions in sorbent and/or PBS according to the directions (see "Control sera").

4. Pipet 0.2 ml sorbent into a test tube for each test serum.

5. Using a 0.2 ml pipet and measuring from the bottom, add 0.05 ml of the heated test serum into the appropriate tube and mix eight times.

6. Cover the appropriate antigen smears with 0.03 ml of the reactive (4 +), minimally reactive (1 +), and nonspecific control serum dilutions.

7. Cover the appropriate antigen smears with 0.03 ml PBS and 0.03 ml sorbent for nonspecific staining controls.

8. Cover the appropriate antigen smears with 0.03 ml of the test serum dilutions.

9. Prevent evaporation by placing slides within a moist chamber.

10. Place slides in an incubator at 35-37° C for 30 min.

11. Rinse slides as follows:

   a. Place slides in slide carriers and rinse slides with running PBS for approximately 5 sec.

   b. Place slides in staining dish containing PBS for 5 min.

   c. Agitate slides by dipping them in and out of the PBS at least 10 times.

   d. Using fresh PBS, repeat steps b and c.

   e. Rinse slides in running distilled water for approximately 5 sec.

12. Gently blot slides with bibulous paper to remove all water drops.

13. Dilute conjugate to its working titer in PBS containing 2% Tween 80.

14. Place approximately 0.03 ml diluted conjugate on each smear. Spread uniformly with a glass rod to cover entire smear.

15. Repeat steps 9-12.

16. Mount slides immediately by placing a small drop of mounting medium on each smear and applying a coverslip.

17. Examine slides as soon as possible. If a delay in reading is necessary, place slides in a darkened room and read within 4 hr.

18. Study smears microscopically by using an ultraviolet light source and a high-power dry objective. A combination of BG 12 exciting filter, not more than 3 mm in thickness, and OG 1 barrier filter (or equivalents)* has been found to be satisfactory for routine use.

19. Check nonreactive smears by using illumination from a tungsten light source to verify the presence of treponemes.

20. Using the minimally reactive (1 +) control slide as the reading standard, record the intensity of fluorescence of the treponemes according to Table 35-8.

The FTA-ABS reporting scheme is illustrated in Table 35-9. For additional information on borderline test results, see boxed material that is shown on p. 1048.

---

*Exciting filter equivalent is as follows: BG 12 = 0 = AO 702. Barrier filter equivalents are as follows: OG 1 = 0 = A(724 or 1124); = 0 = B&L Y-8; = 0 = Zeiss 50/-(II/O).

Table 35-8. Recording of fluorescence

Reading	Intensity of fluorescence	Report*
2+ to 4+	Moderate to strong	R
1+	Equivalent to minimally reactive (1+) control	R†
<1+	Weak but definite; less than minimally reactive (1+) control	B†
—	None or vaguely visible	N

*R = Reactive; B = borderline; N = nonreactive.
†Retest all specimens with intensity of fluorescence of 1+ or less. When a specimen initially read as 1+ is retested and is subsequently read as 1+ or greater, the test is reported as reactive. All other results on retests are reported as borderline. It is not necessary to retest nonfluorescent (nonreactive) specimens.

Table 35-9. Reporting scheme

Test reading	Repeat	Report*
4+		R
3+		R
2+		R
1+	1+ or greater	R
	<1+ or −	B
<1+	1+, <1+, or −	B
−		N

*R = Reactive; B = borderline; N = nonreactive.

SUGGESTED ATTACHMENT TO REPORTS OF BORDERLINE TEST RESULTS

The borderline report of the FTA-ABS test performed in our laboratory on the specimen obtained from (patient's name) means that the results cannot be interpreted as either reactive or nonreactive.

If this is the first specimen you have submitted for FTA-ABS testing on this patient, another specimen should be submitted for FTA-ABS testing.

If this is a second specimen from this patient on which an FTA-ABS test has been made and the report is again borderline, it is impossible to state definitely that the patient does or does not have serologic evidence of syphilitic infection. A careful review of the patient's history and physical findings is suggested, and diagnosis will necessarily rest on the clinical evidence in view of the borderline serologic findings.

SEROLOGY IN THE DIAGNOSIS OF OTHER INFECTIOUS DISEASES

Streptococcal infections and their antibodies

Group A β-hemolytic streptococci are responsible for a large number of infections not only in the very young and elderly but also in older children and adults. These disease processes include pharyngitis (with or without scarlet fever), impetigo, pyoderma, cellulitis, erythema nodosum, and puerperal sepsis. There are two important nonsuppurative sequelae of group A streptococcal infections:

1. Acute poststreptococcal glomerulonephritis, which may follow 1-4 weeks after throat and skin infections with nephritogenic strains (mostly types 1, 2, 12, and 49)[84]
2. Rheumatic fever, which occurs 3-4 weeks after throat infections in 2-3% of patients[85] and is rarely followed by Sydenham's chorea. The pathogenesis of these sequelae is not quite clear but probably involves an immune complex phenomenon.

Group A β-hemolytic streptococci produce numerous intracellular and extracellular antigens, which lead to the production of antibodies in the infected patient.[86] Some of the cell wall proteins are antigenic, such as the M, T, and R proteins as well as the group-specific carbohydrates and cytoplasmic membrane antigens.[87,88] Many of the extracellular products are enzymes, which are toxic and antigenic and include erythrogenic toxins, streptolysins, diphosphopyridine nucleotidase, streptokinases, deoxyribonucleases, and hyaluronidase. The most commonly used serologic tests detect antistreptolysin O (ASO), antihyaluronidase (AH), and antideoxyribonuclease B (ADN-B). The performance of these tests may be preceded by a 2 min screening multienzyme slide test, Streptozyme (Wampole Laboratories, Cranbury, N.J.), which detects antibodies to a number of streptococcal extracellular antigens. The antibodies include ASO, AH, ADN-B, and antistreptokinase.

Antistreptolysin O test[86]

In the investigation of disease processes related to streptococcal infections, the antistreptolysin O (ASO) test is unique in that it is widely accepted and has good reproducibility, and the antigen is commercially available and is produced by most group A streptococci.

Principle: Streptolysin O (SLO) is an enzyme produced by many strains of streptococci of groups A, C, and G. When released into tissues in the course of a streptococcal infection it stimulates the production of antistreptolysin antibodies, which in vitro block the hemolytic properties of their antigen. If in the test system the patient's serum containing antistreptolysin antibody is added to streptolysin, an antigen-antibody reaction takes place, which, depending on the antibody level, completely or partially neutralizes the hemolytic action of streptolysin. A constant quantity of streptolysin (antigen) is added to progressively decreasing amounts of serum, and if the antibody present is sufficient to neutralize the antigen, no hemolysis will occur when red cells are subsequently added. When the antigen exceeds the antibody, the excess streptolysin will cause hemolysis. The ASO antibody titer is the reciprocal of the highest serum dilution that prevents hemolysis of the cells. The ASO titer is measured in Todd units, the reciprocal of the highest dilution of serum showing no hemolysis.[89]

A number of test procedures are available, the most commonly used method is the macrotechnic of Rantz and Randall,[90] which is also adopted by commercial suppliers. It is carried out in tubes containing constant volumes of SLO reagent and various dilutions of patient's serum. After 15 min incubation at 37° C a constant volume of 5% erythrocyte suspension is added. After reincubation and centrifugation the end point (highest dilution showing absence of hemolysis) is observed.

Reagents: Reagents are commercially available (Difco Laboratories, Detroit).

1. SLO reagent, desiccated in reduced form, standardized, so that 0.5 ml will combine with 1 unit of antistreptolysin O
2. SLO buffer
3. ASO control of known titer
4. Patient's serum
5. Washed human red cells (type O, Rh negative) or rabbit cells
   Suspend 5 ml of washed packed cells in 95 ml SLO buffer.

Procedure: Prepare serum dilutions as follows:

1. 1:10 = 0.5 ml serum + 4.5 SLO buffer
2. 1:100 = 1 ml 1:10 + 9.0 ml SLO buffer
3. 1:500 = 2 ml 1:100 + 8.0 ml SLO buffer

Varying amounts of these dilutions are pipetted into 100 × 13 ml tubes according to Table 35-10. The serum dilutions are as follows: 1:12, 1:50, 1:100, 1:125, 1:166, 1:250, 1:333, 1:500, 1:625, 1:833, 1:1250, and 1:2500.

Add 0.5 ml SLO buffer to each tube. Add 0.5 ml red cell suspension to each tube. Incubate at 37° C for 45 min. Centrifuge (Table 35-10).

Controls:

1. Red cell control (1.5 ml SLO buffer solution used as diluent plus 0.5 ml cell suspension)
   The supernatant after centrifugation or 2 hr standing should be without hemolysis. This tube may be used to aid in determining slight amounts of hemolysis in other tubes.
2. Streptolysin control (1.0 ml SLO buffer solution, 0.5 ml of reconstituted lysin, and 0.5 ml cell suspension)
   This tube should show marked to complete hemolysis.
3. ASO Standard (having a titer of 166 Todd units is recommended as a control of the conditions of the test)
   Rehydrated Bacto-ASO standard is used without further dilution as the 1:100 serum dilution in the range of 100 through 333 Todd units (tubes 3-7), as indicated in Table 35-10. If desired, sera with known low or high titers may also be included as controls. These additional control sera are treated in the same manner as are unknown sera. The person performing the test should consistently reproduce a stated titer within +1 dilution.

Results: The ASO titer, expressed in Todd units, is

Table 35-10. Methodology for the titration of antistreptolysin O titers

| | Serum dilution | | | | | | | | | | | | Red cell control | Strepto-lysin control |
	1:10		1:100					1:500						
Tube no.	1	2	3	4	5	6	7	8	9	10	11	12	13	14
Diluted serum (ml)	0.8	0.2	1.0	0.8	0.6	0.4	0.3	1.0	0.8	0.6	0.4	0.2	—	—
Streptolysin buffer (ml)	0.2	0.8	0.0	0.2	0.4	0.6	0.7	0.0	0.2	0.4	0.6	0.8	1.5	1.0
Shake gently to mix.														
Streptolysin (ml)	0.5	0.5	0.5	0.5	0.5	0.5	0.5	0.5	0.5	0.5	0.5	0.5	—	0.5
Shake gently to mix. Incubate at 37° C for 15 min.														
Red cell suspension, 5% (ml)	0.5	0.5	0.5	0.5	0.5	0.5	0.5	0.5	0.5	0.5	0.5	0.5	0.5	0.5
Shake gently. Incubate at 37° C for 45 min, shaking after first 15 min. Centrifuge tubes for 1 min at 1000-1500 rpm.														
Unit value*	12	50	100	125	166	250	333	500	625	833	1250	2500	Control	Control

*The entire range from 12-2500 Todd units is seldom used for a serum titration. Generally, for the initial titration, the first seven dilutions covering the range of 12-333 Todd units are employed. This range will indicate normal or elevated titers, and subsequent titration dilutions may be based on the previous titers.

the reciprocal of the highest dilution of serum showing no hemolysis. For example, the ASO titer of a serum showing no hemolysis in tubes 1-4, a trace of hemolysis in tube 5, and complete hemolysis in other tubes would be 125.

Normal range: The normal range is 0-200 Todd units. This wide range is explained by the fact that most patients have experienced streptococcal infections at one time or the other. A single titer is difficult to interpret and should be followed by titration of a second specimen obtained 10-14 days later.

Discussion: A titer of 400 Todd units or higher is strong evidence for recent streptococcal infection. In suspected streptococcal sequelae the titer may have returned to normal by the time they manifest clinical symptoms. In addition, only about 80% of streptococcal infections are associated with a rise in ASO titer. Streptococcal skin infections and their sequelae (glomerulonephritis) produce very low ASO titers,[91] and in these cases the ADN-B or AH test is preferred. The ASO tube test has a number of disadvantages. False positive results may result from (1) oxidation of the SLO reagent by shaking the vial during rehydration or (2) inhibition of low titer of SLO by lipoprotein, cholesterol, normal sera, or bacterial growth products in the serum. The irregular spacing of the dilution intervals is also a bothersome feature.

Antistreptolysin O microtitration test

The ASO microtitration test[92] has the advantage of reduced cost over the tube test, because a larger number of tests can be run per unit time, requiring less reagents.

Equipment and reagents (commercially available from Beckman Instruments, Fullerton, Calif.):
1. Microtitration equipment: microdiluters (0.05 ml), disposable U plates (0.025 and 0.05 ml), and calibrated dropper pipets
2. Centrifuge
3. Microdiluter testers
4. Test reading mirror
5. Vibratory mixer (Syntron paper jogger)
6. Serologic pipets
7. Gelatin-barbital buffer (GB)
8. SLO
9. Suspension of sheep or rabbit red cells, 2.5%
10. Cold distilled water
11. Ice
12. Standard antiserum
13. Test sera

Preparation of 2.5% red cell suspension:
1. Pipet 3-4 ml citrated rabbit or sheep blood through two layers of clean gauze into 15 ml graduated centrifuge tube. Add 2 or 3 volumes of GB to each volume of blood. Centrifuge at 600 × g for 5 min.
2. Remove supernatant and layer of white cells. Fill centrifuge tube with GB. Resuspend cells by mixing gently with pipet. Centrifuge at 600 × g for 5 min. Repeat washing process twice. If supernatant is not colorless after two washings, cells are too fragile and should not be used.

3. After second washing, add GB to packed cells up to 10 ml graduated mark. Resuspend cells with pipet. Centrifuge at $600 \times g$ for 10 min. Record column of packed cells and remove supernatant. Prepare 2.5% suspension by adding 3.9 ml buffered diluent to each 0.1 ml packed cells.

4. Store cell suspension at 4° C. Discard at first sign of hemolysis or contamination.

Preparation of initial serum dilutions: The initial serum dilutions of 1:10, 1:60, and 1:85 are prepared in test tubes. Subsequent dilutions are prepared in U plates. Both serum and GB should be at room temperature when preparing dilutions. Include standard serum of known titer in each day's run to serve as positive control. Prepare dilutions as shown below. Mix thoroughly.

Tube no.	Initial dilution	GB	Undiluted serum	1:10 serum
1	1:10	0.9 ml	0.1 ml	0.2 ml
2	1:60	1.0 ml	—	0.2 ml
3	1:85	1.5 ml	—	0.2 ml

Procedure[4]: Label microtiter U plate as indicated in plate pattern (Fig. 35-10), so that each specimen is assigned two rows (a 1:60 row and a 1:85 row), with six wells per row. Label six wells on bottom row of each plate as specimen hemolysis controls. Also label a well for streptolysin control and a well for red cell control on one plate in each run (not for each plate).

Add GB at room temperature as follows:

1. 0.05 ml (0.05 ml dropper) to wells 2-6 of each row assigned to specimens and to SLO control well

2. 0.025 ml (0.025 ml dropper) to each serum hemolysin control well

3. 0.075 ml (0.025 dropper) to red cell control well

Pipet (with 0.2 ml pipet) 0.1 ml of each 1:60 serum dilution into labeled test well. Pipet 0.1 ml of each 1:85 serum dilution into labeled test well and 0.05 ml into serum hemolysin control wells. Test 0.05 ml microdiluter for accuracy. Transfer 0.05 ml from first well to second well. Prepare serial twofold dilutions through sixth well. Serum dilutions for each serum are as follows: first row—1:60, 1:120, 1:240, 1:480, 1:960, and 1:1920; second row—1:85, 1:170, 1:340, 1:680, 1:1360, and 1:2720. Check microdiluters for accuracy and place in distilled water for rinsing. Repeat any dilution series that gives an inaccurate diluter check.

Reconstitute SLO reagent according to package directions with cold distilled water. Mix gently to avoid aeration. Keep reconstituted reagent in ice water. Add 0.025 ml cold SLO reagent to all wells except red cell and serum hemolysin controls.

Turn on vibrator. Place plate on vibrator for 20 sec. Remove plate before stopping vibrator. CAUTION: Extended agitation may cause oxidation and inactivation of SLO.

Cover plate with empty plate. If there is more than one test plate, three plates may be stacked, with a cover placed on top. Place covered plate in 37° C incubator for 15 min. Remove plate from incubator and add 0.025 ml (with 0.025 ml dropper) of cold 2.5% red

cells to all wells. Do not add red cells to more than six plates at a time before mixing on vibrator, because red cells will settle out and will be more difficult to resuspend.

Mix on vibrator for 15-20 sec or until all cells are in suspension. Restack and cover plates. Incubate at 37° C for 15 min. Remove plates from incubator.

Mix on vibrator for 15-20 sec or until all cells are in suspension. Restack and/or cover plates. Reincubate at 37° C for 30 min. Centrifuge plates for 2 min at 250 $\times$ g to pack red cells (1200 rpm in size 2 international centrifuge with no. 976 head).

Read for presence or absence of hemolysis by using reading mirror and fluorescent lamp.

Reading of test:
1. Examine streptolysin control for presence of complete hemolysis.
2. Examine cell control for absence of hemolysis.
3. Examine serum control for absence of hemolysis.
4. For validity repeat the test on all sera in the run if:
   a. Titer of reference serum is not as stated by manufacturer
   b. SLO control does not show complete hemolysis of red cells
   c. Red cell control shows any hemolysis
5. If there is hemolysis in serum hemolysin control, test on that specimen is not valid unless there is at least one well above 1:85 dilution in test (for that particular serum) that has no hemolysis. Hemolysis in serum hemolysin control well indicates presence of natural hemolysin for red cells in patient's serum. This hemolysin is usually diluted out at dilutions above 1:85 and does not interfere with determination of end point.

Reporting results: The titer may be expressed in Todd units (TU) if the potency of the SLO used in the test has been adjusted against the Todd standard or in international units (IU) if the potency of the SLO used in the test has been adjusted against the WHO international standard. For practical purposes, these two units are equivalent.

Precautions and suggestions:
Streptolysin:
1. Avoid shaking or aeration of streptolysin solution. Mix gently when reconstituting; oxidation reduces hemolytic activity.
2. Discard leftover streptolysin solution; it is not reusable.

Red cell suspension:
1. Do not use same pipet dropper for red cells that was used for streptolysin solution; trace of streptolysin in dropper can cause some lysis of cells.
2. Do not add cells to more than six plates at a time before mixing plates; cells settle out and are difficult to resuspend.

Incubation:
1. To ensure proper incubation temperature for all plates, do not put more than three plates (plus cover) in a stack.
2. Keep a pan of water in incubator to provide a moist atmosphere to prevent evaporation from plates.

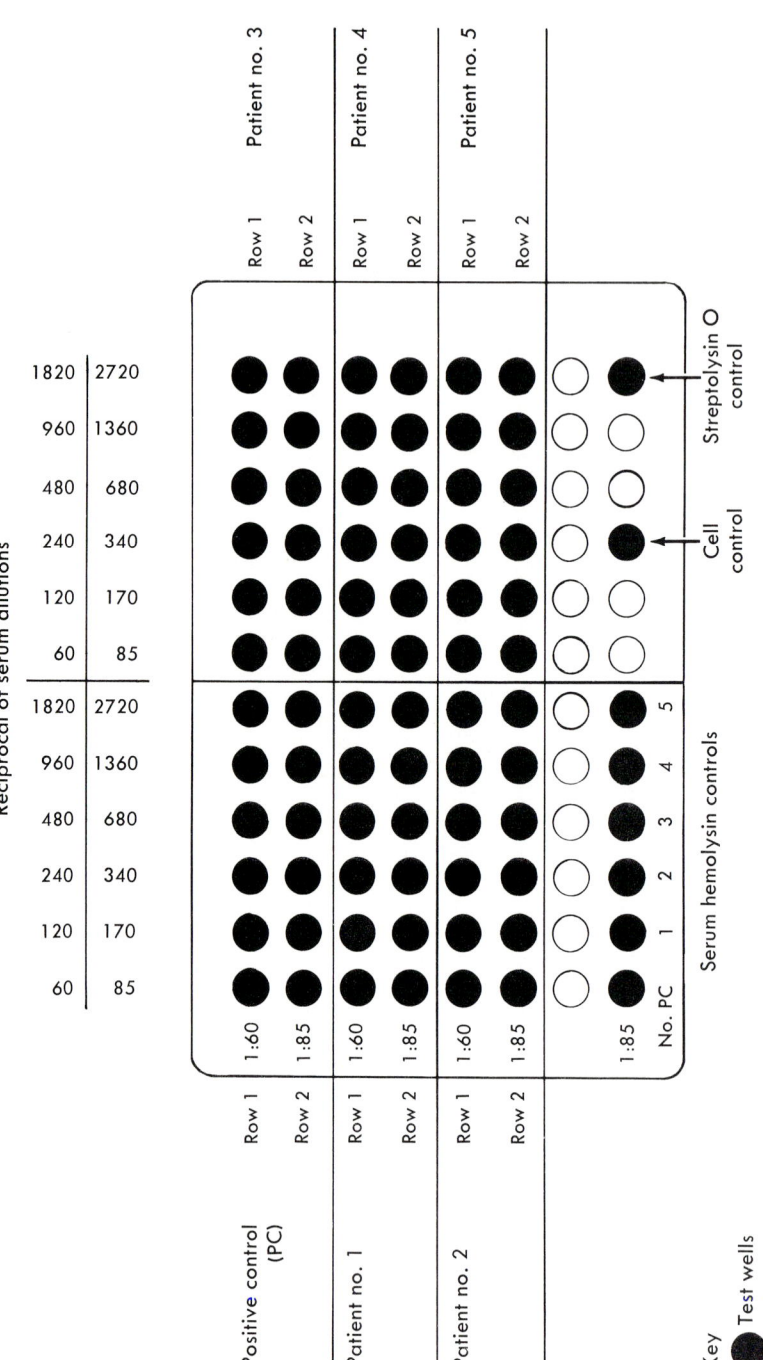

Fig. 35-10. ASO titration plate pattern. (From Palmer, D.F., Cavallaro, J.J., and Galt, R.H.: Laboratory diagnosis by serology methods, Atlanta, 1975, Centers for Disease Control.)

Antistreptolysin O latex agglutination test

Principle: The antistreptolysin O (ASO) latex agglutination test employs an immunologic reaction that has two phases: (1) The serum (containing ASO) is adsorbed by the antigen (streptolysin O [SLO]), which is designed to neutralize approximately 200 Todd units (TU), since only titers exceeding this value are of interest to physicians treating adult patients. (2) Subsequent addition of ASO reagent coating the surface of biologically inert latex particles results in agglutination if any ASO remains unneutralized.

Equipment and reagents (commercially available from Calbiochem-Behring Corp., San Diego):
1. Test tubes
2. Pipets, 0.5 ml and 0.1 ml
3. Serofuge
4. Black test slide
5. Pasteur pipets
6. Slide rotator
7. Stirring rod
8. High-intensity light
9. SLO (β-hemolytic streptococci C), lyophilized, reconstituted according to manufacturer's specifications
10. ASO reagent (suspension of latex particles coated with SLO, pH 8.2, in glycine buffer)
11. ASO positive control (serum containing ASO exceeding 200 TU [IU/ml])
12. ASO negative control (serum containing ASO below 100 TU [IU/ml])
13. Normal saline

Procedure:

Qualitative determinations: Bring all reagents and serum samples to room temperature. Add normal saline as indicated on label to a vial of lyophilized SLO. Shake gently to dissolve.

Pipet 0.3 ml solution into three small test tubes. Add 0.1 ml patient's serum to first tube, 0.1 ml ASO positive control to second tube, and 0.1 ml ASO negative control to third tube. Mix by shaking. Let tubes stand for 15 min at room temperature.

Place 1 drop (0.05 ml)* of each mixture on three separated fields on test slide. Shake ASO latex reagent to obtain uniform suspension. Expel contents of dropper, refill, and add 1 drop to each field containing sample to be tested. Mix well with stirring rod, spreading mixture over most of field. Tilt slide through several planes for 5 min. Rotary shaker may also be used.

Examine for agglutination immediately using direct light (e.g., high-intensity lamp) at a distance of approximately 10-15 cm from surface of slide. Suitable equipment for analysis of agglutination tests may also be used. Reaction of test serum is compared to ASO positive and negative control sera.

Quantitative determinations: The ASO latex agglutination test may be modified to quantitate the ASO concentration (latex kit titration). For procedure see Sonnenwirth.[109]

Results: No agglutination is reported if the ASO titer is less than 200 TU. Agglutination of the latex particle

suspension indicates that ASO is present in the serum in a concentration exceeding 200 TU (IU/ml). Positive or negative results may be caused by 200-230 IU/ml. Agglutination by the slide test should be followed by the tube test.

Discussion: Bach et al.[93] compared an ASO latex kit (qualitative method) with the tube dilution hemolysis method of Rantz and Randall[90] in measurement of ASO antibody levels. Although the latex procedure is standardized on the basis of international units,[94] the results they presented with their study were expressed in Todd units. All sera with 250 TU or above were positive with the ASO latex reagent.[93] At ASO titers of 166 TU, a frequently used upper limit of normal,[95] 10% of the sera tested were negative by latex agglutination. Specimens with titers in the range of 100-125 TU showed variable agglutination patterns. All of the sera with an ASO titer below 100 TU were negative. Prozone reactions may be responsible for false negative results. In general, the strength of the agglutination does not reflect the ASO concentration.[93]

Multienzyme test (Streptozyme) for detection of antibodies to streptococcal extracellular antigens[96]

The Streptozyme (Wampole Laboratories, Cranbury, N.J.) test described below is a qualitative test, but it can also be used for determining a quantitative Streptozyme antibody titer. Streptozyme (STZ) offers a simple, rapid screen or titration method for detection of antibodies to the extracellular antigens of streptococcus A, such as may develop in streptococcal pharyngitis, rheumatic fever, pyoderma, glomerulonephritis, and other related conditions. Since streptolysin is only one of several streptococcus A exoenzymes, the antistreptolysin O (ASO) test will not detect the other antibodies to exoenzymes of streptococcus A that are discovered by the Streptozyme test.

Examinations of over 1000 sera[96-100] have shown that approximately 80% of the sera positive by Streptozyme at a 1:100 dilution (100 STZ units) have an ASO titer of 166 Todd units (TU) or above, whereas an additional 10% showed an antistreptokinase (ASK) and/or antihyaluronidase (AH) titer also above 166. Positive agglutination in the other 10% is speculated to be caused by the presence of antibodies to other streptococcal extracellular antigens[98,101] or to the combined effect of several antibodies, which individually would fall below the 166 titer. Practically no sera with an elevated ASO titer are missed by the Streptozyme slide test. Thus the accuracy of detection of antibodies to extracellular antigens of streptococcus A is superior for Streptozyme as compared to the conventional ASO test used alone.[100,101]

Streptozyme detects more positive specimens than any single test for streptococcal exoenzyme antibodies.[97,100] It is recognized that a single determination of antibodies to streptococcal A extracellular antigens is not as significant as serial titrations performed at weekly or biweekly intervals for up to 6 weeks following the streptococcal infection. Positive sera should be further diluted to determine the titer. Sequential determinations can give the trend of the patient's antibody

---

*If a Pasteur pipet is used to dispense serum-SLO mixture, 2 drops may have to be used to obtain required volume (0.05 ml).

production to allow clinical conclusions with regard to the progress of the disease and treatment.

Cholesterol and β-lipoproteins that may cause false positive titers with the classic ASO test do not interfere with the Streptozyme test.[97]

Principle: The Streptozyme reagent consists of a standardized suspension of aldehyde-fixed sheep cells sensitized with streptococcus A extracellular antigens, including some of the classic exoenzymes, e.g., streptolysin, streptokinase, hyaluronidase, DNase, and NADase, that will react with antibodies to these antigens to give a positive agglutination reaction.

Reagents:
1. Streptozyme reagent (standardized sheep cells sensitized with streptococcus A extracellular antigens); cell concentration = 3-5%; contains buffer and preservative
2. Positive control serum (human); contains preservative; reconstitute to 1.0 ml

PRECAUTIONS: Before use, read instructions carefully. For indications of deterioration, read instructions.

Specimen collection and preparation:
1. Fresh or inactivated serum or plasma as well as peripheral blood from fingertip or earlobe may be used.
2. If serum is to be tested, fresh serum should be used. If serum cannot be tested within 24 hr after collection, it should be stored frozen. If sample to be tested is to be mailed, a preservative such as 0.1% sodium azide or thimerosal (1:10,000) should be added. In frozen state, serum may be kept for extended periods.
3. When performing test with blood, a heparinized capillary or the plain capillary supplied in the kit may be used.

Materials:
1. Reagent
2. Positive control serum
3. Calibrated capillary tubes and bulbs
4. Mirrored glass slide
5. Isotonic saline (0.85% sodium chloride)
6. Stirrers
7. Pipets or syringes with large hypodermic needles
8. Conventional test tubes

Procedure for qualitative determinations with serum or plasma: To obtain accurate and reproducible results, the test procedure must be carefully followed.
1. Dilute serum sample 1:100 with isotonic saline.
2. Fill capillary to mark (0.05 ml) with diluted serum and expel into section of slide.
3. Add 1 drop of reagent.
4. Using disposable stirrer, thoroughly mix fluids. Use clean stirrer for each mixture.
5. Rock mirror slide back and forth gently and evenly for 2 min at rate of 8-10 times per minute; then stop rocking and gently place slide on flat surface and observe for agglutination within 10 sec.

NOTE: Direct light source above slide facilitates reading.

Procedure for peripheral blood:
1. Draw blood from fingertip, earlobe, or other suitable area.

2. Allow capillary supplied to fill to line (0.05 ml).
3. Without allowing blood to clot and using bulb supplied, expel sample into tube containing 2.5 ml isotonic saline. On a basis of a 50% hematocrit, this 1:50 blood dilution is equivalent to a 1:100 serum dilution.
4. Proceed as with steps 2-5 under "Procedure for qualitative determinations with serum or plasma."

Positive results with Streptozyme, compared with positive results for ASO, antideoxyribonuclease B, and antihyaluronidase individually tested, agreed in over 96% of the cases; overall agreement was approximately 93% for both positive (elevated) and negative (nonelevated) titers.[96] The accuracy of Streptozyme in a group of 76 patients with streptococcal disease, including acute rheumatic fever, acute glomerulonephritis, pharyngitis, and pyoderma was found to be 95%.[97]

Results: Positive sera show readily visible agglutination. Negative sera are uniformly turbid or slightly granular.

Procedure for quantitative determinations with serum or plasma: To obtain the level of Streptozyme antibody (STZ titer), dilutions of the serum or plasma are prepared.[2] The results of the dilution test should not be reported in Todd units, since Streptozyme detects antibodies to multiple streptococcal extracellular antigens, only one of which is SLO. For the same reason it is possible for a patient to have a significant STZ titer while showing a negative ASO response.

Antihyaluronidase test

Most group A streptococci produce the enzyme hyaluronidase. Many individuals, after a group A streptococcal infection, develop an increasing titer of antihyaluronidase (AH), an antibody that inhibits the activity of the enzyme.

Principle: The antihyaluronidase test (AHT) is an enzyme neutralization test based on the mucin clot prevention test for hyaluronidase[102] in which streptococcal hyaluronidase is used as antigen[103] and the patient's AH is the antibody. If AH is present in the patient's serum, it inhibits the streptococcal hyaluronidase from hydrolyzing its substrate, potassium hyaluronate, which in the presence of acetic acid, forms a mucin clot. The test materials are commercially available (Difco Laboratories, Detroit).

Procedure: Add constant volume of standardized hyaluronidase to serial doubling dilutions of the patient's serum in water. Incubate the mixture at 37° C for 15 min; then refrigerate for 10 min.

Add constant volume of potassium hyaluronate (hyaluronidase substrate) to each tube, and incubate the mixture at 37° C for 20 min; then refrigerate for 30 min. Add 0.1 ml of 2N acetic acid to each tube, and mix by vigorous shaking.

Observe the tubes for presence or absence of clot formation. Negative or positive controls must be included.

Interpretation: If AH is present in the patient's serum, it inactivates its antigen, hyaluronidase, which is unable to interact with potassium hyaluronate, its substrate. On addition of acetic acid the potassium hyaluronate forms a clot. If the hyaluronidase is not neutralized by AH, it splits the potassium hyaluronate, so that on addition of acetic acid no clot forms. The end point is the highest dilution of serum that gives a definite clot. The AHT titer is the reciprocal of this value.

Normal range: Titers up to 250.

Discussion: The AH test is useful as a second test accompanying the ASO titer, since in acute glomerulonephritis following streptococcal skin infections, the ASO levels are usually low, and the factors that may lead to false positive ASO tests do not influence the AH (or the antideoxyribonuclease B) test.

Antideoxyribonuclease B test[104,105]

Streptococci produce a number of deoxyribonucleases; however, DNase B is found only among group A β-hemolytic streptococci and a few strains of groups C and G organisms. An increasing titer of antideoxyribonuclease B (ADN-B) is therefore a good indicator of infection with group A streptococci.

Principle: The ADN-B antibody in the serum inactivates the streptococcal DNase B antigen that is added to the system and is thus prevented from depolymerizing the DNA methyl green substrate, which is included as an indicator of the anti–DNase B activity. All materials are commercially available (Beckman Instruments, Fullerton, Calif.), and the test is performed with microtitration equipment.

Procedure: Add a constant volume of DNase B to various dilutions of patient's and control sera prepared with a special buffer. During the ensuing period of incubation the DNase B interacts with its antibody (ADN-B) in the serum. At the completion of the incubation, add a constant volume of deoxyribonucleic acid (DNA) to the serum (antibody–DNase B mixture), which is reincubated. The DNA acts as an indicator of the antigen-antibody reaction. If the DNase-B has been inactivated by the specific antibody (ADN-B) in the serum, it will not depolymerize the DNA substrate. In the microtitration test, methyl green is added as an indicator of DNA polymerization. It remains green when linked to polymerized DNA, but it loses its color if combined with depolymerized DNA.[106]

Results: Results are reported in units, as the reciprocal of highest dilution with at least a 3 + reaction. Reference values given by Peacock and Tomar[3] are as follows: adults, 75%, (less than 680 units); school-aged children, 80% (less than 680 units); and preschool children, 90% have no titer. The upper limits of normal values quoted by Klein, Baker, and Jones[105] are as follows: adults, 85 units; school-aged children, 170 units; and preschool children, 60 units.

Discussion: The ADN-B test is probably the best single test for the serologic detection of recent hemolytic streptococcal infection.[92] Compared to the ASO titer the rise of the ADN-B test occurs later and lasts longer.

C-reactive protein

C-reactive protein (CRP) is an abnormal glycoprotein that appears in blood in the acute stages of various inflammatory disorders but is undetectable in the blood of healthy persons. The name of the protein is derived from the fact that it forms a precipitate with the non-type-specific somatic C polysaccharide of the *Pneumococcus*. It is probably an α-globulin, consisting of at least 2 components, and its production is stimulated by bacterial infections or the products of injured tissue. CRP is an acute-phase reactant, which becomes elevated in the serum several days after the onset of an inflammatory event and declines rapidly as the inflammatory process abates. It is elevated in acute rheumatic fever, bacterial infections, myocardial infarcts, rheumatoid arthritis, carcinomatosis, gout, and viral infections.

The clinical indications of CRP overlap with those of an equally nonspecific test, the sedimentation rate, but there are advantages of the CRP test over the erythrocyte sedimentation rate: (1) The sedimentation rate may be elevated without the presence of an inflammatory process, as in anemia, pregnancy, the convalescent stage of an infectious disease, nephrotic syndrome, and hyperglobulinemia; and (2) the sedimentation rate may be normal in patients with frank rheumatic activity in the presence of congestive heart failure. In such cases, CRP, which is present only in inflammatory conditions, is a valuable adjunct or substitute for the sedimentation test.

In rheumatic patients treated with ACTH and cortisone, CRP reappears when the treatment is discontinued. In most cases this is caused by the so-called rebound phenomenon, which disappears within days. When CRP is present in such cases for a period of longer than 2 weeks, treatment is renewed, since the persistence of CRP is considered evidence of the persistence of rheumatic activity.

CRP in spinal fluid: Corrall et al.[106a] report that CRP in cerebrospinal fluid is more sensitive in differentiating bacterial from nonbacterial meningitis than any other single test.

Excellent discussions and reviews of CRP were published by Hedlund[107] and Fischel.[108]

CRP is measured by means of an antibody to purified CRP by capillary precipitin reaction, radial immunodiffusion, and a latex slide test, (the recommended test procedure).

Rapid latex slide test

The rapid latex slide test is much more rapid and convenient than the capillary precipitin test and others. It is also more sensitive than the capillary precipitin tests. It can be employed as a screening test to detect the presence of CRP or as a quantitative test to determine its level in the patient's serum. A kit is commercially available (Hyland Laboratories, Costa Mesa, Calif.).

Qualitative procedure: Inactivate test serum at 56° C for 30 min. Prepare a 1:5 dilution of serum under test by adding 0.1 ml serum to 0.4 ml glycine-saline buffer diluent.

Using one of the capillary pipets supplied, place a drop of diluted serum in one section of a divided slide. Using same pipet, place a drop of undiluted serum in another section of slide. The same capillary pipet may be used for transferring both samples, provided it is used for the diluted one first and then emptied as com-

Table 35-11. Interpretation of rapid slide latex test

Undiluted serum	Diluted serum	Interpretation
0 to 2+	2+ to 4+	Strongly positive
3+ to 4+	0 to 2+	Positive
1+ to 2+	Negative	Weakly positive
Negative	Negative	Negative

Courtesy Hyland Laboratories, Costa Mesa, Calif.

pletely as possible before it is used for the undiluted sample.

Add 1 drop of latex anti-CRP reagent* to each section. With a wooden applicator or toothpick, mix each reaction mixture (diluted sample first) and spread over are approximately 20 × 25 mm.

Tilt slide slowly from side to side for 1-2 min and observe for macroscopic clumping.

Interpretation: The test is an antigen-antibody reaction, which is most marked when the reactants are in optimal concentrations. Prozones may be encountered, in which case flocculation will be seen with diluted serum and a weak or negative reaction with undiluted serum. Visible flocculation in either or both sections indicates the presence of CRP. Serum devoid of this abnormal protein will give a smooth suspension with no visible flocculation in either section. Interpretation of results may be made as shown in Table 35-11.

Quantitative procedure: Prepare dilutions of serum in glycine-saline buffer diluent. Serum specimens are tested at dilutions of 1:2, 1:4, 1:8, 1:16, 1:32, and 1:64. Occasionally greater dilutions may be necessary.

Using a capillary pipet, transfer 1 drop of each serum dilution to successive sections of divided slide. The same capillary pipet may be used for a series of dilutions if the transfer is started with the highest dilution and continued toward the lowest dilution. Add 1 drop of latex–anti-CRP reagent to each drop of serum dilution. Using wooden applicator or toothpick and starting with highest serum dilution, mix each reaction mixture and spread it over an area approximately 20 × 25 mm.

Tilt slide slowly from side to side for 1-2 min and observe for macroscopic agglutination.

Interpretation: The highest serum dilution showing visible flocculation is taken as the CRP titer of the specimen.

Febrile agglutination tests[109]

Agglutination tests have been widely used for the detection of antibodies in the patient's serum against various disease-producing microorganisms. The early example of such procedures was the **Widal test,** devised for the diagnosis of typhoid fever, It employed as antigen a suspension of killed *Salmonella typhi* organisms.

Essentially the same technic is used in many other diseases; the antigen used is a suspension of the bacteria causing the suspected disease. The tests, commonly

referred to as febrile agglutination tests, are employed in the indirect diagnosis of various enteric fevers (typhoid and paratyphoid), brucellosis, tularemia, pertussis, glanders, leptospirosis, and various rickettsial diseases, e.g., Rocky Mountain spotted fever and typhus.

The *Proteus* antigens listed below have been widely used in a procedure known as the **Weil-Felix reaction** for the diagnosis of diseases caused by rickettsiae. *Proteus* organisms possess antigens in common with the rickettsiae and thus have been used to detect rickettsial antibodies.

Certain rules are essential in the performance and evaluation of febrile agglutination tests:

1. A single agglutination test is of little value. At least two and prefereably more tests should be performed every 3-5 days after the onset of the disease to demonstrate a change in antibody titer. Many individuals possess agglutinins in their sera to several of the antigens commonly used. These agglutinins are usually of low titer (with *Salmonella* antigens, usually 20-80 or occasionally 160). Others have agglutinins caused by immunization. A definite change, usually a significant rise, occurs in the first 8-15 days of the illness. A progressive increase in titer is the prime evidence of infection. If the tests are performed late in the disease, a gradual decline in the titer will be noted over a period of time.

2. Antibodies are occasionally produced through stimulation by a new and unrelated infection (**anamnestic reaction** caused by group bacterial antigens).

3. The tests have usually been performed as a battery. Such a battery includes titrations with a number of antigens. Slide agglutination tests are used as screening procedures. Any positive or doubtful reaction should be repeated with the macroscopic tube agglutination test. In recent years the battery usually includes the following antigens[109]:

Salmonella group A	Paratyphoid A (a)
Salmonella group B	Paratyphoid B (b, 1, 2)
Salmonella group C (C₁ and C₂)	Paratyphoid C (c, 1, 5)
Salmonella group D (typhoid)	Typhoid H (d)
Salmonella group E	*Brucella abortus*
Proteus OX-19	*Francisella tularensis*

The *Salmonella* group antigens are somatic (O) antigens, and the paratyphoid and typhoid (d) antigens are flagellar (H) antigens; both should be used.

Value of and discrepancies in Salmonella and other febrile agglutination tests

The value of the *Salmonella* agglutination tests has declined as (1) the incidence of typhoid fever has decreased, at least in the developed world, (2) the general use of vaccines has increased, and (3) ever-increasing numbers of antigenically related serotypes of *Salmo-*

---

*Latex particles precoated with anti-CRP (serum hyperimmune to CRP).

nella have been recognized. The sensitivity of the *Salmonella* agglutination test is poor, and the titers of antibody against O and H antigens at times have been misleading and lacking correlation with (cultural) diagnosis.

The value of the **Weil-Felix** (*Proteus*) **test** for diagnosis of Rocky Mountain spotted fever has recently been challenged by Hechemy et al.,[110] who found very extensive differences in results obtained by the classic Weil-Felix procedure and by the recently described specific microimmunofluorescence test employing rickettsial antigens.[111]

On the other hand, there is little doubt about the value of agglutination tests in suspected cases of brucellosis, tularemia, or leptospirosis. Antibodies to these organisms can usually be demonstrated with considerably higher specificity and sensitivity than those against *Salmonella*.

Slide agglutination test

A number of investigators have claimed that a simple quantitative slide agglutination test for the detection of exclusion of serum agglutinins developed during certain febrile infections is as informative as the tube agglutination procedure. The rapid slide agglutination test is used as a screening procedure. (Some commercial tularemia antigens are to be used only for tube agglutination tests.) The technic described is based on the use of commercial antigens; the technic for the use of antigens of various manufacturers is, with minor variations, generally the same.

Procedure*: Use commercial antigens. Most commercial antigen bottles contain droppers standardized to deliver approximately 0.03 ml antigen. Conduct tests on a large sheet of plate glass (30 × 41 cm) that has been ruled into 3.8 cm squares with a diamond point or wax pencil.

Using a 0.2 ml pipet, deliver 0.08, 0.04, 0.02, 0.01, 0.005, and 0.002 ml quantities of serum to squares or rings of one row, from left to right. Do this with serum to be tested for as many rows as there are antigens to be used. Use clear, unheated serum. Mix antigen vials by shaking. With dropper of antigen vial place 1 drop of antigen on each quantity of serum on each row, from left to right.

When the antigen (1 drop) is mixed with quantities of serum indicated the test will approximate the results of the conventional tube dilution test in the following dilutions: 1:20, 1:40, 1:80, 1:160, and 1:320. Further dilutions may be prepared by using a 1:10 dilution of serum in physiologic saline and the volumes described above.

Proceeding from right to left, mix contents of each square of one horizontal row with wooden applicator stick or glass rod. Use new applicator or wipe glass rod clean before mixing contents of squares of another horizontal row.

Hold glass plate near an adequate light source. Slowly rock and tilt and observe for a period not to exceed 3 min. Record all observed degrees of agglutination as follows:

Complete (100%) agglutination	4 plus(+ + + +)
Approximately 75% agglutination	3 plus (+ + +)
Approximately 50% agglutination	2 plus (+ +)
Approximately 25% agglutination	1 plus (+)
No agglutination	Negative (−)

The smallest quantity of serum that exhibits a 2 plus (+ +) or 50% agglutination is considered the end point of serum reactivity or serum titer. Therefore if a serum specimen showed the pattern given in Table 35-12, it would be reported as the following serum titers:

Antigen X	1:160
Antigen Y	1:80
Antigen Z	1:80

Interpretation: It is important that there be close communication between the physician and the laboratory. Results should always be interpreted with reference to clinical data.

A single test result is not diagnostically significant unless the titer is unusually high. In the unvaccinated patient a serologic diagnosis is usually made if there is fourfold rise in O antigen titer or if the titer for O antigen is higher than 1:50 or 1:100 on a single specimen taken in the first 2-3 weeks of infection. Antibiotic treatment in typhoid fever often prevents a rise in titer, or it may inhibit the development of detectable antibody.

Negative results: Negative results may be caused by the absence of the agglutinin sought (i.e., the patient does not have the infection for which the test was made) or because the blood was taken too early in the disease (before the appearance of sufficient agglutinin in the serum). It should be remembered that a positive result following a negative one after several days (rise in titer) is usually significant. Negative results do not necessarily rule out infection, and such results are best used as baselines for subsequent comparative titrations.

Positive results: Past history of immunization or infection is important in the correct interpretation of positive results.

In **brucellosis** a titer of 1:160 is suggestive of recent infection. Persistently low titers are significant if previous tests were negative. Individuals who had brucellosis may be nonspecifically restimulated by subsequent nonbrucellar infections, with their *Brucella* titer rising

Table 35-12. Agglutination pattern of a serum against three different antigens

Serum (ml)	Equivalent dilution	Antigen X	Antigen Y	Antigen Z
0.08	1:20	4+	4+	3+
0.04	1:40	4+	3+	2+
0.02	1:80	4+	2+	2+
0.01	1:160	2+	1+	−
0.005	1:320	−	−	−
0.002	1:640	−	−	−

---

*Condensed from *Clinical laboratory aids manual*, Pearl River, N.Y., 1968, Lederle Laboratories (now out of print).

rapidly (1:160) and then dropping precipitously in 10-15 days.

In suspected **acute brucellosis,** the following should be noted[4]:

1. Little or no titer may develop during the first 10 days of illness.
2. Acute- and convalescent-phase serum specimens, taken 2-4 weeks apart and tested in the same test run, are essential for demonstration of active infection. A fourfold rise in titer is significant.
3. The titer may decline after the sixth week or may persist as high as 1:160 for years after apparent clinical recovery; therefore a titer of 1:160 or above is indicative of *Brucella* infection at some time but not necessarily of current or recent infection.

In **chronic brucellosis** there is no definite criterion whereby the significance of an agglutination test titer may be judged. No diagnostic question is likely to be raised about persons yielding high titers (titers higher than 1:160) and clinical findings that are compatible with modern knowledge of brucellosis while showing no symptoms of tularemia. Even though a titer of 1:20 is obtained, infection with *Brucella* cannot be ruled out on the basis of agglutination tests alone. In fact, some individuals, although infected, do not develop agglutinins.

Persons who have recovered from brucellosis may have *Brucella* antibodies restimulated nonspecifically by any subsequent febrile illness. In such instances agglutination tests may rise to 1:160 or sometimes higher in a few days and drop to negative or 1:20 within 10 days. Such reactions confuse test interpretation.

In **tularemia,** serum agglutinin titers of 1:80 or 1:160 usually appear in the second week of the disease and increase considerably during the fourth to seventh week (1:640-1:10,240), with a gradual dropping in titer at the end of 1 year. Uninfected individuals may have titers of 1:40. If only a single specimen is available, a titer of 1:160 or above is indicative of a *Francisella* infection at some time but not necessarily of current or recent infection. Agglutinins decline slowly but may be detectable for life.

Cross-reactions often occur and must be considered. Vaccinations with typhus (rickettsial) antigen will evoke the formation of *Proteus* OX-19 antibodies. Cholera vaccine may produce *B. abortus* antibodies. Tularemia agglutinins may agglutinate *B. abortus,* whereas *Brucella* agglutinins may react with *P. tularensis.*

Tube agglutination test

The macroscopic tube agglutination test represents more work than the rapid slide agglutination test. However, it is the definitive procedure in confirming or ruling out results of the slide test. False positive slide tests are usually ruled out by the tube test. It is useful in clarifying erratic or equivocal agglutination or prozone reactions obtained in the slide test and in the accurate determination of the variations in serum antibody titers that occur during the various stages of infection.

Procedure: See Sonnenwirth.[109]

Serologic tests for Mycoplasma infections

Three methods are available for the detection of antibody to *Mycoplasma pneumoniae:* complement fixation, metabolic inhibition, and fluorescent antibody technic.[112,113] The first two procedures measure antibody to lipid determinants of the organism and are of about equal sensitivity.[114]

Complement-fixation test

The complement-fixation test procedure uses paired sera and a standard microtiter complement-fixation technic. Whole organism antigens are commercially available, although lipid extracts are preferred. The titration is set up in such a way that twofold dilutions of antigen are tested against twofold dilutions of human serum. Paired sera should be collected at the onset of the infection and then again after 3 weeks and sould exhibit a fourfold rise in antibody titer.[115] For microtiter complement-fixation procedure see reference 6.

Cold agglutinin test

The cold agglutinin test has long been used for the diagnosis of *M. pneumoniae* infections, because an increase in antibodies is found in 34-68% of *M. pneumoniae* infections.[115] However, the test is not specific for *M. pneumoniae,* a variety of other diseases will also produce a fourfold rise.

Procedure: The cold agglutinin test of Schmidt et al.[116] is recommended.

Blood to be tested for cold agglutinins should be stored at room temperature before separation of the clot. Storage at 4° C will result in absorption of antibodies onto red cells but warming to 37° C will release cold agglutinins.[117]

Prepare twofold serial dilutions of serum in saline and dispense in 0.1 ml volumes into test tubes. Add to each tube a 0.1 ml volume of 1.0% human O erythrocytes. Incubate tubes at 4° C for 1 hr.

Read tests immediately on removal from cold. A positive test will result in a button on the bottom of the tube that is difficult to disrupt by gentle shaking. Reversibility of agglutination is tested by incubation at 37° C for 15-30 min.

Highest dilution of antibody that agglutinates red cells and that is reversible at 37° C is termed the end point of the test.

Interpretation: A fourfold or greater rise in cold agglutinins is suggestive of a recent *M. pneumoniae* infection. High titers (greater than 1:32) may indicate infection with *M. pneumoniae* but are frequently present in the absence of such infection.

Indirect fluorescent antibody test for Legionnaires' disease

The indirect fluorescent antibody (IFA) test was applied to Legionnaires' disease studies by McDade et al.[117] The demonstration of titers in the sera of patients with Legionnaires' disease established the newly isolated bacterium as the causative agent of the disease.

The IFA test for the detection of antibodies in human serum to the Legionnaires' disease bacterium (LDB) appears to be specific; however, if possible, all positive results should be accompanied by isolation[117] or direct demonstration of the LDB.[118,119] Until recently LDB isolates were serologically similar, and only one representative antigen was needed for competent IFA screening. The discovery of distinct serogroups (four at the time of this writing) means that several antigens are now required for IFA screening and that even more may be required later when more serogroups are defined.

The IFA test[120] for the LDB is the primary diagnostic tool.

Procedure: See Philip et al.[111]

Latex agglutination test for Cryptococcus neoformans antigen[121-125]

Cryptococcosis is a systemic infection caused by the pathogenic fungus *Cryptococcus neoformans*. The organism gains entrance to the body by causing a brief, inflammatory lung infection. From there it rapidly disseminates and shows a preference for the central nervous system. *C. neoformans* is usually a secondary invader, which coexists with tuberculosis, hematologic malignant diseases, and diabetes. Therapy with corticosteroids, other immunosuppressive agents, or broad-spectrum antibiotics may also reduce a patient's resistance to this disease. Thus the symptoms of cryptococcosis may be masked by those of the primary affliction.

Until recently, the sole method of diagnosis of cryptococcosis was the culturing of *C. neoformans* from blood or cerebrospinal fluid (CSF). Cryptococcosis, however, is one of the diseases in which antigens of the infective agent circulate within the host, and the latex agglutination (LA) test for *Cryptococcus* (Crypto LA Kit, International Biological Laboratories, Cranbury, N.J.) detects these antigens.[6]

The LA test provides a technic for detecting the polysaccharide antigen of *C. neoformans* in serum or CSF. This technic gives more rapid results than isolation of *C. neoformans* from serum or CSF, and antigen is occasionally detected in patients from whom no organism can be isolated. Rheumatoid factor in the patient's serum may interfere with the test.

The test is an **indirect agglutination procedure** that uses latex particles sensitized with either normal or anticryptococcal rabbit globulin. When the anticryptococcal globulin–sensitized latex comes in contact with the polysaccharide antigen of *C. neoformans* in the specimen, the globulin-polysaccharide complex reacts, causing the sensitized latex to agglutinate. Latex sensitized with normal rabbit globulin should not be agglutinated by the polysaccharide antigen. Serum or CSF specimens that show agglutination with both the anticryptococcal globulin–sensitized latex and the normal globulin–sensitized latex usually show interference caused by rheumatoid factor (RF) in the sample. Any samples that show agglutination with both the sensitized latex reagents should be titrated with both reagents through a series of twofold dilutions. If the titer of the serum when tested with anticryptococcal globulin–sensitized latex is at least fourfold higher than when tested with normal globulin–sensitized latex, cryptococcosis is suspected, although a positive diagnosis cannot be made because of the interference. Nearly equal titers with the two reagents give an equivocal test, and subsequent samples should be tested for a rising titer with the anticryptococcal globulin–sensitized latex.

Agar-gel immunodiffusion test for histoplasmosis[4,126-134]

Histoplasmosis is caused by a yeastlike fungus, *Histoplasma capsulatum*. Because of the varying clinical manifestations of histoplasmosis, laboratory procedures are essential for diagnosis. Dermal sensitivity to histoplasmin persists for years after recovery and may be of little use in an endemic area because of the high incidence of positive but otherwise healthy reactors. The skin test is also complicated by frequent cross-reactions with other mycoses, e.g., blastomycosis and coccidioidomycosis. Culturing of *H. capsulatum* is probably the most conclusive laboratory procedure, but it is not always easy to accomplish. The agar-gel precipitin test in conjunction with other serologic procedures, e.g., the complement-fixation test,[6] is of considerable value in the diagnosis and prognosis of histoplasmosis. It can be performed with relative ease and in most cases will distinguish hypersensitivity and chronic infection from an active case of histoplasmosis. It is especially useful when the complement-fixation test is negative or the patient's serum is anticomplementary.

Principles:
1. Homologous antigen and antibody, diffusing toward each other through a semisolid medium, will mix at some point in optimal or near optimal proportions to form a visible band of precipitate.
2. *Histoplasma* antibodies in a patient's serum will precipitate one or more antigens present in a histoplasmin preparation.
3. *Histoplasma* antibodies in a patient's serum can be identified by allowing the patient's serum and the known histoplasmin antigen to diffuse toward each other through a semisolid medium and then comparing the resulting bands of precipitation with those of a reference antiserum.

Procedure: See Sonnenwirth.[109]

Serology of Epstein-Barr virus and infectious mononucleosis

Henle, Henle, and Horwitz[135] have firmly established the etiologic relation of Epstein-Barr virus (EBV) to infectious mononucleosis (IM). Henle's investigations are also discussed in Chapter 9. Several groups of EBV-associated antigens have been identified by the indirect immunofluorescence (IF) technic, e.g., the viral capsid antigen (VCA), which is antigenic and leads to the production of corresponding antibodies. IgG antibodies to VCA can be detected in sera from all individuals who have become infected with EBV in the past and have remained carriers.[136] IgM antibodies to EBV are found only in primary EBV infection,[136] and IgA antibodies are encountered in nasopharyngeal carcinoma. Antibodies to the EBV–early induced antigens (EA) are strikingly disease specific, and an antibody to the D variant of EA is found in IM. Whenever a patient with IM has anti-VCA antibodies, he also has anti-EBV-associated nuclear antigen (EBNA) antibodies. The EBV-specific antibody responses in IM are presented in Fig 9-26, but EBV-specific serodiagnosis is not often indicated in patients with IM, because the differential absorption test of Davidsohn and the rapid slide test are specific for the disease. EBV-specific serodiagnostic procedures are indicated in patients who are heterophile antibody negative and present a clinical picture like IM, which may be due to *Toxoplasma*, cytomegalovirus, or other viruses.[137] Serodiagnostic procedures are also indicated when patients present IM-associated complications, e.g., Guillain-Barré syndrome,[138] but lack the clinical and hematologic features of IM.

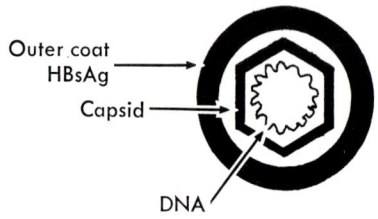

Fig. 35-11. The hepatitis B virus (Dane particle).

Serologic tests for hepatitis

The term *viral hepatitis* includes at least three diseases: type A (infectious, short incubation hepatitis); type B (serum or transfusion hepatitis, homologous serum jaundice, long incubation hepatitis); and type C (non-A, non-B hepatitis), which may include hepatitis caused by cytomegalovirus, Epstein-Barr virus, rubella virus, herpes simplex virus, and enteroviruses.[139]

Hepatitis A

The virus of hepatitis A (HAV) has only one antigen, which 2-4 weeks after exposure to the HAV may be responsible for IgM antibodies, which after 4 weeks are replaced by IgG antibodies. The antigen can be detected in stool specimens by immunofluorescence[140] and by enzyme-linked immunosorbent assay (ELISA).[141] In the acute phase of the disease, IgM anti-HAV antibodies can be demonstrated by radioimmunoassay or by ELISA in the serum of the patient.

Hepatitis B

The hepatitis B virus (HBV), the Dane particle, consists of a number of components: the inner core antigen (HBcAg), the e antigen (HBeAg), and double-stranded DNA (Fig. 35-11). The outer envelope surrounding the core is designated hepatitis B surface antigen, HBsAg,

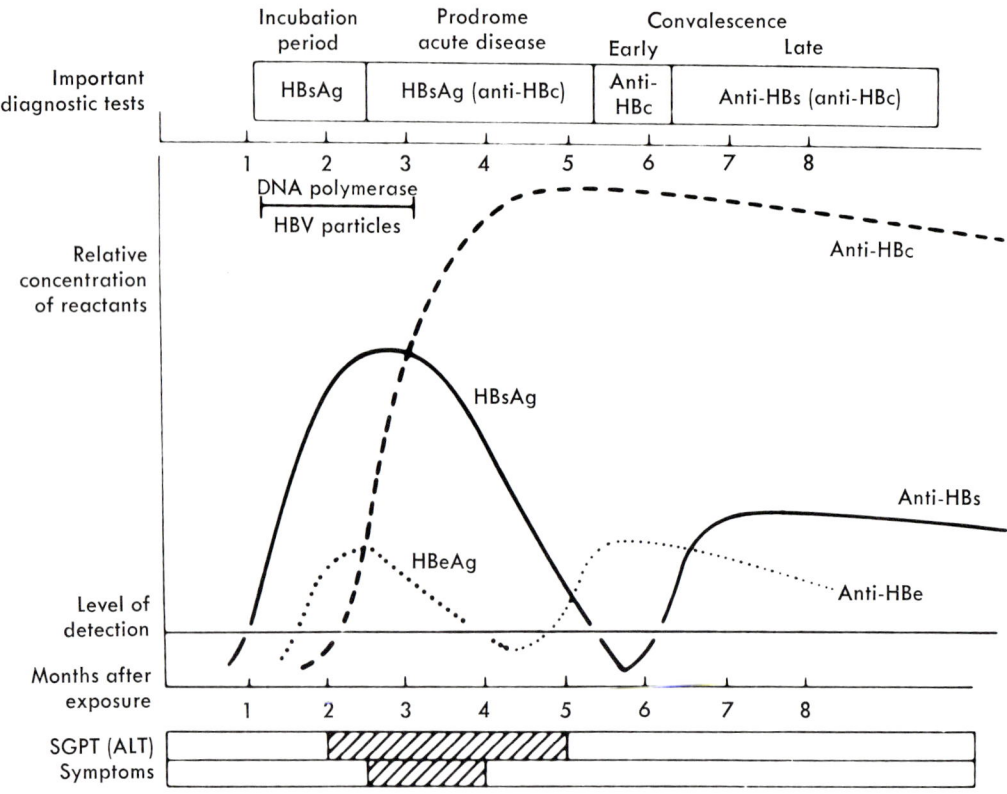

Fig. 35-12. Serologic and clinical patterns observed during acute hepatitis B viral infection. (From Hollinger, F.B., and Dreesman, G.R.: In Rose, N.R., and Friedman, H., editors: Manual of clinical immunology, ed. 2, Washington, D.C., 1980, American Society for Microbiology.)

previously known as Australia antigen or hepatitis-associated antigen. Antibodies to the core, surface, and e antigens are designated anti-HBc, anti-HBs, and anti-HBe antibodies.

Exposure to HBV may produce a complex serologic (and clinical) picture (Fig. 35-12). HBsAg appears 2-4 weeks before demonstrable liver disease, peaks at the onset of the clinical disease, and declines within 4-6 months to undetectable levels. As the liver disease progresses, HBeAg, endogenous DNA polymerase activity, and HBcAg appear in the serum. After clearance of HBsAg and before anti-HBs antibodies make their appearance, anti-HBc may be the only indicator of HBV activity. Anti-HBs and anti-HBc may persist for many years. Anti-HBe develops after anti-HBc and before anti-HBs. Numerous serologic procedures are available for the demonstration of the antigens and antibodies just described. The original studies on HBsAg were done by agar gel immunodiffusion. It was replaced by the more sensitive counterimmunoelectrophoresis[142] and complement-fixation[6] tests. Radioimmunoassay technic provides the most specific and sensitive methods for detecting HBsAg, anti-HBs, and anti-HBc.[143,144]

Non-A, non-B hepatitis (hepatitis C)

About 90% of all transfusion-associated hepatitides are of the non-A, non-B type and are probably the result of infection with a number of viruses. Since serologic markers of this disease are not known at present, the diagnosis of hepatitis C is one of exclusion.

REFERENCES

1. Barrett, J.T.: Textbook of immunology, ed. 3, St. Louis, 1978, The C.V. Mosby Co.
2. Sonnenwirth, A.C., and Neter, E.: In Sonnenwirth, A.C., and Jarett, L., editors: Gradwohl's clinical laboratory methods and diagnosis, ed. 8, St. Louis, 1980, The C.V. Mosby Co., vol. 2.
3. Peacock, J.E., and Tomar, R.H.: Manual of laboratory immunology, Philadelphia, 1980, Lea & Febiger.
4. Palmer, D.F., Cavallaro, J.J., and Galt, R.H.: Laboratory diagnosis by serology methods, Atlanta, 1975, Centers for Disease Control.
5. Sever, J.L.: J. Immunol. **88:**320, 1962.
6. Conrath, T.B., and Coupe, N.B., editors: Handbook of manual microtiter procedures, ed. 2, Place du Commerce, Guernsey, 1978, Dynatech Publications.
7. Cooper, H.A., Bowie, E.J.W., and Owen, C.A., Jr.: Am. J. Clin. Pathol. **57:**332, 1972.
8. Gavan, T.L., and Town, M.A.: Am. J. Clin. Pathol. **53:**880, 1970.
9. Oudin, J.: Comptes Rendu Acad. Sci. **222:**115, 1946.
10. Hayward, B.J., and Augustin, R.: Int. Arch. Allergy **11:**192, 1957.
11. Ouchterlony, Ö.: Handbook of immunodiffusion and immunoelectrophoresis, Ann Arbor, Mich., 1968, Ann Arbor Science Publishers, Inc.
12. Mancini, G., Carbonara, A.O., and Heremans, J.F.: Immunochemistry **2:**235, 1965.
13. Fahey, J.L., and McKelvey, E.M.: J. Immunol. **94:**84, 1965.
14. Laurell, C.-B.: Anal. Biochem. **15:**45, 1966.
15. Laurell, C.-B.: Anal. Biochem. **10:**358, 1965.
16. Cejka, J., Conway, T.P., and Poulik, M.D.: In Sonnenwirth, A.C., and Jarett, L., editors: Gradwohl's clinical

laboratory methods and diagnosis, ed. 8, St. Louis, 1980, The C.V. Mosby Co., vol. 2.
17. Milford-Ward, A.: In Thompson, R.A., editor: Techniques in clinical immunology, London, 1977, Blackwell Scientific Publications, Ltd.
18. Weeke, B.: Scand. J. Clin. Lab. Invest. **22:**107, 1968.
19. Scheidegger, J.J.: Int. Arch. Allergy **7:**103, 1955.
20. Ganrot, P.O.: Scand. J. Clin. Lab. Invest. **29**(suppl. 124):39, 1972.
21. Axelsen, N.H., Bock, E., and Krøll, J.: Scand. J. Immunol. **2**(suppl.):101, 1973.
22. Crowle, A.J.: J. Immunol. Methods **14:**197, 1977.
23. Crowle, A.J.: In Rose, N.R., and Friedman, H. editors: Manual of clinical immunology, ed. 2, Washington, D.C., 1980, American Society for Microbiology.
24. Versey, J.M.B., Slater, L., and Hobbs, J.R.: J. Immunol. Methods **3:**63, 1973.
25. Rytel, M.W.: Hosp. Pract. **10**(10):75, 1975.
26. Farmer, S.G., and Tilton, R.C.: In Lennette, E.H., et al., editors: Manual of clinical microbiology, ed. 3, Washington, D.C., 1980, American Society for Microbiology.
27. Cikes, M.: J. Immunol. Methods **8:**89, 1975.
28. Delaat, A.N.C.: Can. J. Med. Tech. **26:**35, 1964.
29. Delaat, A.N.C.: Primer of serology, New York, 1976, Harper and Row, Publishers, Inc.
30. Standardized diagnostic complement fixation method and adaption to microtest, Atlanta, 1974, Centers for Disease Control.
31. Riggs, J.L., et al.: Am. J. Pathol. **34:**1081, 1958.
32. Faulk, W.P., and Hijmans, W.: Prog. Allergy **16:**9, 1972.
33. Kawamura, A., Jr., editor: Fluorescent antibody techniques and their applications, ed. 2, Baltimore, 1977, University Park Press.
34. Hirst, G.K.: J. Exp. Med. **75:**49, 1942.
35. Stevens, R.W.: In Friedman, H., Linna, T.J., and Prier, J.E., editors: Immunoserology in the diagnosis of infectious diseases, Baltimore, 1979, University Park Press.
36. Bird, G.W.G., and Wingham, J.: In Thompson, R.A., editor: Techniques in clinical immunology, London, 1977, Blackwell Scientific Publications, Ltd.
37. Sever, J.L., Krasny, M.A., and Ley, A.C.: In Friedman, H., Linna, T.J., and Prier, J.E., editors: Immunoserology in the diagnosis of infectious diseases, Baltimore, 1979, University Park Press.
38. Yalow, R.S., and Berson, S.A.: J. Clin. Invest. **39:**1157, 1960.
39. Ogle, J.D., and Ogle, C.K.: In Natelson, S., Pesce, A.J., and Dietz, A.A., editors: Clinical immunochemistry, Washington, D.C., 1978, American Association of Clinical Chemistry.
40. Engvall, E., and Perlmann, P.: J. Immunol. **109:**129, 1972.
41. Engvall, E., and Perlmann, P.: Immunochemistry **8:**871, 1971.
42. Wide, L., Bennich, H., and Johansson, S.G.O.: Lancet **2:**1105, 1967.
43. Miles, L.E.M., and Hales, C.N.: Nature **219:**186, 1968.
44. Addison, G.M., and Hales, C.N.: In Kirkham, K.E., and Hunter, W.M., editors: Radioimmunoassay methods, Baltimore, 1971, The Williams & Wilkins Co.
45. Rubenstein, K.E., Schneider, R.S., and Ullman, E.F.: Biochem. Biophys. Res. Commun. **47:**846, 1972.
46. Greenwood, H.M., and Schneider, R.S.: In Natelson, S., Pesce, A.J., and Dietz, A.A., editors: Clinical immunochemistry, Washington, D.C., 1978, American Association of Clinical Chemistry.
47. Lizana, J., and Hellsing, K.: Clin. Chem. **20:**1181, 1974.

48. White, R.M., et al.: Ann. Clin. Lab. Sci. **6:**525, 1976.
49. Brown, W.J., et al.: Syphilis and other venereal diseases, Cambridge, Mass., 1970, Harvard University Press.
50. Olansky, S.: In Samter, M., and Alexander, H.L., editors: Immunological diseases, Boston, 1965, Little, Brown & Co.
51. Nicholas, L.: In Friedman, H., Linna, T.J., and Prier, J.E., editors: Immunoserology in the diagnosis of infectious diseases, Baltimore, 1979, University Park Press.
52. Wallace, A.L., and Harris, A.: Bull. WHO **36** (suppl. 2):1, 1967.
53. Willcox, R.R., and Guthe, T.: Bull. WHO **35:**1, 1966.
54. Jaffe, H.W.: Ann. Intern. Med. **83:**846, 1975.
55. Hunter, E.F., Deacon, W.E., and Meyer, P.E.: Public Health Rep. **79:**410, 1964.
56. Coffey, E.M., et al.: Appl. Microbiol. **24:**26, 1972.
57. Hunter, E.F., et al.: Bull. WHO **39:**873, 1968.
58. Shore, R.N., and Faricelli, J.A.: Arch. Dermatol. **113:**37, 1977.
59. McKenna, C.H., et al.: Mayo Clin. Proc. **48:**545, 1973.
60. Cohen, P., Stout, G., and Ende, N.: Arch. Intern. Med. **124:**364, 1969.
61. Tomizawa, T., and Kasamatsu, S.: Jpn. J. Med. Sci. Biol. **19:**305, 1966.
62. Rathlev, T.: Br. J. Vener. Dis. **43:**181, 1967.
63. Sparling, P.F.: N. Engl. J. Med. **284:**642, 1971.
64. Sever, J.L.: J. Pediatr. **75:**1111, 1969.
65. Scotti, A.T., and Logan, L.: J. Pediatr. **73:**242, 1968.
66. Sepetjian, M., et al.: Br. J. Vener. Dis. **46:**18, 1970.
67. Escobar, M.R., Dalton, H.P., and Allison, M.J.: Am. J. Clin. Pathol. **53:**886, 1970.
68. Hooshmand, H., Escobar, M.R., and Kopf, S.W.: J.A.M.A. **219:**726, 1972.
69. Robertson, R.G., and Walsh, W.T.: In Friedman, H., Linna, T.J., and Prier, J.E., editors: Immunoserology in the diagnosis of infectious diseases, Baltimore, 1979, University Park Press.
70. Manual of tests for syphilis, Atlanta, 1969, Centers for Disease Control.
71. Bodily, H.L., Updyke, E.L., and Mason, J.O.: Diagnostic procedures for bacterial, mycotic and parasitic infections, ed. 5, New York, 1970, American Public Health Association.
72. Wallace, A.L.: Am. J. Clin. Pathol. **44:**712, 1965.
73. Portnoy, J., Garson, W., and Smith, C.A.: Public Health Rep. **72:**761, 1957.
74. Portnoy, J., et al.: Public Health Rep. **76:**933, 1961.
75. Portnoy, J.: Am. J. Clin. Pathol. **40:**473, 1963.
76. Portnoy, J., and Garson, W.: Public Health Rep. **75:**985, 1960.
77. Technique for the automated reagin test (ART), Atlanta, 1970, Centers for Disease Control.
78. Falcone, V.H., Stout, G.W., and Moore, M.B., Jr.: Public Health Rep. **79:**491, 1964.
79. Portnoy, J.: Public Health Lab. **23:**43, 1965.
80. Harris, A., Rosenberg, A., and Del Vecchio, E.R.: J. Ven. Dis. Inform. **29:**72, 1948.
81. Deacon, W.E., Lucas, J.B., and Price, E.V.: J.A.M.A. **198:**624, 1966.
82. Stout, G.W., et al.: Health Lab. Sci. **4:**5, 1967.
83. Staff of the Venereal Disease Research Laboratory: Health Lab. Sci. **5:**23, 1968.
84. Lewy, J.E.: Pediatr. Clin. North Am. **23:**751, 1976.
85. Wannamaker, L.W.: Circulation **48:**9, 1973.
86. Klein, G.C.: In Rose, N.R., and Friedman, H., editors: Manual of clinical immunology, ed. 2, Washington, D.C., 1980, American Society for Microbiology.
87. Zabriskie, J.B., Hsu, K.C., and Seegal, B.C.: Clin. Exp. Immunol. **7:**147, 1970.
88. Shulman, S.T., and Ayoub, E.M.: J. Clin. Invest. **54:**990, 1974.
89. Todd, E.W.: J. Exp. Med. **55:**267, 1932.
90. Rantz, L.A., and Randall, E.: Proc. Soc. Exp. Biol. Med. **59:**22, 1945.
91. Kaplan, E.J., et al.: J. Clin. Invest. **49:**1405, 1970.
92. Klein, G.C., et al.: Am. J. Clin. Pathol. **53:**159, 1970.
93. Bach, G.L., et al.: Am. J. Clin. Pathol. **52:**126, 1969.
94. Spaun, J.M., et al.: Bull. WHO **24:**271, 1961.
95. Davidsohn, I., and Nelson, D.A.: In Davidsohn, I., and Henry, J.B., editors: Todd-Sanford clinical diagnosis by laboratory methods, ed. 15, Philadelphia, 1974, W.B. Saunders Co.
96. Klein, G.C., and Jones, W.L.: Appl. Microbiol. **21:**257, 1971.
97. Bisno, A.L., and Ofek, I.: Am. J. Dis. Child. **127:**676, 1974.
98. Janeff, J., et al.: Lab. Med. **2:**32, 1971.
99. Collins, O.D., III.: Am. J. Clin. Pathol. **57:**598, 1972.
100. Dodge, W.F., et al.: N. Engl. J. Med. **286:**273, 1972.
101. Ofek, I., et al.: Clin. Pediatr. **12:**341, 1973.
102. Quinn, R., and Liao, S.: J. Clin. Invest. **29:**1156, 1950.
103. Harris, T.N., and Harris, S.: Am. J. Med. Sci. **217:**174, 1949.
104. Nelson, J., Ayoub, E., and Wannamaker, L.: J. Lab. Clin. Med. **71:**867, 1968.
105. Klein, G.C., Baker, C.N., and Jones, W.L.: Appl. Microbiol. **21:**999, 1971.
106. Kurnick, N.B.: Arch. Biochem. **29:**41, 1950.
106a. Corrall, C.J., et al.: J. Pediatr. **99:**365, 1981.
107. Hedlund, P.: Acta Med Scand. **169**(suppl. 361):1, 1961.
108. Fischel, E.E.: In Cohen, A.S., editor: Laboratory diagnostic procedures in the rheumatic diseases, ed. 2, Boston, 1975, Little, Brown & Co.
109. Sonnenwirth, A.C.: In Sonnenwirth, A.C., and Jarett, L., editors: Gradwohl's clinical laboratory methods and diagnosis, ed. 8, St. Louis, 1980, the The C.V. Mosby Co., vol. 2.
110. Hechemy, K.E., et al.: J. Clin. Microbiol. **9:**292, 1979.
111. Philip, R.N., et al.: J. Clin. Microbiol. **3:**51, 1976.
112. Kenny, G.E.: In Sonnenwirth, A.C., and Jarett, L., editors: Gradwohl's clinical laboratory methods and diagnosis, ed. 8, St. Louis, 1980, The C.V. Mosby Co., vol. 2.
113. Kenny, G.E.: In Rose, N.R., and Friedman, H., editors: Manual of clinical immunology, ed.2, Washington, D.C., 1980, American Society for Microbiology.
114. Senterfit, L.B., Pollack, J.D., and Somerson, N.L.: Proc. Soc. Exp. Biol. Med. **140:**1294, 1972.
115. Grayston, J.T., Foy, H.M., and Kenny, G.E.: In Hayflick, L., editor: The mycoplasmatales and L. phase of bacteria, New York, 1969, Appleton-Century-Crofts.
116. Schmidt, N.J., et al.: J. Immunol. **97:**95, 1966.
117. McDade, J.E., et al.: N. Engl. J. Med. **297:**1197, 1977.
118. Chandler, F.W., Hicklin, M.D., and Blackmon, J.A.: N. Engl. J. Med. **297:**1218, 1977.
119. Cherry, W.B., et al.: J. Clin. Microbiol. **8:**329, 1978.
120. Jones, G.L., and Hebert, G.A., editors: "Legionnaires": the disease, the bacterium and the methodology, Atlanta, May 1978 (revised October 1978), Centers for Disease Control.
121. Bennett, J.E., and Bailey, J.W.: Am. J. Clin. Pathol. **56:**360, 1971.
122. Bloomfield, N., Gordon, M.A., and Elmendorf, D.F., Jr.: Proc. Soc. Exp. Biol. Med. **114:**64, 1963.
123. Goodman, J.S., Kaufman, L., and Koenig, M.G.: N. Engl. J. Med. **285:**434, 1971.
124. Gordon, M.A., and Vedder, D.K.: J.A.M.A. **197:**961, 1966.

125. Kaufman, L., and Blumer, S.: Appl. Microbiol. **16:**1907, 1968.
126. Bennett, D.E.: South. Med. J. **59:**922, 1966.
127. Busey, J.F., and Hinton, P.F.: Am. Rev. Respir. Dis. **92:**637, 1965.
128. Burnett, G.W., and Scherp, H.W.: Oral microbiology and infectious disease, ed. 2, Baltimore, 1962, The Williams & Wilkins Co.
129. Heiner, D.C.: Pediatrics **22:**616, 1958.
130. Kaufman, L.: Public Health Rep. **81:**177-185, 1966.
131. Kaufman, L., Brandt, B., and McLaughlin, D.: Am. J. Hyg. **79:**181, 1964.
132. Schubert, J.H., Lynch, H.J., and Ajello, L.: Am. Rev. Respir. Dis. **84:**845, 1961.
133. Wiggins, G.L., and Schubert, J.H.: J. Bacteriol. **89:**589, 1965.
134. Manual of standardized serodiagnostic procedures for systemic mycosis. Part I. Agar immunodiffusion tests, 1972, Pan American Health Organization.
135. Henle, W., Henle, G., and Horwitz, C.A.: Hum. Pathol. **5:**551, 1974.
136. Henle, W.: In Friedman, H., Linna, T.J., and Prier, J.E., editors: Immunoserology in the diagnosis of infectious diseases, Baltimore, 1979, University Park Press.
137. Klemola, E., et al.: J. Infect. Dis. **121:**608, 1970.
138. Grose, C., et al.: N. Engl. J. Med. **292:**392, 1975.
139. Hollinger, F.B., and Dreesman, G.R.: In Rose, N.R., and Friedman, H., editors: Manual of clinical immunology, ed. 2, Washington, D.C., 1980, American Society for Microbiology.
140. Mathiesen, L.R., et al.: Infect. Immun. **18:**524, 1977.
141. Mathiesen, L.R., et al.: J. Clin. Microbiol. **7:**184, 1978.
142. Dreesman, G.R., Hollinger, F.B., and Melnick, J.L.: Appl. Microbiol. **24:**1001, 1972.
143. Purcell, R.H., et al.: Intervirology **2:**231, 1973/74.
144. Ling, C.M., and Overby, L.R.: J. Immunol. **109:**834, 1972.

Clinical immunology

Clinical immunology is a rapidly expanding and evolving field in the modern clinical laboratory that is

The author is indebted to Lii-Mei Tsai, M.D., Stanford T. Roodman, Ph.D., and Janet C. Kister, M.T.(A.S.C.P.) and I.(A.S.C.P.), for their suggestions and technical help in the preparation of this manuscript.

directly and indirectly related to patient care. The emergence of laboratories devoted to clinical immunology in most large medical centers and several community hospitals has steadily increased during the past decade. Clinical immunology is no longer and should not be limited to the "serology section" in clinical microbiology; nor should it be placed in the special chemistry division in clinical chemistry.

This chapter is intended to convey relatively comprehensive up-to-date laboratory information regarding the rapidly increasing knowledge in the field of medical immunology. Because of the great diversity in immunologic reactions and variable instrumental applications of immunologic technics, the scope of this chapter will be limited to the practice and readily applicable immunologic methodology in most medical centers and hospital laboratories.

LABORATORY INVESTIGATION OF IMMUNE DEFICIENCY DISEASES

Immune deficiency diseases may be caused by defects in quality or quantity of lymphocytes and may be either congenital or acquired.[1,2] The congenital defects are rare but tend to be more severe than the acquired deficiencies, which are fairly common and vary in their clinical expression. Both are responsible for an increased susceptibility to repeated bacterial, viral, and fungal infections and for frequent lack of response to therapy.

Immunoglobulin (Ig) disorders involve the plasma cell–lymphocyte–macrophage system responsible for the defense and the immune responses of the body. Immunoglobulin disorders may be the result of (1) defective immunoglobulin synthesis, either congenital or acquired; (2) excessive protein loss; (3) increased immunoglobulin catabolism; or (4) immunoglobulin overproduction, either benign or malignant. The first three defects are responsible for the immune deficiency diseases, while the fourth abnormality results in the production of polyclonal or monoclonal (M proteins) gammopathies.

For convenient classification and approach, immune deficiencies are divided into (1) humoral (immunoglobulins [B-lymphocyte] and complement components), (2) cell mediated (cellular [T-lymphocyte], and (3) combined (T and B cell). Actually, it has been found that complex interaction and cooperation between T- and B-lymphocytes are required for immune competence in humans.

Classification of immune deficiency diseases[1-5]

I. Congenital deficiencies
  A. B cell defects (humoral)
    1. Infantile X-linked agammaglobulinemia (Bruton's agammaglobulinemia)[6]
    2. Selective immunoglobulin deficiencies: IgA, IgG, IgM, and IgE[7,8]
  B. T cell defects (cellular, cell mediated)
    1. Thymic hypoplasia (DiGeorge's syndrome, pharyngeal pouch syndrome)[9]
    2. Lymphopenia with normal immunoglobulins (Nezelof's syndrome)[10]
  C. Combined T and B cell defects
    1. Agammaglobulinemia with thymoma[11]
    2. Ataxia-telangiectasia[12]
    3. Severe combined immunodeficiency (stem cell defect,[13] Swiss-type agammaglobulinemia, thymic alymphoplasia, adenosine-deaminase deficiency)[13-15]
    4. Immunodeficiency with short-limbed dwarfism[16]

II. Acquired deficiencies
  A. B cell defects (humoral immune deficiencies)
    1. Transient hypogammaglobulinemia of infancy (prematurity, delayed maturity)[17]
    2. Hypogammaglobulinemia and agammaglobulinemia
    3. Variable immunoglobulin deficiencies (dysgammaglobulinemias, selective decreased synthesis of various immunoglobulins)
    4. Steroid and immunosuppressive therapy
    5. Autoimmune disorders
      a. Systemic lupus erythematosus
      b. Lymphocytic thyroiditis
      c. Rheumatoid arthritis
    6. Lymphoproliferative disorders[18-20]
      a. Non-Hodgkin's lymphomas
      b. Leukemias
      c. Multiple myeloma
      d. Waldenström's macroglobulinemia
    7. Bone marrow disorders (e.g., myelosclerosis)
    8. Protein loss
      a. Protein-losing enteropathy (ulcerative colitis, Whipple's disease, Menetrier's disease)
      b. Burns (exfoliative dermatitis)
    9. Nephrotic syndrome
      a. Diabetes
      b. Lupus erythematosus
      c. Chronic glomerulonephritis
      d. Lipoid nephrosis
      e. Amyloidosis
    10. Intestinal lymphangiectasia
    11. Hypercatabolism
  B. T cell defects (cellular immune deficiencies)[21]
    1. Mycosis fungoides and Sézary's syndrome
    2. Hodgkin's disease
    3. Chronic lymphocytic leukemia
    4. Systemic lupus erythematosus
    5. Immunosuppressive therapies
  C. Combined T and B cell defects[21-23]
    1. Intestinal lymphangiectasia[22]
    2. Wiskott-Aldrich syndrome[24]
    3. Immunosuppressive therapies

Laboratory tests for immune deficiency diseases

The suggested laboratory tests for the investigation of immunodeficiencies are as follows:

1. Complete blood count
2. Serum protein electrophoresis
3. Serum IgG (and subclasses), IgM, IgD, IgE, and IgA quantitation
4. Secretory IgA level
5. Immunoglobulin catabolic rates
6. Bone marrow and/or lymph node examination
7. Quantitation of antibodies to widely distributed antigens, e.g., titration of isohemagglutinins and antistreptolysin O antibodies
8. B cell quantitation by immunofluorescence
9. Tests involving effectors of B cell function
  a. Complement assay
  b. Phagocytic function tests
10. T cell quantitation by E (erythocyte) rosette technic
11. Lymphocyte function studies

Complete blood count

The first evidence of a defect responsible for repeated infections may be an absolute neutrophil count below 1800 cells/mm^3, an absolute lymphocyte count below 1500 cells/mm^3, or a thrombocytopenia below 50,000 platelets/mm^3 (Wiskott-Aldrich syndrome).[24] Lymphopenia is found (1) in congenital B cell deficiencies such as lymphopenic agammaglobulinemia and dysgammaglobulinemia, (2) in T and B cell deficiencies such as severe combined immunodeficiency (SCID) and intestinal lymphangiectasia,[22] and (3) in T cell deficiencies such as thymic hypoplasia (also known as DiGeorge's syndrome). Since 75-80% of the peripheral blood lymphocytes are T cells, the lymphocyte count is of special importance in the evaluation of these cells.

Serum protein electrophoresis

Hypogammaglobulinemia is seen in congenital and acquired B cell deficiencies and in some lymphoproliferative disorders, notably in light-chain disease and chronic lymphocytic leukemia. It may also be seen in bronchiectasis, sprue, thymomas, pernicious anemia, protein-losing enteropathies, and space-occupying bone marrow lesions. A normal serum protein electrophoretogram may at times hide functionally deficient immunoglobulins.

Quantitation of serum immunoglobulins (immunoelectrophoresis, radial immunodiffusion, or laser nephelometry)

Deficiencies of all immunoglobulins are found in infantile agammaglobulinemia, delayed or transient hypogammaglobulinemia of infancy, combined immunodeficiencies, toxic suppression of immunoglobulins (uremia, lymphomas), increased loss (nephrosis, etc.), and certain infections.

Selective IgG deficiency may be seen in prematurity, delayed maturity, hypercatabolism of IgG (shortened half-life and often decreased production), and protein loss. It is rarely the only deficiency and may be combined with IgA deficiency and increased or decreased IgM levels. The presence of M proteins in immunoelectrophoresis is usually emphasized by the depression of the normal immunoglobulins.

Selective IgA deficiency is seen in about 0.5% of normal individuals. It also occurs in most cases of ataxia-telangiectasia, with IgG deficiency, and with T cell defects.

Selective IgM deficiency is most commonly secondary to uremia and to lymphoreticular neoplasms.[20] In Wiskott-Aldrich syndrome the depressed IgM level contrasts with the increased IgA level.

Secretory IgA level

IgA is a major immunoglobulin of exocrine secretions. Saliva is a suitable test material to demonstrate IgA activity. In selective IgA deficiency, serum and secretory IgA are usually deficient.

Catabolism of immunoglobulins

IgG is normally gradually broken down with a half-life of about 24 days. Hypercatabolism of IgG leading to IgG deficiency has been reported in association with an anti-IgG antibody (IgM)[25] as seen in paroxysmal nocturnal hemoglobinuria.[26]

Bone marrow or lymph node examination

Since the plasma cells are the terminal cells of the B-lymphocyte transformation and are responsible for immunoglobulin production, bone marrow or lymph node examination is a useful method of their quantitation. In agammaglobulinemia and hypogammaglobulinemia they are absent or markedly reduced.

Quantitation of antibodies to widely distributed antigens

B cell function can be evaluated by assaying the titer of universal or widely distributed antibodies, e.g., isohemagglutinins or antistreptolysins.

B cell quantitation by immunofluoresence

The number of B cells can be estimated by the demonstration of surface immunoglobulins using antisera to whole immunoglobulins (IgG, IgM, IgA, and IgD) and to κ- and λ-light chains. The B cells are decreased in the B cell deficiencies mentioned on p. 1065. See also "Isolation and characterization of human lymphocytes," p. 1070.

Evaluation of effectors of B cell function

B cell function can be mediated by several effectors, e.g., complements, and by phagocytosis. The complement concentration is reduced in the complementopathies, and the phagocytic function of granulocytes is impaired in the granulocytopathies.

Laboratory evaluation of complement system

The complement system consists of a group of interacting glycoproteins present in fresh serum that aid or "complement" the activity of antibodies in defense and immunologic reactions.[27,28] A total of more than 11 complement components are recognized and are symbolized by the letter C and a number. A bar over the number indicates an activated component. C1 consists of three subfragments, which are suffixed with lowercase letters. Discounting these subfragments, the components in order of their reactivity are C1, C4, C2, C3, C5, C6, C7, C8, and C9. Each of these components exists in the inactive form until activated by either of two mechanisms: (1) the classic, or intrinsic, pathway and (2) the properdin, extrinsic, or alternate pathway. The initial activation is followed by a series of sequential reactions and interactions that transform inactive precursors into active proteolytic enzymes and join some of the cleavage products to each other or to other complement components.[29] The complement system also includes at least three inhibitors, which inhibit certain steps in the complement activation scheme.[30] The classic complement pathway is activated by antigen-antibody complexes of IgG and IgM acting on C1, which is cleaved and acts on its substratum, C4 and C2, the activation product of which acts on C3, which is cleaved into a number of fragments, which act on C5, C6, and C7. The activated complexes of C5, C6, and C7 act on C8 and C9.

The alternate pathway of complement activation does not require an antigen-antibody interaction but involves the properdin system, which acts on C3 and is activated by microbial polysaccharides.[31,32] The system of serum proteins includes properdin (P) itself and two factors designated D and B. The activated forms are symbolized by bars over the numbers (e.g., $\overline{C42}$). This properdin pathway can also be activated by IgA or IgE immune complexes.

Complement activity is associated with a number of biologic phenomena. It enhances the phagocytic activity of granulocytes and monocytes by producing increased vascular permeability and stimulating opsonization, immune adherence, chemotaxis, and lysis. It is therefore closely associated with inflammatory responses and host defense against pathogenic organisms (see discussion of granuloctye function tests elsewhere).

In the so-called immune complex diseases (lupus erythematosus, acute and subacute glomerulonephritis) complement activation is the result of tissue-bound antigen-antibody complexes and is directly related to the tissue injury produced by these complexes and their complement by-products.

Complement is also involved in anaphylaxis, since it increases vascular permeability and causes degranulation of mast cells, or basophils.

Complements play a role in the antibody (B cell) mediated lysis of bacteria and thus in the host defense against infection.[5,33] Complement is associated with the initial phases of phagocytosis, e.g., chemotaxis, opsonization, immune adherence, and bacterial inactivation. A number of approaches can be utilized to measure complement: (1) a functional approach to quantitate the total hemolytic activity of complement, (2) a quantitative approach to measure the concentration of individual proteins of the complement system, or (3) the demonstration of complement fixation in tissues by immunofluorescence (p. 1111). Most clinical laboratories are able to investigate complement levels by immunochemical methods (radial immunodiffusion or laser nephelometry), which in recent years because of their accuracy and ease of performance have found wider use than the functional hemolytic assays. The complementopathies of clinical importance are the congenital or acquired deficiencies.

Congenital complement deficiencies[34]: Individuals heterozygous for a deficient complement component usually have 20-40% of the normal complement component level, whereas the homozygous absence of the genes controlling the complement synthesis leads to a total absence of the complement component. Individuals who have defects in the early phases of the classic pathway of C3 activation are usually free of clinical evidence of disease because the defect in C3 activation is compensated for by an intact alternate pathway of C3 activation.[35] On the other hand, patients with a C3 de-

ficiency are subject to frequent pyogenic infections because of the pivotal position of C3 in the opsonization of bacteria.[35,36] C5-C9 deficiencies do not lead to recurrent infections but may be responsible for connective tissue or collagen disease–like states (Table 36-1).

Two inherited abnormalities of the complement inhibitor system are clinically important. The first is hereditary angioneurotic edema, which results from the defective synthesis of C1 esterase inhibitor.[37] Patients with this abnormality experience recurrent episodes of edema of sudden onset. The serum of heterozygous patients contains 10-30% of the normal inhibitor level. The clinical diagnosis is supported by the immunochemical demonstration of low C4, C2, and C1 esterase inhibitor levels. C4 concentration is abnormally low during and between attacks. In some cases the concentration of the inhibitor is normal but the molecule is functionally deficient.[38] The functionally deficient inhibitor molecule usually exhibits abnormal electrophoretic mobility.[39]

A second inactivator deficiency involves the C3 inactivator the homozygous deficiency of which leads to increased susceptibility to infections.[40]

Table 36-1. Complement deficiency states of humans*

Component	Number of patients†	Clinical findings
Classic pathway		
C1r	3	Glomerulonephritis (1), LLS (2)
C1s	5	SLE (2), LLS (1), normal (2)
C4	3	SLE (2), normal (1)
C2	42	Normal (18), SLE, DLE, or LLS (16), other (8)‡
C3	5	Recurrent pyogenic infections (4), LLS (1)
C5	2	LLS (1), normal (1)
C6	2	Raynaud's phenomenon and recurrent gonococcal septicemia, recurrent meningococcal meningitis
C7	5	Raynaud's phenomenon and sclerodactyly normal (2), unclassified renal disease, ankylosing spondylitis
C8	3	SLE, xeroderma pigmentosum, disseminated recurrent gonococcal infections
C9	1	Normal§
Alternative pathway		
None known		
Inhibitors		
C1 inhibitor	Many	HAE, SLE, or DLE and HAE (6)
C3b inactivator	2	Recurrent infections
More complex deficiency states		
C1q	Many	Hypogammaglobulinemia
C5 dysfunction	15-20	Leiner's syndrome (gram-negative infections and eczema)
Factor B	Many	Sickle cell anemia

From Atkinson, J.P., and Frank, M.M.: In Parker, C.W., editor: Clinical immunology, Philadelphia, 1980, W.B. Saunders Co., vol. 1.
*Abbreviations: LLS, lupus-like syndrome; SLE, systemic lupus erythematosus; DLE, discoid lupus erythematosus; HAE, hereditary angioedema.
†The number of patients with known genetically controlled homozygous deficiency of complement components is growing rapidly. These numbers are included to indicate relative numbers of patients at the time this review was written.
‡Anaphylactoid purpura (3), dermatomyositis (1), Hodgkin's disease (1), CLL and dermatitis herpetiformis (1), recurrent infections (2), and idiopathic membranous glomerulonephritis (1).
§Of note is the fact that this one patient had a low (approximately 30% of normal) total hemolytic complement activity. Complement-mediated lysis occurs at a reduced rate if C9 is missing, and this fact probably accounts for the lysis observed. This defect would be difficult to detect by CH_{50} assay.

Acquired complement deficiencies: Complement is decreased in a limited number of conditions, e.g., active systemic lupus erythematosus (depression of C4 and C3), acute poststreptococcal glomerulonephritis (depression of C3),[39] and membranoproliferative glomerulonephritis and hypocomplementemic glomerulonephritis (depression of C3).[41] Depressed complement levels are also encountered in malaria, hepatitis B, hemolytic anemias, and rheumatoid arthritis.

Acquired increased complement concentration: Complement may be increased in inflammatory and necrotizing disorders since it represents one of the acute-phase reactants.[39] Elevated values are encountered in infections (C3), acute-phase plasma protein responses (C3), and rheumatoid arthritis (C3).

It is clear from the foregoing enumeration that in clinical practice the quantitation of C3, C4, and C5 by radial immunodiffusion can be substituted for the hemolytic complement assay. On the other hand, if the hemolytic complement assay is performed as a screening test and is found to be low, the following complement components should be quantitated by radial immunodiffusion or by electroimmunodiffusion.

Quantitation of C3, C4, and C3 activator[42] by radial immunodiffusion, electroimmunodiffusion, or laser nephelometry: For the technic see "Quantitation of serum immunoglobulins."

Assay of serum hemolytic complement activity:

Principle: The serum hemolytic complement activity evaluates the functional adequacy of the complement hemolytic system as a whole. The test measures the ability of complement in serum or other fluids to lyse 50% of a standard suspension of sheep red cells coated (sensitized) with rabbit anti-sheep-red-cell antibody and evaluates all components of complement and their inhibitors present in the sample. Varying dilutions of the unknown sample are incubated with sensitized sheep red cells for 30 min at 37° C. After centrifugation the degree of hemolysis is determined spectrophotometrically and the amount of serum containing 1 CH_{50} unit corresponding to 50% hemolysis is read off a graph. From this figure the number of CH_{50} units per milliliter of sample is calculated. Normal fresh human serum contains about 30 or 40 CH_{50} units/ml.

The serum must be used within 1 hr after drawing the blood or stored frozen below 140° C until used.

Reagents:
1. Stock diluent buffer
   Dissolve 83.8 g NaCl, 2.52 g $NaHCO_3$, and 3.0 g sodium diethyl barbiturate in about 1 L water. Dissolve 4.6 g diethylbarbituric acid, 1.0 g $MgCl_2 \cdot 6H_2O$, and 0.14 g anhydrous $CaCl_2$ in about 5 dl hot water. Mix the two solutions, cool, and dilute to 2 L. Store buffer in the refrigerator. The buffer may also be obtained from Cordis Laboratories, Miami, Fla.
2. Working buffer
   Accurately dilute 1 volume of the stock buffer with 4 volumes of distilled water.
3. Sensitized sheep erythrocytes
   These may be obtained from Cordis Laboratories, Miami, Fla. The sensitized sheep cells are suspended in the working buffer to a concentration

of 10^9 cells/ml (1,000,000 cells/mm³). The concentration of the cells may be checked by measuring the absorbance of the suspension at 541 nm. A suspension of 10^9 cells/ml should give an absorbance of 0.680 when read in a cuvet with a 5 mm light path. If a cuvet of this light path is not available, an aliquot of the suspension can be further diluted 1:2 and read in a 10 mm cuvet. Alternately, one can measure the absorbance at 541 nm of a suspension of known concentration (as determined by actual counting) with the cuvets available, and this absorbance may be used to check other suspensions. For example, if a suspension containing 1.23×10^9 cells/ml gave an absorbance of 0.792 in the cuvet used, then the desired concentraion should have an absorbance of 0.792/1.23 = 0.644. The suspension is made up to be slightly more concentrated than desired, the absorbance is measured, and then the suspension is diluted to the required value. For example, if a suspension as measured gave an absorbance of 0.785 in 5 mm cuvets, then to 10 ml of this suspension one would add exactly (0.785 − 0.680)/0.680 × 10 = 1.54 ml buffer to give the required suspension.

Procedure: Dilute serum 1:40 with the working buffer. Set up 12 tubes as outlined in Table 36-2. To each tube add 0.5 ml of well-mixed sensitized cell suspension, diluted serum, buffer, or water as given in Table 36-2. If desired, the tubes may be set up in duplicate. Incubate the tubes at 37° C for 1 hr with gentle shaking. Add 3.5 ml diluent buffer to each tube, mix well, and centrifuge for 15 min at 1800 rpm. Decant the supernatant from the tubes and read absorbance of all tubes at 412 nm.

Calculation: Tube 1 corresponds to zero hemolysis and tube 2 to complete hemolysis. Then if A_3 is the absorbance reading of the third tube, calculate the percent hemolysis for tubes 3-12 as follows:

$$\text{Percent hemolysis} = \frac{A_3 - A_1}{A_2 - A_1} \times 100$$

Table 36-2. Tube arrangement for assay of serum hemolytic complement activity

Tube no.	Diluted serum (ml)	Working buffer (ml)	H₂O (ml)
1	0	1.0	0
2	0	0	1.0
3	0.1	0.9	0
4	0.2	0.8	0
5	0.3	0.7	0
6	0.4	0.6	0
7	0.5	0.5	0
8	0.6	0.4	0
9	0.7	0.3	0
10	0.8	0.2	0
11	0.9	0.1	0
12	1.0	0	0

Plot the percent hemolysis against the amount of diluted serum added to the respective tubes (0.1-1.0 ml) on log paper. Obtain from the curve the amount of the diluted serum that corresponds to exactly 50% hemolysis. Call this value Y. Then the titer of the serum is as follows:

$$\text{Titer} = D/Y \text{ units}$$

where Y is read from the curve and D is the original dilution factor for the serum. In the directions as given above, D = 40, but for serum with very high or low titers it may be necessary to repeat the test using a different initial dilution.

Normal values: Normal values are between 30-40 CH_{50} units/ml and 70-150 CH_{50} units/ml. Normal range should be established in each laboratory.

Interpretation: The hemolytic complement may be normal even if there are significant (50%) reductions in the concentration of some of the individual complement components, e.g., C1, C2, C3, C6, and C7. The concentration of only a few components critically affects the hemolytic assay.

Depression of complement: There are a number of inherited complement deficiencies, e.g., hereditary angioneurotic edema (C1 inhibitor),[43] and deficiencies of C2, C3, and C5.[44-46] Acquired complement deficiencies are found in immune complex diseases[47,48] such as lupus erythematosus (C3 and C4), poststreptococcal glomerulonephritis (C3 and C5), membranoproliferative glomerulonephritis (C3 and C5), diffuse intravascular coagulation (C3),[28] and agammaglobulinemia.[28] Low complement values are seen in some autoimmune hemolytic anemias (C3) during the hemolytic episode, especially if associated with cold antibodies, and in paroxysmal cold hemoglobinuria (C3).[49]

Laboratory investigation of phagocytosis

Methods developed for the investigation of granulocytopathies are described in Chapter 9 and are utilized in the investigation of patients with recurrent bacterial infections. The functional activities of phagocytic cells include chemotaxis, phagocytosis, and bactericidal capacity.

The first step in the investigation of phagocytosis is a total leukocyte and differential count, since, even if the neutrophils are functionally and morphologically normal, a certain number of these cells are required to control infection. The Rebuck skin window[50] and the Boyden chamber technics test for[51] overall defects in the inflammatory response because they are sensitive to abnormalities of chemotaxis and to complement deficiencies.

Chemotactic defects are seen in newborns[52] and in patients with the ''lazy'' leukocyte syndrome,[53] Chédiak-Higashi syndrome,[51] rheumatoid arthritis,[54] diabetes mellitus,[55] cirrhosis,[56] complementopathies,[34] and severe infections characterized by Döhle bodies and toxic granulation.[57] The chemotactic defect does not involve phagocytosis and bactericidal activity, both of which may be normal.

The qualitative, quantitative, or stimulated nitroblue tetrazolium (NBT) tests[58] are used to demonstrate defects in phagocytic function. Such defects are seen in congenital agammaglobulinemia,[59] chronic granulomatous disease,[60] and complement deficiency[34] and in patients receiving cortisone, aspirin, and antibiotic therapy.[61,62] The NBT test stmulated with endotoxin differentiates the effect of antibiotics from that of phagocytic dysfunction.[63]

Phagocytic killing is measured by bactericidal or fungicidal tests.[64] In some patients catalase-producing bacteria are normally phagocytosed but are not killed by the intracellular enzyme system. Such defects are seen in chronic granulomatous disease,[59] myeloperoxidase deficiency,[65] and lysosomal defects of Chédiak-Higashi syndrome.

T cell quantitation by E rosette technic

Since the majority (70-80%) of peripheral blood lymphocytes are T-lymphocytes, lymphocytopenia as discovered by white cell and differential counts is a significant finding in patients with deficient cell-mediated immunity. Special attention must be paid to the number of small lymphocytes, which may be low even in the presence of a normal total lymphocyte count, which may consist mainly of large and medium-sized forms. The high normal absolute lymphocyte count of infants and children must be kept in mind to correctly interpret the functional aspects of the differential count in young patients.[66] In the congenital T cell deficiencies the failure of the development of the thymus and parathyroids, derivatives of the third and fourth brachial arches, leads to hypocalcemia. Peripheral blood T cells can be identified and quantitated by the use of sheep red cells, which adhere to T-lymphocytes forming spontaneous T rosettes, a sensitive T cell marker.

The absence of normal T cell function can be demonstrated by the absence of blastoid transformation when peripheral blood lymphocytes are cultured with phytohemagglutinin or with specific T antigens. The buffy coat lymphocytes can also be tested for failure to release the macrophage migratory inhibitory factor (MIF) (see ''Isolation and characterization of human lymphocytes,'' p. 1070, for a detailed discussion).

Primary T cell deficiency is seen in congenital thymic hypoplasia (DiGeorge's syndrome)[67] and in combination with B cell deficiency in most immunodeficiency states, except the ones that are caused by pure B cell defects (Bruton's agammaglobulinemia). Acquired T cell deficiencies are found in systemic lupus erythematosus, Hodgkin's disease, lymphomas, and immunosuppressive therapy.

General lymphocyte function studies[73,74]

T- and B-lymphocyte quantitation and functional characterization are important laboratory parameters in a number of diseases. B cells are lymphocytes that can synthesize and secrete immunoglobulins, i.e., IgM, IgG, and IgA, on specific challenge by antigens. They have surface immunoglobulins (sIg), which are normally polyclonal, i.e., kappa (κ) and lambda (λ) light chains are present on the cytoplasmic membrane of B cells. Mu (μ) and delta (δ) heavy chains are found usually with either the κ or λ chains on any one cell surface. Gamma (γ) and alpha (α) are rarely found on the surface of properly prepared normal lymphocytes.

T cells are lymphocytes that do not have sIg and do not secrete immunoglobulins but are involved in all other lymphocyte functions through helper or supressor effects. T cells are thymus dependent for maturation into lymphocytes involved in cell-mediated immunity. T cells respond to antigen by dividing and are responsible for delayed hypersensitivity, graft rejection, bacterial and viral killing, and elimination by direct cytotoxic effects or by release of soluble mediators. T cells are enumerated by the formation of spontaneous rosettes with sheep red cells (E rosette).

Normal peripheral blood lymphocytes contain approximately 8-12% (0.25×10^6) B cells per milliliter and 60-75% (1.55×10^6) T cells per milliliter by the tests described in this chapter. These numbers can vary in certain diseases. In acute lymphocytic leukemia, proliferation of T cells or null cells, i.e., lymphocytes with neither sIg or sheep red cell rosette formation, is increased dramatically.[68] Since these two cell types can only be distinguished by immunologic tests and the prognoses for the T and null leukemia are statistically different, knowledge of the particular type of leukemia can be a valuable aid to the physician.

Chronic lymphocytic leukemia is usually a proliferation of monoclonal B cells. Determination of the light- and heavy-chain specificity can often help the physician in observing course of treatment. IgM-κ is the most common sIg in these patients.

Many immunodeficiency diseases exist in which a decrease of T or B cells or both occurs.[1,2] Therefore determination of the actual number of circulating T- and B-lymphocytes can confirm the clinical diagnosis. Wiskott-Aldrich and DiGeorge's diseases are examples of diseases in which T cells are decreased; decreased B cells are found in infantile sex-linked agammaglobulinemia and common variable immunodeficiency; and both T and B cell deficiencies are described in severe combined immunodeficiency.[69] Other diseases are listed in other immunology textbooks and reviews.[70,71]

Selected markers for T- and B-lymphocytes: Lymphocytes can be classified in many different ways: according to size, basophilia of cytoplasm (pyroninophilia), membrane characteristics,[68,72] scanning electron microscopic appearances, life span, and function.[73] Experimentally, they can be divided into B-lymphocytes, which are derived from the bone marrow or the bursa equivalent organ in humans, and T-lymphocytes, which are derived from the thymus. Morphologically, using Wright-Giemsa stain, one cannot distinguish T- and B-lymphocytes, but functionally, histochemically (see "Leukocyte acid phosphatase stain," Chapter 5), immunologically, and experimentally one can distinguish between the two. Lymphocytes that lack both T and B cell markers are classified as null cells. The study of T- and B-lymphocytes has provided new insight into lymphoproliferative disorders, immunodeficiency diseases, cell-mediated immunity, and humoral antibody formation. The following outline gives selected markers used in lymphocyte function studies:

A. B-lymphocytes
   1. Method described: surface immunoglobulins (sIg)[74]
   2. Other methods

a. Receptor sites for activated C3 component complement[75]
b. Receptor sites for aggregated immunoglobulin (Fc receptor)[75,76]
c. Receptor sites for Fc portion of IgG[77]
d. Receptor sites for complement; erythrocytes coated with antibody and complement (EAC) rosette formation[78]
e. Receptor site for mouse red cells[79]

B. T-lymphocytes
   1. Methods described
      a. E receptor for sheep red cells (nonimmune E rosettes)[80]
      b. Mitogen-induced lymphocyte transformation[81]
      c. Migration inhibition factor (MIF) assay[82]
   2. Other methods
      a. Cytotoxicity assay (complement dependent)[83]
      b. Receptor sites for ox red cell coated with IgG antibody (Tγ)[84]
      c. Receptor sites for ox red cell coated with IgM antibody (Tμ)[85]

ISOLATION AND CHARACTERIZATION OF HUMAN LYMPHOCYTES
Isolation of lymphocytes[86]

Principle: Lymphocytes and some monocytes from diluted heparinized blood are purified by banding in a layer after centrifugation on a Ficoll-Hypaque discontinuous gradient. Separation is based on the density difference between denser red cells and polymorphic nuclear cells and less dense lymphocytes and platelets. The cells are washed by centrifugation and counted and are then ready for the various tests.

Reagents:
1. Sterile deionized distilled water
   Maintain aseptic conditions.
2. Phosphate buffered saline (PBS)
   Use Dulbecco's PBS (free of calcium and magnesium). Dilute $10\times$ commercial solution (stored at room temperature) with sterile water before use (1 part $10\times$ stock to 9 parts water).
3. Fetal calf serum (FCS)
   Inactivate by heating for 1 hr at $56°$ C. Store at $-20°$ C.
4. PBS and 5% FCS
   Dilute fresh PBS with FCS (19:1). Make up only needed amount. Prepare fresh every time test is run.
5. Ficoll
   Ficoll (mol. wt. 400,000; 9% w/v solution) is commercially available (Sigma Chemical Co., St. Louis or Pharmacia Laboratories, Piscataway, N.J.). Dissolve 14.4 g in 160 ml H_2O and stir gently for 3 hr at room temperature to dissolve completely. Store at $4°$ C.
6. Hypaque, 50%
   Hypaque is commercially available (Winthrop Laboratories, New York). Protect from light with aluminum foil. Keep sterile.
7. Ficoll (6.35%) and Hypaque (10%) solution
   Store at $4°$ C covered with aluminum foil.

Final concentration		
9% Ficoll	160 ml	6.35%
50% Hypaque	45.4 ml	10.0%
Sterile water	21.4 ml	
	226.8 ml	

Density should be 1.077 g/cc. Check by weighing 0.20 ml in tared micropipet tips. Adjust with water or Hypaque if necessary. Finally, filter and sterilize through 0.22 μm pore filter. Keep sterile.

8. Preservative-free heparin

   Heparin is commercially available (Sigma Chemical Co., St. Louis). Keep sterile.

9. Absorbed FCS

   Add heat-inactivated FCS (see above) to washed packed sheep red cells to 5% v/v (2.5 ml of packed cells to 50 ml of FCS). Mix frequently over 30 min incubation time at 37° C and store overnight at 4° C. Centrifuge at 400 × g for 15 min. Pour off supernatant (red cell free) and recentrifuge. Using sterile technic filter through 0.22 μm filter. Store at −20° C.

10. Falcon (Falcon Co., Oxnard, Calif.) 15 ml centrifuge tube, polystyrene, sterile (no. 2095)

Procedure: Draw blood in plastic syringe and immediately place in 15 ml disposal plastic centrifuge tube containing 300 units heparin. Mix well immediately. Approximately 10-20 ml of blood is needed for complete study depending on lymphocyte count. Store at room temperature for 1 day if necessary.

NOTE: Save 1.5 ml of blood from syringe for small EDTA tube for hematology section for Coulter count and differential. Record volume of blood remaining. It is essential to have the number of lymphocytes per milliliter and the total volume of blood used in the purification.

Record volume of blood used after removing aliquot for hematology section's cell count and differential.

Dilute blood with equal (or 2) volumes of PBS. Mix. Dispense 12 ml into each Falcon centrifuge tube.

Add 3 ml of Ficoll-Hypaque solution to bottom of centrifuge tube with blood with sterile 3 in. (or longer) needle attached to 5 ml syringe. Slowly push out solution when needle is at bottom. Blood will rise.

Centrifuge tubes at 400 × g (at interface) for 40 min at room temperature with brake off. Use 1440 rpm in IEC's PRJ centrifuge (International Equipment Co., Needham, Mass.) with 269 head and 320 tube holder. After centrifugation, lymphocytes plus monocytes (10%) and platelets will be in a white layer above the red cells.

Carefully insert sterile Pasteur pipet into layer with slight pressure to prevent premature uptake of plasma. Remove white cell and aggregates by rimming tip of pipet while sucking out cells. Usually remove 2-3 ml. Place in sterile plastic (12 ml) graduated centrifuge tube.

Add 2 volumes of PBS. Mix well. Centrifuge at 200 × g for 1 min at room temperature. Platelets will not pellet at this and lower speeds. Pour off supernatant containing platelets and resuspend pellet gently in 5 ml of fresh PBS and 5% FCS mixture with sterile Pasteur pipet. Centrifuge at 100 × g for 5 min. Repeat wash

and centrifugation steps one additional time for a total of three centrifugations. Resuspend final pellet in 1 ml of PBS-FCS (absorbed).

Count lymphocytes by removing 0.020 ml, adding 0.080 ml PBS and 0.100 ml trypan blue (0.4%), mixing, and placing in a Neubauer hemocytometer counter using a 40× objective. The number of lymphocytes in 16 large squares $\times 10^4 \times 10^1$ = the number of cells per milliliter. Count dead lymphocyte cells separately from those with blue dye. Red cells are perfectly round and have a glossy sheen and no nuclear material as seen by irregularities in the center of the cell. Dilute cell suspension to 5.0×10^6 lymphocytes/ml with PBS-FCS (absorbed). Cells are now ready for use. Record final volume and cell number. Calculate percent recovery of lymphocytes.

$$\frac{\text{Final volume} \atop \text{of purified} \atop \text{lymphocytes} \times {\text{No. of} \atop \text{lymphocytes} \atop \text{per milliliter}}}{\text{White cells} \atop {(\text{Coulter} \atop \text{count})} \times {\text{Lymphocytes} \atop (\%) \atop (\text{differential})} \times {\text{Blood} \atop \text{used} \atop (\text{ml})}} = {\text{Recovery} \atop (\%)}$$

Laboratory assays for B-lymphocytes

B cells are short-lived, predominantly small lymphocytes, which, on antigenic[38] stimulation, become immunoglobulin-producing lymphocytes and precursors of plasma cells. By scanning electron microscopy their surfaces appear to be studded with villi, probably representing redundant cell membrane. B-lymphocytes carry surface markers that are not present on T cells and are therefore used to identify this group of cells in suspensions of live lymphocytes or in frozen sections of lymphoid tissues:

1. Immunoglobulin surface markers can be detected by the use of polyspecific antisera against all immunoglobulin classes.

2. Subclasses of lymphocytes with specific surface markers are identified by the use of monospecific antisera directed against specific immunoglobulins, e.g., IgG and IgM.

3. Some lymphocytes possess receptor sites for complement. These cells are able to bind antibody-coated sheep red blood cells (SRBC) or erythrocytes (E) and complement to their surface to form immunorosettes (EAC rosettes). The sheep red cells are treated with rabbit anti-sheep-red-cell antibodies (usually IgM) and incubated with live lymphocytes in fresh human or mouse serum, which supplies the complement (C3).

4. B-lymphocytes also exhibit receptor sites for heat-aggregated γ-globulin, which are identified by labeling IgG aggregates with fluorescein. These sites probably bind the Fc portion of the IgG molecule and appear to be identical with the receptor sites for immunoglobulins and for antigen-antibody complexes.

Detection of surface immunoglobulins by immunofluorescence

Principle: Immunoglobulins on the surface of lymphocytes can be demonstrated by a number of technics, e.g., fluorescein labeling, radioimmunolabeling, fluorescein-labeled, aggregated γ-globulin, and demonstration of receptor sites for antigen-antibody complexes and for Fc fragments of immunoglobulins.

Mononuclear cells (90% lymphocytes, 10% monocytes) are isolated on a Ficoll-Hypaque gradient. Surface immunoglobulin molecules are detected by fluorescein-labeled antihuman immunoglobulin, either polyvalent or monospecific. The surface immunoglobulins are synthesized by the lymphocytes, normally only one class by a single cell or clone. All known classes of immunoglobulins (IgG, IgA, IgM, IgD, and IgE) have been identified as surface immunoglobulins.

Reagents:
1. Fluorescein isothiocyanate conjugated [F(ab′)₂] and goat anti-immunoglobin (IgG, IgA, IgM) polyvalent (Fl-Ab)*
   Reconstitute the lyophilized powder (stored at 4° C) by adding sterile water. Centrifuge for 1 hr at 100,00 × g in Ti50 Rotor (International Equipment Co. [IEC], Needham, Mass.). Carefully pipet off supernatant (all but pellet) and dispense in 0.050 ml aliquots and freeze at −20° C. Before use, centrifuge for 1 hr at 19,000 rpm in Serval or Microfuge. Do not refreeze thawed materials.
2. PBS-glycerol (1:9 v/v)
3. Slides, 1.0 mm thick, and no. 1½ coverslips (20 × 40 mm)
4. Sodium azide, 1%
   Prepare fresh daily: 0.1 g in 10 ml PBS.
5. PBS-FCS and 0.05% NaN₃ (cold)
   Use 5 ml NaN₃ per 95 ml of PBS-FCS.

Procedure: Determine optimal amount of Fl-Ab. Mix 0.1 ml of lymphocytes at 5×10^6 cells/ml with 2, 5, 10, 15, and 20 μl of Fl-Ab in plastic 12 × 75 mm tube on ice. Add 10 ml of 1% NaN₃. Incubate for 30 min at 4° C. Keep tubes covered from light. After 30 min, add 2.0 ml PBS-FSC-NaN₃ buffer.

Centrifuge at 200 × g for 5 min. Remove liquid without disturbing pellet with Pasteur pipet attached to water vacuum. Resuspend pellet in 3.0 ml of PBS-FCS-NaN₃ and recentrifuge. Repeat for total of three centrifugations. Resuspend final pellet in 0.03 ml PBS-FCS.

Resuspend in 0.03 ml of PBS and 5% FCS gently— avoid bubbles. Transfer entire amount with Pasteur pipet to center of 10 mm thick slide (95% alcohol prewiped). Allow to air dry. Cover slide with 95% alcohol and allow to air dry. Cover with 2 drops of 9:1 glycerol-PBS. Cover with coverslip and seal with nail polish. Store at 4° C.

Use Leitz (E. Leitz, Inc., Rockleigh, N.J.) Orthrolux Fluorescence microscope with phase 100× oil objective. Count the number of lymphocytes per field under normal light. Lymphocytes are small, irregularly round cells with very little or no cytoplasm of uniform grainy appearance (but no definite granules). They have a definite edge and must not touch other lymphocytes or have tiny cells (platelets) surrounding them. Then shift

to ultraviolet light and count number of lymphocytes with yellow-green fluorescent spots on the surface or edge. If a cell has a solid uniform fluorescence, it is a dead cell—do not count it. Do not count cells in clumps or larger monocytes.

$$\text{B cells (\%)} = \frac{\text{No. of fluorescent lymphocyte cells}}{\text{Total lymphocytes}}$$

Use an amount of fluorescent antibody that gives a maximal response. For a negative control, use fluorescein-conjugated goat antirabbit immunoglobulin.

Examine under fluorescent microscope and enumerate total number of cells (remove barrier filter) and number of fluorescent cells. It is important that only small lymphocytes be counted, since monocytes may also accept anti-IgG antibodies through the Fc receptor and, if included in the total count, lead to a spuriously high B cell percentage. Monocytes are much larger than small lymphocytes and can also be identified by the α-naphthyl butyrate histochemical method, which does not stain lymphocytes. Fc and C3 receptors are also found on monocytes.

Result and calculation: The average value of surface immunoglobulin–positive lymphocytes is 20-30% (our laboratory results are somewhat lower, 10-12%); IgG-positive lymphocytes, 11-19% (average 15%) IgA-positive lymphocytes, 3-8% (average 6%); IgM-positive lymphocytes, 3-11% (average 8%); κ-positive lymphocytes, 12-24%; and λ-positive lymphocytes, 2-14% (usually a 2:1 ratio of κ-positive lymphocytes to λ-positive lymphocytes).

On the basis of the total lymphocyte count and the percentage of B (or T) cells, the absolute number of B (or T) cells can be calculated according to the formula:

Absolute number of B (or T) cells =

$$\text{Total lymphocyte count} \times \frac{\text{No. of cells}}{100}$$

Interpretation: Peripheral blood has 20-30% B-lymphocytes, spleen contains about 41%, and lymph nodes about 31%. Lymphoreticular neoplasms primarily involving B cells are chronic lymphatic leukemia (about 80% B=lymphocytes),[87] lymphosarcoma (leukosarcoma), macroglobulinemia of Waldenström, immunoblastic sarcoma, Burkitt's lymphoma,[88] and follicular center cell lymphoma.[89] Patients with hypogammaglobulinemia show a marked decrease in B-lymphocytes,[74] and some acute lymphocytic leukemia cells are also deprived of the surface markers for B-lymphocytes.[90] In the monoclonal gammopathy of malignant lymphoreticular disorders, the majority of lymphocytes are of the B cell type and carry one single type of heavy and light chain of immunoglobulin,[91] while in benign secondary lymphocytosis the B-lymphocytes are not increased and show the usual polyclonal immunoglobulin pattern.[92]

The technic of quantitation of B-lymphocytes is difficult to standardize because of a number of factors: (1) variations in the harvesting of lymphocytes, (2) variable specificity of the reagents, (3) difficulty in the identification of the immunofluorescent cells, and (4) nonspecific staining reactions.

---

*Available from Kallestad Laboratories, Chaska, Minn., or N.L. Cappel Laboratories, Cochranville, Pa.

Mouse red cell rosettes for detecting B-lymphocytes

Principle: It has been reported that by using mouse red cells in an E rosette technic certain B cell proliferative disorders can be identified according to their possession of mouse red cell receptors.[79] Some cases of B-lymphocyte chronic lymphocytic leukemia are characterized by weak surface immunoglobulin staining and formation of mouse cell rosettes. Other B cell disorders, e.g., prolymphocytic leukemia, exhibit intense surface immunoglobulin staining and negative mouse rosettes. It has been proposed that the mouse rosette test measures young B-lymphocytes (pre-B-lymphocyte);[79] thus the receptor for mouse cells may be a differentiation marker.

Reagents: See reagents sections under "Isolation of lymphocytes."

Mouse red cells:

Procedure: Obtain fresh mouse red cells: Place 15 λ of heparin (heparin concentration = 10,000 units/ml) into a small plastic tube. Anesthetize a mouse with ether and remove 1-2 ml of blood by severing the brachial artery. Place the blood into the heparin tube and mix well. Place heparinized blood into a 15 ml centrifuge tube and add 10 ml of PBS or veronal buffer. Centrifuge for 5 min at 1800 rpm. Remove buffer and white cells from blood and wash two more times. Mouse red cells may then be stored for 1 week in veronal buffer (see E, EA, and EAC procedures) at 4° C.

Perform rosette technic: Take mouse red cells and remove buffer until volume in tube is 1 ml. Count the cells in 16 small squares on hemocytometer after making a 1:1000 dilution in PBS. Using an aliquot of the 1 ml mouse red cells make a tube containing a suspension of 4×10^8 mouse red cells following the same instructions as those for sheep red cells in the total T cell rosette procedure (p. 1074). Using the same amounts and concentrations as outlined for total T rosettes, perform mouse rosette technic except use mouse red cells wherever the total T procedure calls for sheep red cells. Incubate tubes for 154 hr or overnight at 4° C.

Read rosettes as for total T rosettes and record the percentage of rosettes.

Interpretation: Normal range is 3-20% but depends on the individual laboratory's own control.

Results greater than 20% showing a rise in normal B-lymphocytes or especially pre-B-lymphocytes may indicate a leukemic process if no other membrane receptors can be identified.

IgM EAC rosette (complement receptors) for B-lymphocytes[78]

Principle: Circulating B-lymphocytes as well as B-lymphocytes in tissue contain receptors for complement. These receptors are identified by coating sheep red cells with IgM antibody against sheep red cells. With the addition of complement attaching to the Fc portion of the IgM anti-sheep red cells, the B-lymphocytes are identified by rosette formation of the EAC cells around the B-lymphocytes. A count of three or more EAC cells in a rosette is considered positive.

Reagents and procedure: Prepare EACs as defined in the section on EAC rosettes (p. 1112). Use a 50:1 ratio of EACs to white cells of patient.

$$EACs = 4 \times 10^8$$

$$\text{Patient's lymphocytes} = 0.05 \times 10^8$$

$$\frac{4 \times 10^8}{0.05 \times 10^8} = 80:1 \text{ ratio}$$

$$\frac{80}{1} = \frac{50}{X}$$

where X = 63 λ. Use 63 EACs to every 100 λ of lymphocytes or use 31.5 λ EACs to every 50 λ of lymphocytes.

Incubate with gentle shaking for 45 min at room temperature. Add 100 λ trypan blue to EAC tube. Count percent of rosettes out of 100 cells.

Results: Normal range is 5-20% but depends on the individual laboratory's own control.

Laboratory assays for T-lymphocytes

T-lymphocyte reactivity can be tested by two groups of substances:

1. Up to 90% normal T-lymphocytes in short-term tissue culture may be stimulated by a variety of nonspecific mitogens to blast transformation. Suitable mitogens are phytohemagglutinin (PHA), a kidney bean extract, pokeweed mitogen (PWM), and concanavalin A.

2. Specific stimulants that also lead to lymphocyte transformation are (1) antigens to which the lymphocyte donor is sensitized and (2) lymphocytes of a phenotypically unrelated donor. In a mixed leukocyte culture, lymphocytes from two unrelated individuals cause reciprocal blast transformation of the two cell populations. The later observation forms the basis of one group of histocompatibility tests. Specific antigens do not stimulate unsensitized lymphocytes. If the lymphocytes are sensitized, about 35% of the lymphocytes are transformed.

Sheep erythrocyte (E) rosette for T-lymphocytes[80,93,94]

Principle: The rosette technic exposes identical receptors (E receptors) on test cells (lymphocytes) and on "signal" cells (sheep red cells). T-lymphocytes form spontaneous non-immunoglobulin-mediated rosettes with sheep red cells. A rosette-forming T cell is defined as a lymphocyte that has three or more red cells adhering to its surface (Fig. 36-1). The method described by Hepburn et al.[95] uses glass slide–smear preparations of fixed stained cells, which are evaluated morphologically. The slides can be stored and reviewed when convenient. Other technics utilize unstable wet preparations that need to be examined after completion of the test.

Reagent: Sheep red cells, Colorado Serum.

Use cells within 3 weeks. Remove 2 ml of cells and dilute with 8 ml of PBS. Centrifuge at 200 x *g* for 5 min. Siphon off supernatant and top layer of sheep red cells (to remove any sheep white cells) and resuspend pellet in PBS to around 5% (0.5 ml packed volume of cells to 10 ml of solution). Repeat washing and centrif-

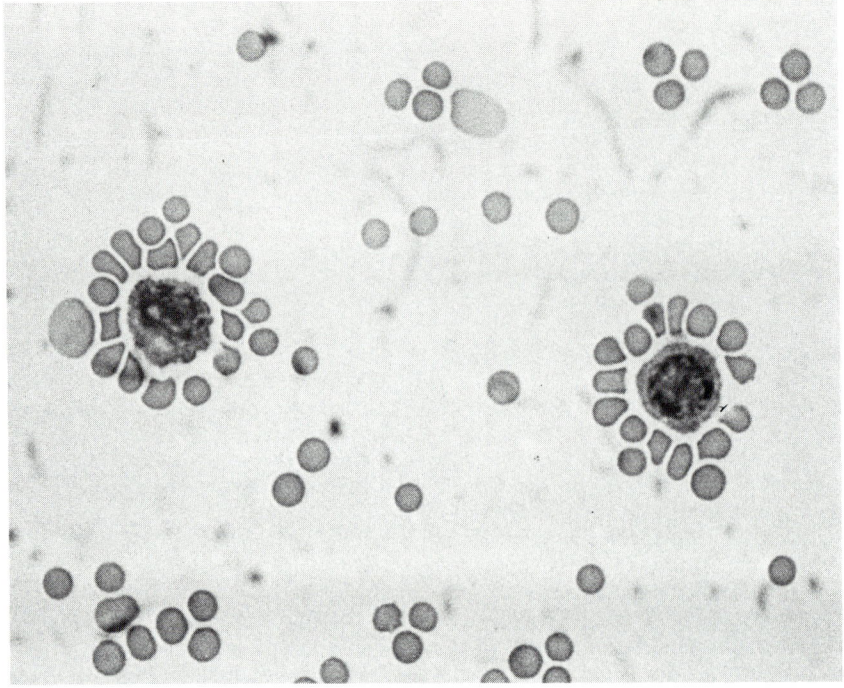

Fig. 36-1. E rosette in Giemsa-stained cytocentrifuge preparation from a normal adult peripheral blood sample. (×650.)

ugation two times. Resuspend cells in 1 ml Hank's 10% FCS absorbed. Titrate by diluting $1:10^3$ (100 λ to 9.9 ml mix or 100 λ to 0.9 ml mix). In hemocytometer count number of cells in 16 squares $\times 10^7$, which is equal to the number of cells per milliliter. Adjust to 4 $\times 10^8$ cells in 1 ml by using the following equation:

$$\text{Vol. of cells} = \frac{4 \times 10^8}{\text{SRBC titer}}$$

Adjust to final volume of 1.0 with Hank's 10% FCS (absorbed). Mix and transfer 0.1 ml to 0.9 ml of PBS to yield 4×10^7 cells/ml for active E rosettes.

Procedure:

Total rosette[94]: Mix 0.05 ml washed lymphocytes with 0.025 ml of sheep red cells (4×10^8 cells/ml) and 0.050 ml Hank's 10% FCS (absorbed) in 12 × 75 mm plastic tube. Ratio of sheep red cells to lymphocytes should be 40:1. Do duplicates.

Centrifuge at $50 \times g$ for 5 min (500 rpm). Carefully remove tube and leave at room temperature for 1½ hr. Do not mix or pour off supernatant. Incubate at 4° C for 2 hr or overnight.

To count rosettes, very gently resuspend cell pellet by rocking back and forth several times. Also, gently tilt tube toward horizontal plane in order to just resuspend pellet. Gently add 0.2 ml trypan blue. Add suspension to hemocytometer with Pasteur pipet. With 40× objective count lymphocytes surrounded by three or more red cells (rosette) and separate live lymphocytes with two or less red cells (nonrosettes).

$$\text{T cells (\%)} = \frac{\text{No. in rosettes}}{\text{No. in rosettes} + \text{No. not in rosettes}}$$

Use care in distinguishing human red cells with uniform sheen from free lymphocytes, which are approximately the same size. Lymphocytes are not perfectly round and have an irregular light-reflecting center because of the nucleus. Count total of 200 cells from each duplicate. Do not count clumped lymphocytes, cells with visible cytoplasm, or cells larger than small lymphocytes.

Active rosette[96,97]: Conditions are adjusted so that only those lymphocytes with a higher affinity for sheep red cells can form rosettes. Conditions modified are shorter incubation, lower ratio of sheep red cells to lymphocytes, and different media.

Mix 0.05 ml of purified lymphocytes (5×10^6 cells/ml) with 005 ml FCS (absorbed). Incubate for 60 min at 37° C. Add 0.05 ml of washed sheep red cells (4×10^7 cells/ml) in PBS. Sheep red cell/lymphocyte ratio is 8:1. Mix gently and centrifuge at $50 \times g$ (500 rpm) for 5 min. Gently resuspend pellet, add 0.15 ml trypan blue, and count rosettes as described above.

Calculation: The percent of T-and B-lymphocytes per milliliter of blood is calculated as follows:

$$10^3 \times \frac{\text{WBCs*}}{\text{mm}^3} \times \frac{\text{Lymphocytes (\%)}}{\text{(differential)}} \times \frac{\text{T cells (\%)}}{\text{(from rosettes)}} =$$
$$\text{No. of T-lymphocytes per milliliter}$$

$$10^3 \times \frac{\text{WBCs*}}{\text{mm}^3} \times \frac{\text{Lymphocytes (\%)}}{\text{(differential)}} \times \frac{\text{B cells (\%)}}{\text{(from sIg)}} =$$
$$\text{No. of B-lymphocytes per milliliter}$$

---

*By Coulter Counter (Coulter Electronics, Hialeah, Fla.).

Interpretation: Cord blood lymphocytes show the same proportion of B cells as do lymphocytes of adults, but using the E binding technic the cord T cells are reduced in number.[98] In newborns the B- and T-lymphocyte distribution is similiar to that in adults, although their absolute number is increased in keeping with the neonatal lymphocytosis. In the aged there is a progressive increase in B cells and a decrease in T cells,[98] a phenomenon that may be related to the increased incidence of carcinoma in older age groups because of impairment in cell-mediated immunity. The results obtained by the use of anti-T-cells era and by the rosette formation test are not identical in a number of conditions.

Normal value: In excess of 70% of peripheral blood lymphocytes are T cells.

If the above method for identification of T cells is combined with the immunofluorescein staining method for B cells, the following distribution of T and B cells is found in the peripheral blood of normal adult individuals:

Noncommitted null cells: 0.5-1%
B cells: 7-23%
T cells: 70-90%

Mitogen and antigen stimulation studies of lymphocytes

Principle and background: A large proportion of lymphocytes respond to certain plant proteins called mitogens in a nonimmunologic, i.e., nonspecific, polyclonal manner by mitosis and cell division.[99,100] During this process of cell transformation, DNA synthesis occurs, and it has been found that the amount of DNA synthesis correlates with cell division and the percent of cells becoming blastlike. DNA synthesis is measured by the incorporation of ^{3}H-thymidine into water-insoluble nuclear material. The ^{3}H-thymidine is taken up by the cells and converted first into water-soluble ^{3}H-thymidine triphosphate and then into DNA in the nucleus (water soluble).

Antigen stimulation, e.g., with purified protein derivative (PPD) or *Candida*, affects specifically only prechallenged or preimmunized (sensitized) lymphocytes. T cells respond to antigens by mitosis and cell division as with the mitogens, but only a smaller number of cells so respond and the maximal DNA synthesis period is increased from 3-4 days for the mitogens to 6-7 days for most antigens.

The stimulation index is the relative increase in ^{3}H-thymidine incorporation into DNA in the presence of mitogen or antigen compared to the control without the addition of the mitogen or antigen. The stimulation index is 50-200 for mitogens and over 3 for antigens.

Reagents and procedures:

1. Phytohemagglutinin, purified (PHA-P)
   Phytohemagglutinin is commercially available (Wellcome Reagents HA-17, Burroughs Wellcome & Co., Research Triangle Park, N.C.) Make stock solution of 1.0 mg/ml, use PBS to filter and sterilize through 0.22 μm filter, and freeze at 20° C in 0.05 ml aliquots. For use, thaw aliquot and add 0.45 ml media; do not save diluted material.

2. Concanavalin A
   Concanavalin A is commercially available (Sigma C2010, Sigma Chemical Co., St. Louis). Prepare a stock solution with sterile water of 0.5 mg/ml and filter and sterilize as above. Store at −20° C in 0.10 ml aliquots. To use add 0.150 media to thawed aliquot to five 100 μg/ml solution.

3. Pokeweed mitogen (PWM)
   Pokeweed mitogen is commmercially available (GBCO 670-5360, Gibco Diagnostics, Chagrin Falls, Ohio). Dissolve contents of sterile bottle in sterile water according to directions on the bottle. Store in 0.1 ml aliquots at −20° C. For use, thaw aliquot and add 0.4 ml media.

4. Purified protein derivative (PPD)
   PPD is available as a lyophilized powder from Ministry of Agriculture, Fisheries and Food, Central Veterinary Laboratory, Weybridge Surrey, England as lyophilized powder. Store at −20° C. Prepare a 0.40 mg/ml stock solution with sterile water. Filter sterilize. Store 0.1 ml aliquots at −20° C. For use, thaw aliquot and use directly.

5. Streptokinase-streptodornase (SK-SD)
   SK-SD is commercially available as Varidase (Lederle Laboratories, Pearl River, N.Y.). One vial contains 10,000 units SK and 5000 units SD. Add 1 ml Dulbecco's PBS and using freshly boiled dialysis bags, dialyze two times against 1 dl PBS for 12 hr at 4° C with stirring to remove the preservative. Aseptically remove the SK-SD and store in 20 λ aliquots at −20° C. To use add 0.18 ml media to thawed aliquot. Add 2 ml PBS to vial. Dialyze and sterilize. Store in 40 λ aliquots. Add 0.16 ml media.

6. Bacterial vaccine (MRV)
   Bacterial vaccine is commercially available (Hollister-Stier Labs., Spokane, Wash.). Remove approximately 2 ml aliquots and add to freshly boiled dialysis bags and dialyze against 2 dl PBS as in no. 5 above. Store cloudy suspension at 4° C. Shake well before use. Dilute 50 λ with 100 λ of media for use.

7. *Candida* extract (Dermatophytin "O"; allergenic extract)
   Candida extract is commercially available (Hollister-Stier Labs., Spokane, Wash.). Dialyze extract as in no. 6 above. Store at 4° C. Keep sterile. Dilute 50 λ with 50 λ of media for use.

8. RPMI 1640 media + NaHCO$_3$ − Glutamine*
   Store media at 4° C. Add normal human serum (heat inactivated for 30 min at 56° C) to 10%, glutamine to 2 mmole from 200 mmole stock, and penicillin (10,000 units/ml) and streptomycin (5000 units/ml) mixture to 1%. EXAMPLE: For 30 ml of media use 3 ml human serum, 0.3 ml glutamine, 0.3 ml Pen-Strep (Associated

---

*Commercially available from K.C. Biological, Lenexa, Kan.; Gibco Diagnostics, Chagrin Falls, Ohio; and Associated Biomedic Systems, Buffalo, N.Y.

Biomedics System, Buffalo, N.Y.), and 24.6 ml RPMI 1640 1 × media. pH should be 7.4, and color should be light cherry pink.

9. Scintillation Cocktail Toulene
   This is commercially available (Fisher no. 313, Fisher Scientific Co., Pittsburgh) and contains 0.05% PPO (2,5 Diphenyloxazole) and 0.04% POPOP (1,4-bis[2(4-methyl-5-phenyl-oxazolyl]-benzene).

10. Purified lymphocytes
    Purified lymphocytes, 5 × 10⁶ cells/ml, are used. They are sterile in PBS-FSC till used.

11. Tissue Culture II Microtiter Plate and Lid
    The Tissue Culture II Microtiter Plate and Lid are available from Falcon (3040 and 3041, Falcon Co., Oxnard, Calif.). The plate has a sterile flat bottom.

12. ³H-Thymidine
    ³H-Thymidine (5 c/mmole; 1 mCi/ml stock solution, sterile in saline) is commercially available (NET-027, New England Nuclear, Boston). Store at 4° C; shelf life is approximately 6 months.

Table 36-3 summarizes the amounts of mitogens and antigens determined experimentally as giving optimal stimulation with several normal lymphocytes. As new batches or lots of mitogens or antigens are used, the optimal amount can be rechecked using 6, 8, 10, 12, and 14 μl of the diluted stock per well as described above.

For each mitogen or antigen, use triplicates and also include controls of no mitogen or antigen. Additional controls used are a zero time control in which the ³H-thymidine is added to the cells plus mitogen immediately before the harvesting. For each well add 20 μl of purified lymphocytes (5 × 10⁶ cells/ml), 170 μl of media, plus 10 μl of mitogen or antigen. Media and the cells can be precombined by determining the total number of wells needed (n) and adding 190 λ per well of the mixture containing n × 0.19 ml media + n × 0.02 ml cells. At 72 hr for mitogens, or 6 days for antigens, add 50 μl ³H-thymidine (0.5 μCi) to each well. The ³H-thymidine (1 mCi/ml) is diluted 1:100 with unused sterile media to give 10 μCi/ml. Incubate overnight for 16-18 hr.

At the end of the labeling period, the ³H-thymidine incorporated into cellular DNA is measured by collecting water-lysed cells on a Whatman Glass Fiber Filter (934AH; Whatman Inc., Clifton, N.J.) using the Multiple Automated Sample Harvester (Microbiological Associates, Walkersville, Md.). The wells are filled five times with water for washing and transferring to the filter. The filter strip is dried under a heat lamp and after cooling (or overnight at room temperature), the filter disk is placed in a small vial (no. 7475-1, Rochester Scientific Co., Rochester, N.Y.) followed by 1 ml of scintillation cocktail. Numbered vials are placed in a glass carrier and counted in the liquid scintillation counter.

$$\text{Stimulation index} = \frac{\text{Mean of } (+\text{mitogen}) \text{ samples} - \text{mean of zero time controls}}{\text{Mean of } (-\text{mitogen}) \text{ controls} - \text{Mean of zero time controls}}$$

Interpretation: Compare patient and normal control run simultaneously. The normal control with the mitogens should have a stimulation index of 50-100 depending on the mitogen used. If the normal is greater than 2 standard deviations from the mean control, the experimental data should be examined carefully and repeated if necessary. For antigenic stimulation a stimulation index greater than 3.0 is considered positive. A positive individual thus has been exposed and immunologically challenged by that particular antigen and has competent functional T-lymphocytes. Phytohemagglutinin (PHA)-stimulated lymphocytes reveal 90% blastogenesis, or if tritiated thymidine is used as an indicator of blastoid transformation they exceed 100 times the normal unstimulated control. Significantly defective T-lymphocytes show less than 5% blast formation.

Congenital immunologic defects with defective lymphocyte reactivity are rare and include combined immunodeficiency disease, DiGeorge's syndrome (thymic agenesis), ataxia-telangiectasia, Wiskott-Aldrich syndrome, and chronic mucocutaneous candidiasis. The acquired conditions of defective lymphocyte transformation form a long list and include neoplastic diseases, Hodgkin's disease, old age, sarcoidosis, liver diseases, chemotherapy, hypogammaglobulinemia, viral infections, autoimmune diseases, including lupus erythematosus, and serum factors, which may be specific or nonspecific for lymphocytes and suppress lymphocytic reactivity.

Lymphocyte transformation in response to an antigen may be used as a sensitive tool to detect prior exposure to this antigen. T cell malignancies are mycosis fungoides, Sézary's syndrome, Sternberg sarcoma, and some forms of chronic lymphocytic leukemia.

Table 36-3. Summary of mitogens and antigens

	Stock solution	Diluted stock	Amount used in assay	Final concentration in assay
PHA	1 mg/ml	0.1mg/ml	10 λ	5 μg/ml
Con A	0.5 mg/ml	0.2 mg/ml	10 λ	10 μg/ml
PWM	Undiluted	1/5	10 λ	1:10 dilution
PPD	0.4 mg/ml	N/A	10 λ	10 μg/ml
SK-SD	25,000 units/ml	2500 units/ml	10 λ	125 units/ml
Bacterial vaccine	Undiluted	1/3	10 λ	1:60 dilution
Candida	Undiluted	1/4	10 λ	1:80 dilution

Quality controls in human lymphocyte isolation and stimulation studies
Lymphocyte isolation quality controls

Always run a "normal" control with every patient test or tests. The normal control should be an adult who is not on medication such as antibiotics, corticosteroids, or aspirin when his blood is drawn.

The normal control lymphocytes should be processed and handled in exactly the same manner as the patient's lymphocytes and the results recorded. If the normal control results differ significantly from that of the established normal range, the patient results are questionable unless some reason can be found to cause this difference in the normal control results (i.e., the normal control develops a viral illness such as a cold subsequent to his blood donation, which may have caused alteration in his white cells).

Normal range*:

	%	No. × 10 ^{3}/ml
Total T-lympho-cytes	60% ± 7.5%	1.55 ± 0.42
Active T-lympho-cytes	26% ± 8.5%	0.64 ± 0.25
Florescent B cells	8% ± 3.7% (n = 24)	0.167 + 0.105
Mouse rosettes	6 + 2.8 (n = 7)	Not done
EAC rosettes	8-10%	Not done

Lymphocyte stimulation quality controls

As directed in the section on lymphocyte differential controls, always run a normal control with lymphocyte stimulations, following the directions given in the control section for differentials.

Normal range*:

Mitogens: stimulation index	
PHA	193 ± 69
Con A	127 ± 52
PWM	67 ± 38
Antigens: stimulation index	
PPD	>3
SK-SD	>3
Candida	>3
Bacterial vaccine	>3

Macrophage migration inhibition test[82]

Principle: Antigen-stimulated sensitized lymphocytes release a number of soluble substances (lymphokines) that affect other cell populations. One such factor is the migration inhibitory factor (MIF), which inhibits the migration of normal guinea pig peritoneal macrophages. Related to the MIF is the leukocyte inhibitory factor (LIF), which inhibits the migration of human buffy coat leukocytes (mononuclear and polymorphonuclear leukocytes) from a capillary tube into a tissue culture medium.[95] These factors are found in the cell-free supernatant of sensitized lymphocyte cultures exposed to the specific antigen. The method presented has two phases[101-103]:

1. Sensitized lymphocytes are cultured with the specific antigen and are thus stimulated to produce the MIF, which is found in the supernatant.

2. The MIF is assayed on leukocytes in capillary tubes embedded in the supernatant tissue culture me-

dium. The inhibition of migration is read at 18-24 hr. Under the conditions of the test, normal leukocytes migrate from the capillary tube into tissue culture medium for a visible distance. This migration area is measured after 24 hr (control) and is compared with the inhibited migration area when, in a repeat experiment, the leukocytes are confronted with the culture-produced MIF. The migration inhibition is the result of MIF produced by sensitized and challenged T-lymphocytes and is an indicator of the acquisition of cellular immunity to an antigen. The migration inhibition is expressed as percent inhibition or as migration index.

Reagents:
1. Ammonium chloride, 0.83%
2. Lactated Ringer's solution
3. Plachette (clear plastic chamber with a volume of 0.5 ml with circular sterile coverslip)
4. Microcapillary tubes (75 mm length and 1.1-1.2 mm diameter)
5. Eagle's minimal essential medium (MEM) in Eagle's basic salt solution with L-glutamine, vitamins, penicillin, streptomycin, and mycostatin (Gibco Diagnostics, Chagrin Falls, Ohio)
6. Clay
7. Silicone grease

Procedure: Draw 30 ml venous blood into a heparinized plastic syringe. Allow to stand in an upright position until the red cells and plasma separate. Aspirate leukocyte-rich plasma, centrifuge at 150 g for 10 min and aspirate plasma. Wash cell pellet once in 0.83% ammonium chloride and four times in lactated Ringer's solution. Suspend leukocytes in MEM to obtain a final suspension of 10,000,000 cells/ml. Determine viability of cells with trypan blue stain. Draw final suspension of cells into microhematocrit tube to 20 μl mark and seal with clay. Centrifuge capillary tube in microhematocrit centrifuge at 600 g for 5 min.

Edge capillary with file and break at the level of the culture medium and cell interphase. Place the cell portion in a planchette, holding it in place by a drop of silicone grease. Add tissue culture medium (MEM) to planchette via injection port and cover planchette with round cover slip held in place by silicone grease; seal port. Incubate at 37° C for 24 hr under 5% CO_2. Project area of migration onto paper, outline the area, and measure with a planimeter. Repeat test by injecting MIF-containing MEM into chamber and measure migration area. Set up three or four chambers for each test group and average results.

Results: Relate average migration area of MIF-containing cultures to average migration area of control cultures without antigen and express as migration index.

$$\text{Migration index} = \frac{\text{Average area of migration with antigen}}{\text{Average area of migration without antigen}}$$

The material containing the MIF is found in supernatants of stimulated lymphocyte cultures as described for the lymphocyte transformation test. After incubation of 12-24 hr the culture is centrifuged for 15 min at 500 g and the supernatant is filtered through 45 μ Millipore filter.

Interpretation: Sensitized T-lymphocytes in the

---

*Individual laboratories should establish their own normal ranges.

presence of the corresponding antigen produce MIF, which inhibits migration of leukocytes from capillary tubes. Immune-deficient lymphocytes fail to release MIF, as seen in Hodgkin's disease, sarcoidosis, and collagen diseases. The migration inhibition system has also been used to study various tissue antigens that stimulate sensitized lymphocytes to produce mediator substances; e.g., lymphocytes of patients suffering from Guillain-Barré syndrome produce MIF in response to peripheral nerve antigens.[104]

LABORATORY INVESTIGATION OF IMMUNOGLOBULINS

Immunoglobulins are the secretory protein product of B-lymphocytes and of their terminal differentiation, the plasma cells, in response to immunogenic stimulation. Despite the fact that these cells form numerous classes and subclasses of immunoglobulins with distinctive biological functions and properties, the immunoglobulins share the same basic molecular-structural design. Each immunoglobulin molecule is composed of four polypeptide chains, which, according to their amino acid sequences, are divided into two identical light (L) chains and two identical heavy (H) chains. The latter are joined together at their center by two or more interchain disulfide bonds. The L chains are attached to the hinge area of the H chains by a single interchain disulfide bond. The distinctive biologic function of each immunoglobulin is located in the variable regions (V-regions) or the N-terminal segments of each immunoglobulin molecule, which occupy one half of each light chain (V_L) and one fourth of each heavy chain (V_H). The remaining immunoglobulin molecule consists of L and H chain constant (C) regions (C_L, C_H) which show a marked similarity in amino acid sequences.

Based on the polypeptide composition of the constant regions, the heavy chains are divided into five classes: γ (gamma), α (alpha), μ (mu), δ (delta), and ε (epsilon). The heavy chains determine the immunoglobulin classes, which are designated IgG (γ-chain), IgA (α-chain), IgM (μ-chain), IgD (δ-chain), and IgE (ε-chain). Four subclasses of IgG are described IgG[1], IgG[2], IgG[3], and IgG[4]) and two subclasesses of IgA (IgA[1] and IgA[2]). The light chains are of two types: κ (kappa) and λ (lambda). Since immunoglobulins contain either two light chains of the κ-type or two of the λ-type and since each immunoglobulin consists of two identical H and two identical L chains, the molecular formula of each immunoglobulin can be written as follows: IgG may be $\gamma_2\kappa_2$ or $\gamma_2\lambda_2$, IgA may be $\alpha_2\kappa_2$ or $\alpha_2\lambda_2$, etc. (Table 36-4). The subclasses increase the number of H chains, e.g., $\gamma1$, $\gamma2$, $\gamma3$, $\gamma4$, and $\alpha1$, $\alpha2$, so that the molecular formula may read $\gamma_2\kappa_2$ or $\gamma_2\lambda_2$, etc. Even though the synthesis of the light chains is independent of the production of the heavy chains, the normal plasma cells, and even some myeloma cell groups, produce equal numbers of heavy and light chains. On the other hand, 75% of plasma cell neoplasias produce excess numbers of light or heavy chains. The variable regions are the site of the antigen binding of the immunoglobulin molecule, while the constant regions are responsible for the class characteristics and physiologic properties, e.g., complement binding or placental transfer (Table 36-5).

The immunoglobulin molecule can be cleaved by proteolytic enzymes (papain, pepsin) acting on the hinge areas of the H chains into three fragments, two of which are designated the Fab fragments, are identical, and consist of one light chain and one N-terminal half of the heavy chain (Fab stands of antigen-binding fragments). The remaining fragment, called Fc fragment, consists of the terminal halves of the two heavy chains (Fc stands for fragment that crystallizes). The Fc fragments contain the functional units of the H chains.[105]

IgG and most IgA circulate in the body in the monomer form, but the other immunoglobulins circulate as aggregates, forming disulfide-linked dimers, trimers, and pentamers, so that the basic formula for immunoglobulins should read (H2L2)n. Ten percent of IgA is dimeric (9S) or trimeric (13S), and almost all IgM is pentameric (19S).

Laboratory evaluation of overproduction of immunoglobulins

The overproduction of immunoglobulins (dysgammaglobulinemia) is either polyclonal or monoclonal. The polyclonal gammopathies include liver diseases such as hepatitis and cirrhosis, infections such as tuberculosis and infectious mononucleosis, collagen diseases such as lupus erythematosus and rheumatoid arthritis, and sarcoidosis. The monoclonal gammopathies include malignant conditions such as multiple myeloma, plasma cell leukemia, Waldenström's macroglobulinemia, heavy-chain disease, amyloidosis, rarely non-Hodgkin's lymphomas and chronic lymphatic leukemia, and benign idiopathic forms of unknown significance, probably not related to B cell disorders, e.g., carcinoma and aging.

The investigative procedures follow this protocol[110-112]:
1. Complete blood count including platelet count
2. Urinalysis
3. Quantitation of total protein in serum and urine
4. Protein electrophoresis of serum and urine to detect monoclonal proteins
5. Immunoelectrophoresis of serum and urine to identify the monoclonal proteins
6. Radial immunodiffusion or laser nephelometry of serum and urine to quantitate the immunoglobulins
7. Bone marrow aspiration, Wright-Giemsa stain, direct immunofluorescence if nonsecretory forms of monoclonal gammopathy are considered
8. Tests of cryoglobulins and pyroglobulins
9. Evaluation of serum viscosity (If an immune complex disease is suspected, also perform quantitation of circulating immune complex.)
10. Complement assay
11. Immunofluorescent studies, bone marrow smear, or biopsy tissue
12. C1q precipitin reaction

A large number of laboratory findings, e.g., hypercalcemia, hyperproteinemia and hypoproteinemia, hypergammaglobulinemia, pancytopenia, lymphocytosis, lymphopenia, and plasmacytosis, suggest additional diagnostic studies to discover possible abnormalities in the concentration and distribution of immunoglobulins

Table 36-4. Composition of immunoglobulins

Immunoglobulin	Heavy chain	Light chain	Molecular structure	Designation
IgG	2γ	2κ or 2λ	$\gamma_2\kappa_2$ or $\gamma g_2\lambda_2$	κIgG or λIgG
IgA	2α	2κ or 2λ	$\alpha_2\kappa_2$ or $\alpha_2\lambda_2$	κIgA or λIgA
IgD	2δ	2κ or 2λ	$\delta_2\kappa_2$ or $\delta_2\lambda_2$	κIgD or λIgD
IgM	2μ	2κ or 2λ	$\mu_2\kappa_2$ or $\mu_2\lambda_2$	κIgM or λIgM
IgE	2ε	2κ or 2λ	$\varepsilon_2\kappa_2$ or $\varepsilon_2\lambda_2$	κIgE or λIgE

Table 36-5. Characteristics of immunoglobulins

Characteristics	IgG[105]	IgA[106]	IgM[107]	IgD[108]	IgE[109]
Molecular weight	150,000	170,000 (serum) 390,000 (secretions)	900,000	180,000	196,000
Sedimentation constant	7S	7S	19S	7S	8S
Percent of total serum immunoglobulin	80	19	10	<0.2	0.0002
Plasma concentration (mg/dl) (adult average)*	1200	210	140	3	0.03
Half-life (days)	23	6	6	2.8	2.3
Crosses placenta	+	−	−	−	−
Function	Antibody to viruses and to bacterial toxins of gram-positive bacteria; warm autoimmune antibodies	Found in all body secretions; antibacterial and antiviral antibodies; attached to "secretory piece"	Antibody to endotoxins of gram-negative bacteria, to I antigen, and to ABO group; heterophile antibodies, cold agglutins, and hemolysins	?	Affinity to mast cells and basophil reaginic antibodies
Complement fixation	IgG4 − IgG1 − 3 +	−	4 +	−	?
Electrophoretic migration	γ	slow β	$\beta - \gamma$	$\beta - \gamma$	slow β

*Varies with age, sex and race (see Fig. 36-5).

and in existing antibodies. The immunoglobulin abnormalities or dysproteinemias may be of three types: (1) a heterogeneous diffuse increase of a great number of various immunoglobulins (polyclonal gammopathy), (2) an abnormal increase of a specific homogeneous immunoglobulin, often at the expense of the other immunoglobulins (monoclonal gammopathy), and (3) an absence or decrease of immunoglobulins (agammaglobulinemia or hypogammaglobulinemia).

Hypergammaglobulinemia

Polyclonal gammopathy: The increased production of a large number of different immunoglobulin classes (clones) is responsible for the polyclonal gammopathy pattern that is characterized by a diffuse, broad increase in γ-globulins and is encountered in collagen diseases, chronic liver diseases, chronic infections, and rheumatoid arthritis. The selective marked increase of IgG of both κ- and λ-types, which is seen in some forms of liver disease–associated polyclonal gammopathy, is called oligoclonal gammopathy. Unless it is clinically warranted, further investigation of the immunoglobu-

lins responsible for the polyclonal gammopathies is usually not indicated, although there are instances when the polyclonal pattern and even a normal γ-globulin pattern require immunoelectrophoretic investigation.

Monoclonal gammopathy: Monoclonal gammopathy is a group of disorders characterized by an abnormal proliferation of a simple clone of B-lymphocytes and/ or plasma cells that produce a homogeneous monoclonal immunoglobulin. The term *monoclonal gammopathy* has been used synonymously with dysgammaglobulinemia, immunoglobulinopathy, and plasma cell dyscrasia. The monoclonal protein commonly consists of one class of heavy polypeptide chain and one type of light chain (κ or λ). It is encountered in multiple myeloma, plasmacytoma, plasma cell leukemia, macroglobulinemia, non-Hodgkin's lymphoma, and other malignant neoplasms. A relatively benign form of monoclonal gammopathy has been used for its absence of association with the above neoplastic processes. In some instances the plasma cells excrete excessive quantities of only heavy chains (heavy-chain diseases) or light chains (light-chain diseases).

Laboratory investigation of monoclonal gammopathy or plasma cell dyscrasia

Principle: In monoclonal gammopathy one clone or colony of plasma cells proliferates and is responsible for the production of one class of homogeneous immunoglobulins or rarely of light chains only (light-chain disease) or heavy chains only (heavy-chain disease). In the serum protein electrophoretogram the homogeneous immunoglobulins form a single, narrow-based spike, most frequently in the globulin region, less commonly in the γ-β region, and rarely in the β-α$_2$–and α$_1$-areas. These homogeneous immunoglobulins are designated "abnormal immunoglobulins," "paraproteins," or "M proteins" since they are frequently found in lymphocyte–plasma cell disorders such as multiple myeloma, macroglobulinemia, and malignant lymphomas. Waldenström is responsible for the term *monoclonal gammopathy*.[113] Since M proteins have been shown to have specific antibody activity, they are not "abnormal immunoglobulins" except in quantity and etiology.[114] The detection of small M protein spikes in the β- and α-regions may require careful scrutiny of the serum protein electrophoretogram since densitometric results may completely gloss over and miss these diagnostic features. The sera containing M proteins usually show varying degrees of reciprocal hypogammaglobulinemia caused by depression of the immunoglobulin not involved in the spike. If the proliferating plasma cells produce only light or heavy chains, the M protein spike is absent and only the flat curve of the accompanying hypogammaglobulinemia is seen. M protein–like spikes have been recorded in conditions other than the malignant disorders mentioned, e.g., in old age and in a variety of nonreticular neoplasms and inflammatory diseases.[115-117] The presence of a homogeneous protein spike is an invitation to further investigate by immunoelectrophoresis and radial immunodiffusion the identity and quantity of the immunoglobulin responsible for the peak to aid in the diagnosis and follow-up of the underlying pathologic condition. If the total serum protein, the A/G ratio, and the serum protein electrophoretogram are normal, a monoclonal gammopathy is unlikely, but since light-chain disease may be accompanied by hypogammaglobulinemia and heavy-chain disease by normal γ-globulin levels, the latter two conditions may also have to be further investigated if clinically indicated.[118]

Cellulose acetate electrophoresis also allows identification of urinary proteins and can be utilized to distinguish global proteinuria from Bence-Jones proteinuria, although immunoelectrophoresis of urine is the preferred method for the demonstration of the latter.

Serum protein electrophoresis

The serum protein electrophoretogram is the result of the separation of serum proteins into five fractions (if the cellulose acetate method is employed) on the basis of their rate of migration in an electric field. The methodology is discussed in detail in the section on protein chemistry.

Interpretation: Serum protein electrophoresis allows an initial classification of the γ-globulin fraction, which contains most immunoglobulins, into hypergamma-globulinemia, either polyclonal or monoclonal, agammaglobulinemia, or hypogammaglobulinemia.

Serum immunoelectrophoresis

Principle: Immunoelectrophoresis (IEP) consists of two phases: electrophoresis and gel diffusion. In the first phase the proteins to be analyzed are deposited in a circular well and are electrophoretically separated along one axis of the support medium (agarose) into the γ, β, α$_2$, α$_1$, and albumin fractions. In the second phase these fractions are allowed to act as antigens and to interact with the corresponding antibodies deposited in an antibody trough (Fig. 36-2). Diffusion of both the antigens and the antibodies toward each other results in antigen-antibody complexes made visible by precipitin lines, each one of which represents one specific protein. The antibody diffuses as a uniform band parallel to the antibody trough while the antigen diffuses in a circle if the protein is homogeneous and in an ellipse if the protein is heterogeneous. The antigen-antibody precipitation line of the former forms a segment (arc) of a circle while the precipitation line of the latter has an elliptic shape. Because homogeneous proteins, e.g., albumin, vary only as far as concentration is concerned from patient to patient, their electrophoretic mobility and position are constant and they are best identified and quantitated by radial immunodiffusion. By contrast, immunoglobulins show significant structural variations (the different variable regions), so that their electrophoretic mobility and concentration must be evaluated. This is best achieved by immunoelectrophoresis and analysis of the precipitation lines. The constant regions are responsible for the general electrophoretic mobility of various classes of immunoglobulins, but the variant regions determine the position within the class.

Equipment and reagents: The method described utilizes the (Bioware Inc., Wichita, Kan.) technic and equipment.[112,119,120]

1. Cool Pack (Bioware) or other suitable electrophoretic cell and power supply, 100-160 V
2. Incubation chamber (Bioware) or the protective plastic trays in which the gels are packaged for shipment
3. Precut, prebuffered rehydratable agarose IEP gels (Bioware cat. no. 70-722-0-11)
4. Multi-Media camera with 4 in. lens and Land-pack (optional for photography)
5. Immuno-Glo (darkfield illumination) (optional for photography)
6. Immuno Electric Dryer or compatible hot forced air dryer, 50° C
7. Film support
8. Barbital buffer, pH 8.6, 0.05M Store at 4-8° C.
9. Normal saline, 0.85% (w/v)
10. Protein stain: 0.5% brilliant blue R in 10% acetic acid/45% methanol
11. Destaining solution: 10% acetic acid in 50% reagent alcohol
12. Marking dye: bromphenol blue–albumin
13. Mercaptoethanol, 1:10 dilution
14. Antisera

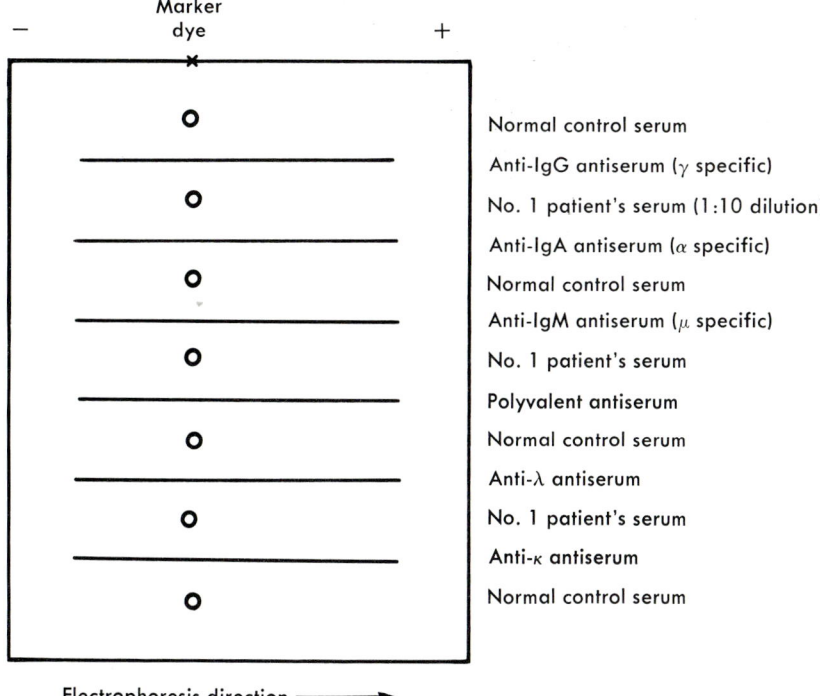

Marker
dye

−   +

	Normal control serum
	Anti-IgG antiserum (γ specific)
	No. 1 patient's serum (1:10 dilution)
	Anti-IgA antiserum (α specific)
	Normal control serum
	Anti-IgM antiserum (μ specific)
	No. 1 patient's serum
	Polyvalent antiserum
	Normal control serum
	Anti-λ antiserum
	No. 1 patient's serum
	Anti-κ antiserum
	Normal control serum

Electrophoresis direction ⟶

Fig. 36-2. Suggested sequence of antigen-antiserum combinations employed in immunoelectrophoresis (IEP).

Polyvalent antihuman antisera contain antibodies against most serum proteins, e.g., antialbumin, anti-complement, and antitransferrin. Polyvalent antiimmunoglobulin antisera contain antibodies against IgG, IgA, and IgM. Monospecific anti-IgG, -IgA, and -IgM antisera may react with the whole protein molecule (H and L chains) in which case the anti-L-chain fraction of the antiserum will also react with other immunoglobulins that have the same L chains. Other monospecific antiglobulin sera react only with the H chains. Anti-κ-chain and anti-λ-chain antisera should also be included in the test protocol. All sera are commercially available. The exact nature and activity of each antiserum must be quality controlled.

Procedure:
1. Sample preparation
   a. Fresh, fasting serum is the sample of choice; however, aged serum or plasma can be used.
   b. Sample size of 1 ml is adequate.
   c. Prepare a 1:10 solution of serum by adding 1 part serum to 9 parts 0.85% sodium chloride or barbital buffer, pH 8.6, ionic strength, 0.05.
2. Inoculation and electrophoresis
   a. Remove precut gels from pouch and rehydrate in water for 1 hr and subsequently in barbital buffer for 15 min.
   b. Lift out of buffer tank and blot.
   c. Inoculate antigen wells from left to right with 3 units of antigen (serum, urine, and cerebrospinal fluid), alternating full strength and 1:10 dilution. The 1:10 dilution is suggested to prevent abnormal curves caused by antigen

excess. The remaining wells are occupied by normal controls according to the same procedure as for patient's serum.
   d. Dip applicator stick into marker dye and lightly insert into edge of gel at the level of the antigen wells.
   e. Fill electrophoresis cell with barbital buffer, 150 ml buffer/tank, 4-8° C.
   f. Place gel into chamber, gel side up, so that the proteins migrate parallel to the long sides of the antisera troughs and electrophorese at 90 V/agarose plate for about 55 min until the stained albumin has reached a migration mark 3.2 cm anodic from the application point.
   g. Remove the IEP gel from the electrophoretic cell and place on the film support.
3. Development of immunoelectrophoretogram
   a. Fill the antisera trenches of the gels with 100 μl specific antisera.
   b. Place the IEP gel in the incubation chamber for 16-18 hr at room temperature or in the protective plastic trays the gels are packaged in for shipment. Optimal diffusion and formation of precipitation lines may require 24-48 hr incubation.
4. Photography
   a. Remove the IEP gel from the incubation chamber and place in 5 in. × 7 in. film hangers. The precipitant bands may be intensified by placing gel in 1% tannic acid for 5-10 min.
   b. Immediately place in saline solution until ready to photograph.
   c. The immunoelectrophoretogram is then pho-

tographed with the Multi-Media camera with the 4 in. lens and the Immuno-Glo (darkfield illumination).

d. The Polaroid print may be used for interpretation, and a duplicate print may be attached to the report. The actual immunoelectrophoretogram may be discarded or, if desired, processed for staining.

5. Staining

a. Place the IEP gel, agarose surface up, on a film support; cover with 1-2 cm layer of Whatman no. 1 filter paper and apply even pressure (2 kg) for 30 min. Carefully remove filter paper. (Apply a single sheet of filter paper first making sure there are no air pockets between gel and filter paper or that there are no wrinkles in the filter paper. Then apply remaining filter paper.)

b. Soak in 0.85% saline for 30 min and repeat step 1 above.

c. Place in Immuno Electric Dryer until dry.

d. After the plate is completely dry, stain with protein stain for 20 min, destain, and dry as for serum protein electrophoretograms.

NOTES: The dilution of the serum can serve as a rough quantitative measurement of the amount of serum immunoglobulins or other antigens present.

The addition of β-mercaptoethanol to serum is occasionally needed if high concentrations of IgM (19S) are present since IgM becomes tightly bound in the gel and neither migrates nor forms a definite precipitate band. To reduce the disulfide bonds (19S-7S), mix 0.1 ml of the patient's serum with 0.01 ml of 1:10 dilution of mercaptoethanol and incubate for 60 min at 37° C. Inoculate the patient's unreduced serum in antigen wells 2 and 6 and the patient's reduced serum (mercaptoethanol-treated serum) in antigen well 4. Process as for regular immunoelectrophoresis.

Interpretation:

Normal patterns: The immunoprecipitin bands (Fig. 36-3) should be of normal curvature, symmetry, length, position, intensity, and distance from the antigen well and antibody trough. In normal serum, IgG, IgA, and IgM are present in sufficient concentration (10 mg/ml, 2 mg/ml, and 1 mg/ml, respectively) to produce precipitin lines, while normal IgD and IgE concentrations are too low to be detected by IEP. The normal IgG precipitin band is elongated, elliptic, slightly curved, and clearly visible in undiluted and 1:10 diluted serum. The normal IgM and IgA bands disappear at a 1:10 dilution. The IgG band is located cathodic to the antigen well in the γ-area of the electrophoretogram and, if monospecific sera are used, fuses with a thin precipitin line positioned midway between antigen well and antibody trough and extends into the β-area. The IgA line is a flattened thin arc, slightly cathodic to the well in the γ-β position. The IgM line is a barely visible thin line, slightly cathodic to the antigen well. The normally low serum concentration of IgM is responsible for the difficulty in its visualization.

Abnormal patterns: Protein abnormalities (Fig. 36-4)[112] are detected by evaluating the following features of the precipitin bands: (1) position of the band in relation to the electrophoretically identified protein fraction; (2) its position between the antigen well and the antibody trough; (3) thickening (density) and elongation; (4) shortening (inhibition), thinning, or doubling; and (5) distortion of the curvature or "arc" formation.

Polyvalent antisera confirm the presence or absence of major protein fractions, while antisera monospecific

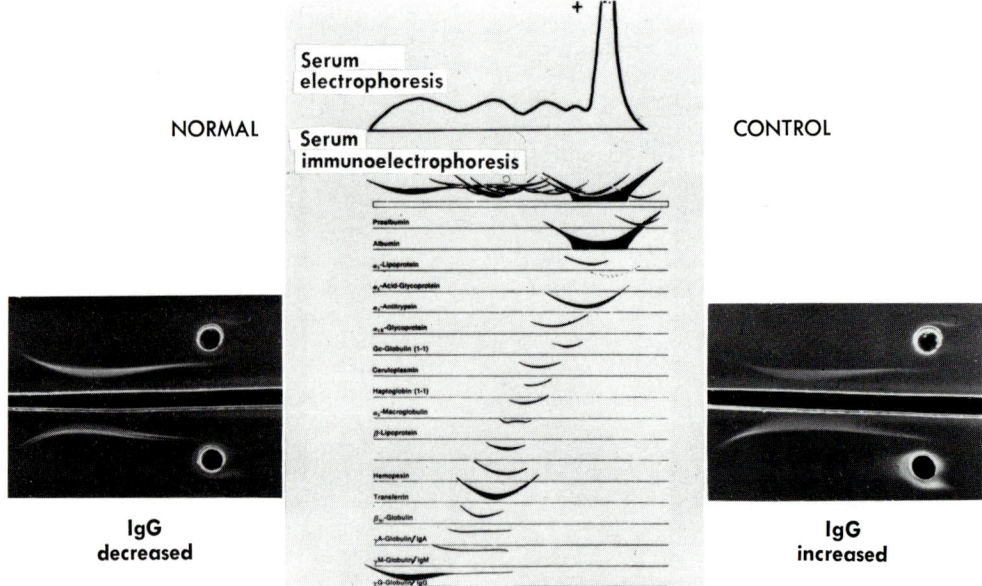

Fig. 36-3. Immunoelectrophoresis patterns. *Left,* Hypogammaglobulinemia pattern (IgG). *Middle,* Individual serum proteins. *Right,* Polyclonal gammopathy pattern (IgG). (From Ritzmann, S.E., and Daniels, J.C.: Serum protein abnormalities: diagnostic and clinical aspects, Boston, 1975, Little, Brown & Co. Copyright © 1975.)

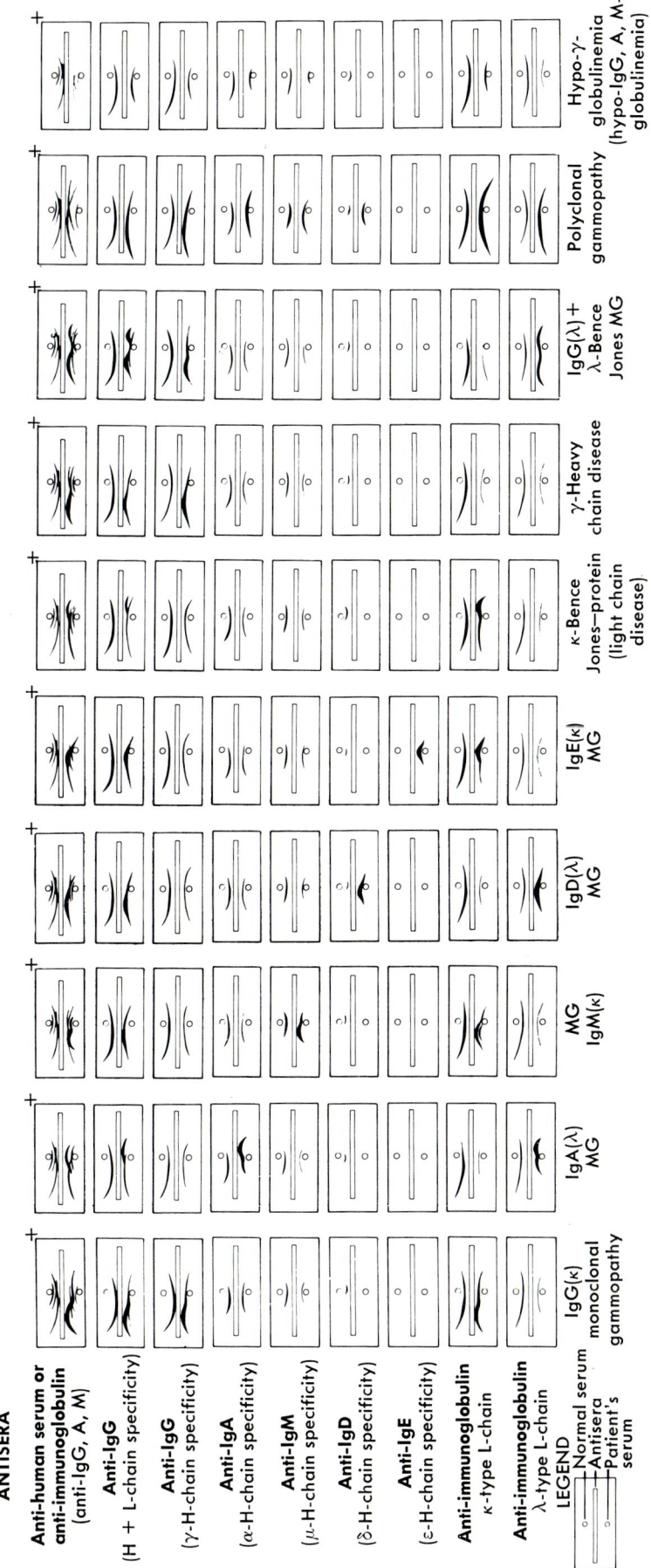

Fig. 36-4. Abnormal immunoglobulin pattern (IEP). (From Ritzman, S.E., and Daniels, J.C.: Laboratory notes—serum proteins. No. 3, Somerville, N.J., 1973, Behring Diagnostics/Hoechst Pharmaceuticals, Inc.)

for individual immunoglobulins identify only the corresponding proteins. If the monospecific antisera have combining sites for H and L chains, the combining sites will react with L chains of other immunoglobulins or with the free L chains of Bence Jones protein. H chain–specific sera do not cross react with other proteins. The anti-κ and anti-λ antisera are necessary for complete typing of the immunoglobulins for the evaluation of the ratio and for the diagnosis of monoclonal M proteins.

Quantitative abnormalities of protein antigen: Although IEP is not a good quantitative method, it allows certain quantitative considerations.

INCREASED CONCENTRATION OF ANTIGEN: The precipitin line is situated closer to the antibody trough since the highly concentrated antigen diffuses a greater distance. It is also thicker, longer, and broader than the normal control precipitation. M proteins lead to an antigen excess, which is responsible for an abnormal curvature of the precipitin line.

The monoclonal IgG line shows an arc of a circle rather than the elongated, elliptic shape of the normal line, since it reflects the homogeneous nature and the limited electrophoretic mobility of the abnormal protein. The line is dense and touches the antiserum trough.

The monoclonal IgA line is denser than the normal line and closer to the antibody trough.

The normal IgM line is hardly visible, but the monoclonal IgM line is dense and represents a skewed arc of a circle.

The diagnosis of monoclonal gammopathies is aided by the absence or reduction of the other two immunoglobulin precipitin lines and by the use if anti-κ or anti-λ sera to show a change in the κ/λ ratio, since the M proteins are either λ or κ in type. There are twice as many κ monoclonal gammopathies as there are λ. The light-chain precipitin lines (either κ or λ) are symmetric with the line of the monoclonal H chain to which they belong and are often of similar density.

The monoclonal IgD line forms a thickened, skewed arc in the area of the antigen well extending to the cathodal side. In the normal immunoelectrophoretogram the IgD precipitin line is not visible. Monoclonal IgD proteins are usually of λ-type so that the λ-precipitin line is symmetric with the IgD line. IgG, IgM and IgA lines are just visible, because these immnoglobulins are depressed.

Monoclonal IgE elevation leads to a short, thick arc in the antigen well area extending to the anodal side. The IgM and IgA lines are not visible, and the IgG line is thinned. In most cases, the κ-precipitin line is symmetric with the IgE line.

DECREASED CONCENTRATION OF ANTIGEN: The precipitin line is found closer to the electrophoresis pathway, since the antigen diffuses only a short distance. It is shortened, thinned, and at times represented by two parallel lines of the L chains only.

Qualitative abnormalities of protein antigen: The precipitin band may be displaced compared to its normal position in the control serum, since molecular changes in the abnormal protein may affect its speed of migration in the electrophoretic phase of IEP. It may also be shortened and incomplete because of "inhibi-

tion" of a segment, since the antibody may react only with a portion of the abnormal protein. Structurally abnormal immunoglobulins have been described in some plasma cell dyscrasias,[121] but in the majority of these disorders the immunoglobulin structure is not altered.[114]

Immunoelectrophoresis of urine

Principle: The most important application of IEP of urine lies in the demonstration of Bence Jones proteinuria, since this method detects very low concentrations of Bence Jones protein (BJP) (about 1-2 mg/dl).

Procedure: Using the Amicon Minicon B-15 (Amicon Corp., Lexington, Mass.) concentration device, the urine is concentrated about 50-fold and electrophoresis is performed against anti-κ and anti-λ light-chain antisera. It may also be concentrated 10 times and applied 5 times.

Results: If BJP is present in the urine, precipitin lines will form with either the one or the other anti-light-chain serum because BJP is composed of homogeneous light chains of a single antigenic type, either κ or λ. Normal light chains are heterogeneous and include equal concentrations of κ- and λ-types.

Evaluation of Bence Jones protein

Principle: Bence Jones protein (BJP) is a homogeneous monoclonal protein produced by a single colony of plasma cells and lymphocytes and is frequently seen in patients with multiple myeloma, Waldenström's macroglobulinemia, and primary amyloidosis[117,122] but may also occur in some lymphoreticular neoplasms and very rarely in patients with benign monoclonal gammopathies.[123] It is frequently (50-70%) found in association with IgG, IgA, and IgM monoclonal gammopathies, and it is found in about 90% of patients with IgD monoclonal proteins[117] or with Waldenström's macroglobulinemia. The light-chain production is either of κ- or λ-type. The κ-form is primarily monomeric and, because of its small size, is rapidly filtered by the glomeruli but easily and rapidly reabsorbed and catabolized by the kidneys, so that in the early stages of abnormal plasma cell hyperplasia it can be detected in the urine but not in the serum. In the later stages it is found in both. The λ-proteins occur as dimers and trimers and are the most frequently encountered types of BJP.[124] Because of their large size, they may be confined to the serum and fail to appear in the urine.[125] A number of tests can be utilized to discover BJP, e.g., (1) tests for proteinuria (e.g., sulfosalicylic acid in conjunction with "dipsticks"), (2) heat test, (3) electrophoresis, (4) immunoelectrophoresis, and (5) radial immunodiffusion. The technics of these tests are described in other sections; only their relative merits are discussed here.

Sulfosalicylic acid test: Sulfosalicylic acid (20%) precipitates most Bence Jones and non–Bence Jones proteins while the dipstick (Albustix, Ames Co., Elkhart, Ind.) is specific for albumin. A strongly positive sulfosalicylic acid test accompanied by a negative or weakly positive dipstick test is highly suggestive of BJP. The sulfosalicylic acid test is sensitive enough to detect about 40 mg BJP/dl.

Heat test: The heat test is based on the peculiar solubility and thermal characteristics of BJP, which precipitates when heated to 50-60° C but resolubilizes at 90-100° C to precipitate again on cooling, whereas other urinary proteins precipitate at a higher temperature and remain insoluble. Because these precipitated proteins may obscure the BJP, the boiling urine should be filtered and the test repeated. The reappearance of the precipitate after cooling to 56° C is the diagnostic phase of the test. The heat test is relatively insensitive, requiring 150 mg BJP/dl to be positive,[126] and furthermore, not all BJP reacts with this test.[127] Other drawbacks include the necessity to strictly control the pH and buffer and the fact that false positive and false negative results have been documented by comparing the heat test results with those obtained by immune methods.

Electrophoresis: The BJP may be responsible for a monoclonal spike in the γ- or β-region of the cellulose acetate electrophoretogram of concentrated urine.[124] The test is cumbersome and unreliable.[112]

Immunoelectrophoresis: Immunoelectrophoresis is the method of choice for the detection of BJP in urine and serum, using monospecific antisera to κ- and λ-light chains. The method is sensitive to 1-2 mg BJP/dl.[128] If BJP is present, immunoelectrophoresis reveals an increase in one or the other light-chain arc and a decrease in the uninvolved light chain.[129] A short, thickened precipitin arc situated at the level of the antigen well extending to the anodal side is suggestive of BJP. If anti-IgG (H and L chain specificity) antiserum is used, the BJP arc fuses with the anodal end of the IgG precipitin line.

Radial immunodiffusion: Radial immunodiffusion (RID) quantitates BJP, so that serial measurements of BJP (and of immunoglobulins) allow the evaluation of success or failure of any therapeutic regimen, since an increase in their concentration indicates an increased tumor load while a decrease coincides with response to therapy. The method is sensitive and is able to detect 1-2 mg BJP/dl.

Radial immunodiffusion (RID)

Principle: Immunoelectrophoresis is essentially a qualitative procedure, while RID provides qualitative as well as quantitative information. The method is relatively rapid (18-24 hr) and fairly sensitive (10-20 mg protein/dl, depending on the protein).

A quantitative relationship exists between the concentration of a protein deposited in a well, cut into a thin agarose layer containing the corresponding monospecific antiserum in uniform concentration, and the size of the resulting precipitin ring. The wells are filled with the unknown serum and suitable standards and are incubated in a moist environment at room temperature. After the end point of the diffusion has been reached, the diameters of the precipitin rings are proportional to the concentration of the immunoglobulin (Mancini technic).[130]

Equipment and reagents:
1. RID plates, commercially available
2. Three standard serum dilutions
3. Microliter dispenser
4. Semilog and linear graph paper
5. Measuring ruler

Procedure: Remove plate from envelope and allow

to stand open for about 5 min to evaporate any moisture that may have collected in the wells.

Note numbering system of the wells or turn plate agarose surface down and, using a permanent marker, number wells counterclockwise at the outer margin of the plate and on a card identify sera and controls to be deposited into the wells.

Turn plate agarose surface up and, depending on the specific protein assayed, fill three wells with 2-20 μl (in accordance with manufacturer's instructions) with the standards supplied.

Fill the remaining groups of two or three wells with diluted or undiluted patient's sera (follow manufacturer's instructions). IgM, for instance, is determined by using an undiluted erum.

Tightly close plate and place into envelope that is sealed with tape to prevent loss of moisture.

Store plate in a horizontal position at room temperature for a minimum of 6-12 hr (Fahey-McKelvey early readout technic)[131] or for about 50 hr (end point technic of Mancini),[130] depending on the type of immunoglobulin assayed.

After the appropriate time (see below) measure the diameter (D) of the precipitin ring (in millimieters) of unknown and standards to an accuracy of 0.1 mm using a calibrated magnifier and a light source beneath the plate. Square the diameter readings (D^2) and construct a standard curve.

The rings may be photographed (see immunoelectrophoresis technic) and measured on the print.

Calculations: Two methods are available for the construction of the standard curve and the calculation of the patient's values.

Method A: The **Mancini technic**[130] is based on the fact that after a certain time, which depends on the concentration and the molecular weight of the protein, a precipitin ring reaches a maximal value and further incubation fails to increase its size. The area of the precipitin ring (square of its diameter) is linearly proportional to the antigen concentration in the well, so that the plotting of these values on linear graph paper results in a straight line. The maximal ring diameter is obtained in about 24 hr by IgG in normal concentration and in about 50 hr by IgM of normal concentration. The linear relationship beween the area (in square millimeters) and concentration is not established until the rings (standards and unknown) reach their maximal size.[132] The end point method has a high degree of accuracy, reproducibility, and sensitivity but requires time.

1. Plot the squared diameter (D^2) of the precipitin rings obtained from the three standards on the ordinate of linear graph paper and enter the corresponding concentrations of the standards (in milligrams per deciliter) on the abscissa. Connecting the three reference points should result in a straight line. The patient's value is obtained by reference to this calibration curve.
2. If diluted patient's serum is used, multiply the concentration must be by the dilution factor to obtain the value for whole serum.

Method B: The early readout method of Fahey measures the precipitin rings (unknown and standards) before they reach maximal size, after about 6-12 hr. In this method the logarithm of the antigen concentration is proportional to the area of the precipitin ring (D^2). The determination can be carried out as early as 6-12 hr after the start of diffusion.

1. Plot the squared diameter (D^2) of the precipitin rings obtained from three standards on the ordinate of semilog graph paper and enter the corresponding concentrations of the standards (in milligrams per deciliter) on the abscissa. Since the concentrations are plotted on semilog paper, a straight line is obtained.
2. Calculate the patient's value from the curve and multiply by the dilution factor.

Technical notes pertaining to radial immunodiffusion: Inaccuracies occur if the standard and unknown immunoglobulins vary in their degree of polymerization and aggregation. IgA, IgM, and light chains (BJP) polymerize readily, diffuse more slowly, and will therefore be underestimated. Quantitation of monoclonal immunoglobulins may be abnormally high if they contain antigenic determinants that fail to react with the antiserum incorporated in the agar,[133-135] or if low molecular forms that diffuse rapidly are present.[136] Technical errors include spilling of the antigen, inadequate filling of the wells, and damage to the gel.

Electroimmunodiffusion

Principle: In the one-dimensional electroimmunodiffusion (EID) technic electrophoresis of the antigen is performed in a support medium of cellulose acetate or agarose containing the appropriate antiserum. The method combines the speed of electrophoresis with the accuracy and sensitivity of immunodiffusion.[132,137] The precipitin lines flank the lateral borders of the moving antigen until the exhaustion of the antigen as a result of precipitation causes the precipitin lines to converge and to finally meet in the middle of the leading edge of the antigen path when all the antigen is precipitated. The precipitate pattern resembles the outline of a rocket (rocket electrophoresis). EID allows quantitation of all proteins that have a negative charge that differs from that of the antibody. Immunoglobulins must be modified by special alkaline buffers to increase their negative charge and thus their anodic migration. The method is not suitable for quantitation of M proteins of monoclonal gammopathies, since their variations are responsible for abnormal electrophoretic mobilities that may stop short of the expected end point. (See discussion of limitations of radial immunodiffusion.)

The support medium contains 16 application sites. Two dilutions of the patient's serum are applied to two sites, and three or four increasing dilutions of the protein standards are applied to other sites. after electrophoresis a standard curve is constructed relating the migration distance (height of rockets) to the protein concentration of the standards. The concentration of the unknown is determined from the standard curve.

Reagents and equipment: The method presented utilizes Helena (Helena Laboratories, Beaumont, Tex.) equipment and cellulose acetate technic. The equipment is the same as that used for serum protein electrophoresis, although a constant current power supply is preferred.

1. Titan III cellulose acetate plates wetted in a buffer containing antibodies in an antiserum buffer ratio of 1:20
2. Hamilton 1 μl syringe, dispensing in volumes of 0.25 μl
3. Teflon applicator tips
4. PO_4 buffer
   a. Stock and chamber buffer, 1:1000 dilution
   b. Soaking buffer, 1:8 dilution of stock buffer
5. Diluted antisera
   The antisera must be of high titer, prepared from rabbits, and free of azide. They are diluted 1:20 in PO_4 stock buffer.
6. Stock Ponceau S: 3 mg/L in 5% acetic acid
   For working stain use 1 ml stock solution in 1 dl 5% acetic acid.
7. Patient's serum, diluted with stock buffer as follows:

IgA quantitation	1:16 and 1:32
IgM quantitation	1:8 and 1:16
IgG quantitation	1:64 and 1:128

Serum dilutions should be in the range of standard dilutions.

8. Standards, diluted with stock buffer
   Standard sera are available from Helena Laboratories (Beaumont, Tex.) in a standardized lyophilized form (Kemtrol Normal).
9. Template
   A plastic plate with holes drilled in a straight line can be obtained from Helena Laboratories (Beaumont, Tex.). The specifications are as follows: 16 holes of 0.9 mm diameter, 3.5 mm apart, 1.6 mm from the sides of the membrane, and 2.4 mm from the end of the membrane.

Procedure:

1. Dilution of antisera
   a. After preparing the phosphate stock buffer dilute it 1:3 with distilled water.
   b. Dilute antisera according to Table 36-6 in a shallow disposable dish and make sure mixing is complete before wetting plates.
   c. Store stock and diluted buffers at 4° C.
2. Wetting of cellulose acetate plates
   a. Since the initial wetting is critical, follow manufacturer's instructions.
   b. Soak the plate in the antiserum-buffer solution for 20-25 min at 22° C.
3. Standards (see reagent 6)
4. Application of samples
   a. After soaking place plates with Mylar surface down on a piece of blotting paper soaked in buffer and proceed to blot the cellulose acetate side firmly.
   b. Cover with template, which must be accurately centered.
   c. Apply 0.25 μl of sample through guide holes, using a 1 μl Hamilton syringe fitted with a Teflon tube tip. Barely crack the surface of the plate and slowly and evenly dispense material into the membrane.
   d. After the sample application, draw water into

Table 36-6. Protocol of immunodiffusion

Antisera	Dilution of antisera	Buffer	Dilution of standard sera	Time (min)	mA
IgG	1:20	PO$_4$	1:64 to 1:512	60	4
IgA	1:20	PO$_4$	1:16 to 1:128	35	4
IgM	1:20	PO$_4$	1:8 to 1:64	60	5
IgD	1:12	Barbital	1:1 to 1:8	45	6

tip, eject onto blotter, and continue with the next sample.
  e. After application of all samples allow membrane to rest for 3-4 min to achieve complete absorption.
5. Electrophoresis
  a. Fill electrophoresis chambers with undiluted chamber buffer (1 dl each) and place membrane, cellulose acetate side down, onto sponge electrodes.
  b. Close cover, allow to equilibrate for 1 min, and perform electrophoresis at 4-5 mA/strip for 35-60 min.
6. After electrophoresis is completed, wash off excess protein in diluted soaking buffer for 15 min.
7. Stain membrane in dilute Ponceau S for 10 min and destain in successive rinses of 5% acetic acid.
8. Air dry before quantitating.

Calculation: Hold the plate up to a light source and mark tops of peaks with marking pencil. Then place plate on a flat surface and, using a measuring magnifier, measure the height of the precipitin peak to the closest 0.1 mm. The precipitin lines are rather faint.

Construct standard curve on linear graph paper by plotting the length (in millimeters) of the precipitin peaks of the standard solutions on the ordinate and the respective protein concentrations on the abscissa.

Determine the concentration of the unknown by reference to the calibration curve.

Automated immunoprecipitation

Principle: The quantitation of the immunoglobulins (and of other proteins such as complement) is accomplished by mixing diluted antiserum of known titer and activity with dilute antigen and determining the degree of turbidity produced by the antigen-antibody precipitin complexes. The light-scattering effect of these complexes is measured in a nephelometer and is proportional to the protein concentration. If the titer of the diluted specific antiserum is kept constant and the concentration of the diluted standard antigen is varied, a standard curve can be established for each protein relating the light-scattering effect of the complex to the protein concentration. The concentration of the unknown protein is obtained from the standard curve by relating its percent of light scattering to its concentration. Newer instruments, some of which employ a laser beam as the light source, allow quantitation of immunoglobulins in seconds and minutes as compared to hours and days required for diffusion methods.

Radioimmunoassay

Radioimmunoassay (RIA) allows the quantitation of a large number of proteins with great accuracy. It is the method of choice (1) for the quantitation of IgE of normal concentration and (2) for the quantitation of the other immunoglobulins in fluids other than serum, e.g., cerebrospinal fluid. The RIA technic is described in the chemistry section.

Laser nephelometry: Laser nephelometry is discussed in the clinical chemistry section.

Normal values of immunoglobulins

Normal immunoglobulin values are age and race dependent (Fig. 36-5 and Table 36-7).

Immunoglobulin concentrations in newborns, infants, and children[112,139,140] (Fig. 36-6)

The serum IgG level of the newborn is that of the mother because of its placental transfer. In the first 6 months of life the maternal IgG decreases rapidly in the infant's blood and the lowest levels (about 400 mg/dl) are seen between 3-6 months of age. They then gradually rise to about 800 mg/dl or over at the end of the first year, reflecting the infant's own IgG synthesis. Adult levels are reached at about 5 years of age.

The IgA level at birth is less than 5 mg/dl, since IgA does not cross the placenta and its own synthesis is slow. At the end of the first year it reaches about 30 mg/dl or over and slowly climbs to about 60 mg/dl in about 5 years. Secretory IgA is supplied in the mother's milk.

The IgM level at birth is 10 mg/dl and rises rapidly to about 100 mg/dl at the end of the first year. Because the maternal IgM does not cross the placenta, the cord blood IgM level reflects the infant's own synthesis. Increased IgM cord blood levels over 19 mg/dl have been accepted as evidence of intrauterine infection by such organisms as cytomegalovirus, toxoplasma, and rubella virus.[140] The adult value is not reached until 15-20 years of age.

IgD is absent from cord blood or present in very low concentrations and reaches adult levels after about 5 years.

IgE is less than 1 mg/dl in cord blood and reaches adult levels at about 10-12 years.

Laboratory investigation of thermoproteins

Thermoproteins are serum or urine proteins that exhibit physical changes at temperatures below or above 37° C and can be divided into (1) cryoglobulins or cryoimmunoglobulins, which form reversible or irreversible precipitates, gels, or crystals at temperatures

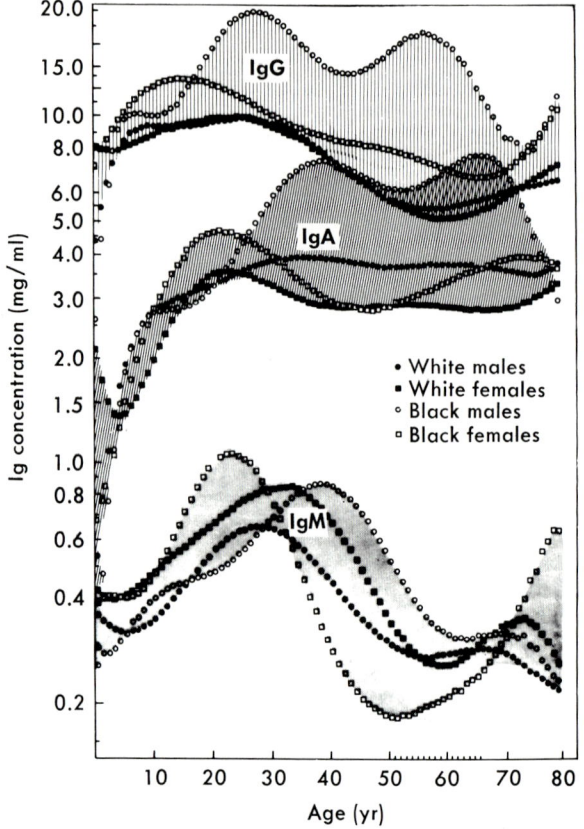

Fig. 36-5. Serum immunoglobulins in 800 apparently healthy patients. Comparison of ages at which race and sex differences in serum immunoglobulin concentration are most significant. (From Buckley, C.E., III, and Dorsey, F.C.: Ann. Intern. Med. **75:**673, 1971.)

Table 36-7. Adult immunoglobulin levels (average values)

Immunoglobulin	Average value (mg/dl)
IgG	1250
IgA	210
IgM	140
IgD	3
IgE	0.03

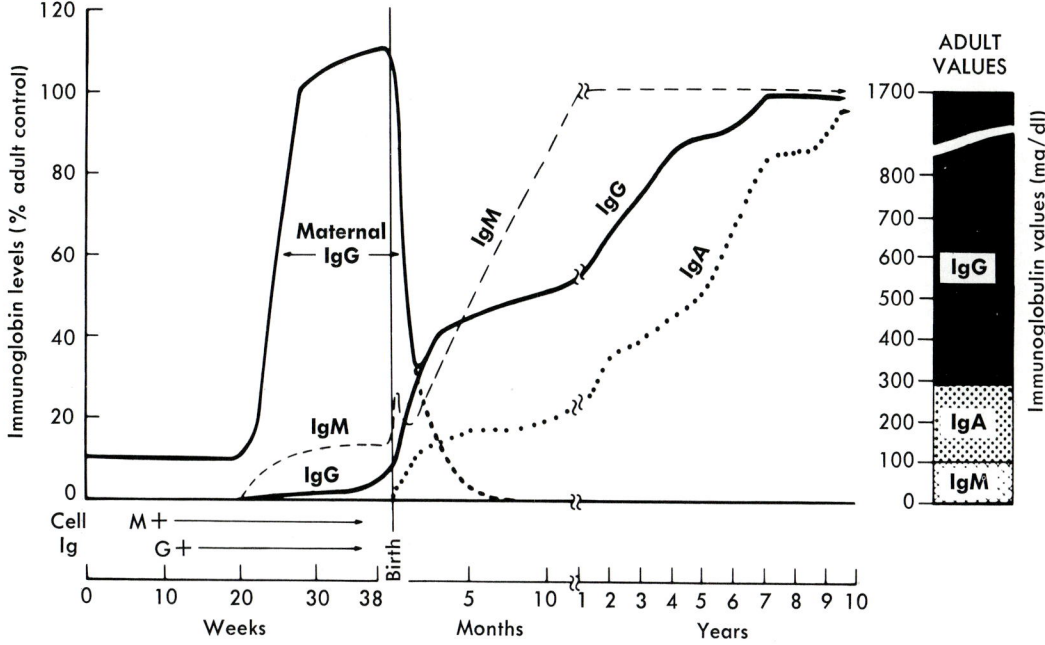

Fig. 36-6. Immunoglobulin concentration in newborns, infants, and children. (From Alford, C.A., Jr.: Pediatr. Clin. North Am. **18:**99, 1971.)

below 37° C; (2) pyroglobulins, which irreversibly precipitate at 56° C; and (3) Bence Jones proteins, which not only reversibly precipitate at 40° C but also include some cold insoluble forms.[141,142]

The majority of cryoglobulins are monoclonal immunoglobulins or mixed cryoglobulins that usually consist of IgM complexed with IgG. Cryoglobulins are usually associated with plasma cell–lymphocytic disorders, but they have also been demonstrated in collagen diseases (systemic lupus erythematosus), in infections (infectious mononucleosis and cytomegalovirus disease), in an essential form not related to any underlying disorder, and in low concentrations in apparently normal individuals. In the latter condition the highest level is 80 μg/ml.[143] Cryoproteins that are not of an immunoglobulin nature can be demonstrated in essential or primary cryoglobulinemia[144] in which high levels of cryofibrinogen are associated with cryoglobulins.[145] As pointed out by Grey and Kohler, the cryoglobulins encountered in plasma cell–lymphocytic proliferative disorders should be called cryoimmunoglobulins.[142] Monoclonal cryoimmunoglobulins G are encountered in about 5% of patients with multiple myeloma, and the cryoimmunoglobulinemia may precede the clinically identifiable plasma cell neoplasia by several years. Monoclonal cryoimmunoglobulinemia M is found in about 7% of patients with Waldenström's macroglobulinemia and is associated with elevated serum or plasma viscosity. The clinical consequences of cryoimmunoglobulins are mainly cold intolerance (ischemia), Raynaud's phenomenon, and various immune complex diseases such as vasculitis, glomerulonephritis, purpura, and arthritis.

Demonstration of cryoimmunoglobulins and cryofibrinogen

***Principle*:** Precipitate is formed on exposure to cold.
***Procedure*:**
1. Collect whole blood in a warmed (37° C) syringe and needle and immediately transfer to a prewarmed test tube held upright in a 37° C heating block.
2. Allow the blood to clot at 37° C and transfer serum into a microhematocrit tube.
3. Allow the tube to stand at room temperature for 4 hr and then transfer to a 4° C refrigerator for 12 hr to 3 days.
4. Remove microhematocrit tube, centrifuge at 4° C, and examine for precipitate for gel formation, the vol % of which can be read directly from microhematocrit reader (Cryocrit).[146]
5. The precipitate will dissolve on warming.
6. If serum clots at 37° C, addition of a chelating agent such as EDTA may be tried to prevent clotting at 37° C.

NOTE: To measure cryofibrinogen, use plasma instead of serum (see step 6 above).

***Normal values and interpretation*:** See "Laboratory investigation of thermoproteins."

Demonstration of pyroglobulins

***Principle*:** Precipitation occurs at 56° C.
***Procedure*:** Allow whole blood to clot at room temperature. Transfer serum to microhematocrit tube and heat to 56° C for 30 min. Centrifuge microhematocrit tube at room temperature and measure pyroprecipitate in microhematocrit reader.

Interpretation: See "Laboratory investigation of thermoproteins." Pyroglobulins are seen in association with M protein–producing plasma cell–lymphocyte disorders, in some collagen diseases, and in primary idiopathic hypergammaglobulinemia.[147, 148] Pyroglobulins are asymptomatic and are usually discovered when complement is inactivated.

Laboratory demonstration of hyperviscosity

The viscosity of blood may be altered by (1) an increase in the number of red cells (polycythemia) and white cells (leukemia), (2) lack of deformability of red cells (sickle cell anemia), and (3) abnormal immunoglobulins.[149, 150] The blood viscosity is the result of the interplay of the red cells and the plasma proteins. The latter have a characteristic intrinsic viscosity that depends on their molecular weight and shape. IgM molecules in high concentrations significantly raise the blood viscosity since they are large, polymerized, and have a five-pronged structure. The IgM-dependent hyperviscosity syndrome has been demonstrated in almost 90% of patients with Waldenström's macroglobulinemia, next in frequency in multiple myeloma, and lastly in collagen diseases. In Waldenström's macroglobulinemia the high viscosity is caused by the high concentration of IgM; in multiple myeloma it is related in some cases to the polymerization of IgA and in others to very high IgG and in a third group to IgG3 aggregates,[151] while in connective tissue diseases aggregates of the rheumatoid factor are responsible for the increased viscosity.

Measurement of viscosity

Principle: The viscosity is determined with an Ostwald viscosimeter, which is a U-shaped tube, one limb of which is relatively wide and opens into a reservoir before it joins the other limb, which is a capillary expanded into one bulb, above and below which measuring lines are etched. The time required for the top of the fluid column to pass between these two measuring lines expresses the viscosity of the fluid.

Equipment:
1. Ostwald viscosimeter (disposable capillary and pipet viscosimeters also available)
2. Water bath, 37° C
3. Stopwatch
4. Stand with clamp to hold viscosimeter

Procedure:
1. Suspend the Ostwald viscosimeter tube in a 37° C glass water bath by means of a special clamp so that the lower half of the tube is immersed in the water.
2. Centrifuge serum for 15 min to remove any particulate matter.
3. Allow 5 ml serum to flow down the wide receiving tube into the reservoir bulb and to warm to 37° C.
4. Attach a suction rubber tubing to the top of the capillary measuring tube and apply suction until the upper meniscus of the serum is above the top mark.
5. Release the suction and allow the fluid to flow back into the reservoir.

6. With a stopwatch measure the time required for the upper meniscus of the serum to travel the distance from the upper mark to the lower mark.
7. Rinse viscosimeter with saline and distilled water.
8. Repeat steps 1-6 using distilled water.

Calculation:

$$\text{Relative viscosity at } 37° C = \frac{\text{Flow time of serum (sec)}}{\text{Flow time of water (sec)}}$$

Normal values: 1.6-1.9.[152]

Discussion: A relative viscosity of 4 or above is indicative of hyperviscosity. The abnormal proteins (see "Laboratory investigation of thermoproteins") responsible for it are often thermoproteins, which render the serum viscosity temperature dependent.[153, 154]

Sia test for macroglobulins and euglobulins[155]

Principle: When serum is diluted with water so that the ionic strength of the serum is decreased, euglobulins and macroglobulins are precipitated.

Procedure: Add 1-2 drops of serum to 10 ml distilled water.

Results: Normal serum proteins diffuse throughout the water. A white cloudy precipitate forms if euglobulins, macroglobulins, or both are present. According to some observers, the pH of the water determines which protein precipitates: at pH 7.2 macroglobulins precipitate; at pH 5 euglobulins do so.[156] Macroglobulins dissolve in saline solution.

The Sia test is a screening test only, and results should be confirmed by quantitative radical immunodiffusion.

Titration of anti-A or anti-B isoantibodies (qualitative assay of humoral immunity)

The lymphoid system and its immunologic expression undergo changes with age. At birth anti-A and anti-B antibodies may be just demonstrable and they remain low for the first 1-2 years, after which time the anti-A titer reaches a level of 1:32 or over, and the anti-B titer climbs to 1:16 or over.[157-159] The titer remains at the adult levels for about 50 years, after which time it may gradually decline. Patients with agammaglobulinemia and hypogammaglobulinemia exhibit deficiencies in immunoglobulins and in the naturally occurring isoantibodies (IgM).

Principle: Saline suspensions of washed group A or B cells are added to equal volumes of serially saline-diluted serum. After 2 hr incubation at room temperature, the highest serum dilution giving a definitely positive although weak agglutination reaction when examined microscopically represents the agglutination titer, expressed as the reciprocal of the serum dilution.

Reagent: 2% suspension of washed group A and B red cells, Rh negative.

Procedure: Prepare nine 65 × 10 mm test tubes. Add 0.2 ml saline to each test tube. Add 0.2 ml serum to first tube and mix. Transfer 0.2 ml of mixture from first to second tube, mix, and continue transfer until the eighth tube is reached. Discard 0.2 ml of mixture in eighth tube.

The ninth tube contains 0.2 ml saline only (control).

Add 0.2 ml 2% red cell suspension to each serum dilution and to the saline control. Mix and allow to stand at room temperature for 2 hr. Look for agglutination microscopically.

Result: The agglutination titer is the reciprocal of the highest serum dilution that gives a positive weak agglutination.

Interpretation: See above.

LABORATORY DIAGNOSIS OF CONNECTIVE TISSUE DISEASES AND AUTOIMMUNE DISORDERS

Systemic lupus erythematosus (SLE) is a diffuse connective tissue disorder that has many features of a complement-dependent autoimmune disease characterized by a variety of antibodies, e.g., antinuclear, anticytoplasmic, anti-IgG, and antierythrocytic, and by such plasma proteins as lymphocytotoxins and circulating anticoagulants.[160]

Hematologic findings

A mild to moderate hypochromic microcytic anemia is seen in almost every patient with SLE. It can be classified as an anemia of chronic disorders since both the serum iron concentration and the total iron-binding capacity are low. The anemia is multifactorial in origin. There may be some difficulty in iron absorption, a mild degree of hemolysis, some blood loss because of hemorrhages, and bone marrow depression because of kidney involvement. A frank autoimmune hemolytic anemia is found in about 5% of the patients and is often combined with an immune thrombocytopenia. The autoimmune anemia is Coombs positive, reacting best with broad-spectrum anticomplement–anti-γ-globulin antisera, and may precede by weeks and months the development of SLE. The erythrocyte sedimentation rate is elevated mainly because of the dysproteinemia and can therefore be used as a rough indicator of disease activity. If the hemolysis is a significant factor, it may be responsible for a mild leukocytosis (less than 40,000 cells/mm^3), which contrasts with the moderate leukopenia seen in about 80% of the patients with SLE.[161] The differential count may be normal but frequently shows an absolute lymphopenia, and fewer than 5% of the patients have a moderate eosinophilia. Thrombocytopenia (less than 100,000/mm^3) is seen in about 25% of the patients and is thought to be caused by an immune mechanism, even though antiplatelet antibodies cannot be demonstrated in all cases,[161] but the giant young platelets found in the peripheral smear and the megakaryocytic hyperplasia of the bone marrow are reminiscent of idiopathic thrombocytopenic purpura, which may precede SLE by months or years.

The bleeding tendency in SLE is caused by a number of factors, the thrombocytopenia being one of the least important contributors. The development of lupoid hepatitis is responsible for the hypofibrinogenemia and the depression of the vitamin K–depending factors. Lupoid nephritis adds a vascular component, and the dysproteinemia is responsible for the development of circulating anticoagulants, which may be antithrombins or specifically directed against factor X[162] and against activation of factors VIII and IX.[163]

In the early stages the bone marrow is cellular and may show myeloid and megakaryocytic hyperplasia.[164] As the disease progresses necrobiosis of various cell groups leads to a reduction in the normal marrow elements and to an increase in plasma cells, tissue mast cells, and phagocytic reticulum cells, which may contain iron and normoblastic nuclei. Free and phagocytosed hematoxylin bodies represent an in vivo LE cell phenomenon.

Antibodies to many different nuclear antigens occur in SLE and in other collagen diseases (Table 36-8), but they vary in their diagnostic and clinical significance depending on their role in the disease process. Some of the nuclear antigens are (1) native DNA (deoxyribonucleic acid) or double-stranded DNA, (2) denatured DNA, (3) nuclear proteins (deoxyribonucleoproteins), (4) nucleolar (RNA) antigen, and (5) extractable nuclear antigen (ENA). A variety of diagnostic tests for antinuclear antibodies are used in the clinical laboratory. They vary in specificity and ease with which they can be performed.[165-167] In general the more sensitive the less specific they are and vice versa (a detailed individual test is discussed later).

LE cell test

Principle: An IgG 7S complement-fixing antibody (LE plasma factor) reacts with the nuclear antigen deoxyribonucleic acid–histone nucleoprotein complex of some white cell nuclei, which are freed and damaged by the test procedure. The antibody depolymerizes the nuclear DNA resulting in nuclear swelling and homogenization (hematoxylin body). This antibody-coated nuclear material in the presence of complement is phagocytosed by polymorphonuclear leukocytes and by monocytes resulting in the formation of the LE cell.

Procedure of glass bead method[168]: Draw 5 ml of venous blood into a heparinized tube and allow to stand for 30-60 min. Rotate with four to eight 4 mm glass beads for 20-30 min in Shen-type rotator. Centrifuge the tube for 5-10 min at 1500 rpm. Transfer the buffy coat from the test tube to a Wintrobe tube. Centrifuge for 5 min at 2500 rpm. Using a Pasteur pipet remove supernatant and transfer buffy coat to a watch glass. Prepare coverslip preparations from the combined buffy coat material (see discussion of preparation of bone marrow smears), stain with Wright-Giemsa stain, and examine for LE cells under high power and oil immersion.

Results: LE cells (Fig. 36-7) are monocytes and polymorphonuclear leukocytes that have phagocytosed, homogeneous, pale, lavender-colored material that lacks nuclear characteristics and displaces the nucleus to the periphery. The formation of the LE cells is accompanied by the production of free LE (hematoxylin) bodies and rosettes (polymorphonuclear cells surrounding LE bodies), morphologic configurations that by themselves are not diagnostic of SLE. Tart (patient's name in whom the cell was first discovered) cells or pseudo-LE cells must not be confused with LE cells. They are polymorphonuclear cells containing phagocytosed nuclei that have retained their chromatin pattern.

Interpretation: Two or more LE cells per coverslip preparation are considered positive.[169] Strict criteria for

Table 36-8. Clinical use of antinuclear antibodies

Antibody	Clinical use	Antibody	Clinical use
Anti-DNA*			
Positive	Antibody to native DNA essentially *diagnostic*, indicates *probability of active nephritis;* antibody to denatured DNA less diagnostic, seen in other inflammatory diseases	Negative	Rarely if ever negative except after long high-dose steroids; *negative result strongly against SLE diagnosis;* repeat only if laboratory error suspected
Negative	Not useful in diagnosis—negative in one half to one third of SLE patients; suggests *absence of active nephritis*	**Antibody to ENA‡**	
		Positive	Reported to indicate probability of more favorable response in anti-DNA-positive SLE nephritis
Antinucleoprotein			
LE cell test			
Positive	Not in itself diagnostic of SLE; *confirms clinical diagnosis*	Negative	Reported to indicate probability of less favorable response in anti-DNA-positive SLE nephritis
		Total ANA§	
Negative	May be negative in SLE; therefore negative test does not exclude diagnosis; perform serologic test if negative	Positive	Not strongly confirmatory; positive results relatively common in variety of chronic diseases and in the aged
Serologic test†			
Positive	Not in itself diagnostic of SLE; *confirms clinical diagnosis;* somewhat less specific than LE cell test—more common in rheumatoid arthritis and conditions related to SLE; positive results infrequent in other medical conditions	Negative	Rarely if ever negative except after long high-dose steroids; *negative result strongly against SLE diagnosis;* repeat only if laboratory error suspected

From Friou, G.J., In Hollander, J.L., and McCarty, D.J., Jr., editors: Arthritis and allied conditions, Philadelphia, 1972, Lea & Febiger.
*Tests using pure DNA as antigen; also shaggy or peripheral immunofluorescent patterns.
†Tests using deoxyribonucleoprotein as antigen; also homogeneous immunofluorescent pattern.
‡Tests using extractable nuclear antigen or nuclear ribonucleoprotein as antigen; also speckled immunofluorescent pattern.
§Tests using whole nuclei without distinguishing antigens or patterns.

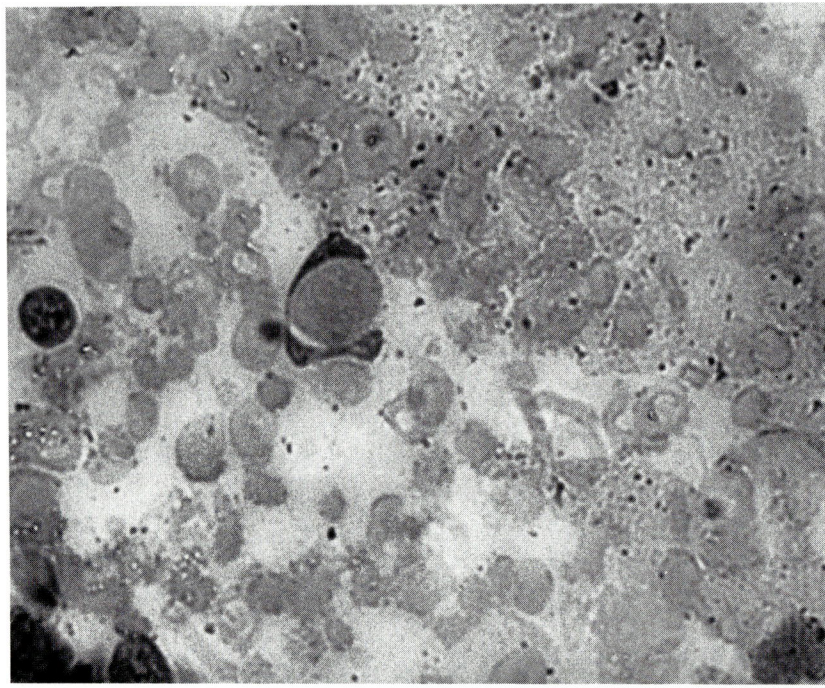

Fig. 36-7. LE cell in peripheral blood sample of a patient with systemic lupus erythematosus. (Giemsa stain, ×650.)

the identification of LE cells must be established. A number of variables affect the LE cell test. If the patient's blood is leukopenic, homologous white cells may be used instead of the patient's cells. To allow the LE factor to penetrate the white cells, they must be damaged. The injury can be inflicted by a number of methods, and enough time must be allowed for the factor to act and for phagocytosis to take place. Inadequate amounts of complement interfere with phagocytosis, and too much heparin inhibits the LE phenomenon.

Discussion: The LE cell test is easy to perform but difficult to standardize and impossible to titrate or quantitate. Since it is positive in only 50-75% of proven cases of SLE, it cannot be used as a screening test to exclude cases of SLE. The LE cell is also found in diseases other than SLE, e.g., rheumatoid arthritis, drug-induced lupus, chronic active (lupoid) hepatitis, scleroderma, dermatomyositis, Sjögren's syndrome,[170] and chronic discoid lupus erythematosus.

Antinuclear antibody

Antinuclear antibodies (ANA) are a heterogeneous group of three immunoglobulin classes present simultaneously (polyclonal pattern). IgG antinuclear antibody is demonstrated in 96% of patients with SLE, while IgM and IgA antinuclear antibodies are found in 81% and 51%, respectively.

Indirect immunofluorescent technic[171]

Principle: The detection of autoantibodies by immunofluoresence has become extremely valuable. The detection of antinuclear antibodies, for example, is extremely sensitive and may be frequently positive in cases where tests for complement fixing or precipitating antinuclear antibodies are negative. Detection of antinuclear antibody is found in a variety of diseases, in elderly individuals without disease, and in 10% of healthy nonelderly individuals.

The antigen, located in the substrate tissue, is fixed to slides for testing purposes. ANA is not specific for a particular organ, and therefore any tissue containing nuclei may be used as substrate[172] The most commonly used tissues are rat or mouse liver or kidney or cell-cultured fibroblasts grown on slides. Unlabeled antibody from the patient's serum, if it is present, will attach to the nuclei in the substrate. After the substrate is washed in buffer, it is incubated with fluorescein-tagged goat antihuman immunoglobulin. If the antibody is present from the first step, the anti-immunoglobulin will attach to it and fluoresce when examined under an ultraviolet light.

At present, the immunofluorescent method is the most widely used technic for ANA screening. Its greatest value is as a laboratory screening test for active SLE, since it is positive in more than 95% of such cases. The ANA test provides the laboratory with a simple and sensitive technic for detecting and measuring these antibodies. The significance of ANA in a patient must be assessed in relationship to the patient's age, sex, clinical history, and other laboratory findings.

Equipment and supplies:
1. Cryostat, adjustable to 4 μ
2. Darkfield fluorescence microscope assembly

3. Kimwipes (Kimberly-Clark Co., Neenah, Wis.) or gauze
4. Diamond point pen
5. Slide racks
6. Slide drainer
7. Slide folders
8. Microscope slides, 1 × 3 in., frosted end, 1 mm thick
9. Coverslips, no.1, 22 mm square
10. Staining dishes and slide carriers

Reagents:
1. Acetone
2. Phosphate buffered saline (PBS): pH 7.2 ± 0.10
   The following formula is for 4 L: 30.6 g NaCl, 2.9 g Na_2HPO_4, 0.84 g KH_2PO_4. Add salts to demineralized or distilled water bringing total volume to 4 L. Stir on magnetic stirrer to ensure adequate mixing. Check pH of each batch of PBS prepared. Discard PBS outside the range of pH 7.2 ± 0.10. Store PBS at 4° C in 4 L glass bottles with screw-cap lids.
3. Glycerin/PBS
   To 9 ml of reagent-quality glycerin in a small dropper bottle add 1 ml of PBS. Shake gently until the two reagents are mixed.
4. Ether, anesthesia grade
5. Fluorescein-labeled conjugates, antihuman globulin, IgG, and IgM Purchase commercially. Determine the working titer of these conjugates following the instruction under "Check-testing anti-DNA slides and fluorescein-labeled antihuman immunoglobulin." Prepare aliquots of the conjugates in 0.3 ml quantities when received and store at −70° C. When conjugate is thawed for use, do not refreeze, but store at 4° C and use as long as satisfactory results are obtained with controls, or follow manufacturer's directions.

Technic:
Preparation of tissue sections:
1. Antinuclear antibody (ANA) requires normal mouse kidney sections.
   a. Select normal mouse from colony (1-6 months of age; if female, use virgins only).
   b. Anesthetize mouse with ether in anesthetizing jar. Bleed animal out and remove both kidneys. Do not allow tissue to dry out.
   c. Cut kidneys in half, remove fat, and replace in labeled glass screw-capped vials. Drop vial into liquid nitrogen. Store at −70° C.
2. Prepare slides for indirect testing by first marking the back (unfrosted side) of the slide with a diamond point pen. Use the serum slide rack as a template and place a small mark on the slide to coincide with the marks on the rack. Place two sections on each slide. Slides may be cut and fixed and then frozen at −78° C until needed for testing. They should be stored in closed plastic boxes and labeled and dated. They are good as long as the controls work properly.
3. Place a section on the frosted side of the slide over the etched mark. Cut enough sections for testing at 4 μ in a −20° C cryostat (see instruction manual on top of cryostat [International Equipment Co., Needham, Mass.]).

4. After the sections are cut, fix them for 10 min in acetone. Allow those slides fixed in acetone to air dry thoroughly.

Preparation of sera: Store and use control sera as given in "Control sera for indirect immunofluorescence."

POSITIVE CONTROL: Positive rim and diffused pattern ANA show a strong positive reaction when diluted 1:100 or greater with PBS.

Using a 2.0 ml pipet, add 1.00 ml of PBS to a small test tube. Using an Eppendorf pipet, add 0.01 ml (10 λ) of the positive control into the tube. Mix well.

NEGATIVE CONTROL: Negative serum should show no fluorescence when diluted 1:20 in PBS.

NONSPECIFIC CONTROL: A tissue section stained with buffer and conjugate only should show no fluorescence. Use this when titrating conjugates.

Use the first slide as a control slide and identify it by marking on the frosted end of the slide. EXAMPLE: Slide 1 should have the positive control on the A spot and the negative control on the B spot.

Procedure:

1. To test sera for ANA screening with globulin, dilute all samples 1:20 with PBS. Add 0.05 ml of serum to 0.95 ml of PBS in a tube.
2. Identify previously prepared slides by marking the frosted end of the slide with a lead pencil.
3. To test sera for ANA testing for IgG and IgM antibodies, dilute sera 1:20 with PBS for IgG testing and 1:20 with PBS for globulin testing (contains IgM).
4. Identify slides as in step 2.
5. With a disposable transfer pipet, drop approximately 0.2 ml of the control and test serum dilutions on the serum slide rack corresponding to the location of the slides.
6. Carefully place the labeled slide (tissue side down) on the dilutions on the rack.
7. Stain at room temperature for 30 min.
8. At the end of the time, place the slides in a slide carrier, which is immersed in cold PBS for 5 min. Agitate slides while rinsing. Repeat this step using fresh PBS.
9. While slides are rinsing, prepare dilutions of conjugates to be used by adding PBS to produce the working titer previously determined.
10. Using an Eppendorf pipet, add 0.025 ml (use 50 ml pipet and divide between two spots) to the appropriate locations on the conjugate slide rack. ANA screening utilizes globulin; routine ANA uses globulin and IgG.
11. Remove slides one by one from slide rack and let drain for a moment. Gently blot the excess PBS from around the sections. **Do not allow tissue to dry out.** Place slides on rack as described in step 6.
12. Stain at room temperature for 30 min.
13. Repeat step 8 and let slides drain as in step 11.
14. Mount slides by placing a coverslip (to which a drop of glycerin-PBS has been added) on the sections.
15. Place slides in folder and store at 4° C until time to view. Viewing should be done within 4 hr of completion of the test.

16. Study sections microscopically using mercury arc illumination and 250X dry objective with darkfield condenser. Use a BG12 exciting filter and OG1 barrier filter.
17. For ANA screening tests, sections showing no fluorescence are reported as negative. For those sections showing fluorescence of nuclei, determine titer as follows:

Intensity of fluorescence	Titer
Weak fluorescence	1:40 and 1:80
Moderate fluorescence	1:100 and 1:200
Strong fluorescence	1:400, 1:800, and 1:1600

18. For ANA testing for IgG and IgM antibodies, determine titer for all positive combined globulin and IgG fluorescence as in step 17. For positive globulin fluorescence but negative IgG fluorescence, determine titer for sera as in step 17 but use IgM conjugate.
19. Note patterns of nuclear staining as follows: A diffused pattern is indicated by homogeneous staining of the nuclei; speckled staining shows clumps or granules of fluorescence in the nuclei; a rim pattern shows a halo of fluorescence at the periphery of the nuclei; and a nucleolar pattern shows only one or two clumps of staining in the nuclei. Results are reported as negative or positive. If positive, report the immunoglobulin used (IgG or IgM), the titer, and the pattern. EXAMPLE: ANA positive, IgM, 1:200, speckled.

Titration of ANA serum: Make up ANA controls and titer dilutions as required. Make up the initial dilution and set up the required serial dilutions. EXAMPLE: For 1:400 add 0.01 ml (10λ) to 3.99 ml PBS. Make 1:800 and 1:1600 by serial dilution of the 1:400 solution.

Follow the procedure outlined in the previous section for ANA testing.

Read results by determining the titer. The titer is the highest dilution at which weak fluorescence is definitely noted. Determine any change in pattern.

Report the results as positive, including IgG or IgM class, the titer, and pattern. EXAMPLE: ANA positive, IgG class, titer of 1:100, diffused pattern. If the pattern should change in dilution, report the pattern associated with the highest titer.

Interpretation of staining patterns[173-175]: ANAs are groups of immunoglobulins (antibodies) that react with the whole nucleus or with nuclear components such as nuclear proteins, DNA, or histone so that a number of reaction patterns are produced, which reflect the distribution of the various antigens witin the nuclei (Figs. 36-8 and 36-9).

The diffused or homogeneous pattern results from anti–deoxyribonucleic acid–nucleoprotein antibodies and is characteristic of SLE but may also be seen in rheumatoid arthritis. The whole nucleus fluoresces evenly, although vacuoles may be seen.[176]

The peripheral (marginal or rim) pattern results from antibodies to DNA and is seen in SLE and Sjögren's syndrome. The central portion of the nucleus is only lightly stained or not stained at all, while the nuclear margins fluoresce strongly and appear to extend into the cytoplasm.[177]

The speckled pattern occurs in the presence of antibodies to an extractable nuclear antigen (ENA) devoid of DNA or histone[178] and may indicate a connective tissue disease (mixed connective tissue disease [MCTD])[179] with a relatively better prognosis than SLE and is usually observed in rheumatoid arthritis, Sjögren's syndrome, scleroderma, and dermatomyositis, although it is also seen in SLE. Numerous round dots of nuclear fluorescence are seen against a brown-red background. The antibody is directed against saline extractable nuclear antigens (anti-RNP and anti-Sm). See section on anti-ENA (p. 1106).

The nucleolar pattern reflects an antibody to nucleolar RNA and occurs in about 50% of patients with scleroderma (progressive systemic sclerosis),[176,180] in Sjögren's syndrome, and in SLE. Multiple round, smooth nucleoli that vary in size light up under the ultraviolet light.

Figs. 36-8 and 36-9 are simplified illustrations of the patterns just described.

Horseradish peroxidase conjugated antibody technic[181-183]

Principle: The horseradish peroxidase (HRP) conjugated antibody technic involves overlaying the substrate tissue section (rat liver or kidney devoid of peroxidase) with an unknown serum. The binding of the serum ANA to the substrate nuclei is detected by reacting the section with antihuman immunoglobulin conjugated to HRP. The enzyme is localized and demonstrated by its ability to catalyze the oxidation of diaminobenzidine to an insoluble product that stains the nuclei dark brown.

The sensitivity of the method and the patterns observed correspond to those of the fluorescent method, but the HRP technic has the advantages of requiring only a light microscope and of providing permanent sections.

Reagents: The reagents are commercially available from Bioware (Wichita, Kan.) and allow some degree of standardization and reproducibility.[181]

Results: Examine slides for light to dark reddish brown staining nuclear material against a light pink background using the medium and high-dry objectives of a light microscope.

Interpretation of staining patterns: See the following discussion of the ANA immunofluorescent test.

General discussion of ANA test[173-175]

In the evaluation of patients with connective tissue diseases, the ANA must be interpreted with caution. The significance of a positive ANA depends on the titer and observed pattern. ANA is not commonly found in young healthy individuals; however, increasing age often leads to low titer ANA in "normal" men and women. ANA is almost invariably present in high titer in patients with untreated active SLE. The absence of ANA in a serum almost excludes the diagnosis of SLE. ANA titers of 10-80 usually have little significance but may be seen in patients with rheumatoid arthritis or scleroderma.

There is no general agreement on the significance of the various patterns. Some patterns may mask other patterns in high concentration. For example, a diffused pattern at 1:20 may obscure a speckled pattern which can be seen when the end point titer of the sample is determined. Since a diffused pattern is so common, a titer of 100 or above should be considered strong circumstantial evidence for a connective tissue disorder. ANA is often found in liver disease associated with autoimmunity such as chronic active hepatitis, primary biliary cirrhosis, and cryptogenic cirrhosis. No diagnosis should be based solely on nuclear patterns in a patient's serum. Clinical data, antibody titer, and other laboratory findings should all be reviewed before a definite diagnosis is made.

Significance: The following significance may be attached to titers obtained in our laboratory:

20-40: Not significant unless patient's history suggests evidence of connective tissue disease
80-200: Suggestive of connective tissue disorder
200 or higher: Strong evidence for connective tissue disorder

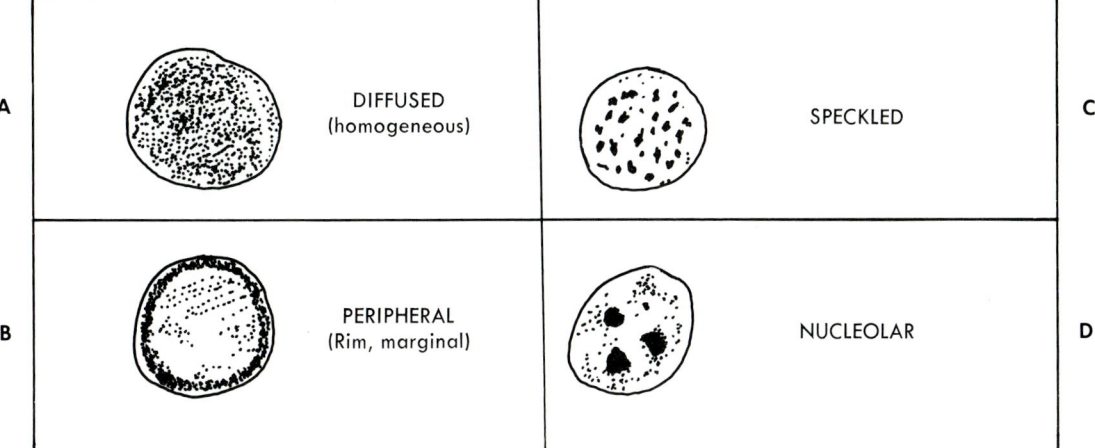

Fig. 36-8. Schematic drawings of four different patterns of antinuclear antibodies, **A, B, C,** and **D,** which correspond to the immunofluorescent patterns in Fig. 36-9.

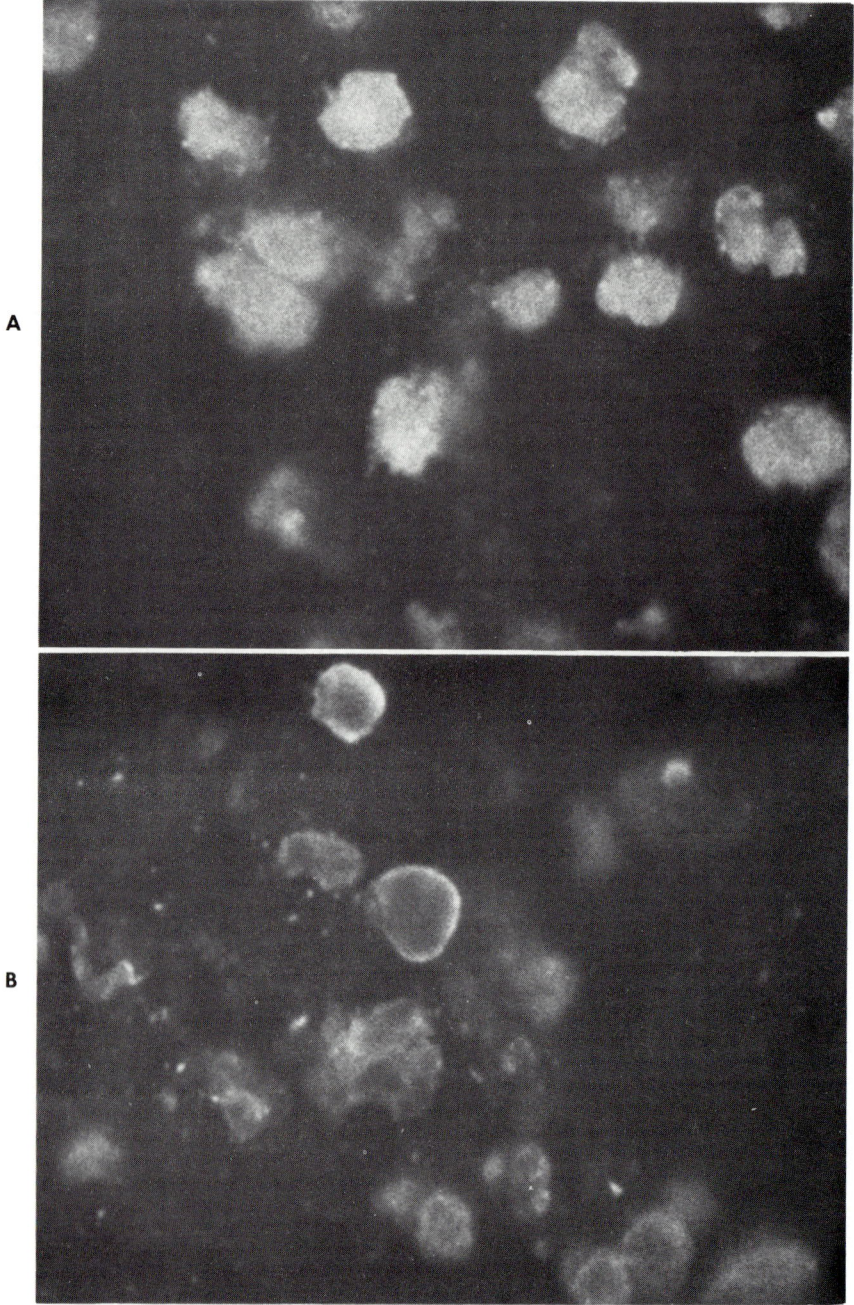

Fig. 36-9. Immunofluorescent patterns of ANA. Mouse kidney sections. **A,** Diffused. **B,** Rim. **C,** Speckled. **D,** Nucleolar. (×500.)

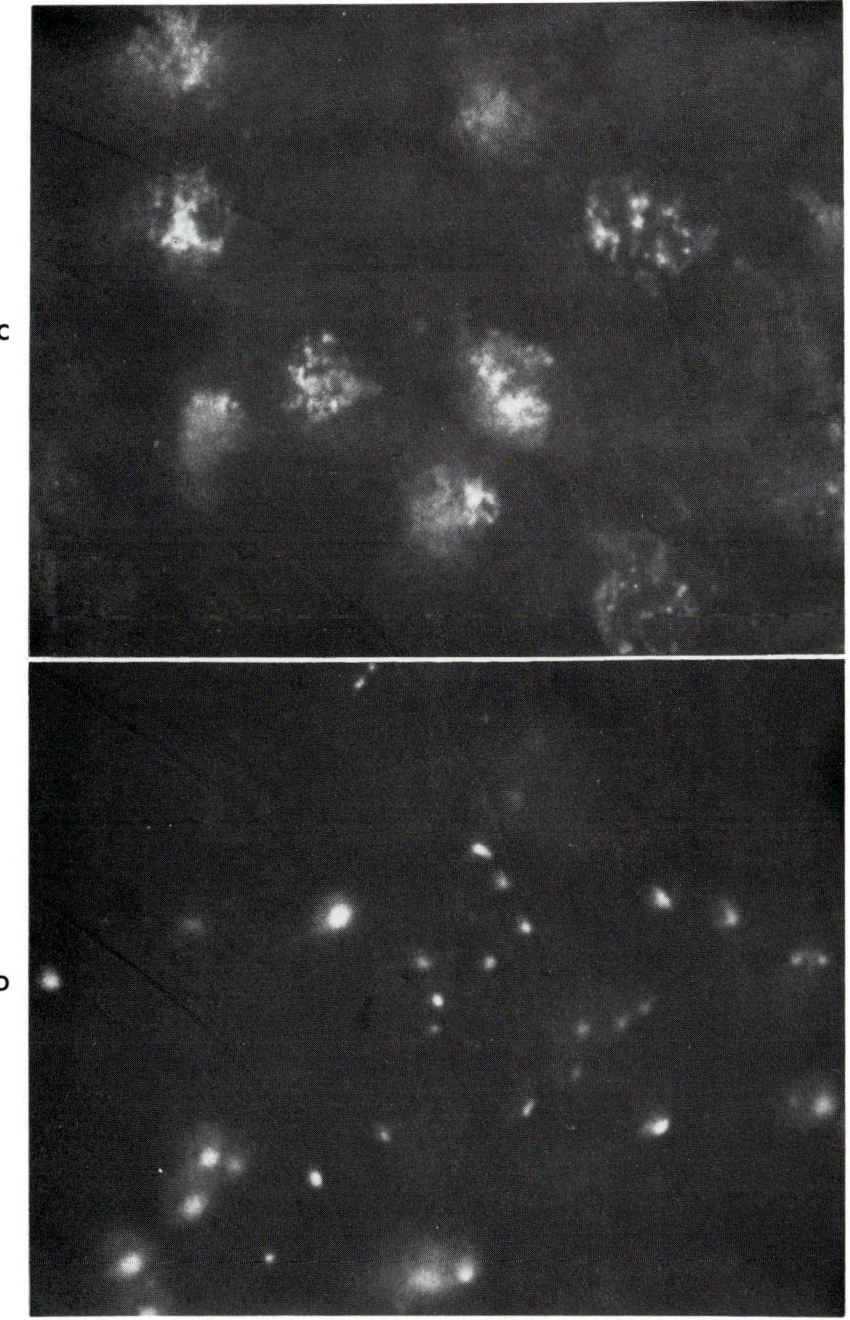

Fig. 36-9, cont'd, For legend see opposite page.

ANA titers of 1:80 and over can be demonstrated in about 95% of patients with SLE, but they are not specific for SLE. If the ANA test is negative, SLE can usually be excluded provided the patient is not under treatment and false negative reactions have been excluded. If the ANA test is positive, it should be confirmed by the anti-DNA antibody test. The LE cell test is not useful as a confirmatory test since it is positive in only 75% of patients with confirmed SLE.[184]

Generally, the antinuclear antibody has no organ or species specificity and the nuclear material from a variety of organs of human or animal origin can be used as antigens, e.g., human leukocytes,[185] chicken erythrocytes,[186] frozen rat liver,[177] tissue culture cells,[187] rat and mouse kidney,[188] and spots of nuclear protein and DNA.[189] Human leukocytes are quite adequate and sensitive, eliminate the need for cryostat procedures, and can be concentrated in buffy coat preparations.[190] The spot-antigen technic shares many of the advantages of the leukocyte method. The advantage of the rat tissue is the fact that it is widely used and results are therefore comparable.

False negative reactions may occur if the ANAs happen to be specific for an antigen other than the one used in the procedure, e.g., specific antihuman leukocyte antinuclear antibodies have been reported. False negative results may also occur if the substrate is fixed in acetone and is inadequately washed.[191]

On the other hand, without fixation some soluble nuclear antigens may be lost.[191] False negative ANA tests may also be related to the binding of the antinuclear factor to circulating antigens forming immune complexes and to too low an antibody titer.[169]

False positive reactions may occur when the speckled pattern predominates.[170]

Sera may be screened at standardized dilutions, e.g., 1:100. Lower dilutions should not be used, since 1% of the normal population are positive at these dilutions.[165] If the serum is positive at 1:10 dilution, it should be retested at dilutions from 1:20 to 1:320. Changes in the antibody titer can be used to observe the disease activity.

The incidence of ANA in SLE is 95% or greater, in Sjögren's syndrome 68%, in scleroderma 40%, and in rheumatoid arthritis 15-25%.[192] The higher the ANA titer, the more likely is the diagnosis of SLE.[165]

Nonspecific staining reactions occur whenever the conjugate or the serum contains antibodies to other tissue antigens and must be differentiated from the ANA patterns. Careful rinsing and removal of excess fluoresceinated conjugate minimizes some of the nonspecific staining reactions.

Detection of antibodies to deoxyribonucleic acid: anti-DNA

In contrast to the antinucleoprotein antibodies, which are not diagnostic of SLE, the antibodies to double-strained (native) DNA are specific for SLE if present in high concentrations.[193] In low concentrations they may be found in other collagen diseases. They disappear from the serum during the chronic phase of SLE to emerge again during exacerbations. The fall of the anti-DNA titer in response to treatment and its rise in the acute phase allow it to be used to monitor the clinical course of SLE. Since anti-DNA–DNA–complement complexes are etiologically involved in lupus nephritis, a rising anti-DNA titer associated with a fall in complement points to renal involvement.[194] Most SLE sera also react with heat denatured (single-stranded) DNA,[195] but the reaction has the same specificity as the ANA test. A number of methods are available for the demonstraton of anti–native DNA antibodies. Because commercial DNA usually contains both native and denatured DNA—but usually more of the first—the spot test can be utilized to demonstrate anti–native DNA antibodies.[189] Other methods include agarose gel diffusion,[196] hemagglutination,[197,198] complement fixation, and radioimmunoassay.[199] The latter method is the most sensitive technic for the demonstration of anti-DNA (native and denatured) antibodies and is highly reproducible. The agarose double diffusion precipitin test[196] for anti-DNA is relatively insensitive, while the more sensitive complement-fixation test is handicapped by the fact that many LE sera are anticomplementary. The hemagglutination test[197,198] is sensitive and uses tanned formalized erythrocytes onto which DNA is absorbed.

Radioimmunoassay for antibodies to deoxyribonucleic acid[199]

Introduction and discussion: Radioimmunoassay measures the direct binding of radioactive DNA to antibody. The serum complement, which may nonspecifically bind nucleic acid, is destroyed by heating and the serum is then incubated with the radioactive DNA at 37° C and at 4° C to allow the formation of radioactive immune complexes. The radiolabeled DNA is commercially available as DNA complexed with radioactive actinomycin D or as DNA labeled with ^{14}C or ^{3}H. The radioactive immune complexes are detected by the **ammonium sulfate method**[200-202] or by the **cellulose ester filter technic**.[203] The ammonium sulfate method is based on the fact that uncomplexed DNA is soluble in 50% saturated ammonium sulfate, while the DNA–anti-DNA complexes are not soluble and are therefore precipitated. The unbound free antigen and the complexed antigen can thus be separated by centrifugation. A comparison of the radioactivity in the supernatant and the precipitate gives the DNA binding activity.[201] The sensitivity of the ammonium sulfate technic is 1:10,000 to 1:25,000 compared to a hemagglutination sensitivity of 1:512 and a complement-fixation sensitivity of 1:1000.

The filter method of assaying the radioactive immune complexes is accomplished by trapping the complexes on cellulose ester filters and measuring their radioactivity in scintillation counters.[203] The amount of radioactivity reflects the antibody concentration. The free, unbound DNA passes through the filters.

Indirect immunofluorescent test for anti-DNA

Principle: Anti–native deoxyribonucleic acid (nDNA) antibodies are frequently found in sera from patients with active spontaneous systemic lupus erythematosus (SLE) and some drug-induced syndromes.[196] The presence of nDNA antibodies indicates active SLE and correlates closely with the onset of lupus nephritis.[194] The specificity of nDNA antibodies for SLE is much greater than antinuclear antibodies. Therefore detection of nDNA antibodies provides valuable diagnostic as well as prognostic information for the differential diagnosis of SLE. The presence of nDNA antibodies in known SLE sera is considered an indication of recurrent active disease or poor response to therapy. Consequently, periodic monitoring of nDNA antibodies in SLE patients aids in evaluating the clinical course of the disease and its response to therapy.[193,196]

The test for anti-DNA is an indirect immunofluorescence procedure using *Crithidia luciliae* as the substrate.[204] The kinetoplast of this protozoan hemoflagellate contains a high concentration of nDNA that is double-stranded DNA without any nicks or other types of degradation. If the patient's serum contains antibodies to nDNA they will react with the nDNA in the kinetoplast. When floreoscein-labeled antihuman γ-globulin is added in the second step, a positive apple-green fluorescent staining in the small kinetoplasts of *C. luciliae* will be observed.

Equipment and supplies:
1. *C. luciliae* antigen slides
2. Darkfield fluorescence microscope assembly
3. Bibulous paper
4. Wet box
5. Coverslips, no. 1.5, 25 × 50 mm
6. Slide folder
7. Staining dish and slide carrier

Reagents:
1. Phosphate buffered saline (PBS), pH 7.2 ± 0.10 See ANA section for formula.
2. Glycerin-PBS See ANA section for formula.
3. Fluorescein-labeled antihuman γ-globulin See ANA section.

Procedures:
Preparation of serum:
1. For positive control select known positive high titer serum for positive anti-DNA control. Dilute serum 1:10 with PBS. Divide into aliquots of 50 λ units per microvial and store at −78° C.
2. For negative control select serum with a negative anti-DNA and ANA as negative control. Dilute 1:10 with PBS. Negative control for ANA test can be used as negative anti-DNA control.
3. Dilute all patients' sera 1:10 with PBS.
Procedures for anti-DNA:
1. Remove slides from freezer, tear open the protective envelope, and remove slides containing *C. luciliae*. Allow slides to reach room temperature. Label slides numerically if using more than one slide.
2. Prepare control and patient's sera at 1:10 dilution in PBS. Do not use hemolyzed specimens.
3. Identify each well with the appropriate patient's sera and controls.
4. Cover each well with approximately 10 λ of either patient's serum or control serum.
5. Place the slides, with the well up, in a covered moist chamber and incubate at room temperature for 30 min.

6. After incubation, wash slide in two 5 min changes of PBS.
7. Dry slide between bibulous paper and cover each well with approximately 10 λ of the conjugate. Incubate in covered moist chamber for 30 min at room temperature.
8. Repeat step 6.
9. Dry slide between bibulous paper. Place a small drop of PBS-glycerol on a 22 × 50 mm slide for each well and apply coverslip to slide.
10. Read slides within 4 hr using fluorescent microscope.

Quality controls for anti-DNA test:
Tolerance limits: The positive control serum should show bright staining of only the kinetoplast of *C. luciliae*. The negative serum should show no fluorescent staining of the kinetoplast or nucleus of *C. luciliae*.
Check-testing anti-DNA slides and fluorescein-labeled antihuman immunoglobulin:
1. Cross check new lot number of DNA slides in parallel with old lot of DNA slides three times using 1:100 dilution of positive and negative controls and selected patients' sera. Results should be identical for old and new lot numbers.
2. Cross check new lot number of fluorescein-labeled antihuman immunoglobulin at 1:20, 1:40, 1:80, and 1:160 with the 1:10 dilution of the positive control sera. Cross check the fluorescein-labeled antihuman immunoglobulin at 1:20 with the 1:10 dilution of the negative control sera. Run the old lot number of fluorescein-labeled antihuman immunoglobluin at a 1:10 dilution with the positive and negative controls diluted 1:10. Repeat cross check with the old and new lot numbers of fluorescein-labeled antihuman immunoglobulin three times in parallel. The end point of the titration is the highest dilution giving a strongly positive result with the positive control DNA serum. The working titer of the conjugate is one doubling dilution below the end point. The conjugate should not stain nonspecifically at two doubling dilutions below the working titer of the conjugate.

Interpretation:[194,196] Any observed apple-green staining of the small kinetoplast of the *C. luciliae* substrate organisms (Fig. 36-10) at a 1:10 dilution based on a 1+ to 4+ scale is considered positive. All sera positive at 1:10 should be titrated to the end point dilution by making a 1:20, 1:40, 1:80, etc., serial dilution of all positive sera. The end point is the highest dilution that produces a positive reaction. Staining of both the small kinetoplast and the adjacent larger *C. luciliae* nuclcus simultaneously should be interpreted as a positive test. Polar staining at the base of the flagella is not significant. Staining of the nucleus only should be interpreted as a positive test.

Some limitations to the test are that SLE patients undergoing steroid therapy may have negative test results and some drugs, particularly hydralazine, may induce nDNA antibody production. The detection of nDNA antibodies by the indirect fluorescent technic is a diagnostic aid. Therefore it is imperative that any results be interpreted in light of the patients' clinical condition.

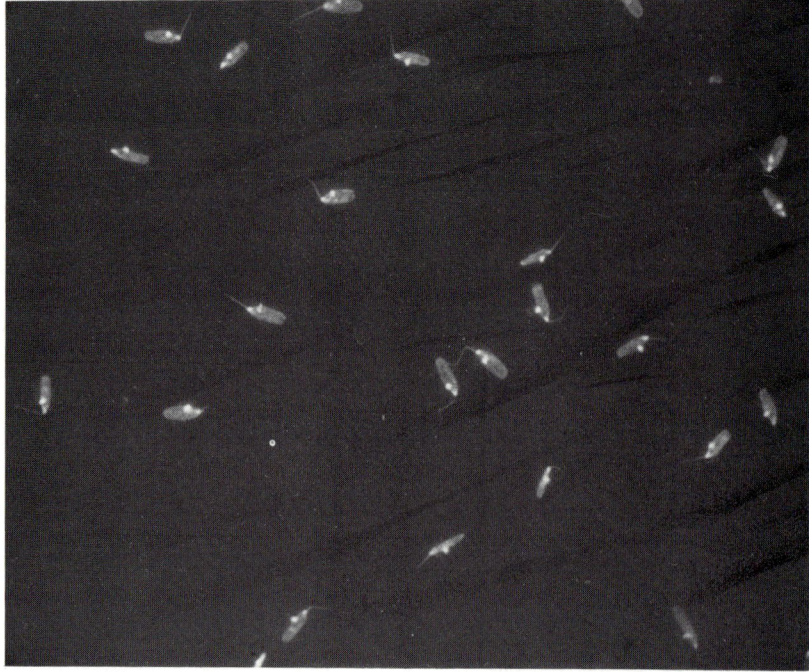

Fig. 36-10. Anti-nDNA shown by indirect immunofluorescence. Staining of both the small kinetoplast and the adjacent larger nucleus of *Crithidia luciliae* occur simultaneously. (×500.)

Significance:
1. Titers less than 1:10 are considered negative.
2. Titers positive at 1:10 or above with a high titer ANA are highly suggestive of SLE.
3. Titers positive at 1:10 to 1:20 with a low titer ANA are probably suggestive of another disease state rather than SLE.

Normal range: Negative.

Antimitochondrial antibody

Principle: Most of the autoantibodies demonstrated in the serum of patients with liver disease are non-organ-specific antibodies that are directed against antigens shared by the liver and other organs. Liver disease may show positive results in the ANA, antimitochondrial antibody (AMA), and anti-smooth-muscle antibody tests. The different immunofluorescence tests for these antibodes can be a diagnostic aid in differentiating chronic active hepatitis, primary biliary cirrhosis, and cryptogenic cirrhosis from other diseases.[205]

Antibodies to mitochondria have been found in high titer in approximately 92% of patients with primary biliary cirrhosis and are not normally found in patients with extrahepatic biliary obstructions,[206] drug-associated hepatitis, or viral hepatitis. AMA has been found in patients with chronic active hepatitis and cryptogenic cirrhosis. ANA is found in all the liver disorders associated with autoimmunity, especially in chronic active hepatitis and primary biliary cirrhosis.[207]

The antigen used for AMA is most commonly rat or mouse kidney. The technic is that of indirect immunofluorescence similar to the ANA procedure (Fig. 36-11). The antigen is a lipoprotein of the inner mitochon-

drial membrane. It is likely that antibodies to other components of cell organelles may occur as well, especially to a membrane antigen or granular endoplasmic reticulum and to the outer nuclear membrane. Using the distal kidney in immunofluorescence tests as the site of the strongest reaction for primary biliary cirrhosis provides reasonably clear-cut results.

Equipment and supplies: See ANA section on equipment and supplies.

Reagents: See reagents under ANA section.

The fluorescein-labeled conjugate is the antihuman immunoglobulin, which is the same as that for the ANA test.

Technics:

Preparation of tissue sections:
1. AMA requires normal mouse kidneys. Collect and prepare tissue as for ANAs.
2. After the sections are cut, they may be frozen at −78° C or used immediately. Fixation is not necessary.

Preparation of serum:
1. The positive control for AMA is diluted 1:100 or 1:200 depending on the control sample and should show 3+ fluorescence at this dilution. The negative control should be diluted 1:20 and show no fluorescence at this dilution.
2. All patients' sera are tested at 1:20 and 1:80 dilutions in PBS for AMA.

Procedure: See ANA section.

Quality controls:

TOLERANCE LIMITS: Moderate to strong fluorescence in the mitochondria of the distal tubules indicates a positive reaction (note whether a prozone phenomenon ex-

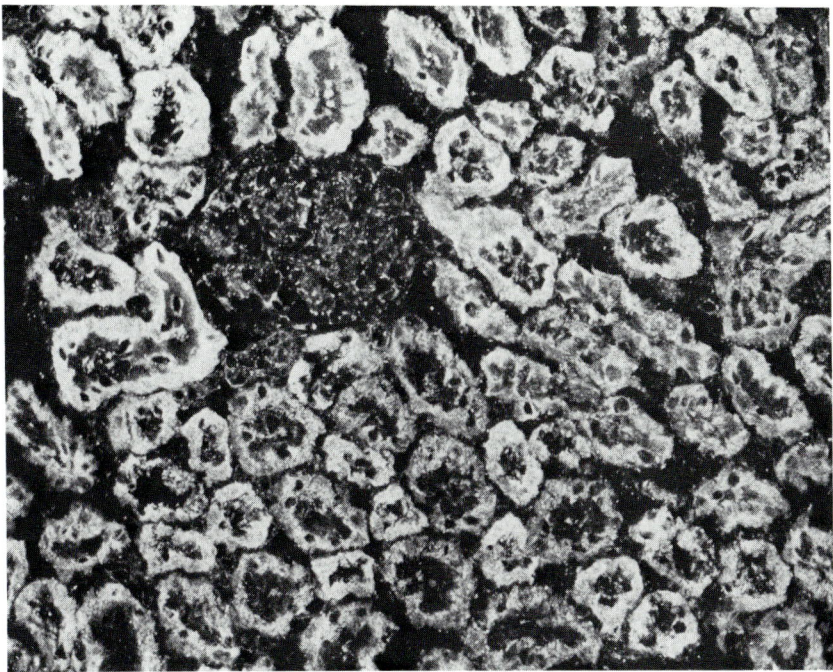

Fig. 36-11. Antimitochondrial antibody (AMA) in mouse kidney section shown by indirect immunofluorescence. (×500.)

ists at the 1:20 dilution). No fluorescence at 1:20 indicates a negative result. Results are reported as positive or negative.

CONTROL SERA FOR INDIRECT IMMUNOFLUORESCENCE: Prepare and store control sera as indicated in ANA section.

CHECK-TESTING FLUORESCEIN-LABELED CONJUGATE: See ANA section.

Interpretation: Primary biliary cirrhosis (PBC) is characterized by a chronic inflammatory destruction of the small intrahepatic biliary ducts and tubules.[205] It is found most frequently in women aged 30-60 years. AMA has been found to be of diagnostic value in differentiating PBC from extrahepatic biliary tract obstruction and from drug-induced cholestatic jaundice.[206,207]

Titers of AMA in PBC have been reported in the range of 20-6000. Positive fluorescence at 1:20 is considered positive for mitochondrial antibodies. There is no correlation between titer and activity of disease. The occurrence of AMA is very rare in healthy individuals (<1%).

Significance: The following significance may be related to results obtained in our laboratory:

Positive at 1:20, negative at 1:80: Suggestive of PBC; report as positive and less than 1:80
Positive at 1:20 and 1:80: Strong evidence for PBC; report as positive and greater than 1:80

Normal range: Negative.

Anti-smooth-muscle antibody

Principle: As described in the section on antimitochondrial antibody, the test for anti-smooth-muscle an-

tibody (ASMA) is often positive in patients with chronic active hepatitis, primary biliary cirrhosis, and cryptogenic cirrhosis.[205] The highest incidence of smooth muscle antibodies has been found in patients with chronic active hepatitis (lupoid hepatitis) and has been estimated to be of value in confirming 70% of the cases of this disease.[208] ASMA has been found in 50% of biliary cirrhosis cases and 28% of cryptogenic cirrhosis cases.

The antigen that is used in ASMA testing is rat or mouse stomach, human stomach, and human or monkey uterus (Fig. 36-12). Again, this test serves to help to differentiate active chronic hepatitis, biliary cirrhosis, and cryptogenic cirrhosis from other liver diseases.

Equipment and supplies: See ANA section.

Reagents: See reagent under ANA section.

The fluorescein-labeled conjugate is the antihuman immunoglobulin, which is the same as that for ANAs.

Technics:

Preparation of tissue sections:

1. ASMA requires normal mouse stomach. Follow the procedure outlined for mouse kidney (ANA) except remove the stomach. Rinse it well in cold PBS and roll it up jelly roll fashion. Freeze in vials as for mouse kidney.
2. Cut sections to run control sera and two dilutions of each patient's serum. Do not fix these slides before use.
3. Slides may be cut and stored at −78° C if desired.

Preparation of serum:

1. The positive control for ASMA is diluted 1:20

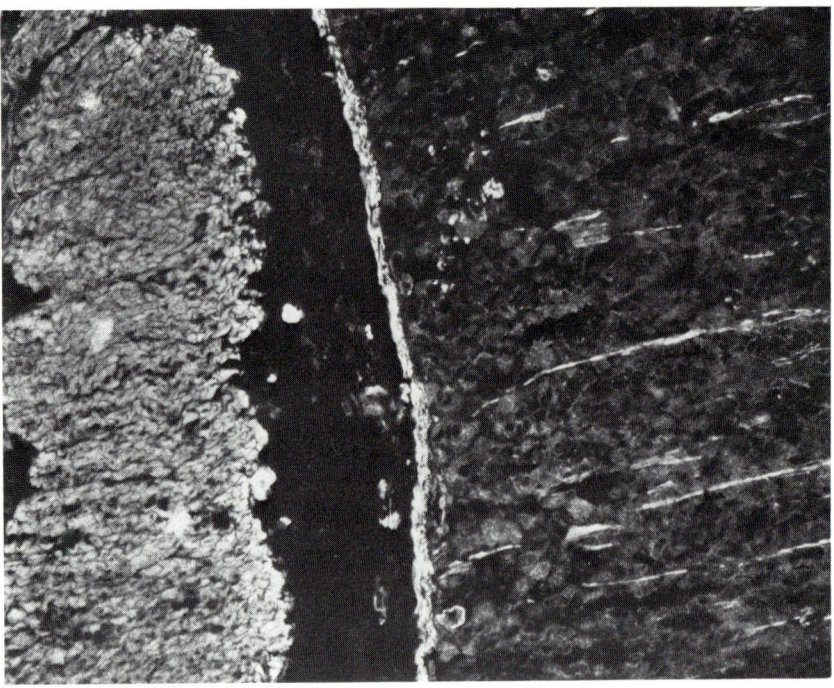

Fig. 36-12. Anti-smooth-muscle antibody (ASMA) in mouse stomach section shown by indirect immunofluorescence. (×500.)

and should show 3-4+ fluorescence at this dilution in the muscle fibers of the mouse stomach. The negative control should be diluted 1:20 and show no fluorescence at this dilution.
2. All patients' sera are tested at 1:20 and 1:80 dilutions in PBS for ASMA.

Procedure: See ANA section.

Quality controls:

TOLERANCE LIMITS: Strong fluorescence in the muscle fibers of the mouse stomach indicates a positive reaction. No fluorescence at 1:20 indicates a negative result. Results are reported as positive or negative.

Interpretation: Chronic active hepatitis (CAH), also called plasma cell hepatitis, lupoid hepatitis, and juvenile cirrhosis, is a chronic disease usually affecting young females. Liver function deteriorates because of progressive necrosis of hepatic parenchymal cells in areas of lymphocytic and plasma cell infiltrate. In the past ASMA was considered specific for CAH, however, these antibodies are not confined to CAH or other liver diseases.[205] ASMAs are found in 40-70% of patients with CAH, in 50% of patients with biliary cirrhosis, and in 28% of patients with cryptogenic cirrhosis. ASMA has also been found in patients with infectious mononucleosis,[209,210] asthma, malignant diseases,[210] and yellow fever. ASMA titers are usually in the range of 80-320 and persist for many years. Lower titers may be seen in viral hepatitis and biliary cirrhosis. ASMA has been reported to be of aid in confirming the diagnosis of approximately 70% of CAH cases.

Significance: The following significance may be found in results obtained in our laboratory:

ASMA positive at 1:20, negative at 1:80: Suggestive of CAH; report as positive, less than 1:80
ASMA positive at 1:20 and 1:80: Strong evidence for CAH; report as positive, greater than 1:80

Normal range: Negative.

Antithyroid antibodies

Principle: Thyroid antibodies (TAs) are a characteristic finding in patients with Hashimoto's thyroiditis and Graves' disease.[211] They may also be found in the serum of patients with other diseases such as myxedema, granulomatous thyroiditis, nontoxic nodular goiter, and thyroid carcinoma.[212] TAs are also found in most cases of lymphocytic thyroiditis in children and rarely in patients with pernicious anemia and Sjögren's syndrome. Most TAs are of the IgG class; however, IgA and IgM TAs have been observed. Two distinct antibodies to thyroid antigens are routinely detected by immunofluorescence. These are (1) antibodies to thyroglobulin and the thyroid follicles and (2) antibodies to thyroid microsomal components of thyroid epithelial cells.

The antigen used for antithyroid antibody (ATA) is human or monkey thyroid tissue (Fig. 36-13). The technic is that of indirect immunofluorescence similar to the ANA procedure.

Equipment and supplies: See ANA section on equipment and supplies.

Reagents: See reagents under ANA section. The fluorescein-labeled conjugate is the antihuman polyvalent immunoglobulin used in the ANA procedure.

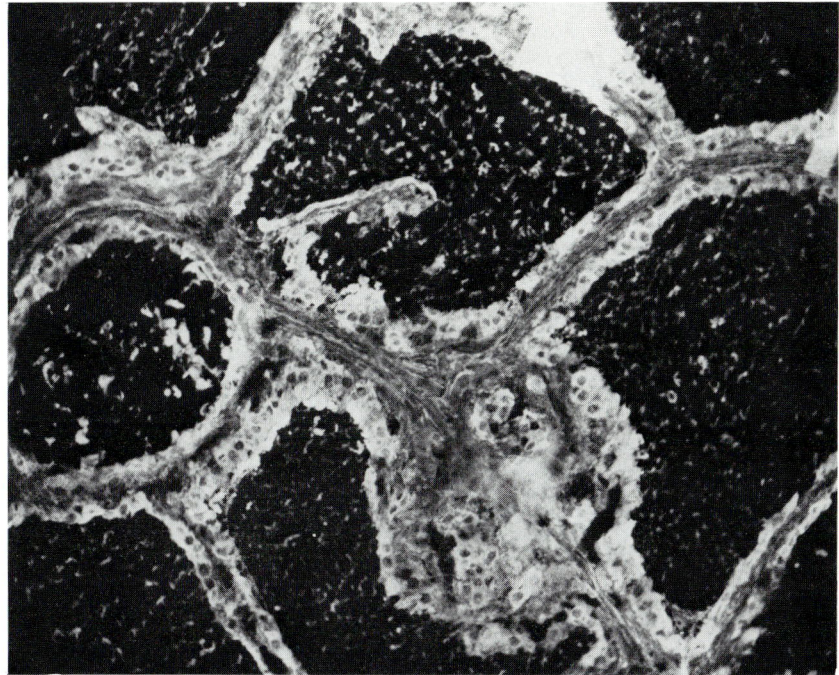

Fig. 36-13. Antithyroid antibodies (ATA) in human thyroid section shown by indirect immunofluorescence. Both antithyroglobulin and antithyroid microsomal antibodies are seen in this patient. ($\times$ 500.)

Technics:

Preparation of tissue sections:

1. ATA requires normal human or monkey thyroid tissue. For ATA using human thyroid, go to an autopsy of a "normal" person (15-40 year old, having died suddenly by accident or homicide). The autopsy should be done within 4 hr of death. Take thyroid (as much as possible) and cut into 1 cm square chunks and freeze in liquid nitrogen as for mouse tissue. Label and store at $-78°$ C.

2. After the sections are cut, fix in acetone for 10 min. Air dry slides and then use immediately or store at $-78°$ C until ready to use.

Preparation of serum:

1. The positive control (positive thyroglobulin and positive microsomal staining) and negative control are both diluted 1:20 with PBS. The positive control should show 3-4 + staining for thyroglobulin and microsomal components. The negative control should show no fluorescence.

2. All patients' sera are tested in duplicate at 1:20.

Procedure: See ANA section.

Quality controls:

TOLERANCE LIMITS: Moderate to strong fluorescence in the epithelial cell or thyroglobulin indicates a positive reaction. No fluorescence at 1:20 indicates a negative result. Results are reported as positive or negative for thyroglobulin or microsomal (epithelial) components.

CONTROL SERA FOR INDIRECT IMMUNOFLUORESCENCE: Prepare and store control sera as indicated in ANA section.

CHECK-TESTING FLUORESCEIN-LABELED CONJUGATE: See ANA section.

Interpretation: Immunofluorescence for ATA (Fig. 36-13) helps in distinguishing Hashimoto's disease from simple nontoxic goiters and thyroid carcinomas, de Quervain's disease, and Riedel's disease (fibrous thyroiditis).[213] In interpreting the results of thyroid antibody tests, three factors should be kept in mind:

1. Thyroid antibodies occur in up to 15% of "normal" control subjects. This normal incidence increases in older age groups and is higher in females than in males.[212]

2. In three major types of thyroid disorders (Hashimoto's disease, primary hypothyroidism, and Graves' disease), the incidence of elevated levels of thyroid antibodies is significantly higher than in "normal" control subjects.[212]

3. Thyroid autoimmunity overlaps with other diseases. High titers of thyroid antibodies have been reported in patients with nonthyroid disorders, e.g., pernicious anemia, Addison's disease, myasthenia gravis, liver disease, diabetes mellitus, and various connective tissue disorders.[213]

The incidence of all thyroid antibodies has been determined as follows:

Hashimoto's disease	99%
Primary myxedema	93%
Graves' disease	85%
Nontoxic goiter	49%
Carcinoma of thyroid	45%
de Quervain's disease	53%

Significance: Positive titers at 1:20 or greater for antithyroglobulin and/or antimicrosomal components are significant. Report as positive indicating which antibody or antibodies are positive.

Normal range: Negative.

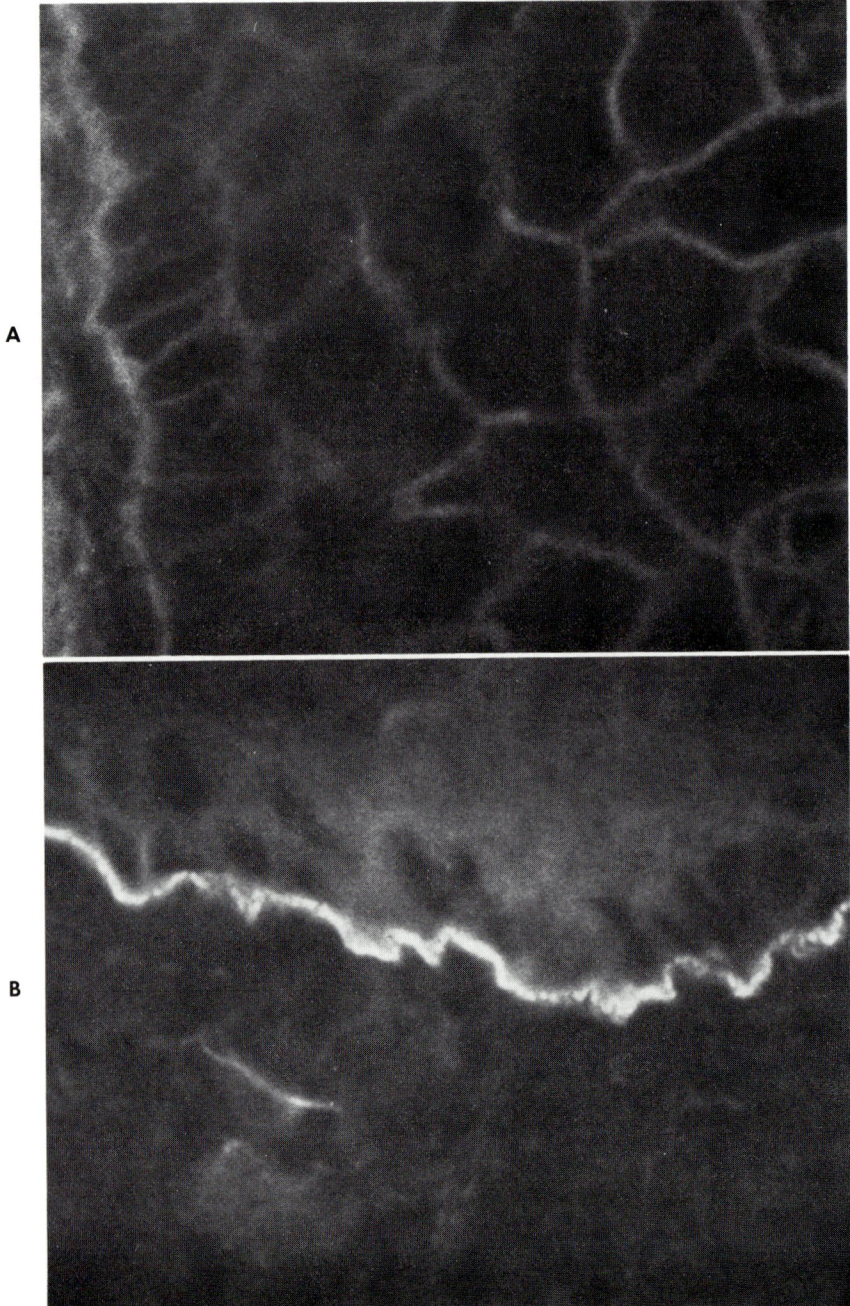

Fig. 36-14. Antiskin antibodies. **A,** Pemphigus antibody. **B,** Pemphigoid antibody. Mouse esophagus section shown by indirect immunofluorescence. (×500.)

Antiskin antibodies

Principle: Indirect immunofluorescence reveals that the serum of patients with pemphigus vulgaris and pemphigus foliaceus contains antibodies (ASAs) against the intercellular substance of stratified epithelium of skin or mucosa. In addition, the titer of the antibody is in general proportional to the severity of the disease and may be used in evaluating treatment.[214,215] Bullous pemphigoid has been noted to have specific antibodies for the subepithelial basement zone of the skin and mucosa. Since this disease is the only one with subepidermal bullae in which antibodies are present in the serum, this test is very helpful in differentiating bullous pemphigoid from erythema multiforme and dermatitis herpetiformis.[214,215] Again, the titer is generally proportional to the severity of the disease. The substrate for pemphigus antibody can be human skin, rat or mouse mucosa, or human, monkey, or mouse esophagus (Fig. 36-14).

Equipment and supplies: See ANA section on equipment and supplies.

Reagents: See reagents under ANA section.

The fluorescein-labeled conjugate is the antihuman inmmunoglobulin that is used for ANAs.

Technics:

Preparation of tissue sections:

1. Two substrate tissues are utilized: mouse esophagus and human esophagus. The mouse esophagus tissue is prepared in the same manner as the kidney is for ANA except that the mouse esophagus is removed, cut into smaller pieces, and frozen in liquid nitrogen. Human esophagus should be obtained from autopsy, cut in pieces, and also frozen in liquid nitrogen.
2. Cut 4 μm sections of both substrate tissues (mouse and human esophagus) for running the test and include a slide for each control (pemphigus and pemphigoid) and for two dilutions of the patient's serum.
3. Fix the human esophagus slides in acetone for 10 min. Do not fix the mouse esophagus slides.
4. Slides may be frozen and stored at −78° C if desired.

Preparation of serum:

1. The positive control for pemphigus is diluted 1:20 and should show 3+ fluorescence in the intercellular substance of the human esophagus. The negative control at 1:20 should show no fluorescence in this area.
2. The positive control for pemphigoid is diluted 1:10 or greater as determined by titration and should show 3-4+ fluorescence in the basement membrane of the mouse esophagus. The negative control at 1:20 should show no fluorescence in this area.
3. All patients' sera are tested at 1:20 and 1:80 dilutions on both substrate tissues. Positive sera should be titrated.

Procedure: See ANA section.

Quality controls:

TOLERANCE LIMITS: Strong fluorescence should be observed in the intercellular space and basement membrane of the appropriate tissue. No fluorescence at 1:20 indicates a negative result.

CONTROL SERA FOR INDIRECT IMMUNOFLUORESCENCE: Prepare and store control sera as indicated in the ANA section.

CHECK-TESTING FLUORESCEIN-LABELED CONJUGATE: See ANA section.

Interpretation: Indirect immunofluorescence is a valuable screening tool for the detection of pemphigus and pemphigoid antibodies.[214,215] Titers of pemphigus antibodies often reflect disease activity and may be used in the assessment of therapy. This is often not true with pemphigoid antibodies. Pemphigus antibodies have occasionally been reported to be positive in burn patients, possibly because of thermal alteration of skin components.

In pemphigus, patients with severe lesions usually show a titer of 1:120 or higher. Patients with moderate disease have a titer of 1:20 to 1:80, while the titer of early-stage patients may be negative. Pemphigoid patients with extensive lesions of more than 1 month's duration usually have titers above 1:120, whereas patients with fewer lesions and less than 1 month's duration may have negative titers.

> ASA positive at 1:100 or greater: Good evidence for pemphigus or pemphigoid; report as positive, give titer

Normal range: Negative.

Miscellaneous autoantibody tests

Principles: There are several additional autoantibodies that have been associated with various diseases.

1. Anti-parietal-cell antibodies have been found in up to 90% of patients with pernicious anemia.[216,217] They will react only with the parietal cell cytoplasm of the gastric mucosa. Parietal cell antibodies have also been found in patients with Hashimoto's thyroiditis, myxedema, gastric ulcer, and myasthenia gravis. The test uses human, rat, or mouse gastric fundal mucosa. The test has been shown to be a diagnostic aid in distinguishing autoimmune pernicious anemia from other megaloblastic anemias of adults and juveniles.

2. There appears to be a significant association between antimyocardial antibodies and cardiac disease, especially in patients after cardiac surgery, in myocardial infarct, in rheumatic fever, and rarely with streptococcal infection.[218] This test may aid in the differential diagnosis of coronary heart disease in detecting minimal myocardial infarction. It utilizes mouse heart tissue as substrate.

3. Anti-glomerular-basement-membrane (GBM) antibody has been detected in patients with Goodpasture's syndrome.[219,220] It uses human kidney as substrate and may aid in the diagnosis of renal disease caused by Goodpasture's syndrome.

4. Antiadrenal antibody has been associated with Addison's disease[221,222] and uses human adrenal gland as substrate.

Equipment and supplies: See ANA section on equipment and supplies.

Reagents: See reagents under ANA section.

The fluorescein-labeled conjugate is the antihuman immunoglobulin, which is the same as that for ANAs.

Technics:

Preparation of tissues for miscellaneous autoantibodies:

1. Anti-parietal-cell antibody requires mouse stomach and mouse kidney. The same tissues as in the AMA and ASMA are used. Cut enough mouse kidney slides to run AMA on each patient's serum. Also cut enough mouse stomach to run control sera at 1:20 dilutions. No fixation is needed.
2. Antimyocardial antibodies require mouse heart. Remove heart in the same manner as described for mouse kidney (ANA). Cut enough slides to run control and patient's sera. No fixation is needed.
3. Anti-GBM antibodies and antiadrenal antibodies use human autopsy kidney and adrenal gland, respectively. Prepare tissue as described in antithyroid antibody section on "Preparation of tissues." Cut enough slides for control and patient's sera. No fixation is needed.
4. The above slides (1-3) may be cut and stored at −78° C.

Preparation of control serum:

1. The positive control sera for each test should be diluted according to determined titers in order to show 2-3+ fluorescence when examined. The negative control should be diluted 1:20 and show no fluorescence at this dilution.
2. All patients' sera are tested at 1:20 in PBS for these tests.

Procedure: See ANA section.

Quality controls:

TOLERANCE LIMITS: Moderate to strong fluorescence in the appropriate tissue indicates a positive reaction. No fluorescence at 1:20 indicates a negative result. AMA should also be run at the same time to verify that the anti-parietal-cell antibody is not the result of AMA.

CONTROL SERA FOR INDIRECT IMMUNOFLUORESCENCE: Prepare and store control sera as directed in ANA section.

CHECK-TESTING FLUORESCEIN-LABELED CONJUGATE: See ANA section.

Interpretation: Since these specialized antibody tests have not been widely evaluated, a positive result may indicate the possibility of the disease corresponding to the antibody. However, these results should be evaluated in the light of the patient's clinical history.

Significance:

Positive at 1:20: Suggestive of disease associated with the autoantibody; report as positive, 1:20 or greater

Normal range: Negative.

Anti-ENA
Hemagglutination technic

Principle: Studies by many investigators have demonstrated that antibodies were present in the sera of patients with autoimmune disease which reacted with nuclear antigens of other chemical specificities. Anti-ENA (extractable nuclear antigens) utilizes a hemagglutination technic that detects antibodies to two saline-soluble nuclear antigens, one called Sm and the other called RNP (ribonucleoprotein).[223]

Antibody to Sm is present almost exclusively in SLE, perhaps indicating that this is a marker for this disease.[224] Antibody to RNP occurs in a number of rheumatic diseases such as SLE, DLE, and PSS.[224] Most often high titer RNP antibodies are associated with "mixed connective tissue," which has a relatively low prevalence in renal disease and good response to treatment with corticosteroids.[225-227]

Sm is saline soluble and easily extracted from the nucleus and is a nonhistone nuclear protein that is devoid of nucleic acids. Its antigenicity is not destroyed by RNase. RNP is also saline soluble and is thought to consist of a complex of ribonucleic acids and protein whose antigenicity is destroyed by RNase. Sensitivity (RNP) or resistance (Sm) to RNase is the basis for distinguishing between antibodies to RNP and Sm in the hemagglutination test.[223]

Tanned sheep erythrocytes are coated with an extract of rabbit thymus containing RNP (RNase-sensitive) antigens and Sm (RNase-resistant) antigens. A portion of the treated cells is incubated with RNase to selectively remove the RNP antigen. A passive hemagglutination test is performed in a microtiter system with the use of parallel dilutions of the patient's serum against both the untreated and treated cells. A positive hemagglutination test with the untreated cells and a negative one with the treated cells indicate antibody to RNP.[226]

Reagents:

1. Phosphate buffered saline (PBS), pH 7.2 ± 0.10
   Add 30.6 g NaC1 (0.1M), 2.9 g Na_2HOP, and 0.84 g KH_2PO_4 (0.01M PO_4) to demineralized or distilled water bringing total volume to 4 L. Stir on magnetic stirrer to ensure adequate mixing. Check pH of each batch of PBS prepared. Store at 4° C.
2. McIlvaine buffered saline, pH 7.8
   Add 1.13 g of 0.02M Na_2HOP_4 and 3.50 g of 0.15M NaC1 to demineralized or distilled water bringing volume to 4 dl. Adjust pH to 7.8 with 0.1M citric acid (1.92 g in 1 dl H_2O).
3. Tannic acid, 0.0012% (w/v)
   Prepare fresh just before use. Weigh 0.012 g (12 mg) of tannic acid and add to 1 dl PBS. Warm to 37° C and then dilute to 0.0012% tannic acid with warm (37° C) PBS (90 ml PBS + 10 ml 0.012% tannic acid).
4. Fetal calf serum (FCS)
   Inactivate fetal calf serum at 56° C for 30 min and absorb with sheep red cells (FCS-ABS), 1% (v/v). Add 1 ml of FCS-ABS to 99 ml PBS.
5. Normal human serum (NHS),
   Inactivate normal human serum at 56° C for 30 min and absorb with sheep red cells in the same manner as FCS-ABS. Add 0.4 ml NHS-ABS to 19.6 ml PBS (Microbiological Associates, Walkersville, Md.)
6. RNase solution (Worthington Biochemical Co., Freehold, N.J.)
   One milligram of RNase in 1 ml of 1% FCS will treat cells for one set of plates.
7. Rabbit thymus acetone powder (Pel-Freez Biologicals, Rogers, Ark.)
   a. To each 60 mg of rabbit thymus powder add 1 ml of PBS.

b. Extract for 4-12 hr at 4° C on a magnetic stirrer using a very low speed to avoid denaturation (a rheostat aids in decreasing the speed of the stirrer).

c. Centrifuge at 10,000 × g for 2 min (9300 rpm on Sorvall SS34 rotor head).

d. Determine the protein concentration of the supernatant fluid. Adjust the concentration of antigen to 1 mg/ml and store in aliquots.

e. This saline extract of rabbit thymus, which contains Sm and RNP antigens, can be stored in aliquot portions at −70° C and is stable for at least 10 weeks.

f. Always clear extract containing antigens by centrifugation before use for coupling to sheep red cells.

NOTE: Care must be taken to keep reagents cold to avoid enzymatic digestion of the antigens.

8. Sheep erythrocytes in Alsever solution (Colorado Serum Co., Denver)

Equipment and supplies:

1. Pipet droppers, 0.025 ml calibration
2. Microdiluters, 0.025 ml calibration
3. Disposable V-shaped microtiter plates
4. Centrifuge tubes, 15 ml
5. Plate sealers
6. Go-no-go blotters
7. Water bath (adjustable to 37° C and 56° C)
8. Centrifuge (PRJ)

Procedure (Fig. 36-15): Prepare a 1:10 (v/v) dilution of the patient's sera and control sera in PBS (0.05 ml of serum + 0.45 ml of PBS). Inactivate samples at 56° C for 30 min. Meanwhile wash four times with PBS enough sheep erythrocytes to give a packed volume of 0.5 ml for serum and 0.5 ml for tannic acid treatment (2 ml of sheep erythrocytes will yield a packed cell volume of 0.5 ml).

Absorb each serum with an equal volume (0.5 ml) of packed cells for 30 min at room temperature. Centrifuge samples and remove supernatant serum for use in testing. Resuspend the remaining 0.5 ml packed cells in PBS to give a 2.5% (v/v) suspension (0.5 ml of packed sheep cells + 19.5 ml of PBS).

Mix gently equal volumes of the 2.5% suspension (20 ml) of sheep erythrocytes and 0.0012% tannic acid in PBS (20 ml). Incubate for 10 min in a 37° C water bath with gentle swirling at 5 and 10 min. Centrifuge and wash twice with PBS (this should be at least 20 times the volume of packed sheep erythrocytes). Resuspend to 2.5% suspension.

Remove 2 ml of tanned sheep erythrocytes into each of three centrifuge tubes designated control, test, and RNase. Centrifuge and discard supernatant. Resuspend each packed cell volume with 10 ml McIlvaine saline buffer.

Add 2 ml of McIlvaine saline buffer to the tube containing the control cells. Add 2 ml of antigen solution to the test and RNase cells for each 0.05 ml of packed sheep erythrocytes. (Prepare sufficient antigen in McIlvaine saline buffer to have 1 mg of rabbit thymus extract in 2 ml). Mix gently and incubate at 37° C for 30 min. Swirl or shake gently at 10 min intervals to even by coat cells.

Centrifuge and wash cells three times with 1% FCS in PBS. Add 5 ml of 2% NHS (normal human serum) in PBS for each 0.05 ml of control cells and test cells. These cells are ready to use. Add 4 ml of 2% NHS in PBS and 1 ml of ribonuclease solution containing 1 mg of RNase/ml for each 0.05 ml of packed sheep erythrocytes to the RNase cells. Incubate at 37° C in water bath for 30 min with gentle mixing at 10 min intervals. These RNase-treated cells are now ready to use.

Test performance:

1. Label plates, allowing 24 wells for each antigen. Therefore each patient's sera will need two rows of 24 wells (one for RNP and one for Sm). Sera are titrated to 23 wells. The last well is labeled antibody control. Three wells are labeled for cell controls—tanned cells, test cells, and RNase-treated cells.

2. Add with the pipet dropper 0.025 ml of diluent (1% FCS in PBS) to each well.

3. Add with a diluter 0.025 ml of patient's and/or control serum to the proper antibody well (serum control).

4. Mix well by twirling about 10 times.

5. Remove and blot.

6. Add 0.025 ml of the patient's and/or control serum to the first well of the plate using the same diluter.

7. Repeat this procedure until all sample diluters are in the first wells.

8. Make serial dilutions of these samples simultaneously. Mix well by twirling about 10 times in each well.

9. Blot the loops when the dilutions are finished, rinse in distilled water, flame to incandescence, and plunge into distilled water. Blot again and prewet in diluent.

10. Add 0.025 ml of control cells with a pipet dropper to the row of antibody control (serum control) wells and to the cell control for tanned sheep cells.

11. Add 0.025 ml of the test cells with a pipet dropper to the appropriate serum dilutions and to the cell control labeled for test cells.

12. Add 0.025 ml of RNase-treated cells with a pipet dropper to appropriate serum dilutions and to cell control labeled for RNase test cells.

13. Tap plates gently to mix. Cover with plate sealers.

14. Allow cells to settle for at least 2 hr at room temperature and observe hemagglutination reaction.

Quality controls:

1. A positive serum for both Sm and RNP antibodies should be run each time the test is performed. The titer of each antibody should be 10,480 or greater and at least dilutions from 1:20 to 1:20,480 should be performed with each test.

2. A positive serum for RNP only should be run each time the test is performed. Again the titer should be 1:20,480 or greater and dilutions of 1:20 to 1:20,480 should be run.

3. A negative control serum should show no agglutination with either type of cell (RNP and Sm).

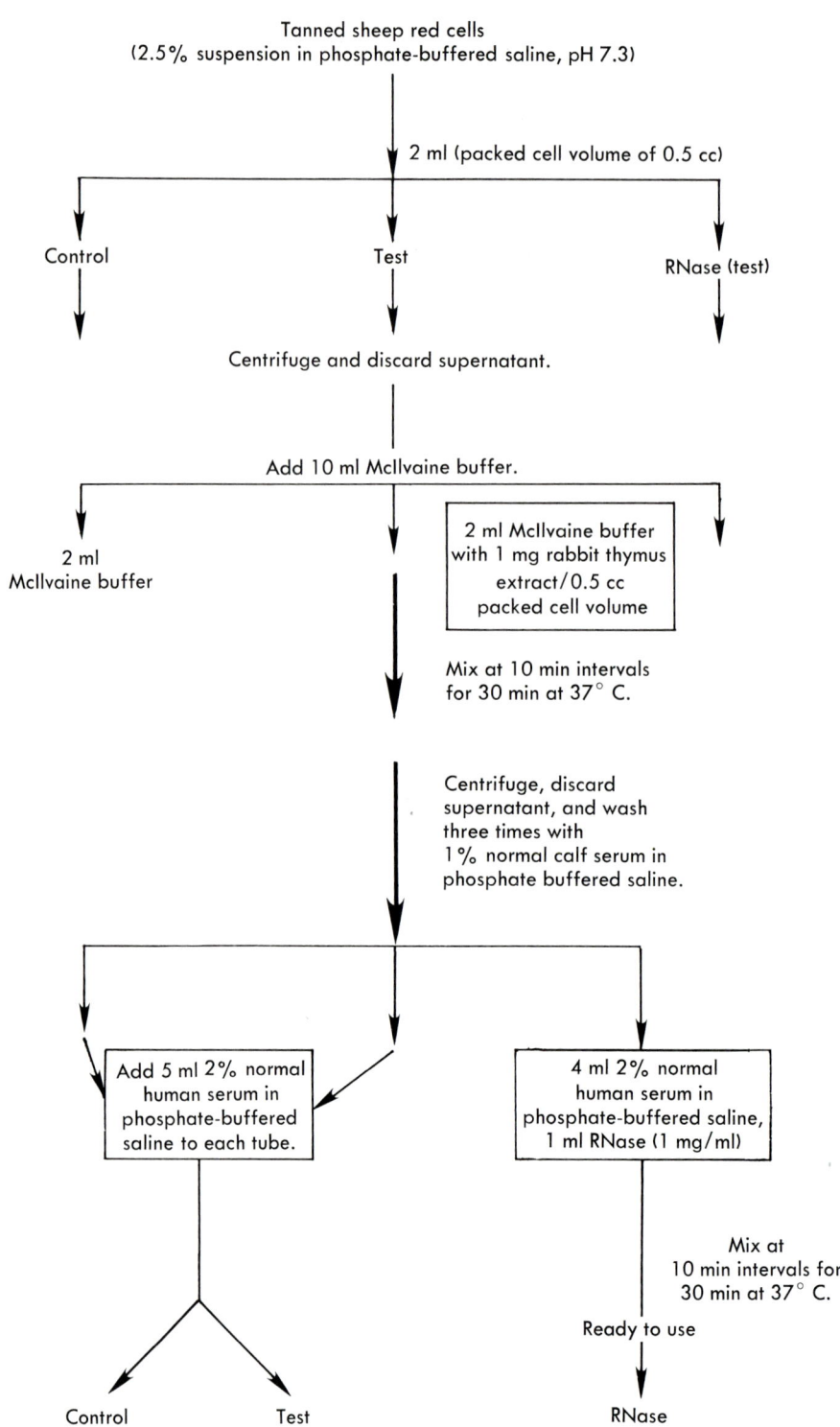

Fig. 36-15. Cell preparation for anti-ENA procedure—antigen coupling.

4. Antibody controls on each patient's and control serum should be run. This requires running a 1:20 and 1:40 dilution of serum with untreated cells to rule out nonspecific agglutination. Results should be negative on these samples.
5. Cell controls should be run. Untreated cells and cells with and without RNase treatment should show no agglutination when diluted in buffer.

Tolerance limits: If the above conditions are not met, the test should be repeated.

Cross-checking ENA antigen: Each time a new batch of ENA is made, it is cross-checked with the old batch. This is done by running the two batches simultaneously using the same control and patient's sera. The titer results using the new batch should be within ± 2 dilutions of the titers obtained using the old batch. The results should be recorded in the cross-checking book.

Interpretation:

Results positive: A smooth mat of cells covering the bottom of the well (+)
Results negative: A clearly defined button in the bottom of the well (−)
Results intermediate: Incomplete settling of cells with no clearly defined button (The reactions are noted [±] but not reported.)
End point: Highest dilution giving a positive reaction

If hemagglutination is present in wells with test cells and RNase-treated cells, this indicates antibody to RNase-resistant antigens (Sm). There could also be RNase-sensitive antigens (RNP) in lower titers. If hemagglutination is present only with test cells this shows antibody to RNase-sensitive antigen (RNP) only. This is considered, especially in high titers, to be highly suggestive of MCTD (mixed connective tissue disease).[227] No hemagglutination with both antigens indicates a negative test (Fig. 36-16).

Significance:

Normal range: If the test is negative for Sm and RNP antibodies, report as negative. Positive results for only RNP antibodies greater than 160 indicate the possibility of MCTD.

High titer RNP antibodies (10,000 or greater) indicate MCTD.

Positive results for both Sm and RNP antibodies greater than 160 may indicate the presence of SLE.

High titer Sm and RNP antibodies, 10,000 or greater, indicate SLE.

NOTE: If the cell control is positive with the patient's serum, the results are not reportable and the physician should be instructed to draw another sample.

Notes:
1. The serum preparation (absorption) may be done one or more days before testing. These sera can be frozen at −20° C or colder for future use.
2. Tanned sheep erythrocytes are stable for 1 week at 4° C.
3. The plates may be left overnight before reading with no appreciable change in results.
4. Sensitivity and specificity of the test are influenced by many variables. Cell and antigen concentration can reduce the sensitivity if in excess.
5. Serum is always used, since various anticoagulants may give different results that are not comparable.
6. The pH of 7.8 gives optimal coating of both Sm and RNP, and the concentration of the RNase allows for proper digestion of the RNP for differentiation.

Guidelines for reporting values of anti-ENA: A saline extract of rabbit thymus is coupled to red cells and used to test for the presence of antibodies to it in the patient's serum. The antigenic material in the calf thymus extract is called ribonucleoprotein (RNP). In addition, the RNP is treated with RNase after coupling to the red cells. The remaining antigenic substances, which are RNase resistant, are called RNase-resistant ENA, which acknowledges that they represent a collection of antigens. In quantitation of these antigens the following three cases can occur.

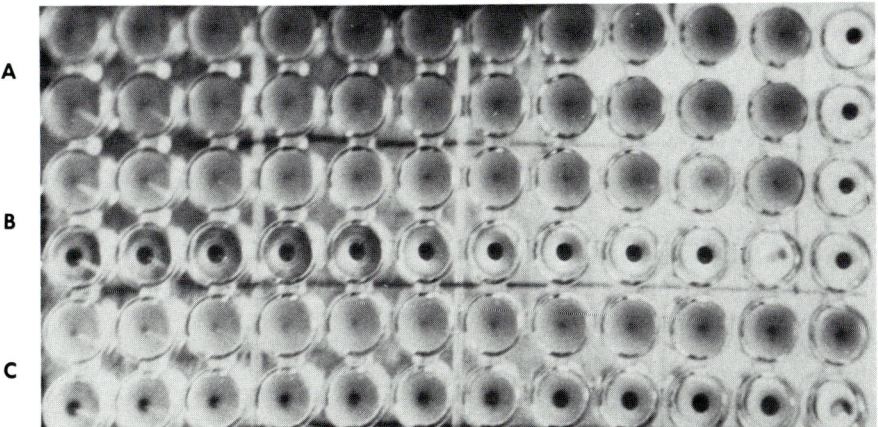

Fig. 36-16. Anti-ENA (extractable nuclear antigens). Hemagglutination test with (lower row) and without (upper row) ribonuclease (Rnase) digestion. *Serum A* contained antibody to Sm *or* Sm and RNP in equal amounts, the titers remain the same with and without RNase treatment. *Serum B* had antibody to RNP only because of its complete sensitivity to enzyme digestion. *Serum C* contained antibodies to both nuclear RNP and Sm, with anti-RNP titer higher than anti-Sm.

CASE 1: The RNP titer is positive and the RNase-resistant ENA is negative. Therefore, the antibodies are only to the RNP antigens, and the RNP titer is reported as positive and RNase-resistant ENA titer is reported as negative.

CASE 2: The RNP and the RNase-resistant ENA titer are the same. In this case, the RNP titer is impossible to evaluate by the hemagglutination technic. The RNase-resistant titer can be reported as the titer obtained, but the RNP titer should be reported as unknown.

CASE 3: The RNase-resistant ENA titer is less than the RNP titer. In this case, the existence of both antibodies is demonstrated. The larger RNP titer is reported as found, as also is the RNase-resistant ENA titer. Since the titer of antibodies determined by hemagglutination tests is not additive, if both are present at the same time, the actual titer can be used.

For example:

	Titer	Report
Case 1:		
RNP	1:25,000	RNP 1/25,000
RNase-resistant ENA	0	RNase-resistant ENA; none
Case 2:		
RNP	1:50,000	RNP unknown
RNase-resistant ENA	1:50,000	RNase-resistant ENA; 1:50,000
Case 3:		
RNP	1:50,000	RNP 1:50,000
RNase-resistant ENA	1:10,000	RNase-resistnat ENA; 1:10,000

Quantitation of circulating immune complexes
Introduction and principles

Circulating DNA−anti−DNA complexes are implicated in the etiology of nephritis in SLE.[228] They are preformed in the circulation carrying with them complement and are deposited as granular precipitates along the glomerular and vascular basement membranes. They are thus thought to be responsible for the main manifestations of immune complex diseases: glomerulonephritis, vasculitis, serositis, and hypocomplementemia. Circulating immune complexes may be demonstrated by a number of technic, such as Clq component of complement,[229] rheumatoid factor (19S anti-IgG),[230] platelets,[231] and Raji cells.[232] They all react with complexes of immunoglobulins but not with the single immunoglobulin molecule. The principles of these methods are outlined.

Two test systems utilize Clq, one employs gel diffusion and the other a radioimmunoassay method. In the **gel diffusion method**[229] Clq forms precipitin lines with immune complexes at the optimal pH of 7.2 in agarose gel of low concentration. The undiluted specimens and the solution of Clq are deposited in wells and allowed to diffuse toward each other while the plates are incubated at room temperature for 48 hr and subsequently at 0° C for 72 hr. Positive and normal controls must be run at the same time as the unknown specimens are processed. Positive specimens are rerun at dilutions of 1:2 to 1:16.

In the radioimmunoassay method[233] radiolabeled Clq is allowed to react with the soluble immune complexes

and the remaining free Clq is separated from the complex bound ^{125}I Clq by selective precipitation of the latter with polyethylene glycol. In low concentrations polyethylene glycol precipitates the large-sized soluble antigen-antibody complexes while free labeled Clq remains in solution. After suitable incubation the tubes are centrifuged and the radioactivity measured in the precipitates. The results are expressed as percent ^{125}I Clq precipitated. Normal value is less than 10% ^{125}I Clq. In SLE the ^{125}I Clq precipitation is related to disease activity, being increased in the acute phase (lupus nephritis) and decreased in remissions. In most instances Clq activity closely parallels the hemolytic complement concentration.

The method utilizing **polyclonal rheumatoid factor** (pRF)[230] is based on the inhibition by soluble serum immune complexes of the binding of pRF (IgM) to ^{125}I-labeled aggregated IgG.[234,235] Normal sera do not inhibit this reaction while sera from patients with certain connective tissue diseases may show 50% inhibition at a 1:500 dilution.

The method utilizing **platelet aggregation**[231] is based on the observation that antigen-antibody complexes interact with the surface of platelets, a reaction that does not require complement and is a sensitive indicator of IgG immune complexes.[236,237] This interaction can be monitored by platelet aggregation since it increases the adhesive properties of the platelet surface, which in the proposed system is insensitive to some of the other factors that produce platelet aggregation. Platelets are separated from blood bank blood in saline, resuspended, and adjusted to a concentration of 200,000/mm^3 monitored by the optimal density of the solution. The platelets from three donors are collected and must be used the same day. Preliminary titration must be carried out using various known antigen-antibody concentrations. The test sera are inactivated and using microtiter pipets and disposable U plates serial twofold dilutions are made. To each well 0.05 ml platelet suspension is added and the plates are incubated at 5-8° C overnight. The sedimentation patterns are read against a dark background, and the titer represents the highest dilution giving a positive sedimentation pattern. Positive and negative controls must be run with the test. To quantitate the immune complexes the sedimentation titer must be compared with that of known immune complexes.

Complement-fixing immune complexes can also be detected and quantitated by the Raji cell **radioimmune method**.[232] Raji cells, cultured human lymphoblastoid cells derived from Burkitt's lymphoma, lack membrane-bound immunoglobulins but have receptors for complement at which sites they are able to bind immune complexes. The uptake of immune complexes by the Raji cells is quantitated by ^{125}I antihuman IgG. The amount of radioactivity bound to the washed cells is determined and plotted on a standard curve of radioactive antibody uptake by cells incubated with increasing amounts of aggregated human γ-globulin.

Solid phase Clq RIA method for detection of circulating immune complexes

Principle: The following procedure for quantitation of circulating immune complexes is based on developmental work done at St. Louis University[238] as well as that of I.M. Roitt[239] and S.E. Svehag in other laboratories.[240,241] The method is based on the unique ability of the first component of complement, Clq, to bond immune complexes selectively. Quantitation of the complexes bound to solid-phase Clq is accomplished through the use of a ^{125}I antihuman IgG antibody, which binds to the IgG portion of the immune complex. In principle it is a simple sandwich RIA procedure.

Supplies and equipment:
1. Polystyrene balls absorbed with Clq
2. Plastic tubes (polystyrene with caps)
3. [125]I antihuman IgG (absorbed) (RAH [rabbit-anti-human])
4. γ-Counter
5. Automatic shaker

Reagents:
1. Polystyrene balls adsorbed with Clq
   Mix the balls with a pure solution of Clq and buffer A (below). Adsorption proceeds at room temperature for 1 hr with circular mixing. Typically, adsorption is carried out in a Sigma NAD vial (Sigma Chemical Co., St. Louis). At the end of the adsorption period, the balls are washed with two vial volumes of PBS. They are then ready for use.
2. Buffer A: 0.05M sodium chloride and, 0.01M phosphate at a pH of 7.5
3. Buffer B: 1.5% Tween 20, 2% bovine serum albumin (BSA), and 0.3M sodium chloride at a pH of 7.5.
4. Aggregated human γ-globulin
   Weigh 6.5 mg/ml of Sigma Cohn II γ-globulin (Sigma Chemical Co., St. Louis) and dissolve in 1 ml buffer A. Then heat to 63° C for 20 min followed by rapid cooling in ice. The centrifuge at 5000 × g for 9 min before use to remove large unsoluble aggregates.

Procedure:
1. Place a Clq polystyrene ball into each tube for the test with 0.5 ml of buffer B.
2. Add aggregated human γ-globulin in 1-20 μg amounts for control tubes.
3. Add test serum to other tubes in 1-20 μg amounts.
4. Incubate for 1 hr at room temperature with constant shaking.
5. Then wash tubes by first aspirating the 0.5 ml reaction solution, adding one tube volume of buffer B, and aspirating. Repeat one more time.
6. Add 10 μg of RAH-IgG ^{125}I to each tube in 0.5 ml of buffer B (may be added before antibody addition).
7. Incubate for 1 hr at room temperature with constant shaking.
8. Repeat wash procedure as in step 5.
9. Cap tubes and count for 1 min in a γ-counter.
10. Plot standard curve and calculate test results from graph.

Direct immunofluorescence of tissues

Principle: Biopsy materials, e.g., renal tissue, of patients with connective tissue diseases, immune complex disease, or a variety of other antibody-mediated diseases will show deposition of these antibody-antigen complexes in the tissue when stained with appropriate fluorescein-labeled antihuman conjugates.[241] Demonstration of these deposits can allow an immunopathologist to make a diagnosis of disease or to do follow-up studies on these patients.[242,243]

Equipment and supplies:
1. Cryostat, adjustable to 4 μm
2. Fluorescence microscope assembly
3. Diamond point pen
4. Kimwipes or gauze
5. Slide rack for conjugates
6. Microscope slides, 1 × 3 in., frosted on one end, 1 mm thick
7. Coverslips, no. 1, 22 mm square
8. Staining dishes and slide carriers
9. Slide drainer
10. Slide folders

Reagents:
1. Ether, anesthesia grade: 95% ethanol, USP
2. Acetone, PBS, and glycerin-PBS
   These reagents are the same as required for indirect fluorescent antibody tests (see reagents under indirect fluorescent antibody tests).
3. Fluorescein-labeled conjugates
   Antihuman albumin, IgG, IgM, IgA, and IgE are purchased commercially (Meloy Laboratories, Springfield Va.). C3, Clq, and fibrinogen are also purchased commercially (Calbiochem-Behring Corp., San Diego). Determine the working titer using positive and negative tissue and using the method outlined for indirect fluorescent antibody tests. The positive and negative tissues for biopsy controls are stored in tightly capped plastic bottles at −70° C. Divide the conjugates into aliquots of 0.3 ml when received and store at −70° C. When the conjugate is thawed for use, do not refreeze, but store at 4° C and use as long as satisfactory results are obtained with test controls.

Procedure:
Preparation of biopsy tissues:
1. All biopsy tissue must be frozen immediately in liquid nitrogen and never allowed to thaw. Do not allow biopsy material to dry out before freezing. Use gauze moist with PBS to protect tissue if necessary.
2. For **renal biopsy specimens,** after splitting the sample lengthwise and obtaining enough tissue for histology, immunofluorescence, and electron microscopy (if desired), place renal tissue on a small piece of cork for immunofluorescence. Place cork in small screw-capped vial and drop into liquid nitrogen. The tissue for histology should be placed into formalin, and the tissue for electron microscopy should be placed in 4% glutaraldehyde. Excessive exposure to air both before and after freezing should be avoided.

   For **skin and muscle biopsy specimens,** place these tissues directly into a small glass vial and freeze. Make sure tissue is obtained for histology also.

   For **synovial biopsy specimens** taken by needle, keep small pieces moist on gauze with PBS. When the procedure is over, divide the small pieces equally for histology and immunofluorescence. Place the pieces for immunofluorescence in one clump and freeze on the side of a glass vial as for the other biopsy specimens.

NOTE: Biopsy tissue may be kept moist with PBS or saline if there is a delay. For longer periods of time (not to exceed 2 hr) tissue may be kept moist on gauze and stored at 4° C (not frozen in freezer!) until it can be frozen in liquid nitrogen.

3. Store biopsy material in Revco (Revco, Inc., W. Columbia, S.C.) at −70° C until it is cut.
4. Cut tissue at 4 μm in cryostat at −20° C. Kidney tissue should contain glomeruli for definitive diagnosis. See operation manual (on top of cryostat) for instructions on use of the cryostat.
5. Tissue sections should be placed on ''A'' spot area of slide (see procedure for indirect immunofluorescence antibody tests). Circle sections with diamond point pen and label with patient's name and conjugate to be used. Nine slides are needed: one for hematoxylin-eosin and one each for antialbumin, IgG, IgM, IgA, IgE, C3, Clq, and fibrogen.
6. When enough slides have been obtained, fix sections as follows: PBS—3 min; ether (95% ethanol [1:])—10 min; 95% ethanol—20 min; PBS—two washes, 5 min each. Biopsy material can be processed the same day the sections are cut, or sections may be frozen (unfixed) at −70° C for not more than 1 week.

Preparation of control tissues:
1. The control tissue is a biopsy or autopsy material that is judged by an immunopathologist to be adequate for positive staining in each of the conjugates used. This tissue is labeled and stored at −70° C. It is cut as needed for biopsy testing, usually an autopsy of a lupus patient.
2. Negative control tissue is obtained from ''normal'' (i.e., sudden death or accident) autopsy material. It is stored at −70° C.
3. Cut, circle, and label tissue sections from control material as needed. Fix as for biopsy material.

Staining procedure: While slides are rinsing in last PBS wash (see step 6 in Preparation of biopsy tissues), place 0.05 ml of each conjugate on appropriately labeled conjugate slide rack using enough spaces for each biopsy and control tissue.

Remove slides from PBS and allow to drain in slide drainer. **Do not allow tissue to dry out.** Wipe excess PBS carefully from around the tissue section on the slide and place the tissue section side of the slide onto the prepared drops of conjugate on the slide rack. Stain for 45 min in conjugate at room temperature. Remove slides from conjugate, place in slide carrier, and wash in PBS two times for 5 min.

Lay out sufficient coverslips and place 1 drop of glycerin-PBS on each coverslip. Drain and wipe slides as before and pick up coverslip with tissue side of slide.

Store slides a 4° C in a folder until they are viewed by the immunopathologist. They should be viewed within 24 hr. The pathologist will decide if any sections need to be recut because of a problem in reading the specimen or if the entire specimen is negative. Repeat specimens will be viewed again and the results determined by the pathologist. Write results in a workbook. The pathologist will write the report from these results.

Immunologic studies on trypsin digestion of paraffin-embedded tissue sections

Principle: It is occasionally necessary to perform immunofluorescence on tissue that has been formalin fixed and embedded in paraffin.[244,245]This procedure allows the performance of the test by using trypsin to restore tissue to a state in which regular immunofluorescent reagents may be used.

Procedure: Prepare clean glass slides by washing in acetone. Prepare celloidin solution by diluting 1:150 in absolute alcohol and store for use at 4° C. Prelabel slides if possible and then dip them briefly in celloidin solution. Let air dry for 10 min. Slides may be stored in a box at 4° C if desired.

Cut 4 μm thick neutral formalin-fixed, paraffin-embedded sections floated briefly on a 43° C water bath and mounted to glass slides coated with celloidin. Dry sections for 15 min at 43° C and then 15 min at 68° C (or 65° C for 1 hr) and store at room temperature if desired. Place the slides in two changes of cold (4° C) xylene, 5 min for each change. Rehydrate with graded alcohol. Wash in distilled water.

Prepare trypsin solution. Add solid ingredients, i.e., 0.1% trypsin (Sigma no. T-8253 [Sigma Chemical Co., St. Louis]), 0.2 g/2 dl, and 0.1% $CaCl_2.2H_2O$ (Fisher no. C-79 [Fisher Scientific Co., Pittsburgh]), 0.266 g/2 dl, to distilled water and adjust to pH 7.8 with 0.1N sodium hydroxide. Warm to 37° C.

Place slides in trypsin solution in Coplin jar and let digestion proceed for 2 hr. Wash slides five times in distilled water and place in 4° C PBS, pH 7.2, for 30 min to 2 hr. Air dry and process tissue as for direct or indirect immunofluorescence (no fixation necessary).

For leukemic tissues or lymphoma, stain slides with F(ab′)2 fluorescein-labeled antihuman IgG, IgM, IgA, and K- and λ-chains. For kidney biopsy specimens stain slides with regular fluorescein-labeled antihuman IgG, IgM, IgA, C3, fibrinogen, and Clq. For tissues in which a specific antigen is desired, use the indirect immunofluorescence method or the direct method if labeled conjugate is available for the antigen.

Results: The diagnosis should be made by a qualified immunopathologist as stated in the regular direct immunofluorescent procedure.

IDENTIFICATION AND CHARACTERIZATION OF MONONUCLEAR CELLS

Identification and characterization of the type of mononuclear cells present in frozen sections of tissues such as lymph node, spleen, thymus, or tumor may be carried out by the use of the following four methods: membrane receptor study of frozen tissue section; complement receptor by IgM EAC rosettes—B-lymphocyte; Fc receptor by IgG EA rosettes—monocyte, machrophage, and tissue histiocyte; and E receptor by neuraminidase and AET-E (2-aminoethylisothiouranium bromide hydrobromide) rosettes—T-lymphocyte.

Principle: Human T cells bind sheep red cells to form rosettes.[246,247] This marker is called the E (erythrocyte) rosette and can be used on frozen sections of tissues such as tumors or lymphoid elements to determine the relative quantity of T cell.[248] Human B cells contain surface receptors for complement. B cell marker is demonstrated by a rosetting technic using EAC (erythrocyte-antibody-complement) rosettes, which are sheep red cells coated with IgM anti–sheep red cells and complement. Again, the presence of EAC adhering to tissue sections indicates the presence of B cells.[249] Tissue macrophages have surface Fc receptors that can be detected by EA (erythrocyte-amboceptor) rosettes. In this case sheep red cells are coated with IgG anti–sheep red cells. Macrophage present in tissue can be seen by aggregates of red cells adhering to the tissue section. Therefore this technic gives an assessment of normal or abnormal histology as well as cellular classification. Perhaps the area in which an immunologic profile of a frozen section is most useful is in non-Hodgkin's lymphoma.[247,250]

Supplies and equipment:
1. Cryostat
2. Liquid N_2
3. Antiserum: 19S antibodies to sheep red cells (Cordis Laboratories, Miami, Fla.); 7S antibodies to sheep red cells (Cordis Laboratories)
4. Neuraminidase (Sigma Chemical Co., St. Louis)
5. Mouse complement (fresh serum)

Reagents:
A. Stock reagents
   1. 5X Stock veronal buffer
      a. Sodium chloride, 41.5 g
      b. 4.1 g Na-5,5-diethyl barbiturate
      c. Glass-distilled water
      Dissolve a and b in 9 dl glass distilled water. Adjust pH to 7:35 with IN hydrochloric acid. Add water up to 1 L and check pH again. Store stock buffer at 4° C. It is usable for 6 months if it remains sterile.
   2. Gelatin
      a. Gelatin, 2 g
      b. Water, 1 dl
      Heat to dissolve gelatin. Store at 4° C in 10 ml aliquots.
   3. Calcium-magnesium stock solution
      a. Anhydrous calcium chloride, 0.03 M, 0.33 g
      b. $MgCl_2.6H_2O$, 0.10M, 2.03 g
      Add glass distilled water up to 1 dl. Sterilize through 0.2 μm filter and store at 4° C.
   4. Dextrose, monohydrate powder
B. Dextrose-gelatin-veronal buffer (DGVB) Make 2 dl of DGVB (5 g dextrose, 2 ml calcium-magnesium stock solution, 10 ml gelatin [heated to 56° C], and 20 ml 5x stock veronal buffer). Add glass-distilled water up to 200 ml; mix well. Buffer is good for 1 day.
C. Mouse complement
   1. Anesthetize mouse with ether.
   2. Collect blood by cutting the axillary vessels.
   3. Allow blood to clot at room temperature for 10 min and then place in ice for 60 min.

4. Centrifuge for 10 min at 700 G at 4° C.
5. Preferably use fresh or store at −70° C until use.
D. Stock neuraminidase, 10 units/ml
E. Sheep red cells
   Wash 2 cc of sheep red cells three times in DGVB (2 cc sheep red cells = 0.5 ml packed cells). Adjust concentration to 4×10^9 cells/ml.

$$20\% \ (1/5) \times \text{Vol.} = \text{Packed vol.}$$
$$\text{Vol.} = \text{Packed vol.} \times 5$$

EXAMPLE: If packed vol. = 0.35 ml,

$$\text{Vol.} = 0.35 \times 5 = 1.75 \ ml$$

Add DGVB to 1.75 ml. This approximately equals a 20% suspension. Count cells in 16 squares $\times \ 10^7$ to see if they have appropriate dilution. EXAMPLE:

$$370 \times 10^7 = 3.7 \times 10^9$$

This is an adequate cell count for running the test. EXAMPLE: 470 cells in 16 squares $\times \ 10^7$. To get 4×10^9

$$4.7 \times \text{Vol. of RBCs} = 4 \times \text{Diluted vol.}$$

F. Fresh tissue frozen immediately in liquid N_2 and kept at −70° C until cut on cryostat

Procedure:
Positive controls:
1. **E rosette control.** Use human thymus as E rosette control for T cells. When treated with neuraminidase-labeled sheep red cells, the fresh cut thymus should demonstrate 2+ adherence over the entire section by the cells when viewed by the pathologist. A negative thymus control should also be run. This is a frozen section that has been allowed to air dry before being coated with cells. The negative slide should have little or no attached red cells.
2. **EA rosette control.** Use a human tissue that has been shown to have high macrophage contents, e.g., inflamed lymph node or necrotic tumor sections. When treated with EAs the tissue should demonstrate 3+ aggregation with the red cells in the areas of macrophage residency as determined by the pathologist.
3. **EAC rosette control.** Use human spleen that has been shown to have normal germinal centers with adequate numbers of B cells. When treated with EACs the germinal centers should exhibit 3+ aggregation of red cells.

Tolerance limits: The presence of no adhering rosettes or very few rosettes indicates a negative or borderline result. If the above controls do not indicate 2−3+ adherence in the appropriate areas of sections, the test should be repeated.

Rosette cell preparations:
EA AND EAC ROSETTES:
1. For EA rosette make a 1:40 dilution (10 λ 7S IgG = 390 λ DGVB) of 7S IgG anti–sheep red cells.
2. For EAC rosette make a 1:5 dilution (20 λ 19S

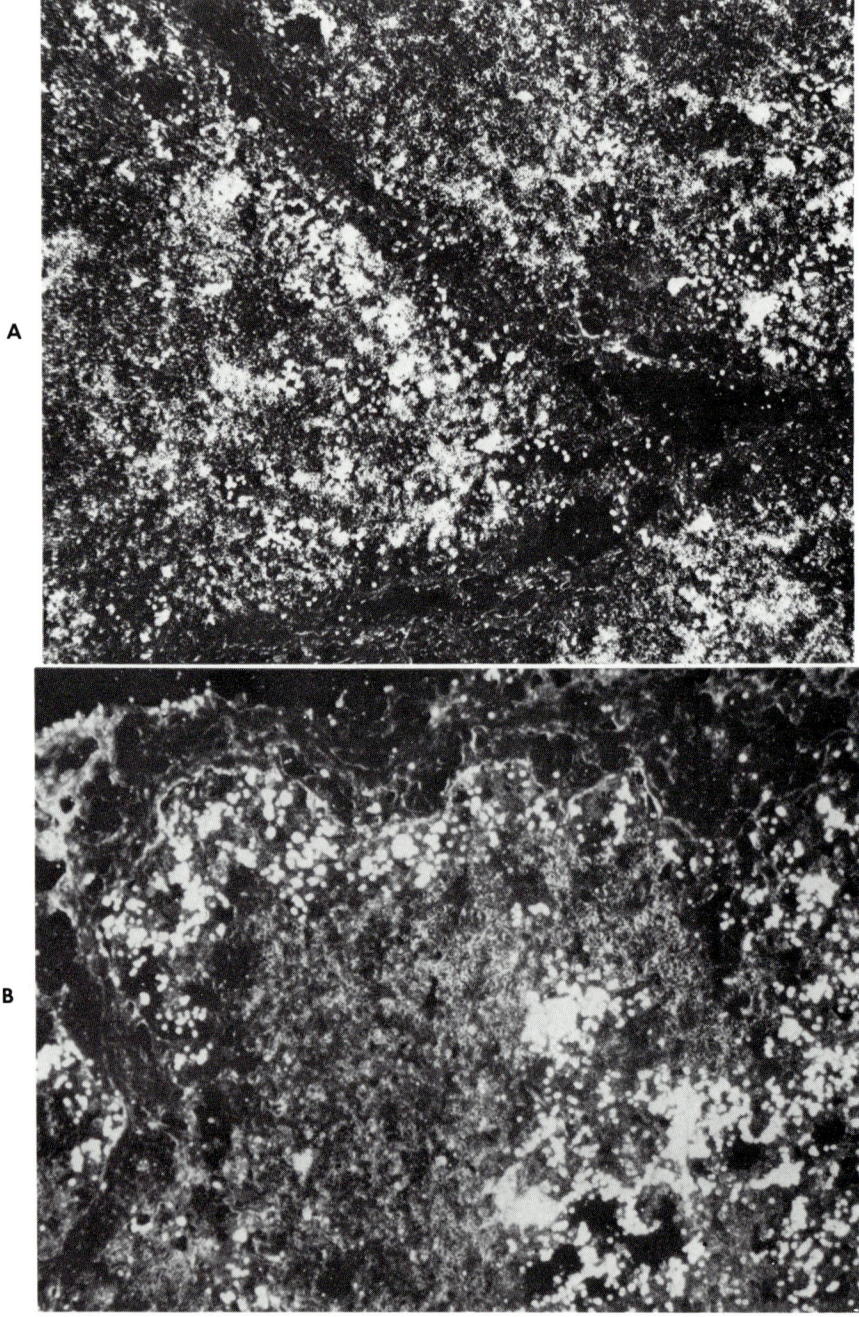

Fig. 36-17. Surface membrane receptor studies of frozen tissue sections. **A,** E rosette in normal thymus gland. **B,** IgG EA rosette in human lymph node biopsy specimen. IgG Fc receptors were seen in the marginal sinus histiocytes.

IgM + 80 λ DGVB) of 19S IgM anti–sheep red cells.

3. Label two tubes, one with EA and one with EAC.
4. In the tube labeled EAC, place 0.3 ml of 4 × 10^9 sheep red cells + 0.3 ml DGVB and 10.1 λ of IgM dilution (6.7 λ for each 0.1 ml sheep red cells).
5. In tube marked EAS, place 3 ml of 4 × 10^8 sheep red cells (0.3 ml of 4 × 10^9 cells + 2.7 ml DGVB) + 3 ml of DGVB and 180 λ of IgG dilution.
6. Incubate both tubes for 15 min at 37° C. Shake frequently.
7. Wash three times with DGVB at 1200 rpm for 5 min.
8. Resuspend EA rosette in 3 ml DGVB. It is now ready to use.
9. Resuspend EAC rosette in 0.3 ml DGVB, and 0.3 ml mouse C (diluted 1:5 of fresh or −70° C frozen mouse serum absorbed with sheep red cells (60 λ C + 240 λ DGVB).
10. Incubate for 30 min at 37° C. Shake frequently.
11. Wash twice in DGVB, and resuspend EAC rosette in 3 ml DGVB. It is now ready to use.

E ROSETTE: For neuraminidase treatment follow these steps:

1. Use 1 × 10^9 sheep red cells; therefore make a 1:4 dilution of stock (0.25 ml stock cells + 0.75 ml DGVB).
2. To 1 ml of 1 × 10^9 cells add 20 λ of 10 units/ml neuraminidase.
3. Incubate for 1 hr at 37° C. Shake every 10 min.
4. Wash three times with DGVB at 1200 rpm for 5 min.

5. Resuspend in 5 ml DGVB to give a final concentration of 2 × 10^8 cells/ml.
6. Keep at 37° C until ready to use.

If desired, sheep red cells may be treated with AET (2-aminoethylisothiouronium bromide hydrobromide) instead of neuraminidase (E rosette).

1. Add 0.5 g of AET solution to 10 ml distilled water. Adjust the pH to 9.0 using concentrated sodium hydroxide. Make the final volume 12 ml by adding distilled water. Check pH to be sure it is 9.0. This solution must be made fresh each time it is used.
2. Centrifuge the washed sheep red cells in DGVB or PBS after having removed aliquots for EA and EAC rosettes. To each 0.15 ml packed volume of red cells add 0.4 ml of the AET solution. Allow mixture to stand at room temperature for 15 min.
3. Wash four times in PBS. To each 0.1 ml packed volume of red cells add 0.9 ml of 1640 RPM1 medium with 10% FCS (fetal calf serum—see DNA section on reagents) to give a 10% final suspension. Dilute this 10% suspension 1:20 with media-FCS to give a final 0.5% AET suspension. Use 200 λ of this solution per section. The slides may be cut and dried for this method. Follow steps 3-7 under "Test performance" below.

Test performance:

1. Cut frozen tissues at 6-8 μm according to the section on controls (one control slide for each test)
2. Each patient's sample should be cut at 6-8 μm in duplicate for each test. For example, a biopsy of lymph node would require seven slides: two for E rosettes (cut and kept frozen until ready to use) and one slide cut and air dried (negative control);

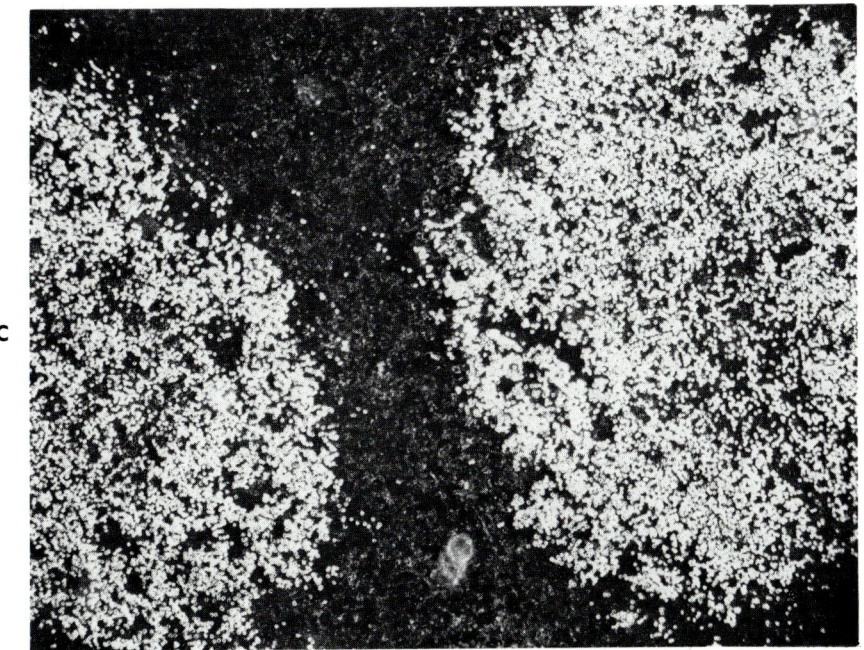

Fig. 36-17, cont'd. C, IgM EAC rosette in human normal spleen. Complement receptors were seen in the germinal centers of white pulp.

two slides for EA rosettes (cut and air dried); and two slides for EAC rosettes (cut and air dried).

3. Overlay each tissue section on slide with respective red cell preparation. Use 200 λ of each cell preparation per slide. Place in wet box and incubate for 30 min at room temperature. NOTE: With the cold E rosette slides wait 45 sec or until chill leaves slide before adding cells.

4. Wash in cold PBS. Use two containers and dip three times in each (six dips total).

5. Fix in 3% glutaraldehyde for 30 min.

6. Stain with hematoxylin-eosin (skip formalin step).

7. View slides by darkfield microscopy.

Interpretation: Positive areas (rosetting) appear as white spheres because of highly refractive sheep red cells (Fig. 36-17). One can examine the slides under a darkfield microscope or view with a regular light microscope after counterstaining with hematoxylin-eosin or another stain.

The pathologist will view the slides and made a diagnosis on the basis of the findings. Again, the controls should demonstrate adequate staining upon viewing. The presence of E, EA, or EAC rosettes in particular areas or in certain quantities in the tissue may indicate the proliferating cell type.

Biopsy specimens from normal or uninvolved tissue should show only normal histologic organization in lymph nodes, spleen, thymus, etc.

REFERENCES

1. Cooper, M.D., et al.: N. Engl. J. Med. **288**:960, 1973.
2. Stiehm, E.R., and Fulginiti, V.A., editors: Immunologic disorders in infants and children, Philadelphia, 1973, W.B. Saunders Co.
3. Smith, L.G., and Louria, D.: Med. Clin. North Am. **57**:409, 1973.
4. Clough, J.D.: Cleve. Clin. Q. **42**:49, 1975.
5. Johnston, R.B., Jr., Lawton, A.R., and Cooper, M.D.: Med. Clin. North Am. **57**:421, 1973.
6. Bruton, O.C.: Pediatrics **9**:722, 1952.
7. Fudenberg, H.H., et al.: N. Engl. J. Med. **283**:656, 1970.
8. Polmar, S.H., et al.: J. Clin. Invest. **51**:326, 1972.
9. Freedom, R.M., Rosen, F.S., and Nadas, A.A.: Circulation **46**:165, 1972.
10. Nezelof, C., et al.: Arch. Fr. Pediatr. **21**:897, 1964.
11. Good, R.A.: Bull. Univ. Minn. Hosp. **26**:1, 1954.
12. Peterson, R.D.A., Kelly, W.D., and Good, R.A.: Lancet **1**:1189, 1964.
13. Hitzig, W.H., et al.: Helv. Paediatr. Acta **13**:551, 1958.
14. Gitlin, D., and Craig, J.M.: Pediatrics **32**:517, 1963.
15. Giblett, E.R., et al.: Lancet **2**:1967, 1972.
16. Gatti, R.A., et al.: J. Pediatr. **75**:675, 1969.
17. Hobbs, J.R., and Davis, J.A.: Lancet **1**:757, 1967.
18. Waldman, T.A., Strober, W., and Blaese, K.M.: Ann. Intern. Med. **77**:605, 1972.
19. Miller, D.G.: In Samter, M., editor: Immunological deficiency diseases, Boston, 1971, Little, Brown & Co.
20. Stoelinga, G.B.A., van Munster, P.J.J., and Slooff, J.P.: Acta Paediatr. Scand. **58**:352, 1969.
21. Soothill, J.F.: In Gell, P.G.H., Coombs, R.R.A., and Lachmann, P.J., editors: Clinical aspects of immunology, ed. 3, Oxford, England, 1975, Blackwell Scientific Publications.
22. Stiehm, E.R., and Fudenberg, H.H.: Am. J. Med. **40**:805, 1966.

23. Seligmann, M., Fudenberg, H.H., and Good, R.A.: Am. J. Med. **45**:817, 1968.
24. Edelson, P.J.: Calif. Med. **116**:19, 1972.
25. Stoelinga, G.B.A., van Munster, P.J.J., and Slooff, J.P.: Pediatr. Res. **3**:233, 1969.
26. Kaplan, M.E., et al.: Blood **28**:446, 1966.
27. Tucker, E.S., III, and Nakamura, R.M.: In Ritzmann, S.E., and Daniels, J.C., editors: Serum protein abnormalities: diagnostic and clinical aspects, Boston, 1975, Little, Brown & Co.
28. Alper, C.A., and Rosen, F.S.: In Vyas, G.N., Stites, D.P., and Brecher, G., editors: Laboratory diagnosis of immunologic disorders, New York, 1975, Grune & Stratton, Inc.
29. Polley, M.J., and Bearn, A.G.: Am. J. Med. **58**:105, 1975.
30. Nelson, R.H., Jr., et al.: Immunochemistry **3**:111, 1966.
31. Goodkofsky, I., and Lepow, I.H.: J. Immunol. **107**:1200, 1971.
32. Hunsicker, L.G., et al.: N. Engl. J. Med. **287**:835, 1972.
33. Frank, M.M., and Atkinson, J.P.: D.M., January 1975.
34. Ruddy, S., Gigli, I., and Austen, K.F.: N. Engl. J. Med. **287**:489, 545, 592, 642, 1972.
35. Polley, M.J., and Bearn, A.G.: Am. J. Med. **58**:105, 1975.
36. Alper, C.A., et al.: N. Engl. J. Med. **282**:349, 1970.
37. Donaldson, V.H., et al.: J. Clin. Invest. **48**:642, 1969.
38. Rosen, F.S., et al.: Science **148**:957, 1965.
39. Alper, C.A., and Rosen, F.S.: In Vyas, G.N., Sites, D.P., and Brecher, G., editors: Laboratory diagnosis of immunologic disorders, New York, 1975, Grune & Stratton, Inc.
40. Alper, C.A., Rosen, F.S., and Lachmann, P.J.: Proc. Natl. Acad. Sci. U.S.A. **69**:2910, 1972.
41. Gotoff, S.P., et al.: N. Engl. J. Med. **273**:524, 1965.
42. Gotze, O., and Muller-Eberhard, H.J.: J. Exp. Med. **134**(suppl.):90, 1971.
43. Rosen, R.S., et al.: J. Clin. Invest. **50**:2143, 1971.
44. Klemperer, M.R., et al.: J. Clin. Invest. **45**:880, 1966.
45. Alper, C.A.: Lancet **2**:1179, 1972.
46. Rosenfeld, S.I., and Leddy, J.P.: J. Clin. Invest. **53**:67, 1974 (abstract).
47. Alper, C.A., and Rosen, F.S.: J. Clin. Invest. **46**:2021, 1976.
48. Ruddy, S., Gigli, I., and Austen, K.F.: N. Engl. J. Med. **287**:489, 545, 592, 642, 1972.
49. Dacie, J.V., and Worlledge, S.M.: In Dacie, J.V., and Lewis, S.M.: Practical haematology, Edinburgh, 1975, Churchill Livingstone.
50. Rebuck, J.W., and Crowley, J.H.: Ann. N.Y. Acad. Sci. **59**:757, 1955.
51. Clark, R.A., and Kimball, H.R.: J. Clin. Invest. **50**:2645, 1971.
52. Miller, M.E.: Pediatr. Res. **5**:487, 1971.
53. Miller, M.E., Oski, F.A., and Harris, M.B.: Lancet **1**:665, 1971.
54. Mowat, A.G., and Baum, J.: J. Clin. Invest. **50**:2541, 1971.
55. Perillie, P.E., Nolan, J.P., and Finch, S.C.: J. Lab. Clin. Med **59**:1008, 1962.
56. DeMeo, A.N., and Anderson, B.R.: N. Engl. J. Med. **286**:735, 1972.
57. McCall, C.E., et al.: J. Infect. Dis. **124**:68, 1971.
58. Baehner, R.L., and Nathan, D.G.: N. Engl. J. Med. **278**:971, 1968.
59. Park, B.H., et al.: Pediatr. Res. **4**:463, 1970.
60. Johnston, R.B., Jr., and Baehner, R.L.: Pediatrics **48**:730, 1971.

61. Douwes, F.R.: N. Engl. J. Med. **287:**822, 1972.
62. Park, B.H., and Good, R.A.: Proc. Natl. Acad. Sci. U.S.A. **69:**371, 1972.
63. Park, B.H., and Good, R.A.: Lancet **1:**616, 1970.
64. Kaplan, E.L., Laxdal, T., and Quie, P.G.: Pediatrics **41:**591, 1968.
65. Lehrer, R.I., and Cline, M.J.: J. Clin. Invest. **48:**1478, 1969.
66. Hong, R.: Diseases of delayed hypersensitivity. In Kegen, B.M., and Stiehm, E.R., editors: Immunologic incompetence, Chicago, 1971, Year Book Medical Publishers, Inc.
67. Gajl-Peczalska, K.J., et al.: J. Clin. Invest. **52:**919, 1973.
68. Robbins, D., and Gershwin, M.D.: Semin. Arthritis Rheum. **7:**245, 1978.
69. Kohout, E., and Dutz, W.: Prog. Clin. Pathol. **7:**197, 1978.
70. Chess, L., and Schlossman, S.F.: Adv. Immunol. **25:**213, 1977.
71. International Union of Immunological Societies (IUIS) Report, Clin. Immunol. Immunopathol. **3:**584, 1975.
72. Mehrishi, J.N., and Zeiller, K.: Br. Med. J. **1:**360, 1974.
73. Kay, H.E.M.: Br. J. Haematol. **20:**139, 1971.
74. Seligmann, M., Preud'Homme, J.L., and Brouet, J.C.: Transplant Rev. **16:**85, 1973.
75. Bianco, C., Patrick, R., and Nussenzweig, V.: J. Exp. Med. **132:**702, 1970.
76. Basten, A., et al.: J. Exp. Med. **135:**610, 1972.
77. Shevach, E.M., Jaffe, E.S., and Green, I.: Transplant Rev. **16:**3, 1973.
78. Schevach, E.M., Herberman, R., and Frank, M.M.: J. Clin. Invest. **51:**1933, 1972.
79. Catousky, D.: Br. J. Haematol. **33:**173, 1976.
80. Jondal, M., Holm, G., and Wigzell, H.: J. Exp. Med. **136:**207, 1972.
81. Oppenheim, J.J., et al.: In Vyas, G.N., Stites, D.P., and Brecher, G., editors: Laboratory diagnosis of immunologic disorders, New York, 1975, Grune & Stratton, Inc.
82. Rocklin, R.E.: In Vyas, G.N., Stites, D.P., and Brecher, G., editors: Laboratory diagnosis of immunologic disorders, New York, 1975, Grune & Stratton, Inc.
83. Bobrove, A.M., et al.: J. Immunol. **112:**520, 1974.
84. Haegart, D.G., Hallberg, T., and Coombs, R.R.A.: Int. Arch. Allergy Appl. Immunol. **46:**525, 1974.
85. Moretta, L.O., et al.: Eur. J. Immunol. **5:**561, 1975.
86. Boyum, A.: Scand. J. Immunol. **5:**9, 1976.
87. Grey, H.M., Rabellino, E., and Priofsky, B.: J. Clin. Invest. **50:**2368, 1971.
88. Binder, R.A., et al.: Cancer **36:**161, 1975.
89. Lukes, R.J., and Collins, R.D.: Cancer **34:**1488, 1974.
90. Catovsky, D., et al.: Br. Med. J. **2:**643, 1974.
91. Wilson, J.D., and Nossal, G.J.V.: Lancet **1:**788, 1971.
92. Aiuti, F., et al.: Infect. Immun. **8:**110, 1973.
93. Weiner, M.S., Bianco, C., and Nussenzweig, V.: Blood **42:**939, 1973.
94. Small, P.: Ann. Allergy **34:**345, 1975.
95. Hepburn, B., and Ritts, R.E.: Mayo Clin. Proc. **49:**866, 1974.
96. Fudenberg, H.H., Wybran, J., and Robbins, D.: N. Engl. J. Med. **292:**475, 1975.
97. Horowitz, S., et al.: Clin. Immunol. Immunopathol. **4:**405, 1975.
98. Bentiwich, Z., et al.: Clin. Immunol. Immunopathol. **1:**511, 1973.
99. MacDermott, R.P., Chess, L., and Schlossman, S.F.: Clin. Immunol. Immunopathol. **4:**415, 1975.
100. Keightley, R., Cooper, M., and Lawton, A.: J. Immunol. **117:**1538, 1976.
101. Diaz-Jouanen, E., Strockland, R.G., and Williams, R.C., Jr.: Am. J. Med. **58:**610 1975.
102. Rocklin, R.E.: J. Immunol. **112:**1461, 1974.
103. Bloom, B.R.: Adv. Immunol. **13:**122, 1971.
104. David, J.R., and David, R.A.: Prog. Allergy **16:**300, 1972.
105. Cohen, S., and Porter, R.R.: Adv. Immunol. **4:**287, 1964.
106. Tomaski, T.B., Jr., and Bienenstock, J.: Adv. Immunol. **9:**1, 1968.
107. Metzger, H.: Adv. Immunol. **12:**57, 1970.
108. Spiegelberg, J.L.: In Inman, F.P., editor: Contemporary topics in immunochemistry, New York, 1972, Plenum Press.
109. Bennich, H., and Johansson, S.G.O.: Adv. Immunol. **13:**1, 1971.
110. Solomon, A., and McLaughlin, C.L.: Med. Clin. North Am. **57:**499, 1973.
111. Delaney, W.E.: Ann. Clin. Lab. Sci. **2:**75, 1972.
112. Ritzmann, S.E., and Daniels, J.C.: Serum protein abnormalities: diagnostic and clinical aspects, Boston, 1975, Little, Brown & Co.
113. Ritzman, S.E., et al., Tex. Med. **68:**91, 1972.
114. Seligmann, M., and Brouet, J.C.: Semin. Hematol. **10:**163, 1973.
115. Isobe, T., and Osserman, E.F.: Ann. N.Y. Acad. Sci. **190:**507, 1971.
116. Williams, R.C., Jr., Bailly, R.C., and Howe, R.B.: Am. J. Med. Sci. **257:**275, 1969.
117. Solomon, A.: N. Engl. J. Med. **294:**91, 1976.
118. Franklin, E.C.: In Vyas, G.N., Stites, D.P., and Brecher, G., editors: Laboratory diagnosis of immunologic disorders, New York, 1975, Grune & Stratton, Inc.
119. Cawley, L.P.: Electrophoresis and immunoelectrophoresis, Boston, 1969, Little, Brown & Co.
120. Cawley, L.P., et al.: Basic electrophoresis, immunoelectrophoresis and immunochemistry, Chicago, 1972, American Society of Clinical Pathologists.
121. Frangione, B., and Franklin, E.C.: Semin. Hematol. **10:**53, 1973.
122. Solomon, A.: N. Engl. J. Med. **294:**17, 1976.
123. Dammacco, F., and Waldenstrom, J.: Acta Med. Scand. **184:**403, 1968.
124. Solomon, A., and Fahey, J.L.: Am. J. Med. **37:**206, 1964.
125. Grey, H.M., and Kohler, P.F.: Clin. Exp. Immunol. **3:**277, 1968.
126. Lindstrom, F.D., et al.: J. Lab. Clin. Med. **71:**812, 1968.
127. Putman, F.W., et al.: Arch. Biochem. Biophys. **83:**115, 1959.
128. Perry, M.C., and Kyle, R.A.: Mayo Clin. Proc. **50:**234, 1975.
129. Tan, M., and Epstein, W.V.: J. Lab. Clin. Med. **66:**344, 1965.
130. Mancini, G., Carbonara, A.O., and Heremans, J.F.: Immunochemistry **2:**235, 1965.
131. Fahey, J.L., and McKelvey, E.M.: J. Immunol. **94:**84, 1965.
132. Gilliland, B.C., and Mannik, M.: In Vyas, G.N., Stites, D.P., and Brecher, G., editors: Laboratory diagnosis of immunologic disorders, New York, 1975, Grune & Stratton, Inc.
133. Morrell, A., Skvarid, F., and Barandun, S.: Clin. Immunol. Immunopathol. **13:**293, 1973.
134. Grubb, A.: Scand. J. Clin. Lab. Invest. **31:**465, 1973.
135. Daniels, J.C., et al.: Clin. Chem. **21:**243, 1975.

136. Solomon, A.: J. Immunol. **102**:496, 1969.
137. Ritzmann, S.E., Fischer, C.L., and Nakamura, R.M.: In Ritzmann, S.E., and Daniels, J.C., editors: Serum protein abnormalities: diagnostic and clinical aspects, Boston, 1975, Little, Brown & Co.
138. Gill, C.W., Fischer, C.L., and Holleman, C.L.: Clin. Chem. **17**:501, 1971.
139. Buckley, R.H., Dees, S.C., and O'Fallon, W.M.: Pediatrics **41**:600, 1968.
140. Alford, C.A., Jr.: Pediatr. Clin. North Am. **18**:99, 1971.
141. Zinneman, H.H., Levi, D., and Seal, U.S.: J. Immunol. **100**:594, 1968.
142. Grey, H.M., and Kohler, P.F.: Semin. Hematol. **10**:87, 1973.
143. Cream, J.J.: Clin. Exp. Immunol. **10**:17, 1972.
144. Ritzmann, S.E., and Levin, W.C.: Arch. Intern. Med. **107**:754, 1961.
145. Zoltnick, A., Shahin, W., and Rachmilewitz, E.A.: Acta Haematol. **42**:8, 1969.
146. Stastny, P., and Ziff, M.: N. Engl. J. Med. **280**:1367, 1969.
147. Martin, W.J., Mathieson, D.R., and Eigler, J.O.C.: Proc. Staff Meetings Mayo Clin. **34**:95, 1959.
148. Wolf, R.E., Levin, W.C., and Ritzmann, S.E.: In Ritzmann, S.E., and Daniels, J.C., editors: Serum protein abnormalities: diagnostic and clinical aspects, Boston, 1975, Little, Brown & Co.
149. Bloch, K.J., and Maki, D.G.: Semin. Hematol. **10**:113, 1973.
150. Wells, R.: N. Engl. J. Med. **283**:183, 1970.
151. Capra, J.D., and Kunkel, H.G.: J. Clin. Invest. **49**:610, 1970.
152. Fahey, J.L. Barth, W.F., and Solomon, A.: J.A.M.A. **192**:464, 1965.
153. Constanzi, J.J., et al.: Am. J. Med. **39**:163, 1965.
154. Ritzmann, S.E., et al.: Arch. Intern. Med. **105**:939, 1960.
155. Hartmann, W., Farin, R., and Yokoyama N.: Hawaii Med. J. **26**:531, 1967.
156. Franglen, G.: Clin. Chim. Acta **14**:559, 1966.
157. Gartner, O.T., et al.: J.A.M.A. **201**:206, 1967.
158. Taylor, W.F., et al.: Ann. Allergy **29**:377, 1971.
159. Davis, S.D., Schaller, J., and Wedgewood, R.J.: In Kagen, M.B., and Stiehm, E.R., editors: Immunologic incompetence, Chicago, 1971, Year Book Medical Publishers, Inc.
160. Hughes, G.R.V.: Br. J. Haematol. **25**:409, 1973.
161. Harvey, A.M., et al.: Medicine **33**:291, 1954.
162. Wall, R.L., Haq, A., and Moore, D.: J. Lab. Clin. Med. **70**:8861, 1967.
163. Bithell, T.C., and Bunting, D.L.: Clin. Res. **15**:103, 1967.
164. Burkhardt, R.: Semin. Hematol. **2**:29, 1965.
165. Nakamura, R.M.: In Cawley, L.P., et al., editors: Clinical immunology and immunochemistry, Chicago, 1972, American Society of Clinical Pathologists.
166. Friou, G.J., and Quismorio, F.P.: In Cohen, A.S., editor: Laboratory diagnostic procedures in the rheumatic diseases, Boston, 1975, Little, Brown & Co.
167. Nakamura, R.M.: Immunopathology: clinical laboratory concept and methods, Boston, 1974, Little Brown & Co.
168. Zinkham, W.H., and Conley, C.L.: Bull. Johns Hopkins Hosp. **98**:102, 1956.
169. Koller, S.R., et al.: Am. J. Clin. Pathol. **66**:495, 1976.
170. Niejadlik, D.C.: Postgrad. Med. **50**:273, 1971.
171. Rothfield, N.F.: In Rose, N.R., and Friedman, H., editors: Manual of clinical immunology, Washington, D.C., 1976, American Society for Microbiology.
172. Bigazzi, P.E., and Rose, N.R.: In Rose, N.R., and Friedman, H., editors: Manual of clinical immunology, Washington, D.C., 1976, American Society for Microbiology.
173. Tan, E.M., Northway, J.D., and Pinnas, J.L.: Postgrad. Med. **54**:143-150, 1973.
174. Husain, M., et al.: Am. J. Clin. Pathol. **61**:59-65, 1973.
175. Tan, E.M.: J. Lab. Clin. Med. **70**:800-812, 1967.
176. Beck, J.S.: Lancet **1**:1203, 1961.
177. Casals, S.P., Friou, G.J., and Teague, P.O.: J. Lab. Clin. Med. **62**:625, 1963.
178. Lachmann, P.J., and Kinkel, H.G.: Lancet **2**:436, 1961.
179. Sharp, G.C., et al.: Am. J. Med. **52**:148, 1972.
180. Ritchie, R.F.: N. Engl. J. Med. **282**:1174, 1970.
181. Cawley, L.P.: In Cawley, L.P., et al., editors: Clinical immunology and immunochemistry, Chicago, 1972, American Society of Clinical Pathologists.
182. Benson, M.D., and Cohen, A.S: Ann. Intern. Med. **73**:943, 1970.
183. Kawaoi, A., and Nakane, P.K.: Fed. Proc. **32**:840, 1973.
184. Friou, G.J., and Quismario, F.P.: In Cohen, A.S., editor: Laboratory diagnostic procedures in the rheumatic diseases, ed. 2, Boston, 1975, Little, Brown & Co.
185. Alexander, W.R.M., and Duthie J.J.R.: Br. Med. J. **2**:1565, 1958.
186. Ten Veen, J.H., and Feltkamp, T.E.W.: Clin. Exp. Immunol. **5**:673, 1969.
187. Muna, N.M., Verner, J.L., and Hammond, D.F.: Am. J. Clin. Pathol. **45**:117, 1966.
188. Tan, E.M.: J. Lab. Clin. Med. **70**:800, 1967.
189. Friou, G.J.: Arthritis Rheum. **5**:407, 1962.
190. Elling, P.: Acta Pathol. Microbiol. Scand. **68**:281, 1966.
191. Cleymaet, J.E., and Nakamura, R.M.: Am. J. Clin. Pathol. **58**:388, 1972.
192. Beck, J.S.: Scott. Med. J. **8**:373, 1963.
193. Casals, S.P., Friou, G.J., and Myers, L.L.: Arthritis Rheum. **7**:379, 1964.
194. Koffler, D., Schur, P.H., and Kunkel, H.G.: J. Exp. Med. **126**:607-627, 1967.
195. Stollar, D., and Levine, L.: J. Immunol. **87**:477, 1961.
196. Tan, E.M., Schur, P.H., and Carr, R.I.: J. Clin. Invest. **45**:1732, 1966.
197. Koffler, D., et al.: Fed. Proc. **28**:486, 1969.
198. Inami, Y.H., and Nakamura, R.H.: In Rose, N.R., and Friedman, H., editors: Manual of clinical immunology, Washington, D.C., 1976, American Society for Microbiology.
199. Wold, R.T., et al.: Science **161**:896, 1968.
200. Hughes, G.R.V., Cohen, S.A., and Christian, C.L.: Ann. Rheum. Dis. **30**:259, 1971.
201. Pincus, T.: Arthritis Rheum. **14**:623, 1971.
202. Carr, R.I., et al.: Clin. Exp. Immunol. **4**:527, 1969.
203. Talal, N., and Pillarisetty, R.: In Rose, N.R., and Friedman, H., editors: Manual of clinical immunology, Washington, D.C., 1976, American Society for Microbiology.
204. Aarden, L.A., DeGroot, E.R., and Feltkamp, T.E.W.: Proc. N.Y. Acad. Sci. **254**:505, 1975.
205. Doniach, D., et al.: Clini. Exp. Immunol. **1**:237, 1966.
206. Lam, K.C., Mistilis, S.P., and Perrott, M.: N. Engl. J. Med. **286**:1400-1401, 1972.
207. Doniach, D., et al.: N. Engl. J. Med. **282**:86, 1970.
208. Whittingham, S., et al.: Gastroenterology **5**:499, 1966.
209. Holboron, E.J.: Proc. R. Soc. Med. **65**:481, 1972.
210. Whitehouse, J.M.A., and Holborow, E.J.: Br. Med. J. **4**:511, 1971.
211. Balfour, B.M., et al.: Br. J. Exp. Pathol. **43**:307, 1961.
212. Rose, N.R., and Bigazzi: In Laskin, A.I., and Lechevalier, H.A., editors: Handbook of microbiology, vol. 4, Cleveland, 1974, C.R.C. Press, Inc.

213. Delespesse, G., et al.: Thyroid autoimmunity. In Basteine, P.A. and Evans, A.M., editors: Thyroditis and thyroid function, Oxford, England, 1972, Pergamon Press, Ltd.
214. Jordon, R.E.: In Rose, N.R., and Friedman, H., editors: Manual of clinical immunology, Washington, D.C., 1976, American Society for Microbiology.
215. Jablanska, S., Chorzelski, T.P., and Buetner, E.H.: In Buetner, E.H., et al., editors: Immunopathology of the skin: labeled antibody studies, Stroudsburg, Pa., 1973, Dowden, Hutchinson & Ross, Inc.
216. Goldberg, L.S., and Fudenberg, H.H.: Am. J. Med. **46:**489, 1969.
217. Bernhardt, H., et al.: Ann. Intern. Med. **63:**635, 1965.
218. Engle, M.A., et al.: Circulation **49:**401, 1974.
219. Wilson, C.B., and Dixon, F.J.: Kidney Int. **3:**74, 1973.
220. McPhaul, J.J., Jr., and Dixon, F.J.: J. Immunol. **103:**1168, 1968.
221. Andrada, J.A., et al.: J.A.M.A. **206:**1535, 1968.
222. Irvine, W.J., Stewart, A.G., and Scarth, L.: Clin. Exp. Immunol. **2:**31, 1967.
223. Tan, E.M., and Peebles, C.: In Rose, N.R., and Friedman, H., editors: Manual of clinical immunology, Washington, D.C., 1978, American Society for Microbiology.
224. Notman, D., Kurata, N., and Tan, E.M.: Ann. Intern. Med. **83:**464-469, 1975.
225. Reichlin, M., and Mattioli, M.: N. Engl. J. Med. **286:**908-911, 1972.
226. Sharp, G.C., et al.: J. Clin. Invest. **50:**350, 1971.
227. Sharp, G.C., et al.: Am. J. Med. **52:**148-159, 1972.
228. Koffler, D., et al.: J. Exp. Med. **134**(suppl.):169, 1971.
229. Agnello, V., Winchester, R.J., and Kunkel, H.G.: Immunology **19:**909, 1970.
230. Winchester, R.J., Kunkel, H.G., and Agnello, V.: J. Exp. Med. **134:**2865, 1971.
231. Penttinen, K., et al.: Acta Pathol. Microbiol. Scand. **77:**309, 1969.
232. Theofilopoulos, A.M., Wilson, C.B., and Dixon, F.J.: J. Clin. Invest. **57:**169, 1976.
233. Hay, F.C., Nineham, L.J., and Roitt, I.M.: Clin. Exp. Immunol. **24:**396, 1976.
234. Cowdery, J.S., Jr., Tredwell, P.E., and Fritz, R.B.: J. Immunol. **114:**5, 1975.
235. Luthra, H.S., et al.: J. Clin. Invest. **54:**458, 1975.
236. Wager, O., et al.: Clin. Exp. Immunol. **15:**393, 1973.
237. Penttinen, K., and Myllyla, G.: Bull. WHO **42:**980, 1970.
238. Pohl, D., Tsai, C.C., and Roodman, S.T.: J. Immunol. Methods **40:**313, 1981.
239. Riott, I.M., Nineham, L.J., and Hay, F.C.: Clin. Exp. Immunol. **24:**396, 1976.
240. Svehag, S.E.: Scand. J. Immunol. **4:**687, 1975.
241. Svehag, S.E., Farrell, C., and Sogaard, H.: Scand. J. Immunol. **4:**673, 1975.
242. Wilson, C.B.: In Rose, N.R., and Friedman, H., editors: Manual of clinical immunology, Washington, D.C., 1976, American Society for Microbiology.
243. Jordon, R.E.: In Rose, N.R., and Friedman, H., editors: Manual of clinical immunology, Washington, D.C., 1976, American Society for Microbiology.
244. Qualman, S.J., et al.: Lab. Invest. **41:**483-489, 1979.
245. Choi, Y.J., et al.: Am. J. Clin. Pathol. **73:**116-119, 1980.
246. Kohnt, E., and Dutz, W.: Prog. Clin. Pathol. **7:**198, 1977.
247. Lukes, R.J., and Collins, R.D.: Br. J. Cancer **31:**1, 1975; Am. J. Pathol. **90:**461, 1978.
248. Nussenzwig, V., et al.: In Bloom, B.R., and David, J.R., editors: In vitro methods in cell-mediated immunity, New York, 1976, Academic Press Inc.
249. Brubaker, D.B., and Whiteside, T.L.: Am. J. Pathol. **8:**323, 1977.
250. Jaffe, E.S., and Green, I.: In Green, I., Cohen, S., and McCluskey, R.T., editors: Mechanisms of tumor immunity, New York, 1977, John Wiley & Sons, Inc.

Normal values

CHEMISTRY

Alanine aminotransferase (ALT)	Serum	7-30 units/L
Albumin	Serum	4.0-5.5 g/dl (40-55 g/L)
Alcohol (ethyl)	Blood	<0.1 g/L (2.2 mmol/L)
Aldolase	Serum	Male, 8.5-20 units/L, female, 7.0-14 units/L
Aldosterone	Urine	2-26 μg/24 hr. (6-72 nmol/24 h)
Amino acid nitrogen	Plasma	3.5-7.0 mg/dl (2.5-5.0 mmol/L)
	Urine	50-200 mg/24 hr. (3.6-7.2 mmol/24 h)
Ammonia	Blood	18-60 μg/dl (10-30 μmol/L)
Amniotic fluid		Net absorbance at 540 nm < 0.020, billirubin, <0.25 mg/dl (4.3 μmol/L); L/S ratio > 2
Amylase	Serum	60-180 Somogyi units (110-330 U/L)
	Urine	35-260 units/hr; 80-5000 units/24 hr
Antistreptolysin titier	Serum	<200 Todd units; absence of rising titer
Ascorbic acid	Plasma	0.5-2.0 mg/dl (30-120 μmol/L)
Aspartate aminotransferase (AST)	Serum	12-30 units/L
Arsenic	Urine	<100 μg/L (1.3 μmol/L)
Barbiturates (therapeutic range)	Serum	
Short acting		0.05-0.15 mg/dl (0.5-1.5 mg/L)
Intermediate acting		0.1-0.5 mg/dl (1-5 mg/L)
Long acting		1.5-3.0 mg/dl (15-30 mg/L)
Bilirubin	Serum	Total, 0.2-1.3 mg/dl (3.4-22 μmol/L); direct, 0.1-0.4 mg/dl (1.7-7.0 μmol/L)
Blood urea nitrogen (BUN)	Serum	10-18 mg/dl (3.6-6.5 mmol/L as urea)
Bromide	Serum	<3 mg/dl (0.12 mmol/L)
Bromsulfphthalein (BSP)	Serum	<6% remaining after 45 min
Calcium	Serum	8.5-10.5 mg/dl (2.1-2.6 mmol/L)
	Urine	60-400 mg/24 hr (1.5-10 mmol/24 h)
Calcium, ionic	Serum	4.6-5.4 mg/dl (1.15-1.35 mmol/L
Carbon dioxide (CO_2) content	Serum	24-32 mmol/L
	Venous blood	23-30 mmol/L
	Arterial blood	21-28 mmol/L
Carbon dioxide pressure (P_{CO_2})	Blood	38-49 mm Hg (torr) (5.1-6.5 kPa)
Carboxyhemoglobin	Blood	<5% of total hemoglobin
Cardio-Green (liver function)	Serum	<4% remaining after 20 min; disappearance rate of 18-26%/min
Carotene	Serum	50-250 μg/dl (0.93-4.7 μmol/L)
Catecholamines (total)	Urine	30-70 μg/24 hr (175-420 nmol/L as norepinephrine)

NOTE: Normal values, particularly those of enzymes, may vary with the method used for their determination. The values listed are those for adults (those differing for children are specifically mentioned) and have been obtained by the methods used in this book or, where no method is given, by commonly used methods. Caution should be used in interpreting these normal values in children (except where specifically noted) and in individuals over the age of 60. These differences in normal values are discussed in the interpretations given with the specific procedures. Therapeutic levels are given only for some of the most commonly used drugs. A more complete listing is found in the review by Winek (Winek, C.L.: Clin. Chem. **22**:832, 1976).

Ceruloplasmin (see Ferroxidase)		
Chloride	Serum	98-109 mEq/L (mmol/L)
	Spinal fluid	122-132 mEq/L (mmol/L)
	Sweat	10-35 mEq/L (mmol/L)
Cholesterol (total)	Serum	150-270 mg/dl (39-70 mmol/L)
Cholesterol esters	Serum	68-74% of total
Cholinesterase (pseudo)	Serum	9-12 units/L
Cold agglutinin	Serum	<1:32 dilution
Concentration test	Urine	Specific gravity of 1.025 or higher
Copper	Serum	75-155 μg/dl (12-25 μmol/L)
Coproporphyrin	Urine	20-100 μg/24 hr (30-150 nmol/24 h)
Corticosteroids, total (hydroxysteroids as cortisol)	Urine	Male, 5-14 mg/24 hr (14-39 μmol/24 hr); female, 4-13 mg/24 hr (11-36 μmol/24 hr)
Cortisol	Plasma	8 AM, 10-25 μg/dl (300-700 nmol/L); 8 PM, 4-13 μg/dl (110-350 nmol/L)
	Urine	Male, 110-410 μg/24 hr (0.3-1.1 μmol/24 h); female, 80-360 μg/24 hr (0.22-0.90 μmol/24h)
Creatine phosphokinase (CPK)	Serum	Male, 20-50 units/L; female, 10-40 units/L
Creatinine	Serum	0.6-1.2 mg/dl (53-106 μmol/L)
	Urine	Male, 1.0-1.4 g/24 hr (8.8-12.4 mmol/24 h); female, 0.8-1.2 g/24 hr (7.1-10.6 mmol/24 h)
Creatinine clearance		Males, 113-167 ml/min (1.88-2.78 ml/s); females, 92-132 ml/min (1.53-2.20 ml/s)
C'3 component	Serum	123-167 mg/dl (1.23-1.67 g/L)
Digoxin (therapeutic level)	Serum	1.0-2.25ng/ml (1.3-2.9 nmol/L)
Diphenylhydantoin (phenytoin) (therapeutic level)	Serum	1-2 mg/dl (40-80 μmol/L)
Epinephrine	Urine	10-40% of the total catecholamines
Estrogens	Pregnancy urine	Gradually increasing from 3-7 mg/24 hrs (11-18 mmole/d) at 20 weeks to 15-45 mg/24 hrs (33-100 mmol/d) at term
Fat	Feces	<5 g/24 hr on normal diet
Fatty acids	Serum	
Esterified		7-14 mmol/L
Free		0.15-1.2 mmol/L
Fibrinogen	Plasma	0.2-0.4 g/dl (2-4 g/L)
Follicle-stimulating hormone	Urine	6-60mU/24 hr
Gastric analysis		Free acidity 0-40 mmole/L, total acidity, 10-50 mmole/L, pH 1.5-4.0; volume, 30-100 ml
Globulins - (see protein fractionation and Immunoglobulins)		
Glucose	Serum	85-110 mg/dl (4.4-6.0 mmol/L)
	Spinal fluid	40-80 mg/dl (2.2-4.4 mmol/L
Glucose tolerance (oral)	Serum	Fasting, 80-110 mg/dl (4.4-6 mmol/L);1 hr <180 mg/dl (8.3 mmol/L);2 hr, <140 mg/dl (7.8 mmol/L)
Glucose-6-phosphate dehydrogenase	Blood	5-10 U/g hemoglobin
Glutamic oxalacetic transaminase (see Alanine aminotransferase)		
Glutamic pyruvic transaminase (see Aspartate aminotransferase)		
Glutamyl transpeptidase	Serum	Males 10-50 units/L; females, about 20% lower
Haptoglobin	Serum	70-140 mg/dl (9.7-1.4 g/L)
Hydroxybutyric dehydrogenase	Serum	50-125 units/L
5-Hydroxyindole acetic acid (5-HIAA)	Urine	2-14 mg/24 hr (11-75 μmol/d)
Hydroxysteroids (see corticosteroids)		
Immunoglobulins	Serum	IgA, 100-400 mg/dl (1-4 g/L); IgG, 650-1600 mg/dl (6.5-16 g/L); IgM, 30-120 mg/dl (0.3-1.2 g/L)
Iron	Serum	Male, 80-160 mg/dl (14-28 μmol/L); female, 60-136 mg/dl (11-24 μmol/L)
Iron-binding capacity (total)	Serum	250-350 mg/dl (45-63 μmol/L)
Isocitric dehydrogenase (ICDH)	Serum	240-690 units/L

17-Ketosteroids (calculated as dehydroepiandrosterone)	Urine	Male, 10-18 mg/24 hr (35-63 μmol/24 h); female, 6-15 mg/24 hr (21-52 μmol/24 hr)
ACTH stimulation		Increase of 50% or more in ketosteroids; 100% increase in ketogenic steroids
Metyrapone test		Increase of 50% in ketosteroids; 100% increase in ketogenic steroids
Lactate	Blood	5-12 mg/dl (0.56-1.3 mmol/L)
Lactate dehydrogenase (LDH)	Serum	95-200 unitsL
	Spinal fluid	10-30 units/L
	Urine	60-240 units/hr in overnight specimen
Lead	Blood	<40 μg/dl (1.9 μmol/L)
Leucine aminopeptidase (LAP)	Serum	11-30 units/L
	Urine	Male, 0.8-6.2 units in overnight specimen; female, 0.2-4.7 units/L in overnight specimen
Lipase	Serum	<1.0 units (<280 mU/L)
Lipids (total)	Serum	400-850 mg/dl (4.0-8.5 g/L)
Lithium (therapeutic range)	Serum	0.5-1.2 mEq/L (mmol/L)
Lysozyme (muramidase)	Serum	3-8 μg/ml (mg/L)
Magnesium	Serum	1.6-2.1 mEq/L (0.8-1.05 mmol/L)
Methemoglobin	Blood	<1.5% of total hemoglobin
3-Methoxy-4-hydroxymandelic acid (see VMA)		
Metyrapone test (see 17-Ketosteroids)		
Norepinephrine	Urine	60-90% of total catecholamines
Osmolality	Serum	275-295 mOsm/kg
	Urine	400-1000 mOsm/kg
Oxygen pressure (Po_2)	Arterial blood	60-80 mm Hg (torr) (8.0-10.7 kPa)
	Venous blood	30-50 mm Hg (torr) (4.0-6.3 kPa)
Oxygen saturation	arterial blood	90-95% (0.90-0.95)
	Venous blood	60-85% (0.60-0.85)
pH	Arterial blood	7.32-7.42
	Venous blood	7.35-7.45
	Urine	4.8-7.6 (average 6.0)
Phenolsulfonphthalein (PSP)	Urine	25 50% excreted in first 15 min; 15-25% more in next 15 min; 10-15% in next 30 min; 60-85% total excreted in 1 hr
Phosphatase		
Acid	Serum	Male, 2.5-11 units/L; female, 0.3-9 units/L
Total		
Tartaric acid labile		Male, 0.2-3.5 units/L; female, 0.0-0.8 units/L
Alkaline	Serum	Adults, 20-90 units/L; children, 40-200 units/L
Heat labile, bone		> 60% of total
Phospholipids	Serum	150-300 mg/dl (1.9-4.5 mmol/L)
Phosphorus (inorganic)	Serum	Adults, 2.5-4.8 mg/dl (0.8-1.55 mmol/L); children, 3.5-6.0 mg/dl (1.1-1.9 mmol/L)
Porphobilinogen synthase (aminolevulinate dehydratase)	Red cells	4-20 mmole/min/ml red cells
Porphyrins	Urine	Uroporphyrin <40 μg/24 hr (50 nmol); coproporphyrin < 200 μg/24 hr (250 nmol)
Potassium	Serum	3.5-5.6 mEq/L (mmol/L)
	Urine	25-100 mEq/L (mmol/L)
Protein (total)	Serum	6-8 g/dl (60-80 g/L)
	Spinal fluid	15-45 mg/dl (150-450 mg/L)
Protein fractionation		
Prealbumin	Serum	—
	Spinal fluid	2-7% of total
Albumin	Serum	52-68%
	Spinal fluid	52-72%
α_1-Globulin	Serum	2-6%
	Spinal fluid	1-7%
α_2-Globulin	Serum	5-11%
	Spinal fluid	3-12%
β-Globulin	Serum	8-16%
	Spinal fluid	7-23%
γ-Globulin	Serum	10-22%
	Spinal fluid	3-13%
Prothrombin time	Plasma	70-100% or 11-13 sec
Protoporphyrin	Red cells	15-100 μg/dl red cells (0.27-1.78 μmol/L)
Quinidine (therapeutic level)	Serum	0.2-0.5 mg/dl (6-15 μmol/L)

Renin level		
Normal diet	Plasma	Upright, 0.3-3.6 ng/ml; supine, 0.3-1.9 ng/ml
Low salt diet		Upright, 4.1-9.1 ng/ml; supine, 0.9-4.5 ng/ml
Salicylate (therapeutic level)	Serum	15-30 mg/dl (110-220 μmol/L)
Serotonin (see 5-Hydroxyindolacetic acid)		
Sodium	Serum	125-145 mEq/L (mmol/L)
	Sweat	5-35 mEq/L
	Urine	130-260 mEq/24 hr
Sulfhemoglobin	Blood	<1% of total hemoglobin
T3, T4, TBI (see thyroid function tests)		
Testosterone	Serum	Male, 400-1000 μg/dl (14-35 μmol/L); female, 40-120 μg/dl (1.4-2.2 μmol/L)
Thyroid funtion tests	Serum	
Thyroxine (by column)		3.5-7.5 μg thyroxine iodine/dl = 5.5-11.6 μg thyroxine/dl (70-150 μmol/L)
Thyroxine (by CPB* or RIA†)		5.5-11.5 μg/dl (70-150 μmol/L)
T3 uptake		25-35%
TBI		1.10-0.90
Triglycerides	Serum	50-145 mg/dl (0.57-1.66 mmol/L)
Trypsin	Duodenal contents	150-600 μg/ml
Urea (see Blood urea nitrogen)		
Uric acid	Serum	Male, 3.5-8.0 mg/dl (210-475 μmol/L); female, 2.5-7.0 mg/dl (150-415 μmol/L)
Urobilinogen	Urine	0.4-1.0 mg/24 hr (0.7-1.7 μmol/24 h)
	Feces	40-280 mg/24 hr (68-475 μmol)
Vitamin A	Serum	25-75 μg/dl (0.85-2.65 μmol/L)
Vitamin C (see Ascorbic acid)		
VMA	Urine	2-14 mg/dl (10-70 μmol/L)
Xylose excretion	Urine	25 g dose, 16-36% excreted in 4 hr; 5 g dose, 20-45% excreted

HEMATOLOGY

Hemoglobin	Male, 14-18 g/dl (140-180 g/L); female, 12-16 g/dl (120-160 g/L)
Hematocrit	Male, 40-54% (0.40-0.54); female, 37-47% (0.37-0.47)
Red cell count	Male, 4.6-6.2 mil/mm^3 (4.6-6.2 $\times$ 10^{12}/L); female, 4.2-5.4 mil/mm^3 (4.2-5.4 $\times$ 10^{12}/L)
White cell count	5000-10,000/mm^3 (5-10 $\times$ 10^9/L)
Differential leukocyte count	
Neutrophils	60-70%) (0.60-0.70)
Lymphocytes	20-30% (0.20-0.30)
Monocytes	2-6% (0.06-0.10)
Eosinophils	1-4% (0.01-0.04)
Basophils	0-0.5% (0.00-0.005)
Platelet count	150,000-350,000 (150-350 $\times$ 10^6/L)
Blood indices	
MCH	27-31 $\mu\mu$g (27-31 pg [picograms])
MCV	82-92 μm^3 (82-92 fl [femtoliters])
MCHC	32-36% (0.32-0.36 pg/fl)
Eosinophil count	100-300 mm^3 (100-300 $\times$ 10^6/L)

*Competitive protein binding.
†Radioimmunoassay.

Index

Page numbers in *italics* indicate illustrations. Page numbers followed
by *t* indicate tables.

Azides, safety precautions for, 21-22
Azurophilic granules in white blood cell, 125

B

B antigen, 353, 358
  acquired, 359
B cell function, evaluation of effectors of, in immune deficiency diseases, 1066
B cell quantitation by immunofluorescence in immune deficiency diseases, 1066
Babesiosis, 986
Bacillaceae, 882-886
Bacillus(i), 882-883
  definition of, 804
  maintenance conditions for, 17*t*
Bacillus anthracis, 882-883
Bacillus cereus, 883
Bacillus subtilis, 883
  for stock cultures, 17*t*
Bacitracin, sensitivity to, for group A streptococci, 837-838
Back pain in hemolysis, 432
Bacteremia, definition of, 906
Bacteria
  anaerobic, standardized single disk method for antibiotic susceptibility testing of, 835
  antibody-coated, in urine, 829
  appearance of, stained with Sternheimer-Malbin stain, 714
  colonies of, 807
  division of, 806
  growth factors for, 807
  infections from
    acute, leukocyte alkaline phosphatase values in, 116
    acute pure red cell aplasia in, 227
    hemolytic anemias caused by, 208, 221
      laboratory findings in, 226
    lymphocytic leukocytosis caused by, 236
    monocytic leukocytosis caused by, 236
    neutropenia caused by, 237
    neutrophilic leukocytosis caused by, 235
  L-phase variants of, 807
  methods for estimating number of, in urine, 829
  morphologic classification of, 804-806
  oxygen requirements of, in incubation for anaerobic cultures, 815
  radiometric detection of, 825-826
  selection of media for, 813-816
  staining methods of, 810-813
  sterilization in, 807-808
  structure of, 806
  in urinary sediment analysis, 718-719
Bacterial endocarditis, subacute, monocytic leukocytosis from, 236
Bacterial enzymes and toxins, 806
Bacterial inhibition test for blood phenylalanine, 693
Bacterial meningitis, diagnosis of, by counterimmunoelectrophoresis, 844
Bacterial reactions, 436
Bacterial stains in cerebrospinal fluid examination, 761
Bactericidal mechanisms of phagocytosis, tests for, 174
Bacteriologic material, examination of, 809-810
Bacteriologic methods, 808-809
Bacteriologic specimens, collection, handling, and shipment of, 829
Bacteriology, clinical, introduction to, 804-809
Bacteriology laboratory
  quality control for, 15-17
  safety in, 808
  safety rules for, 15
Bacteroides, 869-870
Bacteroides fragilis, 869
Bacteroides melaninogenicus, 869-870

Bacto-agar, 69
Baginski, phosphorus method of, for phospholipid determination, 548-549
Balantidium coli, 974
Band cells
  in myelogram of children, 271*t*
  naphthol AS-D chloroacetate staining of, 118
  Sudan black B staining of, 117
Band granulocyte(s), *129*
  basophilic, in myelogram of adult, 270*t*
  degenerated, *129*
  eosinophilic, in myelogram of adult, 270*t*
  morphology of, 152, *153*
  in myelogram of adult, 270*t*
  neutrophilic
    in multiple myeloma, *257*
    in myelogram of adult, 270*t*
  in polycythemia vera, 231
Bands, oligoclonal, in cerebrospinal fluid examination, 757
Banti's syndrome, lymphocytic leukocytosis from, 236
Barbital buffer
  0.1M, pH 6.8-9.4, preparation of, 560
  0.075 mole/L, pH 8.6 in factor VIII assay, 307
  preparation of, 560
Barbital-buffered saline in factor VIII assay, 307
Barbiturate(s), 657-659
  analysis of
    calculation in, 658-659
    procedure for, 658
  analytic procedures for, 631*t*
  concentrations of, in blood serum, interpretation of, 659*t*
  differentiation of, 659
  F and R values of, 658*t*
  $R_f \times 100$ of, in TLC, 637*t*
  in visualizing procedure for TLC, 638*t*
Barbiturate buffer, 50 mmole/L, pH 7.5 in 5'-nucleotidase, 584
Barbiturate control in barbiturate analysis, 658
Barium hydroxide
  0.15 mole/L in Somogyi filtrate, 469
  in nonglucose reducing sugar determination, 481
Barium sulfate–adsorbed normal citrated plasma in calibration curve, 297
Barium sulfate–adsorbed plasma in coagulation procedures, 288
Barium sulfate eluate, coagulation factors in, 288*t*
Barr body(ies)
  morphologic variations of, *156*
  size and number of, and sex chromatic patterns, relationship between, *157*
Barr body buccal smear technic of nuclear sexing, 154, *156*, 157
Bartonella, hemolytic anemias from, 221
Bartonellosis, hemolytic anemias caused by, 226
Basal secretion in gastric analysis, 780
Base(s)
  dilution of concentrated, 563*t*
  standard solutions of, 561
  strengths of concentrated, 563*t*
Basidiospore(s), 912
  definition of, 946
  formation of, *914*
Basidium, definition of, 946
Basket cells in polymorphonuclear leukocytes, 161
Basophil(s)
  in chronic granulocytic leukemia, 247-248
  counting of, absolute, manual, 204
  in glycogen, PAS staining of, 120
  granules of
    Sudan black B staining of, 117
    Wright-Giemsa staining of, 111

Secretory IgA level for immune deficiency diseases, 1066
Sediment
  in gastric juice examination, 782
  urinary, 713-724
    Addis count in, 714
    amorphous sediment in, 719
    bacteria in, 718-719
      crystals in, 691, 719, 724
      epithelial cells in, 718
      erythrocytes in, 715
      exfoliative cytology and, 718
      foreign material in, 724
      hemosiderin in, 724
      identification of, cytocentrifuge-Papanicolaou technic in, 714
      leukocytes in, 714-715
      metachromatic granules in, 724
      mucous strands or threads in, 718
      parasites in, 719
      semen in, 719
      stained with Sternheimer-Malbin stain, appearance of 714
      telescoped, 718
      urinary casts in, 715-718
      viruses and other inclusions in, 719
      yeast in, 719
Sedimentation
  in blood preparation, 381-382
  of erythrocytes, rate of, 194-195
    measurement of, 194-195
    mechanism of, 194
Sedimentation rate
  in cold agglutinin disease, 224
  in multiple myeloma, 258
  in polycythemia vera, 230
  in systemic lupus erythematosus, 262
  in Waldenström's macroglobulinemia, 259
Segmented cells in myelogram of children, 271t
Segmented granulocytes
  eosinophilic, in myelogram of adult, 270t
  morphology of, 152, 153, 154
  in myelogram of adult, 270t
  neutrophilic, in myelogram of adult, 270t
Segmenters, definition of, 976
Selective media, 813
Selectivity of protein excretion, 686-687
Selectivity measuring, technics of pore sizing and, 687
Selenite F broth, use of, in microbiology, 821
Sellvanoff test for fructose, 699
Semen
  average normal values for, 736
  collection of, 736
  definition of, 736
  fructose determination of, 738-739
  gross examination of, 737
  lower limits of normal of, 737
  microscopic examination of, 737
  in urinary sediment analysis, 719
Semiautomatic micropipets, 446
Semiquantitative catalase test for Mycobacteria analysis, 877
Semisolid motility medium technic
  in bacteria analysis, 812
  in bacteriologic material examination, 809
Semistupor from elevated methemoglobin in blood, 44
Senile purpura, 336
Sensitivity
  antibiotic, 830-835
  to bacitracin for group A streptococci, 837-838
  to Optocin, 836
Sensitize, definition of, 907
Sensitized antibodies, 413

Sepsis, definition of, 907
Septicemia, definition of, 907
Septate, definition of, 947
Septate hyphae, definition of, 912
Septicemia
  granulocytosis in, 235
  meningococcal, hemolytic anemia caused by, 226
  neutropenia from, 237
Septum, definition of, 947
Serial dilutions, 1026-1027
Serodiagnosis
  of Leishmania donovani, 972
  of syphilis, technics of, 1037-1042
Serofibrinous pleural effusion, 753
Serologic heterogeneity of immunoglobulins, 413t
Serologic kits
  commercial, quality control for, 12
  and immunologic determinations, 466-467
Serologic test(s)
  in bacteriology, 16
  definition of, 907
  in fungi culture, 921
  for hepatitis, 1060-1061
  interpretation of, for syphilis, 1035-1036
  for Mycoplasma infections, 1058
Serology
  in congenital syphilis diagnosis, 1036-1037
  of Epstein-Barr virus and infectious mononucleosis, 1059-1060
  in infectious disease diagnosis, 1049-1061
  in neurosyphilis diagnosis, 1037
  quality control in, 12
Serotonin, determination of, 626-628
Serous cavities, fluids from, 827
Serous fluid(s)
  differentiation of transudate and exudate from, 752t
  normal, characteristics of
    in pericardial effusion, 750-751
    in peritoneal effusion, 750-751
    in pleural effusion, 750-751
Serous pleural effusions, 753
Serratia, 856-857
  species of, differentiation of, 856
Sertoli cell, definition of, 748
Serum(a)
  ABO, compatible with patient's red cells, for sucrose hemolysis test for paroxysmal nocturnal hemoglobinuria, 218
  adsorbed, 407
    coagulation factors in, 288t
  aged
    in coagulation procedures, 288
    in mixing tests for single factor deficiency identification, 293
    in thromboplastin generation test, 299
  analysis for, 443, 468
  antilymphocytic, lymphopenia from, 238
  in bacteria examination by capsule stain method, 810
  calcium in
    colorimetric determination of, 506-507
    normal values and interpretation of, 508-509
  chloride determination in, with chloridometer, procedure for, 522
  copper in, determination of, 516
    without precipitation, 517
  creatinine in, procedure for, 489, 490
  deproteinization of, using Folin-Wu filtrate, 469
  drug screen of, by ultraviolet spectrophotometry, 655-656
  estrogens in, 616
  ferritin in, radioimmunoassay of, 83